Oxford Textbook of
Clinical Nephrology

Project Administration Newgen Imaging Systems (P) Ltd
Project Manager Kate Martin
Indexer Newgen Imaging Systems (P) Ltd
Design Manager Andrew Meaden
Publisher Helen Liepman

Editors

Alex M. Davison

Emeritus Professor of Renal Medicine, St James's University Hospital, Leeds, UK

J. Stewart Cameron

Emeritus Professor of Renal Medicine, Guy's, King's and St Thomas' School of Medicine, London, UK

Jean-Pierre Grünfeld

Professor of Nephrology, Hôpital Necker, Faculté de Médecine de Paris 5, Paris, France

Claudio Ponticelli

Professor and Director, Division of Nephrology and Dialysis, Istituto Scientifico Ospedale Maggiore Milano, Milan, Italy

Eberhard Ritz

Emeritus Professor of Nephrology, Department of Internal Medicine, Division of Nephrology, Heidelberg, Germany

Christopher G. Winearls

Consultant Nephrologist, Oxford Radcliffe Hospital, Oxford, UK

Charles van Ypersele

Professor of Medicine, Universite Catholique de Louvain, Cliniques Universitaires Saint-Luc, Brussels, Belgium

Subject Editors

Martin Barratt

Emeritus Professor of Paediatric Nephrology, Institute of Child Health, University College London, London, UK

James M. Ritter

Professor of Clinical Pharmacology, Guy's, King's and St Thomas' School of Medicine, London, UK

Jan Weening

Professor of Renal Pathology, University of Amsterdam, The Netherlands

volume **3**

Oxford Textbook of
Clinical
Nephrology
Third Edition

Edited by

Alex M. Davison

J. Stewart Cameron

Jean-Pierre Grünfeld

Claudio Ponticelli

Eberhard Ritz

Christopher G. Winearls

and Charles van Ypersele

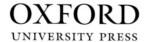

OXFORD
UNIVERSITY PRESS

OXFORD
UNIVERSITY PRESS

Great Clarendon Street, Oxford OX2 6DP

Oxford University Press is a department of the University of Oxford.
It furthers the University's objective of excellence in research, scholarship,
and education by publishing worldwide in

Oxford New York

Auckland Cape Town Dar es Salaam Hong Kong Karachi
Kuala Lumpur Madrid Melbourne Mexico City Nairobi
New Delhi Shanghai Taipei Toronto

With offices in

Argentina Austria Brazil Chile Czech Republic France Greece
Guatemala Hungary Italy Japan South Korea Poland Portugal
Singapore Switzerland Thailand Turkey Ukraine Vietnam

Oxford is a registered trade mark of Oxford University Press
in the UK and in certain other countries

Published in the United States
by Oxford University Press Inc., New York

© Oxford University Press, 2005

British Library Cataloguing in Publication Data

Data available

Library of Congress Cataloging in Publication Data

ISBN 0 19 856796 0 (volume 1)
0 19 856797 9 (volume 2)
0 19 856798 7 (volume 3)
0 19 850824 7 (set)
available as a set only

10 9 8 7 6 5 4 3 2 1

Typeset by Newgen Imaging Systems (P) Ltd, Chennai, India
Printed in Italy
on acid-free paper by Lego Print

Summary of contents

Contents

Preface to the third edition

Seven years after the publication of the second edition of this clinical text many advances in clinical practice justify the publication of a third edition. The text remains primarily a reference for the practising clinician. The chapters of the second edition have been carefully and critically reviewed. The overall framework of the book has been retained. Several previous chapters have been changed and some additions have been made. In line with our previous policy, the Editors have also modified the authorship of several chapters so as to keep the text as fresh as possible. As with previous editions we have, wherever possible, limited authors to two for each chapter. It is not surprising that a new view on a subject brings a different approach but this maintains vitality. In addition, where new concepts develop and new information becomes available, we have included such material—as illustrated by the information about the influence of smoking on renal diseases.

In this edition we have encouraged authors to add appropriate illustrations and to include pathological illustrative material. Wherever possible we have tried to avoid duplication in text, tables, and figures in an effort to maintain a reasonable overall size to the text. Some repetitions are unavoidable, but they have been included to avoid unnecessary cross-references.

In the production of a text of this size there are a number of people to thank for their hard work and devotion. There has been a change in Editors in that Claudio Ponticelli and Charles van Ypersele have joined the Editorial Board in place of David Kerr who has retired. We would like to thank David Kerr most sincerely for his encouragement in the production of this third edition and his invaluable help with the first two editions. Once again thanks go to the Subject Editors who have provided much useful critical advice which has gone a long way in securing authority and currency. Finally our thanks to the production team at Oxford University Press for all they have done towards launching this third edition.

Alex M. Davison
J. Stewart Cameron
Jean-Pierre Grünfeld
Claudio Ponticelli
Eberhard Ritz
Christopher G. Winearls
Charles van Ypersele
October 2004

Preface to the second edition

We have been gratified by the sales and published reviews of the first edition of our clinical text, published in 1992. During the preparation of this second edition all chapters in the first edition were subjected to review by practising nephrologists who were given the specific task of critically commenting on the content and practical value of each chapter. The authors were asked to revise their chapters in the light of the comments and the advances in clinical science since the production of the first edition. In some areas, such as molecular medicine, there have been very significant advances in our understanding of renal disease while in other areas there have been few changes. The challenge was readily accepted by the contributors and we hope that the final result is a thoroughly revised and up-to-date text.

We have retained the prime aim of the first edition—to produce a text of value to those with clinical responsibility for patients with renal disease. The changes we have introduced have been made in order to keep the text fresh; as a matter of policy we have introduced some new chapters and some new authors for existing chapters. The overall structure is unchanged: each section is centred on the patient with a particular disease or syndrome but the order of the sections has been slightly changed to a more logical sequence.

A major change has been the introduction of colour illustrations throughout the text, wherever possible. We greatly appreciate the efforts of chapter authors in finding suitable clinical and pathological illustrative material. We hope that the clinical illustrations will be of particular value to those in training.

It is with great sadness that we record the deaths of four distinguished authors, Professor Claude Amiel of Paris, Dr Ross R. Bailey of Christchurch, New Zealand, Dr A. Gordon Leitch of Edinburgh, and Professor Tony Raine of London. Claude and Tony died after tragic illnesses borne with supreme courage, Ross while swimming, and Gordon suddenly by drowning while trying to save the life of a fellow holiday-maker. Their chapters are a fitting memorial to their lives. We are all diminished by their loss.

The revision of the text could not have been undertaken without the enthusiastic support of a number of people. We would like to record our thanks to our Subject Editors, Martin Barratt (paediatrics), Michael Dunnill (pathology), Rainer Greger (physiology), and James Ritter (pharmacology) and to our Associate Editors, Claudio Ponticelli, Andy Rees, and Charles van Ypersele de Strihou without whose help and expertise this revised text would not have been completed. In addition our thanks are due to Marion Davison for secretarial support and to the staff of Oxford University Press for their devotion in seeing this venture to conclusion.

Alex M. Davison
J. Stewart Cameron
Jean-Pierre Grünfeld
David N.S. Kerr
Eberhard Ritz
and Christopher Winearls
June 1997

Preface to the first edition

Why another large text of nephrology? Because this one is *different*. It begins not with the anatomy of the nephron, but with the approach to the renal patient. It is intended as a text on *clinical nephrology*, of primary use to those caring for patients with renal disease. Not that we do not value the science that underlies our clinical practice—far from it. In each section the basic science relevant to the problem under discussion will be found incorporated at the appropriate point in the text for the clinician. In this area we have had the assistance of one of the foremost renal physiologists.

We deal in this book with many of the rarer renal problems and renal manifestations of systematic disease that are not dealt with in other texts—as a glance at the index and that of other similar volumes will show. A unique feature of the book is that at the end we have provided a guide to the book from the point of view of other specialist physicians—gastroenterologists, rheumatologists, neurologists, and so on—so that both they and generalists can enter the complex world of nephrology more easily. We have paid special attention to the handling of drugs by the kidney, and to the effects of drugs upon the kidney and renal tract. In this we have been assisted by our distinguished editor in clinical pharmacology.

We have tried to look at nephrology in a global context, remembering that the great majority of patients with renal diseases live in the developing world. Several chapters deal specifically with nephrology as it is seen in the tropics. We have also included chapters which deal with renal disease at the extremes of life. Paediatric nephrology has been blended into the text throughout with the assistance of our able paediatric editor, and several chapters deal with the special problems of the growing number of elderly patients with renal disease.

Finally, we hope that these volumes will be, as well as for day-to-day use when needed, a useful and pleasurable source for browsing when the pressure is off. Above all we hope that these volumes will be a literate as well as a comprehensive guide to diseases of the kidney, and diseases affecting the kidney. We thank our Associate Editors Luis Hernando, Claudio Ponticelli, Andy Rees, Charles van Ypersele de Strihou, and C.J. Winearls without whom these volumes could never have been completed.

Stewart Cameron
Alex M. Davison
Jean-Pierre Grünfeld
David Kerr
Eberhard Ritz

Contributors

Daniel Abramowicz Departement Medico-Chirurgical de Nephrologie, Dialyse et Transplantation, Hopital Erasme, Brussels, Belgium
13.2.2 Immunosuppression for renal transplantation

Horacio J. Adrogué Chief, Renal Section, The Methodist Hospital, Professor of Medicine, Baylor College of Medicine, Houston, Texas, USA
2.1 Hypo–hypernatraemia: disorders of water balance
5.4 Renal tubular acidosis

Dwomoa Adu Department of Nephrology, University Hospital Birmingham, Birmingham, UK
4.9 The patient with rheumatoid arthritis, mixed connective tissue disease, or polymyositis
6.3 Non-steroidal anti-inflammatory drugs and the kidney

J.-R. Allenberg Department of Vascular Surgery, University of Heidelberg School of Medicine, Heidelberg, Germany
9.7 Renovascular hypertension

Alessandro Amore Professor of Nephrology, Nephrology Dialysis Transplantation Unit, Ospedale Regina Margherita, Turin, Italy
4.5.2 The nephritis of Henoch–Schönlein purpura
11.3.11 Effect on the immune response

Corinne Antignac INSERM U574 and Department of Genetics, Hôpital Necker—Enfants Malades, Paris, France
16.3 Nephronophthisis

Pierre Aucouturier INSERM E209, Hopital Saint-Antoine, Batiment Raoul Kourilsky 184, Paris, France
4.3 Kidney involvement in plasma cell dyscrasias

Manuel Urrutia Avisrror Professor of Urology, Department of Surgery, University of Salamanca, Salamanca, Spain
18.1 Renal carcinoma and other tumours

Giovanni Banfi Vice-Director, Division of Nephrology, Instituto Scientifico, Ospedale Maggiore di Milano, Milan, Italy
4.7.2 Systemic lupus erythematosus (clinical)

Rashad S. Barsoum Professor of Internal Medicine, Cairo Kidney Center, Antikhana, Bab-El-Louk, Cairo, Egypt
7.4 Schistosomiasis

Chris Baylis Professor of Physiology and Medicine, University of Florida, Gainsville, Florida, USA
15.1 The normal renal physiological changes which occur during pregnancy
15.3 Pregnancy in patients with underlying renal disease

Michel Beaufils Department of Internal Medicine, Hopital Tenon, Paris, France
10.7.2 Pregnancy

Gordon M. Bell Consultant Nephrologist and Clinical Director of Nephrology, Royal Liverpool University Hospital, Liverpool, UK
4.12.1 Substance misuse, organic solvents and kidney disease

Rinaldo Bellomo Department of Intensive Care, Austin & Repatriation Medical Centre, Heidelberg, Victoria, Australia
10.4 Renal replacement methods in acute renal failure

Jo H.M. Berden Professor of Nephrology, Department of Nephrology 545, University Medical Center St Radboud, Nijmegen, The Netherlands
1.8 Immunological investigation of the patient with renal disease

Jaap J. Beutler Consultant Nephrologist, Department of Nephrology and Hypertension, University Medical Centre Utrecht, Utrecht, The Netherlands
1.6.1.vii Isotope scanning

Daniel G. Bichet Professor of Medicine, Universite de Montreal, Canada Research Chair, Genetics in Renal Diseases, Director, Clinical Research Unit, Hospital du Sacre-Coeur de Montréal, Montréal, Québec, Canada
5.6 Nephrogenic diabetes insipidus

Carol M. Black Professor of Rheumatology, Centre for Rheumatology, Royal Free & University College London Medical School, Royal Free Campus, London, UK
4.8 The patient with scleroderma—systemic sclerosis

Guillaume Bobrie Unite d'hypertension arterielle, Hopital Europeen Georges Pompidou, Paris, France
16.4.3 Nail-patella syndrome and other rare inherited disorders with glomerular involvement

Paola Boccardo Mario Negri Institute for Pharmacological Research, Bergamo, Italy
11.3.12 Coagulation disorders

Jürgen Bommer Klinikum der Universitat Heidelberg, Sektion Nephrologie, Heidelberg, Germany
11.3.3 Sexual disorders

Michael Boulton-Jones Renal Unit, Walton Building, Royal Infirmary, Glasgow, UK
4.2.1 Amyloidosis

J. Douglas Briggs 48 Kingsborough Gardens, Glasgow, UK
13.3.3 Long-term medical complications

J. Trevor Brocklebank Reader in Paediatric Nephrology, Department of Paediatrics, Clinical Science Building, St James's University Hospital, Leeds, UK
10.7.1 Infants and children

Nilufer Broeders Hopital Erasme, Brussels, Belgium
13.2.2 Immunosuppression for renal transplantation

Alison L. Brown Consultant Nephrologist, Freeman Hospital, High Heaton, Newcastle-upon-Tyne, UK
9.2 Clinical approach to hypertension

Michael Broyer Group Hospitalier, Hopital Necker-Enfants Malades, Paris, France
16.5.1 Cystinosis

Vincenzo Cambi Cattedra di Nefrologia, Ospedale Maggiore, Parma, Italy
12.1 Dialysis strategies

J. Stewart Cameron Emeritus Professor of Renal Medicine, Guy's, King's, and St Thomas' School of Medicine, London, UK
1.5 The ageing kidney
3.3 The patient with proteinuria and/or haematuria
3.4 The nephrotic syndrome: management, complications, and pathophysiology
6.4 Uric acid and the kidney
14.2 Chronic renal failure in the elderly
16.5.3 Inherited disorders of purine metabolism and transport
16.7 Some rare syndromes with renal involvement
17.5 Medullary sponge kidney

José M. Campistol Renal Transplant Unit, Hospital Clinic, University of Barcelona, Barcelona, Spain
10.6.4 Acute renal failure in liver disease

Marco Cappelletti Radiologist, Viale Scarampo, Milan, Italy
1.6.2.v Living donor workup

Ruggero Caputo Director, Institute of Dermatological Sciences, University of Milan, IRCCS Osperdale Maggiore, Milan, Italy
11.3.13 Dermatological disorders

Andrés Cárdenas Instructor in Medicine, Division of Gastroenterology and Hepatology, Beth Israel Deaconess Medical Center, Harvard Medical School, Boston, Massachusetts, USA
10.6.4 Acute renal failure in liver disease

D.J.S. Carmichael Consultant Nephrologist, Southend General Hospital, Pricklewood Chase, Westcliff on Sea, Essex, UK
19.2 Handling of drugs in kidney disease

Ralph Caruana Professor of Medicine, Vice Dean for Clinical Affairs, Medical College of Georgia, Augusta, Georgia, USA
4.11 The patient with sickle-cell disease

Michael J.D. Cassidy Clinical Director, Renal and Transplant Unit, Nottingham City Hospital NHS Trust, Nottingham, UK
11.2 Assessment and initial management of the patient with failing renal function

W.R. Cattell 30 Tavistock Terrace, London, UK
7.1 Lower and upper urinary tract infections in the adult

Daniel Cattran University Health Network, Toronto General Hospital, Toronto, Ontario, Canada
3.7 Membranous nephropathy

Dominique Chauveau Service de Néphrologie, Hôpital Necker, Paris, France
16.2.2 Autosomal-dominant polycystic kidney disease

Paramit Chowdhury Department of Nephrology, King's College London, London, UK
9.5 Ischaemic nephropathy
10.6.5 Ischaemic renal disease

Y. Chrétien Radiotherapie, Hopital europeen Georges-Pompidou, Paris, France
1.6.1.iii Percutaneous nephrostomy and ureteral stenting

Kirpal S. Chugh Emeritus Professor of Nephrology, National Kidney Clinic and Research Centre, Chandigarh, India
3.14 Glomerular disease in the tropics
10.7.3 Acute renal failure in the tropical countries

Pierre Cochat Professor of Pediatrics/Head Renal Unit, Department of Pediatrics, Hopital Edouard Herriot, Universite Claude-Bernard, Lyon, France
16.5.2 The primary hyperoxalurias

Fredric L. Coe Professor of Medicine and Physiology, University of Chicago School of Medicine, Chicago, Illinois, USA
8.2 The medical management of stone disease

Eric P. Cohen Professor of Medicine, Nephrology Division, Medical College of Wisconsin, Milwaukee, Wisconsin, USA
6.6 Radiation nephropathy

Rosanna Coppo Ospedale Regina Margherita, Nefrologia, Dialisi e Trapianto, Turin, Italy
3.6 IgA nephropathies
4.5.2 The nephritis of Henoch–Schönlein purpura
11.3.11 Effect on the immune response

Catherine M. Corbishley Consultant Histopathologist, Department of Cellular Pathology, St George's Hospital, London, UK
7.3 Renal tuberculosis and other mycobacterial infections

François Cornud Consultant Radiologist, Hospital Cochin, Paris, France
1.6.1.iii Percutaneous nephrostomy and ureteral stenting

Jean-Michel Correas Vice Chairman, Service de Radiologie, Hôpital Necker, Paris, France
1.6.1.i Ultrasound
1.6.2.ii Hypertension and suspected renovascular disease
1.6.2.iv Renal masses
1.6.2.vi Transplant dysfunction

J.P. Cosyns Professor of Clinical Pathology, Department of Pathology, Medical School, Cliniques Universitaires Saint-Luc, Universite Catholque de Louvain, Brussels, Belgium
6.7 Balkan nephropathy
6.8 Chinese herbs (and other rare causes of interstitial nephropathy)

Malcolm G. Coulthard Department of Paediatric Nephrology, Royal Victoria Infirmary, Newcastle-upon-Tyne, UK
7.2 Urinary tract infections in infancy and childhood

Vincenzo D'Intini Divisione Nefrologia, Ospedale San Bortolo, Vicenza, Italy
10.4 Renal replacement methods in acute renal failure

André Noël Dardenne Associate Professor of Radiology, Universite Catholique de Louvain, Cliniques Universitaires Saint-Luc, Brussels, Belgium
1.6.1.v CT scanning and helical CT

Markus Daschner Pediatric Nephrologist, University Children's Hospital, Heidelberg, Germany
11.3.2 Endocrine disorders

Andrew Davenport Consultant Nephrologist/Honorary Senior Lecturer, Centre for Nephrology, Royal Free Campus, Royal Free and University College Medical School, London, UK
11.3.14 Neuropsychiatric disorders

Salvatore David Cattedra di Nefrologia, Ospedale Maggiore, Parma, Italy
12.1 Dialysis strategies

Alex M. Davison Emeritus Professor of Renal Medicine, St James's University Hospital, Leeds, UK
1.1 History and clinical examination of the patient with renal disease
3.12 Infection related glomerulonephritis
3.13 Malignancy-associated glomerular disease

John M. Davison School of Surgical and Reproductive Sciences, Department of Obstetrics & Gynaecology, Medical School, Newcastle-upon-Tyne, UK
15.1 The normal renal physiological changes which occur during pregnancy
15.2 Renal complications that may occur in pregnancy
15.3 Pregnancy in patients with underlying renal disease

Marc E. De Broe Department of Nephrology, University Hospital Antwerp, Edegem/Antwerp, Belgium
6.2 Analgesic nephropathy
6.5 Nephrotoxic metals
19.1 Drug-induced nephropathies

John M.H. De Klerk Consultant in Nuclear Medicine, Department of Nuclear Medicine, University Centre Utrecht, Utrecht, The Netherlands
1.6.1.vii Isotope scanning

Rita De Smet Department of Nephrology, University Hospital, Ghent, Belgium
11.3.1 Uraemic toxicity

Peter R.F. Dear Regional Neonatal Intensive Care Unit, St James's University Hospital, Leeds, UK
1.4 Renal function in the newborn infant

Christopher P. Denton Clinical Research Fellow, Academic Unit of Rheumatology, Royal Free Hospital School of Medicine, University of London, London, UK
4.8 The patient with scleroderma—systemic sclerosis

Robert J. Desnick Professor and Chairman, Department of Human Genetics, Mount Sinai School of Medicine, New York, USA
16.4.2 Fabry disease

Olivier Devuyst Division of Nephrology, UCL Medical School, (Universite Catholique de Louvain), Brussels, Belgium
16.2.2 Autosomal-dominant polycystic kidney disease

Ralf Dikow Sektion Nephrologie, Heidelberg, Germany
4.1 The patient with diabetes mellitus
9.6 Hypertension and unilateral renal parenchymal disease
9.8 Malignant hypertension
11.3.4 Hypertension
14.3 The diabetic patient with impaired renal function

John H. Dirks Chair, ISN COMGAN, President, The Gairdner Foundation, Senior Fellow, Massey College, University of Toronto, Toronto, Ontario, Canada
2.5 Hypo–hypermagnesaemia

Ciaran Doherty Regional Nephrology Unit, Belfast City Hospital, Belfast, UK
10.1 Epidemiology of acute renal failure
11.3.6 Gastrointestinal effects

Raymond A.M.G. Donckerwolcke Professor and Chairman, Department of Paediatrics, University Hospital Maastricht, Maastricht, The Netherlands
3.4 The nephrotic syndrome: management, complications, and pathophysiology

Sven Dorph Department of Radiology, Helsingor Hospital, Helsingor, Denmark
1.6.2.i Haematuria, infection, acute renal failure, and obstruction

Dominique Droz Service d'Anatomie Pathologique, Hopital Saint-Louis, Paris, France
10.6.2 Acute tubulointerstitial nephritis

Tilman B. Drüeke INSERM Unit 507 and Division of Nephrology, Hopital Necker, Paris, France
11.3.9 Skeletal disorders

I. Dulau-Florea Schwabing General Hospital, Ludwig Maximilians University, Munich, Germany
9.7 Renovascular hypertension

John B. Eastwood Consultant Renal Physician and Reader in Medicine, Department of Renal Medicine, and Transplantation, St George's Hospital, London, UK
7.3 Renal tuberculosis and other mycobacterial infections

Kai-Uwe Eckardt Department of Nephrology and Medical Intensive Care, Charité, Campus Virchow Klinikum, Berlin, Germany
11.3.8 Haematological disorders

Lisette El Hajj Hôpital de Rangueil, Service Central d Radiologie, Toulouse, France
1.6.1.iv Renal arteriography

A. Meguid El Nahas Professor of Nephrology, Sheffield Kidney Institute, Sheffield teaching Hospitals NHS Trust, Northern General Hospital, Sheffield, UK
11.1 Mechanisms of experimental and clinical renal scarring

Marlies Elger Abteilung Nephrologie, Forschungszentrum der Medizinischen Hochschule, am Oststadtkrankenhaus, Hannover, Germany
3.1 The renal glomerulus—the structural basis of ultrafiltration

Paul Emery ARC Professor of Rheumatology, Molecular Medicine Unit, School of Medicine, Leeds, UK
4.9 The patient with rheumatoid arthritis, mixed connective tissue disease, or polymyositis

Karlhans Endlich Assistant Professor, Department of Anatomy and Cell Biology, University of Heidelberg, Heidelberg, Germany
9.1 The structure and function of blood vessels in the kidney

John Feehally Department of Nephrology, Leicester General Hospital, Leicester, UK
3.2 Glomerular injury and glomerular response

Terry Feest The Richard Bright Renal Unit, Southmead Hospital, Westbury-on-Trym, Bristol, UK
1.9 The epidemiology of renal disease

J.D. Firth Consultant Physician and Nephrologist, Addenbrooke's Hospital, Cambridge, UK
10.3 The clinical approach to the patient with acute renal failure

Maggie Fitzpatrick Consultant Paediatric Nephrologist, Department of Paediatrics Nephrology, St James's Hospital, Leeds, UK
1.1 History and clinical examination of the patient with renal disease
10.7.1 Infants and children

Jürgen Floege Medizinische Klinik II der RWTH, Aachen, Germany
3.2 Glomerular injury and glomerular response

Giovanni B. Fogazzi Divisione di Nefrologia e Dialisi, Oespedale Maggiore, IRCCS, Milan, Italy
1.2 Urinalysis and microscopy

Robert N. Foley Department of Medicine, Hennepin County Medical Center, Minneapolis, Minnesota, USA
11.3.5 Cardiovascular risk factors

Gérard Friedlander Professor and Chief, INSERM U 426, Department of Physiology, Xavier Bichat Medical Faculty, Paris, France
1.3 The clinical assessment of renal function
2.4 Hypo–hyperphosphataemia

Marie-France Gagnadoux Pediatric Nephrologist, Necker-Enfants Malades, Paris, France
16.2.1 Polycystic kidney disease in children

Gillian Gaskin Renal Section, Division of Medicine, Faculty of Medicine, Imperial College, Hammersmith Hospital, London, UK
4.5.3 Systemic vasculitis

Pere Ginès Associate Professor of Medicine, Liver Unit, Institut de Malalties Digestives, Hospital Clinic, University of Barcelona, Barcelona, Spain
10.6.4 Acute renal failure in liver disease

Matthias Girndt Assistant Professor of Internal Medicine and Nephrology, Medical Department IV, University of Saarland, Homburg, Germany
11.3.7 Liver disorders

Sven Glaesker Department of Nephrology, Clinics of the Albert Freiburg University, Freiburg, Germany
16.6 Renal involvement in tuberous sclerosis and von Hippel–Lindau disease

Griet Glorieux Nephrology Department, University Hospital Ghent, Ghent, Belgium
11.3.1 Uraemic toxicity

Ram Gokal Consultant Nephrologist, Honorary Professor of Medicine, Manchester Royal Infirmary, Manchester, UK
12.4 Peritoneal dialysis and complications of technique

David S. Goldfarb Associate Professor of Medicine and Physiology, New York University School of Medicine, Nephrology/111G, NY Department of Veterans Affairs Medical Centre, New York, USA
8.2 The medical management of stone disease

John M. Grange Visiting Professor, Royal Free and University College Medical School, Windeyer Institute for Medical Science, London, UK
7.3 Renal tuberculosis and other mycobacterial infections

Ian A. Greer Deputy Dean—Faculty of Medicine, Regius Professor—Obstetrics and Gynaecology, University of Glasgow, Glasgow Royal Infirmary, Glasgow, UK
15.4 Pregnancy-induced hypertension

Rainer Greger Physiologisches Institut, Albert-Ludwigs-Universität, Freiburg, Germany
19.3 Action and clinical use of diuretics

Jean-Pierre Grünfeld Professor of Nephrology, Hôpital Necker, Faculté de Médecine de Paris 5, Paris, France
1.1 History and clinical examination of the patient with renal disease
16.4.1 Alport's syndrome
16.4.2 Fabry disease
16.4.3 Nail-patella syndrome and other rare inherited disorders with glomerular involvement
16.7 Some rare syndromes with renal involvement

Marie-Claire Gubler INSERM U574, Hôpital Necker—Enfants Malades, Paris, France
16.3 Nephronophthisis
16.5.1 Cystinosis

Sanjeev Gulati Department of Nephrology, Sanjay Gandhi Postgraduate Institute of Medical Sciences, Lucknow, India
3.8 Mesangiocapillary glomerulonephritis

Krishan Lal Gupta Additional Professor of Nephrology, Postgraduate Institute of Medical Education and Research, Chandigarh, India
7.5 Fungal infections and the kidney

Suresh K. Gupta 46 Glebe Avenue, Grappenhal, Warrington, UK
8.3 The surgical management of renal stones

Kenneth R. Hallows Assistant Professor, Renal-Electrolyte Division, Department of Medicine, University of Pittsburgh School of Medicine, Pittsburgh, Pennsylvania, USA
2.2 Hypo–hyperkalaemia

Neveen A.T. Hamdy Head Clinic Section, Department of Endocrinology & Metabolic Diseases, Leiden University Medical Center, Leiden, The Netherlands
2.3 Hypo–hypercalcaemia

Barrie Hartley Department of Pathology, St James's University Hospital, Leeds, UK
3.13 Malignancy-associated glomerular disease

George B. Haycock Consultant in Paediatrics, Guy's, King's, and St Thomas' Hospital, London, UK
5.2 Isolated defects of tubular function

August Heidland Department of Internal Medicine, University of Wurzburg, Kuratorium für Dialysis und Nierentransplantation, Wurzburg, Germany
19.3 Action and clinical use of diuretics

Olivier Hélénon Chairman, Service de Radiologie, Hôpital Necker, Paris, France
1.6.1.i Ultrasound
1.6.1.iii Percutaneous nephrostomy and ureteral stenting
1.6.2.ii Hypertension and suspected renovascular disease
1.6.2.iv Renal masses
1.6.2.vi Transplant dysfunction

Udo Helmchen Department of Pathology, Universitätsklinikum Hamburg-Eppendorf, Hamburg, Germany
9.4 The effects of hypertension on renal vasculature and structure

Elizabeth Petri Henske Fox Chase Cancer Center, 7701 Burholme Avenue, Philadelphia, Pennsylvania, USA
16.6 Renal involvement in tuberous sclerosis and von Hippel–Lindau disease

Lukas B. Hilbrands University Medical Centre Nymegen, Department of Nephrology, Nijmegen, The Netherlands
13.1 Selection and preparation of the recipient

Friedhelm Hildebrandt Professor of Pediatrics and Human Genetics, Huetwell Professor for the Cure and Prevention of Birth Defects, Department of Pediatrics, University of Michigan, Ann Arbor, Michigan, USA
16.1 Strategies for the investigation of inherited renal disease

Andries J. Hoitsma Division of Nephrology, University Medical Center St Radboud, Nijmegen, The Netherlands
13.1 Selection and preparation of the recipient

Christer Holmberg Hospital for Children and Adolescents, University of Helsinki, Helsinki, Finland
16.4.4 Congenital nephrotic syndrome

Matthew L.P. Howse Link 6C, Royal Liverpool University Hospital, Liverpool, UK
4.12.1 Substance misuse, organic solvents and kidney disease

Othon Iliopoulos MGH Cancer Center, Massachusetts General Hospital, Boston, Massachusetts, USA
16.6 Renal involvement in tuberous sclerosis and von Hippel–Lindau disease

Enrico Imbasciati Director, Division of Nephrology, Ospedale Maggiore di Lodi, Lodi, Italy
1.7 Renal biopsy: indications for and interpretation

David A. Isenberg Centre for Rheumatology, Royal Free and University College Hospital, London, UK
4.7.1 The pathogenesis of systemic lupus erythematosus

Claude Jacobs Groupe hospitalier Pitié-Salpêtrière, Service de nephrologie, Paris, France
12.6 Medical management of the dialysis patient

Michel Jadoul Cliniques Universitaires St Luc, Department of Nephrology, Brussels, Belgium
11.3.10 β2M Amyloidosis

Hannu Jalanko Hospital for Children and Adolescents, University of Helsinki, Helsinki, Finland
16.4.4 Congenital nephrotic syndrome

Vivekanand Jha Associate Professor, Department of Nephrology, Postgraduate Institute of Medical Education and Research, Chandigarh, India
3.14   Glomerular disease in the tropics
10.7.3 Acute renal failure in the tropical countries

Francis G. Joffre Hôpital de Rangueil, Service Central d Radiologie, Toulouse, France
1.6.1.iv Renal arteriography

Kate Verrier Jones KRUF Children's Kidney Centre for Wales, University of Wales, College of Medicine, Heath Park, Cardiff, UK
17.2 Vesicoureteric reflux and reflux nephropathy

Nicola Joss Renal Unit, Walton Building, Royal Infirmary, Glasgow, UK
4.2.1 Amyloidosis

Islam Junaid Consultant Urologist and Transplant Surgeon, Department of Renal Medicine & Transplantation, The Royal London Hospital, Whitechapel, London, UK
17.3 The patient with urinary tract obstruction

Brian Junor Consultant Nephrologist, Renal Unit, Western Infirmary, Glasgow, UK
13.3.5 Outcome of renal transplantation

Cees G.M. Kallenberg Department of Clinical Immunology, University Hospital Groningen, Groningen, The Netherlands
4.5.1 Pathogenesis of angiitis

John A. Kanis Sheffield Metabolic Bone Unit, Sheffield, UK
2.3 Hypo–hypercalcaemia

Alexandre Karras Service de Néphrologie et Transplantation Rénale, Hopital Saint-Louis, Paris, France
10.6.2 Acute tubulointerstitial nephritis

Akira Kawashima Professor of Radiology, Mayo Clinic College of Medicine, Department of Radiology, Mayo Clinic, Rochester, Minnesota, USA
1.6.1.ii Plain radiography, contrast radiography, and excretion radiography
1.6.1.vi Magnetic resonance imaging

Vijay Kher Department of Nephrology, Indraprastha Apollo Hospitals, New Delhi, India
3.8 Mesangiocapillary glomerulonephritis

Bernard F. King, Jr. Mayo School of Graduate Medical Education, Department of Radiology, Mayo Clinic, Rochester, Minnesota, USA
1.6.1.vi Magnetic resonance imaging

Bertrand Knebelmann Hôpital Necker, Paris, France
16.4.1 Alport's syndrome

Nine V.A.M. Knoers University Hospital Nijmegen, Nijmegen, The Netherlands
5.5 Hypokalaemic tubular disorders

Karl-Martin Koch Medizinische Hochschule Hannover, Zentrum Innere Medizin und Dermatologie, Abteilung Nephrologie, NHH, Hannover, Germany
12.3 Haemodialysis, haemofiltration, and complications of technique

Hans Köhler Universitätskliniken des Saarlandes, Medizinische Klinik und Poliklinik, Medical Department IV, University of Saarland, Homburg, Germany
11.3.7 Liver disorders

Hein A. Koomans Professor of Nephrology and Head of Department of Nephrology and Hypertension, Department of Nephrology, University Centre Utrecht, Utrecht, The Netherlands
1.6.1.vii Isotope scanning

Stephen M. Korbet Professor of Medicine, Rush University Medical Center, Chicago, Illinois, USA
4.2.2 Fibrillary and immunotactoid glomerulopathy

Wilhelm Kriz Professor and Chairman, Institute of Anatomy and Cell Biology, University of Heidelberg, Heidelberg, Germany
3.1 The renal glomerulus—the structural basis of ultrafiltration

B. Krumme Department of Nephrology, Deutsche Klinik fur Diagnostick, Wiesbaden, Germany
9.7 Renovascular hypertension

Heather J. Lambert Department of Paediatric Nephrology, Royal Victoria Infirmary, Newcastle-upon-Tyne, UK
7.2 Urinary tract infections in infancy and childhood

Norbert Hendrik Lameire Renal Division, University Hospital Ghent, Ghent, Belgium
10.2   Acute renal failure: pathophysiology and prevention
10.7.4 The elderly
11.3.1 Uraemic toxicity

Florian Lang Department of Physiology, University of Tubingen, Tubingen, Germany
19.3 Action and clinical use of diuretics

Andrew J. LeRoy Associate Professor of Radiology, Mayo Clinic College of Medicine, Department of Radiology, Mayo Clinic, Rochester, Minnesota, USA
1.6.1.ii Plain radiography, contrast radiography, and excretion radiography

Philippe Lesavre Service de Nephrologie, Hôpital Necker, Paris, France
3.12 Infection related glomerulonephritis

Jeremy Levy Consultant Nephrologist and Physician, Imperial College, Hammersmith Hospital, London, UK
3.10 Crescentic glomerulonephritis

Edmund J. Lewis Professor of Medicine, Rush University Medical Center, Chicago, Illinois, USA
4.2.2 Fibrillary and immunotactoid glomerulopathy

Gerhard Lonnemann Department of Nephrology, Medical School, Hannover, Germany
12.3 Haemodialysis, haemofiltration, and complications of technique

Iain C. Macdougall The Renal Unit, King's College Hospital, London, UK
11.3.8 Haematological disorders

Nicolaos E. Madias Chairman, Department of Medicine, Caritas St Elizabeth's Medical Center and Professor of Medicine, Tufts University School of Medicine, Boston, Massachusetts, USA
2.1 Hypo–hypernatraemia: disorders of water balance
5.4 Renal tubular acidosis

J.F.E. Mann Krankenhaus Monchen Schwabing, Munich, Germany
9.7 Renovascular hypertension

A.M. Marinaki Purine Research Unit, Guy's Hospital, London Bridge, London, UK
16.5.3 Inherited disorders of purine metabolism and transport

Frank Martinez Service de Néphrologie et Transplantation Rénale, Hopital Saint-Louis, Paris, France
10.6.2 Acute tubulointerstitial nephritis

Angelo Valerio Marzano Assistant Dermatologist, Institute of Dermatological Sciences, University of Milan, IRCCS Osperdale Maggiore, Milan, Italy
11.3.13 Dermatological disorders

L.J. Mason Research Assistant, Centre for Rheumatology, University College London, Windeyer Institute of Medical Sciences, London, UK
4.7.1 The pathogenesis of systemic lupus erythematosus

Philip D. Mason Consultant Nephrologist, Oxford Kidney Unit, Churchill Hospital, Headington, Oxford, UK
10.6.1 Glomerulonephritis, vasculitis, and the nephrotic syndrome

Arnaud Méjean Service d'Urologie, Paris, France
1.6.2.iv Renal masses
1.6.2.vi Transplant dysfunction

Jean-Philippe Méry 59 rue Madame, Paris, France
4.4 The patient with sarcoidosis

Alain Meyrier Hôpital Europeen Georges-Pompidou, Paris, France
3.5 Minimal change and focal–segmental glomerular sclerosis

Michael J. Mihatsch Director, Institute for Pathology, University of Basel, Basel, Switzerland
1.7 Renal biopsy: indications for and interpretation

Robert D. Mills Consultant Urologist, Norfolk & Norwich University Hospital, Norwich, UK
18.4 Tumours of the bladder

Christopher Mitchell Paediatric Haematology/Oncology Unit, The John Radcliffe Hospital, Headington, Oxford, UK
18.2 Wilms' tumour

Leo A.H. Monnens Department of Pediatrics, University Hospital Nijmegen, Nijmegen, The Netherlands
5.5 Hypokalaemic tubular disorders

Emmanuel Morelon Department on Transplantation, Hôpital Necker, Universite Paris V, Paris, France
1.6.2.vi Transplant dysfunction

Stephen H. Morgan Basildon Hospital, Nether Mayne, Basildon, UK
16.4.2 Fabry disease

Gabriella Moroni Assistant Nephrologist, Division of Nephrology, Instituto Scientifico, Ospedale Maggiore di Milano, Milan, Italy
4.7.2 Systemic lupus erythematosus (clinical)

Béatrice Mougenot Pathologist, Hôpital Tenon, Paris, France
4.3 Kidney involvement in plasma cell dyscrasias

Claudia A. Müller Section Transplantation Immunology, ZMF, Tubingen, Germany
6.1 Mechanisms of interstitial inflammation

Gerhard A. Müller Universitätsklinikum/Innere Medizin, Abteilung für Nephrologie und Rheumatologie, Göttingen, Germany
6.1 Mechanisms of interstitial inflammation

Robert G. Narins Director of Postgraduate Education, American Society of Nephrology, Washington, DC, USA
2.6 Clinical acid–base disorders

Guy H. Neild Institute of Urology and Nephrology, Middlesex Hospital, London, UK
10.6.3 Acute renal failure associated with microangiopathy (haemolytic–uraemic syndrome and thrombotic thrombocytopenic purpura)

Hartmut P.H. Neumann Medizinische Universitätsklinik, Freiburg im Breisgau, Germany
16.6 Renal involvement in tuberous sclerosis and von Hippel–Lindau disease

Simon J. Newell Regional Neonatal Intensive Care Unit, St James's University Hospital, Leeds, UK
1.4 Renal function in the newborn infant

Chas G. Newstead Department of Renal medicine, St James's University Hospital, Leeds, UK
13.3.4 Recurrent disease and de novo disease

Patrick Niaudet Nephrologie Paediatrique, Hospital Necker-Enfants Malades, Paris, France
3.5 Minimal change and focal–segmental glomerular sclerosis

Michael Nicholson Division of Transplant Surgery, Leicester General Hospital, Leicester, UK
13.3.1 Surgery and surgical complications

Juan F. Macías-Núñez Unidad de Hipertension, Hospital Universitario de Salamanca, Salamanca, Spain
1.5 The ageing kidney
14.2 Chronic renal failure in the elderly

Christopher Olbricht Klinik fur Nieren-und Hochdruckkrankheiten, Katharine Hospital, Stuttgart, Germany
12.3 Haemodialysis, haemofiltration, and complications of technique

Stephan R. Orth Dialysis Centre Schwandorf, Schwandorf, Germany
4.12.2 Smoking and the kidney

Kazuo Ota Director, Ota Medical Research Institute, Chouo-ku, Tokyo, Japan
12.2 Vascular access

Edgar Otto Research Investigator, Department of Pediatrics, University of Michigan, Ann Arbor, Michigan, USA
16.1 Strategies for the investigation of inherited renal disease

Biff F. Palmer Professor of Internal Medicine, Department of Internal Medicine, Division of Nephrology, University of Texas Southwestern Medical School, Dallas, Texas, USA
2.6 Clinical acid–base disorders

Vicente Arroyo Pérez Institute of Digestive Diseases, Hospital Clinic 1 Provincial de Barcelona, Barcelona, Spain
10.6.4 Acute renal failure in liver disease

Phuong-Chi T. Pham Assistant Clinical Professor of Medicine, Division of Nephrology, Department of Medicine, David Geffen School of Medicine at UCLA, Los Angeles, California, USA
13.3.2 The early management of the recipient

Phuong-Thu T. Pham Assistant Clinical Professor of Medicine, Division of Nephrology, Kidney Transplant Program, David Geffen School of Medicine at UCLA, Los Angeles, California, USA
13.3.2 The early management of the recipient

Yves Pirson Department of Nephrology, University of Louvain Medical School, Cliniques Universitaires St Luc, Faculté de médecine, Brussels, Belgium
16.2.2 Autosomal-dominant polycystic kidney disease

Wolfgang Pommer Director, Department of Internal Medicine—Nephrology, Vivantes Humboldt Klinikum, Berlin, Germany
6.2 Analgesic nephropathy

Claudio Ponticelli Professor and Director, Division of Nephrology and Dialysis, Istituto Scientifico Ospedale Maggiore Milano, Milan, Italy
1.6.2.iii Renal biopsy—procedure and complications
1.6.2.v Living donor workup
1.7 Renal biopsy: indications for and interpretation
4.7.2 Systemic lupus erythematosus (clinical)
11.3.13 Dermatological disorders

Dominique Prié Assistant Professor INSERM U 426, Department of Physiology, Xavier Bichat Medical Faculty, Paris, France
1.3 The clinical assessment of renal function

Charles D. Pusey Renal Section, Division of Medicine, Imperial College, Hammersmith Hospital, London, UK
3.10 Crescentic glomerulonephritis

Uwe Querfeld Director, Pediatric Nephrology, Department of Pediatric Nephrology, Charité Campus, Virchow Klinkum Children's Hospital, Berlin, Germany
14.1 Chronic renal failure in children

Wolfgang Rascher Professor of Pediatrics, Head and Chairman, Department of Pediatrics, Erlangen, Germany
9.9 The hypertensive child
17.4 Congenital abnormalities of the urinary tract

Andrew J. Rees Regius Professor of Medicine, University of Aberdeen, Institute of Medical Sciences, Foresterhill, Aberdeen, UK
3.11 Antiglomerular basement disease

Giuseppe Remuzzi Division of Nephrology and Dialysis, Ospedali Riuniti di Bergamo, Mario Negri Institute for Pharmacological Research, Bergamo, Italy
11.3.12 Coagulation disorders

Eberhard Ritz Emeritus Professor of Nephrology, Department of Internal Medicine, Division of Nephrology, Heidelberg, Germany
4.1 The patient with diabetes mellitus
9.8 Malignant hypertension
11.3.4 Hypertension
11.3.5 Cardiovascular risk factors
11.3.9 Skeletal disorders
14.3 The diabetic patient with impaired renal function

Paul J. Roderick Senior Lecturer in Public Health Medicine, Applied Clinical Epidemiology Group, Community Clinical Sciences Research Division, School of Medicine, University of Southampton, Southampton, UK
1.9 The epidemiology of renal disease

Bernardo Rodríguez-Iturbe Professor of Medicine and Chief of Nephrology, Hospital Universitario, Universidad del Zulia and Director, Instituto de Investigaciones Biomedicas, Maracaibo, Venezuela
3.9 Acute endocapillary glomerulonephritis

Marie-Odile Rolland Laboratoire de Biochimie Pediatrique, Hospitalk Debrousse, Lyon, France
16.5.2 The primary hyperoxalurias

Claudio Ronco Director, Department of Nephrology, St Bortolo Hospital, Vicenza, Italy
10.4 Renal replacement methods in acute renal failure

Pierre M. Ronco Renal Department and INSERM, Unité 489, Hôpital Tenon, Paris, France
4.3 Kidney involvement in plasma cell dyscrasias

Wolfgang H. Rösch Kinderurologische Abteilung der Universität Regensburg, In der Klinik St Hedwig, Regensburg, Germany
17.4 Congenital abnormalities of the urinary tract

Luis M. Ruilope Univdad de Hipertension, Hospital 12 de Octubre, Madrid, Spain
9.3 The kidney and control of blood pressure

Rémi Salomon INSERM U574 and Department of Pediatric Nephrology, Hôpital Necker—Enfants Malades, Paris, France
16.3 Nephronophthisis

John Savill Professor of Medicine, Vice Principal and Head of the College of Medicine & Veterinary Medicine, University of Edinburgh, Edinburgh, UK
3.2 Glomerular injury and glomerular response

Franz Schaefer Division of Pediatric Nephrology, University Children's Hospital, Heidelberg, Germany
11.3.2 Endocrine disorders

Francesco Paolo Schena University of Bari, Renal Unit, Policlinico, Bari, Italy
3.6 IgA nephropathies

Michael Schömig Sektion Nephrologie, Heidelberg, Germany
9.6 Hypertension and unilateral renal parenchymal disease

Melvin M. Schwartz Professor of Pathology, Rush University Medical Center, Chicago, Illinois, USA
4.2.2 Fibrillary and immunotactoid glomerulopathy

John E. Scoble Department of Renal Medicine and Transplantation, Guy's Hospital, London, UK
9.5 Ischaemic nephropathy
10.6.5 Ischaemic renal disease

Katarina Sebekova Institute of Preventive and Clinical Medicine, Bratislava, Slovakia
19.3 Action and clinical use of diuretics

Günter Seyffart Head, Dialysis Center, Bad Homburg, Germany
10.5 Dialysis and haemoperfusion treatment of acute poisoning

David G. Shirley Research Fellow and Honorary Reader, Royal Free & University College Medical School, London, UK
5.1 The structure and function of tubules

Caroline Silve Senior Investigator, INSERM U 426, Department of Physiology, Xavier Bichat Medical Faculty, Paris, France
2.4 Hypo—hyperphosphataemia

H. Anne Simmonds Purine Research Unit, Guy's Hospital, London Bridge, London, UK
6.4 Uric acid and the kidney
16.5.3 Inherited disorders of purine metabolism and transport

Visith Sitprija Director, Queen Saovabha Memorial Institute, Thai Red Cross Society, Patumwan, Bangkok, Thailand
10.7.3 Acute renal failure in the tropical countries

Philip H. Smith 2 Creskeld Lane, Bramhope LS16 9AW, UK
18.5 Tumours of the prostate

John S. Smyth Department of Renal Medicine, Guy's, St Thomas' NHS Trust, London, UK
10.6.5 Ischaemic renal disease

Patrick G.J.F. Starremans Department of Paediatrics & Cell Physiology, University of Nijmegen, Nijmegen, The Netherlands
5.5 Hypokalaemic tubular disorders

Vladisav Stefanović Professor of Medicine, Institute of Nephrology and Haemodialysis, University School of Medicine, University of Niš, Niš, Yugoslavia
6.7 Balkan nephropathy

Coen A. Stegeman Associate Professor of Nephrology, Department of Nephrology, University Hospital Groningen, Groningen, The Netherlands
4.5.1 Pathogenesis of angiitis

Henk Stevens Consultant in Nuclear Medicine, Department of Nuclear Medicine, University Centre Utrecht, Utrecht, The Netherlands
1.6.1.vii Isotope scanning

Terry B. Strom Professor of Medicine, Harvard Medical School, Chief, Division of Immunology, BI-Deaconess Medical Center, Boston, Massachusetts, USA
13.2.1 The immunology of transplantation

Frank Strutz Universitätsklinikum/Innere Medizin, Abteilung für Nephrologie und Rheumatologie, Göttingen, Germany
6.1 Mechanisms of interstitial inflammation

Manikkam Suthanthiran Chief, Nephrology and Transplantation Medicine, Stanton Griffis Distinguished Professor of Medicine, Cornell University Medical College, New York, USA
13.2.1 The immunology of transplantation

Dante Tagliavini Cattedra di Nefrologia, Ospedale Maggiore, Parma, Italy
12.1 Dialysis strategies

Richard L. Tannen University of Pennsylvania School of Medicine, Philadelphia, Pennsylvania, USA
2.2 Hypo–hyperkalaemia

Antonio Tarantino Divisione Di Nefrologia, Ospedale Maggiore, IRCCS, Milan, Italy
4.6 The patient with mixed cryoglobulinaemia and hepatitis C infection

James Tattersall Department of Nephrology, St James's University Hospital, Leeds, UK
12.5 Adequacy of dialysis

C. Mark Taylor Department of Nephrology, Birmingham Children's Hospital, Birmingham, UK
10.6.3 Acute renal failure associated with microangiopathy (haemolytic–uraemic syndrome and thrombotic thrombocytopenic purpura)

Hans-Göran Tiselius Professor of Urology, Department of Urology, Huddinge University Hospital, Stockholm, Sweden
8.1 Aetiological factors in stone formation

Wai Y. Tse Department of Nephrology, Derriford Hospital, Plymouth, UK
6.3 Non-steroidal anti-inflammatory drugs and the kidney

A. Neil Turner Professor of Nephrology, University of Edinburgh, Renal & Autoimmunity Group, Royal Infirmary, Edinburgh, UK
3.2 Glomerular injury and glomerular response
3.11 Antiglomerular basement disease

William H. Turner Consultant Urologist, Addenbrooks NHS Trust, Cambridge, UK
18.4 Tumours of the bladder

Robert J. Unwin St Peter's Professor of Nephrology, Centre for Nephrology, Royal Free and University College Medical School, London, UK
5.1 The structure and function of tubules

Seppo Vainio Department of Biochemistry, University of Oulu, Linnanmaa, Finland
17.1 The development of the kidney and renal dysplasia

Bernard E. Van Beers Professor of Radiology, Universite Catholique de Louvain, Cliniques Universitaires Saint-Luc, Brussels, Belgium
1.6.1.v CT scanning and helical CT

Nele Van Den Noortgate Department of Internal Medicine, Division of Geriatric Medicine, Ghent University Hospital, Ghent, Belgium
10.7.4 The elderly

Charles van Ypersele Professor of Medicine, Universite Catholique de Louvain, Cliniques Universitaires Saint-Luc, Brussels, Belgium
6.8 Chinese herbs (and other rare causes of interstitial nephropathy)
10.6.6 Hantavirus infection
11.3.10 β2M Amyloidosis

William G. van't Hoff Consultant Paediatric Nephrologist, Great Ormond Street Hospital for Children, NHS Trust, London, UK
5.3 Fanconi syndrome
8.5 Renal and urinary tract stone disease in children

Raymond Camille Vanholder Nephrology Department, University Hospital Ghent, Ghent, Belgium
10.2 Acute renal failure: pathophysiology and prevention
10.7.4 The elderly
11.3.1 Uraemic toxicity

Patrick J.W. Venables Kennedy Institute of Rheumatology, Faculty of Medicine, The Charing Cross Hospital Campus, Arthritis Research Campaign Building, London, UK
4.10 The patient with Sjögren's syndrome and overlap syndromes

Christoph Wanner Department of Medicine, Division of Nephrology, University Hospital, Würzburg, Germany
11.3.4 Hypertension

Richard P. Wedeen Professor of Medicine, Professor of Preventive Medicine and Community Health, UMDNJ—New Jersey Medical School and Associate Chief of Staff for Research and Development, Department of Veterans Affairs New Jersey Health Care System, East Orange, New Jersey, USA
6.5 Nephrotoxic metals

Pieter M. Ter Wee Department of Nephrology, Vrije Universiteit Academic Medical Center, Amsterdam, The Netherlands
11.2 Assessment and initial management of the patient with failing renal function

Richard B. Weiner Clinical Assistant Professor of Psychiatry, SUNY Health Sciences Center at Brooklyn and Director, Children's Psychiatric Impatient Unit, Division of Child and Adolescent Psychiatry, Kings County Hospital Center, Brooklyn, New York, USA
12.7 Psychological aspects of treatment for renal failure

Ulrich Wenzel Department of Medicine, Division of Nephrology, Universitätsklinikum Hamburg-Eppendorf, Hamburg, Germany
9.4 The effects of hypertension on renal vasculature and structure

Jack F.M. Wetzels University Medical Center St Radboud, Division of Nephrology 545, Nijmegen, The Netherlands
1.8 Immunological investigation of the patient with renal disease

Peter Whelan Department of Urology, St James's University Hospital, Leeds, UK
18.3 Tumours of the renal pelvis and ureter

Hugh Whitfield Department of Urology, Battle Hospital, Reading, Berkshire, UK
8.3 The surgical management of renal stones

Alan H. Wilkinson Professor of Medicine, Director Kidney & Kidney/Pancreas Transplantation, David Geffen School of Medicine, University of California at Los Angeles, Los Angeles, California, USA
13.3.2 The early management of the recipient

Robert Wilkinson Department of Nephrology, The Freeman Hospital, High Heaton, Newcastle-upon-Tyne, UK
9.2 Clinical approach to hypertension

K. Martin Wissing Departement Medico-Chirurgical de Nephrologie, Dialyse et Transplantation, Hopital Erasme, Brussels, Belgium
13.2.2 Immunosuppression for renal transplantation

Oliver Wrong University College London, Department of Nephrology, Middlesex Hospital, London, UK
8.4 Nephrocalcinosis

Muhammad Magdi Yaqoob Professor and Lead Consultant in Nephrology, Department of Renal Medicine & Transplantation, The Royal London Hospital, Whitechapel, London, UK
17.3 The patient with urinary tract obstruction

Jerry Yee Division Head, Division of Nephrology and Hypertension, Department of Medicine, Henry Ford Hospital, Detroit, Michigan, USA
2.6 Clinical acid–base disorders

Michael Zellweger Nephrology Fellow, Research Center, Hôpital du Sacré-Coeur de Montréal, Montréal, Québec, Canada
5.6 Nephrogenic diabetes insipidus

Carla Zoja Mario Negri Institute for Pharmacological Research, Bergamo, Italy
11.3.12 Coagulation disorders

11

The patient with failing renal function

11.1 Mechanisms of experimental and clinical renal scarring

A. Meguid El Nahas

Definition of chronic kidney disease

Chronic kidney failure (CKF) refers to a progressive and irreversible loss of renal function. This usually occurs when the glomerular filtration rate (GFR) is reduced to at least 50–60 ml/min. The recent Kidney Disease Outcomes Quality Initiative (K/DOQI 2002) guidelines have classified chronic kidney diseases (CKD) into five stages;

Stage 1: Patients with normal GFR but with some evidence of kidney damage such as microalbuminuria/proteinuria, haematuria, or histological changes

Stage 2: Mild CKD with a GFR ranging from 89 to 60 ml/min/1.73 m^2

Stage 3: Moderate CKD with a GFR ranging from 59 to 30 ml/min

Stage 4: Severe CKD with a GFR ranging from 29 to 15 ml/min

Stage 5: Kidney failure when GFR is less than 15 ml/min (K/DOQI 2002). This stage is when renal replacement therapy (RRT) in the form of dialysis or transplantation has to be considered.

Epidemiology and natural history of chronic kidney failure in humans

Epidemiology

In the United States, the third National Health and Nutrition Examination Survey (NHANES III: 1988–1994) estimated that 3 per cent of the population (5.6 million individuals) had an elevated serum creatinine 1.4–1.6 mg/dl (Coresh et al. 2001) and of these, 70 per cent are hypertensive. The study also found the prevalence of proteinuria (raised albumin to creatinine ratio) to be around 11.7 per cent (19.2–20.2 million Americans) (Jones et al. 1998; Coresh et al. 2001, 2003; K/DOQI 2002). However, on repeat testing, only 54 per cent had persistent proteinuria (3.3 per cent of the US population; 5.9 million adults) (Coresh et al. 2003). Such a high prevalence may reflect the increased albumin excretion rate in those aged over 70 years (prevalence around 30 per cent) and in individuals with diabetes mellitus (>50 per cent). It remains to be determined what percentage of these individuals will progress to CKF or to endstage renal failure (ESRF).

In the United Kingdom, the incidence of endstage renal disease (ESRD), as measured by the number of patients commencing renal replacement treatment, varies between 80 and 110 new patients per million of population (pmp) per year (93.2 pmp in 2001) (UK Renal Registry 2002). In the United States, the incidence of ESRD is much higher at around 315 pmp in 1999 (USRDS 2001). In general, the incidence of ESRD increases with age, reaching around 1300 pmp per year in patients aged over 65 years. A projected analysis undertaken in the United States suggests that the incidence of ESRD will continue to increase until 2010 at a rate of 6–7 per cent per year (Xue et al. 2001).

As the majority of patients with CKF do not develop uraemic symptoms until the GFR is less than 25–20 ml/min, it is difficult to ascertain the prevalence of CKF within a community. Screening of individuals for CKD would have to rely on clinical examination, biochemical investigations, and/or urinalysis of at risk individuals. Of relevance, the recently launched KEEP (Kidney Early Evaluation Program) of the National Kidney Foundation (USA) showed that when screened for kidney diseases, up to 71.4 per cent of at risk individuals have at least one abnormality (Brown et al. 2003).

Natural history of chronic kidney disease

The proportion of patients with stages 1 and 2 CKD who progress to ESRD remains to be determined. Progression is more common in patients with significantly impaired kidney function at presentation, as the majority of patients with stages 3–5 CKD progress relentlessly. The decline in renal function has been described in most patients as constant with a straight-line plot of the reciprocal of serum creatinine (1/sCr) against time. However, a significant proportion of patients have breakpoints in their progression slopes suggesting an acceleration or decceleration of their progressing insufficiency due to either spontaneous or secondary events such as infections, dehydration, obstruction, or changes in blood pressure control.

The rate of progression of CKF varies according to the underlying nephropathy and between individual patients (for review, see Locatelli and Del Vecchio 2000; K/DOQI 2002). The rate of progression of untreated diabetic nephropathy (DN) has an annual loss of GFR of around −10 ml/min. The rate of progression depends on the quality of the control of both the glycaemia and systemic hypertension (discussed below). It has been suggested that the rate of decline is faster in polycystic kidney diseases (PKD) and chronic glomerulonephritis (CGN) compared with chronic interstitial nephropathies or hypertensive nephrosclerosis (HNS) (Hunsicker et al. 1997). On the other hand, in a large European study, the rate of progression of CKF was 2.5 times greater in patients with CGN compared with those with CIN and 1.5 times faster than those with HNS or PKD. In this study, the type of nephropathy was the most significant predictor of progression, with proteinuria the only continuous variable identified as an independent risk factor (discussed below) (for review, see Locatelli and Del Vecchio 2000).

Pathogenesis and pathology

Experimental kidney scarring

Experimental models

Understanding of progressive CKF and scarring comes from the study of a range of experimental models. Most bear some similarities to clinical nephropathies, but none is fully representative.

Renal ablation

This experimental model, extensively used over the last 25 years, is based on a reduction of the functional renal mass by 40–80 per cent. Following renal ablation, adaptive changes take place in the remnant kidney in proportion to the amount of tissue resected and are characterized by hypertrophy and hyperfunction. The early glomerular haemodynamic adaptive changes (glomerular hyperperfusion, hyperfiltration, and hypertension) have been implicated in the pathogenesis of glomerulosclerosis (for review, see Dworkin and Weir 2000) (discussed below).

Histologically, the remnant kidney model evolves in two stages: an early stage of adaptive renal growth with glomerular and proximal tubular hypertrophy, and a late stage of progressive glomerulosclerosis and tubulointerstitial scarring (Rennke 1986) evolving over 60–180 days depending on the extent of the intial reduction in renal mass. This model is primarily one of severe systemic hypertension, which, in the absence of effective autoregulation of the remnant glomeruli, is freely transmitted to the glomerular capillary bed (reviewed in Dworkin and Weir 2000).

Extensive renal ablation has been studied in many species, rats, mice, rabbits, dogs, and baboons. The course of the nephropathy in these varies, with rabbits developing a predominantly tubulointerstitial nephropathy, dogs preserving renal function up to 4 years after a 75 per cent nephrectomy, and baboons showing a progressive decline in GFR when fed a 25 per cent protein diet.

This model has been extensively studied as it is easily reproduced and bears similarities to the progression of CKF in man. A wide range of dietary and pharmacological manipulations has been studied in rats submitted to extensive renal ablation.

Models of glomerulosclerosis

Models of glomerulonephritis

Nephrotoxic serum nephritis The nephrotoxic serum nephritis model, first described by Masugi in Japan, is induced in rats by a single injection of an anti-glomerular basement membrane antibody (anti-GBM) which leads to an initial monocyte-mediated, necrotizing or crescentic glomerulonephritis with proteinuria and impaired renal function. In some rats, in particular, those with severe nephrotoxic nephritis, the glomerulonephritis is progressive and leads to ESRF. Progression is independent of the initial immune response as the transplantation of kidneys affected by nephrotoxic serum nephritis into non-immunized syngeneic recipients does not alter the course of the disease (El Nahas *et al.* 1985).

Histologically, the acute (autologous) phase is characterized in the rat by a proliferative and necrotizing glomerulonephritis that progresses to a mesangiocapillary glomerulonephritis and ultimately to glomerulosclerosis (El Nahas *et al.* 1985). The element of tubulointerstitial scarring in this model is mild and takes place late in the course of the nephropathy, and systemic hypertension is rare. In the absence of systemic hypertension and severe tubulointerstitial scarring,

progression to CKF in this model is variable. The superimposition of systemic hypertension accelerates the course of nephrotoxic nephritis.

The standard model of acute nephrotoxic serum nephritis bears similarities to acute necrotizing and crescentic glomerulonephritis in man. Chronic nephrotoxic serum nephritis resembles mesangiocapillary glomerulonephritis, with progression in some instances to glomerulosclerosis. The limitation of this model of nephrotoxic nephritis is its varied and unpredictable nature and outcome.

Heymann nephritis (autologous immune-complex glomerulonephritis)
This is an experimental model of membranous nephropathy induced in rats by a single injection of a heterologous (rabbit) anti-rat proximal tubular brush border antigen. The antibody directed against the F×1A antigen cross-reacts with antigenic sites [glycoprotein (gp) 330] on the glomerular epithelial foot processes leading to the formation of *in situ* immune complexes (Kerjaschki 1995). The ensuing membranous nephropathy is characterized by heavy proteinuria associated with mild glomerulosclerosis and minimal interstitial fibrosis. The absence of systemic hypertension may explain the non-progressive nature of this experimental nephropathy. Superimposition of systemic hypertension in rats with Heymann nephritis leads to an exacerbation of the glomerulosclerosis.

This model has proved useful in the study of immunological aspects of membranous nephropathy. It has also being used to study the behaviour of podocytes during the course of experimental nephrosis (Petermann *et al.* 2003) and to test the efficacy of antiproteinuric and lipid-reducing interventions and their interactions with respect to minimizing renal scarring (Zoja *et al.* 2002).

Anti-thy-1 glomerulonephritis This model has, in recent years, come to the forefront of research and is induced in rats by a single injection of an antibody to the mesangial cell-membrane antigen thy 1.1. It is characterized by an acute, complement-dependent mesangiolysis followed by a mesangioproliferative glomerulonephritis leading to glomerulosclerosis. Migration and proliferation of residual mesangial cells, as well as that of haematopoietic precursors migrating into the injured glomerular tufts, contribute within a few weeks from injury to the repopulation of the damaged glomeruli (Hugo *et al.* 1997). Ultimately, and within 28 days from the initiation of the glomerulonephritis, the proliferative and sclerotic changes resolve.

This model is not associated with systemic hypertension or with significant tubulointerstitial changes. This may explain the fact that it is self-limiting and does not progress to CKF. A progressive variant of the anti-thy-1 model has been produced by repeated injections of the inducing antibody (Yamamoto *et al.* 1994).

Models of nephrotic syndrome

Puromycin aminonucleoside nephrosis The single injection of the aminonucleoside puromycin leads to glomerular epithelial injury and nephrotic syndrome. Administration of puromycin to rats leads to severe proteinuria and histological lesions resembling those of minimal-change nephropathy in man. The model is not associated with systemic or intraglomerular hypertension.

Puromycin nephrosis is characterized by mild focal and segmental glomerulosclerosis (FSGS) and stable renal function. By contrast, the repeated subcutaneous, intravenous, or intraperitoneal injection of puromycin aminonucleoside leads to progressive kidney failure, glomerulosclerosis, and tubulointerstitial fibrosis (van Goor *et al.* 1993). This appears to be associated with a progressive depletion of glomerular visceral epithelial cells (podocytes) and denudement of the underlying GBM (Kim *et al.* 2001a).

Adriamycin nephrosis This experimental model of nephrotic syndrome is induced by a single intravenous injection of adriamycin. The severity of the ensuing glomerulosclerosis depends on the dose injected. In the mild, single-dose variant (5 mg/kg body weight), adriamycin nephropathy is characterized by heavy and sustained proteinuria appearing within a few days of the injection. Histological changes are minimal and similar to those described in the puromycin model. The single-dose model is not associated with systemic hypertension, although an increase in intra-glomerular capillary pressure (Pgc) has been described (O'Donnell *et al.* 1985), neither is the nephrosis progressive, as renal function is maintained and glomerulosclerosis is minimal. By contrast, the injection of adriamycin, 7.5 mg/kg body weight, or the repeated injection of adriamycin, leads to systemic hypertension, tubulointerstitial scarring, and progressive glomerulosclerosis. Accelerated variants of adriamycin nephropathy have been induced in spontaneously hypertensive rats and in rats submitted to extensive renal ablation (Fries *et al.* 1989).

The adriamycin model, as well as the puromycin model described above, have been valuable in determining the contribution of nephrotic syndrome (heavy proteinuria and hyperlipidaemia) to the progression of FSGS. They have highlighted the key role played by podocytes injury in the development of glomerulosclerosis and proteinuria (Endlich *et al.* 2001a).

Podocyte dysfunction A growing literature has attributed a central role to podocytes in the pathogenesis and progression of experimental proteinuria and glomerulosclerosis (Endlich *et al.* 2001a; Antignac 2002). In a variety of experimental models, associations have been observed between podocytes depletion (podocytopenia) and the severity of proteinuria as well as the progression of glomerulosclerosis.

Advances in cellular and molecular biology have identified a range of cell surface proteins and markers associated with podocytes and involved in maintaining their integrity and function (Endlich *et al.* 2001a), such as nephrin, podocin, α-actinin 4, and CD2-associated protein (CD2AP). Mutations associated with the depletion of these podocytic proteins in mice have been associated with the nephrotic syndrome and progressive FSGS (Endlich *et al.* 2001a). These insights have opened the way to the detection of similar mutations for nephrin (NPHS1, 19q), podocin (NPHS2, 1p), as well as α-actinin-4 (19q) associated with congenital and familial forms of steroid-resistant nephrotic syndrome and FSGS in humans (Endlich *et al.* 2001a).

Diabetic nephropathy

Type 1 diabetes Diabetes mellitus can be induced in experimental animals by a single injection of agents capable of destroying pancreatic β-cells, such as streptozotocin and alloxan. Streptozotocin-induced diabetes has been extensively applied to the study of DN in rats. Following the induction of diabetes, the nephropathy evolves in three stages. The first is characterized by early renal and glomerular hypertrophy as well as glomerular hyperperfusion, hyperfiltration, and hypertension (Hostetter 1986). This is followed within 1–3 months by progressive mesangial expansion and associated proteinuria. The final stage occurs after 12–18 months, when some degree of glomerular sclerosis develops. However, these lesions are not representative of the typical nodular hyalinosis observed in patients with advanced DN. Renal function is maintained in streptozotocin-induced diabetes and animals are normotensive.

An acceleration of the course of DN in rats has been induced by concomitant uninephrectomy and subtotal nephrectomy (reviewed in Hostetter 1986). The superimposition of systemic hypertension accelerates the development of glomerulosclerosis. The strict control of glycaemia in diabetic rats prevents the development of microangiopathy and nephropathy (Jensen *et al.* 1987).

The diabetic renal lesions induced in dogs or monkeys are more representative of those observed in man, but take years to develop and are, therefore, more difficult to study (reviewed in Steffes and Mauer 1984).

Recently, interest has focused on models of diabetes mellitus occurring spontaneously in inbred strains of rodents. The BB (Bio-Breeding) rat develops a genetically determined, autoimmune destruction of pancreatic β-cells, thus reproducing human type 1 diabetes (Kempe *et al.* 1993). The non-obese diabetic (NOD) mouse also develops spontaneous, immune-mediated, insulin-dependent diabetes mellitus (Kempe *et al.* 1993).

Transgenic mice overexpressing the human receptor of advanced glycation end products (RAGE) develop a severe form of experimental DN when crossbred with another transgenic mouse strain that develops insulin-dependent diabetes after birth (Yamamoto *et al.* 2001). This double transgenic mouse model reproduces the diabetic renal lesions seen in humans.

Type 2 diabetes and obesity The development of FSGS has been studied in the obese Zucker (OZR) strain of rats (Kasiske *et al.* 1993). These animals are obese, insulin-resistant, and hyperlipidaemic: mimicking the metabolic profile of patients with non-insulin-dependent diabetes mellitus, but they do not develop significant systemic hypertension.

Other models of type 2 diabetes have been described in Cohen, Obese spontaneous hypertensive rat (SHR), Wistar fatty and Goto Kakizaki (GK) rats (Kempe *et al.* 1993). The GK rat has sustained hyperglycaemia without the confounding effects of systemic hypertension, dyslipidaemia, or obesity (Riley *et al.* 1999). The structural renal changes in this model resemble those of longstanding type 2 diabetes in man with thickening of the GBM, mesangial expansion and activation, podocyte injury as well as interstitial inflammatory, monocytic, infiltrate. However, this model is not associated with progressive kidney insufficiency, unless systemic hypertension is superimposed.

Systemic hypertension

Many spontaneous and experimental models of systemic hypertension have been studied (reviewed in Dworkin and Weir 2000). Hypertension can be induced in rats by the administration of mineralocorticoids (deoxycorticosterol acetate), by salt loading, as well as by inducing unilateral stenosis of the renal artery (reviewed in Mann and Luft 1993). In models such as the Milan hypertensive or the young, spontaneously hypertensive rat, systemic hypertension is not transmitted to the glomeruli and glomerulosclerosis does not develop (Olson *et al.* 1986). The glomeruli are, therefore, protected through autoregulation and afferent arteriolar vasoconstriction (Olson *et al.* 1986). By contrast, when systemic hypertension is allowed to reach the glomerular capillaries through defective autoregulation, as in old or uninephrectomized, spontaneously hypertensive rats and Dahl salt-sensitive rats, Pgc increases and glomerulosclerosis occurs (Dworkin and Feiner 1986).

The superimposition of systemic hypertension in models of experimental glomerulonephritis and nephrosis, as well as in the streptozotocin-induced model of DN, leads to accelerated glomerulosclerosis (reviewed in Baldwin and Neugarten 1986).

Experimental hypertensive renal injury has been induced in rats by the chronic inhibition of the nitric oxide (NO) system (Zatz and Baylis 1998; Klahr 2001) associated with the activation of the renin–angiotensin system and the sympathetic nervous system. It has been suggested that an imbalance between NO and angiotensin II can be instrumental in the development of systemic hypertension (Reviewed in Klahr 2001; Leclercq et al. 2002).

Overexpression of a wide range of hypertension mediators such as renin and angiotensin II is associated with experimental hypertension (reviewed in Luft 2000). The Tsukuba hypertensive mouse, overexpressing both renin and angiotensin, displays fibrinoid vascular lesions, cardiac hypertrophy, and glomerulosclerosis. Of interest, mice overexpressing endothelin-1 develop cystic renal lesions and interstitial fibrosis in the absence of systemic hypertension (Hocher et al. 1997; Theuring et al. 1998).

Models of tubulointerstitial injury and fibrosis

Cyclosporin-induced renal scarring The administration of high doses (10–25 mg/kg/day) of cyclosporin A (CsA) to rats causes mild tubulo-interstitial changes. These are characterized by tubular vacuolation and striped interstitial fibrosis (Porter et al. 1999). A body of experimental evidence suggests that superimposed salt-depletion accelerates the progression of the interstitial fibrosis induced by the chronic administration of CsA (a dose as low as 5 mg/kg/day) (Porter et al. 1999). Salt-depletion reproduces many of the lesions induced by CsA in humans including afferent arteriolar hyalinosis, tubular atrophy, and striped interstitial fibrosis (Porter et al. 1999).

More recently, the chronic administration of another calcineurin antagonist, FK506 (Tacrolimus), to rats has resulted in interstitial fibrosis similar to that observed with chronic CsA administration (Bennett 1998).

Protein overload nephropathy The chronic administration of protein and in particular large amounts of bovine serum albumin (BSA; 5 g/day injected intraperitoneally) to rats has long been known to be associated with heavy proteinuria, tubular protein overload and subsequently injury (Lawrence and Brewer 1981). Protein overload induces severe interstitial inflammatory (monocytic) infiltrate that precedes the onset of progressive interstitial fibrosis.

This model has been used to study chronic interstitial inflammation and fibrosis and the contribution of albuminuria to the initiation and progression of chronic tubulointerstitial lesions. Data derived from the study of this model suggest a role for apoptosis in albumin-induced tubular cell atrophy (Thomas et al. 1999). Changes in the synthesis of extracellular matrix under the influence of fibrogenic mediators including growth factors as well as a decrease in renal collagenolytic activity has been identified as key events leading to interstitial fibrosis in this model (reviewed in Jernigan and Eddy 2000).

Obstructive nephropathy Obstructive nephropathy, induced in rodents by the ligation of the ureter, has been used as a model of tubulo-interstitial injury and damage leading to renal interstitial fibrosis. Within a few days of unilateral ureteric obstruction (UUO), tubular cell deletion takes place through apoptosis. Tubular cell deletion is associated with progressive increase in interstitial extracellular collagenous matrix (ECM) culminating in interstitial fibrosis (reviewed in Klahr 2000).

The advantage of this experimental model is that interstitial fibrosis is initiated within hours of UUO and progresses rapidly over a short period of time (days). This takes place in the absence of proteinuria or significant hypertension. Further, relief of the UUO allows an estimate of the reversibility of the functional and histological changes (reviewed in Klahr 2000).

Genetically modified animal models

The technical progress made over the last decade in molecular biology and genetics has allowed the development of mice over- (transgenes) or under- (knockout) expressing genes thought to be involved in renal scarring (reviewed in Anders and Schlondorff 2000; Terzi et al. 2000).

Mice with transgenes for a range of proinflammatory cytokines have been studied. Those with the interleukin (IL)-6 gene develop a plasma-cell dyscrasia bearing similarities to multiple myeloma associated with the development of a diffuse mesangioproliferative glomerulonephritis (Suematsu et al. 1989). IL-4 transgenic mice develop glomerulosclerosis independently from immunoglobulin deposition (Ruger et al. 2000).

Overexpression of pro-fibrogenic growth factors such as platelet-derived growth factor (PDGF) and transforming growth factor-β1 (TGF-β1) has also been explored. The transfection of the human TGF-β1 gene into rat glomerular mesangial cells leads to the expression of smooth muscle-cell characteristics and progressive glomerulosclerosis (Isaka et al. 1993). By contrast, rats whose glomeruli are transfected with the human PDGF B-chain gene develop a proliferation of mesangial cells with minimal sclerosis (Isaka et al. 1993; Imai et al. 1994).

Transgenic mice overexpressing TGF-β1 develop mesangial expansion, glomerulosclerosis, and interstitial fibrosis (reviewed in Kopp et al. 1997). On the other hand, mice overexpressing decorin, a small molecular weight proteoglycan known to antagonize TGF-β1 are protected against the development of renal scarring (Isaka et al. 1996). Transgenic mice overexpressing hepatocyte growth factor (HGF) develop cystic tubular changes as well as glomerulosclerosis (Takayama et al. 1997). Mice with transgenes for profibrotic hormones and autacoids have also been studied to evaluate the contribution to renal scarring of hormones such as growth hormone (GH) (Doi et al. 1988, 1991), growth hormone releasing hormone (GHRH), insulin-like growth factor-1 (IGF-1) (Doi et al. 1988) and its binding protein1 (IGFBP-1) (Doublier et al. 2000), as well as autacoids such as angiotensin II and endothelin-1 (reviewed in Anders and Schlondorff 2000).

In addition, targeted mutations of putative receptors such as the angiotensin II types 1 (ATR1) and 2 (ATR2) receptors have allowed studies of the respective roles of different activation pathways in the pathogenesis of renal fibrosis (Suzuki et al. 2001). For example, experimental interstitial fibrosis is attenuated in AT1-deficient mice (Suzuki et al. 2001) and accelerated in mice deficient in the AT2 receptor (Ma et al. 1998).

Mice with transgenes for a variety of virus and virus-related proteins have been shown to be prone to glomerulosclerosis. Those transgenic for the simian virus 40 or the human immune deficiency virus (reviewed in Kopp 1997) display glomerular hypertrophy and mesangial proliferation. Mice transgenic for a gag-pol-deleted HIV-1 develop FSGS associated with heavy proteinuria and kidney failure (Shrivastav et al. 2000).

Genetic manipulation of metabolic and enzymatic targets has also been studied to determine the relevance of various metabolic pathways to the pathogenesis of glomerulosclerosis. Lecithin cholesterol acyltransferase (LCAT)-deficient mice are prone to develop atherosclerosis and glomerulosclerosis (Lambert et al. 2001). Transgenic mice overexpressing human RAGE develop a severe form of DN when crossbred with insulin-dependent mice (Yamamoto *et al.* 2001). The mutant mouse strain Mpv17−/− that carries a retroviral germline that inactivates the Mpv17 gene is prone to glomerulosclerosis highlighting the importance of this peroxisomal protein and the role of antioxidant enzymes in the prevention of glomerulosclerosis (O'Bryan *et al.* 2000).

In summary, experimental models of kidney scarring have highlighted the importance of systemic hypertension and tubulointerstitial scarring, as well as their mediators, as determinants of progressive renal insufficiency. In few models is that progression in the absence of systemic hypertension. Similarly, progression is often associated with tubulointerstitial scarring.

Mechanisms of progressive kidney scarring

Numerous hypotheses have attempted to explain the mechanisms underlying the relentless progression of CKF. Some have focused on the progression of glomerulosclerosis, others have examined the mechanisms underlying the progression of tubulointerstitial scarring or vascular sclerosis. Many have been exclusive whilst others have attempted to incorporate all aspects of kidney scarring.

Renal adaptation to injury

Adaptative glomerular changes

The role of adaptive glomerular haemodynamic changes This hypothesis proposed by Brenner, Hostetter, and their associates in the early 1980s attributed a key role in the initiation and progression of glomerulosclerosis to the adaptive changes in glomerular haemodynamics, that take place after a reduction in functional renal mass (Hostetter *et al.* 1981; Brenner *et al.* 1982; Brenner 1985). They suggested that glomerular hyperperfusion and hyperfiltration, as well as hypertension, lead to the stretching of the glomerular capillary wall, resulting in endothelial and epithelial injury together with the transudation of macromolecules into the mesangium (Olson *et al.* 1985), leading to mesangial overload and dysfunction.

Morphological changes attributed to glomerular hypertension include glomerular microaneurysms, endothelial detachment, glomerular transudation of proteins, the formation of platelet aggregates and microthrombi within glomerular capillaries, epithelial stretching with secondary denudation of the GBM and mesangial expansion (Olson *et al.* 1985; Rennke 1986). These changes evolve with time to progressive mesangial sclerosis, and ultimately to glomerulosclerosis (Rennke 1986). It was therefore suggested that the early compensatory changes taking place within remnant glomeruli were maladaptive, as they resulted eventually in glomerular scarring and loss of renal function (reviewed in Dworkin and Weir 2000).

This hypothesis also attempted to explain the progression of proteinuria and renal failure in individuals born with oligomeganephronia, unilateral renal agenesis, or following unilateral nephrectomy, as well as in patients with diabetic and non-diabetic nephropathies. It highlighted the nephrotoxicity of a high intake of dietary protein (Brenner *et al.* 1982). The therapeutic implication of this hypothesis was that the reduction of glomerular hypertension would prevent the progression of glomerulosclerosis. This could be achieved by both dietary protein restriction and angiotensin-converting enzyme (ACE) inhibition (reviewed in Anderson 2000). This hypothesis suggested that ACE inhibitors had a therapeutic advantage over conventional antihypertensive agents as they reduced both systemic and glomerular hypertension (reviewed in Dworkin and Weir 2000).

In spite of its limitations (Reviewed in El Nahas 1998), the glomerular hyperperfusion/hyperfiltration/hypertension hypothesis highlighted the importance of haemodynamic changes and the renin–angiotensin–aldosterone (RAA) system in the glomerular microcirculation to the development of glomerulosclerosis.

Evidence for the hyperperfusion/hyperfiltration hypothesis in human disease is limited. It has been suggested that the early increase in renal blood flow and GFR characteristic of early diabetes mellitus may initiate DN (Hostetter *et al.* 1981). Hyperfiltration was shown to be an independent predictor of DN (Rudberg *et al.* 1992).

The role of adaptive glomerular hypertrophy Although questioning the pathogenic role of glomerular hypertension, some investigators have suggested that adaptive glomerular hypertrophy (enlargement) is relevant to the initiation and progression of experimental glomerulosclerosis (reviewed in Fogo and Ichikawa 1991; Johnson 1994; Fogo 2001a), but failed to observe a correlation between the degree of glomerular hyperfunction detected by micropuncture and the subsequent sclerosis. On the other hand, Fogo *et al.* (1990) observed, in rats and patients, a close correlation between glomerular enlargement and early glomerulosclerosis. Support for the argument comes from mice transgenic for the bovine GH gene in which glomerular hypertrophy precedes the onset of accelerated, age-related mesangial sclerosis (Doi *et al.* 1991). Furthermore, the study of glomerulosclerosis in SV40 transgenic mice showed a close correlation between glomerular size and the severity of glomerulosclerosis.

Conversely, in PVG/c rats the limited adaptive glomerular hypertrophy that follows renal ablation may explain the resistance of this strain to the development of glomerulosclerosis (reviewed in Weening *et al.* 1986; Grond *et al.* 1989).

These observations notwithstanding, glomerular hypertrophy is unlikely to be the sole determinant of the development of glomerulosclerosis in rats. Mice transgenic for the IGF-1 gene develop glomerular hypertrophy without glomerulosclerosis and certain strains of mice (C57/Os+) predisposed to oligomeganephronia (reduced number of nephrons and large glomeruli) seem resistant to ablation-induced glomerulosclerosis (Esposito *et al.* 1999). These observations imply that genetic predisposition to glomerulosclerosis prevails over glomerular size.

An association between glomerular hypertrophy and sclerosis has been put forward to explain the glomerulosclerosis that occurs in diabetic, obese, and elderly individuals, and in those with oligomeganephronia (reviewed in Brenner and Chertow 1994).

Adaptive tubular changes

As with compensatory glomerular changes, tubular functional changes may be 'maladaptive' and have been implicated in the pathogenesis of tubulointerstitial scarring.

The role of adaptive tubular growth and hypermetabolism A feature of compensatory renal growth is increased sodium reabsorption and oxygen consumption by the proximal tubules. A threefold increase in oxygen consumption by the remnant kidney can be demonstrated *in vitro* using the isolated, perfused kidney technique and *in vivo* using nuclear magnetic resonance. Schrier *et al.* (1994) suggested that the increase in tubular sodium reabsorption and the activation of sodium/hydrogen exchange not only led to proton extrusion and increased cellular pH, but also increases the generation and utilization of Na^+–K^+ ATP, which could lead to excessive generation of oxygen free radicals, causing peroxidation and damage to tissue lipids.

Oxidative stress Recent evidence links the hypertrophy of the proximal tubules to the generation of reactive oxygen species (ROS) and subsequent tubular injury. Angiotensin II is likely to be one of the major mediators of proximal tubular hypertrophy either directly or indirectly through the stimulation of proximal tubular release of TGF-β1 (Wolf 2001), increased generation of ROS (Hannken *et al.* 2000), and NO production. Interactions between ROS and NO lead to the formation of peroxynitrite (ONOO$^-$); with loss of NO homeostatic effects and peroxynitrite-induced cytotoxicity (Welch *et al.* 2000).

ROS have also been shown to play an important role in tubulointerstitial inflammation and fibrosis. The generation of ROS is capable of the activation of the transcription factor nuclear factor-κB (NF-κB), leading to the synthesis of a range of proinflammatory cell adhesion molecules, cytokines and chemokines (Wardle 2000, 2002). Of note, inhibition of NF-κB protects against proteinuria-induced interstitial scarring (Rangan *et al.* 1999). Beside their well-known cytotoxicity, and their proinflammatory effects, ROS may also have a direct fibrogenic effect (Houglum *et al.* 1991).

The role of oxygen free radicals in kidney scarring is supported by the observation that the lipid peroxidation product malondialdehyde accumulates progressively within the cortex of remnant kidneys (Nath *et al.* 1994; Haugen and Nath 1999). Recent evidence also points to the upregulation of oxidative stress mediators and nitric oxide synthase (NOS) in diabetic kidneys as well as those of spontaneously hypertensive rat kidneys (Onozato *et al.* 2002). Similar observations have been made in an experimental model of PKD where expression of heme oxygenase-1 (HO-1) mRNA, an inducible marker of oxidative stress, was shown to be increased (Maser *et al.* 2002). By contrast, there was a decrease in the mRNA and protein levels of a wide range of antioxidant enzymes including glutathione peroxidase, superoxide dismutase, catalase, and glutathione S-transferase during disease progression (Maser *et al.* 2002).

Many interventions that reduce the severity of experimental CKF and scarring, including dietary protein and phosphate restriction, thyroidectomy, and chronic treatment with calcium antagonists, also reduce oxygen consumption (Schrier *et al.* 1988). Indirect evidence derived from experiments with weaning rats fed a diet deficient in antioxidants (vitamin E and selenium) suggests that ROS stimulate renal growth and promote injury (Haugen and Nath 1999). Experimental data in diabetic and non-diabetic models of renal scarring have shown that the antioxidant vitamin E supplementation reduces proteinuria, glomerulosclerosis, and renal scarring (Gorgun *et al.* 1999; Hahn *et al.* 1999). The antioxidant amino acid taurine and the drug probucol have been shown to be protective in experimental models of proteinuria and kidney scarring (Trachtman *et al.* 1992; Modi *et al.* 1993). The protective effect of taurine in age-related glomerulosclerosis appears to involve the downregulation of ROS as well as TGF-β1 and the synthesis of ECM. Also, reduction of oxidative stress with a bioflavonoid, quercetin, attenuates the functional and structural renal abnormalities induced by CyA in rats (Satyanarayana *et al.* 2001).

The scope for antioxidants preventing tubulointerstitial fibrosis is considerable and warrants clinical investigation.

The role of adaptive tubular ammoniagenesis In remnant nephrons, the proximal tubules increase the secretion of acid through both the enhanced reabsorption of bicarbonate and the generation of ammonia. Nath and coworkers (1985) have postulated that increased concentrations of ammonia can initiate chronic tubulointerstitial inflammation through the activation of the alternate pathway of the complement system (reviewed in Nath *et al.* 1991).

Proteinuria has been implicated in the pathogenesis of tubulointerstitial inflammation and fibrosis (discussed below). Excessive reabsorption of proteins by the proximal tubular cells and their catabolism would, of course, stimulate ammoniagenesis. Similarly, angiotensin II, which stimulates ammoniagenesis, may also be involved in the pathogenesis of tubulointerstitial inflammation and fibrosis. Of relevance, ACE inhibition has recently been shown to reduce both proteinuria and renal ammoniagenesis in chronic allograft nephropathy (Rustom *et al.* 1998, 2001). Thus, ammoniagenesis may be one of the explanations for the nephrotoxicity of both proteinuria and angiotensin II.

The relevance of these observations to patients with CKF is unknown. Patients with diabetic and non-diabetic nephropathies excrete C5b–C9 in their urine (Schulze *et al.* 1991). The progression of membranous nephropathy has been correlated with the urinary excretion of this membrane-attack complex (Kon *et al.* 1995). Rustom *et al.* (2001) demonstrated that the correction of metabolic acidosis with oral sodium bicarbonate in patients with CKF reduced proximal renal tubular protein catabolism as well as ammoniagenesis along with a decrease in the release of surrogate markers of proximal tubular injury.

The role of systemic hypertension

Systemic hypertension is one of the causes of ESRD and has long been recognized to accelerate the progression of chronic nephropathies in experimental animals and in humans (reviewed in Dworkin and Weir 2000).

Many of the discrepancies regarding the development of glomerulosclerosis in various experimental nephropathies, described above, can be attributed to the development of systemic hypertension (El Nahas 1989). Progressive glomerulosclerosis develops in experimental nephropathies associated with systemic hypertension. On the other hand, glomerulosclerosis is slow to develop and often mild and functionally insignificant in the absence of hypertension.

An understanding of the mechanism by which systemic hypertension initiates glomerular scarring comes from the study of experimental models of hypertension in the rat. Wilson and Byrom (1941), and more recently Hill and Heptinstall (1968), suggested that the transmission of systemic hypertension to the glomerular capillary bed, normally prevented by autoregulation, determines the severity of glomerular scarring. In experimental models of hypertension where effective autoregulation and afferent vasoconstriction protect glomeruli from the transmission of systemic hypertension, glomerulosclerosis does not occur. On the other hand, when autoregulation is impaired, glomerular hypertension and glomerulosclerosis occur.

Experimental data suggests that systemic hypertension in rats may act synergistically with glomerular hypertension and hypertrophy. When systemic hypertension is transmitted to the glomeruli, the severity of glomerular scarring may depend on the degree of enlargement of these glomeruli and the dilatation of their capillary loops. According to Laplace's law, the degree of tension generated within a sphere depends on the product of the pressure inside it and its radius. It was therefore suggested by Fries *et al.* (1989) that, for any given level of Pgc, the tension on the glomerular capillary wall is proportional to the glomerular size/volume: enlarged glomeruli with dilated capillary loops would therefore be more susceptible to hypertensive injury. Such hypertension may account for some of the age-, strain-, and ablation-related susceptibility to hypertensive injury in rats (reviewed in Dworkin and Weir 2000).

The harmful effect of hypertension on renal function in patients with chronic nephropathies contrasts with the condition in essential hypertension, where renal dysfunction is rarely progressive (Rostand *et al.* 1989). In patients with essential hypertension, the incidence of significant kidney functional impairment rarely exceeds 15 per cent. Further, ESRF rarely occurs (<0.5 per cent) in the absence of an accelerated phase in these patients.

The role of proteinuria

Glomerulosclerosis Proteinuria is one of the major risk factors for the progression of CKF in experimental animals and humans. Proteinuria is also likely to play a significant part in the initiation of glomerulosclerosis (Remuzzi and Bertani 1990). The reduction of proteinuria by dietary or pharmacological interventions often leads to an attenuation of experimental glomerulosclerosis.

The transudation of plasma proteins into the endothelial and subendothelial space can initiate glomerular hyalinosis (Olson *et al.* 1985), which may, in turn, narrow and ultimately occlude glomerular capillaries. Increased traffic of macromolecules into the glomerular mesangium may also contribute to the pathogenesis of glomerulosclerosis (Remuzzi and Bertani 1990). Mesangial overload and activation may lead to the release of ROS including hydrogen peroxide with activation of proinflammatory as well as profibrotic pathways. ROS activate the transcription factor NF-κB in mesangial cells with the subsequent upregulation of mesangial transcription of a wide range of proinflammatory cytokines (Wardle 2000, 2002). Also, ROS upregulate mesangial synthesis of ECM through TGF-β1-dependent pathways (Iglesias-De La Cruz *et al.* 2001).

Increased glomerular permeability to proteins may also affect glomerular epithelial cells, leading to structural and functional changes; this may in turn further increase the passage of macromolecules across glomerular capillaries (reviewed in Rennke and Klein 1989; Gassler *et al.* 2001).

Proteinuria is unlikely to be the sole determinant of progressive glomerular scarring. As discussed above, rats treated with adriamycin develop sustained, heavy proteinuria without concomitant progressive glomerulosclerosis. Conversely, the Nagase analbuminaemic rat develops severe glomerulosclerosis when injected with adriamycin, in spite of the absence of albuminuria, although other proteins are excreted in the urine of these animals (Okuda *et al.* 1992).

In experimental animals, certain dietary and pharmacological interventions can dissociate proteinuria from the development of glomerulosclerosis. Supplementation of the diet of subtotally nephrectomized rats with tryptophan reduces proteinuria, but functional and histological deterioration continues to progress (Kaysen and Kropp 1983). Conversely, verapamil given to rats with renal ablation prevents progressive glomerular scarring without reducing proteinuria (Harris *et al.* 1988). In puromycin-induced nephrotic syndrome, treatment with a hepatic hydroxymethylglutaryl coenzyme-A (HMG-CoA) reductase inhibitor (statin) corrects the hyperlipidaemia and attenuates the glomerulosclerosis without reducing proteinuria (Harris *et al.* 1990). Similar observations were made in experimental DN where lovastatin reduced glomerulosclerosis without affecting proteinuria (Inman *et al.* 1999).

It remains to be determined whether proteinuria itself contributes to the pathogenesis of glomerular scarring or whether it merely reflects its severity. Arguments have been put forward to suggest that, as in experimental animals, it may be the quality of proteinuria and

the associated fatty aciduria that determines its nephrotoxicity (reviewed in Harris 2000).

Tubulointerstitial inflammation and scarring An association has been observed between experimental proteinuria and tubulointerstitial inflammation and scarring (reviewed in Eddy 2001).

Proteinuria may lead to tubulointerstitial scarring and fibrosis through direct and indirect pathways. Increased uptake, reabsorption, and trafficking of proteins by proximal tubular cells is thought to be associated with the activation of lysosomal enzymes leading to tubular cell injury. Evidence derived from tissue culture experiments suggests that exposure of proximal tubular cells to high concentrations of albumin stimulates their proliferation (reviewed in Harris 2000). Proteinuria has also been shown to be instrumental in the development of tubular cell apoptosis in experimental models of tubulointerstitial scarring such as protein overload nephropathy (Thomas *et al.* 1999).

It is likely that proteinuria can lead to tubular dysfunction, including stimulation of the synthesis and release of a variety of cytokines, chemokines, and growth factors (reviewed in Harris 2000; Eddy 2001). This may be mediated by the albumin-induced activation of NF-κB (Wang *et al.* 1999), initiating interstitial inflammation, a forerunner of fibrosis. Inhibition of NF-κB attenuates proteinuria-induced renal injury (Rangan *et al.* 1999; Wardle 2002). Further, the gene transfer of a truncated form of the NF-κB inhibitor (IκBα) into the renal arteries of rats with protein overload nephropathy reduced proteinuria and tubulointerstitial injury (Takase *et al.* 2003).

It remains uncertain whether proteinuria/albuminuria *per se* is the sole factor in the interstitial tubulointerstitial scarring associated with proteinuric states. Other filtered substances such as transferrin, complement components, growth factors and lipoproteins have all been implicated (they will be discussed below).

The role of lipids

Glomerulosclerosis The hyperfiltration hypothesis emphasized the nephrotoxicity of protein and its role in the progression of experimental and clinical renal scarring (Brenner *et al.* 1982), whereas the lipid hypothesis focused on the nephrotoxicity of lipids (Moorhead *et al.* 1982). It established that feeding rodents with cholesterol-supplemented diets accelerates age-related (Kasiske *et al.* 1991) and experimental (Modi *et al.* 1993; Keane 2000) nephropathies. Conversely, reduction of hyperlipidaemia by dietary or pharmacological means is protective in models of spontaneous and experimental glomerulosclerosis (reviewed in Keane 2000).

The mechanisms postulated to account for the glomerular toxicity of lipids have included an increase in Pgc as well as functional and structural endothelial and mesangial changes. Glomerular endothelial and mesangial cells have receptors for both low-density lipoprotein (LDL) and oxidized-LDL (ox-LDL). Under conditions of glomerular oxidative stress such as inflammation, deposited LDL undergo oxidative modifications. This would, in turn, induce further inflammatory changes through the release of monocyte chemoattractant protein-1 (MCP-1). This would stimulate the influx of monocytes to the glomeruli and exacerbate glomerular injury. Such infiltration often precedes glomerulosclerosis in inflammatory as well as non-inflammatory models (reviewed in Floege and Grone 1997).

Similarly, it has been suggested that LDL accumulate in the mesangial cells and matrix of dyslipidaemic states (Schlondorff 1993). Modified LDL exert cytotoxic effects on endothelial, mesangial, and epithelial cells and stimulate *in vitro* the proliferation of mesangial cells (Wasserman *et al.* 1989; Nishida *et al.* 1999). The interaction of these lipoproteins with the mesangial LDL receptors activates Ras and mitogen activated protein kinase (MAPK) as well as that cyclin/cyclin dependent kinases (CDK) (Kamanna 2002). These signal transduction pathways lead to mesangial DNA synthesis and cellular proliferation (Kamanna 2002). Recent data suggest an initial proliferative response followed in the later stages of experimental DN by a tendency of mesangial cells expressing high TGFβ1 levels to synthesize ECM (Okada *et al.* 2002). Such a functional switch in mesangial cells from proliferation to ECM synthesis may contribute to the development of glomerulosclerosis in DN.

It has been suggested that qualitative changes in LDL contribute to their nephrotoxicity. Large LDL in the plasma of cholesterol-fed rabbits may contribute to glomerular injury. By contrast, the large amounts of circulating, structurally normal, LDL observed in spontaneously hyperlipidaemic Watanabe rabbits are not associated with nephrotoxicity (Schlondorff 1993). Experimental evidence supporting this assumption has been reported. A subset of LCAT knockout mice accumulated lipoprotein X and developed proteinuria and glomerulosclerosis with mesangial lipid accumulation, proliferation, and sclerosis (Lambert *et al.* 2001). These observations might also explain why patients with familial hyperlipidaemia do not develop renal diseases. On the other hand, patients with an inherited deficiency of LCAT have abnormal lipoproteins, leading to glomerulosclerosis (Gjone *et al.* 1974). Lipoprotein thrombi have occasionally been described within the glomerular capillaries of dyslipidaemic patients (Sato *et al.* 1993) and have been attributed to an abnormality of apolipoprotein E (apoE) (Saito *et al.* 1989, 1999). Further, mutations in the apoE gene have been reported in patients with lipoprotein glomerulopathy characterized by abnormal lipoprotein profiles similar to those in type III hyperlipoproteinaemia (Saito *et al.* 1999). Similarly, the accumulation of apolipoproteins a and B100 has been observed in the glomeruli of patients with CGN (Sato *et al.* 1993). Finally, a protective effect has been attributed to apoE as this apolipoprotein has been shown to inhibit mesangial proliferation as well as apoptosis of mesangial cells induced by LDL (Chen *et al.* 2001). These data suggest that apoE deficiency rather than hyperlipidaemia may contribute to mesangial expansion.

Tubulointerstitial scarring That lipids might be toxic to the tubules was suggested by Moorhead, El Nahas and their colleagues (1982).

Recent experimental evidence supports the notion that lipids play a role in the initiation and progression of tubulointerstitial scarring. Human proximal tubular cells are capable of the uptake and oxidization of LDL *in vitro*; these lipoproteins stimulate the proliferation of proximal tubular cells in culture as well as the synthesis of ECM components such as fibronectin. In addition, LDL induces phenotypic changes in proximal tubular cells in culture including the expression of α-smooth muscle actin (α-SMA). In contrast, the accumulation of particles of native LDL within tubular cells is not toxic. It was, therefore, suggested that the balance of oxygen free radicals and antioxidants might determine the fate of LDL reabsorbed by proximal tubular cells and ultimately their nephrotoxicity (Ong and Moorhead 1994). This would lead to a unified concept linking lipid nephrotoxicity with adaptive tubular hypermetabolism and the production of oxygen free radicals (reviewed in Schrier *et al.* 1994), ischaemia and hypoxia (reviewed in Fine *et al.* 2000), haematuria (Hill *et al.* 1989), and proteinuria/transferrinuria with tubular iron overload (Alfrey 1994).

Another explanation for the nephrotoxicity of lipids relates to the reabsorption by proximal tubular cells of fatty acids linked to albumin. It was suggested that free fatty acids lead to the generation of a novel lipid chemotactic factor which attracts monocytes and initiates tubulointerstitial inflammation. In support of this concept is the observation in protein (BSA)-loaded rats of a monocytic infiltrate surrounding proximal tubular cells within days of the initiation of the nephropathy (Thomas *et al.* 1999). On the other hand, the administration of fatty acid-depleted albumin failed to induce the same interstitial inflammatory reaction (Thomas *et al.* 1999). In addition, apoptosis was a major feature of the injury associated with overloading rats with fatty acid-replete albumin (Thomas *et al.* 1999). Fatty acids interact with peroxisome proliferator-activated receptors (PPAR) in primary cultures of human proximal tubule cells and result in enhanced apoptosis (Arici *et al.* 2003). Of interest in this respect, diets deficient in essential fatty acids protect against tubulointerstitial inflammation and scarring in experimental nephrosis (reviewed in Harris 2000).

Arguments against an exclusive role for lipids in the initiation and progression of human renal disease are based on the observation that very few individuals with primary hyperlipidaemia develop renal disease and that persistent hyperlipidaemia in some nephrotic patients is not invariably associated with progression. However, this may be explained by the nature of circulating lipids. It has also been suggested that a genetic predisposition, in addition to a renal insult or environmental factors, is required for the initiation of lipid-associated nephropathies (Matsunaga *et al.* 1999).

Similarities between glomerulosclerosis and atherosclerosis

Research on the pathogenetic role of lipids in glomerulosclerosis has prompted some to find similarities between atherosclerosis and glomerulosclerosis. The term glomerulatherosis was coined in 1983, and the hypothesis was further developed by Grond *et al.* (1986), El Nahas (1988), and Diamond and Karnovsky (1988), who highlighted the similarities between the pathogenesis of glomerulosclerosis and atherosclerosis. It was claimed that both processes involved endothelial injury, smooth-muscle cell/mesangial proliferation, extracellular matrix deposition within the vascular wall, and ultimately sclerosis. This one hypothesis accommodates many of those discussed above and is the basis of current thought on the pathogenesis of glomerulosclerosis. For instance, an initial haemodynamic or mechanical insult is common to glomerulosclerosis and atherosclerosis. Further, they are both accelerated by systemic hypertension. This hypothesis also incorporates a role for lipids as they are implicated in the pathogenesis of atherosclerosis. Synergy between hyperlipidaemia and hypertension in the initiation of experimental (Tolins *et al.* 1992) and clinical (Attman *et al.* 1999) glomerular injury has been postulated as it has in the pathogenesis of atherosclerosis. This hypothesis has also drawn attention to the contribution of cytokines, chemokines, and growth factors to glomerulosclerosis in view of their involvement in atherosclerosis. Similarly, a role for oxygen free radicals (Haugen and Nath 1999) and NO (Cattell 2002) in both processes is well established.

The role of calcium and phosphorus, oxalate, and urate crystals

As with glomerulosclerosis, the injury to tubular cells may be initiated either through direct insult or, as previously discussed, indirectly through adaptive changes. Such injury leads to the accumulation of calcium within the cytoplasm and mitochondria of tubular cells (Caulfield and Schrag 1964; Ibels *et al.* 1980). An increase in tubulointerstitial calcium occurs early in the course of experimental and clinical chronic renal failure (CRF) (Gimenez *et al.* 1987). In rats with renal ablation, the extent of renal calcification varies considerably with changes in dietary protein and phosphate intake (reviewed in Kleinknecht and Laouari 1986). Renal calcification occurs early in the course of chronic nephropathies in man and correlates with the serum phosphate (Gimenez *et al.* 1987). As renal insufficiency progresses, the interstitial deposition of calcium may be facilitated by hyperparathyroidism and the concomitant increase in the serum calcium × phosphate product (reviewed in Lau 1989).

The intratubular deposition of oxalate has also been observed in scarred kidneys of animals and patients with chronic uraemia. It has been suggested that such deposits might lead to tubular obstruction and cystic dilatation, contributing, along with calcium deposition, to progressive tubulointerstitial scarring.

Recent attention has focused on the potential nephrotoxicity of uric acid (Johnson *et al.* 1999). Chronic mild hyperuricaemia has been shown to induce hypertension and renal fibrosis in rats (Johnson *et al.* 1999). Hyperuricaemia appears to exacerbate experimental cyclosporin-induced nephrotoxicity through crystal-independent pathways involving the activation of the renin–angiotensin system (Mazzali *et al.* 2002). The relevance of hyperuricaemia to the progression of CKF in humans remains uncertain.

The role of iron
Along with albuminuria, transferrinuria has been implicated in the pathogenesis of tubulointerstitial inflammation and fibrosis. Filtered transferrin releases its iron content in the acidic environment of tubular fluid. Free iron (Fe^{2+}) ions are known to be cytotoxic and may therefore damage tubular cells. Iron is present in the tubular fluid and parenchyma of experimental animals (reviewed in Alfrey 1994) and humans (Nankivell *et al.* 1992) with the nephrotic syndrome. It has been suggested that free iron within the lumen catalyzes the formation of toxic oxygen free radicals, which, in turn, destroy the adjacent tubules and accelerate the tubulointerstitial scarring (reviewed in Alfrey 1994).

Exposure of tubular cells to transferrin-iron, but not transferrin alone, leads to an increase in lactic dehydrogenase release and lipid peroxidation (for review see Harris 2000). Transferrin has been shown to stimulate the synthesis of MCP-1 by proximal tubular cells (Wang *et al.* 1997), which has been implicated in the pathogenesis of the interstitial inflammatory reaction induced by albumin, transferrin, and endothelin. Data on the effect of transferrin and transferrin-iron on tubular cells production of extracellular matrix in culture has been conflicting. Some experiments show stimulation at very high doses while others showing no effect at physiological concentrations (reviewed in Harris 2000).

In vivo rat studies showed a positive correlation between urinary iron excretion and tubulointerstitial scarring. In this model, iron deficiency attenuates tubulointerstitial scarring and prevents deterioration of kidney function (reviewed in Alfrey 1994). Iron deposition within proximal tubular cells has been linked to HO-1 depletion, a key regulating enzyme for the prevention of abnormal intracellular iron accumulation (Ishizaka *et al.* 2002). It has recently been postulated that iron may mediate angiotensin II-induced tubular injury. Angiotensin II infusion leads to the accumulation of tubular iron in rats (Ishizaka *et al.* 2002). Angiotensin-induced tubular injury has been prevented by the coadministration of the iron chelator desferrioxamine (Ishizaka *et al.* 2002).

In addition to iron itself, heme protein is nephrotoxic and can induce severe inflammatory changes when injected into susceptible animals (Nath *et al.* 2000, 2001). This proinflammatory effect of heme protein appears to be mediated by the activation of the key transcription factor NF-κB with the consequent upregulation of renal chemokines initiating inflammation (Nath *et al.* 2001). The chronic interstitial fibrosis induced by heme protein may also be due to the oxidative stress-mediated activation of TGF-β1 (Nath *et al.* 2000). These experimental data may provide some explanations, along with the nephrotoxicity of iron, for the potential harmful effects of sustained haematuria in CKD (Hill *et al.* 1989).

The role of intrinsic renal cells in the pathogenesis of kidney scarring

Glomerular cells

The role of the endothelium Endothelial cells play an important part in preserving the structural and functional integrity of vascular beds including the glomeruli. They are likely to have anticoagulant, vasoactive, anti-inflammatory, and antiproliferative properties (reviewed in Savage 1994; Stewart and Marsden 1994). Within glomerular capillaries, endothelial cells are the first to be exposed to injurious insults such as mechanical (haemodynamic/shear stress), immunological, or metabolic factors.

Glomerular endothelial injury is characterized by swelling, cell-surface protrusions, and detachment from the underlying basement membrane. Functional endothelial changes include the loss of anticoagulant properties, the expression of cell-adhesion molecules as well as the release of chemotactic, growth-promoting, and fibrogenic mediators (reviewed in Stewart and Marsden 1994).

An important factor in the loss of glomerular endothelial anticoagulant and anti-inflammatory properties may be the decreased NO-synthase activity of damaged endothelium. The loss of NO-mediated anticoagulant properties would contribute to the adhesion and aggregation of platelets within the damaged glomeruli of experimental animals and humans. NO also inhibits leucocyte adhesion to the glomerular capillaries and thus has anti-inflammatory effects (reviewed in Cattell 2002). The loss of such a protective factor along with the expression of cell adhesion molecules would facilitate the infiltration of glomerular capillaries by inflammatory cells. Of relevance, NOS knockout mice develop an accelerated form of experimental nephrotoxic nephritis characterized by increased glomerular capillary thrombosis and neutrophil infiltration (Cattell 2002). Angiotensin II suppresses NO generation through its AT1 receptor. The imbalance between angiotensin II and NO will lead to the stimulation of the proinflammatory transcription factor NF-κB and the subsequent synthesis and release of a wide range of proinflammatory cytokines and chemokines and the upregulation of cell adhesion molecules (Wardle 2000, 2002; Leclercq *et al.* 2002).

Recent experimental evidence attributes a role for apoptosis in the deletion of endothelial cells observed after injury (reviewed in Kang *et al.* 2002). Evidence derived from tissue culture experiments suggests that the sphingolipid-derived second messenger ceramide and oxidative stress are intimately involved in the induction of glomerular endothelial cells apoptosis (Huwiler *et al.* 2001).

Regeneration of the glomerular capillary endothelium may rely on angiogenesis. Impaired glomerular endothelial angiogenesis has been reported after subtotal nephrectomy and implicated in the development of glomerulosclerosis in remnant kidneys (reviewed in Kang *et al.* 2002).

Normal glomerular endothelium is capable of releasing angiogenic factors such as vascular endothelial growth factor (VEGF) and fibroblast growth factor-2 (FGF-2). Glomerular endothelial cells also express VEGF receptors. VEGF is thought to mediate reactive endothelial proliferation in damaged glomeruli. In an experimental model of glomerulonephritis, the administration of VEGF165 enhanced glomerular capillary repair and accelerated the resolution of the extensive endothelial damage (reviewed in Kang et al. 2002).

The role of the mesangium Mesangial cells play an important part in the development and progression of glomerulosclerosis. These specialized pericytes have contractile, phagocytic, and metabolic functions indispensable to the maintenance of glomerular integrity (Schlondorff 1987). In experimental and clinical models of glomerular injury, mesangial changes are noted early and include mesangiolysis, apoptosis, proliferation, expansion, and sclerosis (Rennke and Klein 1989). Changes in the phenotype of mesangial cells are also observed, with the expression of smooth-muscle cell characteristics such as cytoplasmic α-SMA (Johnson et al. 1991; Alpers et al. 1992). This may contribute to the migration and contraction of mesangial cells during the glomerular healing process and may also contribute to glomerular scarring (discussed below).

Functional mesangial changes are also observed in rats with experimental nephropathies. These are characterized by the accumulation of macromolecules, including lipids, within the mesangium (Raij and Keane 1985; Elema and Grond 1988), which is associated with glomerulosclerosis (Grond and Weening 1990). Accumulation of macromolecules in the subendothelial area may contribute to glomerular hyalinosis (Olson et al. 1985), with the narrowing and ultimately the occlusion of glomerular capillaries and their sclerosis (Rennke 1994). By contrast, when mesangial uptake/clearance of macromolecules is normal, glomerulosclerosis and CKF do not seem to develop (Raij and Keane 1985). However, others have shown that mesangial dysfunction is not a prerequisite for the development of glomerulosclerosis in subtotally nephrectomized rats (Schwartz and Bidani 1991).

Mesangial hypercellularity often precedes the development of mesangial sclerosis. It is thought to result from the stimulation of mesangial proliferation by growth factors such as platelet-derived growth factor (PDGF) and basic FGF (bFGF) (discussed below). A variety of kinases has been shown to mediate mesangial proliferation in response to various stimuli. A role for MAP kinases, p44/42 MAP kinase and Jun N-terminal kinase/stress-activated protein kinase have all been implicated in the initiation of mesangial proliferation (Krepinsky et al. 2002). The nuclear translocation of some of these kinases and their binding to activating protein-1 (AP-1) leads to DNA synthesis and cellular proliferation. In addition, the PPARs are nuclear receptors involved in the regulation of mesangial cell cycle and ECM processing (reviewed in Guan and Breyer 2001). The turnover of mesangial cells *in vivo* appears to be regulated by a complex interplay of CDKs and their cyclin kinase inhibitors (CKI) (reviewed in Shankland 1999).

The balance between proliferative and antiproliferative factors may determine the fate of mesangioproliferative changes. The resolution of mesangial proliferation in experimental glomerulonephritis has been attributed to apoptosis (Baker et al. 1994). The balance between mesangial cell proliferation and apoptosis may determine the outcome of an acute glomerulonephritis (Savill 2001).

Mesangial survival depends on a constant supply of survival factors, also the cell surface receptors integrins, and in particular α1β1 integrin, are also thought to promote mesangial survival. Mesangial cell α1β1 integrin expression appears to be a critical determinant of mesangial cell phenotype, growth, and collagen remodelling capacity (Kagami et al. 2000). Collagen IV and laminin, the normal constitutents of the mesangial and GBM matrix have mesangial survival promoting properties mediated through a β(1) integrin-mediated, but arg-gly-asp (RGD)-independent mechanism (Mooney et al. 1999). On the other hand, collagen I, fibronectin, and osteonectin/secreted protein acidic and rich in cysteine (SPARC), which are overexpressed in diseased glomeruli do not promote rat mesangial cell survival thus potentially contributing to their apoptosis during the course of glomerulosclerosis (Mooney et al. 1999).

Recent evidence suggests that a significant proportion of new mesangial cells repopulating glomeruli after injury may be bone marrow-derived (Ito et al. 2001). The capacity of these cells to migrate and differentiate into mesangial cells could be a key factor in the resolution of mesangial injury and the restoration of normal glomerular cellularity (Hugo et al. 1997; Ito et al. 2001). The bone marrow origin of mesangial cells has been used in experimental IgA nephropathy, where transplantation of bone marrow from normal mice to those prone to IgA nephropathy attenuates the severity of mesangial IgA deposition and the associated sclerosis (Imasawa et al. 1999). Conversely, when mice resistant to glomerulosclerosis (ROP+/+) were transplanted with the bone marrow of glomerulosclerosis-prone congenic mice (ROP Os/+), they developed glomerulosclerosis (Cornacchia et al. 2001). These observations suggest that the development of glomerulosclerosis may depend on the bone marrow phenotype and that of the derived mesangium (reviewed in El Nahas 2003). They also open the way to therapeutic manipulations of mesangial cells through the transplantation of bone marrow/stem cells (reviewed in Imasawa and Utsunomiya 2002).

Mesangial expansion and sclerosis is thought to be due to the stimulation by fibrogenic growth factors, such as TGF-β1, of mesangial synthesis of extracellular matrix (reviewed in Basile 1999; Yu et al. 2002). TGF-β1 may also induce the changes in mesangial phenotype observed in experimental glomerulonephritis and in transfected glomeruli (Imai et al. 1994). The transdifferentiation of mesangial cells into myofibroblasts under the influence of TGF-β1 is also associated with the synthesis by these cells of interstitial type III collagen (Imai et al. 1994). While mesangial cells release collagenases (matrix metalloproteinases, MMPs) capable of breaking down glomerular type IV collagen, they are devoid of collagenolytic activity against type III. Thus, the release by activated and transdifferentiated mesangial cells of collagen III may contribute to irreversible glomerulosclerosis.

Strong correlations have been described in DN (Drummond and Mauer 2002) and in CGN (Hattori et al. 1997) between mesangial expansion and volume, and the development of glomerulosclerosis. In DN, a causative role has been attributed to mesangial expansion in glomerular ischaemia and obsolescence (Mauer et al. 1984). Mesangial activation/transdifferentiation into myofibroblasts has been reported in a wide range of human glomerular diseases (Alpers et al. 1992; Goumenos et al. 1994, 1998). This may contribute in humans, as in experimental animals, to quantitative but also qualitative changes in the glomerular ECM.

The role of the epithelium The glomerular visceral epithelial layer consists of highly differentiated cells; the podocytes. They represent a glomerular pericyte holding the glomerular capillary wall together against the centrifugal hydrostatic force driving glomerular filtration.

These cells appear to be unable to replicate. It has been argued that changes in cell cycle regulatory proteins with the upregulation of CKI may underlie the low proliferative capacity of the glomerular epithelial cells in response to immune injury (Reviewed in Shankland 1999). Thus, degenerated podocytes cannot be replaced. Occasionally, in response to extreme stimulation, these cells undergo mitosis but in the absence of cell division they become binucleated cells (Kriz and Lemley 1999; Endlich *et al.* 2001). One exception to this rule is observed in collapsing glomerulopathies where podocytes lose their differentiated phenotype and proliferate.

Changes in glomerular visceral epithelial cells occur in rats with experimental nephropathies (reviewed in Kriz and Lemley 1999; Endlich *et al.* 2001). These changes are characterized by the formation of cytoplasmic blebs, as well as the focal retraction, simplification, and flattening of foot processes. Epithelial changes do not merely reflect heavy proteinuria as they are also observed in analbuminaemic rats. Fusion and retraction of epithelial podocytes, which is also characteristic of the glomeruli of patients with nephrotic syndrome, are likely to affect glomerular permeability. This may be due to the denudation of areas of the basement membrane following the stretching and rearrangement of foot processes facilitating, in the presence of glomerular hypertension, the hydraulic flux, trafficking, and permeability of macromolecules, and hence proteinuria (Rennke 1994). This has been observed in experimental models of proteinuria and nephrotic syndrome (reviewed in Endlich *et al.* 2001).

There is increasing evidence pointing to a crucial role for podocyte depletion in the pathogenesis of glomerulosclerosis. In the puromycin nephrosis model, podocytes depletion is proportional to the severity of the initial insult and to the subsequent development of glomerulosclerosis (Kim *et al.* 2001b). In the OZR rat, early podocytes damage precedes the onset of glomerulosclerosis in the absence of any mesangial abnormalities (Gassler *et al.* 2001). Podocytes apoptosis also precedes the onset of glomerulosclerosis in transgenic mice overexpressing TGF-β1 (Schiffer *et al.* 2001). HGF, on the other hand, attenuates podocyte apoptosis (Fornoni *et al.* 2001). Another mechanism of podocyte depletion may be the shedding of viable podocytes into the urine (Petermann *et al.* 2003).

Podocyte abnormalities with foot process effacement have also been observed in the hypertrophied glomeruli of type 2 diabetic patients and implicated in defects in the GBM size permselectivity and the subsequent development of 'macromolecular shunts' through the glomerular barrier (Lemley *et al.* 2000). The same group reported that the number of podocytes per glomerulus was the strongest predictor of disease progression, fewer cells predicting rapid progression. Similar observations were made in patients with IgA nephropathy (Lemley *et al.* 2002).

Areas/gaps in the podocytes' cover of the GBM have been implicated in the pathogenesis of glomerulosclerosis (Kim *et al.* 2001b). The denuded GBM would adhere to the parietal epithelium and the Bowman's capsule to form capsular adhesions which may initiate segmental glomerulosclerosis. It has been postulated that such adhesions would form bridges between the glomeruli and the surrounding periglomerular interstitium, thus facilitating the migration of interstitial myofibroblasts into scarred glomeruli (El Nahas 1996). This may also misdirect the glomerular ultrafiltrate into the periglomerular interstitium (Endlich *et al.* 2001).

Recent years have seen major advances in the understanding of the biology of the podocyte. A wide range of cytoplasmic, cell surface and slit diaphragm-associated proteins and their role in the maintenance of the integrity of the podocyte and the glomerular barrier have been identified. These include nephrin, which forms the backbone of the slit diaphragm, and CD2AP which is an adaptor protein that binds to the cytoplasmic domain of nephrin (Reviewed in Shaw and Miner 2001). Podocin is an integral podocyte membrane protein. α-Actinin-4 is also localized to podocytes and might serve to crosslink cytoplasmic actin filaments. Nephrin is the product of the gene NPHS1 and mutations of this gene account for the vast majority of cases of congenital nephrotic syndrome of the Finnish type which is associated with FSGS (reviewed in Tryggvason 2001; Antignac 2002). Mutations of NPHS2 coding for podocin is associated with another form of familial recessive steroid-resistant nephrotic syndrome and FSGS (for review Antignac 2002). Knockout mice lacking CD2AP exhibit defects in epithelial foot processes, mesangial hypercellularity and progressive glomerulosclerosis resulting in early death from kidney failure (reviewed in Shaw and Miner 2001).

Epithelial cells may also contribute to glomerulosclerosis through the expression of class II antigens of the major histocompatibility complex, the release of chemotactic factors such as complement components, and the uptake of lipids, as well as by the synthesis of cytokines and growth factors such as PDGF (Pavenstadt 2000).

The link between glomerulosclerosis and tubulointerstitial fibrosis
Numerous pathways link glomerular damage and sclerosis to the development of tubulointerstitial fibrosis (Kuncio *et al.* 1991). First, glomerular injury leads to the sustained release into the glomerular ultrafiltrate of a variety of cytokines, chemokines, and growth factors (Wang *et al.* 2000). These are likely to be taken up by tubular cells through receptor-dependent and independent pathways leading to the production of further proinflammatory and fibrogenic mediators as well as the synthesis of components of ECM (Wang *et al.* 2000). Second, glomerular injury and the associated changes to the tone of the efferent arterioles and the postglomerular capillaries may contribute to reduce peritubular perfusion and initiate local ischaemia and hypoxia causing tubular atrophy and interstitial fibrosis (Fine *et al.* 2000). Third, proteinuria resulting from glomerular damage has been implicated in the initiation of tubulointerstitial inflammation and fibrosis. Fourth, glomeruli with epithelial injury and focal capsular adhesions may be disconnected from their tubules leading to atubular glomeruli (Javaid *et al.* 2001). This would lead to misdirected filtration into the periglomerular interstitium initiating a fibrotic reaction (Gassler *et al.* 2001).

Tubular epithelial cells In the past, tubular cells were considered innocent bystanders in the process of renal scarring. Recent evidence attributes an active and important role to these cells in the initiation and progression of tubulointerstitial scarring.

Proximal tubular cells respond to injury by the expression of cell-adhesion molecules and HLA class II antigens (reviewed in Brady 1994). The expression of these would convert proximal tubules to antigen-presenting cells whilst that of cell-adhesion molecules would stimulate interactions between tubular cells and the interstitial inflammatory infiltrate. The proinflammatory action of proximal tubular cells is also likely to be due to their release of chemotactic factors such as complement (Eddy 2001), NO (reviewed in Cattell 2002), fatty acid-derived chemotactins as well as chemokines such as MCP-1 (reviewed in Harris 2000; Zeisberg *et al.* 2000; Eddy 2001; Anders *et al.* 2003). As discussed previously, it has also been postulated that ammoniagenesis by the proximal tubule has a role in interstitial complement activation and inflammation (Nath *et al.* 1985; Nath 1993). Similarly, proteinuria apears to play an important role in the activation of proximal tubular cells and in altering their phenotype and structure, thought to be a major pathway of the pathogenesis of tubulointerstitial inflammation and scarring (reviewed in Harris 2000; Zeisberg et al. 2000; Eddy 2001).

Proximal tubular cells are capable of the synthesis and release of fibrogenic growth factors such as PDGF and TGF-β1 (reviewed in Zeisberg et al. 2000, 2001). They are also capable of generating potent vasoactive and profibrotic autacoids such as angiotensin II and endothelin-1. Proximal tubular cells express angiotensin II AT1 receptors. It has been demonstrated in vitro that proximal tubular cells incubated with angiotensin II (reviewed Wolf 2001) or a high-glucose medium release TGF-β1. The angiotensin II-mediated hypertrophy of proximal tubular cells has been attributed to their release of TGF-β1 (Wolf 2001).

Tubuloepithelial cells respond to a variety of stimuli, including albumin, transferrin, and LDL/ox-LDL, by overproduction of components of the extracellular matrix. Both angiotensin II and endothelin-1 are capable of increasing the synthesis of collagen IV by proximal tubular cells (reviewed in Wolf 2001). Growth factors such as TGF-β1 lead to an increased synthesis of collagen by rat tubulo-epithelial cells (Grande et al. 2002). In addition, tubular epithelial cells are also capable of the synthesis of both MMPs (gelatinases/collagenases) as well as their inhibitors, tissue inhibitor of tissue metalloproteinases (TIMPs). Thus, the balance between epithelial cells' synthesis and breakdown of ECM may be key to the progression of tubulointerstitial fibrosis.

Tubulointerstitial fibrosis is characterized by the deletion of tubular epithelial cells and their replacement by the expanding ECM. Recent evidence attributes a major role to apoptosis in the pathogenesis of tubular cell depletion (Thomas et al. 1998). Tubular atrophy through apoptosis or necrosis is likely to be a major factor in the progression of experimental and clinical renal fibrosis (Javaid et al. 2001). Disruption of the glomerular tubular junction has been shown to be associated with the presence of amorphous material separating damaged tubular cells from the basement membrane. These findings suggest that local extension of glomerular injury to destroy the tubule neck is an important cause of loss of kidney function in experimental nephrosis (Javaid et al. 2001).

The link between tubular cell death and the associated interstitial fibrosis is speculative. Unlike necrosis, cell death through apoptosis is not conventionally associated with inflammation. Recent data link tubular apoptosis, and in particular the activation of the proapoptotic caspase pathway, with the activation of proinflammatory mediators such as IL-1, thought to be a key renal fibrogenic cytokine (Burns 2002; Vesey et al. 2002).

A novel pathway mechanism has been put forward to explain the contribution of tubuloepithelial cells to fibrogenesis; the epithelial–mesenchymal transformation (EMT). This hypothesis was put forward by Strutz and Neilson (Strutz et al. 1995; Strutz and Muller 2000) after the cloning and characterization of a fibroblast-specific protein (FSP-1). They suggested that tubuloepithelial cells can transdifferentiate into fibroblasts acquiring a fibroblast phenotype and markers such as FSP-1 and α-SMA (Strutz et al. 1995; Okada et al. 2000).

As with glomerular cellular integrity, the architecture of the basement membrane appears to play an important role in the maintenance of tubular epithelial phenotype. Changes in basement membrane architecture may lead to the upregulation of TGF-β1 (Zeisberg et al. 2001). FGF-2 makes an important contribution to the mechanisms of EMT by stimulating microenvironmental proteases (MMP 2 and 9)

essential for basement membrane disintegration and facilitating tubular epithelial cell motility (Strutz et al. 2002). Conversely, HGF has been shown to inhibit EMT, explaining some of its antifibrotic effects (Liu 2002).

Although the transdifferentiation of proximal tubular cells may be an additional pathway for the progression of tubulointerstitial fibrosis, there may be a different explanation for these observations. The majority of tubular epithelial cells including proximal tubules are derived, like interstitial renal cells, from metanephric mesenchymal cells. De-differentiation of mature epithelial cells is known to occur in response to injury. Injury to epithelial cells is often associated with a regression to a de-differentiated embryonic phenotype until repair takes place and injury resolves. It is therefore possible that the expression of mesenchymal markers by injured tubular cells merely reflects their de-differentiation rather than transdifferentiation in response to injury. The true contribution of tubular epithelial cells to the fibroblastic/myofibroblastic pool remains uncertain.

Fibroblasts and myofibroblasts A role has been attributed to interstitial fibroblasts and myofibroblasts in the pathogenesis of renal fibrosis. The activation of quiescent fibroblasts is associated with the acquisition of new phenotypic features including in some case the expression of α-SMA (myofibroblasts). The activation of renal fibroblasts is likely to follow one of four key pathways: stimulation by growth factors ('auto- and paracrine'), by direct cell–cell contacts, by extracellular matrix via integrins, and by environmental conditions such as hyperglycaemia or hypoxia in renal disease (reviewed in Zeisberg et al. 2000). The activation of renal fibroblasts can be driven by the release of cytokines and growth factors by glomerular cells, tubular cells as well as interstitial inflammatory cells. In addition, renal fibroblasts are capable of releasing growth factors such as IL-1 and FGF-2 capable of autocrine stimulation (reviewed in Zeisberg et al. 2000). They are believed to synthesize fibrogenic growth factors such as TGF-β1 and PDGF (Yamamoto et al. 1994) and produce fibrillar collagen (Wiggins et al. 1993). In addition, renal fibroblasts are known to produce and release MMPs and TIMPs (Norman and Lewis 1996). Therefore, renal fibroblasts/myofibroblasts are capable of controlling the turnover of surrounding ECM. Their regulation and source may provide the key to the prevention of the progression of renal scarring and fibrosis.

Myofibroblasts have been detected in the interstitium of experimental animals and humans (Johnson et al. 1991; Alpers et al. 1992; Goumenos et al. 1994) with progressive glomerulonephritis. In man, their presence within the interstitium is a sensitive marker of progressive renal disease (Goumenos et al. 1994). These cells may infiltrate the glomeruli through adhesions or holes in Bowman's capsule, thus contributing to glomerulosclerosis (Lan et al. 1992). In that respect, capsular adhesions would form bridges between the glomerular tufts and the periglomerular interstitium facilitating fibroblastic infiltration of the glomeruli (El Nahas 1996).

Fibroblasts derived from scarred kidneys display marked heterogeneity with a tendency to phenotypic changes associated with heightened proliferation (Rodemann and Muller 1990) and ECM production (Muller and Rodemann 1991; Rodemann and Muller 1991). The proliferation of interstitial renal fibroblasts derived from patients with renal fibrosis, unlike those derived from normal kidneys, appears to be dependent on IL-1 and independent of bFGF (Lonnemann et al. 1995). Furthermore, fibrosis-derived fibroblasts produce IL-1 capable of acting in a paracrine fashion (Lonnemann et al. 1995). It has also been suggested that a small fraction of renal fibroblasts derived from diseased kidneys may be resistant to normal regulatory influences and may contribute to ongoing renal fibrosis well after inflammatory-driven fibroblastic proliferation and activation has subsided (Sommer et al. 1999).

The proliferation of fibroblasts/myofibroblasts within the renal interstitium is associated with their increased synthesis of interstitial collagens and is a forerunner of established renal fibrosis. It has been argued that healing would take place when myofibroblastic infiltration of wounds resolves through the apoptosis of these cells. Scarring, on the other hand, would proceed when they continue to proliferate and cause tissue fibrosis.

Interventions aimed to control the activation of renal fibroblasts may open the way to the prevention of progressive renal fibrosis (reviewed in Strutz 2001; Imai and Isaka 2002a). The administration of potentially antifibrogenic growth factors such as HGF, epidermal growth factor (EGF), VEGF, or bone morphogenic protein-7 has afforded some protection and reduction of interstitial fibrosis (Imai and Isaka 2002b).

Attention has recently shifted to the inhibition of intracellular and nuclear signalling pathways mediating renal fibrosis. Inhibition of PDGF-mediated tyrosine kinase activation has showed promise (Cybulsky 2000). The Rho-associated coiled-coil forming protein kinase (Rho-ROCK) has been implicated in the development of tissue fibrosis (Sharpe and Hendry 2003). The administration of Y-27632, an inhibitor of the Rho-ROCK signalling pathway, has shown a therapeutic potential in preventing interstitial fibrosis in progressive renal disease of mice with unilateral ureteral obstruction (Nagatoya et al. 2002). The overexpression of Smad7 in proximal tubular cells results in a marked inhibition of TGF-β-induced transdifferentiation into myofibroblasts (Li et al. 2002). The up-regulation of the early growth response gene 1 (Egr-1) has been shown to precede the expression of α-SMA in renal fibroblasts in obstructed kidney with interstitial fibrosis. The introduction by retrograde electroporation-mediated gene transfer of a DNA enzyme for Egr-1 (ED5) into interstitial fibroblasts has inhibited their α-SMA expression and collagen synthesis in obstructed rat kidneys (Nakamura et al. 2002).

Vascular sclerosis

In addition to the progressive scarring of glomeruli and renal tubules, sclerosis and hyalinosis of intrarenal arterioles are common in patients with chronic renal disorders which has, in the past, been attributed to systemic hypertension. However, in most forms of CGN, these vascular structural changes are observed well before the onset of CRF and hypertension (reviewed in Baldwin and Neugarten 1986), suggesting that intrarenal vascular disease is a primary feature in glomerulonephritis and not merely a secondary phenomenon of sustained hypertension. However, an effect of early, nocturnal, or labile hypertension on the renal vasculature cannot be excluded. The presence of vascular sclerosis in such patients indicates a poor prognosis (Gallo et al. 1978). A role was also attributed to arteriolar hyalinosis in the development of glomerulosclerosis in diabetic patients (Harris et al. 1991), in whom the early lesions of arteriolar hyalinosis developed in the absence of overt hypertension and correlated with the severity of glomerulosclerosis. In patients with systemic lupus erythematosus, the presence of vascular lesions was associated with a significantly lower kidney survival rate at 5 and 10 years when compared to those without vascular lesions (reviewed in Zuchelli and Zuccala 1993). The severity of the renal arteriolar changes in chronic kidney disorders contrasts with those of essential hypertension.

Renal ischaemia is associated with tubulointerstitial hypoxia which may itself be a renal fibrogenic stimulus (reviewed in Fine et al. 2000). Fine, Norman and their colleagues showed that the exposure of renal proximal tubular cells as well as renal fibroblasts to hypoxia stimulates their release of TGF-β1, as well as their synthesis of ECM (Norman et al. 2000).

Peritubular and microvascular injury and angiogenesis Large- and small-vessel changes are likely to contribute to renal interstitial fibrosis through ischaemia and hypoxia. Recent attention has focused on the severe and progressive depletion of peritubular capillaries during the course of experimental renal scarring and interstitial fibrosis. This was first described by Bohle and colleagues who implicated the loss of peritubular capillaries in the progression of interstitial fibrosis (Bohle et al. 1981, 1987). Experimental observations in a range of models show that an initial phase of peritubular endothelial proliferation is followed by a loss of cells and peritubular rarefaction (reviewed in Kang et al. 2002).

Thrombospondin-1 (TSP-1) is known to inhibit endothelial cell proliferation and induce apoptosis. TSP-1 expression correlates with the loss of the microvasculature endothelium (Hugo et al. 1997; Kang et al. 2002). Like many profibrotic substances, TSP-1 is expressed by tubular cells, macrophages, and fibroblasts. Another antiangiogenic factor, SPARC is also upregulated in remnant kidneys (Wu et al. 1997). SPARC also stimulates the synthesis by mesangial of TGF-β1 as shown by the downregulation of this growth factor in SPARC null mice (Francki et al. 1999). Furthermore, the increase in antiangiogenic and angiotoxic factors is associated with a down regulation in angiogenic factors such as VEGF. This has been observed in a variety of experimental models of interstitial fibrosis associated with the loss of peritubular capillaries (reviewed in Kang et al. 2002).

Extrinsic cells

The role of platelets and coagulation Platelets play an important part in the initiation and progression of glomerulosclerosis (reviewed in Johnson 1994). Endothelial injury and dysfunction and the associated loss of endothelial anticoagulant properties and the acquisition of proaggregatory functions attract platelets and stimulate their adhesion and aggregation within damaged glomerular capillary loops. Platelets and platelet-release products have been detected in a wide range of experimental nephropathies and in patients with CKD (Cameron 1984). In these patients, platelet activation has been suggested by their shortened half-life, increased aggregation, and increased circulating β-thromboglobulin and platelet factor 4 (Cameron 1984). Interactions between platelets, monocytes, and mesangial cells within glomeruli may determine the extent of glomerular microthrombosis. Infiltrating monocytes may aggravate this process through the stimulation of glomerular procoagulant activity and fibrin deposition (Tipping and Holdsworth 1986). The subsequent outcome may depend on the glomerular fibrinolytic capacity. *In vitro*, mesangial cells synthesize and release both a tissue-type plasminogen activator and a plasminogen-activator inhibitor related to plasminogen-activator inhibitor-1 (PAI-1). Mesangial injury and dysfunction could therefore affect glomerular fibrinolytic activity and accelerate intraglomerular coagulation.

A growing body of evidence implicates changes in coagulation cascade products in glomerulosclerosis. Mesangial cells express thrombin receptors (protease activator receptor-1/PAR1) (Sraer and Rondeau 1996). Thrombin stimulates ECM production by mesangial cells in culture. Further, thrombin is also capable of inducing mesangial synthesis of TIMP-1 (Kaizuka *et al.* 1999). These thrombin-induced changes in mesangial cells are thought to be mediated by TGF-β1 (Kaizuka *et al.* 1999). Similarly, thrombin also stimulates glomerular epithelial cell production of TGF-β1 (Tsunoda *et al.* 2001). Thus thrombin, through the stimulation of TGF-β1 release by glomerular cells, is capable of inducing changes in ECM turnover conducive to the development of glomerulosclerosis.

Plasmin is likely to have opposing effects on glomerulosclerosis. Plasmin, like thrombin, is a potent activator of TGF-β1 and may therefore be involved in its activation within scarred glomeruli but, on the other hand, is a proteolytic enzyme capable of breaking down glomerular ECM directly and indirectly through its activation of MMPs.

It has been suggested that the progression of glomerulosclerosis after glomerular endothelial injury may reflect the balance between thrombotic/antiproteolytic and anticoagulant/proteolytic activities with a key role played by PAI-1 in modulating thrombosis and mediating progression from glomerular thrombosis to sclerosis (reviewed in Fogo 2001a). PAI-1 expression in normal glomeruli is minimal but it is upregulated with glomerular injury (Hamano *et al.* 2002). In addition to its role in thrombosis, PAI-1 has important effects on ECM turnover as it inhibits plasmin which is known to have proteolytic activities either directly or indirectly through the activation of MMPs (Fogo 2001a). Of relevance, PAI-1 deficiency attenuates the renal fibrogenic response to unilateral ureteral obstruction in PAI-1 deficient ($-/-$) mice (Oda *et al.* 2001). In human glomerulonephritis, an upregulation of PAI-1 mRNA was reported in patients with membranous nephropathy as well as those with FSGS (Hamano *et al.* 2002), and this correlated with the severity of proteinuria.

In support of a role for platelets and the coagulation system in the pathogenesis of glomerular cellular proliferation and sclerosis are the studies where platelet depletion, antiplatelet agents, or anticoagulants, inhibitors of thromboxane synthesis, as well as antibodies against PDGF, prevent cellular proliferation and glomerulosclerosis (reviewed in Klahr *et al.* 1986). Heparin has potent glomerular antiproliferative and antifibrotic effects, although this may not be solely due to its anticoagulant effect.

Monocytes/macrophages

Glomerulosclerosis Monocytes have been identified within the glomeruli of experimental animals with immune- and non-immune-mediated nephropathies (reviewed in Erwig *et al.* 2001; Rodriguez-Iturbe *et al.* 2001). Whilst their presence and role in experimental glomerulonephritis has long been established, their detection in the early stages of non-immune renal disease is more recent. They have been detected in the glomeruli of rats with a variety of kidney diseases (reviewed in Rodriguez-Iturbe *et al.* 2001). In these models, the infiltration of glomeruli by monocytes is often associated with mesangial proliferation. The release by injured glomeruli of chemotactic factors such as complement components, cytokines, chemokines, and of lipid-derived factors such as leukotrienes and platelet-activating factor, are likely to attract monocytes to the glomerular capillaries (reviewed by Segerer *et al.* 2000). As discussed above, endothelial cells play an important part in this process through the neo-expression of adhesion molecules such as ICAM-1 : CD54 (Stewart and Marsden 1994).

There is increasing evidence that macrophages infiltrating various tissues behave differently according to the microenvironment in which they find themselves. The type and severity of glomerular injury could

also affect macrophage function. It would appear that macrophage programming and behaviour are affected by the initial cytokine contact and not the sum of cytokines activities they may encounter later (reviewed in Erwig *et al.* 2001), suggesting phenotypic and functional changes in macrophages infiltrating inflamed glomeruli that may determine very early in the process the fate of these cells.

The relevance of monocytes to the initiation and progression of experimental renal scarring has been supported by studies in which their depletion by antibodies, X-irradiation, liposome-encapsulated diphosphonates, or an essential fatty acid-deficient diet have all proved protective (reviewed in Erwig *et al.* 2001).

The prevention of interactions between monocytes and endothelium with anti-ICAM-1 or LFA-1 antibodies was also protective in the acute phase of crescentic nephritis in rabbits. However, the blockade of Mac-1 that binds to ICAM-1, did not reduce the degree of macrophage infiltration in the same experimental model in spite of a significant reduction in proteinuria (Wu *et al.* 1996). Of interest, the administration to rats with nephrotoxic serum nephritis, of neutralizing antibodies to the very late antigen-4, the macrophage counter receptor of VCAM-1, attenuated renal injury without reducing the number of macrophages infiltrating the injured glomeruli. Blockade of VCAM-1 in the same study had little effect on macrophage infiltration. Chemoadhesins such as fractalkine and Gro-α that may play an important role in the localization of macrophages to inflamed glomeruli. Blockade of these cell surface receptors have proved promising in limiting the ability of macrophages to localize to glomeruli in rats with nephrotoxic nephritis (reviewed in Erwig *et al.* 2001).

The modulation of macrophage function may be as important as their number in glomerulonephritis. IL-4 and IL-10 knockout mice develop severe glomerular inflammation with an increased number of infiltrating glomerular macrophages in nephrotoxic serum nephritis. Of interest, IL-4 infusion in this model reduces the severity of the injury by affecting the phenotype of the macrophages and increasing the number of NOS-positive cells without affecting the total count.

New approaches based on gene transfer and macrophage-delivered anti-inflammatory cytokines have been applied for the control of experimental glomerular inflammation (Kluth *et al.* 2000); macrophages transfected with the cDNA coding for IL-1 receptor antagonist localize in the glomeruli of mice with nephrotoxic serum nephritis and preserve function (Yokoo *et al.* 1999), IL-4 transfected macrophages in nephrotoxic serum nephritis leads to a reduction in infiltrating macrophages and decrease proteinuria (Kluth *et al.* 2001), and 15-lipoxygenase gene transfer to the glomeruli of rats with nephrotoxic serum nephritis decreases the severity of the glomerulonephritis (Munger *et al.* 1999).

There is now a shift in the perception of the role of macrophages in renal disease. While initial observations have attributed a predominant, if not exclusive, role to macrophages in the initiation and progression of glomerular inflammation and sclerosis, more recent research has highlighted the contribution of these cells in the termination of inflammation and the resolution of glomerular injury. Studies in genetically modified mice showed that prevention of macrophage infiltration can exacerbate the severity of experimental glomerulonephritis (Rovin 2000).

Tubulointerstitial fibrosis Monocytes are thought to be one of the most important components of the tubulointerstitial infiltrate in experimental animals and humans (reviewed in Harris 2000; Eddy 2001). In animals, the interstitial monocytic infiltrate correlates with the severity of the proteinuria and predicts progression to CRF. Monocytes attracted by the release of chemotactic factors by tubular cells, such as MCP-1, RANTES and complement components are likely to be instrumental (reviewed in Anders *et al.* 2003).

Proximal tubular cells are capable of synthesizing as well as activating components of the complement system (Song *et al.* 1998). In the remnant kidney model of progressive renal scarring, the initial interstitial changes are complement-independent and largely reversible, whereas progressive interstitial fibrosis is mediated predominantly by C5b-9 (Nangaku *et al.* 2002). Renal scarring is attenuated in this model in C6-deficient mice (Nangaku *et al.* 2002). Inhibition of complement activation by depletion (cobra venom factor) or antagonism (complement type I receptor) decreases the severity of interstitial monocytic infiltrate in experimental models (Nomura *et al.* 1997).

The mechanism of monocyte-induced renal fibrosis might be by the release by monocytes of fibrogenic growth factors such as TGF-β1 or to changes in the homeostasis of the extracellular matrix. In a variety of rat experimental models, a close association was described between the severity of the tubulointerstitial monocytic infiltrate and the amount of TGF-β1 mRNA in the kidney (reviewed in Jernigan and Eddy 2000).

Monocytes are capable of the synthesis and release of components of the extracellular matrix such as fibronectin and collagen (reviewed in Erwig *et al.* 2001). Further, macrophages are likely sources of ECM-regulating enzymes. They can release TIMP-1, thus contributing to a decrease in the breakdown of collagen. In Heymann nephritis, parallel changes in the numbers of interstitial monocytes and amounts of renal TIMP-1 mRNA were demonstrated by Eddy *et al.* (1991) (for review Jernigan and Eddy 2000; Eddy 2001).

Experimental interventions known to reduce the interstitial monocytic infiltrate, such as dietary protein restriction, an essential fatty acid-deficient diet, and methylprednisolone, also attenuate the severity of renal fibrosis and scarring (reviewed in Jernigan and Eddy 2000; Harris 2000).

The progression of interstitial inflammation may depend on the balance between the recruitment, *in situ* activation, and proliferation of the macrophages in the interstitium and their depletion through migration out of the kidney or death through apoptosis (reviewed in Rodriguez-Iturbe *et al.* 2001).

Lymphocytes In experimental models of renal fibrosis, a brisk interstitial inflammatory infiltrate often precedes the onset of the fibrotic changes. This infiltrate consists predominantly of monocytes, T lymphocytes and to a lesser degree B lymphocytes. Both T-helper and T-cytotoxic cells have been identified in experimental models of interstitial fibrosis (Reviewed in Rodriguez-Iturbe *et al.* 2001). In albumin overload nephropathy, a transient T-helper infiltrate decreases after 3 weeks while T-cytotoxic cells persists throughout the experimental time course (7 weeks). Of interest, T-cell depletion does not prevent the accumulation of monocytes in this experimental model suggesting a T-cell-independent influx of mononuclear cells. On the other hand, mizoribine, an immunosuppressive agent capable of inhibiting T-cell proliferation, has been shown to prevent experimental interstitial fibrosis in rats with UUO (Sato *et al.* 2001).

Beside the inflammatory role of Th1 lymphocytes, it is likely that Th2 lymphocytes and their anti-inflammatory release products may play a modulating role in the progression of renal inflammation and injury. The balance between Th1 and Th2 lymphocytes has been suggested to be a key factor in the progression as well as resolution of renal inflammation (Lim *et al.* 2001).

Mast cells

Studies on mast cells have shown their presence in significant numbers within scarred interstitium in experimental animals and humans. In animals, these cells have been shown to infiltrate the interstitium in immune- and non-immune models of renal scarring, including DN. In humans, scarred native and transplanted kidneys contain a significant number of mast cells. The number of these cells often correlates with the severity of the interstitial fibrosis. Of relevance, clinical and experimental observations have shown the upregulation of stem cell factor (SCF), a potent mast cell chemoattractant, in damaged tubular cells (El-Koraie *et al.* 2001).

Mast cells are potent fibrogenic cells through their release of a wide range of profibrotic mediators including chymase and tryptase as well as histamine. These mediators are known to stimulate the proliferation of renal fibroblasts as well as their production of ECM. Of note, fibroblasts are also able to attract and interact with mast cells through their release and expression of SCF. In addition, mast cells stimulate the release of eotactin by fibroblasts which is a potent chemotactin for eosinophils. Eosinophils are also potentially fibrogenic through their interactions with fibroblasts.

Plasticity of renal cells

While intrinsic and extrinsic renal cells undoubtedly play important roles in the pathogenesis of renal scarring, advances in cell biology suggest more complex interactions. In particular, considerable interest has recently been given to the plasticity of renal cells with intrinsic cells having the potential to transdifferentiate whilst extrinsic haematopoietic cells showing potential to invade the kidneys and replace damaged renal cells. Within the glomeruli, both mesangial and epithelial cells respond to injury by a transformation into a mesenchymal phenotype, reminiscent of the embryonic one and that of myofibroblasts with expression of cytoskeletal proteins and the acquisition of a network of stress fibres (reviewed in El Nahas 2003). Such a transformation of glomerular cells may contribute to glomerulosclerosis through the release of interstitial collagens (types I and III) that the glomeruli are unable to clear due to lack of specific collagenases. Similarly, injury to tubular cells leads to their transformation and regression to an embryonic, metanephric, mesenchymal/myofibroblastic phenotype contributing to interstitial fibrosis (discussed above and reviewed in Strutz and Muller 2000 and El Nahas 2003).

On the other hand, a growing body of evidence suggests that haematopoietic cells contribute to renal healing and possibly scarring. Glomerular repair appears to require the migration of progenitor haematopoietic cells to the mesangium (Hugo *et al.* 1997). Similarly, haematopoietic stem cells have been shown to contribute to the repair of tubular cells in humans (Poulsom *et al.* 2001) and experimental animals (Gupta *et al.* 2002). Preliminary data suggest that bone marrow-derived mesenchymal cells may also contribute to the renal interstitial fibroblastic pool. The fate of bone marrow-derived cells in the kidney may determine the outcome of renal remodelling to either healing or scarring. Healing would depend on the transformation of these cells into mature renal cells while scarring may result from their transformation into mesenchymal, fibroblastic cells (reviewed in El Nahas 2003). In addition, genetically manipulated bone marrow-derived cells may be used therapeutically to deliver to the kidney anti-inflammatory and antifibrotic mediators (Yamagishi *et al.* 2001).

Mediators of kidney scarring (Table 1)

The role of growth factors

Glomerulosclerosis

Chemokines and cytokines Chemotactic cytokines, chemokines, released by glomerular cells play a major role in the attraction and recruitment

Table 1 List of major pro- and antifibrotic mediators based on experimental data from studies of experimental kidney scarring

Mediators	Agonists	Antagonists
Hormones/ autacoids	GH	Octreotide
	Aldosterone	Spironolactone
	Angiotensin II	ACE inhibitors/ARBs
	Endothelin	ECE inhibitors/ERBs
	PAI-1	ACE inhibitors/ antagonists
Growth factors (harmful)	PDGF	SPARC
		Neutralizing antibodies
		Aptamers
		Antisense oligonucleotides
	TGF-β1	Decorin
		Neutralizing Abs
		Antireceptor antibodies
		Smad7
		PPAR gamma
		Antisense oligonucleotides
	TGF-β2	
	CTGF	
	BFGF	
	FGF-2	
	Thrombospondin1	
	Osteopontin	
Growth factors (beneficial)	IGF-I	
	OP-1	
	VEGF	
	HGF	
	Nitric oxide	
Miscellaneous antifibrotic interventions		Pirfenidone
		AGE inhibitors
		GAG/heparinoids/ sulodexide
		Relaxin
		AST 120

GH, growth hormone; PAI-1, plasminogen activator inhibitor-1; ACE, angiotensin converting enzyme; EC, endothelin converting enzyme; ARBs, angiotensin receptor blockers; ERBs, endothelin receptor blockers; PDGF, platelet derived growth factor; TGF-β1, transforming growth factor-β1; TGF-β2, transforming growth factor-β2; CTGF, connective tissue growth factor; bFGF, basic fibroblast growth factor; FGF-2, fibroblast growth factor 2; PPAR, peroxisome proliferator-activated receptors; SPARC, serine proteinase acidic and rich in cysteine; IGF-I, insulin-like growth factor-I; OP-1, osteogenic protein-1; VEGF, vascular endothelial growth factor; HGF, hepatocyte growth factor; AGE, advanced glycation end products; GAG, glycosaminoglycans; Abs, antibodies.

of inflammatory cells into the injured glomeruli. The initial inflammatory response, driven by chemokines, leads to negative and positive feedback reactions that either terminate the initial inflammatory response or amplify it and lead to glomerular cell proliferation and glomerulosclerosis (reviewed in Segerer *et al.* 2000; Anders *et al.* 2003).

A wide range of stimuli including cytokines (IL-1β and TNF-α), immunoglobulins, ROS, and lipopolysaccharides can induce the synthesis and release of chemokines such as MCP-1 and RANTES from mesangial cells in culture. In addition, growth factors (PDGF and bFGF) and autacoids such as angiotensin II and endothelin can induce chemokine production by glomerular cells. Many induce chemokine synthesis through the activation of NF-κB. On the other hand, TGF-β1 and prostaglandins have the capacity to inhibit production of chemokines.

Cytokines bind to specific receptors on renal cells and induce the activation of a range of intracellular signal transduction pathways. This leads to the recruitment of adaptor kinases leading to the activation of downstream pathways such as the Ras extracellular signal-regulated kinase pathway, JAK-Stat pathway, Smads and others including MAPK (reviewed in Cybulsky 2000). These pathways will activate transcription factors which will in turn bind to DNA binding sites leading to the synthesis of a range of cyclins and cyclin-dependent kinases and their inhibitors which will in turn regulate renal cell turnover (reviewed in Shankland 1999).

Platelet-derived growth factor Mesangial cells respond to the majority of chemokines, cytokines, and growth factors in culture by proliferation. Silver *et al.* (1989) suggested that cytokines and growth factors stimulate the release of PDGF by mesangial cells, thus initiating positive-feedback autocrine loops. Mesangioproliferative glomerulonephritides are associated in experimental animals and humans with an upregulation of glomerular PDGF (reviewed in Johnson *et al.* 1993 and Cybulsky 2000). The infusion of PDGF into rats (Floege *et al.* 1993) or the transfection of their glomeruli with the PDGF B-chain gene (Isaka *et al.* 1993) induces mesangial proliferation *in vivo*. PDGFs as well as FGF-induced mesangial proliferation is regulated by specific cell-cycle proteins/cyclin kinases and their inhibitors such as p27 (reviewed in Shankland 1999). The reduction of the levels of the cyclin kinases inhibitor p27 leads to an enhanced mesangial proliferative response to PDGF and FGF.

Inhibition of the effects of PDGF by neutralizing antibodies, high-affinity oligonucleotide aptamers, antisense nucleotides, or signal transduction inhibitors decreases the mesangioproliferative changes observed in experimental glomerulonephritis (reviewed in Cybulsky 2000; Floege and Ostendorf 2001).

In response to injury, PDGF may have a role in the glomerular repair process, as it appears to be a key factor in the migration of mesangial cells and their repopulation of the glomerular tuft (Haseley *et al.* 1999).

Transforming growth factor-β1 TGF-β1, possibly the single most important fibrogenic growth factor in the pathogenesis of glomerulosclerosis (reviewed in Basile 1999), has been shown to be upregulated in the glomeruli and tubules of rats with a range of diabetic and non-diabetic nephropathies (reviewed in Basile 1999; Yu *et al.* 2002). TGF-β1 is a multifunctional growth factor with contrasting functions depending on the microenvironment it finds itself in. It can be both pro- and antiproliferative as well as pro- and anti-inflammatory. TGF-β1 exerts its various effects within the glomeruli through interactions with two receptors (type I and II) expressed on glomerular endothelial and mesangial cells.

Two intracellular signal pathways have been implicated to mediate the effects of TGF-β1 on renal cells. These consist of the Smad family of proteins as well as the MAPK family (Poncelet *et al.* 1999). Recent data has shown Smad2 and Smad3 activation by TGF-β1 in human mesangial cells with resultant increased collagen transcription (Poncelet and Schnaper 2001).

TGF-β1 has been shown to induce phenotypic changes in mesangial cells including their expression of α-SMA (Isaka *et al.* 1993; Imai *et al.* 1994) and mediates glomerulosclerosis through the stimulation of the synthesis of ECM and the inhibition of its breakdown. TGF-β1 is thought to inhibit the release of MMPs and stimulate the synthesis of their inhibitors (TIMPs). This would favour irreversible ECM deposition.

The fibrogenic effect of TGF-β1 has been attributed to the stimulation by this growth factor of another fibrogenic growth factor, connective tissue growth factor (CTGF) (reviewed in Gupta *et al.* 2000). The upregulation of this growth factor in mesangial as well as tubular cells has been shown to follow TGF-β1-dependent and -independent pathways. In mesangial cells and fibroblasts, CTGF mediates some of TGF-β1 induced increased ECM production by autocrine modes of action.

Therapeutic interventions aimed at reducing TGF-β1 by neutralizing antibodies, antisense oligonucleotides as well as natural antagonists such as decorin have been shown to attenuate experimental glomerulosclerosis (reviewed in Yu *et al.* 2002).

It is important to appreciate that TGF-β1 is potentially beneficial by its antiproliferative and anti-inflammatory effects postulated as key mechanisms in the resolution of glomerular inflammation and injury; glomerular self-defence (Kitamura and Fine 1999).

Fibroblast growth factor-2 FGF-2 is another pleomorphic growth factor capable of inducing glomerulosclerosis. Glomerular cells express FGF-2 receptors (FGFR-1 and FGFR-3) (Floege *et al.* 1999). The infusion of a high dose of FGF-2 casues mesangial proliferation as well as glomerulosclerosis (Floege *et al.* 1993, 1998). Conversely, the inhibition of FGF-2 reduces the severity of glomerular injury in an experimental model of mesangioproliferative glomerulonephritis (Floege *et al.* 1998).

Of note, the progression of glomerular injury, proliferation, and sclerosis is likely to depend on the balance between the action of proinflammatory, mitotic, and fibrogenic growth factors and their antagonists. Natural antagonists to growth factors such as SPARC for PDGF and decorin for TGF-β1 may play a modulating role. A reduction in the glomerular content of decorin, a natural proteoglycan antagonist of TGF-β1 appears to precede the development of experimental glomerulosclerosis (Yu *et al.* 2002).

Potentially beneficial growth factors A range of potentially beneficial growth factors has been identified. These include HGF, VEGF, and bone morphogenic protein-7 (BMP-7). The HGF receptor c-Met is expressed on glomerular cells (endothelial, mesangial, and epithelial). In addition, macrophages are also potential sources of HGF. VEGF receptors are also expressed on glomerular, endothelial, and mesangial cells (VEGFR-1 and VEGFR-2). VEGFR-2 is upregulated in mesangioproliferative glomerulonephritis (reviewed in Kang *et al.* 2002). A role has been put forward for VEGF in the resolution of glomerular endothelial injury. Inhibition of VEGF-165 by aptamers delays the resolution of glomerular injury in rats with anti-thy1-mediated glomerulonephritis (Ostendorf *et al.* 1999).

Tubulointerstitial fibrosis As in glomerulosclerosis, an important role has been attributed to cytokines and growth factors in the pathogenesis of tubulointerstitial scarring. Tubulointerstitial growth factors may be derived from the glomerular effluent (Wang *et al.* 2000), from infiltrating inflammatory cells, and from the renal tubular cells themselves. Growth factors are likely to be released by infiltrating lymphocytes, monocytes, and mast cells, which are capable of releasing a wide range of mitotic, proinflammatory, and fibrogenic factors.

Chemokines and cytokines As discussed above, the activation/injury of tubular epithelial cells stimulate their release of chemokines, cytokines and growth factors (Anders *et al.* 2003). In addition, exposure of proximal tubular cells in culture to albumin activates NF-κB which in turn stimulate the synthesis by these cells of a wide range of NF-κB-dependent cytokines and chemokines (reviewed in Wardle 2000, 2002). Tubular activation and overexpression of NF-κB and AP-1 has been associated in a variety of proteinuric human nephropathies with the parallel tubular upregulation of chemokines (MCP-1, RANTES), cytokines and profibrogenic growth factors (TGF-β1) (Mezzano *et al.* 2001). The release by tubular cells of these proinflammatory mediators initiates and propagates tubulointerstitial inflammation (reviewed in Eddy 2001).

Platelet-derived growth factor PDGF from tubular cells stimulates the proliferation of renal fibroblasts *in vitro* (Knecht *et al.* 1991). In addition, treatment of rats with recombinant PDGF leads to tubulointerstitial cellular proliferation and interstitial fibrosis. The effect of PDGF on interstitial fibrosis may be mediated through its stimulation of fibroblast proliferation, their transformation into myofibroblasts as well as the stimulation of ECM production (Floege and Johnson 1995).

Transforming growth factor-β1 The most potent of profibrogenic growth factors implicated in interstitial fibrosis is TGF-β1 (reviewed in Basile 1999; Yu *et al.* 2002) derived from tubular cells, infiltrating macrophages and renal fibroblasts. Once activated, TGF-β1 is fibrogenic through the stimulation of renal tubular as well as fibroblast synthesis of ECM as well as the capacity of this growth factor to inhibit ECM breakdown through the stimulation of TIMPs.

Many of the fibrogenic effects of TGF-β1 appear to be mediated through CTGF (reviewed in Gupta *et al.* 2000) by downregulation of the CKI p27 and the subsequent stimulation of renal fibroblast proliferation (Kothapalli and Grotendorst 2000). TGF-β1 is also capable to induce the upregulation of FGF-2 in renal fibroblasts. This growth factor, like CTGF, induces renal fibroblast proliferation through the induction of cdk2 protein and the downregulation of p27 (Strutz *et al.* 2001).

As with glomerulosclerosis, TGF-β1 has been implicated in the apoptosis of tubular cells. The administration of an anti-TGF-β1 neutralizing antibody has been shown to diminish the severity of tubular apoptosis in a model of unilateral ureteric obstruction in rats (Miyajima *et al.* 2000).

Potentially beneficial growth factors In addition to harmful growth factors, a range of growth factors has been noted to have potential beneficial and protective effects. These include HGF, [BMP-7]/osteogenic protein-1 [OP-1], VEGF, IGF-1, and EGF (reviewed in Imai and Isaka 2002a,b).

In a number of experimental models, a reduction in tissue HGF has coincided with the increase in TGF-β1 and fibrosis. It has been suggested that HGF counteracts TGF-β and vice versa (Mizuno *et al.* 2000). In rats submitted to subtotal nephrectomy, treatment with a neutralizing anti-HGF antibody led to an exacerbation of renal injury and scarring (reviewed in Liu 2002). The protective effect of HGF was attributed to the activation by this growth factor of matrix degradation pathways. Conversely, the administration of HGF has proved protective in experimental models of interstitial fibrosis (reviewed in Liu 2002).

HGF prevents tubular epithelial cell death, enhances regeneration after injury, and has recently been shown to inhibit epithelial–mesenchymal transdifferentiation (reviewed in Yang and Liu 2002).

BMP-7 is a member of the TGF-β superfamily and has been localized to the collecting ducts. The administration of BMP-7 in rats with unilateral ureteral obstruction preserved tubular epithelial integrity, inhibited tubular cell apoptosis, and prevented interstitial fibrosis (reviewed in Hruska 2002).

VEGF is a member of the heparin-binding growth factors family. In the ageing kidney, cyclosporin-, and subtotal nephrectomy-induced interstitial fibrosis, a reduction in VEGF expression coincides with the progression of interstitial fibrosis and the rarefaction of the peritubular microvasculature. Administration of VEGF121 reverses these changes and protects against the progression of experimental interstitial scarring (reviewed in Kang et al. 2002).

Hormones Circulating concentrations of most peptide hormones are increased in CRF; some have been implicated in the progression of kidney scarring (Egido 1996). A chronic increase in circulating GH leads to glomerular hypertrophy and sclerosis in transgenic mice (Doi et al. 1988, 1991; Yang et al. 1997). Conversely, dwarf GH-deficient rats appeared resistant to the development of progressive glomerulosclerosis after subtotal nephrectomy (El Nahas et al. 1991). Similarly, mice overexpressing a GH antagonist are immune to glomerulosclerosis (Chen et al. 1997). It is interesting in this respect, that mice overexpressing IGF-1 develop glomerular hypertrophy without glomerulosclerosis (Doi et al. 1988). Those overexpressing IGFBP-1 are, on the other hand, prone to glomerulosclerosis (Doublier et al. 2000).

A role for GH in the progression of experimental DN was suggested by the outcome of experiments where the treatment of diabetic rats with octreotide (a somatostatin analogue) decreased the severity of proteinuria (Flyvbjerg et al. 1992; Landau et al. 2001). Similar observations have been made of a protective effect of the GH receptor antagonist in experimental DN (Flyvbjerg 2001). Diabetic dwarf mice transgenic for a mutated GH have less glomerulosclerosis in spite of increased glomerular synthesis of TGF-β1 (Esposito et al. 1996). Also, mice with a disruption of the GH receptor/binding protein gene appear to be resistant to the development of experimental DN (Bellush et al. 2000).

Other pituitary hormones may also have a permissive role in the development of glomerular scarring. Hypophysectomy reduced age-related (Wyndham et al. 1987) and ablation-induced glomerulosclerosis. Protection from progressive kidney scarring was reported in subtotally nephrectomized rats treated with antidiuretic hormone (ADH) receptor antagonists (Yamamura et al. 1994).

The effect of hyperparathyroidism on progression is uncertain as parathyroidectomy does not prevent progressive glomerulosclerosis in rats with glomerulonephritis. Thyroidectomy reduced proteinuria, corrected hypertriglyceridaemia, and prevented progressive uraemia and renal scarring in rats with glomerulonephritis, although the reported effects of thyroidectomy in rats with remnant kidneys are conflicting (reviewed in Alfrey 1986). Of relevance, recent data shows that the kidney is capable of expressing thyroid-specific genes; thyroid stimulating hormone receptor and thyroglobulin (Sellitti et al. 2000) which could conceivably mediate the effects of thyroid disease in the kidney.

An excess of glucocorticoids increases the Pgc and accelerates the progression of glomerulosclerosis in rats with remnant kidneys (Garcia et al. 1987). Experiments based on the pharmacological inhibition of glucocorticoids suggested that these hormones mediate some

of the glomerular adaptive haemodynamic changes (glomerular hyperperfusion and hyperfiltration) but were not involved in the pathogenesis of proteinuria or glomerulosclerosis (Cardoso et al. 1997). Pharmacological glucocorticoid blockade by RU-486 failed to attenuate the severity of the renal lesions and the associated kidney failure in rats submitted to subtotal nephrectomy (Cardoso et al. 1997).

A role for oestrogen in the prevention of glomerulosclerosis has been suspected for a long time, as male rats are more susceptible to proteinuria and renal scarring when compared to females (Neugarten 2002; Neugarten et al. 2002). The castration of male rats reduces their proteinuria and estrogens are protective in females (Verhagen et al. 2000). Male rats are more sensitive than female rats to develop proteinuria induced by chronic NO inhibition (Verhagen et al. 2000). In this experimental model of hypertension and proteinuria, oestrogens provided some protection in females, whereas orchidectomy prevented the increase in blood pressure and proteinuria in males (Verhagen et al. 2000).

Recent data suggests that oestrogen upregulates the synthesis of the collagenolytic enzymes MMP-2 and MMP-9 by mesangial cells through interactions with oestrogen receptors (OR α and β) (Guccione et al. 2002; Neugarten et al. 2002). Furthermore, oestrogens have been shown to reduce mesangial proliferation and collagen synthesis (Kwan et al. 1996).

The therapeutic potential of such observations was highlighted by experiments showing that oestrogen receptor modulators (SORMs), that have oestrogen-like actions, such as LY-117018 (an analogue of raloxifen) and tamoxifen inhibits mesangial cells synthesis of type I and type IV collagens (Neugarten et al. 2000).

Autacoids A prominent role for autacoids such as angiotensin II and endothelin-1 has been postulated in the pathogenesis of tubulointerstitial fibrosis.

The role of the renin–angiotensin–aldosterone system The hypotheses discussed above have highlighted the important role of the RAA system in the pathogenesis of systemic as well as glomerular hypertension and the associated renal scarring (reviewed in Ma and Fogo 2001; Fogo 2001b). As described above, besides the well-known role of angiotensin II in the pathogenesis of systemic hypertension, this autacoid has been implicated in the glomerular relative efferent arteriolar vasoconstriction that contributes to raised Pgc (reviewed in Anderson 2000). Angiotensin II also increases the size permselectivity of the glomerular capillary wall, thus favouring proteinuria.

Angiotensin II has proinflammatory, trophic, as well as fibrogenic effects that are likely to mediate glomerular as well as tubulointerstitial scarring. The proinflammatory effect of angiotensin II may be mediated in part by its activation of endothelial NF-κB (reviewed in Ruiz-Ortega et al. 2001).

Angiotensin II stimulates the contraction, hypertrophy, and proliferation of mesangial cells and their synthesis of extracellular matrix (Ma and Fogo 2001; Wolf 2001). Some of these effects may be mediated by the stimulation by angiotensin II of the release of TGF-β1 by renal cells (Gaedeke et al. 2001).

Angiotensin II has proinflammatory and fibrogenic effects on tubular epithelial cells (reviewed in Wolf 2001). These effects are direct and indirect through the activation of NF-κB and TGF-β1, respectively. Infusion of angiotensin II to rats induces tubulointerstitial inflammation and fibrosis (Johnson et al. 1992) by proinflammatory effects and activation of the transcription factor NF-κB as well as the induction within tubular cells of the chemotatic factor osteopontin (Ruiz-Ortega et al. 2001).

Both ACE inhibition and angiotensin receptor blockade (ARB) have been shown to be protective in most experimental models of glomerulosclerosis and/or tubulointerstitial fibrosis (Mackenzie *et al.* 1997; Anderson 2000).

Surprisingly, recent evidence has attributed a potentially protective effect of angiotensin II in experimental proliferative antithymocyte antibody-induced glomerulonephritis (Wenzel *et al.* 2002). This has been attributed to the stimulation of angiotensin II of TGF-β which may protect the glomeruli from inflammatory injury and cellular proliferation through the activation of CKI and the consequent induction of cell cycle arrest of infiltrating and local cells.

Aldosterone Aldosterone has potent fibrogenic effects including the stimulation of vascular smooth muscle cell hypertrophy, the upregulation of angiotensin II receptors and ECM production (Epstein 2001). In addition, aldosterone may promote renal fibrosis through the stimulation of both TGF-β1 and PAI-1 (Epstein 2001). Treatment of spontaneously hypertensive rats with an aldosterone receptor antagonist spironolactone reduces proteinuria and attenuates the severity of the renal scarring process (Rocha *et al.* 1999). On the other hand, aldosterone antagonists do not seem to prevent the progression of kidney scarring in rats submitted to subtotal nephrectomy in spite of a significant reduction in left ventricular hypertrophy.

Endothelin-1 Endothelin-1 is a potent proinflammatory autacoid (Chatziantoniou and Dussaule 2000), the effects of which may, at least in part, be mediated through the activation of NF-κB and the consequent synthesis and release of cytokines and chemokines (Wardle 2000, 2002). This may take place in glomerular endothelial (mediated by the ETB receptor) and proximal tubular epithelial (mediated by the ETA receptor) cells. Endothelin-1 is capable of stimulating the proliferation as well as ECM synthesis by mesangial cells through its type A receptor (ETA). Blockade of ETA as well as combined type A and B receptor blockades control hypertension, reduce proteinuria and attenuate kidney scarring in immune and non-immune models of experimental renal scarring (reviewed in Benigni *et al.* 2000).

Endothelin-1 has been shown to be proinflammatory and fibrogenic within the kidney (Chatziantoniou and Dussaule 2000; reviewed in Benigni 2000). Exposure of proximal tubular cells to high concentrations of albumin stimulates their synthesis of endothelin-1 (Zoja *et al.* 1999) with subsequent activation of NF-κB and the conseqent proinflammatory response (reviewed in Ruiz-Ortega *et al.* 2001). Endothelin-1 is fibrogenic through the stimulation of fibroblast chemotaxis, proliferation, and synthesis of ECM (Benigni 2000).

Extracellular matrix turnover
Glomerulosclerosis Matrix degradation depends on the activity of two collagenolytic systems, the MMPs and the plasminogen–plasmin system. The MMPs are zinc- and calcium-dependent enzymes. TIMP1, 2, 3, and 4 inhibit the activity of the MMPs by covalently binding to these enzymes' catalytic site. The glomerular ECM is regulated by the synthesis of its components by all three lines of glomerular cells as well as its breakdown by a range of metalloproteinases/collagenases (MMP-1, -2, and -9).

The increased synthesis by glomerular cells of extracellular matrix components such as collagens, fibronectin, and proteoglycans is thought to contribute to glomerulosclerosis. Mesangial cells release metalloproteinases capable of breaking down extracellular matrix. Further, glomerular cells synthesize and release TIMP-1, -2, and -3.

Glomerulosclerosis may result from an imbalance between mesangial MMPs and TIMPs. The incubation of mesangial cells with high concentrations of glucose and TGF-β1, reproducing the DN milieu (Singh *et al.* 2001), or with endothelin-1 (Yao *et al.* 2001) downregulate their release of MMP-2 and upregulate TIMP-2. By contrast, the incubation of mesangial cells with oestrogen upregulates their synthesis of MMP-9 and MMP-2 (Potier *et al.* 2001; Guccione *et al.* 2002). Such an upregulation of collagenolytic enzymes by oestrogens may contribute to the relative resistance of female rodents to glomerulosclerosis.

In IgA nephropathy, an overexpression of MMP-9 was reported in mesangial proliferative lesions (Wang *et al.* 2002). On the other hand, sclerotic glomeruli showed an upregulation of TIMP-1 and a downregulation of MMP-9 (Wang *et al.* 2002). In patients with type 2 DN, urinary MMP-9 and MMP-2 releases were shown to be significantly increased (reviewed in Zaoui *et al.* 2000).

Decreased glomerular collagenolytic activity has been described in ageing rats and in experimental glomerulonephritis (reviewed in Heidland *et al.* 1997). The progression of glomerulosclerosis in the antithy-1 model of mesangioproliferative glomerulonephritis is associated with a significant increase in the synthesis of TIMPs (Yamamoto *et al.* 1994). Others have shown that glomerulosclerosis in this model is associated with the inhibition of the plasmin protease system. Upregulation of glomerular PAI-1 by TGF-β1 has been implicated (Fogo 2001a). These observations suggest that local MMP/TIMP imbalance is involved in renal remodelling.

Finally, qualitative changes in the type of extracellular matrix synthesized and deposited within scarred glomeruli might also affect the outcome. Collagen types I and III have been detected in experimental and clinical nephropathies (Striker *et al.* 1984) and attributed to the infiltration of scarred glomeruli by interstitial fibroblasts/myofibroblasts (Striker *et al.* 1984; El Nahas 1996). Qualitative changes of the glomerular extracellular matrix have been described in diabetic rats and humans (Costigan *et al.* 1995). Upregulation of the expression of glomerular collagens V and VI has been reported (Groma 1998; Moriya *et al.* 2001). Qualitative changes in the glomerular extracellular matrix may modify the proliferative response of mesangial cells, as the culture of these cells *in vitro* on collagen type I enhanced their proliferative response to growth factors (Ruef *et al.* 1992). Changes in the ECM substrate may also affect the survival of mesangial cells (Mooney *et al.* 1999).

In addition, recent evidence suggests that some of the ECM qualitative changes taking place within scarred glomeruli may render the ECM resistant to the proteolytic actions of MMPs (Johnson *et al.* 1997; Skill *et al.* 2001). In experimental DN, the upregulation of the crosslinking enzyme tissue transglutaminase has been implicated in mesangial matrix crosslinking and resistance to breakdown (Johnson *et al.* 1997).

Tubulointerstitial fibrosis As in glomerulosclerosis, tubulointerstitial fibrosis is likely to result from an inbalance between the synthesis and breakdown of extracellular matrix. Tubular cells and infiltrating macrophages and interstitial fibroblasts are all capable of ECM synthesis and release (reviewed in Harris 2000).

Increased synthesis of components of the interstitial extracellular matrix has been described in a wide range of experimental nephropathies (reviewed in Jernigan and Eddy 2000; Eddy 2001). In a number of models, the increased deposition of interstitial collagen is associated with an increased synthesis of TIMP-1 by the kidney (Jones *et al.* 1991, 1995; Yamamoto *et al.* 1994). TIMP-1 mRNA is upregulated in tubular cells and fibroblasts during the course of protein-overload nephropathy (reviewed in Jernigan and Eddy 2000). However, TIMP-1 knockout mice are not protected from the development of interstitial fibrosis (Eddy *et al.* 2000; Kim *et al.* 2001a), possibly due to a compensatory upregulation of TIMP-2 and -3.

A prominent role has been attributed to ischaemia and the resulting hypoxia in the pathogenesis of interstitial fibrosis (reviewed in Fine *et al.* 2000). *In vitro* experiments suggest that hypoxia is a potent fibrogenic stimulus leading to an upregulation of collagen and TIMPs synthesis as well as the downregulation of that of MMPs in both tubular cells and renal fibroblasts (Norman *et al.* 2000).

The second major matrix degradation pathway is the plasminogen–plasmin system. It is inhibited by PAI-1 which is upregulated in various experimental models of interstitial fibrosis. PAI-1 synthesis is increased by fibrotic mediators such as angiotensin II and TGF-β1 (reviewed in Fogo 2001b). Mice genetically deficient in PAI-1 are less prone to interstitial fibrosis (Oda *et al.* 2001). Tubulointerstitial fibrosis is likely to result from increased synthesis as well as decreased breakdown of extracellular matrix.

Summary of mechanisms of kidney scarring

The progression of both glomerulosclerosis (Figs 1–3) and tubulointerstitial fibrosis (Figs 4–6) follow similar pathways. An initial injury leads to induction of fibrogenesis by the activation of glomerular/tubular cells and their release of chemokines and cytokines attracting inflammatory cells. This initial stage of inflammation leads to interactions between infiltrating cells and resident renal cells mediated by cell–cell contact or through the release of a range of mediators including vasoactive peptides, cytokines growth factors, and ROS. A proliferative phase ensues characterized by the activation and proliferation of mesenchymal mesangial and fibroblastic cells. It also leads to the epithelial–mesenchymal transdifferentiation of tubular cells and their involvement in the fibrosis process and their synthesis of components of the ECM. The resolution or progression of fibrosis could be halted at the initial inflammatory stage by anti-inflammatory factors including anti-inflammatory cytokines and TGF-β1. The proliferative phase may be checked by antiproliferative factors such as SPARC and calponin. Apoptosis may also play a role in the resolution of injury and the death of infiltrating and proliferating cells. The final fibrotic phase is likely to result from an imbalance between the synthesis and degradation of ECM leading to irreversible fibrosis.

Modulating factors of progressive kidney disease

The progression of chronic kidney damage is influenced by a variety of factors (Fig. 7). *Susceptibility* factors determining predisposition to the development of a specific nephropathy are predominantly genetic and

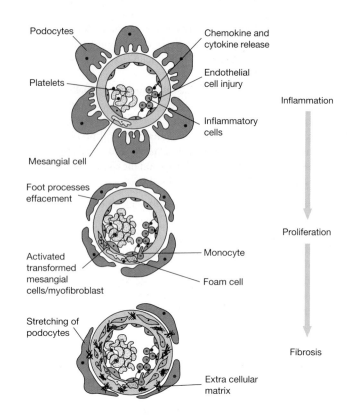

Fig. 2 Schematic representation of the stages of glomerulosclerosis.

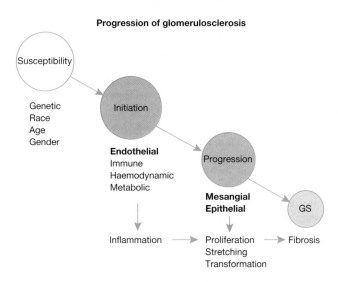

Fig. 3 Diagrammatic representation of the stages of glomerulosclerosis (GS).

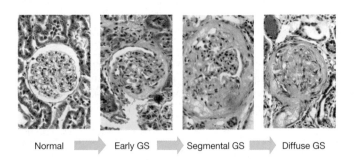

Fig. 1 Histological features of progressive glomerulosclerosis.

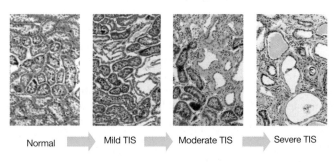

Fig. 4 Histological features of tubulointerstitial scarring.

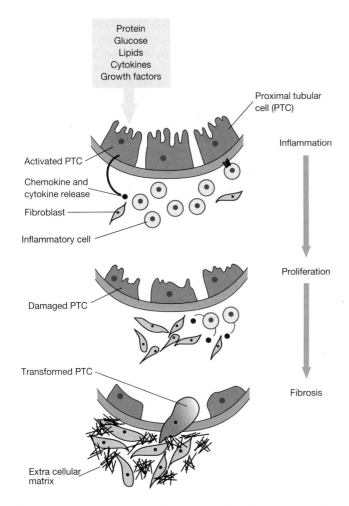

Fig. 5 Schematic representation of proximal tubular cell activation and the initiation of tubulointerstitial inflammation and fibrosis.

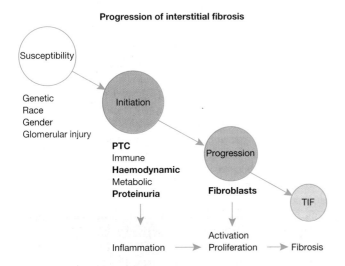

Progression of interstitial fibrosis

Fig. 6 Diagrammatic representation of the stages of tubulointerstitial fibrosis (TIF).

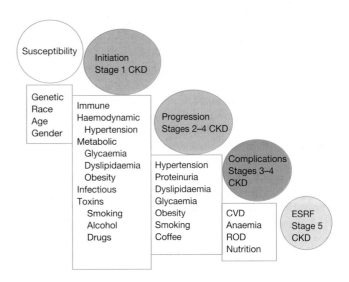

Fig. 7 Diagrammatic representation of the stages of CKD.

gender. Modifiable factors include systemic hypertension, proteinuria, dyslipidaemia, and lifestyle factors such as smoking, alcohol, caffeine, and the use of recreational drugs.

Non-modifiable risk factors

Genetic factors

Genetic factors are known to affect the susceptibility of both animals and man to various nephropathies, but they influence the natural history and progression of CKD too.

In the rat, the development of age-related and disease-induced glomerulosclerosis is strain dependent. Sprague–Dawley, Wistar, and Lewis rats are prone to develop progressive, age-related glomerular lesions. Three rat strains, Wistar–Kyoto, PVG/c, and ACI/MN, are known to be resistant to the development of age-related glomerulosclerosis (Weening *et al.* 1986; Grond *et al.* 1989).

The C57/Os+ mice predisposed to oligomeganephronia (reduced number of nephrons and large glomeruli) are resistant to ablation-induced glomerulosclerosis. This contrasts with the ROP/Os+ mutant strain of mice which have enlarged glomeruli and are prone to spontaneous as well as ablation-induced glomerulosclerosis (Esposito *et al.* 1999). These observations imply that the genetic predisposition to glomerulosclerosis prevails over glomerular size. Of interest, the transplantation of bone marrow of glomerulosclerosis-prone mice to those glomerulosclerosis-resistant leads to glomerulosclerosis highlighting the importance of genetic influences on mesangial phenotypes and the development of glomerulosclerosis (Cornacchia *et al.* 2001). The development of diabetic glomerulosclerosis is also strain-dependent with the ROP/Os+ mice susceptible and the C57/Os+ resistant (Zheng *et al.* 1998). Furthermore, the glucose-induced changes in collagen synthesis in culture were reversible in mesangial cells derived from sclerosis-resistant mice and permanent in those obtained from sclerosis-prone (ROP) mice highlighting the importance of the interplay between genetic and metabolic factors (Fornoni *et al.* 2002).

Rennke *et al.* (1987) have reported interstrain variations in the development of proteinuria and glomerulosclerosis in rats with immune-complex nephritis; progressive proteinuria is severe in Wistar–Kyoto rats and glomerulosclerosis is negligible in Brown– Norway and Sprague–Dawley rats. Wistar–Kyoto rats are also very susceptible to the

racial. *Progression* factors affect the rate of decline of renal insufficiency after the onset of the renal disease. Progression factors are divided into the modifiable and non-modifiable. Non-modifiable factors include the patient's genetic and racial background, age and development of rapidly progressive necrotizing glomerulonephritis when injected with an anti-GBM antibody (Kanno et al. 1998).

Other strains, such as the OZR and Fawn-Hooded rats, are prone to develop accelerated forms of glomerular scarring. In the obese, hyperphagic, and hyperlipidaemic Zucker and Koletsky rats, this leads to renal failure and a significant reduction in lifespan. The Fawn-Hooded rat develops hypertension and progressive glomerular scarring (Kuijpers and de Jong 1987); these animals also display defective platelet aggregability, and the combination of hypertension and abnormal platelet function is likely to contribute to the development of the glomerular lesions. At least five genetic loci (Rf-1–Rf-5) have been linked to the development of renal impairment and glomerulosclerosis in Fawn-Hooded rats (Brown et al. 1998). Of these five, renal failure (Rf)-1 appears to play a major role. Transfer of the Rf-1B region of chromosome 1 of susceptible Fawn-Hooded rats to the genome of normotensive August × Copenhagen Irish (ACI) rat confers the susceptibility to progressive renal failure when hypertension is superimposed (Provoost et al. 2002). These observations suggest that genetic traits might affect the progression of renal disease through changes in metabolic, clotting, and haemodynamic factors.

In rats, age-related and disease-induced proteinuria and glomerulosclerosis tend to be more severe in males (Zeier and Gretz 1993; Neugarten et al. 2002). The relative resistance of female rats to proteinuria and glomerulosclerosis can be reversed by the administration of androgens; the susceptibility of males can be lessened by castration.

The increased male susceptibility to glomerulosclerosis in the rat is likely to be multifactorial in origin. Although male rats have larger kidneys than females, they do not seem to have larger glomeruli to account for their increased susceptibility. On the other hand, male Munich–Wistar rats have lower renal vascular and afferent arteriolar resistance than females. Consequently, they have a higher Pgc after renal ablation. Gender-related differences in the permeability of the GBM have also been described in the Munich–Wistar Fromter rat (MWF/Ztm), a strain in which hydraulic membrane permeability is greater in males than females, leading to heavy proteinuria.

As discussed above, oestrogens are potentially protective against glomerulosclerosis through inhibition of mesangial cell proliferation as well as their synthesis of ECM. Oestrogens also upregulate mesangial synthesis of MMPs, thus facilitating ECM breakdown (Potier et al. 2001) (discussed above).

Immunogenetics and the progression of chronic kidney diseases in humans

Genetic factors also affect the susceptibility to, and the natural history of, chronic nephropathies in man. Investigations have been undertaken based on immunogenetic as well as the study of genetic polymorphism.

Immunogenetics

Investigation has been undertaken in patients with CKD by serological and genetic methods. Associations have been observed between HLA-related antigens and molecules and the susceptibility to progressive renal insufficiency.

A race-controlled investigation of HLA phenotype and the predisposition to ESRD was undertaken in the United States based on a renal transplant registry. This study showed a link between HLA-DR3 and the predisposition to ESRD in African-Americans with HNS, diabetic, and membranous nephropathies. In Caucasians, HLA-DR3 was also associated with ESRD in patients with membranous and diabetic nephropathies. On the other hand, HLA-DR3 was not associated with ESRD in FSGS or IgA nephropathy.

A wide range of HLA haplotypes have been associated with the predisposition to, and the progression of, most types of chronic nephropathies (reviewed in Locatelli and Del Vecchio 2000). This includes HLA-DR3, DR5, and DR3–B18–Bf*F in idiopathic membranous nephropathy. Patients with IgA nephropathy carrying the HLA-BW35 (France), DR4 (Japan), B27 and DR1 (United States) antigens as well as the complement phenotype C3FF (homozygous for BfFF) (Germany) were said to have a faster rate of progression. A strong association was reported between HLA-DQB1*0301 and the progression of IgA nephropathy. In patients with IgA nephropathy the complement protein 4A deficiency has been linked to a higher incidence of ESRF (for review, see Locatelli and Del Vecchio 2000).

In mesangiocapillary glomerulopathy, the presence of the extended haplotype B8–DR3–SCO1–GLO2 has been linked with a somewhat poorer prognosis. In Goodpasture's syndrome, carriers of the antigen DR2 (DRW15 allele) have an increased susceptibility to the disease, and those with the HLA-DR2–B7 haplotype have a worse prognosis.

Genetic polymorphisms and the progression of chronic kidney failure

The newer genetic techniques are proving powerful tools to investigate the links between genetic susceptibility and the progression of chronic kidney diseases. Two research strategies have been applied. The first is the candidate gene approach aiming to detect an association with a particular polymorphic DNA marker. The second is the genome wide search of unknown genes potentially associated with progressive CKF.

The first approach based on polymorphic changes in candidate genes has been applied to genes coding for angiotensin, NO, kallikrein, cytokines, and growth factors. The polymorphism that has received the most interest is the angiotensin I converting enzyme gene located on chromosome 17. A 287 bp insertion/deletion (I/D) polymorphism of intron 16 of this gene has been the subject of investigation in relation to the susceptibility to cardiovascular diseases as well as the development and progression of CKD.

In DN, it has been suggested that the development of nephropathy is influenced by the ACE I/D polymorphism; homozygotes for the D allele may be at increased risk of developing DN. In one study, a stronger association was also reported with the polymorphism of the allele designed as DdeI '=' in intron 7 of the ACE gene. Type 1 diabetic patients carrying the susceptibility haplotype combining deletions in intron 16 and 7 had a fourfold increased risk of developing DN. In type 2 DM Asian, but not Caucasian, carriers of the D allele are at increased risk of developing DN (OR = 1.88). The D allele of the ACE gene has not only been associated with suceptibility to DN but also to its progression. Further, it has been suggested that the response to treatment (ACE inhibition) may also be influenced by the ACE gene polymorphism with resistance to treatment in those who are homozygous for the D allele (reviewed by Locatelli and Del Vecchio 2000).

In other nephropathies, the D allele of the ACE gene has been associated with a faster rate of decline in renal function in IgA nephropathy, FSGS, reflux nephropathy and PKD. Recent data suggest that the influence of the ACE genotype on the progression of CKF may be influenced by the genotype of a cytoskeletal protein (adducin). Synergy between the ACE (DD) polymorphism and the ATR1 receptor gene has also been postulated. Similarly, interactions between the ACE gene and that coding for angiotensinogen (AGT) have been reported. In IgA nephropathy, a study suggested that patients with the ACE/DD polymorphism had a poor prognosis only in the presence of the AGT/MM genotype. Interactions between the polymorphism (4G4G) of the PAI-1 promoter gene with the ACE DD genotype have been implicated in the pathogenesis of macrovascular complications in patients with type 2 DN. Many of these associations have been based on studies with a small number of patients and warrant further validation (for review, see Locatelli and Del Vecchio 2000).

Polymorphism in the growth factors genes coding for PDGF-B chain and TGF-β1 have been investigated. Preliminary data suggest susceptibility to CKD is associated with TGF-β1 polymorphism in C homozygotes at codon 10 (Leu10Pro). Polymorphism of (C-509T) of the promoter of the TGF-β1 gene on the long arm of chromosome 19 has been linked to susceptibility to renal diseases as well as a faster rate of progression of CKF. Carriers of the T allele were found to have a faster rate of progression compared to others. On the other hand, African-Americans with ESRD did not have an association between their PDGF-B or TGF-β1 genotypes and the susceptibility to progressive renal insufficiency (Freedman et al. 1997).

The human homologue of the rat kidney failure gene has been localized on chromosome 10q. In African-Americans with ESRF caused by a variety of underlying nephropathies, an association between two markers (D10S1435 and D10S249) spanning 21 polymorphic regions of chromosome 10 approached significance in non-diabetic patients (Yu et al. 1999). However, the human homologue of the Rf-1 gene is unlikely to contribute significantly to the progression of CKF in African-Americans (Yu et al. 1999).

Racial factors

Genetic factors are likely to explain the race-related differences in susceptibility and outcome of nephropathies. In the United States, most studies relying on univariate analysis showed a faster rate of progression of diabetic and other nephropathies in Blacks compared to Whites (K/DOQI 2002). Of note, only one study confirmed the faster progression in black Americans by multivariate analysis. The Multiple Risk Factor Intervention Trial (MRFIT) demonstrated a higher incidence of ESRD for all causes in African-Americans compared to Whites at all levels of blood pressure (Klag et al. 1997).

There are similar observations of an increased incidence of ESRD in native Americans (Feldman et al. 1992), who have a higher rate of diabetic ESRD than either White or Black Americans (Smith et al. 1991). As with African-Americans the increased incidence of ESRD is explained by type II diabetes (Smith et al. 1991).

A large single-centre study in the United Kingdom of 771 patients with ESRD showed a higher incidence of DN in patients from the Indian subcontinent, while hypertensive renal disease was more common in individuals of Caribbean and African descent (Pazianas et al. 1991). This was confirmed by a study in which Indo-Asians were shown to have higher susceptibility to DN and non-DN (Buck and Feehally 1997). Furthermore, UK Asians with DN may have a faster rate of decline of GFR when compared to Caucasians (Earle et al. 2001). Whether these differences in the rate of progression are related to race-related genetic factors remains to be determined.

The influence of race on the susceptibility and progression of non-diabetic/hypertensive nephropathies is less well defined (reviewed in Locatelli and Del Vecchio 2000).

The underlying mechanism for the race-related susceptibility to hypertensive renal injury in African-Americans remains unknown, but might reflect genetically determined variations in glomerular size, filtration surface, or number (reviewed in Brenner and Chertow 1994). It might also be attributable to the numerous renal, hormonal, and physiological differences between Black and White individuals. Socioeconomic factors, as well as access to and compliance with treatment, might also affect the outcome of kidney disease in some ethnic minorities.

Gender-related factors

ESRF is more common in males (USRDS 2001; K/DOQI 2002). The incident rate in the United States in 1999 was 380 pmp/year in males compared to 266 pmp in females (USRDS 2001). Eighteen major studies have investigated to date the association of gender with progression of CKF and suggested a faster rate of decline in GFR in males (K/DOQI 2002).

Many of the studies described above relied on univariate analysis of risk factors. Multivariate analyses have not always confirmed an independent gender-related risk factor. One study from Japan suggested that females had a faster rate of progression (reviewed K/DOQI 2002). Also, a very high incidence of diabetic kidney failure has been described in postmenopausal African-American women.

Age-related factors

The incidence of ESRF increases with age (USRDS 2001; UK Registry 2002). The aetiology of CKF is different in the elderly with a higher incidence of hypertension (including renovascular hypertension), diabetes (type 2), and obstructive uropathy accounting for 40–60 per cent of patients with CKD.

The rate of decline of CKF is also influenced by age. The K/DOQI review of 21 studies suggested that age was a risk factor for the progression of CKD (K/DOQI 2002). One notable exception is type 1 DN where young age at diagnosis is associated with a faster rate of GFR decline. The faster rate of progression of CKF in the elderly may be influenced by higher levels of blood pressure, underlying atherosclerotic renal ischaemia as well as the associated nephropathy. In addition, the underlying age-related glomerulosclerosis and interstitial fibrosis as well as the reduced kidney functional reserve may affect outcome of renal diseases in the elderly.

Modifiable risk factors

Whilst nothing can be done to influence the non-modifiable risk factors, increasing attention has been paid to the modifiable factors affecting the rate of progression of CKF. These include systemic hypertension, proteinuria, metabolic factors such as hyperglycaemia, dyslipidaemia, obesity and possibly hyperuricaemia. In addition, recent interest has focused on the contribution of cigarette smoking, alcohol and caffeine consumption as well as recreational drugs to the risk of development of ESRD.

Hypertension

Systemic hypertension has been shown to be both an initiation and progression factor for diabetic and other nephropathies (Fig. 8).

NHANES III 1988–1994 undertaken in the United States suggested that there were around 30 million individuals with hypertension in 1994 (Coresh et al. 2001). Assuming that 2.5–5 per cent of all cases of hypertension were secondary to underlying renal diseases, it was estimated that between 700,000 and 1,400,000 Americans were affected. MRFIT

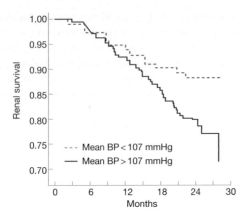

Fig. 8 Actuarial renal survival rates according to baseline mean arterial blood pressure in patients with CKD (Locatelli *et al.* 1996).

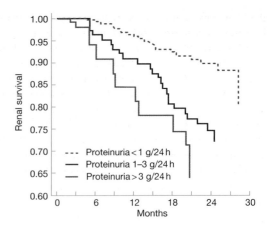

Fig. 9 Actuarial renal survival rates according to baseline 24 h proteinuria in patients with CKD (Locatelli *et al.* 1996).

studied the relationship between hypertension and ESRD in 332,544 American men aged between 35 and 57 (Klag *et al.* 1997), and observed a strong positive correlation between the severity of both systolic as well as diastolic hypertension and the incidence of ESRD. Even patients with stage 1 hypertension (BP = 140–159/90–99 mmHg) had a threefold increased risk of ESRD compared to normotensives (Klag *et al.* 1997).

Strong evidence links the progression of CKD to systemic hypertension (reviewed in Adamczak *et al.* 2002). The recent K/DOQI review (2002) reported a positive association between hypertension and the progression of CKD by univariate as well as multivariate analysis in a large number of studies. Some have suggested that nocturnal hypertension (loss of night-time fall/dip) may be an independent risk factor for the progression of renal failure. Others suggest that the elevation of pulse pressure may be an additional factor in the initiation and progression of CKD in DN and non-DN.

Proteinuria

The K/DOQI has reviewed 24 studies investigating the link between proteinuria and the progression of CKD (K/DOQI 2002). The majority of studies showed an association between heavy proteinuria and a fast rate of GFR decline by univariate analysis. Eleven studies confirmed, by multivariate analysis, that heavy proteinuria was associated with a faster rate of progression of CKD (reviewed in K/DOQI 2002). In a wide range of glomerulonephritis, the severity of proteinuria predicts the outcome (Locatelli *et al.* 1996; Jafar *et al.* 2001a) (Fig. 9). The modification of diet in renal disease (MDRD) and other studies showed that baseline proteinuria was a strong predictor of subsequent decline in renal function (Klahr *et al.* 1994; Locatelli *et al.* 1996; Jafar *et al.* 2001a). In a European study, synergism between the severity of proteinuria and hypertension on the rate of progression of CKD was suggested (Locatelli *et al.* 1996, Fig. 10).

Intervention studies have shown that the reduction of proteinuria by diet (El Nahas *et al.* 1984) or ACE inhibition (Gansevoort *et al.* 1997) predicts a better outcome in diabetic as well as other nephropathies. Further, both dietary (El Nahas *et al.* 1984) and pharmacological (GISEN 1997) interventions showed an improvement in renal function proportional to the extent of the reduction in proteinuria.

In addition, proteinuria and albuminuria have been associated with increased cardiovasular morbidity and mortality in patients with diabetic and other nephropathies (Hebert *et al.* 2002).

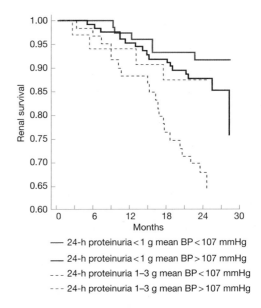

— 24-h proteinuria < 1 g mean BP < 107 mmHg
— 24-h proteinuria < 1 g mean BP > 107 mmHg
--- 24-h proteinuria 1–3 g mean BP < 107 mmHg
--- 24-h proteinuria 1–3 g mean BP > 107 mmHg

Fig. 10 Actuarial renal survival rates in patients with CKD with baseline proteinuria greater than 1 g/24 h and mean arterial blood pressure greater than 107 mmHg (Locatelli *et al.* 1996).

Metabolic factors

Glycaemia There is little doubt that poor blood glucose control is a major factor in the initiation of nephropathy in susceptible diabetics, but evidence for a role in progression is conflicting. Of the 13 major studies reviewed by K/DOQI, six showed an association by multivariate analysis while a similar number showed no association between hyperglycaemia and the rate of progression of diabetic kidney disease (K/DOQI 2002). The faster rate of decline of GFR in diabetic patients with poor glycaemic control in some of the larger studies lends support to an association (Breyer *et al.* 1996; Rossing *et al.* 2002).

Intervention studies show convincingly that tight glycaemia was associated with improved prognosis (DCCT 1995). Similarly, the United Kingdom Prospective Diabetes Study (UKPDS) showed that the progression to DN in patients with type 2 diabetes was also improved by better control of glycaemia (Turner 1998).

Lipids Lipids may contribute to the initiation and progression of CKD as data from the Atherosclerosis Risk in Communities (ARIC) study in the United States has shown that hyperlipidaemia (triglyceridaemia) is associated with an increased risk of ESRF (Muntner *et al.* 2000).

In patients with CKD, an association has been proposed between lipoproteins and the progression of CKD (Attman *et al.* 1999). The K/DOQI review of 15 major studies reported that seven of these studies confirmed by multivariate analysis that dyslipidaemia is a risk factor for a faster rate of progression (K/DOQI 2002). In DN, hypercholesterolaemia has been associated with a faster rate of decline in GFR (Krowleski *et al.* 1993; Bonnet and Cooper 2000). Similarly, in nephropathies other than diabetes, elevated plasma cholesterol and triglycerides appear to be associated with a faster rate of progression compared with those without hyperlipidaemia (Attman *et al.* 1999).

Hyperuricaemia Experimental data suggests a link between uric acid concentrations and the progression of hypertensive and toxic nephropathies. In humans, a link between hyperuricaemia and the development of systemic hypertension, cardiovascular and renal diseases has been postulated (Johnson *et al.* 1999).

Obesity In patients with IgA nephropathy, a recent report showed that individuals with excessive body weight and a raised body mass index (BMI) have a faster rate of progression of CKF (Bonnet *et al.* 2001). In this study, hypertension-free survival was also considerably shorter in overweight patients.

Miscellaneous

Smoking (see also Chapter 4.12.2) Over the last decade, accumulating evidence has suggested a detrimental effect of smoking on the progression of diabetic and non-diabetic nephropathies (reviewed in Orth 2002). Cigarette smoking causes an increase in systemic blood pressure and affects renal haemodynamics. In a study of men with CKD, smoking was reported to increase the risk of developing ESRF by a factor of 1–6 proportional to the amount of cigarette smoked. In patients treated with ACE inhibitors the odds ratios were around 3 increasing to 10 in those on other antihypertensive agents. Further, following renal transplantation smokers have a lower survival rate and poorer functional outcome (Kasiske and Klinger 2000). Histologically, smokers with glomerulonephritis appear to have more severe vascular pathology compared to non-smokers (Lhotta *et al.* 2002).

Alcohol Epidemiological data links heavy alcohol consumption to progressive renal insufficiency (Parekh and Klag 2001). Patients with CKD consuming more than two alcohol drinks a day appear to have increased odds ratio (2–4) for the development of ESRF compared to those drinking less (Parekh and Klag 2001), perhaps linked to the effect of alcohol on blood pressure. A Japanese study showed that men who habitually drank more than 46 g/day (five to six drinks per day) have over twice the risk of developing hypertension compared to those who drank less (Tsuruta *et al.* 2000). It is therefore advisable for patients with CKD to reduce their daily alcohol intake to less than two units/day (Parekh and Klag 2001).

Caffeine Experimental data suggest a link between excessive caffeine consumption and the progression of renal scarring (Tofovic *et al.* 2002).

There is no clinical data yet to confirm the relevance of this association in humans, although a US survey of a cohort of 1017 White male former medical students suggested that chronic coffee drinking is associated with small increases in blood pressure (Klag *et al.* 2002).

Recreational drugs (see also Chapter 4.12.1) In the United States, a case control study in the general population showed that recreational drugs are risk factors for the development of ESRF (Perneger *et al.* 2001). In this study, individuals who consumed heroin or opiates (any amount) were at increased risk of ESRF (odds ratio of 19.1). After adjustment for confounding and sociodemographic factors, the use of cocaine or crack and psychedelic drugs were also associated with ESRF, although this association could not be dissociated from the influence of heroin use (Perneger *et al.* 2001).

Management of chronic kidney disease

The improved understanding of the pathophysiology of CKD and some of the factors that affect its progression suggests new therapeutic approaches. It also sheds some light on the mechanisms of action of dietary and pharmacological interventions aimed at preventing renal scarring and progressive CRF.

Dietary intervention in chronic kidney failure

Dietary protein restriction

A reduction in dietary protein intake is beneficial in virtually all animal models of CKF (reviewed in Modi *et al.* 1993). The protective effect of dietary protein restriction on glomerular scarring is likely to be multifactorial (reviewed in Anderson 2000). Dietary protein restriction affects renal trophic and haemodynamic change in response to injury (reviewed in Dworkin and Weir 2000). A low-protein intake might also exert a protective effect through changes in glomerular permeability and macromolecular trafficking, and a reduction of proteinuria (Remuzzi and Bertani 1990). A low protein diet (LPD) also affects some of the factors thought to be involved in the progression of renal scarring such as hyperlipidaemia, renal thromboxane excretion, the renin–angiotensin system, endothelin and TGF-β1 (reviewed in Eddy 2001; Sawashima *et al.* 2002).

Early clinical trails of LPD on the progression of CKF in patients were flawed and inconclusive (El Nahas and Coles 1986). More recent, large-scale, multicentre, randomized studies have also failed to establish convincingly that there is a beneficial effect from a LPD on the progression of CKF. The largest of these trials, the MDRD involved 840 patients followed prospectively over 3 years and failed to show convincingly that an LPD slowed the progression of chronic renal diseases (Klahr *et al.* 1994). However, subsequent analyses suggested that there was a positive correlation between dietary protein intake and the rate of progression of renal insufficiency in patients with a GFR between 13 and 24 ml/min/1.73 m^2; in this group, a daily reduction of 0.2 g/kg in protein intake appeared to lead to a slowing of the decline in GFR by 1.15 ml/min/year (Teschan *et al.* 1998).

A meta-analysis of the major controlled LPD trials in diabetic and non-diabetic nephropathies suggested that the relative risk of renal failure was 0.67 in favour of an LPD (Pedrini *et al.* 1996). This was despite the heterogeneity of the trials included in the analysis; different outcome measures, diets, and compliance. The authors calculated that a trial of 1000 or more patients would be necessary to show a 33 per cent ESRF risk reduction with dietary protein restriction. Other meta-analyses reported conflicting results (reviewed in Aparicio *et al.* 2001). One showed undoubted benefit with an odds ratio for renal death on LPD compared to control of 0.54 (Fouque *et al.* 1992). Of interest, this meta-analysis did not include the MDRD trial. This meta-analysis was recently updated reviewing data involving seven clinical trials selected from 40 studies since 1975 involving 1494 non-diabetic patients with CKD (Fouque *et al.* 2000). There was a 39 per cent relative risk reduction in renal death in favour of a LPD. The largest meta-analysis of trials of LPD in CKD, comprising 13 randomized and 11 non-randomized clinical trials involving 2248 patients, showed a marginal benefit for LPD (Kasiske *et al.* 1998). The apparent differences among the major meta-analyses can be attributed to differences in their objectives as the first three meta-analyses focused on the prevention of ESRF, while the fourth assessed the risk of decline in renal function.

The K/DOQI Nutrition Guideline recommends consideration of a reduction of dietary protein intake (DPI) to 0.6 g/kg/day for individuals with a GFR less than 25 ml/min (CKD stages 4 and 5) (NKF/DOQI 2002). At least 50 per cent of the protein intake should consist of high biological value protein. Close nutritional monitoring is also recommended if protein restriction is implemented.

The prescription of dietary protein restriction to patients with advanced kidney insufficiency warrants careful nutritional monitoring by an experienced dietitian. Undernutrition in these patients can be compounded by the fact that spontaneous reductions in dietary protein intake also take place in patients with progressive CKD (Ikizler *et al.* 1995). Around 50 per cent of patients starting RRT have some degree of protein-calorie malnutrition that carries a high risk of increased morbidity and mortality.

Dietary salt

A high salt intake has been shown to be detrimental to the progression of experimental renal scarring in a limited number of studies. Dietary salt may accelerate renal scarring through TGF-β-dependent pathways (Ying and Sanders 1998).

Clinical evidence suggests that salt restriction optimizes both the antihypertensive and antiproteinuric effects of ACE inhibitors, angiotensin receptor blockers, and non-dihydropyridine calcium channel blockers (NDCCB) (Heeg *et al.* 1987; Bakris *et al.* 1996). The National Kidney Foundation (NKF) Task Force on Cardiovascular Disease in Chronic Renal Disease recommends a reduction in dietary salt to individuals within the general population with borderline hypertension (140/90 mmHg) as well as to those with stages 1–4 CKD in conjunction with antihypertensive agents (Bakris *et al.* 2000). These recommendations are based on those of the JNC-6 for the control of blood pressure. A goal of NaCl of 80–120 mmol/day has been suggested. In the absence of compliance to a salt restricted diet, diuretic therapy would potentiate the antiproteinuric effect of ACE inhibitors and ARBs (Buter *et al.* 1998).

The Dietary Approaches to Stop Hypertension (DASH) study showed that dietary potassium supplementation is also beneficial in reducing systemic blood pressure in humans (Conlin *et al.* 2000; Hermansen 2000). However, in patients with CKD, such a diet runs the risk of hyperkalaemia, in particular, in patients receiving ACE inhibitors.

Dietary lipids

In experimental animals, diets low in saturated fat and supplemented with polyunsaturated fatty acids have reduced the severity of age-related and disease-induced glomerular sclerosis (Reviewed in Modi *et al.* 1993).

Diets supplemented with polyunsaturated fatty acids are likely to have multiple effects on renal scarring: they reduce systemic hypertension and proteinuria, may affect renal haemodynamics through their effects on eicosanoids, inhibit platelet aggregation, correct hyperlipidaemia, and interfere with the inflammatory response (Donadio 2001).

Dietary supplementation with fish oil improved the hyperlipidaemia and reduced systemic hypertension and whole-blood viscosity in uraemic patients. Preliminary reports suggested a beneficial effect of eicosapentanoic acid on the progression of IgA nephropathy in Japanese patients, not confirmed in a larger study of Australian patients treated with eicosapentanoic acid for 2 years. A meta-analysis of all the major studies of fish oil supplementation in CKD failed to confirm a statistically significant beneficial effect (Dillon 2001). The therapeutic potential of manipulating dietary lipids in the management of progressive CKF in man remains subject of controversy. However, both the Australian and Canadian Societies of Nephrology recommend fish oil supplementation for patients with IgA nephropathy.

Pharmacological interventions in chronic kidney failure

Until recently, such interventions were mainly restricted to the treatment of systemic hypertension and renal osteodystrophy. However, recent advances in our understanding of the pathophysiology of renal scarring open the way to new developments in this field.

Blood pressure control

As discussed previously, systemic hypertension seems to be one of the major factors in the initiation and progression of experimental and clinical CRF (reviewed in Dworkin and Weir 2000; Adamczak *et al.* 2002). Consequently, control of systemic hypertension is likely to play a part in the prevention of the development and progression of severe renal insufficiency, but only recently have some experimental and clinical data substantiated this possibility.

Experimental evidence

The control of systemic hypertension has proved beneficial in a wide range of experimental nephropathies in the rat: reduction of systemic blood pressure in rats with renal ablation, CGN, and DN reduced proteinuria, preserved renal function, and attenuated the severity of glomerulosclerosis (reviewed in Anderson 2000). Some argued that an additional therapeutic advantage is obtained when hypertension is treated with drugs that simultaneously reduce systemic and intraglomerular hypertension (reviewed in Anderson 2000; Dworkin and Weir 2000). On the other hand, Griffin *et al.* (1994) observed by radiotelemetric monitoring of blood pressure in subtotally nephrectomized rats that the protective effect of antihypertensive agents was proportional to their antihypertensive efficacy regardless of their class (Bidani *et al.* 2000; Bidani and Griffin 2002).

Clinical evidence

In patients with DN and non-DN, there is little doubt that blood pressure control slows the rate of decline in GFR (reviewed in Marcantoni *et al.* 2000; Adamczak *et al.* 2002). The next consideration is the blood pressure target levels and the type of antihypertensive agents used.

Few studies addressed blood pressure goals in relation to progressive kidney disease. The MDRD study suggested a lower target (mean arterial pressure, MAP ~ 92 mmHg) in patients with heavy proteinuria compared with those with mild/moderate proteinuria (MAP ~ 97 mmHg) (Peterson *et al.* 1995; Hebert 1999). The same study also implied that lower targets (MAP ~ 92 mmHg) should be sought in hypertensive African-Americans with progressive CRF compared with their

White counterparts (MAP ~ 97 mmHg). A pooled analysis of antihypertensive intervention studies in major studies in diabetic and non-diabetic nephropathies suggest a slowing of the rate of decline in GFR proportional to the reduction in MAP. A study of aggressive blood pressure control (~128/75 mmHg) in normotensive type 2 diabetic patients showed this to be protective against the progression of incipient and overt DN, decreasing the severity of retinopathy and diminishing the incidence of strokes (Schrier et al. 2002). This study highlights the importance of an aggressive reduction of blood pressure, beyond values previously considered to be normotensive, in order to prevent macrovascular and microvascular complications in at risk diabetic patients. This was achieved regardless of the antihypertensive drug used (enalapril or nisoldipine) (Schrier et al. 2002).

The NKF Task Force on Cardiovascular Disease in Chronic Renal Disease has suggested different blood pressure targets depending on the stage of kidney disease (Levey et al. 1998). In the general population, with normal kidney function and no proteinuria a blood pressure goal of 140/90 mmHg is recommended. In patients with CKD stage 1–4 with proteinuria less than 1 g/day the recommended target is <135/85 mmHg. By contrast in those (CKD stages 1–4) with proteinuria in excess of 1 g/day, a blood pressure goal of less than 125/75 mmHg is suggested (Levey et al. 1998). These recommendations have been endorsed by the recent K/DOQI guidelines (DOQI 2002). Thus, the level of proteinuria in patients with progressive CRD should be used as a guide to define the target blood pressure levels. Hypertension target levels being significantly lower in proteinuric patients at risk of a faster rate of decline of GFR compared to those with no or mild proteinuria known to have a better prognosis.

Angiotensin-converting enzyme inhibitors/angiotensin receptor blockers

The next consideration is the type of antihypertensive agent used to achieve these goals.

As discussed above, the potential nephrotoxic effects of angiotensin II are multiple. ACE inhibition has been shown to be protective in a wide range of experimental models of CKD (reviewed in Anderson 2000; Dworkin and Weir 2000; Fogo 2001b). In addition, a growing body of experimental evidence suggests that ARBs are equally effective (Mackenzie et al. 1997; Komers and Anderson 2000).

In patients with CKF, a growing body of clinical evidence suggests that control of hypertension without the concomitant reduction of proteinuria limits the efficacy of the intervention (Locatelli et al. 1996; Locatelli and Del Vecchio 2000; Jafar et al. 2001a). Therefore, attention has focused on antihypertensive agents capable of reducing both systemic hypertension and proteinuria. Data in hypertensive and proteinuric diabetic and non-diabetic patients showed that for comparable reduction in blood pressure, ACE inhibitors have superior antiproteinuric effects (Gansevoort et al. 1997). It is worth noting that amongst calcium channel blockers dihydropyridines (DHCCBs) are the least antiproteinuric while the non-DHCCBs have been shown in some studies of type 2 diabetic patients to be as effective as ACE inhibitors (for review see Sheinfeld and Bakris 1999; Koshy and Bakris 2000).

ACE inhibitors have been reported to be advantageous in slowing progressive CKF when compared to other antihypertensive drugs in patients with diabetic (Lewis et al. 1993) as well as non-diabetic (Maschio et al. 1996; GISEN 1997; Ruggenenti et al. 1999; Jafar et al. 2001b) kidney diseases. Most of the early studies comparing ACE inhibitors to conventional antihypertensive agents were flawed. Some, in type 1 diabetic patients, failed to randomize patients properly such that the control

group had higher baseline proteinuria, biasing the outcome in favour of the ACE inhibitor (Captopril) treated group (Lewis et al. 1993). Differences in blood pressure levels between patients with CKF treated with ACE inhibitors compared to other agents is a feature of most clinical trials with the authors at loss to establish that such differences do not explain the better outcome (Lewis et al. 1993; Maschio et al. 1996). More recently, the Ramipril Efficacy In Nephropathy (REIN) study of non-diabetic proteinuric patients with progressive CRF showed that Ramipril was more protective than other agents with equal blood pressure control (GISEN 1997; Ruggenenti et al. 1999). The beneficial effect was more evident in patients with heavy proteinuria. The protective advantage of the ACE inhibitor was most obvious at high levels of blood pressure (MAP ~ 100–110 mmHg). Equal protection was obtained with other antihypertensive agents when the mean arterial blood pressure was lowered to values less than 100 mmHg. Also, protection was more apparent in patients who were DD homozygous for the ACE gene (Ruggenenti et al. 2000). A recent post hoc analysis of the REIN study suggested that renoprotection by ACE inhibitors is maximized when ACE inhibitors are started early in the course of CKF and that longterm treatment may result in GFR stabilization and the prevention of ESRF (Ruggenenti et al. 2001). A meta-analysis of 11 studies of non-diabetic nephropathies suggested that ACE inhibitors reduced the relative risk of ESRD by 31 per cent (Giatras et al. 1997; Jafar et al. 2001b). However, this meta-analysis could not dissociate the protective effect of ACE inhibition on progressive CRF from its antihypertensive effect (Giatras et al. 1997).

It has to be noted that in all the studies comparing ACE inhibitors with other hypotensive agents, blood pressure measurements were made casually with no data given on the overall 24-h blood pressure control or even peak : trough ratios. Thus, it is possible that the therapeutic advantage of ACE inhibitors is sometimes due to superior overall blood pressure control.

Although experimental data suggest that ATR1 antagonists are as effective as ACE inhibitors in reducing proteinuria and protection from progressive renal insufficiency, recent clinical trials have avoided head to head comparisons (Brenner et al. 2001; Lewis et al. 2001; Parving et al. 2001). There are hypothetical explanations to suggest therapeutic advantages and disadvantages of these drugs compared with ACE inhibitors (for review, see Komers and Anderson 2000; Noris and Remuzzi 2002).

An additive antihypertensive, and to a lesser extent antiproteinuric, effect of ACE inhibition and receptor blockade has been described in patients with DN, although neither agent was given alone in its maximum dose to ascertain their full potential when given individually (Mogensen 2000). This has prompted some to suggest that combination therapy may have practical as well as theoretical advantages (reviewed in Komers and Anderson 2000; Noris and Remuzzi 2002). With this data in mind, the NKF Force on Cardiovascular Disease in Chronic Renal Disease suggest the use of ACE inhibitors and ARBs as first line therapies for patients with CKD (stages 1–4) in association with dietary salt restriction and diuretics (Levey et al. 1998; K/DOQI 2002).

Some studies in diabetic and other nephropathies have suggested that a similar antihypertensive and antiproteinuric effect can be achieved with other agents (for review Koshy and Bakris 2000). This is the case in type 2 diabetes of non-DHCCB, such as diltiazem and verapamil (for review, see Sheinfeld and Bakris 1999; Koshy and Bakris 2000). DHCCBs are less protective probably because they reduce afferent arteriolar tone without a concomitant reduction in the efferent arteriolar resistance. Beta blockers appear to be less effective than ACE inhibitors in reducing proteinuria and in slowing the rate of progression of CKF in diabetic patients. It has been suggested that the combination of ACE inhibitors and non-DHCCB may be an effective way of achieving the aggressive reduction of blood pressure needed to slow the progression of DN (Sheinfeld and Bakris 1999) (Table 2, Fig. 11).

Table 2 Interventions and objectives aimed at slowing the progression of CKD

Parameters	Interventions/target
Diet	Moderate protein restriction: 0.6–0.75 g/kg/day Low salt: 80–120 mmol/day (~4–6 g NaCl intake)

Blood pressure control	BP < 130–135/80–85 mmHg (MAP ~ 92 mmHg)
	   if proteinuria <1g/24 h
	BP < 125/75 mmHg (MAP ~ 90 mmHg)
	   if proteinuria >1 g/24 h
	Initially with an ACE inhibitor
	Add salt restriction/diuretic
	Add
	   Angiotensin-2 receptor blocker (ARB)
	   Non-dihydropyridine calcium channel blocker
	   (NDHCCB)

Proteinuria	Reduce to <1 g/24 h Use an ACE inhibitor/ARB
Glycaemia control in DM	HbA1c < 8%
Dyslipidaemia	Total cholesterol < 5 mmol/l (200 mg/dl) LDL cholesterol < 2 mmol/l (120 mg/dl) Use an HMG-CoA reductase inhibitor (statin)
Smoking	No cigarette smoking

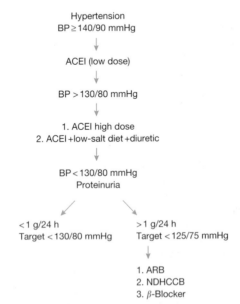

ACEI = Angiotensin converting enzyme inhibitors
NDHCCB = Non-dihydropyridine calcium channel blocker
ARB = Angiotensin receptor blocker

Fig. 11 Algorithm for the management of hypertension/proteinuria in CKD.

The administration of ACE inhibitors to patients with impaired renal function and the elderly warrants careful monitoring, as these agents have the potential to lead to some deterioration in renal function. A mild to moderate (10–30 per cent) increase in serum creatinine is to be expected as these agents reduce the hyperfiltration of remnant glomeruli. Such an increase in serum creatinine does not justify the discontinuation of the treatment as it may reflect the fall in filtration fraction considered to be the basis for the underlying protective effect of the ACE inhibition. However, any further increment in serum creatinine or significant hyperkalaemia warrants the replacement of the ACE inhibitor by a different class of antihypertensive drug (reviewed in Tamimi and El Nahas 2000).

Lipid-lowering agents

Hyperlipidaemia may contribute to the progression of experimental CKD and control by dietary manipulation prevents progressive renal scarring in rats (Keane *et al.* 1988). The reduction of serum lipids with agents such as cholestyramine, halofenate, clofibric acid, and the 3-hydroxy-3-methylglutaryl coenzyme-A (HMG CoA) reductase inhibitor lovastatin reduces the severity of age-related and ablation-induced glomerular sclerosis in animals with CKD. Of interest, HMG CoA reductase inhibitors are likely to be protective through both lipid-lowering and other mechanisms of action (Keane 2000). Statins have well-established immunomodulatory, antiproliferative, anti-inflammatory, as well as antifibrotic properties (reviewed in Martin-Ventura and Egido 2003). Recent data in rats with Heymann nephritis and progressive renal insufficiency suggests that treatment with a statin potentiates the protective effect of ACE inhibition and ARB (Zoja *et al.* 2002).

So far there is no convincing evidence that a reduction in hyperlipidaemia during the course of CKD is associated with an improvement in renal function. Numerous trials of lipid-lowering agents have proved inconclusive in that respect. A clinical trial of simvastatin, an HMG CoA reductase inhibitor, reduced proteinuria but failed to slow the progression of CKD over a 2-year period in a relatively small number of patients (Thomas *et al.* 1993). A meta-analysis of 12 lipid lowering interventions including 362 patients has shown only a marginal protective effect on the rate of progression of CKD (Fried *et al.* 2001).

Antiplatelet agents and anticoagulants

Intraglomerular platelet aggregation and microthrombosis is likely to play a part in the pathogenesis of progressive glomerulosclerosis and therefore antiplatelet agents as well as anticoagulants may protect against progressive renal scarring and insufficiency.

Treatment of rats with renal insufficiency with antiplatelet agents and anticoagulants has proved beneficial (Klahr *et al.* 1986). The beneficial effect of heparin in rats with renal ablation can be reproduced by *N*-desulfated/acetylated heparin, which is almost completely devoid of anticoagulant properties. An oral heparinoid, Pentosan polysulfate (PPS) reduced glomerulosclerosis in a variety of experiments undertaken in mice predisposed to glomerulosclerosis by attenuating cellular proliferation and ECM synthesis (Striker *et al.* 1997) and the severity of tubulointerstitial inflammation and fibrosis (Bobadilla *et al.* 2001).

These observations suggest that the protective effect of heparinoids on progressive glomerular scarring could be independent of their anticoagulant properties. Heparin, a polyanion, may affect the negative electrical potential of the GBM and suppresses the proliferation of mesangial cells in culture. Heparin has, through the activation of serum lipases, lipid-lowering effects. Data also suggest a suppressive effect of heparin on the synthesis of glomerular growth factors. More recently, it was observed that heparin-like glycosaminoglycans (GAG) inhibit glucose-induced mesangial upregulation of TGF-β1 expression (Ceol *et al.* 2000). These findings indicate a potential for GAG and heparinoids in the prevention of diabetic glomerulosclerosis (Ceol *et al.* 2000). The protective effects of anticoagulants, as well as non-anticoagulant heparinoids and glycosaminoglycans, on experimental progressive renal insufficiency are clearly multifactorial.

Data on the use of antiplatelets and anticoagulants agents to prevent the progression of CKD in humans is inconclusive (reviewed Coles and El Nahas 2000). Caution has to be exerted in the administration of these agents to uraemic patients who have an underlying bleeding diathesis.

Miscellaneous interventions

In experimental animals a range of new interventions suggest potential benefits in slowing the progression of CKF (reviewed in Fukagawa *et al.* 1999). These include the administration of antifibrogenic growth factors such as HGF, EGF, IGF-1, and OP-1. Of these, IGF-1 has been tested in patients with progressive CRF/ESRF and has shown some promise in delaying the requirement of RRT (Miller and Rabkin 1997; Vijayan *et al.* 1999). Other experimental interventions have relied on the administration of proangiogenic factors such as VEGF (Kang *et al.* 2002). Many of the growth factors listed above such as IGF-1, HGF, and VEGF are potent NO stimulators. NO donors have also been shown to protect against experimental nephrosclerosis (Fukada *et al.* 2001). This intervention has been associated with the remodelling of the glomerular as well as the peritubular microvasculature and the preservation of renal function in numerous experimental models (Kang *et al.* 2002). The administration of antifibrogenic hormones/autacoids such as relaxin has been shown to preserve renal function and attenuate interstitial fibrosis in rats injected with bromo-ethylamine (Garber *et al.* 2001). Treatment with agents as diverse as aminoguanidine/advanced glycation end products (AGE) inhibitors, heparinoids/glycosaminoglycans and miscellaneous antifibrotic agents such as perfenidone have also been tested in experimental animals with diabetic and non-diabetic nephropathies with some success (reviewed in Fukagawa *et al.* 1999).

A wide range of anecdotal interventions in patients with CKF have claimed benefit (reviewed in Coles and El Nahas 2000). These include the administration of a dopamine analogue (ibopamine), Chinese herbal extracts, oral sorbents (AST-120), and the infusion of prostaglandin E$_1$. The anecdotal nature of these reports precludes useful conclusions. More interesting are the observations of renal functional improvement in patients with moderate and even ESRF when injected with IGF-1 (Miller and Rabkin 1997; Vijayan *et al.* 1999), a hormone known to have acute renal haemodynamic effects.

General recommendations

The following general recommendations can be made for the management of patients with progressive CKD (Pereira 2000; Hebert *et al.* 2001).

1. Frequent clinic follow-up is required with particular attention to the detection, monitoring, and treatment of hypertension and a simultaneous reduction of proteinuria (Table 2).

2. Advise patients with progressive CKD to avoid a high-protein diet, but caution should be exerted when recommending dietary protein restriction (0.6 g/kg/day) with its inherent risk of under-nutrition.

3. Hypertensive and proteinuric patients with CKD should reduce their dietary salt intake (no added salt—sodium ~80–120 mmol/day, or 4–6 g NaCl/day). This is all the more relevant when these patients are treated with an ACE inhibitor or ARB (evidence-based statement).

4. Advise patients with CKD to reduce their saturated fat intake and control hypercholesterolaemia with a statin.

5. Patients with CKD should stop cigarette smoking.

6. Early management of the complications of CKD including anaemia, metabolic acidosis, hypocalcaemia, and hyperphosphataemia with the associated renal osteodystrophy.

7. Avoidance of potential nephrotoxins, including nonsteroidal anti-inflammatory agents, nephrotoxic antibiotics as well as intravenous radiographic contrast media.

References

Adamczak, M., Zeier, M., Dikow, R., and Ritz, E. (2002). Kidney and hypertension. *Kidney International* **61** (Suppl. 80), 62–67.

Alfrey, A. C. (1986). Thyroid and parathyroid hormones in experimental renal failure. *Contemporary Issues in Nephrology* **14**, 37–44.

Alfrey, A. C. (1994). Role of iron and oxygen radicals in the progression of chronic renal failure. *American Journal of Kidney Diseases* **23**, 183–187.

Alpers, C. E., Hudkins, K. L., Gown, A. M., and Johnson, R. J. (1992). Enhanced expression of 'muscle-specific' actin in glomerulonephritis. *Kidney International* **41**, 1134–1142.

Anders, H. and Schlondorff, D. (2000). Murine models of renal disease: possibilities and problems in studies using mutant mice. *Experimental Nephrology* **8**, 181–193.

Anders, H.-J., Vielhauer, V., and Schlondorff, D. (2003). Chermokines and chemokine receptors are involved in the resolution or progression of renal disease. *Kidney International* **63**, 416–426.

Anderson, S. Glomerulosclerosis: insights into pathogenesis and treatment. In *Mechanisms and Management of Progressive Renal Failure* (ed. A. M. El Nahas, S. Anderson, and K. P. G. Harris), pp. 80–103. London: Oxford University Press, 2000.

Antignac, C. (2002). Genetic models: clues for understanding the pathogenesis of idiopathic nephrotic syndrome. *Journal of Clinical Investigation* **109**, 447–449.

Aparicio, M., Chauveau, P., and Combe, C. (2001). Low protein diets and outcome of renal patients. *Journal of Nephrology* **14**, 433–439.

Arici, M., Chana, R., Lewington, A., Brown, J., and Brunskill, N. (2003). Stimulation of proximal tubular cell apoptosis by albumin-bound fatty acids mediated by peroxisome proliferator activated receptor-gamma. *Journal of the American Society of Nephrology* **14**, 17–27.

Attman, P. O., Alaupovic, P., and Samuelsson, O. (1999). Lipoprotein abnormalities as a risk factor for progressive nondiabetic renal disease. *Kidney International* **71**, S14–S17.

Baker, A. J., Mooney, A., Hughes, J., Lombardi, D., Johnson, R. J., and Savill, J. (1994). Mesangial cell apoptosis: the major mechanism for resolution of glomerular hypercellularity in experimental mesangial proliferatie nephritis. *Journal of Clinical Investigation* **94**, 2105–2116.

Bakris, G. L., Copley, J. B., Vicknair, N., Sadler, R., and Leurgans, S. (1996). Calcium channel blockers versus other antihypertensive therapies on progression of NIDDM associated nephropathy. *Kidney International* **50**, 1641–1650.

Bakris, G. L. *et al.* (2000). Preserving renal function in adults with hypertension and diabetes: a consensus approach. National Kidney Foundation

Hypertension and Diabetes Executive Committees Working Group. *American Journal of Kidney Diseases* **36**, 646–661.

Baldwin, D. S. and Neugarten, J. (1986). Blood pressure control and progression of renal insufficiency. *Contemporary Issues in Nephrology* **14**, 81–110.

Basile, D. P. (1999). The transforming growth factor beta system in kidney disease and repair: recent progress and future directions. *Current Opinion in Nephrology and Hypertension* **8**, 21–30.

Bellush, L. L., Doublier, S., Holland, A. N., Striker, L. J., Striker, G. E., and Kopchick, J. J. (2000). Protection against diabetes-induced nephropathy in growth hormone receptor/binding protein gene-disrupted mice. *Endocrinology* **141**, 163–168.

Benigni, A. (2000). Tubulointerstitial disease mediators of injury: the role of endothelin. *Nephrology, Dialysis, Transplantation* **15** (Suppl. 6), 50–52.

Benigni, A., Perico, N., and Remuzzi, G. (2000). Endothelin antagonists and renal protection. *Journal of Cardiovascular Pharmacology* **35**, S75–S78.

Bennett, W. M. (1998). The nephrotoxicity of new and old immunosuppressive drugs. *Renal Failure* **20**, 687–690.

Bidani, A. K. and Griffin, K. A. (2002). Long-term renal consequences of hypertension for normal and diseased kidneys. *Current Opinion in Nephrology Hypertension* **11**, 73–80.

Bidani, A. K., Griffin, K. A., Bakris, G., and Picken, M. M. (2000). Lack of evidence of blood pressure-independent protection by renin–angiotensin system blockade after renal ablation. *Kidney International* **57**, 1651–1661.

Bobadilla, N. A. *et al.* (2001). Pentosan polysulfate prevents glomerular hypertension and structural injury despite persisting hypertension in 5/6 nephrectomy rats. *Journal of the American Society of Nephrology* **12**, 2080–2087.

Bohle, A., von Gise, H., Mackensen-Haen, S., and Stark-Jakob, B. (1981). The obliteration of postglomerular capillaries and its influence upon the function of both glomeruli and tubuli. *Klinisch Woschenchrift* **59**, 1043–1051.

Bohle, A., Mackenson-Haen, S., and Gise, H. (1987). Significance of tubulo-interstitial changes in the renal cortex for the excretory function and concentration ability of the kidney: a morphometric contribution. *American Journal of Nephrology* **7**, 421–433.

Bonnet, F. and Cooper, M. E. (2000). Potential influence of lipids in diabetic nephropathy: insights from experimental data and clinical studies. *Diabetes Metabolism* **26**, 254–264.

Bonnet, F. *et al.* (2001). Excessive body weight as a new independent risk factor for clinical and pathological progression in primary IgA nephritis. *American Journal of Kidney Diseases* **37**, 720–727.

Brady, H. R. (1994). Leukocyte adhesion molecules and kidney diseases. *Kidney International* **45**, 1285–1300.

Brenner, B. M. (1985). Nephron adaptation to renal injury or ablation. *American Journal of Physiology* **249**, F324–F337.

Brenner, B. M. and Chertow, G. M. (1994). Congenital oligonephropathy and the etiology of adult hypertension and progressive renal injury. *American Journal of Kidney Diseases* **23**, 171–175.

Brenner, B. M., Meyer, T. W., and Hostetter, T. H. (1982). Dietary protein intake and the progressive nature of kidney disease. *New England Journal of Medicine* **307**, 652–660.

Brenner, B. M. *et al.* (2001). Effects of losartan on renal and cardiovascular outcomes in patients with type 2 diabetes and nephropathy. *New England Journal of Medicine* **345**, 861–869.

Breyer, J. A. *et al.* (1996). Predictors of the progression of renal insufficiency in patients with insulin-dependent diabetes and overt diabetic nephropathy. The collaborative study group. *Kidney International* **50**, 1651–1658.

Brown, D. M. *et al.* (1998). Genetic control of susceptibility for renal damage in hypertensive fawn-hooded rats. *Renal Failure* **20**, 407–411.

Brown, W. W. *et al.* (2003). Identification of persons at high risk for kidney disease via targeted screening: the NKF Kidney Early Evaluation Program. *Kidney International* **63** (Suppl. 83), S50–S55.

Buck, K. and Feehally, J. (1997). Diabetes and renal failure in Indo-Asians in the UK—a paradigm for the study of disease susceptibility. *Nephrology, Dialysis, Transplantation* **12**, 1555–1557.

Burns, K. D. (2002). Interleukin-1β as a mediator of tubulointerstitial fibrosis. *Kidney International* **62**, 346–347.

Buter, H., Hemmelder, M. H., Navis, G., de Jong, P. E., and de Zeeuw, D. (1998). The blunting of the antiproteinuric efficacy of ACE inhibition by high sodium intake can be restored by hydrochlorothiazide. *Nephrology, Dialysis, Transplantation* **13**, 1682–1685.

Cameron, J. S. (1984). Platelets in glomerular disease. *Annual Review of Medicine* **35**, 175–190.

Cattell, V. (2002). Nitric oxide and glomerulonephritis. *Kidney International* **61**, 816–821.

Cardoso, L. R. *et al.* (1997). Effect of the antiglucocorticoid RU-486 on glomerular hemodynamics in remnant nephrons. *Experimental Nephrology* **5**, 217–224.

Caulfield, J. and Schrag, E. (1964). Electron microscopic study of renal calcification. *American Journal of Pathology* **44**, 365–381.

Ceol, M. *et al.* (2000). Glycosaminoglycan therapy prevents TGF-beta1 overexpression and pathologic changes in renal tissue of long-term diabetic rats. *Journal of the American Society of Nephrology* **11**, 2324–2336.

Chatziantoniou, C. and Dussaule, J. C. (2000). Endothelin and renal vascular fibrosis: of mice and men. *Current Opinion in Nephrology and Hypertension* **9**, 31–36.

Chen, N. Y., Chen, W. Y., Striker, L. J., Striker, G. E., and Kopchick, J. J. (1997). Co-expression of bovine growth hormone (GH) and human GH antagonist genes in transgenic mice. *Endocrinology* **138**, 851–854.

Chen, G., Paka, L., Kako, Y., Singhal, P., Duan, W., and Pillarisetti, S. (2001). A protective role for kidney apolipoprotein E. Regulation of mesangial cell proliferation and matrix expansion. *Journal of Biological Chemistry* **276**, 49142–49147.

Coles, G. A. and El Nahas, A. M. Clinical interventions in chronic renal failure. In *Mechanisms and Management of Progressive Renal Failure* (ed. A. M. El Nahas, S. Anderson, and K. P. G. Harris), pp. 401–423. Oxford: Oxford University Press, 2000.

Conlin, P. R. *et al.* (2000). The effect of dietary patterns on blood pressure control in hypertensive patients: results from the Dietary Approaches to Stop Hypertension (DASH) trial. *American Journal of Hypertension* **13**, 949–955.

Coresh, J., Wei, G. L., McQuillan, G., Brancati, F. L., Levey, A. S., Jones, C., and Klag, M. J. (2001). Prevalence of high blood pressure and elevated serum creatinine level in the United States: findings from the third National Health and Nutrition Examination Survey (1988–1994). *Archives of Internal Medicine* **161**, 1207–1216.

Coresh, J., Astor, B. C., Greene, T., Eknoyan, G., and Levey, A. S. (2003). Prevalence of chronic kidney disease and decreased kidney function in the adult US population: Third National Health and Nutrition Examination Survey. *American Journal of Kidney Diseases* **41**, 1–12.

Cornacchia, F. *et al.* (2001). Glomerulosclerosis is transmitted by bone marrow-derived mesangial cell progenitors. *Journal of Clinical Investigation* **108**, 1649–1656.

Costigan, M., Chambers, D.A., and Boot-Handford, R. P. (1995). Collagen turnover in renal disease. *Experimental Nephrology* **3**, 114–121.

Cybulsky, A. V. (2000). Growth factor pathways in proliferative glomerulonephritis. *Current Opinion in Nephrology and Hypertension* **9**, 217–223.

DCCT (1995). Effect of intensive therapy on the development and progression of diabetic nephropathy in the Diabetes Control and Complications Trial (DCCT) Research group. *Kidney International* **47**, 1703–1720.

Diamond, J. R. and Karnovsky, M. J. (1988). Focal and segmental glomerulosclerosis: analogies to atherosclerosis. *Kidney International* **33**, 917–924.

Dillon, J. J. (2001). Treating IgA nephropathy. *Journal of the American Society of Nephrology* **12**, 846–847.

Doi, T. *et al.* (1988). Progressive glomerulosclerosis develops in transgenic mice chronically expressing growth hormone and growth hormone releasing factor but not those expressing insulin-like growth factor-1. *American Journal of Pathology* **131**, 398–403.

Doi, T., Striker, L. J., Kimata, K., Peter, E. P., Yamada, Y., and Striker, G. (1991). Glomerulosclerosis in mice transgenic for growth hormone. Increased mesangial extracellular matrix is correlated with kidney mRNA levels. *Journal of Experimental Medicine* **173**, 1287–1290.

Donadio, J. V. (2001). n-3 Fatty acids and their role in nephrologic practice. *Current Opinion in Nephrology and Hypertension* **10**, 639–642.

Doublier, S. *et al.* (2000). Glomerulosclerosis in mice transgenic for human insulin-like growth factor-binding protein-1. *Kidney International* **57**, 2299–2307.

Drummond, K. and Mauer, M. (2002). The early natural history of nephropathy in type 1 diabetes: II. Early renal structural changes in type 1 diabetes. *Diabetes* **51**, 1580–1587.

Dworkin, L. D. and Feiner, H. D. (1986). Glomerular injury in uninephrectomized spontaneously hypertensive rats. A consequence of glomerular capillary hypertension. *Journal of Clinical Investigation* **77**, 797–809.

Dworkin, L. D. and Weir, M. R. Hypertension in renal parenchymal disease: Role in progression. In *Mechanisms and Management of Progressive Renal Failure* (ed. A. M. El Nahas, S. Anderson, and K. P. G. Harris), pp. 173–210. London: Oxford University Press, 2000.

Earle, K. K., Porter, K. A., Ostberg, J., and Yudkin, J. S. (2001). Variation in the progression of diabetic nephropathy according to racial origin. *Nephrology, Dialysis, Transplantation* **16**, 286–290.

Eddy, A. (2001). Role of cellular infiltrates in response to proteinuria. *American Journal of Kidney Diseases* **37** (Suppl. 2), S25–S29.

Eddy, A. A., McCulloch, L., Liu, E., and Adams, J. (1991). A relationship between proteinuria and acute tubulointerstitial disease in rats with experimental nephritic syndrome. *American Journal of Pathology* **138**, 1111–1123.

Eddy, A. A., Kim, H., Lopez-Guisa, J., Oda, T., and Soloway, P. D. (2000). Interstitial fibrosis in mice with overload proteinuria: deficiency of TIMP-1 is not protective. *Kidney International* **58**, 618–628.

Egido, J. (1996). Vasoactive hormones and renal sclerosis. *Kidney International* **49**, 578–597.

Elema, J. D. and Grond, J. (1988). Mesangial overloading and glomerular sclerosis in some proteinuric models of experimental glomerulopathy. *Nephrology* **1**, 574–583.

El-Koraie, A. F., Baddour, N. M., Adam, A. G., El Kashef, E. H., and El Nahas, A. M. (2001). Role of stem cell factor and mast cells in the progression of chronic glomerulonephritides. *Kidney International* **60**, 167–172.

El Nahas, A. M. (1988). Glomerulosclerosis: a form of atherosclerosis. In *Nephrology* (ed. A. M. Davison), pp. 1206–1218. London: Bailliere Tindall, 1988.

El Nahas, A. M. (1989). Glomerulosclerosis: insights into pathogenesis and treatment. *Nephrology, Dialysis, Transplantation* **4**, 843–853.

El Nahas, A. M. (1996). Glomerulosclerosis: intrinsic and extrinsic pathways. *Nephrology, Dialysis, Transplantation* **11**, 773–777.

El Nahas, A. M. Mechanisms of experimental and clinical renal scaring. In *Oxford Textbook of Clinical Nephrology* Vol. 3 (ed. A. M. Davison, J. S. Cameron, J.-P. Grunfeld, D. N. S. Kerr, E. Ritz, and C. G. Winearls), pp. 1749–1788. Oxford: Oxford University Press, 1998.

El Nahas, A. M. (2003). Plasticity of kidney cells: role in kidney remodeling and scarring. *Kidney International* **64**, 1553–1563.

El Nahas, A. M. and Coles, G. A. (1986). Dietary treatment of chronic renal failure: ten unanswered questions. *Lancet* **i**, 597–600.

El Nahas, A. M. *et al.* (1984). Selective effects of low protein diets in chronic renal failure. *British Medical Journal* **289**, 1337–1340.

El Nahas, A. M., Lechler, R., Zoob, S. N., and Rees, A. J. (1985). Progression to renal failure after nephrotoxic nephritis in rats studied by renal transplantation. *Clinical Science* **68**, 15–21.

El Nahas, A. M., Bassett, A. H., Cope, G. H., and Le Carpentier, J. E. (1991). Role of growth hormone in the development of experimental renal scarring. *Kidney International* **40**, 29–34.

Endlich, K., Kriz, W., and Witzgall, R. (2001). Update in podocyte biology. *Current Opinion in Nephrology and Hypertension* **10**, 331–340.

Epstein, M. (2001). Aldosterone as a mediator of progressive renal disease: pathogenetic and clinical implications. *American Journal of Kidney Diseases* **37**, 677–688.

Erwig, L. P., Kluth, D. C., and Rees, A. J. (2001). Macrophages in renal inflammation. *Current Opinion in Nephrology and Hypertension* **10**, 341–347.

Esposito, C. *et al.* (1996). Inhibition of diabetic nephropathy by a GH antagonist: a molecular analysis. *Kidney International* **50**, 506–514.

Esposito, C., He, C. J., Striker, G. E., Zalups, R. K., and Striker, L. J. (1999). Nature and severity of the glomerular response to nephron reduction is strain-dependent in mice. *American Journal of Pathology* **154**, 891–897.

Feldman, H. I., Klag, M. J., Chiapella, A. P., and Whelton, P. K. (1992). End stage renal disease in US minority groups. *American Journal of Kidney Diseases* **19**, 397–410.

Fine, L. G., Bandyopadhay, D., and Norman, J. T. (2000). Is there a common mechanism for the progression of different types of renal diseases other than proteinuria? Towards the unifying theme of chronic hypoxia. *Kidney International* **75**, (Suppl.) S22–S26.

Floege, J. and Johnson, R. J. (1995). Multiple roles for platelet-derived growth factor in renal disease. *Mineral and Electrolyte Metabolism* **21**, 271–282.

Floege, J. and Grone, H. J. (1997). Glomerular cells in the progression of human and experimental nephropathies. *Advances in Nephrology Necker Hospital* **27**, 15–37.

Floege, J. and Ostendorf, T. (2001). Platelet-derived growth factor: a new clinical target on the horizon. *Kidney International* **59**, 1592–1593.

Floege, J. *et al.* (1993). Infusion of platelet-derived growth factor or basic fibroblast growth factor induces selective glomerular mesangial proliferation and matrix accumulation in rats. *Journal of Clinical Investigation* **92**, 2952–2962.

Floege, J. *et al.* (1998). Endogenous fibroblast growth factor-2 mediates cytotoxicity in experimental mesangioproliferative glomerulonephritis. *Journal of the American Society of Nephrology* **9**, 792–801.

Floege, J. *et al.* (1999). Localization of fibroblast growth factor-2 (basic FGF) and FGF receptor-1 in adult human kidney. *Kidney International* **56**, 883–897.

Flyvbjerg, A. (2001). Potential use of growth hormone receptor antagonist in the treatment of diabetic kidney disease. *Growth Hormone and IGF Research* **11** (Suppl. A), S115–S119.

Flyvbjerg, A., Marshall, S. M., Frystyk, J., Hansen, K. W., and Osterby, R. (1992). Six months octreotide treatment in diabetic rats: effects on kidney growth and urinary albumin excretion. *Kidney International* **41**, 805–812.

Fogo, A. B. (2001a). Progression and potential regression of glomerulosclerosis. *Kidney International* **59**, 804–819.

Fogo, A. B. (2001b). Renal fibrosis and the renin–angiotensin system. *Advances in Nephrology Necker Hospital* **31**, 69–87.

Fogo, A. and Ichikawa, I. (1991). Evidence for a pathogenic linkage between glomerular hypertrophy and sclerosis. *American Journal of Kidney Diseases* **17**, 666–669.

Fogo, A. *et al.* (1990). Glomerular hypertrophy in minimal change disease predicts subsequent progression to focal glomerular sclerosis. *Kidney International* **38**, 115–123.

Fornoni, A., Lenz, O., Tack, I., Potier, M., Elliot, S. J., Striker, L. J., and Striker, G. E. (2000). Matrix accumulation in mesangial cells exposed to cyclosporine A requires a permissive genetic background. *Transplantation* **70**, 587–593.

Fornoni, A., Li, H., Foschi, A., Striker, G. E., and Striker, L. J. (2001). Hepatocyte growth factor, but not insulin-like growth factor I, protects podocytes against cyclosporin A-induced apoptosis. *American Journal of Pathology* **158**, 275–280.

Fornoni, A., Striker, L. J., Zheng, F., and Striker, G. E. (2002). Reversibility of glucose-induced changes in mesangial cell extracellular matrix depends on the genetic background. *Diabetes* **51**, 499–505.

Fouque, D., Laville, M., Boissel, J. P., Chifflet, R., Labeeuw, M., and Zech, P. Y. (1992). Controlled low protein diets in chronic renal insufficiency: meta-analysis. *British Medical Journal* **304**, 216–220.

Fouque, D., Wang, P., Laville, M., and Boissel, J. P. (2000). Low protein diets delay end-stage renal disease in non-diabetic adults with chronic renal failure. *Nephrology, Dialysis, Transplantation* **15**, 1986–1992.

Francki, A., Bradshaw, A. D., Bassuk, J. A., Howe, C. C., Couser, W. G., and Sage, E. H. (1999). SPARC regulates the expression of collagen type I and transforming growth factor-beta1 in mesangial cells. *Journal of Biological Chemistry* **274**, 32145–32152.

Freedman, B. I., Yu, H., Spray, B. J., Rich, S. S., Rothschild, C. B., and Bowden, D. W. (1997). Genetic linkage analysis of growth factor loci and end-stage renal disease in African Americans. *Kidney International* **51**, 819–825.

Fried, L. F., Orchard, T. J., and Kasiske, B. L. (2001). Effect of lipid reduction on the progression of renal disease: a meta-analysis. *Kidney International* **59**, 260–269.

Fries, J. U. *et al.* (1989). Glomerular hypertrophy and epithelial cell injury modulate progressive glomerulosclerosis in the rat. *Laboratory Investigation* **60**, 205–209.

Fukada, J. *et al.* (2001). Nitric oxide donor FK409 attenuates the development of neointimal hyperplasia in a rat aortic allograft model. *Transplantation Proceedings* **33**, 536–537.

Fukagawa, M., Noda, M., Shimizu, T., and Kurokawa, K. (1999). Chronic progressive interstitial fibrosis in renal disease—are there novel pharmacological approaches? *Nephrology, Dialysis, Transplantation* **14**, 2793–2795.

Gaedeke, J., Peters, H., Noble, N. A., and Border, W. A. (2001). Angiotensin II, TGF-beta and renal fibrosis. *Contributions to Nephrology* **135**, 153–160.

Gallo, G. R. *et al.* (1978). Role of intrarenal vascular sclerosis in progression of post-streptococcal glomerulonephritis. *Clinical Nephrology* **13**, 49–57.

Gansevoort, R. T., Navis, G. J., Wapstra, F. H., de Jong, P. E., and de Zeeuw, D. (1997). Proteinuria and progression of renal disease: therapeutic implications. *Current Opinion in Nephrology and Hypertension* **6**, 133–140.

Garber, S. L. *et al.* (2001). Relaxin decreases renal interstitial fibrosis and slows progression of renal disease. *Kidney International* **59**, 876–882.

Garcia, D. L., Rennke, H. G., Brenner, B. M., and Anderson, S. (1987). Chronic glucocorticoid therapy amplifies glomerular injury in rats with renal ablation. *Journal of Clinical Investigation* **80**, 867–874.

Gassler, N. *et al.* (2001). Podocyte injury underlies the progression of focal segmental glomerulosclerosis in the fa/fa Zucker rat. *Kidney International* **60**, 106–116.

Giatras, I., Lau, J., and Levey, A. S. (1997). Effect of angiotensin-converting enzyme inhibitors on the progression of nondiabetic renal disease: a meta-analysis of randomized trials. Angiotensin-Converting-Enzyme Inhibition and Progressive Renal Disease Study Group. *Annals of Internal Medicine* **127**, 337–345.

Gimenez, L. F., Solez, K., and Walker, W. G. (1987). Relation between renal calcium content and renal impairment in 246 human renal biopsies. *Kidney International* **31**, 93–99.

GISEN Group (Gruppo Italiano di Studi Epidemiologici in Nefrologia) (1997). Randomised placebo-controlled trial of effect of ramipril on decline in glomerular filtration rate and risk of terminal renal failure in proteinuric, non-diabetic nephropathy. *Lancet* **349**, 1857–1863.

Gjone, E., Blomhoff, J. P., and Skarbovik, A. J. (1974). Possible associations between an abnormal low density lipoprotein and nephropathy in lecithin : cholesterol acyltransferase deficiency. *Clinica Chemica Acta* **54**, 11–18.

Gorgun, M., Erdogan, D., Abban, G., Turkozkan, N., and Elbeg, S. (1999). Effect of vitamin E on adriamycin-induced nephrotoxicity at the ultrastructural level in guinea pigs. *Nephron* **82**, 155–163.

Goumenos, D., Brown, C. B., Shortland, J., and El Nahas, A. M. (1994). Myofibroblasts, predictors of progression in IgA nephropathy. *Nephrology, Dialysis, Transplantation* **9**, 1418–1425.

Goumenos, D., Tsomi, K., Iatrou, C., Oldroyd, S., Sungur, A., Papaioannides, D., Moustakas, G., Ziroyannis, P., Mountokalakis, T., and El Nahas, A. M. (1998). Myofibroblasts and the progression of crescentic glomerulonephritis. *Nephrology, Dialysis, Transplantation* **13**, 1652–1661.

Grande, J. P. *et al.* (2002). TGF-beta1 is an autocrine mediator of renal tubular epithelial cell growth and collagen IV production. *Experimental Biology and Medicine (Maywood)* **227**, 171–181.

Griffin, K. A., Picken, M., and Bidani, A. K. (1994). Radiotelemetric BP monitoring, antihypertensives and glomeruloprotection in remnant kidney model. *Kidney International* **46**, 1010–1018.

Groma, V. (1998). Demonstration of collagen type VI and alpha-smooth muscle actin in renal fibrotic injury in man. *Nephrology, Dialysis, Transplantation* **13**, 305–312.

Grond, J. and Weening, J. J. (1990). Mesangial cell injury, glomerulosclerosis, and therapeutic interventions. *Contributions to Nephrology* **81**, 229–239.

Grond, J., van Goor, H., Erkelens, D. W., and Elema, J. D. (1986). Glomerular sclerotic lesions in the rat. Histochemical analysis of their macromolecular and cellular composition. *Virchows Archives B Cell Pathol* **51**, 521–534.

Grond, J., Muller, E. W., and Weening, J. J. (1989). Genetic differences in susceptibility to glomerulosclerosis. *American Journal of Medicine* **87**, 5–30.

Guan, Y. and Breyer, M. D. (2001). Peroxisome proliferator-activated receptors (PPARs): novel therapeutic targets in renal disease. *Kidney International* **60**, 14–30.

Guccione, M., Silbiger, S., Lei, J., and Neugarten, J. (2002). Estradiol upregulates mesangial cell MMP-2 activity via the transcription factor AP-2. *American Journal of Physiology* **282**, F164–F169.

Gupta, S., Clarkson, M. R., Duggan, J., and Brady, H. R. (2000). Connective tissue growth factor: potential role in glomerulosclerosis and tubulointerstitial fibrosis. *Kidney International* **58**, 1389–1399.

Gupta, S., Verfaille, C., Chmielewski, D., Kim, Y., and Rosenberg, M. E. (2002). A role for extrarenal cells in the regeneration following acute renal injury. *Kidney International* **62**, 1285–1290.

Hahn, S. *et al.* (1999). Vitamin E suppresses oxidative stress and glomerulosclerosis in rat remnant kidney. *Pediatric Nephrology* **13**, 195–198.

Hamano, K., Iwano, M., Akai, Y., Sato, H., Kubo, A., Nishitani, Y., Uyama, H., Yoshida, Y., Miyazaki, M., Shiiki, H., Kohno, S., and Dohi, K. (2002). Expression of glomerular plasminogen activator inhibitor type 1 in glomerulonephritis. *American Journal of Kidney Diseases* **39**, 695–705.

Hannken, T., Schroeder, R., Zahner, G., Stahl, R. A., and Wolf, G. (2000). Reactive oxygen species stimulate p44/42 mitogen-activated protein kinase and induce p27(Kip1): role in angiotensin II-mediated hypertrophy of proximal tubular cells. *Journal of the American Society of Nephrology* **11**, 1387–1397.

Harris, D. C., Chan, L., and Schrier, R. W. (1988). Remnant kidney hypermetabolism and progression of chronic renal failure. *American Journal of Physiology* **254**, 267–276.

Harris, K. P. G. Proteinuria: implications for progression and management. In *Mechanisms and Management of Progressive Renal Failure* (ed. A. M. El Nahas, S. Anderson, and K. P. G. Harris), pp. 146–172. London: Oxford University Press, 2000.

Harris, K. P. G., Lefkowith, J. B., Klahr, S., and Schreiner, G. F. (1990). Essential fatty acid deficiency ameliorates acute renal dysfunction in the rat after the administration of the aminonucleoside of puromycin. *Journal of Clinical Investigation* **86**, 1115–1123.

Harris, R. D., Steffes, M. W., Bilous, R. W., Sutherland, D. E. R., and Mauer, S. M. (1991). Global glomerular sclerosis and glomerular arteriolar hyalinosis in insulin dependent diabetes. *Kidney International* **40**, 107–114.

Haseley, L. A., Hugo, C., Reidy, M. A., and Johnson, R. J. (1999). Dissociation of mesangial cell migration and proliferation in experimental glomerulonephritis. *Kidney International* **56**, 964–972.

Hattori, M., Horita, S., Yoshioka, T., Yamaguchi, Y., Kawaguchi, H., and Ito, K. (1997). Mesangial phenotypic changes associated with cellular lesions in primary focal segmental glomerulosclerosis. *American Journal of Kidney Diseases* **30**, 632–638.

Haugen, E. and Nath, K. A. (1999). The involvement of oxidative stress in the progression of renal injury. *Blood Purification* **17**, 58–65.

Hebert, L. A. (1999). Target blood pressure for antihypertensive therapy in patients with proteinuric renal disease. *Current Hypertension Reports* **1**, 454–460.

Hebert, L. A., Wilmer, W. A., Falkenhain, M. E., Ladson-Wofford, S. E., Nahman, N. S., Jr., and Rovin, B. H. (2001). Renoprotection: one or many therapies? *Kidney International* **59**, 1211–1226.

Hebert, L. A., Spetie, D. N., and Keane, W. F. (2002). The urgent call of albuminuria/proteinuria. Heeding its significance in early detection of kidney disease. *Postgraduate Medicine* **111**, 23.

Heeg, J. E., de Jong, P. E., van der Hem, G. K., and de Zeeuw, D. (1987). Reduction of proteinuria by angiotensin converting enzyme inhibition. *Kidney International* **32**, 78–83.

Heidland, A. *et al.* (1997). Renal fibrosis: role of impaired proteolysis and potential therapeutic strategies. *Kidney International* **52**, S32–S35.

Hermansen, K. (2000). Diet, blood pressure and hypertension. *British Journal of Nutrition* **83** (Suppl. 1), S113–S119.

Hill, G. S. and Heptinstall, R. H. (1968). Steroid-induced hypertension in the rat: a microangiographic and histologic study on the pathogenesis of hypertensive vascular and glomerular lesions. *American Journal of Pathology* **52**, 1–10.

Hill, P. A., Davies, D. J., Kincaid-Smith, P., and Ryan, G. B. (1989). Ultrastructural changes in renal tubules associated with glomerular bleeding. *Kidney International* **36**, 992–997.

Hocher, B. *et al.* (1997). Endothelin-1 transgenic mice develop glomerulosclerosis, interstitial fibrosis, and renal cysts but not hypertension. *Journal of Clinical Investigation* **99**, 1380–1389.

Hostetter, T. H. Pathogenesis of diabetic nephropathy. In *The Progressive Nature of Renal Disease* (ed. W. E. Mitch, B. M. Brenner, and J. H. Stein), pp. 149–166. New York: Churchill Livingstone, 1986.

Hostetter, T. H. *et al.* (1981). Hyperfiltration in remnant nephrons: a potentially adverse response to renal ablation. *American Journal of Physiology* **241**, F85–F93.

Houglum, K., Brenner, D. A., and Chojkier, M. (1991). D-α-tocopherol inhibits collagen 1(I) gene expression in cultured human fibroblasts. Modulation of constitutive collagen gene expression by lipid peroxidation. *Journal of Clinical Investigation* **87**, 2230–2235.

Hruska, K. A. (2002). Treatment of chronic tubulointerstitial disease: a new concept. *Kidney International* **61**, 1911–1922.

Hugo, C., Shankland, S. J., Bowen-Pope, D. F., Couser, W. G., and Johnson, R. J. (1997). Extraglomerular origin of the mesangial cell after injury. A new role of the juxtaglomerular apparatus. *Journal of Clinical Investigation* **100**, 786–794.

Hunsicker, L. G. *et al.* (1997). Predictors of the progression of renal disease in the Modification of Diet in Renal Disease Study. *Kidney International* **51**, 1908–1919.

Huwiler, A. *et al.* (2001). Superoxide potently induces ceramide formation in glomerular endothelial cells. *Biochemistry Biophysics Research Communications* **284**, 404–410.

Ibels, L. S. *et al.* (1980). Calcification in end stage kidney. *American Journal of Medicine* **71**, 33–39.

Iglesias-De La Cruz, M. C. *et al.* (2001). Hydrogen peroxide increases extracellular matrix mRNA through TGF-beta in human mesangial cells. *Kidney International* **59**, 87–95.

Ikizler, T. A., Greene, J. H., Wingard, R. L., Parker, R. A., and Hakim, R. M. (1995). Spontaneous dietary protein intake during progression of chronic renal failure. *Journal of the American Society of Nephrology* **6**, 1386–1391.

Imai, E. and Isaka, Y. (2002a). Gene electrotransfer: potential for gene therapy of renal diseases. *Kidney International* **61** (Suppl. 1), 37–41.

Imai, E. and Isaka, Y. (2002b). Targeting growth factors to the kidney: myth or reality? *Current Opinion in Nephrology and Hypertension* **11**, 49–57.

Imai, E. *et al.* (1994). Phenotypic change of the mesangial cells induced by overexpression of the TGF-β in *in vivo* glomerulus. *Journal of the American Society of Nephrology* **5**, 782 (abstract).

Imasawa, T. and Utsunomiya, Y. (2002). Stem cells in renal biology: bone marrow transplantation for the treatment of IgA nephropathy. *Experimental Nephrology* **10**, 51–58.

Imasawa, T., Nagasawa, R., Utsunomiya, Y., Kawamura, T., Zhong, Y., Makita, N., Muso, E., Miyawaki, S., Maruyama, N., Hosoya, T., Sakai, O., and Ohno, T. (1999). Bone marrow transplantation attenuates murine IgA nephropathy: role of a stem cell disorder. *Kidney International* **56**, 1964–1966.

Inman, S. R. *et al.* (1999). Lovastatin preserves renal function in experimental diabetes. *American Journal of Medical Science* **317**, 215–221.

Isaka, Y., Fujiwara, Y., Ueda, N., Kaneda, Y., Kamada, T., and Imai, E. (1993). Glomerulosclerosis induced by *in vivo* transfection of TGF-β or PDGF gene into the rat kidney. *Journal of Clinical Investigation* **92**, 2597–2601.

Isaka, Y. *et al.* (1996). Gene therapy by skeletal muscle expression of decorin prevents fibrotic disease in rat kidney. *Nature Medicine* **2**, 418–423.

Ishizaka, N. *et al.* (2002). Abnormal iron deposition in renal cells in the rat with chronic angiotensin II administration. *Laboratory Investigation* **82**, 87–96.

Ito, T., Suzuki, A., Imai, E., and Hori, M. (2001). Bone marrow is a reservoir of repopulating mesangial cells during glomerular remodelling. *Journal of the American Society of Nephrology* **12**, 2625–2635.

Jafar, T. H. *et al.* (2001a). Proteinuria as a modifiable risk factor for the progression of non-diabetic renal disease. *Kidney International* **60**, 1131–1140.

Jafar, T. H. *et al.* (2001b). Angiotensin-converting enzyme inhibitors and progression of non-diabetic renal disease. A meta-analysis of patient-level data. *Annals of Internal Medicine* **135**, 73–78.

Javaid, B., Olson, J. L., and Meyer, T. W. (2001). Glomerular injury and tubular loss in adriamycin nephrosis. *Journal of the American Society of Nephrology* **12**, 1391–1400.

Jensen, P. K., Christiansen, J. S., Steven, K., and Parving, H. H. (1987). Strict metabolic control and renal function in the streptozotocin diabetic rat. *Kidney International* **31**, 47–51.

Jernigan, S. M. and Eddy, A. A. Experimental insights into the mechanisms of tubulointerstitial scarring. In *Mechanisms and Management of Progressive Renal Failure* (ed. A. M. El Nahas, S. Anderson, and K. P. G. Harris), pp. 104–145. Oxford: Oxford University Press, 2000.

Johnson, R. J. (1994). The glomerular response to injury: progression or resolution? *Kidney International* **45**, 1769–1782.

Johnson, R. J. *et al.* (1991). Expression of smooth muscle cell phenotype by rat mesangial cells in immune complex nephritis. *Journal of Clinical Investigation* **87**, 847–858.

Johnson, R. J. *et al.* (1992). Renal injury from angiotensin II-mediated hypertension. *Hypertension* **19**, 464–474.

Johnson, R. J., Floege, J., Couser, W. G., and Alpers, C. E. (1993). Role of platelet-derived growth factor in glomerular disease. *Journal of the American Society of Nephrology* **4**, 119–128.

Johnson, R. J., Kivlighn, S. D., Kim, Y. G., Suga, S., and Fogo, A. B. (1999). Reappraisal of the pathogenesis and consequences of hyperuricemia in hypertension, cardiovascular disease, and renal disease. *American Journal of Kidney Diseases* **33**, 225–234.

Johnson, T. S. *et al.* (1997). The role of transglutaminase in the rat subtotal nephrectomy model of renal fibrosis. *Journal of Clinical Investigation* **99**, 2950–2960.

Jones, C. A. *et al.* (1998). Serum creatinine levels in the US population: third National Health and Nutrition Examination Survey. *American Journal of Kidney Diseases* **32**, 992–999.

Jones, C. L., Buch, S., Post, M., McCulloch, L., Liu, E., and Eddy, A. A. (1991). Pathogenesis of interstitial fibrosis in chronic purine aminonucleoside nephrosis. *Kidney International* **40**, 1020–1031.

Jones, C. L., Fecondo, J., Kelynack, K., Forbes, J., Walker, R., and Becker, G. (1995). Tissue inhibitor of the metalloproteinases and renal extracellular matrix accumulation. *Experimental Nephrology* **3**, 80–86.

Kagami, S., Kondo, S., Urushihara, M., Loster, K., Reutter, W., Saijo, T., Kitamura, A., Kobayashi, S., and Kuroda, Y. (2000). Overexpression of alpha1beta1 integrin directly affects rat mesangial cell behaviour. *Kidney International* **58** (3), 1088–1097.

Kaizuka, M., Yamabe, H., Osawa, H., Okumura, K., and Fujimoto, N. (1999). Thrombin stimulates synthesis of type IV collagen and tissue inhibitor of metalloproteinases-1 by cultured human mesangial cells. *Journal of the American Society of Nephrology* **10**, 1516–1523.

Kamanna, V. S. (2002). Low density lipoproteins and mitogenic signal transduction processes: role in the pathogenesis of renal disease. *Histology and Histopathology* **17**, 497–505.

Kang, D. H. *et al.* (2002). Role of the microvascular endothelium in progressive renal disease. *Journal of the American Society of Nephrology* **13**, 806–816.

Kanno, K., Okumura, F., Toriumi, W., Ishiyama, N., Nishiyama, S., and Naito, K. (1998). Nephrotoxic serum-induced nephritis in Wistar–Kyoto rats: a model to evaluate antinephritic agents. *Japanese Journal of Pharmacology* **77**, 129–135.

Kasiske, B. L. and Klinger, D. (2000). Cigarette smoking in renal transplant recipients. *Journal of the American Society of Nephrology* **11**, 753–759.

Kasiske, B. L., O'Donnell, M. P., Schmitz, P., and Keane, W. F. (1991). The role of lipid abnormalities in the pathogenesis of chronic progressive renal disease. *Advances in Nephrology* **20**, 109–126.

Kasiske, B. L., O'Donnell, M. P., and Keane, W. F. The obese Zucker rat model of chronic progressive glomerular injury. In *Experimental and Genetic Rat Models of Chronic Renal Failure* (ed. N. Gretz and M. Strauch), pp. 90–99. Basel: Karger, 1993.

Kasiske, B. L., Lakatua, J. D., Ma, J. Z., and Louis, T. A. (1998). A meta-analysis of the effects of dietary protein restriction on the rate of decline in renal function. *American Journal of Kidney Diseases* **31**, 954–961.

Kaysen, G. A. and Kropp, J. (1983). Dietary tryptophan supplementation prevents proteinuria in the seven-eighths nephrectomized rat. *Kidney International* **23**, 473–479.

K/DOQI (2002). Clinical practice guidelines for chronic kidney disease: evaluation, classification, and stratification. Kidney Disease Outcome Quality Initiative. *American Journal of Kidney Diseases* **39** (2 Suppl. 2), S1–S246.

Keane, W. F. (2000). The role of lipids in renal disease: future challenges. *Kidney International* **75**, S27–S31.

Keane, W. F., Kasiske, B. L., and O'Donnell, M. P. (1988). Hyperlipidemia and the progression of renal disease. *American Journal of Clinical Nutrition* **47**, 157–160.

Kempe, H. P., Engelmann, K., Gretz, N., and Hasslacher, C. Models of diabetes for studying diabetic nephropathy. In *Experimental and Genetic Rat Models of Chronic Renal Failure* (ed. N. Gretz and M. Strauch), pp. 148–155. Basel: Karger, 1993.

Kerjaschki, D. (1995). Epitopes and radicals: early events in glomerular injury in membranous nephropathy. *Experimental Nephrology* **3**, 1–8.

Kim, H. *et al.* (2001a). TIMP-1 deficiency does not attenuate interstitial fibrosis in obstructive nephropathy. *Journal of the American Society of Nephrology* **12**, 736–748.

Kim, Y. H. *et al.* (2001b). Podocyte depletion and glomerulosclerosis have a direct relationship in the PAN-treated rat. *Kidney International* **60**, 957–968.

Kitamura, M. and Fine, L. G. (1999). The concept of glomerular self-defense. *Kidney International* **55**, 1639–1671.

Klag, M. J., Whelton, P. K., Randall, B. L., Neaton, J. D., Brancati, F. L., and Stamler, J. (1997). End-stage renal disease in African-American and white men. 16-year MRFIT findings. *Journal of the American Medical Association* **277**, 1293–1298.

Klag, M. J. *et al.* (2002). Coffee intake and risk of hypertension: the Johns Hopkins precursors study. *Archives of Internal Medicine* **162**, 657–662.

Klahr, S. (2000). Obstructive nephropathy. *Internal Medicine* **39**, 355–361.

Klahr, S. (2001). The role of nitric oxide in hypertension and renal disease progression. *Nephrology, Dialysis, Transplantation* **16** (Suppl. 1), 60–62.

Klahr, S., Heifets, M., and Purkerson, M. L. (1986). The influence of anticoagulation on the progression of experimental renal disease. *Contemporary Issues in Nephrology* **14**, 45–64.

Klahr, S. *et al.* (1994). The effects of dietary protein restriction and blood pressure control on the progression of chronic renal disease. *New England Journal of Medicine* **330**, 877–884.

Kleinknecht, C. and Laouari, D. (1986). The influence of dietary components on experimental renal disease. *Contemporary Issues in Nephrology* **14**, 17–35.

Kluth, D. C., Erwig, L. P., Pearce, W. P., and Rees, A. J. (2000). Gene transfer into inflamed glomeruli using macrophages transfected with adenovirus. *Gene Therapy* **7**, 263–270.

Kluth, D. C. *et al.* (2001). Macrophages transfected with adenovirus to express IL-4 reduce inflammation in experimental glomerulonephritis. *Journal of Immunology* **166**, 4728–4736.

Knecht, A., Fine, L. G., Kleinman, K. S., Rodemann, H. P., Muller, G. A., Woo, D. D., and Norman, J. T. (1991). Fibroblasts of rabbit kidney in culture. II. Paracrine stimulation of papillary fibroblasts by PDGF. *American Journal of Physiology* **261**, F292–F299.

Komers, R. and Anderson S. (2000). Optimal strategies for preventing progression of renal disease: should angiotensin converting enzyme inhibitors and angiotensin receptor blockers be used together? *Current Hypertension Reports* **2**, 465–472.

Kon, S. P. *et al.* (1995). Urinary C5b-9 excretion and clinical course in idiopathic membranous nephropathy. *Kidney International* **48**, 1953–1958.

Kopp, J. B. (1997). Gene expression in kidney using transgenic approaches. *Experimental Nephrology* **5**, 157–167.

Koshy, S. and Bakris, G. L. (2000). Therapeutic approaches to achieve desired blood pressure goals: focus on calcium channel blockers. *Cardiovascular Drugs and Therapeutics* **14**, 295–301.

Kothapalli, D. and Grotendorst, G. R. (2000). CTGF modulates cell cycle progression in cAMP-arrested NRK fibroblasts. *Journal of Cell Physiology* **182**, 119–126.

Krepinsky, J. *et al.* (2002). 17beta-Estradiol modulates mechanical strain-induced MAPK activation in mesangial cells. *Journal of Biological Chemistry* **277**, 9387–9394.

Kriz, W. and Lemley, K. V. (1999). The role of the podocyte in glomerulosclerosis. *Current Opinion in Nephrology and Hypertension* **8**, 489–497.

Krolewski, A. S., Warram, H. J., and Christlieb, A. R. (1993). Hypercholesterolemia—a determinant of renal function loss and deaths in IDDM patients with nephropathy. *Kidney International* **45**, S125–S131.

Kuijpers, M. H. and de Jong, W. (1987). Relationship between blood pressure level, renal histopathological lesions and plasma renin activity in fawn-hooded rats. *British Journal of Experimental Pathology* **68**, 179–187.

Kuncio, G. S., Neilson, E. G., and Haverty, T. (1991). Mechanisms of tubulointerstitial fibrosis. *Kidney International* **39**, 550–556.

Kwan, G., Neugarten, J., Sherman, M., Ding, Q., Fotadar, U., Lei, J., and Silbiger, S. (1996). Effects of sex hormones on mesangial cell proliferation and collagen synthesis. *Kidney International* **50**, 1173–1179.

Lambert, G. *et al.* (2001). Analysis of glomerulosclerosis and atherosclerosis in lecithin cholesterol acyltransferase-deficient mice. *Journal of Biological Chemistry* **276**, 15090–15098.

Lan, H. Y., Nikolic-Paterson, D. J., and Atkins, R. C. (1992). Involvement of activated periglomerular leucocytes in the rupture of Bowman's capsule and crescent progression in experimental glomerulonephritis. *Laboratory Investigation* **67**, 743–751.

Landau, D. *et al.* (2001). A novel somatostatin analogue prevents early renal complications in the nonobese diabetic mouse. *Kidney International* **60**, 505–512.

Lau, K. (1989). Phosphate excess and progressive renal failure: the precipitation–calcification hypothesis. *Kidney International* **36**, 918–937.

Lawrence, G. M. and Brewer, D. B. (1981). Effect of strain and sex on the induction of hyperalbuminaemic proteinuria in the rat. *Clinical Science* **61**, 751–756.

Leclercq, B., Jaimes, E. A., and Raij, L. (2002). Nitric oxide synthase and hypertension. *Current Opinion in Nephrology and Hypertension* **11**, 185–189.

Lemley, K. V., Abdullah, I., Myers, B. D., Meyer, T. W., Blouch, K., Smith, W. E., Bennett, P. H., and Nelson, R. G. (2000). Evolution of incipient nephropathy in type 2 diabetes mellitus. *Kidney International* **58**, 1228–1237.

Lemley, K. V., Lafayette, R. A., Safai, M., Derby, G., Blouch, K., Squarer, A., and Myers, B. D. (2002). Podocytopenia and disease severity in IgA nephropathy. *Kidney International* **61**, 1475–1485.

Levey, A. S. *et al.* (1998). Controlling the epidemic of cardiovascular disease in chronic renal disease: what do we know? What do we need to learn? Where do we go from here? National Kidney Foundation Task Force on Cardiovascular Disease. *American Journal of Kidney Diseases* **32**, 853–906.

Lewis, E., Hunsicker, L. G., Barin, R. P., and Rohde, R. D. (1993). The effect of angiotensin converting enzyme inhibitor on diabetic nephropathy. *New England Journal of Medicine* **329**, 1456–1462.

Lewis, E. J. *et al.* (2001). Renoprotective effect of the angiotensin-receptor antagonist irbesartan in patients with nephropathy due to type 2 diabetes. *New England Journal of Medicine* **345**, 851–860.

Lhotta, K., Rumpelt, H. J., Konig, P., Mayer, G., and Kronenberg, F. (2002). Cigarette smoking and vascular pathology in renal biopsies. *Kidney International* **61**, 648–654.

Li, J. H. *et al.* (2002). Smad7 inhibits fibrotic effects of TGF-b on renal tubular epithelial cells by blocking Smad2 activation. *Journal of the American Society of Nephrology* **13**, 1464–1472.

Lim, C. S. *et al.* (2001). Th1/Th2 predominance and proinflammatory cytokines determine the clinicopathological severity of IgA nephropathy. *Nephrology, Dialysis, Transplantation* **16**, 269–275.

Liu, Y. (2002). Hepatocyte growth factor and the kidney. *Current Opinion in Nephrology and Hypertension* **11**, 23–30.

Locatelli, F. and Del Vecchio, L. Natural history and factors affecting the progression of chronic renal failure. In *Mechanisms and Management of Progressive Renal Failure* (ed. A. M. El Nahas, S. Anderson, and K. P. G. Harris), pp. 20–79. Oxford: Oxford University Press, 2000.

Locatelli, F. *et al.* (1996). Proteinuria and blood pressure as causal components of progression to end-stage renal failure. *Nephrology, Dialysis, Transplantation* **11**, 461–467.

Lonnemann, G., Shapiro, L., Engler-Blum, G., Muller, G. A., Koch, K. M., and Dinarello, C. A. (1995). Cytokines in human renal interstitial fibrosis. I. Interleukin-1 is a paracrine growth factor for cultured fibrosis-derived kidney fibroblasts. *Kidney International* **47**, 837–844.

Luft, F. C. (2000). Molecular genetics of human hypertension. *Current Opinion in Nephrology and Hypertension* **9**, 259–266.

Ma, J., Nishimura, H., Fogo, A., Kon, V., Inagami, T., and Ichikawa, I. (1998). Accelerated fibrosis and collagen deposition develop in the renal interstitium of angiotensin type 2 receptor null mutant mice during ureteral obstruction. *Kidney International* **53**, 937–944.

Ma, L. and Fogo, A. B. (2001). Role of angiotensin II in glomerular injury. *Seminars in Nephrology* **21**, 544–553.

Mackenzie, H. S., Ots, M., Ziai, F., Lee, K. W., Kato, S., and Brenner, B. M. (1997). Angiotensin receptor antagonists in experimental models of chronic renal failure. *Kidney International* **63** (Suppl.), S140–S143.

Mann, J. F. E. and Luft, F. C. Hypertension induced models of nephrosclerosis in the rat. In *Experimental and Genetic Models of Chornic Renal Failure* (ed. N. Gretz and M. Strauch), pp. 141–147. Basel: Karger, 1993.

Marcantoni, C., Jafar, T. H., Oldrizzi, L., Levey, A. S., and Maschio, G. (2000). The role of systemic hypertension in the progression of nondiabetic renal disease. *Kidney International* (Suppl.) **75**, S44–S48.

Martin-Ventura, L. and Egido, J. (2003). Anti-inflammtory and immunomodulatory effects of statins. *Kidney International* **63**, 12–23.

Maschio, G. *et al.* (1996). Effect of the angiotensin-converting-enzyme inhibitor benazepril on the progression of chronic renal insufficiency. The Angiotensin-Converting-Enzyme Inhibition in Progressive Renal Insufficiency Study Group. *New England Journal of Medicine* **334**, 939–945.

Maser, R. L., Vassmer, D., Magenheimer, B. S., and Calvet, J. P. (2002). Oxidant stress and reduced antioxidant enzyme protection in polycystic kidney disease. *Journal of the American Society of Nephrology* **13**, 991–999.

Matsunaga, A. *et al.* (1999). A novel apolipoprotein E mutation, E2 (Arg25Cys), in lipoprotein glomerulopathy. *Kidney International* **56**, 421–427.

Mauer, S. M., Steffes, M. W., Ellis, E. N., Sutherland, D. E., Brown, D. M., and Goetz, F. C. (1984). Structural-functional relationships in diabetic nephropathy. *Journal of Clinical Investigation* **74**, 1143–1155.

Mazzali, M. *et al.* (2002). Hyperuricemia induces a primary renal arteriolopathy in rats by a blood pressure-independent mechanism. *American Journal of Physiology* **282**, F991–F997.

Mezzano, S. A., Barria, M., Droguett, M. A., Burgos, M. E., Ardiles, L. G., Flores, C., and Egido, J. (2001). Tubular NF-kappaB and AP-1 activation in human proteinuric renal disease. *Kidney International* **60**, 1366–1377.

Miller, S. B. and Rabkin, R. (1997). The use of growth factors to increase glomerular filtration rate in chronic renal failure patients. *Current Opinion in Nephrology and Hypertension* **6**, 401–404.

Miyajima, A. *et al.* (2000). Antibody to transforming growth factor-beta ameliorates tubular apoptosis in unilateral ureteral obstruction. *Kidney International* **58**, 2301–2313.

Mizuno, S., Matsumoto, K., Kurosawa, T., Mizuno-Horikawa, Y., and Nakamura, Y. (2000). Reciprocal balance of hepatocyte growth factor and transforming growth factor-beta 1 in renal fibrosis in mice. *Kidney International* **57**, 937–948.

Modi, K. S., O'Donnell, M. P., and Keane, W. F. Dietary interventions for progressive renal disease in experimental animal models. In *Prevention of Progressive Chronic Renal Failure* Vol. 1 (ed. A. M. El Nahas, N. P. Mallick, and S. Anderson), pp. 117–122. Oxford: Oxford University Press, 1993.

Mogensen, C. E. Diabetic nephropathy: natural history and management. In *Mechanisms and Management of Progressive Renal Failure* (ed. A. M. El Nahas, S. Anderson, and K. P. G. Harris), pp. 211–240. London: Oxford University Press, 2000.

Mooney, A. *et al.* (1999). Type IV collagen and laminin regulate glomerular mesangial cell susceptibility to apoptosis via beta(1) integrin-mediated survival signals. *American Journal of Pathology* **155**, 599–606.

Moorhead, J. F., El Nahas, A. M., Chan, M. K., and Varghese, Z. (1982). Lipid nephrotoxicity in chronic progressive glomerular and tubulo-interstitial disease. *Lancet* **ii**, 1309–1312.

Moriya, T., Groppoli, T. J., Kim, Y., and Mauer, M. (2001). Quantitative immuno-electron microscopy of type VI collagen in glomeruli in type I diabetic patients. *Kidney International* **59**, 317–323.

Muller, G. A. and Rodemann, H. P. (1991). Characterization of human renal fibroblasts in health and disease: I. Immunophenotyping of cultured tubular epithelial cells and fibroblasts derived from kidneys with histologically proven interstitial fibrosis. *American Journal of Kidney Diseases* **6**, 680–683.

Munger, K. A. *et al.* (1999). Transfection of rat kidney with human 15-lipoxygenase suppresses inflammation and preserves function in experimental glomerulonephritis. *Proceedings of the National Academy of Sciences USA* **96**, 13375–13380.

Muntner, P., Coresh, J., Smith, J. C., Eckfeldt, J., and Klag, M. J. (2000). Plasma lipids and risk of developing renal dysfunction: the atherosclerosis risk in communities study. *Kidney International* **58**, 293–301.

Nagatoya, K. *et al.* (2002). Y-27632 prevents tubulointerstitial fibrosis in mouse kidneys with unilateral ureteral obstruction. *Kidney International* **61**, 1684–1695.

Nakamura, H. *et al.* (2002). Introduction of DNA enzyme for Egr-1 into tubulointerstitial fibroblasts by electroporation reduced interstitial alpha-smooth muscle actin expression and fibrosis in unilateral ureteral obstruction (UUO) rats. *Gene Therapy* **9**, 495–502.

Nangaku, M., Pippin, J., and Couser, W. G. (2002). C6 mediates chronic progression of tubulointerstitial damage in rats with remnant kidneys. *Journal of the American Society of Nephrology* **13**, 928–936.

Nankivell, B. J., Boadle, R. A., and Harris, D. C. (1992). Iron accumulation in human chronic renal disease. *American Journal of Kidney Diseases* **20**, 580–584.

Nath, K. A. The role of tubulo-interstitial processes in progressive renal disease. In *Prevention of Progressive Chronic Renal Failure* Vol. 1 (ed. A. M. El Nahas, M. P. Mallick, and S. Anderson), pp. 62–97. Oxford: Oxford University Press, 1993.

Nath, K. A., Hostetter, M. K., and Hostetter, T. H. (1985). Pathophysiology of chronic tubulo-interstitial disease in rats. Interactions of dietary acid load, ammonia, and complement component C3. *Journal of Clinical Investigation* **76**, 667–675.

Nath, K. A., Hostetter, M. K., and Hostetter, T. H. (1991). The role of ammonia in progressive renal injury. *Contributions to Nephrology* **92**, 78–82.

Nath, K. A., Fischereder, M., and Hostetter, T. H. (1994). The role of oxidants in progressive renal injury. *Kidney International* **45** (Suppl. 45), S111–S115.

Nath, K. A., Croatt, A. J., Haggard, J. J., and Grande, J. P. (2000). Renal response to repetitive exposure to heme proteins: chronic injury induced by an acute insult. *Kidney International* 57, 2423–2433.

Nath, K. A. *et al.* (2001). Heme protein-induced chronic renal inflammation: suppressive effect of induced heme oxygenase-1. *Kidney International* 59, 106–117.

National Kidney Foundation/DOQI Kidney Disease Outcome Quality Initiative (2002). *American Journal of Kidney Diseases* 39 (Suppl. 1), S1–S266.

Neugarten, J. (2002). Gender and the progression of renal disease. *Journal of the American Society of Nephrology* 13, 2807–2809.

Neugarten, J., Acharya, A., Lei, J., and Silbiger, S. (2000). Selective estrogen receptor modulators suppress mesangial cell collagen synthesis. *American Journal of Physiology* 279, F309–F318.

Neugarten, J., Kasiske, B., Silbiger, S. R., and Nyengaard, J. R. (2002). Effects of sex on renal structure. *Nephron* 90, 139–144.

Nishida, Y., Oda, H., and Yorioka, N. (1999). Effect of lipoproteins on mesangial cell proliferation. *Kidney International* 71, S51–S53.

Nomura, A. *et al.* (1997). Role of complement in acute tubulointerstitial injury of rats with aminonucleoside nephrosis. *American Journal of Pathology* 151, 539–547.

Noris, M. and Remuzzi, G. (2002). ACE inhibitors and AT1 receptor antagonists: is two better than one? *Kidney International* 61, 1545–1547.

Norman, J. T. and Lewis, M. P. (1996). Matrix metalloproteinases (MMPs) in renal fibrosis. *Kidney International* 54, S61–S63.

Norman, J. T., Clark, I. M., and Garcia, P. L. (2000). Hypoxia promotes fibrogenesis in human renal fibroblasts. *Kidney International* 58, 2351–2366.

O'Bryan, T., Weiher, H., Rennke, H. G., Kren, S., and Hostetter, T. H. (2000). Course of renal injury in the Mpv17-deficient transgenic mouse. *Journal of the American Society of Nephrology* 11, 1067–1074.

Oda, T., Jung, Y. O., Kim, H. S., Cai, X., Lopez-Guisa, J. M., Ikeda, Y., and Eddy, A. A. (2001). PAI-1 deficiency attenuates the fibrogenic response to ureteral obstruction. *Kidney International* 60, 587–596.

O'Donnell, M. P. *et al.* (1985). Adriamycin-induced chronic proteinuria: a structural and functional study. *Journal of Laboratory and Clinical Medicine* 106, 62–67.

Okada, H., Ban, S., Nagao, S., Takahashi, H., Suzuki, H., and Neilson, E. G. (2000). Progressive renal fibrosis in murine polycystic kidney disease: an immunohistochemical observation. *Kidney International* 58, 587–597.

Okada, M., Takemura, T., Yanagida, H., and Yoshioka, K. (2002). Response of mesangial cells to low-density lipoprotein and angiotensin II in diabetic (OLETF) rats. *Kidney International* 61, 113–124.

Okuda, S. *et al.* (1992). Albuminuria is not an aggravating factor in experimental focal glomerulosclerosis and hyalinosis. *Journal of Laboratory and Clinical Medicine* 119, 245–253.

Olson, J. L., de Urdaneta, A. G., and Heptinstall, R. H. (1985). Glomerular hyalinosis and its relation to hyperfiltration. *Laboratory Investigation* 52, 387–398.

Olson, J. L., Wilson, S. K., and Heptinstall, R. H. (1986). Relation of glomerular injury to preglomerular resistance in experimental hypertension. *Kidney International* 29, 849–856.

Ong, A. C. M. and Moorhead, J. F. (1994). Tubular lipidoses; epiphenomenon or pathogenetic lesion in human renal disease? *Kidney International* 45, 753–762.

Onozato, M. L., Tojo, A., Goto, A., Fujita, T., and Wilcox, C. S. (2002). Oxidative stress and nitric oxide synthase in rat diabetic nephropathy: effects of ACEI and ARB. *Kidney International* 61, 186–194.

Orth, S. R. (2002). Smoking and the kidney. *Journal of the American Society of Nephrology* 13, 1663–1672.

Ostendorf, T. *et al.* (1999). VEGF(165) mediates glomerular endothelial repair. *Journal of Clinical Investigation* 104, 913–923.

Parekh, R. S. and Klag, M. J. (2001). Alcohol: role in the development of hypertension and end-stage renal disease. *Current Opinion in Nephrology and Hypertension* 10, 385–390.

Parving, H. H. *et al.* (2001). The effect of irbesartan on the development of diabetic nephropathy in patients with type 2 diabetes. *New England Journal of Medicine* 345, 870–878.

Pavenstadt, H. (2000). Roles of the podocyte in glomerular function. *American Journal of Physiology* 278, F173–F179.

Pazianas, M., Eastwood, J. B., MacRae, K. D., and Phillips, M. E. (1991). Racial origin and primary renal diagnosis in 771 patients with end stage renal disease. *Nephrology, Dialysis, Transplantation* 6, 931–935.

Pedrini, M. T., Levey, A. S., Lau, J., Chalmers, T. C., and Wang, P. H. (1996). The effect of dietary protein restriction on the progression of diabetic and nondiabetic renal diseases: a meta-analysis. *Annals of Internal Medicine* 124, 627–632.

Pereira, B. J. (2000). Optimization of pre-ESRD care: the key to improved dialysis outcomes. *Kidney International* 57, 351–365.

Perneger, T. V., Klag, M. J., and Whelton, P. (2001). Recreational drugs: a neglected risk factor for end-stage renal disease. *American Journal of Kidney Diseases* 38, 49–56.

Petermann, A. T. *et al.* (2003). Podocytes that detach in experimental membranous nephropathy are viable. *Kidney International* 64, 1222–1231.

Peterson, J. C., Adler, S., Burkart, J. M., Greene, T., Hebert, L. A., Hunsicker, L. G., King, A. J., Klahr, S., Massry, S. G., and Seifter, J. L. (1995). Blood pressure control, proteinuria, and the progression of renal disease. The Modification of Diet in Renal Disease Study. *Annals of Internal Medicine* 123, 754–762.

Poncelet, A. C. and Schnaper, H. W. (2001). Sp1 and Smad proteins cooperate to mediate transforming growth factor-beta 1-induced alpha 2(I) collagen expression in human glomerular mesangial cells. *Journal of Biological Chemistry* 276, 6983–6992.

Poncelet, A. C., de Caestecker, M. P., and Schnaper, H. W. (1999). The transforming growth factor-beta/SMAD signaling pathway is present and functional in human mesangial cells. *Kidney International* 56, 1354–1365.

Porter, G. A., Andoh, T. F., and Bennett, W. M. (1999). An animal model of chronic cyclosporine nephrotoxicity. *Renal Failure* 21, 365–368.

Potier, M., Elliot, S. J., Tack, I., Lenz, O., Striker, G. E., Striker, L. J., and Karl, M. (2001). Expression and regulation of estrogen receptors in mesangial cells: influence on matrix metalloproteinase-9. *Journal of the American Society of Nephrology* 12, 241–251.

Poulsom, R. *et al.* (2001). Bone marrow contributes to renal parenchymal turnover and regeneration. *Journal of Pathology* 195, 229–235.

Provoost, A. P., Shiozawa, M., Van Dokkum, R. P., and Jacob, H. J. (2002). Transfer of the Rf-1 region from FHH onto the ACI background increases susceptibility to renal impairment. *Physiology and Genomics* 8, 123–129.

Raij, L. and Keane, W. F. (1985). Glomerular mesangium: its function and relationship to angiotensin II. *American Journal of Medicine* 79 (Suppl. 3C), 24–30.

Rangan, G. K., Wang, Y., Tay, Y. C., and Harris, D. C. (1999). Inhibition of nuclear factor-kappaB activation reduces cortical tubulointerstitial injury in proteinuric rats. *Kidney International* 56, 118–134.

Remuzzi, G. and Bertani, T. (1990). Is glomerulosclerosis a consequence of altered glomerular permeability to macromolecules? *Kidney International* 38, 384–394.

Rennke, H. G. (1986). Structural alterations associated with glomerular hyperfiltration. *Contemporary Issues in Nephrology* 14, 111–131.

Rennke, H. G. (1994). How does glomerular epithelial cell injury contribute to progressive glomerular damage? *Kidney International* 45, S58–S63.

Rennke, H. G. and Klein, P. S. (1989). Pathogenesis and significance of nonprimary focal and segmental glomerulosclerosis. *American Journal of Kidney Diseases* 13, 443–456.

Rennke, H. G. *et al.* (1987). Inter-strain variations in urinary protein excretion rates and progressive glomerulosclerosis in immune complex nephritis in the rat. *Kidney International* 31, 392.

Riley, S. G., Steadman, R., Williams, J. D., Floege, J., and Phillips, A. O. (1999). Augmentation of kidney injury by basic fibroblast growth factor or platelet-derived growth factor does not induce progressive diabetic nephropathy in the Goto Kakizaki model of non-insulin-dependent diabetes. *Journal of Laboratory and Clinical Medicine* **134**, 304–312.

Rocha, R., Chander, P. N., Zuckerman, A., and Stier, C. T., Jr. (1999). Role of aldosterone in renal vascular injury in stroke-prone hypertensive rats. *Hypertension* **33**, 232–237.

Rodemann, H. P. and Muller, G. A. (1990). Abnormal growth and clonal proliferation of fibroblasts derived from kidneys with interstitial fibrosis. *Proceedings of the Society of Experimental Biology and Medicine* **195**, 57–63.

Rodemann, H. P. and Muller, G. A. (1991). Characterization of human renal fibroblasts in health and disease. II. *In vitro* growth, differentiation, and collagen synthesis of fibroblasts from kidneys with interstitial fibrosis. *American Journal of Kidney Diseases* **17**, 684–686.

Rodriguez-Iturbe, B., Pons, H., Herrera-Acosta, J., and Johnson, R. J. (2001). Role of immunocompetent cells in nonimmune renal diseases. *Kidney International* **59**, 1626–1640.

Rossing, P., Hougaard, P., and Parving, H. H. (2002). Risk factors for development of incipient and overt diabetic nephropathy in type 1 diabetic patients: a 10-year prospective observational study. *Diabetes Care* **25**, 859–864.

Rostand, S. G. *et al.* (1989). Renal insufficiency in treated essential hypertension. *New England Journal of Medicine* **320**, 684–688.

Rovin, B. H. (2000). Chemokine blockade as a therapy for renal disease. *Current Opinion in Nephrology and Hypertension* **9**, 225–232.

Rudberg, S., Persson, B., and Dahlquist, G. (1992). Increased glomerular filtration rate as a predictor of diabetic nephropathy—results from an eight year prospective study. *Kidney International* **41**, 822–828.

Ruef, C., Kashgarian, M., and Coleman, D. L. (1992). Mesangial cell–matrix interactions. Effects on mesangial growth and cytokine secretion. *American Journal of Pathology* **141**, 429–439.

Ruger, B. M., Erb, K. J., He, Y., Lane, J. M., Davis, P. F., and Hasan, Q. (2000). Interleukin-4 transgenic mice develop glomerulosclerosis independent of immunoglobulin deposition. *European Journal of Immunology* **30**, 2698–2703.

Ruggenenti, P. *et al.* (1999). Renoprotective properties of ACE-inhibition in non-diabetic nephropathies with non-nephrotic proteinuria. *Lancet* **354**, 359–364.

Ruggenenti, P., Perna, A., Zoccali, C., Gherardi, G., Benini, R., Testa, A., and Remuzzi, G. (2000). Chronic proteinuric nephropathies. II. Outcomes and response to treatment in a prospective cohort of 352 patients: differences between women and men in relation to the ACE gene polymorphism. Gruppo Italiano di Studi Epidemiologici in Nefrologia (Gisen). *Journal of the American Society of Nephrology* **11**, 88–96.

Ruggenenti, P., Perna, A., and Remuzzi, G. on behalf of GISEN (2001). ACE inibitors to prevent end-stage renal disease: when to start and why possibly never to stop: a post hoc analysis of the REIN trial results. *Journal of the American Society of Nephrology* **12**, 2832–2837.

Ruiz-Ortega, M., Lorenzo, O., Suzuki, Y., Ruperez, M., and Egido, J. (2001). Proinflammatory actions of angiotensins. *Current Opinion in Nephrology and Hypertension* **10**, 321–329.

Rustom, R. *et al.* (1998). Tubular peptide hypermetabolism and urinary ammonia in chronic renal failure in man: a maladaptive response? *Nephron* **79**, 306–311.

Rustom, R. *et al.* (2001). Renal tubular peptide catabolism in chronic vascular rejection. *Renal Failure* **23**, 517–531.

Saito, T. *et al.* (1989). Lipoprotein glomerulopathy; glomerular lipoprotein thrombi in a patient with hyperlipoproteinemia. *American Journal of Kidney Diseases* **13**, 148–153.

Saito, T., Oikawa, S., Sato, H., and Sasaki, J. (1999). Lipoprotein glomerulopathy: renal lipidosis induced by novel apolipoprotein E variants. *Nephron* **83**, 193–201.

Sanders, P. W. *et al.* (2001). Increased dietary salt accelerates chronic allograft nephropathy in rats. *Kidney International* **59**, 1149–1157.

Sato, H. *et al.* (1993). Localization of apolipoprotein(a) and B-100 in various renal diseases. *Kidney International* **43**, 430–435.

Sato, N. *et al.* (2001). Mizoribine ameliorates the tubulointerstitial fibrosis of obstructive nephropathy. *Nephron* **89**, 177–185.

Satyanarayana, P. S., Singh, D., and Chopra, K. (2001). Quercetin, a bioflavonoid, protects against oxidative stress-related renal dysfunction by cyclosporine in rats. *Methods Find Experimental and Clinical Pharmacology* **23**, 175–181.

Savage, C. O. S. (1994). The biology of the glomerulus: endothelial cells. *Kidney International* **45**, 314–319.

Savill, J. (2001). Phagocyte clearance of cells dying by apoptosis and the regulation of glomerular inflammation. *Advances in Nephrology from the Necker Hospital* **31**, 21–28.

Sawashima, K., Mizuno, S., Mizuno-Horikawa, Y., Kudo, T., and Kurosawa, T. (2002). Protein restriction ameliorates renal tubulointerstitial nephritis and reduces renal transforming growth factor-beta expression in unilateral ureteral obstruction. *Experimental Nephrology* **10**, 7–18.

Schiffer, M. *et al.* (2001). Apoptosis in podocytes induced by TGF-beta and Smad7. *Journal of Clinical Investigation* **108**, 807–816.

Schlondorff, D. (1987). The glomerular mesangial cell: an expanding role for a specialized pericyte. *FASEB Journal* **1**, 272–281.

Schlondorff, D. (1993). Cellular mechanisms of lipid injury in the glomerulus. *American Journal of Kidney Diseases* **22**, 72–82.

Schrier, R. W., Harris, D. C., Chan, L., Shapiro, J. I., and Caramelo, C. (1988). Tubular hypermatabolism as a factor in the progression of chronic renal failure. *American Journal of Kidney Diseases* **12**, 243–249.

Schrier, R. W., Shapiro, J. I., Chan, L., and Harris, D. C. H. (1994). Increased nephron oxygen consumption: potential role in progression of chronic renal disease. *American Journal of Kidney Diseases* **23**, 176–182.

Schrier, R. W., Estacio, R. O., Esler, A., and Mehler, P. (2002). Effects of aggressive blood pressure control in normotensive type2 diabetic patients on albuminuria, retinopathy and strokes. *Kidney International* **61**, 1086–1097.

Schulze, M. *et al.* (1991). Elevated urinary excretion of the C5b-9 complex in membranous nephropathy. *Kidney International* **40**, 533–538.

Schwartz, M. M. and Bidani, A. K. (1991). Mesangial structure and function in the remnant kidney. *Kidney International* **40**, 226–237.

Segerer, S., Nelson, P. J., and Schlondorff, D. (2000). Chemokines, chemokine receptors, and renal disease: from basic science to pathophysiologic and therapeutic studies. *Journal of the American Society of Nephrology* **11**, 152–176.

Sellitti, D. F. *et al.* (2000). Renal expression of two 'thyroid-specific' genes: thyrotropin receptor and thyroglobulin. *Experimental Nephrology* **8**, 235–243.

Shankland, S. J. (1999). Cell cycle regulatory proteins in glomerular disease. *Kidney International* **56**, 1208–1215.

Sharpe, C. C. and Hendry, B. M. (2003). Signalling: focus on Rho in renal disease. *Journal of the American Society of Nephrology* **14**, 261–264.

Shaw, A. S. and Miner, J. H. (2001). CD2-associated protein and the kidney. *Current Opinion in Nephrology and Hypertension* **10**, 19–22.

Sheinfeld, G. R. and Bakris, G. L. (1999). Benefits of combination angiotensin-converting enzyme inhibitor and calcium antagonist therapy for diabetic patients. *American Journal of Hypertension* **12**, 80S–85S.

Shrivastav, S., Cusumano, A., Kanno, Y., Chen, G., Bryant, J. L., and Kopp, J. B. (2000). Role of T lymphocytes in renal disease in HIV-transgenic mice. *American Journal of Kidney Diseases* **35**, 408–417.

Silver, B. L., Jaffer, J. E., and Abboud, H. E. (1989). Platelet-derived growth factor synthesis in mesangial cells: induction by multiple peptide mitogens. *Proceedings of the National Academy of Sciences USA* **86**, 1056–1060.

Singh, R., Song, R. H., Alavi, N., Pegoraro, A. A., Singh, A. K., and Leehey, D. J. (2001). High glucose decreases matrix metalloproteinase-2 activity in rat mesangial cells via transforming growth factor-beta1. *Experimental Nephrology* **9**, 249–257.

Skill, N. J. *et al.* (2001). Increases in renal epsilon-(gamma-glutamyl)-lysine crossline result from compartment-specific changes in tissue transglutaminase in early experimental diabetic nephropathy pathologic implications. *Laboratory Investigation* **81**, 705–716.

Smith, S. R., Svetkey, L. P., and Dennis, V. W. (1991). Racial differences in the incidence and progression of renal disease. *Kidney International* **40**, 815–822.

Sommer, M. *et al.* (1999). Abnormal growth and clonal proliferation of fibroblasts in an animal model of unilateral ureteral obstruction. *Nephron* **82**, 39–50.

Song, D., Zhou, W., Sheerin, S. H., and Sacks, S. H. (1998). Compartmental localization of complement component transcripts in the normal human kidney. *Nephron* **78**, 15–22.

Sraer, J. D. and Rondeau, E. (1996). Role of thrombin and its receptor in the pathogenesis of severe forms of human glomerulonephritis with fibrin deposits. *Bulletin de l'academie Nationale de Medecine* **180**, 1609–1623.

Steffes, M. W. and Mauer, S. M. (1984). Diabetic glomerulopathy in man and experimental animal models. *International Review of Experimental Pathology* **26**, 147–160.

Stewart, R. J. and Marsden, P. A. (1994). Vascular endothelial cell activation in models of vascular and glomerular injury. *Kidney International* **45** (Suppl. 45), S37–S44.

Striker, L. M.-M., Killen, P. D., Chi, E., and Striker, G. E. (1984). The composition of glomerulosclerosis: 1. Studies in focal sclerosis, crescentic glomerulonephritis and membranoproliferative glomerulonephritis. *Laboratory Investigation* **51**, 181–192.

Striker, G. E. *et al.* (1997). Glomerulosclerosis, arteriosclerosis, and vascular graft stenosis: treatment with oral heparinoids. *Kidney International* **63**, S120–S123.

Strutz, F. (2001). Potential methods to prevent interstitial fibrosis in renal disease. *Expert Opinion in Investigation Drugs* **10**, 1989–2001.

Strutz, F. and Muller, G. A. (2000). Transdifferentiation comes of age. *Nephrology, Dialysis, Transplantation* **15**, 1729–1731.

Strutz, F. *et al.* (1995). Identification and characterisation of a fibroblast marker: FSP1. *Journal of Cell Biology* **130**, 393–405.

Strutz, F. *et al.* (2001). TGF-beta 1 induces proliferation in human renal fibroblasts via induction of basic fibroblast growth factor (FGF-2). *Kidney International* **59**, 579–592.

Strutz, F. *et al.* (2002). Role of basic fibroblast growth factor-2 in epithelial-mesenchymal transformation. *Kidney International* **61**, 1714–1728.

Suematsu, S. *et al.* (1989). IgG1 plasmacytosis in interleukin 6 transgenic mice. *Proceedings of the National Academy of Sciences USA* **86**, 7547–7551.

Suzuki, Y. *et al.* (2001). Renal tubulointerstitial damage caused by persistent proteinuria is attenuated in AT1-deficient mice: role of endothelin-1. *American Journal of Pathology* **159**, 1895–1904.

Takase, O. *et al.* (2003). Gene transfer of truncated IkBa prevents tubulointerstitial injury. *Kidney International* **63**, 501–513.

Takayama, H., LaRochelle, W. J., Sabnis, S. G., Otsuka, T., and Merlino, G. (1997). Renal tubular hyperplasia, polycystic disease, and glomerulosclerosis in transgenic mice overexpressing hepatocyte growth factor/scatter factor. *Laboratory Investigation* **77**, 131–138.

Tamimi, N. and El Nahas, A. M. (2000). Angiotensin-converting enzyme inhibition: facts and fiction. *Nephron* **84**, 299–304.

Terzi, F., Burtin, M., and Friedlander, G. (2000). Using transgenic mice to analyze the mechanisms of progression of chronic renal failure. *Journal of the American Society of Nephrology* **11** (Suppl. 16), S144–S148.

Teschan, P. E. *et al.* (1998). Effect of a ketoacid-aminoacid-supplemented very low protein diet on the progression of advanced renal disease: a reanalysis of the MDRD feasibility study. *Clinical Nephrology* **50**, 273–283.

Theuring, F. *et al.* (1998). Pathophysiology in endothelin-1 transgenic mice. *Journal of Cardiovascular Pharmacology* **31** (Suppl. 1), S489–S491.

Thomas, G. L., Yang, B., Wagner, B. E., Savill, J., and El Nahas, A. M. (1998). Cellular apoptosis and proliferation in experimental renal fibrosis. *Nephrology, Dialysis, Transplantation* **13**, 2216–2226.

Thomas, M. E. *et al.* (1993). Simvastatin therapy for hypercholesterolemic patients with nephrotic syndrome or significant proteinuria. *Kidney International* **44**, 1124–1129.

Thomas, M. E. *et al.* (1999). Proteinuria induces tubular cell turnover: a potential mechanism for tubular atrophy. *Kidney International* **55** (3), 890–898.

Tipping, P. G. and Holdsworth, S. R. (1986). The participation of macrophages, glomerular procoagulant activity and factor VIII in glomerular fibrin deposition. *American Journal of Pathology* **124**, 10–17.

Tofovic, S. P., Kost, C. K., Jackson, E. K., and Bastacky, S. I. (2002). Long-term caffeine consumption exacerbates renal failure in obese, diabetic, ZSF1 (fa-facp) rats. *Kidney International* **61**, 1433–1444.

Tolins, J. P., Stone, B. G., and Raij, L. (1992). Interactions of hypercholesterolemia and hypertension in initiation of glomerular injury. *Kidney International* **41**, 1254–1261.

Trachtman, H. *et al.* (1992). Taurine attenuates renal disease in chronic puromycin aminonucleoside nephropathy. *American Journal of Physiology* **262**, F117–F123.

Tryggvason, K. (2001). Nephrin: role in normal kidney and in disease. *Advances in Nephrology from the Necker Hospital* **31**, 221–234.

Tsunoda, S., Yamabae, H., Osawa, H., Kaizuka, M., Shirato, K., and Okumura, K. (2001). Cultured rat glomerular epithelial cells show gene expression and production of transforming growth factor-beta: expression is enhanced by thrombin. *Nephrology, Dialysis, Transplantation* **16**, 1776–1782.

Tsuruta, M., Adachi, H., Hirai, Y., Fujiura, Y., and Imaizumi, T. (2000). Association between alcohol intake and development of hypertension in Japanese normotensive men: 12-year follow-up study. *American Journal of Hypertension* **13**, 482–487.

Turner, R. C. (1998). The U. K. Prospective Diabetes Study. A review. *Diabetes Care* **21** (Suppl. 3), C35–C38.

UK Renal Registry: The fifth annual report. December 2002.

US Renal Data System: USRDS 2001 Annual Data Report (2001). The National Institutes of Health, National Institute of Diabetes and Digestive and Kidney Diseases, Bethesda, MD. Incidence and prevalence of ESRD. *American Journal of Kidney Diseases* **38** (Suppl. 3), S17–S36.

van Goor, H., Diamond, J. R., and Grond, J. Renal disease induced in rats by puromycin aminonucleoside. In *Experimental and Genetic Rat Models of Chronic Renal Failure* (ed. N. Gretz and M. Strauch), pp. 68–81. Basel: Karger, 1993.

Verhagen, A. M., Attia, D. M., Koomans, H. A., and Joles, J. A. (2000). Male gender increases sensitivity to proteinuria induced by mild NOS inhibition in rats: role of sex hormones. *American Journal of Physiology* **279** (4), F664–F670.

Vesey, D. A. *et al.* (2002). Interleukin-1b induces human proximal tubule cell injury, α-smooth muscle actin expression and fibronectin production. *Kidney International* **62**, 31–40.

Vijayan, A., Franklin, S. C., Behrend, T., Hammerman, M. R., and Miller, S. B. (1999). Insulin-like growth factor-1 improves renal function in patients with endstage chronic renal failure. *American Journal of Physiology* **276**, 929–934.

Wang, J., Chen, X., Shi, S., Zhang, Y., and Tian, Y. (2002). Expression of matrix metalloproteinase-9 and tissue inhibitor of metalloproteinase-1 in IgA nephropathy. *Zhonghua Nei Ke Za Zhi* **41**, 75–78.

Wang, S. N., LaPage, J., and Hirschberg, R. (1999). Pathophysiologic glomerulotubular growth factor link. *Mineral Electrolyte and Metabolism* **25**, 234–241.

Wang, S. N., LaPage, J., and Hirschberg, R. (2000). Role of glomerular ultrafiltration of growth factors in progressive interstitial fibrosis in diabetic nephropathy. *Kidney International* **57**, 1002–1014.

Wang, Y., Chen, J., Chen, L., Tay, Y. C., Rangan, G. K., and Harris, D. C. (1997). Induction of monocyte chemoattractant protein-1 in proximal tubule cells by urinary protein. *Journal of the American Society of Nephrology* **8**, 1537–1545.

Wardle, E. N. (2000). Nuclear factor kappaB for the nephrologist. *Nephrology, Dialysis, Transplantation* **16**, 764–768.

Wardle, E. N. (2002). Antagonism of nuclear factor kappa B. *Nephron* **90**, 239–240.

Wasserman, J., Santiago, A., Rifici, V., Holthofer, H., Scharschmidt, L., Epstein, M., and Schlondorff, D. (1989). Interactions of low density lipoprotein with rat mesangial cells. *Kidney International* **35**, 1168–1174.

Weening, J. J., Beukers, J. J. B., Grond, J., and Elema, J. D. (1986). Genetic factors in focal segmental glomerulosclerosis. *Kidney International* **29**, 789–798.

Welch, W. J., Tojo, A., and Wilcox, C. S. (2000). Roles of NO and oxygen radicals in tubuloglomerular feedback in SHR. *American Journal of Physiology* **278**, F769–F776.

Wenzel, U., Thaiss, F., Helmchen, U., Stahl, R. A. K., and Wolf, G. (2002). Angiotensin II infusion ameliorates the early phase of a mesangial mesangioproliferative glomerulonephritis. *Kidney International* **61**, 1020–1029.

Wiggins, R. C., Goyal, M., Merritt, S. E., and Killen, P. D. (1993). Vascular adventitial cell expression of collagen I messenger ribonucleic acid in anti-glomerular basement membrane antibody-induced crescentic nephritis in the rabbit. A cellular source for interstitial collagen synthesis in inflammatory renal disease. *Laboratory Investigation* **68**, 557–565.

Wilson, C. and Byrom, F. B. (1941). The vicious circle in chronic Bright's disease. Experimental evidence from the hypertensive rat. *Quarterly Journal of Medicine* **38**, 65–93.

Wolf, G. (2001). Angiotensin II as a renal growth factor. *Contribution to Nephrology* **135**, 92–110.

Wu, J. C., Fan, G. M., Kitazawa, K., and Sugisaki, T. (1996). The relationship of adhesion molecules and leukocyte infiltration in chronic tubulointerstitial nephritis induced by puromycin aminonucleoside in Wistar rats. *Clinical Immunology and Immunopathology* **79**, 229–235.

Wu, L. L., Cox, A., Roe, C. J., Dziadek, M., Cooper, M. E., and Gilbert, R. E. (1997). Secreted protein acidic and rich in cysteine expression after sub-total nephrectomy and blockade of the renin–angiotensin system. *Journal of the American Society of Nephrology* **8**, 1373–1382.

Wyndham, J. R., Everitt, A. V., Eyland, A., and Major, J. (1987). Inhibitory effect of hypophysectomy and food restriction on glomerular basement membrane thickening, proteinuria and renal enlargement in ageing male Wistar rats. *Archives of Gerontology and Geriatrics* **6**, 323–337.

Xue, J. L., Ma, J. Z., Liu, T. A., and Collins, A. J. (2001). Forecast of the number of patients with end stage renal disease in the United States to the year 2110. *Journal of the American Society of Nephrology* **12**, 2753–2758.

Yamagishi, H., Yokoo, T., Imasawa, T., Mitarai, T., Kawamura, T., and Utsunomiya, Y. (2001). Genetically modified bone marrow-derived vehicle cells site specifically deliver an anti-inflammatory cytokine to inflamed interstitium of obstructive nephropathy. *Journal of Immunology* **166**, 609–616.

Yamamoto, T., Noble, N. A., Miller, D. E., and Border, W. A. (1994). Sustained expression of TGF-β_1 underlies development of progressive kidney fibrosis. *Kidney International* **45**, 916–927.

Yamamoto, Y. *et al.* (2001). Development and prevention of advanced diabetic nephropathy in RAGE-overexpressing mice. *Journal of Clinical Investigation* **108**, 261–268.

Yamamura, Y. *et al.* (1994). Oral non-peptide vasopressin antagonists attenuate the progression of chronic renal failure in the rat. *Journal of the American Society of Nephrology* **5**, 674.

Yang, C. W., Striker, G. E., Chen, W. Y., Kopchick, J. J., and Striker, L. J. (1997). Differential expression of glomerular extracellular matrix and growth factor mRNA in rapid and slowly progressive glomerulosclerosis: studies in mice transgenic for native or mutated growth hormone. *Laboratory Investigation* **76**, 467–476.

Yang, J. and Liu, Y. (2002). Blockage of tubular epithelial to myofibroblast transition by hepatocyte growth factor prevents renal interstitial fibrosis. *Journal of the American Society of Nephrology* **13**, 96–107.

Yao, J., Morioka, T., Li, B., and Oite, T. (2001). Endothelin is a potent inhibitor of matrix metalloproteinase-2 secretion and activation in rat mesangial cells. *American Journal of Physiology* **280**, F628–F635.

Yard, B. A., Chorianopoulos, E., Herr, D., and van der Woude, F. J. (2001). Regulation of endothelin-1 and transforming growth factor-beta1 production in cultured proximal tubular cells by albumin and heparan sulphate glycosaminoglycans. *Nephrology, Dialysis, Transplantation* **16**, 1769–1775.

Ying, W. Z. and Sanders, P. W. (1998). Dietary salt modulates renal production of transforming growth factor-beta in rats. *American Journal of Physiology* **274**, 635–641.

Yokoo, T. *et al.* (1999). Prophylaxis of antibody-induced acute glomerulo-nephritis with genetically modified bone marrow-derived vehicle cells. *Human Gene Therapy* **10**, 2673–2678.

Yu, H., Sale, M., Rich, S. S., Spray, B. J., Roh, B. H., Bowden, D. W., and Freedman, B. I. (1999). Evaluation of markers on human chromosome 10, including the homologue of the rodent Rf-1 gene, for linkage to ESRD in black patients. *American Journal of Kidney Diseases* **33**, 294–300.

Yu, L., Noble, N. A., and Border, W. A. (2002). Therapeutic strategies to halt renal fibrosis. *Current Opinion in Pharmacology* **2**, 177–181.

Zaoui, P. *et al.* (2000). Role of metalloproteases and inhibitors in the occurrence and progression of diabetic renal lesions. *Diabetes and Metabolism* **26** (Suppl. 4), 25–29.

Zatz, R., and Baylis, C. (1998). Chronic nitric oxide inhibition model six years on. *Hypertension* **32**, 958–964.

Zeier, M. and Gretz, N. The influence of gender on the progression of renal failure. In *Experimental and Genetic Models of Chronic Renal Failure* (ed. N. Gretz and M. Strauch), pp. 250–257. Basel: Karger, 1993.

Zeisberg, M., Strutz, F., and Muller, G. A. (2000). Role of fibroblast activation in inducing interstitial fibrosis. *Journal of Nephrology* **13** (Suppl. 3), S111–S120.

Zeisberg, M., Strutz, F., and Muller, G. A. (2001). Renal fibrosis: an update. *Current Opinion in Nephrology and Hypertension* **10**, 315–320.

Zheng, F., Striker, G. E., Esposito, C., Lupia, E., and Striker, L. J. (1998). Strain differences rather than hyperglycemia determine the severity of glomerulosclerosis in mice. *Kidney International* **54**, 1999–2007.

Zoja, C., Benigni, A., and Remuzzi, G. (1999). Protein overload activates proximal tubular cells to release vasoactive and inflammatory mediators. *Experimental Nephrology* **7**, 420–428.

Zoja, C. *et al.* (2002). How to fully protect the kidney in a severe model of progressive nephropathy: a multidrug approach. *Journal of the American Society of Nephrology* **13**, 2898–2908.

Zuchelli, P. and Zuccala, A. Mechanisms of progression: the role of vascular injury/sclerosis. In *Prevention of Progressive Chronic Renal Failure* Vol. 1 (ed. A. M. El Nahas, N. P. Mallick, and S. Anderson), pp. 98–116. Oxford: Oxford University Press, 1993.

11.2 Assessment and initial management of the patient with failing renal function

Michael J.D. Cassidy and Pieter M. Ter Wee

In the United Kingdom, it is estimated that the dialysis population will double in the next 15 years. Elderly patients with diabetes mellitus and hypertension will account for the majority of the increase. The extent of the problem is illustrated by a recent study reporting a prevalence of renal impairment (a serum creatinine of >120 μmol/l) of 6.1 per cent in known hypertensives, 12.6 per cent in known diabetics, and 16.9 per cent in patients with both these conditions in the age group 50–75 years (Ellis and Cairns 2001). These patients were detected by routine screening in a primary health care setting. It is possible that there may be a reduction in the estimation of this gloomy prediction with early prevention of progression of renal disease. Future recommendations will include early referral of patients found to have impaired renal function to a nephrologist to establish a diagnosis, to recommend initial treatment and to draw up joint management plans with the primary care physician. Future recommendations are likely to suggest referral to a nephrologist when serum creatinine exceeds 150 μmol/l in men and 120 μmol/l in women corresponding to a glomerular filtration rate (GFR) of 50–60 ml/min. As it has been estimated that 12.3 per cent of the population of the United States has a GFR of less than 60 ml/min (Jones *et al.* 1998), there will have to be considerable investment in nephrological services to achieve this goal. In practice, the stage of renal failure and the extent of prior investigation at the time of referral vary widely.

Most patients are sent in a stable state to the renal outpatient clinic. At the first visit a thorough medical history and physical examination are obtained and the patient's previous case records are carefully scrutinized. Additional investigations are carried out to fill in the gaps. Thus, a diagnosis can be established and decisions about management may be made. The general practitioner is kept closely informed and should play an important part in follow-up.

Some patients present as an 'acute uraemic emergency' with a short history and no diagnosis; they are first resuscitated and then investigated to detect or exclude an acute renal condition which will require specific treatment. Thereafter, establishing a diagnosis can proceed at leisure in those countries where there are adequate facilities for the treatment of chronic renal failure.

This chapter is divided into two sections. The first section describes the initial assessment, the purpose of which is to establish the primary diagnosis when possible and in all cases to detect or exclude reversible causes of renal failure and those which affect decisions about renal transplantation or require family screening and genetic counselling; to detect acute-on-chronic renal failure; and to recognize involvement of other systems by the primary disease or concomitant illnesses. The second section describes the initial treatment and follow-up of the patient with renal insufficiency.

Establishing a diagnosis

In a uraemic emergency

In an uraemic emergency, the history is focused on the mechanisms that cause acute renal failure. These are conventionally divided into prerenal, renal, and postrenal (Table 1) (see also Section 10).

Prerenal causes

The prerenal causes of renal failure result from insufficient perfusion of the kidneys. This may be caused by a decreased (effective) circulating blood volume, or renal vascular disease (Chapter 9.7). An absolute decrease in blood volume occurs with blood loss due to trauma or gastrointestinal bleeding, or dehydration, due to diarrhoea, severe burns, hyperglycaemia, or overuse of diuretics. In the absence of such an evident cause, hypovolaemia should be suspected if there is thirst and dizziness due to postural hypotension.

A decreased effective circulating volume is characterized by a diminished intravascular volume despite an increase in total body sodium and water, which are sequestered in the intercellular space (oedema), abdominal cavity (ascites), or thorax (pleural effusion). This can be caused by cardiac failure as a result of myocardial infarction, myocardial ischaemia, long-standing hypertension, or cardiomyopathy. A history of chest pain, orthopnoea, effort dyspnoea, and weight gain due to oedema may indicate renal insufficiency secondary to cardiac failure. Another cause of a decreased effective circulating volume is the hepatorenal syndrome. This may occur in acute liver failure, in which general discomfort, fever, and jaundice may be present, or in liver cirrhosis when it is often accompanied by ascites, haematemesis due to gastric ulcers or oesophageal varices, and/or coma (Chapter 10.6.4). A severe form of decreased effective circulating volume is septic shock. This may complicate pneumonia, meningitis, peritonitis, and pyelonephritis (Chapter 7.1); fever and rigors are frequently present. The overuse of antihypertensive agents may cause hypotension resulting in renal hypoperfusion. Measurement of urinary sodium, osmolality, urea, and creatinine is useful in distinguishing prerenal uraemia from acute tubular necrosis; a concentrated urine with a sodium content less than 10 mmol/l and a fractional sodium, excretion of less than 1 per cent are usual in the former.

Renal causes

Almost any of the renal causes listed in the next section can present as a uraemic emergency, but often when the kidneys are already largely destroyed after a long insidious illness. The urgent task is to detect reversible forms of acute renal disease. Acute interstitial nephritis

(Chapter 10.6.2) is suggested by a history of ingestion of drugs that cause it, notably non-steroidal anti-inflammatory agents and penicillins, and by skin rash and eosinophilia; Hantavirus infection (Chapter 10.6.6) by exposure to carriers such as voles and rats and by haemorrhagic lesions; Weil's disease by exposure to rat-infested water,

Table 1 Mechanisms underlying the development of both acute and chronic renal failure

Prerenal causes (that aggravate pre-existing chronic renal failure)
Absolute decrease in blood volume
    Gastrointestinal bleeding
    Trauma
    Dehydration
Decreased effective circulating volume
    Cardiac failure
    Hepatorenal syndrome
    Septic shock
    Overuse of antihypertensive agents
Renal artery stenosis

Renal causes
Functional change
    NSAIDs, ACE inhibitors
Renal diseases
    Postinfectious glomerulonephritis
    Other primary glomerulopathies (membranous, mesangiocapillary, etc.)
Interstitial nephritis
    Acute, allergic [numerous drugs (Chapter 10.6.3)]
    Chronic—reflux nephropathy
    Secondary pyelonephritis
    Analgesic nephropathy
    Chinese herb nephropathy
Hereditary diseases
    Autosomal dominant polycystic kidney disease
    Alport's disease
    Many rarer congenital diseases (Section 16, Chapter 17.3)
Systemic disease with renal involvement
    Diabetes mellitus
    Essential hypertension
    Systemic lupus erythematosus
    Systemic sclerosis
    Amyloidosis
        Primary
        Secondary (rheumatoid arthritis, tuberculosis, etc.)
    Vasculitis
        Wegener's granulomatosis
        Polyarteritis
        Isolated renal vasculitis
    Goodpasture's syndrome
Microangiopathic syndromes
    Haemolytic uraemic syndrome
        Drug induced
        Postpartum
    Disseminated intravascular coagulation
    Accelerated hypertension
    Antiphospholipid syndrome

Postrenal causes
Prostatic hypertrophy
Retroperitoneal fibrosis/tumours
Renal calculi

jaundice, and haemorrhage. Rapidly progressive glomerulonephritis (Chapters 3.10 and 3.11) is recognized by the very active urinary deposit with numerous red cell casts and by the features of the diseases causing it such as lung haemorrhage in Goodpasture's syndrome and systemic vasculitis (Chapters 3.11 and 4.5.3), skin lesions (Fig. 1), splinter haemorrhages (Fig. 2), and retinal haemorrhages in the latter; Wegener's granulomatosis by purulent secretion from the nose, epistaxis, and rarely a saddle nose (Fig. 3). Systemic lupus (Chapter 4.7.2) may be suggested by butterfly rash (easily overlooked in the dark-skinned races), joint pains, and fever. Drugs and toxins must always be considered and a careful history, including the use of over-the-counter medication or visits to traditional healers when appropriate, may disclose a potential cause.

Postrenal causes

Obstruction of both ureters, or the ureter to the single functioning kidney, must always be excluded as a cause of an unexplained acute uraemic emergency. Ultrasonography of the renal tract is an essential investigation but clinical clues should also be sought. Pelvic examination (for carcinoma of the cervix), rectal examination, and urine

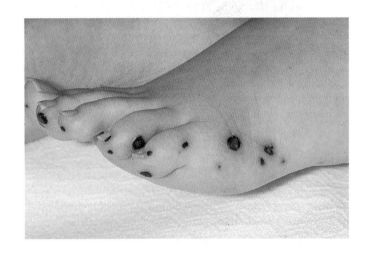

Fig. 1 Skin infarcts caused by systemic vasculitis.

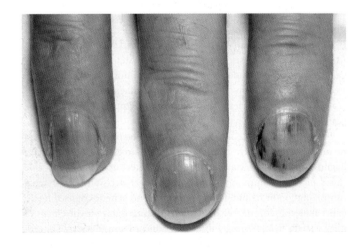

Fig. 2 Splinter haemorrhages in a patient with systemic vasculitis.

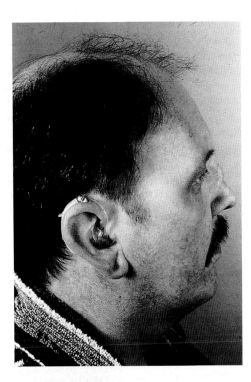

Fig. 3 A 40-year-old man with Wegener's granulomatosis who presented with a rapidly progressive glomerulonephritis. Two clinical clues to the underlying diagnosis can be seen in this photograph; a hearing aid and the collapsed bridge of his nose.

cytology (for bladder tumours) are often omitted, with embarrassing or serious consequences, and the vague presenting symptoms of retroperitoneal fibrosis (Chapter 17.3) ensure that it is still one of the diagnoses missed even by experienced clinicians.

In chronic renal disease

When the patient presents with chronic renal disease and is referred early in the course of the disease, the need for a diagnosis is self-evident. The difficulty of obtaining a precise diagnosis increases as the patient approaches endstage and the rewards diminish. Consequently, a substantial proportion of patients starting dialysis have no more precise a diagnosis than 'chronic renal failure, cause unknown'. Although we acknowledge the difficulty of establishing a firm diagnosis in some patients presenting in late renal failure with small fibrotic kidneys, we advocate a vigorous diagnostic approach in all others, since a precise diagnosis is valuable in identifying the groups of diseases causing renal failure which affect patient management. In addition, this approach has identified an over-representation of certain histopathological conditions such as idiopathic interstitial nephritis and focal segmental sclerosis in the UK Indo-Asian population.

Renal causes

Renal insufficiency can ensue from a primary renal disease or a systemic disease which affects the kidneys. In the glomerulonephritides, renal involvement may manifest as haematuria, signs of a nephrotic syndrome (tiredness, weight gain, oedema, susceptibility to infection, hyperlipidaemia), and/or hypertension. With more frequent, regular

health screening in well women and men clinics, one of the most common presentations of chronic glomerulonephritis, of which IgA nephropathy is the most frequent (Chapter 3.6), is the detection of dipstix proteinuria and or haematuria, hypertension or an elevated serum creatinine in an asymptomatic patient. The variable and usually prolonged natural history of IgA nephropathy has made it difficult to predict progression to end stage renal failure on an individual basis. There are well-known poor prognostic indicators (D'Amico 2000) and recently these have been refined (Bartosik *et al.* 2001). Enquiry should be made about recent infections and the duration between any infection and the development of symptoms suggestive of renal disease. Especially in childhood, a non-specific infection may be followed by a combination of haematuria, purpura, arthritis of the large joints, and abdominal symptoms (pain, melaena, haematemesis) characteristic of Henoch–Schönlein nephritis (Chapter 4.5.2). Poststreptococcal glomerulonephritis follows a β-haemolytic streptococcal infection, usually 10–21 days after acute tonsillitis in developed countries or up to 6 weeks after impetigo, often complicating scabies, in tropical countries. Postinfectious glomerulonephritis may also develop as a result of many other infections (Chapter 3.12) including endocarditis, during which fever together with a cardiac murmur as well as systemic symptoms usually exist. HIV-associated nephropathy (HIVAN) is a major problem in certain geographical locations. This is well known to be the case in sub-Saharan Africa, for example. It is also a major problem in large urban communities in the United States with high Black and Hispanic populations; HIVAN is the third leading cause of endstage renal failure (ESRF) in the United States in Blacks aged 20–64 years (Winston *et al.* 1998).

Reflux nephropathy (Chapter 17.2) is usually diagnosed in childhood during investigation of urinary infection or screening in families with the condition. It may, however, escape discovery until adult life when it is detected during investigation of urinary infection, especially in pregnancy, hypertension, or renal failure. Though often silent, there may be a history of recurrent episodes of flank pain, dysuria, fever, and rigors. Renal failure from this cause in adult life peaks in the twenties and thirties and is uncommon after the age of 50. The long-term renal prognosis is excellent in patients presenting with a serum creatinine of less than 90 μmol/l (Goodship 2000). Secondary chronic pyelonephritis should be suspected in patients with renal failure and a history of stone disease, obstruction, or neuropathic bladder, for example, following spina bifida or spinal injury.

In Western Europe, renal tuberculosis is rare but its incidence is increasing due to the enlarging immigrant population. Multidrug-resistant tuberculosis also is becoming more prevalent, especially in Eastern Europe, Iran, and China. Classically, it presents with dysuria, fever, and sterile pyuria and is confirmed by urine culture and renal imaging (Chapter 7.4). Occasionally, the classical form presents with renal failure, in the absence of symptoms pointing to the urinary tract, following silent irreversible destruction of renal parenchyma, recognized on renal imaging by the calcified renal substance, or, more commonly, reversible bilateral ureteric obstruction (Lazarus and Peraino 1984). In the British immigrant population from the Indian subcontinent, interstitial renal tuberculosis causes renal failure with small kidneys on imaging, and without the tell-tale renal calcification, the diagnosis is made by renal biopsy or inferred from evidence of tuberculosis in other systems (Lightstone *et al.* 1995). Other infections associated with ESRF that show a geographic variation include schistosomiasis, which is an important cause of end-stage renal failure in

Egypt and HIVAN, which may present as a nephritic syndrome and rapidly progressive renal failure accounting for up to 38 per cent of patients on dialysis programmes in some US inner-city communities (Pastan and Bailey 1998).

The medication history should include agents bought over the counter as well as those prescribed and used recreationally. An example of particular importance in view of its silent onset and often irreversible nature is Chinese herb nephropathy (Chapter 6.9). Fibrosis and tubulointerstitial changes persist for months or years after discontinuation of the toxin though slow recovery may occur if the agent is stopped. This condition is also of particular importance as the toxic culprit (*Aristolochia fangchi*) is also carcinogenic, patients should therefore have regular follow-up to exclude urothelial tumours. Some authors have recommended the prophylactic removal of native kidneys and ureters and annual cystoscopy in these patients once on dialysis or transplanted (Nortier *et al.* 2000). Non-steroidal anti-inflammatory agents have been mentioned as a cause of acute renal failure, often accompanied by the nephrotic syndrome. They also cause an acute reduction in GFR in patients with primary and secondary glomerulonephritis, due to inhibition of vasodilatory prostaglandins, which is reversed on withdrawal of the drug (Murray and Brater 1993). Selective COX-2 agents have also been associated with adverse effects on renal function in susceptible individuals as well as causing acute interstitial nephritis. Whether they also cause a nephrotic syndrome or papillary necrosis is not yet known. The term analgesic nephropathy is usually reserved for the chronic interstitial nephritis caused by prolonged high consumption of analgesics (Chapter 6.2). It remains an important cause of renal failure in some parts of the world, for example in Queensland, Australia the incidence increased to 10 per cent of new patients in 1999, primarily in the 65–74 year age group [ANZDATA (2000) 23rd Annual Report]. The great majority of cases are caused by consumption of mixtures of analgesics; single drugs such as aspirin and paracetamol are seldom incriminated as opposed to regular use of NSAIDs (Perneger *et al.* 1994; De Broe and Elseviers 1998). Long-term regular use of both paracetamol and aspirin have also been associated with increasing the risk of developing chronic renal failure from whatever cause by a factor of 2.5 (Fored *et al.* 2001). Detection of analgesic abuse is sometimes difficult, since it is often denied by the patient, but a history can often be obtained by judicious questioning, concentrating on chronic pain and inserting the question of analgesic intake sympathetically in that context, or by interviewing relatives. There may be a history of flank pain or haematuria due to a sloughed papilla. There is frequently a concomitant history of heavy smoking and alcohol intake, minor or major personality disorders, and symptoms of peptic ulcer if the analgesics contain aspirin. Pyuria, with or without infection, is almost universal at the stage of renal failure. Methaemoglobinaemia may be detected if the analgesic contains phenacetin. Again, urothelial malignancy is more common in this group of patients so annual urine cytology is recommended.

Angiotensin-converting enzyme (ACE) inhibitors are being used more frequently in elderly patients. Impressive results in recent studies, such from the PROGRESS (Perindopril Protection Against Recurrent Stroke Study) collaborative in secondary prevention of stroke recommends consideration of use of perinderopril and indapamide routinely in all patients whether hypertensive or not who have had a stroke or transient ischaemic attack. Similarly, the HOPE (Hypertension Outcomes Prevention Evaluation) study demonstrated a significant reduction in risks of further cardiac events reducing mortality. Despite their common use, progressive renal failure secondary to ACE inhibition, frequently in high risk patients, is uncommon. They and angiotensin II receptor antagonists may cause renal insufficiency in the presence of bilateral renal artery stenosis or renal artery stenosis in subjects with a single kidney due to renal hypoperfusion. This is especially the case when there is a history of atherosclerotic vascular disease and in those at high risk such as an elderly diabetic with angina pectoris and intermittent claudication, and in such cases it is essential to check renal function within one week of commencing an ACE inhibitor and carefully monitor renal function thereafter. It is also important to warn the patient and the general practitioner that dehydration (either by the addition of diuretic therapy or an episode of gastroenteritis) may precipitate renal failure. Early withdrawal of the drug in such situations usually reverses renal insufficiency. Interestingly, in the SOLVD (Studies of Left Ventricular Dysfunction) study, there was a renoprotective effect when β-blockers were used in conjunction with ACE inhibitors. This, and the concern regarding uraemia with their use is reviewed by Bar (1999).

Substance abuse is becoming more common (it is estimated that over 40 per cent of young people have tried illicit drugs at sometime in the United Kingdom); these drugs may affect the kidney in a variety of different ways including the development of progressive renal failure (Crowe *et al.* 2000). Though heroin-associated nephropathy was an important cause of ESRF in New York, there has been a significant decline of this cause of ESRF as the purity of the street drug has improved (Friedman and Tao 1995).

A family history may give diagnostic clues. The most frequent hereditary cause of renal failure is autosomal dominant polycystic kidney disease (APKD). Renal failure usually occurs in the third to fifth decade, and the family history is positive in about 75 per cent of the cases. The diagnosis is frequently made prior to the onset of renal insufficiency, either during the screening of family members, or at presentation with haematuria, flank pain, urinary tract infection, or hypertension. Similarly, a positive family history is usual in the more rare types of renal cystic disease such as tuberous sclerosis and medullary cystic disease (Fick and Gabow 1994). Another important hereditary condition is Alport's syndrome (Chapter 16.4.1), which is characterized by progressive nephritis with haematuria and sensori-neural hearing loss in successive generations of a family. Affected children have microscopic haematuria and 50 per cent manifest gross haematuria often before age 5. Opthalmoscopy may reveal lenticonus. Genetic diseases should be sought assiduously in infants and children with renal failure; the numerous causes are described in Section 16. Diagnoses of other genetic conditions such as Fabry's disease may be missed because of their sometimes obscure symptomatology and their rarity. (In Fabry's disease, the incidence has been calculated in two separate studies as 1 in 1,17,000 and 1 in 4,76,000 live births.) It is now important not to miss this condition because there is effective enzyme replacement therapy and the potential for cure with gene therapy. A valuable resource increasingly used by patients and their relatives are internet sites devoted to the condition. The physician would do well to visit these also; examples relating to this paragraph include http://www.pkdcure.org (for polycystic kidney disease) and http://www.tuberous-sclerosis.org.

Systemic diseases

The most frequent cause of renal involvement in a disease affecting other organs is diabetes mellitus (Chapter 4.1). Renal involvement occurs at least as frequently in type II as in type I diabetes. The increasing prevalence of renal failure in the developed world in particular is predominantly accounted for by type II diabetics (Hostetter 2001). The number is certain to increase with the expected doubling of the prevalence of diabetes in the world over the next 10 years. Type II diabetes is also occurring earlier and even in childhood. Proteinuria due to diabetic nephropathy in type II diabetes is a strong predictor of death from associated macrovascular disease, and many patients die from cardiovascular events before commencing dialysis. Renal insufficiency in subjects with insulin-dependent diabetes mellitus and a disease duration exceeding 5 years together with heavy proteinuria, hypertension and retinopathy is highly suspicious of diabetic nephropathy. Once developed, a progressive deterioration in GFR is relentless, though highly variable (median loss 12 ml/min/year, range 1–24 ml/min/year). Accelerated essential hypertension characteristically causes acute renal failure. The clinical clues include papilloedema on fundal examination, anaemia with fragments on the blood film, a raised serum LDH, and hypokalaemia. Long-standing 'benign' hypertension is also an important cause of chronic renal failure, particularly in the elderly age group, but is difficult to differentiate from occult renal diseases with secondary hypertension except by renal biopsy. In systemic lupus erythematosus (SLE) (Chapter 4.7.2), a renal biopsy should be performed in any patient with proteinuria or an abnormal urinary sediment, and therefore most patients should have had one by the time of their initial assessment for renal insufficiency. Secondary amyloidosis should be suspected when chronic renal failure complicates long-standing inflammatory diseases, for example, severe rheumatoid arthritis or chronic infections such as destructive lung disease due to tuberculosis; it often presents as a nephrotic syndrome. Making the diagnosis is important, as regression and clinical improvement may occur by treating the underlying disease (Iggo et al. 2000). Primary amyloidosis, due to the proliferation of a single clone of plasma cells, frequently presents silently in middle and old age with renal insufficiency and proteinuria. The majority of patients with AL amyloidosis have a monoclonal protein in their serum or urine. Treatment remains unsatisfactory; the key will come with elimination of the plasma cell clone. In patients with plasma cell dyscrasias, renal failure may also result from myeloma cast nephropathy, light chain deposition disease, or the hyperviscosity syndrome (Chapter 4.3). A group of diseases characterized by systemic vasculitis may cause rapidly progressive renal failure (Chapters 4.5.3). A history of haemoptysis and dyspnoea, together with rapidly deteriorating renal function and an active urine sediment, suggest antiglomerular basement membrane disease (Goodpasture's syndrome) but can also occur in systemic vasculitis. Rapidly progressive renal failure in association with symptoms of persistent sinusitis (epistaxis, rhinorrhoea, nasal discomfort) or otitis, together with dyspnoea, cough, and haemoptysis, are suspect for Wegener's disease. Commonly, general discomfort, weight loss, and fever are present. If symptoms of respiratory tract disease are lacking, a diagnosis of microscopic polyarteritis nodosa is more likely, although considerable overlap exists. Finally, renal failure may result from a thrombotic microangiopathy caused by disseminated intravascular coagulation, primary antiphospholipid syndrome, haemolytic uraemic syndrome, or thrombotic thrombocytopenic purpura.

There are few recognized occupational renal diseases, but lead toxicity is worth excluding. Since the introduction of higher industrial standards, chronic lead intoxication has virtually disappeared in Europe but there is a high prevalence of elevated body lead in patients with varying degrees of renal failure, partly reflecting occupational exposure before these precautions were imposed (Staessen et al. 1992). It is particularly important to think of covert lead intoxication in patients with hyperuricaemia, hypertension, and small kidneys. The diagnosis is best made by demonstrating an increase in urinary lead excretion following an infusion of EDTA. More recently, long-term occupational or environmental exposure to relatively low levels of cadmium has been shown to contribute to the development of chronic renal failure (Hellström et al. 2001).

Postrenal causes

Obstruction of the lower urinary tract is common in elderly males and is usually symptomatic. The diagnostic problem is that 40 per cent of men over the age of 65 have some of the symptoms of prostatic hypertrophy: hesitancy, slow and forked stream, urgency with or without urge incontinence, frequency, intermittency, nocturia, and terminal dribbling (Gofin 1982). The severity of symptoms and prostate size both correlate poorly with the degree of obstruction which can only be accurately assessed by urodynamic studies. Pressure-flow measurements have shown that two-thirds of patients with such symptoms have some degree of outflow obstruction and are at risk of urinary retention (Jacobsen et al. 1995). A useful clinical clue to serious outflow obstruction is palpation of a distended bladder after micturition; this can be confirmed more reliably by ultrasonography before and after micturition.

Obstruction due to retroperitoneal fibrosis, sloughed papillae, and renal calculi induces hydronephrosis and a deterioration of renal function.

Physical examination

At the patient's first visit, body height and weight, temperature, central venous pressure, pulse rate, and blood pressure, with the patient lying and standing, should be recorded. Postural hypotension suggests a low central blood volume, overdosing of antihypertensives or autonomic neuropathy, particularly in diabetics; signs of depleted extracellular volume should be sought. Reduced skin turgor and eye ball pressure are unreliable signs of dehydration, especially in the elderly, compared to postural hypotension and a low jugular venous pressure. The more common problem in stable chronic renal failure is oedema which should be sought in the orbits, ankles and, in patients in bed, the sacrum, and backs of thighs. It is found in the nephrotic syndrome and in late chronic renal failure from sodium and water overload or from cardiac failure. The presence of fever, unexplained by an obvious infection, should alert the nephrologist to the possibility of endocarditis, shunt nephritis, systemic vasculitis, SLE, and urinary infection complicating reflux nephropathy, stones, or polycystic disease.

A full standard physical examination, as taught at medical school, but seldom practised in busy outpatient clinics, pays dividends. The nephrologist must be alert for a wide variety of clinical features of primary diseases, a few of which are illustrated here. General observation may provide clues such as the body habitus of Lawrence Moon Biedl syndrome (a rare cause of chronic renal failure) or the dyed hair and nicotine-stained fingers associated with analgesic nephropathy in some cultures. Purulent secretion of the nose with epistaxis and, rarely, a saddle nose (Fig. 3) may be present in Wegener's disease. Deafness in young males indicates Alport's disease. Careful examination of the skin provides many clues. SLE may be suspected from the classical butterfly rash, gingival ulcers, changes in the nail fold capillaries, best viewed through a high power lens or skin microscope, or polyarthropathy. Skin infarcts (Fig. 1), splinter haemorrhages (Fig. 2), and retinal haemorrhages and exudates, not explained by severe hypertension, should suggest systemic vasculitis. Livedo reticularis is found in cholesterol embolization, oxalosis, and some autoimmune diseases. Characteristic nail changes are seen in the nail-patella syndrome. The striking facial appearances of adenoma sebaceum (Fig. 4) should raise the suspicion of tuberosclerosis.

Cardiac examination may detect the murmurs of endocarditis as well as the effects of hypertension and fluid overload (functional murmurs of mitral and aortic incompetence in late renal failure) or the friction rub of pericarditis in endstage renal disease. Chest examination may reveal the râles and rhonchi accompanying Goodpasture's syndrome, Wegener's granulomatosis, Churg–Strauss syndrome, and microscopic polyarteritis nodosa which must be distinguished from more common causes such as fluid overload, bronchitis, and pneumonia. Examination of the abdomen should focus on the presence of ascites, distended bladder after voiding (Fig. 5), palpation of the kidneys for masses (polycystic disease, hydronephrosis, bladder tumours), or tenderness. An enlarged hard liver suggests polycystic disease among other possibilities and, splenomegaly or lymphadenopathy are clues to amyloidosis, lymphomas or AIDS. Pelvic examination may reveal an enlarged prostate or a pelvic mass causing urinary obstruction.

The neurological examination may detect the neuropathies associated with diabetes, polyarteritis, Wegener's granulomatosis, and primary amyloidosis. Full examination of the eyes is important. Dilatation of the pupils is essential in the presence of diabetes or hypertension. In late renal failure it may reveal complications such as corneal calcification, best seen with a slit lamp or an ophthalmoscope with a +20 leans at right angles to the line of vision, pingueculae which are more unsightly than symptomatic, or rarely the 'uraemic red eye' of acute hypercalcaemia usually precipitated by overdose of vitamin D analogues (Fig. 6).

Laboratory investigations (Table 2)

Urine

Careful investigation of urine is essential. Dipstix analysis, urine microscopy, and quantitative analysis of a urine sample, and 24-h urine volume should be performed.

Dipstix examination

The dipstix examination of a fresh urine sample is the preferred step to assess the urinary pH and screen for the presence of leucocyturia, proteinuria, haematuria, and glucosuria. The pH is usually low in chronic renal failure, unless the patient is on a very low protein diet. A high pH raises suspicion of urinary infection with organisms

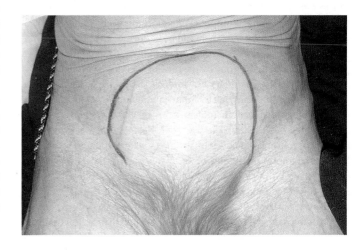

Fig. 5 Distended bladder after voiding in an elderly man. The absence of pain when the bladder contained well over a litre of urine indicated chronic obstruction.

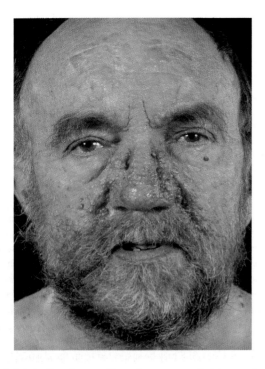

Fig. 4 Epiloia is often diagnosed from the presence of adenoma sebaceum.

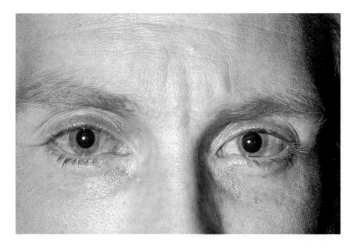

Fig. 6 'Uraemic red eye' that accompanied acute hypercalcaemia after immobilization for a pathological fracture of the femur caused by aluminium osteodystrophy.

Table 2 Laboratory investigations performed at the initial assessment of the patient with renal insufficiency

Test	Measurement (purpose)
Urine	
Dipstix	pH—detect infection, monitor diet
	Proteinuria ⎫
	Haematuria ⎬ Screening tests
	Glucosuria ⎪
	Pyuria ⎭
Urine sediment	Confirm pyuria
	Detect bacteriuria (confirm by culture)
	Confirm erythrocyturia
	Define red cell morphology
	Identify casts and crystals
Urine sodium	Sodium concentration
(acute uraemic presentation)	Fractional excretion of sodium
24-h urine	Quantify proteinuria
	Measure creatinine clearance (for GFR)
	Measure urinary urea (for protein intake)
	Measure urinary sodium (confirm intake)
Random urine	Bence Jones protein (detect paraproteinaemia)
	Protein to creatinine ratio (monitor proteinuria)
Midstream urine culture	Confirm infection
Blood	
Full blood count and reticulocytes,	Define type of anaemia
% hypochromic red cells	
Autoanalyser profile	Urea, creatinine (degree of uraemia)
	Bicarbonate (degree of acidosis)
	Ca, PO_4, alkaline phosphatase (detect bone disease)
	Glucose, HbA1c—detect/monitor diabetes
Serology	HBsAg (detect hepatitis B carrier)
	HBsAb (need for vaccination)
	HCAb Hepatitis C mRNA (detect hepatitis C carrier)
	HIV (determine HIV status)
	C3, C4, CH-50 (detect/monitor SLE, MCGN, etc.)
	ANF, anti-ds-DNA (detect SLE)
	ANCA, anti-GBM (detect/differentiate systemic
	vasculitis, anti-GBM disease)
	cryoglobulins (detect cryoglobulinaemia)
	Electrophoresis (detect paraproteins)
Imaging	
Chest radiograph	Assess cardiac size and volume status
	Document coincidental or related chest disease
Renal ultrasound	Document kidney size, cortical thickness, echogenicity
	Detect hydronephrosis, cystic diseases
	Detect stones
Plain radiograph of renal tract	Detect stones, nephrocalcinosis, vascular calcification
IVU, CT scan, MRI, renogram, angiogram	For specific indications
Electrocardiogram	Detect LVH and arrhythmias
Echocardiogram	Determine left ventricular function, assess valves, pericardium
Renal biopsy	For specific indications

ANCA, antineutrophil cytoplasmic antibody; ANF, antinuclear factor; ds, double-stranded; GBM, glomerular basement membrane; IVU, intravenous urogram; LVH, left ventricular hypertrophy; MCGN, mesangiocapillary glomerulonephritis; SLE, systemic lupus erythematosus; other abbreviations as in text.

that split urea. A false positive test for proteinuria may be seen in the presence of lysosymuria, which may occur in acute myeloid leukaemia. If the urine contains non-albumin proteinuria, then the dipstix will be negative, yet a 24-h protein will record protein. This can be confirmed by a simple side-room investigation of mixing urine with sulfosalicylic acid in equal quantities and looking for turbidity. This is a useful test in the early detection of myeloma. The test for blood is very sensitive and may give false positives if the sample is contaminated with some cleansing agents; this is best avoided by collecting the urine in a disposable plastic container.

Urine sediment

Microscopy of urine sediment may reveal erythrocytes, leucocytes, and casts. Careful examination of the erythrocytes' morphology with a phase contrast microscope can indicate whether they are of glomerular (dysmorphic, irregular size) or non-glomerular origin (monomorphic) (Fig. 7). Red cell casts are seen in glomerulonephritis (IgA, postinfectious, and SLE and in cases of vasculitis (Wegener's granulomatosis, polyarteritis nodosa, renal limited vasculitis). White cell casts identify pyuria as coming from the kidney and are found in stone disease, tuberculosis, analgesic nephropathy, and other causes of chronic interstitial nephritis. Crystals may be present to assist with the diagnosis of stone disease. Amorphous phosphates may interfere with the microscopy, and can be dissolved by a drop of acetic acid. Occasionally, the observer may be rewarded by a finding that clinches the diagnosis such as that seen in Fig. 8. An inactive urine sediment also provides valuable information, suggesting a diagnosis of obstruction or atheroembolic renal disease.

Quantitative analysis of 24-h urine volume

The 24-h urine is used to measure proteinuria, calculate creatinine clearance, and estimate daily protein and sodium chloride intake. Although proteinuria is almost universal in chronic renal failure, proteinuria in the nephrotic range is uncommon when serum creatinine concentration exceeds 800 mol/l. Its presence suggests one of a few diagnoses: diabetes, mesangiocapillary glomerulonephritis, amyloid, and the 'malignant' subtype of focal sclerosing glomerulonephritis. Compliance is checked by total urinary creatinine, which is fairly constant in individuals and varies in the range 10–14 mmol/24 h in females and 12–18 mmol/24 h in males of average build. If compliance is poor despite repeated instruction, proteinuria can be judged by the protein/creatinine ratio on a spot urine sample; a good correlation has been shown between this measurement and 24-h urinary protein (Kristal *et al.* 1988). The correlation is less good at the extremes of

creatinine excretion, for example, in muscular men and cachextic patients who will have high and low urinary creatinine concentrations, respectively.

Blood

Full blood count

A full blood with a reticulocyte count is important to establish the type of anaemia. Reticulocytosis and an elevated serum lactate dehydrogenase suggest haemolysis; a Coomb's test should be performed to exclude autoantibody-induced haemolysis, as can be present in SLE, usually associated with leucocytopenia. A peripheral blood smear may demonstrate the characteristic abnormalities of microangiopathic haemolytic anaemia (fragmented red cells, helmet-shaped erythrocytes, burr cells), which, in combination with thrombocytopenia is suggestive of the haemolytic uraemic syndrome or thrombotic thrombocytopenic purpura.

Autoanalyser

An autoanalyser profile is run to record the uraemic state. Serum creatinine concentration depends on the production and elimination of creatinine. With deteriorating GFR, tubular secretion of creatinine increases. A slightly elevated serum creatinine may be associated with a 50 per cent reduction in GFR, especially in older people with reduced muscle mass. Consequently, serum creatinine provides only a rough approximation of GFR (Levey *et al.* 1988). Because of the risk of arrhythmias, serum potassium is checked and the serum sodium provides information about the patient's fluid balance. In addition, clues for underlying diseases such as diabetes mellitus and liver failure are obtained.

Serological tests

Serological tests can give additional support in the assessment of a diagnosis. Which serological tests are performed depends on the case

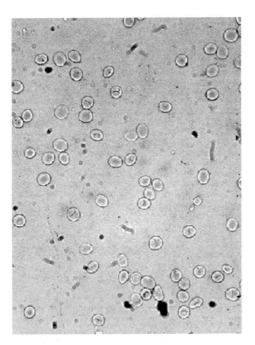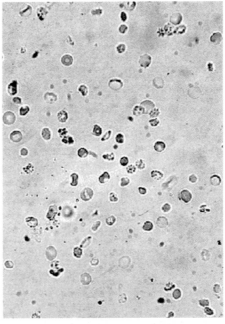

Fig. 7 Microscopy of fresh urine samples illustrating monomorphic red cells in a case of non-glomerular haematuria (on the left) and dysmorphic red cells from a patient with glomerulonephritis (on the right).

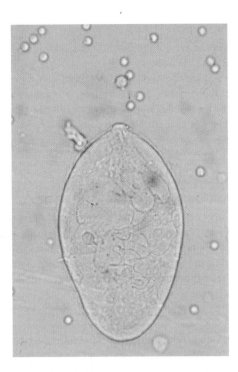

Fig. 8 Microscopy of a fresh urine sample from a 15-year-old boy with episodes of macroscopic haematuria revealed this schistosomal egg. An idea of the size can be determined from the surrounding red cells.

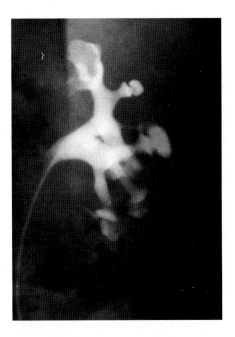

Fig. 9 Retrograde pyelogram in a patient with chronic renal failure due to analgesic nephropathy showing a 'ring sign' around a sloughed papilla in the upper pole and cavitated papillae opening into the other calyces. These features are usually shown by intravenous urography at an earlier stage of the disease.

history and the patient's urinalysis. Serum total haemolytic complement and C_3 can be decreased in mesangiocapillary glomerulonephritis, post-infectious glomerulonephritis (including endocarditis), cryoglobulinaemia, and lupus erythematosus. Elevated titres of serum antinuclear factor and anti-double-stranded DNA support the diagnosis lupus. In rapidly progressive renal failure with an active urine sediment, anti-glomerular basement membrane antibodies confirm a diagnosis of Goodpasture's disease. Antineutrophil cytoplasmic antibodies support a diagnosis of systemic necrotizing vasculitis. With ELISA techniques, these antibodies can be further characterized as being directed against antiproteinase 3, which is specific for Wegener's granulomatosis or against myeloperoxidase, which is more frequently associated with microscopic polyarteritis nodosa. HBsAg is associated with membranous glomerulopathy, IgA nephropathy, and mixed cryoglobulinaemia in areas of high endemicity. Hepatitis C virus (HCV) infection is associated with type 1 membranoproliferative glomerulonephritis and cryoglobulinaemia (see Chapter 3.8). Over 95 per cent of patients with mixed essential cryoglobulinaemia have evidence of HCV infection if looked for carefully, by testing for anti-HCV antibodies and examining the cryoprecipitate for polyclonal IgG anti-HCV antibodies and HCV RNA.

Radiological investigations

Of the radiological investigations that may help in the assessment of the patient with renal insufficiency, renal ultrasonography is particularly valuable. With this technique, renal size, thickness of renal cortex, and echogenicity can be determined, and cysts and hydronephrosis can be demonstrated. Its sensitivity for renal stones is less, and for this purpose, it is combined with straight radiography of the urinary tract. Calcified papillae of analgesic nephropathy are revealed by their sound shadow but that disease is more often detected by IVU (Fig. 9). Unlike

ultrasound, intravenous urography, computerized tomography with intravenous contrast, and arteriography, may be complicated by nephrotoxicity as well as the risks of iodine sensitivity. With the recent advances in diagnostic imaging, in particular, spiral computerized tomography and magnetic resonance imaging, angiography is required less frequently though it still has a place in diagnosing classical polyarteritis and renovascular disease. Magnetic resonance imaging is the gold standard in diagnosing renal vein thrombosis and is taking over from computerized tomography in assessing renal cell carcinoma. It has over 90 per cent sensitivity and also high specificity, though it may miss accessory renal arteries. Angiography remains the 'gold standard' for diagnosing renovascular disease. There is no necessity to admit patients, there is no arterial puncture, and the gadolinium used as a contrast agent is not nephrotoxic; these are significant advantages (see also Chapter 1.6.2.iv).

Renal biopsy (see also Chapter 1.7)

Many patients with chronic renal failure have had a renal biopsy performed earlier in the course of the disease. In others, it may have been unnecessary because the diagnosis was established on clinical grounds, for example, in diabetes. If the kidneys are small, the hazards of the procedure are increased and have to be weighed against the small chance of finding a reversible cause.

Renal biopsy should be performed in the patient presenting with renal impairment with no apparent cause either on clinical grounds or on review of earlier investigations, and with normal size kidneys, provided that there are no contraindications such as a coagulopathy or severe uncontrolled hypertension. The importance of a biopsy in this type of patient is underscored by renal biopsy findings in 109 patients from St Bartholomew's Hospital with unexplained renal failure and normal sized kidneys where the most common histological findings were interstitial nephritis and glomerulonephritis, including rapidly progressive glomerulonephritis (Farrington *et al.* 1988).

Establishing chronicity

This section deals with the patient who presents in renal failure with no previous medical history to help in distinguishing acute and chronic renal failure. The manifestations of chronicity that are helpful in making a clinical judgement and deciding on the need for renal biopsy are listed in Table 3.

Nocturia

A history of nocturia coming on for the first time a few months or years before the patient's first visit to the renal clinic is often a good indication that the renal failure is chronic. The onset is often attributed to age but readily remembered by the patient or spouse when they are directly questioned. Nocturia is not necessarily accompanied by polyuria and is due to a reversal of the normal circadian pattern of urine flow. The pathogenesis of the impaired concentrating ability and reversal of the normal circadian rhythm is complex and multifactorial. Concentrating urine requires the production of hypertonic interstitial fluid in the medulla of the kidney and regulation of the transfer of water from the distal convoluted tubule and collecting duct to the interstitial fluid by various endocrine and paracrine influences such as vasopressin and prostaglandins E_2. The hypertonic interstitial milieu is maintained by the physiological interactions and anatomical relationships between the vasa recta, collecting ducts, and loops of Henle. Factors that might interfere with urinary concentration are listed in Table 4.

Table 3 Factors suggesting chronicity

Duration of symptoms for months
Nocturia
Absence of severe symptoms in the face of very high urea and creatinine
Anaemia of chronic disorders
Bone disease
Sexual dysfunction
Skin disorders, nail changes, pruritus
Neurological complications
Small kidneys on renal imaging

Table 4 Mechanisms that may interfere with urinary concentration

Increased solute load
Wash-out of normal medullary concentration gradient
Destruction of normal medullary architecture
Augmented rate of vasa recta blood flow
Impaired function of loop of Henle
Impaired intrarenal urea recycling
Defective tubular cell function
Impaired responsiveness to ADH

Anaemia (see Chapter 11.3.8)

Because anaemia is present in many diseases causing acute renal failure (e.g. SLE and the haemolytic uraemic syndrome), it cannot be relied on as a marker of chronicity (Table 5). It is often possible, however, to identify the normochromic, normocytic anaemia of chronic renal failure by the blood film, reticulocyte count, and other investigations. The degree of anaemia tends to parallel the degree of uraemia, but there is a wide range at any level of GFR. It is uncommon, however, for the haemoglobin to be less than 6 g/dl in adults with chronic renal failure.

Sexual dysfunction (see Chapter 11.3.3)

Erectile dysfunction in men and dysfunctional uterine bleeding, amenorrhoea, and anovulatory cycles are common in women with chronic renal failure. Both sexes suffer from reduced libido and reduced fertility. In men, gonadal dysfunction predominates and disturbances of the hypothalamic–pituitary axis are more subtle, whereas the opposite is true in women (Palmer 1999). The patient may not complain of these symptoms, and therefore, they may go unnoticed unless specifically asked for. Primarily organic in nature, when due to uraemia alone, these symptoms usually appear in the last few months before dialysis. Recent onset, therefore, in a patient presenting with advanced renal failure strongly suggests chronicity. However, they can also be due to the primary disease, particularly diabetes mellitus, or side-effects of drugs, some of which are commonly used in renal failure, for example β-blockers and thiazide diuretics.

Skin manifestations (see Chapter 11.3.13)

Pruritus is a common symptom of uraemia. Provided skin diseases and drug side-effects can be excluded, its onset during the course of chronic renal failure, particularly when accompanied by scratching leading to excoriated skin with a bleeding maculopapular rash is a good indication that the time for dialysis is near. Other skin manifestations that are helpful in indicating that uraemia is chronic include yellowish-brown discoloration of the skin in Caucasians, deepening pigmentation in other races, brown nail arcs ('half-and-half nails') (Fig. 10), and dry

Table 5 Differential diagnosis of anaemia in patients with renal insufficiency

Defective erythropoiesis
Functional iron deficiency

Gastrointestinal bleeding and true iron deficiency
    Oesophageal tears from vomiting
    Erosions from uraemic gastritis
    Angiodysplasia
    Uraemic colitis

Autoimmune haemolysis in SLE

Microangiopathic haemolytic anaemia
    Malignant hypertension
    Haemolytic uraemic syndrome

Folic acid deficiency in malnourished patients

Bone marrow infiltration
    Myeloma
    Myelodysplasia and myelofibrosis

Splenomegaly

flaky skin. Each of these has a list of other causes, but their occurrence together in a uraemic patient is strong evidence of chronicity.

Neurological manifestations (see Chapter 11.3.14)

Peripheral neuropathy is rare in acute renal failure except when due to the primary disease. Consequently, the presence of a neuropathy suggests chronic renal failure, unless it can be explained by the primary disease (e.g. diabetes, amyloidosis, and polyarteritis), drug therapy affected by loss of renal excretion (e.g. nitrofurantoin), or a coincidental condition (e.g. alcoholism). However, the absence of neuropathy is of no diagnostic help because the symptoms are rare even when the GFR is less than 12 ml/min (Coomes *et al.* 1965), and the physical signs are not detected in one-third of patients starting dialysis, even when carefully examined (Raskin and Fishman 1976). The restless limbs syndrome is more specific for chronic renal failure and in the past was present in about 40 per cent of patients starting dialysis.

The encephalopathy of renal failure is of little help in distinguishing acute and chronic renal failure. However, the patient with slowly progressive renal failure has time to adapt and so a useful clinical sign that sometimes helps in recognizing chronicity is the surprising mental clarity of a patient with a grossly elevated serum creatinine. Causes of impaired mentation in chronic renal failure are listed in Table 6.

Other aspects of the initial assessment

A first assessment of the patient's social circumstances including the distance from the renal clinic, and the cost and difficulty of travel, determines the distribution of medical care between the renal clinic, the local hospital, and the general practitioner. Help from the social worker may be needed in rehousing, in anticipation of future dialysis, and in negotiation with the employer regarding time off work for clinical visits, or lighter work in keeping with their physical condition.

The occupational history is of great importance in judging the patient's suitability for the various types of renal replacement therapy and the possible need for a change in occupation.

At the end of the assessment, a problem list is drawn up, summarizing the primary disease causing renal failure and its effects on other systems, the presence of coincidental diseases, the complications of renal failure and hypertension, and social problems. In many renal centres, this forms the basis of the computerized record that will follow the patient through conservative treatment, dialysis, and transplantation.

Acute-on-chronic renal failure

If a patient with stable renal insufficiency or steadily deteriorating kidney function shows a sudden accelerated decline in renal function without symptoms or signs of an exacerbation of the original renal disease, non-renal aggravating factors can usually be found (Table 7).

Table 6 Differential diagnosis of impaired mentation in patients with renal insufficiency

Drug accumulation, for example, opiates, methyldopa, cimetidine

Primary disease, for example, malignant hypertension, cerebral lupus, AIDS

Steroid psychosis

Uraemia

Hyponatraemia

Hypoglycaemia

Severe hyperkalaemia

Aluminium encephalopathy

Hypercalcaemia

Hypermagnesaemia

Table 7 Causes of acute-on-chronic renal failure

Dehydration, acute tubular necrosis

Hypotension, often iatrogenic due to overuse of antihypertensive drugs

Accelerated hypertension

Cardiac failure

Drugs, especially tetracyclines

Contrast media

Poisons and toxins

Infection
    Urinary tract
    Septicaemia
    Bacterial endocarditis

Obstruction

Renal papillary necrosis

Atheroembolic disease

Renal vein thrombosis

Crescentic conversion of glomerulonephritis

Acute interstitial nephritis

Flare of primary systemic disease

Hypercalcaemia

Acute hyperuricaemia

Cardiac tamponade

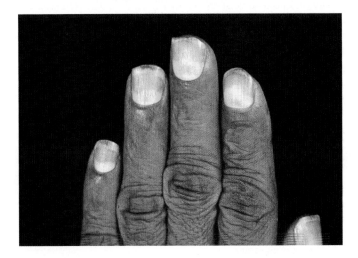

Fig. 10 The distal pigmentation of the nails in chronic renal failure. This 59-year-old man had polycystic kidney disease and a serum creatinine of 1203 μmol/l.

Careful investigation is mandatory, and if identified must be eliminated in order to prevent irreversible loss of residual renal function.

Volume depletion

Absolute volume depletion is characterized by loss of intravascular and extracellular fluid, causing thirst, physical signs of dehydration, and a reduction in GFR. Because of the inability to produce sufficiently concentrated urine, this is seen with gastrointestinal fluid loss and in those with insufficient fluid intake because of anorexia or unconsciousness. A common cause of volume depletion is low sodium intake in combination with vigorous diuretic therapy or a salt-wasting nephropathy. Finally, absolute volume depletion will occur with haemorrhagic shock. Replacement of fluids, either orally or intravenously, is imperative to re-establish renal function and to prevent acute tubular or cortical necrosis.

Decreased effective circulating blood volume can result in deterioration of renal function because of inadequate renal perfusion. Extracellular volume may be normal, and is often elevated. Common causes of decreased effective circulating blood volume are congestive heart failure, cirrhosis of the liver, and hypoalbuminaemia: the latter may be the result of either excessive albumin loss, as in severe proteinuria and nephrotic syndrome, or insufficient albumin synthesis, as in severe liver cirrhosis. Drugs that improve cardiac output will help in cases of congestive heart failure, and intravenous albumin may be necessary to reverse hypoalbuminaemia.

Accelerated hypertension

The risk of transition into the malignant form of hypertension is particularly common in patients with chronic renal failure. Malignant hypertension is characterized by severely elevated diastolic and systolic blood pressures, retinal haemorrhages, exudates and papilloedema, with subsequent deterioration of vision, and rapid decline in renal function. This may be associated with headache, disturbed consciousness, and seizures. Renin concentrations are high and histologically, necrotizing arteriolar and glomerular lesions are present. Admission to hospital is necessary, where immediate, effective antihypertensive therapy is required in order to prevent further deterioration of renal function. Too rapid a reduction in blood pressure must be avoided (>30 mmHg in 24 h) as hypoperfusion of end organs may cause irreversible damage, including blindness, 'watershed' zone cerebral infarction, myocardial infarction, and acute tubular necrosis (Kaplan 1994). The chances of partial recovery of renal function are reasonably good with treatment.

Urinary tract infections (see also Section 7)

Urinary tract infection in the absence of reduced urine flow (due to urological or neurological causes) is a rare cause of deterioration of renal function except in diabetics. If infection is suspected, urine should be examined by microscopy and a midstream urine sample cultured. Predisposing factors should be looked for, including renal or bladder stones, or, in males, chronic prostatitis. Ultrasonography of the urinary bladder before and after voiding should also be performed to detect and measure residual urine in patients with recurrent infection. If residual volume after voiding exceeds 100 ml, investigations to differentiate between motor bladder disturbances and outflow obstruction are indicated.

Urinary tract obstruction (see also Chapter 17.3)

An accelerated decline of renal function may be the first clue to obstruction and the recurrent urinary tract infection to which it predisposes.

Common causes of lower urinary tract obstruction, which may therefore complicate other renal diseases are prostatic hypertrophy and stenosis of the bladder neck. Causes of upper urinary tract obstruction include stones, malignancy, retroperitoneal fibrosis, and, especially in analgesic nephropathy or diabetic patients, sloughed papillae.

Intratubular obstruction, for example, by Bence Jones protein in multiple myeloma or by uric acid crystals in some malignancies after the initiation of treatment, is an occasional cause of sudden deterioration of renal function.

Extrarenal infections

Patients with chronic renal failure are susceptible to systemic infections such as pneumonia, a consequence of impaired leucocyte function, with diminished chemotaxis and deranged immunoregulation (see Chapter 11.3.11). Other factors, including acidosis, poor glycaemic control (in diabetic patients), malnutrition, defective mucosal barriers, and use of immunosuppressive drugs may contribute to this susceptibility. Infections may cause a further decline in renal function if complicated by volume depletion or septic shock. Unfortunately, diagnosis may be difficult since uraemia can blunt the pyrexial response.

Drugs and toxins

Renal function can be affected adversely by several drugs as a result of allergic reactions or toxic effects. An unexpected deterioration of renal function should prompt an enquiry of recent changes in medication.

A decline of renal function occasionally arises due to volume depletion in patients on diuretics. Overenthusiastic antihypertensive treatment may also occasionally affect renal function adversely by reducing renal perfusion, particularly in older patients with advanced atherosclerosis. Though this should not stand in the way of reducing blood pressure to the recommended limits, it should be remembered that hypertension is best defined as that level of blood pressure above which treatment does more good than harm. ACE inhibitors can cause deterioration of renal function in patients with or even without renal artery stenosis (Henin et al. 1989): renal function is usually restored after withdrawal of these drugs. A 20–30 per cent non-progressive increase in the serum creatinine concentration occurring in the context of better blood-pressure control however is not an indication to stop the ACE inhibitor as this indicates that intra-glomerular hypertension has been successfully reduced (Palmer 2002). Non-steroidal anti-inflammatory drugs and other inhibitors of prostaglandin synthesis can also cause deterioration of renal function, particularly in patients with glomerulonephritis, the nephrotic syndrome, heart failure, and in those taking high doses of diuretics.

Allergic interstitial nephritis may be caused by drugs such as penicillin and thiazide diuretics in patients with pre-existing renal disease. Microscopic examination of urine may reveal eosinophils. A firm diagnosis can only be made by renal biopsy, but this is not practical if the kidneys are small. A presumptive diagnosis can be made if withdrawal of the causative drug restores kidney function to its previous level.

Several drugs have direct toxic effects on the kidney, resulting in further loss of renal function. The risk is particularly high for drugs that accumulate in renal failure, including antimicrobial drugs such as the aminoglycosides, vancomycin, and amphotericin B. If these drugs have to be used, careful monitoring of their blood levels and dose adjustment is necessary.

It is well known that radiographic contrast materials can induce acute renal failure. Parfrey et al. (1989) demonstrated that the intravascular administration of radiographic contrast agents induced acute on chronic renal failure (defined as an increase in serum creatinine by more than 25 per cent) in 7 per cent of patients with pre-existing renal insufficiency. Patients with diabetic nephropathy were particularly at risk. The incidence of nephrotoxicity is not influenced by the osmolarity of radiographic contrast materials, or the ionic nature of the contrast medium (Schwab *et al.* 1989). Loss of renal function after the administration of contrast medium may be prevented by careful maintenance of hydration with isotonic saline before, and especially after, the diagnostic procedure. Administration of calcium channel blockers may be protective. More recently, an oral dose of the antioxidant acetylcysteine along with hydration prior to the procedure has been shown to be protective (Tepel *et al.* 2000).

Metabolic disorders

Poor glycaemic control can accelerate the decline in renal function in patients with diabetes mellitus. Hypercalcaemia, whether spontaneous or a result of vitamin D therapy, may cause a sudden decline in renal function. This may in part be the reversible result of volume depletion, arising from nausea, vomiting, and polyuria. Irreversible loss of renal function may be due to nephrocalcinosis. The disturbances of calcium and phosphorus metabolism in patients with chronic renal failure are discussed in more detail in Chapter 11.3.9.

Mild to moderate hyperuricaemia accompanying chronic renal failure needs no treatment, provided symptoms of gout are absent. It is, however, a powerful predictor of all cardiovascular risk in patients with normal renal function. If a severely hyperuricaemic patient becomes dehydrated, deposition of uric acid crystals may cause tubular obstruction. This can be prevented by sufficient fluid intake. Allopurinol should only be administered to patients with recurrent gout or severe persistent hyperuricaemia (plasma concentration $\geq 650\ \mu$mol/l). Since allopurinol and its metabolite oxopurinol accumulate in renal failure, a dose of 100 mg/day allopurinol should not be exceeded, except in patients with uric acid overproduction (Hanoke *et al.* 1984).

Follow-up assessment and treatment

The aims of follow-up are to monitor the progression to endstage renal failure and slow or arrest it where possible; to detect and treat the complications of chronic renal failure and the primary disease; to detect those symptoms of uraemia that call for dialysis and transplantation; and to plan and implement an orderly preparation for renal replacement therapy (Table 8). The ability to predict confidently the rate of progression of chronic renal failure is valuable in making these plans. Timely vascular access or CAPD catheter placement allows

Table 8 Predialysis assessment checklist

From previous follow-up visits

Full blood count	Other appropriate tests, e.g. complement,	Midstream urine
Calcium, magnesium, phosphate	VDRL, HBsAg, C-reactive protein, protein	Radiography
Alkaline phosphatase	electrophoresis, HbA$_1$C 24-h urinary protein	Renal ultrasound
Liver function tests		ECG
Blood sugar		

Test	Reason for test
In preparation for dialysis and transplant	
Ferritin, iron, and transferrin	Iron status, particularly important when considering treatment by erythropoietin
Folate and vitamin B$_{12}$	To rule out another cause of anaemia
Parathyroid hormone, vitamin D	To assess degree of renal osteodystrophy and to act as a baseline
Aluminium level	As a baseline for future tests on dialysis and to assess toxicity
Glucose tolerance test	If fasting blood sugar is abnormal, to assess diabetic status
HIV status	If positive, will affect decisions regarding management. Special precautions with blood letting
Hepatitis C status	If positive, special precautions with blood letting
Blood group, tissue typing and cytotoxic antibodies	Relevant for future transplant
Fasting lipids	Patients are at risk of hyperlipidaemia
CMV serology	Relevant to future transplant and donor CMV serology
Skeletal survey	To assess renal osteodystrophy
Micturating cystourethrogram	A routine in some centres to assess the bladder and exclude reflux before transplant
Dental assessment	To look for occult dental sepsis pretransplant and for dental treatment predialysis
Ophthalmology assessment	In diabetics
Urological assessment	In certain conditions, e.g. reflux or stone disease
Family planning	In females of child-bearing age regarding contraception and in males for consideration of sperm banking
Assessment by gastroenterologist	It is routine in some centres to examine pretransplant patients by endoscopy
Assessment by cardiologist	For ischaemic heart disease
Assessment by social worker	To assess need for social support and counselling
Assessment by dialysis administrator	To assess need for home adaptation for home haemodialysis
Family interview	For education and to assess possible family donors
Assessment by dialysis nursing staff	To assess suitability for CAPD/haemodialysis and counselling

CAPD, continuous ambulatory peritoneal dialysis; CMV, cytomegalovirus; ECG, electrocardiogram; VDRL, Veneral Diseases Research Laboratory (test); other abbreviations as in text.

a smooth transition to dialysis. This is largely, though not exclusively, dependent on early referral to a nephrologist (Astor *et al.* 2001).

The factors most likely to speed progression that can be modified include control of blood pressure, diet, avoidance of unnecessary drugs, and, in some instances, control of the underlying disease. Partial correction of anaemia with erythropoeitin may also slow progression. Care can be shared with the general practitioner in monitoring some of these parameters such as blood pressure.

Monitoring decline in GFR

Serum creatinine concentration (see Chapter 1.3)

Serum creatinine is much the most widely used serial measurement of GFR but has important limitations.

When GFR declines, serum creatinine initially changes only slightly (Fig. 11). Minor changes in serum creatinine may, therefore, reflect major changes in GFR and they have to be distinguished from the transient increase in serum creatinine that follows the consumption of cooked meat. When GFR declines to less than 40 ml/min/1.73 m^2, the loss of nephrons over-rides the effects of enhanced tubular secretion and decreased generation of creatinine, and large increases in serum creatinine correspond to small changes in GFR (Fig. 11). Thus, serum creatinine concentration is a poor indicator of renal function in patients with renal impairment and cannot be used to assess GFR accurately. In addition, serum creatinine concentration is affected by other factors such as changes in muscle mass and nutritional status, physical activity and gut metabolism of creatinine (Perrone *et al.* 1992). Any reduction in serum creatinine in late renal failure may well reflect a loss in muscle mass rather than improvement in renal function. Another more suitable endogenous marker for GFR is the protein cystatin C

which is produced by all nucleated cells and which is almost exclusively eliminated from the circulation by glomerular filtration (Nilsson and Grub 1994). High cost precludes its routine use in clinical practice.

Most clinicians use a calculation based on serum creatinine to estimate GFR in the clinic as this is a simple practical method. The Cockcroft–Gault formula is reasonably accurate in mild renal impairment with a GFR of around 50 ml/min but can overestimate GFR by up to 100 per cent when GFR is less than 10 ml/min. The MDRD formula (Levey *et al.* 1999) is more accurate especially at low clearance and we recommend this be used in preference to the Cockcroft and Gault method. A caveat is that this method has only been validated in Black and White Americans and not in other racial groups.

Reciprocal of serum creatinine

In the chronic renal failure clinic the reciprocal of the serum creatinine against time should be plotted (Fig. 12). Linear regression of this produces a straight line in most patients making it possible to predict the time when dialysis will be required. Several limitations of the reciprocal creatinine plot must be kept in mind. The accuracy of this prediction increases with the number of observations of serum creatinine. Also, a proportion of patients do not have a linear decline in renal function; Mitch *et al.* (1976) reported that 9 per cent of adults, and Leumann (1978) reported 13 per cent of children, deviated significantly from a straight line. Even among those that do follow a straight line, 20 per cent deviate from it at least once during their follow-up (Rutherford *et al.* 1977). Finally, although most creatinine production is from muscle, some is derived from ingested meat; a change from a normal to a low protein diet may therefore cause an upward bend in the reciprocal creatinine plot giving a short term misleading impression of benefit (Gretz *et al.* 1986). However, if account is taken of these limitations, the plot is useful in drawing attention to episodes of acute-on-chronic renal failure, monitoring response to treatment, and predicting when end-stage will be reached.

Clearance of endogenous creatinine

Because creatinine is excreted into the urine by tubular secretion as well as glomerular filtration, measurement of endogenous creatinine

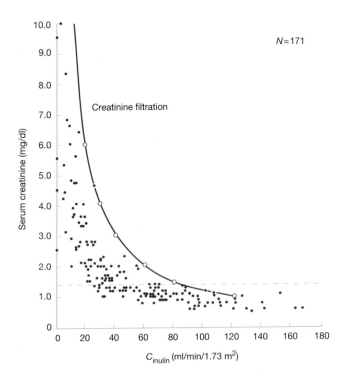

Fig. 11 Relation between serum creatinine and GFR in 171 patients with glomerular disease. (Reproduced with permission from Shemesh *et al.* 1985.)

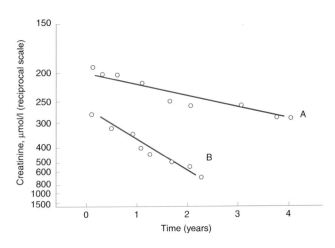

Fig. 12 The reciprocal plots of two patients being followed in our clinic illustrating a linear progression in decline in renal function. The limitations and caveats of such plots are discussed in the text and in Chapter 1.3.

clearance overestimates the true GFR. This is especially the case in patients with chronic renal failure and severe proteinuria (Bauer *et al.* 1982). The coefficient of variation of creatinine clearance is rather high (Florijn *et al.* 1994), mostly due to the unreliability of 24-h urine collections. There is a small extra renal loss of creatinine in faeces of about 2 ml/min. Thus, the endogenous creatinine clearance is notoriously unreliable for accurate assessment of the GFR. In everyday practice, however, it can be used as a screening tool, provided that the limitations of the method are taken into account.

Treatment with cimetidine on the day before and the day of 24-h urine collection reduces the coefficient of variation of intraindividual determinations of the endogenous creatinine clearance to 6.4 per cent (Florijn *et al.* 1994). In patients with a GFR less than 60 ml/min/1.73 m^2, treatment with cimetidine resulted in a ratio of creatinine clearance over GFR that approached 1. Thus, creatinine clearance measured during cimetidine treatment could provide a convenient and reproducible method to assess the GFR accurately. The GFR estimated by averaging the urea and creatinine clearance also correlates well with the gold standard of inulin clearance in patients with a GFR of less than 20 ml/min (Lubowitz *et al.* 1967).

Renal Kt/V_{urea} and nPNA

The National Kidney Foundation-Dialysis Outcomes Quality Initiative (NKF-DOQI) provide two clinical guidelines on when to start dialysis. The first recommends that dialysis is initiated when the failing kidney is unable to eliminate toxins as effectively as dialysis. This is mathematically equivalent to a weekly renal Kt/V of less than 2, extrapolated from the recommended target dose of dialysis in CAPD patients where a weekly Kt/V of less than 2 is associated with an increased mortality rate. The guideline is based on opinion only.

$$\text{Renal } Kt/V = \frac{\text{Urea clearance (ml/min)} \times 10{,}080 \text{ (minutes/week)}}{\text{Body water content (ml)}}$$

where:

$$\text{Urea clearance} = \frac{\text{Urine volume (ml)} \times \begin{array}{c} \text{urine urea} \\ \text{concentration} \\ \text{(mmol/dl)} \end{array} \times 1.73 \text{ (m}^2\text{)}}{\begin{array}{c} \text{Collection} \\ \text{period (min)} \end{array} \times \begin{array}{c} \text{serum urea} \\ \text{(mmol/dl)} \end{array} \times \begin{array}{c} \text{body surface} \\ \text{area (m}^2\text{)} \end{array}}$$

$$\text{Body water content} = \text{Volume of distribution of urea}$$

$$= \begin{cases} \text{Men: } 2.447 - (0.09516 \times \text{age in years}) \\ \qquad + (0.1074 \times \text{height in cm}) \\ \qquad + (0.3362 \times \text{weight in kg}) \\ \text{Women: } -2.097 + (0.1069 \times \text{height in cm}) \\ \qquad + (0.2446 \times \text{weight in kg}) \end{cases}$$

A weekly r-Kt/V of 2 equates to a urea clearance of 7 ml/min, a creatinine clearance of between 9 and 14 ml/min/1.73 m^2 and a mean urea, creatinine clearance of 10.5 ml/min/1.73 m^2. The validity of using this parameter to initiate dialysis was recently examined by Kuhlmann *et al.* (2001). These authors report that the measurement of r-Kt/V has poor sensitivity but acceptable specificity in deciding when dialysis is necessary and should be used in conjunction with other parameters such as the averaged urea, creatinine clearance.

The second guideline is based on the level of protein intake estimated by the normalized protein catabolic rate (nPNA).

$$\text{nPNA (g/kg/day)} = \left[\frac{\begin{array}{c} [6.49 \times \text{UUN (g/day)}] \\ + 0.294 \text{ (g/l/day)} \times V_{\text{urea}} \text{ (l)} \end{array}}{V_{\text{urea}} \text{ (l)}/0.58 \text{ (l/kg)}} \right]$$

The recommendation is that dialysis should start once the nPNA falls to below 0.8 g/kg per day. Again these data were derived from studies in CAPD patients. It has been suggested that these guidelines, derived from one population group, are not necessarily valid in other populations (Jansen *et al.* 2001).

Inulin, iohexol clearance, and radioisotope methods

Steady-state inulin clearance has been the 'gold standard' for measuring GFR. However, it requires constant delivery of inulin after a bolus injection to assure a constant plasma concentration, water loading to achieve sufficient urine flow, and accurate timing of the urine collections. Urine collections without catheterization may be unreliable, and alternative techniques that do not require urine collection introduce other sources of error. Since the determination of inulin in plasma and urine is difficult and time consuming, it is not a suitable method for estimating renal function in daily practice. Constant infusions or single dose techniques utilizing (^{125}I)iothalamate, (^{51}Cr)EDTA, or (^{99}Tcm)DTPA have been developed to overcome some of the problems encountered. Although these methods are much simpler than measuring inulin clearance, they are time consuming, particularly when GFR is low, and require specific laboratory facilities. Therefore, they are useful for research, but not for routine practice. They also expose the patient to a small amount of radiation, equivalent to a chest radiograph. Iohexol clearance, on the other hand, which is virtually identical to inulin clearance, is an easily accessible method for accurately measuring GFR (Nilsson-Ehle and Grub 1994).

It has been suggested that these guidelines, which derived from one population group, are not necessarily valid in other populations (Jansen *et al.* 2001).

Monitoring uraemic symptoms and when to start dialysis

Monitoring the patient to assess when dialysis will be required is one of the main aims of follow-up and one of the most difficult. The timing of the start of dialysis is controversial, not least because of financial and practical implications, consequently practice varies widely. Recently there has been a general trend in the developed world to initiate dialysis at an earlier stage of renal failure which would be in line with the DOQI recommendations that dialysis should be commenced once the GFR declines to less than 10.5 ml/min/1.73 m^2 or the creatinine clearance is in the range of 9–14 ml/min. This guideline is based on opinion only. Though many studies indicate a better survival in patients who start dialysis early, it is difficult to correct for lead-time bias (the earlier stage of the overall disease at the time of dialysis) and for late-referral bias, which may be an independent predictor of mortality. One recent study, taking into account lead-time bias showed no difference in survival between patients starting dialysis with a GFR of 6 and 10 ml/min (Korevaar *et al.* 2001). In practice initiation of dialysis according to biochemical markers varies widely. This is highlighted by the data of Malangone *et al.* (1989) who retrospectively analysed the clinical and laboratory features in 402 patients at the start of dialysis and noted the very wide range in creatinine (3.5–35 mg/dl; 308–3080 μmol/l) and blood urea nitrogen (35–345 mg/dl; 12.5–123 mmol/l of urea). A decade later, a comprehensive study by Obrador et al. (1999), this time in the United States, showed a similar wide variation in renal function at the start of dialysis (predicted GFR ranged from >15 to <2 ml/min/ 1.73 m^2) in 90,897 patients. In our view, the decision of when to start dialysis should involve a combination of clinical acumen in assessing symptomatology, discussed below, and identifying early signs of malnu- trition in association with measurements of declining GFR discussed above. Evidence currently would also suggest that delaying dialysis till the GFR is less than 6 ml/min irrespective of symptoms is unsafe.

Much has been written about the prevalence of uraemic symptoms during regular dialysis and their value in assessing dialysis adequacy, yet there is remarkably little documentation of the value of individ- ual symptoms in judging that the time for dialysis has come during conservative treatment. Prominent among the complaints of patients at the start of dialysis in the study of Malangone et al. (1989) were anorexia–nausea–vomiting (76 per cent), fatigue-weakness (72 per cent), pruritus (40 per cent), dyspnoea-orthopnoea (26 per cent), insomnia (14 per cent), bleeding tendency (14 per cent), apathy—mental changes (12 per cent), asterixis-muscle twitching-cramps (11 per cent), and dys- guesia (8 per cent). The authors found that none of these symptoms had a significant relationship to biochemical measurements reflecting GFR (creatinine clearance, serum creatinine, and urea) except bleed- ing tendency. Unfortunately, this extensive study devoted little space to the analysis of symptoms and the prevalence in any study is bound to reflect the diligence with which the authors enquired about particular symptoms; for instance, Malagnone et al. (1989) made no mention of sexual dysfunction.

The onset of pericarditis or symptomatic peripheral neuropathy, with no alternative explanation, is an indication that dialysis is already late and should be started at once. Nausea and vomiting are signs that dialysis is needed very soon. Restless limbs (a symptom which patients have difficulty in describing and often refer to as pain, itching, or dis- comfort until questioned closely) are usually a sign that dialysis is needed soon; a more generalized restlessness syndrome is an uncommon but dramatic indication that it is overdue. Severe pruritus and excoriated rash is an indication for early dialysis if not explained by drug allergy or coincidental skin disease. Other warnings that uraemia is becoming troublesome are myoclonic jerks (particularly on falling asleep), sleep disturbance, severe lethargy, mental clouding, loss of concentration and sexual dysfunction in younger adults, unexplained by drug therapy. In a significant minority of our patients, the trigger to starting dialysis is dif- ficulty in controlling fluid balance and blood pressure rather than the symptoms or biochemical evidence of severe uraemia. A check for ankle oedema, crepitations at the lung bases, a raised jugular venous pressure and the presence of cardiomegaly, a third heart sound and functional cardiac murmurs is therefore a routine part of the follow-up assessment.

Attenuation of progression

Blood pressure control

The importance of the control of blood pressure in patients with renal disease is highlighted in Chapter 11.1. Systemic hypertension is com- mon in patients with chronic renal disease, the rate of decline in renal function increases with increasing blood pressure (Brazy 1989; Rambausek 1989), and also reduction in blood pressure attenuates the

deterioration of renal function. The latter was convincingly demon- strated at first in patients with diabetic nephropathy (Parving et al. 1983, 1987; Chapter 14.3). Two important factors contribute to the rise in blood pressure of patients with chronic renal failure. First, most renal diseases are associated with sodium retention, which results in an increase in extracellular fluid volume and an increase in peripheral vas- cular resistance. Second, activation of the renin–angiotensin–aldosterone system results in increased circulating angiotensin II, which in addition to being a potent vasoconstrictor, also enhances sodium retention by the kidney. Consequently, it can be argued that the two initial steps in the treatment of hypertension in the majority of patients with chronic renal failure should consist of a reduction in sodium intake, with or without the use of diuretics, and treatment with agents that block the effects of angiotensin II, that is, ACE inhibitors or blockers of the angiotensin II receptor (AT$_1$).

Regular follow-up is essential as it has been demonstrated that patient compliance, efficacy of antihypertensive treatment, and retarda- tion of renal failure are clearly related to the number of outpatient visits (Bergstrom et al. 1986).

Target blood pressure

A pragmatic view is that the target blood pressure is best defined as a level which treatment does more good than harm (Bulpitt 2000). There is currently no definite information available about the target blood pressure, which will maximally ameliorate progression of renal failure. In patients with early diabetic nephropathy, reduction of blood pressure to values within the normal range slowed the decline in renal function. The same is true in patients with other renal diseases and proteinuria of over 1 g/day (Klahr et al. 1994). These observations resulted in the recommendation of aiming for a blood pressure within the normal range (120/70 mmHg) by the authors of the JNC-VI (1997), especially in patients with proteinuria greater than 1 g per day.

Non-pharmacological treatment

These measures are advised as the sole, initial therapeutic step in patients with mild hypertension, as they may be sufficient to achieve normotension. The effects of non-pharmacological treatment should be evaluated over a period of 2–3 months.

Sodium restriction

In patients with chronic renal failure, the ability to excrete sodium usu- ally is limited. Thus, a sodium-restricted diet of 6 g/day is a useful initial step in the treatment of hypertension. Determining a 24 h urinary sodium excretion can check compliance with the sodium restricted diet.

Obesity is clearly associated with hypertension, and reduction of body weight should be recommended to obese patients. Increasing physical exercise and reducing calorie intake may achieve this. Some caution is advised in patients with advanced renal failure because of the risk of catabolism. Alcohol abuse can also contribute to hypertens- ion and may also interfere with adherence to antihypertensive or other therapy. It is anyway advisable to limit alcohol intake to less than 21 units in men and 14 units in women.

Pharmacological treatment

A diuretic, β-blocker, ACE inhibitor, angiotensin II receptor antago- nist, or calcium-entry blocker may be chosen as initial therapy. Individual factors should be considered in the selection of the initial drug: these may be related to the response (e.g. Black subjects respond less well to monotherapy with β-blockers and ACE inhibitors; older people generally respond well to diuretics) or associated medical problems (e.g. β-blockers in coexistent coronary artery disease; ACE inhibitors in associated congestive heart failure, and no β-blockers in asthma).

Diuretics

Thiazide diuretics can be used as long as GFR is greater than 30 ml/min, but these drugs usually become ineffective, at least as monotherapy, once the GFR is less than this. Loop diuretics (e.g. frusemide) should then be used. Coadministration of metolazone in a dose of 5–10 mg daily can provoke a marked diuresis and other thiazide diuretics have additive effects even in advanced renal failure (Fliser *et al.* 1994). Dehydration and sodium depletion may result from vigorous diuretic therapy, particularly when combined with dietary sodium restriction, presenting as a sudden deterioration of renal function (prerenal failure) and low blood pressure or postural hypotension. Hypokalaemia is another hazard of diuretic therapy. However, the use of potassium-sparing diuretics (spironolactone, amiloride, and triamterene) is usually contraindicated in chronic renal failure, and potassium supplementation should also be used with caution because of the risk of hyperkalaemia.

ACE inhibitors and angiotensin II receptor blockers

There is now compelling evidence that patients with proteinuria should be treated with agents that offset the effects of angiotensin II (i.e. ACE inhibitors or ARBs) in order to delay the progression of chronic renal failure. Whereas initially it was demonstrated that the development and progression of microalbuminuria could be postponed in insulin-dependent diabetic patients by treatment with the ACE inhibitor captopril (Lewis *et al.* 1993), it more recently became clear that this could also be achieved with angiotensin II receptor blockers in patients with non-insulin dependent diabetes mellitus (Brenner *et al.* 2001; Lewis *et al.* 2001). In non-diabetic nephropathy and overt proteinuria, the Italian researchers of the GISEN group (Ruggenenti *et al.* 1999a,b) also demonstrated the beneficial effects of ACE inhibition in retarding progression of renal disease. Treatment with the ACE inhibitor ramipril reduced proteinuria and resulted in a reduction in the decline in renal failure (Ruggenenti *et al.* 1999a; Fig. 13). The greater the reduction in proteinuria, the greater the retardation in progression of renal failure. The achieved blood pressure levels were the same in ACE inhibitor-treated and the control patients. Because of the impressive effects of ACE inhibition in patients with greater than 3 g of proteinuria per day already present at the second interim analysis, the randomization code was broken and the control patients were also treated with an ACE inhibitor. This resulted in a retardation in their progression of renal failure (Ruggenenti *et al.* 1999b). In patients that continued to use ACE inhibition the decline in renal function was abated (Fig. 14) and in some patients GFR even improved. In patients with heavy proteinuria (>3 g/day), progression of renal failure was slowed compared to controls (Ruggenenti *et al.* 1999b). As yet, data on angiotensin II receptor blockers and the progression of non-diabetic renal failure are lacking. In a few short-term studies it has been demonstrated that angiotensin II receptor antagonists reduced proteinuria to the same extent as ACE inhibitors (Gansevoort *et al.* 1994; Perico *et al.* 1998). In several meta analyses, ACE inhibitors have a superior antiproteinuric effect compared to other antihypertensive agents (Gansevoort *et al.* 1995; Jafar *et al.* 2001). From observations such as these it is our opinion that ACE inhibitors or angiotensin II antagonists should be the first line antihypertensive agents in patients with chronic

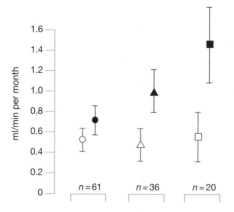

Fig. 13 The average rate of decline in GFR after 2 years of treatment with the ACE inhibitor ramipril (open symbols) or placebo in patients with 3.0–4.5 g/day (circles), 4.5–7.0 g/day (triangles), or 7.0 g/day (squares) proteinuria. Note that the decline in GFR increases with higher rates of proteinuria and, second, that treatment with ramipril reduced the decline in GFR in all groups to the same extent (adapted from Ruggenenti *et al.* 1999a).

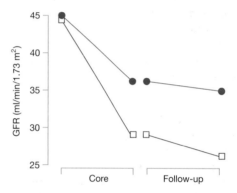

Fig. 14 GFR in the patients treated with the ACE inhibitor ramipril (solid symbols) and in the placebo-treated patients during the core study and the follow-up period during which all patients were treated with ramipril. Note that during the core period, GFR had fallen less in the ACE inhibitor-treated patients than in the placebo-treated patients and that during the follow-up period, the decline in GFR was attenuated in the placebo group and virtually halted in the group continuously treated with the ACE inhibitor (adapted from Ruggenenti *et al.* 1999b).

renal failure and overt proteinuria where there is no contraindication to their use. It is important to emphasize that patients who are treated with ACE inhibitors or angiotensin II receptor antagonists should adhere to a sodium restricted diet (approximately 6 g NaCl per day) and/or be treated with a diuretic as it has been demonstrated that the effects of ACE inhibition on proteinuria and GFR can be offset by a high sodium intake.

Well-known side-effects of ACE inhibitors are non-productive cough, hyperkalaemia, and a sudden reduction in GFR in patients with atherosclerotic renovascular disease and rarely angioneurotic oedema. The angiotensin II receptor antagonists are well tolerated and have few side-effects, but hyperkalaemia is frequently seen and angioneurotic oedema has also been described.

Calcium channel blockers

Despite their potent antihypertensive effects, the dihydropyridine calcium channel blockers in general do not reduce proteinuria

(Ter Wee *et al.* 1994). This may be due to the preglomerular vasodilation they cause which offsets the fall in systemic blood pressure resulting in an unaffected glomerular capillary pressure. On the other hand, the non-dihydropyridine calcium channel blockers not only induce pre-glomerular vasodilation, but also efferent arteriolar vasodilation. Consequently, these agents do reduce proteinuria and might be preferably used as additional antihypertensive agents in patients with chronic renal failure and proteinuria (Bakris 1990).

Although this class of antihypertensive agents is frequently used, relative little data on their effect on the progression of renal failure are available. In a few prospective studies in patients with non-diabetic failure, progression of renal failure was retarded (Eliahou *et al.* 1988; Zucchelli *et al.* 1992; Ecder *et al.* 2000). A few recently published studies also report dihydropyridine calcium channel blockers reduce the rate of progression in patients with diabetic nephropathy (Fogari *et al.* 1999; Tarnow *et al.* 2000; Baba 2001). In addition, a subanalysis of large intervention studies, recently demonstrated that dihydropyridine calcium antagonists could protect against progression of proteinuria and loss of creatinine clearance (Voyaki *et al.* 2001). Finally, in recently published papers, the combination of an ACE inhibitor with a dihydropyridine calcium channel blocker has been demonstrated to be more effective in retarding progression of renal failure compared to monotherapy (Taylor and Sunthornyothin 1999; Petersen *et al.* 2001). The overall conclusion is that (dihydropyridine) calcium channel blockers do retard the progression of renal failure despite a less favourable effect on proteinuria, and might be added preferentially to ACE inhibitors in controlling blood pressure in patients with renal failure and hypertension.

Pretibial oedema is a common side-effect of calcium channel blockers and must not be mistaken for evidence of sodium retention. Lacidipine, which is predominantly cleared by the liver, may have fewer side-effects in renal failure. Some calcium channel blockers have negative inotropic effects and should be used with caution in patients with congestive heart failure. The combination of non-dihydropyridine calcium entry blockers (verapamil or diltiazem) and a β-blocker should be avoided due to the potential risk of fatal cardiac conductance disturbances such as atrioventricular block.

β-Blockers

These may be chosen as initial therapy, particularly in patients with coronary artery disease. β-Blockers are contraindicated in patients with chronic airway obstruction because of the risk of bronchospasm. In patients with diabetes mellitus, β-blocker-induced impairment of hypoglycaemic awareness and counter-regulation may be a problem, and in patients with peripheral vascular disease cutaneous perfusion may be reduced. They may also aggravate hyperkalaemia.

Vasodilators and other agents

The α-adrenoceptor blocking agent doxazosin is a useful adjunct to treatment. The postural hypotension is largely overcome by using the modified release formula though it often still is a problem in diabetics. It also indicated in patients with bladder outflow obstruction and benign prostatic hypertension. Hydrallazine and prazocin are often effective though prazocin, in particular, is associated with tachyphylaxis. Methyldopa should not be used in advanced renal failure as accumulation invariably leads to significant drowsiness. It is, however, useful in mild renal insufficiency and also safe in pregnancy.

Minoxidil is reserved for cases that have not responded to the above drugs, no dose adjustment for renal impairment is necessary. The adverse side-effect of hirsutism is particularly distressing for young women, in whom it should be avoided. It must be used with a diuretic to off set the fluid accumulation it causes. An uncommon side-effect but one worth noting is the development of pericardial effusions on treatment. Another cardiac abnormality is T-wave inversion on electrocardiogram in about half of patients treated; this tends to regress with continued therapy.

Adverse effects of antihypertensive treatment

If blood pressure is decreased abruptly in patients with severe or accelerated phase hypertension, hypoperfusion of several organs can produce severe adverse effects: cerebrovascular accidents, myocardial infarction, amaurosis secondary to optical nerve atrophy, ischaemic colitis, and decline in renal function. Such side-effects are particularly common in patients with advanced atherosclerosis. Elevated blood pressure should, therefore, only be lowered gradually. As previously mentioned in patients with suspected or proven ischaemic heart disease, diastolic blood pressure should not be reduced to less than 85 mmHg since the prevalence of myocardial infarction and mortality may increase below this level (Cruickshank *et al.* 1987; Kaplan 1998).

Lowering of blood pressure can cause a decline in GFR: this is usually transient and may be explained by perturbed autoregulation. However, since lowering of blood pressure will retard the progression of renal failure, the long-term result will often be prolonged preservation of renal function. The effects of antihypertensive therapy on renal function (i.e. GFR and proteinuria) should therefore be monitored carefully.

The development of postural hypotension is another well-known adverse effect of antihypertensive treatment, particularly in older patients and diabetics. This requires modification of the antihypertensive therapy, often with the result that supine normotension cannot be achieved.

Protein restriction

The aims of dietary protein restriction are to alleviate the symptoms of uraemia in those not being considered for dialysis and to attempt to slow the progression of renal insufficiency without negatively jeopardizing nitrogen balance.

Attenuation of progression

After initial observations in the rat model with reduced renal mass had shown that protein restriction attenuated the development and progression of renal failure, it was claimed from retrospective studies that a low protein diet might have the same effect in humans (Barsotti *et al.* 1983; Maschio *et al.* 1983). In several (but not all) subsequently performed randomized prospective studies, these early retrospective observations were confirmed. Rosman *et al.* (1984) initially reported attenuation of progression of renal failure with a 0.4–0.6 g/kg body weight protein-restricted diet. After a follow-up period of 4 years, however, a beneficial effect of the diet was only observed in patients with chronic glomerulonephritis (Rosman *et al.* 1989). In the initial analysis of the Modification of Diet in Renal Disease (MDRD) Study (Klahr 1994), the largest trial to date on the effect of protein restriction on chronic renal failure in man, the investigators reported a small beneficial effect of the low-protein diets on the course of renal function after an average follow-up period of 2.2 years. When the initial 4 months of low-protein diet [in which haemodynamic changes to the low protein diet reduce GFR (Bilo 1989)] were excluded from the analysis, the decline in GFR of protein-restricted patients was attenuated (Levey *et al.* 1996). This secondary analysis of the MDRD trial patients also revealed a high protein intake was associated with a more rapid decline in GFR (Levey *et al.* 1996). It was calculated that each 0.2 g/kg body weight reduction in protein intake resulted in a 29 per cent reduction in the rate of decline in GFR.

The effect of protein restriction on the progression of chronic renal failure has been analysed in three meta-analyses (Fouque *et al.* 1992; Kasiske *et al.* 1998). Altogether, it can be concluded from these studies that protein restriction causes a modest reduction in the progression of chronic renal failure in man. It was concluded that dietary protein restriction significantly reduced the risk for renal insufficiency or death with a relative risk of 0.67 (95% confidence interval 0.50–0.89) in patients with non-diabetic renal failure and 0.56 (95% confidence interval 0.40–0.77) in patients with diabetic nephropathy. Several questions remain to be answered; for example, to what extent should the protein intake be reduced? At what time should the diet should be implemented? And are the observed untoward effects of protein attributed to red meat only?

Practical considerations

The help of a dedicated renal unit dietitian is essential. Prior to institution of a protein restricted diet, it is necessary to evaluate, and to take into account, the eating habits and protein intake of the patient so that a balanced diet, adjusted to the needs and habits of the individual may be prescribed. Initially, patients should consult the dietitian regularly so that daily protein intake can be assessed, advice can be given on dietary problems, and adequate calorie intake can be ensured. We advise a diet of 30 kcal/kg body weight/day or more with a moderate protein restriction of 0.6 g/kg body weight/day. Dietary compliance may be monitored most readily by measuring the serum urea : creatinine ratio (which should be reduced by treatment) and the 24-h urinary urea excretion. The latter is usually reported in millimoles; a 40 g protein diet should produce about 150 mmol of urea. Daily protein intake can be estimated from urea excretion using the equation

$$[(g\ urea/day) \times 3] + 15 = g\ protein/day$$

In patients with severe liver disease or during gastrointestinal bleeding, this formula cannot be used reliably. As prolonged use of a low-protein diet might result in a negative nitrogen balance and malnutrition, it is necessary to check for loss of muscle mass and other evidence of protein depletion. Simple measurements are mid-arm circumference (to judge muscle mass), triceps skin fold thickness (to correct for changes in subcutaneous fat), and serum albumin.

Smoking

In patients with diabetic and non-diabetic renal failure it has been shown that cigarette smoking enhances the rate of progression of renal failure (Biesenbach *et al.* 1997; Orth *et al.* 1998). Thus, patients with chronic renal failure should be strongly advised to quit smoking.

Hyperlipidaemia

Hyperlipidaemia is often present in patients with chronic renal failure (Attman *et al.* 1993). Nonetheless, there are only a limited number of studies, usually with a small number of patients included, in which the effects of treatment of hyperlipidaemia has been investigated. Therefore, it is only since the recent meta-analysis of Fried *et al.* (2001a,b) that it is clear that treatment of hyperlipidaemia ameliorates the progression of renal failure.

Management of fluid and electrolytes

In renal insufficiency the regulatory capacity of the kidney is progressively reduced (Fig. 15). Both excretion and conservation of electrolytes and water are impaired; when sudden loads of potassium, acid, or fluid has to be handled the limitations of renal functional reserve become apparent and signs of decompensation may occur. Consequently, water and electrolyte intakes must be adapted to renal excretory capacity.

Water

Dehydration occurs easily in patients with inadequate fluid intake, due to persistent diuresis despite fluid deprivation. Defective urinary concentrating ability is particularly common in patients with conditions that predominantly affect the renal medulla, for example, interstitial nephritis, pyelonephritis, and medullary cystic disease. Several mechanisms are responsible for the inability to excrete concentrated urine, including the increased solute load in remnant nephrons resulting in an osmotic diuresis, perturbation of medullary interstitial solute concentrations as a result of the damaged countercurrent exchange system and impaired medullary blood flow. In addition, impaired sensitivity to antidiuretic hormone causes decreased outward water transport in the distal nephron segments. As a result of decreased concentrating capacity, urine osmolality is roughly that of plasma, approximately 300 mOsm/kg H_2O, in patients with chronic renal failure. If the obligatory osmolar production in an adult is around 600 mOsm/kg H_2O, daily urine output will be roughly 2 l per day. Fluid intake should therefore be approximately 2–3 l/day in order to ensure adequate urine flow rates and to prevent dehydration. In some patients who are 'salt losers', fluid requirements may be even greater.

Sodium (see Chapter 2.1)

Subtle abnormalities of renal sodium handling are apparent in early renal failure. Initially, sodium excretion per nephron can be increased to a remarkable extent, maintaining total body sodium content and extracellular fluid volume within normal limits until late in renal failure. Frank sodium retention on a normal diet is more common once GFR falls below 10 ml/min, and in patients with nephrotic syndrome or cardiac failure.

Sodium retention will result in symptoms of expanded extracellular fluid volume, including hypertension, peripheral oedema, elevated central venous pressure, pulmonary congestion, and functional cardiac murmurs. A sodium restricted diet (approximately 3–5 g/day) and loop diuretics are then required for treatment.

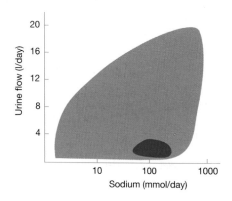

Fig. 15 Renal capacity for water and sodium excretion in healthy individuals (light shading) and in patients with a severely impaired renal function (dark shading).

Sodium depletion may also occur in patients with renal insufficiency, particularly in tubulointerstitial disease such as pyelonephritis, interstitial nephritis, hydronephrosis, and medullary cystic disease. Extrarenal loss of sodium from vomiting, diarrhoea, or fever may also result in extracellular fluid depletion. The clinical symptoms and signs are thirst, dry mucous membranes, orthostatic hypotension, dizziness, vascular collapse, and a reversible deterioration in renal function. In addition to removing the underlying cause, when possible, intravenous administration of isotonic saline may be necessary to correct the sodium and volume depletion and restore renal function. Diuretics, if being used, must be withheld temporarily. In less severe cases of sodium depletion, an increase in oral sodium and water intake together with a temporarily reduced or discontinued intake of diuretics may be sufficient.

Potassium

Patients with chronic renal failure are usually able to maintain serum potassium within normal limits until oliguria occurs or GFR is less than 5 ml/min. Preservation of normokalaemia results from an adaptive increase in potassium excretion by remnant nephrons and increased bowel loss. However, hyperkalaemia may be an early feature of renal failure in patients with (hyperchloraemic) metabolic acidosis and hyporeninaemic hypoaldosteronism, which occur particularly in patients with tubulointerstitial disease and diabetes mellitus. Hyperkalaemia also complicates an acute potassium load (e.g. transfusion of old blood) or administration of medication, which interferes with potassium secretion, for example, potassium sparing diuretics, ACE inhibitors, β-blockers, and NSAIDs. Foods, which contain high levels of potassium, are nuts, chocolate, fruits, wine, and fruit juice. Particularly dangerous are some salt substitutes, available in supermarkets that contain potassium instead of sodium. The endogenous potassium load is increased in states associated with cell lysis and release of intracellular potassium, including haemolysis, rhabdomyolysis, tumour lysis, and following trauma and surgery. Acidosis also results in hyperkalaemia due to exchange of intracellular potassium for extracellular hydrogen ions (every 0.1 unit fall in blood pH causes an increase in serum potassium concentration of about 0.6 mmol/l). Minor electrocardiographic abnormalities (tall-peaked T waves) may be the first indication of hyperkalaemia but by the time serious changes occur (Fig. 16), the patient usually complains of muscle weakness, paraesthesia, and lethargy.

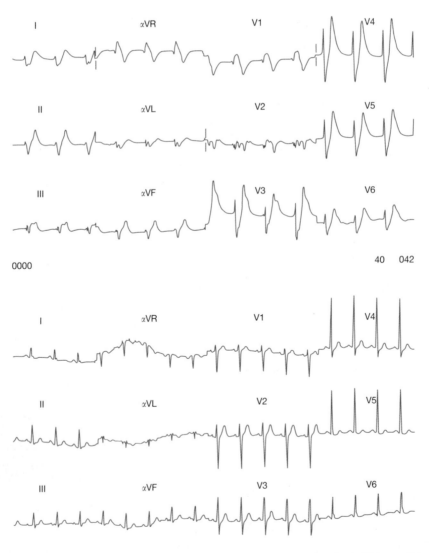

Fig. 16 Two electrocardiograms (ECG) from a patient presenting with renal failure and a serum potassium level of 7.6 mmol/l (top ECG) and after 2 h of dialysis (bottom ECG). The changes of hyperkalaemia are seen to be reversed with dialysis and normokalaemia.

Treatment of acute hyperkalaemia

Acute reduction of serum potassium is required at levels exceeding 7.0 mmol/l, because of the risk of cardiac arrest. Though a rapid reduction in serum potassium concentration is best achieved by acute haemodialysis, this takes time to institute. Emergency treatment should be started by the administration of calcium (10–30 ml of 10 per cent calcium gluconate over 10 min intravenously). Furthermore, intravenous glucose (50 ml dextrose 50 per cent, preferably by central venous infusion) should be given followed by or combined with 10 units of short-acting regular insulin, because combined administration of glucose and insulin results in a greater decline in serum potassium levels (Allon 1995). Successful treatment of hyperkalaemia may also be achieved by β_2-adrenergic agonists (e.g. salbutamol 0.5 mg in 100 ml dextrose 5 per cent intravenously over 15 min) (Lens et al. 1989). Combined use of β_2-adrenergic agonists with glucose and insulin will maximize the reduction in serum potassium (Allon and Copkney 1990). When patients are dialysed subsequently, the removal of potassium during the dialysis session may be reduced, however, resulting in a possible rebound hyperkalaemia several hours after the dialysis session (Allon and Shanklin 1995). In case of metabolic acidosis, correction of acidosis by infusion of intravenous sodium bicarbonate will contribute to the correction of hyperkalaemia but it is contraindicated if the patient is fluid overloaded. After acute hyperkalaemia has been corrected, the more slowly acting ion exchangers may be given orally or rectally (e.g. sodium/calcium polystyrene sulfonate 15–30 g, with an equal amount of sorbitol to prevent faecal impaction). Ion exchangers may also be given in less severe cases of hyperkalaemia in order to preempt a further increase in serum potassium. Reducing the dietary potassium and promoting a diuresis with a loop diuretic should control milder degrees of hyperkalaemia.

Hypokalaemia

Spontaneous hypokalaemia is uncommon in renal insufficiency and occurs only in patients with salt-wasting nephropathy, hereditary or acquired tubulointerstitial diseases, Fanconi syndrome, or renal tubular acidosis. On rare occasions, hypokalaemia is the result of a solitary renal reabsorption defect. Hypokalaemia usually results from a low dietary intake of potassium combined with high doses of diuretics or gastrointestinal loss by vomiting, gastric suction, or more rarely, colonic tumours. Temporary interruption of diuretic treatment and later resumption with lower doses or correction of gastrointestinal losses is usually all that is required to return serum potassium levels to normal. Food rich in potassium should be given. If severe volume depletion is present it may be necessary to correct the sodium chloride deficit by intravenous infusion to reverse metabolic alkalosis and secondary hyperaldosteronism.

Acidosis

Patients with chronic renal failure are at risk of acidosis if GFR is less than 30 ml/min, when the capacity of the kidney to excrete hydrogen ions may no longer be great enough to cope with endogenous acid production or high exogenous acid loads. The main cause of acidosis in patients with renal failure is impaired renal generation of ammonia; bicarbonate threshold may also be lowered as the result of diminished proximal tubular reabsorption, in part due to hyperparathyroidism. Distal proton secretion is usually unaffected.

Chronic metabolic acidosis is usually well tolerated. Severe acidosis may cause dyspnoea on exertion or at rest, particularly in elderly patients

with compromised cardiac function, and may also predispose to pulmonary oedema. This results from depression of cardiac contractility and venoconstriction with fluid shift into the central cardiopulmonary compartment. Metabolic acidosis can enhance protein catabolism, thus contributing to malnutrition in patients with chronic renal failure (Bergstrom et al. 1998). Likewise, metabolic acidosis has been implicated in the genesis of renal osteodystrophy (Kraut 1995). Since excess hydrogen ions are sequestered intracellularly and buffered by bone salts in patients with chronic renal failure, severe acidosis is rare unless other metabolic disturbances are superimposed, for example, diabetic keto-acidosis, lactic acidosis, or loss of bicarbonate ions.

Treatment of acidosis should certainly be started when serum bicarbonate concentrations is less than 15 mmol/l. In view of the role of acidosis in the catabolism of uraemia, treatment of patients with less severe acidosis has become increasingly popular. In order to correct acidosis, calcium carbonate (500–2000 mg thrice daily) can be given: this may simultaneously correct hypocalcaemia and hyperphosphataemia. Alternatively, sodium bicarbonate or sodium citrate (1–2 g thrice daily) can be used. The aim of treatment is to increase serum bicarbonate concentration above 18 mmol/l. Citrate increases the risk of aluminium intoxication in patients who are receiving aluminium-containing phosphate binders, since it promotes the interstitial absorption of aluminium and should not be used with aluminium-containing phosphate-binding gels. It is of note that sodium retention and hypertension occur less readily when sodium is given with bicarbonate instead of chloride as the anion.

Management of other cardiovascular conditions (see Chapter 11.3.5)

Renal insufficiency is independently associated with an increased cardiovascular disease related and all cause mortality rate (Muntner et al. 2002).

Coronary artery disease

Ischaemic heart disease is an almost inevitable accompaniment of chronic renal failure in diabetics and the elderly. Coronary artery disease also develops at a relatively younger age in patients with chronic renal failure (particularly if preceded by a nephrotic syndrome) and is a cause of significant morbidity and mortality. In addition to the recognized risk factors mentioned above, it has been suggested that a 'uraemic factor' may play a role in the pathogenesis of accelerated atherosclerosis. This has recently been reviewed by Parfrey (2000). Clinically, symptoms and signs are similar to the general population though the higher frequency of diabetes increases the prevalence of silent ischaemic events. Patients undergoing coronary angiography with chronic renal insufficiency have a poor long-term prognosis (Hemmelgarn et al. 2001). By electron beam scanning it has recently been shown that patients on haemodialysis manifest significant coronary arteriolar calcification (Goodman et al. 2000). The latter indicates that the disturbances in calcium–phosphorus homeostasis of patients with chronic renal failure, frequently causing secondary hyperparathyroidism with hypercalcaemia and hyperphosphataemia, can result in arteriolar calcifications, thus contributing to the elevated cardiovascular risk of these patients.

Congestive heart failure

Several factors contribute to the development of congestive heart failure in patients with severely impaired renal function. Expansion of extracellular volume, as a result of decreased capacity to excrete sodium and water, increases preload. Increased cardiac workload due to hypertension, anaemia, ischaemic heart disease as a result of coronary artery disease, and myocardial fibrosis and deposits of calcium and phosphate, all contribute to the evolution of congestive heart failure. Treatment with orally or intravenously administered loop diuretics is indicated and ultrafiltration should be considered in advanced cases. Angiotensin converting enzyme inhibitors (in reduced dose) and digoxin should be administered as required.

Pericarditis

Pericarditis is often a sign of terminal uraemia in patients who are not dialysed. Both acute fibrinous pericarditis and a chronic adhesive pericarditis may occur. Acute fibrinous pericarditis usually presents with retrosternal chest pain that is often aggravated by deep breathing and relieved by sitting forward. A low-grade temperature may be present and a friction rub can usually be heard over the praecordium. The electrocardiograph may show typical changes of ST segment elevation in the chest leads. Less well known is a depression of the PR segment in lead 2 and the elevation of this segment in AVR, which, if present, is pathoneumonic of pericarditis. The most serious complication of an effusion is tamponade, caused by a rapidly forming effusion and haemorrhage. The presentation is usually dramatic with severe hypotension, palpable pulsus paradoxus and signs of acute right heart failure. Prompt recognition of the problem and emergency pericardiocentesis can be life saving. As little as 100 ml of blood can cause acute tamponade if it accumulates rapidly. By contrast, a slowly developing effusion may stretch the pericardium and over 1 l of fluid can accumulate with minimal symptoms and signs. The friction rub also is often lost. The ECG reveals small QRS complexes and the chest radiograph a large globular heart shadow (Fig. 17). The diagnosis is most easily confirmed by echocardiography.

Myocardial fibrosis and calcification

Myocardial fibrosis is found at post mortem in a number of conditions that affect the heart including cardiac failure, diabetes, and hypertension. It has also been described in uraemia where its relevance is uncertain, but it may be responsible for the diastolic left ventricular

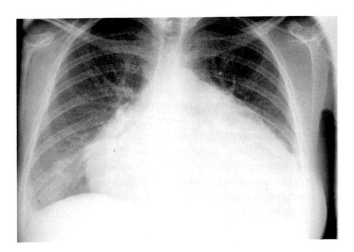

Fig. 17 Chest radiograph from a patient with a large pericardial effusion.

dysfunction and reduced left ventricular compliance so often seen in uraemic patients (Amann *et al.* 1994). Metastatic calcification outside of the coronary arteries (mentioned above), in the conducting system of the heart has also been implicated as a cause of sudden death in some patients with chronic renal failure.

Treatment and monitoring of bone disease (see Chapter 11.3.9)

Skeletal abnormalities occur early in renal failure, well before symptoms develop (Rix *et al.* 1999). A variety of biochemical and radiological investigations are available to assist in the diagnosis and monitoring of renal osteodystrophy. Measurement of serum parathyroid hormone (PTH) remains the single most useful biochemical test in predicting bone histology in an individual patient (Roe and Cassidy 2000). Further developments in assays to measure PTH have resulted in an assay that only measures the whole molecule of PTH (1–84 PTH) (John *et al.* 1999). Other conventional intact assays measure the 1–84 molecule in addition to the 7–84 fragment. Interestingly, the latter fragment competitively inhibits the action of 1–84 PTH. What impact measuring their ratio will further aid in management in renal bone disease remains to be seen.

In early renal failure, it would appear that adynamic bone disease is the principal type of bone lesion with high turnover bone disease developing with more advanced renal failure. As renal insufficiency progresses, higher levels of PTH are necessary for normal bone remodeling. The cause of this 'skeletal resistance' to PTH in uraemia is probably multifactorial. Inhibition of osteoclastic bone resorption appears to be the central mechanism, which, in turn, may be related accumulation of osteoprotegerin as renal function declines. Therefore a plasma PTH of two to three times the normal value is usually required to maintain normal bone turnover. A detailed description of the types of high and low turnover bone disease that forms the spectrum of renal bone disease can be found in Chapter 11.3.9.

If the patient is seen in the early phases of chronic renal insufficiency, the objective is to maintain normal bone turnover by maintaining serum calcium, phosphate, PTH and 1,25-$(OH)_2D3$, and blood pH in the normal range. Ideally, the first four of these, and plasma bicarbonate as an indication of blood pH, should be monitored regularly. In practice, it is usual to monitor plasma bicarbonate, serum calcium, phosphate, and alkaline phosphatase as part of a multichannel biochemical profile at each visit and to measure serum PTH at less frequent intervals. Measurement of vitamin D metabolites are dictated by availability and cost rather than logic.

The dietician should be involved in management early as the mainstay in preventing secondary hyperparathyroidism is strict phosphorus control. Some dietary phosphate restriction is usually required once GFR is less than 50 ml/min. In some patients who are obsessive with dietary compliance, serum phosphate levels remain in the normal range even with a GFR fall of less than 15 ml/min. Care must be taken in maintaining a sufficient protein intake, however, and adequate nutrition must be maintained. Dietary restriction alone is usually inadequate in controlling serum phosphate once GFR is less than 25 ml/min. Phosphate binders are then added to reduce phosphorus absorption from the intestine. Calcium carbonate (500–2000 mg thrice daily) is effective and probably the most widely used phosphate binder. It must be taken with food to give optimal phosphorus binding and to reduce the risk of hypercalcaemia. If hyperphosphataemia persists despite administration of calcium carbonate, excess dietary intake, for example, dairy products, should be excluded, followed by the use of alternative phosphorus binding agents. Other calcium containing binders include calcium acetate and calcium citrate. The latter should not be used in renal failure due to its significant effect in promoting aluminium absorption from the gut. Calcium acetate, on the other hand, is a more effective binder than calcium carbonate and is less likely to be associated with hypercalcaemia. The use of calcium containing phosphate binders carries the risk of a positive calcium balance which in dialysis patients is associated with vascular calcification and a raised calcium phosphate product is associated with a higher relative risk of death. Sevelemar hydrochloride (Renagel®) is an effective phosphate binder with, as yet, only a license for use in haemodialysis patients in the United Kingdom. In this group of patients, its use leads to a significant improvement in the calcium phosphorus product. In some patients, aluminium-containing phosphate binders have to be resorted to. If needed, they should be used only for a limited period of time since aluminium is absorbed to a variable extent and can lead to aluminium overload, manifesting as anaemia and aluminium-mediated bone disease. Other binders still being evaluated include lanthanum carbonate and poly-nuclear iron preparations.

In patients with mild to moderate renal insufficiency, administration of 1,25-$(OH)_2$D3 0.25 μg/day causes a rise in serum calcium, a fall in serum phosphorus and alkaline phosphatase, and retards the development of histological bone abnormalities (Baker et al. 1989). The continued administration of calcium carbonate (1 g/day) and low dose calcitriol (0.25 μg/day) in early renal failure (GFR ~ 50 ml/min has shown to be beneficial (Bianchi et al. 1994). Careful monitoring of serum calcium is required, since hypercalcaemia may accelerate the decline in renal function (for a full discussion, see Chapter 2.3). Though new vitamin D metabolites are available such as 22-oxacalcitriol, para-calcitriol (19 nor-1,25 dihydroxy-vitamin D2), and doxercalciferol (1-hydroxy-vitamin D2), their benefits over conventional calcitriol and alfacalcidol remain to be established (Cunningham 1999).

Bone biopsy is generally reserved for patients with unusual biochemical and radiological evidence of bone disease.

Management of other complications

Hyperlipidaemia

This is common in patients with chronic renal failure and is more severe in patients who are nephrotic, in diabetics, and in some patients with atheroembolic disease. The hyperlipidaemia may be aggravated by thiazides and β-blockers. The common abnormalities are hyper-triglyceridaemia and elevation of LDL cholesterol. Concentrations should be monitored on fasting blood samples, which can be taken by the general practitioner if usual attendance at the renal unit is in the afternoon or evening. Potential adverse effects of hyperlipidaemia include an increased risk of cardiovascular complications and accelerated loss of renal function. Lipid-lowering agents such as the HMG-CoA reductase inhibitors lower serum lipids effectively. Current guidelines indicate that patients with a cardiovascular event should be treated with HMG-CoA reductase to decrease the risk of cardiovascular disease. Patients should be treated to achieve a LDL cholesterol less than 100 mg/dl (<2.6 mmol/l). In patients with LDL cholesterol between 100–129 mg/dl (2.6–3.4 mmol/l), this can be done by therapeutic lifestyle changes for three months. When LDL cholesterol is persistently elevated, treatment with an HMG-CoA reductase inhibitor should be initiated. Patients

with triglycerides greater than 180–499 mg/dl (2.0–5.7 mmol/l) after 3 months of therapeutic lifestyle changes should be treated with an HMG-CoA reductase inhibitor, to achieve a non-HDL cholesterol less than 130 mg/dl.

The pharmacokinetics of some drugs used in the treatment of dyslipidaemia are altered by renal failure; that is, the toxicity of clofibrate may arise due to accumulation. The following drugs are safe and effective in patients with renal failure: cholestyramine (Valeri et al. 1986), gemfibrozil (Pasternack et al. 1987), probucol (Ida et al. 1987), and statins. However, the combination of a fibric analogue with a HmG-CoA reductase inhibitor should be avoided because of the high risk of rhabdomyolysis.

Glucose homeostasis

Glucose intolerance is common in uraemic patients despite the increase in plasma insulin. The sensitivity to insulin of especially the skeletal muscle is impaired. Furthermore, metabolic clearance of insulin and glucose uptake is decreased in preterminal renal failure (DeFronzo and Alvestrand 1980). Blood glucagon concentrations are often increased. The kidney is responsible for the metabolism and clearance of insulin and in the diabetic patient insulin requirements decline as renal mass diminishes, such that in some patients exogenous insulin is no longer needed.

Despite this, glucose intolerance is common in the non-diabetic and in addition to the increased insulin concentrations in the blood, the fasting blood sugar is usually mildly raised. This improves considerably after starting haemodialysis suggesting that a dialyzable factor is responsible. Abnormalities in PTH and 1,25-$(OH)_2$D3 may also be involved. It has been demonstrated that administration of calcitriol result in an increase in insulin secretion and improved glucose tolerance (Mak 1992). Likewise, in uraemic children with severe secondary hyperparathyroidism, glucose intolerance improved after parathyroidectomy (Make et al. 1985). The cellular mechanisms responsible for insulin resistance have yet to be clarified. Insulin receptors and their binding affinity are usually normal or increased and the defect would appear to be at a post-receptor level.

Gout

Urate clearance is significantly reduced in renal insufficiency even before GFR is reduced and subsequently there is a positive correlation between serum urate and creatinine. This may explain the increased frequency of gout in slowly progressive renal disease. The risk of gout complicating hyperuricaemia in chronic renal failure is generally low and does not justify any prophylactic treatment.

Joint pains may also be another manifestation of the underlying disease such as in Wegener's granulomatosis or amyloid secondary to rheumatoid arthritis. Hyperuricaemia should make the physician think of lead toxicity or a familial cause of gout and interstitial nephritis such as familial juvenile gouty nephropathy or more rarely hypoxanthine-guanine-phosphoribosyl-transferase deficiency. The most common cause contributing to a high serum urate in chronic renal failure is diuretic use.

The diagnosis of gout should be confirmed, wherever possible, by joint aspiration as pyrophosphate arthropathy is common, particularly in diabetics with chronic renal disease. Treatment of gout with non-steroidal anti-inflammatory drugs may be associated with a reduction in renal function and the course of treatment should be short. Diarrhoea is also more common in those given colchicine, so a short course of steroids is recommended by some to relieve pain. Follow-up treatment with allopurinol is indicated when there are recurrent attacks of definite gout, tophi, or uric acid stones. The dose must be reduced according to the creatinine clearance.

Anaemia (see Chapter 11.3.8)

Anaemia is a predictable consequence of chronic renal insufficiency and is directly related to its severity. It frequently occurs early in renal failure; in one recent study 45 per cent of patients with a creatinine of 2 mg/dl or less had a haematocrit of less than 36 per cent (Kazmi et al. 2001). Monitoring anaemia is important to determine if it becomes disproportionate to the degree of renal failure. A haemoglobin of less than 6 g/dl is rarely due to renal failure alone. Red cell indices should be scrutinized to detect the onset of iron, folate of B_{12} deficiency. Functional iron deficiency is common and should be confirmed by measurement of percentage hypochromic red cells on a full blood count, serum iron, transferrin and ferritin. As oral iron is often poorly tolerated, intravenous iron is now frequently administered to predialysis patients. Occult gastrointestinal bleeding is common in patients with advanced renal failure and is most commonly due to superficial upper gastrointestinal lesions (Akmal et al. 1994).

Recombinant human erythropoietin is effective in treating anaemia in adults and children with chronic renal failure prior to starting dialysis (Mitwalli et al. 1993; Van Geet et al. 1994; Kazmi et al. 2001). Its wider use in predialysis patients is mainly limited by funding issues. Benefits of correcting anaemia include increased quality of life, reduced morbidity and improved survival. The latter may be related to reduction in left ventricular mass and normalization of cardiac output with partial correction of anaemia. If one can extrapolate from data in dialysis patients, however, normalization of haemaglobin has no effect on all cause mortality. There is also evidence to suggest that erythropoietin therapy may retard the progression of renal failure and delay the onset of dialysis by as much as 6 months (Kuriyama et al. 1997; Jungers et al. 2001).

Haemorrhagic diathesis (see Chapter 11.3.12)

In patients with chronic renal insufficiency, this is predominantly caused by abnormal platelet function, though more recently the role of the endothelium has been implicated (Rabelink et al. 1994). The result is a prolonged bleeding time. The implication of this is that bleeding time must be checked and corrected if necessary, prior to medical interventions, which require normal haemostasis (e.g. neurosurgery, eye surgery, renal biopsy). If appropriate, surgical haemostasis can be obtained, a Mielke's bleeding time of up to 10 min can be accepted. If haemostasis has to be normal, Mielke's bleeding time should be less than 6 min. This may be achieved by the infusion of vasopressin (0.3 μg/kg in 100 ml NaCl 0.9 per cent in 30 min). The effect of vasopressin must be checked 30 min after its administration. If vasopressin corrects the bleeding time, it must be given 1 h before surgery and should be administered three times at intervals of 12 h. If vasopressin fails to correct the bleeding time, correction of anaemia by blood transfusion and administration of cryoprecipitate (1000 U intravenously) can be tried. Cryoprecipitate can be given 1 h before and three times at 12-hourly intervals after surgery, provided that bleeding time is corrected successfully. A more prolonged effect (up to 14 days) can be obtained by intravenous oestrogens in a dose of 0.6 mg/kg daily for

5 days (Livio et al. 1986). These manoeuvres may also stop epistaxis. If these manoeuvres fail, haemodialysis often corrects the defect.

Urinary tract infections

A high fluid intake is recommended. In the community, the most common organism causing uncomplicated urinary tract injection is *Escherichia coli*. Specific antibiotic treatment will depend on local resistance patterns and hospital antibiotic policy. Urinary antiseptics should not be used in patients with significant renal impairment. Nitrofurantoin is absolutely contraindicated in renal failure. Prolonged treatment may be required when infection complicates conditions such as polycystic kidney disease. Some structural abnormalities make it impossible to eradicate infection, for example, infected staghorn calculi.

Sexual dysfunction (see Chapter 11.3.1)

Improvement of sexual function may occur in both sexes with general measures such as correcting anaemia with erythropoietin and by addressing any psychosocial issues. Control of secondary hyperparathyroidism with calcitriol may also lower prolactin in some patients. In men, zinc deficiency has been associated with reduced testosterone production. This can readily be corrected, though the effect is not dramatic. Similarly, supplemental testosterone where levels are low usually is unhelpful unless the only complaint is reduced libido. Bromocriptine will reduce high circulating prolactin though it is of limited value and associated with side-effects. Sildenafil (Viagra), on the other hand, is well tolerated and effective in treating this problem (Sadovsky et al. 2001). Sildenafil clearance has been shown to be reduced and maximum plasma concentrations doubled in patients with creatinine clearances of less than 30 ml/min, so the recommended starting dose is 25 mg. Its use is contraindicated in patients taking nitrates and it should be used with caution in patients with known coronary heart disease.

In women with amenorrhoea who wish to resume menstruation, progesterone may be given in the last days of the monthly cycle to stimulate bleeding. This may aggravate anaemia. It is not known if amenorrhoea predisposes to endometrial hyperplasia or uterine cancer in women with chronic renal failure, so periodic gynaecological review is prudent. Other symptoms related to reduced circulating oestradiol such as vaginal atrophy and dryness that may result in dysparunia can be treated with topical oestrogen and or lubricants. Women who are menstruating are at risk of pregnancy and should be advised about birth control.

Monitoring underlying disease

When the underlying disease is still active and potentially lethal (e.g. diabetes, amyloid, myeloma), its management and monitoring may dominate the follow-up and are unlikely to be overlooked. However, when it is relatively inactive or has received curative treatment (e.g. tuberculosis, schistosomiasis), a recrudescence or relapse may be missed. Any management plan, therefore, should feature these quiescent diseases and ensure that necessary tests for cure are completed.

As renal failure progresses in diabetics, their insulin requirements decline as renal mass diminishes. Special care with the use of oral hypoglycaemic agents is required; long-acting sulfonylureas are contraindicated because of the risk of hypoglycaemia, as is metformin because of the risk of lactic acidosis. Short-acting sulfonylureas, which are metabolized principally by the liver, are preferred, but it should be remembered that diabetics with renal failure can become hypoglycaemic even on diet alone.

Several systemic diseases are prone to relapse long after successful treatment or during maintenance therapy. Relapses are often precipitated by intercurrent infections or changes in drug therapy. The history at each visit should include the vague symptoms of tiredness, fever, weight loss, and aches and pains, which may be the only warnings of a relapse affecting renal function. Routine immunological monitoring at each visit can be helpful in detecting early relapse. Serum C3 and C4 are guides to relapse in systemic lupus, but not in all patients. A raised serum C-reactive protein is an excellent marker for relapse in polyarteritis and other vasculitides, if not explained by infection or other illness. Measurement of antineutrophil cytoplasmic antibody titres can also be helpful.

Pregnancy

Pregnancy does not usually accelerate progression of chronic renal failure, provided blood pressure is well controlled (Section 15). The exception is reflux nephropathy with bilateral scarring (El-Khatib *et al.* 1994). However, approximately 20 per cent of pregnancies in patients with chronic renal insufficiency are complicated by premature delivery, and abortion, stillbirth, or neonatal death in about 25 per cent. Fetal outcome is particularly poor in patients with hypertension, nephrotic range proteinuria, or an increase in serum creatinine of more than 50 per cent during pregnancy. In a study by Bar *et al.* (2000), worse pregnancy outcomes were observed in patients with moderate or severe renal failure. Contraceptive measures are therefore strongly advised for patients with serum creatinine greater than 230 µmol/l (>2.5 mg/dl), hypertension, and proteinuria. None of the contraceptive measures is ideal. Because of increased susceptibility to infections, the use of intrauterine devices carries a certain risk in patients with chronic renal failure, and oestrogen-containing contraceptives may aggravate hypertension.

Predialysis assessment (see Table 9)

A checklist is useful at this stage in the management of the patient (Table 8). The assessment is not complete without an interview with the family and referral to the social worker. Decisions are made about further management and the patient is prepared for dialysis and/or transplantation.

Social assessment (see Chapter 11.3.14)

The patient entering a dialysis and transplant programme has to face many changes in life style due to such factors as dependence and change of body image. The renal unit should function as a multidisciplinary team of which the social worker is a vital member, providing the social assessment on which many decisions hinge and counselling the patient during an extremely stressful period. The social worker assesses patients' grasp of what is happening and establishes good communication. This will depend on their intelligence, level of education, and linguistic skills.

The social report describes the patient's family and social relationships, and assesses the strength of these support systems and others, such as religious faith, church membership and work environment, from which patients can draw strength in their new dependency. Their housing is important in deciding whether peritoneal dialysis or home haemodialysis is a treatment option; rehousing on medical grounds usually takes between 3 months and one year in Britain and may disrupt the support from family and neighbours. The patient's employment record and financial situation are explored so that interruption of employment can be predicted and state and charitable funds mobilized to meet the financial strains of hospital attendance, hospital visits by the family, home adaptations and extra bills for heating and diet at a time of reduced earnings.

During the interviews, the social worker can assess the physical mobility of the patient and advise if transport will be necessary to bring the patient to hospital or if the occupational therapist's help is needed with home adaptations. The attitude of the patient to the illness is assessed: how much denial, incomprehension, depression, and withdrawal are present? Are there features of the illness that the patient is particularly worried about but has not mentioned to the doctor such as loss of libido or impotence?

Interviewing the family is also part of the social assessment, giving a better understanding of the patient and his or her social interrelationships and provides an opportunity to discuss the possibility of a live related transplant. In addition to explaining what is involved, it is important to allow the parent or sibling a way of saying 'no' and supporting them in this decision.

The patient must receive consistent and realistic advice about future treatment options. This demands good communication between the members of the renal team, which is typically ensured by a weekly meeting at which patients are discussed and a team decision arrived at.

The period of adjustment to the loss of freedom that is a part of having renal failure is seldom less than 6–12 months and some patients never adjust. The social worker can help the patient work through this period. Denial and noncompliance with treatment are then less of a problem.

Hepatitis screening

All patients should be screened for hepatitis B and C. Patients who are negative for HBsAg are offered vaccination if they do not have naturally acquired immunity. As chronic renal failure reduces the effectiveness vaccination, it is best to arrange this early. In healthy adults at risk of

Table 9 The predialysis assessment(s)

Objectives
To review database and fill in any gaps in information
To assess the patients' suitability for dialysis and/or transplantation
Guided by the results of (2) above plan:
    Counselling of patient and family
    Vascular access if for haemodialysis
    Screening of live donors
    Home assessment for peritoneal dialysis or home haemodialysis
    Palliative care package

Methods
Complete checklist (see Table 8)
Social survey
Additional clinical and laboratory studies

a suboptimal response, a novel triple antigen vaccine produces a greater degree of protection without the need of a prolonged course (Young et al. 2001) and it would therefore seem reasonable to use this vaccine in patients with chronic renal failure. The preferred injection site is the deltoid in adults and the anterolateral thigh in children because the buttock site is associated with a smaller chance of response. If the patient is HBsAg positive, it should be repeated and tests for HBeAg and anti-HBeAg performed. HbsAg positive patients have the same survival on regular dialysis as HbsAg negative patients but a poorer prognosis and a higher incidence of hepatic disease after renal transplantation (Parfrey et al. 1985).

The prevalence of hepatitis C virus (HCV) infection in ESRF patients varies throughout the world with the highest reported prevalence in Egypt of 22 per cent compared to 1.9 per cent in the United States. Approximately 75 per cent of subjects who are antibody positive also have viral particles in their blood and are therefore infectious. A four-antigen recombinant blot (RIBA) assay is currently the best confirmatory test for detecting hepatitis C antibodies. If patients are hepatitis C antibody positive, mRNA should be sought. Some strains (genotype 1) are less responsive to treatment with interferon alpha. Since blood donor screening for hepatitis C is routine, the risk of transmission by this route has been estimated as 1 in 1,03,000 transfused units. The virulence and outcome of hepatitis C infection in patients with chronic renal failure is yet to be clearly defined.

HIV testing

It is advisable to test for HIV infection prior to dialysis with appropriate counselling when indicated. The AIDS epidemic has a marked geographic distribution; its main impact in nephrology services is in large population centres. In developed economies such as the United States, Blacks and Hispanics are the racial groups with the highest prevalence of AIDS. HIVAN is the third leading cause of ESRF in Blacks in the age group 20–64 after diabetes and hypertension in the United States (Winston et al. 1998). HIV is less infectious than hepatitis B and there is no evidence that social contact or sharing of eating and drinking utensils results in transmission. The most likely mode of transmission to hospital staff is through inoculation of infected blood by needle prick and there is so far no evidence of epidemic spread in dialysis units. The majority of HIV infections are picked up by routine testing and if the patient is known to be HIV positive, continuous ambulatory peritoneal dialysis (CAPD) or home haemodialysis would be the treatment of choice in most cases. A review of the use of antiretroviral drugs in dialysis patients has been published recently (Izzedine et al. 2001). Blood taking should be kept to a minimum—for example, it is not necessary to estimate cytotoxic antibodies regularly since it is inappropriate to transplant HIV-positive patients. Special care should be taken in handling, transporting, and analysing samples. Healthcare workers need to be aware of the need for assessment for postexposure HIV prophylaxis in the event of a needle stick injury. In some dialysis units with a high prevalence of HIV infection, HTLV-1 is also prevalent (Perez et al. 1989).

Cytotoxic antibodies

Leucocytotoxic antibodies are formed against HLA antigens as a result of immunization by blood transfusion, previous pregnancy, or a previous transplant. Patients on the transplant list should have blood sent for panel reactive antibodies periodically. Using established techniques, including more recently developed flow cytometry and ELISA assays

for detecting HLA antibodies, 'false positives' still occur. These may be due to autoantibodies directed at beta 2 microglobulin (part of the structure of the class 1 HLA antigens) developing in, for example, patients with SLE. Infection such as CMV (MacLeod et al. 1987) may be the trigger for cross-reacting non-HLA antibodies. It is worth identifying these autoantibodies which mean a positive cross match may not be a bar to transplantation.

Suitability for haemodialysis and vascular access (see Chapter 12.2)

The planning of vascular access is of great importance for a smooth start to haemodialysis. If a fistula is required for haemodialysis, it should be created at least 3 months before the estimated date of starting dialysis in males and up to 6 months in a female with small veins. This allows time for maturation of the fistula, prepares the patient psychologically for the inevitable and avoids the need for temporary access such as a jugular or femoral vein catheter with all the attendant risks of such procedures viz trauma, septicaemia, venous stenosis, and thrombosis. Because of the high risk of stenosis in the subclavian vein, which seriously jeopardizes future fistula attempts and venous hypertension in the fistula, the use of subclavian catheters should be avoided (Mansfield et al. 1994).

On the other hand, if the patient is to be treated by CAPD and receives an early renal transplant and therefore not likely to require haemodialysis, it is then best not to fashion a fistula, which may thrombose during an acute intercurrent illness which causes hypotension. It is therefore essential that a pathway through the treatment options should be mapped before decisions on access are taken. In arriving at the decision, the state of the blood vessels in the forearm is of major importance. This is especially important in diabetics.

Suitability for continuous ambulatory dialysis

During the predialysis assessment period, we always include a visit by the patient to the CAPD unit to acquaint them and their family with the technique and staff. The unit staff who would train the patient then assess suitability for CAPD. There are few absolute contraindications to CAPD though some, such as a major diaphragmatic defects will only become apparent after CAPD has been started. A colostomy, ileostomy, or nephrostomy is a firm contraindication and previous major abdominal operations relative contraindications. For young children, for those with severe physical handicaps such as blindness, crippling arthritis, paralysis, or severe incoordination and for the mentally handicapped a family member such as the spouse or parent will be trained, and thus the suitability of the helper will need to be assessed. However, blind patients and some with severe arthritis have been trained to perform CAPD successfully themselves.

Obesity and hyperlipidaemia get worse more frequently in CAPD patients than in haemodialysis patients, so they are a relative contraindication to CAPD. Abdominal wall hernias are aggravated by CAPD and should be repaired before CAPD is started. CAPD will also result in an exaggerated lumbar lordosis, and if pre-existing lumbar disc disease is present, this will almost always deteriorate on CAPD.

Suitability for predialysis transplantation

Pre-emptive renal transplantation, if contemplated, should obviously be planned early in the assessment of the patient. When possible, it obviates all the attendant risks and cost of dialysis. It is appropriate in patients with a predictable cause, such as diabetes, so that 'end stage' can be accurately dated. It is also easier to plan when a family donor is available. In recent years, it has also become clear that the outcome of living, unrelated kidney donation is better compared to cadaver donation (Lowell *et al.* 1996). Interestingly, pre-emptive transplantation compared to transplantation from long-term dialysis is associated with better graft survival (Mange *et al.* 2001). In this study, there was a 52 per cent reduction in the risk of allograft loss in the first year in patients transplanted without prior dialysis.

Palliative care

Some patients approaching end stage renal failure do not wish to have renal replacement treatment, and in others it may be inappropriate if multiple other comorbid conditions coexist. In such cases, providing good palliative care at the end of life is essential. Many symptoms can be alleviated with the use of drugs such as erythropoietin and diuretics, analgesics, and later, sedatives. Frequently nephrologists lack appropriate training in palliative care and a multidisciplinary approach should be adopted drawing on facilities such as the local hospice, district nurses, and general practitioners according to local circumstances.

References

Akmal, M., Sawelson, S., Karubian, F., and Gadallah, M. (1994). The prevalence and significance of occult blood loss in patients with predialysis advanced chronic renal failure (CRF), or receiving dialytic therapy. *Clinical Nephrology* **42**, 198–202.

Amann, K., Mall, G., and Ritz, E. (1994). Myocardial interstitial fibrosis in uraemia: is it relevant? *Nephrology, Dialysis, Transplantation* **9**, 127–128.

Allon, M. (1995). Hyperkalemia in end-stage renal disease: mechanisms and management. *Journal of the American Society of Nephrology* **6**, 1134–1142.

Allon, M. and Copkney, C. (1990). Albuterol and insulin for treatment of hyperkalemia in hemodialysis patients. *Kidney International* **38**, 869–872.

Allon, M. and Shanklin, N. (1995). Effect of albuterol treatment on subsequent dialytic potassium removal. *American Journal of Kidney Diseases* **26**, 607–613.

ANZDATA. *Annual Report of the Australian and New Zealand Dialysis and Transplant Registry* 23rd edn. Adelaide: The Queen Elizabeth Hospital, 2000.

Astor, B. C., Eustace, J. A., Powe, N. R., Klag, M. J., Sadler, J. H., Fink, N. E., and Coresh, J. (2001). Timing of nephrologist referral and arteriovenous access use: the CHOICE study. *American Journal of Kidney Diseases* **38**, 494–501.

Attman, P.-O., Samuelsson, O., and Alaupovic, P. (1993). Lipid metabolism and renal failure. *American Journal of Kidney Diseases* **21**, 373–592.

Baba, S. (2001). Nifedipine and enalapril equally reduce the progression of nephropathy in hypertensive type 2 diabetics. *Diabetes Research and Clinical Practice* **54**, 191–201.

Baker, L. R. I. *et al.* (1989). 1,25-$(OH)_2D_3$ administration in moderate renal failure: a prospective double-blind trial. *Kidney International* **35**, 661–669.

Bakris, G. L. (1990). Effects of diltiazem or lisinopril on massive proteinuria associated with diabetes mellitus. *Annals of Internal Medicine* **112**, 707–708.

Bar, B. A. (1999). Concern for azotemia with angiotensin-converting enzyme inhibitors: public health implications and clinical relevance. *American Heart Journal* **138**, 801–803.

Bar, J., Ben-Rafael, Z., Padoa, A., Boner, G., and Hod, M. (2000). Prediction of pregancy outcome in subgroups of women with renal disease. *Clinical Nephrology* **53**, 437–444.

Barsotti, G., Morelli, E., Giannoni, A., Guiducci, A., Lupetti, S., and Giovanetti, S. (1983). Restricted phosphorus and nitrogen intake to slow the progression of chronic renal failure: a controlled trial. *Kidney International* **24** (Suppl. 16), S278–S284.

Bartosik, L. P., Lajoie, G., Sugar, L., and Cattran, D. C. (2001). Predicting progression in IgA nephropathy. *American Journal of Kidney Diseases* **38**, 728–735.

Bauer, J. H., Brooks, C. S., and Burch, R. N. (1982). Clinical appraisal of creatinine clearance as a marker of glomerular filtration rate. *American Journal of Kidney Diseases* **1**, 337–346.

Bergstrom, J., Alvestrand, A., Bucht, H., and Gutierrez, A. (1986). Progression of chronic renal failure in man is retarded with more clinical follow-ups and better blood pressure control. *Clinical Nephrology* **25**, 1–6.

Bergstrom, J., Wang, T., and Lindholm, B. (1998). Factors contributing to catabolism in end-stage renal disease patients. *Mineral and Electrolyte Metabolism* **24**, 92–101.

Bianchi, M. L., Colantonio, G., Campanini, F., Rossi, R., Valenti, G., Ortolani, S., and Buccianti, G. (1994). Calcitriol and calcium carbonate therapy in early chronic renal failure. *Nephrology, Dialysis, Transplantation* **9**, 1595–1599.

Biesenbach, G., Grafinger, P., Janko, O., and Zazgornik, J. (1997). Influence of cigarette-smoking on the progression of clinical diabetic nephropathy in type 2 diabetic patients. *Clinical Nephrology* **48**, 146–150.

Bilo, H. J. G., Schaap, G. H., Blaak, E., Gans, R. O. B., Oe, P. L., and Donker, A. J. M. (1989). Effects of chronic and acute protein administration on renal function in patients with chronic renal insufficiency. *Nephron* **53**, 181–187.

Bulpitt C. J. (2000). Controlling hypertension in the elderly. *Quarterly Journal of Medicine* **93**, 203–206.

Brazy, P. C., Stead, W. W., and Fitzwilliam, J. F. (1989). Progression of renal insufficiency: role of blood pressure. *Kidney International* **35**, 670–674.

Brenner, B. M. *et al.* (2001). Effects of losartan on renal and cardiovascular outcomes in patients with type 2 diabetes and nephropathy. *New England Journal of Medicine* **345**, 861–869.

Coomes, E. N., Berlyne, G. M., and Shaw, A. B. (1965). Incidence of neuropathy in non-dialysed chronic renal failure patients. *Proceedings of the European Dialysis and Transplant Association* **2**, 133–137.

Crowe, A. V., Howse, M., Bell, G. M., and Henry, J. A. (2000). Substance abuse and the kidney. *Quarterly Journal of Medicine* **93** (3), 147–152.

Cruickshank, J. M., Thorp, J. M., and Zacharias, F. J. (1987). Benefits and potential harm of lowering blood pressure. *Lancet* **i**, 581–584.

Cunningham, J. (1999). What is the optimal regimen for vitamin D? *Kidney International* **56**, S59–S64.

D'Amico, G. (2000). Natural history of IgA nephropathy: role of clinical and histological prognostic factors. *American Journal of Kidney Diseases* **36**, 227–237.

De Broe, M. E. and Elseviers, M. M. (1998). Analgesic nephropathy. *New England Journal of Medicine* **338**, 446–452.

DeFronzo, R. A. and Alvestrand, A. (1980). Glucose intolerance in uremia: site and mechanism. *American Journal of Clinical Nutrition* **33**, 1438–1445.

Ecder, T. *et al.* (2000). Effect of antihypertensive therapy on renal function and urinary albumin excretion in hypertensive patients with autosomal dominant polycystic kidney disease. *American Journal of Kidney Diseases* **35**, 427–432.

El-Khatib, M., Packham, D. K., Becker, G. J., and Kincaid-Smith, P. (1994). Pregnancy-related complications in women with reflux nephropathy. *Clinical Nephrology* **41**, 50–54.

Eliahou, H. E. *et al.* (1988). Effect of the calcium channel blocker nisoldipine on the progression of chronic renal failure in man. *American Journal of Medicine* **8**, 285–290.

Ellis, P. A. and Cairns, H. S. (2001). Renal impairment in elderly patients with hypertension and diabetes. *Quarterly Journal of Medicine* **94**, 261–265.

Farrington, K., Levison, D. A., Greenwood, R. N., Cattell, W. R., and Baker, L. R. I. (1988). Renal biopsy in patients with unexplained renal impairment and normal kidney size. *Quarterly Journal of Medicine* **70**, 221–233.

Fick, G. M. and Gabow, P. A. (1994). Hereditary and acquired cystic disease of the kidney. *Kidney International* **46**, 951–964.

Fliser, D., Schroter, M., Neubeck, M., and Ritz, E. (1994). Coadministration of thiazides increases the efficacy of loop diuretics even in patients with advanced renal failure. *Kidney International* **46**, 482–488.

Florijn, K. W., Barendregt, J. N. M., van Saase, J. L. C. M., van Es, L. A., and Chang, P. C. Reproducibility and accuracy of creatinine clearances during oral cimetidine treatment. In *Studies in Autosomal Dominant Polycystic Kidney Disease* (ed. K. W. Florijin), pp. 125–145. The Netherlands: University of Leiden, 1994.

Fogari, R. *et al.* (1999). Long-term effects of ramipril and nitrendipine on albuminuria in hypertensive patients with type II diabetes and impaired renal function. *Journal of Human Hypertension* **13**, 47–53.

Fored, M. C. *et al.* (2001). Acetaminophen, aspirin, and chronic renal failure. *New England Journal of Medicine* **345**, 1801–1808.

Fouque, D. *et al.* (1992). Controlled low protein diets in chronic renal insufficiency: meta-analysis. *British Medical Journal* **304**, 216–220.

Fried, L. F. *et al.* (2001a). Lipid modulation in insulin-dependent diabetes mellitus: effect on microvascular outcomes. *Journal of Diabetes Complications* **15**, 113–119.

Fried, L. F., Orchard, T. J., and Kasiske, B. L. (2001b). Effect of lipid reduction on the progression of renal disease: a meta-analysis. *Kidney International* **59**, 260–269.

Friedman, E. A. and Tao, K. T. (1995). Disappearance of uremia due to heroin-associated nephropathy. *American Journal of Kidney Diseases* **25**, 689–693.

Gansevoort, R. T., de Zeeuw, D., and de Jong, P. E. (1994). Is the antiproteinuric effect of ACE inhibition mediated by interference in the renin–angiotensin system? *Kidney International* **45**, 861–867.

Gansevoort, R. T., Sluiter, W. J., Hemmelder, M. H., de Zeeuw, D., and de Jong, P. E. (1995). Antiproteinuric effect of blood-pressure-lowering agents: a meta-analysis of comparative trials. *Nephrology, Dialysis, Transplantation* **10**, 1963–1974.

Gofin, R. (1982). The health status of elderly men: a community study. *Public Health* **96**, 345–354.

Goodman, W. G. *et al.* (2000). Coronary-artery calcification in young adults with end-stage renal disease who are undergoing dialysis. *New England Journal of Medicine* **342**, 1478–1483.

Goodship, T. H. J. *et al.* (2000). Longterm follow-up of patients presenting to adult nephrologists with chronic pyelonephritis and 'normal' renal function. *Quarterly Journal of Medicine* **93**, 799–803.

Gretz, N., Meisenger, E., and Strauch, M. (1986). Influence of the underlying renal disease on the rate of progression. *Contributions in Nephrology* **53**, 92–101.

Hanoke, R. K., Noone, R. H., and Stone, W. J. (1984). Severe allopurinol toxicity. *American Journal of Medicine* **76**, 47–56.

Hellström, L., Elinder, C.-G., Dahlberg, B., Lundberg, M., Järup, L., Persson, B., and Axelson, O. (2001). Cadmium exposure and end-stage renal disease. *American Journal of Kidney Diseases* **38**, 1001–1008.

Hemmelgran, B. R. *et al.* (2000). Poor long-term survival after coronary angiography in patients with renal insufficiency. *American Journal of Kidney Diseases* **37**, 64–72.

Henin, P., de Plaen, J. F., and van Ypersele de Strihou, C. (1989). Angiotensin converting enzyme inhibitors may reversibly impair renal function in the absence of renal artery stenosis. *Nephrology, Dialysis, Transplantation* **4**, 444.

Hostetter, T. H. (2001). Prevention of end-stage renal disease due to type 2 diabetes. *New England Journal of Medicine* **345**, 910–912.

Ida, H., Izumino, K., Asaka, M., Fujita, M., Nishino, A., and Sasuyoma, S. (1987). Effects of probucol on hyperlipidemia in patients with nephrotic syndrome. *Nephron* **47**, 280–283.

Iggo, N., Littlewood, T., and Winearls, C. G. (2000). Prospects for effective treatment of AL amyloidosis. *Quarterly Journal of Medicine* **93**, 257–260.

Izzedine, H., Launay-Vacher, V., Baumelou, A., and Deray, G. (2001). An appraisal of antiretroviral drugs in hemodialysis. *Kidney International* **60**, 821–830.

Jacobsen, S. J., Oesterling, J. E., and Lieber, M. M. (1995). Community-based population studies on the natural history of prostatism. *Current Opinion in Urology* **5**, 13–17.

Jafar, T. H. *et al.* (2001). Angiotensin-converting enzyme inhibitors and progression of nondiabetic renal disease. A meta-analysis of patient-level data. *Annals of Internal Medicine* **135**, 73–87.

Jansen, M. A. M. *et al.* (2001). Renal function and nutritional status at the start of chronic dialysis treatment. *Journal of the American Society of Nephrology* **12**, 157–163.

JNC-VI The Sixth Report of the Joint National Committee on Prevention, Detection, Evaluation, and Treatment of High Blood Pressure (1997). *Archives of Internal Medicine* **157**, 2413–2446.

John, M. R., Goodman, W. G., Gao, P., Cantor, T. L., Salusky, I. B., and Juppner, H. J. (1999). A novel immunoradiometric assay detects full-length human PTH but not amino-terminally truncated fragments: implications for PTH measurement in renal failure. *Journal of Clinical Endocrinology and Metabolism* **84**, 4287–4290.

Jones, C. A., McQuillan, G. M., Kusek, J. W., Eberhardt, M. S., Herman, W. H., Coresh, J., Salive, M., Jones, C. P., and Agodoa, L. Y. (1998). Serum creatinine levels in the US population: Third National Health and Nutrition Examination Survey. *American Journal of Kidney Diseases* **32**, 992–999.

Jungers, P., Choukroun, G., Oualim, Z., Robino, C., Nguyen, A.-T., and Man, N.-K. (2001). Beneficial influence of recombinant human erythropoietin therapy on the rate of progression of chronic renal failure in predialysis patients. *Nephrology, Dialysis, Transplantation* **16**, 307–312.

Kaplan, N. M. (1994). Management of hypertensive emergencies. *Lancet* **344**, 1335–1338.

Kaplan, N. M. (1998). J-curve not burned off by HOT study. *Lancet* **351**, 1748.

Kasiske, B. L., Lakatua, J. D., Ma, J. Z., and Louis, T. A. (1998). A meta-analysis of the effects of dietary protein restriction on the rate of decline in renal function. *American Journal of Kidney Diseases* **31**, 954–961.

Kazmi, W. H., Kausz, A. T., Khan, S., Abichandani, R., Ruthazer, R., Obrador G. T., and Pereira, B. J. G. (2001). Anemia: an early complication of chronic renal insufficiency. *American Journal of Kidney Diseases* **38**, 803–812.

Klahr, S. *et al.* (1994). The effects of dietary protein restriction and blood-pressure control on the progression of chronic renal disease. *New England Journal of Medicine* **330**, 877–884.

Korevaar, Jr., Jansen, M. A. M., Dekker, F. W., Jager, K. J., Boeschoten, E. W., Krediet, R. T., and Bossuyt, P. M. M. (2001). When to initiate dialysis: effect of proposed US guidelines on survival. *Lancet* **358**, 1046–1050.

Kraut, J. A. (1995). The role of metabolic acidosis in the pathogenesis of renal osteodystrophy. *Advancements in Renal Replacement Therapy* **2**, 40–51.

Kristal, B., Shasha, S. M., Labin, L., and Cohen, A. (1988). Estimation of quantitative proteinuria by using the protein–creatinine ratio in random urine samples. *American Journal of Nephrology* **8**, 198–203.

Kuhlmann, M. K., Heckmann, M., Riegel, W., and Khler, H. (2001). Evaluation of renal Kt/V as a marker of renal function in predialysis patients. *Kidney International* **60**, 1540–1546.

Kuriyama, S., Tomonari, H., Yoshida, H., Hashimoto, T., Kawaguchi, Y., and Sakai, O. (1997). Reversal of anemia by erythropoietin therapy retards the progression of chronic renal failure, especially in nondiabetic patients. *Nephron* **77**, 176–185.

Lazarus, L. and Peraino, R. A. (1984). Reversible uremia due to bilateral ureteral obstruction from tuberculosis. *American Journal of Nephrology* **4**, 322–327.

Lens, X. M., Montoliu, J., Cases, A., Campistol, J. M., and Revert, L. (1989). Treatment of hyperkalaemia in renal failure: salbutamol v. insulin. *Nephrology, Dialysis, Transplantation* **4**, 228–232.

Leumann, E. P. (1978). Progression of renal insufficiency in pediatric patients: estimation from serum creatinine. *Helvetica Paediatrica Acta* **33**, 25–35.

Levey, A. S., Perrone, R. D., and Madias, N. E. (1988). Serum creatinine and renal function. *Annual Review of Medicine* **39**, 465–490.

Levey, A. S. *et al.* (1996). Effects of dietary protein restriction on the progression of advanced renal disease in the Modification of Diet in Renal Disease Study. *American Journal of Kidney Diseases* **27**, 652–663.

Levey, A. S. *et al.* (1999). A more accurate method to estimate glomerular filtration rate from serum creatinine: a new prediction equation. Modification of Diet in Renal Disease Study Group. *Annals of Internal Medicine* **130**, 461–470.

Lewis, E. J., Hunsicker, L. G., Bain, R. P., and Rohde, R. D. (1993). The effect of angiotensin-converting-enzyme inhibition on diabetic nephropathy. The Collaborative Study Group. *New England Journal of Medicine* **329**, 1456–1462.

Lewis, E. J. *et al.* (2001). Renoprotective effect of the angiotensin-receptor antagonist irbesartan in patients with nephropathy due to type 2 diabetes. *New England Journal of Medicine* **345**, 851–860.

Lightstone, L., Rees, A. J., Tomson, C., Walls, J., Winearls, C. G., and Feehally, J. (1995). High incidence of end-stage renal disease in Indo-Asians in the UK. *Quarterly Journal of Medicine* **88**, 191–195.

Livio, M. *et al.* (1986). Conjugated estrogens for the management of bleeding associated with renal failure. *New England Journal of Medicine* **315**, 731–735.

Lowell, J. A. *et al.* (1996). Living-unrelated renal transplantation provides comparable results to living-related renal transplantation: a 12-year single-center experience. *Surgery* **119**, 538–543.

Lubowitz, H. *et al.* (1967). Glomerular filtration rate: determination in patients with chronic renal disease. *Journal of the American Medical Association* **199**, 100–104.

MacLeod, A. M., Kurtz, J., Chapman, J. R., Ting, A., and Morris, P. J. (1987). Autolymphocytotoxins and virus infection in renal transplantation. *Transplantation Proceedings* **19**, 901.

Mak, R. H., Bettinelli, A., Turner, C., Haycock, G. B., and Chantler, C. (1985). The influence of hyperparathyroidism on glucose metabolism in uremia. *Journal of Clinical Endocrinology and Metabolism* **60**, 229–233.

Malangone, J. M., Abuelo, J. G., Pezzullo, J. C., Lund, K., and McGloin, C. A. (1989). Clinical and laboratory features of patients with chronic renal disease at the start of dialysis. *Clinical Nephrology* **31**, 77–87.

Mange, K. C., Joffe, M. M., and Feldman, H. I. (2001). Effect of the use or nonuse of long-term dialysis on the subsequent survival of renal transplants from living donors. *New England Journal of Medicine* **344**, 726–731.

Mansfield, P. F., Hohn, D. C., Fornage, B. D., Gregurich, M. A., and Ota, D. M. (1994). Complications and failures of subclavian-vein cathererization. *New England Journal of Medicine* **331**, 1735–1738.

Maschio, G. *et al.* (1983). Early dietary protein and phosphorus restriction is effective in delaying progression of chronic renal failure. *Kidney International* **24** (Suppl. 16), S273–S277.

Mitch, W. E., Walser, M., Buffington, G. A., and Lemann, J., Jr. (1976). A simple method of estimating progression of chronic renal failure. *Lancet* **ii**, 1326–1328.

Mitwalli, A., Abuaisha, H., al Wakeel, J., al Mohaya, S., Alam, A. A., el Gamal, H., and Fayed, H. (1993). Effectiveness of low-dose erythropoietin in predialysis patients. *Nephrology, Dialysis, Transplantation* **8**, 1085–1089.

Muntner, P., He, J., Hamm, L., Loria, C., and Whelton, P. K. (2002). Renal insufficiency and subsequent deathy resulting from cardiovascular disease in the United States. *Journal of the American Society of Nephrology* **13**, 745–753.

Murray, M. D. and Brater, D. C. (1993). Renal toxicity of the nonsteroidal anti-inflammatory drugs. *Annual Reviews Pharmacology Toxicology* **33**, 435–465.

Nilsson-Ehle, P. and Grub, A. (1994). New markers for the determination of GFR: iohexol clearance and cystatin C serum concentration. *Kidney International* **46** (Suppl. 47), S17–S19.

Norteir, J. L. *et al.* (2000). Urothelial carcinoma associated with the use of a Chinese herb (*Aristolochia fangchi*). *New England Journal of Medicine* **342**, 1686–1692.

Obrador, G. T., Arora, P., Kausz, A. T., Ruthazer, R., Pereira, B. J. T., and Levey, A. S. (1999). Level of renal function at the initiation of dialysis in the US end-stage renal disease population. *Kidney International* **56**, 2227–2235.

Orth, S. R. *et al.* (1998). Smoking as a risk factor for end-stage renal failure in men with primary renal disease. *Kidney International* **54**, 926–931.

Palmer, B. F. (1999). Sexual dysfunction in uremia. *Journal of the American Society of Nephrology* **10**, 1381–1388.

Palmer, B. F. (2002). Renal dysfunction complicating the treatment of hypertension. *New England Journal of Medicine* **347**, 1256–1261.

Parfrey, P. S. (2001). Is renal insufficiency an atherogenic state? Reflections on prevalence, incidence, and risk. *American Journal of Kidney Diseases* **37**, 64–72.

Parfrey, P. S., Farge, D., Forbes, R. D. C., Dandavino, R., Kenick, S., and Guttmann, R. D. (1985). Chronic hepatitis in end-stage renal disease: comparison of HBsAg-negative and HBsAg-positive patients. *Kidney International* **28**, 959–967.

Parfrey, P. S. *et al.* (1989). Contrast material-induced renal failure in patients with diabetes mellitus, renal insufficiency, or both. *New England Journal of Medicine* **320**, 143–149.

Parving, H.-H., Andersen, A. R., Smidt, U. M., Hommel, A., Mathiesen, E. R., and Svendsen, P. A. (1987). Effect of antihypertensive treatment on kidney function in diabetic nephropathy. *British Medical Journal* **294**, 1443–1447.

Parving, H.-H., Anderson, A. R., Smidt, U. M., and Svendsen, P. A. (1983). Early aggressive antihypertensive treatment reduces rate of decline in kidney function in diabetic nephropathy. *Lancet* **i**, 1175–1179.

Pastan, S. and Bailey, J. (1998). Dialysis therapy. *New England Journal of Medicine* **338**, 1428–1437.

Pasternack, A., Vanttinen, T., Solakivi, T., Kuusi, T., and Korte, T. (1987). Normalization of lipoprotein lipase and hepatic lipase by gemfibrozil results in correction of lipoprotein abnormalities in chronic renal failure. *Clinical Nephrology* **27**, 163–168.

Perez, G., Ortiz-Interian, C., Lee, H., de Medina, M., Cerney, M., Allain, J.-P., Schiff, E., Parks, E., Parks, W., and Bourgoignie, J. J. (1989). Human immunodeficiency virus and human T-cell leukemia virus type 1 in patients undergoing maintenance hemodialysis in Miami. *American Journal of Kidney Diseases* **14**, 39–43.

Perico, N. *et al.* (1998). The antiproteinuric effect of angiotensin antagonism in human IgA nephropathy is potentiated by indomethacin. *Journal of the American Society of Nephrology* **9**, 2308–2317.

Perneger, T. V., Whelton, P. K., and Klag, J. M. (1994). Risk of kidney failure associated with the use of acetaminophen, aspirin, and nonsteroidal anti-inflammatory drugs. *New England Journal of Medicine* **331**, 1675–1679.

Perrone, R. D., Madias N. E., and Levey, A. S. (1992). Serum creatinine as an index of renal function: new insights into old concepts. *Clinical Chemistry* **38**, 1933–1953.

Petersen, L. J. *et al.* (2001). A randomized and double-blind comparison of isradipine and spirapril as monotherapy and in combination on the decline in renal function in patients with chronic renal failure and hypertension. *Clinical Nephrology* **55**, 375–383.

Progress Collaborative Group (2001). Randomised trial of a peindopril-based blood pressure-lowering regimen among 6105 individuals with previous stroke or transient ischaemic attack. *Lancet* **358**, 1033–1041.

Rabelink, T. N., Zwaginga, J. J., Koomans, H. A., and Sixma, J. J. (1994). Thrombosis and haemostasis in renal disease. *Kidney International* **46**, 287–296.

Rambausek, M., Rhein, C., Waldherr, R., Goetz, R., Heidland, A., and Ritz, E. (1989). Hypertension in chronic idiopathic glomerulonephritis: analysis of 311 biopsied patients. *European Journal of Clinical Investigation* **19**, 176–180.

Raskin, N. H. and Fishman, R. A. (1976). Neurologic disorders in renal failure. *New England Journal of Medicine* **294**, 143–148.

Rix, M., Andreassen, H., Eskilden, P., Langdahl, B., and Olgaard, K. (1999). Bone mineral density and biochemical markers of bone turnover in patients with predialysis chronic renal failure. *Kidney International* **56**, 1084–1093.

Roe, S. and Cassidy, M. J. D. (2000). Diagnosis and monitoring of renal osteodystrophy. *Current Opinion in Nephrology and Hypertension* **9**, 675–681.

Rosman, J. B., Ter Wee, P. M., Meijer, S., Piers-Becht, T. Ph. M., Sluiter, W. J., and Donker, A. J. M. (1984). Prospective randomized trial of early dietary protein restriction in chronic renal failure. *Lancet* **ii**, 1291–1295.

Rosman, J. B. *et al.* (1989). Protein-restricted diets in chronic renal failure: a four year's follow-up shows limited indications. *Kidney International* **36** (Suppl. 27), S96–S102.

Ruggenenti, P. *et al.* (1999a). In chronic nephropathies prolonged ACE inhibition can induce remission: dynamics of time-dependent changes in GFR. Investigators of the GISEN Group. Gruppo Italiano Studi Epidemiologici in Nefrologia. *Journal of the American Society of Nephrology* **10**, 997–1006.

Ruggenenti, P. *et al.* (1999b). Renoprotective properties of ACE-inhibition in non-diabetic nephropathies with non-nephrotic proteinuria. *Lancet* **354**, 359–364.

Rutherford, W. E., Blondin, J., Miller, J. P., Greenwalt, A. S., and Vavra, J. D. (1977). Chronic progressive renal disease: rate of change of serum creatinine concentration. *Kidney International* **11**, 62–70.

Sadovsky, R., Miller, T., Moskowitz, M., and Hackett, G. (2001). Three-year update of sildenafil citrate (Viagra®) efficacy and safety. *International Journal of Clinical Practice* **55**, 115–128.

Schwab, S. J. *et al.* (1989). Contrast nephrotoxicity: a randomized controlled trial of a nonionic and an ionic radiographic contrast agent. *New England Journal of Medicine* **320**, 149–153.

Shenmesh, O., Golbetz, H., Kriss, J. P., and Myers, B. D. (1985). Limitations of creatinine as a filtration marker in glomerulopathic patients. *Kidney International* **28**, 830–838.

Staessen, J. A. *et al.* (1992). Impairment of renal function with increasing blood lead concentrations in the general population. *New England Journal of Medicine* **327**, 151–156.

Tarnow, L., Rossing, P., Jensen, C., Hansen, B. V., and Parving, H. H. (2000). Long-term renoprotective effect of nisoldipine and lisinopril in type 1 diabetic patients with diabetic nephropathy. *Diabetes Care* **23**, 1725–1730.

Taylor, A. A. and Sunthornyothin, S. (1999). The case for combining angiotensin-converting enzyme inhibitors and calcium-channel blockers. *Current Hypertension Reports* **1**, 446–453.

Tepel, M., van der Giet, M., Schwarzfeld, C., Laufer, U., Liermann, D., and Zidek, W. (2000). Prevention of radiographic-contrast-agent-induced reductions in renal function by acetylcysteine. *New England Journal of Medicine* **343**, 180–184.

Ter Wee, P. M., De Micheli, A. G., and Epstein, M. (1994). Effects of calcium antagonists on renal hemodynamics and progression of nondiabetic chronic renal disease. *Archives of Internal Medicine* **154**, 1185–1202.

The GISEN Group (Gruppo Italiano di Studi Epidemiologici in Nefrologia) (1997). Randomised placebo-controlled trial of effect of ramipril on decline in glomerular filtration rate and risk of terminal renal failure in proteinuric, non-diabetic nephropathy. *Lancet* **349**, 1857–1863.

Valeri, A., Gelfand, G., Blum, C., and Appel, G. B. (1986). Treatment of hyperlipidemia of the nephrotic syndrome. *American Journal of Kidney Diseases* **6**, 388–396.

Van Geet, C., Van Dyck, M., and Proesmans, W. (1994). Subcutaneous recombinant erythropoietin in preterminal renal insufficiency. *European Journal of Pediatrics* **153**, 129–132.

Voyaki, S. M. *et al.* (2001). Follow-up of renal function in treated and untreated older patients with isolated systolic hypertension. Systolic hypertension in Europe (Syst-Eur) trial investigators. *Journal of Hypertension* **19**, 511–519.

Winston, J. A., Burns, G. C., and Klotman, P. E. (1998). The human immunodeficiency virus (HIV) epidemic and HIV-associated nephropathy. *Seminars in Nephrology* **18**, 373–377.

Young, M. D., Schneider, D. L., Zuckerman, A. J., Du, W., Dickson, B., and Maddrey, W. C. (2001). Adult hepatitis B vaccination using a novel triple antigen recombinant vaccine. *Hepatology* **34**, 372–376.

Zucchelli, P., Zuccala, A., Borghi, M. *et al.* (1992). Long-term comparison between captopril and nifedipine in the progression of renal insufficiency. *Kidney International* **42**, 452–458.

11.3 The patient with uraemia

11.3.1 Uraemic toxicity

Raymond Camille Vanholder, Griet Glorieux, Rita De Smet, and Norbert Hendrik Lameire

Introduction

The uraemic syndrome is the result of the retention of solutes, which under normal conditions are cleared by the kidneys, but derangements of hormonal, metabolic, and enzymatic axes also play a role. The impact in renal failure patients is underscored by the clinical improvement resulting from dietary protein restriction, dialysis, and kidney transplantation.

The uraemic syndrome is characterized by a deterioration of biochemical and physiological functions (Table 1), in parallel with the progression of renal failure. This results in various non-specific symptoms, which mimic the picture of exogenous poisoning. Although the link between clinical deterioration and uraemia has long been recognized, our knowledge of the factors responsible remains incomplete.

Table 1 The uraemic syndrome—main clinical alterations

Cardiovascular system
Atheromatosis
Cardiomyopathy
Decreased diastolic compliance
Hyper/hypotension
Pericarditis

Nervous system
Cramps
Dementia
Depression
Fatigue
Headache
Motor weakness
Polyneuritis
Reduced sociability
Restless legs
Sleep disorders
Stupor, coma

Table 1 Continued

Haematological system/coagulation
Anaemia
Bleeding
Hypercoagulability

Immunological system
Inadequate antibody formation
Susceptibility to cancer
Susceptibility to infection

Endocrinology
Dyslipidaemia
Glucose intolerance
Growth retardation
Hyperparathyroidism
Hypogonadism
Impotence, diminished libido

Bone disease
Adynamic bone disease
Amyloidosis (β_2-microglobulin)
Defective calcitriol metabolism
Osteitis fibrosa
Osteomalacia
Osteoporosis

Skin
Melanosis
Pruritus
Uraemic frost

Gastrointestinal system
Anorexia
Dyspepsia
Gastrointestinal ulcers
Hiccup
Nausea, vomiting
Pancreatitis

Pulmonary system
Pleuritis
Pulmonary oedema
Sleep apnoea syndrome

Miscellaneous
Hypothermia
Thirst
Uraemic foetor
Weight loss

General classification of uraemic solutes

Uraemic toxicity is not a simple single-factor process caused by one or two toxins affecting many different metabolic processes. Under normal conditions, the glomerular filter clears molecules with a molecular weight (MW) up to ±58,000 Da. All these substances are likely to be retained in renal failure. An additional role should be attributed to changes in tubular secretion, reabsorption, and metabolic breakdown, which are all altered when renal mass decreases. The molecules metabolized by the kidneys may have a higher MW (>58,000 Da) than those cleared by filtration. Renal and non-renal metabolism of solutes and non-renal clearance may in their turn be inhibited by uraemic retention products.

Uraemic retention products are arbitrarily divided according to their MW and physicochemical characteristics (Table 2) (Vanholder and De Smet 1999). Low MW molecules have a MW less than 500 Da [e.g. urea (MW: 60), creatinine (MW: 113)]. They can further be subdivided into protein-bound and non-protein-bound molecules. Substances with a middle MW range from 500 to 12,000 Da [e.g. parathyroid hormone (PTH) (MW: 9424), β_2-microglobulin (β_2-M) (MW: 11,818)]. Several of the recently defined uraemic retention products, for example, various peptides and advanced glycation end products (AGEs) fall into the category of 'middle molecules' (MMs)

Table 2 Physicochemical characteristics of some of the uraemic retention solutes

Name	Multicompartment[a]	Toxic
Classical 'small' molecules		
Creatinine	−	−
Guanidines	+/−	+
Myo-inositol	?	+/−
Pseudouridine	−	−
Purines	−	+
Organic phosphates	+	+
Oxalate	−	+/−
Urea	−	+/−
Classical 'middle' molecules		
Advanced glycation end products	+	+
β_2-Microglobulin	+	+
Leptin	+	+
Parathyroid hormone	+	+
Peptides	+	+
Small 'protein-bound' solutes		
CMPF[b]	+	+
Hippuric acid	−	+
Homocysteine	+	+
Indoles	+	+
Indoxyl sulfate	+	+
Phenols	+	+
Polyamines	+	+

[a] The term 'Multicompartment' points to multicompartmental behaviour during dialysis.

[b] CMPF = 3-carboxy-4-methyl-5-propyl-2-furanpropionic acid.

Those small molecules scoring + for multicompartmental distribution may behave like larger molecules during dialysis. Many of the classical 'small' solutes are not toxic or toxic only to a limited extent.

(see below). Several compounds of biological significance (e.g. leptin) are in the high MW range viz. greater than or equal to 12,000 Da. The use of high flux dialysis membranes with the capacity to remove MMs have been related to lower mortality, a slower loss of residual renal function, and a lower prevalence of the carpal tunnel syndrome. However, these membranes are also less complement activating than unmodified cellulose. The relative importance of the removal of MMs versus biocompatibility in the proposed benefits is unresolved. Recent studies, however, have pointed to an independent benefit of large molecule removal (Port *et al.* 2001).

Small compounds such as hippuric acid or p-cresol, which are protein bound, behave during dialysis like MMs. Their removal by classical haemodialysis systems, even with large pore membranes, remains disappointingly low (Lesaffer *et al.* 2000), which may be attributed to the complex distribution and intradialytic kinetics of these compounds. Alternative removal strategies, such as adsorption, changes in timeframes, use of 'protein-leaking' membranes, and/or stimulation of metabolic pathways need to be considered.

Peritoneal dialysis (PD) is a better remover of protein-bound compounds than haemodialysis, because the peritoneal pore size allows the transfer of substantial quantities of albumin together with its bound moieties. The continuous nature of PD might also explain the enhanced removal of these compounds.

Main uraemic retention products

Several uraemic retention solutes definitely influence biological functions while others, although having no proven direct toxicity, may be useful markers of uraemic retention. A review of the most currently known uraemic retention solutes with their MW is given in Table 3. It must be remembered that non-organic compounds such as water and potassium exert 'toxicity' as well.

Advanced glycation end products

As first described by Maillard, glucose and other reducing sugars react non-enzymatically with free amino groups to form reversible Schiff base adducts (in days) and stable Amadori products (in weeks), which are then converted into AGEs through chemical rearrangements and degradation reactions. Several AGE compounds are peptide-linked degradation products, although the baseline AGE products such as pentosidine, 2-(2-fuoryl)-4(5)-(2-furanyl)-1H-imidazole (FFI), imidazolone, 3-deoxyglucosone, pyrrole aldehyde, and N^ε–(carboxymethyl) lysine have a substantially lower MW (Table 3).

AGEs are retained not only in renal failure, but also in diabetes mellitus and ageing, where they are held responsible for tissular damage and functional disturbances. The production of AGE in endstage renal disease (ESRD) has been related to oxidative and carbonyl stress, rather than to reactions with glucose. Not all AGE generation is oxidative, however.

AGEs provoke monocyte activation, as well as the induction of interleukin (IL)-6, tumour necrosis factor (TNF)-α, and interferon-γ generation (Imani *et al.* 1993). AGE-modified β_2-M may play a role in the generation of dialysis-associated amyloidosis (see below). AGEs can react with, and chemically inactivate nitric oxide (NO) (Bucala *et al.* 1991), the potent endothelium-derived vasodilator, antiaggregant, and antiproliferative factor. Conversely, NO inhibits the formation

Table 3 Major uraemic retention solutes and their molecular weight (Da)

Compound	MW	Compound	MW	Compound	MW
ADMA/SDMA	202	γ-Guanidinobutyric acid	145	Oxalate	90
Adrenomedullin	5729	Glomerulopressin	500	p-Cresol	108
ANF	3080	GIP I	28,000	p-OH-Hippuric acid	195
Benzylalcohol	108	GIP II	25,000	Pentosidine	135
β-Endorphin	3465	Guanidine	59	Phenylacetylglutamine	264
β-Guanidinopropionic acid	131	Guanidinoacetic acid	117	Phenol	94
β₂-Microglobulin	11,818	Guanidinosuccinic acid	175	Phosphate	96
CGRP	3789	Hippuric acid	179	Pseudouridine	244
Cholecystokinin	3866	Homoarginine	188	Putrescine	88
CIP	8500	Homocysteine	135	Retinol binding protein	21,200
Clara cell protein	15,800	Hyaluronic acid	25,000	Spermine	202
CML	188	Hypoxanthine	136	Spermidine	145
CMPF	240	Imidazolone	203	Thymine	126
Complement factor D	23,750	Indole-3-acetic acid	175	Trichloromethane	119
Creatine	131	Indoxyl sulfate	251	Tryptophan	202
Creatinine	113	Leptin	16,000	Urea	60
Cystatin C	13,300	Melatonin	126	Uric acid	168
Cytidine	234	Methylguanidine	73	Uridine	244
DIP I	14,400	Myoinositol	180	Xanthine	152
DIP II	24,000	Neuropeptide Y	4272		
3-Deoxyglucosone	162	Orotic acid	156		
Endothelin	4283	Orotidine	288		

The underlined compounds conform with the definition of MM (MW above 500 and 12,000 Da).

ADMA, asymmetrical dimethylarginine; SDMA, symmetrical dimethylarginine; ANF, atrial natriuretic factor; CGRP, calcitonin gene related peptide; CIP, chemotaxis inhibiting protein; CMPF, 3-carboxy-4-methyl-5-propyl-2-furanpropionic acid; CML, carboxymethyllysine; DIP I, degranulation inhibiting protein I; DIP II, degranulation inhibiting protein II; GIP I, granulocyte inhibiting protein I; GIP II, granulocyte inhibiting protein II.

of AGEs. 3-Deoxyglucosone inactivates glutathione peroxidase, a key enzyme in the neutralization of hydrogen peroxide. Transferrin and lysozyme, after contact with AGE-modified albumin, lose their immune-enhancing property. In a recent study, it was demonstrated that AGEs accumulate in atheromatous plaque of the aortic wall of subjects with ESRD, where they may contribute to a more rapid progression of atherosclerosis (Sakata *et al.* 1998). To our knowledge, there is however no observational study in uraemia, linking AGEs directly to atherogenesis.

Most of the biological actions of AGEs that have been registered up to now have not been obtained with AGEs recovered from uraemic or diabetic serum, but with AGEs artificially prepared in the laboratory. Uraemic human serum albumin, collected from patient blood, appeared to be only minimally AGE modified. It remains unclear which AGEs exert toxicity *in vivo*, and to what extent.

Concentrations in ESRD patients might be attributed to increased uptake, production, and/or retention. During industrial food processing, cooking procedures, and storage of foods, food proteins are modified by carbohydrates, and those are absorbed via the gastrointestinal tract. In spite of continuous contact with glucose via the dialysate, continuous ambulatory peritoneal dialysis (CAPD) patients do not have higher serum AGEs than haemodialysis patients, but protein glycation has been demonstrated in the peritoneal membrane. The heat sterilization of glucose-containing peritoneal dialysate induces the formation of glucose degradation products (GDPs), which are precursors of AGEs. GDPs inhibit leucocyte response, and this effect is attenuated when heat sterilization is replaced by alternative procedures (e.g. filter sterilization) (Wieslander *et al.* 1995).

Removal of AGEs is significantly more important with high flux haemodialysis than with conventional dialysis with low flux membranes (Makita *et al.* 1994). Even then steady state serum levels remain substantially above normal. It is of note that there is a marked heterogeneity in the removal pattern of AGEs, even during high flux dialysis. It is unclear which compounds should serve as a marker for the overall group of AGEs.

β₂-Microglobulin

β₂-M (MW approximately 12,000 Da) is a component of the major histocompatibility antigen. Uraemia-related amyloid is to a large extent composed of β₂-M. It is usually found in the osteoarticular system and in the carpal tunnel, although deposition can be systemic as well. Uraemia-related amyloidosis becomes most often clinically apparent after several years of chronic renal failure and/or in the aged. Recent data, however, have shown that amyloidosis develops earlier than previously suspected (Jadoul *et al.* 1998), even in patients not yet maintained by dialysis. The exact pathophysiology of this disease remains largely unknown. The relationship between β₂-M serum concentrations and the development of β₂-M amyloidosis is weak.

AGEs (see above) and β₂-M amyloidosis are closely connected. AGE-modified β₂-M has been identified in amyloid of haemodialysed patients. AGE-modified β₂-M enhances monocytic migration and cytokine secretion, suggesting that foci containing AGE–β₂-M may initiate inflammatory response, leading to bone and joint destruction. Recent studies, however, suggest that macrophage infiltrates might be a secondary phenomenon.

Other modifications have been proposed to participate in amyloid generation, such as proteolysis of the N-terminus of β_2-M and deamination of the Asn 17. Some arguments, such as the lack of a higher clinical incidence of β_2-M-amyloidosis in diabetic dialysis patients, who generate large quantities of AGEs in the presence of hyperglycaemia, cast a doubt on the pathophysiological role of AGEs in amyloid formation. Long-term haemodialysis with large pore membranes results in a progressive decrease of predialysis β_2-M concentrations. The concentrations remain, however, far above normal, even after intensive removal therapy. Long-term dialysis with large-pore dialysers results in a lower prevalence of dialysis-related amyloidosis and/or carpal tunnel syndrome (Locatelli et al. 1999). Whether this benefit is attributable to a better removal of β_2-M, to lower complement and leucocyte activating capacity, or to protection against the transfer of dialysate impurities into the blood stream (e.g. lipopolysaccharides) is not decided, since most of the dialysers associated with a lower incidence of amyloidosis have all three of the above mentioned properties.

3-Carboxy-4-methyl-5-propyl-2-furanpropionic acid

3-Carboxy-4-methyl-5-propyl-2-furanpropionic acid (CMPF) is one of the urofuranic acids, a lipophilic and strongly protein-bound uraemic solute, and one of the major inhibitors of the protein binding of drugs and of bilirubin. The clearance of CMPF is strongly reduced in renal failure. CMPF inhibits the renal uptake of p-amino hippuric acid (PAH) in rat kidney cortical slices, and causes a decrease in renal excretion of several drugs, of their metabolites, and of endogenously produced organic acids which are removed via the PAH pathway. CMPF inhibits hepatic glutathione-S-transferase, deiodination of T_4 and T_3 by cultured hepatocytes, and ADP-stimulated oxidation of NADH-linked substrates in isolated mitochondria.

CMPF concentrations are lower in CAPD than in haemodialysis. The strong protein binding of CMPF (Lesaffer et al. 2000) hampers its removal during haemodialysis (Lesaffer et al. 2000). Alternative removal strategies, such as adsorption, or strategies that modify generation, should be considered. Protein leaking haemodialysis induces a reduction of CMPF, and has been associated with an increase in predialysis haematocrit (Niwa et al. 1995).

Complement factor D

Plasmatic concentrations of complement factor D rise in uraemia, because of a decrease in renal catabolism. Complement factor D activates the alternative complement pathway, which might contribute to the inflammatory state observed in chronic renal disease (Deppisch et al. 2001). Furthermore, complement factor D suppresses stimulated polymorphonuclear (PMNL) function. High flux dialysis membranes remove complement factor D, and this is at least in part attributed to adsorption. Also high flux haemodiafiltration removes more complement factor D than high flux haemodialysis.

Creatinine

Creatinine belongs to the large group of guanidines (see below). Because it is used as a marker of renal function, it deserves special attention.

Creatinine itself has been held responsible for only a few uraemic effects, such as chloride channel blocking. Injection of creatinine in uraemic rats shortens their life span. Creatinine is a precursor of methylguanidine.

Serum creatinine is not only the resultant of uraemic retention but also of muscular break-down; therefore, a high serum creatinine may be the consequence of high muscular mass, and hence an indicator of metabolic well being, rather than underdialysis.

Cytokines

In view of the strong associations between atherosclerosis, malnutrition, and inflammation, it is possible that factors associated with malnutrition and inflammation may contribute to the excess prevalence of cardiovascular disease in renal failure. The proinflammatory cytokine system is activated in ESRD patients, and various lines of evidence suggest that decreased renal clearance might play an important role in cytokine retention.

Guanidines

The guanidines include several structural metabolites of arginine. Among them are well-known uraemic retention solutes, such as creatinine and guanidine, and newly detected moieties such as asymmetrical and symmetrical dimethylarginine (ADMA and SDMA). The concentration of four guanidino compounds [creatinine, guanidine, guanidinosuccinic acid (GSA), and methylguanidine (MG)] are greatly increased in uraemia.

Several guanidino compounds modify key biological functions. GSA inhibits the production of calcitriol by 1α-hydroxylase, and interferes with activation of ADP-induced platelet factor 3. A mixture of guanidino compounds suppresses free radical production by neutrophils. Several guanidines induce seizures after systemic and/or cerebroventricular administration to animals (De Deyn and MacDonald 1990). This effect is attributable to competitive antagonism at the transmission site of the γ-aminobutyric acid$_A$ receptor. GSA probably also acts as a selective agonist at the N-methyl-D-aspartate (NMDA) receptor.

Arginine, another guanidine, enhances NO production, an effect which might be counterbalanced by arginine analogues, such as ADMA. ADMA is the most specific endogenous inhibitor of NO synthesis. ADMA accumulates in the body during the development of renal failure, in proportion to decreased renal excretion but possibly also because of suppressed enzymatic degradation. The increase of SDMA is more pronounced, but this compound is biologically less active. In the brain, ADMA is a vasoconstrictive agent. MG, another endogenous guanidine, also shows a limited capacity to inhibit NO synthesis.

In haemodialysis patients, ADMA is a strong and independent predictor of overall and cardiovascular mortality (Zoccali et al. 2001).

In contradiction of the hypothesis of inhibition of NO synthesis in uraemia, Noris et al. (1993) described enhanced NO production in patients susceptible to uraemic bleeding tendency. This effect is probably limited to a subgroup of the uraemic population.

Dialytic removal of guanidino compounds is very variable, possibly because tissue distribution or protein binding are relevant. In spite of a low molecular weight, removal by haemodialysis of ADMA is only in the range of 20–30 per cent.

Hippuric acid

Hippuric acid interferes with the transport of a variety of organic acids, with the protein binding of drugs, and with glucose tolerance.

The protein binding of hippuric acid tends to increase during dialysis. Procentual dialytic removal is, however, close to that of urea (Lesaffer *et al.* 2000), possibly because protein binding is only moderate.

Homocysteine

Homocysteine (Hcy), a sulfur-containing amino acid, is produced by the demethylation of dietary methionine. Retention results in the cellular accumulation of S-adenosyl homocysteine (AdoHcy), an extremely toxic compound, which competes with S-adenosyl-methionine (AdoMet) and inhibits methyltransferase. Moderate hyperhomocysteinaemia is an independent risk factor for cardiovascular disease in the general population.

Patients with chronic renal failure have total serum Hcy levels two- to fourfold above normal. The serum concentration depends not only on the degree of renal failure, but also on nutritional intake (e.g. of methionine), vitamin status (e.g. of folate), genetic factors, and decreased renal metabolization. Detoxification of Hcy by remethylation to methionine is inhibited in haemodialysis patients, possibly due to folate resistance.

Hcy induces the proliferation of vascular smooth muscle cells, and involves endothelial dysfunction and reactive oxygen species generation. The administration of excess quantities of the Hcy precursor methionine to rats induces atherosclerosis-like alterations in the aorta. Hcy also disrupts several anticoagulant functions in the vessel wall, which results in thrombosis.

Hyperhomocysteinaemia is the most prevalent cardiovascular risk factor in ESRD (Bostom *et al.* 1995), and is also present in kidney transplant recipients with cardiovascular disease. In dialysis patients, there is a direct correlation between plasma Hcy and the odds ratio for vascular complications. In a study by Suliman *et al.* (2000), however, total plasma Hcy was lower in haemodialysis patients with cardiovascular disease. Direct clinical proof of the benefit of lowering Hcy concentration in uraemia has not been produced.

Hcy is partly bound to albumin, which hampers removal by haemodialysis. Hyperhomocysteinaemia is more pronounced in haemodialysis patients, than in those on PD, but even PD fails to normalize total plasma Hcy.

Hcy can be reduced by folic acid, vitamin B_6, and vitamin B_{12}. Oral supplementation with high doses of folic acid and pyridoxine in haemodialysis patients reduces Hcy, but does not restore levels to normal. Extremely high doses of 30–60 mg folic acid per day have no additional impact.

The disappointing efficiency of folic acid might be related to an impairment of the metabolization of folic acid to 5-methyltetrahydrofolate (MTHF), which is the active compound (Touam *et al.* 1999). Touam *et al.* (1999) showed a reduction of total Hcy to normal in approximately 80 per cent of the studied population, by the administration of folinic acid, a precursor of MTHF. The folinic acid was administered intravenously and combined with pyridoxine so that it is uncertain which element of this therapeutic strategy is responsible for the decrease.

Hyaluronic acid

Hyaluronic acid is increased above normal in the majority of patients with chronic renal failure. The basic entity is a non-polymerized molecule of 25 kDa, but the compound may be present in a polymerized form as well. High values are found especially in patients in a poor clinical state. In haemodialysis patients, hyaluronic acid is a strong independent negative predictor of long-term survival.

Hyaluronic acid enhances the expression of the adhesion molecule VCAM-1 and of monocyte chemoattractant protein-1.

Indoles

Indoles are found in various plants and herbs, and are produced by the intestinal flora. Several indolic metabolites are retained in uraemia. Indoxyl sulfate, tryptophan, melatonin, and indole-3-acetic acid are all indoles. Indoxyl sulfate and melatonin are discussed under separate headings (see below).

As a protein-bound compound, indole-3-acetic acid competes for drug protein binding, and inhibits tubular secretion. After oxidation, it becomes cytotoxic. Quinolinic acid is an endogenous excitotoxic agonist of NMDA receptors, and an inhibitor of hepatic phosphoenolpyruvate carboxykinase and gluconeogenesis.

Not all indoles show a similar kinetic behaviour. Tryptophan does not even conform with the strict definition of uraemic retention solutes, as its global concentration in ESRD is low rather than high (e.g. tryptophan). The decrease in plasma tryptophan is related to shifts in metabolic pathways that at the same time result in an increase of concentration of other related metabolites, which may exert neurotoxicity.

Indoxyl sulfate

Indoxyl sulfate is metabolized by the liver from indole, which is produced by the intestinal flora as a metabolite of tryptophan. It competes with acidic drugs at the protein binding sites, inhibits the active tubular secretion of these compounds, and inhibits deiodination of thyroxin 4 by cultured hepatocytes. The oral administration of indole or indoxyl sulfate to uraemic rats causes progression of glomerular sclerosis and of renal failure (Niwa and Ise 1994), and this effect is refrained by the administration of adsorbants of indole. Intraintestinal absorption of indoxyl sulfate also reduces uraemic itching.

Compared to removal of creatinine during one haemodialysis session of approximately 50 per cent, removal of indoxyl sulfate is (because of protein binding) only 0–20 per cent. Removal by CAPD is more effective. Sophisticated haemodialysis strategies such as high flux dialysis do not enhance removal (Lesaffer *et al.* 2000). Alternative extracorporeal removal procedures such as haemoperfusion should be considered.

Melatonin

The pineal hormone melatonin plays a role in the regulation of the hypothalamic–pituitary axis, sleep pattern, mood changes, cellular immunity, antibody response, and skin pigmentation, all of which are altered in ESRD. Melatonin inhibits lipopolysaccharide induced NO synthase, and acts as a free radical scavenger, although some authors attribute pro-oxidant activity to this compound. In contrast to Vaziri *et al.* (1993), Viljoen *et al.* (1992) demonstrated elevated melatonin levels in patients with chronic renal failure. Haemodialysis has no effect on concentration.

Methylamines

Methylamine, dimethylamine, and trimethylamine are retained in uraemia, especially intracellularly. Methylamine generation increases after intake of fish, seafood, and certain vegetables (tomatoes, pears, peas).

Methylamines might play a role in central nervous disturbances and in the inhibition of fibroblast cellular function. Increased deamination of methylamines might play a role in oxidative stress and atherogenesis.

At supraphysiological concentrations, for example, in the renal medulla, methylamines counteract the biological effects of urea (Burg et al. 1999). This protective effect might be at play in uraemia as well, although no direct proof for this hypothesis has been delivered as yet.

Myo-inositol

An increased concentration of myo-inositol has been found in uraemic nervous tissue. Sciatic nerve conduction velocity is decreased in rats after administration of myo-inositol. Myo-inositol also inhibits proliferation of Schwann cells.

o- and p-Hydroxyhippuric acid

In spite of their low MW, these compounds are characterized by a middle molecular intradialytic behaviour, because of protein binding. They interfere with the albumin binding of acidic drugs. Possible precursors of o-hippuric acid are compounds from the tyrosine–dopa–catecholamine pathway, and salicylate. Use and abuse of salicylate was a cause of ESRD at the moment of the detection of o-hydroxyhippuric acid as a so-called uraemic toxin, which has cast some doubts on its endogenous origin. p-Hydroxyhippuric acid inhibits cellular Ca^{2+}-ATPase.

Oxalate

In ESRD patients without primary hyperoxaluria, plasma oxalate is increased approximately 40-fold. This secondary oxalosis is complicated by deposition of calcium oxalate in various tissues, especially if dialysis is inefficient, or in the presence of excessive intake of oxalate precursors (ascorbic acid, green leafy vegetables, rhubarb, tea, chocolate, or beets) or in the presence of inflammatory bowel disease. Pyridoxine at 800 mg/day caused a decrease of oxalate in haemodialysis patients, but at the expense of gastrointestinal side-effects.

Peritoneal clearance of oxalate is less than 10 per cent of the normal renal clearance, which results in oxalate accumulation in CAPD patients. Also in haemodialysis, oxalate levels are not restored to normal because removal does not match generation.

Oxidation products

Oxidative capacity is increased in uraemia, even before dialysis treatment is started. Hydroxyl radicals subsequently react with proteins, causing structural modifications and irreparable damage. Uraemic patients also show an impaired antioxidant response.

The concentrations of advanced oxidation protein products (AOPPs) are increased in the plasma of uraemic patients (Witko-Sarsat et al. 1998). AOPPs act in their turn as mediators of oxidative stress and monocyte respiratory burst (Witko-Sarsat et al. 1998). Structural modification of albumin alters its binding capacity.

Low-density lipoprotein (LDL) from uraemic patients is more susceptible to oxidation than that from control subjects. This oxidized LDL is more readily accumulated in macrophages, and results in the development of foam cells, an early event in atherogenesis. Oxidative modification of the protein moiety of LDL is a trigger of macrophage respiratory burst.

Malondialdehyde is increased in ESRD. The capacity of malonaldehyde to form DNA adducts may play a pathophysiological role in carcinogenesis.

Small molecular compounds might also be modified by free radical species. Organic chloramines are generated by the chemical binding of hypochlorite to retained organic compounds. In as far as binding occurs with liposoluble compounds, for example, spermine or spermidine, removal by haemodialysis will be hampered, whereas the capacity to penetrate cellular membranes will be enhanced.

Preliminary data with haemolipodialysis, a strategy which incorporates liposomes and antioxidants, suggest an attenuation of oxidation with this procedure.

Parathyroid hormone

Parathyroid hormone (PTH) is generally recognized as a uraemic toxin, although its increased concentration during ESRD is merely attributable to enhanced glandular secretion. Excess PTH gives rise to an increase in intracellular calcium, which results in functional disturbances of virtually every organ system.

Paradoxically, moderate hyperparathyroidism improves the bone response of uraemic patients. If PTH remains in the lower range, patients may suffer from relative hypoparathyroidism, which results in aplastic bone, and redistribution of body calcium stores leading to metastatic tissue calcification. The current test methods for the determination of PTH levels overestimate true concentrations, as they react as well with intact PTH as with functionally inactive fragments. New test methods have been developed that estimate only intact PTH.

Downregulation of PTH–PTHrP receptor mRNA expression is observed in various tissues. Parathyroidectomy does not entirely prevent this downregulation. Calcium receptors also show abnormal function.

The increased PTH concentration in uraemia is the result of a number of compensatory homeostatic mechanisms. Hyperparathyroidism results from phosphate retention, decreased production of calcitriol [1,25(OH)$_2$ vitamin D3], and/or hypocalcaemia.

Only dialysis membranes with a large pore size remove PTH. Differences in concentration at the end of the dialysis session are, however, subtle. A more efficient way to correct PTH hypersecretion is the correction of the plasma calcium, provision of calcitriol, and removal of phosphorus (Lau et al. 1998). Therapy with calcitriol or its analogues also restores the secretory reserve of the parathyroid gland during hypocalcaemia. Uraemia is, however, not only characterized by a depressed production of calcitriol, but also by resistance to this hormone (Patel et al. 1995). If pharmacological interventions remain ineffective, parathyroidectomy is the ultimate therapeutic resort. In the future, it might become possible to obviate the side-effects of hyperparathyroidism, such as hypercalcaemia, by the administration of calcimimetics. New vitamin D analogues which have less calcaemic and phosphataemic effects are also under development.

Peptides

Peptides constitute a heterogeneous group of typical MMs.

Granulocyte inhibiting protein I (GIP I—28 kDa) suppresses PMNL killing of invading bacteria. It has structural analogy with the variable part of kappa light chains. Free immunoglobulin light chains

(25 kDa) increase the number of viable neutrophils by inhibiting spontaneous apoptotic cell death. Another peptide with granulocyte inhibitory effect (GIP II—9.5 kDa) is partially homologous with β_2-M (Haag-Weber et al. 1994). A degranulation inhibiting protein (DIP—24 kDa), identical to angiogenin, has been isolated from uraemic ultrafiltrate. The structure responsible for the inhibition of degranulation is different from the angiogenic sites. A structural variant of ubiquitin inhibits PMNL chemotaxis (chemotaxis inhibiting protein—CIP—8.5 kDa).

Atrial natriuretic peptide (ANP—3.1 kDa) and endothelin (3.5 kDa) play a role in the regulation of blood pressure. ANP correlates with fluid overload, and systemic clearance. Endothelin causes peripheral insulin resistance, and may play a role in uraemic hypertension. Progression of renal failure, myocardial fibrosis, as well as left ventricular dysfunction are prevented by endothelin receptor blockade.

Neuropeptide Y is a 36-amino acid orexigen with renal vasoconstrictive properties.

Adrenomedullin, a 52-amino acid hypotensive peptide, activates inducible NO synthase. Apart from inducing hypotension, this factor may be involved in mechanisms protecting the cardiovascular system. Cystatin C (13.3 kDa), Clara cell protein (CC16) (15.8 kDa), and retinol binding protein (21.2 kDa) are elevated in renal failure. Cystatin C is an inhibitor proteinases and cathepsins. CC16 is an α-microprotein, playing an immunosuppressive role in the airways.

Leptin, a 16 kDa plasma protein that suppresses appetite, induces weight reduction in mice and may play a role in the decreased appetite of uraemic patients. The increase in serum leptin is mostly attributed to decreased renal elimination. Increased leptin is associated with low protein intake and loss of lean tissue in chronic renal failure patients. In CAPD patients, serum leptin showed a progressive rise only in those patients losing body weight (Stenvinkel et al. 2000).

However, leptin is also elevated in obesity and is, hence, not necessarily related to reduced appetite. Body fat and serum leptin also correlate in uraemia. Several authors have found no correlation between leptinaemia and markers of protein malnutrition. The administration of cytokines, such as IL-1β and TNF-α, has been shown to increase serum leptin levels. In ESRD patients, however, leptin may be depressed during inflammation. The biochemical role of leptin in renal failure remains inadequately defined.

Phenols

p-Cresol, a phenolic volatile compound with a MW of only 108.1 Da blocks several vital functions (Vanholder et al. 1999). p-Cresol inhibits various metabolic processes that are involved in the destruction of invading bacteria. Aluminium uptake by hepatocytes and the toxic effect of aluminium on these cells is increased in the presence of p-cresol. p-Cresol and phenol inhibit platelet-activating factor (PAF) synthesis by phagocytic leucocytes, and p-cresol inhibits detoxification of arsenic.

p-Cresol is produced by the intestinal flora, as a result of the metabolism of tyrosine and phenylalanine, but might be generated from environmental sources as well.

p-Cresol is lipophilic and protein-bound, and its removal by haemodialysis is markedly lower than that of urea. In haemodialysis, the removal of p-cresol and that of urea are not correlated (Lesaffer et al. 2000), showing that this marker is not representative for the intradialytic behaviour of protein-bound p-cresol. p-Cresol levels are markedly lower in PD than haemodialysis patients.

Phosphate

High phosphate levels are associated with pruritus and the development of secondary hyperparathyroidism. They affect PTH levels indirectly by decreasing plasma Ca^{2+} and calcitriol synthesis, but also by direct stimulation of PTH secretion. In 2000, 60 per cent of the haemodialysis patients in the United States were shown to have serum phosphate levels higher than 5.5 mg/dl. Hyperphosphataemia is directly correlated to mortality (Block et al. 1998), which appears to be linked to a high Ca $\times$ P product, and enhanced tissue deposition of Ca-containing complexes, for example, in the vessel walls (Block et al. 1998).

Hyperphosphataemia is not only a direct cause of hyperparathyroidism, but is also the result of the action of excessive PTH on the bone. The administration of calcitriol in an attempt to control PTH aggravates hyperphosphataemia.

The blood phosphate concentration is the result of protein catabolism and protein intake, and ingestion of other sources (e.g. cola drinks). Until recently, oral phosphate binders consisted mainly of aluminium or calcium salts. The efficacy of the latter, however, is often insufficient. The presence of a high calcium phosphate product results in tissue deposition of calcium. New phosphate binders such as sevelamer hydrochloride, lanthanum carbonate, and trivalent iron-containing compounds offer the advantage that they contain no calcium, so that the risk of hypercalcaemia is reduced. Whether these compounds are more efficient phosphate binders remains to be proved. Sevelamer hydrochloride has a lipid lowering effect. Lanthanum is a cationic trace element and could if absorbed into the body, create similar problems as aluminium.

Phosphate shows a retention and removal pattern unlike that of any other molecule. Cellular clearance during haemodialysis is much less than that of urea, resulting in a substantial postdialysis rebound. Removal seems to be effective only during the initial phase of a haemodialysis session. Alternative dialytic strategies such as daily dialysis, slow prolonged dialysis sessions, or haemodiafiltration might all improve phosphate removal. The application of daily dialysis even results in a decreased need for peroral phosphate binders (Kooistra et al. 1998).

Polyamines

Polyamines (e.g. spermine, spermidine, putrescine) have long been thought to inhibit erythropoiesis. They have a high affinity for body proteins and cells. Putrescine inhibits cell growth in vitro, and causes irreversible cell degeneration. Several polyamines interfere with the NMDA receptor, which plays a role in channel conductance and Ca^{2+} permeability of brain cells, but spermine might induce neurotoxicity by other pathways too. Spermine reduces intracellular free calcium in permeabilized pancreatic islets, and inhibits NO synthase. Polyamines antagonize platelet aggregation. Oxidation of polyamines results in cytotoxic compounds, with a potential role in brain damage.

Purines

The purines disturb calcitriol metabolism. Administration of purines to animals results in a net decrease of serum calcitriol and of the binding of vitamin D receptor to DNA chromatin. An allopurinol-induced decrease of uric acid results in a rise of plasma calcitriol levels. Purines are involved in the resistance to calcitriol of immune competent cells, by a reduction of the expression of the lipopolysaccharide receptor CD14 on the surface of monocytes. Xanthine and hypoxanthine have been implicated as modulators of neurotransmission, may be related to poor appetite and weight loss, induce vasoconstriction, and disturb endothelial barriers.

In spite of a markedly diminished urinary secretion of uric acid in renal failure, the rise in plasma uric acid levels is only moderate, because of net intestinal secretion. Erythrocyte hypoxanthine formation, as an index of adenine nucleotide metabolism, is higher in chronic renal failure than in controls.

Uric acid is a small water soluble compound that is removed by haemodialysis in a similar way to urea, but removal from the intracellular compartment is far less efficient. Dialytic removal of xanthine and hypoxanthine shows no correlation with that of urea and creatinine.

Urea

In spite of the extensive number of toxicity studies to which urea has been submitted, there are few well-defined reports of an adverse impact attributable to concentrations encountered in uraemia. In the classic study by Johnson *et al.* (1972) comparing long-lasting dialysis against dialysate containing high urea concentrations, there was no consistent impact on uraemic symptoms. It has been suggested that *in vivo*, urea toxicity is counterbalanced by the methylamines (Lee *et al.* 1991).

Urea inhibits NaK_2Cl cotransport in human erythrocytes. A heat shock response is elicited by urea in human neuroblastoma cells, which might be a factor in uraemic neurotoxicity. Urea induces macrophage proliferation by inhibition of inducible nitric oxide synthesis. Urea shortens the life-span of bilaterally nephrectomized rats. This might be attributed to an osmotic effect. Overall, for the impressive number of studies during which the biological impact of urea was addressed, the yield of studies demonstrating an impact was deceivingly low, and the large majority of them was *in vitro*.

Urea is a precursor of some of the guanidines (see above), which by themselves induce biochemical disturbances. Urea is also a source of cyanate and isocyanic acid, which are at the origin of carbamoylation, resulting in structural and functional changes of amino acids and proteins. As the uraemic retention solute with the highest net contributor to osmolality, urea may also be involved in dialysis disequilibrium.

Urea is unequivocally recognized as a marker of solute retention and removal in dialysed patients. It is one of the few solutes that have been correlated convincingly with clinical outcome of dialysis. Dynamic urea kinetic parameters, reflecting dialytic removal (total clearance normalized for distribution volume—Kt/V) are valuable indices of dialysis adequacy. Nevertheless, high blood concentrations of urea do not necessarily relate to poor outcome if removal is sufficient, since urea concentration is not only influenced by dialytic removal but also by dietary protein intake, an indicator of good nutrition. This observation is further evidence against the toxicity of urea *per se*. The relation of urea removal with survival is probably only related to the removal of another water soluble compound, for example, potassium.

One might question the validity of urea as a marker for the retention and the removal of other solutes because biochemical systems are at least in part affected by compounds with a kinetic behaviour very different from that of urea (e.g. MMs, protein bound solutes).

Factors influencing uraemic solute concentration (Table 4)

Dialysis-related factors

Removal pattern

Conventional haemodialysis easily removes small water-soluble compounds, such as urea and creatinine, which are the usual markers of uraemic retention and removal. Urea removal is linked to dialysis-related mortality (Bloembergen *et al.* 1996). Removal pattern of urea and creatinine is markedly different from that of many other uraemic solutes with proven toxicity. MMs are better removed by high flux haemodialysers, and by convection (e.g. haemodiafiltration), which affects morbidity and mortality independant of urea removal. CAPD allows a relatively more efficient removal of MMs.

Protein bound molecules behave during dialysis like larger (middle) molecules, but their removal is not greatly influenced by an increase in pore size, unless the carrier proteins (mainly albumin) are removed at the same time. Lower plasma levels are found in patients treated by PD.

Adsorption

Adsorption on specifically designed devices may be a more promising solution for the elimination of difficult to remove molecules, such as the protein-bound compounds (Winchester *et al.* 2001). Adsorption occurs on most current haemodialysis membranes, but the surface is insufficient to allow adequate removal. The most acceptable option is the development of chemical polymers that contain structures on to which the targeted molecules could fit. As most small water-soluble molecules are easily removed by diffusion, it is of more relevance to develop devices with high adsorptive surface area (>200 m^2) for large and/or lipophilic molecules. The question arises whether the adsorptive capacity of such devices will be sufficient, especially if confronted with toxins with a multicompartmental distribution.

Sorbent techniques can be used to extract compounds from dialysate, from ultrafiltrate whereby regenerated ultrafiltrate is returned to the blood stream, from plasma if combined with plasmafiltration, or directly from blood.

Removal of protein-bound compounds during haemodialysis could perhaps be increased by the addition of albumin to the dialysate.

Change in dialysis duration

Even under optimal conditions, Kt/V_{urea} in PD patients is low compared to haemodialysis, but the clinical status for both modalities is similar. This suggests that other compounds than urea, presumably with dissimilar physical characteristics, play a role in uraemic toxicity, and/or that the slow toxin removal by PD and/or its capacity to remove protein-bound moieties may cause an additional benefit. Because removal is more gradual with continuous strategies, more compounds will be cleared, especially those with low clearance rates. Continuous haemodialysis strategies, slow low-efficiency dialysis applied over prolonged time periods, or daily dialysis might therefore result in better toxin removal.

Phosphate plasma levels are similar or lower with daily haemodialysis, compared to classical alternate day haemodialysis, in spite of a lower intake of phosphate binders (Kooistra *et al.* 1998). The clinical state of patients improves if they are submitted to daily and/or slow

Table 4 Factors influencing solute concentration in dialysed patients

Solute-related factors
Compartmental distribution
Intracellular concentration
    Resistance of cell membrane
Protein binding
Electrostatic charge
Steric configuration
Molecular weight
Hydrophilicity/lipophilicity

Patient-related factors
Distribution volume and body weight
Intake and generation
    Solute
    Metabolic precursors
Residual renal function
Access quality
Metabolic generation
Metabolic degradation
Absorption from the intestine
Haematocrit
Blood viscosity
Serum albumin concentration

Dialysis related factors
Dialysis time
Interdialytic intervals
Blood flow
    Mean blood flow
    Blood flow pattern
    Shear in dialyser
Blood distribution
Dialysate flow
Dialysate distribution
Dialysate processing (single pass/batch)
Dialyser surface
Dialyser volume
Dialyser membrane resistance
Dialyser pore size
Dialyser hydrophilicity/hydrophobicity
Adsorption
    On the membrane
    On other constituents of the circuit
Ultrafiltration rate
Intradialytic changes in efficacy
Changes with a direct impact on solute related factors
    Blood pH
    Heparinization
    Free fatty acid concentration
    Haemodynamic stability during dialysis

prolonged haemodialysis. AGE levels are lower in patients treated by daily dialysis than they are when on an alternate day scheme, in spite of identical weekly dialysis time and *Kt/V*.

Intracellular shifts and removal

Uraemic solutes accumulate not only in the plasma but also within the cell, where most of the biological activity is exerted. Removal of intracellular compounds across the cell membrane may be delayed during dialysis, resulting in multicompartmental kinetics, as removal is largely limited to the plasma compartment. Even small water-soluble compounds, such as urea, which are not subjected to resistance during their passage through the cell membrane, may display a multicompartmental behaviour, due to haemodynamic sequestration in certain body compartments. One of the consequences is a rebound at the end of the dialysis session.

Non-dialytic factors

Nutritional and environmental effects

Most toxins or their precursors enter the body via the gastrointestinal route and some are generated by the intestinal flora. Inhibition of intestinal absorption, and modifications in the composition of the intestinal flora could therefore influence solute concentration. A specific oral sorbent (AST120) decreases serum indoxyl sulfate and *p*-cresol in uraemic rats. A few potassium and phosphate binders are applied in the clinical setting today, but in general, the techniques to decrease intestinal delivery of uraemic solutes have not been fully explored.

A number of toxins are produced from protein breakdown or from metabolization of amino acids. Protein restriction might therefore reduce toxicity, were it not that protein malnutrition increases morbidity and mortality by itself.

Several toxins or their precursors, such as AGEs, trace elements, conservation agents (e.g. benzylalcohol as a precursor of hippuric acid), or vitamin C (precursor of oxalate), are present in food; these compounds are not necessarily linked to protein intake. Other rarely considered sources are contact with volatile precursors (e.g. toluene), which are inhaled or swallowed, the intake of herbal medicines and psychedelic drugs, or contact with environmental noxae, leached from elements of the dialysis system (e.g. GDPs present in heat-sterilized glucose-containing PD solutions).

Pharmacological interaction

One of the future aspects of the treatment of uraemia will consist of influencing toxin metabolization by drugs or other compounds. Allopurinol decreases uric acid. Vitamin C increases urinary excretion of CMPF. Hcy can be lowered in uraemic patients by supplementation of folic acid, pyridoxine, and/or vitamin B_{12}. Pyridoxine reduces oxalate levels. Aminoguanidine has the presumed property to reduce AGE generation. The *in vivo* effect of aminoguanidine is not entirely convincing, but other inhibitors of AGE formation, which might turn out to be more efficient, will become available in the future.

Residual renal function

The impact of residual renal function on removal and retention of uraemia-related molecules is substantial. This relative contribution is particularly important for larger molecules and those with multicompartmental behaviour, which are removed less efficiently by the dialysis procedure. Therefore, the longer preservation of residual renal function with CAPD and high flux biocompatible dialysers, compared to conventional haemodialysis, may have a substantial impact on toxicity. Uraemic retention solutes have been held responsible for a faster deterioration of residual renal function. At least one of these compounds, indoxyl sulfate, is removed more efficiently by CAPD.

Conclusions

The uraemic syndrome is the consequence of a complex set of biochemical and pathophysiological disturbances, causing malaise and organ dysfunction. It is related to the retention of a host of compounds, many of which exert a negative impact on key functions of the body, and have, therefore, been identified as uraemic toxins. Up to now, the toxic action of single solutes has repeatedly been studied, but the interference between compounds has rarely been considered. Although solute retention is one of the major pathophysiological events, deficiencies are functionally important as well.

The effect of many compounds with proven biological or biochemical impact, especially toxins that are hydrophobic and/or not generated from protein breakdown, cannot be predicted from the intradialytic behaviour of urea, a current marker with relatively little biological impact.

Solute clearance eventually reaches a plateau as dialyser blood flow and/or dialysate flow are increased; this plateau is reached much sooner for molecules with a higher MW. As a result, clearance of MMs stricto sensu is relatively blood and dialysate flow independent. Only an increase of dialysis time, dialyser surface area, ultrafiltration rates, and/or dialyser pore size can enhance their removal.

Removal of solutes that behave like larger molecules because of their protein binding, multicompartmental distribution and/or lipophilicity will be less affected by the use of high flux dialysers and/or dialysers with a larger pore size. To improve the clearances of these 'new definition MM', it may be necessary to develop renal replacement systems with different characteristics, for example, specific adsorption systems and/or procedures that allow a slower exchange of solutes.

Earlier concepts of charcoal adsorption, now largely abandoned, should perhaps be reconsidered, especially for the removal of organic acids. More specific and/or more efficient adsorptive systems may be needed, however. As an alternative, adsorption of toxins or of their precursors may be pursued at the intestinal level. Another alternative is dialysis against recycled albumin-containing dialysate, allowing a better diffusion of protein-bound toxic compounds (Abe et al. 2001). Another option would be the use of protein permeable membranes, to remove larger molecules as well as protein-bound substances. The amount of removal sufficient to reduce uraemic toxicity would have to be balanced against the possibility of enhancing or inducing protein malnutrition, and the cost of the procedures. Even if solute removal is improved by alternative strategies, mass transfer may be limited if the compounds of interest are distributed over multiple compartments.

The next option is to pursue more specific removal. Before this can be realized, we need to know more about the responsible toxic compounds. Although some progress has been made during the last few years, a structural approach comparing a large panel of putative toxins, at well-defined concentrations and with well-defined test methods, is still lacking. The next step would be to launch controlled studies so that therapeutic strategies that remove the characterized toxins could be tested for their impact on morbidity and mortality.

The approach to enhancing uraemic toxin removal needs to be changed. Increasing pore size, alone or in combination with adaptations in dialyser geometry, is not the solution, and might have come close to its maximal capacity.

References

Abe, T. et al. (2001). A new method for removal of albumin-binding uremic toxins: efficacy of an albumin-dialysate. Therapeutic Apheresis 5, 58–63.

Block, G. A., Hulbert-Shearon, T. E., Levin, N. W., and Port, F. K. (1998). Association of serum phosphorus and calcium × phosphate product with mortality risk in chronic hemodialysis patients: a national study. American Journal of Kidney Diseases 31, 607–617.

Bloembergen, W. E. et al. (1996). Relationship of dose of hemodialysis and cause-specific mortality. Kidney International 50, 557–565.

Bostom, A. G. et al. (1995). Hyperhomocysteinemia and traditional cardiovascular disease risk factors in end-stage renal disease patients on dialysis: a case–control study. Atherosclerosis 114, 93–103.

Bucala, R., Tracey, K. J., and Cerami, A. (1991). Advanced glycosylation products quench nitric oxide and mediate defective endothelium-dependent vasodilatation in experimental diabetes. Journal of Clinical Investigation 87, 432–438.

Burg, M. B., Peters, E. M., Bohren, K. M., and Gabbay, K. H. (1999). Factors affecting counteraction by methylamines of urea effects on aldose reductase. Proceedings of the National Academy of Science USA 96, 6517–6522.

De Deyn, P. P. and MacDonald, R. L. (1990). Guanidino compounds that are increased in cerebrospinal fluid and brain of uremic patients inhibit GABA and glycine responses on mouse neurons in cell culture. Annals of Neurology 28, 627–633.

Deppisch, R. M., Beck, W., Goehl, H., and Ritz, E. (2001). Complement components as uremic toxins and their potential role as mediators of microinflammation. Kidney International 59 (Suppl. 78), S271–S277.

Haag-Weber, M., Mai, B., and Horl, W. H. (1994). Isolation of a granulocyte inhibitory protein from uraemic patients with homology of beta 2-microglobulin. Nephrology, Dialysis, Transplantation 9, 382–388.

Imani, F. et al. (1993). Advanced glycosylation endproduct-specific receptors on human and rat T-lymphocytes mediate synthesis of interferon gamma: role in tissue remodeling. Journal of Experimental Medicine 178, 2165–2172.

Jadoul, M. et al. (1998). Prevalence of histological beta2-microglobulin amyloidosis in CAPD patients compared with hemodialysis patients. Kidney International 54, 956–959.

Johnson, W. J., Hagge, W. W., Wagoner, R. D., Dinapoli, R. P., and Rosevear, J. W. (1972). Effects of urea loading in patients with far-advanced renal failure. Mayo Clinic Proceedings 47, 21–29.

Kooistra, M. P., Vos, J., Koomans, H. A., and Vos, P. F. (1998). Daily home haemodialysis in The Netherlands: effects on metabolic control, haemodynamics, and quality of life. Nephrology, Dialysis, Transplantation 13, 2853–2860.

Lau, A. H., Kuk, J. M., and Franson, K. L. (1998). Phosphate-binding capacities of calcium and aluminum formulations. International Journal of Artificial Organs 21, 19–22.

Lee, J. A., Lee, H. A., and Sadler, P. J. (1991). Uraemia: is urea more important than we think? Lancet 338, 1438–1440.

Lesaffer, G., de Smet, R., Lameire, N., Dhondt, A., Duym, P., and Vanholder, R. (2000). Intradialytic removal of protein-bound uraemic toxins: role of solute characteristics and of dialyser membrane. Nephrology, Dialysis, Transplantation 15, 50–7.

Locatelli, F., Marcelli, D., Conte, F., Limido, A., Malberti, F., and Spotti, D. (1999). Comparison of mortality in ESRD patients on convective and diffusive extracorporeal treatments. The Registro Lombardo Dialisi E Trapianto. Kidney International 55, 286–293.

Makita, Z. et al. (1994). Reactive glycosylation endproducts in diabetic uraemia and treatment of renal failure. Lancet 343 (8912), 1519–1522.

Niwa, T. and Ise, M. (1994). Indoxyl sulfate, a circulating uremic toxin, stimulates the progression of glomerular sclerosis. Journal of Laboratory and Clinical Medicine 124, 96–104.

Niwa, T., Asada, H., Tsutsui, S., and Miyazaki, T. (1995). Efficient removal of albumin-bound furancarboxylic acid by protein-leaking hemodialysis. American Journal of Nephrology 15, 463–467.

Noris, M. *et al.* (1993). Enhanced nitric oxide synthesis in uremia: implications for platelet dysfunction and dialysis hypotension. *Kidney International* **44**, 445–450.

Patel, S. R., Ke, H. Q., Vanholder, R., Koenig, R. J., and Hsu, C. H. (1995). Inhibition of calcitriol receptor binding to vitamin D response elements by uremic toxins. *Journal of Clinical Investigation* **96**, 50–59.

Port, F. K. *et al.* (2001). Mortality risk by hemodialyzer reuse practice and dialyzer membrane characteristics: results from the USRDS dialysis morbidity and mortality study. *American Journal of Kidney Diseases* **37**, 276–286.

Sakata, S. *et al.* (1998). The relationship between pentosidine and hemodialysis-related connective tissue disorders. *Nephron* **78**, 260–265.

Stenvinkel, P., Lindholm, B., Lonnqvist, F., Katzarski, K., and Heimburger, O. (2000). Increases in serum leptin levels during peritoneal dialysis are associated with inflammation and a decrease in lean body mass. *Journal of the American Society of Nephrology* **11**, 1303–1309.

Suliman, M. E. *et al.* (2000). Hyperhomocysteinemia, nutritional status, and cardiovascular disease in hemodialysis patients. *Kidney International* **57**, 1727–1735.

Touam, M., Zingraff, J., Jungers, P., Chadefaux-Vekemans, B., Drueke, T., and Massy, Z. A. (1999). Effective correction of hyperhomocysteinemia in hemodialysis patients by intravenous folinic acid and pyridoxine therapy. *Kidney International* **56**, 2292–2296.

Vanholder, R. and de Smet, R. (1999). Pathophysiologic effects of uremic retention solutes. *Journal of the American Society of Nephrology* **10**, 1815–1823.

Vanholder, R., De Smet, R., and Lesaffer, G. (1999). *p*-Cresol: a toxin revealing many neglected but relevant aspects of uraemic toxicity. *Nephrology, Dialysis, Transplantation* **14**, 2813–2815.

Vaziri, N. D., Oveisi, F., Wierszbiezki, M., Shaw, V., and Sporty, L. D. (1993). Serum melatonin and 6-sulfatoxymelatonin in end-stage renal disease: effect of hemodialysis. *Artificial Organs* **17**, 764–769.

Viljoen, M., Steyn, M. E., van Rensburg, B. W., and Reinach, S. G. (1992). Melatonin in chronic renal failure. *Nephron* **60**, 138–143.

Wieslander, A. P., Kjellstrand, P. T., and Rippe, B. (1995). Heat sterilization of glucose-containing fluids for peritoneal dialysis: biological consequences of chemical alterations. *Peritoneal Dialysis International* **15**, S52–S59.

Winchester, J. F. *et al.* (2001). Sorbent augmented dialysis: minor addition or major advance in therapy? *Blood Purification* **19**, 255–259.

Witko-Sarsat, V. *et al.* (1998). Advanced oxidation protein products as novel mediators of inflammation and monocyte activation in chronic renal failure. *Journal of Immunology* **161**, 2524–2532.

Zoccali, C. *et al.* (2001). Plasma concentration of asymmetrical dimethylarginine and mortality in patients with end-stage renal disease: a prospective study. *Lancet* **358**, 2113–2117.

11.3.2 Endocrine disorders

Markus Daschner and Franz Schaefer

Pathomechanisms of endocrine disorders in uraemia

Many endocrine systems are regulated in a complex, cascade-like manner by a variety of signalling molecules produced by different organs (e.g. hypothalamic releasing factors → pituitary peptide hormones → steroid and non-steroid hormone release from peripheral glands), involving multiple-level feedback loops. This functional organization permits both precise short-term adjustments to maintain whole body homeostasis under different conditions as well as long-term adaptation to induce developmental changes.

Uraemia can interfere with the metabolism and regulation of hormones at each level of the regulatory cascade by various mechanisms. Since only a minority of these changes can be accurately detected by routine laboratory tests, the interpretation of clinical and laboratory findings in uraemic patients may be extremely difficult.

Alterations of steady-state hormone concentrations

Increased hormone concentrations

The kidney is a major catabolic site of many polypeptide hormones, and it is these which accumulate in renal failure.

Renal catabolism accounts for about one- to two-thirds of the metabolic clearance of various polypeptide hormones. In early renal failure, hormone clearance declines in parallel with renal blood flow. When renal failure progresses, the tubular and peritubular uptake of polypeptide hormones decreases, causing a disproportionate increase in serum concentrations.

In addition to renal clearance, *extrarenal elimination* may also be reduced in renal failure. There is experimental evidence that degradation of insulin in skeletal muscle tissue is diminished in uraemia (Rabkin *et al.* 1979). Reduced hepatic catabolism of biologically active PTH has also been described in uraemia (Hruska *et al.* 1981).

Finally, *hypersecretion* of hormones may either constitute an appropriate response to secretory stimuli resulting from the altered internal milieu (e.g. low Ca^{2+} in secondary hyperparathyroidism), or it may occur without an apparent homeostatic signal (e.g. prolactin).

Decreased hormone concentrations

The kidney is an endocrine organ involved in the regulation of red cell production and mineral metabolism via the production of erythropoietin and 1,25-dihydroxy vitamin D_3 [$1,25(OH)_2D_3$]. The reduction of functional renal mass is assumed to be the main cause for decreased concentrations of these hormones in progressive renal failure. Decreased extrarenal hormones may be observed especially when the hormone-producing gland is the final effector organ of a complex hormonal axis (e.g. testis—testosterone and ovary—oestradiol). In this case, insufficient production of hormones may result either from direct toxic damage to the endocrine gland, from insufficient stimulatory input from the superior part of the hormonal axis, or from hyporesponsiveness of the gland.

Disorders of hormonal action

Disturbed activation of prohormones

Concentrations of certain prohormones are elevated in uraemia, for example pro-insulin-like growth factor (pro-IGF)-IA (a precursor of IGF-I), which is not detectable in normal serum (Powell *et al.* 1987), or proinsulin, which is not converted peripherally to insulin and C-peptide in patients with terminal renal failure (Zilker *et al.* 1988). Similarly, peripheral conversion of thyroxine (T_4) to tissue-active triiodothyronine (T_3) is impaired (Lim *et al.* 1977). Some prohormones may block hormone action by competitively inhibiting receptor binding in tissue.

Multimolecular forms of variable bioactivity

Abnormal glycosylation and sialysation (Kishore *et al.* 1983) or a diminished metabolic clearance of less glycosylated isoforms may shift the isohormone spectrum towards less bioactive forms [e.g. luteinizing hormone (LH)] (Schaefer *et al.* 1991).

Hormone binding to plasma proteins

Excessively high concentrations of several IGF-binding proteins are found in patients with chronic renal failure (Blum *et al.* 1989; Lee *et al.* 1989). Binding proteins can compete for the hormone with target organ receptors, and this may explain the reduced somatomedin bioactivity in the presence of normal total serum IGF. Abnormal concentrations of other polypeptide binding proteins may similarly be related to abnormal hormone action in uraemia.

Alteration of target tissue sensitivity

Diminished target organ responsiveness is observed in various endocrine systems in uraemia. Mechanisms for altered target tissue sensitivity include reduced cellular receptor due to:

(1) the presence of inhibitory substances;

(2) accumulation of molecules inhibiting hormone (e.g. IGF-I, Blum *et al.* 1989);

(3) structural changes of either the hormone or its receptor; and finally,

(4) defects of hormone–receptor complex dependent intracellular signalling. Such postreceptor events seem to play a key role in the pathogenesis of insulin (Smith and Defronzo 1982) or growth hormone (Schaefer *et al.* 2001) resistance in uraemia (see Fig. 1).

Disorders of thyroid function

Clinical findings

The incidence of goitre is increased in patients with endstage renal disease (ESRD) (Kaptein *et al.* 1988). High-resolution ultrasound scanning shows increased thyroid gland volumes in about 50 per cent of euthyroid patients with chronic renal failure (CRF) without clinical evidence of thyroid enlargement (see Fig. 2) (Hegedus *et al.* 1985).

The prevalence of hypothyroidism in ESRD ranges between 0 and 9.5 per cent. Primary hypothyroidism was observed 2.5 times more frequently in dialysis patients than in patients with other chronic non-renal disease, while the prevalence of hyperthyroidism was not different (Kaptein *et al.* 1988). However, such epidemiological surveys may be biased by inclusion of patients with diabetes mellitus and other autoimmune diseases, which may independently affect thyroid function. In fact, Kaptein *et al.* (1988) found antithyroid antibody titres in 6.7 per cent of uraemic patients, but in only 1.4 per cent of those with non-renal disease.

The exclusion of the diagnosis of hypothyroidism on clinical grounds may be extremely difficult in a patient with uraemia, since some manifestations of hypothyroidism, such as pallor, hypothermia, and asthenia may also occur in CRF. Therefore, investigation of the hormonal status of a patient is essential for the diagnosis of an accompanying thyroidal disorder.

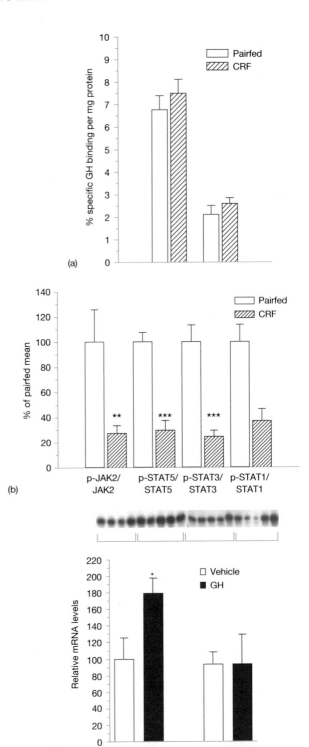

Fig. 1 (a) Specific binding of radiolabelled bGH to receptors in purified liver plasma membranes and microsomes from uraemic (CRF) and pairfed (PF) rats. (b) Relative phosphorylation of the signal-transducing proteins JAK2 and STAT proteins 10 min after bGH bolus in CRF and PF control animals. (c) Decreased mRNA levels of IGF-I in CRF and PF rats after 7-day treatment with vehicle or GH (adapted from Schaefer *et al.* 2001).

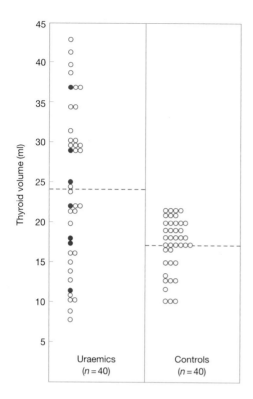

Fig. 2 Thyroid gland volume in 40 subjects with CRF and 40 sex-, age-, and weight-matched healthy controls. Open circles: subjects not on haemodialysis; closed circles: subjects on haemodialysis. Broken horizontal lines indicate the median thyroid volume. (Reprinted with permission from Hegedus *et al.* 1985.)

Thyroid hormone metabolism

As inorganic iodine is normally excreted by the kidney, plasma iodine increases as renal function decreases (Koutras *et al.* 1972). Low basal radioiodine uptake by the thyroid (Ramirez *et al.* 1973) may result from an expanded iodine pool.

Plasma thyroid hormones

Most studies of thyroid hormones in renal patients showed decreased plasma total T_4 (thyroxine) and T_3 (tri-iodothyronine). Usually, there is a more distinct suppression of T_3 than of T_4 (Lim 1986). In endstage renal failure, on average, diminished T_4 is found in 29 per cent and diminished T_3 in 55 per cent of patients (Ramirez *et al.* 1973; Spector *et al.* 1976; De-Marchi *et al.* 1987).

Binding proteins

The thyroid hormones in plasma are bound to thyroid hormone-binding globulin, albumin, and prealbumin. Thyroid hormone-binding globulin concentrations are usually normal in haemodialysis patients (Pagliacci *et al.* 1987) and low or normal in those on continuous ambulatory peritoneal dialysis (Pagliacci *et al.* 1987), who lose thyroxin-binding proteins via the peritoneum (Robey *et al.* 1989). Only the free T_4 (fT_4) and T_3 (fT_3) fractions are biologically active. Using equilibrium dialysis, normal fT_4 and fT_3 were found in ESRD (Spector *et al.* 1976; Kaptein *et al.* 1987). However, this method is prone to interference by free fatty acids arising *in vitro*, and may thus overestimate fT_4 and fT_3 (Liewendahl *et al.* 1987; Hardy *et al.* 1988). Conversely, direct measurements of fT_4 and fT_3 by radioimmunoassay yields low plasma concentrations for both hormones (Hardy *et al.* 1988; Goffin *et al.* 1993), and normal dissociation constants for specific T_4 and T_3 binding (Beckett *et al.* 1983).

Kinetics of thyroid hormones

The production rates of thyroid hormones are normal (Kaptein *et al.* 1983, 1987). Metabolic clearance rates of the hormones may (Faber *et al.* 1983) or may not (Kaptein *et al.* 1987) be increased in patients with ESRD. Peripheral deiodination of T_4 to T_3 is impaired (Faber *et al.* 1983); this finding is consistent with the more pronounced decrease of T_3 than of T_4 in progressive renal failure. Instead, there is preferential diversion to inactive metabolites (Faber *et al.* 1983). In contrast to other non-thyroidal illnesses, production and metabolic clearance rate of the inactive T_4 metabolite reverse T_3 (rT_3) are normal (Kaptein *et al.* 1983), and there is increased extravascular binding of rT_3, resulting in low normal plasma values (Kaptein *et al.* 1987).

Hypothalamo-pituitary–thyroid axis

Despite low total and probably also free T_4 and T_3, thyroid-stimulating hormone (TSH) concentrations are usually normal (Weissel *et al.* 1979; Davis *et al.* 1982; Beckett *et al.* 1983; Hardy *et al.* 1988). Normal TSH in the face of low fT_3 and fT_4 points to altered regulation of the hypothalamo-pituitary–thyroid axis. Experimental data suggest that sensitivity of the thyrotroph to feedback inhibition is increased in the uraemic rat. In addition, a blunted, delayed increase of TSH in response to exogenous thyrotrophin-releasing hormone administration was found by most investigators (Lim *et al.* 1977; Weissel *et al.* 1979; Beckett *et al.* 1983; Giordano *et al.* 1984). As expected, the duration of the TSH response is prolonged due to decreased metabolic clearance and increased half-lives of both thyrotrophin-releasing hormone and TSH (Davis *et al.* 1982; Duntas *et al.* 1992). While basal iodine uptake is low (Ramirez *et al.* 1973), thyroid responsiveness to stimulation by TSH is normal (Silverberg *et al.* 1973).

The most convincing evidence for a primary hypothalamic defect comes from studies on the temporal organization of TSH release. The physiological nocturnal TSH surge is frequently blunted in patients with endstage CRF (Wheatley *et al.* 1989; Bartalena *et al.* 1990), and the pattern of pulsatile TSH secretion is altered towards low-amplitude, high-frequency pulses (Wheatley *et al.* 1989).

In conclusion, alterations of secretory activity and responsiveness to stimulation and feedback inhibition occur at multiple levels in the hypothalamo-pituitary–thyroid axis. They are compatible with a resetting of the central thyrostat towards lower circulating thyroid hormone concentrations.

Thyroid hormone action

Clinically, patients with CRF usually appear euthyroid. Measurements of basal metabolic rates and rough clinical indices yield normal results (Spector *et al.* 1976). Normal TSH concentrations suggest that euthyroidism is also present in pituitary thyrotrophs.

In uraemia, thyroid hormones act efficiently at the nuclear level, but other actions of the thyroid hormones are compromised. Patients with CRF show a marked resistance to thyroid hormones with regard to thermogenesis. Serum T_3 is inversely related to serum protein concentrations. Consequently, reduced T_3 may be beneficial by lowering protein breakdown (Verger et al. 1987). In contrast to normal controls, T_3 supplementation results in a negative nitrogen balance in uraemic patients (Lim 2001), similar to patients with chronic illness or malnutrition (Spaulding et al. 1976).

On the basis of these observations, part of the changes of the thyroid axis in uraemia has been interpreted as a physiological adaptation to conserve energy in an adverse metabolic environment. Supplementary thyroid hormone treatment might, therefore, not only be useless but even harmful. On the other hand, the impaired in vitro activation of mononuclear cells of patients with uraemia can be improved by addition of T_3, suggesting that low circulating free thyroid hormone levels may contribute to the impairment of cell-mediated immune functions in uraemia (Blaehr et al. 1992).

Thyroid hormones in uraemia and other chronic illnesses

The characteristic changes of the thyroidal axis in uraemia, primary hypothyroidism, and other states of chronic illness are compared in Table 1. Chronic non-thyroidal diseases are characterized by a low T_3 syndrome. In this so-called 'sick euthyroid syndrome' increased rT_3 results from impaired peripheral conversion of T_4 to T_3. In chronic renal failure, T_3 is low as in the low T_3 syndrome, but rT_3 is normal or even low. This has been explained by a redistribution of rT_3 into extravascular compartments in uraemia.

The thyroid in continuous ambulatory peritoneal dialysis

Continuous ambulatory peritoneal dialysis (CAPD) treatment leads to loss of serum proteins including thyroid hormone-binding globulin (Pagliacci et al. 1987) in the dialysis fluid. Thyroid hormones are translocated across the peritoneum predominantly in their protein-bound forms (Herrmann et al. 1973). As a consequence, low total T_3 and T_4,

Table 1 Changes of thyroid hormone concentrations in endstage chronic renal failure (CRF), primary hypothyroidism, and other chronic non-thyroidal illness ('sick euthyroid' syndrome) (see text for sources)

	CRF	Primary hypothyroidism	'Sick euthyroid' syndrome
tT_3	↓	↓	↓
tT_4	↓	↓	↓
rT_3	=	↓	↑
fT_3 (RIA)	↓	↓	↓
fT_4	↓	↓	↓
TBG	CAPD: ↓ HD: =	=	=
TSH	=	↑	=
TRH test	= or ↓	↑	=

RIA, radioimmunoassay; TBG, thyroid hormone-binding globulin; CAPD, continuous ambulatory peritoneal dialysis; HD, haemodialysis; TSH, thyroid stimulating hormone; TRH, thyrotrophin releasing hormone.

together with normal free hormone, are found in patients undergoing CAPD (Pagliacci et al. 1987). Some studies found only a slight or no decrease of thyroid hormone in these patients, in contrast to haemodialysed patients (Ross et al. 1985; Verger et al. 1987). The greater carbohydrate intake of patients undergoing CAPD may explain the difference.

Clinical management of thyroid disorders in chronic renal failure

The prevalence of hypothyroidism is increased in CRF. Risk factors are female sex, insulin-dependent diabetes mellitus, and age greater than 50 years (Kaptein et al. 1988), increased iodine intake (Takeda et al. 1993), and extensive haemosiderosis (Shirota et al. 1992). Since the clinical features of uraemia and hypothyroidism may be indistinguishable, all patients with ESRD should be screened for potential hypothyroidism. In a patient with uraemia, hypothyroidism should only be diagnosed if the total and free T_4 (measured by radioimmunoassay) are distinctly low in the presence of normal thyroid hormone-binding globulin. Basal TSH must be clearly elevated (>20 µU/ml), as normal TSH concentrations are a valid indicator of tissue euthyroidism.

In haemodialysis patients, heparin may interfere with methods used to evaluate thyroid hormone status. Heparin competes with T_4 at intra- and extravascular binding sites, thus increasing total and free serum T_4 for at least 24 h postdialysis (van Leusen and Meinders 1982). Heparin may also elevate concentrations of free fatty acids in vivo and in vitro, resulting in artefactually high fT_4 measured by equilibrium dialysis (Rochiccioli et al. 1986). Other substances can cause similar artefacts, for example, high-dose frusemide (Liewendahl et al. 1987). Therefore, strict standardization of the timing of investigations in relation to dialysis is essential. Blood should be sampled before heparin administration at the beginning of the dialysis session.

Patients with CRF who undergo repeated radiological investigations with iodinated contrast agents may be at increased risk of developing acute iodine-induced hyperthyroidism because of reduced iodine clearance. Primary hyperthyroidism is extremely rare in patients with CRF. So far, only eight patients have been reported (Soffer et al. 1980; Foley and Hammer 1985; McKillop et al. 1985; Alarcon et al. 1992; Nibhanupudy et al. 1993). These patients have been treated successfully with iodine isotopes, antithyroid drugs, or thyroidectomy. The treatment of hyperthyroidism in a patient with uraemia is complicated by the reduced renal clearance of antithyroid agents (e.g. metamizole). Radioiodine may also accumulate. Due to the expansion of the iodine pool in uraemia, high doses must be administered. As a consequence, the preferred procedure is usually thyroid surgery after a short course of antithyroid medication.

Growth hormone–somatomedin axis

During normal childhood, the somatotrophic hormone axis plays a key role in the regulation of body growth. In addition, growth hormone is part of a complex system of counter-regulatory hormones maintaining the homeostasis of carbohydrate metabolism.

Growth hormone

Plasma values and kinetics

Fasting growth hormone concentrations are elevated in uraemic children and adults in proportion to the extent of renal failure

(Davidson *et al.* 1976; Ramirez *et al.* 1978) (Fig. 3). Basal growth hormone and responses to glucose or tolbutamide are not affected by the nutritional state in uraemic patients (Allegra *et al.* 1988).

The kidney is a major site of growth hormone degradation (Johnson and Maack 1977). In patients with endstage renal failure, the metabolic clearance rate of growth hormone is reduced by approximately 50 per cent (Haffner *et al.* 1994; Schaefer *et al.* 1996). Deconvolution studies of plasma growth hormone concentration profiles in adolescents with uraemia disclosed that the increase in mean plasma growth hormone concentrations is due to a consistent increase in plasma half-life, whereas the pituitary growth hormone secretion rate was found to be variable between patients and studies. A high-normal calculated GH secretion rate and an amplified number of GH secretory bursts were reported in prepubertal children with ESRD, presumably resulting from attenuated bioactive IGF-I feedback of the somatotropic axis (Tönshoff *et al.* 1995b). In adult patients on haemodialysis, the GH secretion rate was clearly elevated (Veldhuis *et al.* 1994), whereas in pubertal patients with advanced CRF reduced GH secretion rates were observed, indicating an altered sensitivity of the somatotropic hormone axis to the stimulatory effect of sex steroids at least in this developmental stage (Schaefer *et al.* 1994).

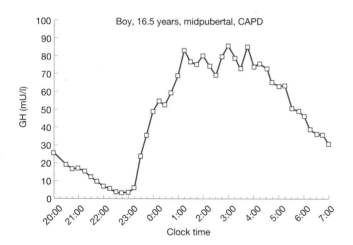

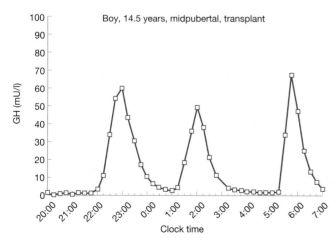

Fig. 3 Spontaneous nocturnal growth hormone secretion profiles in a patient on haemodialysis treatment (upper panel) and in a transplant recipient (lower panel). (Reprinted from Schaefer *et al.* 1991.)

Neuroendocrine control of growth hormone release

Dysregulation of growth hormone secretion may be related to abnormalities of central neuroendocrine control mechanisms. Evidence for this is provided by several hypothalamic–pituitary function tests. The growth hormone response to intravenous growth hormone-releasing hormone is augmented and prolonged, at least in children (Bessarione *et al.* 1987). Exogenous thyrotrophin-releasing hormone, which does not affect growth hormone release in normal individuals, markedly enhances growth hormone secretion in subjects with uraemia (Ramirez *et al.* 1978; Weissel *et al.* 1979; Giordano *et al.* 1984). However, the exaggerated pituitary response to growth hormone-releasing hormone and thyrotrophin-releasing hormone may be secondary to the reduced metabolic clearance of these releasing hormones in uraemia (Duntas *et al.* 1992). Patients with uraemia respond to acute hyperglycaemia by a paradoxical increase in growth hormone secretion (Ramirez *et al.* 1978; Alvestrand *et al.* 1989). Stimulation tests such as arginine infusion and insulin-induced hypoglycaemia lead to a sustained, exaggerated increase of growth hormone, which is more pronounced in patients undergoing haemodialysis than in those on CAPD (Ramirez *et al.* 1978; Marumo *et al.* 1979; Rodger *et al.* 1986a). However, the altered metabolic clearance rates of growth hormone as well as of the provocative agents in renal failure make a meaningful clinical interpretation of such tests virtually impossible.

Plasma binding and peripheral action

About 50 per cent of circulating growth hormone is bound to two plasma proteins, one of which is produced by proteolytic cleavage of the growth hormone membrane receptor mainly from liver tissue and is thought to reflect growth hormone receptor expression (Leung *et al.* 1987). Reduced concentrations of this high-affinity binding protein have been reported in patients with CRF (Baumann *et al.* 1989; Postel-Vinay *et al.* 1991). Decreased binding protein concentrations in the presence of increased plasma growth hormone would implicate a marked elevation of the free hormone fraction at the target tissues. On the other hand, reduced phosphorylation of intracellular tyrosine kinases in cultured chondrocytes from uraemic rats after growth hormone stimulation despite normal growth hormone receptor binding (Schaefer *et al.* 2001) suggests that impaired intracellular signal transduction may be a limiting factor for the peripheral action of growth hormone in uraemia.

Somatomedins

Plasma insulin-like growth factor

The effect of growth hormone on longitudinal growth is partially mediated by stimulating the production of somatomedins, the two most important of which are IGF-I and II. Serum IGF-I and IGF-II levels in children with preterminal CRF are in the normal range, whereas in ESRD mean age-related serum IGF-I levels are slightly, but significantly decreased and IGF-II levels slightly, but significantly elevated (Tönshoff *et al.* 1995a). Hence, total immunoreactive IGF levels in CRF serum are normal, but IGF bioactivity measured by sulfate incorporation into porcine costal cartilage is markedly reduced. Similarly, the level of free IGF-I is reduced by 50 per cent in relation to the degree of renal dysfunction (Frystyk *et al.* 1999). This finding is one of the key abnormalities of the GH/IGF axis in children with CRF.

Somatomedin bioactivity

The discrepancy between low somatomedin activity by bioassay and normal or elevated IGF by radioimmunossay or radioreceptor assay suggests the presence of circulating somatomedin inhibitors in uraemia. Uraemic serum contains low-molecular weight (about 1 kDa) IGF inhibitors whose molecular structure, however, has not yet been defined (Phillips *et al.* 1984).

The most likely explanation for the inhibition of somatomedin action in uraemia has emerged from the identification of six insulin-like growth factor-binding proteins (IGFBP1–6) of which IGFBP3 appears to be the most abundant in humans, constituting more than 95 per cent of total circulating IGFBP. In children with chronic renal failure, the serum concentrations of IGFBP1, IGFBP2, IGFBP4, and IGFBP6 are increased (Blum *et al.* 1989; Lee *et al.* 1989; Tönshoff *et al.* 1995a; Powell *et al.* 1997, 1999) (Fig. 4). Ligand blotting shows that the elevation of radioimmunoassayable IGFBP3 is due to an increase in low molecular weight forms mainly in the range 14–19 kDa, whereas intact IGFBP 3 (38 and 41 kDa) is markedly reduced (Liu *et al.* 1989; Lee *et al.* 1994).

IGFBP1, IGFBP2, and IGFBP6 inhibit somatomedin bioactivity *in vitro* (Kiepe *et al.* 2002). Somatomedin bioactivity in uraemic serum can be returned to normal by removing unsaturated IGFBP (Blum *et al.* 1991). An important question is whether the imbalance between normal total IGF and the excess of unsaturated IGFBPs contributes to growth failure in the setting of clinical CRF. Serum levels of IGFBP1, IGFBP2, and IGFBP4 correlate significantly and inversely with standardized height in CRF children, implying that these IGFBPs contribute to the growth failure in these children (Tönshoff *et al.* 1995a; Powell *et al.* 1997; Ulinski *et al.* 2000). The potential role of serum IGFBP3 for longitudinal growth appears to be more complex. There is neither a positive relationship between immunoreactive IGFBP3 and standardized height in CRF, as observed under normal conditions in healthy children, nor a negative correlation, which would be expected if IGFBP3 acted merely as an IGF inhibitor in CRF. On the other hand, GH therapy in CRF induced an increase in serum IGFBP3 levels in correlation to the improved growth of these children (Powell *et al.* 1997), suggesting a potential growth stimulatory effect of intact IGFBP3 in this setting.

Growth hormone–somatomedin axis and body growth

Prepubertal, and to a major part also pubertal, body growth is mainly mediated by the growth hormone–somatomedin axis. Poor body growth and reduced final height are well-known complications of CRF in childhood. The reported elevation of growth hormone levels in the face of low somatomedin activity suggests that growth failure in uraemia is due to end-organ hyporesponsiveness to growth hormone. Nevertheless, treatment of uraemic children with pharmacological doses of exogenous recombinant human growth hormone results in marked stimulation of growth (Tönshoff *et al.* 1990).

Growth hormone–somatomedin axis and carbohydrate metabolism

Growth hormone normally counteracts the effects of insulin in carbohydrate metabolism. Pharmacological doses of growth hormone can significantly affect glucose tolerance (Bratusch-Marrain *et al.* 1982). Daily treatment by recombinant human growth hormone in supraphysiological doses did not change glucose tolerance in children with uraemia, but induced an increase in stimulated insulin secretion (Tönshoff *et al.* 1990).

Growth hormone–somatomedin axis and kidney function

GFR and renal plasma flow can be increased by administration of growth hormone in healthy individuals (Christiansen *et al.* 1981). Infusion studies in rats confirmed that IGF-I increases GFR and renal plasma flow by an eicosanoid- and nitric oxide-dependent mechanism (Hirschberg and Kopple 1989; Tsukahara *et al.* 1994). In view of the concept that progression of renal failure is related to glomerular hyperfiltration (Brenner *et al.* 1982), this effect of growth hormone has caused some concern with respect to the long-term consequences of growth hormone treatment in children with CRF. However, there is experimental evidence from animal studies that in CRF growth hormone no longer increases GFR. Haffner *et al.* (1989) confirmed this observation in men with uraemia.

Pituitary–adrenal axis

Clinical findings

Analogous to thyroid disorders, dysfunction of the pituitary–adrenal axis may be difficult to diagnose in patients with CRF. Uraemia shares many clinical signs and symptoms with Cushing's syndrome, such as osteopenia, proximal muscle weakness with atrophy, glucose intolerance, and hypertension (Sharp *et al.* 1986); therefore, Cushing's syndrome may easily be overlooked if it occurs concomitantly with renal

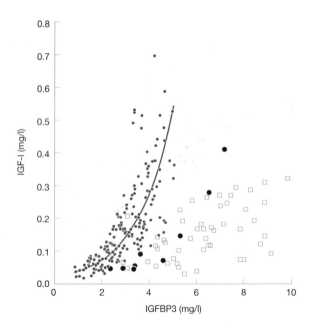

Fig. 4 Correlation of IGF-I versus IGFBP3 in normal children (dots) and children with CRF (squares). (Reprinted with permission from Blum *et al.* 1989.)

failure. Conversely, adrenal insufficiency may also present with symptoms which are not uncommon in renal failure, for example hypotension, weakness, and hyperkalaemia. To confirm or reject the diagnoses of Cushing's syndrome or adrenal failure, the clinician has to rely on the evaluation of the patient's hormonal status under basal and stimulated conditions. For intelligent interpretation of the results, the changes of the hypothalamo-pituitary–adrenal axis induced by uraemia *per se* must be kept in mind.

Plasma concentrations of pituitary–adrenal axis hormones

Cortisol is conjugated by the liver to water-soluble metabolites, which are predominantly excreted via the kidney and accumulate in renal failure. This may explain why discrepant results are reported regarding basal cortisol levels in uraemia (Nolan *et al.* 1981). Wallace *et al.* (1980) demonstrated that in contrast to *basal levels* measured at 8 a.m. which were *still* in the *normal range*, integrated *24-hour total and free cortisol* in patients with uraemia were *elevated by 100 per cent*. Cortisol binding to plasma proteins was found to be unchanged in uraemia (McDonald *et al.* 1979; Wallace *et al.* 1980). The diurnal rhythm and the pulsatile mode of cortisol secretion is retained in renal failure, although the half-life of the endogenous secretory peaks is prolonged (Cooke *et al.* 1979; Wallace *et al.* 1980; Ramirez *et al.* 1982); in haemodialysis patients, the secretory activity is shifted towards the hours of dialysis, but a normal pattern is observed on days off dialysis.

Basal ACTH is normal (Ramirez *et al.* 1988; Siamopoulos *et al.* 1988) or elevated (McDonald *et al.* 1979; Luger *et al.* 1987) in uraemia. The finding of increased ACTH in the presence of normal cortisol has raised the speculation that the bioactivity of the ACTH-like activity may be reduced.

Pituitary–adrenal function tests

Glucocorticoids

A clinical synopsis of function tests to assess disorders of glucocorticoid metabolism is given in Table 2.

Cortisol profile

The normal range of serum cortisol is 5.6–20 µg/dl at 8 a.m. and 5–10 µg/dl (or 50 per cent of morning levels) at 6 p.m. Pituitary hypersecretion predominantly leads to increased evening levels, hypopituitarism in decreased morning levels. Increased evening levels are also associated with stress or acute psychosis. Diurnal rhythmicity is lost in patients with autonomous adrenocortical adenoma. Assay cross reaction with predniso(lo)ne may occur in patients receiving high-dose corticosteroids.

Dexamethasone suppression test

The dexamethasone suppression test is performed to confirm the diagnosis of Cushing's syndrome, to distinguish between central and peripheral hypercortisolism and to confirm the diagnosis of dexamethasone-suppressible hyperaldosteronism (a rare genetic defect resulting in hyperactivity of the ACTH-inducible form of 11-hydroxylase).

Basal serum cortisol levels are measured in the morning, then 5 mg/m^2 body surface area of dexamethasone are given in the evening of day 1. A decrease of serum cortisol levels to less than 3 µg/dl the next morning excludes the diagnosis of Cushing's syndrome. No decrease of serum cortisol levels occurs in patients with adrenal cortical adenoma or ectopic ACTH secretion.

In patients with CRF, ACTH secretion is not suppressible by standard oral doses of dexamethasone (McDonald *et al.* 1979; Rosman *et al.*

Table 2 Clinical synopsis of function tests to assess disorders of glucocorticoid metabolism (details in Forest 1996)

Parameter		Normal range	Cushing's		Addison		Uraemia	Post-transplant
			Central	Peripheral	Primary	Secondary		
Serum cortisol profile		8 a.m.: 5.6–20 µg/dl 6 p.m.: 5–10 µg/dl	Evening cortisol ↑	Loss of diurnal rhythmicity	Morning cortisol ↓	Morning cortisol ↓	=/↑	↓
Dexamethasone suppression test	Cortisol decrease	<3 µg/dl	↓	↓	Not useful	Not useful	= t 1/2 ↑	Not useful
Metyrapone test	ACTH increase	>120 pg/ml	↑	↓	=	=/↓	↓	=/↓
	11-Desoxycortisol increase	>7 µg/dl	↑	↓	↓	↓	↓	↓
Basal ACTH			↑	↓	↑	↓	=/↑	↓
ACTH test	Cortisol increase	By >10 µg/dl or >two-fold of basal; absolute levels <40 µg/dl	Not useful	Not useful	↓↓	=/↓	=	=/↓
CRF test	ACTH increase	2–3 fold of basal	=	↓↓	=/↑	=/↓	=	↓
	Cortisol increase	>50% of basal	=	↓↓	↓		↓	↓

1982). However, oral absorption of dexamethasone is reduced in uraemia (Ramirez *et al.* 1982), and suppression is seen with high doses (Ramirez *et al.* 1982, 1988). Delayed suppression of plasma cortisol is seen after intravenous administration of dexamethasone, but this may be due to reduced metabolic clearance of cortisol in renal failure (Workman *et al.* 1986). Thus, a 2-day dexamethasone suppression test is suggested in uraemic patients. Adequate suppression of cortisol secretion can only be expected when serum dexamethasone levels exceed 200 ng/dl. Dexamethasone kinetics can also be altered in obese subjects.

Under normal conditions, serum *aldosterone* levels remain unchanged after administration of dexamethasone. In patients with dexamethasone-suppressible hyperaldosteronism, a marked decrease of serum aldosterone levels is found.

Metyrapone test

Metyrapone is an inhibitor of 11-hydroxylase, the rate limiting enzyme of cortisol synthesis. In healthy subjects, cortisol depletion results in a stimulation of CRH and ACTH. In the metyrapone test, serum levels of ACTH, cortisol, and 11-desoxy-cortisol are measured. After a basal blood sample in the morning, 30 mg/kg body weight of metyrapone is given in the evening and a second sample is collected the next morning. Under normal conditions, ACTH should rise to more than 120 pg/ml and 11-desoxy-cortisol should increase to more than 5.6 μg/dl, whereas serum cortisol levels should decrease to less than 8 μg/dl to confirm adequate 11-hydroxylase inhibition. This response is absent in patients with autonomous adreno-cortical adenoma or ectopic ACTH secretion. In patients with hypopituitarism, ACTH and 11-desoxy-cortisol exhibit only a small increase. In patients with adrenocortical insufficiency, the increase of 11-desoxy-cortisol is blunted, whereas the increase of serum ACTH levels is not. A very high increase of both parameters is found in patients with hypoplasia of the adrenal cortex or Cushing's disease. The response to metyrapone is blunted in uraemia (McDonald *et al.* 1979). The metabolism of metyrapone is increased by enzyme-inducing drugs (e.g. phenobarbital, phenytoin, rifampin, etc.). The test should not be performed in infants due to an increased risk of hypoglycaemia.

CRH test

The CRH test is performed to diagnose an insufficiency of the anterior pituitary gland. Blood samples are withdrawn 30 min and immediately before injection of 1 μg/kg body weight of CRH and 15, 30, and 60 min thereafter to determine ACTH and serum cortisol levels. Under normal conditions, ACTH levels increase to two to three fold of basal concentrations, whereas serum cortisol should increase by at least 50 per cent. In the case of adrenal Cushing's syndrome, ACTH and cortisol levels do not change upon application of CRH. The pharmacokinetics of corticotrophin-releasing hormone is unaltered in patients with end-stage renal failure. Compared to controls, the pituitary response to corticotrophin-releasing hormone infusion occurs earlier but is blunted (Luger *et al.* 1987; Siamopoulos *et al.* 1988). When renal anaemia is partially corrected by recombinant human erythropoietin, the corticotroph responsiveness to corticotrophin-releasing hormone may improve (Watschinger et al. 1991).

ACTH test

The ACTH test is performed to diagnose or exclude adrenocortical insufficiency. Systemic glucocorticoid medication must be stopped at least 24 h before the test. In females, the test should be performed between the 3rd and 8th day after menstruation. Blood samples to determine serum cortisol levels are withdrawn prior and 1 h after injection of 0.25 mg synthetic ACTH after an overnight fast. Adrenocortical insufficiency can be excluded when serum cortisol levels rise two-fold from normal basal levels (normal range 5.6–20 μg/dl in the morning) or increase by more than 10 μg/dl (normal range after ACTH: <40 μg/dl). Excessively increased cortisol levels are found in adrenocortical hyperplasia. Fifty per cent of patients with an autonomous adrenocortical adenoma respond with a moderate increase of serum cortisol levels, in the remaining 50 per cent serum cortisol levels do not change after ACTH administration.

A reduced stimulated cortisol secretion in response to recombinant CRH despite prolonged elevation of ACTH has been observed in patients on haemodialysis (Grant *et al.* 1993). This finding contrasts with the normal cortisol response observed with low doses of exogenous ACTH (Zager *et al.* 1985). Zona glomerulosa steroids (aldosterone,18-OH-corticosterone) are stimulated normally in patients undergoing CAPD (Zager *et al.* 1983, 1985) but not in haemodialysis patients (Williams *et al.* 1973). Transient hyporesponsiveness to ACTH was found in the majority of patients who returned to dialysis after transplant failure (Rodger *et al.* 1986b).

Mineralocorticoids

Captopril test

The captopril test permits to distinguish primary from secondary hyperaldosteronism. Diuretics and antihypertensive drugs should be stopped at least 1 week before the test. The patient should rest in a horizontal position for at least 2 h before the beginning of the test. Blood samples are collected after an overnight fast before and 30, 60, 90, and 120 min after oral application of 25 mg of captopril for the determination of serum aldosterone and renin levels. The test is contraindicated with bilateral renal arteries stenosis.

In secondary hyperaldosteronism, serum aldosterone decreases after application of captopril, whereas serum renin levels increase by approximately 50 per cent. In primary hyperaldosteronism, serum aldosterone levels and renin levels remain unchanged after captopril. Elevated renin levels and a blood pressure drop in response to captopril were found in 60 per cent out of 68 uraemic patients with arterial hypertension (Schohn *et al.* 1988).

Other function tests performed in the diagnostic work-up of primary or secondary hyperaldosteronism may produce invalid results under uraemic conditions. The orthostasis test, which measures changes of renal renin secretion after postural changes, can be influenced by electrolyte imbalances, which are frequently present in patients with CRF. The furosemide test, which measures the stimulation of renin secretion by an increase of renotubular sodium concentration, may be influenced by a reduced susceptibility to diuretics in advanced renal failure.

References

Alarcon, R. D., Groover, A. M., and Jenkins-Ross, C. S. (1992). Organic anxiety disorder secondary to hyperthyroidism in a hemodialysis patient. *Psychosomatics* **33**, 214–217.

Allegra, V. *et al.* (1988). Growth hormone secretion abnormalities in uremic patients: which is the role of impaired glucose hypothalamic sensitivity? *Nephron* **48**, 76–77.

Alvestrand, A. *et al.* (1989). Glucose intolerance in uremic patients: the relative contributions of impaired beta-cell function and insulin resistance. *Clinical Nephrology* **31**, 175–183.

Bartalena, L. *et al.* (1990). Lack of nocturnal serum thyrotropin (TSH) surge in patients with chronic renal failure undergoing maintenance hemofiltration: a case of central hypothyroidism. *Clinical Nephrology* **34**, 30–34.

Baumann, G., Shaw, M. A., and Amburn, K. (1989). Regulation of plasma growth hormone-binding proteins in health and disease. *Metabolism* **38**, 683–689.

Beckett, G. J. *et al.* (1983). Thyroid status in patients with chronic renal failure. *Clinical Nephrology* **19**, 172–178.

Bessarione, D. *et al.* (1987). Growth hormone response to growth hormone-releasing hormone in normal and uraemic children: comparison with hypoglycemia following insulin administration. *Acta Endrocrinologica (Copenhagen)* **114**, 5–11.

Blaehr, H., Bregengaard, C., and Povlsen, J. V. (1992). Triiodothyronine stimulates growth of peripheral blood mononuclear cells in serum-free cultures in uremic patients. *American Journal of Nephrology* **12**, 148–154.

Blum W. F. *et al.* Excess of IGF-binding proteins in chronic renal failure: evidence for relative GH resistance and inhibition of somatomedin activity. In *Insulin-Like Growth Factor Binding Proteins* (ed. S. L. S. Drop and R. L. Hintz), pp. 93–99. Amsterdam: Elsevier Science, 1989.

Blum, W. F. *et al.* (1991). GH resistance and inhibition of somatomedin activity by excess of insulin-like growth factor binding protein in uremia. *Pediatric Nephrology* **5**, 539–544.

Bratusch-Marrain, P. R., Smith, D., and Defronzo, R. A. (1982). The effect of growth hormone on glucose metabolism and insulin secretion in man. *Journal of Clinical Endrocrinology and Metabolism* **55**, 973–982.

Brenner, B. M., Meyer, T. W., and Hostetter, T. H. (1982). Dietary protein intake and the progressive nature of kidney disease. *New England Journal of Medicine* **307**, 652–659.

Christiansen, S. J. *et al.* (1981). Kidney function and size in normal subjects before and during growth hormone administration for one week. *European Journal of Clinical Investigation* **11**, 487–490.

Cooke, C. R. *et al.* (1979). Dissociation of the diurnal variation of aldosterone and cortisol in anephric patients. *Kidney International* **15**, 669–675.

Davidson, M. B. *et al.* (1976). Effect of protein intake and dialysis on the abnormal growth hormone, glucose, and insulin homeostasis in uremia. *Metabolism* **25**, 455–464.

Davis, F. B. *et al.* (1982). Comparison of pituitary-thyroid function in patients with end-stage renal disease and in age- and sex-matched controls. *Kidney International* **21**, 362–364.

De-Marchi, S. *et al.* (1987). Serum reverse T3 assay for predicting glucose intolerance in uremic patients on dialysis therapy. *Clinical Nephrology* **27**, 189–198.

Duntas, L. *et al.* (1992). Tyrotropin-releasing hormone: pharmacokinetic and pharmacodynamic properties in chronic renal failure. *Clinical Nephrology* **38**, 214–218.

Faber, J. *et al.* (1983). Simultaneous turnover studies of thyroxine, 3,5,3′- and 3,3′,5′-triiodothyronine, 3,5-, 3,3′-, and 3′,5′-diiodothyronine, and 3′-monoiodothyronine in chronic renal failure. *Journal of Clinical Endrocrinology and Metabolism* **56**, 211–217.

Foley, R. J. and Hammer, R. W. (1985). Hyperthyroidism in end stage renal disease. *American Journal of Nephrology* **5**, 292–295.

Forest, M. G. Adrenal function tests. In *Diagnostics of Endocrine Function in Children and Adolescents* (ed. M. B. Ranke), p. 370. Heidelberg, Leipzig: J. Ambrosius Barth Verlag, 1996.

Frystyk, J. *et al.* (1999). Serum-free insulin-like growth factor I correlates with clearance in patients with chronic renal failure. *Kidney International* **56**, 2076–2084.

Giordano, C. *et al.* (1984). TSH response to TRH in hemodialysis and CAPD patients. *The Journal of Artificial Organs* **7**, 7–10.

Goffin, E. *et al.* (1993). Assessment of the thyroid function of patients undergoing regular haemodialysis. *Nephron* **65**, 568–572.

Grant, A. C. *et al.* (1993). Hypothalamo-pituitary–adrenal axis in uremia: evidence for primary adrenal dysfunction? *Nephrology, Dialysis, Transplantation* **8**, 307–310.

Haffner, D. *et al.* (1989). The acute effect of growth hormone on GFR is obliterated in chronic renal failure. *Journal of Clinical Investigation* **32**, 266–269.

Haffner, D. *et al.* (1994). Metabolic clearance of recombinant human growth hormone in health and chronic renal failure. *Journal of Clinical Investigation* **93**, 1163–1171.

Hardy, M. J., Ragbeer, S. S., and Nascimento, L. (1988). Pituitary-thyroid function in chronic renal failure assessed by a highly sensitive thyrotropin assay. *Journal of Clinical Endocrinology and Metabolism* **66**, 233–236.

Hegedus, L. *et al.* (1985). Thyroid gland volume and serum concentrations of thyroid hormones in chronic renal failure. *Nephron* **40**, 171–174.

Herrmann, J., Schmidt, H. J., and Krüskemper, H. L. (1973). Thyroxine elimination by peritoneal dialysis in experimental thyrotoxicosis. *Hormone and Metabolic Research* **5**, 180–183.

Hirschberg, R. and Kopple, J. D. (1989). Evidence that insulin-like growth factor I increases renal plasma flow and glomerular filtration rate in fasted rats. *Journal of Clinical Investigation* **83**, 326–330.

Hruska, K. A. *et al.* (1981). Peripheral metabolism of intact parathyroid hormone. *Journal of Clinical Investigation* **67**, 885–892.

Johnson, V. and Maack, T. (1977). Renal extraction, filtration, absorption, and catabolism of growth hormone. *American Journal of Physiology* **233**, F185–F196.

Kaptein, E. M. *et al.* (1983). Serum reverse triiodothyronine and thyroxine kinetics in patients with chronic renal failure. *Journal of Clinical Endocrinology and Metabolism* **57**, 181–189.

Kaptein, E. M. *et al.* (1987). Thyroxine transfer and distribution in critical nonthyroidal illnesses, chronic renal failure, and chronic ethanol abuse. *Journal of Clinical Endocrinology and Metabolism* **65**, 606–616.

Kaptein, E. M. *et al.* (1988). The thyroid in end-stage renal disease. *Medicine (Baltimore)* **67**, 187–197.

Kiepe, D., Ulinski, T., Powell, D. R., Durham, S. K., Mehls, O., and Tönshoff, B. (2002). Differential effects of insulin-like growth factor binding proteins-1, -2, -3, and -6 on cultured growth plate chondrocytes. *Kidney International* **62**, 1591–1600.

Kishore, B. K., Arakawa, M., and Geiyo, F. (1983). Altered glycosylation and sialisation of serum proteins and lipid bound sialic acids in chronic renal failure. *Postgraduate Medical Journal* **59**, 551–555.

Koutras, D. A. *et al.* (1972). Iodine metabolism in chronic renal insufficiency. *Nephron* **9**, 55–65.

Lee, D. *et al.* (1994). Alteration in insulin-like growth factor-binding proteins (IGFBPs) and IGFBP-3 protease activity in serum and urine from acute and chronic renal failure. *Journal of Clinical Endocrinology and Metabolism* **79**, 1376–1382.

Lee, P. D. *et al.* (1989). IGF binding proteins in growth-retarded children with chronic renal failure. *Pediatric Research* **26**, 308–315.

Leung, D. W., Spencer, S. A., and Cachianes, G. (1987). Growth hormone receptor and serum binding protein: purification, cloning and expression. *Nature* **330**, 537–543.

Liewendahl, K. *et al.* (1987). Concentrations of iodothyronines in serum of patients with chronic renal failure and other nonthyroidal illnesses: role of free fatty acids. *Clinical Chemistry* **33**, 1382–1386.

Lim, V. S. (1986). Renal failure and thyroid function. *International Journal of Artificial Organs* **9**, 385–386.

Lim, V. S. (2001). Thyroid function in patients with chronic renal failure. *American Journal of Kidney Diseases* **38**, S80–S84.

Lim, V. S. *et al.* (1977). Thyroid dysfunction in chronic renal failure. *Journal of Clinical Investigation* **60**, 522–534.

Liu, F., Powell, D. R., and Hintz, R. L. (1989). Characterization of insulin-like growth factor-binding proteins in human serum from patients with chronic renal failure. *Journal of Clinical Endocrinology and Metabolism* **70**, 620–628.

Luger, A. *et al.* (1987). Abnormalities in the hypothalamic–pituitary–adrenocortical axis in patients with chronic renal failure. *American Journal of Kidney Diseases* **9**, 51–54.

Marumo, F., Sakai, T., and Sato, S. (1979). Response of insulin, glucagon and growth hormone to arginine infusion in patients with chronic renal failure. *Nephron* **24**, 81–84.

McDonald, W. J. *et al.* (1979). Adrenocorticotropin–cortisol axis abnormalities in hemodialysis patients. *Journal of Clinical Endocrinology and Metabolism* **48**, 92–95.

McKillop, J. H., Leung, A. C. T., and Wilson, R. (1985). Successful management of Graves' disease in a patient undergoing regular dialysis therapy. *Archives of Internal Medicine* **145**, 337–339.

Nibhanupudy, J. R. *et al.* (1993). Iodine-131 treatment of hyperthyroidism in a patient on dialysis for chronic renal failure. *American Journal of Nephrology* **13**, 214–217.

Nolan, G. O. *et al.* (1981). Spurious overestimation of plasma cortisol in patients with chronic renal failure. *Journal of Clinical Endocrinology and Metabolism* **52**, 1242–1245.

Pagliacci, M. C. *et al.* (1987). Thyroid function tests in patients undergoing maintenance dialysis: characterization of the 'low-T4 syndrome' in subjects on regular hemodialysis and continuous ambulatory peritoneal dialysis. *Nephron* **46**, 225–230.

Phillips, L. S. *et al.* (1984). Somatomedin inhibitor in uremia. *Journal of Clinical Endocrinology and Metabolism* **59**, 764–772.

Postel-Vinay, M. C. *et al.* (1991). Plasma growth-hormone binding is low in uremic children. *Pediatric Nephrology* **5**, 545–547.

Powell, D. *et al.* (1997). Modulation of growth factors by growth hormone in children with chronic renal failure. *Kidney International* **51**, 1970–1979.

Powell, D. R. *et al.* (1987). Antiserum developed for the E peptide region of insulin-like growth factor IA prohormone recognizes a serum protein by both immunoblot and radioimmunoassay. *Journal of Clinical Endocrinology and Metabolism* **65**, 868–875.

Powell, D. R. *et al.* (1997). Insulin-like growth factor-binding protein-6 levels are elevated in serum of children with chronic renal failure: a report of the Southwest Pediatric Nephrology Study Group. *Journal of Clinical Endocrinology and Metabolism* **82**, 2978–2984.

Powell, D. R. *et al.* (1999). Effects of chronic renal failure and growth hormone on serum levels of insulin-like growth factor-binding protein-4 (IGFBP-4) and IGFBP-5 in children: a report of the Southwest Pediatric Nephrology Study Group. *Journal of Clinical Endocrinology and Metabolism* **84**, 596–601.

Rabkin, R., Unterhalter, S. A., and Duckworth, W. C. (1979). Effect of prolonged uremia on insulin metabolism by isolated liver and muscle. *Kidney International* **16**, 433–439.

Ramirez, G., Brueggemeyer, C., and Ganguly, A. (1988). Counterregulatory hormonal response to insulin-induced hypoglycemia in patients on chronic hemodialysis. *Nephron* **49**, 231–236.

Ramirez, G. *et al.* (1973). Thyroid abnormalities in renal failure. A study of 53 patients on chronic hemodialysis. *Annals of Internal Medicine* **79**, 500–504.

Ramirez, G. *et al.* (1978). Abnormalities in the regulation of growth hormone in chronic renal failure. *Archives of Internal Medicine* **138**, 267–271.

Ramirez, G. *et al.* (1982). Evaluation of the hypothalamic hypophyseal adrenal axis in patients receiving long-term hemodialysis. *Archives of Internal Medicine* **142**, 1448–1452.

Robey, C., Shreedhar, K., and Batuman, V. (1989). Effects of chronic peritoneal dialysis on thyroid function tests. *American Journal of Kidney Diseases* **13**, 99–103.

Rochiccioli, P. *et al.* (1986). Partial somatotropin deficiency in a case of chronic renal insufficiency with renal transplantation. Efficacy of treatment with human growth hormone. *Archives Francaises de Pediatrie* **43**, 51–53.

Rodger, R. S. C. *et al.* (1986a). Anterior pituitary dysfunction in patients with chronic renal failure treated by hemodialysis or continuous ambulatory peritoneal dialysis. *Nephron* **43**, 169–172.

Rodger, R. S. C. *et al.* (1986b). Hypothalamic–pituitary–adrenocortical suppression and recovery in renal transplant patients returning to maintenance dialysis. *The Quarterly Journal of Medicine* **61**, 1039–1046.

Rosman, P. M. *et al.* (1982). Pituitary-adrenocortical function in chronic renal failure: blunted suppression and early escape of plasma cortisol levels after intravenous dexamethasone. *Journal of Clinical Endocrinology and Metabolism* **54**, 528–533.

Ross, R. J. *et al.* (1985). Alteration of pituitary–thyroid function in patients with chronic renal failure treated by haemodialysis or continuous ambulatory peritoneal dialysis. *Annals of Clinical Biochemistry* **22**, 156–160.

Schaefer, F. H. (1991). Cooperative and study on pubertal development in chronic renal failure. Pulsatile growth hormone secretion in peripubertal patients with chronic renal failure. *The Journal of Pediatrics* **119**, 568–577.

Schaefer, F. *et al.* (1991). Pulsatile immunoreactive and bioactive luteinizing hormone secretion in pubertal patients with chronic renal failure. *Pediatric Nephrology* **5**, 566–571.

Schaefer, F. *et al.* (1994). Alterations in growth hormone secretion and clearance in peripubertal boys with chronic renal failure and after renal transplantation. *Journal of Clinical Endocrinology and Metabolism* **78**, 1298–1306.

Schaefer, F. *et al.* (1996). Multifactorial control of the elimination kinetics of unbound (free) growth hormone (GH) in the human: regulation by age, adiposity, renal function, and steady state concentrations of GH in plasma. *Journal of Clinical Endocrinology and Metabolism* **81**, 22–31.

Schaefer, F. *et al.* (2001). Impaired JAK-STAT signal transduction contributes to growth hormone resistance in chronic uremia. *Journal of Clinical Investigation* **108**, 467–475.

Schohn, D. C., Jahn, H. A., and Schmitt, R. L. (1988). Predictability of a standardized captopril test in hypertension in end-stage renal failure. *Kidney International* **34** (Suppl. 25), S145–S148.

Sharp, N. A., Devlin, J. T., and Rimmer, J. M. (1986). Renal failure obfuscates the diagnosis of Cushing's disease. *The Journal of American Medical Association* **256**, 2564–2565.

Shirota, T. *et al.* (1992). Primary hypothyroidism and multiple endocrine failure in association with hemochromatosis in a long-term hemodialysis patient. *Clinical Nephrology* **38**, 105–109.

Siamopoulos, K. C. *et al.* (1988). Ovine corticotropin-releasing hormone stimulation test in patients with chronic renal failure: pharmacokinetic properties, and plasma adrenocorticotropic hormone and serum cortisol responses. *Hormone Research* **30**, 17–21.

Silverberg, D. S. *et al.* (1973). Effects of chronic hemodialysis on thyroid function in chronic renal failure. *Canadian Medical Association Journal* **189**, 282–286.

Smith, D. and Defronzo, R. A. (1982). Insulin resistance in uremia mediated by postbinding defects. *Kidney International* **22**, 54–62.

Soffer, O., Chary, K. R., and Hall, W. D. (1980). Clinical hyperthyroidism in a patient receiving long term hemodialysis. *Archives of Internal Medicine* **140**, 708–709.

Spaulding, S. W. *et al.* (1976). Effect of caloric restriction and dietary composition on serum T3 and reverse T3 in man. *Journal of Clinical Endocrinology and Metabolism* **42**, 197–200.

Spector, D. A. *et al.* (1976). Thyroid function and metabolic state in chronic renal failure. *Annals of International Medicine* **85**, 724–730.

Takeda, S., Michigishi, T., and Takazakura, E. (1993). Iodine-induced hypothyroidism in patients on regular dialysis treatment. *Nephron* **65**, 51–55.

Tönshoff, B. *et al.* (1990). Growth-stimulating effects of recombinant human growth hormone in children with end-stage renal disease. *Journal of Pediatrics* **116**, 561–566.

Tönshoff, B. *et al.* (1995a). Serum insulin-like growth factors (IGFs) and IGF binding proteins 1, 2 and 3 in children with chronic renal failure: relationship to height and glomerular filtration rate. *Journal of Clinical Endocrinology and Metabolism* **80**, 2684–2691.

Tönshoff, B. *et al.* (1995b). Deconvolution analysis of spontaneous nocturnal growth hormone secretion in prepubertal children with chronic renal failure. *Pediatric Research* **37**, 86–93.

Tsukahara, H. *et al.* (1994). Direct demonstration of insulin-like growth factor-I-induced nitric oxide production by endothelial cells. *Kidney International* **45**, 598–604.

Ulinski, T. *et al.* (2000). Serum insulin-like growth factor binding protein IGFBP-4 and IGFBP-5 in children with chronic renal failure: relationship to growth and glomerular filtration rate. *Pediatric Nephrology* **14**, 589–597.

van Leusen, R. and Meinders, A. E. (1982). Cyclical changes in serum thyroid hormone concentrations related to hemodialysis: movement of hormone into and out of the extravascular space as a possible mechanism. *Clinical Nephrology* **18**, 193–199.

Veldhuis, J. D. *et al.* (1994). Neuroendocrine alterations in the somatotropic and lactotropic axes in uremic men. *European Journal of Endocrinology* **131**, 489–498.

Verger, M. *et al.* (1987). Relationship between thyroid hormones and nutrition in chronic failure. *Nephron* **45**, 211–215.

Wallace, E. Z. *et al.* (1980). Pituitary-adrenocortical function in chronic renal failure: studies of episodic secretion of cortisol and dexamethasone suppressibility. *Journal of Clinical Endocrinology and Metabolism* **50**, 46–51.

Watschinger, B. *et al.* (1991). Effect of recombinant human erythropoietin on anterior pituitary function in patients on chronic hemodialysis. *Hormone Research* **36**, 22–26.

Weissel, M. *et al.* (1979). Basal and TRH-stimulated thyroid and pituitary hormones in various degrees of renal insufficiency. *Acta Endocrinologica (Copenhagen)* **90**, 23–32.

Wheatley, T. *et al.* (1989). Abnormalities of thyrotrophin (TSH) evening rise and pulsatile release in the hemodialysis patients: evidence for hypothalamic-pituitary changes in chronic renal failure. *Clinical Endocrinology* **31**, 39–50.

Williams, G. H., Bailey, G. L., and Hampers, C. L. (1973). Studies on the metabolism of aldosterone in chronic renal failure and anephric man. *Kidney International* **4**, 280–288.

Workman, R. J., Vaughn, W. K., and Stone, W. J. (1986). Dexamethasone suppression testing in chronic renal failure: pharmacokinetics of dexamethasone and demonstration of a normal hypothalamic-pituitary-adrenal axis. *Journal of Clinical Endocrinology and Metabolism* **63**, 741–746.

Zager, P. G., Frey, H. J., and Gerdes, B. G. (1983). Plasma 18-hydroxycorticosterone during continuous ambulatory peritoneal dialysis. *Journal of Laboratory and Clinical Medicine* **102**, 604–612.

Zager, P. G. *et al.* (1985). Low dose adrenocorticotropin infusion in continuous ambulatory peritoneal dialysis patients. *Journal of Clinical Endocrinology and Metabolism* **61**, 1205–1210.

Zilker, T. R. *et al.* (1988). Kinetics of biosynthetic human proinsulin in patients with terminal renal insufficiency. *Hormone and Metabolism Research Supplement Series* **18**, 43–48.

11.3.3 Sexual disorders

Jürgen Bommer

Introduction

The sexual problems caused by chronic renal failure are common and affect the quality of life of patients adversely. They seldom receive the same attention as other complications.

Males

Erectile impotence

Sexual dysfunction is found in about two-thirds or more of both haemo- and peritoneal-dialysis patients (Abram *et al.* 1975; Bommer *et al.* 1976; Karacan and Salis 1980; Diemont *et al.* 2000).

Sexual activity decreases to occasional sexual intercourse at the time of starting dialysis, but improves after effective maintenance haemodialysis (Bommer *et al.* 1976). In transplant patients sexual problems are significantly less prevalent, but still occur in nearly 50 per cent (Diemont *et al.* 2000).

Dialysis patients with sexual dysfunction complain predominantly of reduction or loss of fertility, libido, erectile potency, but also inadequate satisfaction and ejaculation. In male dialysis patients about 50–60 per cent report reduced libido (Toorians *et al.* 1997). Partial and complete erectile impotence is found in 40–80 per cent of haemodialysis patients (Abram *et al.* 1975; Bommer *et al.* 1976; Karacan and Salis 1980; Toorians *et al.* 1997; Diemont *et al.* 2000). During the early era of dialysis therapy psychological factors seem to play a dominant role in the loss of libido and potency. If these problems are improved or solved and effective dialysis therapy improves physical fitness and ability to work, increased libido and potency can be expected in the first 2 years of haemodialysis therapy (Bommer 1976).

In patients on maintenance haemodialysis various factors may contribute to the loss of libido and potency including psychological factors, reduced arterial blood flow, venous leakage due to venous shunts, altered penile smooth muscle function, hormonal disturbances, side-effects of medication, and neurogenic dysfunction. Optimal treatment of sexual problems in the individual patient requires a careful assessment of these factors. Most diagnostic algorithms start with the differentiation between psychogenic and organic impotence. In clinical practice, however, psychogenic and organic causes of impotence are not the ends of a one-dimensional diagnostic scale but rather represent two interwoven dimensions. In most, if not all, dialysis patients sexual dysfunction results from both psychological and organic problems.

Vascular factors of impotence

Arterial blood flow

Adequate arterial blood flow and pressure in penile arteries are prerequisites for correct penile erection. An intracavernosal arterial blood pressure greater than 80 mmHg is essential for erection that is sufficient to allow penetration. During erection, the intracavernosal pressure is about 20 mmHg less than the blood pressure of pelvic arteries such as the internal iliac artery. A further increase of intracavernosal pressures above systemic blood pressure, causing maximal penile rigidity, occurs by contraction of the *m. bulbus spongiosus* and *m. ischiocavernosus*. Therefore, a blood pressure of 80–100 mmHg in the pelvic arteries is necessary to maintain an intracavernosal pressure of 80 mmHg. In patients with arterial occlusive disease, claudication is observed in the lower extremities only if intra-arterial blood pressure is less than 70 mmHg. Therefore, erectile dysfunction often precedes symptomatic arterial occlusive disease of the lower extremity.

Penile erection is the consequence of accumulation of blood under pressure. This results from:

(1) dilatation of the penile arteries enhancing blood flow and pressure to the corpora cavernosa;

(2) relaxation of the trabecular smooth muscle followed by the expansion of the intracavernous lacunar space and trapping of blood by compression of the peripheral draining venules (veno-occlusion mechanism). In this respect, insufficient intracavernous pressure can result not only from a decreased arterial perfusion pressure but also from insufficient dilatation of helicine arteries.

Impotence results from vascular problems in about 60 per cent of non-uraemic patients (May *et al.* 1969; Virag 1984). Detailed data regarding pelvic arteries are not available for dialysis patients, but the high prevalence of vascular problems with markedly advanced arteriosclerosis in such patients suggest that arterial occlusions play an important role in erectile dysfunction.

Arteriosclerosis of the aorto-iliac arteries is a common finding in long-term haemodialysis patients, with an increasing prevalence and severity over time. Vascular erectile dysfunction also progresses with time in these patients. Delayed erection, followed by reduced penile rigidity, and decreased nocturnal penile tumescence (NPT) is followed by decreasing incidence of erection until total erectile impotence is reached.

The precise aetiological significance of renal insufficiency in arterial vascular impotence has not yet been clarified. Age, diabetes mellitus, smoking, hypertension, hyperlipidaemia, homocysteinaemia, and disturbed calcium/phosphate metabolism are probably the main factors favouring arterial causes of impotence, not only in uraemic patients but also in those without renal insufficiency. In non-uraemic patients (age 56–70), the probability of complete impotence increased from near zero to 16 per cent as high density lipoprotein (HDL) cholesterol decreased from 90 to 30 mg/dl (Virag *et al.* 1985; Feldman *et al.* 1994). Low blood HDL cholesterol is found in many haemodialysis patients. Most dialysis patients have been hypertensive for many years before the onset of uraemia, and even after initiation of maintenance haemodialysis 50–80 per cent require continuous antihypertensive therapy. During 1999–2001, 20–30 per cent of incident dialysis patients in Europe and 46 per cent in the United States had diabetes mellitus (DOPPS, unpublished data). In addition to diabetic micro- and macroangiopathy and fibrotic thickening of the walls of penile arteries, neuropathy is present in 30–80 per cent of diabetic patients. Neurological factors can also alter penile blood circulation (McConnell and Benson 1982) (see below).

A diagnosis of arteriogenic penile impotence requires:

(1) an abnormal blood pressure index (ratio between blood pressure in the penile arteries and *A. brachialis*, normal >0.6);

(2) evaluation of erection following intracavernosal injection of vasodilating drugs, which mimics the haemodynamic changes during erection and documents the vasomotor reserve of penile arteries;

(3) colour duplex Doppler ultrasonography of penile arteries before and after intracavernosal injection of vasodilating substances (sensitivity of 90 per cent compared with angiography);

(4) angiography (digital subtraction angiography), if arterial reconstruction is planned.

Venous leakage

In impotent uraemic patients with absent NPT, defective venous occlusion with normal arterial function has been reported (Bellinghieri *et al.* 1992). The frequent complaint of incomplete or insufficiently persisting erection suggests a dysfunction of smooth muscle followed by impaired veno-occlusion in dialysis patients.

During penile erection, venous efflux is reduced by the expansion of penile smooth muscle against the inflexible tunica albuginea, resulting in a compression of subtunical veins (*Vv. emissariae*). Impaired relaxation of penile smooth muscle is the main reason for insufficient reduction of venous efflux from the cavernosal space, resulting in erectile impotence. Neural and neurohumoral disturbances are the primary causes of smooth muscle dysfunction. Furthermore, precocious ageing and enhanced fibrosis which diminish the fibroelastic compliance of smooth muscle trabeculae, are common in long-term haemodialysis patients. During ageing of collagen, increasing intermolecular cross-links mediated by the advanced glycation reaction as well as the increase of a pentose-mediated protein cross-link named pentosidine have been reported (Sell and Monnier 1990). Pentosidine concentrations are 22 times greater in plasma, skin, and other tissues of patients with chronic renal failure. After kidney transplantation, plasma pentosidine remained three- to fourfold elevated compared to healthy controls (Hricik *et al.* 1993). Pentosidine is also present in cavernosal smooth muscle and tunica albuginea. Hypoxia induced overexpression of TGF-β1 may also play a role in the fibrosis of the corpus cavernosum. In this context it has been postulated that NPTs may serve to periodically oxygenate the corpus cavernosum and that a decrease in the quality and number of NPT can indirectly affect erectile function (Tarcan *et al.* 1998).

Venous leakage or corpus cavernosum insufficiency can be documented by:

(1) incomplete or briefly lasting erections after intracavernosal injection of vasodilating substances; or

(2) high diastolic blood flow in penile arteries in duplex Doppler ultrasonography after intracavernosal injection of vasodilating substances;

(3) cavernosometry, after intracavernosal injection of vasodilating substances (sensitivity of >95 per cent);

(4) cavernosography, after intracavernosal injection of vasodilating substances; smooth muscle contraction and relaxation can be evaluated by recording cavernosus electromyography (Gerstenberg *et al.* 1992; Truss *et al.* 1993).

Neurogenic and psychogenic impotence

There are different neurogenic processes involved in erection. (a) Psychogenic erection results from visual and auditory stimuli or phantasy and are mediated by cerebral pulses and transmitted by the thoracocolumbar and sacral centres to the cavernosus nerves. (b) Reflexogenic erection results from sensory cutaneous receptors of the shaft of the penis and somatic nerves carry afferent impulses and efferent distribution is by the sacral parasympathetic at the S2–S4 level. (c) The mechanism of nocturnal erection—which occurs during rapid eye movement (REM) sleep—is unknown, but it seems to be more sensitive to low androgen levels than to psychogenic and reflexogenic causes (Levy *et al.* 2000). Central nervous system regulation of sexual function is very complex and involves specific groups of neurons.

In general, erection is a very complex process influenced by several humoral, neural, and local substances in addition to central effects. Enhancing factors are: androgens, oestrogen, corticosteroids, acetylcholine, nitric oxide (NO), calcitonin gene related peptide, vasoactive intestinal polypeptide, substance P, prostaglandins (PGE 1), and local ATP. Inhibiting factors are: catecholamines (adrenaline, noradrenaline), vasopressin, neuropeptide Y, endothelin 1, thromboxane A2, and angiotensin II. In the periphery the tone of cavernosal and helicine arteries and smooth muscle is controlled by adrenergic, cholinergic and non-adrenergic, non-cholinergic neurotransmitters (Blanco *et al.* 1988; Saenz de Tejada *et al.* 1988). Relaxation of penile blood vessels and smooth muscle is primarily regulated by cholinergic and non-cholinergic–non-adrenergic neurotransmitters. The resulting NO formation plays a crucial role in smooth muscle relaxation (Burnett *et al.* 1992). Sacral parasympathetic stimulation initiates vasodilatation of the arterial bed, increasing blood flow and increasing intracavernosal blood oxygen. In this oxygen enhanced environment, autonomic dilator nerves and endothelium are better able to synthesize NO, resulting in smooth muscle relaxation, with progressive entrapment of blood in the corpora cavernosa (Kim *et al.* 1993). In response to sexual stimulation NO is released from non-adrenergic–non-cholinergic nerves and endothelial cells, which activates guanylyl cyclase resulting in an increased formation of cyclic guanosine-monophosphate (cGMP), thereby reducing intracellular Ca^{2+} inducing relaxation of smooth muscle and increasing blood flow to the penis (Rajfer *et al.* 1992).

This pathway can also be activated by nitrovasodilators such as sodium nitroprusside and electrical nerve stimulation. Sildenafil reduces cGMP-clearance and enhances, but does not initiate, the erectile response to erotic stimuli by inhibiting cGMP-specific phosphodiesterase type 5 (PDE5). As neuronal NO release is necessary to initiate tumescense the erectile dysfunction that results from non-nerve sparing radical prostatectomy is not responsive to sildenafil (Marks *et al.* 1999; Merrick *et al.* 1999). In addition to this cGMP pathway, intracavernosal vasoactive drugs such as PGE1 and vasoactive intestinal peptide (VIP) activate adenylate cyclase, which increases the intracellular cAMP resulting in muscle relaxation. Both cGMP and cAMP are metabolized by PDE isoforms.

Adrenergic stimulation results in contraction of the helicine arteries and trabecular smooth muscle followed by a decrease in blood pressure within the cavernosal sinuses and brings the penis to a flaccid state.

Penile erection can be initiated by direct local sensory and central psychogenic stimulation inducing reflex erection through a spinal reflex via the dorsal penile nerve, sacral parasympathetic centres, and the cavernosal nerve. Direct nerve destruction, for example after surgery (radical prostatectomy, proctocolectomy, or other pelvic surgery), can cause neurogenic impotence.

Autonomic neuropathy, a frequent complication in chronic renal failure, plays a prominent role in erectile impotence of many uraemic patients and a significantly abnormal Valsalva ratio corresponds to abnormalities in NPT and reduced frequency of intercourse (Campese *et al.* 1982). Parasympathetic dysfunction was found in 65.9 per cent of older dialysis patients (>65 years of age) and 33.3 per cent of younger dialysis patients and in 11.8 and 0 per cent of the older and younger control subjects, respectively. Combined parasympathetic and sympathetic dysfunction was seen in 41.5 and 11.9 per cent of older or younger dialysis patients but not in any of the control groups (Jassal *et al.* 1998). Improved autonomic nerve function has been reported after several months of haemodialysis (Roeckel *et al.* 1979; Zucchelli *et al.* 1985; Solders 1986). In this context polyneuropathy due to diabetes mellitus or alcoholism may play an additional role in dialysis patients.

The role of psychological problems cannot be overestimated in impotent men. In the Massachusetts Male Aging Study in non-uraemic men, moderate or complete impotence was found in 90 per cent of men with severe depression, compared to 25 per cent of them with minimal

depression (Feldmann *et al.* 1994). The pathway of psychogenic effects on penile erection is less clear, but various central stimuli, hypothalamic nuclei, and peripheral sympathetic and parasympathetic nerve fibres are involved. Psychogenic stimuli to the sacral cord may inhibit reflex erections and, therefore, activation of the parasympathetic dilator nerves to the penis. Excessive sympathetic stimulation, elevated blood catecholamine, or both, may also increase penile smooth muscle tone, opposing the smooth muscle relaxation necessary for erection. Insufficient relaxation of trabecular smooth muscle may, therefore, occur in stressed, anxious patients with excessive adrenergic reactions, or in patients with impaired parasympathetic tone. Patients with chronic uraemia suffer from many physical and psychological stresses. Psychological tests have documented an increased rate of depression in haemodialysis patients compared to transplanted patients or healthy controls. The time lost to dialysis treatment, whether haemodialysis, chronic ambulatory peritoneal dialysis, or intermittent peritoneal dialysis, and the physical and psychological implications of such a severe disease and its therapy produce problems and increased stress at home and at work. Alternative social roles at home and in marriage may influence self-confidence, resulting in a more passive behaviour of the male patient, which in itself favours performance anxiety (Glass *et al.* 1987).

In male haemodialysis patients, reduced NPT, commonly 3–5 times per night, during REM sleep, has been reported concomitantly with impotence and low plasma testosterone (Massry *et al.* 1980; Muir *et al.* 1983). The lack of such nocturnal erections has been used as a reliable parameter for organic erectile impotence: in patients with psychogenic erectile dysfunction, NPT are preserved. Patients with organic dysfunction of the dorsal nerve, cortical centres, and brain stem may have normal nocturnal tumescence but impaired sexual erection. The frequency and duration of nocturnal erection is reduced by age, depression, exhaustion, insufficient sleep, and nightmares; in particular, dream anxiety may totally or partially suppress nocturnal erection (Karacan *et al.* 1966).

Impotence induced by drugs or other agents

Disturbed libido and potency are well-known side-effects of various drugs (see Table 1). Some substances interfere with central neuroendocrine regulation or neurovascular control of penile arteries and

Table 1 Drugs with a negative effect on erection

Hormones	Antiandrogens, oestrogens, progesterone
β-Blockers	Propranolol, atenolol, pindolol
Sympatholytics	Methyldopa, clonidine, guanethidine phenoxybenzamine, reserpine
Vasodilators	Hydralazine
Diuretics	Thiazide, spironolactone
Antihyperlipidaemics	Clofibrate, gemfibrozil
Sedatives	Various barbiturates, bromides
Psychotropic drugs	Lithium with benzodiazepine, benzodiazepines, phenothiazines, tricyclic antidepressants, monoamino-oxidase inhibitors, diazepam with opiates
Others	Immunosuppressive substances, digoxin, cimetidine, ranitidine, anticholinergic drugs

smooth muscle. Drugs with central neurological effects can also reduce libido. Tobacco and alcohol reduce sexual function in all subjects and also in patients with renal failure (Mannino *et al.* 1994). Monoamino oxidase (MAO) inhibitors and tricyclic antidepressants have been reported to inhibit both erection and ejaculation. Lithium monotherapy has only little effect, but if combined with benzodiazepines, is more likely to cause sexual dysfunction. Conflicting data have been reported about the potential impairment of sexual function due to antihypertensive therapy. A direct correlation between erectile potency and blood pressure can be observed in patients with arterial occlusive disease receiving antihypertensive therapy.

In the Treatment of Mild Hypertension Study (Grimm *et al.* 1997), erectile dysfunction in non-renal patients with mild hypertension was significantly increased compared to placebo in chlorthalidone treated patients but not in patients treated with acebutolol, amlodipine, enalapril, or doxazosin.

In dialysis patients, impaired erectile potency may be a side-effect of sympatholytics, for example methyldopa, clonidine, adrenergic receptor blocking agents, for example prazosin, β-blockers, for example propranolol, and vasodilators, for example hydralazine. α-Adrenergic agents such as clonidine may also act via constriction of the cavernosal artery regulated by α2-adrenergic receptors (Hedlund and Andersson 1985). It has not been proved whether vasodilating antihypertensive drugs markedly impair sexual function if no severe arterial stenosis coexists. At least angiotensin-converting enzyme (ACE) inhibitors seem to impair sexual behaviour to a lesser degree. Reduction of serum testosterone and oestrogen has been observed after long-term digoxin treatment.

Hormonal abnormalities

Hypothalamo–hypophyseal function luteinizing hormone (LH) and LH-releasing hormone

Pulsatile secretion of LH-releasing hormone (LHRH) every 90– 120 min is essential for effective hypophyseal gonadotrophin secretion and is reflected by corresponding LH pulses. This physiological hypothalamic secretion of LHRR which regulates hypophyseal production of gonadotrophins is controlled by various substances such as adrenergic, dopaminergic sustances, endorphins, oxytocin, neuropeptide Y, leptin, and others. Since uraemia may alter the metabolism and efficacy of such compounds, hormones may be influenced in dialysis patients by various mechanisms, for example, it was shown recently that in experimental studies uraemia influenced the local amino acid neurotransmitter outflow and milieu in the hypothalamus (Schaefer *et al.* 2001).

Some authors report a delayed and blunted gonadotrophin response to exogenous gonadotrophin-releasing hormone (GnRH) (Schaefer *et al.* 1994c). In the majority of cases, a normal pituitary secretory response of LH to LHRH was reported following exogenous GnRH stimulation (Distiller *et al.* 1975; Holdsworth *et al.* 1977; LeRoith *et al.* 1980; Handelsman 1985; Veldhuis *et al.* 1993).

Plasma LH is elevated in maintenance haemodialysis patients. LH is increased about 1.5-fold using a LH-Bioassay and twofold using a radio immunoassay, compared with healthy controls, approaching concentrations detected in patients with primary hypogonadism (Rodger *et al.* 1985; Mastrogiacomo *et al.* 1988; Talbot *et al.* 1990; Veldhuis 1993). A two- to fourfold prolongation of plasma half-life of immunoreactive and bioactive LH has been reported. The basal secretion of immunoreactive but not bioactive LH seems to be increased (Veldhuis *et al.* 1993; Schaefer *et al.* 1994b).

In uraemic men, the pulsatile rhythm of LH secretion is reduced by about 50 per cent. Absence or low frequency of LH peaks have been reported (Talbot 1990). A more detailed study documented a rather normal frequency of LH peaks but the maximal levels and, predominantly, the duration of LH peaks were reduced (Veldhuis *et al.* 1993). Assuming prolonged half-life of LH and normal LH response to exogenous GnRH, it can be concluded that in uraemic patients a significantly reduced pulsatile secretion rate of LH follows inadequate hypothalamic pulsatile secretion of LHRH, as has been demonstrated in the uraemic rat model.

The effect of peripheral testosterone or oestradiol on the negative feedback control of LH secretion may also be disturbed. Normal or low testosterone levels have been reported in uraemic men (Bommer *et al.* 1990; Talbot *et al.* 1990), serum oestradiol is normal (Sawin *et al.* 1973; Muir *et al.* 1983) or elevated (Rodger *et al.* 1985; Veldhuis *et al.* 1993), and total oestrogens are elevated (Lim and Fang 1975). Exogenous testosterone produces a diminished (Daubresse *et al.* 1972; Coppola and Cuomo 1990) or normal (Barton *et al.* 1982) feedback suppression of LH. Clomiphene, a synthetic oestrogen analogue, blocks hypothalamic oestradiol receptors, leading to maximal secretion of LHRH. After chronic administration of clomiphene, increased LH levels, with a consequent increase in plasma testosterone, have been reported (Lim and Fang 1976). This was paralleled by improved potency in uraemic men, which persisted for several months after cessation of clomiphene therapy.

Endogenous opiates are known to be involved in the negative feedback control of pulsatile LH release in normal humans (Swamy *et al.* 1979), and LH levels in uraemic patients increase after administration of the endorphin antagonist naloxone (Grzeszczak *et al.* 1987; Tay *et al.* 1993; Verhelst *et al.* 1995). Plasma β-endorphin and β-lipotropin are normal and unchanged during haemodialysis sessions (Elias *et al.* 1986). This, however, does not exclude a potential benefit from the recently available apomorphine sublingual. The effects of iron and aluminium deposition in the hypothalamic nuclei of dialysis patients is unknown. Furthermore, a potential effect of increased cytokine release in dialysed patients may play a role. In healthy men, intravenous injection of recombinant tumour necrosis factor (TNF)-α was followed by a transient increase of LH and reduction of testosterone, whereas follicle-stimulating hormone (FSH) levels remained unchanged (Van der Poll *et al.* 1993). TNF increased the release of prolactin and LH from rat pituitary cells *in vitro* (Yamaguchi *et al.* 1991), but it reduced the LH release after GnRH in other studies (Gaillard 1990).

Follicle-stimulating hormone

FSH concentrations in uraemic men are in the upper normal range or elevated (Lim *et al.* 1980; Rodger *et al.* 1985; Rudolf *et al.* 1988). This hormone stimulates spermatogenesis, and is regulated by a negative feedback via the testicular peptide inhibin. Inhibin serum levels were increased in haemodialysis males, but did not correlate with either LH or FSH (Sasagawa 1998) Secretion of FSH is also suppressed by oestrogen or oestradiol (Rodger *et al.* 1985), which may account for the normal or only mildly elevated levels of FSH in uraemic men, despite decreased spermatogenesis.

Prolactin

About 40–70 per cent of dialysed males have an elevated serum prolactin (Bommer *et al.* 1979; Lim *et al.* 1979; Muir *et al.* 1983), and the biological activity of this hormone is also increased (Smith *et al.* 1989). As renal failure progresses, elevation of serum prolactin levels seems to correlate with serum creatinine (Biasioli et al. 1988). The normal circadian rhythm of prolactin secretion is disturbed in that the characteristic sleep-induced secretory bursts are not found, although episodic secretion occurs during daytime (Biasioli et al. 1988).

Hyperprolactinaemia in uraemic patients cannot be explained by slightly diminished prolactin clearance. A primary mechanism seems to be the inadequate dopaminergic inhibition of prolactin release from the pituitary lactotrophs (Lim et al. 1979). Other authors (Bommer et al. 1979; Muir et al. 1983) reported that basal and stimulated prolactin concentrations became subnormal after the long-term administration of dopaminergic agonists such as bromocriptine, suggesting that prolactin secretion in uraemic patients can be suppressed at least by chronic dopaminergic stimulation. Characteristic stimuli such as thyrotrophin-releasing hormone, chlorpromazine, metoclopramide, and arginine or insulin-induced hypoglycaemia result in a blunted prolactin response in dialysed patients (Ramirez et al. 1977; Schmitz and Moller 1983; Rodger et al. 1986).

In non-uraemic men, hyperprolactinaemia is associated with sexual dysfunction, loss of libido, impaired erection potency, and infertility (Franks et al. 1978; Spark et al. 1982). It is not known whether the exact mechanism of this disturbed sexual function results from a gonadal effect of prolactin or from a hypothalamic hypophyseal effect. In uraemic patients, the hypothalamic LHRH release is apparently suppressed, and high prolactin levels may be implicated in this abnormality. However, the diminished peripheral clearance of LH prevents the association of hyperprolactinemia with low LH levels.

Testicular hormones

The exact mechanisms by which hormones affect sexual function are still unknown. In the 'Massachusetts Male Aging Study' only the adrenal androgen metabolite dehydroepiandrosterone sulfate but not total or free testosterone levels showed an age-adjusted correlation with impotence (Feldman et al. 1994). Androgen receptors in the sacral parasympathetic nucleus, hypothalamus, and limbic system suggest a possible hormonal regulation of centres involved in erection (Sar and Stumpf 1977; Rees and Michael 1982). However, normal erection can be observed after castration, despite extremely low serum and tissue testosterone (Bancroft and Wu 1983; Kwan et al. 1983).

Most male uraemic patients have low serum testosterone (Ramirez et al. 1987), although there is a wide overlap with age-corrected normal concentrations. Since testosterone binding capacity is normal (Muir et al. 1983; De Vries et al. 1984; Ramirez et al. 1987), free testosterone (Ramirez et al. 1987) as well as salivary testosterone concentrations are also low. These low testosterone levels have been explained by a depressed testosterone production rate or elevated metabolic clearance of testosterone (Corvol et al. 1974; Stewart-Bentley et al. 1974). Other authors, however, reported normal or at least low normal testosterone levels and free testosterone levels (Rodger et al. 1985; Bommer et al. 1990; Talbot et al. 1990). The normal circadian rhythm of plasma testosterone, with a peak at 4–8 a.m. and a nadir at 8–12 p.m., is maintained in uraemic patients (Zadeh et al. 1975).

Normal testosterone concentrations in the presence of high levels of LH suggest resistance of the Leydig cells to LH. In men, there is a delayed subnormal response to acute administration of LH analogue (human chorionic gonadotrophin) (Stewart-Bentley et al. 1974; Ramirez et al. 1987).

Discrepant plasma concentrations of testosterone metabolites have been reported, with an increase in 5-α-dihydrotestosterone and

androstendiol (Van Kammen et al. 1978), and low levels of dihydrotestosterone, androstenedione, or dihydroepiandrosterone sulfate (Van Coevorden et al. 1988). The concentration of the adrenal androgen dihydroandrosterone and its sulfate ester also seems to be low (Ferraris et al. 1980). Some, but not all, authors report a correlation between circulating testosterone levels and sexual activity in dialysis patients. Limited information is available on the action of testosterone on androgen-sensitive tissues.

Receptors for 1,25-dihydroxyvitamin D3 have been detected on the adrenal basophils. It is of note that 1,25-$(OH)_2$D3 also influences prolactin secretion (Wark 1985) and lowers prolactin in uraemic patients (Verbeelen et al. 1983).

Hyperparathyroidism may interact with abnormalities of the pituitary–gonadal axis (Massry et al. 1977; Fioretti et al. 1986); however, diminished serum testosterone and impaired sexual function resulting from severe secondary hyperparathyroidism were not shown to improve with 1,25-$(OH)_2$D3 therapy in placebo-controlled trials (Blumberg et al. 1979). The potential effect of phthalate-containing plasticizers from haemodialysis tubing has not been adequately studied. In experimental animals, phthalate causes decreased testosterone, impaired spermatogenesis, and progressive testicular atrophy, with diminished zinc concentrations in the testes (Wams 1987). The effect of zinc deficiency on testosterone production and spermatogenesis is not clear (Mahajan et al. 1985). Zinc acetate inhibits prolactin synthesis and release with and without LHRH stimulation in vitro (Judd et al. 1984). Malnutrition or protein deficiency are likely to lead to reduced serum testosterone. In uraemic males on a low protein diet, supplementation with essential amino acids and ketone analogues raised low serum testosterone levels, while pituitary hormones remained unchanged (Fioretti et al. 1986). In non-uraemic mice, interleukin 2 and TNF-α reduce plasma testosterone concentration with and without LH stimulation (Meikle 1992). A similar effect of TNF has been reported in porcine Leydig cells and in rats (Mealy et al. 1990; Mauduit et al. 1993). TNF also stimulated PRL secretion in pituitary cells (Koike et al. 1991; Yamaguchi 1991; Nolten et al. 1993) and in cancer patients (Nolten et al. 1993). Furthermore, hypothyroidism as well as hyperthyroidism may impair sexual function in dialysis patients.

Diagnostic procedure: a careful medical history of sexual problems should be taken, in particular, whether this concerns libido, erection, potency, or fertility problems. Psychological factors such as depression, anxiety, or stress should be evaluated. Mild organic disturbances may cause severe psychological problems, followed by sexual dysfunction. Other diseases complicated by polyneuropathy such as diabetes, alcoholism, or vascular problems with arteriosclerosis, claudication, and various medications must be considered for their potential effects on sexual function. All severe illnesses, which result in a poor physical condition, also impair sexual behaviour.

Basal hormonal analysis should include first: assays of testosterone, prolactin, and LH, and secondly, measurement of prolactin, LH, and FSH before, 30 and 60 min (for a potentially delayed increase) after simultaneous intravenous injection of 100 μg LHRH and 200 μg thyrotrophin-releasing hormone.

Measurements of NPT have been recommended to differentiate between psychogenic and organic causes of impotence. This can be done by stamp test, snap gauge band, or special strain transfusers, which register the intensity and frequency of tumescence during the night. The increase of the penile circumferences varies between 1.36 and 4.8 cm in healthy men (Karacan et al. 1970). During erection, the rigidity of the penis should also be documented to exclude simple circumferential changes without complete erection. Using the Rigiscan system and Tumistore (LifeTec Inc., Texas), penile tumescence can be studied in special sleep laboratories with parallel measurement of electro-oculographic, electroencephalographic, and electromyographic activity. Nocturnal penile erection depends on the intensity and quantity of sleep, which suggests recording of penile tumescence over several nights.

For the limited reliability and validity of the time-consuming and expensive measurement of NPT, penile erection was evaluated under visual sexual stimulation (VSS) with and without vibrotactile stimulation of the penis (Janssen et al. 1994) in a laboratory setting. Penile tumescence and rigidity were monitored continuously when the patient was exposed to visual stimulation by videotaped erotic material (Morales 1990; Katlowitz et al. 1993; Toorians et al. 1997). A rather good agreement has been reported between NPT and VSS penile response. VSS tests are not only easier to perform but are also more reproducible and cost effective for differentiating between psychogenic and organic impotence (Slob et al. 1990).

Sildenafil inhibits the metabolism of vasodilating NO resulting from sexual stimulation. Oral ingestion is followed after 15–30 min by penile erection if neurological stimulation is given and vascular factors are not operating. The starting dose is 25 mg sildenafil with obligatory sexual stimulation. This dose can be increased to 100 mg. When such tests are positive, many patients do not accept further detailed diagnostic procedures but prefer to use sildenafil for effective therapy, which is well tolerated (see section 'Sildenafil').

If detailed vascular diagnosis is required, systolic blood pressure of the penile artery can be measured using a small sphygmomanometer cuff and Doppler sonography, and this provides rough information on the A. iliaca and A. pudenda interna. A penile blood pressure index (ratio of blood pressure in the penile artery and A. brachialis) of less than 0.6 indicates arteriogenic impotence. In most cases, the decreased penile blood pressure index reflects obstructive aortoiliac disease, but arterial dysplasias, which may involve the penile arteries, may also contribute to diminished penile blood pressure.

Measurement of penile systolic blood pressure does not give accurate information about vascular causes of impotence. Intracavernosal injection of a vasodilating agent is a much more reliable method to evaluate vascular or neurological causes. The arterial blood flow after such injection mimics the haemodynamics during penile erection. In patients without major vascular disease, intracavernosal injection of vasodilating agents such as 10 μg PGE1, is followed by a full rigid erection within 10–15 min lasting for at least 30 min. If patients respond normally to intracavernous injection of vasodilating agents, relevant vascular problems can be excluded and severe neurological or psychological problems have to be excluded.

An incomplete or low erectile response 30 min or later after injection of vasodilating agents suggests arterial disorders. A rapid but only short-lasting erection of limited rigidity indicates disturbed smooth muscle function and veno-occlusive dysfunction. Increase of sympathetic tone under central nervous and psychological influences reduces cavernous smooth muscle relaxation after injection of vasodilating agents. In patients without fully rigid erection following intracavernosal injection of vasodilating agents, additional manual self-stimulation or additional VSS has been recommended. If the patient does not respond with a complete erection, vascular disorders must be suspected and duplex Doppler ultra sonography of all penile arteries (Aa. dorsalis penis, Aa. penis profundae) before and after intracavernosal injection of vasodilating agents is useful. The reflection of Doppler signals is inversely related to the velocity of blood flow within the penile arteries. The frequency of sound reflects flow velocity while the intensity of sound reflects the flow volume.

The proximal and distal parts of all four penile arteries must be studied to exclude distal artery dysplasia. After injection of vasodilating agents, the blood flow velocity is doubled in normal penile arteries with an increase in all four penile arteries. A simultaneous dilation of Aa. pudenda and Aa iliaca interna has been documented by selective angiography of Aa. iliaca interna (Zorgniotti and Lefleur 1985). Vasodilatation raises the peak systolic velocity of blood flow to more than 30 cm/s in the penile artery and increases the vessel diameter by 75 per cent which can be visualized by colour duplex Doppler sonography. Careful Doppler sonography before and after injection of vasodilating agents has a sensitivity of about 90 per cent. For this reason, arteriography is only required if arterial vascular reconstruction is planned. The amount and concentration of contrast medium required for angiography of aortic iliacal pudendal and penile arteries can be reduced, followed by a lower incidence of vasospasm and painful erection, if the subtraction angiography technique is used. If surgical correction of venous abnormalities are planned, cavernosometry and cavernosography are useful. In dialysis patients, infusion cavernosometry should be performed after maximal relaxation of smooth muscle by injection of vasodilating agents to reduce saline load in anuric patients.

If single or repeated vasoactive pharmacotherapy cannot induce complete erection, venous insufficiency must be suspected (Bähren et al. 1986), and the dose of PGE1 can be increased stepwise (Wang et al. 1992). If increasing doses of a vasodilating agent are used (Bähren et al. 1986), a minimal diastolic blood velocity of more than 3 cm/s suggests the presence of venogenic impotence. Venous leakage is paralleled by arteriogenic impotence in most patients. Cavernosography identifies pathological venous drainage from V. dorsalis penis profunda or Vv. profundae penis to the Vv. pudendae internae or plexus vesicoprostaticus, or between the corpus cavernosum and corpus spongiosum. This requires insertion of a needle into one of the corpora cavernosa and perfusion with warm (37°C) sodium chloride solution containing a non-ionic contrast medium. Under continuous infusion, venous reflux of the medium can be observed on a monitor or video. In the early phase, venous collaterals, increased venous drainage by shunts, disturbed structure of tunica albuginea, defects due to rare small tumours, or diverticula can be seen. The severity of venous leakage can be quantified by increasing the rate of infusion.

Damage to the pudendal nerve can be detected by measurement of latency of the bulbus cavernous reflex. Autonomic nerve dysfunction can be documented by orthostatic hypotension, Valsalva ratio, and cold pressure hand tests.

Treatment of impotence (Fig. 1)

Extensive interviews with patients and their partners are mandatory to establish psychological causes of impotence. If patients and/or their partners recognize the psychological problems and learn to solve or manage them, sexual function may improve. In this context it should be acknowledged that increased age commonly reduces male sexual activity and function. In some cases, psychotherapy may be of benefit. Sometimes, temporary restraint from genital sexual activity is recommended. When intercourse is forbidden, the patient's preoccupation with failure decreases or disappears. As a consequence of the patient's

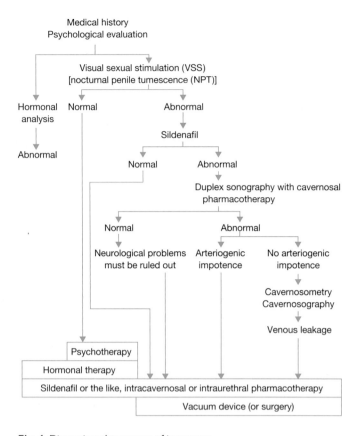

Fig. 1 Diagnosis and treatment of impotence.

restored confidence, both the patient and his partner have the opportunity to experience orgasm. Alcohol consumption and in particular smoking must be avoided, since both reduce sexual function.

Furthermore quality of dialysis should be maximized because improved general well being and fitness will also improve sexual function.

Hormonal treatment

A beneficial effect of testosterone undecanoate on sexual function has been reported in uraemic patients, even in the presence of normal hormone levels (Van Coevorden *et al.* 1986). No or little benefit, however, was seen in other studies (Barton *et al.* 1982; Stuart 1984; Lawrence *et al.* 1998). Testosterone therapy may increase libido without improving potency, augmenting the patient's dilemma. Furthermore, priapism is a well-recognized complication of testosterone therapy in anaemic dialysis patients. Oral DHEA treatment may improve sexual function in patients with erectile dysfunction who have hypertension or patients with erectile dysfunction without organic aetiology (Reiter *et al.* 2001).

Administration of clomiphene (100 mg/day) (Lim and Fang 1976) or human chorionic gonadotrophin (500 IU/week) (Canale *et al.* 1984) has improved sexual function in dialysis patients, but long-term results have not been reported. Clomiphene treatment was followed by a reduction in LH, an increase in testosterone, and a decrease in plasma prolactin. The latter was found in both healthy and kidney transplant recipients (Martin-Malo *et al.* 1993). Improved libido and sexual activity have been reported in haemodialysis patients when haematocrit levels increased during erythropoietin therapy (Schaefer *et al.* 1989b; Bommer *et al.* 1990). Whether such improved sexual function just parallels improved well-being and fitness without hormonal changes

(Bommer *et al.* 1990; Steffensen and Aunsholt 1993), or whether it is mediated by hormonal changes, such as decreased serum prolactin (Schaefer *et al.* 1988, 1989a; Kokot *et al.* 1989; Ramirez *et al.* 1992), or whether it is due to improvement of hypothalamic GnRH secretion and partial restoration of a pulsatile plasma LH pattern (Schaefer *et al.* 1994c; Lawrence *et al.* 1997) is not resolved.

Bromocriptine and dopaminergic agonists

Administration of dopaminergic agonists such as bromocriptine or lisuride (lisuride maleate), has been followed by a decrease in prolactin levels to the low normal range and by a moderate increase of plasma testosterone levels, leading to improved sexual function and a higher frequency of intercourse (Bommer *et al.* 1979; Muir *et al.* 1983; Bommer 1986). Many patients (30–50 per cent) do not tolerate bromocriptine therapy because of side-effects, including hypotension and nausea. Such complications seem to be less frequent during lisuride therapy.

Bromocriptine improves sexual function without significant normalization of LH, FSH, and testosterone. It has been reported that patients responding to bromocriptine therapy have higher LH, FSH, and testosterone levels than non-responders. Bromocriptine therapy also improves sexual function in uraemic patients without severe hyperprolactinaemia (Muir *et al.* 1983), suggesting that mechanisms other than decreasing serum prolactin are involved. Since the penile erection is influenced by activation of catecholaminergic receptors (Kedia and Markland 1975) and bromocriptine lowers plasma noradrenaline (Degli-Esposti *et al.* 1985), a direct dopaminergic effect cannot be excluded. Bromocriptine is also used as an antidepressant (Waehrens and Gerlach 1981) and may improve both mood and potency. Serum testosterone may increase during bromocriptine therapy (Vircburger *et al.* 1985). This increase is greater in hyperprolactinaemic patients than in lisuride-treated normoprolactinaemic patients (Ruilope *et al.* 1985).

Other drugs

In some studies, administration of zinc via the dialysate (Antoniou *et al.* 1977) or orally (50 mg zinc acetate for 6 months) increased plasma testosterone, lowered plasma LH or FSH, and improved spermatogenesis, potency, libido, and frequency of intercourse (Mahajan *et al.* 1985). However, in a controlled double-blind study, zinc therapy had no significant effect on serum levels of testosterone, LH or FSH, or on libido and NPT (Brook *et al.* 1980).

Optimistic reports suggest improved sexual function in non-renal patients with psychogenic impotence during treatment with yohimbine hydrochloride (3×36 mg per day) which has properties of two adrenoreceptor antagonists (Reid *et al.* 1987). No reliable data are available on the use of such substances in haemodialysis patients, and altered drug metabolism must be considered in uraemic patients. Since endomorphines influence sexual behaviour by central nervous regulation, sublingual application of apomorphine hydrochloride has been used in non-renal patients with erectile dysfunction. No experience in dialysis patients has been reported. Perhaps this compound may be used synergistically with drugs acting in the periphery.

Sildenafil

By inhibiting cGMP-specific PDE5, sildenafil reduces cGMP-clearance and enhances, but does not initiate, the erectile response to erotic stimuli. Its efficacy depends on the integrity of local nerve supply as a source of NO.

Sildenafil is rapidly absorbed after oral administration and an erection can be expected after 15–20 min lasting for up to 2–3 h maximum (Rosas *et al.* 2001). Sildenafil has a bioavailability of 40 per cent and is cleared by hepatic metabolism. In healthy subjects as well as in dialysis patients plasma concentrations were comparable with a maximal concentration after 30–120 min and a half-life of 4–5 h. About 50–60 per cent of dialysis patients reported an erection after sildenafil (Ayub and Fletcher 2000; Türk *et al.* 2001). As neuronal NO release is necessary to initiate tumescence, the erectile dysfunction that results from severe nerve dysfunction, for example after non-nerve sparing radical prostectomy, is not amenable to sildenafil (Marks *et al.* 1999). Reduced arterial function does not exclude the beneficial effect of sildenafil, explaining why 60 per cent of diabetics reported at least one successful attempt at intercourse after sildenafil (Rendell *et al.* 1999).

Sildenafil is metabolized by cytochrome P450. In consequence, simultaneous treatment with tacrolimus prolongs the effect of sildenafil. However, the maximal serum level remained unchanged.

In general the drug is well tolerated by about 90 per cent of males 1 year after initiation. In dialysed patients side-effects were comparable to that found in non-renal patients: headache (~20 per cent), dizziness (≥14 per cent), nasal congestion (≤10 per cent), and facial flushing (5–10 per cent) (Goldstein *et al.* 1998; Siegel 2001). As PDE5 is present in the gastroesophageal junction muscle cells, sildenafil can also induce dyspepsia (Holmes 2000). Alteration in colour vision occurs rarely (3 per cent in normal subjects and up to 14 per cent in dialysis patients in various trials) and is due to a limited inhibition of PDE6 by sildenafil.

In general sildenafil reduces the blood pressure by about 5–10 mmHg. Sildenafil taken 2 h before or after dialysis does not increase the incidence of hypotensive episodes (Siegel 2001). This mild hypotensive effect is also found in addition to the effect of antihypertensive therapies. Only the simultaneous use of any nitrate drug or NO donor drug results in a precipitous drop of blood pressure due to their synergistic action. The use of sildenafil is therefore contraindicated in patients taking any form of nitrate drug. Sildenafil is also contraindicated in hypotensive patients, patients with severe hepatic impairment (since the drug is metabolized by hepatic cytochrome P450), and in rare cases of retinitis pigmentosa (Cheitlin *et al.* 1999). Furthermore it has been reported that sildenafil lowers the pulse wave reflexion, which may reduce physical endurance/stamina (Mahmud *et al.* 2000). But in patients with myocardial insufficiency (NYHA II–III) physical endurance and oxygen uptake at maximum workload increased after 50 mg sildenafil (Bocchi *et al.* 2001). Serious side-effects such as myocardial infarction, or significant cardiovascular events were initially reported. However, such complications are probably not due to sildenafil therapy itself, they may more likely be related to the exercise involved in sexual activity particularly since the myocardium contains PDE isoforms other than PDE5.

More recently, novel inhibitors of phosphodiesterase type 5 (Vardenafil, Tadalafil) has been studied like. Vardenafil is characterized by very high potency *in vitro*. The time to maximum plasma concentration of Vardenafil was 0.7–0.9 h. The absorption of Vardenafil is delayed, if taken after a meal containing greater than 30 per cent fat. Administration of 5.10 or 20 mg doses improved erectile function in 66–80 per cent of patients with Vardenafil compared to 30 per cent with placebo. The most frequent side effect was flushing in about 10 per cent of patients, headache, rhinitis which were in most patients only transient but caused discontinuation of treatment in 3–4 per cent of patients (Montorsi *et al.* 2003a).

Another novel phosphodiesterase type 5 inhibitor is Tadalafil. In contrast to Sildenafil and Vardenafil, this drug has a maximun serum peak of 2 hours and a half-life of 17.5 h. In consequence, this drug can be used as a chronic drug. 36 h after 20 mg Tadalafil, 59.2 per cent of intercourse attempts were successful (Porst *et al.* 2003). In phase III studies, 10 and 20 mg Tadalafil improved erection in 56 or 64 per cent of patients, which was significantly better than the placebo treatment which improved the erection in 25 per cent of patients (Saenz de Tejada *et al.* 2002). The long half-life of Tadalafil has been associated with an erectogenic potential of the drug, lasting for 24 h which might contribute to a better spontaneity during sexual activity when using Tadalafil.

Apomorphine SL

Two small hypothalamic nuclei the paraventricular nucleus and medial preoptic area play a key role in erectile function. A number of central neurotransmitters are involved in the initiation of erection. One main neurotransmitter is Dopamin, Dopamin receptors are divided in two main families D^1 and D^2 like receptors. Apomorphine SL (sublingual) has a high affinity to the D^2 like receptor, that are thought to be the main site for the induction of erections in the paraventricular nucleus. Apomorphine SL is therefore postulated to increase erectile responses by adding a conditioner increasing the response to sexual stimuli resulting in an enhanced erection induced in the periphery.

The beneficial effect of Apomorphine SL, was shown in many trials including more than 5000 men with various underline causes of erectile dysfunction (Mirone *et al.* 2001). The Apomorphine SL was efficacious particularly in patients with mild or moderate erectile dysfunction. Approximately two-third of patients reported positive erectile response within the first 20 min after sublingual application of the drug, however also later effect has been reported. Optimal effect has been reported mostly after 2–3 mg dose, 4 mg did not result in a significant better response (Montorsi 2003b). Dizziness, headaches, nausea when present, were often mild and transient. Another adverse event with Apomorphine SL was a transient vasovagal syncope (Dula *et al.* 2001; Mulhall *et al.* 2001).

Nitroglycerin ointment or plaster

In 1977, Mudd stated that sublingual nitroglycerin taken for angina improved erectile impotence. In the following years, improvement of psychogenic and vasculogenic impotence was reported to occur 2–6 h after the topical application of a nitroglycerin patch (release of 10 mg/24 h) or 1.5 in of 2 per cent nitroglycerin ointment in nonuraemic patients. The sexual partner should be protected by the use of latex condom. Nitrates probably induce dilatation of cavernosal and helicine arteries, and relaxation of trabecular smooth muscle (Mudd 1977; Nunez and Anderson 1993). The alternative application of 1 ml of a 2 per cent solution of minoxidil at the glans penis was more successful than 2.5 g of a 10 per cent nitroglycerin ointment applied to the penis shaft (Cavallini 1991).

Intracavernosal, intraurethral pharmacotherapy

Intracavernosal injection of various drugs results in smooth-muscle relaxation. This has been observed after injection of papaverin which is a general PDE-inhibitor but now prostaglandin E1 or synthetic analogue alprostatil is used. The drug acts via a specific surface receptor of smooth-muscle cells via the adenylate cyclase system in using relaxation and opening of both the vascular spaces of the erectile tissue and the feeding vascular arterioles (Linet and Ogrinc 1996). Erection occurs about 5–10 min after injection and lasts for 15 min to 2 h. The intracavernosal injection of PGE1 is successful in 75–80 per cent of patients and similar efficacy has been reported for a combination of VIP and phentolamine (Lee *et al.* 1989; Virag *et al.* 1991; Junemann *et al.* 1996).

Ultra-thin needles, 26 or 28.5 G, are recommended for the injection, which should be made in the middle of the corpora cavernosa, about 1–2 cm from the base of the penis. Immediate local problems include penile pain reported in up to 30 per cent of patients after PGE2. Furthermore, urethral bleeding, bruising, and corporal fibrosis have been reported both as a result of the injection technique and the frequency of use.

There is a risk of systemic hypotension which may explain rare cases of syncope and vasovagal reaction. Increases in transaminases after papaverine injection have been reported (Levine *et al.* 1989). More dangerous complications are long-lasting penile erection or even priapism. About 70 per cent of such complications respond to appropriate therapy (see section 'Priapism'). In general, intracavernosal pharmacotherapy has a high dropout rate of more than 50 per cent during the first year in some studies.

As an alternative to such intracavernosal injection, prostaglandin has been applied intraurethrally. PGE2 can be administered as a pellet through a specific delivery device prior to intercourse. After voiding urine, the patient inserts a device to release a pellet and then massages the penis to enhance dissolution of the drug which is absorbed by the urethral mucosa. The intraurethral application of PGE2 requires a dose which, in the majority of patients, is up to 1000 μg. In non-renal patients, a success rate has been reported between 40 and 65 per cent. Using this method, penile pain was reported in one-third of the patients but priapism is much less frequently reported compared to intracavernosal injection of phentolamine.

Vacuum device

In 1917, Lederer described the first vacuum constrictor device to treat erectile impotence. The penis, generously treated with a water soluble lubricant, is placed in the cylindrical chamber. When a vacuum of about 100–180 mm mercury, created by an electric or hand-operated mechanical pump, results in a rigid penile erection within a few minutes, a rubber band or O-ring is put in place to grip the base of the penis. In this way, sufficient rigidity can be maintained for 30 min. When the vacuum was limited to 180 mmHg and correct banding was used, no serious injuries were reported. Particularly in men taking aspirin or other anticoagulant drugs, painless ecchymosis can occur but this disappears within a few days. The success rate of this method is about 70–80 per cent and the dropout rate was quite low at 16 per cent at 1 year, compared with 50–60 per cent using intracavernosal pharmacotherapy (Lawrence *et al.* 1998).

Surgical treatment of erectile impotence

Arterial erectile dysfunction has been treated by various surgical procedures, including a saphenous graft between *A. femoralis* and cavernosum, anastomosis between *A. epigastrica* inferior and the dorsal penile arteries, or end-to-side anastomosis between *A. epigastrica* inferior and *A. dorsalis* penis and *V. dorsalis penis profunda*. The concomitant arterialization of penile veins is preferred if veno-occlusion is also defective. Success rates between 30 and 80 per cent have been reported. In general, this procedure should be restricted to young patients without arteriosclerosis. Limited results are available from balloon dilation of the pelvic arteries. Various forms of penile prostheses have been used, including semiflexible prostheses and inflatable penile prostheses with two silicone or polyurethane cylinders and a fluid reservoir at the cavum Retzii and a small pump at the scrotum.

Spermatogenesis

Spermatogenesis is already impaired in patients with moderate renal insufficiency (serum creatinine 3–500 μmol/l) (Vollrath *et al.* 1976). But procreation is by no means impossible even in patients on long-term dialysis. Commonly in uraemic patients, ejaculate volume is low with a diminished fructose and acid phosphatase content; sperm count is markedly decreased, and sperm abnormalities (asthenospermia, teratospermia) are frequent (Lim and Fang 1975; Holdsworth *et al.* 1978; Tharandt *et al.* 1980). Sperm motility is also severely diminished. Normospermia is found in only 20 per cent of dialysis patients (Vollrath *et al.* 1976). Testicular biopsies show arrest of maturation with a lack of mature sperm (De Kretser *et al.* 1974; Holdsworth *et al.* 1977). This is a typical result of hormone deficiency, in contrast to toxic effects which affect earlier stages of spermatogenesis (Meistrich 1986). Other authors have reported atrophy of sertoli cells and seminiferous tubules, interstitial fibrosis, and calcification and thickening of tubular basement membrane (Lim and Fang 1975). These morphological changes are partly reversible after transplantation (Toorians *et al.* 1997; De Celis and Pedron-Nuevo 1999; Malavaud *et al.* 2000). In this context, it may be relevant that TNF-α antagonizes the FSH effect in cultured sertoli cells including a 90 per cent reduction of inhibin production (Mauduit *et al.* 1993).

Treatment of impaired fertility of dialysis patients

There is little or no correlation between circulating FSH or plasma testosterone and sperm count or sperm motility. Some authors reported a slightly increased sperm count, but no increase in motility after treatment with clomiphene citrate. If patients want to have children, sexual activity should be restricted to the time of maximal probability of conception, since this will increase the chance of ejaculating sufficiently viable sperm. Frequent intercourse at the expected time of ovulation should be avoided: this exhausts spermatogenesis and decreases the sperm count. Testes should not be exposed to elevated temperature, this includes tight-fitting trousers or steam baths. In some patients with erectile impotence, electrostimulation can promote ejaculation and recovery of sperm for subsequent artificial insemination. There is little evidence that hormonal intervention improves spermatogenesis. Alternatively, the patient should postpone family planning until successful renal transplantation has been completed.

Priapism

Priapism is a not infrequent and severe complication of maintenance haemodialysis: some authors estimate that one in 70 young males on dialysis have had an episode of priapism (Port *et al.* 1974; Sale and Cameron 1974). Priapism is not related to sexual activity and can also result from erection during REM sleep. Androgen therapy for anaemia, polycythemia, particularly in patients with polycystic kidney disease seems to be a risk factor (Fassbinder *et al.* 1975). The majority of cases of priapism occur during intravenous heparinization while on haemodialysis (Port *et al.* 1974; Sale and Cameron 1974); other cases occur after ingestion of the vasodilator prazosin (Block *et al.* 1988). Most recent cases of priapism followed cavernosal pharmacotherapy.

Withdrawal of 20 ml of blood from the corpus cavernosum followed by intracavernosal injection of 200 μg phenylephrine diluted in saline or intracavernosal injection of metaraminol (2–5 mg) satisfactorily releases priapism in many patients (Branger *et al.* 1985). In others, surgical treatment, such as thrombectomy or venous anastomosis is necessary, although long-term penile dysfunction often results from venous anastomosis.

Gynaecomastia

Gynaecomastia, sometimes painful, was not uncommon in dialysis patients in the past. In recent years, the incidence of gynaecomastia has decreased, possibly as a result of improved dialysis or more likely, initiation of dialysis at an earlier stage of endstage renal failure. Gynaecomastia usually occurs during the initial months of dialysis and spontaneously regresses during the first 2 years of treatment. No relationship has been found between prevalence of gynaecomastia (Nagel *et al.* 1973) and plasma prolactin or androgen to oestrogen ratio. In some dialysis patients, gynaecomastia may be related to the refeeding gynaecomastia observed in malnourished patients. Primary hypothyroidism may also induce gynaecomastia, with hyperprolactinaemia and galactorrhoea. This occurs when low thyroid hormone levels increase thyrotrophin-releasing hormone secretion which, in turn, stimulates thyroid stimulating hormone and prolactin release ('overlap syndrome').

Transplantation

Transplanted patients commonly reported marked improvement of sexual function within a few weeks or months after successful transplantation. Within 2–3 months after transplantation, plasma testosterone increases to the normal range and levels of LH and FSH decrease. Compared to the dialysis period, a marked increase of sperm count was reported 9–16 months after transplantation in four of five patients (Phadke *et al.* 1970; Gonzales *et al.* 1981; Handelsman *et al.* 1981). It is worth noting that the increase in the sperm count was not observed less than 6 months after transplantation. Sperm motility was improved at the same time, and FSH decreased as sperm count improved (Lim and Fang 1975). In most patients, the sperm count did not reach normal levels and FSH remained elevated, suggesting that hypothalamic/hypophyseal regulation improved but did not return to normal after successful renal transplantation (De Celis and Pedron-Nuevo 1999).

Gonadal resistance to gonadotrophins present in haemodialysed patients is also improved after successful renal transplantation. Human gonadotrophin induces a higher but not normal testosterone response in transplanted patients compared to haemodialysed patients. Successful transplantation normalizes plasma prolactin. Suppression of serum prolactin after L-dopa (0.5 g orally) or dopamine (4 g/kg/min for 3 h) is normal in patients with a successful transplant. In good agreement with this finding, infusion of thyrotrophin-releasing hormone (500 μg) induces an increase in prolactin. This response is slightly less than in normal subjects, but much greater than in haemodialysed patients.

Sexual activity and erectile potency also improve after successful transplantation, but normal function is not usually achieved. Erectile dysfunction may continue in more than 80 per cent of men despite normalization of hormonal laboratory values and improved physiology (Witherington 1990). The psychological problems are not completely solved by transplantation. Transplanted patients suffer from increased anxiety. In addition, anastomosis between *A. iliaca interna* and the transplanted renal artery diminishes penile blood flow (Burns *et al.* 1979; Gittes and Waters 1979). Particularly, if a second transplantation has been performed using the same anastomosis technique on the contralateral side, impotence results frequently. For this reason, some authors recommended side-to-end anastomosis between *A. iliaca communis* and the transplanted renal artery, at least for the second transplanted kidney. Increasing age and progressive arteriosclerosis must also be considered. In most transplanted patients, antihypertensive therapy is required. Age, hypertension, diabetogenic effects of steroids, and lipid disorders favour arteriosclerosis, thereby enhancing

arteriogenic impotence. In a few patients, after renal transplantation, increased collateral formation may improve penile blood flow followed by normal penile blood pressure (Nghiem *et al.* 1983).

Females

The limited information about sexual behaviour in dialysed female patients indicates a diminution of sexual activity with progression of renal failure: 33 per cent of patients reported no sexual activity and 44 per cent only one episode of intercourse per week or less (Levi 1973). While 63 per cent of female patients reported regular orgasm during intercourse prior to uraemia, only 33 per cent of chronically dialysed women had regular orgasm during intercourse. However, one-third of female patients did not answer the questions in this study. A recent assessment by questionnaires and interview in selected patients gave similar results (Toorians *et al.* 1997; Diemont *et al.* 2000).

Gonadotrophins

The hypothalamic pulse generation of GnRH is influenced by many factors such as interleukin 1, β-endorphine, epinephrine, norepinephrine, oxytocin, serotonin, VIP, neuropeptide Y, γ-amino-butyric acid, glutamate, and others. Several factors are disturbed in women receiving maintenance dialysis, for example, the tonic and pulsatile secretion of gonadotrophin is inhibited by increased stress and followed by infertility (Chatterton 1990; Schenker *et al.* 1992). Gonadotrophin secretion is calcium-dependent (Naor and Catt 1980) and calcium-phosphate homeostasis is disturbed in dialysis patients. Leukotrienes, which are stimulated during dialysis may also stimulate gonadotrophin secretion (Kiesel and Catt 1984).

Serum LH is significantly elevated in most premenopausal patients. The response to stimulation with LHRH is delayed, but normal or supranormal concentrations of LH are achieved (Swamy *et al.* 1979). In uraemic patients, clomiphene stimulation for 5 days significantly increases LH and FSH, suggesting that the negative feedback effect of oestrogens on the hypothalamus and the storage and release of gonadotrophins from the pituitary are intact.

Physiological pulsatile release of LHRH is followed by pulsatile release of gonadotrophins. In normal women, short-term peaks of these hormones occur about every 90 min during the follicular phase of the menstrual cycle. This pulsatile hormone release is modified by a positive and negative feedback mechanism via oestradiol and progesterone. Oestradiol lowers the amplitude of LH pulses whereas progesterone increases the amplitude and lowers the frequency of these pulses (Djanhanbakhch *et al.* 1984; Soules *et al.* 1984). This spontaneous pulsatile LH secretion is disturbed in uraemic women. Some data indicate that it is absent in female dialysis patients (Swamy *et al.* 1979). The diurnal pulsatile secretion of LH and a high preovulatory peak of LHRH and, consequently, LH required for ovulation, are not found in most patients. Exogenous oestrogen (ethinyl oestradiol 2.5 μg/kg body weight every 4 h orally for 4 days) does not induce the LH surge (Lim *et al.* 1980), suggesting an impaired positive feedback mechanism.

FSH is usually within the normal range found during the follicular and luteal phase in normal women; LHRH induces only a moderate increase in FSH. The decreased ratio of FSH to LH argues against primary ovarian failure and suggests a hypothalamic–hypophyseal dysregulation. It may be of further interest that cytokines such as TNF-α and interleukins are involved in ovulation and follicle maturation and also endorphins can inhibit ovulation (Sancho-Tello and Terranova 1991; Brannstrom *et al.* 1994).

Prolactin

Hyperprolactinaemia is common in female as well as in male dialysis patients (Rudolf *et al.* 1983; Ferraris *et al.* 1987). Compared to healthy controls, the increase of serum prolactin is blunted after thyrotrophin-releasing hormone stimulation (Rudolf *et al.* 1983). Hyperprolactinaemia is a well-known cause of galactorrhoea and gonadal disturbances with menstrual irregularities, commonly amenorrhoea, in non-uraemic patients. In women without renal failure, the menstrual disturbance is inversely correlated with the serum prolactin. Amenorrhoea is found in patients with maximal prolactin levels, and the lowest prolactin levels are found in patients with regular menstruation (Michaelides and Humke 1993). Other menstrual irregularities, including anovulatory cycles or oligomenorrhoea, are more frequent in hyperprolactinaemic patients than galactorrhoea, which is the classical symptom of hyperprolactinaemia (L'Hermite *et al.* 1977).

Sexual hormones

Normal oestradiol (E2) concentrations have been reported in premenopausal uraemic women. E2 levels are lower in uraemic women with hyperprolactinaemia (Gomez *et al.* 1980). The typical cyclic variations of E2 are not found in female dialysis patients. Luteinization of follicles (Morley *et al.* 1979) is absent or very rare, as indicated by indirect measures of progestional status (vaginal cytology, basal body temperature, luteal endometrial biopsies). As a consequence, the increase in progesterone which normally occurs in the second half of the menstrual cycle is absent. Non-luteal progesterone levels are normal or low, and testosterone also tends to be low (Hubinont *et al.* 1983).

Vaginal and menstrual abnormalities

In half of the dialysed women, low plasma oestrogen is associated with atrophic vaginitis, pruritus, and reduced pubic hairs (Michaelides and Humke 1993). Vaginal cytology documents disturbed hormonal status. The normal midcyclic increase of karyopyknosis index is absent. The presence of malignant cells is not increased. The prevalence and spectrum of vaginal infections are not different in preuraemic or dialysis patients.

Menstrual irregularities develop along with uraemia. Amenorrhoea has been reported in 50–100 per cent of female patients with endstage renal failure (Goodwin *et al.* 1968; Huriet *et al.* 1974; Espersen *et al.* 1988). In many patients, amenorrhoea changes to irregular menstruation during maintenance haemodialysis, but the majority of patients suffer from continuous amenorrhoea. Of those patients who do menstruate, 50–80 per cent suffer from hypermenorrhoea, menorrhagia, or oligomenorrhoea (Larsen 1972; Huriet *et al.* 1974; Rice 1978; Morley *et al.* 1979; Michaelides *et al.* 1993).

In the early years of dialysis the midcycle increase in basal body temperature, which is normally an indicator of ovulation, was not observed in 95 per cent of female dialysis patients. Recently, perhaps because of correction of renal anaemia with erythropoietin, more frequent ovulatory cycles have been reported (Schaefer *et al.* 1989b). In women with anovulatory cycles progesterone deficiency results in incomplete maturation of the endometrium, followed by hypermenorrhoea and dysfunctional bleeding, that is, the menstrual abnormalities common in many dialysed women result predominantly from disturbed hypothalamic–hypophyseal regulation and gonadal dysfunction. Uraemic coagulopathy and heparinization during haemodialysis may intensify menstrual bleeding. In uraemic women, menstrual abnormalities may also be the consequence of hyper- and hypothyroidism, severe diabetes mellitus, Addison's disease, or severe diseases such as carcinoma, tuberculosis, and immunological disorders.

Increased ovarian cyst formation has been noted in menstruating uraemic women (Thaysen *et al.* 1975). This must be distinguished from polycystic ovarian syndrome (Yen 1980) or androgen producing tumours, which can be identified by elevated serum testosterone or dehydroepiandrosterone sulfate, sonography, and computed tomography of ovary and adrenals. Non-uraemic patients with anovulation and insufficiency of corpus luteum have an increased risk of endometrial cancer.

Treatment of menstrual abnormalities

Before epoetin was available amenorrhoea and oligomenorrhoea were welcome symptoms in many anaemic female patients on maintenance haemodialysis. If menstrual bleeding is required, the common failure of follicle luteinization can be treated with progesterone (4 mg medroxyprogesterone/day between days 14 and 25 of the cycle); this induces endometrial transformation and normal menstruation. In view of the increased risk of endometrial cancer in patients with anovulation and corpus luteum insufficiency, application of such intermittent progesterone therapy every half a year should be considered. Alternatively regular monthly oestrogen/progesterone combination therapy can be used, as in non-uraemic patients. Low oestrogen containing preparations are preferred to avoid potential effects on blood pressure. Oestrogen/progesterone combinations are beneficial for bone disease in dialysis patients. Weisinger reported that mineral density in the trabecular bone was significantly less in the amenorrhoic women when compared with regularly menstruating dialysis patients. Lumbar spine bone mineral density and total oestradiol concentrations correlate significantly in the amenorrhoic women (Weisinger *et al.* 2000).

Hypermenorrhoea can be stopped within 1 or 2 days by application of high doses of progesterone (100 mg medroxyprogesterone/day). In patients with chronic hypermenorrhoea, or if menstruation in general is undesired, perhaps due to anaemia, endometrial atrophy can be induced by continuous administration of high doses of progesterone: 25–100 mg medroxyprogesterone/day, starting with a dose of 75–100 mg which can be reduced to the lowest dose suppressing menstrual bleeding. Alternatively, intermittent intramuscular injection of progesterone (medroxyprogesterone acetate 500–1000 mg intramuscularly every 2–3 months) may prevent menstrual bleeding. However, such long-term exclusive progesterone therapy increases bone problems in dialysis patients. For this reason intermittent oestrogen therapy or oestrogen/progesterone combinations for some months are particularly recommended. As a last resort, a hysterectomy can be performed.

Galactorrhoea

Galactorrhoea has been reported to occur with varying frequency, ranging from 0 to 40 per cent of women on maintenance haemodialysis. Increased plasma prolactin probably plays a major role. If the typical combination of galactorrhoea/amenorrhoea syndrome is present, prolactinoma must be excluded by appropriate radiographic and computed tomography examination. Galactorrhoea must also be distinguished from abnormal breast secretions: mammography and cytology of nodules may be required. If malignant breast secretion is excluded, galactorrhoea due to hyperprolactinaemia can be treated with prolactin inhibitors such as bromocriptine (2.5–5 mg/day) or lisuride (0.2–0.5 mg/day). Primary hypothyroidism with constantly elevated thyrotrophin-releasing hormones may induce hyperprolactinaemia, and consequently, galactorrhoea ('overlap syndrome'). In such patients, galactorrhoea of 100–200 ml/day has been observed; this disappears after replacement with thyroxine.

Fertility

Basal body temperature, vaginal cytology, and luteal endometrial biopsies indicate that anovulatory cycles are common (>90 per cent) in women on maintenance haemodialysis (Huriet et al. 1974; Michaelides and Humke 1993). However, general infertility cannot be assumed. Ovulation in 45 per cent of cycles have been reported, although with a slightly atypical hormonal pattern. More frequent ovulatory cycles have been reported not only with bromocriptine therapy (Wass et al. 1979), but also with epoetin therapy. In dialysed patients some authors also reported a reduction of hyperprolactinaemia on epoetin, but this was not confirmed by others. It is recommended that during the reproductive age sexually active dialysis women should use contraception to avoid unwanted pregnancies.

If improved fertility is desired, bromocriptine therapy (2.5–5 mg) can induce resumption of menstrual bleeding and ovulatory cycles in some patients (Wass et al. 1979). Disappearance of amenorrhoea and the onset of ovulation have also been reported when anaemia was improved after recombinant human erythropoietin therapy (Schaefer et al. 1989b).

Moderate ovarian hyperstimulation syndrome occurred with GnRH agonist (leuprolide acetate) in an anephric dialysis woman (Hampton et al. 1991). Information is lacking about the efficacy of pulsatile GnRH given subcutaneously or intravenously in dialysis patients, although this is a successful therapy in non-uraemic women with hypogonadotropic hypogonadism.

For pregnancy in patients receiving dialysis or following transplantation see Chapter 15.3.

References

Abram, H. S., Hester, L. R., Sheridan, W. F., and Epstein, G. M. (1975). Sexual functioning in patients with chronic renal failure. *Journal of Nervous and Mental Disease* **166**, 220–226.

Antoniou, L. D., Sudhaker, T., Shalhoub, R. J., and Smith, J. C. (1977). Reversal of uraemic impotence by zinc. *Lancet* **ii**, 895–898.

Ayub, W. and Fletcher, S. (2000). End-stage renal disease and erectile dysfunction. Is there any hope? *Nephrology, Dialysis, Transplantation* **15**, 1525–1528.

Bähren, W., Stief, Ch., Scherb, W., Gall, H., Gallwitz, A., and Altwein, J. E. (1986). Rationelle Diagnostik der erektilen Dysfunktion unter Anwendung eines pharmakologischen Tests. *Acta Urologica Belgica* **4**, 177–178.

Bancroft, J. and Wu, C. F. (1983). Changes in erectile responsiveness during androgen replacement therapy. *Archives of Sexual Behaviour* **12**, 59–66.

Barton, C. H., Mirahamadi, M. K., and Vairi, N. D. (1982). Effects of long-term testosterone administration on pituitary-testicular axis in end-stage renal failure. *Nephron* **31**, 61–64.

Bellinghieri, G., Lo Forti, B., and Savica, V. (1992). The penile c.w. Doppler test in the study of uraemic impotence. *Medical Science Research* **20**, 95.

Biasioli, S., Mazzali, A., Foroni, R., D'Andrea, G., Feriani, M., Chiaramonte, S., Cesaro, A., and Micieli, G. (1988). Chronobiological variations of prolactin (PRL) in chronic renal failure (CRF). *Clinical Nephrology* **30**, 86–92.

Blanco, R., Saenz de Tejada, I., Goldstein, I., Krane, R. J., Wotiz, H. H., and Cohen, R. A. (1988). Cholinergic neurotransmission in human corpus cavernosum. II. Acetylcholine synthesis. *American Journal of Physiology* **254**, H468–H472.

Block, T., Sturm, W., Ernst, G., Stähler, G., and Schmiedt, E. (1988). Metamarinol in therapy of various forms of priapism. *Urologe A* **27**, 225–229.

Blumberg, A., Wildbolz, A., Descouedres, C., Hennes, V., Dambacher, M. A., Fischer, J. A., and Weidmann, P. (1979). Influence of 1,25-dihydroxy-cholecalciferol (1,25 OH) on sexual dysfunction and related endocrine parameters in patients on maintenance hemodialysis. *Clinical Nephrology* **13** (5), 208–214.

Bocchi, E. A. et al. (2001). Beneficial effects of a phosphodiesterase type 5 inhibitor (sildenafil) on exercise, neurohumoral activation, and erectile dysfunction in patients with congestive heart failure—a double-blind placebo-controlled cross-over randomized study. *Journal of American College of Cardiology* **37** (Suppl. 2), 163A.

Bommer, J. (1986). Management of uraemic patients with sexual difficulties. *Contributions to Nephrology* **50**, 139–152.

Bommer, J., Tschöpe, W., Ritz, E., and Andrassy, K. (1976). Sexual behaviour of haemodialyzed patients. *Clinical Nephrology* **6**, 315–318.

Bommer, J., Kugel, M., Schwöbel, B., Ritz, E., Barth, H. P., and Seelig, R. (1990). Improved sexual function during recombinant human erythropoietin therapy. *Nephrology, Dialysis, Transplantation* **5**, 204–207.

Bommer, J. et al. (1979). Improved sexual function in male haemodialysis patients on bromocriptine. *Lancet* **ii**, 496–498.

Branger, B. et al. (1985). Metaraminal for haemodialysis-associated priapism. *Lancet* **i**, 641.

Brannstrom, M., Norman, R. J., Seamark, R. F., and Robertson, S. A. (1994). Rat ovary produces cytokines during ovulation. *Biology of Reproduction* **50** (1), 88–94.

Brook, A. C., Johnston, D. G., Ward, M. K., Watson, M. J., Cook, D. B., and Kerr, D. N. S. (1980). Absence of therapeutic effect of zinc in the sexual dysfunction of haemodialysis patients. *Lancet* **ii**, 618–619.

Burnett, A. L., Lowenstein, C. J., Bredt, D. S., Chang, T. S. K., and Snyder, S. H. (1992). Nitric oxide: a physiologic mediator of penile erection. *Science* **257**, 401–403.

Burns, J. R., Houttin, E., Gregory, J. G., Hawatmeh, I. S., and Sullivan, T. R. (1979). Vascular-induced erectile impotence in renal transplant recipients. *Journal of Urology* **121**, 721–723.

Campese, V. M., Procci, W. R., Levitan, D., Romoff, M. S., Goldstein, D. A., and Massry, S. G. (1982). Autonomic nervous system dysfunction and impotence in uraemia. *American Journal of Nephrology* **2**, 140–143.

Canale, D. et al. (1984). Human chorionic gonadotropin treatment of male sexual inadequacy in patients affected by chronic renal failure. *Journal of Andrology* **5**, 120–124.

Cavallini, G. (1991). Minoxidil versus nitroglycerin: a prospective double-blind controlled trial in transcutaneous erection fascilitation for organic impotence. *Journal of Urology* **146**, 50–53.

Chatterton, R. T. (1990). The role of stress in female reproduction: animal and human considerations. *International Journal of Fertility* **35** (1), 8–13.

Cheitlin, M. D. et al. (1999). ACC/AHA expert consensus document. Use of sildenafil (Viagra) in patients with cardiovascular disease. *Journal of American College of Cardiology* **33**, 273–282.

Coppola, A. and Cuomo, G. (1990). Pituitary–testicular assays in patients with chronic renal failure undergoing haemodialysis treatment. *Minerva Medica* **81** (6), 461–464.

Corvol, B., Bertagna, X., and Bedrossian, J. (1974). Increased steroid metabolic clearance rate in anephric patients. *Acta Endocrinologica* **75**, 756–761.

Daubresse, J. C., Palem-Vliers, M., Gyselinck-Mambourg, A. M., and Franchimont, P. (1972). Etude de la secretion de gonadotrophines au cours de l'insuffisance renal chez l'homme. *Proceedings of the European Dialysis and Transplantation Association* **9**, 555–558.

De Celis, R. and Pedron-Nuevo, N. (1999). Male fertility of kidney transplant patients with one to ten years of evolution using a conventional immunosuppressive regimen. *Archives of Andrology* **42**, 9–20.

De Kretser, D. M., Atkins, R. C., and Hudson, B. (1974). Disordered spermatogenesis in patients with chronic renal failure undergoing maintenance haemodialysis. *Australian and New Zealand Journal of Medicine* 4, 178–781.

Degli-Esposti, E., Sturani, A., Santoro, A., Zuccala, A., Chiarini, C., and Zuchelli, P. (1985). Effects of bromocriptine treatment on prolactin, noradrenaline and blood pressure in hypertensive haemodialysis patients. *Clinical Science* 69, 51–56.

DeVries, C. P., Gooren, L. J. G., and Oe, P. L. (1984). Haemodialysis and testicular function. *International Journal of Andrology* 7, 97–103.

Diemont, W. L. *et al.* (2000). Sexual dysfunction after renal replacement therapy. *American Journal of Kidney Diseases* 35 (5), 845–851.

Distiller, L. A. *et al.* (1975). Pituitary-gonadal function in chronic renal failure: the effect of luteinizing hormone-releasing hormone and the influence of dialysis. *Metabolism* 24, 711–720.

Djanhanbakhch, G., Warner, P., McNeilly, A. S., and Baird, D. T. (1984). Pulsatile release of LH and estradiol during the preovulatory period in women. *Clinical Endocrinology* 20, 576–589.

Dula, E., Bukofzer, S., Perdok, R., and George, M. (2000). Double-blind, crossover comparison of 3 mg apomorphine SL with placebo and with 4 mg apomorphine SL in male erectile dysfunction. *European Urology* 558–564.

Elias, A. N., Vaziri, N. D., and Maksy, M. (1986). Plasma beta-endorphin and beta-lipotropin in patients with end-stage renal disease effects of hmodialysis. *Nephron* 43, 173–176.

Espersen, T., Schmitz, O., Hansen, H. E., Moller, J., and Klebe, J. G. (1988). Ovulation in uraemic women: the reproductive cycle in women on chronic hemodialysis. *International Journal of Fertility* 33, 103–106.

Fassbinder, W., Frei, U., and Issantier, R. (1975). Factors predisposing to priapism in hemodialysis patients. *Proceedings of the European Dialysis and Transplantation Association* 12, 380–386.

Feldman, H. A., Goldstein, I., Hatzchristou, D. G., and Krane, R. L. (1994). Impotence and its medical and psychosocial correlates: results of the Massachusetts male aging study. *Journal of Urology* 151, 54–61.

Ferraris, J. *et al.* (1980). Delayed puberty in males with chronic renal failure. *Kidney International* 8, 344–350.

Ferraris, J. R., Domene, H. M., Escobar, M. E., Caletti, M. G., Ramirez, J. A., and Rivarola, M. A. (1987). Hormonal profile in pubertal females with chronic renal failure: before and under haemodialysis and after renal transplantation. *Acta Endocrinologica* 115, 289–296.

Fioretti, P. *et al.* (1986). Parathyroid function and pituitary-gonadal axis in male uraemics: effect of dietary treatment and of maintenance hemodialysis. *Clinical Nephrology* 25, 155–158.

Franks, S., Jacobs, H. S., Martin, N., and Nabarro, J. D. (1978). Hyperprolactinemia and impotence. *Clinical Endocrinology* 8, 277–287.

Gaillard, R. C. (1990). Tumor necrosis factor alpha inhibits the hormonal response of the pituitary gland to hypothalamic releasing factors. *Endocrinology* 127, 101–106.

Gerstenberg, T. C., Metz, P., Ottesen, B., and Fahrenkrug, J. (1992). Intracavernous self-injection with vasoactive intestinal polypeptide and phentolamine in the management of erectile failure. *Journal of Urology* 147 (5), 1277–1279.

Gittes, R. F. and Waters, W. B. (1979). Sexual impotence: the overlooked complication of a second renal transplant. *Journal of Urology* 121, 719–720.

Glass, C. A., Fielding, D. M., Evans, C., and Ashcroft, J. B. (1987). Factors related to sexual functioning in male patients undergoing hemodialysis and with renal transplants. *Archives of Sexual Behaviour* 16, 189–207.

Goldstein, I. *et al.* (1998). Oral sildenafil in the treatment of erectile dysfunction. *New England Journal of Medicine* 388, 1397–1404.

Gomez, F., de la Cueva, R., Wauters, J.-P., and Lemarchand-Berand, T. (1980). Endocrine abnormalities in patients undergoing long-term hemodialysis. *American Journal of Medicine* 68, 522–530.

Goodwin, N. J., Valenti, C., Hall, J. E., and Friedman, E. A. (1968). Effects of uraemia and chronic hemodialysis on the reproductive cycle. *American Journal of Obstetrics and Gynaecology* 100, 528–535.

Grimm, R. H., Jr. *et al.* (1997). Longterm effects on sexual function of 5 antihypertensive drugs and nutritional hygenic treatment in hypertensive men and women. Treatment of Mild Hypertension Study (TOMHS). *Hypertension* 29, 8.

Grzeszcak, W., Kokot, F., and Dulawa, J. (1987). Effects of naloxone administration on endocrine abnormalities in chronic renal failure. *American Journal of Nephrology* 7, 93–100.

Handelsman, D. J. (1985). Hypothalamic-pituitary gonadal dysfunction in renal failure, dialysis and renal transplantation. *Endocrine Reviews* 6, 151–182.

Handelsman, D. J., Ralec, V. L., Tiller, D. J., Horvath, J. S., and Turtle, J. R. (1981). Testicular function after renal transplantation. *Clinical Endocrinology (Oxford)* 14, 527–538.

Hedlund, H. and Andersson, K. E. (1985). Comparison of the responses to drugs acting on adrenoceptors and muscarinic receptors in human isolated corpus cavernosum and cavernous artery. *Journal of Autonomic Pharmacology* 5, 81–88.

Herrmann, H. C., Chang, G., Klughere, B. D., and Mahoney, P. D. (2000). Hemodynamic effects of sildenafil in men with severe CAD sildenafil citrate in men with severe coronary artery disease. *New England Journal of Medicine* 342 (22), 1622–1626.

Holdsworth, S. R., Atkins, R. C., and de Kretser, D. M. (1977). The pituitary–testicular axis in men with chronic renal failure. *New England Journal of Medicine* 296, 1245–1249.

Holdsworth, S. R., de Kretser, D. M., and Atkins, R. C. (1978). A comparison of hemodialysis and transplantation in reversing the uraemic disturbance of male reproductive failure. *Clinical Nephrology* 10, 146–150.

Holmes, S. (2000). Treatment of male sexual dysfunction. *British Medical Bulletin* 56 (3), 798–808.

Hricik, D. E., Schulak, J. A., Sell, D. R., Fogarty, J. F., and Monnier, M. (1993). Effects of kidney-pancreas transplantation on plasma pentosidine. *Kidney International* 43, 398–403.

Hubinont, C., Vanherweghem, J. L., Mockel, J., Franckson, M., and Schwers, J. (1983). Hormonal profile in women undergoing hemodialysis. *Kidney International* 24, S335.

Huriet, J. C. *et al.* (1974). Profil clinique et cytologique de la femme en hemodialyse. *Journal d'Urologie et Nephrologie* 14 (5), 369–375.

Janssen, E. E., Van Lunsen, R. H. W., and Oelermans, S. (1994). Visual stimulation facilitates penile responses to vibration in men with and without erectile disorders. *Journal of Consulting and Clinical Psychology* 62, 1222–1228.

Jassal, S. V. *et al.* (1998). Prevalence of central autonomic neuropathy in elderly dialysis patients. *Nephrology, Dialysis, Transplantation* 13, 1702–1708.

Judd, A. M., MacLeod, R. M., and Login, R. S. (1984). Growth hormone releasing factor increases growth hormone release from MtTW15 pituitary tumors. *Brain Research* 308, 137–140.

Junemann, K. P., Manning, M., Krautsch, A., and Alken, P. (1996). 15 Years of injection therapy in men with erectile dysfunction. *International Journal of Impotence Research* 8, A60.

Karacan, I. and Salis, P. J. (1980). Diagnosis and treatment of erectile impotence. *Psychiatric Clinics of North America* 3, 97–111.

Karacan, I., Goodenough, D. R., and Shapiro, A. (1966). Erection during sleep in relation to dream anxiety. *Archives of General Psychiatry* 15, 183–189.

Karacan, I., Goodenough, D. R., and Shapiro, A. (1970). Nocturnal erection, differential diagnosis of impotence and diabetes. *Biological Psychiatry* 12, 373–380.

Katlowitz, N. M., Albano, G. J., Morales, P., and Golimbu, M. (1993). Potentiation of drug-induced erection with audiovisual sexual stimulation. *Urology* 41 (5), 431–434.

Kedia, K. and Markland, C. (1975). The effect of pharmacological agents on ejaculation. *Journal of Urology* 114, 569–574.

Kiesel, L. and Catt, K. J. (1984). Phosphatidic acid and the calcium-dependent actions of gonadotropin-releasing hormone in pituitary gonadotrophs. *Archives of Biochemistry and Biophysics* 231, 202–210.

Kim, N., Vardi, Y., Padma-Nathan, H., Daley, J., Goldstein, I., and Saenz de Tejada, I. (1993). Oxygen tension regulates the nitric oxide pathway: physiological role in penile erection. *Journal of Clinical Investigation* 91, 437–442.

Koike, K., Hirota, K., Ohmichi, M., Kadowaki, K., Ikegami, H., Yamaguchi, M., Miyake, A., and Tanizawa, O. (1991). Tumor necrosis factor-alpha increases release of arachidonate and prolactin from rat anterior pituitary cells. *Endocrinology* **128** (6), 2791–2798.

Kokot, F., Wiecek, A., Grzeszczak, W., Klepacka, J., Klin, M., and Lao, M. (1989). Influence of erythropoietin treatment on endocrine abnormalities in hemodialyzed patients. *Contributions to Nephrology* **76**, 257–272.

Kwan, A., Greenleaf, W. J., Mann, J., Crapo, L., and Davison, J. M. (1983). The nature of androgen action on male sexuality: a combined laboratory and self-report study on hypogonadal men. *Journal of Clinical Endocrinology and Metabolism* **12**, 59–66.

Larsen, N. A. Sexual problems of patients on RDT and after renal transplantation. In *Proceedings of the European Dialysis and Transplantation Association* (ed. J. S. Cameron), p. 271. Baltimore, MD: Williams & Wilkins, 1972.

Lawrence, I. G., Price, D. E., Howlett, T. A., Harris, K. P., Feehally, J., and Walls, J. (1997). Erythropoietin and sexual dysfunction. *Nephrology, Dialysis, Transplantation* **12**, 741–747.

Lawrence, I. G. *et al.* (1998). Correcting impotence in the male dialysis patient: experience with testosterone replacement and vacuum tumescence therapy. *American Journal of Kidney Diseases* **31** (2), 313–319.

Lee, L. M., Stevenson, R. W., and Szasz, G. (1989). Prostaglandin E1 versus phentolamine/papaverine for the treatment of erectile impotence: a double-blind comparison. *Journal of Urology* **141**, 549–550.

LeRoith, D., Danovitz, G., Trestian, S., and Spitz, J. M. (1980). Dissociation of pituitary glycoprotein response to releasing hormones in chronic renal failure. *Acta Endocrinologica* **93**, 277–282.

Levi, N. B. (1973). Sexual adjustment of maintenance hemodialysis and renal transplantation. National Survey by Questionnaire; Preliminary Report. *Transactions of the American Society for Artificial Internal Organs* **19**, 138–143.

Levine, S. B., Althof, S. E., and Turner, L. A. (1989). Side effects of self-administration of intracavernous papaverine and phentolamine for treatment of impotence. *Journal of Urology* **141**, 54–57.

Levy, A., Crowley, T., and Gingell, C. (2000). Non-surgical management of erectile dysfunction. *Clinical Endocrinology* **52** (3), 253–260.

L'Hermite, M., Cauffriez, A., and Robyn, C. Pathophysiology of human prolactin secretion with special reference to prolactin secreting pituitary adenomas and isolated galactorrhea. In *Prolactin and Human Reproduction* (ed. P. G. Crosignani and C. Robyn), p. 179. New York, NY: Academic Press, 1977.

Lim, V. S. and Fang, V. S. (1975). Gonadal dysfunction in uraemic men. A study of hypothalamo-pituitary-testicular axis before and after renal transplantation. *American Journal of Medicine* **58**, 655–662.

Lim, V. S. and Fang, V. S. (1976). Restoration of plasma testosterone levels in uraemic men with clomiphene citrate. *Journal of Clinical Endocrinology and Metabolism* **43**, 1370–1377.

Lim, V. S., Henriquez, C., Sievertsen, G., and Frohman, L. A. (1980). Ovarian function in chronic renal failure: evidence suggesting hypothalamic anovulation. *Annals of Internal Medicine* **93**, 21–27.

Lim, V. S., Kathpalia, S. C., and Frohman, L. A. (1979). Hyperprolactinemia and impaired pituitary response to suppression and stimulation in chronic renal failure: reversal after transplantation. *Journal of Clinical Endocrinology and Metabolism* **48**, 101–107.

Linet, O. I. and Ogrinc, F. G. (1996). Efficacy and safety of intracavernosal alprostadil in men with erectile dysfunction. *New England Journal of Medicine* **334**, 873–877.

Mahajan, S. K., Hamburger, R. J., Flamenbaum, W., Prasad, A. S., and McDonald, F. D. (1985). Effect of zinc supplementation on hyperprolactinaemia in uraemic men. *Lancet* **ii**, 750–751.

Mahmud, A., Hennessy, M., and Feely, J. (2000). Effect of sildenafil on blood pressure and arterial stiffness. *British Journal of Clinical Pharmacology* **49**, 510.

Malavaud, B., Rostaing, L., Rischmann, P., Sarramon, J. P., and Durand, D. (2000). High prevalence of erectile dysfunction after renal transplantation. *Transplantation* **69**, 2121–2124.

Mannino, D. H., Klevens, R. M., and Flaanders, W. D. (1994). Cigarette-smoking: an independent risk factor for impotence. *American Journal of Epidemiology* **140**, 1003.

Marks, L. S., Duda, C., Dorey, F. J., Macairan, M. L., and Santos, P. B. (1999). Treatment of erectile dysfunction with sildenafil. *Urology* **53**, 19–24.

Martin-Malo, A., Benito, P., Castillo, D., Espinosa, M., Burdiel, L. G., Perez, R., and Aljama, P. (1993). Effect of clomiphene citrate on hormonal profile in male hemodialysis and kidney transplant patients. *Nephron* **63**, 390–394.

Massry, S. G., Goldstein, D. A., Procci, W. R., and Kletsky, O. A. (1977). Impotence in patients with uraemia. A possible role for parathyroid hormone. *Nephron* **19**, 305–310.

Massry, S. G., Goldstein, D. A., Procci, W. R., and Kletsky, O. A. (1980). On the pathogenesis of sexual dysfunction of the uraemic male. *Proceedings of the European Dialysis and Transplantation Association* **17**, 139–146.

Mastrogiacomo, I. *et al.* (1988). Male hypogonadism of uraemic patients on hemodialysis. *Archives of Andrology* **20**, 171–175.

Mauduit, C., Jaspar, J. M., Poncelet, E., Charlet, C., Revol, A., Franchimont, P., and Benahmed, M. (1993). Tumor necrosis factor-alpha antagonizes follicle-stimulating hormone action in cultured sertoli cells. *Endocrinology* **133** (1), 69–76.

May, A. G., DeWeese, J. A., and Rob, C. G. (1969). Changes in sexual function following operation on the abdominal aorta. *Surgery* **65**, 41–44.

McConnell, J. and Benson, G. S. (1982). Enervation of human penile blood vessels. *Neurology, Urology and Urodynamics* **1**, 199–210.

Mealy, K., Robinson, B., Millette, C. F., Majzoub, J., and Wilmore, D. W. (1990). The testicular effects of tumor necrosis factor. *Annals of Surgery* **211**, 470–475.

Meikle, A. W., Cardoso de Sousa, J. C., Dacosta, N., Bishop, D. K., and Samlowski, W. E. (1992). Direct and indirect effects of murine interleukin-2, gamma interferon, and tumor necrosis factor on testosterone synthesis in mouse Leydig cells. *Journal of Andrology* **13** (5), 437–443.

Meistrich, M. L. (1986). Relationship between spermatologonial stem cell survival and testis function after cytotoxic therapy. *British Journal of Cancer* **7** (Suppl.), 89–101.

Merrick, G. S., Butler, W. M., Lief, J., Stipetich, R. L., Abel, L. J., and Dorsey, A. (1999). Efficacy of sildenafil citrate in prostate brachytherapy patients with erectile dysfunction. *Urology* **53** (6), 1112–1116.

Michaelides, N. and Humke, W. (1993). Erfahrungen bei der gynäkologischen Betrteuung von Patientinnen mit chronischer Niereninsuffizienz. *Nieren-und Hochdruckkrankheiten* **22**, 187–192.

Mirone, V. G. and Stief, C. G. (2001). Efficacy of apomorphine SL in erectile dysfunction. *British Journal of Urology International* **88** (Suppl. 3), 25–29.

Montorsi, F., Salonia, A., Deho, F., Cestari, A., Guazzoni, G., Rigatti, P., and Stief, C. (2003a). Pharmacological management of erectile dysfunction. *British Journal of Urology International* **91**, 446–454.

Montorsi, F. (2003b). Tolerability and safety of apomorphine SL [Ixense (TM)]. *International Journal of Impotence Research* **15** (Suppl. 2), 7–9, 10–15.

Morales, A. (1990). The role of nocturnal penile tumescence monitoring in the diagnosis of impotence: a review. *Journal of Urology* **143**, 441–446.

Morley, J. E. *et al.* (1979). Menstrual disturbances in chronic renal failure. *Hormone and Metabolic Research* **11**, 68–72.

Mudd, J. W. (1977). Impotence responsive to glyceryl trinitrate. *American Journal of Psychology* **134**, 922–925.

Mulhall, J. P., Bukofzer, S., Edmonds, A. L., George, M., Apomorphine SL Study Group (2001). An open-label, uncontrolled dose-optimization study of sublingual apomorphine in erectile dysfunction. *Clinical Therapy* **23**, 1260–1271.

Muir, J. W. *et al.* (1983). Bromocriptine improves reduced libido and potency in men receiving maintenance hemodialysis. *Clinical Nephrology* **20** (3), 8–14.

Nagel, T. C., Freinkel, N., Bell, R. H., Friesen, H., Wilber, J. F., and Metzger, B. E. (1973). Gynecomastia, prolactin, and other peptide hormones in patients undergoing chronic hemodialysis. *Journal of Clinical Endocrinology and Metabolism* **36**, 428–432.

Naor, Z. and Catt, K. J. (1980). Independent actions of gonadotropin-releasing hormone upon cGMP production and luteinizing hormone release. *Journal of Biological Chemistry* **255**, 342–344.

Nghiem, D. D., Corry, R. J., Picon-Mendez. G., and Lee, H. M. (1983). *Urology* **21**, 49–52.

Nolten, W. E., Goldstein, D., Lindström, M., McKenna, M. V., Carlson, I. H., Trump, D. L., Schiller, J., Borden, E. C., and Ehrlich, E. N. (1993). Effects of cytokines on the pituitary-adrenal axis in cancer patients. *Journal of Interferon Research* **13** (5), 349–357.

Nunez, B. D. and Anderson, D. C., Jr. (1993). Nitroglycerin ointment in the treatment of impotence. *Journal of Urology* **150**, 1241–1243.

Phadke, A., MacKinnon, K., and Dossetos, J. (1970). Male fertility in uraemia: restoration by renal allografts. *Canadian Medical Association* **102**, 607–608.

Porst, H., Padma-Nathan, H., Giuliano, F., Anglin, G., Varanese, L., and Rosen, R. (2003). Efficacy of tadalafil for the treatment of erectile dysfunction at 24 and 36 hours after dosing: a randomized controlled trial. *Urology* **62** (1), 121–125.

Port, F. K., Fiegel, P., Hecking, E., Köhler, H., and Distler, A. (1974). Priapism during regular haemodialysis. *Lancet* **ii**, 1287–1288.

Rajfer, J., Aronson, W. J., Bush, P. A. Dorey, F. J., and Ignarro, L. J. (1992). Nitric oxide as a mediator of relaxation of the corpus cavernosum in response to nonadrenergic, noncholinergic neurotransmission. *New England Journal of Medicine* **326**, 90–94.

Ramirez, G., Bittle, P. A., Sanders, H., and Bercu, B. B. (1992). Hypothalamo-hypophyseal thyroid and gonadal function before and after erythropoietin therapy in dialysis patients. *Journal of Clinical Endocrinology and Metabolism* **73/3**, 517–524.

Ramirez, G., Butcher, D., Brüggemeyer, C. D., and Ganguly, A. (1987). Testicular defect: the primary abnormality in gonadal dysfunction of uraemia. *Southern Medical Journal* **80**, 698–701.

Ramirez, G., O'Neill, W. M., Bloomer, H. A., and Jubiz, W. (1977). Abnormalities in the regulation of prolactin in patients with renal failure. *Journal of Clinical Endocrinology and Metabolism* **45**, 658–661.

Rees, H. D. and Michael, R. P. (1982). Brain cells of the Rhesus monkey accumulate iH-testosterone or its metabolites. *Journal of Comparative Neurology* **206**, 273–277.

Reid, K., Morales, A., Harris, C., Surridge, D. H. C., Condra, M., and Owen, J. (1987). Double-blind trial of Yohimbine in treatment of psychogenic impotence. *Lancet* **ii**, 421–423.

Reiter, W. J. *et al.* (2001). Dehydroepiandrosterone in the treatment of erectile dysfunction in patients with different organic etiologies. *Urological Research* **29** (4), 278–281.

Rendell, M. S., Rajfer, J., Wicker, P. A., and Smith, M. D. for the Sildenafil Diabetes Study Group (1999). Sildenafil for treatment of erectile dysfunction in men with diabetes: a randomized controlled trial. *Journal of the American Medical Association* **281**, 421–426.

Rice, C. G. (1978). Hypermenorrhea in the young dialysis patient. *American Journal of Obstetrics and Gynaecology* **116**, 539–543.

Rodger, R. S. C., Morrison, L., Dewar, J. H., Wilkinson, R., Ward, M. K., and Kerr, D. N. S. (1985). Loss of pulsatile luteinising hormone secretion in men with chronic renal failure. *British Medical Journal* **291**, 1598–1600.

Rodger, R. S. C., Dewar, J. H., Turner, S. J., Watson, M. J., and Ward, M. K. (1986). Anterior pituitary dysfunction in patients with chronic renal failure treated by hemodialysis or continuous peritoneal ambulatory dialysis. *Nephron* **43**, 169–172.

Roeckel, A., Henneman, H., Sternagel-Haase, A., and Heidland, A. (1979). Uraemic sympathetic neuropathy after hemodialysis and transplantation. *European Journal of Clinical Investigation* **9**, 23–27.

Rosas, S. E., Wasserstein, A., Kobrin, S., and Feldman, H. I. (2001). Preliminary observations of sildenafil treatment for erectile dysfunction in dialysis patients. *American Journal of Kidney Diseases* **37** (1), 134–137.

Rudolf, K., Rudolf, H., Rüting, M., and Falkenhagen, D. (1983). Verhalten basaler und stimulierter Sermspiegel von Prolaktin, Wachstumshormon and Gonadotropinen bei Frauen mit chronischer Urämie. *Zeitschrift für die Gesamte Innere Medizin und Ihre Grenzgebiete* **43**, 542–543.

Rudolf, K., Kunkel, S., Rudolf, H., Falkenhagen, D., and Rüting, M. (1988). Basal and gonadotropin releasing hormone-stimulated gonadotropin secretion in patients with chronic uraemia. *Zentralblatt für Gynäkologie* **110**, 683–688.

Ruilope, L. *et al.* (1985). Influence of lisuride, a dopaminergic agonist, on the sexual function of male patients with chronic renal failure. *American Journal of Kidney Diseases* **5**, 182–185.

Saenz de Tejada, I., Emmick, J., Anglin, G., Fredlund, P., and Pullman, W. (2001). The effect of as-needed tadalafil (IC351) treatment of erectile dysfunction in men with diabetes. *International Journal of Impotence Research* **13**, A128.

Saenz de Tejada, I. *et al.* (1988). Cholinergic neurotransmission in human corpus cavernosum. I. Responses of isolated tissue. *American Journal of Physiology* **254**, H459–H467.

Sale, D. and Cameron, J. S. (1974). Priapism during regular dialysis. *Nephron* **ii**, 1567–1568.

Sancho-Tello, M. and Terranova, P. F. (1991). Involvement of protein kinase in regulating tumor necrosis factor alpha-stimulated progesterone production in rat preovulatory follicles *in vitro*. *Endocrinology* **128** (3), 1223–1228.

Sar, M. and Stumpf, W. E. (1977). Distribution of androgen target cells in rat forebrain and pituitary after (3H)-dihydotestosterone administration. *Journal of Steroid Biochemistry* **8**, 1131–1135.

Sasagawa, I., Tateno, T., Suzuki, Y., Yazawa, H., Ichiyanagi, O., Nakada, T., and Miura, H. (1998). Circulating levels of inhibin in hemodialysis males. *Archives of Andrology* **41**, 167–171.

Sawin, C. T., Longcope, C., Schmitt, G. W., and Ryan, R. J. (1973). Blood levels of gonadotropins and gonadal hormones in gynecomastia associated with chronic haemodialysis. *Journal of Clinical Endocrinology and Metabolism* **36**, 988–990.

Schaefer, R. M., Kokot, F., Kürner, B., Zech, M., and Heidland, A. (1988). Normalization of elevated prolactin levels in hemodialysis patients on erythropoietin. *Nephron* **50**, 400–401.

Schaefer, F., Stanhope, R., Scheil, H., Schönberg, D., Preece, M. A., and Schärer, K. (1989a). Pulsatile gonadotropin secretion in pubertal children with chronic renal railure. *Acta Endocrinologica* **120**, 14–19.

Schaefer R. M., Kokot, F., Wernze, H., Geiger, H., and Heideland, A. (1989b). Improved sexual function in hemodialysis patients on recombinant erythropoietin: a possible role for prolactin. *Clinical Nephrology* **31** (1), 1–5.

Schaefer, F., Daschner, M., Veldhuis, J. D., Oh, J., Qadri, F., and Schärer, K. (1994a). *In vivo* alterations in the gonadotropin-releasing hormone pulse generator and the secretion and clearance of luteinizing hormone in the uraemic castrate rat. *Neuroendocrinology* **59**, 285–296.

Schaefer, F., Veldhuis, J. D., Robertson, W. R., Dunger, D., Schärer, K., and The Cooperative Study Group on Pubertal Development in Chronic Renal Failure (1994b). Immunoreactive and bioactive luteinizing hormone in pubertal patients with chronic renal failure. *Kidney International* **45**, 1465–1476.

Schaefer, F., van Kaick, B., Veldhuis, J. D., Stein, G., Schärer, K., Robertson, W. R., and Ritz, E. (1994c). Changes in the kinetics and biopotency of luteinizing hormone in hemodialyzed men during treatment with recombinant human erythropoietin. *Journal of the American Society of Nephrology* **5**, 1208–1215.

Schaefer, F., Vogel, M., Kerkhoff, G., Woitzik, J., Daschner, M., and Mehls, O. (2001). Experimental uraemia affects hypothalamic amino acid neurotransmitter milieu. *Journal of the American Society of Nephrology* **12** (6), 1218–1227.

Schenker, J. G., Meirow, D., and Schenker, E. (1992). Stress and human reproduction. *European Journal of Obstetrics, Gynecology, and Reproductive Biology* **45** (1), 1–8.

Schmitz, O. and Moller, J. (1983). Impaired prolactin response to arginine infusion and insulin hypoglycemia in chronic renal failure. *Acta Endocrinologica* **102**, 486–491.

Sell, D. R. and Monnier, V. M. (1990). End-stage renal disease and diabetes catalyze the formation of pentose derived cross-link from aging human collagen. *Journal of Clinical Investigation* **85**, 380–384.

Siegel, R. (2001). Timing of sildenafil therapy in dialysis patients. *Nephrology, Dialysis, Transplantation* **16**, 1719–1730.

Slob, A. K., Blom, J. H. M., and van der Werf ten Bosch, J. J. (1990). Erection problems in medical practice: differential diagnosis with relatively simple method. *Journal of Urology* **143**, 46–50.

Smith, C. R., Butler, J., Iggo, N., and Norman, M. R. (1989). Serum prolactin in uraemia correlation between bioactivity and activity in two immuno-assays. *Acta Endocrinologica* **120**, 295–300.

Solders, G. (1986). Autonomic function test in healthy controls and in terminal uraemia. *Acta Neurologica Scandinavica* **73**, 638–642.

Soules, M. R., Steiner, R. A., Clifton, D. K., Cohen, N. L., Aksel, S., and Bremner, W. J. (1984). Progesterone modulation of pulsatile luteinizing hormone secretion in normal women. *Journal of Clinical Endocrinology and Metabolism* **58**, 378–383.

Spark, R. E. *et al.* (1982). Hyperprolactinemia in males with and without pituitary macroadenomas. *Lancet* **ii**, 129–131.

Steffensen, G. and Aunsholt, N. A. (1993). Does erythropoietin cause hormonal changes in haemodialysis patients? *Nephrology, Dialysis, Transplantation* **8** (11), 1215–1218.

Stewart-Bentley, M., Gans, D., and Horton, R. (1974). Regulation of gonadal function in uraemia. *Metabolism* **23**, 1065–1072.

Stuart, R. C. (1984). Prevalence and pathogenesis of impotence in one hundred uraemic men. *Uraemia Investigation* **8**, 89–92.

Swamy, A. P., Woolf, P. D., and Cestero, R. V. M. (1979). Hypothalmic pituitary-ovarian axis in uraemic women. *Journal of Laboratory and Clinical Medicine* **93**, 1066–1072.

Talbot, J. A., Rodger, R. S., and Robertson, W. R. (1990). Pulsatile bioactive luteinizing hormone secretion in men with chronic renal failure and following renal transplantation. *Nephron* **56**, 66–72.

Tarcan, T., Azadzoi, K. M., Siroky, M. B., Goldstein, I., and Krane, R. J. (1998). Age-related erectile and voiding dysfunction: the role of arterial insuffi-ciency. *British Journal of Urology* **82** (Suppl. 1), 26–33.

Tay, C. C., Glasier, A. F., Illingworth, P. J., and Baird, D. T. (1993). Abnormal twenty-four hour pattern of pulsatile luteinizing hormone secretion and the response to naloxone in women with hyperprolactinaemic amenorrhoea. *Clinical Endocrinology (Oxford)* **39**, 599–606.

Tharandt, L. *et al.* (1980). Effects of prolactin suppression on hypogonadism in patients on maintenance hemodialysis. *Proceedings of the European Dialysis and Transplantation Association* **17**, 323–327.

Thaysen, J. H., Olgaard, K., and Jensen, H. G. (1975). Ovarian cysts in women on chronic intermittent haemodialysis. *Acta Medica Scandinavica* **197**, 433–437.

Toorians, A. W. F. T. *et al.* (1997). Chronic renal failure and sexual function-ing: clinical status versus objectively assessed sexual response. *Nephrology, Dialysis, Transplantation* **12**, 2654–2663.

Truss, M. C., Djamilian, M. H., Tan, H.-K., Hinrichs, H., Feistner, H., Stief, Ch. G., and Jonas, U. (1993). Single potential analysis of cavernous electrical activity. *European Urology* **24**, 358–365.

Türk, S. *et al.* (2001). Erectile dysfunction and the effects of sildenafil treatment in patients on heamodialysis and continuous ambulatory peritoneal dia-lysis. *Nephrology, Dialysis, Transplantation* **16**, 1818–1822.

Van Coevorden, A., Stolear, J. C., Dhaene, M., van Herweghem, J. L., and Mockel, J. (1986). Effect of chronic oral testosterone undecanoate admin-istration on the pituitary–testicular axes of hemodialyzed male patients. *Clinical Nephrology* **26** (1), 48–54.

Van Coevorden, A., Stolear, J.-C., Dhaene, M., van Herweghem, J.-L., and Mockel, J. (1988). Effect of chronic oral testosterone on the pituitary–testicular axes of hemodialyzed male patients. *Journal of Clinical Nephrology* **26**, 48–54.

Van der Poll, T., Romijn, J. A., Endert, E., and Sauerwein, H. P. (1993). Effects of tumor on the hypothalamic-pituitary-testicular axis in healthy men. *Metabolism* **42** (39), 303–307.

Van Kammen, E., Thijssen, J. H. H., and Schwarz, F. (1978). Sex hormones in male patients with chronic renal failure. 1. The production of testosterone and of androstenedione. *Clinical Endocrinology* **8**, 7–12.

Veldhuis, J. D., Wilkowski, M. J., Zwart, A. D., Urban, R. J., Lizarralde, G., Iranmanesh, A., and Bolton, W. K. (1993). Evidence for attention of hypo-thalamine gonadotropin-releasing hormone (GnRH) impulse strength with preservation of GnRH pulse frequency in men with chronic renal fail-ure. *Journal of Clinical Endocrinology and Metabolism* **76**, 648–654.

Verbeelen, D., Vanhaelst, L., van Steirteghem, A. C., and Sennesael, J. (1983). Effect of 1,25-dihydroxyvitamin D3 on plasma proteins in patients with renal failure on regular dialysis treatment. *Journal of Endocrinological Investigation* **6**, 359–362.

Verhelst, J., Beckcers Al., and Abs, R. (1995). The effect of naloxone and metoclopramide on the secretion of luteinizing hormone in a hyperpro-lactinemic hypogonadotropic postmenopausal woman. *Fertility and Sterility* **64**, 969–971.

Virag, R. (1984). Impotence: a new field in angiology. *International Angiology* **13**, 217.

Virag, R., Bouilly, R., and Frydman, D. (1985). Is impotence an arterial disorder? *Lancet* **i**, 181–184.

Virag, R., Shourky, K., Floresco, F., Nollet, F., and Greco, E. (1991). Intracaver-nous self-injection of vasoactive drugs in the treatment of impotence: 8-year experience with 615 cases. *Journal of Urology* **145**, 287–293.

Vircburger, M. L., Prelevic, G. M., Peric, L. A., Knezevic, J., and Djukanovic, L. (1985). Testosterone levels after bromocriptine treatment in patients under-going long-term hemodialysis. *Journal of Andrology* **6**, 113–116.

Vollrath, P. *et al.* (1976). Sexualverhalten hämodialysierter Patienten. *Innere Medizin* **3**, 349–356.

Waehrens, J. and Gerlach, J. (1981). Bromocriptine and imipraine in endogen-ous depression. *Journal of Affective Disorders* **3**, 193–202.

Wams, T. J. Diethylhexylphthalate as an environmental contaminant review. In *Science of the Total Environment* (ed. E. J. Hamilton and J. O. Nriagu), pp. 1–16. Amsterdam: Elsevier Science, 1987.

Wang, C.-J., Wu, C.-C., Hunag, C.-H., and Chiang, C.-P. (1992). A comparat-ive study with intracavernous injection of prostaglandin E1 versus papaverine for the diagnostic assessment of erectile impotence. *Journal of Medical Science* **8**, 585–590.

Wark, J. D. Regulation by 1,25-dihydroxyvitamin D3 (1,25(OH)$_2$D3) of specific gene expression in GH pituitary cells. In *Vitamin D, A Chemical, Biochemical and Clinical Update* (ed. A. W. Norman, K. Schaefer, H. G. Grigolet, and D. V. Herrath), pp. 901–902. Berlin: Walter de Gruyter, 1985.

Wass, V. J., Wass, J. A., Rees, L., Edwards, C. R. W., and Ogg, C. S. (1979). Sex hormone changes underlying menstrual disturbances on hemodia-lysis. *Proceedings of the European Dialysis and Transplantation Association* **15**, 178–186.

Weisinger, J. R. *et al.* (2000). Role of persistent amenorrhea in bone mineral metabolism of young hemodialyzed women. *Kidney International* **58**, 331–335.

Winters, S. J. and Troen, P. (1984). Altered pulsatile secretion of luteinising hormone in hypogonadal men with hyperprolactinemia. *Clinical Endocrinology* **21**, 257–263.

Witherington, R. (1990). External penile appliances for management of impot-ence. *Seminars in Urology* **8**, 124–128.

Wu, S. C., Lin, S. L., and Jeng, F. R. (2001). Influence of erythropoietin treat-ment on gonadotropic hormone levels and sexual function in male uremic patients. *Scandinavian Journal of Urology and Nephrology* **35**, 136–140.

Yamaguchi, M., Koike, K., Yoshimoto, Y., Ikegami, H., Miyake, A., and Tanizawa, O. (1991). Effect of TNF-alpha on prolactin secretion from rat pituitary and dopamine release from the hypothalamus. Comparison with the effect of interleukin-1 beta. *Endocrinology Japan* **38** (4), 357–361.

Yen, S. S. (1980). The polycystic ovary syndrome. *Clinical Endocrinology* **12**, 177–207.

Zadeh, J. A., Koutsaimanis, K. G., Roberts, A. P., Curtis, J. R., and Daly, J. R. (1975). The effect of maintenance haemodialysis and renal transplanta-tion on the plasma testosterone levels of male patients in chronic renal failure. *Acta Endocrinologica* **80**, 577–582.

Zorgniotti, A. W. and Lefleur, R. S. (1985). Autoinjection of the corpus caver-nosum with a weather active drug combination for vasculogenic impotence. *Journal of Urology* **133**, 39–42.

Zucchelli, P., Turani, A., Zuccala, A., Santoro, A., Degli Esposti, E., and Chiarini, C. (1985). Dysfunction of the autonomic nervous system in patients with end-stage renal failure. *Contributions to Nephrology* **45**, 69–81.

11.3.4 Hypertension

Ralf Dikow, Christoph Wanner, and Eberhard Ritz

Why is blood pressure important for the clinical nephrologist?

In patients with renal disease blood pressure increases very early, first within the range of normotensive values. The increase in blood pressure starts even before the glomerular filtration rate (GFR) decreases. In later stages frank hypertension is extremely common. It is found in more than 90 per cent of patients with terminal renal failure requiring renal replacement therapy. Hypertension is an important problem for the nephrologist because it has a major impact both on progression of renal failure and on cardiovascular risk, that is, left ventricular hypertrophy, myocardial infarction, and congestive heart failure.

The problem is so important because today hypertension is an eminently treatable condition. Correct blood pressure management requires correct assessment of blood pressure, selection of the appropriate antihypertensive agents, and monitoring of outcome. The two outcome measures are blood pressure values and urinary protein excretion.

To interfere with progression of renal failure, reduction of blood pressure is the single most important intervention. It is for this reason that clinical nephrologists should be well informed about the points covered in this chapter.

Investigations (see also Table 1)

Blood pressure measurements

Casual blood pressure measurements should be taken both in the supine and upright positions to identify orthostatic hypotension, which is often the consequence of overenthusiastic diuretic treatment or ultrafiltration. In dialysed patients, blood pressure must obviously be assisted both pre- and post-dialysis.

In dialysed patients, the blood pressure measurements should be taken in the non-fistula bearing arm. If blood pressure has to be measured in the lower limb, it is important to remember that it is higher in the leg. If the patient has anaemia, Korotkow-Phase V-values are extremely low and phase IV values (muffling) must be taken to define the diastolic blood pressure value.

In cases of severe vascular sclerosis, sphygmomanometric measurements may yield spuriously high values because excessive cuff pressure is required to compress the stiffened artery (so-called pseudohypertension). This phenomenon is not uncommon in elderly diabetic patients as a result of arterial calcification or vascular sclerosis. It has been suggested that Osler's sign, that is, palpable radial arteries even when the cuff pressure has been increased above the systolic blood pressure, is a reliable indicator of pseudohypertension (Messerli 1986). In our experience, however, this sign is unreliable.

Blood pressure of the right and left arm should be compared, particularly in patients with arterio-occlusive disease and in elderly diabetic patients, in order to recognize stenosis of the upper arm arteries at their origin in the aortic arc.

Marked variability and absence of a nocturnal decline of blood pressure are common in renal patients. Twenty-four hour ambulatory blood pressure monitoring (ABPM) may be necessary to assess nocturnal blood pressure and to judge the adequacy of blood pressure control. An elevated nocturnal pressure or even an attenuated nocturnal decline of blood pressure, is a predictor of the onset of nephropathy in diabetics (Lurbe *et al.* 2002). It also predicts a high rate of progression of renal failure (Goldsmith *et al.* 1997; Ritz *et al.* 2001) and is a powerful predictor of death in diabetic and non-diabetic patients (Nakano *et al.* 1998; Schernthaner *et al.* 1999).

Funduscopy

The main purposes of funduscopy is to assess the severity of arteriolar wall thickening and wall irregularity and to recognize the features of malignant hypertension, that is, striated haemorrhage, cotton wool exudates, and swelling of the papilla. In contrast to punctate haemorrhage, striated haemorrhage indicates that the bleeding had occurred in the innermost layer of the retina. Striation indicates that extravasated blood followed the direction of the optic neurons. Cotton wool exudates represent retinal microinfarcts, and swelling of the papilla reflects ischaemic injury to the optic nerve.

Cardiological assessment

Since in the renal patient, blood pressure tends to be volume-dependent, circulatory congestion must be excluded by thoracic radiography, echocardiography, and sonography of the retrohepatic segment of the inferior vena cava (measurement of diameter and inspiratory collapse). Peripheral oedema is unreliable as an index of overhydration.

In our view, full cardiological assessment is an essential component of the initial examination of the hypertensive patient with chronic renal disease. The main features to look for are left ventricular hypertrophy

---

Table 1 Investigation of the hypertensive patient with renal disease

Blood pressure measurement
Casual blood pressure (in the dialysed patient pre- and post-dialysis)
Supine
Upright
Osler's sign (pseudohypertension)
Ambulatory 24-h blood pressure
Fundoscopy
Physical examination of the heart and peripheral arteries
Thoracic radiography (heart size, pulmonary congestion)
ECG (electric axis, Sokolof index, strain pattern, QT duration)
Echocardiography (M-mode, two-dimensional, and Doppler)
Left ventricular hypertrophy
Regional contraction abnormalities (usually ischaemic heart disease)
Valvular stenosis
Valvular incompetence; relative, i.e. from overhydration, or absolute
Disturbed left ventricular compliance (transmitral Doppler)
Sonography of vena cava (diameter and inspiratory collapse to assess vascular filling)
Evaluation of peripheral vessels
Abdominal aorta (sonography or CT; calcified plaques and aneurysm formation)
Carotid/limb (B image (wall thickness, plaques), duplex Doppler (turbulence, stenosis), radiography (calcification of intima plaques or media)

(asymmetric or symmetric, concentric or eccentric), assessment of systolic pumping function (ejection fraction, circumferential fibre shortening), left ventricular compliance (transmitral inflow pattern using echo-Doppler, particularly the E/A-ratio i.e. early diastolic inflow/atrial contraction), regional contraction abnormalities (as potential indicators of ischaemia), and valvular disease. Relative aortic and mitral incompetence is not infrequent in patients with circulatory congestion. Auscultation may be problematic if functional murmurs (hypervolaemia) or continuous venous hums (anaemia and propagated murmurs from the av-fistula) are heard. The functional importance of valvular regurgitation can only be fully assessed after overhydration has been corrected. A particularly difficult problem is the assessment of clinically silent calcifying aortic stenosis (Raine 1994).

When one is faced with a patient showing signs of circulatory congestion, it is often difficult to decide whether one is dealing with volume expansion, impaired cardiac pumping function, or a combination of both. Signs of systolic pumping dysfunction, for example, low ejection fraction or regional contraction abnormalities, are helpful pointers to congestive heart failure.

Nevertheless it is often wise to reserve final judgement until overhydration has been reversed by vigorous diuretic treatment or ultrafiltration. This manoeuvre often causes dramatic reversal of systolic dysfunction.

Evaluation of peripheral vessels

It is important to recognize vascular problems, such as aneurysms of the abdominal aorta, ischaemic nephropathy, advanced calcification and plaque-formation of the iliac arteries (these may also be a potential impediment to renal transplantation) and stenosis of carotid arteries and limbs. These investigations should be done before vigorous lowering of blood pressure is attempted, since blood pressure lowering is hazardous if stenosing lesions of carotid or peripheral arteries are present. The same is true for vigorous ultrafiltration on dialysis, which may lead to vascular catastrophes, for example, amaurosis from optic nerve ischaemia or non-thrombotic mesenteric artery infarction (Zeier et al. 1995). Full assessment of the vascular status includes imaging of carotid artery wall with measurement of wall thickness and search for plaques (B-image and two-dimensional image), assessment of turbulent flow in the carotid and leg arteries (Duplex Doppler), and measurement of pressure in the leg arteries (although this may yield artefacts in the presence of vascular calcification).

If doubts remain, angiography should be performed, preferably magnetic resonance angiography to avoid contrast media and the resulting risk to residual renal function. This consideration is particularly persistent in the patient who is not dialysis dependent and in whom angiography of the coronary or peripheral arteries is planned. The risk can be reduced by selection of a low dosage of radiocontrast medium, adequate hydration, and temporary withdrawal of diuretics [and possibly of angiotensin-converting enzyme (ACE) inhibitors as well].

Pathogenesis of renoparenchymal hypertension

Based upon experimental evidence, Guyton (1987) proposed the hypothesis that whenever blood pressure increases for prolonged periods, the mechanism which finally maintains elevated blood pressure is a shift to the right of the blood pressure/natriuresis relationship so that higher perfusion pressure is required to eliminate the daily sodium load via the kidney. This does not imply that all forms of hypertension are caused by renal disease, but it implies that a renal functional

abnormality is a *sine-qua-non* for the development and persistance of hypertension (Adamczak et al. 2002).

The important role of the kidney in the induction and maintenance of hypertension is illustrated by experimental studies which showed that 'blood pressure goes with the kidney'. As shown in Fig. 1, transplantation of the kidney taken from a genetically hypertension prone donor rat causes a progressive increase of blood pressure in a recipient which had been genetically manipulated to prevent rejection of the graft (Rettig et al. 1990). There is also analogous evidence in humans. Patients who had become dialysis dependent because of renal injury became normotensive after they had received a well-functioning kidney of a normotensive donor (Curtis et al. 1983).

In patients with renal disease, it had been accepted for a long time that renal damage is the cause of hypertension. But the relation between renal disease and hypertension is somewhat more complex. There is increasing evidence that a genetic predisposition to hypertension increases also the risk to develop renal disease. This has for instance been shown in patients with glomerulonephritis (Schmid et al. 1990a,b); blood pressure values were higher in the parents of patients with glomerulonephritis than in parents of matched controls. The same is true for diabetic nephropathy: the blood pressure values were higher in parents of type 1 diabetic patients compared to parents of patients without nephropathy (Fagerudd et al. 1998). Blood pressure values were also higher in offspring of parents with type 2 diabetes and nephropathy compared with offspring of diabetic parents without nephropathy (Strojek et al. 1997). The latter is shown in Table 2.

In the past it had been thought that impaired renal function, reflected by a decrease in GFR, was a *sine-que-non* condition for the increase in blood pressure. This is definitely not the case. In children with a nephrotic syndrome, Küster et al. (1990), found that the blood pressure values remained within the range of normotension, but nevertheless were systematically higher during the nephrotic episode than after remission of the disease. That a reduction of whole kidney GFR is not a prerequisite for an increase in blood pressure was also shown by Stefanski et al. (1996) in patients with mesangial IgA-glomerulonephritis and normal inulin clearance (Table 3).

In the past it had been thought that hypertension caused renal damage only when it induced arteriolonecrosis resulting in target organ ischaemia ('malignant hypertension'), but not when it caused

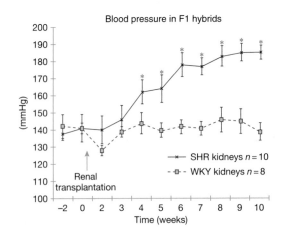

Fig. 1 Development of progressive hypertension after transplantation of a kidney from an SHR, but not WKY rat in F1 hybrids which are unable to launch a rejection reaction (courtesy Dr Rettig, Greifswald, Germany).

hyalinosis and intimal thickening of arterioles (arteriolohyalinosis, so-called 'benign hypertension'). There is no doubt that in malignant hypertension, that is, accelerated hypertension with arteriolonecrosis, renal function deteriorates rapidly (Byrom 1974). Indeed renal failure was a frequent cause of death in such patients before antihypertensive treatment had become available. There is increasing evidence, however, that even in the absence of malignant hypertension, renal failure may develop in hypertensive patients without primary renal disease. This is a slow process, however, requiring decades to develop. Decades ago Perera (1955) had noted that during long-term follow-up of patients with essential hypertension, renal failure developed in about 20 per cent. More recently, Klag *et al.* (1996) as well as Perry *et al.* (1995) noted a relation between baseline blood pressure and endstage renal disease in patients without *a priori* evidence of renal disease. The age-dependent decrease in GFR is to a large extent due to high blood pressure (Fliser *et al.* 1997a,b). Since hypertension is more prevalent with advancing age, hypertension explains to a large extent the progressively higher incidence of terminal renal failure with increasing age (Feest *et al.* 1990). It also explains why renal failure may be found in some elderly hypertensive individuals without primal renal disease. In such individuals histology shows only uncharacteristic nephrosclerosis. In countries where renal biopsies are performed only in a minority of patients, a highly inflated rate of 'hypertensive nephropathy' has been reported as the cause of endstage renal failure, but there is no doubt that this condition does occur, particularly in the elderly and in severely hypertensive patients.

The nephrologist who wishes to treat hypertension must know the pathomechanisms underlying the hypertension of patients with renal failure in order to select the appropriate medication. The most relevant pathomechanisms are summarized in Table 4 and are discussed in the following paragraph.

Table 2 Blood pressure and urinary albumin excretion in offspring of parents with type 2 diabetes according to absence or presence of diabetic nephropathy in the parents

	Parents type 2 diabetes	
	Without nephropathy offspring ($n = 30$)	With nephropathy offspring ($n = 26$)
Ambulatory blood pressure (mmHg systolic)	117 ± 12.9	125 ± 16.9
Albumin excretion rate (μg ml^{-1})	4.8 (0.36–17.5)	7.8 (1.04–19.0)
Increase in urinary albumin after ergonometry	6.3-fold (1.5–231)	16-fold (1.2–236)

Salt/volume retention

The blood pressure of patients with chronic renal disease is salt-sensitive. As pointed out above, Guyton (1987) proposed that a disturbance of the blood pressure/natriuresis relationship ('renal function curve') is largely responsible for the blood pressure elevation when renal function is impaired. According to this concept, the 'gain' of the blood pressure/natriuresis relationship is so high that it overrides all other regulatory systems.

Consequently, whatever the primary pathogenesis, the ultimate determinant of blood pressure is resetting of the renal handling of sodium. This view does not imply that hypertension is a renal disease, but it indicates that a renal functional abnormality, that is, a disturbed blood pressure/natriuresis relationship, is a prerequisite for the development of any type of hypertension.

The exchangeable sodium is increased very early in renal disease. Table 5 shows, for instance, that the exchangeable sodium is increased in young patients with autosomal dominant polycystic kidney disease (ADPKD) although their GFR is still normal (Harrap *et al.* 1991). A state of sodium retention is also suggested by the observation that compared to healthy controls they have higher concentrations of atrial natriuretic factor (ANF) as a consequence of the distension of the atrium. This is seen both on low and high salt intake. The ANF response to changes in sodium intake is greater than in controls (Schmid *et al.* 1990a,b).

There is also evidence in patients with chronic kidney disease, that hypertension is causally related to sodium chloride intake and the resulting volume expansion. Koomans *et al.* (1986) showed that mean arterial blood pressure (MAP) (Fig. 2a) and blood volume (Fig. 2b) increase in parallel with progressive expansion of the extracellular fluid space. Sodium retention and hypervolaemia cannot fully explain hypertension, however. For instance in pregnancy there is marked sodium retention, yet blood pressure does not increase. Sodium retention increases blood pressure only when peripheral vascular resistance is inappropriately high. This explains the finding illustrated in Fig. 3. In renal patients, an increase in sodium intake causes a consistent and marked increase in MAP. In contrast, in healthy controls an even more pronounced increase of sodium intake fails to affect MAP. This observation illustrates that renal patients are particularly susceptible to the hypertensinogenic effect of sodium loading and hypervolaemia.

The blood pressure response to an increased intake of sodium chloride follows a characteristic time course. As illustrated schematically in Fig. 4, when the intake of sodium elevation is increased, sodium retention causes hypervolaemia and this increases cardiac output. Because of an acute compensatory decrease in vascular resistance (MacAllister and Vallance 1996), blood pressure changes only modestly, if at all. In the long run, however, vascular resistance increases progressively as a result of a poorly understood process, so-called 'autoregulation', that is, a homeostatically useful response to keep tissue

Table 3 Blood pressure status in patients with IgA-glomerulonephritis and normal inulin clearance (after Stefanski *et al.* 1997)

	Casual BP (mmHg)		24-h BP		Day-time BP		Night-time BP	
	Systolic	Diastolic	Systolic	Diastolic	Systolic	Diastolic	Systolic	Diastolic
Glomerulonephritis ($n = 20$)	125 (110–140)	80 (70–90)	124.5 (107–135)	76.5 (69–84)	129 (107–141)	82 (73–88)	111 (97–129)	64.8 (56.5–72)
Matched controls ($n = 20$)	120 (105–130)	72.5 (60–85)	114.5 (106–135)	70.5 (62–79)	119 (108–144)	75 (66–87)	103 (91–117)	58 (48–70)
p	0.04	0.04	0.007	0.0006	0.012	0.003	0.003	0.001

perfusion constant. The underlying mechanisms are complex and comprise blood flow autoregulation independent of reflex-control (Baylis-effect), endothelium-independent pressure-dependent myogenic regulation and opening of non-specific cation-channels. The delayed blood pressure response to hypervolaemia is important to explain the so-called 'lag phenomenon', that is, the observation that it takes several weeks before hypervolaemia causes hypertension in dialysis patients (Charra *et al.* 1998a,b).

Table 4 also lists some additional factors, which underly the inappropriately elevated peripheral vascular resistance in patients with chronic kidney disease, for example, inappropriate activity of the

Table 4 Factors involved in the genesis of hypertension in chronic renal disease

Salt/volume retention (shifted pressure–natriuresis relationship)

Inappropriate activity of the renin–angiotensin system

Activation of the sympathetic nerve system

Inhibition of NO-synthase; ADMA; scavengering of NO by reactive oxygen species

Loss of renal vasodepressor factors ('medullipin')?

Circulating inhibitors of Na^+,K^+-ATPase?

Increased intracellular Ca^{2+}?

Increased endothelin activity?

Other

Table 5 Findings relevant to blood pressure regulation in young patients with autosomal dominant kidney disease

	Unaffected (n = 20)	Affected (n = 19)	p-value
Systolic blood pressure (mmHg)	115 (±11)	123 (±13)	<0.02
RPF (ml/min/1.73 m²)	605 (±118)	532 (±86)	<0.05
Exchangeable sodium (mmol/kg)	38 (±4)	41 (±2)	<0.05
Plasma volume (ml/kg)	40 (±9)	42 (±5)	NS
Active plasma renin (μU/ml)	14 (±11)	26 (±15)	<0.05

renin–angiotensin system (RAS), activation of the sympathetic nerve system, and impaired vasodilatation. Apart from these functional factors, structural causes such as wall-thickening of resistance vessels also help to maintain the elevated peripheral vascular resistance (Amman *et al.* 1994).

Inappropriate activity of the renin–angiotensin system

Inappropriate activity of the RAS is a hallmark of chronic renal failure. At baseline, plasma renin activity (PRA) is increased in relation to elevated blood pressure and high exchangeable sodium, both of which should decrease PRA. PRA is also not adequately suppressed in response to sodium loads (Schalekamp *et al.* 1973). Inappropriate PRA is demonstrable very early in renal disease. As illustrated in Fig. 5 postcaptopril PRA is higher in patients with ADPKD compared to blood-pressure-matched patients with essential hypertension (Chapman *et al.* 1990). Table 5 illustrates increased basal PRA despite increased exchangeable sodium in normotensive patients with ADPKD (Harrap *et al.* 1991). Why is the renin system activated? Guyton (1987) postulated that renin is continuously released from the juxtaglomerular apparatus in patchy areas of renal ischaemia. Here the lumen of preglomerular vessels is reduced so that the baroreceptor mechanism is 'fooled', since the baroreceptor measures a low perfusion pressure despite a high systemic pressure. This reproduces in some nephrons the situation which entire kidney experiences in the two-kidney model of Goldblatt hypertension. As a result, the non-ischaemic regions of the kidney are exposed to a combination of high pressure and high circulating renin.

Ectopic synthesis of renin outside the juxtaglomerular apparatus has also been documented for instance in ADPKD (Zeier *et al.* 1992). Finally, in the model of the subtotally nephrectomized rat, increased synthesis of angiotensinogen and ANG II have been documented in the activated proximal tubular endothelial cells (it).

Navar *et al.* (1999) and Kobori *et al.* (2002) showed that activation of the local RAS outside the juxtaglomerular apparatus caused high ANG II-concentrations in the interstitial and in the tubular fluid. The urinary excretion of angiotensinogen was shown to reflect the activity of the intrarenal RAS. In the tubular fluid, ANG II is produced from angiotensinogen via ACE. ANG II in the tubular fluid increases sodium reabsorption in the collecting duct by activating the Na-channel (ENaC). It is currently unresolved whether aldosterone further contributes to sodium retention and hypertension in renal disease, although recent evidence very clearly documents that it plays an important role in progression (Hostetter *et al.* 2001; Stier *et al.* 2002).

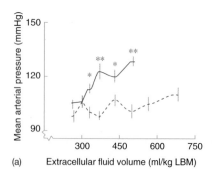

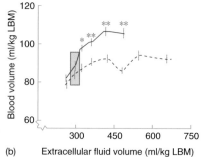

Fig. 2 Dependence of extracellular fluid volume (per kg lean body mass) on (a) mean arterial pressure and (b) blood volume in patients with nephrotic syndrome (dotted curve) and renal failure (solid curve). Note the marked increase of blood pressure in patients with renal failure compared with those with nephrotic syndrome.

In renal failure, not only the plasma renin system, but also the tissue renin systems are activated as documented in the perfused hindlimb preparation of the subtotally nephrectomized rat (Kuczera *et al.* 1991). Prior to the availability of modern antihypertensive agents, 'resistant'

hypertension, that is, resistant to volume subtraction by ultrafiltration and characterized by pronounced activation of the RAS, was found in 5–10 per cent of dialysis patients. In these patients, blood pressure was promptly normalized by bilateral nephrectomy (Vertes *et al.* 1969).

The role of activation of the sympathetic nerve system

It has been shown a long time ago that pharmacological blockade of the autonomous nerve system (McGrath *et al.* 1977; Schohn *et al.* 1985) reduces the blood pressure in patients with chronic kidney disease. Meanwhile, sympathetic overactivity has been well documented using microneurography as the methodological gold-standard (Converse *et al.* 1992; Ligtenberg *et al.* 1999). Such overactivity does not occur in patients with bilateral nephrectomy. This observation suggests that the kidney is the source of excitatory signals and this concept is also supported by experimental studies. Bigazzi *et al.* (1994) found high noradrenaline turnover in the posterior hypothalamic nuclei and locus coeruleus of subtotally nephrectomized rats. This was abrogated by section of the dorsal roots, that is, deafferentiation and this also blunted the increase of blood pressure (Fig. 6) (Campese and Kojosov 1995). Sympathetic overactivity is important not only in the genesis of hypertension, but also as a factor contributing progression of renal disease (Amann *et al.* 2000a,b) and to cardiac problems, particularly arrhythmia (Zuanetti *et al.* 1997).

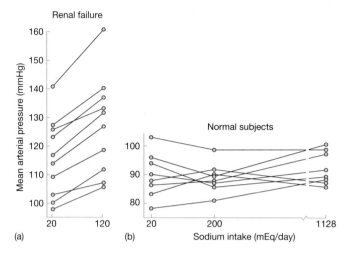

Fig. 3 Mean arterial pressure on low (20 mmol/day) and high (120, 200, and 1128 mmol/day) sodium intake in (a) patients with renal failure and (b) normal subjects. Note the consistent increase in mean arterial pressure in patients with renal failure and the absence of change in normal subjects even at extremes of sodium intake.

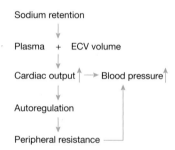

Fig. 4 The interaction of salt retention, extracellular volume expansion and the resulting increase in blood pressure (after Guyton 1987).

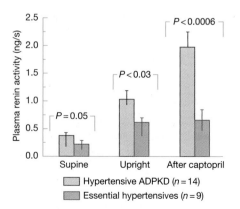

Fig. 5 Comparison of plasma renin activity under baseline conditions and after stimulatory manoeuvres in hypertensive patients with autosomal dominant polycystic kidney disease and in blood-pressure-matched patients with essential hypertension (after Chapman *et al.* 1990).

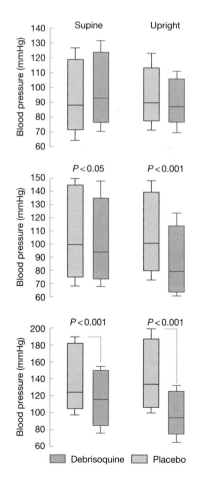

Fig. 6 Effect of debrisoquine and placebo on supine and upright blood pressure in controls and in normotensive or hypertensive dialysis patients (after Schohn *et al.* 1985).

Endothelial-cell-dependent vasodilatation

In patients with chronic kidney disease, flow-dependent vasodilatation is impaired. This type of vasodilatation is dependent on the bioavailability of nitric oxide (NO). There are indications that the generation of NO is diminished in chronic kidney disease (Schmidt and Baylis 2000), possibly because synthesis via NO-synthase is inhibited by circulating asymmetric dimethyl-L-arginine (ADMA) (Kielstein et al. 2002). In addition, because of oxidative stress, the bioavailability of NO is reduced, since NO is scavenged by reactive oxygen species. The importance of this mechanism is illustrated by the fact that a cell permeable analogue of superoxide dismutase, tempol, reduces elevated blood pressure in animals with subtotal nephrectomy (Schnackenberg et al. 1998; Vaziri et al. 1998; Hasdan et al. 2002).

Reduced aortic compliance

The hypertension of patients with chronic kidney disease is characterized by an abnormal profile of pulse pressure (Fig. 7). London et al. (1990, 1992) and Barenbrock et al. (1994) showed that the compliance of elastic arteries is impaired increasing pulse wave velocity and causing earlier return of the reflected wave. In dialysed patients, pulse wave velocity is a major determinant of left ventricular hypertrophy and a major predictor of cardiovascular death (Guerin et al. 2001). How does an altered pulse profile explain the high cardiovascular risk in chronic kidney disease? Figure 7 illustrates that if the aortic elasticity is diminished in renal patients, the blood pressure amplitude will increase. As a consequence, the peak systolic pressure will be increased and the trough diastolic pressure will be decreased. This has the twin adverse consequences that the left ventricular stroke work index is increased while at the same time the coronary perfusion is decreased. This is the obvious result of the fact that perfusion of the coronary arteries occurs only during diastole and is reduced when the diastolic pressure in the aorta is low. This problem is rendered even worse, since the end-diastolic pressure of the non-compliant left ventricles is increased so that the trans-coronary pressure gradient is further reduced.

As a consequence, because of the higher stroke work, oxygen demand is increased while oxygen supply is decreased. The aortic compliance becomes progressively worse with increasing duration of dialysis treatment (London et al. 1990), presumably because of fragmentation of elastic fibres, because of cross-linking of collagen fibers, by advanced glycation products, and because of calcification of the vascular wall (Blacher et al. 2001). A role for inflammatory mechanisms has also been documented (Drueke et al. 2002). Because peak systolic pressure is increased and diastolic pressure is decreased, the blood pressure amplitude (pulse pressure) is increased in patients with chronic kidney disease, similar to what is seen in ageing individuals, suggesting that uraemia is a state of accelerated and premature ageing of the vasculature.

Other factors

Raine et al. (1993) showed a correlation between blood pressure and platelet Ca^{2+} concentrations and the latter was related to elevated parathyroid hormone (PTH). In acute experiments PTH increased blood pressure (Fliser et al. 1997a,b). Hypercalcaemia per se also increases blood pressure to a certain extent and this has also been documented in dialysis patients.

It is known that remodelling of resistance vessels with luminal narrowing contributes to the maintenance of elevated vascular resistance and high blood pressure in different forms of hypertension (Folkow 1993). In this context it is relevant that wall thickening of resistance vessels, that is, arterioles (Amann et al. 1995) and even of veins is observed. The latter observation suggests that non-haemodynamic factors also play a pathogenetic role (Fig. 8). Finally, when the haemoglobin concentration rises rapidly in patients with chronic kidney disease receiving recombinant human erythropoietin (rhEPO), severe hypertension may occur. This was frequent in the early days, but has now become rare because the major role of hypervolaemia has been recognized. The pronounced effect of hypervolaemia is explained by the fact that vessels which had been vasodilated during anaemia and

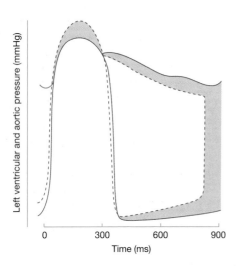

Fig. 7 Intracardiac and aortic pressures in a hypothetical normal patient (——) and uraemic patient (- - - - -) (by courtesy of Dr London, Paris). Note excessive peak systolic pressure and exaggerated rate of decline of diastolic pressure in the uraemic patient. The pressure gradient for coronary perfusion during diastole is reduced not only because of lower aortic pressure, but also because of higher left ventricular end-diastolic pressure.

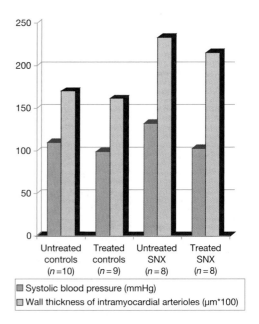

Fig. 8 Vessel wall thickness in subtotally nephrectomized rats (SNX) with or without antihypertensive treatment (hydralazine plus frusemide) (after Amann et al. 1995).

hypoxia, will constrict after reversal of anaemia (posthypoxic vaso-constriction). If hypervolaemia is well controlled, hypertension after rhEPO is no longer a major problem.

Consequences of hypertension in patients with chronic kidney disease

In patients with chronic kidney disease hypertension is important (first) because it accelerates progression (loss of renal function) and (second) because it increases the cardiovascular risk (e.g. left ventricular hypertrophy, congestive heart failure, acceleration of artherogenesis).

Impact of hypertension on progression

Decades ago Volhard (1923) had postulated that a relation existed between high blood pressure and progressive loss of renal function. As early as 1923, he postulated: 'I doubt very much whether hypertension has any useful purpose. We are confronted with a vicious circle which is responsible for progression of hypertensive renal disease with the final outcome of renal insufficiency'. It took decades before the correlation between hypertension and progression was confirmed first in observational studies in diabetic (Mogensen 1982; Parving et al. 1983) and later in non-diabetic patients with renal disease (Brazy et al. 1989). In order to prove that there was a causal relationship, interventional trials were necessary to document that lowering of blood pressure attenuated progression (Klahr et al. 1994).

It is remarkable that this point was first proven by diabetologists (Mogensen 1982; Parving et al. 1983). They showed that when blood pressure was lowered by administration of diuretics, β-blockers, and hydralazine, the progressive decrease of GFR was attenuated. Parving showed that it took several years before the full effect of lowering of blood pressure became apparent. This is illustrated in Fig. 9 which shows the effect of treatment in a small cohort of type 1 diabetic patients with nephropathy. It illustrates that the rate of loss of GFR was progressively reduced from 0.94 ml/min/month to no more than 0.1 ml/min/month. Meanwhile, the beneficial effect of blood pressure lowering on progression has also been documented in patients with advanced non-diabetic renal disease (Klahr et al. 1994; Petersen et al. 1995). This is shown in Table 6. Patients in whom blood pressure was

reduced only to the conventional threshold of normotension by the past WHO criteria, that is, 140/90 mmHg equivalent to a MAP of 107 mmHg, the rate of progression was significantly faster than in patients in whom blood pressure values were further lowered within the range of normotensive blood pressure values. More detailed analysis (see below) showed that at least in patients with urinary protein excretion greater than 1 g/24 h, a continuous relation existed between the achieved MAP and the yearly rate of loss of GFR. As shown in Fig. 10, in patients with 140/90 mmHg (equivalent to a MAP of 107 mmHg) the rate of loss of GFR was approximately 9 ml/min/year, whilst in patients with an achieved blood pressure of 120/70 mmHg (MAP 85 mmHg) the rate of loss was only 3 ml/min/year. This observation illustrates the powerful effect of further lowering blood pressure within the range of normotensive values, but only in patients with heavy proteinuria, that is, exceeding 1g/24 h.

Impact of hypertension on the cardiovascular system

Blood pressure, including blood pressure values in the range of normotension, are powerful predictors of cardiac and cerebrovascular events (Lewington et al. 2002) even in the general population. Because of the higher event rate in patients with chronic kidney disease and particular patients on renal replacement therapy, the absolute risk conferred by high blood pressure values is much greater in renal patients. This was documented early on by the French Diaphane Study in dialysis patients. Cardiovascular mortality, particularly stroke mortality was related to both systolic and diastolic pressure (Fig. 11). There is, however, much discussion in recent times about which blood pressure is optimal for the patient with terminal renal failure. This discussion was started when short-term observation in dialysed patients showed that predialysis systolic blood pressure values in the hypertensive range

Table 6 Blood pressure and progression—MDRD (Modification of Diet in Renal Disease)-study (after Klahr et al. 1994)

Blood pressure control	Target pressure (mean arterial pressure)	Loss of GFR (ml/min/year)
Ordinary	107 mmHg	3.4 (2.6–4.1)
Intensified	91 mmHg	1.9 (1.1–2.7)

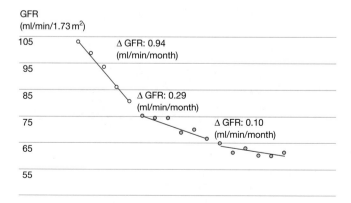

Fig. 9 Progressive attenuation of GFR loss in patients with type 1 diabetic nephropathy on aggressive antihypertensive treatment (after Parving et al. 1994).

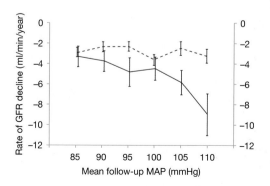

Fig. 10 Rate of glomerular filtration rate (GFR) decline, as a function of proteinuria and achieved mean arterial pressure (MDRD-study; after Petersen et al. 1995).

conferred surprisingly little risk of overall and cardiovascular death, whilst low blood pressure values were associated with a significantly increased risk (Zager *et al.* 1998; Port *et al.* 1999). This paradoxical relationship presumably reflects the phenomenon of 'reversed causality': if a patient has developed heart disease, possibly as a result of pre-existing hypertension, hypotension is a marker of impaired cardiac function which in and by itself is associated with extremely high mortality. That this interpretation is correct is supported by the finding that in short-term observations over 2–3 years, low blood pressure values predict a high rate of death. Beyond the third year, however, a continuous positive linear relationship is found between systolic blood pressure and cardiovascular death (Mazzuchi *et al.* 2000). These observations are in line with the intriguing experience of the centre in Tassin where a particularly low prevalence of hypertension is seen. According to Table 7 (Charra *et al.* 1992) a 24 per cent difference of actual survival rate of 15 years was noted in patients with an MAP below the median of 99 mmHg compared with those with a MAP greater than 99 mmHg. A MAP of 99 mmHg corresponds to approximately 130/80 mmHg. The observation of a graded increase of risk within the range of normotensive blood pressure values corresponds to what has been found with respect to progression (Petersen *et al.* 1995) and is also in line with recent observations in the general population (Lewington *et al.* 2002). Obviously substantially lower target blood pressure values than recommended in the past should be aimed for in the patient with chronic kidney disease. In uraemic patients, the problem is compounded by the fact that casual blood pressure measurements are a particularly poor reflection of the 24 h blood pressure load to target organs. This is the result of an abnormal circadian blood pressure profile with an attenuation or even loss of the nocturnal decline of blood pressure, so-called 'non-dipping' (Timio *et al.* 1995; Schwenger *et al.* 1998).

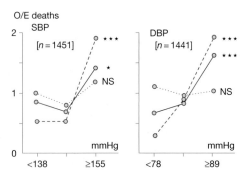

Fig. 11 Risk of death (O/E; observed/expected) in the three tertiles of systolic (SBP) and diastolic (DBP) blood pressure: (———) cardiovascular mortality (⋯⋯⋯) non-cardiovascular mortality (------) stroke mortality (after Degoulet *et al.* 1982).

Table 7 Survival of dialysis patients as a function of mean arterial blood pressure (after Charra *et al.* 1992)

Mean arterial blood pressure (mmHg)	Actuarial survival (%)			
	5 years	10 years	15 years	20 years dialysis
<99 (N = 222)	93	85	67	53
>99 (N = 223)	81	65	43	

What is the appropriate target blood pressure?

Target blood pressure for attenuation of progression

The renal risk increases progressively with increase in blood pressure without any definite threshold. In an observational study Opelz *et al.* (1998) found that in renal graft recipients (as one model of renal damage) graft survival is progressively worse for increasingly higher systolic blood pressure values (Fig. 12). This relationship has recently been confirmed by a meta-analysis of controlled intervention trials in patients with non-diabetic renal disease. The best renal prognosis was found in individuals with systolic blood pressure less than 110 mmHg (Jafar *et al.* 2002). It is likely, but currently not definitely proven, that ABPM is more predictive than office blood pressure. Particularly predictive is an attenuated decrease of blood pressure at nigh-time (Ritz *et al.* 2001). In patients with IgA-glomerulonephritis (Csiky *et al.* 1999) as well as in patients with advanced diabetic (Farmer *et al.* 1998) or non-diabetic renal disease (Timio *et al.* 1995) a greater rate of loss of endogenous creatinine clearance was found in patients in whom the night-time decrease of blood pressure was attenuated (non-dippers) than in patients in whom the nocturnal decrease of blood pressure was preserved (dippers). Nakano *et al.* (1998a,b) found that in type 2 diabetic patients without a night-time decrease of blood pressure, had a twofold higher risk of death and also a much higher risk to progress to endstage renal disease (Nakano *et al.* 1999).

Several boards recommend to lower blood pressure to 130/85 mmHg in diabetic patients without evidence of renal involvement and to 125/75 mmHg in diabetic and non-diabetic patients with proteinuric renal disease (Petersen *et al.* 1995; WHO ISH Guidelines subcommittee 1999). Presumably there is no definite threshold. Rather, analogous to what is seen in observational studies in the general population (Lewington *et al.* 2002) and in interventioanl studies in proteinuric renal disease (Petersen *et al.* 1995), a continuous and progressive reduction of the risk of progression can be achieved by progressively more intensive reduction of systolic blood pressure values.

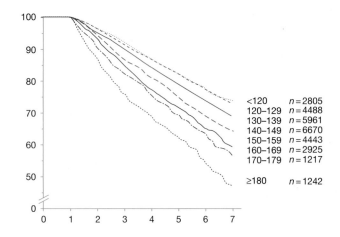

Fig. 12 Systolic blood pressure 1 year after transplantation predicts graft survival in recipients of first cadaver kidney transplants (after Opelz *et al.* 1998).

In the past there has been much discussion about the so-called J-phenomenon, that is, the paradoxical finding that cardiovascular mortality decreased until a diastolic pressure of approximately 80 mmHg was reached, only to increase if diastolic blood pressure values were lowered further (Cruickshank *et al.* 1987). This was interpreted as evidence of cardiac ischaemia in patients with pre-existing coronary artery stenosis. The J-curve is apparently a biostatistical artefact. Even in the placebo arms of intervention trials and in observational studies of the general population, low diastolic pressures predicted cardiovascular death (Bullpitt *et al.* 1992). In major intervention trials (Petersen *et al.* 1995; Brenner *et al.* 2001; Lewis *et al.* 2001) no evidence for a J-curve-phenomenon was found in renal patients. This does not of course exclude the possibility that lowering of blood pressure may provoke critical ischaemia in individual patients with critical stenosis of the intracerebral carotid or peripheral arteries. It is therefore, necessary to examine the patient before blood pressure is lowered in order to exclude stenoses. In view of the impaired endothelial cell function (Zoccali 2002), particularly impaired endothelial-cell-dependant vasodilatation and autoregulation in renal patients, it is important to lower blood pressure slowly and to examine the patient repeatedly for evidence of ischaemic organ damage.

A potential problem is orthostatic hypotension. This is common in patients with hypovolaemia secondary to overaggressive diuretic treatment and is particularly frequent in patients with autonomic polyneuropathy and impaired baroreflex function. In the IDNT trial on type 2 diabetic patients, the risk of progression was greater in patients with frequent episodes of orthostatic hypotension; possibly in diabetes the kidney is more susceptible to ischaemic injury (Melin *et al.* 1997). Avoidance of hypotension is a particular problem in the patient on dialysis. Koch *et al.* (1993) showed that repeated hypotensive episodes with a decrease of systolic BP below 90 mmHg, that is, below the threshold of autoregulation in the coronary system, increased cardiovascular mortality by a factor of 3.

There has been an issue whether systolic, mean, or diastolic pressure, or blood pressure amplitude predicts progression and cardiovascular events. With respect to progression, Opelz *et al.* (1998) showed that systolic blood pressure was a more potent predictor of progression than diastolic or mean blood pressure and blood pressure amplitude. This finding is plausible because in the damaged kidney afferent arterioles are vasodilated so that a higher proportion of peak systolic pressure in the aorta is transmitted into the glomerular microcirculation giving rise to 'glomerular hypertension'. It is therefore quite clear that in order to prevent progression, systolic blood pressure is the appropriate target.

The matter is more complex with respect to cardiovascular endpoints. According to the recent meta-analysis on non-renal subjects (Lewington *et al.* 2002) systolic blood pressure is highly predictive for cardiovascular events as well. In many patients with chronic kidney disease, however, loss of elasticity of central arteries (aortic stiffening) causes an increase in the blood pressure amplitude (see above). In such patients, diastolic blood pressure may decrease to very low values. If diastolic pressure is decreased further by antihypertensive medication, it may compromise coronary perfusion which occurs only during diastole. Consequently, although no definite information is available on this point, it may be wise not to lower the systolic pressure excessively in the patient with chronic kidney disease and a high blood pressure amplitude if this has to be done at the expense of excessive lowering of diastolic pressure or at the risk of causing orthostatic hypotension.

Does selection of the antihypertensive agents matter?

The evidence is overwhelming that angiotensin II aggravates progression both by haemodynamic and by non-haemodynamic mechanisms (Wolf 1999). Pharmacological blockade of the RAS is reno-protective even in states where the RAS in the circulation is suppressed, as indicated by low PRA and by an attenuated hypotensive effect. This paradox can be explained by recent observations that not only the RAS in the juxtaglomerular apparatus is activated, but also the local RAS in tubular endothelial cells (Gilbert *et al.* 1999). This has been shown in the ablation model, but is also seen in diabetes mellitus and in ageing. In type 2 diabetic patients Price *et al.* (1999) found a greater increment in renal plasma flow than in controls after administration of an angiotensinogen receptor blocker. This observation suggests greater angiotensin II dependency of renal vascular tone in diabetic patients despite low PRA (Fig. 13). It has also been shown that such suprasensitivity to angiotensin receptor blockade was only present under hyperglycaemic, but not under normoglycaemic conditions (Miller 1999). Today there is no more doubt that pharmacological blockade of the RAS by administration of ACE inhibitors or angiotensin receptor blockers (ARB) provides blood pressure independant renoprotection. The major studies are the AIPRI (Maschio *et al.* 1996) and REIN (The GISEN group 1997) trials in patients with non-diabetic renal disease and the Captopril trial in type I (Lewis *et al.* 1993) as well as the IDNT (Lewis *et al.* 2001) and RENAAL (Brenner *et al.* 2001) trials in type 2 diabetic patients with nephropathy. The results are summarized in Table 8. The side-effect profile of ACE inhibitors is summarized in Table 9.

Ancillary measures

Recently it has been postulated that sympathetic nerve system plays a role in the progression of renal disease. In experimental animals (Campese and Kojosov 1995) as well as in humans with renal disease (Converse *et al.* 1992), increased sympathetic efferent sympathetic nerve traffic has been documented. In experimental studies sympathetic overactivity contributes to progression independently of any effect on blood pressure: non-hypotensive doses of the central sympatheticoplegic agent Moxolidine reduced albuminuria and the development of glomerulosclerosis in subtotally nephrectomized rats (Amann *et al.* 2000a,b) and the same was seen with Metoprolol (Amann *et al.* 2001) and after renal denervation. That these observations are relevant

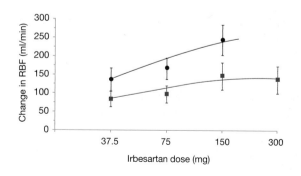

Fig. 13 Relationship between Irbesartan dose and peak renal blood flow (RBF) response in healthy subjects and patients with type 2 diabetes mellitus (after Price *et al.* 1999).

Table 8 Selected studies showing renoprotection properties of angiotensin-converting enzyme (ACE) inhibitors or angiotensin II receptor type 1 antagonists (AT-1-RB)

Study	AIPRI	REIN	Lewis et al. (1993, 2001)		IDNTRENAAL
Study group	Various nephropathies	Non-diabetic nephropathy	Nephropathy type 1 diabetes	Nephropathy type 2 diabetes	Nephropathy type 2 diabetes
Sample size	583	323	409	1715	1513
Planned duration of follow-up (years)	3.0	2.2	3.0	2.6	4.5
Study medication (ACE inhibitors or AT-1-RB)	Benazepril	Ramipril	Captopril	Irbesartan	Losartan
Dosage of study medication (mg/day)	10	1.25–5.0	75	75–300	50–100
Baseline serum creatinine concentration (μmol/l)	186	194	115	148	168
Relative risk (95% CI) of ESRD in the treated group	0.89 (0.06–14.2)	0.51 (0.30–0.87)	0.50 (0.18–0.70)	0.83 (0.62–1.11)	0.75
Relative risk (95% CI) of doubling serum creatinine concentration in the treated group	0.44 (0.27–0.70)	0.47 (0.29–0.77)	0.48 (0.16–0.69)	0.71 (0.54–0.92)	0.72

Table 9 Side-effects of ACE inhibitors in renal patients

Decrease of glomerular filtration rate/oliguria
   Renal artery stenosis
      Bilateral
      Single kidney (including renal graft)
   Hyper-reninaemic states due to accompanying conditions
      Preceding diuretic treatment
      Congestive heart failure
      Liver cirrhosis
   Specific primary renal diseases
      Haemolytic uraemic syndrome/scleroderma crisis
      Malignant hypertension
      Autosomal dominant polycystic kidney disease

Hyperkalaemia
   Hyporeninaemic hypoaldosteronism (elderly type 2 diabetics)
   Hyperchloraemic metabolic acidosis (tubulointerstitial disease)
Aggravation of metabolic acidosis
Aggravation of hyporegenerative anaemia (decreased erythropoietin)
Anaphylactoid symptoms in patients treated with synthetic dialysis
   membranes/devices
   (inhibition of kinin degradation in the presence of increased generation
   of kinins)

for humans as well is documented by the observation of Strojek et al. (2001) who showed in normotensive microalbuminuric type 1 diabetic patients that Moxonidine at doses that did not affect blood pressure lowered albumin excretion in the morning urine.

When antihypertensive treatment is administered in isolation, the effect on cardiac mortality is disappointingly modest. This finding illustrates the necessity of reversing all accessible risk factors for coronary heart disease and not to just lower blood pressure. Further risk factor interventions include cessation of smoking (Orth et al. 1998)

and vigorous treatment of dyslipidaemia (Wanner et al. 1999). There are good arguments that the excessive sympathetic activity in renal patients contributes to the high rate of cardiac death. Cardioselective β-blockers are highly effective in secondary cardiac prevention. In a prospective trial, Koch et al. (1993) found that only 3 per cent of diabetic patients who had died from cardiac causes were on β-blockers whereas 13 per cent of the survivors were taking β-blockers. Meanwhile controlled prospective evidence is available that at least in dialysed patients with heart failure, Carvedilol was superior to placebo in lowering the NYHA-category and improving the ejection fraction (Cice et al. 2001). In addition in an observational study, dialysed patients receiving β-blockers had 17 per cent lower overall mortality (Bragg et al. 2002). These observations reinforce the postulate (Zuanetti et al. 1997) that β-blockers should be used more liberally in patients with chronic kidney disease.

Apart from the classical risk factors, several non-classical risk factors have recently been identified, particularly low haematocrit values (which can be reversed by rhEPO) and hyperphosphataemia (Block et al. 1998). Aggressive efforts are justified to keep phosphate concentrations in the normal, possibly even better in the mid-normal range, that is, 2.5–5.5 mg/dl (Block and Port 2000).

Practical points

Combination therapy versus monotherapy

It is rarely possible to achieve the above target blood pressures using antihypertensive monotherapy. In our outpatient clinic, on average four different antihypertensive drugs are required to normalize blood pressure in patients when serum creatinine is on average 4 mg/dl (354 μmol/l) (Schwenger et al. 1998). Combination offers the further advantage that side-effects of drug monotherapies may cancel out. For instance, diuretic therapy which is a corner stone of antihypertensive treatment in renal disease, causes dyslipidaemia and increases the concentration of angiotensin II (which is undesirable because angiotensin II promotes progression). Both effects are prevented by concomitant treatment with ACE inhibitors. Calcium-channel blockers reduce coughing induced by ACE inhibitors, and conversely the ACE inhibitors reduce oedema caused by calcium-channel blockers (Stefanski et al. 1995). Since angiotensin II plays a role in progression, a combination of ACE inhibitors and calcium-channel blockers appears attractive (Stefanski et al. 1995; Münter et al. 1996), as it combines diminished generation of angiotensin II (ACE inhibition) with diminished responsiveness to angiotensin II at the post-receptor-level (calcium-channel blockers). This hypothesis is supported by clinical observations of more intense reduction of proteinuria by this combination (Bakris and Williams 1995; Stefanski et al. 1995).

There has recently been much concern that the administration of calcium-channel blockers increases cardiovascular mortality particularly in diabetic patients but the retrospective analysis of the EUROSYSTEUR study (Tuomilehto et al. 1999) and particularly the large ALLHAT Study (2002) failed to show evidence of an increased cardiovascular risk for dihydropyridine calcium-channel blockers. In patients with progressive renal disease the renal haemodynamic effects of calcium-channel blockers are a definite problem. Calcium-channel blockers dilate preferentially the afferent arterioles, thus exposing the glomeruli to the risk of glomerular hypertension. It is therefore, not surprising that in the AASK trial (Wright et al. 2002) monotherapy with the calcium channel blocker amlodipine caused greater loss of GFR than monotherapy with the ACE inhibitor Ramipril. Consequently pharmacological blockade of the renin system must remain the first line treatment in patients with progressive renal disease. It must be emphasized, however, that when ACE inhibitors are combined with calcium-channel blockers, and when target MAP values of less than 100 mmHg are reached, no more evidence of an adverse effect of calcium-channel blockers on progression could be found in the REIN trial (Ruggenenti et al. 1998). Similarly, in the IDNT-trial (Lewis et al. 2001) there was no evidence that amlodipine accelerated the rate of loss of GFR in type 2 diabetic patients in whom very low blood pressure values had been achieved.

Altered pharmacokinetics

As shown in Table 10, when treating patients with chronic kidney disease it must be remembered that some antihypertensive agents (or their active metabolites) accumulate in renal failure. Since antihypertensive agents are usually prescribed according to blood pressure response, cumulation does not usually cause problems of hypotension, but complications such as bradycardia (β-blockers), hyperkalaemia (potassium-sparing diuretics which are strictly contraindicated) and sedation or depression (alpha-Methyldopa or Clonidin) may arise.

Control of sodium retention

Because of the overriding role of volume retention and hypervolaemia in the genesis of hypertension in renal disease, restriction of the dietary intake of sodium chloride as well as diuretic treatment are the cornerstones of antihypertensive management of the renal patient. It is advisable to reduce daily NaCl-intake to approximately 5–7 g and to monitor NaCl-intake by occasionally measuring Na excretion in 24-h urine collections. The efficiency of ACE inhibitors or ARBs depends on the sodium balance. The full nephroprotective action of ACE inhibitors or ARBs is only seen when mild sodium depletion is achieved by reducing sodium intake or administering diuretics. A negative sodium balance activates the RAS and makes it more susceptible to inhibition by ACE inhibitors or ARBs.

In contrast to sodium chloride, sodium bicarbonate, which is often used to treat metabolic acidosis, does not increase blood pressure.

It is commonly stated, that at a serum creatinine concentration of 2 mg/dl (177 μmol/l) thiazide diuretics are ineffective and contraindicated. This statement is incorrect. At that stage thiazides still increase fractional sodium excretion. Because the absolute rate of sodium excretion is low, however, it takes longer time until a negative sodium balance is achieved. Undoubtedly loop diuretics are the diuretics of choice in advanced renal failure. It has recently been shown (Fliser et al. 1994), however, that a combination of loop diuretics and thiazides increases their efficiency. Thiazides interfere with compensatory stimulation of sodium transport in the distal nephron which limits the effect of loop diuretic monotherapy. Furthermore, thiazides block the so-called rebound-phenomenon, that is, the compensatory increase of sodium reabsorption when the natriuretic effect of loop diuretics has waned.

The high efficiency of thiazides is explained by their long half-lives which allow using once daily administration to maintain a modestly negative sodium balance over 24 h without the risk of rebound sodium retention. In contrast, rebound occurs with once daily (or even twice daily) administration of short-acting loop diuretics (e.g. frusemide).

Side-effects of antihypertensive treatment

The patients should be monitored regularly to detect potential side-effects of antihypertensive treatment.

Potassium-sparing diuretics are contraindicated in patients with reduced GFR. Recently following the spectacular results of the Rales-trial (Pitt et al. 1999) administration of aldosterone-antagonists has become popular for patients with cardiac disease even when serum creatinine concentration is elevated. This approach, however, makes it necessary to

Table 10 Comparison of the accumulation of antihypertensive drugs in renal failure and in normal function

Drug	Half-life (h)	
	Normal renal function	**Impaired renal function**
Amiloride[a]	6	8–144
Triamterene	2–3	—[b]
Atenolol	6–9	15–35
Nadolol	12–24	45
Sotalol	5–8	30–50
Doxazosin	22	22
Clonidine	6–23	39–42
Hydralazine	2–5	7–16
Captopril	0.5–2	12–40
Enalapril	10–12	15–35

[a] Contraindicated in renal failure.

[b] Also accumulation of an active metabolite.

closely monitor the patient and to limit the dose of spironolactone, for example, to a maximum of 25 mg daily. There has also been recent evidence that aldosterone blockade further attenuates proteinuria (as a surrogate marker for progression), even when the RAS has been blocked by ACE inhibitors. Again, the safety of this measure has not been documented in patients with impaired renal function.

Hyperkalaemia may also occur after administration of ACE inhibitors but the frequency is rather low (Lewis *et al.* 2001). The risk of hyperkalaemia is particularly high in patients with hyporeninaemic hypoaldosteronism which is not infrequent in elderly type 2 diabetics as well as in patients with tubulointerstitial disease and hyperchloraemic acidosis, for example, in patients with analgesic nephropathy.

Conversely there may be a risk of hypokalaemia after administration of diuretics. The risk can be reduced by decreasing the dietary intake of sodium chloride, thus reducing the delivery of sodium to the Na^+,K^+-exchange site in the distal nephron. A further possibility is the combination of diuretics with an ACE inhibitor.

In renal patients ACE inhibitors pose some specific problems (Table 10) in addition to the known side-effects of cough (approximately 20 per cent of patients) and angioneurotic oedema. Acute deterioration of renal function and even oliguria may occur in hyperreninaemic patients, for example, patients with unrecognized renal artery stenosis affecting both the kidneys or a solitary kidney. The risk of occult renal artery stenosis is higher in patients with a history of smoking and arterio-occlusive disease. In elderly patients with type 2 diabetes, the risk is also somewhat higher, but according to the IDNT study it is not excessive (Lewis *et al.* 2001). Caution is required, however, if renal ultrasonography shows asymmetry of renal size and parenchymal width (although these signs are obviously not specific).

Deterioration of renal function after ACE inhibition or angiotensin receptor blockade is also not uncommon when the RAS has been stimulated by intense diuretic treatment. Therefore it is advisable to reduce the dose of diuretics, or to interrupt diuretic treatment temporarily, prior to the administration of a test-dose of an ACE inhibitor or ARB. Since side-effects usually occur early on, it is advisable to monitor urine output, serum creatinine, and serum potassium, 1 and 3 days after the first dose of an ACE inhibitor. ACE inhibitors aggravate metabolic acidosis (because proximal tubular bicarbonate reabsorption is reduced) and anaemia (because EPO secretion is reduced). Serious anaphylactic side-effects (hypotension, bronchoconstriction, and increased kinin concentrations) have been reported in patients who were dialysed with synthetic AN 69 membranes. Those membranes have a high electronegative charge and activate the Hagemann-factor and the kinin system. On top of this, ACE inhibitors interfere with the breakdown of kinins and amplify the response to increased kinin concentrations.

Hypertension in the dialysed patient

Most studies show a high prevalence of systolic, less so of diastolic, hypertension in patients who are dialysed three times weekly for 3–5 h (Mailloux and Haley 1998). This is illustrated in Fig. 14, which shows that most patients have systolic pressure values between 150 and 159 mmHg, that is, are above the definitions of WHO/ISH of normal (130/85 mmHg) or ideal blood pressure (120/80 mmHg) (WHO ISH Guidelines subcommittee 1999), whilst the same patients have diastolic pressure values within the normotensive range. This pattern of isolated systolic hypertension is an exaggeration of what is seen in the

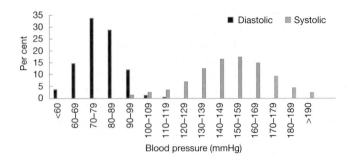

Fig. 14 Distribution of systolic and diastolic blood pressure values in dialysed patients (after Mailloux and Haley 1998).

predialytic phase and results from impaired elasticity ('stiffening') of the central arteries (London *et al.* 2002).

What are the causes of hypertension? The most important factor is undoubtedly hypervolaemia. This was noted as early as 1960 by Scribner *et al.* who have stated 'As in the case of nephrectomized dogs, hypertension appears to be influenced by the size of the extracellular space. The combination of dietary sodium restriction and ultrafiltration during dialysis permits regulation of extracellular volume. In time, it may be possible to clarify the importance of the size of the extracellular space in the aetiology of hypertension and the effects it may have on modifying the response to antihypertensive therapy' (Scribner *et al.* 1960).

There is no doubt that hypovolaemia is a crucial factor for the development of hypertension. According to the concepts of Guyton (1987), sodium retention causes an expansion of the plasma and extracellular volumes (Fig. 4), raising venous return and cardiac output and tending to raise blood pressure. The increase is not a major one, however, unless a second factor intervenes, that is increased peripheral vascular resistance. In experimental studies, a slow process called autoregulation raises the resistance to organ perfusion, that is, the vascular resistance, thus increasing total peripheral resistance and causing a major increase in blood pressure. This is reminiscent of what has been described as the 'lag phenomenon' (Charra *et al.* 1998a,b), that is, the notion that it takes weeks or months before volume expansion causes an increase and conversely volume reduction a decrease in blood pressure in the dialysed patients, reflecting the slow readjustment of peripheral vascular resistance. Vascular resistance in dialysed patients tends to be elevated for the reasons described before, that is, inappropriate activation of the local and vessel wall RAS, sympathetic overactivity, impaired endothelial-cell-dependent vasodilatation and remodelling of resistance vessels with luminal narrowing.

Blood pressure in the dialysis patient is characterized by several peculiarities including an abnormal circadian blood pressure profile with insufficient lowering during night-time, even when patients are normotensive (Chazot *et al.* 1997), a high frequency of sleep apnoea (Zoccali *et al.* 2001, 2002) and marked seasonal variability with higher blood pressure values during winter (Argiles *et al.* 1998).

Against the background of a high prevalence of systolic hypertension (Fig. 14), it is of note that remarkably low frequencies of hypertension have been reported from centres providing long/slow dialysis sessions (Charra *et al.* 1998a,b; McGregor *et al.* 1999) or schedules with more frequent dialysis sessions, that is, daily nocturnal (Pierratos *et al.* 1998) or daily home haemodialysis (Kooistra *et al.* 1998). In some of the reports, the frequency of hypertension was even lower than in the general population. Although several factors may be responsible for this observation, the most plausible explanation is that slow and/or frequent dialysis permits better volume control, although additional factors, for example, removal of pressor agents or of inhibitors of vasodilatation are not completely excluded. The difficulty of convective fluid removal with the conventional high efficiency $3 \times 3–5/h$ week schedules relates to the fact that ultrafiltration causes contraction of the plasma volume which can be held in check only by re-filling of the plasma volume, that is, return of fluid from the extracellular space into the plasma space. If the rate of ultrafiltration exceeds the rate of re-filling, vasoconstriction and eventually hypotension occur, thus limiting the rate of fluid removal. Such patients are then obviously predisposed to persisting overhydration.

Additional factors influencing cardiovascular stability during ultrafiltration include dialysate temperature (low temperature favours blood pressure stability), autonomic polyneuropathy (interrupting the baroreceptor reflex and predisposing to intradialytic hypotension), left ventricular hypertrophy, and impaired left ventricular compliance (necessitating higher filling pressures and predisposing patients to hypotension when preload is lowered).

The crucial importance of volume control is illustrated by the fact that treatment strategies are successful which comprise three elements, that is, dietary sodium restriction, aggressive ultrafiltration to reach 'dry weight' and slow reduction in dialysate sodium concentration. This strategy had originally been proposed by Scribner et al. (1998). It has subsequently been proven to be effective by authors using conventional 3×5 h/week dialysis sessions (Krautzig et al. 1998; Özkahya et al. 1998), illustrating that it is volume control rather than duration of dialysis which is the crucial factor.

Why is dietary sodium restriction important? Thirst is controlled by osmotic pressure. If the anuric dialysis patient ingests 9 g of sodium chloride per day, the thirst mechanism will force the patients to ingest 1 l of osmotically free water. With the usual salt intake of approximately 15 g/day in Western countries, this means automatically that the weight gain in the interdialytic interval will be at least 1.8 kg per day. The recommended daily consumption of sodium chloride is 6 g/day and this can be achieved without undue dietary restrictions.

A second problem is the achievement of dry weight. In the early days of dialysis it was naively thought that fluid control was achieved once the patient had lost oedema. It was Thomson et al. (1967) who coined the term 'dry weight'. He gave the following definition: 'the reduction of blood pressure to hypotensive levels during ultrafiltration and unassociated with other causes represents the achievement of a "dry weight" status'. Others (Vertes et al. 1969) stated that 'dry weight is characterised not merely by the absence of edema, but the body sodium content and the volume of body water below which further reduction results in hypotension'. Unfortunately thoracic X-rays are not sufficiently sensitive. Despite the availability of more sophisticated technology such as vena cava ultrasonography, bioimpedance measurements, and others, there are no fail safe clinical parameters to recognize the point when dry weight has been achieved, apart from measurements of atrial natriuretic peptide (ANP) which is not routinely available. The clinician is therefore, forced to use the trial and error approach. It is crucial, however, that the lowering of body weight to the presumed dry weight is done slowly and under supervision.

A third component is to lower dialysate sodium concentration gradually, in the course of weeks. The dialysate sodium concentration must be lower than the sodium concentration in plasma water to prevent diffusive net transfer of sodium into the patient downhill across the membrane. Detailed calculations and measurements by Locatelli et al. (1984) showed that the appropriate correction factor is 0.967. We and others have shown that gradual slow lowering of dialysate serum concentration from 140 to 135 mmol/l, reducing the concentration by steps of 1 mmol/l per 3–4 weeks, is well tolerated, fails to cause side-effects, but effectively lowers blood pressure.

The most important impediment to achievement of dry weight is the administration of antihypertensive agents which will cause hypotensive episodes during ultrafiltration. It has been advised to gradually take off antihypertensive agents and at the very least omit antihypertensive medication on the day of dialysis if this can be justified. It would be unrealistic, however, to assume that all patients become normotensive without antihypertensive medication. Furthermore, blood pressure-independent benefits are derived from B-blockers (Zuanetti et al. 1997) and ACE inhibitors.

Recently there has been much discussion about which blood pressure level is optimal for survival. Charra et al. (1992) (Fig. 14) had reported that in a population of dialysis patients of whom less than 5 per cent had hypertension defined as greater than or equal to 140/90 mmHg, the median value of MAP was 99 mmHg. As shown in Fig. 14, after an interval of up to 5 years there was progressive separation of patients with MAP below versus above an MAP of 99 mmHg. The authors came to the conclusion that blood pressure as low as compatible with well being and absence of hypotensive episodes during dialysis is optimal for survival.

More recently, considerable uncertainty has arisen because, contraintuitively, in short-term observations on two large samples of haemodialysis patients high blood pressure values were not found to be predictive of mortality, whereas low blood pressure values were tightly correlated to poor survival (Zager et al. 1998; Port et al. 1999). As shown in Fig. 15, patients with predialysis blood pressure less than 110 mmHg had a two-fold higher risk to die within a relatively short period of time, whilst pressure values up to 180 mmHg and more had relatively little impact on survival. There has been some discussion

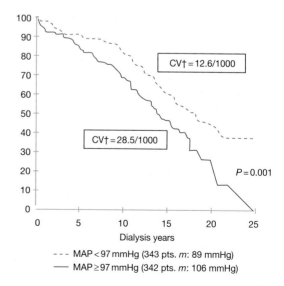

Fig. 15 Relation of actuarial survival and mean arterial pressure (medium value 97 mmHg) in the Tassin population of dialysis patients (Charra B, personal communication).

concerning which blood pressure is optimal (London 2001; Schömig *et al.* 2001), but today there is consensus (Zocalli 2003) that the explanation for the contraintuitive relation between blood pressure and survival is explained by the so-called 'reverse causality'. Low blood pressure is a marker for poor cardiac function. It is easy to see that patients with cardiac malfunction will have a high short-term mortality. Indeed Mazzuchi *et al.* (2000) showed that in the first years of observation, dialysis patients with low systolic blood pressure had high mortality, whilst in the long run, survival was best in patients with low blood pressure values.

There is consensus that in principle predialytic blood pressure values as low as possible are desirable. This postulate must be tempered, however, by one consideration. As had been shown in Fig. 7, the pulse curve of the dialysis patient is characterized by higher peak systolic, but lower trough diastolic pressure values. Since coronary perfusion takes place only during diastole, a low diastolic blood pressure will expose the patient to the risk of coronary underperfusion. It is well known that high blood pressure amplitude (as a surrogate marker of reduced elasticity of the central arteries) is correlated with high mortality in the general population and this has also been shown in dialysis patients (Zoccali 2003). In the effort to achieve low blood pressure values, one should tolerate borderline high blood pressure values if diastolic pressure values are very low.

References

Adamczak, M., Zeier, M., Dikow, R., and Ritz, E. (2002). Kidney and hypertension. *Kidney International* **80**, S62–S67.

ALLHAT study (2002). ALLHAT Officers and Coordinators for the ALLHAT Collaborative Research Group. The Antihypertensive and Lipid-Lowering Treatment to Prevent Heart Attack Trial (ALLHAT). Major outcomes in high-risk hypertensive patients randomized to angiotensin-converting enzyme inhibitor or calcium channel blocker vs diuretic. *Journal of the American Medical Association* **288**, 2981–2997.

Amann, K., Wiest, G., Klaus, G., Ritz, E., and Mall, G. (1994). The role of parathyroid hormone in the genesis of interstitial cell activation in uremia. *Journal of the American Society of Nephrology* **4**, 1814–1819.

Amann, K., Törnig, J., Fletchenmacher, C., Nabokov, A., Mall, G., and Ritz, E. (1995). Blood pressure independent wall thickening of intramyocardial arterioles in experimental uremia—evidence for a permissive action of PTH. *Nephrology, Dialysis, Transplantation* **10**, 2043–2048.

Amann, K. *et al.* (2000a). Effects of low dose sympathic inhibition on glomerulosclerosis and albuminuria in subtotally nephrectomized rats. *Journal of the American Society of Nephrology* **11**, 1469–1478.

Amann, K., Rump, L. C., Simonaviciene, A., Oberhauser, V., Wessels, S., Orth, S. R., Gross, M. L., Koch, A., Bielenberg, G. W., Van Kats, J. P., Ehmke, H., Mall, G., and Ritz, E. (2000b). Effects of low dose sympathic inhibition on glomerulosclerosis and albuminuria in subtotally nephrectomized rats. *Journal of the American Society of Nephrology* **11**, 1469–1478.

Amann, K. *et al.* (2001). Glomerulosclerosis and progression: effect of subantihypertensive doses of α and β blockers. *Kidney International* **60**, 1309–1323.

Argiles, A., Mourad, G., and Mion, C. (1998). Seasonal changes in blood pressure in patients with end-stage renal disease treated with hemodialysis. *New England Journal of Medicine* **339**, 1364–1370.

Bakris, G. L. and Williams, B. (1995). ACE inhibitors and calcium antagonists alone or combined: is there a difference on progression of diabetic renal disease? *Journal of Hypertension* **13**, 95–101.

Barenbrock, M., Spieker, C., Laske, V., Heidenreich, S., Bachmann, H. H. J., Hocks, A. P. G., and Rahn, K. H. (1994). Studies of the vessel wall properties in hemodialysis patients. *Kidney International* **45**, 1397–1400.

Bigazzi, R., Kogosov, E., and Campese, V. M. (1994). Altered norepinephrine turnover in the brain of rats with chronic renal failure. *Journal of the American Society of Nephrology* **4**, 1901–1907.

Blacher, J., Guerin, A. P., Pannier, B., Marchais, S. J., and London, G. M. (2001). Arterial calcifications, arterial stiffness, and cardiovascular risk in end-stage renal disease. *Hypertension* **38**, 938–942.

Block, G. A. and Port, F. K. (2000). Re-evaluation of risks associated with hyperphosphatemia and hyperparathyroidism in dialysis patients: recommendations for a change in management. *American Journal of Kidney Diseases* **35**, 1226–1237.

Block, G. A., Hulbert-Shearon, T. E., Levin, N. W., and Port, F. K. (1998). Association of serum phosphorus and calcium × phosphate product with mortality risk in chronic hemodialysis patients: a national study. *American Journal of Kidney Diseases* **31**, 607–617.

Bragg, J. L., Mason, N. A., Maroni, B. J., Held, P. J., and Young, E. W. Beta-adrenergic antagonist utilization among hemodialysis patients. Data from the DOPPS study. Lecture from the Annual Meeting of the American Society of Nephrology, Philadelphia, 2002.

Brazy, P. C., Stead, W. W., and Fitzwilliam, J. F. (1989). Progression of renal insufficiency: role of blood pressure. *Kidney International* **35**, 670–674.

Brenner, B. M., Cooper, M. E., De Zeeuw, D., Keane, W. F., Mitch, W. E., Parving, H. H., Remuzzi, G., Snapinn, S. M., Zhang, Z., and Shahinfar, S. (2001). Effects of losartan on renal and cardiovascular outcomes in patients with type 2 diabetes and nephropathy. *New England Journal of Medicine* **345**, 861–869.

Bullpitt, C. J. *et al.* (1992). Relation between treated blood pressure and death from ischemic heart disease at different ages: a report from the Department of Health Hypertension Care Computing Project. *Journal of Hypertension* **10**, 1273–1278.

Byrom, F. B. (1974). The evolution of acute hypertensive arterial disease. *Progress in Cardiovascular Diseases* **17**, 31–37.

Campese, V. and Kojosov, E. (1995). Renal afferent denervation prevents hypertension in rats with chronic renal failure. *Hypertension* **25**, 878–882.

Chapman, A. B., Johnson, A., Gabow, P. A., and Schrier, R. W. (1990). The renin angiotensin aldosterone system and autosomal dominant polycystic kidney disease. *New England Journal of Medicine* **323**, 916–920.

Charra, B., Calemard, E., Ruffet, M., Chazot, C., Terrat, J. C., Vanel, T., and Laurent, G. (1992). Survival as an index of adequacy of dialysis. *Kidney International* **41**, 1286–1291.

Charra, B., Bergström, J., and Scribner, B. H. (1998a). Blood pressure control in dialysis patients: importance of the lag phenomenon. *American Journal of Kidney Disease* **32**, 720–724.

Charra, B., Laurent, G., Chazot, C., Jean, G., Terrat, J. C., and Vanel, T. (1998b). Hemodialysis trends in time, 1989 to 1998, independent of dose and outcome. *American Journal of Kidney Diseases* **32**, S63–S70.

Chazot, C., Charra, B., Laurent, G., Didier, C., Vo Van, C., Terrat, J. C., Calemard, E., Vanel, T., and Ruffet, M. (1997). Interdialysis blood pressure monitoring in renal dialysis and transplant patients. *American Journal of Kidney Diseases* **29**, 593–600.

Cice, G., Ferrara, L., Di Benedetto, A., Russo, P. E., Marinelli, G., Pavese, F., and Iacono, A. (2001). Dilated cardiomyopathy in dialysis patients—beneficial effects of carvedilol: a double-blind, placebo-controlled trial. *Journal of the American College of Cardiology* **37**, 407–411.

Converse, R. L., Jacobsen, T. N., Toto, R. D., Jost, C. M. T., Cosentino, F., Fouad-Tarazi, F., and Victor, R. G. (1992). Sympathetic overactivity in patients with CRF. *New England Journal of Medicine* **327**, 1912–1918.

Cruickshank, J. M., Thorp, J. M., and Zacharias, F. J. (1987). Benefits and potential harm of lowering high blood pressure. *Lancet* 581–584.

Csiky, B. *et al.* (1999). Ambulatory blood pressure monitoring and progression in patients with IgA nephropathy. *Nephrology, Dialysis, Transplantation* **14**, 86–90.

Curtis, J. J. *et al.* (1983). Remission of essential hypertension after renal transplantation. *New England Journal of Medicine* **309**, 1009–1014.

Degoulet, P., Legrain, M., Roach, I., Aime, F., Devries, C., Rojas, P., and Jacobs, C. (1982). Mortality risk factors in patients treated by chronic hemodialysis. *Nephron* **31**, 103–110.

Drueke, T., Witko-Sarsat, V., Massy, Z., Descamps-Latscha, B., Guerin, A. P., Marchais, S. J., Gausson, V., and London, G. M. (2002). Iron therapy, advanced oxidation protein products, and carotid artery intima-media thickness in end-stage renal disease. *Circulation* **106**, 2212–2217.

Fagerudd, J. A. *et al.* (1998). Predisposition to essential hypertension and development of diabetic nephropathy in IDDM patients. *Diabetes* **47**, 439–444.

Farmer, C. K. T. *et al.* (1988). Progression of diabetic nephropathy—is diurnal pressure rhythm as important as absolute blood pressure level. *Nephrology, Dialysis, Transplantation* **13**, 635–639.

Feest, T. G., Mistry, C. D., Grimes, D. S., and Mallick, N. P. (1990). Incidence of advanced chronic renal failure and the need for end stage renal replacement treatment. *British Medical Journal* **301**, 897–900.

Fliser, D., Schröter, M., Neubeck, M., and Ritz, E. (1994). Coadministration of thiazides increases the efficacy of loop diuretics even in patients with advanced renal failure. *Kidney International* **46**, 482–488.

Fliser, D., Pacini, G., Engelleiter, R., Kautzky-Willer, A., Prager, R., Franek, E., and Ritz, E. (1997a). Renal function in the elderly: impact of hypertension and cardiac function. *Kidney International* **51**, 1996–1204.

Fliser, D., Franek, E., Fode, P., Stefanski, A., Schmitt, C. P., Lyons, M., and Ritz, E. (1997b). Subacute infusion of physiological doses of parathyroid hormone raises blood pressure in humans. *Nephrology, Dialysis, Transplantation* **12**, 933–938.

Folkow, B. (1993). Early structural changes in hypertension: pathophysiology and clinical consequences. *Journal of Cardiovascular Pharmacology* **22**, S1–S6.

Gilbert, R. E. *et al.* (1999). Pathological expression of renin and angiotensin II in the renal tubule after subtotal nephrectomy. Implications for the pathogenesis of tubulo-interstitial fibrosis. *American Journal of Pathology* **155**, 429–440.

Goldsmith, D. J., Covic, A. C., Venning, M. C., and Ackrill, P. (1997). Ambulatory blood pressure monitoring in renal dialysis and transplant patients. *American Journal of Kidney Diseases* **29**, 593–600.

Guerin, A. P., Blacher, J., Pannier, B., Marchais, S. J., Safar, M. E., and London, G. M. (2001). Impact of aortic stiffness attenuation on survival of patients in end-stage renal failure. *Circulation* **103**, 987–992.

Guyton, A. C. (1987). Renal function curve: a key to understanding the pathogenesis of hypertension. *Hypertension* **10**, 1–6.

Harrap, S. B., Davies, D. L., Macnicol, A. N., and Watson, M. L. (1991). Renal, cardiovascular and hormonal characteristics of young adults with autosomal dominant polycystic kidney disease. *Kidney International* **40**, 501–508.

Hasdan, G., Benchetrit, S., Rashid, G., Green, J., Bernheim, J., and Rathaus, M. (2002). Endothelial dysfunction and hypertension in 5/6 nephrectomized rats are mediated by vascular superoxide. *Kidney International* **61**, 586.

Hostetter, T. H., Rosenberg, M. E., Ibrahim, H. N., and Juknevicius, I. (2001). Aldosterone in progressive renal disease. *Seminars in Nephrology* **21**, 573–579.

Jafar, T. H., Schmid, C. H., and Levey, A. S. (2002). Effect of angiotensin-converting enzyme inhibitors on progression of nondiabetic renal disease. *Annals of Internal Medicine* **137**, 298–299.

Kielstein, J. T., Boger, R. H., Bode-Boger, S. M., Frölich, J. C., Haller, H., Ritz, E., and Fliser, D. (2002). Marked increase of asymmetric dimethylarginine in patients with incipient primary chronic renal disease. *Journal of the American Society of Nephrology* **13**, 170–176.

Klag, M. J. *et al.* (1996). Blood pressure and end-stage renal disease in men. *New England Journal of Medicine* **334**, 13–18.

Klahr, S., Levey, A. S., Beck, G. J., Caggiula, A. W., Hunsicker, L., Kusek, J. W., and Striker, G. (1994). The effects of dietary protein restriction and blood-pressure control on the progression of chronic renal disease. *New England Journal of Medicine* **330**, 877–884.

Kobori, H., Harrison-Bernard, L. M., and Navar, L. G. (2002). Urinary excretion of angiotensinogen reflects intrarenal angiotensinogen production. *Kidney International* **61**, 579–585.

Koch, M., Thomas, B., Tschöpe, W., and Ritz, E. (1993). Survival and predictors of death in dialysed diabetic patients. *Diabetologia* **36**, 1113–1117.

Kooistra, M. P., Vos, J., Koomans, H. A., and Vos, P. F. (1998). Daily home hemodialysis in the Netherlands: effect on metabolic control, hemodynamics and quality of life. *Nephrology, Dialysis, Transplantation* **13**, 2853–2860.

Koomans, H. A., Braam, B., Geers, A. B., Roos, J. C., Dorhout, and Mees, E. J. (1986). The importance of plasma protein for blood volume and blood pressure homeostasis. *Kidney International* **30**, 730–735.

Krautzig, S., Janssen, U., Koch, K. M., Granolleras, C., and Shaldon, S. (1998). Dietary salt restriction and reduction of dialysate sodium to control hypertension in maintenance haemodialysis patients. *Nephrology, Dialysis, Transplantation* **13**, 552–553.

Kuczera, M., Hilgers, K. F., Lisson, C., Ganten, D., Hilgenfeld, U., Ritz, E., and Mann, J. F. E. (1991). Local angiotensin formation in hindlimbs of uremic hypertensive and renovascular hypertensive rats. *Journal of Hypertension* **9**, 41–48.

Küster, S., Mehls, O., Seidel, C., and Ritz, E. (1990). Blood pressure in minimal change and other types of nephrotic syndrome. *American Journal of Nephrology* **10**, S76–S80.

Lewington, S., Clarke, R., Qizilbash, N., Peto, R., Collins, R., and Prospective Studies Collaboration (2002). Age-specific relevance of usual blood pressure to vascular mortality: a meta-analysis of individual data for one million adults in 61 prospective studies. *Lancet* **360**, 1903–1913.

Lewis, E. J., Hunsicker, L. G., Bain, R. P., and Rohde, R. D. (1993). The effect of angiotensin-converting-enzyme inhibition on diabetic nephropathy. *New England Journal of Medicine* **329**, 1456–1462.

Lewis, E. J., Hunsicker, L. G., Clarke, W. R., Berl, T., Pohl, M. A., Lewis, J. B., Ritz, E., Atkins, R. C., Rohde, R., and Raz, I. (2001). Renoprotective effect of the angiotensin-receptor antagonist irbesartan in patients with nephropathy due to type 2 diabetes. *New England Journal of Medicine* **345**, 851–860.

Ligtenberg, G., Blankestijn, P. J., Oey, P. L., Klein, I. H., Dijkhorst-Oei, L. T., Boomsma, F., Wieneke, G. H., van Huffelen, A. C., and Koomans, H. A. (1999). Reduction of sympathetic hyperactivity by enalapril in patients with chronic renal failure. *New England Journal of Medicine* **340**, 1321–1328.

Locatelli, F. *et al.* (1984). Sodium kinetics across dialysis membranes. *Nephron* **38**, 174–177.

London, G. M. (2001). Controversy on optimal blood pressure on haemodialysis: lower is not always better. *Nephrology, Dialysis, Transplantation* **16**, 475–478.

London, G. M. *et al.* (1990). Aortic and large artery compliance in end-stage renal failure. *Kidney International* **37**, 137–142.

London, G. M., Pannier, B., Marchais Benetos, B., and Safar, M. (1992). Increased systolic pressure in chronic uremia. Role of arterial wave reflection. *Hypertension* **20**, 10–19.

London, G. M., Marchais, S. J., Guerin, A. P., Metivier, F., and Adda, H. (2002). Arterial structure and function in end-stage renal disease. *Nephrology, Dialysis, Transplantation* **17**, 1713–1724.

Lurbe, E., Redon, J., Kesani, A., Pascual, J. M., Tacons, J., Alvarez, V., and Batlle, D. (2002). Increase in nocturnal blood pressure and progression to microalbuminuria in type 1 diabetes. *New England Journal of Medicine* **347**, 797–805.

MacAllister, R. J. and Vallance, P. (1996). Systemic vascular adaption to increases in blood volume: the role of the blood-vessel wall. *Nephrology, Dialysis, Transplantation* **11**, 231–240.

Mailloux, L. and Haley, W. E. (1998). Hypertension in the ESRD patient: pathophysiology, therapy, outcomes and future directions. *American Journal of Kidney Diseases* **32**, 705–710.

Maschio, G. *et al.* (1996). Effect of angiotensin-converting enzyme inhibitor benazepril on the progression of chronic renal insufficiency. *New England Journal of Medicine* **334**, 939–945.

Mazzuchi, N., Carbonel, E., and Fernandez-Cean J. (2000). Importance of blood pressure control in hemodialysis patient survival. *Kidney International* **58**, 2147–2154.

McGrath, B. P., Tiller, D. J., Bune, A., Chalmers, J. P., Korner, P. I., and Athr, J. B. (1977). Autonomic blockade and the valsalva maneuver in patients with on maintenance hemodialysis: a hemodynamic study. *Kidney International* **12**, 279.

McGregor, D. O., Buttimore, A. L., Nicholls, M. G., and Lynn, K. L. (1999). Ambulatory blood pressure monitoring in patients receiving long, slow home haemodialysis. *Nephrology, Dialysis, Transplantation* **14**, 2676–2679.

Melin, J., Hellberg, O., Akyurek, L. M., Kallskog, O., Larsson, E., and Fellstrom, B. C. (1997). Ischemia causes rapidly progressive nephropathy in the diabetic rat. *Kidney International* **52**, 985–991.

Messerli, F. H. (1986). Osler's maneuver, pseudohypertension, and true hypertension in the elderly. *American Journal of Medicine* **80**, 906–910.

Miller, J. A. (1999). Impact of hyperglycemia on the renin angiotensin system in early human type 1 diabetes mellitus. *Journal of the American Society of Nephrology* **10**, 1778–1785.

Mogensen, C. E. (1982). Long-term antihypertensive treatment inhibiting progression of diabetic nephropathy. *British Medical Journal* **285**, 685–688.

Münter, K., Hergenröder, S., Jochims, K., and Kirchengast, M. (1996). Individual and combined effects of verapamil or trandolapril on attenuating hypertensive glomerulopathic changes in the stroke-prone rat. *Journal of the American Society of Nephrology* **7**, 1–6.

Nakano, S. *et al.* (1998a). Reversed circadian blood pressure rhythm is associated with occurences of both fatal and nonfatal vascular events in NIDDM subjects. *Diabetes* **47**, 1501–1506.

Nakano, S., Fukuda, M., Hotta, F., Ito, T., Ishii, T., Kitazawa, M., Nishizawa, M., Kigoshi, T., and Uchida, K. (1998b). Reversed circadian blood pressure rhythm is associated with occurences of both fatal and nonfatal vascular events in NIDDM subjects. *Diabetes* **47**, 1501–1506.

Nakano, S. *et al.* (1999). Reversed circadian blood pressure rhythm independently predicts endstage renal failure in non-insulin-dependent diabetes mellitus subjects. *Journal of Diabetes and its Complications* **13**, 224–231.

Navar, L. G., Harrison-Bernard, L. M., Imig, J. D., Wang, C. T., Cervenka, L., and Mitchell, K. D. (1999). Intrarenal angiotensin II generation and renal effects of AT1 receptor blockade. *Journal of the American Society of Nephrology* **10**, S266–S272.

Opelz, G., Wujciak, T., and Ritz, E. (1998). Association of chronic kidney graft failure with recipient blood pressure. *Kidney International* **53**, 217–222.

Orth, S. R., Stockmann, A., Conradt, C., Ritz, E., Ferro, M., Kreusser, W., Piccoli, G., Rambausek, M., Roccatello, D., Schafer, K., Sieberth, H. G., Wanner, C., Watschinger, B., and Zucchelli, P. (1998). Smoking as a risk factor for end-stage renal failure in men with primary renal disease. *Kidney International* **54**, 926–931.

Özkahya, M., Ok, E., Cirit, M., Aydin, S., Akcicek, F., Basci, A., Dorhout, and Mees, E. J. (1998). Regression of left ventricular hypertrophy in hemodialysis patients by ultrafiltration and reduced salt intake without antihypertensives drugs. *Nephrology, Dialysis, Transplantation* **13**, 1489–1493.

Parving, H. H., Andersen, A. R., Smidt, U. M., and Svendsen, P. A. (1983). Early aggressive antihypertensive treatment reduces rate of decline in kidney function in diabetic nephropathy. *Lancet* **28**, 1175–1179.

Perera, G. A. (1955). Hypertensive vascular disease description and natural history. *Journal of Chronic Diseases* **1**, 33–42.

Perry, H. M. *et al.* (1995). Early predictor of 15-year end-stage renal disease in hypertensive patients. *Hypertension* **25**, 587–594.

Petersen, J. C. *et al.* (1995). Blood pressure control, proteinuria, and the progression of renal disease. *Annals of Internal Medicine* **123**, 754–762.

Pierratos, A., Ouwendyk, M., Francoeur, R., Vas, S., Raj, D. S., Ecclestone, A. M., Langos, V., and Uldall, R. (1998). Nocturnal hemodialysis: three-year experience. *Journal of the American Society of Nephrology* **9**, 859–868.

Pitt, B., Zannad, F., Remme, W. J., Cody, R., Castaigne, A., Perez, A., Palensky, J., and Wittes, J. (1999). The effect of spironolactone on morbidity and mortality in patients with severe heart failure. Randomized Aldactone Evaluation Study Investigators. *New England Journal of Medicine* **341**, 709–717.

Port, F. K., Hulbert-Shearon, T. E., Wolfe, R. A., Bloembergen, W. E., Golper, T. A., Agodoa, L. Y., and Young, E. W. (1999). Predialysis blood pressure and mortality risk in a national sample of maintenance hemodialysis patients. *American Journal of Kidney Diseases* **33**, 507–517.

Price, D. A. *et al.* (1999). The paradox of the low-renin state in diabetic nephropathy. *Journal of the American Society of Nephrology* **10**, 2382–2391.

Raine, A. E. G. (1994). Acquired aortic stenosis in dialysis patients. *Nephron* **68**, 159–168.

Raine, A. E. G., Bedford, L., Simpson, A. W. M., Ashley, C. C., Brown, R., Woodhead, J. S., and Ledingham, J. G. G. (1993). Hyperparathyroidism, platelet intracellular free calcium and hypertension in chronic renal failure. *Kidney International* **43**, 700–705.

Rettig, R. *et al.* (1990). Role of the kidney in primary hypertension: a renal transplantation study in rats. *American Journal of Physiology* **258**, F606–F611.

Ritz, E., Schwenger, V., Zeier, M., and Rychlik, I. (2001). Ambulatory blood pressure monitoring: fancy gadgetry or clinical useful exercise? *Nephrology, Dialysis, Transplantation* **16**, 1550–1554.

Ruggenenti, P., Perna, A., Benini, R., and Remuzzi, G. (1998). Effects of dihydropyridine calcium channel blockers, angiotensin-converting enzyme inhibition, and blood pressure control on chronic, nondiabetic nephropathies. Gruppo Italiano di Studi Epidemiologici in Nefrologia (GISEN). *Journal of the American Society of Nephrology* **9**, 2096–2101.

Schalekamp, M. A. *et al.* (1973). Hypertension in chronic renal failure. An abnormal relation between sodium and the renin–angiotensin system. *American Journal of Medicine* **55**, 379.

Schernthaner, G., Ritz, E., Philipp, T., and Bretzel, R. G. (1999). Night time blood pressure in diabetic patients—the submerged portion of the iceberg? *Nephrology, Dialysis, Transplantation* **14**, 1061–1064.

Schmid, M. *et al.* (1990a). Natriuresis–pressure relationship in polycystic kidney disease. *Journal of Hypertension* **8**, 277–283.

Schmid, M., Meyer, S., Wegner, R., and Ritz E. (1990b). Increased genetic risk of hypertension in glomerulonephritis? *Journal of Hypertension* **8**, 573–577.

Schmidt, R. J. and Baylis, C. (2000). Total nitric oxide production is low in patients with chronic renal disease. *Kidney International* **58**, 1261–1266.

Schnackenberg, C. G., Welch, W. J., and Wilcox, C. S. (1998). Normalization of blood pressure and renal vascular resistance in SHR with a membrane-permeable superoxide dismutase mimetic: role of nitric oxide. *Hypertension* **32**, 59–64.

Schohn, D., Weimann, P., Jahn, H., and Beretta-Piccoli, C. (1985). Norepinephrin-related mechanism in hypertension accompanying renal failure. *Kidney International* **28**, 814–822.

Schwenger, V. and Ritz, E. (1998). Audit of antihypertensive treatment in patients with renal failure. *Nephrology, Dialysis, Transplantation* **13**, 3091–3095.

Schömig, M., Eisenhardt, A., and Ritz, E. (2001). Controversy on optimal blood pressure on haemodialysis: normotensive blood pressure values are essential for survival. *Nephrology, Dialysis, Transplantation* **16**, 469–474.

Scribner, B. H., Buri, R., Caner, J. E. Z., Hegstrom, R., and Burnell, J. M. (1960). The treatment of chronic uremia by means of intermittent hemodialysis: a preliminary report. *Transaction of American Society for Artificial Internal Organs* **6**, 114–122.

Scribner, B. H., Buri, R., Caner, J. E., Hegstrom, R., and Burnell, J. M. (1998). The treatment of chronic uremia by means of intermittent hemodialysis: a preliminary report. 1960. *Journal of the American Society of Nephrology* **9**, 719–726.

Stefanski, A., Amann, K., and Ritz, E. (1995). To prevent progression: ACE inhibitors, calcium antagonists or both? *Nephrology, Dialysis, Transplantation* **10**, 151–153.

Stefanski, A., Schmidt, K. G., Waldherr, R., and Ritz, E. (1996). Early increase in blood pressure and diastolic left ventricular malfunction in patients with glomerulonephritis. *Kidney International* **50**, 1321–1326.

Stier, C. T., Jr., Chander, P. N., and Rocha, R. (2002). Aldosterone as a mediator in cardiovascular injury. *Cardiology in Review* **10**, 97–107.

Strojek, K. *et al.* (1997). Nephropathy of type II diabetes: evidence for hereditary factors? *Kidney International* **51**, 1602–1607.

Strojek, K. *et al.* (2001). Lowering of microalbuminuria in diabetic patients by a sympathoplegic agent: a novel approach to prevent progression of diabetic nephropathy? *Journal of the American Society of Nephrology* **12**, 602–605.

The GISEN Group (Gruppo Italiano Di Studi Epidemiologici In Nefrologia) (1997). Randomized placebo-controlled trial of effect of ramipril on decline in glomerular filtration rate and risk of terminal renal failure in proteinuric: non-diabetic nephropathy. *Lancet* **349**, 1857–1863.

Thomson, G. E., Waterhouse, K., McDonald, H. P. J., and Friedman, E. A. (1967). Hemodialysis for chronic renal failure. *Archieves of Internal Medicine* **120**, 153–167.

Timio, M., Venanzi, S., Lolli, S., Lippi, G., Verdura, C., Monarca, C., and Guerrini, E. (1995). 'Non-dipper' hypertensive patients and progressive renal insufficiency. A 3-year longitudinal study. *Clinical Nephrology* **43**, 382–387.

Tuomilehto, J., Rastenyte, D., Birkenhager, W. H., Thijs, L., Antikainen, R., Bulpitt, C. J., Fletcher, A. E., Forette, F., Goldhaber, A., Palatini, P., Sarti, C., and Fagard, R. (1999). Effects of calcium-channel blockade in older patients with diabetes and systolic hypertension. Systolic Hypertension in Europe Trial Investigators. *New England Journal of Medicine* **340**, 677–684.

Vaziri, N. D., Oveisi, F., and Ding, Y. (1998). Role of increased oxygen free radical activity in the pathogenesis of uremic hypertension. *Kidney International* **53**, 1748–1754.

Vertes, V., Cangiano, J. L., Berman, L. B., and Gould, A. (1969). Hypertension in end-stage renal disease. *New England Journal of Medicine* **280**, 978–981.

Volhard, F. (1923). Der arterielle Blutdruck. *Verhandlungen der Deutschen gesellschaft fur Innere Medizin* **35**, 134–184.

Wanner, C., Krane, V., Ruf, G., Marz, W., and Ritz, E. (1999). Rationale and design of a trial improving outcome of type 2 diabetics on hemodialysis. Die Deutsche Diabetes Dialyse Studie Investigators. *Kidney International* **71**, S222–S226.

WHO ISH Guidelines Subcommittee (1999). WHO-ISH guidelines for the management of hypertension. *Journal of Hypertension* **17**, 151–183.

Wolf, G. (1999). Angiotensin II: a pivotal factor in the progression of renal diseases. *Nephrology, Dialysis, Transplantation* **14**, 42–44.

Wright J. T., Jr., Bakris, G., Greene, T., Agodoa, L. Y., Appel, L. J., Charleston, J., Cheek, D., Douglas-Baltimore, J. G., Gassman, J., Glassock, R., Hebert, L., Jamerson, K., Lewis, J., Phillips, R. A., Toto, R. D., Middleton, J. P., Rostand, S. G., and African American Study of Kidney Disease and Hypertension Study Group (2002). Effect of blood pressure lowering and antihypertensive drug class on progression of hypertensive kidney disease: results from the AASK trial. *Journal of the American Medical Association* **288**, 2421–2431.

Zager, P. G., Nikolic, J., Brown, R. H., Campbell, M. A., Hunt, W. C., Peterson, D., Van Stone, J., Levey, A., Meyer, K. B., Klag, M. J., Johnson, H. K., Clark, E., Sadler, J. H., and Teredesai, P. (1998). 'U' curve association of blood pressure and mortality in hemodialysis patients. *Kidney International* **54**, 561–569.

Zeier, M., Fehrenbach, P., Geberth, S., Mohring, K., Waldherr, R., and Ritz, E. (1992). Renal histology in polycystic kidney disease with incipient and advanced renal failure. *Kidney International* **42**, 1259–1265.

Zeier, M., Wiesel, M., Rambausek, M., and Ritz, E. (1995). Non-occlusive mesenteric infarction in dialysis patients: the importance of prevention and early intervention. *Nephrology, Dialysis, Transplantation* **10**, 771–773.

Zoccali, C. (2002). Endothelial damage, asymmetric dimethylarginine and cardiovascular risk in end-stage renal disease. *Blood Purification* **20**, 469–472.

Zoccali, C. (2003). Arterial pressure components and cardiovascular risk in end-stage renal disease. *Nephrology, Dialysis, Transplantation* **18**, 249–252.

Zoccali, C., Mallamaci, F., and Tripepi, G. (2001). Sleep apnea in renal patients. *Journal of the American Society of Nephrology* **12**, 2854–2859.

Zoccali C., Mallamaci, F., and Tripepi, G. (2002). Nocturnal hypoxemia predicts incident cardiovascular complications in dialysis patients. *Journal of the American Society of Nephrology* **13**, 729–733.

Zuanetti, G., Maggioni, A. P., Keane, W., and Ritz, E. (1997). Nephrologists neglect administration of betablockers to dialysed diabetic patients. *Nephrology, Dialysis, Transplantation* **12**, 2497–2500.

11.3.5 Cardiovascular risk factors
Eberhard Ritz and Robert N. Foley

Epidemiology

The frequency of fatal and non-fatal cardiovascular events is increased even in the earliest stages of chronic kidney disease (Ruilope *et al.* 2001a,b; Ritz 2003) and in dialysis patients cardiovascular events are the most frequent cause of death (Table 1). According to the Annual Report 2001 of the United States Renal Data System (USRDS), the incidence of new myocardial infarction in the first year of renal replacement therapy was 7.0 per cent, of cerebrovascular accidents 7.1 per cent, and of surgery for peripheral vascular disease 8.4 per cent. As a crude comparison, the Framingham Heart Study reported that the annual risk of re-infarction in subjects surviving a first recognized myocardial infarction was 4 per cent per year, almost half the risk of new myocardial infarction in dialysis patients (Berger *et al.* 1992). In the recent HEMO study, the most common cause of death in dialysed patients was ischaemic heart disease (20.4 per cent) followed by cardiac rhythm disorder (10.4 per cent), cerebrovascular disease (8.6 per cent), and infections (7.7 per cent) (Rocco *et al.* 2002). The Prospective Canadian Study had reported an incidence of approximately 10 per cent per year for both ischaemic heart disease and cardiac failure in incident patients, significantly greater than the values seen in the

Table 1 Adjusted cause-specific death rates per 1000 patient years in the period from 1999 to 2001

	Death per 1000 dialysis patient years			
	Total	(%)	Male	Female
Acute myocardial infarction	19.9	(8.4)	20.5	19.2
Carrdiac arrest	51.9	(21.9)	50.6	53.2
Cardiomyopathy	8.4	(3.6)	9.3	7.4
Cardic arrhythmia	11.2	(4.7)	11.3	11.1
Valvular disease	1.4	(0.6)	1.3	1.5
Cerebrovascular disease	12.3	(5.2)	10.3	14.7
Septicaemia/infection	26.4	(11.6)	23.3	29.9
Other causes	105	(44.0)	109.9	100.4
Total	236.5	(100.0)	229.3	244.8

Ref.: Annual Report USRDS (www.usrds.org).

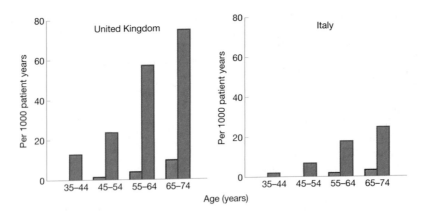

Fig. 1 Incidence of death from ischaemic heart disease in dialysis patients. The age-specific death rate from myocardial ischaemia and infarction is given for males, commencing renal replacement therapy between 1985 and 1990 in the United Kingdom and Italy compared with that of males in the general population. In all renal replacement therapy groups the death rate in Italy is one-third to one-fourth of that in the United Kingdom. Note that the death rate from ischaemic heart disease in each age group in the general population is also markedly less in Italy than in the United Kingdom (Raine *et al.* 1992).

general population (Churchill *et al.* 1992) and considerably beyond the notional threshold value of 20 per cent risk per decade. Not only is the incidence excessive, but also the acute death rate as well as death in the 3 years following myocardial infarction (Herzog *et al.* 1998).

A problem which had to some extent been neglected in the past was cardiac failure as a cause of death. Cohort studies indicate that admission for cardiac failure is a common and frequently lethal occurrence (Harnett *et al.* 1995). This is also true particularly after renal transplantation, where cardiac failure occurred as frequently as ischaemic heart disease with a similar impact on survival. The frequency was markedly higher than in the Framingham cohort. Renal transplantation is apparently more a state of 'accelerated heart failure' than 'accelerated atherosclerosis' (Rigatto *et al.* 2002).

In Europe there are interesting regional differences. When one compares the mortality from cardiovascular causes in patients with endstage renal failure in Northern Europe and in Southern Europe, the mortality rates from stroke, heart failure, and sudden death are relatively similar, whereas the incidence of death from ischaemic heart disease is three to four times greater in North European patients (Fig. 1). However, relative to the general population, age, gender, and country-specific rates of death from myocardial infarction are relative to that of the general population and are equally increased by a factor of approximately 18 both in Northern and Southern Europe. It appears that uraemia acts to amplify the incidence of fatal ischaemic heart disease by a constant factor irrespective of the baseline incidence in the general population (Raine *et al.* 1992).

When maintenance haemodialysis was introduced by Scribner in March 1960, the naive view prevailed that if one removed uraemic toxins sufficiently well by dialysis, life expectancy would approach that in the general population. This view was shattered by the report of Lindner *et al.* (1974) documenting a strikingly increased rate of death from myocardial infarction which led the authors to suggest that atherogenesis was accelerated in uraemia. Meanwhile there is good experimental evidence to suggest that even minor renal dysfunction causes greatly accelerated atherogenesis (Buzello *et al.* 2003). In agreement with this notion both autopsy studies (Clyne *et al.* 1986) and studies using coronary angiography (Ikram *et al.* 1983) or electron-beam computed tomography (Braun *et al.* 1996; Goodman *et al.* 2000;

Table 2 Syndromes presented by uraemic patient

Congestive heart failure/hypervolaemia

Ischaemic heart disease ($\pm$congestive heart failure)

Left ventricular hypertrophy, concentric or eccentric

Acquired valvular heart disease

Arrhythmia

Oh *et al.* 2002) documented an excessive prevalence of coronary atherosclerosis in dialysis patients.

Clinical syndromes

Uraemic patients may present with one of five syndromes (Table 2).

Since there is considerable overlap, the general management of renal patients with these cardiac syndromes are summarized below in the section 'management of the renal patient with cardiac problems'.

Cardiovascular risk and its prevention

Risk factors

Hypertension

In non-renal patients hypertension and left ventricular (LV) hypertrophy are closely related, but this relationship is less marked in patients with renal failure (Huting *et al.* 1988; Amann *et al.* 1996). LV hypertrophy develops in uraemic animals despite normalization of blood pressure by administration of angiotensin-converting enzyme (ACE) inhibitors, α- and β-blockers or diuretics (Rambausek *et al.* 1985). In patients, LV hypertrophy progresses with time on dialysis even when patients are kept normotensive (Huting *et al.* 1988; Parfrey *et al.* 1990; Foley *et al.* 1998). In the study of Parfrey, 71 per cent of non-diabetic dialysis patients without dilated cardiomyopathy had LV hypertrophy and in the majority of patients this progressed over a period of 3–4 years. Progression was not predicted by blood pressure, hyperparathyroidism or anaemia (although these factors are definitely involved), suggesting that additional factors may play a part. The role of angiotensin II, possibly acting locally, is suggested by observations suggesting that LV hypertrophy is ameliorated by administration of ACE inhibitors independent of blood pressure (Cannella *et al.* 1993, 1998) and the role of anaemia is suggested by numerous observations that increasing haematocrit by administration of erythropoietin (EPO) improves (London *et al.* 1989b), or at least prevents LV hypertrophy (Foley *et al.* 2000) but certainly fails to fully normalize LV mass.

It is not only systolic and diastolic blood pressure which determine LV work and LV mass. It has recently been recognized that in renal failure stiffening of the aorta and the associated increased impedance make a major contribution to LV hypertrophy. High pulse pressure, that is, blood pressure amplitude, which is a surrogate marker for aortic stiffness and pulse wave velocity is a potent predictor of LV mass and cardiovascular events (Blacher *et al.* 2002, 2003; Klassen *et al.* 2002; Tozawa *et al.* 2002).

Anaemia

Sustained anaemia leads to vasodilatation, increased venous return, cardiac enlargement and increased cardiac output (Foley *et al.* 1995; Muirhead *et al.* 1995). These compensatory mechanisms lead to maladaptive tradeoffs. Numerous observational studies documented that anaemia is associated with increased LV mass in patients with chronic kidney disease and this is true even for apparently trivial degrees of anaemia (Levin *et al.* 1999). Observational studies have also suggested that anaemia is an independent predictor of mortality (Foley *et al.* 1996; Madore *et al.* 1997; Ma *et al.* 1999), although this association does not necessarily imply causality. Partial correction of anaemia partly corrects LV hypertrophy (London *et al.* 1989a,b; Macdougall *et al.* 1990). Although this would appear intuitively plausible, there is no controlled evidence that reversal of anaemia reduces cardiovascular mortality. The United States Normal Hematocrit Trial assigned patients to haematocrit targets of 30 or 42 per cent. Assignment did not significantly affect death or first non-fatal myocardial infarction which remained similar in both groups (Besarab *et al.* 1998). Several critiques can be raised against this study, however (Macdougall and Ritz 1998). It is apparently easier to prevent, than to reverse, cardiac abnormalities by treating anaemia. In the Canadian Normalisation of Hemoglobin Trial, haemodialysis patients with asymptomatic echocardiographic enlargement were randomly treated to a haemoglobin (Hb) of 10 or 13.5 g/dl. The higher Hb failed to regress left ventricles that were already dilated, but a normal Hb at least prevented the development of new LV dilatation (Foley *et al.* 2000). In a randomized double-blind cross-over study performed in Australian patients, quality of life, LV dilatation and systolic hyperfunction improved, when Hb concentrations of 10 and 14 g/dl were compared (McMahon *et al.* 1999, 2000).

Diabetes mellitus

As discussed elsewhere (Chapter 4.1) diabetic patients with endstage renal failure have particularly high cardiovascular morbidity and mortality. Even diabetic patients without nephropathy have major abnormalities of sympathetic innervation, vasodilatory reserve, and cardiac structure (Standl and Schnell 2000). In observational studies, when compared to non-diabetic individuals, diabetic patients have more severe LV

hypertrophy and also develop more frequently ischaemic heart disease (Foley *et al.* 1997; Dikow and Ritz 2003) as shown in Table 3.

Sympathetic overactivity

Sympathetic overactivity is consistently found in renal failure (Converse *et al.* 1992; Campese and Kogosov 1995; Klein *et al.* 2001) although α- and β-adrenergic end-organ response is attenuated (Rascher *et al.* 1982; Mann *et al.* 1986; Leineweber *et al.* 2002). Increased sympathetic activity has important consequences on the heart: for instance, it contributes to hypertrophy and impairs capillary growth and this can be reversed by sympathoplegic agents (Tornig *et al.* 1996). Renal failure is characterized not only by sympathetic overactivity, but also autonomic polyneuropathy with denervation suprasensitivity. This constellation presumably predisposes to arrhythmia and sudden death. Catecholamines are a strong predictor of cardiac death (Zoccali *et al.* 2002) in dialysed patients and conversely administration of β-blockers is associated with less mortality in observational (Koch *et al.* 1993) and interventional (Cice *et al.* 2003) studies.

Arteriovenous fistula

Cardiomegaly is a well-known complication of large arteriovenous shunts. The fistulas used for vascular access in haemodialysis are usually located in the periphery thus causing relatively little increase of cardiac output. Nevertheless, in the study of London cardiac output was one of the determinants of LV mass. The importance of this factor may be higher for patients with large proximal fistulas which cause marked hypercirculation and eccentric LV hypertrophy (London *et al.* 1987).

Hypervolaemia

Chronic volume overload in the uraemic patient increases cardiac filling pressures and venous return, thus imposing an increased work load on the left ventricle. Ultimately, such increased preload results in LV dilatation and LV hypertrophy. A correlation is found between LV volume and blood volume. In patients with fluid overload the heart diameters usually return to normal a few hours after ultrafiltration, but chronic overload may lead to eccentric LV hypertrophy and irreversible dilatation. The importance of hypervolaemia is illustrated by the observation of Ozkahaya *et al.* (1998, 2002) that volume control by

Table 3 Diabetic patients on dialysis—cardiac findings

	Diabetic patients (*n* = 317) %	Non-diabetic patients (*n* = 317) %	*p*
Baseline			
Concentric left ventricular hypertrophy	50	38	0.04
Ischaemic heart disease	32	18	0.003
Cardiac failure	48	25	0.00001
Follow-up	Adjusted relative risk (diabetic versus non-diabetic)		
Ischaemic heart disease	3.2		0.0002
Overall mortality	2.3		0.0001
Cardiovascular mortality	2.6		0.0001

After (Foley *et al.* 1997).

low salt diet and aggressive ultrafiltration reversed LV dilatation and hypertrophy despite no administration of antihypertensive agents.

Secondary hyperparathyroidism

Several authors have suggested that secondary hyperparathyroidism plays a role in the genesis of LV hypertrophy and dysfunction. Parathyroid hormone (PTH) acts directly on cardiomyocytes to enhance calcium entry; it increased inotropy, but also causes accelerated cell death. It has been found (London *et al.* 1987) that excess PTH caused inappropriate LV hypertrophy, that is, less hypertrophy than anticipated on the basis of LV end-diastolic diameter. This implies some inhibitory effect of PTH on the increase in LV mass.

The issue whether hyperparathyroidism results in increased or impaired systolic function (Lai *et al.* 1985; Sato *et al.* 1995) has not been resolved. PTH is a permissive factor in the genesis of cardiac fibrosis (Amann *et al.* 1994) and wall thickening of cardiac arteries (Amann *et al.* 1995b).

Prevention

Unfortunately, there is next to no controlled evidence to guide the clinician in the prevention of the cardiovascular complications of renal disease. Table 4 lists the main points that have to be considered.

It is important that an increased risk of cardiovascular disease is not unique to endstage renal failure, but is seen with even borderline decrease of glomerular filtration rate (GFR) (Ruilope *et al.* 2001a,b; Ritz 2003). Following observations in the Framingham study, this has been shown in the general population (Henry *et al.* 2002), in patients with hypertension (Ruilope *et al.* 2001a,b), in patients at high cardiovascular risk (Mann *et al.* 2001) and in patients with congestive heart failure (Hillege *et al.* 2000). Even borderline reduction in GFR causes a dramatic increase in the mortality of ischaemic cardiac events (Shlipak *et al.* 2002; Wright *et al.* 2002) and increases mortality after coronary interventions (Reinecke *et al.* 2003).

As shown in Fig. 2, hypertension is an important risk factor and the low blood pressure values recommended in the United States by the Joint National Committee's Report (1997) of less than 130/85 mmHg for patients without and less than 125/75 mmHg for renal patients with proteinuria more than 1 g/24 h are appropriate not only for interfering with progression, but also for cardioprotection. In large trials, for example, the MDRD trial, no evidence for a J-curve phenomenon was noted, that is, for the concept that lowering blood pressure to values less than a threshold value, would cause a paradoxical increase of cardiac mortality.

The HOPE study (Yusuf *et al.* 2000) showed that ACE inhibitors have blood-pressure-independent cardioprotective effects or at least effects which are not fully explained by blood pressure lowering. At least with respect to stroke prevention, the same has been shown for angiotensin receptor blockers (Dahlof *et al.* 2002).

Dyslipidaemia is common in renal patients even at early stages of renal dysfunction. The magnitude of the lipid-related cardiovascular risk cannot be assessed from total cholesterol and total triglyceride concentrations and not even from additional measurements of high density and low density lipoprotein (HDL and LDL, respectively) cholesterol. Uraemia is characterized by the appearance of highly atherogenic lipid subfractions, for example, persisting chylomicrons, highly atherogenic intermediate density lipoproteins (IDL) and small dense LDL as well as HDL modified by an acute phase reaction (Attman 1993; Wanner and

Table 4 Factors influencing left ventricular function and mass in uraemia

Haemodynamic factors
Hypertension
Fluid retention
Renal anaemia
Arteriovenous fistula
Acquired valvular disease
Constrictive pericarditis

Non-haemodynamic factors
Ischaemic heart disease
Diabetic cardiomyopathy
Autonomic dysfunction
Excess PTH
Aluminium overload
Hypocalcaemia
Myocardial calcification
   (calcium–phosphorus product)
Metabolic acidosis
Iron overload
β2m amyloidosis
Thiamine deficiency, carnitine
   deficiency (?)

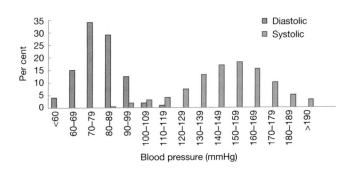

Fig. 2 Percentage risk factor versus blood pressure values.

Krane 2002; Kronenberg *et al.* 2003). In addition, there are changes in the relative contributions of apolipoprotein subfractions (Moberly *et al.* 1999) and finally an increase of Lpa (Kronenberg *et al.* 1996). The cardiovascular risk of the latter depends on the apolipoprotein genotype.

In a retrospective analysis, dialysis patients who have received statins had an approximately 10 per cent better survival (Seliger *et al.* 2002), but one has to wait for the definite controlled evidence in the ongoing 4D trial (Wanner *et al.* 1999) to assess the impact of statins in endstage renal disease. This point is important because conceivably alternative causes that are susceptible to treatment with statines, for instance, vascular calcification, may play an overriding role. Matters are somewhat different for earlier stages of renal failure. Subgroup analysis of patients with impaired renal function in three major studies (Holdaas *et al.* 2003; Sever *et al.* 2003; Tonelli *et al.* 2003) showed uniformly that renal patients were benefitted by the administration of statins with respect to cardiovascular risk.

A relatively novel insight is the observation that even a slight decrease of anaemia increases the cardiovascular risk. Levin *et al.* (1999) noted that an Hb concentration lower by only 0.5 g/dl increased by 30 per cent the relative risk of a gain in LV mass. Whether this translates into higher mortality is currently not proven, but this is likely in view of the correlation between LV mass and survival that is found in dialysed patients (Silverberg *et al.* 2001). In patients with congestive heart failure uncontrolled observational studies (Silverberg *et al.* 2001; Ezekowitz *et al.* 2003) suggest that the outcome is worse when anaemia is present, but again controlled prospective evidence is not available.

Smoking is a potent cardiovascular risk factor in the non-renal patient. In renal patients as well, there is overwhelming evidence that smoking increases the risk of cardiovascular events (Foley *et al.* 2003).

It has long been assumed that since uraemia is associated with thrombocyte dysfunction, the administration of platelet aggregation inhibitors was not indicated. In a sizeable proportion of uraemic patients, increased rather than decreased platelet aggregation was noted in our studies. Although controlled evidence is again not available, it seems sensible to administer low doses of aspirin, for example, 50 mg/day (unless there are contraindications) given the relative safety and the overwhelming evidence in non-renal patients.

In renal patients, a correlation has been found, although not uniformly so (Suliman *et al.* 2003) between homocysteine concentration and cardiovascular events (Chauveau *et al.* 1993; Jungers *et al.* 1997). It is well documented that administration of 5 mg folate per day lowers plasma homocystein concentrations (Perna *et al.* 1997), but higher doses of folate do not result in further lowering. Despite some reports (Schnyder *et al.* 2001) prospective evidence for a beneficial effect of lowering homocysteine is still wanting. Nevertheless, given the fact that folate is safe and inexpensive, most nephrologists prefer to administer this on a routine basis.

In large studies in non-renal patients administration of vitamin E did not reduce cardiovascular events. In contrast, a small study (Boaz *et al.* 2000) showed less cardiovascular events in dialysed patients, although hard endpoints were not evaluated. Animal studies are also encouraging (Amann *et al.* 2002). It may well be that uraemia as a state of high reactive oxidant stress is particularly responsive to the administration of this antioxidant. This issue is currently under investigation in a prospective trial.

Left ventricular hypertrophy

Epidemiology and causal factors

LV hypertrophy is more frequent in early stages of chronic kidney disease and increases progressively, so that it is found in approximately 70 per cent of patients starting renal replacement therapy (Levin *et al.* 1999). Initially concentric LV hypertrophy is seen, while in later stages more frequently eccentric LV hypertrophy prevails. LV hypertrophy tends to be associated with hypertension, anaemia, high arteriovenous fistula flow and poor control of volume overload (London *et al.* 1989a,b). At an early stage systolic function is usually normal or even increased, but evidence of diastolic malfunction—including reduced compliance and abnormal passive filling of the LV—can be found even in asymptomatic patients. Diastolic filling problems are strongly associated with LV hypertrophy of the concentric or asymmetrically (septal) type. LV hypertrophy is not an innocent academic finding: Silberberg *et al.* (1989) had clearly documented that it was an independent predictor of death on dialysis (Fig. 3).

Some important factors influence LV function as well as LV mass and some of these factors will be discussed below.

Left ventricular structure

Increased LV mass is accompanied by increased size of individual cardiomyocytes as seen in other settings of cardiac hypertrophy and this is associated with increased cytosolic calcium and abnormal cycling of calcium (Kennedy *et al.* 2003). In the past LV hypertrophy was thought to be a useful adaptive phenomenon reducing LV wall stress per structural element. It is triggered as a response to increased afterload (parallel deposition of sarcomers leading to concentric hypertrophy) or as a compensatory response to volume overload (causing deposition of sarcomers in series and leading to eccentric hypertrophy). It has recently been recognized, however, that LV hypertrophy has maladaptive structural and functional features (Amann and Ritz 2001). In contrast to the 'athlete's heart' with increased LV mass but normal interstitium, LV hypertrophy of hypertensive or renal patients is associated with cardiac fibrosis (see below). It also predisposes to dilated cardiomyopathy resulting from increased myocyte death as proven experimentally (Amann *et al.* 2003a,b). It also associated with expression of fetal gene programmes. These features are summarized in Fig. 4.

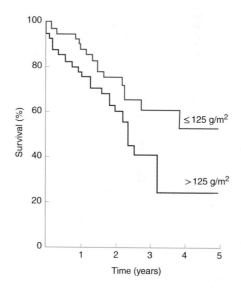

Fig. 3 LV hypertrophy reduces actuarial survival in dialysis patients. Cumulative survival according to echocardiographic LV hypertrophy defined as LV mitral inflow greater than 125 g/m². This cut-off point corresponds to the 95th centile of the normal population.

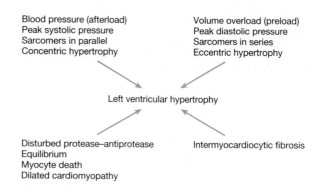

Fig. 4 Factors involved in LV hypertrophy.

Cardiac fibrosis in uraemic patients had been shown decades ago. It is common in patients on dialysis (Mall *et al.* 1990) and can be reproduced in uraemic animals (Mall *et al.* 1988). Ultrastructural analysis (Fig. 5) shows activation of interstitial cells. Activation selectively concerns interstitial, but not endothelial cells. Interstitial cell activation is accompanied by increased expression of cytokines, particularly transforming growth factor β. In subtotally nephrectomized rats, interstitial fibrosis is not consistently prevented by antihypertensive treatment (Tornig *et al.* 1996), but is significantly reduced by parathyroidectomy (Amann *et al.* 1994) and abrogated by endothelin receptor blockers (Nabokov *et al.* 1999). Cardiac fibrosis was found in the right as well as in the left ventricle documenting that factors other than haemodynamic overload must play a role.

A further structural abnormality observed in the heart of uraemic patients is metastatic calcification, most closely related to an elevated calcium phosphate product (Maher and Curtis 1985; Rostand *et al.* 1994).

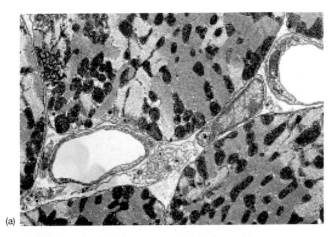

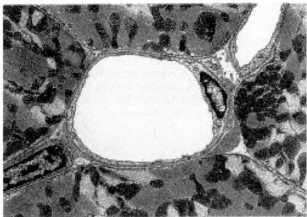

Fig. 5 Ultrastructural evidence of interstitial cell activation in experimental uraemia. (a) Ultrastructure of cardiac myocytes and the vascular and non-vascular interstitium in short-term (14 days) uraemia (subtotally nephrectomized rats). Note the normal morphology of the myocytes and capillaries whilst in the non-vascular interstitium signs of interstitial cell activation are found (electron micrograph stained with uranyl acetate and lead citrate; magnification 7560×). (b) Ultrastructure of the myocardium of a control rat. No interstitial cell activation can be seen. Electron micrograph stained with uranyl acetate and lead citrate, magnification 10,000×).

Structural changes in the heart, that is, LV hypertrophy, cardiac fibrosis, and metastatic calcification, have major implications for cardiac function. LV hypertrophy and fibrosis are associated with impaired LV compliance. As shown by Doppler echocardiography (Fig. 6), the reduction of LV compliance impairs early LV filling: the relative contribution of passive protodiastolic filling is decreased, whilst the relative contribution of active atrial contraction to LV filling is increased (low E/A ratio). This explains why dialysed patients develop heart failure so easily when atrial fibrillation supervenes. Reduction of LV compliance has also an impact on the relation between LV volume and pressure (Fig. 7). As a result hypervolaemia will be less well tolerated because the given increase in LV volume will cause a more marked increase of LV end-diastolic pressure. This increases the risk of pulmonary oedema during hypervolaemia. Conversely, a marked reduction in LV filling, for example, during ultrafiltration, will produce an exaggerated reduction of end-diastolic LV pressure resulting in diminished cardiac output and hypotension. This explains why intradialytic hypotension is much more frequent in patients with LV hypertrophy (Ruffmann *et al.* 1990).

LV hypertrophy also adversely affects the coronary reserve, that is, the ability of coronary arteries to dilate when myocardial demand is increased. Because of the increased extravasal resistance, coronary reserve is reduced as illustrated in the patient with aortic valve stenosis. They suffer from angina pectoris despite patent arteries. Similarly the uraemic patient with LV hypertrophy may have ischaemia intolerance when oxygen demand is increased. Finally, the disruption of cardiac anatomy by fibrotic tissue predisposes to arrhythmogenesis, particularly re-entrant arrhythmias. This results from the fact that interposition of high resistance fibrotic tissue impairs the propagation of the action potential and creates re-entry pathways.

Against this background, it is not surprising that LV hypertrophy is an independent predictor of cardiac death in dialysis patients (Silberberg *et al.* 1989), as illustrated in Fig. 8.

Diagnosis of LV hypertrophy

Clinical methods such as evaluation of apex beat, third and fourth heart sound and increased cardiothoracic ratio on chest radiography may be misleading, since they may also be abnormal because of hypervolaemia. The electrocardiogram (ECG) lacks sensitivity. The method of choice to assess LV geometry is echocardiography [or for investigational purposes magnetic resonance tomography (MRT)]. It is important that a standardized approach is used with initial location of the echo beam through the mitral valve apparatus, and subsequent identification and measurement of a septum and the posterior wall by M-mode recording. The usual procedure is to derive LV mass by the Penn convention (Devereux and Reichek 1977). By using MRT it has recently been shown that the underlying geometrical assumptions are not met and may cause major errors (Stewart *et al.* 1999). Figures 9–12 show typical findings.

Ischaemic heart disease

Pathogenesis of the coronary lesion

Ischaemic heart disease is common in uraemia, but it is noteworthy (Table 1) that myocardial infarction is only the second most frequent cause of cardiovascular death in the dialysis patient. The most frequent cause is sudden death. Accelerated atherogenesis, as postulated by Lindner *et al.* (1974) has meanwhile been confirmed in experimental

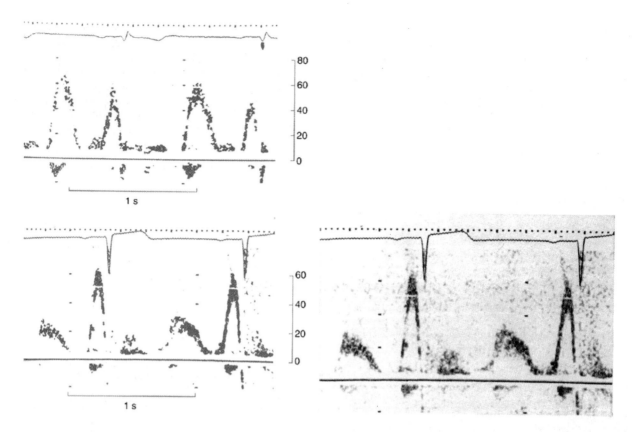

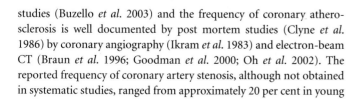

Fig. 6 Doppler echocardiograms showing mitral inflow velocities in a control (upper panel) and a dialysis patient (lower panel). The first peak is due to protodiastolic filling, and the second is due to atrial contraction. The relative contribution of protodiastolic filling to mitral inflow is decreased in the dialysis patient.

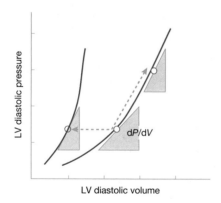

Fig. 7 Left ventricular compliance in uraemic patients. Compliance is indicated by the volume to pressure relationship in the left ventricle during diastolic filling. In patients with endstage renal disease, the pressure–volume relationship of the left ventricle is typically shifted to the left indicating that myocardial compliance is decreased.

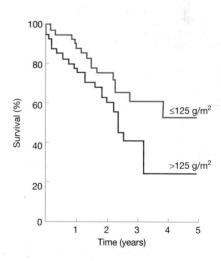

Fig. 8 LV hypertrophy reduces actuarial survival in dialysis patients. Cumulative survival according to echocardiographic LV hypertrophy defined as LV mitral inflow greater than 125 g/m^2. This cut-off corresponds to the 95th centile of the normal population.

studies (Buzello *et al.* 2003) and the frequency of coronary athero-sclerosis is well documented by post mortem studies (Clyne *et al.* 1986) by coronary angiography (Ikram *et al.* 1983) and electron-beam CT (Braun *et al.* 1996; Goodman *et al.* 2000; Oh *et al.* 2002). The reported frequency of coronary artery stenosis, although not obtained in systematic studies, ranged from approximately 20 per cent in young

non-diabetic haemodialysis patients to 85 per cent in elderly uraemic patients with type 1 diabetes (Manske *et al.* 1993).

It appears that ischaemic heart disease is not fully explained by the classical risk factors for cardiovascular disease (Himmelfarb *et al.* 2002).

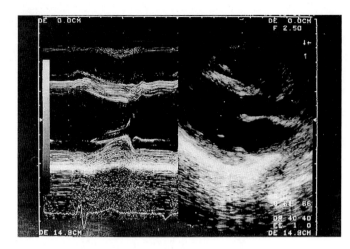

Fig. 9 Long-axis parasternal echocardiogram of a normal LV with normal LV systolic function, normal wall thickness (<12 mm), and normal cavity dimensions (LV end-systolic diameter < 56 mm). The M-mode echocardiogram is shown on the left, with the two-dimensional on the right. Note the echoes immediately anterior to the posterior LV wall, which are from the mitral valve apparatus (posterior chordae) and should be differentiated from the endocardial echoes.

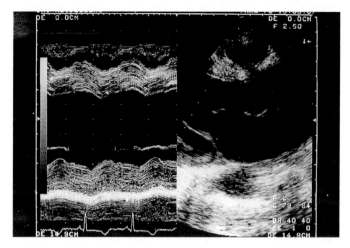

Fig. 11 Concentric left ventricular hypertrophy with marked thickening of the septal and posterior wall and normal systolic function on M-mode (left) and two-dimensional (right) echocardiograms in the long-axis parasternal view.

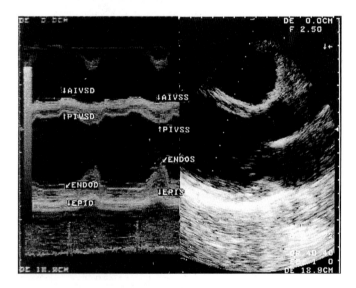

Fig. 10 Left ventricular dilatation with normal systolic function in the long-axis parasternal view on M-mode (left) and two-dimensional (right) echocardiograms: AIVSD, anterior interventricular septum in diastole; PIVSD, posterior interventricular septum in diastole; AIVSS, anterior interventricular septum in systole; PIVSS, posterior interventricular septum in systole; ENDOD, endocardial margin of the posterior wall in diastole; EPID, epicardial margin of the posterior wall in diastole; ENDOS, endocardial margin of the posterior wall in systole; EPIS, epicardial margin of the posterior wall in systole.

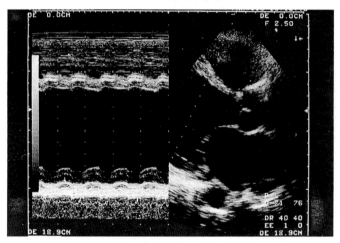

Fig. 12 Global systolic dysfunction with left ventricular dilatation on M-mode (left) and two-dimensional (right) echocardiograms in the long-axis parasternal view. Note that the walls move poorly. The left ventricle diameter varies little from diastole to systole. Opening of the mitral valve is decreased with a typical increased distance between the interventricular septum and the anterior mitral valve leaflet.

Recognized risk factors in renal patients are hypertension, dyslipidaemia (which is not fully reflected by total cholesterol, total triglycerides, HDL and LDL cholesterol and requires more detailed analysis of lipid subfractions and apolipoprotein patterns), increased LpA, increased homocysteine concentration and microinflammation as reflected by concentrations of high sensitivity C reactive protein (hs CRP), IL-6 (Kaysen *et al.* 2001) and many other cytokines (Kimmel *et al.* 1998). High CRP concentrations predict poor survival in dialysis patients (Zimmermann *et al.* 1999) as shown in Fig. 13.

It has recently been recognized that high predialytic serum phosphate concentrations also predict mortality (Block *et al.* 1998) and specifically cardiovascular mortality (Ganesh *et al.* 2001) in dialysis patients. One potential explanation is the propensity of coronary plaques (Schwarz *et al.* 2000) to calcify as recently amply documented by electron-beam CT (Braun *et al.* 1996; Goodman *et al.* 2000; Oh *et al.* 2002). Vascular calcification can no longer be considered as process of passive precipitation of calcium phosphate, in the form of

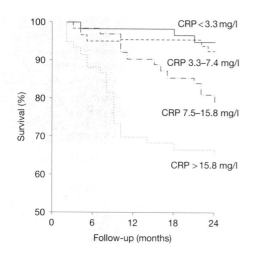

Fig. 13 Percentage survival versus follow-up duration at different CRP concentration in dialysis patients (Zimmermann et al. 1999).

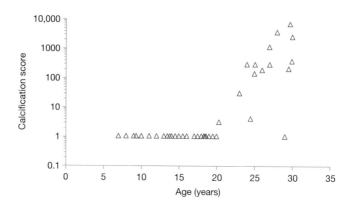

Fig. 14 Prevalence of calcified plaques with age in dialysed patients (Goodman et al. 2000).

hydroxyapatite crystals. Rather it involves active processes (Chen et al. 2002; Demer and Tintut 2003; Giachelli 2003; Moe et al. 2002, 2003). For instance, when vascular smooth muscle cell cultures are exposed to high phosphate concentrations, the cells develop an osteoblastic phenotype. Nevertheless not all adverse cardiovascular effects of hyperphosphataemia are mediated by plaque calcification. Promotion of cardiac fibrosis and arteriolar thickening by hyperphosphataemia has been documented in subtotally nephrectomized rats (Amann et al. 2003a).

It has recently been shown that the concentration of endothelial cell precursor stem cells are closely related to the Framingham risk score (Hill et al. 2003). In this context, it is of interest that in preliminary studies a decreased number of endothelial stem cells has been noted in renal failure and this may provide an additional pathomechanism underlying aggravated atherogenesis.

An important point is the recent finding that coronary atheroma is not a static structure, but an extremely dynamic lesion. Acute events (e.g. myocardial infarction) are often preceded by fissure of the plaque, particularly its 'shoulder', that is, the point of transition to the surrounding endothelium. In advanced lesions covered by a fibrous cap, a delicate balance exists between protease action and antiprotease defence. Inflammatory processes increase protease activity and decrease antiprotease defence. Small lipid-laden plaques appear to carry the greatest risk of rupture (Zaman et al. 1999; Libby et al. 2002). This may explain why there is only a rather loose correlation between coronary stenosis by angiography and cardiac events. Small non-stenosing plaques may be metabolically very active, whilst stenosing plaques may be metabolically quiescent. The prevalence of calcified plaques is very high in dialysed patients (Braun et al. 1996; Goodman et al. 2000; Schwarz et al. 2000), (Fig. 14). There is some controversy whether calcified plaques are inert lesions or—as some studies suggest (Topoleski and Salunke 2000; Huang et al. 2001)—or a locus minorus resistenciae predisposed to rupture when high mechanical forces act upon the transition zone between the calcified and non-calcified vessel wall. Prospective studies showed that hyperphosphataemia control with non-calcium-containing agents, specifically Sevelamer, halted the progressive increase in coronary calcification, but whether this translates into less coronary morbidity and mortality is currently unclear (Chertow et al. 2002).

Ischaemia tolerance

It is obvious that atheromatous coronary stenosis, that is, epicardial macrovessel disease, is only one factor in the genesis of the clinical symptoms of ischaemic heart disease in the renal patient. Clinical symptoms arise as a complex result of a disturbed relation between oxygen demand and oxygen supply. The coronary reserve may be reduced by microvessel disease at the level of the arterioles (Amann et al. 1995a,b; Amann and Ritz 2001) and capillaries (Amann et al. 1998), or by functional imbalance between endothelium derived vasoconstricting and vasodilating substances (e.g. NO and endothelin) causing arterial spasms. In this context, it is important that in uraemia arteries undergo exuberant intimal hyperplasia, potentially imposing further restriction to blood flow distal to the atheroma-induced narrowing of the coronary artery. LV hypertrophy increases the extravascular resistance and further limits the vasodilatory reserve. Finally, insufficient collateralization further aggravates the consequences of ischaemia.

The ischaemia tolerance of the heart in uraemia may also be compromised by abnormal myocardial metabolism. We found decreased expression of insulin-dependent glucose transporter (Glut 4) in the plasma membrane of cardiomyocytes in uraemic rats. Insulin-dependent glucose uptake by the heart was significantly diminished in uraemic animals (Ritz and Fliser 1993; Matthias et al. 1995). Raine et al. (1993) used the isolated perfused Langendorf preparation and recorded ^{32}P NMR spectra. They found decreased phosphocreatine concentrations in the heart of uraemic animals, particularly under conditions of low flow. This was accompanied by release of the nucleotide degradation product adenosine (Fig. 15). This finding is remarkable since a low phosphocreatine/ATP ratio is a useful clinical index of heart failure (Conway et al. 1991). In addition, impaired recovery of cytosolic calcium after stimulation secondary to impaired uptake by the sarcoplasmatic reticulum was found in cardiac myocytes of uraemic animals (Kennedy et al. 2003). This may cause impaired diastolic relaxation, impaired gain of inotropy with increasing heart rate and predispose to arrhythmia.

It follows that many factors disrupt the myocardial oxygen demand/supply balance (Table 5). Such an imbalance is mostly due to an absolute reduction in coronary blood flow (e.g. obstruction by atheroma), but may also be due to an increase in myocardial oxygen demand exceeding the maximal oxygen transport capacity even of non-obstructed coronary vessels. Such imbalance may be aggravated by LV, hypertrophy by episodes of hypotension or by anaemia, that is,

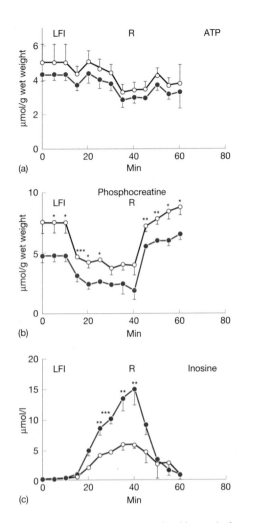

Fig. 15 Disturbed cardiac metabolism in the isolated Langendorf preparation. Effects is of low-flow ischaemia on phosphocreatine and ATP concentrations in uraemic (○) and control (●) rat hearts. Low-flow ischaemia (LFI) was produced by decreasing the perfusion pressure from 70 cm H_2O to 15–20 cm H_2O for 30 min followed by reperfusion for 20 min (R). Concentrations of phosphocreatine and ATP were measured using ^{32}P–NMR (reproduced with permission from Raine *et al.* 1993).

Table 5 Potential non-coronary problems associated with myocardial ischaemia in endstage renal failure

Demand factors
Muscle mass
Wall stress

Supply factors
Anaemia
Diffusion problems (hypertrophy, fibrosis)
Abnormal diastolic relaxation
Compromised subendocardial microcirculation
Small vessel disease
Small vessel dysfunction (endothelial cell
   dependent vasodilatation)

inadequate oxygen carrying capacity of the blood. In uraemic patients, Roig *et al.* (1981) and Rostand *et al.* (1984) had documented that symptoms of ischaemic heart disease, and even myocardial infarction may occur in patients with patent coronary arteries.

Further factors increasing oxygen demand are hyperdynamic circulation (fluid overload, AV fistula, anaemia) or stimulated inotropy (sympathetic activity, ionized calcium).

Clinical presentation

Because symptoms may occur even in the absence of coronary stenosis, the prevalence of coronary artery disease is overestimated in dialysis patients, if the diagnosis is based only on angina pectoris or electrocardiographic changes. The issue is confounded by the fact that coronary spasm may be superimposed upon a fixed obstruction (dynamic stenosis) and that in conditions of increased oxygen demand coronary artery calcification may become flow-limiting even in the absence of significant stenosis.

Myocardial infarction is frequent, as shown in Table 1. Myocardial infarction appears to be associated with a particularly high mortality in the dialysed patient, particularly the diabetic dialysed patient (Herzog *et al.* 1998). It is noteworthy that sudden death continues to be the most common cause of death in the dialysed patient, but there is very little autopsy information on the underlying anatomical abnormalities. Ischaemia, sympathetic overactivity, disturbed propagation of action potentials because of interstitial fibrosis, electrolyte abnormalities, particularly hyperkalaemia, may be contributory causes. It has been shown that hypotensive episodes during haemodialysis may cause critical coronary underperfusion and predispose to arrhythmia and sudden death, particularly in the hours following dialysis sessions. Cardiac death is also particularly common after the long weekend, possibly because of overhydration and/or hyperkalaemia. Overhydration may trigger clinical signs and symptoms of ischaemic heart disease in dialysis patients.

Congestive heart failure

The difficulties of distinguishing congestive heart failure from circulatory congestion have been discussed above. In a cross-sectional study congestive heart failure (defined by persistent or recurrent heart failure when patients were considered to be at dry weight), was found in 10 per cent of non-diabetic dialysis patients (Parfrey *et al.* 1990, 1996; Foley and Parfrey 1997; Parfrey and Foley 1999; Parfrey 2000). Non-specific ancillary findings in patients with congestive heart failure are a history of dyspnoea or peripheral oedema, cardiomegaly, increased jugular venous pressure, basal crepitations, pulmonary venous hypertension or interstitial oedema on chest radiography. A third of the patients had developed their congestive heart failure before reaching endstage renal disease; 53 per cent of these had dilated cardiomyopathy and 47 per cent had hypertrophic hyperkinetic disease. The most common cause of congestive heart failure in these patients is ischaemic heart disease, but other factors (see Table 4), for example, diabetic cardiomyopathy, myocardial calcification, iron overload, and thiamine deficiency may also be involved. Important differential diagnoses with potential consequences for intervention are valvular heart disease and particularly pericardial constriction. Congestive heart failure carries a poor prognosis; actuarial 2-year survival is no more than 33 per cent as compared with 80 per cent in patients without congestive heart failure (Parfrey *et al.* 1990).

In non-uraemic patients with congestive heart failure, cardiomyocyte drop-by apoptosis or necrosis is an important element. It is therefore of interest that cardiomyocyte loss has been documented in experimental uraemia as well (Amann *et al.* 2003a,b). The typical echocardiographic appearance of global systolic dysfunction is shown in Fig. 12.

Management of the renal patient with cardiac problems

Diagnostic procedures

Physical examination

A detailed history gives important clues. This is because many possible causes of chest pain or of cardiac failure must be considered including coronary heart disease, coronary microvascular disease, LV hypertrophy, pericarditis, valvular heart disease, tachyarrhythmia or bradycardia, as well as pure fluid overload. When taking the history one should evaluate the site, duration, severity, and radiation of any pain, and establish whether or not associated symptoms such as palpitations or syncope have been present. Appearance of the symptoms after long weekends are particularly suspicious. Information on nocturnal or postural dyspnoea as well as on exercise tolerance is helpful. Examination should include an assessment of fluid status (which is notoriously misleading), auscultation for third and fourth heart sounds (produced by rapid filling of a poorly compliant left ventricle) and systolic or diastolic murmurs. A late systolic murmur due to papillary muscle dysfunction may be a manifestation of ischaemia and must be distinguished from non-specific early systolic murmurs over the upper left sternal border. The latter is common in chronic renal failure and results from a hypercirculatory state caused by anaemia and the presence of arteriovenous shunt; it may also be related to sclerotic changes or calcification of aortic valves.

Assessment of circulatory congestion

In the setting of impaired renal handling of salt and fluid, particularly in functionally anephric patients, it is crucial to determine whether circulatory congestion is due to volume overload, intrinsic heart dysfunction, or a combination of both. Even a thorough patient history and physical examination will not always allow this differentiation to be made, and additional technical procedures are required.

ECG, chest radiography as well as M-mode, two-dimensional and Doppler echocardiography will be informative. It has been shown that ANP concentrations are a sensitive marker of fluid overload and BNP concentrations more of left heart dysfunction (Nishikimi *et al.* 2001; Osajima *et al.* 2002; McCullough and Sandberg 2003). Troponin T concentrations are a predictor of high cardiac risk (Deegan *et al.* 2001; Zoccali 2003) and are reliable even in the presence of renal failure (Aviles *et al.* 2002). Echocardiography or (when available) MRT will yield useful information on LV size and function, potential regional contraction abnormalities or the presence of valvular disease. Sonography of the retrohepatic segment of the vena cava is abnormal in patients with volume overload (Cheriex *et al.* 1989), but abnormal heart function is a powerful confounder (Mandelbaum *et al.* 1993). Patients with impaired diastolic filling of the left ventricle, particularly in the presence of LV hypertrophy, may experience pulmonary congestion even if LV systolic function is normal. This possibility should be considered when the heart size (on radiography or by echocardiography) is normal despite pulmonary congestion. Measurement of LV inflow velocity across the mitral valve by Doppler echocardiography as well as radionuclide ventriculography are useful to define diastolic filling problems further.

Electrocardiography

Electrocardiographic changes at rest are of limited diagnostic value in patients with chronic renal failure, because repolarization disturbances are a common non-specific finding. The ECG may be modified further by electrolyte abnormalities.

Echocardiography

Two-dimensional echocardiography is a useful non-invasive technique. The findings of impaired LV performance in patients with coronary artery disease may be of value in determining management and prognosis. Since left LV function is a major prognostic factor in coronary artery disease, such patients will require more careful volume restriction, and possibly shorter interdialytic intervals as well as volume-controlled ultrafiltration. Regional disturbances of contractility may point to coronary artery disease.

Exercise testing

Electrocardiographic exercise testing is seldom possible because of reduced exercise capacity of the patients, so that the appropriate heart rate cannot be achieved. Thallium scans are not a useful alternative: although they are correlated with the risk of cardiovascular death (Brown *et al.* 1989; Holley *et al.* 1991; Rostand *et al.* 1991; Rabbat *et al.* 2003) they are very poor in predicting coronary lesions which are susceptible to intervention. Dobutamine stress echocardiography has good sensitivity and specificity (Wilson *et al.* 1994; Brennan *et al.* 1997; Rabbat *et al.* 2003); shortcomings are often limited capacity in the cardiological unit and high observer dependency.

Coronary angiography

It is clear from the above that the diagnostic sensitivity and specificity of non-invasive procedures is much less in uraemic than in non-uraemic patients. Thus the clinician is forced to rely more heavily on coronary angiography in the diagnostic work-up of renal patients, although non-invasive procedures may be valuable for follow-up to monitor treatment results. The demonstration of coronary calcification is no substitute for coronary angiography, because electron-beam CT and multislice CT show vascular calcification, but cannot pick up stenosing lesions.

Coronary angiography should only be performed when its results will have therapeutic consequences. It is indicated when there is a high clinical suspicion of coronary artery disease. It should be performed in all symptomatic dialysis patients who do not respond to medical therapy and in patients in whom non-invasive tests indicate myocardial dysfunction or ischaemia. Furthermore, it is useful to screen diabetic transplant candidates older than 45 years because of the high prevalence of asymptomatic coronary heart disease in this population (Manske *et al.* 1993). Several algorithms have been proposed to identify patients in whom the likelihood of coronary heart disease is low and in whom angiography is unlikely to yield important information (Rutsky and Rostand 1992; Manske *et al.* 1993). In patients with residual renal function, the patient should be adequately pretreated to avoid acute renal failure.

Medical treatment in the patient with renal failure and heart failure, coronary heart disease, or both

Measures to control preload and afterload

Treatment of uraemic patients with circulatory congestion aims to remove excess fluid to reduce preload and at the same time to lower blood pressure, thus reducing afterload. A second aim is correction of anaemia, if present, in order to improve oxygen transport to the myocardium and to reduce the compensatory increase in cardiac output. Antihypertensive therapy and correction of anaemia will be discussed elsewhere. Here we shall deal with control of hypervolaemia.

Prevention of volume overload and maintenance of euvolaemia are helped by restriction of the intake of sodium chloride (3–6 g/day) and water. In the anuric patient, the osmotic drive forces the patient to drink one liter of osmotically free water whenever he or she ingests 9 g of sodium chloride. This underlines the importance of restricting the intake of sodium chloride. Loop diuretics, such as frusemide or torasemide, can be administered orally (or exceptionally intravenously) if there is still residual urinary production. To avoid ototoxicity, a maximum dose of frusemide of 1500 mg or an infusion rate of 1 mg/min should not be exceeded. Frusemide may no longer be effective in advanced renal failure, and uncontrolled volume overload is then a valid indication for haemodialysis.

If coronary heart disease is present, it is particularly important to prevent overhydration. This will reduce pre- and afterload (and in parallel wall stress and oxygen demand of the dilated LV). The efficacy of reducing overhydration has been illustrated by the finding that this manoeuvre caused normotension and reversal of LV hypertrophy despite no administration of antihypertensive agents (Ozkahya et al. 1998, 2002). As mentioned above, overt pulmonary congestion may occur in patients with LV hypertrophy and diastolic left ventricular malfunction, even though the heart is not enlarged by X-ray and systolic function is supranormal. Volume subtraction must be applied cautiously in patients with diastolic malfunction and high LV filling pressures, since rapid reduction of preload may cause an abrupt decrease in cardiac output, similar to that observed in patients with hypertrophic hypertensive cardiomyopathy.

Effect of dialysis modalities on circulatory function

Several parameters of cardiac function, including cardiac filling pressure, vascular resistance, electrolyte concentration and sympathetic drive change during the course of haemodialysis (Wizemann 1996). Therefore, the overall effect of haemodialysis on intrinsic myocardial contractility is difficult to predict. Haemodialysis may exert a positive inotropic effect on LV contractility via an increase in ionized calcium concentration (Henrich et al. 1984). The cardiac index is not necessarily altered during dialysis sessions. However, it increases consistently in patients with depressed baseline LV ejection fraction, presumably as a result of more favourable loading conditions (Hung et al. 1980).

The use of haemofiltration has been proposed in selected patients because of its haemodynamic advantages over haemodialysis. It has been shown that peripheral resistance increases during haemofiltration, whereas it tends to decrease in haemodialysis thus predisposing to intradialytic hypotension. Recent studies showed, however, that the reputed advantage of haemofiltration is exclusively the result of the infusion of cooler substitution fluid preventing a positive

thermobalance (Barendregt et al. 1999; Keijman et al. 1999; van der Sande et al. 2001).

Continuous ambulatory peritoneal dialysis (CAPD) avoids rapid shifts of fluid and electrolytes that occur with haemodialysis. This advantage is counteracted, however, by the tendency to develop hypervolaemia once residual renal function has ceased (Amann et al. 1996; Van Biesen et al. 2002; Wang et al. 2002; Konings et al. 2003). There is no clear indication that the long-term outcome is more favourable in patients on CAPD (Keshaviah et al. 2002; Ganesh et al. 2003).

Drug therapy

Digitalis

We believe that the use of cardiac glycosides is clearly indicated only for the treatment of supraventricular tachyarrhythmia. Special precautions are appropriate in patients with renal failure. We recommend using digitoxin which is metabolized in the liver, so that the half-life is only slightly prolonged (in uraemia 8.5 days). A maintenance dose of 0.07 mg/day with an intravenous loading dose of 0.25 mg if necessary, is usually adequate. Others prefer digoxin because of its shorter half-life, which is 1.6 days in normal patients and 4.4 days in anephric patients. In this instance, the dose has to be reduced, however, to avoid accumulation. In the treatment of heart failure with sinus rhythm, administration of digitalis is an ancillary measure at best (Digitalis Investigation Group 1997). It is potentially fraught with serious side-effects, particularly arrhythmia. If digitalis is used, serum potassium should be kept in the mid-normal range and postdialytic hypokalaemia should be avoided by adjusting the dialysate potassium concentration. If digitalis toxicity develops, haemodialysis is ineffective in removing the drug from the plasma. In emergency situations, haemoperfusion with charcoal or removal of digoxin from its binding site using Fab fragments of monoclonal antibodies should be considered.

Diuretics (Wilcox 2002)

Monotherapy with thiazide diuretics is not effective once GFR is below approximately 30 ml/min. It has been found, however, that thiazides potentiate the diuretic action of loop diuretics, even in advanced renal failure, presumably by sequential blockade of sodium reabsorption along the nephron (Fliser et al. 1999). Potassium-sparing agents must be avoided in patients with renal failure because of the risk of hyperkalaemia. If diuretics are required, it is usually necessary to use a loop diuretic in high doses, such as frusemide or torasemide. The dose required depends on sodium intake and GFR.

Angiotensin-converting enzyme inhibitors/angiotensin receptor blockers

ACE inhibitors or angiotensin receptor blockers have been widely used in dialysis patients. They appear to be particularly beneficial in patients with impaired systolic LV function, since they reduce afterload without the reflex change of heart rate seen with vasodilators. It has been shown that cardiovascular outcome is better in renal patients in whom LV hypertrophy regressed partially on treatment with ACE inhibitors (London et al. 1994; Guerin et al. 2001). There are uncontrolled retrospective observations that cardiovascular events are less in dialysis patients on ACE inhibitors and there is also evidence that they reduce LV hypertrophy, at least in part, independent of blood pressure (Paoletti et al. 2002). In a proportion of dialysed patients, hypertension is renin-dependent (Vertes et al. 1969); since the introduction of ACE inhibitors, bilateral nephrectomy for uncontrollable hypertension has virtually disappeared as a treatment modality.

In subtotally nephrectomized rats, ACE inhibitors improved cardiac morphology in a bradykinin-dependent fashion (Amann *et al.* 2000). ACE inhibitors may cause an anaphylactoid reaction, caused by an cumulation of kinin, in dialysis patients treated with electronegatively charged AN-69 membranes. They are strictly contraindicated in patients on ACE inhibitors (Verresen *et al.* 1994; Krieter *et al.* 1998). Otherwise, ACE inhibitors are usually well tolerated, but may interfere to some extent with ultrafiltration tolerance in dialysis patients particularly when they suffer from recurrent hypotensive episodes. ACE inhibitors are the treatment of choice in patients with congestive heart failure. They may also be useful in secondary prevention after myocardial infarction, because they interfere with ventricular remodelling and reduce cardiac mortality by reducing the rate of myocardial re-infarction (Frishman and Cheng 1999; Latini *et al.* 2000; Enseleit *et al.* 2001; Dickstein and Kjekshus 2002; Efrati *et al.* 2002; van der Elst *et al.* 2003).

β-Adrenergic blocking agents

In dialysis patients, sympathetic overactivity has been well documented by microneurographic techniques (Converse *et al.* 1992) and there are good arguments that the propensity to develop arrhythmia is increased because of partial cardiac denervation in the wake of patchy LV denervation (denervation suprasensitivity), particularly in diabetic patients (Dikow and Ritz 2003). In the absence of contraindications they are mandatory in the renal patient with ischaemic heart disease, but they are underused (Koch *et al.* 1993) showed that in dialysed type 2 diabetic patients the use of β-blockers was less than in survivors (3 versus 12 per cent). In the DOPPS study, mortality was less by 13 per cent when dialysed patients with ischaemic heart disease were treated with β-blockers. There is also controlled evidence in dialysed patients with systolic malfunction that Carvedilol compared to placebo improved ejection fraction, partially reversed LV dilatation and improved survival (Cice *et al.* 2003). β-Blockade may interfere with reflex autonomic adjustment to fluid removal and abrogate the compensatory increase in heart rate, thus potentially aggravating intradialytic hypotension. Water-soluble β-adrenergic blocking agents are eliminated by renal excretion and should not be used, at least not in full doses. This applies to atenolol, sotalol and nadolol. In renal failure, no dose adjustment or only minor dose reductions are necessary for propranolol, metoprolol, pindolol, and timolol. Sotalol may cause torsade de pointes arrhythmia, even at normal plasma concentrations (Bahrle and Schols 1996).

Calcium channel blockers

Calcium channel blockers are frequently necessary for the control of hypertension in renal failure. Dose reduction is not required for verpamil, diltiazem and the dihydropyridines. Verpamil and diltiazem should not be given to patients with systolic pumping dysfunction because of negative inotropy. They are very useful, however, for the treatment of supraventricular tachycardia. Concomitant administration of β-blocking agents may result in high-grade AV block and should be avoided.

Secondary prevention

Apart from β-blockers and ACE inhibitors, secondary prevention in the patient with ischaemic heart disease should include reduction of cholesterol by statins (see above). Dose adaption is not necessary in renal failure. Fibrates with the exception of gemfibrozil, are not the medication of first choice because of the risk of rhabdomyolysis. Monitoring of creatine kinase, LDH, and transaminases is recommended, however.

In the cardiac patient with renal failure it is particularly important to avoid hyperphosphataemia to prevent myocardial (Rostand *et al.* 1994) and coronary (Block *et al.* 1998; Goodman *et al.* 2000) calcification.

Interventional procedures (PTCA, CABG) for symptomatic coronary heart disease

The rationale of conservative anti-ischaemic treatment is to reduce myocardial oxygen consumption and to increase myocardial blood supply, if possible. The main points of treatment are:

(1) volume control;

(2) reduction of blood pressure;

(3) administration of β-blockers and ACE inhibitors;

(4) correction of anaemia;

(5) avoidance of situations that increase myocardial oxygen demand (e.g. tachycardia, hypertensive crisis, hypercalcaemia);

(6) avoidance of drugs with positive inotropic action (e.g. catecholamines);

(7) administration of organic nitrates. They reduce LV preload without inducing reflex tachycardia at least at low doses. They may reduce ultrafiltration tolerance, however.

There is no controlled evidence for the management of the dialysed patient with symptomatic coronary heart disease. The literature shows that survival after myocardial infarction is abysmal in the dialysed patients, particularly in the dialysed diabetic patient (Herzog *et al.* 1998) and is similarly poor in the coronary patient in preterminal renal failure.

Retrospective analysis of available data show that inhospital mortality is somewhat greater for coronary artery bypass surgery compared to percutaneous transluminal coronary angioplasty (PTCA), but one year survival is better with CABG if mammary arteries (and not peripheral veins) are used for bypass grafting. In the past the re-occlusion rate after PTCA had been catastrophic (Kahn *et al.* 1990; Koyanagi *et al.* 1996; Simsir *et al.* 1998; Haller and Kubler 1999), but recent experience is more favourable (Herzog *et al.* 2002a,b) preliminary evidence indicates that this can be substantially reduced by drug eluting stents and possibly also by brachytherapy.

A large proportion of dialysed patients experience symptomatic relief and improved quality of live after coronary artery bypass graft surgery. To avoid the risks of hypervolaemia and hyperkalaemia during surgery, it is wise to use continuous haemofiltration even during the intraoperative period or in close proximity to the intervention (Ilson *et al.* 1992).

Arrhythmia

Cardiac arrhythmia is common in the uraemic patient. Despite a large number of studies it is still not clear whether haemodialysis *per se* is arrhythmogenic. Haemodialysis has both proarrhythmic (hypokalaemia, increased catecholamines, sympathetic overactivity) and antiarrhythmic effects (reduced preload and wall stress). A multicentre cross-sectional study (Gruppo Emodialisi e Patologie Cardiovascolari 1988) clearly demonstrated that the frequency of higher grade premature ventricular contractions increased during dialysis and for some hours afterwards. This was seen more frequently in elderly patients and those with LV dysfunction. It emerged from this study that 21 per cent of the dialysis patients had Lown class IVa or IVb arrhythmia and that haemodialysis *per se* had an arrhythmogenic effect. The prevalence of complex ventricular tachyarrhythmia in dialysis patients appears to be intermediate between healthy controls and patients with organic heart disease.

The prognostic implications of arrhythmia in dialysis patients were clarified by a follow-up study: only age and ischaemic heart disease correlated independently with mortality, and ventricular arrhythmia *per se* did not predict overall mortality (Sforzini *et al.* 1992). It is obvious that the clinical relevance of Lown classes I to III is uncertain and that even Lown IVa and IVb arrhythmia must be interpreted in the context of LV function as in non-renal patients. If arrhythmia is suspected on clinical grounds, long-term Holter monitoring is advisable.

A study of survivors of myocardial infarction with Lown IVb arrhythmia had demonstrated that antiarrhythmic therapy reduced the frequency of arrhythmia, but increased mortality (Cardiac Arrhythmia Suppression Trial 1989). In view of this study the indication for antiarrhythmic therapy must be cautious. It should be restricted to patients in whom an arrhythmogenic substrate is provided by organic heart disease, and it should be based on the same considerations as in non-renal patients. The pharmacokinetics of antiarrhythmic agents (Table 6) which may necessitate dose adjustment in renal patients must be taken into consideration.

General measures that can be used to reduce arrhythmia in dialysis patients are avoidance of predialysis hyperkalaemia and postdialysis hypokalaemia. Plasma potassium should not decrease to less than 3.5 mmol/l, particularly in patients on digitalis. The occurrence of torsade de pointes after administration of sotalol has been observed in dialysis patients even at normal plasma concentrations (Bahrle and Schols 1996).

The risk of severe ventricular arrhythmia in the setting of coronary heart disease may be potentiated by concomitant severe anaemia, hypotension or hypertension and medical treatment of these conditions is necessary.

If severe ventricular arrhythmia in patients with coronary artery disease does not respond satisfactorily to drug treatment, coronary intervention (CABG or PTCA) must be considered. The use of digitalis

should be restricted to tachycardiac atrial fibrillation. It is important to be aware that atrial fibrillation or atrial flatter may result from hypovolaemia (atrial underfilling) as well as from hypervolaemia (atrial overfilling). Therefore monitoring of fluid status is important.

Valvular heart disease

The risk of accelerated calcific valvular heart disease in the dialysis patients (London *et al.* 2000) had not been adequately appreciated in the past (Raine 1994). Calcific aortic stenosis, mitral valve calcification, and (mostly subclinical) metastatic myocardial calcification are common. A high prevalence of aortic valve calcification and aortic valve stenosis has been documented by recent studies using EBCT (Braun *et al.* 1996; Chertow *et al.* 2002). An Italian survey (Mazzaferro *et al.* 1993) found that mitral valve calcification was completely absent in non-uraemic subjects age less than 60 years, while it was found in 37 per cent of dialysis patients. Since age is a risk factor for the development of valvular calcification, uraemia can be considered as a state of accelerated ageing. Risk predictors are duration of dialysis, hyperphosphataemia, hypercalcaemia, elevated PTH (Maher and Curtis 1985) and inflammatory markers (Wang *et al.* 2003). In some patients, calcific aortic stenosis progresses with extreme rapidity (Raine 1994), particularly in the presence of severe hyperparathyroidism. If one relies only on clinical examination, the severity of aortic stenosis is easily underestimated. It should also be remembered that calcific valvular disease is frequently associated with conduction defects. The patient should be managed to maintain serum phosphate concentrations strictly in the normal range. Overt hyperparathyroidism should be corrected. The transvalvular pressure gradient should be monitored. If valve replacement is eventually indicated, the use of a prosthetic valve is appropriate. It has been claimed that the risk of calcification of bioprostheses is excessive, but this has not been confirmed (Herzog *et al.* 2002a,b).

Uraemic pericarditis and pericardial effusion

In the past, uraemic pericarditis was regarded as one of the final events before death in uraemic coma ensued. Although dialysis has dramatically improved the prognosis of uraemic pericarditis, it continues to be an important, though infrequent, clinical problem. A small proportion of patients on maintenance dialysis suffer single or recurrent episodes of pericarditis. The major causes are intercurrent viral infection or

Table 6 Pharmacokinetics of some antiarrhythmic agents in common use

Substance	Space of distribution (l/kg)	Protein binding (%)	Elimination (%) Hepatic	Renal	Metabolite(s)	Half-life (h)	Minimum elimination fraction Q_0
Chinidine	2.4–3	75–90	60–90	10–40	Active	6–7	0.8
Procainamide	1–2	15	50	50	Active	3	0.3
Disopyramide	0.8	50–80	45	55	Active	5–8	0.5
Lidocaine	1.5	60–80	97	3	Active	1.8	0.95
Mexiletin	6–9	55–70	80–90	10–20	Inactive	7–17	0.8
Propafenon	3.5	95	98	2	Active	3–4	0.95
Amiodarone	9–20	96	90	10	Active	600–720	1.0
Sotalol	1.6–2.4	0	1	99	—	7–12	0.1

underdialysis (due to insufficient fistula flow, duration of dialysis sessions, or efficacy of dialysis).

Diagnosis

The patient with uraemic pericarditis presents often, but not invariably, with precordial pain which may resemble angina pectoris. Cardiac arrhythmia, particularly atrial fibrillation, may also be present. Dyspnoea and other symptoms of congestion occur, when large effusions and/or pericardial constriction develop. On clinical examination a systolic/diastolic pericardial friction rub can be heard which typically comprises three components. This important physical sign often disappears with the development of larger effusions. They cause inspiratory distension of jugular veins instead of inspiratory collapse (Kussmaul sign) and may lead to pulsus paradoxus (decrease of systolic pressure upon inspiration). Hypotension in combination with narrowed pulse pressure is an alarming sign, suggesting imminent cardiac tamponade. However, not all uraemic patients with pericarditis are symptomatic. If pericarditis is suspected, echocardiography should be performed to recognize pericardial effusion (Fig. 13). Repeated echocardiography is mandatory to monitor the response of effusion to therapy. Less precise information is provided by chest radiographs and electrocardiography. The absence of pulmonary congestion, despite enlargement of the heart, distinguishes pericardial effusion from congestive heart failure, but extreme effusions may also compromise LV filling and occasionally lead to pulmonary congestion. The ECG is not reliable in the diagnosis of uraemic pericarditis. A low voltage QRS segment is commonly found in patients with marked pericardial effusion, and beat-to-beat variation of the heart axis (swinging heart) may occur. Long-term sequelae of pericardial effusion, particularly of the haemorrhagic type, are pericardial constriction and calcification.

Therapy (Rutsky and Rostand 1992)

Treatment of uraemic pericarditis varies depending on whether the pericardial involvement is fibrinous, effusive, or constrictive. Acute fibrinous pericarditis with or without a small effusion usually responds to conservative measures. Patients in preterminal renal failure who have fibrinous pericarditis should be dialysed. The use of non-steroidal inflammatory agents or steroids is controversial. If a patient on maintenance dialysis develops pericarditis, the treatment regimen should be reassessed since ineffective dialysis is a common cause of pericarditis. Specific attention should be paid to the adequacy of fistula flow (recirculation test). In the presence of pericarditis the dialysis regimen must be intensified; we perform daily dialysis in such patients. Patients with pericarditis are at high risk of cardiac tamponade when routine heparin anticoagulation is administered during haemodialysis, and strict supervision of heparin anticoagulation or heparin-free dialysis is advisable. Pericarditis usually resolves within 2 weeks of the onset of daily dialysis treatment. Therapeutic strategies in addition to intensified haemodialysis are required if large effusions (250 ml) are resistant to conservative treatment. Refilling of large pericardial effusions is certainly more rapid in patients with fluid overload, but if an attempt to remove fluid by ultrafiltration is made, it must be remembered that ventricular filling depends on a sufficiently high filling pressure.

Choosing the appropriate moment for surgical intervention requires clinical judgement. Pericardial effusions that do not respond to dialysis should be drained, but pericardiocentesis is not without danger, because it may precipitate cardiac arrhythmia. It also carries the risk of coronary artery puncture. Therefore, this manoeuvre

should be reserved for emergency situations of life-threatening cardiac tamponade. Tamponade can set in early, particularly when effusions develop rapidly and pericardial membranes are still poorly compliant. The preferred approach to persistent pericardial effusions is primary surgical fenestration, which may be performed by subxiphoid pericardiotomy under local anaesthesia, or, preferably, pericardiectomy under general anaesthesia. The success of pericardiostomy may be limited in the presence of loculated effusion, particularly surrounding the posterior wall. Pericardiectomy involves extended resection of the pericardial sac and, in the case of constrictive pericarditis, decortication of fibrotic tissue.

Endocarditis

Uraemic patients are at an increased risk of developing endocarditis (Stratton *et al.* 2000; Minga *et al.* 2001; Sexton 2001; Fernandez-Cean *et al.* 2002; Maraj *et al.* 2002; Doulton *et al.* 2003). Bacteriaemia in dialysis patients is often related to infections of the vascular access site. This is particularly true for PTFE grafts (and is often overlooked in nonfunctional PTFE grafts which have not been removed). *Staphylococcus aureus* accounts for 70 per cent of such episodes and *Staphylococcus epidermitis* for most of the rest. Most frequently, *Staphylococcal endocarditis* is accompanied by, or preceded by, osteomyelitis of the spine. Patients may only complain of asthenia, reduced physical fitness, dizziness, and occasional pyrexia. Fever may be absent, since uraemic patients tend to be hypothermic, but dialysis may unmask an underlying subfebrile condition and cause transient postdialysis elevation of temperature. Enlargement of the spleen is suggestive of bacterial endocarditis, and sonography of the upper abdomen should be part of the diagnostic procedure. Leucocytosis, elevated erythrocyte sedimentation rate, and elevated CRP as well as procalcitonin concentrations are helpful for the diagnosis, particularly when sequential values show a progressive increase. A further pointer to the diagnosis may be progression anaemia and resistance to recombinant human EPO treatment. Murmurs are common in dialysis patients. They are difficult to interpret, however. Recent development of a murmur and a change in its character is important. Echocardiography, including transoesophageal echocardiography, is recommended in the patient with suspected endocarditis. Valvular vegetations may be detected, but this is not a constant finding. Valvular destruction may be rapid and detection requires repeated transoesophageal echocardiography. Heart failure due to progressive valvular destruction in the course of endocarditis must be prevented by timely valvular replacement. Choice of the correct timing poses a delicate clinical problem.

Antibiotics, chosen according to the results of resistance tests, are the treatment of choice, and repeated blood cultures should be performed in every dialysis patient in whom the possibility of endocarditis is considered. If these are negative despite a strong suspicion of endocarditis, antibiotic treatment is still justified in view of the high mortality of untreated bacterial endocarditis in uraemic patients. Empirical treatment with cephalosporin, aminoglycosides, and vancomycin should be started in the patient with negative blood cultures.

References

Amann, K. and Ritz, E. (2001). The heart in renal failure: morphological changes of the myocardiogram—new insights. *Journal of Clinical and Basic Cardiology* 4, 109–113.

Amann, K., Ritz, E., Wiest, G., Klaus, G., and Mall, G. (1994). A role of parathyroid hormone for the activation of cardiac fibroblasts in uremia. *Journal of the American Society of Nephrology* 4 (10), 1814–1819.

Amann, K., Gharehbaghi, H., Stephen, S., and Mall, G. (1995a). Hypertrophy and hyperplasia of smooth muscle cells of small intramyocardial arteries in spontaneously hypertensive rats. *Hypertension* 25 (1), 124–131.

Amann, K., Tornig, J., Flechtenmacher, C., Nabokov, A., Mall, G., and Ritz, E. (1995b). Blood-pressure-independent wall thickening of intramyocardial arterioles in experimental uraemia: evidence for a permissive action of PTH. *Nephrology, Dialysis, Transplantation* 10 (11), 2043–2048.

Amann, K., Mandelbaum, A., Schwarz, U., and Ritz, E. (1996). Hypertension and left ventricular hypertrophy in the CAPD patient. *Kidney International Supplement* 56, S37–S40.

Amann, K., Breitbach, M., Ritz, E., and Mall, G. (1998). Myocyte/capillary mismatch in the heart of uremic patients. *Journal of the American Society of Nephrology* 9 (6), 1018–1022.

Amann, K., Gassmann, P., Buzello, M., Orth, S. R., Tornig, J., Gross, M. L., Magener, A., Mall, G., and Ritz, E. (2000). Effects of ACE inhibition and bradykinin antagonism on cardiovascular changes in uremic rats. *Kidney International* 58 (1), 153–161.

Amann, K., Tornig, J., Buzello, M., Kuhlmann, A., Gross, M. L., Adamczak, M., and Ritz, E. (2002). Effect of antioxidant therapy with DL-alpha-tocopherol on cardiovascular structure in experimental renal failure. *Kidney International* 62 (3), 877–884.

Amann, K., Tornig, J., Kugel, B., Gross, M. L., Tyralla, K., El-Shakmak, A., Szabo, A., and Ritz, E. (2003a). Hyperphosphatemia aggravates cardiac fibrosis and microvascular disease in experimental uremia. *Kidney International* 63 (4), 1296–1301.

Amann, K., Tyralla, K., Gross, M. L., Schwarz, U., Tornig, J., Haas, C. S., Ritz, E., and Mall, G. (2003b). Cardiomyocyte loss in experimental renal failure: prevention by ramipril. *Kidney International* 63 (5), 1708–1713.

Attman, P. O. (1993). Hyperlipoproteinaemia in renal failure: pathogenesis and perspectives for intervention. *Nephrology, Dialysis, Transplantation* 8 (4), 294–295.

Aviles, R. J., Askari, A. T., Lindahl, B., Wallentin, L., Jia, G., Ohman, E. M., Mahaffey, K. W., Newby, L. K., Califf, R. M., Simoons, M. L., Topol, E. J., Berger, P., and Lauer, M. S. (2002). Troponin T levels in patients with acute coronary syndromes, with or without renal dysfunction. *New England Journal of Medicine* 346 (26), 2047–2052.

Bahrle, S. and Schols, W. (1996). Torsade de pointes in haemodialysis patients. *Nephrology, Dialysis, Transplantation* 11 (6), 944–946.

Barendregt, J. N., Kooman, J. P., Van Der Sande, F. M., Buurma, J. H., Hameleers, P., Kerkhofs, A. M., and Leunissen, K. M. (1999). The effect of dialysate temperature on energy transfer during haemodialysis (HD). *Kidney International* 55 (6), 2598–2608.

Berger, C. J., Murabito, J. M., Evans, J. C., Anderson, K. M., and Levy, D. (1992). Prognosis after first myocardial infarction. Comparison of Q-wave and non-Q-wave myocardial infarction in the Framingham Heart Study. *Journal of the American Medical Association* 268 (12), 1545–1551.

Besarab, A., Bolton, W. K., Browne, J. K., Egrie, J. C., Nissenson, A. R., Okamoto, D. M., Schwab, S. J., and Goodkin, D. A. (1998). The effects of normal as compared with low hematocrit values in patients with cardiac disease who are receiving haemodialysis and epoetin. *New England Journal of Medicine* 339 (9), 584–590.

Blacher, J., Safar, M. E., Pannier, B., Guerin, A. P., Marchais, S. J., and London, G. M. (2002). Prognostic significance of arterial stiffness measurements in end-stage renal disease patients. *Current Opinion in Nephrology and Hypertension* 11 (6), 629–634.

Blacher, J., Safar, M. E., Guerin, A. P., Pannier, B., Marchais, S. J., and London, G. M. (2003). Aortic pulse wave velocity index and mortality in end-stage renal disease. *Kidney International* 63 (5), 1852–1860.

Block, G. A., Hulbert-Shearon, T. E., Levin, N. W., and Port, F. K. (1998). Association of serum phosphorus and calcium × phosphate product with mortality risk in chronic haemodialysis patients: a national study. *American Journal of Kidney Diseases* 31 (4), 607–617.

Boaz, M., Smetana, S., Weinstein, T., Matas, Z., Gafter, U., Iaina, A., Knecht, A., Weissgarten, Y., Brunner, D., Fainaru, M., and Green, M. S. (2000). Secondary prevention with antioxidants of cardiovascular disease in end-stage renal disease (SPACE): randomised placebo-controlled trial. *Lancet* 356 (9237), 1213–1218.

Braun, J., Oldendorf, M., Moshage, W., Heidler, R., Zeitler, E., and Luft, F. C. (1996). Electron beam computed tomography in the evaluation of cardiac calcification in chronic dialysis patients. *American Journal of Kidney Diseases* 27 (3), 394–401.

Brennan, D. C., Vedala, G., Miller, S. B., Anstey, M. E., Singer, G. G., Kovacs, A., Barzilai, B., Lowell, J. A., Shenoy, S., Howard, T. K., and Davila-Roman, V. G. (1997). Pretransplant dobutamine stress echocardiography is useful and cost-effective in renal transplant candidates. *Transplantation Proceedings* 29 (1–2), 233–234.

Brown, K. A., Rimmer, J., and Haisch, C. (1989). Noninvasive cardiac risk stratification of diabetic and nondiabetic uremic renal allograft candidates using dipyridamole-thallium-201 imaging and radionuclide ventriculography. *American Journal of Cardiology* 64 (16), 1017–1021.

Buzello, M., Tornig, J., Faulhaber, J., Ehmke, H., Ritz, E., and Amann, K. (2003). The apolipoprotein e knockout mouse: a model documenting accelerated atherogenesis in uremia. *Journal of the American Society of Nephrology* 14 (2), 311–316.

Campese, V. M. and Kogosov, E. (1995). Renal afferent denervation prevents hypertension in rats with chronic renal failure. *Hypertension* 25 (4 Pt 2), 878–882.

Cannella, G., Paoletti, E., Delfino, R., Peloso, G., Molinari, S., and Traverso, G. B. (1993). Regression of left ventricular hypertrophy in hypertensive dialyzed uremic patients on long-term antihypertensive therapy. *Kidney International* 44 (4), 881–886.

Cannella, G., Paoletti, E., Barocci, S., Massarino, F., Delfino, R., Ravera, G., Di Maio, G., Nocera, A., Patrone, P., and Rolla, D. (1998). Angiotensin-converting enzyme gene polymorphism and reversibility of uremic left ventricular hypertrophy following long-term antihypertensive therapy. *Kidney International* 54 (2), 618–626.

Chauveau, P., Chadefaux, B., Coude, M., Aupetit, J., Hannedouche, T., Kamoun, P., and Jungers, P. (1993). Hyperhomocysteinemia, a risk factor for atherosclerosis in chronic uremic patients. *Kidney International Supplement* 41, S72–77.

Chen, N. X., O'Neill, K. D., Duan, D., and Moe, S. M. (2002). Phosphorus and uremic serum upregulate osteopontin expression in vascular smooth muscle cells. *Kidney International* 62 (5), 1724–1731.

Cheriex, E. C., Leunissen, K. M., Janssen, J. H., Mooy, J. M., and van Hooff, J. P. (1989). Echography of the inferior vena cava is a simple and reliable tool for estimation of 'dry weight' in haemodialysis patients. *Nephrology, Dialysis, Transplantation* 4 (6), 563–568.

Chertow, G. M., Burke, S. K., and Raggi, P. (2002). Sevelamer attenuates the progression of coronary and aortic calcification in haemodialysis patients. *Kidney International* 62 (1), 245–252.

Churchill, D. N. *et al.* (1992). Canadian hemodialysis morbidity study. *American Journal of Kidney Diseases* 19 (3), 214–234.

Cice, G., Ferrara, L., D'Andrea, A., D'Isa, S., Di Benedetto, A., Cittadini, A., Russo, P. E., Golino, P., and Calabro, R. (2003). Carvedilol increases two-year survival in dialysis patients with dilated cardiomyopathy: a prospective, placebo-controlled trial. *Journal of the American College of Cardiology* 41 (9), 1438–1444.

Clyne, N., Lins, L. E., and Pehrsson, S. K. (1986). Occurrence and significance of heart disease in uraemia. An autopsy study. *Scandinavian Journal of Urology and Nephrology* 20 (4), 307–311.

Converse, R. L., Jr., Jacobsen, T. N., Toto, R. D., Jost, C. M., Cosentino, F., Fouad-Tarazi, F., and Victor, R. G. (1992). Sympathetic overactivity in patients with chronic renal failure. *New England Journal of Medicine* 327 (27), 1912–1918.

Conway, M. A., Allis, J., Ouwerkerk, R., Niioka, T., Rajagopalan, B., and Radda, G. K. (1991). Detection of low phosphocreatine to ATP ratio in failing hypertrophied human myocardium by 31P magnetic resonance spectroscopy. *Lancet* **338** (8773), 973–976.

Dahlof, B., Devereux, R. B., Kjeldsen, S. E., Julius, S., Beevers, G., Faire, U., Fyhrquist, F., Ibsen, H., Kristiansson, K., Lederballe-Pedersen, O., Lindholm, L. H., Nieminen, M. S., Omvik, P., Oparil, S., and Wedel, H. (2002). Cardiovascular morbidity and mortality in the Losartan Intervention For Endpoint reduction in hypertension study (LIFE): a randomised trial against atenolol. *Lancet* **359** (9311), 995–1003.

Deegan, P. B., Lafferty, M. E., Blumsohn, A., Henderson, I. S., and McGregor, E. (2001). Prognostic value of troponin T in haemodialysis patients is independent of comorbidity. *Kidney International* **60** (6), 2399–2405.

Demer, L. L. and Tintut, Y. (2003). Mineral exploration: search for the mechanism of vascular calcification and beyond: the 2003 Jeffrey M. Hoeg award lecture. *Arterioscleloresis, Thrombosis, and Vascular Biology* **23** (10), 1739–1743.

Devereux, R. B. and Reichek, N. (1977). Echocardiographic determination of left ventricular mass in man. Anatomic validation of the method. *Circulation* **55** (4), 613–618.

Dickstein, K. and Kjekshus, J. (2002). Effects of losartan and captopril on mortality and morbidity in high-risk patients after acute myocardial infarction: the OPTIMAAL randomised trial. Optimal Trial in Myocardial Infarction with Angiotensin II Antagonist Losartan. *Lancet* **360** (9335), 752–760.

Dikow, R. and Ritz, E. (2003). Cardiovascular complications in the diabetic patient with renal disease: an update in 2003. *Nephrology, Dialysis, Transplantation* **18** (10), 1993–1998.

Doulton, T., Sabharwal, N., Cairns, H. S., Schelenz, S., Eykyn, S., O'Donnell, P., Chambers, J., Austen, C., and Goldsmith, D. J. (2003). Infective endocarditis in dialysis patients: new challenges and old. *Kidney International* **64** (2), 720–727.

Efrati, S., Zaidenstein, R., Dishy, V., Beberashvili, I., Sharist, M., Averbukh, Z., Golik, A., and Weissgarten, J. (2002). ACE inhibitors and survival of haemodialysis patients. *American Journal of Kidney Diseases* **40** (5), 1023–1029.

Enseleit, F., Hurlimann, D., and Luscher, T. F. (2001). Vascular protective effects of angiotensin converting enzyme inhibitors and their relation to clinical events. *Jorunal of Cardiovascular Pharmacology* **37** (Suppl. 1), S21–S30.

Ezekowitz, J. A., McAlister, F. A., and Armstrong, P. W. (2003). Anaemia is common in heart failure and is associated with poor outcomes: insights from a cohort of 12,065 patients with new-onset heart failure. *Circulation* **107** (2), 223–225.

Fernandez-Cean, J., Alvarez, A., Burguez, S., Baldovinos, G., Larre-Borges, P., and Cha, M. (2002). Infective endocarditis in chronic haemodialysis: two treatment strategies. *Nephrology, Dialysis, Transplantation* **17** (12), 2226–2230.

Fliser, D., Zurbruggen, I., Mutschler, E., Bischoff, I., Nussberger, J., Franek, E., and Ritz, E. (1999). Coadministration of albumin and furosemide in patients with the nephrotic syndrome. *Kidney International* **55** (2), 629–634.

Foley, R. N. and Parfrey, P. S. (1997). Cardiac disease in chronic uremia: clinical outcome and risk factors. *Advances in Renal Replacement Therapy* **4** (3), 234–248.

Foley, R. N., Culleton, B. F., Parfrey, P. S., Harnett, J. D., Kent, G. M., Murray, D. C., and Barre, P. E. (1997). Cardiac disease in diabetic end-stage renal disease. *Diabetologia* **40** (11), 1307–1312.

Foley, R. N., Herzog, C. A., and Collins, A. J. (2003). Smoking and cardiovascular outcomes in dialysis patients: The United States Renal Data System Wave 2 Study. *Kidney International* **63** (4), 1462–1467.

Foley, R. N., Parfrey, P. S., Harnett, J. D., Kent, G. M., Martin, C. J., Murray, D. C., and Barre, P. E. (1995). Clinical and echocardiographic disease in patients starting end-stage renal disease therapy. *Kidney International* **47** (1), 186–192.

Foley, R. N., Parfrey, P. S., Harnett, J. D., Kent, G. M., Murray, D. C., and Barre, P. E. (1996). The impact of anaemia on cardiomyopathy, morbidity, and mortality in end-stage renal disease. *American Journal of Kidney Diseases* **28** (1), 53–61.

Foley, R. N., Parfrey, P. S., Kent, G. M., Harnett, J. D., Murray, D. C., and Barre, P. E. (1998). Long-term evolution of cardiomyopathy in dialysis patients. *Kidney International* **54** (5), 1720–1725.

Foley, R. N., Parfrey, P. S., Morgan, J., Barre, P. E., Campbell, P., Cartier, P., Coyle, D., Fine, A., Handa, P., Kingma, I., Lau, C. Y., Levin, A., Mendelssohn, D., Muirhead, N., Murphy, B., Plante, R. K., Posen, G., and Wells, G. A. (2000). Effect of haemoglobin levels in haemodialysis patients with asymptomatic cardiomyopathy. *Kidney International* **58** (3), 1325–1335.

Frishman, W. H. and Cheng, A. (1999). Secondary prevention of myocardial infarction: role of beta-adrenergic blockers and angiotensin-converting enzyme inhibitors. *American Heart Journal* **137** (4 Pt 2), S25–S34.

Ganesh, S. K., Stack, A. G., Levin, N. W., Hulbert-Shearon, T., and Port, F. K. (2001). Association of elevated serum PO(4), Ca × PO(4) product, and parathyroid hormone with cardiac mortality risk in chronic haemodialysis patients. *Journal of the American Society of Nephrology* **12** (10), 2131–2138.

Ganesh, S. K., Hulbert-Shearon, T., Port, F. K., Eagle, K., and Stack, A. G. (2003). Mortality differences by dialysis modality among incident ESRD patients with and without coronary artery disease. *Journal of the American Society of Nephrology* **14** (2), 415–424.

Giachelli, C. M. (2003). Vascular calcification: *in vitro* evidence for the role of inorganic phosphate. *Journal of the American Society of Nephrology* **14** (9 Suppl. 4), S300–S304.

Goodman, W. G., Goldin, J., Kuizon, B. D., Yoon, C., Gales, B., Sider, D., Wang, Y., Chung, J., Emerick, A., Greaser, L., Elashoff, R. M., and Salusky, I. B. (2000). Coronary-artery calcification in young adults with end-stage renal disease who are undergoing dialysis. *New England Journal of Medicine* **342** (20), 1478–1483.

Gruppo Emodialisi e Patologie Cardiovasculari (1988). Multicentre, cross-sectional study of ventricular arrhythmias in chronically haemodialysed patients. *Lancet* **2** (8606), 305–309.

Guerin, A. P., Blacher, J., Pannier, B., Marchais, S. J., Safar, M. E., and London, G. M. (2001). Impact of aortic stiffness attenuation on survival of patients in end-stage renal failure. *Circulation* **103** (7), 987–992.

Haller, C. and Kubler, W. (1999). The disappointing results of PTCA in the uraemic patient—are stents the answer? *Nephrology, Dialysis, Transplantation* **14** (11), 2582–2584.

Harnett, J. D., Foley, R. N., Kent, G. M., Barre, P. E., Murray, D., and Parfrey, P. S. (1995). Congestive heart failure in dialysis patients: prevalence, incidence, prognosis and risk factors. *Kidney International* **47** (3), 884–890.

Henrich, W. L., Hunt, J. M., and Nixon, J. V. (1984). Increased ionized calcium and left ventricular contractility during haemodialysis. *New England Journal of Medicine* **310** (1), 19–23.

Henry, R. M., Kostense, P. J., Bos, G., Dekker, J. M., Nijpels, G., Heine, R. J., Bouter, L. M., and Stehouwer, C. D. (2002). Mild renal insufficiency is associated with increased cardiovascular mortality: The Hoorn Study. *Kidney International* **62** (4), 1402–1407.

Herzog, C. A., Ma, J. Z., and Collins, A. J. (1998). Poor long-term survival after acute myocardial infarction among patients on long-term dialysis. *New England Journal of Medicine* **339** (12), 799–805.

Herzog, C. A., Ma, J. Z., and Collins, A. J. (2002a). Comparative survival of dialysis patients in the United States after coronary angioplasty, coronary artery stenting, and coronary artery bypass surgery and impact of diabetes. *Circulation* **106** (17), 2207–2211.

Herzog, C. A., Ma, J. Z., and Collins, A. J. (2002b). Long-term survival of dialysis patients in the United States with prosthetic heart valves: should ACC/AHA practice guidelines on valve selection be modified? *Circulation* **105** (11), 1336–1341.

Hill, J. M., Zalos, G., Halcox, J. P., Schenke, W. H., Waclawiw, M. A., Quyyumi, A. A., and Finkel, T. (2003). Circulating endothelial progenitor cells, vascular function, and cardiac risk. *New England Journal of Medicine* **348** (7), 593–600.

Hillege, H. L., Girbes, A. R., de Kam, P. J., Boomsma, F., de Zeeuw, D., Charlesworth, A., Hampton, J. R., and van Veldhuisen, D. J. (2000). Renal function, neurohormonal activation, and survival in patients with chronic heart failure. *Circulation* **102** (2), 203–210.

Himmelfarb, J., Stenvinkel, P., Ikizler, T. A., and Hakim, R. M. (2002). The elephant in uremia: oxidant stress as a unifying concept of cardiovascular disease in uremia. *Kidney International* **62** (5), 1524–1538.

Holdaas, H., Fellstrom, B., Jardine, A. G., Holme, I., Nyberg, G., Fauchald, P., Gronhagen-Riska, C., Madsen, S., Neumayer, H. H., Cole, E., Maes, B., Ambuhl, P., Olsson, A. G., Hartmann, A., Solbu, D. O., and Pedersen, T. R. (2003). Effect of fluvastatin on cardiac outcomes in renal transplant recipients: a multicentre, randomised, placebo-controlled trial. *Lancet* **361** (9374), 2024–2031.

Holley, J. L., Fenton, R. A., and Arthur, R. S. (1991). Thallium stress testing does not predict cardiovascular risk in diabetic patients with end-stage renal disease undergoing cadaveric renal transplantation. *American Journal of Medicine* **90** (5), 563–570.

Huang, H., Virmani, R., Younis, H., Burke, A. P., Kamm, R. D., and Lee, R. T. (2001). The impact of calcification on the biomechanical stability of atherosclerotic plaques. *Circulation* **103** (8), 1051–1056.

Hung, J., Harris, P. J., Uren, R. F., Tiller, D. J., and Kelly, D. T. (1980). Uremic cardiomyopathy—effect of haemodialysis on left ventricular function in end-stage renal failure. *New England Journal of Medicine* **302** (10), 547–551.

Huting, J., Kramer, W., Schutterle, G., and Wizemann, V. (1988). Analysis of left-ventricular changes associated with chronic haemodialysis. A non-invasive follow-up study. *Nephron* **49** (4), 284–290.

Ikram, H., Lynn, K. L., Bailey, R. R., and Little, P. J. (1983). Cardiovascular changes in chronic haemodialysis patients. *Kidney International* **24** (3), 371–376.

Ilson, B. E., Bland, P. S., Jorkasky, D. K., Shusterman, N., Allison, N. L., Dubb, J. W., Parr, G. V., Goebel, T. K., and Stote, R. M. (1992). Intraoperative versus routine haemodialysis in end-stage renal disease patients undergoing open-heart surgery. *Nephron* **61** (2), 170–175.

Joint National Committee (1997). The sixth report of the Joint National Committee on prevention, detection, evaluation, and treatment of high blood pressure. *Archives of Internal Medicine* **157** (21), 2413–2446.

Jungers, P., Chauveau, P., Bandin, O., Chadefaux, B., Aupetit, J., Labrunie, M., Descamps-Latscha, B., and Kamoun, P. (1997). Hyperhomocysteinemia is associated with atherosclerotic occlusive arterial accidents in predialysis chronic renal failure patients. *Mineral and Electrolyte Metabolism* **23** (3–6), 170–173.

Kahn, J. K., Rutherford, B. D., McConahay, D. R., Johnson, W. L., Giorgi, L. V., and Hartzler, G. O. (1990). Short- and long-term outcome of percutaneous transluminal coronary angioplasty in chronic dialysis patients. *American Heart Journal* **119** (3 Pt 1), 484–489.

Kaysen, G. A., Chertow, G. M., Adhikarla, R., Young, B., Ronco, C., and Levin, N. W. (2001). Inflammation and dietary protein intake exert competing effects on serum albumin and creatinine in haemodialysis patients. *Kidney International* **60** (1), 333–340.

Keijman, J. M., van der Sande, F. M., Kooman, J. P., and Leunissen, K. M. (1999). Thermal energy balance and body temperature: comparison between isolated ultrafiltration and haemodialysis at different dialysate temperatures. *Nephrology, Dialysis, Transplantation* **14** (9), 2196–2200.

Kennedy, D., Omran, E., Periyasamy, S. M., Nadoor, J., Priyadarshi, A., Willey, J. C., Malhotra, D., Xie, Z., and Shapiro, J. I. (2003). Effect of chronic renal failure on cardiac contractile function, calcium cycling, and gene expression of proteins important for calcium homeostasis in the rat. *Journal of the American Society of Nephrology* **14** (1), 90–97.

Keshaviah, P., Collins, A. J., Ma, J. Z., Churchill, D. N., and Thorpe, K. E. (2002). Survival comparison between haemodialysis and peritoneal dialysis based on matched doses of delivered therapy. *Journal of the American Society of Nephrology* **13** (Suppl. 1), S48–S52.

Kimmel, P. L., Phillips, T. M., Simmens, S. J., Peterson, R. A., Weihs, K. L., Alleyne, S., Cruz, I., Yanovski, J. A., and Veis, J. H. (1998). Immunologic function and survival in haemodialysis patients. *Kidney International* **54** (1), 236–244.

Klassen, P. S., Lowrie, E. G., Reddan, D. N., DeLong, E. R., Coladonato, J. A., Szczech, L. A., Lazarus, J. M., and Owen, W. F., Jr. (2002). Association between pulse pressure and mortality in patients undergoing maintenance haemodialysis. *Journal of the American Medical Association* **287** (12), 1548–1555.

Klein, I. H., Ligtenberg, G., Oey, P. L., Koomans, H. A., and Blankestijn, P. J. (2001). Sympathetic activity is increased in polycystic kidney disease and is associated with hypertension. *Journal of the American Society of Nephrology* **12** (11), 2427–2433.

Koch, M., Thomas, B., Tschope, W., and Ritz, E. (1993). Survival and predictors of death in dialysed diabetic patients. *Diabetologia* **36** (10), 1113–1117.

Konings, C. J., Kooman, J. P., Schonck, M., Struijk, D. G., Gladziwa, U., Hoorntje, S. J., van der Wall Bake, A. W., van der Sande, F. M., and Leunissen, K. M. (2003). Fluid status in CAPD patients is related to peritoneal transport and residual renal function: evidence from a longitudinal study. *Nephrology, Dialysis, Transplantation* **18** (4), 797–803.

Koyanagi, T., Nishida, H., Kitamura, M., Endo, M., Koyanagi, H., Kawaguchi, M., Magosaki, N., Sumiyoshi, T., and Hosoda, S. (1996). Comparison of clinical outcomes of coronary artery bypass grafting and percutaneous transluminal coronary angioplasty in renal dialysis patients. *Annals of Thoracic Surgery* **61** (6), 1793–1796.

Krieter, D. H., Grude, M., Lemke, H. D., Fink, E., Bonner, G., Scholkens, B. A., Schulz, E., and Muller, G. A. (1998). Anaphylactoid reactions during haemodialysis in sheep are ACE inhibitor dose-dependent and mediated by bradykinin. *Kidney International* **53** (4), 1026–1035.

Kronenberg, F., Lingenhel, A., Neyer, U., Lhotta, K., Konig, P., Auinger, M., Wiesholzer, M., Andersson, H., and Dieplinger, H. (2003). Prevalence of dyslipidemic risk factors in haemodialysis and CAPD patients. *Kidney International Supplement* **84**, S113–S116.

Kronenberg, F., Steinmetz, A., Kostner, G. M., and Dieplinger, H. (1996). Lipoprotein(a) in health and disease. *Critical Reviews in Clinical Laboratory Sciences* **33** (6), 495–543.

Lai, K. N., Ng, J., Whitford, J., Buttfield, I., Fassett, R. G., and Mathew, T. H. (1985). Left ventricular function in uremia: echocardiographic and radionuclide assessment in patients on maintenance haemodialysis. *Clinical Nephrology* **23** (3), 125–133.

Latini, R., Santoro, E., Masson, S., Tavazzi, L., Maggioni, A. P., Franzosi, M. G., Barlera, S., Calvillo, L., Salio, M., Staszewsky, L., Labarta, V., and Tognoni, G. (2000). Aspirin does not interact with ACE inhibitors when both are given early after acute myocardial infarction: results of the GISSI-3 Trial. *Heart Disease* **2** (3), 185–190.

Leineweber, K., Heinroth-Hoffmann, I., Ponicke, K., Abraham, G., Osten, B., and Brodde, O. E. (2002). Cardiac beta-adrenoceptor desensitization due to increased beta-adrenoceptor kinase activity in chronic uremia. *Journal of the American Society of Nephrology* **13** (1), 117–124.

Levin, A., Thompson, C. R., Ethier, J., Carlisle, E. J., Tobe, S., Mendelssohn, D., Burgess, E., Jindal, K., Barrett, B., Singer, J., and Djurdjev, O. (1999). Left ventricular mass index increase in early renal disease: impact of decline in haemoglobin. *American Journal of Kidney Diseases* **34** (1), 125–134.

Libby, P., Ridker, P. M., and Maseri, A. (2002). Inflammation and atherosclerosis. *Circulation* **105** (9), 1135–1143.

Lindner, A., Charra, B., Sherrard, D. J., and Scribner, B. H. (1974). Accelerated atherosclerosis in prolonged maintenance haemodialysis. *New England Journal of Medicine* **290** (13), 697–701.

London, G. M., Fabiani, F., Marchais, S. J., de Vernejoul, M. C., Guerin, A. P., Safar, M. E., Metivier, F., and Llach, F. (1987). Uremic cardiomyopathy: an inadequate left ventricular hypertrophy. *Kidney International* **31** (4), 973–980.

London, G. M., Marchais, S. J., Guerin, A. P., and Metivier, F. (1989a). Contributive factors to cardiovascular hypertrophy in renal failure. *American Journal of Hypertension* **2** (11 Pt 2), 261S–263S.

London, G. M., Zins, B., Pannier, B., Naret, C., Berthelot, J. M., Jacquot, C., Safar, M., and Drueke, T. B. (1989b). Vascular changes in haemodialysis patients in response to recombinant human erythropoietin. *Kidney International* **36** (5), 878–882.

London, G. M., Pannier, B., Guerin, A. P., Marchais, S. J., Safar, M. E., and Cuche, J. L. (1994). Cardiac hypertrophy, aortic compliance, peripheral resistance, and wave reflection in end-stage renal disease. Comparative effects of ACE inhibition and calcium channel blockade. *Circulation* **90** (6), 2786–2796.

London, G. M., Pannier, B., Marchais, S. J., and Guerin, A. P. (2000). Calcification of the aortic valve in the dialyzed patient. *Journal of the American Society of Nephrology* **11** (4), 778–783.

Ma, J. Z., Ebben, J., Xia, H., and Collins, A. J. (1999). Hematocrit level and associated mortality in haemodialysis patients. *Journal of the American Society of Nephrology* **10** (3), 610–619.

Macdougall, I. C. and Ritz, E. (1998). The Normal Haematocrit Trial in dialysis patients with cardiac disease: are we any the less confused about target haemoglobin? *Nephrology, Dialysis, Transplantation* **13** (12), 3030–3033.

Macdougall, I. C., Lewis, N. P., Saunders, M. J., Cochlin, D. L., Davies, M. E., Hutton, R. D., Fox, K. A., Coles, G. A., and Williams, J. D. (1990). Long-term cardiorespiratory effects of amelioration of renal anaemia by erythropoietin. *Lancet* **335** (8688), 489–493.

Madore, F., Lowrie, E. G., Brugnara, C., Lew, N. L., Lazarus, J. M., Bridges, K., and Owen, W. F. (1997). Anaemia in haemodialysis patients: variables affecting this outcome predictor. *Journal of the American Society of Nephrology* **8** (12), 1921–1929.

Maher, E. R. and Curtis, J. R. (1985). Calcific aortic stenosis in chronic renal failure. *Lancet* **2** (8462), 1007.

Mall, G., Rambausek, M., Neumeister, A., Kollmar, S., Vetterlein, F., and Ritz, E. (1988). Myocardial interstitial fibrosis in experimental uraemia—implications for cardiac compliance. *Kidney International* **33** (4), 804–811.

Mall, G., Huther, W., Schneider, J., Lundin, P., and Ritz, E. (1990). Diffuse intermyocardiocytic fibrosis in uraemic patients. *Nephrology, Dialysis, Transplantation* **5** (1), 39–44.

Mandelbaum, A., Link, A., Wambach, G., and Ritz, E. (1993). Vena cava ultrasonography for the assessment of hydration status in kidney insufficiency. *Dtsch Med Wochenschr* **118** (37), 1309–1315.

Mann, J. F., Jakobs, K. H., Riedel, J., and Ritz, E. (1986). Reduced chronotropic responsiveness of the heart in experimental uremia. *American Journal of Physiology* **250** (5 Pt 2), H846–H852.

Mann, J. F., Gerstein, H. C., Pogue, J., Bosch, J., and Yusuf, S. (2001). Renal insufficiency as a predictor of cardiovascular outcomes and the impact of ramipril: the HOPE randomized trial. *Annals of Internal Medicine* **134** (8), 629–636.

Manske, C. L., Thomas, W., Wang, Y., and Wilson, R. F. (1993). Screening diabetic transplant candidates for coronary artery disease: identification of a low risk subgroup. *Kidney International* **44** (3), 617–621.

Maraj, S., Jacobs, L. E., Kung, S. C., Raja, R., Krishnasamy, P., Maraj, R., Braitman, L. E., and Kotler, M. N. (2002). Epidemiology and outcome of infective endocarditis in haemodialysis patients. *American Journal of Medicine Sci* **324** (5), 254–260.

Matthias, S., Hönack, C., Rösen, P., Zebe, H., and Ritz, E. (1995). Glucose uptake and expression of glucose transporters in the heart of uremic rats. *Journal of the American Society of Nephrology* **6**, 1023a (abstract).

Mazzaferro, S. *et al.* (1993). Role of ageing, chronic renal failure and dialysis in the calcification of mitral annulus. *Nephrology, Dialysis, Transplantation* **8** (4), 335–340.

McCullough, P. A. and Sandberg, K. R. (2003). B-type natriuretic peptide and renal disease. *Heart Failure Review* **8** (4), 355–358.

McMahon, L. P., McKenna, M. J., Sangkabutra, T., Mason, K., Sostaric, S., Skinner, S. L., Burge, C., Murphy, B., and Crankshaw, D. (1999). Physical performance and associated electrolyte changes after haemoglobin normalization: a comparative study in haemodialysis patients. *Nephrology, Dialysis, Transplantation* **14** (5), 1182–1187.

McMahon, L. P., Mason, K., Skinner, S. L., Burge, C. M., Grigg, L. E., and Becker, G. J. (2000). Effects of haemoglobin normalization on quality of life and cardiovascular parameters in end-stage renal failure. *Nephrology, Dialysis, Transplantation* **15** (9), 1425–1430.

Minga, T. E., Flanagan, K. H., and Allon, M. (2001). Clinical consequences of infected arteriovenous grafts in haemodialysis patients. *American Journal of Kidney Diseases* **38** (5), 975–978.

Moberly, J. B., Attman, P. O., Samuelsson, O., Johansson, A. C., Knight-Gibson, C., and Alaupovic, P. (1999). Apolipoprotein C-III, hypertriglyceridemia and triglyceride-rich lipoproteins in uremia. *Mineral and Electrolyte Metabolism* **25** (4–6), 258–262.

Moe, S. M., O'Neill, K. D., Duan, D., Ahmed, S., Chen, N. X., Leapman, S. B., Fineberg, N., and Kopecky, K. (2002). Medial artery calcification in ESRD patients is associated with deposition of bone matrix proteins. *Kidney International* **61** (2), 638–647.

Moe, S. M., Duan, D., Doehle, B. P., O'Neill, K. D., and Chen, N. X. (2003). Uremia induces the osteoblast differentiation factor Cbfa1 in human blood vessels. *Kidney International* **63** (3), 1003–1011.

Muirhead, N., Bargman, J., Burgess, E., Jindal, K. K., Levin, A., Nolin, L., and Parfrey, P. (1995). Evidence-based recommendations for the clinical use of recombinant human erythropoietin. *American Journal of Kidney Diseases* **26** (2 Suppl. 1), S1–S24.

Nabokov, A. V., Amann, K., Wessels, S., Munter, K., Wagner, J., and Ritz, E. (1999). Endothelin receptor antagonists influence cardiovascular morphology in uremic rats. *Kidney International* **55** (2), 512–519.

Nishikimi, T., Futoo, Y., Tamano, K., Takahashi, M., Suzuki, T., Minami, J., Honda, T., Uetake, S., Asakawa, H., Kobayashi, N., Horinaka, S., Ishimitsu, T., and Matsuoka, H. (2001). Plasma brain natriuretic peptide levels in chronic haemodialysis patients: influence of coronary artery disease. *American Journal of Kidney Diseases* **37** (6), 1201–1208.

Oh, J., Wunsch, R., Turzer, M., Bahner, M., Raggi, P., Querfeld, U., Mehls, O., and Schaefer, F. (2002). Advanced coronary and carotid arteriopathy in young adults with childhood-onset chronic renal failure. *Circulation* **106** (1), 100–105.

Osajima, A., Okazaki, M., Tamura, M., Anai, H., Kabashima, N., Suda, T., Iwamoto, M., Ota, T., Watanabe, Y., Kanegae, K., and Nakashima, Y. (2002). Comparison of plasma levels of mature adrenomedullin and natriuretic peptide as markers of cardiac function in haemodialysis patients with coronary artery disease. *Nephron* **92** (4), 832–839.

Ozkahya, M., Ok, E., Cirit, M., Aydin, S., Akcicek, F., Basci, A., and Dorhout Mees, E. J. (1998). Regression of left ventricular hypertrophy in haemodialysis patients by ultrafiltration and reduced salt intake without antihypertensive drugs. *Nephrology, Dialysis, Transplantation* **13** (6), 1489–1493.

Ozkahya, M., Toz, H., Qzerkan, F., Duman, S., Ok, E., Basci, A., and Mees, E. J. (2002). Impact of volume control on left ventricular hypertrophy in dialysis patients. *Journal of Nephrology* **15** (6), 655–660.

Paoletti, E., Cassottana, P., Bellino, D., Specchia, C., Messa, P., and Cannella, G. (2002). Left ventricular geometry and adverse cardiovascular events in chronic haemodialysis patients on prolonged therapy with ACE inhibitors. *American Journal of Kidney Diseases* **40** (4), 728–736.

Parfrey, P. S. (2000). Cardiac disease in dialysis patients: diagnosis, burden of disease, prognosis, risk factors and management. *Nephrology, Dialysis, Transplantation* **15** (Suppl, 5), 58–168.

Parfrey, P. S. and Foley, R. N. (1999). The clinical epidemiology of cardiac disease in chronic renal failure. *Journal of the American Society of Nephrology* **10** (7), 1606–1615.

Parfrey, P. S., Harnett, J. D., Griffiths, S. M., Taylor, R., Hand, J., King, A., and Barre, P. E. (1990). The clinical course of left ventricular hypertrophy in dialysis patients. *Nephron* **55** (2), 114–120.

Parfrey, P. S., Foley, R. N., Harnett, J. D., Kent, G. M., Murray, D. C., and Barre, P. E. (1996). Outcome and risk factors for left ventricular disorders in chronic uraemia. *Nephrology, Dialysis, Transplantation* **11** (7), 1277–1285.

Perna, A. F., De Santo, N. G., and Ingrosso, D. (1997). Adverse effects of hyperhomocysteinemia and their management by folic acid. *Mineral and Electrolyte Metabolism* **23** (3–6), 174–178.

Rabbat, C. G., Treleaven, D. J., Russell, J. D., Ludwin, D., and Cook, D. J. (2003). Prognostic value of myocardial perfusion studies in patients with end-stage renal disease assessed for kidney or kidney-pancreas transplantation: a meta-analysis. *Journal of the American Society of Nephrology* **14** (2), 431–439.

Raine, A. E. (1994). Acquired aortic stenosis in dialysis patients. *Nephron* **68** (2), 159–168.

Raine, A. E. *et al.* (1992). Report on management of renal failure in Europe, XXII, 1991. *Nephrology, Dialysis, Transplantation* **7** (Suppl. 2), 7–35.

Raine, A. E., Seymour, A. M., Roberts, A. F., Radda, G. K., and Ledingham, J. G. (1993). Impairment of cardiac function and energetics in experimental renal failure. *Journal of Clinical Investigation* **92** (6), 2934–2940.

Rambausek, M., Ritz, E., Mall, G., Mehls, O., and Katus, H. (1985). Myocardial hypertrophy in rats with renal insufficiency. *Kidney International* **28** (5), 775–782.

Rascher, W., Schomig, A., Kreye, V. A., and Ritz, E. (1982). Diminished vascular response to noradrenaline in experimental chronic uremia. *Kidney International* **21** (1), 20–27.

Reinecke, H., Trey, T., Matzkies, F., Fobker, M., Breithardt, G., and Schaefer, R. M. (2003). Grade of chronic renal failure, and acute and long-term outcome after percutaneous coronary interventions. *Kidney International* **63** (2), 696–701.

Rigatto, C., Parfrey, P., Foley, R., Negrijn, C., Tribula, C., and Jeffery, J. (2002). Congestive heart failure in renal transplant recipients: risk factors, outcomes, and relationship with ischemic heart disease. *Journal of the American Society of Nephrology* **13** (4), 1084–1090.

Ritz, E. (2003). Minor renal dysfunction: an emerging independent cardiovascular risk factor. *Heart* **89** (9), 963–964.

Ritz, E. and Fliser, D. (1993). Hypertension and the kidney—an overview. *American Journal of Kidney Diseases* **21** (6 Suppl. 3), 3–9.

Rocco, M. V., Yan, G., Gassman, J., Lewis, J. B., Ornt, D., Weiss, B., and Levey, A. S. (2002). Comparison of causes of death using HEMO study and HCFA end-stage renal disease death notification classification systems. The National Institutes of Health-funded Hemodialysis. Health Care Financing Administration. *American Journal of Kidney Diseases* **39** (1), 146–153.

Roig, E., Betriu, A., Castaner, A., Magrina, J., Sanz, G., and Navarro-Lopez, F. (1981). Disabling angina pectoris with normal coronary arteries in patients undergoing long-term haemodialysis. *American Journal of Medicine* **71** (3), 431–434.

Rostand, S. G., Kirk, K. A., and Rutsky, E. A. (1984). Dialysis-associated ischemic heart disease: insights from coronary angiography. *Kidney International* **25** (4), 653–659.

Rostand, S. G., Brunzell, J. D., Cannon, R. O. III, and Victor, R. G. (1991). Cardiovascular complications in renal failure. *Journal of the American Society of Nephrology* **2** (6), 1053–1062.

Rostand, S. G., Sanders, P. C., and Rutsky, E. A. (1994). Cardiac calcification in uremia. *Contributions to Nephrology* **106**, 26–29.

Ruffmann, K., Mandelbaum, A., Bommer, J., Schmidli, M., and Ritz, E. (1990). Doppler echocardiographic findings in dialysis patients. *Nephrology, Dialysis, Transplantation* **5** (6), 426–431.

Ruilope, L. M., Salvetti, A., Jamerson, K., Hansson, L., Warnold, I., Wedel, H., and Zanchetti, A. (2001a). Renal function and intensive lowering of blood pressure in hypertensive participants of the hypertension optimal treatment (HOT) study. *Journal of the American Society of Nephrology* **12** (2), 218–225.

Ruilope, L. M., van Veldhuisen, D. J., Ritz, E., and Luscher, T. F. (2001b). Renal function: the Cinderella of cardiovascular risk profile. *Journal of the American College of Cardiology* **38** (7), 1782–1787.

Rutsky, E. A. and Rostand, S. G. The management of coronary artery disease in patients with end stage renal disease. In *Cardiac Dysfunction in Chronic Uremia* (ed. P. Parfrey and U. D. Hamett). Dordrecht: Kluwer Academic, 1992.

Sato, S. *et al.* (1995). Effects of parathyroidectomy on left ventricular mass in patients with hyperparathyroidism. *Mineral and Electrolyte Metabolism* **21** (1–3), 67–71.

Schnyder, G., Roffi, M., Pin, R., Flammer, Y., Lange, H., Eberli, F. R., Meier, B., Turi, Z. G., and Hess, O. M. (2001). Decreased rate of coronary restenosis after lowering of plasma homocysteine levels. *New England Journal of Medicine* **345** (22), 1593–1600.

Schwarz, U., Buzello, M., Ritz, E., Stein, G., Raabe, G., Wiest, G., Mall, G., and Amann, K. (2000). Morphology of coronary atherosclerotic lesions in patients with end-stage renal failure. *Nephrology, Dialysis, Transplantation* **15** (2), 218–223.

Seliger, S. L., Weiss, N. S., Gillen, D. L., Kestenbaum, B., Ball, A., Sherrard, D. J., and Stehman-Breen, C. O. (2002). HMG-CoA reductase inhibitors are associated with reduced mortality in ESRD patients. *Kidney International* **61** (1), 297–304.

Sever, P. S., Dahlof, B., Poulter, N. R., Wedel, H., Beevers, G., Caulfield, M., Collins, R., Kjeldsen, S. E., Kristinsson, A., McInnes, G. T., Mehlsen, J., Nieminen, M., O'Brien, E., and Ostergren, J. (2003). Prevention of coronary and stroke events with atorvastatin in hypertensive patients who have average or lower-than-average cholesterol concentrations, in the Anglo-Scandinavian Cardiac Outcomes Trial—Lipid Lowering Arm (ASCOT-LLA): a multicentre randomised controlled trial. *Lancet* **361** (9364), 1149–1158.

Sexton, D. J. (2001). Vascular access infections in patients undergoing dialysis with special emphasis on the role and treatment of *Staphylococcus aureus*. *Infectious Disease Clinics of North America* **15** (3), 731–742, vii.

Sforzini, S., Latini, R., Mingardi, G., Vincenti, A., and Redaelli, B. (1992). Ventricular arrhythmias and four-year mortality in haemodialysis patients. Gruppo Emodialisi e Patologie Cardiovascolari. *Lancet* **339** (8787), 212–213.

Shlipak, M. G., Heidenreich, P. A., Noguchi, H., Chertow, G. M., Browner, W. S., and McClellan, M. B. (2002). Association of renal insufficiency with treatment and outcomes after myocardial infarction in elderly patients. *Annals of Internal Medicine* **137** (7), 555–562.

Silberberg, J. S., Barre, P. E., Prichard, S. S., and Sniderman, A. D. (1989). Impact of left ventricular hypertrophy on survival in end-stage renal disease. *Kidney International* **36** (2), 286–290.

Silverberg, D. S., Wexler, D., Sheps, D., Blum, M., Keren, G., Baruch, R., Schwartz, D., Yachnin, T., Steinbruch, S., Shapira, I., Laniado, S., and Iaina, A. (2001). The effect of correction of mild anaemia in severe, resistant congestive heart failure using subcutaneous erythropoietin and intravenous iron: a randomized controlled study. *Journal of the American College of Cardiology* **37** (7), 1775–1780.

Simsir, S. A., Kohlman-Trigoboff, D., Flood, R., Lindsay, J., and Smith, B. M. (1998). A comparison of coronary artery bypass grafting and percutaneous transluminal coronary angioplasty in patients on haemodialysis. *Cardiovascular Surgery* **6** (5), 500–505.

Standl, E. and Schnell, O. (2000). A new look at the heart in diabetes mellitus: from ailing to failing. *Diabetologia* **43** (12), 1455–1469.

Stewart, G. A., Foster, J., Cowan, M., Rooney, E., McDonagh, T., Dargie, H. J., Rodger, R. S., and Jardine, A. G. (1999). Echocardiography overestimates left ventricular mass in haemodialysis patients relative to magnetic resonance imaging. *Kidney International* **56** (6), 2248–2253.

Stratton, J., Macdonald, A., and Farrington, K. (2000). Successful treatment of MRSA endocarditis in a haemodialysis patient. *Nephrology, Dialysis, Transplantation* **15** (10), 1719–1720.

Suliman, M. E., Stenvinkel, P., Barany, P., Heimburger, O., Anderstam, B., and Lindholm, B. (2003). Hyperhomocysteinemia and its relationship to cardiovascular disease in ESRD: influence of hypoalbuminemia, malnutrition, inflammation, and diabetes mellitus. *American Journal of Kidney Diseases* **41** (3 Suppl. 1), S89–S95.

The Cardiac Arrhythmia Suppression Trial Investigators (1989). Preliminary report: effect of encainide and flecainide on mortality in a randomized trial of arrhythmia suppression after myocardial infarction. The Cardiac Arrhythmia Suppression Trial (CAST) Investigators. *New England Journal of Medicine* **321** (6), 406–412.

The Digitalis Investigation Group (1997). The effect of digoxin on mortality and morbidity in patients with heart failure. The Digitalis Investigation Group. *New England Journal of Medicine* **336** (8), 525–533.

Tonelli, M., Moye, L., Sacks, F. M., Kiberd, B., and Curhan, G. (2003). Pravastatin for secondary prevention of cardiovascular events in persons with mild chronic renal insufficiency. *Annals of Internal Medicine* **138** (2), 98–104.

Topoleski, L. D. and Salunke, N. V. (2000). Mechanical behavior of calcified plaques: a summary of compression and stress-relaxation experiments. *Zeitschrift für Kardiologie* **89** (Suppl. 2), 85–91.

Tornig, J., Amann, K., Ritz, E., Nichols, C., Zeier, M., and Mall, G. (1996). Arteriolar wall thickening, capillary rarefaction and interstitial fibrosis in the heart of rats with renal failure: the effects of ramipril, nifedipine and moxonidine. *Journal of the American Society of Nephrology* **7** (5), 667–675.

Tozawa, M., Iseki, K., Iseki, C., Oshiro, S., Yamazato, M., Higashiuesato, Y., Tomiyama, N., Tana, T., Ikemiya, Y., and Takishita, S. (2002). Evidence for elevated pulse pressure in patients on chronic haemodialysis: a case–control study. *Kidney International* **62** (6), 2195–2201.

Van Biesen, W., Vanholder, R., Veys, N., and Lameire, N. (2002). Peritoneal dialysis in anuric patients: concerns and cautions. *Seminars in Dialysis* **15** (5), 305–310.

van der Elst, M. E., Buurma, H., Bouvy, M. L., and de Boer, A. (2003). Drug therapy for prevention of recurrent myocardial infarction. *Annals of Pharmacotherapy* **37** (10), 1465–1477.

van der Sande, F. M., Kooman, J. P., Konings, C. J., and Leunissen, K. M. (2001). Thermal effects and blood pressure response during postdilution haemodiafiltration and haemodialysis: the effect of amount of replacement fluid and dialysate temperature. *Journal of the American Society of Nephrology* **12** (9), 1916–1920.

Verresen, L., Fink, E., Lemke, H. D., and Vanrenterghem, Y. (1994). Bradykinin is a mediator of anaphylactoid reactions during haemodialysis with AN69 membranes. *Kidney International* **45** (5), 1497–1503.

Vertes, V., Cangiano, J. L., Berman, L. B., and Gould, A. (1969). Hypertension in end-stage renal disease. *New England Journal of Medicine* **280** (18), 978–981.

Wang, A. Y., Wang, M., Woo, J., Law, M. C., Chow, K. M., Li, P. K., Lui, S. F., and Sanderson, J. E. (2002). A novel association between residual renal function and left ventricular hypertrophy in peritoneal dialysis patients. *Kidney International* **62** (2), 639–647.

Wang, A. Y., Wang, M., Woo, J., Lam, C. W., Li, P. K., Lui, S. F., and Sanderson, J. E. (2003). Cardiac valve calcification as an important predictor for all-cause mortality and cardiovascular mortality in long-term peritoneal dialysis patients: a prospective study. *Journal of the American Society of Nephrology* **14** (1), 159–168.

Wanner, C. and Krane, V. (2002). Uremia-specific alterations in lipid metabolism. *Blood Purification* **20** (5), 451–453.

Wanner, C., Krane, V., Ruf, G., Marz, W., and Ritz, E. (1999). Rationale and design of a trial improving outcome of type 2 diabetics on haemodialysis. Die Deutsche Diabetes Dialyse Studie Investigators. *Kidney International Supplement* **71**, S222–S226.

Wilcox, C. S. (2002). New insights into diuretic use in patients with chronic renal disease. *Journal of the American Society of Nephrology* **13** (3), 798–805.

Wilson, R. A., Norman, D. J., Barry, J. M., and Bennett, W. M. (1994). Noninvasive cardiac testing in the end-stage renal disease patient. *Blood Purification* **12** (1), 78–83.

Wizemann, V. (1996). Points to remember when dialysing the patient with coronary disease. *Nephrology, Dialysis, Transplantation* **11** (2), 236–238.

Wright, R. S., Reeder, G. S., Herzog, C. A., Albright, R. C., Williams, B. A., Dvorak, D. L., Miller, W. L., Murphy, J. G., Kopecky, S. L., and Jaffe, A. S. (2002). Acute myocardial infarction and renal dysfunction: a high-risk combination. *Annals of Internal Medicine* **137** (7), 563–570.

Yusuf, S., Sleight, P., Pogue, J., Bosch, J., Davies, R., and Dagenais, G. (2000). Effects of an angiotensin-converting-enzyme inhibitor, ramipril, on cardiovascular events in high-risk patients. The Heart Outcomes Prevention Evaluation Study Investigators. *New England Journal of Medicine* **342** (3), 145–153.

Zaman, A. G., Helft, G., Osende, J. I., Fuster, V., and Badimon, J. J. (1999). Histopathology and pathogenesis of plaque instability and thrombus formation. *Drugs Today (Barcelona, Spain)* **35** (8), 641–656.

Zimmermann, J., Herrlinger, S., Pruy, A., Metzger, T., and Wanner, C. (1999). Inflammation enhances cardiovascular risk and mortality in haemodialysis patients. *Kidney International* **55** (2), 648–658.

Zoccali, C. (2003). Another marker of cardiac dysfunction in dialysis patients? *Nephron Clinical Practice* **93** (2), C49–C50.

Zoccali, C., Mallamaci, F., Parlongo, S., Cutrupi, S., Benedetto, F. A., Tripepi, G., Bonanno, G., Rapisarda, F., Fatuzzo, P., Seminara, G., Cataliotti, A., Stancanelli, B., Malatino, L. S., and Cateliotti, A. (2002). Plasma norepinephrine predicts survival and incident cardiovascular events in patients with end-stage renal disease. *Circulation* **105** (11), 1354–1359.

11.3.6 Gastrointestinal effects
Ciaran Doherty

Gastrointestinal (GI) symptoms in patients with chronic renal failure may be due to uraemia (anorexia, nausea, vomiting) or the disorder causing the renal failure. Examples include abdominal pain with intracyst haemorrhage in polycystic kidney disease; prescribed drugs (diarrhoea with oral iron supplements, vomiting with digoxin toxicity); diabetic gastropathy; or the dialysis treatment itself (abdominal pain due to icodextrin pseudo-peritonitis).

The frequency with which GI symptoms affect patients with chronic renal failure also reflects the increased prevalence of some GI tract disorders and the occurrence of conditions specific to chronic renal failure (e.g. nephrogenic ascites, dialysis amyloidosis). Some GI tract disorders or their treatment may cause chronic uraemia; in short, bowel syndrome oxalate urolithiasis may result in progressive renal failure (Banerjee and warwicker 2002), while salazopyrine treatment for ulcerative colitis may induce chronic interstitial nephritis.

There are also various disorders of GI tract structure and function in chronic renal failure, the clinical significance of which is unclear. These include elevated levels of gastroenterohepatic hormones (Doherty *et al.* 1978), and alterations in small bowel enzyme activity, absorption, and microbial flora (Simenhoff *et al.* 1978). Other changes such as augmented intestinal potassium excretion (Martin *et al.* 1986) in patients with renal insufficiency (largely due to total potassium secretion in the colon) may represent adaptive change and a role for the large intestine in potassium homeostasis as renal potassium excretion declines. Enhanced intestinal absorption of aluminium in renal failure may, in contrast, contribute to the long-term clinical risks of this metal (Drueke 2002).

Concurrent (unrelated) GI tract disease may have significant implications for clinical management of renal patients. For example, Goransson and Bergrem (2002) reported a renal transplant patient with an ileostomy who developed profuse diarrhoea, completely interrupting enterohepatic recirculation of mycophenolate and rendering the serum level undetectable. Autonomic gastroparesis in diabetic patients may cause erratic absorption of both ingested food and oral medication with adverse effects on control of glycaemia and hypertension.

Upper gastrointestinal tract

The following is a review of the pathophysiology of GI tract disorders in patients with chronic renal failure and on dialysis.

Gastric emptying

Functional alterations of the upper GI tract in chronic renal failure include delayed gastric emptying. De Schoenmakere et al. (2001) using radio-isotope markers found the half-life time for gastric emptying was 83 ± 34 min in 56 haemodialysis patients, compared to 50 ± 15 min in a normal reference population. Delayed gastric emptying in this study was associated with changes in nutritional status as judged by serum albumin and other markers.

Peptic ulcer disease

In the early decades of chronic dialysis treatment programmes, peptic ulcer was reported to occur with increased frequency in regular dialysis patients and GI complications, often severe, were common following renal transplantation (Shepherd et al. 1973; Milito et al. 1983). GI tract disease is now a rare cause of death following renal transplantation, and more recent studies based on endoscopic assessment of large numbers of dialysis patients have found an incidence of duodenal ulcer not different to that of the general population (Andriulla et al. 1985). Progressive improvements in regular dialysis treatment together with the widespread introduction of H2 antagonist and proton pump inhibitor therapy may account for this change.

Despite the increased availability of urea as substrate and an observed increase in the frequency of gastritis and duodenitis in patients with chronic renal failure (Mitchell et al. 1979), the prevalence of Helicobacter pylori infection does not appear to differ from that of control populations (Davenport 1991). There are few studies on the efficacy of H. pylori eradication therapy in patients with endstage renal disease (ESRD) and treatment recommendations are therefore based on general guidelines (Howden and Hunt 1998). Suitable regimens are a combination of proton pump inhibitor (e.g. lansoprazole 30 mg once daily), clarithromycin 500 mg 12 hourly, and either amoxycillin 500 mg 8 hourly or metronidazole 500 mg 12 hourly for 2 weeks. Agents containing bismuth salts should be avoided in the presence of renal failure (Fabrizi and Martin 2000).

Biliary tract disease

Studies of cholecystitis and cholelithiasis in patients with ESRD have found a similar prevalence to that in the normal population (Hojs 1995). One study found that 40 per cent of patients with polycystic kidney disease had common bile duct dilatation of at least 7 mm, compared to 9.1 per cent of matched controls (Ishikawa et al. 1996). The clinical significance of this finding is unknown.

Pancreatitis

There is no convincing evidence that acute or chronic pancreatitis is more common in patients with ESRD despite additional risk factors for the disorder, which include hyperparathyroidism, drug ingestion, and hypertriglyceridaemia. The diagnosis of acute pancreatitis is made difficult by the fact that serum pancreatic amylase and lipase are elevated in chronic renal failure. However, in the absence of acute pancreatitis, the absolute values do not exceed three times the upper limit of normal.

Chronic pancreatitis and small bowel disorders cause increased intestinal oxalate absorption and this may result in oxalate-induced renal failure due to nephrolithiasis and tubulointerstitial injury. Hill et al. (2002) described three patients with alcohol-induced chronic pancreatic insufficiency not receiving adequate enzyme supplements, who developed diabetes mellitus and irreversible renal failure. Renal biopsy showed oxalate crystal deposition with severe tubulointerstitial scarring but only mild background diabetic nephropathy. These three cases suggest that renal dysfunction facilitates supersaturation of urinary oxalate leading to interstitial crystallization and renal damage. Renal failure in patients with diabetes due to chronic pancreatitis should not therefore be ascribed to diabetes without a renal biopsy. Treatment of the malabsorption and steatorrhoea with adequate enzyme supplements may prevent this complication of chronic pancreatic insufficiency.

Gastrointestinal manifestations of polycystic kidney disease

In patients with polycystic kidney disease, GI symptoms may arise from extrarenal complications of the disorder including hepatic cysts, colonic diverticula, umbilical, or inguinal hernias (Fig. 1). Massive hepatic cysts occur predominantly in women with advanced renal disease and may cause compression symptoms such as tolerance of only small meals (stomach compression) or lower limb oedema (inferior vena cava compression). Hepatic cysts may also cause chronic upper abdominal pain, which, if severe, may require ultrasound-guided cyst decompression; acute episodes of upper abdominal pain may result

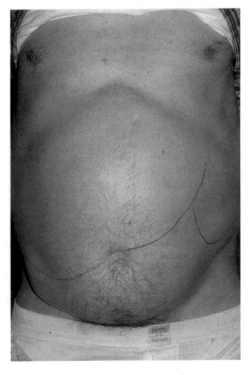

Fig. 1 Massive abdominal distension in a 57-year-old man with adult polycystic kidney and liver disease. This may cause gastric compression symptoms as well as acute and chronic abdominal pain.

from cyst infection, haemorrhage, or, rarely, rupture. Cyst infection may require percutaneous drainage and antibiotic therapy, preferably with a quinolone as this is one of the few antibiotics which achieves bactericidal concentrations within the cyst fluid. Patients with massive symptomatic cysts may be referred to an experienced biliary tract surgeon for consideration of partial hepatic resection (Chauveau 2000).

Colonic diverticulae and umbilical and inguinal hernias are more frequent in patients with polycystic kidney disease than the normal population. Colonic diverticulae may present with abdominal pain (difficult to distinguish from painful renal/hepatic cysts), diarrhoea, and melaena (Scheff 1980). In one series, the incidence of abdominal wall hernias was reported to be 45 per cent in patients with polycystic kidney disease compared with 8 per cent in patients with other causes of chronic renal failure (MorrisStiff 1997).

Lower gastrointestinal tract disorders

Lower GI tract disorders that occur with increased frequency in dialysis patients include ischaemic bowel disease, spontaneous colonic perforation, diverticular disease, angiodysplasia, and faecal impaction. Two important disorders specific to ESRD patients are idiopathic dialysis ascites and dialysis-related amyloidosis.

Ischaemic bowel disease

This condition may cause sudden onset of fever, vomiting, and abdominal pain in elderly dialysis patients, and at laparotomy the findings are those of colonic necrosis and also occasionally small bowel ischaemic change (Zeier et al. 1992). A significant proportion of patients have no gross arterial or venous occlusion, and the disorder is accordingly classified as non-occlusive mesenteric ischaemia/infarction. There is often a prodromal phase characterized by sustained decrease in cardiac output, as may be seen in severe hypovolaemia, congestive heart failure, hypoxic states, or excessive ultrafiltration with intradialytic hypotension. In patients on continuous ambulatory peritoneal dialysis (CAPD), the condition may mimic peritonitis, resulting in delay in diagnosis and initiation of appropriate treatment, and a high mortality rate. Mesenteric angiography is the most important diagnostic test; in non-occlusive mesenteric infarction there will be no evidence of critical stenosis in the major vessels but poor or no flow in the small resistance vessels in the submucosa. A high index of suspicion is therefore required when the symptoms described occur in the setting of ESRD treated with dialysis therapy which triggers hypovolaemia, hypotension, and/or low cardiac output.

Atherosclerosis and low blood flow states are not the only factors which may predispose to ischaemic colitis in patients with chronic renal failure; increased blood viscosity, constipation causing increased intraluminal pressure, and digoxin (which may act as a splanchnic vasoconstrictor) may contribute to increased risk. In addition, Norden and Rabb (2001) recently reported two cases of non-occlusive mesenteric infarction, one of which was due to undiagnosed lymphoma encroaching on mesenteric vessels, and a second due to extensive colonic amyloidosis.

Spontaneous colonic perforation

In non-renal patients, most colonic perforations are due to diverticular disease or obstruction. In patients with ESRD, colonic perforation may also occur in association with barium enema examination (Imai and Satoh 1997), faecal impaction, dehydration, dialysis-related amyloidosis (Min et al. 1997), and aluminium-containing antacids. The diagnosis must be considered in chronic renal failure patients presenting with acute abdominal pain, as the condition has a higher mortality in the uraemic population.

Diverticular disease

The incidence of this disorder is not increased in dialysis patients except for those with polycystic kidney disease. The illness may, however, occur at a younger age and may be more severe with higher rates of haemorrhage (due to uraemic platelet dysfunction and/or iatrogenic anticoagulation), or result in an increased incidence of faecal peritonitis in those undergoing chronic peritoneal dialysis. It is important to detect diverticulitis prior to renal transplantation as post-transplant perforation may occur in patients given high doses of corticosteroids, and this complication is associated with a high mortality rate (Church 1985).

Dialysis-related amyloidosis

β2-Microglobulin amyloid is almost universal in patients undergoing dialysis for extended periods. Although carpal tunnel syndrome is the usual clinical manifestation, visceral involvement has been reported with GI manifestations which may range from decreased motility with gastric dilatation and paralytic ileus, to caecal perforation and/or intestinal necrosis (Borczuk et al. 1995; Min et al. 1997). Maher et al. (1988) reported two patients on dialysis for 17 and 14 years, respectively, one of whom developed melaena, and the other persistent diarrhoea. Both proved to have extensive amyloid deposition affecting the small bowel.

Idiopathic dialysis ascites

The incidence of this disorder is declining due to improvements in nutritional therapy together with better dialysis prescribing and delivery. Patients on maintenance haemodialysis who develop ascites require exclusion of under dialysis and specific disorders such as constrictive pericarditis, cirrhosis, occult infection especially tuberculosis, sclerosing peritonitis (see Chapter 12.4) and neoplastic or granulomatous peritoneal disease. Radiological examination may detect inferior vena cava stenosis due to lymphoma or hepatic cyst. Where no cause can be found, idiopathic dialysis ascites arises as a diagnosis of exclusion. Ascitic fluid in these cases usually shows a straw coloured appearance with a high protein content (3–6 g/dl) and a leucocyte count ranging from 25 to 1600 cells/mm^3. Treatment strategies involve salt and fluid restriction, aggressive ultrafiltration, and intermittent paracentesis. Some patients are improved by switching from haemodialysis to CAPD. Renal transplantation remains the best treatment as complete resolution of ascites usually occurs within 6 weeks of operation (Melero et al. 1995). The prognosis of idiopathic dialysis ascites is poor as one-third of patients will die within a year of diagnosis (Gluck and Nolph 1987).

Intestinal pseudo-obstruction

Normal GI motor function involves extrinsic nerve supply from the brain and spinal cord, the neural plexus within the wall of the stomach and intestine, and locally released transmitters which influence the excitability of intestinal smooth muscle.

Chronic intestinal pseudo-obstruction should be considered when symptoms suggest mechanical bowel obstruction, but no anatomical lesion obstructing the transit of intestinal contents is present. On X-ray, affected bowel segments appear dilated, in contrast to the absence of dilatation in the similar disorder of chronic intestinal dysmotility. Chronic intestinal pseudo-obstruction is usually secondary to an underlying disorder affecting neuromuscular function such as amyloidosis, diabetes mellitus, or scleroderma. It may also be caused by medications that cause neurological dysfunction of the intestine, such as calcium channel blockers and anticholenergic antidepressants. Clinical manifestations include abdominal pain, vomiting, distension, and constipation or diarrhoea. The findings on physical examination are abdominal distension and a succussion splash. Helpful investigations include plain X-ray of abdomen (usually demonstrates air–fluid levels and/or distended loops of small bowel), gastric and small bowel transit testing, by scintigraphy, autonomic testing, and specialized tests such as manometry. The presence of associated steatorrhoea, vitamin B_{12} malabsorption, or folate excess suggests small bowel bacterial overgrowth and should prompt bacteriological culture of a small bowel aspirate to confirm the diagnosis.

Treatment in severe cases may require temporary parenteral nutrition and prokinetic agents such as erythromycin, which may act, in part at least, by stimulation of motilin receptors. Cisapride should be avoided in view of the risk of cardiac arrhythmia and caution is necessary with metoclopromide because of the risk of extra-pyramidal reactions. Antibiotics on a rotating basis are used in patients with confirmed small bowel bacterial overgrowth.

Acute intestinal pseudo-obstruction may develop following renal transplantation. Certain factors are common in patients who develop this syndrome, namely prior chronic constipation, diabetic autonomic neuropathy, retroperitoneal haematoma, and treatment with opioid analgesics, kayexalate, and other drugs. A small percentage of severely affected patients may progress to fatal colonic perforation, and early recognition of the syndrome is therefore important in order to facilitate removal of potentially culpable drug therapy and to consider intervention with colonic decompression.

Management of common gastrointestinal problems in patients with chronic renal failure

Acute abdomen

In this clinical setting, all disorders that affect the non-renal patient may occur, but patients with chronic renal failure face additional risks. Other conditions which may enter the differential diagnosis of the acute abdomen in patients with chronic renal failure are shown in Table 1.

Gastrointestinal bleeding

GI bleeding was a common problem in patients undergoing dialysis and kidney transplantation in the 1970s (Gurland 1973). The incidence and mortality of this disorder in renal transplant patients has greatly decreased as a result of H2 antagonist/proton pump inhibitor treatment, improved dialysis delivery, and reduction in prednisolone dosage used postrenal transplant. GI bleeding in dialysis patients has also declined in recent years, with a changed pattern of causes and requiring

Table 1 Conditions which may enter the differential diagnosis of acute abdomen in patients with chronic renal failure

Diagnosis	Clinical setting
Non-occlusive mesenteric infarction	Ultrafiltration with hypotension in elderly dialysis patients (Zeier et al. 1992)
Acute intestinal obstruction	Opioid analgesia post-renal transplant Excessive use of ion exchange resins
Colonic perforation	High dose corticosteroid treatment post-renal transplant (Stelzner et al. 1997)
Colonic necrosis	Dialysis amyloidosis in long-term haemodialysis patients (Min et al. 1997)
Intussusception	Henoch-Schonlein purpura
Splenic rupture	Primary amyloidosis (Dedi et al. 2001)
Intracyst haemorrhage or infection	Adult polycystic kidney disease
Phlegmonous gastritis	Secondary amyloidosis (Joko et al. 1999)
Pseudomembranous colitis with perforation/abscess/ toxic megacolon	Recent broad spectrum antibiotic therapy
Peritonitis, bacterial	CAPD
Pseudoperitonitis	Icodextrin sensitivity (Heering 2001)
Focal small bowel ischaemia	Malignant hypertension (Padfield 1975)
Campylobacter jejuni gastroenteritis	Subacute abdominal pain and diarrhoea (Adedeji et al. 2000)
Strongyloides stercoralis intestinal infection	(Adedeji et al. 2001)

a different treatment approach. Factors which have contributed to this change include the increased age of the dialysis patient population, the longer years which patients spend undergoing maintenance haemodialysis, and the general decline in the incidence of peptic ulcer disease (Langman 1982).

GI bleeding may be the result of uraemia *per se*, but can also be related to the causative disorder (e.g. gut Kaposi's sarcoma in HIV nephropathy), drug treatment being given (e.g. warfarin, aspirin), the dialysis treatment (excess heparinization), or finally coexistent GI tract disease. If GI bleeding in the dialysis patient falls into the latter category, the pattern of causes differs slightly from the non-uraemic population in that some disorders occur more commonly in uraemic subjects (gastritis, duodenitis), while others are specific to the uraemic state (dialysis amyloidosis). Angiodysplasia is a vascular abnormality which may affect the microcirculation of the GI mucosa and submucosa and cause GI haemorrhage in elderly patients. The condition has been reported to occur with increased incidence in haemodialysis patients; to affect the stomach, duodenum, jejunum, and colon, and to account for 20 per cent of upper GI bleeding in haemodialysis patients (Dave *et al.* 1984). The lesions are invisible on contrast studies, angiographic findings are subtle, and jejunal or ileal lesions may exist beyond the reach of the standard endoscope. Specially designed small bowel enteroscopes may be required to permit visualization of such lesions.

Amyloidosis caused by deposition of β2-microglobulin principally affects periarticular and bony tissues, but more systemic deposition may occur with time and involve the gut causing GI complications including melaena. Campistol (1987) studied 26 patients receiving haemodialysis for a period of over 12 years and found histological evidence of amyloid visceral involvement in 15 (58 per cent). Non-steroidal anti-inflammatory drug (NSAID) induced enteropathy is now known to involve mucosal damage more often in the small intestine than in the stomach (Bjarnason and MacPherson 1989). Up to 70 per cent of patients receiving NSAIDs for more than 6 months may be affected with mucosal damage usually manifested by chronic GI blood loss, and recovery may take up to 18 months after stopping the drug. The pathogenesis of the enteropathy is thought to involve an increase in mucosal permeability which may allow other factors, such as bacteria, bile, and pancreatic proteolytic enzymes to mediate the structural mucosal damage. This condition should be considered in dialysis patients with GI bleeding who have a previous history of rheumatoid or other chronic arthritis or recent treatment with NSAIDs.

Management of bleeding in a dialysis patient should begin by considering if it could be: (a) a direct effect of uraemia (is the patient adequately dialysed?); (b) iatrogenic (aspirin, heparin, warfarin, NSAID); (c) due to underlying systemic disorders; or (d) due to unrelated GI tract disease (Doherty 1993). In the patient who is actively bleeding, initial measures include blood transfusion, intensive care monitoring for elderly hypotensive patients, care to preserve arteriovenous fistula patency, and change of the patient to peritoneal dialysis or heparin-free haemodialysis. Once drugs, uraemia, and underlying systemic disorders have been excluded, the next priority is to establish the underlying cause of the GI bleeding. Practical points of note are the likelihood of angiodysplasia in the older age group, dialysis amyloidosis in the long-term haemodialysis patient, small bowel NSAID-enteropathy in patients with rheumatoid or osteoarthritis, and stercoral ulcers in patients with constipation induced by ion-exchange resins or aluminium hydroxide for phosphate binding. Coagulation abnormalities should always be sought; they may be either the primary cause of the bleeding or an exacerbating factor.

Upper gastrointestinal tract bleeding

Where the diagnosis proves to be a bleeding peptic ulcer, a range of endoscopic therapy options are now available, including laser therapy and injection techniques utilizing adrenaline, ethanol, or polidocanol. It remains prudent to involve a surgeon from the outset in care of the dialysis patient with GI bleeding, but most episodes of haemorrhage from peptic ulcer should now be controllable with endoscopic techniques. Where oesophageal varices are the cause of bleeding, endoscopic sclerotherapy is the treatment of choice, but temporary control of haemorrhage may be achieved using somatostatin or an octreotide infusion. These agents appear at least as effective as balloon tube tamponade. Mallory-Weiss oesophageal tears, which may follow vomiting, usually settle with conservative measures. Haemorrhagic gastritis is often a diffuse lesion and is usually treated with antacid therapy, H2 receptor antagonists, or the cytoprotective agent sucralfate.

Another approach to managing patients with acute bleeding has been to reduce fibrinolysis at the ulcer site, by lessening the tendency of gastric juice to promote clot lysis and rebleeding. Henry and O'Connell (1989) carried out a meta-analysis of randomized, double-blind, placebo-controlled trials comprising 1267 patients with acute upper GI haemorrhage; they found a significant reduction in operation rate

(30 per cent) and mortality (40 per cent) in those treated with tranexamic acid.

Lower gastrointestinal tract bleeding

Antifibrinolytic agents, such as tranexamic acid, may have a role in lower as well as upper GI tract bleeding, but there is little published evidence on their efficacy in this situation. Oestrogen/progesterone preparations have been reported to significantly reduce transfusion requirements in patients with recurrent GI bleeding due to angiodysplasia (Broner 1986), but controlled randomized trials have given conflicting results (Lewis et al. 1992). Other management options for GI tract bleeding due to angiodysplasia include regular blood transfusions, therapeutic endoscopy (electrocoagulation and laser therapy), or surgical resection. Most patients with angiodysplasia, however, are elderly and present a poor surgical risk.

The main problem in lower GI tract bleeding is often one of diagnosis. Barium enema may be of little diagnostic value, and colonoscopy may be impossible because of luminal blood. Selective visceral angiography may reveal the site and sometimes the pathology of colonic bleeding, but the method is dependent on the patient bleeding actively at the time of examination. Radioisotope scanning using labelled red cells is often disappointing as leak of intravenous material into the bowel frequently cannot be localized to the small or large intestine. Fine fibre optic enteroscopes passed with the aid of balloon propulsion into the ileocaecal region and then slowly withdrawn allow visualization of the entire small bowel and are an important diagnostic development. This technique will facilitate diagnosis of small bowel angiodysplasia, NSAID erosions, and other lesions.

In summary, the dialysis patient with GI bleeding requires—in addition to conventional investigation—exclusion of angiodysplasia (older age group), dialysis amyloidosis (especially if on long-term dialysis), and subtle coagulation disturbance. Heparin-free haemodialysis should be considered and drug treatment options include H2 antagonists (peptic ulcer), oestrogen/progesterone (angiodysplasia), somatostatin (oesophageal varices), and sucralfate or tranexamic acid for upper GI lesions (to reduce clot lysis by gastric juice). Therapeutic endoscopy is the treatment of choice for bleeding peptic ulcer and oesophageal varices. Small bowel enteroscopy may be appropriate in difficult cases.

Drug-induced gastrointestinal syndromes in chronic renal failure patients

Some of the common and not so common adverse effects of drug therapy in patients with chronic renal failure are listed in Table 2. Antacid bezoars may occur in the stomach, small bowel, or colon and may cause symptoms ranging from mild flatulence to intestinal obstruction. Angiotensin-converting enzyme (ACE) inhibitors such as captopril may cause severe diarrhoea associated with episodic angioedema (Weinstock et al. 1994). The differential diagnosis of diarrhoea in diabetic patients may prove difficult and requires consideration of autonomic neuropathy, antibiotic-induced pseudo-membranous colitis, non-specific antibiotic-induced diarrhoea, overflow incontinence due to faecal impaction, and the effects on colonic motility of iron supplements, digoxin, phosphate binders, and antihypertensive therapy.

Faecal impaction may complicate the use of phosphate binders, analgesics, and iron, and it can lead to mucosal ulceration, bleeding,

Table 2 Drug-induced gastrointestinal syndromes in chronic renal failure patients

Symptom/syndrome	Commonly implicated drugs
Anorexia, nausea, vomiting	Codeine-containing compound analgesics, antibiotics, oral iron supplements, digoxin, azathioprine, mycophenolate
(Hepatocellular) jaundice	Fucidin
Intestinal obstruction	Antacid bezoars
Intestinal pseudo-obstruction	Calcium channel blockers, anticholinergic antidepressants
Colonic necrosis	Kalexalate enema, especially post surgery
Faecal impaction +/− overflow incontinence, bleeding, perforation	Compound analgesics containing codeine, other opioid analgesics, oral iron supplements, phosphate binders
Diarrhoea	Broad spectrum antibiotics, oral iron supplements, digoxin, phosphate binders, phosphate supplements, ACE inhibitors

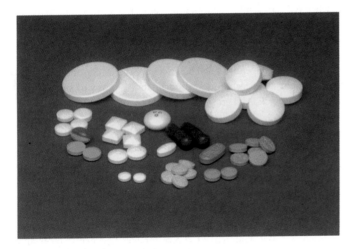

Fig. 2 The average daily medication intake of an patient with endstage renal disease undergoing regular dialysis treatment.

perforation, and/or chronic diarrhoea. Useful laxative preparations include the stool softener sodium docusate in a dose of 100 mg twice daily, osmotic laxatives such as lactulose 20 ml daily, and bisacodyl in a dose of 10 mg daily, either orally or as a suppository (Fig. 2).

Drug induced gastrointestinal syndromes following renal transplantation

Almost all immunosuppressive medications may be associated with adverse GI effects; this topic is reviewed in detail (Helderman 2002).

Infections

Systemic or localized infections (bacterial, viral, fungal, or parasitic) may affect one or more gut segments between the mouth and anus. Cytomegalovirus (CMV) and herpes viruses are very common in transplant recipients especially during the first 6–12 months after transplantation.

Herpes simplex virus usually presents as a reactivation of latent virus within the first 6 weeks of postrenal transplant. Oropharyngeal ulceration is the commonest manifestation, less commonly oesophagitis may occur. Cases almost invariably present during treatment of acute rejection with high-dose steroids and/or antilymphycyte preparations. Untreated herpetic ulcers can progress to haemorrhage or oesophageal perforation. While simple oral ulcers can be treated with a short course of oral aciclovir, more extensive disease may require intravenous aciclovir or ganciclovir if there is concomitant CMV or Epstein–Barr virus (EBV) infection. Non-specific oral ulcers not caused by identifiable pathogens are common in neutropenic patients and may be treated with topical triamcinolone ointment.

Candidiasis postrenal transplant typically presents with oropharyngeal lesions or oesophagitis. Involvement of the oesophagus usually causes dysphagia or odynophagia, less commonly heartburn, epigastric pain, or GI bleeding. The lesions appear as superficial erosions, ulcers, or white plaques, and diagnosis is made by fungal cultures or histopathological examination of appropriate specimens. Treatment is with topical nystatin or amphotericin B lozenges while intravenous antifungal agents may be required for severe cases. Prophylactic dental hygiene and nystatin 1 ml gargle 6 hourly has greatly diminished the incidence of postoperative candida infection.

CMV can affect the GI tract at any point resulting in symptoms which may include dysphagia, odynophagia, vomiting, abdominal pain, GI bleeding, perforation, or diarrhoea. CMV infection can mimic ischaemic colitis, intestinal pseudo-obstruction, toxic megacolon, and colon carcinoma (Bardaxoglou *et al.* 1993). Any patient in the early post-transplant setting or during intensive immunosuppression for rejection, who develops fever, vomiting, or diarrhoea and laboratory findings of leucopenia and/or increased liver enzymes should undergo endoscopy and biopsy to assess the possibility of CMV enteritis. Typical endoscopic findings are shallow, erythematous erosions. Demonstration of CMV in peripheral blood by polymerase chain reaction technique facilitates early diagnosis of active infection requiring treatment with ganciclovir. Current prophylaxis for CMV infection after transplantation has considerably decreased the occurrence of this infectious complication (Patel *et al.* 1996).

Bacterial infections postrenal transplant may include *Clostridium difficile* and *Yersinia enterocolitica*. *C. difficile* colitis, if severe, may cause protracted diarrhoea, pyrexia, intestinal obstruction, abscess, and toxic megacolon. Treatment with oral metronidazole or vancomycin is effective but toxic dilatation may necessitate colectomy.

The prevalence of *H. pylori* infection is not greater than in the general population, but one report has suggested that immunosuppression may decrease the efficacy of eradication therapy (Huwez *et al.* 1997). Microsporidia, an intracellular protozoal parasite, may cause chronic diarrhoea, fatigue, and weight loss post-transplant and may not be detected by routine stool examination. Diagnosis requires that stools are examined with a modified trichrome stain. *Strongyloides stercoralis* may also cause fever, abdominal pain, and diarrhoea in renal transplant recipients (Adedeji *et al.* 2001) and should be considered in patients from endemic areas such as the West Indies or Far East. Microsporidial infections respond well to treatment with metronidazole.

Mucosal ulceration

Ulceration of the upper GI tract in the modern transplant era is uncommon due to the widespread use of prophylaxis with H2 receptor antagonists, proton pump inhibitors, or mucosal protectants.

Cyclosporin concentrations may be altered by concomitant administration of cimetidine, and cimetidine may increase serum creatinine levels by inhibiting tubular creatinine secretion.

Diverticular disease

This disorder has been reported in up to 42 per cent of patients with ESRD, and complications of diverticulitis affect approximately 1 per cent of patients following renal transplantation. However, pretransplant colonic screening of older patients is ineffective in predicting post-transplant complications and is therefore not recommended in asymptomatic patients.

Perforation

Perforations of any part of the GI tract can occur in transplant patients, although the colon is the most usual site. Causative factors include diverticular disease, NSAIDs, corticosteroid, and other immunosuppressive treatment. Early episodes of perforation usually occur in association with intense immunosuppression, particularly with corticosteroids and are largely attributable to diverticulitis or CMV colitis. Perforation in the later years post-transplant is largely attributable to diverticulitis or malignancy, especially lymphoma.

Pancreatitis

Acute pancreatitis has been reported to affect between 1 and 2 per cent of renal transplant patients and be associated with a high mortality rate (Slakey 1997). Common precipitating factors include alcohol, hypercalcaemia, immunosuppression, CMV, and cholelithiasis. The incidence of the condition is higher in azathioprine treated patients compared to those treated with cyclosporin (Soderdahl et al. 1994).

Gastrointestinal malignancy

Lymphomas, skin cancers, and Kaposi's sarcoma occur more often in transplant recipients than in the general population. Post-transplant lymphoproliferative disorder (PTLD) affecting the GI tract is not easily diagnosed and may present late in the disease process with obstruction, perforation, chronic diarrhoea, or GI bleeding. Endoscopy may show raised erythematous lesions with central ulceration. The diagnosis requires demonstration of mono- or oligoclonal populations by cellular or viral markers, and EBV infection of many cells (Paya 1999). Treatment may involve decreasing or stopping immunosuppressive therapy, antiviral agents, and chemotherapy.

Chronic diarrhoea with malnutrition

The author has seen four long-term renal transplant patients who developed chronic diarrhoea resulting in malnutrition. The causative disorders in these four cases were Shigella dysentry (in a patient returned from India), chronic pancreatitis with endocrine insufficiency, chronic CMV enteritis, and small bowel PTLD. In the latter two patients, stool volumes at times exceeded 10 l/day and both required long-term total parenteral nutrition.

Gastrointestinal complications of peritoneal dialysis

Gastrointestinal symptoms may occur in patients undergoing peritoneal dialysis as a result of increased intra-abdominal pressure, which promotes hernia formation, delayed gastric emptying (Brown-Cartwright et al. 1988), and gastro-oesophageal reflux. Other complications may include haemoperitoneum and pain on infusion of dialysate. GI symptoms due to uraemia, medication, and coincident peptic ulcer disease may make diagnosis difficult. If the patient is well dialysed and specific GI causes of the symptoms have been excluded, persistent complaints should prompt consideration of gastro-oesophageal reflux or gastroparesis. If gastro-oesophageal reflux disease is diagnosed, treatment may involve minimizing the supine intraperitoneal fluid volume with adjustment of the overall dialysis prescription to maintain adequate clearance. For severe delay in gastric emptying, oral or intraperitoneal erythromycin may be tried. Haemoperitoneum occurs in over one-half of menstruating women on peritoneal dialysis and is probably caused by ovulation, retrograde menstruation, or endometriosis. The patient should be reassured that the condition is benign and will resolve spontaneously. Rarely, life-threatening haemoperitoneum may occur due to splenic rupture, rupture of a hepatic or renal cyst, or pancreatitis.

Pain associated with infusion of dialysate may occur in the absence of peritonitis and may be due to the acidic pH of conventional lactate dialysate, catheter malposition, or use of hypertonic dialysis solutions. Treatment options include use of bicarbonate dialysis solutions, catheter replacement, slowing the infusion rate, or injecting local anaesthetics (1 per cent lignocaine at 50 mg/exchange).

Abdominal hernias are a significant problem in patients treated with peritoneal dialysis. They may be inguinal, umbilical, or incisional in type. The paramedian approach to catheter insertion has reduced the incidence of exit site and incision hernias. Risk factors for hernia formation include increasing age, duration on peritoneal dialysis, multiparity, and increased number of laparotomies. Complications which may result are intestinal obstruction, incarceration, or strangulation with symptoms of peritonitis.

Scrotal or labial swelling can be caused by dialysis flow through a patent processus vaginalis or by dissection through the peritoneal membrane, followed by tracking of the fluid inferiorly into the scrotal or labial wall. Dialysate fluid leaking into the anterior abdominal wall will cause abdominal wall oedema and decreased peritoneal fluid drainage volumes. Prevention of these complications is helped by paramedian versus midline catheter placement, laxative use to avert constipation, and allowing 2 weeks to elapse before using the catheter postinsertion. Following surgical repair of a hernia, the patient should ideally have interim haemodialysis for 2–4 weeks but if this is not feasible, low volume intermittent peritoneal dialysis may be used. Abdominal wall or genital oedema should be treated with bed rest and temporary haemodialysis. Surgical repair may be difficult if no obvious hernia is present and in this situation, computed tomography scan with contrast in the peritoneal fluid may help localize the defect. Treatment of recurrent genital oedema depends on the cause of the oedema; a patent processus vaginalis should be surgically repaired. This condition can be detected by computed tomography scanning or exploratory laparotomy.

Cloudy effluent, abdominal pain and fever may be caused by infectious peritonitis, or culture-negative peritonitis (sterile, aseptic, or chemical peritonitis) which accounts for 5–50 per cent of all episodes (Mangram et al. 1998). Sterile peritonitis may occur as a result of inappropriate sample handling or culture techniques, infection with fastidious organisms, or previous antimicrobial treatment. Icodextrin 7.5 per cent peritoneal dialysis solution, recommended as a replacement for a single glucose exchange in patients who have lost ultrafiltration on glucose solutions, has been reported to cause sterile peritonitis with cloudy effluent (Heering 2001). Once other possible reasons for cloudy effluent have been excluded, Icodextrin should therefore be stopped and the result of this action evaluated. Peritoneal dialysis may also induce sclerosing peritonitis; this disorder produces a variety of gastrointestinal symptoms and signs, and some patients may have a dramatic response to corticosteroid treatment (see Chapter 12.4).

Diabetic autonomic neuropathy of the gastrointestinal tract

The exact prevalence of enteric neuropathy in diabetics is unknown as a diagnosis based on symptoms alone is unreliable. This diagnosis is an important one to make in the diabetic patient as diabetic gastroparesis may compromise glycaemic control and impair absorption of orally administered drugs. Diabetic gastroparesis is usually suggested on clinical grounds by the combination of suggestive symptoms (bloating, early satiety, episodic vomiting) and the absence of anatomical alterations of the upper GI tract on endoscopy or barium studies. The presence of residual food in the stomach after an overnight fast for upper GI endoscopy supports the diagnosis. Scintigraphic measurement of gastric emptying is the most reliable investigation.

Diabetic gastroparesis

Treatment of delayed gastric emptying involves dietary modification towards a low-fat and low-fibre diet with frequent small meals. Drugs that increase gastric emptying include metoclopramide, domperidone, cisapride, and erythromycin. The first two agents are dopamine antagonists while erythromycin stimulates motilin receptors. All have side-effects which limit their use and only erythromycin is used for chronic administration. In acute exacerbations of diabetic gastroparesis, intravenous erythromycin 250 mg 8 hourly may be used to reduce gastric retention (Janssens *et al.* 1990). Enteral nutrition via a jejunostomy tube may occasionally be required, while parenteral nutrition should be restricted to severe cases in which enteral feeding becomes impossible.

Diabetic enteropathy

Diarrhoea and, on rare occasions, steatorrhoea can occur in diabetic patients, particularly those with advanced disease. The diarrhoea is typically watery and painless, occurs at night, and may be associated with faecal incontinence. The diarrhoea may be episodic with intermittent normal bowel habit and bouts of constipation. The prevalence of diabetic diarrhoea has been estimated at between 8 and 22 per cent. The pathogenesis is not fully understood and multiple factors are probably involved. Diabetic autonomic neuropathy may include vagal nerve dysfunction as well as sympathetic nerve damage. The functional impairment of the enteric nervous system can cause disordered motility of the small bowel and colon which may manifest as either delayed or accelerated small bowel transit. This abnormal small bowel motility may be associated with bacterial overgrowth, resulting in bile acid deconjugation and fat malabsorption. Exocrine pancreatic insufficiency as a further cause for diarrhoea is a rare problem in diabetes mellitus, but there is an association with coeliac disease and serologic markers should be sought (antiendomysial and antigliadin antibodies). Chronic pancreatitis due to alcoholism is an important diagnosis to consider when exocrine and endocrine pancreatic insufficiency coexist.

Because of the multifactorial pathophysiology of diabetic enteropathy, systematic investigation is necessary to assess the underlying

Table 3 Investigation of chronic diarrhoea in a patient with diabetes mellitus

First line
Stool examination for CL difficile, bacterial pathogens, ova and parasites
Barium X-rays—looking for gastric retention, malabsorption pattern, intestinal wall thickness

Second line
Upper GI endoscopy with duodenal biopsy—histology, bacteriology
Colonoscopy with biopsy—histology, bacteriology
Anorectal manometry and sensory testing if faecal incontinence present

Third line
Small intestinal manometry—to rule out intestinal pseudo-obstruction
Small bowel enteroscopy with biopsy
Secretin-pancreazyme test—to exclude exocrine pancreatic insufficiency
(75) SE-HCAT test—to rule out bile acid malabsorption

mechanisms (see Table 3). A combination of factors, for example, small bowel dysmotility, bacterial overgrowth, anorectal dysfunction, and coeliac disease is present in many patients (Valdovinos *et al.* 1993). Chronic treatment should be directed at the identified main cause rather than non-specific treatment on empirical grounds. For accelerated intestinal transit, a trial of antidiarrhoeal agents such as loperamide 2 mg qid may be tried. Walker (1993) has reported successful use of the somatostatin analogue octreotide in treatment of diabetic diarrhoea. Patients with concurrent coeliac disease or exocrine pancreatic insufficiency should receive treatment with a gluten-free diet or pancreatic enzyme supplementation, respectively. For patients with severe gastroparesis unresponsive to medication, alternative treatment approaches include acupuncture and use of gastric electrical stimulators. The role of these treatment techniques at present remains unclear.

References

Adedeji, A. *et al.* (2001). Recurrent *Escherichia coli* bacteraemia in a patient with chronic renal failure. *Nephrology, Dialysis, Transplantation* **16**, 2429–2430.

Andriulla, A. *et al.* (1985). Patients with chronic renal failure are not at a risk of developing chronic peptic ulcers. *Clinical Nephrology* **23**, 245.

Banerjee, A. and Warwicker, P. (2002). Acute renal failure and metabolic disturbances in the short bowel syndrome. *Quarterly Journal of Medicine* **95**, 37–40.

Bardaxoglou, E. *et al.* (1993). Surgical emergencies following kidney transplantation. *Transplant International* **6**, 148–152.

Bjarnason, I. and MacPherson, A. (1989). The changing gastrointestinal side-effect profile on nonsteroidal anti-inflammatory drugs. A new approach for the prevention of a new problem. *Scandinavian Journal of Gastroenterology* **24** (Suppl. 163), 56–64.

Borczuk, A. *et al.* (1995). Intestinal pseudo-obstruction and ischaemia secondary to both $\beta 2$ microglobulin and serum A amyloid deposition. *Modern Pathology* **8**, 577.

Broner, M. H. *et al.* (1986). Oestrogen–progesterone therapy for bleeding gastrointestinal telangiectasias in chronic renal failure: an uncontrolled trial. *Annals of Internal Medicine* **105**, 371.

Brown-Cartwright, D., Smith, H. J., and Feldman, M. (1988). Gastric emptying of an indigestable solid in patients with end stage renal disease on continuous ambulatory peritoneal dialysis. *Gastroenterology* **95**, 49.

Campistol, J. M. *et al.* (1987). Visceryl involvement of dialysis amyloidosis. *American Journal of Nephrology* 7, 390–393.

Chauveau, D., Fakhouri, F., and Grunfeld, J. P. (2000). Liver involvement in autosomal dominant polycystic kidney disease: therapeutic dilemma. *Journal of the American Society of Nephrology* 11, 1767.

Church, M. *et al.* (1985). Perforation of the colon in renal homograft recipients. A report of 11 cases and a review of the literature. *Annals of Surgery* 203, 69.

Dave, P. B. *et al.* (1984). Gastrointestinal telangiectasias: a source of bleeding in patients receiving haemodialysis. *Archives of Internal Medicine* 144, 1781–1783.

Davenport, A. *et al.* (1991). Prevalence of *Helicobacter pylori* in patients with end stage renal failure and renal transplant recipients. *Nephron* 59, 597.

De Schoenmakere, G. *et al.* (2001). Relationship between gastric emptying and clinical and biochemical factors in chronic haemodialysis patients. *Nephrology, Dialysis, Transplantation* 16, 1850–1855.

Doherty, C. C. (1993). Gastrointestinal bleeding in dialysis patients. *Nephron* 63, 132–139.

Doherty, C. C. *et al.* Elevations of gastrointestinal hormones in chronic renal failure. In *Proceedings of the 15th Congress of the European Dialysis and Transplant Association* (ed. B. H. B. Robinson and J. N. Hawkins), pp. 456–465. Pitman Medical, 1978.

Drueke, T. B. (2002). Intestinal absorption of aluminium in renal failure. *Nephrology, Dialysis, Transplantation* 17 (Suppl. 2), 13–16.

Fabrizi, F. and Martin, P. (2000). *Helicobacter pylori* infection in patients with end stage renal disease. *International Journal of Artificial Organs* 23, 157.

Gluck, Z. and Nolph, K. D. (1987). Ascites associated with end stage renal disease. *American Journal of Kidney Diseases* 10, 9.

Goransson, L. G. and Bergrem, H. (2002). Disappearance of measurable mycophenolate mofetil in a patient with a renal transplant and an ileostomy. *Nephrology, Dialysis, Transplantation* 17, 318.

Gurland, H. J. *et al.* (1973). Combined report on regular dialysis and transplantation in Europe. *Proceedings of the European Dialysis and Transplant Association* X, 42.

Heering, P. *et al.* (2001). Peritoneal reaction to icodextrin in a female patient on CAPD. *Peritoneal Dialysis International* 20, 817–822.

Helderman, J. H. and Goral, S. (2002). Gastrointestinal complications of transplant immunosuppression. *Journal of the American Society of Nephrology* 13, 277–287.

Henry, D. A. and O'Connell, D. L. (1989). Effects of fibrinolytic inhibitors on mortality from upper GI haemorrhage. *British Medical Journal* 298, 1442–1146.

Hill, P. *et al.* (2002). Rapid onset irreversible oxalate-induced renal failure in pancreatic insufficiency (abstract). *Nephrology, Dialysis, Transplantation* (in press).

Hojs, R. (1995). Cholecystolithiasis in patients with end stage renal disease treated with haemodialysis: a study prevalence. *American Journal of Nephrology* 15, 15.

Howden, C. and Hunt, R. (1998). Guidelines for the management of *Helicobacter pylori* infection. *American Journal of Gastroenterology* 93, 2330.

Huwez, F. U. *et al.* (1997). Histologically diagnosed *Helicobacter pylori* in heart transplant recipients. *Journal of Heart–Lung Transplant* 16, 596–599.

Imai, H. and Satoh, K. (1997). Perforated diverticulitis after barium enema examination in a patient on CAPD. *Nephrology, Dialysis, Transplantation* 12, 2758–2760.

Ishikawa, I. *et al.* (1996). High incidence of common bile duct dilatation in autosomal dominant polycystic kidney disease patients. *American Journal of Kidney Diseases* 3, 321.

Janssens, J. *et al.* (1990). Improvement of gastric emptying in diabetic gastroparesis by erythromycin. *New England Journal of Medicine* 322, 1028.

Langman, M. J. S. (1982). What is happening to peptic ulcer? *British Medical Journal* 284, 1063–1064.

Lewis, B. *et al.* (1992). Does hormonal therapy have any benefit for bleeding angiodysplasia? *Journal of Clinical Gastroenterology* 15, 99.

Maher, E. R. *et al.* (1988). Gastrointestinal complications of dialysis related amyloidosis. *British Medical Journal* 297, 265–266.

Mangram, A. J. *et al.* (1998). Outbreak of sterile peritonitis among continuous cycling peritoneal dialysis patients. *Kidney International* 54, 1367–1371.

Martin, R. S. *et al.* (1986). Increased secretion of potassium in the rectum of man with chronic renal failure. *American Journal of Kidney Diseases* 8, 105–110.

Melero, M. *et al.* (1995). Idiopathic dialysis ascites in the nineties: resolution after renal transplantation. *American Journal of Kidney Diseases* 26, 668.

Milito, G. *et al.* (1983). Assessment of the upper gastrointestinal tract in patients awaiting renal transplantation. *American Journal of Gastroenterology* 78, 328.

Min, C. H. *et al.* (1997). Dialysis-related amyloidosis (DRA) in a patient on CAPD presenting as haemoperitoneum with colon perforation. *Nephrology, Dialysis, Transplantation* 12 (12), 2761–2763.

Mitchell, C. J. *et al.* (1979). Gastric function and histology in chronic renal failure. *Journal of Clinical Pathology* 32, 208–213.

MorrisStiff, G. *et al.* (1997). Abdominal wall hernia in autosomal dominant polycystic kidney disease. *British Journal of Surgery* 84, 615.

Norden, M. A. and Rabb, H. (2001). Two haemodialysis patients with unclear abdominal symptoms of similar origin. *Nephrology, Dialysis, Transplantation* 16, 2426–2428.

Patel, R. *et al.* (1996). Cytomegalovirus prophylaxis in solid organ transplant recipients. *Transplantation* 61, 1279–1289.

Paya, C. V. *et al.* (1999). Epstein–Barr virus-induced post-transplant lymphoproliferative disorder ASTS/ASTP EBV-PTLD task force and the Mayo Clinic organised international consensus development meeting. *Transplantation* 68, 1517.

Scheff, R. T. *et al.* (1980). Diverticular disease in patients with chronic renal failure due to polycystic kidney disease. *Annals of Internal Medicine* 92, 202.

Shepherd, A. M. M. *et al.* (1973). Peptic ulceration in chronic renal failure. *Lancet* i, 1357–1359.

Simenhoff, M. L. *et al.* (1978). Bacterial populations of the small intestine in uraemia. *Nephron* 22, 63–68.

Slakey, D. P. *et al.* (1997). Management of severe pancreatitis in renal transplant recipients. *Annals of Surgery* 225, 217–222.

Soderdahl, G., Tyden, G., and Groth, C. G. (1994). Incidence of gastrointestinal complications following renal transplantation in the cyclosporin era. *Transplant Proceedings* 26, 1771–1772.

Valdovinos, M. A., Camilleri, M., and Zimmerman, B. R. (1993). Chronic diarrhoea in diabetes mellitus; mechanisms and an approach to diagnosis and treatment. *Mayo Clinic Proceedings* 68, 691.

Walker, J. J. and Kaplan, B. S. (1993). Efficacy of the somatostatin analogue octreotide in the treatment of 2 patients with diabetic diarrhoea. *American Journal of Gastroenterology* 88, 765–767.

Weinstock, L. B., Atkinson, J. P., and Pittman, A. (1994). Episodic angioedema and severe diarrhoea induced by continuous captopril administration. *Illustrated Case Reports in Gastroenterology* 1, 39–43.

Zeier, M., Wiesel, M., and Ritz, E. (1992). Non-occlusive mesenteric infarction (NOMI) in dialysis patients: risk factors, diagnosis, intervention and outcome. *International Journal of Artificial Organs* 15, 387–389.

11.3.7　Liver disorders

Matthias Girndt and Hans Köhler

Viral hepatitis is still an important infectious threat to dialysis patients. The clinically most relevant blood-borne viruses hepatitis B virus (HBV) and hepatitis C virus (HCV) can easily be spread in the dialysis centre where patients are treated together using extracorporeal devices via blood access sites. This situation is aggravated by the influence of uraemia on immune function, which renders patients less able to eliminate viral infections. Precautions against nosocomial transmission should make infection with either hepatitis B or C in the dialysis setting avoidable.

Hepatitis B

Virology

HBV is a small, partially double-stranded DNA virus. Consisting of a virus hull, the hepatitis B surface antigen (HBsAg), and a nucleocapsid, the hepatitis B core antigen (HBcAg). The nucleocapsid contains the viral genome together with enzymes for replication (Lau and Wright 1993). The core antigen is expressed on hepatocytes, while its post-translationally processed form, the HBeAg, together with the HBsAg is found in circulating blood. The seroresponse against the HBV is assessed by assaying antibodies to the structural antigens of the virus: HBsAg, HBcAg, and HBeAg. Among them, anti-HBs is most important for antiviral defense, since only these antibodies eliminate the virus.

Epidemiology

Hepatitis B infection is very common in many parts of the world. An estimated 350 million individuals are infected worldwide. There are large regional differences in the prevalence, with very low rates in Western Europe and Northern America (<1 per cent), higher rates in Eastern Europe (1–5 per cent), and an extremely high prevalence in Asia, Africa, and Central America, where 5–20 per cent of the population are infected. There is a direct link between the prevalence of the virus in the general population and in dialysis patients. The average prevalence in Western European dialysis patients is 3 per cent. It has declined to as low as 0.9 per cent in the United States, while up to 20 per cent of Eastern Europeans are reported to be infected (dialysis patients). Rigorous infection control measures that were put in place after the outbreaks of the late 1960s, decreased the prevalence of HBV from 28 per cent in Western European dialysis centres in 1978 (Ribot *et al.* 1979) to about 3 per cent in 1990 (Valderrabano *et al.* 1996).

Clinical appearance and prognosis

The clinical course of hepatitis B infection in patients with chronic renal failure differs from that in individuals with normal kidney function (London *et al.* 1969). Those with normal renal function experience symptomatic and icteric hepatitis for several weeks until infection is contained and symptoms level off. The prognosis of acute hepatitis B is good, leaving permanent immunity against the virus. Severe cases with life-threatening liver disease are rare (<0.5 per cent). Chronic hepatitis

develops in less than 10 per cent of cases, but impairs prognosis. Up to 20 per cent of patients with chronic hepatitis B will develop liver cirrhosis (Fattovich *et al.* 1991) leading to hepatocellular carcinoma at an annual rate of 2–3 per cent (McMahon *et al.* 1990).

In patients with chronic renal failure, the infection often remains undetected until laboratory values indicate mild hepatitis, or seroconversion is found at routine testing. Jaundice and symptomatic liver disease are rare, transaminases remain normal or only slightly elevated. Chronic hepatitis (HBsAg positive after 6 months) is observed in similar to 60 per cent of individuals (Ribot 1979). Many of them develop the asymptomatic HBsAg carrier state. Since this is very rare in the general population, its prognosis is uncertain. In the largest series which included 317 otherwise healthy patients liver cirrhosis was found in 1.3 per cent within 16 years (Villeneuve *et al.* 1994). The prognosis of chronic HBsAg positive haemodialysis patients without liver disease might be even better. In a small series 30 HBsAg positive dialysis patients were compared to 64 HBsAg negative individuals. No difference in mortality or morbidity over an 8-year follow-up was found (Josselson *et al.* 1987).

Immunity against HBV mainly depends on a cytolytic response by the cellular part of the immune system. Cytolytic CD8+ T lymphocytes that recognize infected hepatocytes are activated (Jung *et al.* 1994). Their destruction blocks further synthesis of virus particles and breaks the replicative cycle of the virus. Liver cell damage in hepatitis B infection is nearly exclusively caused by the host's immune response since the virus itself is not cytolytic. In addition, anti-HBs antibodies able to eliminate free virus from the circulation prevent further infection of hepatocytes (Lee 1997).

Immune defect in chronic renal failure

Chronic renal failure induces a secondary form of immunodeficiency, which leads to impaired activation of a cellular immune response towards the virus. The cytolytic response, which should destroy infected hepatocytes, is weak or even absent. This explains the mild clinical course in dialysis patients since the typical clinical symptoms of HBV infection are a consequence of the immune system's ability to eliminate the virus. Low *in vitro* proliferative responses of lymphocytes from renal failure patients match this clinical observation (Meuer *et al.* 1987; Girndt *et al.* 1993). Furthermore, lymphocytes produce low levels of their auto- and paracrine growth factor interleukin-2, which is needed to enhance clonal expansion of lymphocytes during the immune reaction.

However, T lymphocytes are not the major weakness in the immune system. Antigen-specific activation of T lymphocytes can only occur in the presence of antigen-presenting cells (APCs) that provide the T cell with a set of signals to direct its actions. Recent studies should clarify the important-functional defects of monocytes in renal failure patients (Fig. 1) (Girndt *et al.* 2001). T-cell activation requires at least two separate signals from the APC. The primary signal is derived from the antigen itself and directs the specificity of the cellular response. The T cell recognizes the foreign antigen in conjunction with self-proteins of the MHC molecule on the APC. This primary signal needs to be complemented by a second signal to define the reaction mode of the T cell (Liu and Janeway 1992). Depending on this second signal, the T cell may either be activated for proliferation and effector function, or may be specifically inactivated and become anergic (McAdam *et al.* 1998). The second signal is transmitted by specific

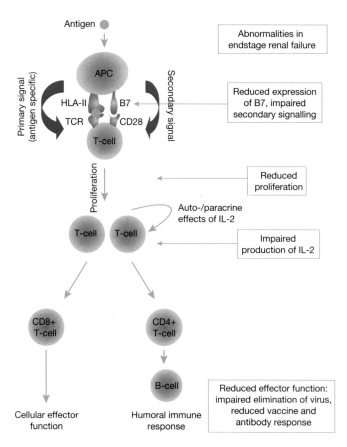

Fig. 1 Altered antigen-specific lymphocyte activation in patients with chronic renal failure. Antigen is processed by antigen-presenting cells (APC) and presented on the HLA class II molecule. This primary signal to the T-cell receptor (TCR) is normally conveyed in dialysis patients. The secondary signal, which should be transmitted from the B7 molecule to its ligand CD28, is insufficiently generated in endstage renal disease. As a consequence, clonal expansion and secretion of IL-2 are diminished. Through reduced activation of CD4+ T helper cells the effector function of cytolytic CD8+ lymphocytes and the production of antibody by B-cells are impaired.

structures on the APC, among them the B7 family of costimulatory molecules.

The constitutive expression of the B7-2 molecule on monocytes is 30–40 per cent lower in dialysis patients than in healthy persons (Girndt *et al.* 2001). Consequently, chronic haemodialysis patients have deficient activation of lymphocytes during primary contact with viral antigens such as the HBV. Activation of CD4+ helper T cells against the virus is crucial for the primary activation of cytotoxic CD8+ lymphocytes which are the effectors for liver cytolysis. In addition, B-cell activation and the humoral response is dependent on CD4+ helper T-cell activation. The costimulatory defect of APCs may thus explain both the reduced liver cytolysis in acute HBV infection as well as the impaired production of anti-HBs both during virus infection and after vaccination.

Further influences on antiviral defence come from the persistent activation of inflammatory processes by uraemia and extracorporal dialysis (Girndt *et al.* 1995). Chronic inflammatory activation has not only several unfavourable consequences for the individual such as malnutrition, amyloidosis, and progressive atherosclerosis (Stenvinkel

et al. 1999), but also immune dysfunction (Girndt *et al.* 1995). Recent studies demonstrate a genetically determined capacity to cope with the load of proinflammatory activation which differs between individuals. The cytokine, IL-10, provides an effective physiological system to limit proinflammatory activation both in healthy persons (Moore *et al.* 2001) and haemodialysis patients (Girndt *et al.* 1995). Production of IL-10 is influenced by a polymorphism in the promoter of its gene. This polymorphism allows the definition of a 'high-producer' and 'low-producer' genotype, which directly influences how the carrier of this gene reacts to proinflammatory challenges (Turner *et al.* 1997). Dialysis patients with the IL-10 'high-producer' genotype show less signs of chronic inflammatory activation than those with the IL-10 'low-producer' genotype. This translates into a close association of the IL-10 'low-producer' genotype with hepatitis B vaccination non-response and vice versa (Girndt *et al.* 2001).

Based on these findings the current hypothesis to explain the low rate of response to hepatitis B in haemodialysis patients includes both, a globally reduced costimulatory function of antigen presenting cells due to uraemia, and the unfavourable influence of a highly activated inflammatory cytokine system, which is controlled by IL-10 in a genetically determined manner.

The immune dysfunction associated with uraemia can be detected early during the course of kidney failure. Even patients with mild or moderate impairment of renal function with a serum creatinine of 250 µmol/l show signs of immune deficiency (Dumann *et al.* 1990). When progressing to endstage renal disease, the uraemia-associated alterations are modified by renal replacement therapy. Haemodialysis treatment introduces biocompatibility issues with blood-dialyser contacts leading to complement and cytokine activation. However, experimental data prove that lymphocyte activation improves in endstage renal failure patients after renal replacement therapy is initiated (Kaul *et al.* 2000).

Diagnosis

The viral antigens can reliably be detected by enzyme immunoassays especially early when there is a high viral load. Serological responses can be monitored by immunoassays detecting anti-HBs, anti-HBc, and anti-HBe (Hoofnagle *et al.* 1991). The first specific marker found during the early period of infection is HBsAg (Fig. 2). In patients with normal renal function anti-HBc is present at the time of the clinical symptoms. The HBeAg is only found during the highly infectious early period, which is then followed by the formation of anti-HBe. Subsequently, anti-HBs appears and initiates the elimination of HBsAg resolving the infection. In the long-term, anti-HBe disappears within months to a few years. The anti-HBs antibody persists longer and may be found after more than 10 years. Thereafter, the only evidence of the healed infection is the persistence of anti-HBc. However, anti-HBc may also be present in chronically replicating hepatitis; these antibodies are not protective and may not eliminate the virus. Acute infection may be distinguished by the presence of IgM type anti-HBc, which remains detectable for up to 6 months.

In addition to antigenaemia and serological response, HBV-DNA may be detected by hybridization or, with higher sensitivity, by the polymerase chain reaction (PCR). The detection of HBV-DNA is useful to determine infectivity in dialysis patients who are positive for HBsAg. Table 1 gives recommendations for the diagnostic approach in chronic dialysis patients.

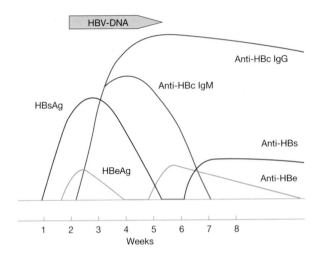

Fig. 2 Time course of immune phenomena in acute hepatitis B virus infection in immunocompetent hosts.

Table 1 Recommendations for virological diagnosis of hepatitis B in dialysis patients (adapted from Centers for Disease Control and Prevention 2001; The EBPG Expert Group on Haemodialysis 2002)

Entry of dialysis patient to a dialysis centre
HBsAg, anti-HBs, anti-HBc

Follow-up of chronic dialysis patients every 12 months
HBsAg, anti-HBs, anti-HBc

Suspected liver disease, after holiday dialysis in endemic areas
HBsAg, anti-HBc
When HBsAg is detected: HBeAg, anti-HBe, anti-HBs, HBV-DNA

Potential indication for interferon treatment
HBV-DNA quantitatively

Prevention

HBV is transmitted parenterally, either by blood, injection-drug abuse, contaminated cannulas, sexual contacts, or perinatally from the mother to the child. While in the 1960s most infections in dialysis patients were caused by blood transfusions, this has become very uncommon. In addition, the number of blood transfusions has sharply decreased since the introduction of recombinant erythropoietin. Prevention of hepatitis B infection is based on hygienic precautions and active vaccination, since the risk of spread of the virus can be reduced by cutting the ways of infection and reducing the susceptibility of the dialysis population (Tokars *et al.* 2001).

Hygienic precautions

Nosocomial transmission of the virus during haemodialysis treatment rarely occurs by direct blood sprinkles from one patient to the other. The dialysis staff are the usual 'vector', and contaminated gloves, equipment, or the outer surfaces of a dialysis monitor may transport the blood. Since the viral load is very high (100–1000 times higher than in hepatitis C infection) (Jalava *et al.* 1992), even low amounts of fluids are sufficient for infection. Dried blood contamination can still be infectious, since the virus may survive on surfaces for up to 7 days

(Bond *et al.* 1981). Therefore, HBsAg positive dialysis patients should be treated separately from those who are susceptible for the infection. This measure is uniformly recommended for hepatitis B, but not for hepatitis C (Centers for Disease Control and Prevention 2001; The EBPG Expert Group on Haemodialysis 2002). The use of dedicated dialysis machines and associated equipment, such as blood pressure cuffs or clamps is essential. Injection cannulas, syringes, heparin vials, dialysis needles, and tubing should be single use only. The dialysis staff must follow 'universal precautions' to prevent transmission of infectious agents, including personal hand hygiene and the use of non-sterile gloves that are changed for each patient (Tokars *et al.* 2001). Dialyser reprocessing for hepatitis B positive patients is strongly discouraged (Council on Dialysis 1997). The use of dedicated dialysis machines mainly refers to the danger of transmitting contaminants via the machine's outer surface, not the internal tubings and valves since the virus cannot cross the dialyser membrane.

Vaccination

Antibodies against HBsAg effectively protect against HBV infection. A successful vaccination with anti-HBs titres greater than 10 U/ml gives almost complete protection (Szmuness *et al.* 1980). Anti-HBs can be induced in more than 95 per cent of healthy adults by a standard vaccination consisting of three intramuscular injections at months 0, 1, and 6 (Szmuness *et al.* 1980). Serological testing for anti-HBs is recommended between months 7 and 9 to allow the determination of an adequate interval for revaccination. Active vaccination in dialysis staff is considered mandatory.

The immune defect of chronic renal failure impairs the response to hepatitis B vaccination. The spectrum of responses ranges from slightly reduced antibody levels to complete nonresponse. Only 50–60 per cent of patients achieved protective anti-HBs levels in the early vaccination studies (Crosnier *et al.* 1981; Köhler *et al.* 1984). The use of double dose vaccine and a fourth injection between months 9 and 12 is generally recommended for chronic renal failure patients. Unfortunately 30 per cent of patients still fail to produce a protective response (Fabrizi *et al.* 1996). More than four injections in complete non-responders are not likely to induce immunity and should thus not be considered. The superiority of fractionated intracutaneous applications instead of the intramuscular injection has not been proven in a prospective randomized study (Charest *et al.* 2000).

Serological monitoring of the response to immunization in endstage renal disease patients is even more important than in healthy individuals. It will identify non-responders who should not be treated near either HBsAg positive patients; patients whose status is unknown, or those returning from holiday dialysis in endemic regions. In contrast, those who mount a sufficient serological response can be treated in the same room as HBsAg positive patients. Monitoring of serological response is also important for the timing of booster immunization, and the decline of antibody titres is fairly similar in dialysis patients and the healthy (Fabrizi *et al.* 1996). A vaccination and monitoring strategy for dialysis patients is described in Fig. 3. The optimal time to start vaccination in patients with progressive renal disease may be 3–6 months prior to the expected initiation of dialysis or at the time of fistula surgery.

Therapy

There is no specific treatment for acute hepatitis B in patients with normal renal function, since this infection generally has a good prognosis.

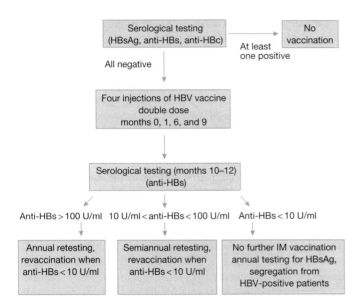

Fig. 3 Suggested strategy for hepatitis B serological testing and vaccination of endstage renal failure patients.

However, after 6 months without elimination of HBsAg, most patients should be treated to prevent the development of liver cirrhosis and hepatocellular carcinoma. Standard therapy uses high dose interferon-α for 4–6 months. A meta-analysis of 15 trials showed that interferon-α led to loss of HBV-DNA in 37 per cent of patients versus 17 per cent in the placebo group. Nevertheless, complete resolution of the infection is rare, long-term elimination of HBsAg occurred in only 7.8 versus 1.8 per cent (Wong *et al.* 1993). Therapy response is usually accompanied by reduced liver enzymes, a decrease in histological changes and a lower risk of liver cirrhosis and hepatocellular carcinoma (Lin *et al.* 1999). Potentially, the introduction of pegylated interferon regimes similar to those used in the treatment of chronic hepatitis C may enhance treatment efficacy.

The nucleoside analogue lamivudine is a therapeutic alternative with less side-effects and a comparable primary efficacy. After a 12-month course of 100 mg lamivudine daily HBV-DNA became undetectable in 44 per cent of patients (16 per cent in the placebo group) (Dienstag *et al.* 1999). However, lamivudine will probably not become first line therapy for chronic hepatitis B because of the very high rate of secondary resistance (15–30 per cent after 1 year and 60 per cent after 3 years). Lamivudine treatment is possible in patients with advanced liver cirrhosis or after organ transplantation. The combination of interferon-α with lamivudine is not effective (Schalm *et al.* 2000). Recently, the nucleoside analogue adefovir was tested as a new agent. It was well tolerated and resulted in a significant suppression of virus replication even in patients with HBeAg negative chronic hepatitis B, who usually do not respond to interferon treatment (Hadziyannis *et al.* 2003).

The use of interferon-α in dialysis patients is hampered by the high rate of side-effects explained by the altered pharmacokinetics of the cytokine. It is filtered by the glomeruli and then metabolized by renal tubular cells. Renal failure prolongs plasma half-life from 6 to 10 h leading to a much higher area under the curve of interferon plasma levels (Rostaing *et al.* 1998). Published therapeutic experience in dialysis patients is mainly confined to the treatment of hepatitis C, but it may be extrapolated to HBV as well. Even with a reduced dose of 3 × 3 million units per week intolerable side effects occur in half of the patients (Degos *et al.* 2001). Single experiences with the drug are

discouraging and show that interferon-α is ineffective. Facing the high rate of side-effects and the lack of proven clinical benefit in chronic hepatitis B, interferon-α cannot be recommended for patients with endstage renal disease. In particular, HBsAg positive patients without clinical signs of liver disease should not be treated.

There is also limited experience with lamivudine in endstage renal failure. This drug is eliminated by the kidneys; the dose has to be adapted to renal function. In a small study it was well tolerated in six haemodialysis patients all of whom eliminated the virus and achieved normalization of transaminases (Ben Ari *et al.* 2000). A general recommendation cannot yet be given and the high rate of resistance during prolonged treatment might limit its use also in endstage renal disease.

Renal transplantation in HBV infected patients

The inadequate activation of HBV specific T lymphocytes in patients with chronic renal failure is responsible for the failure to eliminate the virus completely. It is the balance between lymphocytic response and viral replication that leads to a relatively stable infection. This balance can be disturbed by the administration of immunosuppressive drugs. The risk to develop liver dysfunction during therapeutic immunosuppression depends on the extent of liver disease before transplantation. Fulminant hepatitis in the immunosuppressed HBsAg positive patient is rare but clinical liver disease and long-term complications can occur. A case–control study in 128 HBsAg positive patients showed a significantly reduced survival (55 per cent) compared to non-infected patients (80 per cent) at 10 years after transplantation (Mathurin *et al.* 1999). Differences in survival occurred only after the sixth year of transplantation while the short-term prognosis of infected and non-infected patients was the same.

Chronic infection with the HBV is not a definite contraindication to renal transplantation. However, the decision to list a patient for transplantation should take into account the extent of histological lesions in the liver. Transplantation may be considered in patients without or with only minimum inflammatory liver lesions, however this needs to be decided on the individual case.

European and US American guidelines differ in their recommendations regarding treatment of chronic HBV infection prior to renal transplantation. The European guidelines suggest treatment of transplant candidates with histologically proven chronic hepatitis B with interferon-α or lamivudine (The EBPG Expert Group on Haemodialysis 2002). This recommendation is, however, not very well based since interferon-α treatment is ineffective in most patients and a survival benefit after transplantation has not been shown. The American guidelines recommend starting lamivudine immediately after transplantation with a treatment duration of 18–24 months (Kasiske *et al.* 2002). The problem of this approach is the uncertainty of how to continue thereafter since relapse is very common when discontinuing lamivudine. Interferon-α should not be administered after renal transplantation due to the significant risk of acute rejection (Rostaing *et al.* 1996). For vital indications, lamivudine or the newly introduced adefovir may be an alternative.

Hepatitis C

Virology

HCV is a single strand RNA virus with a very high replication rate (10^{10}–10^{12} viruses per day) (Neumann *et al.* 1998) and a relatively high mutation rate that impairs an effective immune response (Gomez *et al.* 1999). On top of this variability there are six different genotypes causing the same clinical disease (Yotsuyanagi *et al.* 1995), but with a variable response to interferon-α therapy (Simmonds *et al.* 1994). The genotype 1 with lower response rates to therapy is found in more than 60 per cent of cases in Europe and Northern America, followed by genotypes 2 and 3, while the genotypes 4–6 are mainly found in Africa and South-East Asia. The structure and function of the viral RNA genome is partially understood. The entire genome forms a single open reading frame that is translated into a large precursor protein. This more than 3000 amino acids long protein is cleaved into structural and nonstructural proteins.

Epidemiology

Nearly 1–3 per cent of the world's population is infected with HCV, the number of chronic carriers is estimated to be 170 million. The virus is very common in Japan and the southern parts of the United States, in the Mediterranean, Africa, and the Middle East. In contrast, the prevalence is low in Western Europe, the northern part of the United States and Canada. However, this low prevalence still translates into at least 4 million infected people in the United States. In Germany, some 5100 new infections annually add to the already existing count of at least 300,000 chronically infected patients. The prevalence of the virus among dialysis patients depends on the prevalence in the respective population and ranges from 3.0 per cent in the Netherlands to 75 per cent in South-Eastern Europe.

Clinical appearance and prognosis

Acute hepatitis C infection is rarely diagnosed, since it shows a single or non-symptomatic course in 60–70 per cent of infected immunocompetent individuals. Acute hepatitis C develops into chronic infection in up to 80 per cent of cases (Thomas 2000). In most of these patients a certain level of viral replication can be detected by highly sensitive PCR. However, viral load is variable and may evade detection from time to time. Chronic hepatitis C shows a variable course with periods of enhanced disease activity and intermittent elevation of liver enzymes, while at other times no pathological findings can be detected. Histologically, chronic persisting hepatitis is found in the majority of cases, chronic active disease is rare.

HCV does not induce a strong immune reaction of the host. Although both, humoral and cellular reactions can be detected by laboratory methods; they are not usually able to eliminate the virus *in vivo*. The presence of HCV antibodies after infection does not protect against reinfection with the same or another strain (Farci *et al.* 1992). There is only a low-level lymphocyte reaction towards infected liver cells, which explains the lack of symptoms. Similar to HBV, HCV itself does not have a cytopathic effect on hepatocytes. Liver disease and lysis of hepatocytes is dependent on the immune reaction of the host. In chronic infection a balance between immune reaction and viral replication is established, hepatocytes are incompletely lysed and the virus cannot be eliminated. Fulminant hepatitis is very rare (Farci *et al.* 1996), and the acute disease usually does not lead to severe consequences. During the first decade of infection the life expectancy and morbidity of infected patients are comparable to the general population (Harris *et al.* 2002). The long-term prognosis is impaired by the risk of developing liver cirrhosis in 20–30 per cent of cases (Hoofnagle *et al.* 1997) and hepatocellular carcinoma in 1–4 per cent of patients annually (Alter and Seeff 2000).

Although the clinical course can hardly be distinguished between otherwise healthy persons and dialysis patients, recent studies indicated that the rate of patients with intermittent elevation of transaminases is lower and histological alterations are less severe in chronic renal failure (Pol 1995; Luzar *et al.* 2003). Studies with a short follow-up may not detect differences with regard to the prognosis of hepatitis C between both patient groups (Pol *et al.* 2002). A retrospective analysis of the New England Organ Bank register indicated that the presence of HCV infection at the time of listing for renal transplantation predicted an enhanced mortality risk independent from whether the patient was actually transplanted or remained on the waiting list (Pereira *et al.* 1998).

Diagnosis

HCV was first defined by its genomic structure in 1988 (Choo *et al.* 1989). The first generation serological assay detected antibodies against the non-structural C100 protein (Kuo *et al.* 1989). The later immunoassays included more antigens, for example, the core protein (C22) and the non-structural protein C33c (Alter 1992). The first generation assays had a low sensitivity and underestimated the seroprevalence. Current third generation test systems use five different specificities of antibodies (Soffredini 1996) and nearly completely prevent transmission of viral hepatitis by blood transfusions.

The low sensitivity assays severely underestimated the prevalence of hepatitis C in haemodialysis patients. Due to their immunodeficiency, many of these patients do not produce the antibodies used for diagnosis (e.g. only 15 per cent against C100 and 60 per cent against C33c) (Lok *et al.* 1993). Reliable information on seroprevalence of the infection only became available with the introduction of third generation assays. While earlier studies reported up to 10 per cent patients with consistently detectable RNA in the presence of negative serological results (Chan *et al.* 1993), the rate of false-negative serology decreased to 0.8 per cent with the most recent detection systems (de Medina *et al.* 1998). The detection of HCV-RNA in peripheral blood proves the presence of an active replication. In contrast, the presence of HCV antibodies does not allow one to distinguish between acute or chronic infection and does not give information on whether the patient is infectious or not. Indications for screening and follow-up of HCV infection in dialysis patients are listed in Table 2.

Prevention

The routes of transmission for the HCV are nearly the same as for HBV. It can be transmitted by blood, shared cannulas and equipment, and blood transfusions (Jadoul *et al.* 1993). The most important difference from HBV is the much lower concentration of virus particles in the blood, resulting in a lower infection risk by blood aerosols or infected cannulas.

The risk of acquisition by blood transfusions has sharply decreased following to donor testing and the introduction of recombinant erythropoietin. Transmission within a dialysis centre mostly occurs by the dialysis staff who may carry the virus from one patient to another. A recent study detected HCV-RNA in the water that was used by the staff for hand washing. If the nurses cared for HCV-positive patients, RNA was detected in 23 per cent of samples. Interestingly, HCV-RNA was also detected in 8 per cent of water specimens from nurses assigned only to HCV-negative patients in centres caring for both positive and negative patients (AlFurayh *et al.* 2000).

Table 2 Recommendations for virological diagnosis of hepatitis C in dialysis patients (adapted from Centers for Disease Control and Prevention 2001; The EBPG Expert Group on Haemodialysis 2002)

Entry of dialysis patient to a dialysis centre
Anti-HCV (third generation), if positive: HCV-RNA

Follow-up of chronic dialysis patients every 12 months
Anti-HCV

Suspected liver disease, after holiday dialysis in endemic areas
Anti-HCV, HCV-RNA qualitative test

Potential indication for interferon treatment
HCV-RNA quantitative test, genotyping

Nosocomial transmission of hepatitis C infection is prevented by rigorous application of the universal hygienic precautions as recommended by the CDC (Centers for Disease Control and Prevention 2001). A prospective study showed the feasibility to prevent any further transmission in a centre with a nosocomial infection rate of 1.4 per cent by consequent adherence to the hygienic precautions (Jadoul et al. 1998).

As a reflection of the much lower infection risk in HCV compared to HBV, there is no general recommendation to isolate hepatitis C positive patients. They should, however, be assigned to specific dialysis machines to prevent transmission via contamination of the outer surfaces of the monitor. HCV may not permeate through the dialyser membrane into the dialysate (Noiri et al. 2001). CDC guidelines do not explicitly discourage reuse of dialysers in HCV-positive patients (Centers for Disease Control and Prevention 2001).

Antibodies against HCV do not eliminate the virus and do not inhibit virus replication or infectivity. Thus all attempts at active immunization against hepatitis C so far have failed. Not even the infection itself leaves reliable protective immunity in the rare cases of healing (Bukh et al. 1995). Thus, there is neither an active nor a passive vaccine that could be applied to dialysis patients.

Treatment

In patients with normal renal function the acute infection with hepatitis C, if diagnosed, should immediately be treated by interferon-α. Early high-dose therapy may lead to healing of the infection in 98 per cent of cases (Jaeckel et al. 2001). However, diagnosis of hepatitis C in the acute stage is rather infrequent. Most cases are detected by serological testing in the absence of symptoms, often the timing and source of infection are difficult to determine.

Until recently, treatment of chronic hepatitis C was done by standard interferon-α monotherapy. A meta-analysis of 59 controlled clinical trials found the end-point of negative RNA tests at the end of treatment in 40 per cent of cases. However, a sustained virological response (negative RNA 6 months after treatment) was reached in only 17 per cent of cases (Davis 1999). Treatment became more successful after the introduction of the guanosin analog ribavirin in combination with interferon-α. Combination therapy may achieve a sustained virological response in 40 per cent of patients (Poynard et al. 1998). Treatment should last for 6 months in genotypes 2 and 3 and 12 months in genotypes 1 and 4.

The efficacy of interferon-α was enhanced by coupling the cytokine molecule to polyethylene glycol, which alters the pharmacokinetics and enhances the area under the concentration curve by slowing down its metabolism. The first studies with peg-interferon-α monotherapy showed sustained virological responses in 45 per cent of patients (Zeuzem et al. 2000). The current standard therapy for chronic hepatitis C is a combination of pegylated interferon-α together with ribavirin, both drugs dose-adapted to body weight (peg-interferon-α2b at 15 μg/kg once weekly, ribavirin 1000–1200 mg/day) (Manns et al. 2001). Treatment is recommended for patients with elevated liver enzymes, detection of HCV-RNA in the blood and histologically proven chronic hepatitis.

Patients with chronic renal failure can be treated with interferon-α monotherapy. Ribavirin is eliminated by the kidneys and may not be dialysed. There is no general recommendation for its use in patients with advanced renal failure, some authors even consider its use to be contraindicated (Pol et al. 2002) because of a dose-dependent haemolysis that can only be compensated by extremely high doses of erythropoietin. This view might change in the future, since a recent study showed that treatment could safely be administered using reduced ribavirin doses and plasma monitoring (Bruchfeld et al. 2001).

The efficacy of interferon-α monotherapy at 3 $\times$ 3 million units per week in dialysis patients is comparable to individuals with normal renal function. Sustained virological responses can be observed in more than 40 per cent of patients (Campistol et al. 1999; Huraib et al. 1999). However, treatment is not very well tolerated, side-effects include dizziness, myopathy and arthralgia, subfebrile temperatures, bone marrow suppression, and psychiatric symptoms and lead to discontinuation of therapy in 30–40 per cent of patients (Pol et al. 1995). Until now there has been little experience with peg-interferon-α in dialysis patients. Theoretically the modified interferon should have no advantage in terms of side-effects. Preliminary data suggest that the pharmacokinetic data of standard interferon-α and peg-interferon-α are not as different as in patients with normal renal function (Lamb et al. 2001).

Since interferon-α treatment is expensive and hampered by severe side-effects, this therapy cannot be generally recommended for HCV-infected dialysis patients. It should be limited to selected patients who are particularly likely to have a benefit from treatment, such as patients with high disease activity or recent onset, and for genotypes other than one. If interferon-α is considered in a dialysis patient, a liver biopsy should be performed before antiviral therapy is started. Those patients with mild or low-level histological lesions in the absence of elevated liver enzymes will have a low probability of developing severe consequences of the infection and are not therefore good candidates for therapy (Pol et al. 2002). On the other hand, patients with advanced liver cirrhosis should also not be treated with interferon-α because of the risk of liver failure.

Renal transplantation

Chronic hepatitis C is not considered a definite contraindication to renal transplantation. Several short-term reports presented an optimistic picture of the clinical course after transplantation. A small study compared 33 HCV-positive recipients of kidney transplants with 25 HCV-positive dialysis patients listed for transplantation. Overall survival was significantly better in the transplant recipients over a follow-up of at least 2 years (Knoll et al. 1997). Another study with an average observation time of 41 months compared liver histology in

45 transplanted HCV positive patients with 22 patients remaining on dialysis and did not find an overall difference (Glicklich et al. 1999).

However, long-term studies suggests a more cautious position should be adopted. Follow-up liver biopsies in HCV positive patients after transplantation revealed progressive fibrosis in 13 of 36 individuals (Izopet et al. 2000). A retrospective study compared survival of HCV positive and negative patients after transplantation and found a significantly higher survival for HCV negative patients beyond the seventh year after the procedure (Mathurin et al. 1999). A retrospective waiting list based analysis of the data of the New England Organ Bank revealed that HCV positive patients in general had a higher risk of mortality compared to HCV negative patients. This risk was not significantly modified by whether the patient was transplanted or not (Pereira et al. 1998). The decision to list an HCV positive patient for renal transplantation should be based on the observation of the clinical course and liver histology. The risk of transplantation seems to be justified in patients without severe liver dysfunction or extensive histological changes.

It is still a matter of debate whether therapy of chronic hepatitis C before renal transplantation improves the prognosis of the patient. If at all, interferon therapy should be tried before transplantation and cannot be done after the procedure since the risk of acute transplant rejection is intolerably high (Rostaing et al. 1996).

Other hepatitis viruses

Hepatitis A

Hepatitis A is caused by an RNA virus with only one known serotype. Infection occurs orally through water or uncooked meals. The risk is strongly increased by poor hygienic standards and the infection is endemic in developing countries. IgM antibodies indicate acute infection, IgG antibodies neutralize the virus and are protective against reinfection. The acute illness usually resolves and chronic courses virtually unknown. Seroprevalence of hepatitis A in dialysis patients is not different from the general population. The infection is not likely to be transmitted in association with dialysis.

An active vaccination with very good immunogenicity is available. Its use is generally recommended for persons travelling to endemic areas or those who might spread the infection such as employees of food manufacturers. Patients with chronic renal failure do not belong to the high-risk groups unless they intend to travel. Vaccination has been tested and found to be well tolerated and highly effective in this patient group (Fleischmann et al. 2002).

Hepatitis D

The hepatitis D virus (HDV) is an incomplete RNA virus, which forms a replicative virus after inclusion into the surface molecule of HBV. Thus, the chronic HBV carrier state puts the patient at risk for secondary infection by the HD virus. In highly endemic areas such as the Mediterranean, South America, or Asia, up to 60 per cent of chronic HBV carriers are coinfected with the D virus. If the infection with hepatitis B and D occurs concurrently, the clinical course and prognosis are similar to that of HBV. Quite frequently, the D virus superinfects chronic carriers of HBV. This is a more severe condition since liver disease may be promoted and the risk of cirrhosis is greatly enhanced. In patients already cirrhotic, superinfection with the D virus doubles the risk of hepatic decompensation and triples the risk for hepatocellular

carcinoma (Fattovich et al. 2000). The virus can be detected by antibodies against the HDAg. Anti-HDV usually disappears within 1–2 years after resolution of the infection. The detection of viral RNA by RT-PCR is possible, but usually gives no additional information.

Reports on hepatitis D in dialysis patients are rare, even in a highly endemic area with some 35 per cent of HBsAg positive drug addicts and 50 per cent of thalassaemic patients being coinfected, the prevalence of HDV infection was only 9.4 per cent among HBsAg positive haemodialysis patients (Tassopoulos et al. 1986). Nevertheless, in highly endemic areas, dialysis patients should be tested for anti-HDV, and positive patients should be treated separately from HBsAg positives without the coinfection. Hygienic measures for prevention are the same as described for hepatitis B and HBV vaccination protects against HDV infection as well. Long-term follow-up studies on the prognosis of HDV infection in patients with chronic renal failure are lacking, as are studies on the prognosis after renal transplantation, however, an unfavourable influence is likely.

Hepatitis E

The hepatitis E virus (HEV) is found in a number of developing countries, particularly in Asia, India, Africa, and Central America. Its seroprevalence in industrialized countries is low, some 1–2 per cent in European countries. This RNA virus is much like the hepatitis A virus, transmitted via the faecal–oral route and does not induce chronic infection. Diagnosis can be made by anti-HEV antibodies. Outbreaks of the infection have been recorded and a few studies reported fairly high seroprevalences among haemodialysis patients, for example, 30 per cent in India (Agarwal et al. 1999), but the significance of this virus for the patient with chronic renal failure is uncertain.

Hepatitis G

A recently identified RNA virus that was associated with a mild and frequently subclinical hepatitis has been termed hepatitis G virus (HGV). However, it is still uncertain, whether this virus, which may persist in the host for up to several years, does actually cause a relevant disease. The infection can be diagnosed by specific antibodies or by the detection of HGV-RNA by RT-PCR. The prevalence of the virus is high in dialysis patients (25 per cent) but also in health care workers caring for these patients (24 per cent) while being much lower in the respective general population (9 per cent) (Gartner 1999).

References

Agarwal, S. K., Irshad, M., and Dash, S. C. (1999). Prevalence of antibodies against hepatitis E virus in haemodialysis patients in India. Nephron **81**, 448.

AlFurayh, O. et al. (2000). Hand contamination with hepatitis C virus in staff looking after hepatitis C-positive hemodialysis patients. American Journal of Nephrology **20**, 103–106.

Alter, H. J. (1992). New kit on the block: evaluation of second-generation assays for detection of antibody to the hepatitis C virus. Hepatology **15**, 350–353.

Alter, H. J. and Seeff, L. B. (2000). Recovery, persistence, and sequelae in hepatitis C virus infection: a perspective on long-term outcome. Seminars in Liver Disease **20**, 17–35.

Ben Ari, Z. et al. (2000). An open-label study of lamivudine for chronic hepatitis B in six patients with chronic renal failure before and after kidney transplantation. American Journal of Gastroenterology **95**, 3579–3583.

Bond, W. W. et al. (1981). Survival of hepatitis B virus after drying and storage for one week. Lancet 1, 550–551.

Bruchfeld, A. et al. (2001). Ribavirin treatment in dialysis patients with chronic hepatitis C virus infection—a pilot study. Journal of Viral Hepatitis 8, 287–292.

Bukh, J., Miller, R. H., and Purcell, R. H. (1995). Genetic heterogeneity of hepatitis C virus: quasispecies and genotypes. Seminars in Liver Disease 15, 41–63.

Campistol, J. M. et al. (1999). Efficacy and tolerance of interferon-alpha(2b) in the treatment of chronic hepatitis C virus infection in haemodialysis patients. Pre- and post-renal transplantation assessment. Nephrology, Dialysis, Transplantation 14, 2704–2709.

Centers for Disease Control and Prevention (2001). Recommendations for preventing transmission of infections among chronic hemodialysis patients. Morbidity and Mortality Weekly Report 50, 1–43.

Chan, T. M. et al. (1993). Prevalence of hepatitis C virus infection in hemodialysis patients: a longitudinal study comparing the results of RNA and antibody assays. Hepatology 17, 5–8.

Charest, A. F., McDougall, J., and Goldstein, M. B. (2000). A randomized comparison of intradermal and intramuscular vaccination against hepatitis B virus in incident chronic hemodialysis patients. American Journal of Kidney Diseases 36, 976–982.

Choo, Q. L. et al. (1989). Isolation of a cDNA clone derived from a blood-borne non-A, non-B viral hepatitis genome. Science 244, 359–362.

Council on Dialysis, N. K. F. (1997). National Kidney Foundation report on dialyzer reuse. American Journal of Kidney Diseases 30, 859–871.

Crosnier, J. et al. (1981). Randomized placebo-controlled trial of hepatitis B surface antigen vaccine in French hemodialysis units. II. Hemodialysis patients. Lancet I, 797–800.

Davis, G. L. (1999). Combination therapy with interferon alfa and ribavirin as retreatment of interferon relapse in chronic hepatitis C. Seminars in Liver Disease 19 (Suppl. 1), 49–55.

Degos, F. et al. (2001). The tolerance and efficacy of interferon-alpha in haemodialysis patients with HCV infection: a multicentre, prospective study. Nephrology, Dialysis, Transplantation 16, 1017–1023.

de Medina, M. et al. (1998). Detection of anti-hepatitis C virus antibodies in patients undergoing dialysis by utilizing a hepatitis C virus 3.0 assay: correlation with hepatitis C virus RNA. Journal of Laboratory and Clinical Medicine 132, 73–75.

Dienstag, J. L. et al. (1999). Lamivudine as initial treatment for chronic hepatitis B in the United States. New England Journal of Medicine 341, 1256–1263.

Dumann, H. et al. (1990). Hepatitis B vaccination and interleukin 2 receptor expression in chronic renal failure. Kidney International 38, 1164–1168.

Fabrizi, F. et al. (1996). Recombinant hepatitis B vaccine use in chronic hemodialysis patients. Long-term evaluation and cost-effectiveness analysis. Nephron 72, 536–543.

Farci, P. et al. (1992). Lack of protective immunity against reinfection with hepatitis C virus. Science 258, 135–140.

Farci, P. et al. (1996). Hepatitis C virus-associated fulminant hepatic failure. New England Journal of Medicine 335, 631–634.

Fattovich, G. et al. (1991). Natural history and prognostic factors for chronic hepatitis type B. Gut 32, 294–298.

Fattovich, G. et al. (2000). Influence of hepatitis delta virus infection on morbidity and mortality in compensated cirrhosis type B. The European Concerted Action on Viral Hepatitis (Eurohep). Gut 46, 420–426.

Fleischmann, E. H. et al. (2002). Active immunization against hepatitis A in dialysis patients. Nephrology, Dialysis, Transplantation 17, 1825–1828.

Gartner, B. C. et al. (1999). High prevalence of hepatitis G virus (HGV) infections in dialysis staff. Nephrology, Dialysis, Transplantation 14, 406–408.

Girndt, M. et al. (1993). T-cell activation defect in hemodialysis patients: evidence for a role of the B7/CD28 pathway. Kidney International 44, 359–365.

Girndt, M. et al. (1995). Production of interleukin-6, tumor necrosis factor alpha and interleukin-10 in vitro correlates with the clinical immune defect in chronic hemodialysis patients. Kidney International 47, 559–565.

Girndt, M. et al. (2001). Defective expression of B7-2 (CD86) on monocytes of dialysis patients correlates to the uremia-associated immune defect. Kidney International 59, 1382–1389.

Girndt, M. et al. (2001). The interleukin-10 promotor genotype determines clinical immune function in hemodialysis patients. Kidney International 60, 2385–2391.

Glicklich, D. et al. (1999). Comparison of clinical features and liver histology in hepatitis C—positive dialysis patients and renal transplant recipients. American Journal of Gastroenterology 94, 159–163.

Gomez, J. et al. (1999). Hepatitis C viral quasispecies. Journal of Viral Hepatitis 6, 3–16.

Hadziyannis, S. J. et al. (2003). Adefovir dipivoxil for the treatment of hepatitis B e antigen-negative chronic hepatitis B. New England Journal of Medicine 348, 800–807.

Harris, H. E. et al. (2002). Clinical course of hepatitis C virus during the first decade of infection: cohort study. British Medical Journal 324, 450–453.

Hoofnagle, J. H. (1997). Hepatitis C: the clinical spectrum of disease. Hepatology 26, 15S–20S.

Hoofnagle, J. H. and Di Bisceglie, A. M. (1991). Serologic diagnosis of acute and chronic viral hepatitis. Seminars in Liver Disease 11, 73–83.

Huraib, S. et al. (1999). Interferon-alpha in chronic hepatitis C infection in dialysis patients. American Journal of Kidney Diseases 34, 55–60.

Izopet, J. et al. (2000). Longitudinal analysis of hepatitis C virus replication and liver fibrosis progression in renal transplant recipients. Journal of Infectious Diseases 181, 852–858.

Jadoul, M., Cornu, C., and van Ypersele, D. S. (1993). Incidence and risk factors for hepatitis C seroconversion in hemodialysis: a prospective study. The UCL Collaborative Group. Kidney International 44, 1322–1326.

Jadoul, M., Cornu, C., and van Ypersele, D. S. (1998). Universal precautions prevent hepatitis C virus transmission: a 54 month follow-up of the Belgian Multicenter Study. The UCL Collaborative Group. Kidney International 53, 1022–1025.

Jaeckel, E. et al. (2001). Treatment of acute hepatitis C with interferon alfa-2b. New England Journal of Medicine 345, 1452–1457.

Jalava, T. et al. (1992). A rapid and quantitative solution hybridization method for detection of HBV DNA in serum. Journal of Virological Methods 36, 171–180.

Josselson, J. et al. (1987). Hepatitis B surface antigenemia in a chronic hemodialysis program: lack of influence on morbidity and mortality. American Journal of Kidney Diseases 9, 456–461.

Jung, M. C., Diepolder, H. M., and Pape, G. R. (1994). T cell recognition of hepatitis B and C viral antigens. European Journal of Clinical Investigation 24, 641–650.

Kasiske, B. L. et al. (2002). The evaluation of renal transplantation candidates: clinical practice guidelines. American Journal of Transplantation 1 (Suppl. 2), 1–95.

Kaul, H. et al. (2000). Initiation of hemodialysis treatment leads to improvement of T cell activation in patients with end stage renal disease. American Journal of Kidney Diseases 35, 611–616.

Knoll, G. A. et al. (1997). The impact of renal transplantation on survival in hepatitis C-positive end-stage renal disease patients. American Journal of Kidney Diseases 29, 608–614.

Köhler, H. et al. (1984). Active hepatitis B vaccination of dialysis patients and medical staff. Kidney International 25, 124–128.

Kuo, G. et al. (1989). An assay for circulating antibodies to a major etiologic virus of human non-A, non-B hepatitis. Science 244, 362–364.

Lamb, M. W., Marks, I. M., and Wynohradnyk, L. (2001). 40 kDa Peginterferon alpha-2a (Pegasys) can be administered safely in patients with end-stage renal disease. Hepatology 34, 326A (abstract).

Lau, J. Y. and Wright, T. L. (1993). Molecular virology and pathogenesis of hepatitis B. Lancet 342, 1335–1340.

Lee, W. M. (1997). Hepatitis B virus infection. New England Journal of Medicine 337, 1733–1745.

Lin, S. M. *et al.* (1999). Long-term beneficial effect of interferon therapy in patients with chronic hepatitis B virus infection. *Hepatology* **29**, 971–975.

Liu, Y. and Janeway, C. A. (1992). Cells that present both specific ligand and costimulatory activity are the most efficient inducers of clonal expansion of normal CD4 T cells. *Proceedings of the National Academy of Sciences* **89**, 3845–3849.

Lok, A. S. *et al.* (1993). Antibody response to core, envelope and nonstructural hepatitis C virus antigens: comparison of immunocompetent and immunosuppressed patients. *Hepatology* **18**, 497–502.

London, W. T. *et al.* (1969). An epidemic of hepatitis in a chronic hemodialysis unit. *New England Journal of Medicine* **281**, 571–578.

Luzar, B. *et al.* (2003). Does end-stage kidney failure influence hepatitis C progression in hemodialysis patients? *Hepatogastroenterology* **50**, 157–160.

Manns, M. P. *et al.* (2001). Peginterferon alpha-2b plus ribavirin compared with interferon alpha-2b plus ribavirin for initial treatment of chronic hepatitis C: a randomised trial. *Lancet* **358**, 958–965.

Mathurin, P. *et al.* (1999). Impact of hepatitis B and C virus on kidney transplantation outcome. *Hepatology* **29**, 257–263.

McAdam, A. J., Schweitzer, A. N., and Sharpe, A. H. (1998). The role of B7 costimulation in activation and differentiation of CD4+ and CD8+ T cells. *Immunological Reviews* **165**, 231–247.

McMahon, B. J. *et al.* (1990). Hepatitis B-related sequelae. Prospective study in 1400 hepatitis B surface antigen-positive Alaska native carriers. *Archives of Internal Medicine* **150**, 1051–1054.

Meuer, S. C. *et al.* (1987). Selective blockade of the antigen-receptor-mediated pathway of T cell activation in patients with impaired immune responses. *Jorunal of Clinical Investigation* **80**, 743–749.

Moore, K. W. *et al.* (2001). Interleukin-10 and the interleukin-10 receptor. *Annual Review of Immunology* **19**, 683–765.

Neumann, A. U. *et al.* (1998). Hepatitis C viral dynamics *in vivo* and the antiviral efficacy of interferon-alpha therapy. *Science* **282**, 103–107.

Noiri, E. *et al.* (2001). Hepatitis C virus in blood and dialysate in hemodialysis. *American Journal of Kidney Diseases* **37**, 38–42.

Pereira, B. J. *et al.* (1998). Effects of hepatitis C infection and renal transplantation on survival in end-stage renal disease. The New England Organ Bank Hepatitis C Study Group. *Kidney International* **53**, 1374–1381.

Pol, S. (1995). Hepatitis C virus infection in hemodialyzed patients and kidney allograft recipients. *Advances in Nephrology of the Necker Hospital* **24**, 315–330.

Pol, S. *et al.* (1995). Efficacy and tolerance of alpha-2b interferon therapy on HCV infection of hemodialyzed patients. *Kidney International* **47**, 1412–1418.

Pol, S. *et al.* (2002). HCV infection and hemodialysis. *Seminars in Nephrology* **22**, 331–339.

Poynard, T. *et al.* (1998). Randomised trial of interferon alpha2b plus ribavirin for 48 weeks or for 24 weeks versus interferon alpha2b plus placebo for 48 weeks for treatment of chronic infection with hepatitis C virus. *Lancet* **352**, 1426–1432.

Ribot, S. *et al.* (1979). Duration of hepatitis B surface antigenemia (HBsAg) in hemodialysis patients. *Archives of Internal Medicine* **139**, 178–180.

Rostaing, L. *et al.* (1996). Acute renal failure in kidney transplant patients treated with interferon alpha 2b for chronic hepatitis C. *Nephron* **74**, 512–516.

Rostaing, L. *et al.* (1998). Pharmacokinetics of alpha IFN-2b in chronic hepatitis C virus patients undergoing chronic hemodialysis or with normal renal function: clinical implications. *Journal of the American Society of Nephrology* **9**, 2344–2348.

Schalm, S. W. *et al.* (2000). Lamivudine and alpha interferon combination treatment of patients with chronic hepatitis B infection: a randomised trial. *Gut* **46**, 562–568.

Simmonds, P. *et al.* (1994). A proposed system for the nomenclature of hepatitis C viral genotypes. *Hepatology* **19**, 1321–1324.

Soffredini, R. *et al.* (1996). Increased detection of antibody to hepatitis C virus in renal transplant patients by third-generation assays. *American Journal of Kidney Diseases* **28**, 437–440.

Stenvinkel, P. *et al.* (1999). Strong association between malnutrition, inflammation, and atherosclerosis in chronic renal failure. *Kidney International* **55**, 1899–1911.

Szmuness, W. *et al.* (1980). Hepatitis B vaccine. Demonstration of efficiacy in a high-risk population in the United States. *New England Journal of Medicine* **303**, 833–841.

Tassopoulos, N. *et al.* (1986). Serologic markers of hepatitis B virus (HBV) and hepatitis D virus infection in carriers of hepatitis B surface antigen who are frequently exposed to HBV. *Hepatogastroenterology* **33**, 151–154.

The EBPG Expert Group on Haemodialysis (2002). European best practice guidelines for haemodialysis. *Nephrology, Dialysis, Transplantation* **17** (Suppl. 7), 72–87.

Thomas, D. L. (2000). Hepatitis C epidemiology. *Current Topics in Microbiology and Immunology* **242**, 25–41.

Tokars, J. I., Arduino, M. J., and Alter, M. J. (2001). Infection control in hemodialysis units. *Infectious Diseases Clinics of North America* **15**, 797–812, viii.

Turner, D. M. *et al.* (1997). An investigation of polymorphism in the interleukin-10 gene promotor. *European Journal of Immunogenetics* **24**, 1–8.

Valderrabano, F. *et al.* (1996). Report on management of renal failure in Europe, XXV, 1994. The EDTA-ERA Registry. *Nephrology, Dialysis, Transplantation* **11** (Suppl. 1), 2–21.

Villeneuve, J. P. *et al.* (1994). A long-term follow-up study of asymptomatic hepatitis B surface antigen-positive carriers in Montreal. *Gastroenterology* **106**, 1000–1005.

Wong, D. K. *et al.* (1993). Effect of alpha-interferon treatment in patients with hepatitis B e antigen-positive chronic hepatitis B. A meta-analysis. *Annals of Internal Medicine* **119**, 312–323.

Yotsuyanagi, H. *et al.* (1995). Hepatitis C virus genotypes and development of hepatocellular carcinoma. *Cancer* **76**, 1352–1355.

Zeuzem, S. *et al.* (2000). Peginterferon alpha-2a in patients with chronic hepatitis C. *New England Journal of Medicine* **343**, 1666–1672.

11.3.8 Haematological disorders

Iain C. Macdougall and Kai-Uwe Eckardt

Introduction

The close relationship between haematopoiesis and the kidney was first recognized by Richard Bright in 1835 when he described the association between anaemia and chronic renal failure. Much of the morbidity in renal failure patients can be attributed to the consequences of their chronic anaemia. Although other factors may contribute to the development of anaemia, erythropoietin deficiency is the major factor. This is demonstrated by the striking response to administration of recombinant human erythropoietin (see Chapters 11.3.11 and 11.3.12).

Disorders of white cell and platelet function have also been described in renal failure, but these are of secondary importance compared with those related to the red cell. A major part of this chapter is therefore devoted to erythropoiesis, including its control by erythropoietin; how this process is disrupted in uraemia; the consequences of anaemia in renal failure patients; and the effects of recombinant human erythropoietin in treating this condition.

Normal erythropoiesis

The development of the red cell

The erythroid marrow is responsible for the production of red cells to maintain the red cell mass of 30 ± 5 ml/kg in males and 25 ± 5 ml/kg in females. This is more usually assessed by measurement of the red cell count and haemoglobin concentration (for normal values see Table 1). The maintenance of the red cell mass, 1 per cent of which is destroyed each day, depends on continual erythropoiesis with the production of 173,000,000,000 new red cells per day. Pleuripotent stem cells, primitive cells capable of both self-renewal and differentiation, are present in the marrow at low concentrations. These cells give rise to progenitor cells, committed to become myeloid, erythroid, lymphoid, or megakaryocytic cells. This differentiation and multiplication is controlled by an array of growth factors. Differentiation of the committed erythroid precursor into the primitive erythroid progenitor cell, the 'burst forming unit-erythroid' (usually abbreviated to BFU-E), is under the influence of interleukin-3 and granulocyte–macrophage colony-stimulating factor

Table 1 Normal haematological values in adults

Haemoglobin (g/dl)	
Male	13.5–18
Female	11.5–16
Haematocrit	
Male	0.40–0.54
Female	0.37–0.47
Red cell count ($\times 10^{12}$/l)	
Male	4.5–6.5
Female	3.9–5.6
Mean cell volume (MCV) (fl)	81–100
Mean cell haemoglobin (pg)	27–32
Mean cell haemoglobin concentration (g/dl)	32–36
Reticulocyte count (%)	0.8–2.0
Absolute reticulocyte count ($\times 10^9$/l)	25–100
Total blood volume (ml/kg)	70 ± 10
Plasma volume (ml/kg)	45 ± 5
Red cell volume (ml/kg)	
Male	30 ± 5
Female	25 ± 5
Erythron transferrin uptake (μmol/l/day)	60 ± 12
Platelet count ($\times 10^9$/l)	150–400
White cell count ($\times 10^9$/l)	4.0–11.0

Adapted from the *Oxford Textbook of Medicine* 1st edn. (ed. D. J. Weatherall, J. G. G. Ledingham, and D. A. Warrell). Oxford: Oxford University Press. With permission.

(GM-CSF) (Fig. 1). Multiplication and differentiation of the BFU-E and the later 'colony forming unit-erythroid' (CFU-E) requires the presence of erythropoietin. The CFU-E is more sensitive to erythropoietin than the BFU-E, requiring lower concentrations for *in vitro* culture. Apart from erythropoietin, CFU-E growth in culture requires the presence of insulin or insulin-like growth factor 1 (Sawada *et al.* 1989). The CFU-E undergoes successive divisions and gives rise to proerythroblasts and then erythroblasts, which develop into mature red blood cells.

Mode and sites of erythropoietin production

Factors affecting erythropoietin production

Normal serum erythropoietin concentrations in humans are of the order of 10–30 mU/ml as determined by radioimmunoassays, which corresponds to between 2 and 7 pmol/l. Assuming a mean serum half-life of 5–9 h and a mean distribution volume of 0.07 l/kg, as determined in pharmacokinetic studies with recombinant human erythropoietin (see below), it can be estimated that the endogenous production of the hormone normally amounts to about 2–4 U/kg/24 h.

Erythropoietin concentrations are decreased or increased under a variety of conditions largely reflecting alterations of oxygen delivery to tissues (Table 2). Anaemia, of whatever cause, is the most powerful stimulus to an increase in serum erythropoietin, with an inverse relationship between the concentration of erythropoietin and the haemoglobin concentration (Caro *et al.* 1979) (see Fig. 2). In severely anaemic patients up to 1000-fold increases in erythropoietin can be found.

In addition to changes in oxygen delivery, metabolic factors also influence erythropoietin production. Hypophysectomy and starvation are accompanied by decreased concentrations, whereas stimulation of metabolism by thyroxine increases concentrations (Halvorsen *et al.* 1968; Peschle *et al.* 1986). With this latter exception, all the other observations can be summarized in a somewhat simplified way, in that conditions of reduced oxygen supply and increased oxygen demand lead to increased circulating erythropoietin concentrations, whereas decreased concentrations are typical of conditions with increased oxygen supply or reduced oxygen demand.

Production sites of erythropoietin

The body contains no significant stores of erythropoietin, and there is no evidence that the clearance rate of the hormone is subject to any physiological regulation. This has led to the view that any change in serum erythropoietin concentration results from a change in the rate of production. Production in turn has been shown to be primarily determined by the expression level of erythropoietin mRNA in liver and kidneys (Bondurant and Koury 1986; Tan *et al.* 1992) (Fig. 3). The relative contribution of liver and kidneys is primarily age dependent: the liver is the predominant production site during fetal, and in some species also early postnatal life, whereas the kidneys produce most erythropoietin in adults (Eckardt *et al.* 1992c). Nevertheless, in adult animals, the contribution of the liver to erythropoietin production under conditions of severe hypoxia may amount to more than one-third of the total (Tan *et al.* 1992; Eckardt *et al.* 1992c). Despite such a significant production capacity, the liver does not normally

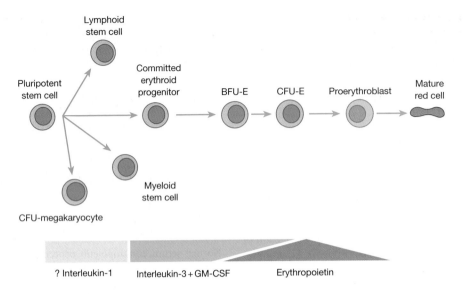

Fig. 1 Normal erythropoiesis.

Table 2 States causing alteration of circulating erythropoietin levels. The influence of changes in oxygen delivery on erythropoietin has been demonstrated in several species including humans. Metabolic influences on erythropoietin formation have so far only been reported in experimental animals

	Increased erythropoietin levels	**Decreased erythropoietin levels**
Oxygen delivery	Anaemia High altitude Cardiopulmonary disorders Carbon monoxide Increased oxygen affinity of haemoglobin	Polycythaemia vera
Metabolism	Thyroxine Growth hormone	Starvation Hypophysectomy
Other	Cobalt	

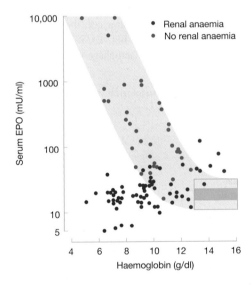

Fig. 2 Relationship between serum immunoreactive erythropoietin (irEPO) levels and haemoglobin concentrations in hypo- and hyper-regenerative non-renal anaemias and in patients with chronic renal failure, excluding patients with polycystic kidneys. The rectangle illustrates interquartile range and 95% confidence range of erythropoietin levels in non-anaemic healthy adults (Eckardt et al. 1991).

compensate for loss or failure of the renal production of erythropoietin (Tan et al. 1991) and in anephric patients serum eythropoietin concentrations are very low (Naets et al. 1986). Small amounts of erythropoietin mRNA have also been detected in brain, testis, lung, spleen, and other organs (Tan et al. 1992; Fandrey and Bunn 1993).

The cells producing erythropoietin in the kidney are peritubular fibroblasts in the renal cortex (Bachmann et al. 1993; Maxwell et al. 1993) (Fig. 4). In the liver, the majority of the cells producing erythropoietin are hepatocytes (Koury et al. 1991; Schuster et al. 1992), but erythropoietin production has also been found in non-epithelial cells in the sinusoidal spaces, most likely the so-called fat-storing or 'Ito'-cells (Maxwell et al. 1994). It is of interest that these cells share several properties with renal fibroblasts, in that they are in close contact with capillaries and parenchymal cells, are involved in matrix synthesis, and transform into myofibroblasts in response to injury.

The oxygen sensor controlling erythropoietin production

Local oxygen sensing and the control of erythropoietin production

The oxygen-dependent control of erythropoietin formation requires sensing mechanisms that perceive changes in oxygen supply and translate them into alterations of erythropoietin gene activity in the liver and kidneys. These mechanisms are key elements in the feedback

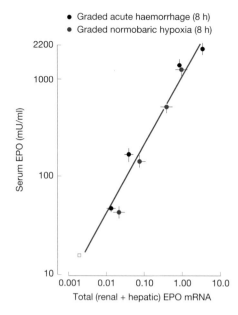

Fig. 3 Relationship between the amount of erythropoietin mRNA in liver and kidneys and the serum hormone level in rats subjected to two different types of acute hypoxia (data from Tan *et al.* 1992).

control of erythropoiesis and their function has therefore attracted considerable interest. These oxygen-sensing mechanisms are sensitive to conditions that affect arterial P_{O_2} and consequently also tissue and venous P_{O_2} (hypoxic hypoxia) as well as conditions in which arterial P_{O_2} is normal and only tissue and venous P_{O_2} are reduced (anaemic hypoxia). Under a variety of clinical and experimental conditions no principal difference in erythropoietin regulation has been found between these two types of hypoxia. Moreover, under normal ambient oxygen tensions and under hypoxic hypoxia the erythropoietin response is attenuated when the haemoglobin concentration increases to above normal. Therefore, it is unlikely that the arterial P_{O_2} can directly influence erythropoietin formation. Rather, it appears to be the tissue oxygen tension that regulates production of the hormone. Several lines of evidence indicate that local tissue oxygen tensions at the sites of erythropoietin production are being sensed.

In the liver, for example, *in situ* hybridization has shown that erythropoietin is preferentially expressed in pericentral areas of the hepatic lobules (Koury *et al.* 1991). Since tissue oxygen tensions in pericentral parts of the hepatic lobule are lower than in periportal areas, this is consistent with local oxygen gradients determining the expression. Furthermore, experiments with isolated liver cells showed that they can directly change the rate of erythropoietin production in response to changes in their oxygenation *in vitro* (Goldberg *et al.* 1991; Eckardt *et al.* 1994), which confirms the presence of cellular oxygen sensing.

In isolated perfused kidneys erythropoietin mRNA and erythropoietin secretion are modulated in response to alterations of the oxygen tension of the perfusate (Ratcliffe *et al.* 1990; Scholz *et al.* 1991). Thus, although humoral signals from extrarenal sensing systems may contribute to the renal control of erythropoietin production under certain conditions, all the events necessary for detection of hypoxia and production of erythropoietin can obviously operate intrarenally. In addition, observations in patients with renal transplants (Rejman

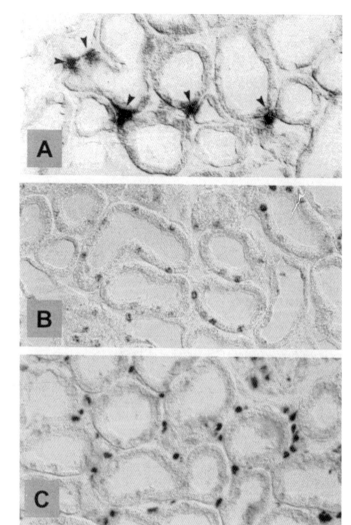

Fig. 4 *In situ* hybridization, demonstrating erythropoietin mRNA in peritubular fibroblasts of the renal cortex.

et al. 1985; Besarab *et al.* 1987) and experimental data (Eckardt *et al.* 1992a) indicate that no essential control of erythropoietin production occurs via the renal nerves.

Intrarenal control of erythropoietin production

Despite much increase in the understanding of cellular oxygen sensing, the intrarenal control of erythropoietin formation remains incompletely understood. So far, attempts to induce erythropoietin formation in isolated renal cell or tissue preparations have failed and therefore the hypothesis that erythropoietin-producing cells are directly oxygen sensitive has not been formally proven. Interestingly, the exponential increase in erythropoietin production in the kidney that occurs with reduction in renal oxygen supply is primarily due to an increase in the proportion of peritubular fibroblasts that express the erythropoietin gene and single cells respond in an almost all-or-none manner (Koury *et al.* 1989; Eckardt *et al.* 1992b) (Fig. 5). This recruitment occurs within the cortical labyrinth and is directed from deep to superficial regions. Under normoxia, erythropoietin is produced by a few cells in the juxtamedullary parts of the

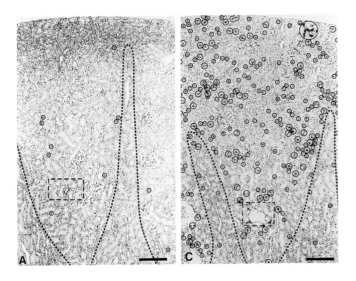

Fig. 5 Distribution of cells expressing erythropoietin mRNA in the renal cortex of rats exposed to two different degrees of hypoxia. Peritubular cells containing erythropoietin mRNA were identified by *in situ* hybridization and are marked with the circles. Note that they are predominantly found in the cortical labyrinth; erythropoietin is rarely expressed in medullary rays and not in the medulla (adapted from Eckardt *et al.* 1992b).

labyrinth, and increasing severity of hypoxia leads to activation of the erythropoietin gene also in midcortical and superficial areas of the cortex. It is tempting to speculate that local oxygen profiles determine this expression pattern of erythropoietin. Although it has been shown that local oxygen gradients exist in the renal cortex (Leichtweiss *et al.* 1969; Schurek *et al.* 1990), it has not been possible yet to align such gradients with the pattern of erythropoietin synthesis.

Oxygen gradients in the kidney cortex presumably result from both a restricted delivery of oxygen and a high rate of oxygen consumption. The major reason for a limited oxygen supply despite a large overall oxygen delivery to the kidney lies in the vascular architecture. Arteries and veins run in parallel over long distances and the close contact between preglomerular arterial and venous vessels allows oxygen to diffuse from arteries into veins before the blood reaches the peritubular capillaries. Therefore, local tissue oxygen tensions in the renal cortex can be much lower than in the renal vein (Leichtweiss *et al.* 1969; Schurek *et al.* 1990).

The major determinant of renal oxygen consumption, on the other hand, is the 'transport work', that is, sodium reabsorption, of the nephron, and this also appears to be relevant for the regulation of erythropoietin production. Tubular sodium reabsorption is proportional to the amount of glomerular filtrate, and glomerular filtration rate (GFR) in turn is linked to renal blood flow. Therefore, changes in renal blood flow can influence both oxygen supply and consumption of the kidney and may have little influence on the ratio of both parameters. This might explain why the kidney is able to adjust erythropoietin production to alterations in blood oxygen content with only a modest confounding influence from changes in renal haemodynamics (Erslev *et al.* 1985). Experimental constriction of the renal arteries, for example, is only a minor stimulus for erythropoietin secretion (Pagel *et al.* 1988), and in patients with renal artery stenosis the incidence of erythrocytosis is low (Luke *et al.* 1965). Among the different nephron segments that contribute to renal oxygen consumption, the convoluted part of the proximal tubule seems to be of particular importance

for erythropoietin regulation. This part of the nephron has almost no capacity for anaerobic glycolysis and is therefore largely oxygen dependent. Erythropoietin production occurs in cells that are located in close proximity to proximal tubular cells, and experimental inhibition of sodium reabsorption of proximal tubules with acetazolamide reduces hypoxia-induced erythropoietin production (Eckardt *et al.* 1989c). Whether it is merely the oxygen consumption of the proximal tubular cells that influences erythropoietin production or whether proximal tubular cells also release paracrine signals that stimulate the peritubular fibroblasts is not clear.

Control of the erythropoietin gene

The final step in the signalling cascade that controls erythropoietin production is an increased expression of the erythropoietin gene. Accumulation of erythropoietin mRNA in erythropoietin-producing cells results mainly from an increase in the transcription rate of the gene, but a specific increase in the stability of erythropoietin mRNA may also contribute (Schuster *et al.* 1989; Goldberg *et al.* 1991).

In general, accurately sited initiation of gene transcription is determined by a promoter region at the 5′ end of a particular gene and the rate of transcription is controlled through the interaction of proteins with regulatory deoxyribonucleic acid (DNA) sequences within or adjacent to the coding sequence of the gene. Due to the unavailability of renal cell preparations producing erythropoietin *in vitro*, studies on the molecular control of erythropoietin gene activity have so far mainly been performed in hepatoma cells and hepatocytes. In addition, erythropoietin gene constructs have been expressed in transgenic animals in order to define regulatory sequences. Both approaches have identified several regulatory elements that stimulate or suppress erythropoietin gene expression and play a role in coordinating the complex tissue- and stimulus-specific expression of the erythropoietin gene. These include certain promoter sequences, which in isolation are able to mediate oxygen-dependent regulation (Blanchard *et al.* 1992). Of major importance, however, for the hypoxic induction of erythropoietin gene activity is a DNA sequence within the immediate 3′ flanking region of the gene. This sequence fulfils criteria of a classical eukaryotic transcriptional enhancer. When it is excised experimentally and linked at a variable distance to other promoters, it confers oxygen-dependent regulation to reporter genes, which are not normally regulated in an oxygen-dependent fashion (Beck *et al.* 1991; Pugh *et al.* 1991).

The search for nuclear proteins interacting with this sequence led to the discovery of a yet unknown transcription factor, called 'hypoxia-inducible factor' (HIF) (Semenza and Wang 1992; Wang and Semenza 1995). Interestingly, although the enhancer sequence was originally identified using transient transfection of erythropoietin gene constructs into erythropoietin-producing hepatoma cells, subsequent studies revealed that it also operates when transfected into a variety of cells that do not normally produce erythropoietin. Furthermore, HIF expression is not confined to erythropoietin producing cells and DNA sequences homologous to the 'erythropoietin enhancer' have meanwhile been found in the vicinity of many other genes that are regulated in an oxygen-dependent fashion. Altogether, these observations demonstrated that a common widespread oxygen-sensing mechanism exists, which controls erythropoietin gene activity in some specialized renal and hepatic cells, and controls an array of other metabolic, inflammatory, and growth-regulating processes in other cells and under other circumstances (reviewed in Semenza 2000; Wenger 2002).

HIF consists of a heterodimer of an oxygen-regulated α-subunit and a constitutive β-subunit (Fig. 6). Both subunits exists as a set of different isoforms, all belonging to the basic-helix-loop-helix PAS protein superfamily. The major regulation of the α-subunit occurs through oxygen-dependent degradation. This was found to be mediated by the von Hippel Lindau protein (pVHL), which acts as a ubiquitin ligase and targets HIFα for proteasomal destruction through the addition of a chain of ubiquitin molecules (Maxwell et al. 1999). pVHL only binds to HIFα in the presence of oxygen and this interaction depends on hydroxylation of prolyl residues of the HIFα protein. HIF prolyl hydroxylation is achieved through a family of prolyl-hydroxylases, which require molecular oxygen as a substrate (Epstein et al. 2001; Jaakola et al. 2001). An additional hydroxylation step was found to regulate HIF transcriptional activity (Lando et al. 2002).

HIF-1α and HIF-2α are the two principal oxygen-regulated HIF subunits. Although both are regulated in a very similar fashion in vitro (Wiesener et al. 1998), their expression in vivo appears to be cell-type specific. In the kidney, HIF-1α is normally expressed in tubular cells and HIF-2α in peritubular endothelial cells and fibroblasts (Rosenberger et al. 2002) (Fig. 4). In the liver, HIF-2α is expressed in hepatocytes and perisinusoidal cells, whereas HIF-1α is expressed in non-parenchymal cells only (Wiesener et al. 2003 and unpublished observations). Thus, HIF-2α rather than HIF-1α is upregulated in cells producing erythropoietin and therefore this isoform appears to be responsible for transcriptional induction of the erythropoietin gene in vivo.

The widespread expression of the HIF transcription factors implies that additional regulatory mechanisms must exist that restrict different oxygen-dependent reactions to certain cell types under certain physiological and pathophysiological conditions. Transgenic animals have revealed that in addition to those sequences that lie in the close vicinity of the erythropoietin gene, other sequences that are located at

a considerable distance of at least 6 kb, but possibly more than 14 kb, from the 5' end to the coding sequence may contribute to this control and that regulatory elements that determine the expression in liver and kidneys are different (Semenza et al. 1991).

Structure of the erythropoietin gene and molecule

The gene encoding human erythropoietin is located on chromosome 7 (Law et al. 1986) and encompasses about 3000 base pairs (Fig. 7). It contains five exons and four introns and encodes for a 193-amino acid polypeptide (Jacobs et al. 1985; Lin et al. 1985). A 27-amino acid leader sequence at the N-terminal part and a carboxy-terminal arginine molecule are cleaved off during secretion, so that the mature protein contains 165 amino acids (Recny et al. 1987). The molecule forms a long loop through a disulfide bridge between residues 7 and 161 and an additional small loop is formed by disulfide bridging between residues 29 and 33. These bridges are of functional significance since the biological activity of erythropoietin is reversibly sensitive to reducing agents (Wang et al. 1985). Before the erythropoietin molecule is released from the cells producing it, four complex, heavily sialylated carbohydrate chains are added to the protein chain at three N- and one O-glycosylation sites (Sasaki et al. 1987; Takeuchi et al. 1988). These sugar side-chains contribute approximately one-third to the relative molecular mass of about 34,000 Da. They are necessary both for normal secretion of the hormone and for its biological activity in vivo, because partially or completely deglycosylated erythropoietin is rapidly cleared from the circulation (Fukuda et al. 1989). However, the sugar side-chains are not required for interaction of the hormone with its target cell receptors (Dordal et al. 1985).

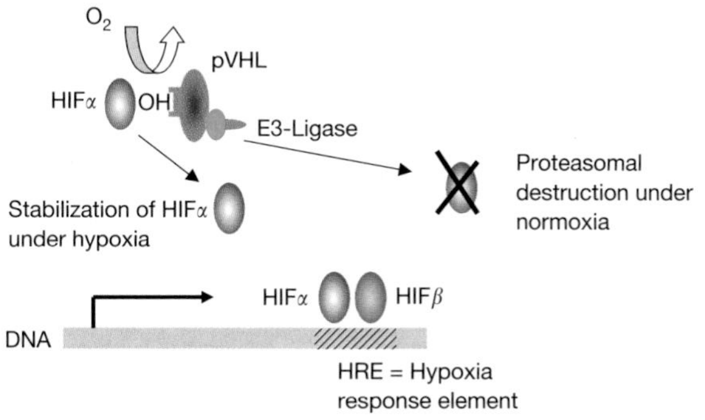

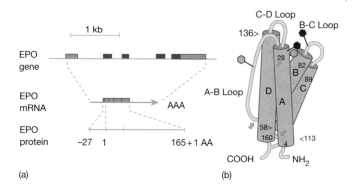

(a)   (b)

Fig. 6 Schematic presentation of the oxygen-sensing mechanism that controls expression of the erythropoietin gene and other hypoxia-inducible genes. The oxygen-regulated α-subunit of the HIF is hydroxylized in the presence of oxygen through specific prolyl- and asparagyl hydroxylases. Prolylhydroxylation of HIFα is required for its binding to the pVHL, which acts as the recognition component of a ubiquitin ligase complex. Following the binding of hydroxylated HIF to pVHL the molecule is rapidly destroyed by the cellular proteasome and thus functionally inactive. Under hypoxia, oxygen required as a substrate for the hydroxylation reactions is lacking and thus binding between HIFα and pVHL is prevented. Together with the constitutive component HIFβ stabilized HIFα can then bind to a DNA recognition sequence, termed 'Hypoxia-Responsive' Element and this binding initiates enhanced transcription of hypoxia-inducible genes (see text for further details).

Fig. 7 Map of the human erythropoietin gene with schematic presentation of its transcription and translation (a) and a model prediction of the three-dimensional structure of the erythropoietin molecule (b). (a) The erythropoietin gene consists of five exons (boxes) and four introns. The exonic regions contain long 5'- and 3'-untranslated regions (open boxes) on either side of the protein coding sequence (black boxes). The arrow indicates the most prominent transcription initiation site. The erythropoietin molecules is synthesized as a proform containing 193 amino acids. A 27-amino acid leader peptide is processed during secretion of the hormone. In addition, a terminal arginine molecule is removed, so that the mature molecule has a protein backbone of 165 amino acids. (b) Two disulfide bridges link both ends of the protein and form an additional small loop. Four complex carbohydrate chains are attached to the molecule. The tertiary structure prediction is that the molecule forms four antiparallel alpha-helices (depicted as cylinders A–D).

Human urinary erythropoietin and recombinant human erythropoietin produced by Chinese hamster ovary cells are identical with respect to primary and secondary structures. The carbohydrate moiety of the recombinant form of erythropoietin is also very similar to that of native erythropoietin purified from human urine (Sasaki *et al.* 1987; Takeuchi *et al.* 1988). Yet, subtle differences have been demonstrated between native erythropoietin isolated from plasma or urine and recombinant erythropoietin as well as between different recombinant erythropoietins (Storring *et al.* 1996; Skibeli *et al.* 1998). More recently, a hyperglycosylated recombinant human erythropoietin molecule has been developed by introduction of amino acids providing additional glycosylation sites (see below).

The action of erythropoietin on red cell progenitors

Erythropoietin acts via specific receptors present on early red cell progenitors. The study of different erythroid precursor cells has revealed between 500 and 1000 erythropoietin receptors per cell (Graber and Krantz 1989; Krantz 1991).

The human erythropoietin receptor molecule is a 508 amino acid polypeptide. It is a member of the cytokine receptor superfamily (Bazan 1990) and consists of a single membrane-spanning domain, an extracytoplasmic *N*-terminal part, which contains the erythropoietin binding site, and a *C*-terminal cytoplasmic domain, which is associated with signal transduction (Jones *et al.* 1990; Yoshimura and Misawa 1998).

Dimerization of the receptor results in autophosphorylation and the activation of several kinases that initiate multiple signal transduction pathways. These include, for example, the Jak/STAT5 pathway, a MAP kinase pathway, and protein kinase C pathways, which overlap or cross-talk to coordinate the expression of genes regulating differentiation and maturation of erythroid precursor cells (reviewed by Chen and Sytkowski 2003). The cellular responses that can be observed following the addition of erythropoietin to erythroid precursor cells include increases in RNA and DNA synthesis, glucose uptake, globin gene expression, transferrin receptor expression, and finally haemoglobin synthesis.

The signalling cascades initiated by binding of erythropoietin to its receptor do not seem to stimulate differentiation and mitosis directly, but rather maintain the cellular viability of erythroid progenitors, which allows these cells to proceed with an endogenous programme of mitosis and terminal differentiation. It has been observed that CFU-Es require erythropoietin for survival irrespective of any effect on mitosis and differentiation (Koury and Bondurant 1988) and that erythropoietin retards the rate of cleavage of DNA, which is characteristic of programmed cell death (apoptosis) (Koury and Bondurant 1990). According to this concept, the majority of CFU-Es do not survive under normal conditions but with increased erythropoietin concentrations; for example, in anaemia, many of the progenitors, which would ordinarily die, are rescued and then progress to red blood cell differentiation.

Although erythropoietin is considered to be a lineage-specific haemopoietic growth factor, it was found to bind to megakaryocytes (Fraser *et al.* 1989), and increased concentrations do, in some studies, stimulate thrombopoiesis *in vivo* (Berridge *et al.* 1988) and *in vitro* (Dessypris *et al.* 1987; Ishibashi *et al.* 1987). Effects of erythropoietin on platelet production could in part be due to structure homologies between erythropoietin and the megakaryocyte growth factor thrombopoietin (Lok *et al.* 1994). Erythropoietin receptors have also been detected in several non-erythroid tissues, including brain and kidney (Westenfelder *et al.* 1999; Brines *et al.* 2000). Erythropoietin receptors have also been demonstrated on several vascular cells, and a proliferative response of endothelial cells *in vitro* has been described (Anagnostou *et al.* 1987; Carlini *et al.* 1995). However, the concentrations of erythropoietin required for these and other extraerythropoietic effects are generally much higher than the serum concentrations achieved under physiological conditions and in patients receiving recombinant erythropoietin therapy.

Additional factors required for normal erythropoiesis

Apart from erythropoietin the production of red cells by the erythroid marrow requires iron, folate, vitamin B_{12}, pyridoxine, ascorbic acid, thyroxine, and various trace elements. Of these, iron is the factor most commonly deficient in patients both with and without renal failure.

Iron absorption and metabolism

A haemoglobin molecule consists of four haem groups linked to four globin chains and can bind four oxygen molecules. Most of the iron in the circulation is destined to be used by developing red cells for haemoglobin synthesis. It is transported in the plasma bound to transferrin, a β-globulin, which binds 1.3 μg of iron/mg of protein at two binding sites capable of binding two ferric iron atoms. Transferrin interacts with a specific receptor to deliver iron to the developing cells.

The average daily iron loss is approximately 1 mg in men and 2 mg in menstruating women. An average Western diet contains about 14 mg daily and, under normal conditions, 5–10 per cent of this is absorbed. Therefore, dietary intake usually provides sufficient iron to balance the daily loss, but is insufficient when daily losses are increased, despite absorption from the intestine being increased. The availability of iron in the food depends on the extent to which it is released by peptic digestion. Absorbed iron that is in excess of cell requirements stimulates the synthesis of ferritin, a soluble protein that is capable of storing iron. In normal subjects in a steady state of erythropoiesis, the plasma ferritin concentration correlates well with iron stores. Premenopausal women have lower mean values (about 30 μg/l) than men (about 100 μg/l). These correspond to total body iron stores of 300 and 1000 mg, respectively.

Pathogenesis of anaemia in chronic renal failure

Characteristics of anaemia in chronic renal failure

The peripheral blood film from a uraemic patient usually reveals a normochromic, normocytic anaemia, occasionally with fragmented red cells or 'burr' cells. The reticulocyte count is low for the degree of anaemia; the white cell count is usually normal. There may be reduced, normal, or increased cellularity of the bone marrow and the myeloid–erythroid ratio may be decreased. There is a reduced red cell mass, but normal total blood volume except in patients who are fluid overloaded (Cotes et al. 1989).

Early work demonstrated that 'uraemic anaemia' was largely the result of depressed erythropoiesis (Desforges 1970), but a reduced red cell lifespan was also found to contribute (Eschbach et al. 1967). The depression of erythropoiesis is primarily due to relative erythropoietin deficiency. Iron or folate deficiency, aluminium toxicity, and marrow fibrosis resulting from hyperparathyroidism can also contribute to renal anaemia, while the existence of 'uraemic inhibitors of erythropoiesis' remains controversial.

Erythropoietin production in renal disease

Chronic kidney disease

Insufficient erythropoietin production is the major reason for the anaemia that develops during chronic renal disease of different aetiology. The plasma erythropoietin concentration is inappropriately low for the degree of anaemia. In anephric subjects, who tend to have more severe anaemia, erythropoietin concentrations are particularly low, but still measurable (Naets et al. 1986); the erythropoietin is probably produced by the liver (Fried 1972).

The mechanisms of inadequate erythropoietin production have not been completely resolved. Focal injury is associated with focal reduction in erythropoietin expression, indicating that the mechanisms involved are predominantly local (Maxwell et al. 1997). Interestingly, renal injury frequently leads to a transformation of peritubular fibroblasts into myofibroblasts, and this switch appears to be associated with a reduced capacity for erythropoietin gene expression (Maxwell et al. 1997). Other evidences suggest that a considerable production capacity for erythropoietin is preserved in chronic renal disease and that the main problem is a blunted response to the signals that stimulate erythropoietin gene expression. Thus, patients with chronic renal failure and anaemia can respond with a significant increase in erythropoietin production in response to an additional hypoxic stimulus (Chandra et al. 1988; Cotes et al. 1989). Animals with experimentally induced kidney failure show a large rise in erythropoietin mRNA and plasma erythropoietin levels in response to severe hypoxic stimulation (Tan et al. 1991, 1996). Possible reasons for this reduced response to low haemoglobin concentrations include: local accumulation of proinflammatory cytokines (Faquin et al. 1992) and a lack of renal oxygen consumption preserving renal tissue Po_2 (Priyadarshi et al. 2002).

Although renal anaemia develops largely independent of the aetiology of kidney disease, there are some exceptions. In some patients with diabetes, anaemia can occur at much lesser degrees of renal failure than in other types of chronic kidney disease (Bosman et al. 2001). Conversely, the degree of anaemia in patients with chronic renal failure caused by autosomal dominant polycystic kidney disease is generally less severe than for other diseases.

Cystic kidney disease

Occasionally, patients with polycystic kidney disease may even become polycythaemic (Maggiore et al. 1986). Haemodialysis patients with acquired renal cysts and single cysts may also develop erythrocytosis (Goldsmith et al. 1982). Serum erythropoietin concentrations in patients with autosomal dominant polycystic kidney disease are, on average, twofold greater than in endstage renal disease of non-cystic origin (Chandra et al. 1985; Besarab et al. 1987) and significant arteriovenous concentration differences for erythropoietin exist in polycystic kidneys (Eckardt et al. 1989b). It is believed therefore that the greater haemoglobin values in these patients result from a comparatively greater production of erythropoietin. The mechanisms by which cysts stimulate erythropoietin production have not been resolved, although it is conceivable that compression and remodelling of pericystic tissue leads to local hypoxia. In the cyst walls of patients with autosomal polycystic kidney disease interstitial cells have been shown to express erythropoietin mRNA, and cysts derived from proximal, but not distal tubules, contain increased concentrations of bioactive erythropoietin (Eckardt et al. 1989b).

Renal allotransplantation

Renal transplantation is usually followed by full correction of renal anaemia (Rejman et al. 1985; Besarab et al. 1987; Sun et al. 1989). Interestingly, a regular increase of erythropoietin formation is not related to the presence of the transplant, but correlates with the onset of graft function (Eckardt et al. 1989a), which provides further evidence for the role of excretory renal function for erythropoietin regulation. Some 10–17 per cent of patients manifest overcorrection and develop erythrocytosis, usually within the first 6 months following transplantation. Selective venous catheterization studies and the response to removal of the native kidneys suggest that increased red cell production in these patients is due to enhanced, dysregulated erythropoietin production by the native kidneys (Thevenod et al. 1983; Aeberhard et al. 1990). Although this clearly indicates that a sufficient production capacity for erythropoietin may be preserved in diseased kidneys, it is unclear how the secretion rate is influenced by transplantation. In other patients with transplant polycythaemia, the circulating erythropoietin concentrations are normal or reduced, and it may be that in these cases there is an increased sensitivity of the erythroid progenitor cells to erythropoietin, or loss of the feedback control mechanisms.

Renal artery stenosis

In patients with renal artery stenosis the oxygen supply to the kidneys is reduced, but the data on erythropoietin production in this situation are contradictory. In experimental animals enhancement of erythropoietin production following renal artery stenosis has been shown by some, but not all, investigators (Jelkmann 1986). This inconsistency is compatible with the rarity of secondary polycythaemia in patients with renal artery stenosis (Luke et al. 1965; Bourgoignie et al. 1968). A study performed in rats revealed that graded reduction of renal blood flow to 10 per cent of the control value caused a maximal threefold increase of serum erythropoietin concentrations (Pagel et al. 1988). In summary, these findings indicate that renal erythropoietin production is rather insensitive to changes in renal blood flow. This may at first seem surprising, but it should be remembered that it is the ratio of oxygen demand to oxygen delivery that governs erythropoietin production, and alterations of renal blood flow can cause simultaneous changes of both parameters (see above).

Renal tumours

Up to 5 per cent of patients with renal carcinomas have an erythrocytosis (Kazal and Erslev 1975) and 35 per cent of tumour-associated erythrocytosis is caused by renal cancer (Hammond and Winnick 1974).

Conflicting data have been reported concerning serum erythro-poietin concentrations in patients with renal tumours, but in some, raised concentrations have been found (Sufrin *et al.* 1977). Furthermore, overexpression of erythropoietin mRNA has been shown in single cases of renal tumours. *In situ* hybridization revealed that accumula-tion of erythropoietin mRNA occurs in epithelial tumour cells, but not interstitial cells of the tumour stroma (DaSilva *et al.* 1990). The recent discovery of the role of the pVHL in the regulation of HIF has renewed interest in the expression of hypoxia-inducible genes in kidney tumours, since the majority of clear cell renal carcinomas—the most frequent type of renal cancer—are associated with mutations of the VHL gene (Motzer *et al.* 1996). Indeed, clear cell renal carcinomas contain high concentrations of HIF, as a consequence of impaired degradation of the transcription factor (Wiesener *et al.* 2001, 2002). Although stabilized HIF in renal tumours appears to be functionally active in inducing HIF-target genes, it is yet unclear why overexpres-sion of erythropoietin is comparatively rare.

Erythropoietin production and drugs

Although the regulation of erythropoietin is obviously due to a complex interaction of various parameters of renal haemodynamics and oxy-genation, few drugs have so far been found to exert a significant influ-ence on erythropoietin production. Acetazolamide has been shown to reduce hypoxia-induced elevations in serum erythropoietin. Depending on the dose, this may be due to a decrease in pH, which is known to sup-press erythropoietin production (Miller *et al.* 1973) or due to inhibition of proximal tubular sodium transport (Eckardt *et al.* 1989c). Inhibition of erythropoietin production is also seen after administration of angiotensin-converting enzyme inhibitors and angiotensin II receptor antagonists, and these drugs have been used successfully to reduce the haematocrit in patients developing erythrocytosis after renal trans-plantation (Gaston *et al.* 1991; Julian *et al.* 1998). Since angiotensin-converting enzyme (ACE) inhibitors reduce efferent arteriolar resistance, it is conceivable that they increase peritubular oxygenation, and hence reduce the signal for erythropoietin production, through a combined effect of increased peritubular blood flow and decreased glomerular filtration (and thus tubular oxygen consumption); altern-atively they may act by enhancing the blood levels of a circulating physiological inhibitor of erythropoiesis: *N*-acetyl-seryl-lysyl-proline (AcSDKP) (Le Meur *et al.* 2001).

A second drug that has been proposed to reduce erythropoietin concentrations in patients with post-transplant erythrocytosis is theo-phylline (Bakris *et al.* 1990). It has been suggested that this effect is due to its role as an adenosine antagonist, but animal experiments failed to show a significant role of adenosine in the regulation of erythropoietin production (Gleiter *et al.* 1997).

Reduced red cell life span

The erythrocyte life span in chronic renal failure decreases with pro-gressive severity of uraemia and may be reduced to one-third of normal. Early experiments, in which red cell survival was found to normalize when cells from uraemic individuals were transfused into non-uraemic recipients and, conversely, red blood cells from non-uraemic donors were prematurely destroyed after transfusion into uraemic patients, suggested that the main reason for shortened red cell survival is extracor-puscular (Loge *et al.* 1958). However, the number of patients enrolled in these studies was small. Many of them were seriously ill, in the

terminal stages of uraemia, so that this conclusion may not generally hold true. In fact, other studies demonstrated that red cells from uraemic patients have an increased susceptibility towards mechanical, oxidative and osmotic stress (Rosenmund *et al.* 1975), suggesting that corpuscular factors also play a role in premature red cell destruction. Several abnormalities of uraemic red cells have been described, includ-ing abnormalities in sodium transport. However, the mechanisms by which uraemia affects red cell metabolism and the precise biochem-ical basis of reduced erythrocyte survival have not been resolved. Actual haemolysis can be caused by toxic contaminants of dialysate, including zinc (Petrie and Row 1977), copper (Manzler and Schreiner 1970), nitrates (Carlson and Shapiro 1970), formaldehyde (Orringer and Mattern 1976), and chloramines (Eaton *et al.* 1973; Richardson *et al.* 1999). In the absence of such water impurities, haemodialysis does not seem to cause significant haemolysis (Lerner *et al.* 1983).

'Uraemic inhibitors' of erythropoiesis (see Chapter 11.3.1)

Whether substances accumulating as a consequence of reduced renal function ('uraemic inhibitors') impair erythropoiesis is controversial. The effect of recombinant human erythropoietin has proven that the action of such inhibitors, if present at all, can usually be overcome. Additional lines of evidence cast doubt upon the relevance of several of the proposed inhibitory mechanisms. First, although serum from uraemic patients may inhibit the growth of murine or canine ery-throid cells *in vitro* (Wallner and Vautrin 1981; McGonigle *et al.* 1984), this inhibition is non-specific. Not only erythropoiesis but also *in vitro* granulopoiesis and megakaryopoiesis are inhibited (Delwiche *et al.* 1986), but leucopenia and thrombocytopenia are not usual con-sequences of chronic renal failure. Second, for none of the putative inhibitors of erythropoiesis, for example, spermine (Radtke *et al.* 1981) has specific and direct inhibition of erythropoiesis been demon-strated. The inhibition of erythropoiesis with parathyroid extracts could not be reproduced with pure parathyroid hormone and the inhibitory effect of hyperparathyroidism is considered to be primarily due to myelofibrosis rather than to a direct inhibitory effect of the hor-mone (Meytes *et al.* 1981; Drueke and Eckardt 2002). Inhibition of erythroid progenitor cells with uraemic serum in the presence of erythropoietin could not be reproduced, when entirely autologous *in vitro* culture systems were employed (Segal *et al.* 1988). Finally, marrow cells from patients with endstage renal disease respond nor-mally to erythropoietin *in vitro* (Delwiche *et al.* 1986). Also the res-ponse to recombinant human erythropoietin *in vivo* was not found to be reduced in patients with chronic renal failure compared with normal volunteers (Eschbach 1992).

On the other hand, the initiation of haemodialysis and peritoneal dialysis is often followed by an improvement in haemoglobin concen-tration (Zappacosta *et al.* 1982; De Paeple *et al.* 1983). Also an increase in the intensity of dialysis can induce a rise in haemoglobin concen-trations in patients with and without recombinant human erythro-poietin therapy (Koch *et al.* 1974; Ifudu *et al.* 1996). Furthermore, lack of cofactors for erythropoiesis, such as iron and folate, and inflam-mation may impair the responsiveness of the bone marrow towards ery-thropoietin and eventually cause erythropoietin resistance. The latter may be due to enhanced T cell production of proinflammatory cytokines such as TNF-alpha and interferon-gamma (Cooper *et al.* 2003), which can suppress erythropoiesis in the bone marrow.

The role of aluminium

Severe aluminium overload in haemodialysis patients is associated with a microcytic anaemia (O'Hare *et al.* 1983; Touam *et al.* 1983), which improves when dialysate aluminium is reduced by deionization of the water supply (O'Hare and Murnaghan 1982) or when the aluminium overload is treated with intravenous desferrioxamine (Tielemans *et al.* 1985). Trials of desferrioxamine therapy for less severe aluminium overload in dialysis patients without microcytosis have also shown an improvement in anaemia (Altmann *et al.* 1988; de La Serna *et al.* 1988). The suggestion is that this improvement is an effect of aluminium binding by desferrioxamine that prevents the aluminium inhibiting the erythroid marrow by interfering with iron transport and/or its utilization or inhibition of haem synthesis.

Iron and folate deficiency

Patients with chronic kidney disease are prone to blood loss caused by the regular dialysis procedure, blood sampling, and gastrointestinal bleeding. It has been estimated that the annual blood loss in haemodialysis patients from dialysers and blood tests alone is between 1 and 4 l (Hocken and Marwah 1971). Although dialyser blood loss has been reduced by modern dialysers and dialysis techniques, it remains significant (Salahudeen *et al.* 1983). In renal patients with unusually severe anaemia, excessive blood loss was identified as the predominant cause (Linton *et al.* 1977). Mild gastrointestinal blood loss is common in patients with chronic renal failure. Significant alimentary losses have been measured, using ^{51}Cr-labelled red cells, even when the routine chemical screening for occult blood in the faeces was negative (Linton *et al.* 1977). In the era of recombinant human erythropoietin, the importance of blood loss is the iron loss associated with it. Because 1 ml of blood with a normal haemoglobin concentration contains 0.5 mg of iron, an annual blood loss of around 2 l corresponds to almost 1 g of iron, exceeding the amount normally absorbed. There is additional, albeit controversial evidence that the physiological increase in iron absorption under conditions of iron deficiency is impaired in patients with renal disease. Thus, regular iron supplementation, mostly via the intravenous route, has become an important part of the management of renal anaemia (Macdougall 1994; Sunder-Plassmann and Hörl 1997).

Folate is required for DNA synthesis, and deficiency results in a megaloblastic erythroid marrow and a macrocytic anaemia. Adequacy of folate supply is best estimated by measuring red cell folate rather than serum folate. Although folate loss through dialysis is greater than by urinary excretion, the losses are usually balanced by a normal Western diet. However, a diagnosis of folate deficiency should be considered in patients with chronic renal insufficiency and a significant elevation in mean cell volume (Hampers *et al.* 1967; Schäefer *et al.* 2002).

Several drugs used in the treatment of malignancy have antagonistic effects on folate, but the use of these in patients with renal failure is uncommon. Anticonvulsant drugs, such as phenytoin, have also been associated with the development of folate deficiency. The mechanism is uncertain, but is probably related either to induction of liver enzymes and increased folate metabolism, or to altered absorption.

Inflammation

Chronic infection and inflammation have long been associated with anaemia, but it is only with the introduction of recombinant human erythropoietin for treatment of anaemia in dialysis patients that the effect of inflammation on anaemia in chronic renal failure has become more clear. It has been observed that surgery, inflammatory disease such as pericarditis or vasculitis, bacterial infections, and malignancy may all reduce the response to recombinant human erythropoietin (Macdougall 1995). The reduced response is characterized by a reduced reticulocyte count and a decline in haemoglobin concentration, and this may not improve for several weeks after resolution of the inflammatory event (Adamson and Eschbach 1989). The mechanism of this effect may be mediated by one or more inflammatory cytokines interacting with erythropoietin and thereby inhibiting its action at the cellular level. Both TNF-α and interferon-γ have been strongly implicated in this process (Means and Krantz 1992). In addition, inflammation impairs iron availability for erythropoiesis.

Other haematological effects associated with chronic renal failure

Leucocyte abnormalities (see Chapter 11.3.11)

In the myeloid lineage, a reduction in the capacity of the bone marrow to generate granulocytes has been documented in renal failure, and there is evidence for accelerated leucocyte apoptosis, as well as enhanced peripheral consumption of neutrophils by the dialyser (Lusvarghi 1994; Jaber *et al.* 2001; Tsuruoka *et al.* 2002). Thus, some dialysis patients may show a borderline neutropenia. Moreover, substances accumulating in uraemia, including so-called granulocyte inhibitory proteins, lead to reduced chemotaxis, oxidative activity, intracellular killing of bacteria, and impaired glucose consumption by polymorphonuclear leucocytes (Hörl 2001). There is also evidence for increased oxidative damage to peripheral blood leucocyte DNA in dialysis patients (Tarng *et al.* 2002). Monocyte function has also been reported to be impaired in dialysis patients, with various studies showing defective antigen presentation, a decrease in chemotactic response (Haniki *et al.* 1979), and a reduction in phagocytic activity (Roccatello *et al.* 1989). *In vitro* production of several cytokines (interleukin-1, interleukin-6, and tumour necrosis factor) from monocytes in uraemic patients is altered, partly affected by the nature of the dialysis membrane (Pertosa *et al.* 1991).

Various abnormalities in the function of T- and B-lymphocytes have been described (Beaurain *et al.* 1989; Alexiewics *et al.* 1990). On the other hand, there is evidence suggesting that the intrinsic function of T- and B-cells is normal when they are provided with normal signalling from antigen-presenting cells. Defective function of costimulation derived from antigen-presenting cells can, however, lead to impaired activation of effector lymphocytes (Girndt *et al.* 2001). In addition, there is increased susceptibility to early activated T-cell apoptosis in association with uraemia, which is enhanced by the dialysis procedure and can account for T-lymphopenia (Meier *et al.* 2002). Furthermore, uraemia is associated with a prevalence of Th1 over Th2 cells and a configuration of cytokine network that depresses cell-mediated immunity (Libetta *et al.* 2001).

These impaired granulocyte, monocyte, and lymphocyte functions contribute to the chronic immunodeficiency state that is characteristic of uraemia. This causes cutaneous anergy, prolonged allograft survival, an increased incidence of infections, in particular due to Gram-negative organisms and mycobacteria, and a reduced efficacy of vaccinations, for example, to hepatitis B. In spite of continuing improvements in haemodialysis techniques, the immune response of uraemic patients remains poor. Paradoxically, however, it is increasingly recognized that uraemia is also associated with enhanced immune activation, causing propagation of proinflammatory cytokines (Kimmel *et al.* 1998).

Platelet abnormalities (see Chapter 11.3.12)

The main defect in the platelets in uraemia relates to abnormalities of their function, causing haemostatic problems characterized by a prolonged bleeding time (Lindsay *et al.* 1975). This seems to be partly due to a defect in the expression and activation of the glycoprotein adhesion receptors, causing both impaired platelet aggregation and adhesion to endothelium (Benigni *et al.* 1993; Salvati 2001). In addition, platelet volume and the circulating platelet mass are reduced in chronic renal failure, possibly due to a reduction in thrombopoietin concentrations or activity (Caster *et al.* 1987). The mean platelet lifespan is reduced in uraemic patients with a GFR of 15–30 ml/min, which is corrected to normal after ~12 months treatment with regular haemodialysis (Lusvarghi *et al.* 1979). The platelet membrane is affected by increased activity of O_2 free radicals and under certain circumstances this can be reversed by vitamin E (Taccone-Gallucci *et al.* 1989). Platelets from uraemic subjects release diminished quantities of ATP, show a selective defect in the pool of deposited serotonin, show increased L-arginine influx, and have an increased ability to synthesize thromboxane A_2 (Barradas *et al.* 1991; Mendes Ribeiro *et al.* 1999).

The functional platelet defect of uraemia has been reported to be transiently reversed by the administration of DDAVP® (desmopressin) (Mannucci *et al.* 1983) or conjugated oestrogens (Livio *et al.* 1986) intravenously. The mechanism by which DDAVP® causes this effect is possibly the release of von Willebrand factor multimers from storage sites into the plasma. Oestrogens may act by inhibiting vascular prostacyclin. Correction of anaemia by blood transfusion or recombinant human erythropoietin also reverses the prolonged bleeding time of uraemia (see below).

Clinical aspects of anaemia management

Prevalence of anaemia in chronic renal failure

The anaemia in patients with chronic kidney disease increases progressively in severity as renal function deteriorates such that, prior to the advent of erythropoietin therapy, patients starting dialysis had haemoglobin concentrations of about 6–8 g/dl. Only about 3 per cent of patients had a normal haematocrit (Charles *et al.* 1981). Traditionally, anaemia was considered as a rather late complication of kidney disease. Although it becomes most evident when GFR is reduced to about one-third of normal, more recent data indicate, however, that the haemoglobin level starts to decline at much lesser degrees of renal impairment and on average is significantly reduced at GFR levels below 60 ml/min/1.73 m^2 (Kazmi *et al.* 2001; Astor *et al.* 2002). It is observed that patients with diabetic nephropathy have more severe anaemia than patients with chronic kidney disease of other aetiologies.

Indeed, some diabetics with very early nephropathy, defined as a normal or mildly reduced GFR, suffer from an erythropoietin-deficient anaemia (Bosman *et al.* 2001).

Before the days of erythropoietin therapy, up to 10 per cent of dialysis patients were transfusion dependent, the risk being greatest in those who were anephric.

As a group, haemodialysis patients tended to have more severe anaemia than those on continuous ambulatory peritoneal dialysis (CAPD). Factors proposed to explain this included a greater degree of blood loss or haemolysis in haemodialysis patients, and better removal of 'uraemic middle molecules'. Sequential comparative studies of changes in haemoglobin concentration after starting dialysis showed a greater initial increase in CAPD patients compared with those on haemodialysis, but after 5 years there was no longer any difference (Fig. 8). Likewise, studies of red cell mass in haemodialysis and CAPD patients suggested that there was little difference between the two modalities of treatment (Salahudeen *et al.* 1983).

The severity of anaemia in dialysis patients is independent of the aetiology of their endstage renal disease, with the exception of patients with adult polycystic kidney disease who tend to have higher haemoglobin concentrations. A marked increase in haemoglobin and even polycythaemia can also occur in dialysis patients who develop acquired cystic disease of the kidneys. The mechanism of this effect is thought to be excessive secretion of erythropoietin from the cyst walls (see above).

Physiological consequences of anaemia in chronic renal failure

In anaemia, there is a reduced delivery of oxygen to the tissues, which causes a variety of signs and symptoms in patients with chronic renal failure which may be difficult to distinguish from the symptoms of uraemia.

Various physiological adaptations occur to compensate for the suboptimal oxygen delivery, and these include modulation of the affinity of haemoglobin for oxygen, an increase in cardiac output, and redistribution of blood flow from the skin to other organs. The symptoms and signs of anaemia include tiredness, lethargy, muscle fatigue, breathlessness at rest or on exertion, angina, palpitations, tachycardia, increased sensitivity to cold, loss of appetite, loss of libido, menstrual irregularity, poor memory and concentration, and impaired cognitive and neurophysiological function.

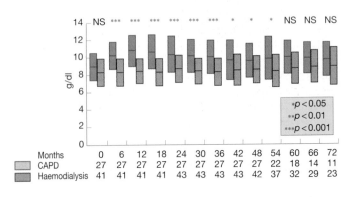

Fig. 8 Changes in haemoglobin concentration in previously untreated patients treated with haemodialysis or CAPD for at least 4 years (mean ± SD) (reproduced with permission from Maiorca *et al.* 1988).

Bleeding diathesis

Severe renal failure is often associated with a bleeding tendency characterized by a prolonged skin bleeding time (Lindsay *et al.* 1975). Although uraemia results in various minor abnormalities of clotting factors and platelet function (see above), the level of haematocrit is of considerable importance. Correction of anaemia usually results in return of the bleeding time to normal; this effect is seen in response to both red cell transfusion (Livio *et al.* 1982; Fernandez *et al.* 1985) and erythropoietin therapy (Moia *et al.* 1987; Macdougall *et al.* 1991a). The mechanisms involved are poorly understood, but improved contact of platelets with the vessel wall, enhanced adenosine diphosphate production, and improved platelet function may all play a part.

Cardiovascular effects

There are various adaptive cardiovascular mechanisms to anaemia including an increase in cardiac output, hypoxia-induced peripheral vasodilatation (which with the decreased viscosity of anaemic blood reduces peripheral vascular resistance). In the long term, the chronic increase in cardiac output leads to a compensatory increase in left ventricular mass and thus contributes to left ventricular hypertrophy in some patients (Fig. 9). It is now recognized that the prevalence of left ventricular hypertrophy increases progressively with declining renal function and up to 75 per cent of patients commencing dialysis treatment have significant left ventricular hypertrophy (Fig. 10) (Levin *et al.* 1996; Parfrey *et al.* 1996). This, along with concomitant atheromatous coronary artery disease which is also present in many renal patients, and the reduced oxygen carrying capacity of anaemic blood, explains the high incidence of myocardial ischaemia and symptoms of angina in such patients. Other cardiac effects include an increase in left ventricular end-diastolic dimensions, impaired myocardial contractility, and both systolic and diastolic dysfunction. Exercise capacity in patients with chronic renal failure is severely impaired, as are measures of respiratory physiology such as the maximum oxygen consumption, anaerobic threshold, and diffusion capacity of the lungs. Many of these effects are reversed with correction of the anaemia by red cell

transfusion (Neff *et al.* 1971), renal transplantation (Himelman *et al.* 1988), or recombinant human erythropoietin (Macdougall *et al.* 1990b; see below), suggesting that anaemia contributes significantly to the cardiac abnormalities of renal failure.

Management of anaemia in chronic renal failure (see Chapter 12.6)

Haematinic supplements

Patients with chronic renal failure are prone to develop haematinic deficiencies as a result of dietary restrictions, poor appetite, and gastrointestinal blood loss. Since these are easy to detect and treat, it is vital that such patients are screened for vitamin B_{12}, folate, and (especially) iron deficiency, and supplements given as required.

Dialysis adequacy

An improvement in anaemia is seen in some patients during the first few months after starting dialysis, and this may be related to the intensity of dialysis treatment and to an enhanced red cell survival (Koch *et al.* 1974). The improvement in haemoglobin concentration is initially greater with CAPD than with haemodialysis (Summerfield *et al.* 1983), but by 3 years of treatment there is little difference between the two modalities (Maiorca *et al.* 1988). Plasma erythropoietin levels are decreased or unchanged on initiating dialysis (Summerfield *et al.* 1983), suggesting that other mechanisms are involved.

A cohort study of over 6000 haemodialysis patients in the United States from 1994 to 1998 showed that the dose requirements for recombinant human erythropoietin decreased as the urea reduction ratio (URR) increased, while the haematocrit increased as the URR increased (Colodonato *et al.* 2002). Similarly, in a study of 68 haemodialysis patients, Movilli *et al.* (2001) found that the weekly dose requirements of erythropoietin decreased as Kt/V increased. Multivariate regression analysis showed that Kt/V was the only independent variable affecting epoetin dose (Fig. 11). Increasing the intensity of dialysis can also improve the haemoglobin response to erythropoietin therapy (Ifudu *et al.* 1996).

Androgen therapy

In Europe and North America, androgens are no longer used in the management of renal anaemia, but they are still prescribed in some parts of the world (such as Turkey and South-East Asia) for their ability to reduce the dose requirements of epoetin (Navarro *et al.* 2003). Androgens

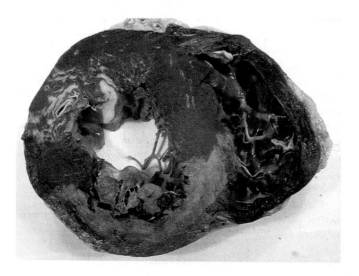

Fig. 9 Autopsy specimen of a section through the left ventricle, showing massive left ventricular hypertrophy as a consequence of longstanding hypertension and anaemia.

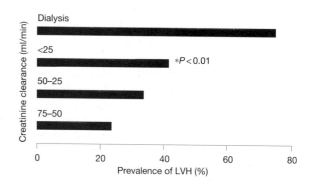

Fig. 10 Prevalence of left ventricular hypertrophy in relation to creatinine clearance (Levin *et al.* 1996).

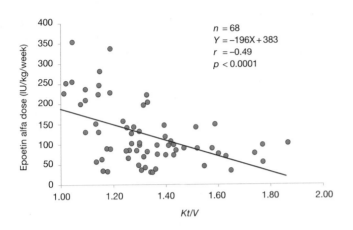

Fig. 11 Correlation between dialysis adequacy (*Kt/V*) and epoetin alfa dose.

increase erythropoiesis by stimulating endogenous erythropoietin production, either from residual renal tissue or from the liver, as well as through direct effects on red cell precursors (Alexanian *et al.* 1967; Koch *et al.* 1974). In some renal patients, androgens may cause partial relief of anaemia with a reduction in transfusion requirements (Eschbach and Adamson 1973), but they tend to be beneficial in mild cases only, and are limited by a high incidence of side-effects such as virilization, muscle and liver damage, and cholestasis (Neff *et al.* 1981).

Blood transfusion

In the era before recombinant erythropoietin many patients with renal failure required repeated blood transfusions in order to avoid the symptoms and complications of severe anaemia. This had several disadvantages (Chapter 12.6). Red cell transfusions are now used in the acute setting in erythropoietin resistant patients and in those with other causes of anaemia.

Erythropoietic agents

The advent of erythropoiesis-stimulating proteins (recombinant human erythropoietin and darbepoetin) is without doubt one of the greatest advances in nephrological practice over the last two decades. The rationale for its use was obvious. It has transformed the management of renal anaemia which previously relied on frequent blood transfusions with considerable disadvantages to the patient (see above).

Since licensing, several million patients worldwide have been treated with recombinant human erythropoietin. More recently, a second-generation erythropoietic protein called darbepoetin alfa has been licensed for the treatment of renal anaemia.

Pharmacokinetics of erythropoietin

In common with other therapeutic protein hormones such as insulin, recombinant human erythropoietin is inactivated by acid in the stomach, and therefore needs to be given parenterally. The early clinical trials in haemodialysis patients used intravenous erythropoietin administered thrice weekly; subsequently, the intraperitoneal, subcutaneous, and intradermal routes of administration were investigated (Boelaert *et al.* 1989; Macdougall *et al.* 1989).

After intravenous administration, erythropoietin levels decay monoexponentially, with an elimination half-life of approximately 4–11 h

(Macdougall *et al.* 1991c); some, but not all authors, found that the half-life was shortened with repeated administration (Egrie *et al.* 1988). The apparent volume of distribution of erythropoietin is about one to two times the plasma volume, and the total body clearance is slower than for other protein hormones such as insulin, glucagon, and prolactin.

The intraperitoneal route was investigated as a potential means of administering erythropoietin to patients on peritoneal dialysis. Following intraperitoneal administration, serum erythropoietin levels begin to rise after 1–2 h, and reach a peak at around 18 h (Macdougall *et al.* 1991c). However, the peak concentrations are only 2–5 per cent of those obtained with the same intravenous dose, and the bioavailability of intraperitoneal erythropoietin is disappointingly low at 3–8 per cent.

With subcutaneous administration, peak serum concentrations of about 4–10 per cent of an equivalent intravenous dose are obtained at around 12 h, and thereafter they decay slowly such that concentrations greater than baseline are still present at 4 days (Macdougall *et al.* 1989). The bioavailability of subcutaneous erythropoietin is about seven times that of intraperitoneal administration, at around 20–25 per cent, which is, however, low compared with insulin, heparin, and growth hormone.

Pharmacodynamics of erythropoietin

Based on pharmacokinetic studies, initial dosage regimens for erythropoietin employed thrice-weekly administration. This has remained the most popular dosage frequency for both intravenous and subcutaneous administration, although once-weekly (Macdougall 2002), twice-weekly, and seven-times-weekly (once-daily) dosing have all been used (Macdougall *et al.* 1992). With intravenous erythropoietin, once-weekly administration is inadequate, and twice- or thrice-weekly dosing is required. Many studies have compared the efficacy and dose requirements of erythropoietin administered intravenously versus subcutaneously, and most suggest that lower doses may be required if the subcutaneous route is used (Kaufman *et al.* 1998; Besarab *et al.* 2002).

Development of darbepoetin alfa

Darbepoetin alfa was created to extend the bioavailability of erythropoietin. The sialic acid residues on the glycosylation chains of human erythropoietin are critical to its metabolic survival *in vivo* (Egrie *et al.* 1993). Furthermore, isomers of erythropoietin containing greater numbers of sialic acid residues were found to be more bioactive *in vivo* and more resistant to metabolic degradation than lower-isomer erythropoietins. Using site-directed mutagenesis, a protein with a further two *N*-linked glycosylation sites, each of which could carry an additional four sialic acid residues, was generated (Egrie and Browne 2001). Thus, the new molecule (called darbepoetin alfa or 'novel erythropoiesis stimulating protein', NESP) contains five *N*-linked and one *O*-linked glycosylation chain(s), and has the capacity to carry up to 22 sialic acid residues, compared to a maximum of 14 sialic acid residues for original recombinant human erythropoietin (Fig. 12). The additional glycosylation on darbepoetin alfa results in a molecule weighing 37.1 kDa compared with 30.4 kDa for erythropoietin.

Pharmacokinetics of darbepoetin alfa

The initial pharmacokinetic study of darbepoetin alfa confirmed both the above hypothesis and the findings in an animal study that this erythropoietic agent had a longer half-life *in vivo* than recombinant

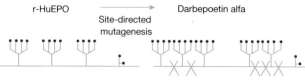

- 3 N-linked CHO chains
- Up to 14 sialic acid residues
- 30,400 Da
- 40% carbohydrate

- 5 N-linked CHO chains
- Up to 22 sialic acid residues
- 37,100 Da
- 51% carbohydrate

Fig. 12 Comparison of structures of recombinant human erythropoietin and darbepoetin alfa.

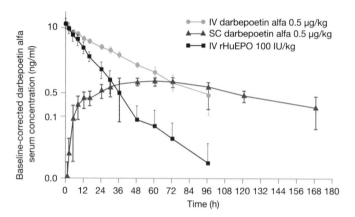

Fig. 13 Pharmacokinetics of intravenous darbepoetin alfa compared with intravenous epoetin alfa (from Macdougall *et al.* 1999).

human erythropoietin. In 11 stable CAPD patients, the elimination half-life of darbepoetin alfa was 25.3 h compared to 8.5 h for an equivalent peptide mass of epoetin alfa (Fig. 13) (Macdougall *et al.* 1999). The serum levels of darbepoetin alfa rose progressively following subcutaneous administration, reaching a peak at 18 h of approximately 10 per cent of that following the same dose administered intravenously. The elimination half-life after subcutaneous administration is around 48 h, which is approximately twice that previously reported for recombinant human erythropoietin.

Pharmacodynamics of darbepoetin alfa

The pharmacokinetic data suggested that darbepoetin alfa may be able to be administered less frequently than epoetin alfa or beta. A number of studies have examined once-weekly and once-every-other-week dosing (summarized in Macdougall 2001). Darbepoetin alfa can both correct and maintain haemoglobin levels at these dosing frequencies, and the side-effect profile is very similar to that of epoetin alfa or beta (Locatelli *et al.* 2001; Macdougall 2001). Several 'conversion' studies suggested that an appropriate conversion factor for switching patients on epoetin alfa or beta to darbepoetin alfa is 200 units of epoetin to 1 μg of darbepoetin alfa. The efficacy of intravenous and subcutaneous darbepoetin alfa dose-for-dose is very similar, in contrast to epoetin alfa or beta where approximately 30 per cent lower doses may be required if the drug is administered subcutaneously compared with intravenously (Kaufman *et al.* 1998).

Haematological effects of erythropoietic proteins

Approximately 90–95 per cent of dialysis patients treated with erythropoietin respond with an improvement in their anaemia (Eschbach *et al.* 1989). Following commencement of regular therapy, a significant increase in the reticulocyte count of around two to three times baseline is usually evident at 1 week, and an increase in haemoglobin concentration is seen by 2–3 weeks. The increase is dose dependent, and most physicians aim for an increment of not more than 1 g/dl/month in order to minimize the risk of adverse effects. There remains some controversy surrounding the optimum target haemoglobin; the European Best Practice Guidelines recommend greater than 11 g/dl while the NKF–DOQI Guidelines suggest 11–12 g/dl, and this is usually attained after 3–6 months of therapy (European Best Practice Guidelines 1999). Several randomized controlled 'normalization of haemoglobin' studies from the United States, Europe, and Canada sought to resolve this issue (Besarab *et al.* 1998; Foley *et al.* 2000; Furuland *et al.* 2003). The US study in high-risk cardiac patients found improved quality of life, but failed to show any benefit from higher haemoglobin levels on cardiac complications and survival, and may even have been harmful (Besarab *et al.* 1998). The Scandinavian and Canadian studies showed no detrimental effects from a higher target haemoglobin, but any benefits seen were fairly modest, considering how much more epoetin was required to achieve the higher haemoglobin levels (Foley *et al.* 2000; Moreno *et al.* 2000; Furuland *et al.* 2003).

The increase in haemoglobin concentration following erythropoietic therapy is associated with an increase in red cell count. No significant changes in white cell or platelet counts are usually seen although a clinically insignificant increase in the platelet count has been documented in a few patients. There is usually a dramatic decline in the serum ferritin concentration and/or the transferrin saturation following commencement of erythropoietin therapy, as large quantities of iron are used up in the manufacture of new red cells.

Radioisotopic blood volume studies confirmed that there is an increase in red cell mass after treatment with erythropoietin, which is associated with a compensatory reduction in plasma volume such that the whole blood volume remains unchanged. Ferrokinetic studies indicated that erythropoietin therapy induces a twofold increase in marrow erythropoietic activity, as evidenced by a doubling of marrow and red cell iron turnover (Cotes *et al.* 1989; Macdougall *et al.* 1990a). There is little or no change in mean red cell life-span after erythropoietin; thus, the increased red cell mass is largely accounted for by the production of greater numbers of red cells, rather than by any significant change in their survival.

Factors affecting response to erythropoietic agents

Many factors can influence the clinical response to erythropoietin (Macdougall 1995). Patients with more severe anaemia (haemoglobin <6 g/dl) at the onset of treatment generally require higher doses than those with mild anaemia (haemoglobin 6–8 g/dl) (Sundal and Kaeser 1989). The conditions which may adversely affect the response to erythropoietin are summarized in Table 3. All these factors should be considered in any patient failing to respond to treatment, or requiring excessive doses of epoetin alfa or beta (e.g. >200–300 U/kg/week) or darbepoetin alfa (e.g. >1–2 μg/kg/week), or losing a previous haemoglobin response. Functional iron deficiency, in particular, has become increasingly apparent in patients on erythropoietic therapy; many individuals who are iron-replete at the start of treatment become deficient under the influence of erythropoietin, and require intensive iron supplementation in order to maintain a haemoglobin response (Macdougall 1994). Dialysis patients often have increased occult gastrointestinal blood loss, partly due to a greater prevalence of gastritis and peptic ulceration, and partly due to an increased bleeding tendency due to both platelet dysfunction and heparin administration during dialysis. The presence of acute or chronic infection, inflammatory disease, or malignancy frequently causes marked inhibition of the response to erythropoietin, even at high doses (Macdougall 1995). This is thought to be mediated via changes in iron metabolism and/or suppression of erythropoiesis by other cytokines and growth factors (Means and Krantz 1992; Cooper *et al.* 2003).

Iron management (see Chapter 12.6) (Table 4)

Secondary effects of anaemia correction

Cardiovascular system

Longstanding severe anaemia has profound effects on the cardiovascular system as detailed above. Many of these effects have been shown to be reversed or improved following correction of anaemia by erythropoietin (Table 5). The increased cardiac output returns towards normal with correction of the anaemia (Teruel *et al.* 1991), the compensatory hypoxic vasodilatation is reversed (producing an increase in peripheral vascular resistance), and the mean arterial blood pressure increases in 20–30 per cent of patients. There are improvements in oxygen delivery to the myocardium, resulting in a reduction in symptoms of angina and in exercise-induced myocardial ischaemia (Macdougall *et al.* 1990b; Wizemann *et al.* 1992). Left ventricular mass also decreases

progressively following erythropoietin therapy, particularly when this is grossly elevated prior to treatment (Macdougall *et al.* 1990b; Löw-Friedrich *et al.* 1991; Pascual *et al.* 1991). This latter finding may have long-term implications for cardiovascular mortality, since left ventricular hypertrophy has been shown to be an independent determinant of survival in dialysis patients (Silberberg *et al.* 1989). The internal dimensions of the left ventricle in both systole and diastole decrease after erythropoietin therapy, and cardiac size therefore progressively diminishes (Löw-Friedrich *et al.* 1991). Finally, there are improvements in exercise physiology following erythropoietin therapy: exercise capacity, maximum oxygen consumption, anaerobic threshold, and carbon monoxide transfer factor have all been shown to increase (Mayer *et al.* 1988; Macdougall *et al.* 1990b).

Non-cardiovascular effects

The list of secondary effects associated with erythropoietin therapy is impressive (Table 6). Studies on the coagulation and haemostatic pathways, prompted by the early observation of possible increased vascular access thrombosis with erythropoietin, have documented a reduction in bleeding time along with improvements in platelet function, both aggregation and adhesion to endothelium (Vigano *et al.* 1991). The standard coagulation tests are unaffected by erythropoietin, as are measurements of the coagulation factors. However, a prothrombotic state may develop, possibly contributed to by increased blood viscosity (Macdougall *et al.* 1991b), reductions in protein C and protein S levels (Macdougall *et al.* 1991a), and increases in thrombin-antithrombin III

Table 3 Factors inhibiting a response to erythropoietic therapy

Major	Minor
Iron deficiency	Hyperparathyroidism (with marrow fibrosis)
Underdialysis	Aluminium toxicity
Infection/inflammation	Vitamin B_{12}/folate deficiency
	Haemolysis
	Marrow disorders
	Haemoglobinopathies
	Blood loss
	Carnitine deficiency
	ACE inhibitors
	Obesity (for subcutaneous epoetin)
	Antierythropoietin antibodies

Table 4 Recommendations for monitoring iron status from European Best Practice Guidelines (Guideline 6)

Recommended levels	Serum ferritin > 100 μg/l
	Hypochromic red cells $< 10\%$
	Transferrin saturation $> 20\%$
Target values to aim for	Serum ferritin 200–500 μg/l
	Hypochromic red cells $< 2.5\%$
	Transferrin saturation 30–40%

Table 5 Cardiovascular effects of erythropoietin therapy

Increased exercise tolerance

Normalization of elevated cardiac output

Increased peripheral vascular resistance

Increased blood pressure (30% of patients)

Decreased symptoms of angina

Reduction in myocardial ischaemia

Reduction in left ventricular hypertrophy

Reduction in left ventricular internal dimensions

Decreased cardiac size on chest radiograph

Table 6 Non-cardiovascular effects of erythropoietin therapy

Improved quality-of-life

Improved brain/cognitive function

Decreased uraemic bleeding tendency

Improved platelet function

Improved sexual function

Improved endocrine function

Enhanced immune function

Decreased uraemic pruritus

levels (Taylor *et al.* 1992), Factor VIII-related activities (Huraib *et al.* 1991), and plasminogen activator inhibitor-1 production following erythropoietin.

The haematocrit is the major determinant of whole blood viscosity, and thus an erythropoietin-induced increase in red cell mass inevitably causes an increase in blood viscosity. Furthermore, the relationship between haematocrit and blood viscosity is exponential, such that a linear increase in the former results in a disproportionate increase in the latter. Detailed rheological studies have indicated that the increase in blood viscosity occurs solely as a result of the larger quantity of circulating red cells, without any change in plasma viscosity or the rheology of the red cells themselves in terms of their deformability or aggregability (Macdougall *et al.* 1991b).

Objective assessments of quality-of-life parameters (Keown 1991; Moreno *et al.* 2000) and of brain and cognitive function (Marsh *et al.* 1991; Nissenson 1992) have also shown improvements following erythropoietin therapy. Patients report subjective improvements in memory, concentration, and other cerebral functions. Electrophysiological studies have shown an increase in amplitude of the P3 component of the brain event-related potential (Marsh *et al.* 1991), and higher scores in various neuropsychological tests have been recorded. These findings suggest that anaemia may be an important factor in the aetiology of uraemic brain dysfunction.

Impaired sexual function is common in dialysis patients; in females this is manifest by anovulation, amenorrhoea, and infertility, while in males impotence, reduced libido, oligospermia, and gynaecomastia are often present. Erythropoietin therapy has been shown to improve libido, potency, and sexual performance in males (Schaefer *et al.* 1989; Bommer *et al.* 1990), and a return of regular menstruation and even pregnancy (Gladziwa *et al.* 1992) has been reported in female dialysis patients. These effects may be partly mediated by changes in prolactin or testosterone levels since reductions in the former and increases in the latter have been found following erythropoietin treatment. Other diverse endocrine effects which have been reported in association with erythropoietin include suppressive effects on the renin–angiotensin system, the pituitary–adrenal axis, growth hormone levels, glucagon, gastrin, follicle stimulating hormone, and luteinizing hormone, while there are reported increases in plasma insulin, parathyroid hormone, and atrial natriuretic peptide (Kokot *et al.* 1989) (see Chapters 11.3.2 and 11.3.3).

Anaemia correction also appears to have effects on the immune system. Levels of circulating cytotoxic antibodies progressively decline in patients receiving erythropoietin therapy (Barany *et al.* 1992) and this effect is only partly due to the avoidance of blood transfusion. There is an increase in immunoglobulin production and proliferation of B cells, and an enhanced seroconversion response to hepatitis B vaccination (Sennesael *et al.* 1991). Phagocytic function in neutrophils is also increased (Veys *et al.* 1992). Uraemic pruritus is lessened following commencement of erythropoietin therapy, possibly due to a reduction in plasma histamine concentrations (De Marchi *et al.* 1992). The nutritional status of patients treated with erythropoietin has also been shown to improve (see Chapter 11.3.11).

Adverse effects of erythropoietic therapy (see Chapter 12.6)

The adverse effects of erythropoietic therapy and the features of epoetin-induced pure red cell aplasia are given in Tables 7 and 8, respectively.

Table 7 Adverse effects of erythropoietin therapy

Hypertension
Seizures/encephalopathy
Vascular access thrombosis
Clotting of dialysis lines
Hyperkalaemia
Myalgia/influenza-like symptoms
Skin irritation
Pure red cell aplasia (with antierythropoietin antibodies)

Table 8 Features of epoetin-induced pure red cell aplasia

Severe transfusion-dependent anaemia despite erythropoietic therapy
Reticulocyte count $< 10 \times 10^9/\text{l}$
Bone marrow shows absence ($<5\%$ erythroblasts) of red cell precursors, but normal white cell and platelet maturation
Normal circulating white cell and platelet counts
Neutralizing antibodies to human erythropoietin (detected by RIP or ELISA)

References

Adamson, J. W. and Eschbach, J. W. (1989). Management of the anaemia of chronic renal failure with recombinant erythropoietin. *Quarterly Journal of Medicine* **73**, 1093–1101.

Aeberhard, J. M., Schneider, P. A., Valloton, M. B., Kurtz, A., and Leski, M. (1990). Multiple site estimates of erythropoietin and renin in polycythemic kidney transplant patients. *Transplantation* **50**, 613–616.

Alexanian, R., Vaughn, W. K., and Ruchelman, M. W. (1967). Erythropoietin excretion in man following androgens. *Journal of Laboratory and Clinical Medicine* **70**, 777–785.

Alexiewics, J. M., Gaciong, Z., Klinger, M., Linker-Israeli, M., Pitts, T. O., and Massry, S. G. (1990). Evidence of impaired T cell function in hemodialysis patients: potential role for secondary hyperparathyroidism. *American Journal of Nephrology* **10**, 495–501.

Altmann, P., Plowman, D., Marsh, F., and Cunningham, J. (1988). Aluminium chelation therapy in dialysis patients: evidence for inhibition of haemoglobin synthesis by low levels of aluminium. *Lancet* **i**, 1012–1015.

Anagnostou, A., Lee, E. S., Kesseimian, N., Levinson, R., and Steiner, M. (1987). *Proceedings of the National Academy of Sciences USA* **87**, 5978–5982.

Astor, B. C. *et al.* (2002). Association of kidney function with anemia: The Third National Health and Nutrition Examination Survey (1988–1994). *Archives of Internal Medicine* **162**, 1401–1408.

Bachmann, S., LeHir, M., and Eckardt, K.-U. (1993). Co-localization of erythropoietin mRNA and ecto-5′-nucleotidase immunoreactivity in peritubular cells of rat renal cortex indicates that fibroblasts produce erythropoietin. *Journal of Histochemistry and Cytochemistry* **41**, 335–341.

Bakris, G. L., Sauter, E. R., Hussey, J. L., Fisher, J. W., Gaber, A. O., and Winsett, R. (1990). Effects of theophylline on erythropoietin production in normal subjects and in patients with erythrocytosis after renal transplantation. *New England Journal of Medicine* **323**, 86–90.

Bárány, P., Fehrman, I., and Godoy, C. (1992). Long-term effects on lymphocytotoxic antibodies and immune reactivity in hemodialysis patients treated with recombinant human erythropoietin. *Clinical Nephrology* **37**, 90–96.

Barradas, M. A. *et al.* (1991). Intraplatelet serotonin, beta-thromboglobulin, and histamine concentrations and thromboxane A2 synthesis in renal disease. *American Journal of Clinical Pathology* **96**, 504–511.

Bazan, J. F. (1990). Structural design and molecular evolution of a cytokine receptor superfamily. *Proceedings of the National Academy of Sciences USA* **87**, 6934–6938.

Beaurain, G. *et al.* (1989). *In vivo* T cell preactivation in chronic uremic hemodialyzed and non-hemodialyzed patients. *Kidney International* **36**, 636–644.

Beck, I., Ramirez, S., Weinmann, R., and Caro, J. (1991). Enhancer element at the 3′-flanking region controls transcriptional response to hypoxia in the human erythropoietin gene. *Journal of Biological Chemistry* **266**, 15563–15566.

Benigni, A. *et al.* (1993). Reversible activation defect of the platelet Glycoprotein IIb–IIIa complex in patients with uremia. *American Journal of Kidney Diseases* **22**, 668–676.

Berridge, M. V., Fraser, J. K., Carter, J. M., and Lin, F. K. (1988). Effects of recombinant human erythropoietin on megakaryocytes and on platelet production in the rat. *Blood* **72**, 970–977.

Besarab, A., Caro, J., Jarrell, B. E., Francos, G., and Erslev, A. J. (1987). Dynamics of erythropoiesis following renal transplantation. *Kidney International* **32**, 526–536.

Besarab, A., Kline Bolton, W., Browne, J. K., Egrie, J. C., Nissenson, A. R., Okamoto, D. M., Schwab, S. J., and Goodkin, D. A. (1998). The effects of normal as compared with low hematocrit values in patients with cardiac disease who are receiving hemodialysis and epoetin. *New England Journal of Medicine* **339**, 584–590.

Besarab, A., Reyes, C. M., and Hornberger, J. (2002). Meta-analysis of subcutaneous versus intravenous epoetin in maintenance treatment of anemia in hemodialysis patients. *American Journal of Kidney Diseases* **40**, 439–446.

Blanchard, K. L., Aquavia, A. M., Galson, D. L., and Bunn, H. F. (1992). Hypoxic induction of the human erythropoietin gene: cooperation between the promoter and enhancer, each of which contains steroid receptor response elements. *Molecular and Cellular Biology* **12**, 5373–5385.

Boelaert, J. R. *et al.* (1989). Comparative pharmacokinetics of recombinant erythropoietin administered by the intravenous, subcutaneous and intraperitoneal routes in continuous ambulatory peritoneal dialysis patients. *Peritoneal Dialysis International* **9**, 95–98.

Bommer, J., Kugel, M., Schwöbel, B., Ritz, E., Barth, H. P., and Seelig, R. (1990). Improved sexual function during recombinant human erythropoietin therapy. *Nephrology, Dialysis, Transplantation* **5**, 204–207.

Bondurant, M. C. and Koury, M. J. (1986). Anemia induces accumulation of erythropoietin mRNA in the kidney and liver. *Molecular and Cell Biology* **6**, 2731–2733.

Bosman, D. R., Winkler, A. S., Marsden, J. T., Macdougall, I. C., and Watkins, P. J. (2001). Anemia with erythropoietin deficiency occurs early in diabetic nephropathy. *Diabetes Care* **24**, 495–499.

Bourgoignie, J. J., Gallagher, N. I., Perry, H. M., Jr., Kurz, L., Warnecke, M. A., and Donati, R. M. (1968). Renin and erythropoietin in normotensive and in hypertensive patients. *Journal of Laboratory and Clinical Medicine* **71**, 523–536.

Brines, M. L., Ghezzi, P., Keenan, S., Agnello, D., de Lanerolle, N. C., Cerami, C., Itir, L. M., and Cerami, A. (2000). Erythropoietin crosses the blood–brain barrier to protect against experimental brain injury. *Proceedings of the National Academy of Sciences USA* **97**, 10526–10531.

Carlini, R. G., Reyes, A. A., and Rothstein, M. (1995). Recombinant human erythropoietin stimulates angiogenesis *in vitro*. *Kidney International* **95**, 740–745.

Carlson, D. J. and Shapiro, F. L. (1970). Methemoglobinemia from well water nitrates; a complication of home dialysis. *Annals of Internal Medicine* **73**, 757–759.

Caro, J., Brown, S., Miller, O., Murray, T., and Erslev, A. J. (1979). Erythropoietin levels in uremic nephric and anephric patients. *Journal of Laboratory and Clinical Medicine* **93**, 449–458.

Caster, U., Bessler, H., Malachi, T., Zevin, D., Djaldetti, M., and Levi, J. (1987). Platelet count and thrombopoietic activity in patients with chronic renal failure. *Nephron* **45**, 207–210.

Chandra, M., Clemons, G. K., and McVicar, M. I. (1988). Relation of serum erythropoietin production in chronic renal failure. *Journal of Pediatrics* **113**, 1015–1021.

Chandra, M., Miller, M. E., Garcia, J. F., Mossey, R. T., and McVicar, M. (1985). Serum immunoreactive erythropoietin levels in patients with polycystic kidney disease as compared with other hemodialysis patients. *Nephron* **39**, 26–29.

Charles, G., Lundin, A. P., III, Delano, B. G., Brown, C., and Friedman, E. A. (1981). Absence of anemia in maintenance hemodialysis. *International Journal of Artificial Organs* **4**, 277–279.

Chen, C. and Sytkowski, A. J. The erythropoietin receptor and its signalling cascade. In *Erythropoietin: Molecular Biology and Clinical Use* (ed. W. F. P. Jelkmann), pp. 165–194. Johnson City, TN, USA: Graham Publishing Co., 2003.

Cooper, A. C., Mikhail, A., Lethbridge, M. W., Kemeny, D. M., and Macdougall, I. C. (2003). Increased expression of erythropoiesis inhibiting cytokines (IFN-gamma, TNF-alpha, IL-10, and IL-13) by T cells in patients exhibiting a poor response to erythropoietin therapy. *Journal of American Society of Nephrology* **14**, 1776–1784.

Cotes, P. M., Pippard, M. J., Reid, C. D. L., Winearls, C. G., Oliver, D. O., and Royston, J. P. (1989). Characterization of the anaemia of chronic renal failure and the mode of its correction by a preparation of human erythropoietin (r-HuEPO). An investigation of the pharmacokinetics of intravenous r-HuEPO and its effect on erythrokinetics. *Quarterly Journal of Medicine* **70**, 113–137.

DaSilva, J. L. *et al.* (1990). Tumor cells are the site of erythropoietin synthesis in human renal cancers associated with polycythemia. *Blood* **75**, 577–582.

De La Serna, F. J., Praga, M., Gilsanz, F., Rodicio, J. L., Ruilope, L. M., and Alcazar, J. M. (1988). Improvement in the erythropoiesis of chronic haemodialysis patients with desferrioxamine. *Lancet* **i**, 1009–1011.

De Marchi, S., Cecchin, E., Villalta, D., Sepiacci, G., Santini, G., and Bartoli, E. (1992). Relief of pruritus and decreases in plasma histamine concentrations during erythropoietin therapy in patients with uremia. *New England Journal of Medicine* **326**, 969–974.

Delwiche, F., Segal, G. M., Eschbach, J. W., and Adamson, J. W. (1986). Hematopoietic inhibitors in chronic renal failure: lack of *in vitro* specificity. *Kidney International* **29**, 641–648.

De Paepe, M. B. J., Schelstraete, K. H. G., Ringoir, S. M. G., and Lameire, N. H. (1983). Influence of continuous ambulatory peritoneal dialysis on the anemia of endstage renal disease. *Kidney International* **23**, 744–748.

Desforges, J. F. (1970). Anemia in uremia. *Archives of Internal Medicine* **126**, 808–811.

Dessypris, E. N., Gleaton, J. H., and Armstrong, O. L. (1987). Effect of human recombinant erythropoietin on human marrow megakaryocyte colony formation *in vitro*. *British Journal of Haematology* **65**, 265–269.

Dordal, M. S., Wang, F. F., and Goldwasser, E. (1985). The role of carbohydrate in erythropoietin action. *Endocrinology* **116**, 2293–2299.

Drüeke, T. B. and Eckardt, K.-U. (2002). Role of secondary hyperparathyroidism in erythropoietin resistance of chronic renal failure patients. *Nephrology, Dialysis, Transplantation* **17** (Suppl. 5), 28–31.

Eaton, J. W., Kolpin, C. F., Swofford, H. S., Kjellstrand, C. M., and Jacob, H. S. (1973). Chlorinated urban water: a cause of dialysis-induced hemolytic anemia. *Science* **181**, 463–464.

Eckardt, K.-U., Frei, U., Kliem, V., Bauer, C., Koch, K. M., and Kurtz, A. (1989a). Role of excretory graft function for erythropoietin formation after renal transplantation. *European Journal of Clinical Investigation* **20**, 564–574.

Eckardt, K.-U. *et al.* (1989b). Erythropoietin in polycystic kidneys. *Journal of Clinical Investigation* **84**, 1160–1166.

Eckardt, K.-U., Kurtz, A., and Bauer, C. (1989c). Regulation of erythropoietin formation is related to proximal tubular function. *American Journal of Physiology* **256**, 942–947.

Eckardt, K.-U., Drüeke, T., Leski, M., and Kurtz, A. (1991). Unutilized reserves: the production capacity for erythropoietin appears to be conserved in chronic renal disease. *Contributions to Nephrology* **88**, 18–31.

Eckardt, K.-U., LeHir, M., Tan, C. C., Ratcliffe, P. J., Kaissling, B., and Kurtz, A. (1992a). Renal innervation plays no role in oxygen dependent control of erythropoietin mRNA levels. *American Journal of Physiology* **263**, F925–F930.

Eckardt, K.-U. *et al.* (1992b). Distribution of erythropoietin producing cells in rat kidneys during hypoxic hypoxia. *Kidney International* **43**, 815–823.

Eckardt, K.-U., Ratcliffe, P. J., Tan, C. C., Bauer, C., and Kurtz, A. (1992c). Age-dependent expression of the erythropoietin gene in rat liver and kidneys. *Journal of Clinical Investigation* **89**, 753–760.

Eckardt, K.-U., Ring, A., Maier, M., Gess, B., Fabbro, D., and Kurtz, A. (1994). Hypoxia induced accumulation of erythropoietin mRNA in isolated hepatocytes is inhibited by protein kinase C. *Pflügers Archives, European Journal of Physiology* **426**, 21–30.

Egrie, J. C. and Browne, J. K. (2001). Development and characterization of novel erythropoiesis stimulating protein (NESP). *Nephrology, Dialysis, Transplantation* **16** (Suppl. 3), 3–13.

Egrie, J. C., Eschbach, J. W., McGuire, T., and Adamson, J. W. (1988). Pharmacokinetics of recombinant human erythropoietin administered to hemodialysis patients. *Kidney International* **33**, 262.

Egrie, J. C., Grant, J. R., Gillies, D. K., Aoki, K. H., and Strickland, T. W. (1993). The role of carbohydrate on the biological activity of erythropoietin. *Glycoconjugate Journal* **10**, 263.

Epstein, A. C. *et al.* (2001). *C. elegans* EGL-9 and mammalian homologs define a family of dioxygenases that regulate HIF by prolyl hydroxylation. *Cell* **107**, 43–54.

Erslev, A. J., Caro, J., and Besarab, A. (1985). Why the kidney? *Nephron* **41**, 213–216.

Eschbach, J. W. and Adamson, J. W. (1973). Improvement in the anemia of chronic renal failure with fluoxymesterone. *Annals of Internal Medicine* **78**, 527–532.

Eschbach, J. W., Downing, M. R., Egrie, J. C., Browne, J. K., and Adamson, J. W. (1989). USA multicenter clinical trial with recombinant human erythropoietin. *Contributions to Nephrology* **76**, 160–165.

Eschbach, J. W., Haley, N. R., Egrie, J. C., and Adamson, J. W. (1992). A comparison of the responses to recombinant human erythropoietin in normal and uremic subjects. *Kidney International* **42**, 407–416.

Eschbach, J. W., Jr., Funk, D., Adamson, J., Kuhn, I., Scribner, B. H., and Finch, C. A. (1967). Erythropoiesis in patients with renal failure undergoing chronic dialysis. *New England Journal of Medicine* **276**, 653–658.

European Best Practice Guidelines for the management of anaemia in patients with chronic renal failure (1999). *Nephrology, Dialysis, Transplantation* **14** (Suppl. 5), 1–50.

Fandrey, J. and Bunn, H. F. (1993). *In vivo* and *in vitro* regualtion of the erythropoietin mRNA: measurement by competitive polymerase chain reaction. *Blood* **81**, 617–623.

Faquin, W. C., Schneider, T. J., and Goldberg, M. A. (1992). Effect of inflammatory cytokines on hypoxia-induced erythropoietin production. *Blood* **79**, 1987–1994.

Fernandez, F. *et al.* (1985). Low haematocrit and prolonged bleeding time in uraemic patients: effect of red cell transfusions. *British Journal of Haematology* **59**, 139–148.

Foley, R. N. *et al.* (2000). Effect of hemoglobin levels in hemodialysis patients with asymptomatic cardiomyopathy. *Kidney International* **58**, 1325–1335.

Fraser, J. K., Tan, A. S., Lin, F.-K., and Berridge, M. V. (1989). Expression of specific high-affinity binding sites for erythropoietin in rat and mouse megakaryocytes. *Experimental Hematology* **17**, 10–16.

Fried, W. (1972). The liver as a source of extrarenal erythropoietin production. *Blood* **40**, 671–677.

Fukuda, M. N., Sasaki, H., Lopez, L., and Fukuda, M. (1989). Survival of recombinant erythropoietin in the circulation: the role of carbohydrates. *Blood* **73**, 90–99.

Furuland, H., Linde, T., Ahlmen, J., Christensson, A., Strombom, U., and Danielson, B. G. (2003). A randomized controlled trial of haemoglobin normalization with epoetin alpha in pre-dialysis and dialysis patients. *Nephrology, Dialysis, Transplantation* **18**, 353–361.

Gaston, R. S., Julian, B. A., Diethelm, A. G., and Curtis, J. J. (1991). Effects of enalapril on erythrocytosis after renal transplantation. *Annals of Internal Medicine* **115**, 954–955.

Girndt, M., Sester, M., Sester, U., Kaul, H., and Kohler, H. (2001). Molecular aspects of T- and B-cell function in uremia. *Kidney International* **78**, S206–S211.

Gladziwa, U., Dakshinamurty, K. V., Mann, H., and Siebert, H.-G. (1992). Pregnancy in a dialysis patient under recombinant human erythropoietin. *Clinical Nephrology* **37**, 215.

Gleiter, C., Brause, M., Delabar, U., and Eckardt, K.-U. (1997). Evidence against a major role of adenosine in oxygen-dependent regulation of erythropoietin in rats. *Kidney International* **52**, 338–344.

Goldberg, M. A., Gaut, C. C., and Bunn, H. F. (1991). Erythropoietin mRNA levels are governed by both the rate of gene transcription and posttranscriptional events. *Blood* **77**, 271–277.

Goldsmith, H. J. *et al.* (1982). Association between rising haemoglobin concentration and renal cyst formation in patients on long-term regular hemodialysis treatment. *Proceedings of the European Dialysis and Transplant Association* **19**, 313–318.

Graber, S. E. and Krantz, S. B. (1989). Erythropoietin: biology and clinical use. *Hematology/Oncology Clinics of North America* **3**, 369–400.

Halvorsen, S., Roh, B. L., and Fisher, J. W. (1968). Erythropoietin production in nephrectomized and hypophysectomized animals. *American Journal of Physiology* **215**, 349–352.

Hammond, D. and Winnick, S. (1974). Paraneoplastic erythrocytosis and ectopic erythropoietins. *Annals of the New York Academy of Sciences* **230**, 219–227.

Hampers, C. L., Streiff, R., Nathan, D. G., Snyder, D., and Merrill, J. P. (1967). Megaloblastic hematopoiesis in uremia and in patients on long-term hemodialysis. *New England Journal of Medicine* **276**, 551–554.

Haniki, Z., Cichocki, T., Komoroswka, Z., Sulowicz, W., and Smolenki, O. (1979). Some aspects of cellular immunity in untreated and maintenance hemodialysis patients. *Nephron* **23**, 273–275.

Himelman, R. B. *et al.* (1988). Cardiac consequences of renal transplantation: changes in left ventricular morphology and function. *Journal of the American College of Cardiology* **12**, 915–923.

Hocken, A. G. and Marwah, P. K. (1971). Iatrogenic contribution to anaemia of chronic renal failure. *Lancet* **i**, 164–165.

Hörl, W. H. (2001). Neutrophil function in renal failure. *Advances in Nephrology from the Necker Hospital* **31**, 173–192.

Huraib, S., Al-Momen, A. K., Gader, A. M. A., Mitwalli, A., Sulimani, F., and Abu-Aisha, H. (1991). Effect of recombinant human erythropoietin (rHuEpo) on the hemostatic system in chronic hemodialysis patients. *Clinical Nephrology* **36**, 252–257.

Ifudu, O., Feldman, J., and Friedman, E. A. (1996). The intensity of hemodialysis and the response to erythropoietin in patients with end-stage renal disease. *New England Journal of Medicine* **334**, 420–425.

Ishibashi, T., Koziol, J. A., and Burstein, S. A. (1987). Human recombinant erythropoietin promotes differentiation of murine megakaryocytes *in vitro*. *Journal of Clinical Investigation* **79**, 286–289.

Jaakkola, P. *et al.* (2001). Targeting of HIF-alpha to the von Hippel–Lindau ubiquitylation complex by O_2-regulated prolyl hydroxylation. *Science* **292**, 468–472.

Jaber, B. L., Cendoroglo, M., Balakrishnan, V. S., Perianayagam, M. C., King, A. J., and Pereira, B. J. (2001). Apoptosis of leucocytes: basic concepts and implications in uremia. *Kidney International* **78**, S197–S205.

Jacobs, K., Shoemaker, C., Rudersdorf, R., Neill, E. F., and Kaufman, R. J. (1985). Isolation and characterisation of genomic and cDNA clones of human erythropoietin. *Nature* **313**, 806–810.

Jelkmann, W. (1986). Renal erythropoietin: properties and production. *Reviews of Physiology, Biochemistry, and Pharmacology* **104**, 139–215.

Jones, S. S., D'Andrea, A. D., Haines, L. L., and Wog, G. G. (1990). Human erythropoietin receptor: cloning, expression and biologic characterization. *Blood* **76**, 31–35.

Julian, B. A., Brantley, R. R. J., Barker, C. V., Stopka, T., Gaston, R. S., Curtis, J. J., Lee, J. Y., and Prchal, J. T. (1998). Losartan, an angiotensin II type 1 receptor antagonist, lowers hematocrit in posttransplant erythrocytosis. *Journal of the American Society of Nephrology* **6**, 1104–1108.

Kaufman, J. S. *et al.* (1998). Subcutaneous compared with intravenous epoetin in patients receiving hemodialysis. Department of Veterans Affairs Cooperative Study Group on Erythropoietin in Hemodialysis patients. *New England Journal of Medicine* **339**, 578–583.

Kazal, L. A. and Erslev, A. J. (1975). Erythropoietin production in renal tumors. *Annals of Clinical and Laboratory Science* **5**, 98–109.

Kazmi, W. H. *et al.* (2001). Anemia: an early complication of chronic renal insufficiency. *American Journal of Kidney Diseases* **38**, 803–812.

Keown, P. A. (1991). Quality of life in end-stage renal disease patients during recombinant human erythropoietin therapy. *Contributions to Nephrology* **88**, 81–86.

Koch, K. M., Patyna, W. D., Shaldon, S., and Werner, E. (1974). Anemia of the regular hemodialysis patient and its treatment. *Nephron* **12**, 405–419.

Kokot, F., Wiecek, A., Grzeszczak, W., Klepacka, J., Klin, M., and Lao, M. (1989). Influence of erythropoietin treatment on endocrine abnormalities in haemodialyzed patients. *Contributions to Nephrology* **76**, 257–272.

Koury, M. J. and Bondurant, M. C. (1988). Maintenance by erythropoietin of viability and maturation of murine erythroid precursor cells. *Journal of Cellular Physiology* **137**, 65–71.

Koury, M. J. and Bondurant, M. C. (1990). Erythropoietin retards DNA breakdown and prevents programmed death in erythroid progenitor cells. *Science* **248**, 378–381.

Koury, S. T., Koury, M. J., Bondurant, M. C., Caro, J., and Graber, S. E. (1989). Quantitation of erythropoietin producing cells in kidneys of mice by *in situ* hybridization: correlation with hematocrit, renal erythropoietin mRNA, and serum erythropoietin concentration. *Blood* **74**, 645–651.

Koury, S. T., Bondurant, M. C., Koury, M. J., and Semenza, G. L. (1991). Localization of cells producing erythropoietin in murine liver by *in situ* hybridization. *Blood* **77**, 2497–2503.

Krantz, S. B. (1991). Erythropoietin. *Blood* **77**, 419–434.

Lando, D., Peet, D. J., Whelan, D. A., Gorman, J. J., and Whitelaw, M. L. (2002). Asparagine hydroxylation of the HIF transactivation domain a hypoxic switch. *Science* **295**, 858–861.

Law, M. L. *et al.* (1986). Chromosomal assignment of the human erythropoietin gene and its DNA polymorphism. *Proceedings of the National Academy of Sciences USA* **83**, 6920–6924.

Leichtweiss, H. P., Lübbers, D. W., Weiss, Ch., Baumgärtl, H., and Reschke, W. (1969). The oxygen supply of the rat kidney: measurement of intrarenal PO_2. *Pflügers Archives* **309**, 328–349.

Le Meur, Y., Lorgeot, V., Comte, L., Szelag, J. C., Aldigier, J. C., Leroux-Robert, C., and Praloran, V. (2001). Plasma levels and metabolism of AcSDKP in patients with chronic renal failure: relationship with erythropoietin requirements. *American Journal of Kidney Diseases* **38**, 510–517.

Lerner, R., Werner, B., Asaba, H., Ternstedt, B., and Elmqvist, E. (1983). Assessment of hemolysis in regular hemodialysis patients by measuring carbon monoxide production rate. *Clinical Nephrology* **20**, 239–243.

Levin, A. *et al.* (1996). Prevalent left ventricular hypertrophy in the predialysis population: identifying opportunities for intervention. *American Journal of Kidney Diseases* **34**, 125–134.

Libetta, C., Rampino, T., and Dal Canton, A. (2001). Polarization of T-helper lymphocytes toward the Th2 phenotype in uremic patients. *American Journal of Kidney Diseases* **38**, 286–295.

Lin, F. K. *et al.* (1985). Cloning and expression of the human erythropoietin gene. *Proceedings of the National Academy of Sciences USA* **82**, 7580–7584.

Lindsay, R. M., Moorthy, A. V., Koens, F., and Linton, A. L. (1975). Platelet function in dialyzed and non-dialyzed patients with chronic renal failure. *Clinical Nephrology* **4**, 52–57.

Linton, A. L., Clark, W. F., Driedger, A. A., Werb, R., and Lindsay, R. M. (1977). Correctable factors contributing to the anemia of dialysis patients. *Nephron* **19**, 95–98.

Livio, E. *et al.* (1986). Conjugated estrogens for the management of bleeding associated with renal failure. *New England Journal of Medicine* **315**, 731–735.

Livio, M., Marchesi, D., Remuzzi, G., Gotti, E., Mecca, G., and De Gaetano, G. (1982). Uraemic bleeding: role of anaemia and beneficial effect of red cell transfusions. *Lancet* **ii**, 1013–1015.

Locatelli, F. *et al.* (2001). Novel erythropoiesis stimulating protein for treatment of anemia in chronic renal insufficiency. *Kidney International* **60**, 741–747.

Loge, J. P., Lange, R. D., and Moore, C. V. (1958). Characterization of the anemia associated with chronic renal insufficiency. *American Journal of Medicine* **24**, 4–18.

Lok, S. *et al.* (1994). Cloning and expression of murine thrombopoietin cDNA and stimulation of platelet production *in vivo*. *Nature* **369**, 565–567.

Löw-Friedrich, I., Grützmacher, P., März, W., Bergmann, M., and Schoeppe, W. (1991). Therapy with recombinant human erythropoietin reduces cardiac size and improves heart function in chronic hemodialysis patients. *American Journal of Nephrology* **11**, 54–60.

Luke, R. G., Kennedy, A. C., Stirling, W. B., and MacDonald, G. A. (1965). Renal artery stenosis, hypertension and polycythaemia. *British Medical Journal* **1**, 164–166.

Lusvarghi, E. (1994). Hematopoiesis in renal failure patients. *Journal of Nephrology* **8**, 79–86.

Lusvarghi, E. *et al.* (1979). Evaluation of platelet kinetics in chronic renal failure (conservative and regular dialysis treatment). *Hematologica* **64**, 747–758.

Macdougall, I. C. (1992). Treatment of renal anemia with recombinant human erythropoietin. *Current Opinion in Nephrology and Hypertension* **1**, 210–219.

Macdougall, I. C. (1994). Monitoring of iron status and iron supplementation in patients treated with erythropoietin. *Current Opinion in Nephrology and Hypertension* **3**, 620–625.

Macdougall, I. C. (1995). Poor response to erythropoietin: practical guidelines on investigation and management. *Nephrology, Dialysis, Transplantation* **10**, 607–614.

Macdougall, I. C. (2001). An overview of the efficacy and safety of novel erythropoiesis stimulating protein (NESP). *Nephrology, Dialysis, Transplantation* **16** (Suppl. 3), 14–21.

Macdougall, I. C. (2002). Once-weekly erythropoietic therapy: is there a difference between the available preparations? *Nephrology, Dialysis, Transplantation* **17**, 2047–2051.

Macdougall, I C. (2002). Once-weekly.

Macdougall, I. C., Roberts, D. E., Neubert, P., Dharmasena, A. D., Coles, G. A., and Williams, J. D. (1989). Pharmacokinetics of recombinant human erythropoietin in patients on continuous ambulatory peritoneal dialysis. *Lancet* **1**, 425–427.

Macdougall, I. C. *et al.* (1990a). The treatment of renal anaemia in CAPD patients with recombinant human erythropoietin. *Nephrology, Dialysis, Transplantation* **5**, 950–955.

Macdougall, I. C. *et al.* (1990b). Long-term cardiorespiratory effects of amelioration of renal anaemia by erythropoietin. *Lancet* **335**, 489–493.

Macdougall, I. C. *et al.* (1991a). Coagulation studies and fistula blood flow during erythropoietin therapy in haemodialysis patients. *Nephrology, Dialysis, Transplantation* **6**, 862–867.

Macdougall, I. C., Davies, M. E., Hutton, R. D., Coles, G. A., and Williams, J. D. (1991b). Rheological studies during treatment of renal anaemia with recombinant human erythropoietin. *British Journal of Haematology* **77**, 550–558.

Macdougall, I. C., Roberts, D. E., Coles, G. A., and Williams, J. D. (1991c). Clinical pharmacokinetics of epoetin (recombinant human erythropoietin). *Clinical Pharmacokinetics* 20, 99–113.

Macdougall, I. C., Gray, S. J., Elston, O., Breen, C., Jenkins, B., Browne, J., and Egrie, J. (1999). Pharmacokinetics of novel erythropoiesis stimulating protein compared with epoetin alpha in dialysis patients. *Journal of the American Society of Nephrology* 10, 2392–2395.

Maggiore, Q., Navalesi, R., and Biagni, M. (1986). Comparative studies on uraemic anaemia in polycystic kidney disease and in other renal disease. *Proceedings of the European Dialysis and Transplant Association* 4, 264–269.

McGonigle, R. J., Wallin, J. D., Shadduck, R. K., and Fisher, J. W. (1984). Erythropoietin deficiency and inhibition of erythropoiesis in renal insufficiency. *Kidney International* 25, 437–444.

Maiorca, R. et al. (1988). CAPD is a first class treatment: results of an eight-year experience with a comparison of patient and method survival in CAPD and hemodialysis. *Clinical Nephrology* 30 (Suppl.), S3–S7.

Mannucci, P. M. et al. (1983). Deamino-8-D-arginine vasopressin shortens the bleeding time in uremia. *New England Journal of Medicine* 308, 8–12.

Manzler, A. D. and Schreiner, A. W. (1970). Copper-induced acute hemolytic anemia. A new complication of hemodialysis. *Annals of Internal Medicine* 73, 409–412.

Marsh, J. T. et al. (1991). rHuEPO treatment improves brain and cognitive function of anemic dialysis patients. *Kidney International* 39, 155–163.

Maxwell, P. H., Ferguson, D. J., Nicholls, L. G., Johnson, M. H., and Ratcliffe, P. J. (1997). The interstitial response to renal injury: fibroblast-like cells show phenotypic changes and have reduced potential for erythropoietin gene expression. *Kidney International* 52, 715–724.

Maxwell, P. H., Wiesener, M., Chang, G.-W., Clifford, S. C., Vaux, E. C., Cockman, M. E., Wykoff, C. C., Pugh, C. W., Maher, E. R., and Ratcliffe, P. J. (1999). The tumour suppressor protein VHL targets hypoxia-inducible factors for oxygen-dependent proteolysis. *Nature* 399, 271–275.

Maxwell, P. H. et al. (1993). Identification of the renal erythropoietin-producing cells using transgenic mice. *Kidney International* 44, 1149–1162.

Maxwell, P. H. et al. (1994). Expression of a homologously recombined erythropoietin-SV 40 T antigen fusion gene in mouse liver: evidence for erythropoietin production by Ito cells. *Blood* 84, 1823–1830.

Mayer, G., Thum, J., Cada, E. M., Stummvoll, H. K., and Graf, H. (1988). Working capacity is increased following recombinant human erythropoietin treatment. *Kidney International* 34, 525–528.

Means, R. T. and Krantz, S. B. (1992). Progress in understanding the pathogenesis of the anemia of chronic disease. *Blood* 80, 1639–1647.

Meier, P., Dayer, E., Blanc, E., and Wauters, J. P. (2002). Early T cell activation correlates with expression of apoptosis markers in patients with end-stage renal disease. *Journal of the American Society of Nephrology* 13, 204–212.

Mendes-Ribeiro, A. C., Brunini, T. M., Yaqoob, M., Aronson, J. K., Mann, G. E., and Ellory, J. C. (1999). Identification of system y + L as the high-affinity transporter for L-arginine in human platelets: up-regulation of L-arginine influx in uraemia. *Pflügers Archives* 438, 573–575.

Meytes, D., Bogin, E., Ma, A., Dukes, P. P., and Massry, S. G. (1981). Effect of parathyroid hormone on erythropoiesis. *Journal of Clinical Investigation* 67, 1263–1269.

Miller, M. E. et al. (1973). pH effect on erythropoietin response to hypoxia. *New England Journal of Medicine* 288, 706–710.

Moia, M., Mannucci, P. M., Vizzotto, L., Casati, S., Cattaneo, M., and Ponticelli, C. (1987). Improvement in the haemostatic defect of uraemia after treatment with recombinant human erythropoietin. *Lancet* ii, 1227–1229.

Moreno, F., Sanz-Guajardo, D., Lopez-Gomez, J. M., Jofre, R., and Valderrabano, F. (2000). Increasing the hematocrit has a beneficial effect on quality of life and is safe in selected hemodialysis patients. Spanish Cooperative Renal Patients Quality of Life Study Group of the Spanish Society of Nephrology. *Journal of the American Society of Nephrology* 11, 335–342.

Movilli, E., Cancarini, G. C., Zani, R., Camerini, C., Sandrini, M., and Maiorca, R. (2001). Adequacy of dialysis reduces the doses of recombinant erythropoietin independently from the use of biocompatible membranes in haemodialysis patients. *Nephrology, Dialysis, Transplantation* 16, 111–114.

Motzer, R. J., Bander, N. H., and Nanus, D. M. (1996). Renal cell carcinoma. *New England Journal of Medicine* 335, 865–873.

Naets, J. P., Garcia, J. F., Tousaaint, G., Buset, M., and Waks, D. (1986). Radioimmunoassay of erythropoietin in chronic uraemia or anephric patients. *Scandinavian Journal of Haematology* 37, 390–394.

Navarro, J. F. (2003). In the erythropoietin era, can we forget alternative or adjunctive therapies for renal anaemia management? The androgen example. *Nephrology, Dialysis, Transplantation* 18, 2222–2226.

Neff, M. S., Kim, K. E., Persoff, M., Oneseti, G., and Swartz, C. (1971). Hemodynamics of uremic anemia. *Circulation* 43, 867–883.

Neff, M. S. et al. (1981). A comparison of androgens for anemia in patients on hemodialysis. *New England Journal of Medicine* 304, 871–875.

Nissenson, A. R. (1992). Epoetin and cognitive function. *American Journal of Kidney Diseases* 20 (Suppl. 1), 21–24.

O'Hare, J. A. and Murnaghan, D. J. (1982). Reversal of aluminum-induced hemodialysis anemia by a low-aluminum dialysate. *New England Journal of Medicine* 306, 654–656.

O'Hare, J. A., Callaghan, N. M., and Murnaghan, D. J. (1983). Dialysis encephalopathy. Clinical, electroencephalographic and interventional aspects. *Medicine* 62, 129–141.

Orringer, E. P. and Mattern, W. D. (1976). Formaldehyde-induced hemolysis during chronic hemodialysis. *New England Journal of Medicine* 294, 1416–1420.

Pagel, H., Jelkmann, W., and Weiss, C. (1988). A comparison of the effects of renal artery constriction and anemia on the production of erythropoietin. *Pflügers Archives* 413, 62–66.

Parfrey, P. S. et al. (1996). Outcome and risk factors for left ventricular disorders in chronic uraemia. *Nephrology, Dialysis, Transplantation* 11, 1277–1285.

Pascual, J., Teruel, J. L., Moya, J. L., Liano, F., Jimenez-Mena, M., and Ortuno, J. (1991). Regression of left ventricular hypertrophy after partial correction of anemia with erythropoietin in patients on hemodialysis: a prospective study. *Clinical Nephrology* 35, 280–287.

Pertosa, G. et al. (1991). Involvement of peripheral blood monocytes in haemodialysis: *in vivo* induction of tumor necrosis factor alpha, interleukin 6 and beta 2-microglobulin. *Nephrology, Dialysis, Transplantation* 6 (Suppl. 2), 18–23.

Peschle, C., Zanjani, E. D., Gidari, A. S., McLaurin, W. D., and Gordon, A. S. (1986). Mechanisms of thyroxine action on erythropoiesis. *Endocrinology* 89, 609–612.

Petrie, J. J. B. and Row, P. G. (1977). Dialysis anaemia caused by subacute zinc toxicity. *Lancet* i, 1178–1180.

Priyadarshi, A., Periyasamy, S., Burke, T. J., Britton, S. L., Malhotra, D., Shapiro, J. I. (2002). Effects of reduction of renal mass on renal oxygen tension and erythropoietin production in the rat. *Kidney International* 61, 542–546.

Pugh, C. W., Tan, C. C., Jones, R. W., and Ratcliffe, P. J. (1991). Functional analysis of an oxygen-regulated transcriptional enhancer lying 3' to the mouse erythropoietin gene. *Proceedings of the National Academy of Sciences USA* 88, 10553–10557.

Radtke, H. W. et al. (1981). Identification of spermine as an inhibitor of erythropoiesis in patients with chronic renal failure. *Journal of Clinical Investigation* 67, 1623–1629.

Ratcliffe, P. J., Jones, R. W., Phillips, R. E., Nicholls, L. G., and Bell, J. I. (1990). Oxygen-dependent modulation of erythropoietin mRNA levels. *Journal of Experimental Medicine* 172, 657–660.

Recny, M., Scoble, H. A., and Kim, Y. (1987). Structural characterization of natural human urinary and recombinant DNA-derived erythropoietin. *Journal of Biological Chemistry* 262, 17156–17163.

Rejman, A. S., Grimes, A. J., Cotes, P. M., Mansell, M. A., and Joekes, A. M. (1985). Correction of anaemia following renal transplantation: serial changes in serum immunoreactive erythropoietin, absolute reticulocyte count and red-cell creatine levels. *British Journal of Haematology* **61**, 421–431.

Richardson, D., Barlett, C., Goutcher, E., Jones, C. H., Davison, A. M., and Will, E. J. (1999). Erythropoietin resistance due to dialysate chloramine: the two-way traffic of solutes in haemodialysis. *Nephrology, Dialysis, Transplantation* **14**, 2625–2627.

Roccatello, D. *et al.* (1989). Functional changes of monocytes due to dialysis membranes. *Kidney International* **35**, 622–631.

Rosenberger, C., Mandriota, S., Jürgensen, J. S., Wiesener, M. S., Hörstrup, J. H., Frei, U., Ratcliffe, P. J., Maxwell, P. H., Bachmann, S., and Eckardt, K. U. (2002). Expression of hypoxia-inducible factor-1α and -2α in hypoxic and ischemic rat kidneys. *Journal of the American Society of Nephrology* **13**, 1721–1732.

Rosenmund, A., Binswanger, U., and Straub, P. W. (1975). Oxidative injury to erythrocytes, cell rigidity, and splenic hemolysis in hemodialysed uremic patients. *Annals of Internal Medicine* **82**, 460–465.

Salahudeen, A. K., Keavey, P. M., Hawkins, T., and Wilkinson, R. (1983). Is anaemia during continuous ambulatory peritoneal dialysis really better than during haemodialysis? *Lancet* **ii**, 1046–1049.

Salvati, F. and Liani, M. (2001). Role of platelet surface receptor abnormalities in the bleeding and thrombotic diathesis of uremic patients on hemodialysis and peritoneal dialysis. *International Journal of Artificial Organs* **24**, 131–135.

Sasaki, H., Bothner, B., Dell, A., and Fukuda, M. (1987). Carbohydrate structure of erythropoietin in Chinese hamster ovary cells by a human erythropoietin cDNA. *Journal of Biological Chemistry* **262**, 12059–12076.

Sawada, K., Krantz, S. B., Dessypris, E. N., Koury, S. T., and Sawyer, S. T. (1989). Human colony-forming units-erythroid do not require accessory cells, but do require direct interaction with insulin-like growth factor 1 and/or insulin for erythroid development. *Journal of Clinical Investigation* **83**, 1702–1709.

Schaefer, R. M., Kokot, F., Wernze, H., Geiger, H., and Heidland, A. (1989). Improved sexual function in hemodialysis patients on recombinant erythropoietin: a possible role for prolactin. *Clinical Nephrology* **31**, 1–5.

Schaefer, R. M., Teschner, M., and Kosch, M. (2002). Folate metabolism in renal failure. *Nephrology, Dialysis, Transplantation* **17** (Suppl. 5), 24–27.

Scholz, H., Schurek, H. J., Eckardt, K.-U., Kurtz, A., and Bauer, C. (1991). Oxygen-dependent erythropoietin production by the isolated perfused rat kidney. *Pflügers Archives* **418**, 228–233.

Schurek, H. J., Host, U., Baumgärtl, H., Bertram, H., and Heckmann, U. (1990). Evidence for a pre-glomerular oxygen diffusion shunt in rat renal cortex. *American Journal of Physiology* **259**, F910–F915.

Schuster, S. J., Badiavas, E. V., Costa-Giomi, P., Weinmann, R., Erslev, A. J., and Caro, J. (1989). Stimulation of erythropoietin gene transcription during hypoxia and cobalt exposure. *Blood* **73**, 13–16.

Schuster, S. J., Koury, S. T., Bohrere, M., Salceda, S., and Caro, J. (1992). Cellular sites of extra-renal and renal erythropoietin production in anaemic rats. *British Journal of Haematology* **81**, 153–159.

Segal, G. M., Eschbach, J. W., Egrie, J. C., Stueve, T., and Adamson, J. W. (1988). The anemia of end-stage renal disease: hematopoietic progenitor cell response. *Kidney International* **33**, 983–988.

Semenza, G. L. (2000). HIF-1: mediator of physiological and pathophysiological responses to hypoxia. *Journal of Applied Physiology* **88**, 1474–1480.

Semenza, G. L. and Wang, G. L. (1992). A nuclear factor induced by hypoxia via *de novo* protein synthesis binds to the human erythropoietin gene enhancer at a site required for transcription activation. *Molecular and Cellular Biology* **12**, 5447–5454.

Semenza, G. L., Koury, S. T., Nejfelt, M. K., Gearhart, J. D., and Antonarakis, S. E. (1991). Cell-type-specific and hypoxia-inducible expression of the human erythropoietin gene in transgenic mice. *Proceedings of the National Academy of Sciences USA* **88**, 8725–8729.

Sennesael, J. J., Van Der Niepen, P., and Verbeelen, D. (1991). Treatment with recombinant human erythropoietin increases antibody titers after hepatitis B vaccination in dialysis patients. *Kidney International* **40**, 121–128.

Silberberg, J. S., Barre, P. E., Prichard, S. S., and Sniderman, A. D. (1989). Impact of left ventricular hypertrophy on survival in end-stage renal disease. *Kidney International* **36**, 286–290.

Skibeli, V., Nissen-Lie, G., and Torjesen, P. (1998). Sugar profiling proves that human serum erythropoietin differs from recombinant human erythropoietin. *Blood* **98**, 3626–3634.

Storring, P. L., Tiplady, R. J., Gaines-Das, R. E., Rafferty, B., and Mistry, Y. G. (1996). Lectin-binding assays for the isoforms of human erythropoietin: comparison of urinary and four recombinant erythropoietins. *Journal of Endocrinology* **150**, 401–412.

Sufrin, G., Mirnad, E. A., Moore, R. H., Chu, T. M., and Murphy, G. P. (1977). Hormones in renal cancer. *Journal of Urology* **117**, 433–438.

Summerfield, G. P., Gyde, O. H. B., Forbes, A. M. W., Goldsmith, H. J., and Bellingham, A. J. (1983). Haemoglobin concentration and serum erythropoietin in renal dialysis and transplant patients. *Scandinavian Journal of Haematology* **30**, 389–400.

Sun, C. H., Ward, H. J., Wellington, L. P., Koyle, M. A., Yanagawa, N., and Lee, D. N. B. (1989). Serum erythropoietin levels after renal transplantation. *New England Journal of Medicine* **321**, 151–157.

Sundal, E. and Kaeser, U. (1989). Correction of anaemia of chronic renal failure with recombinant human erythropoietin: safety and efficacy of one year's treatment in a European multicentre study of 150 haemodialysis-dependent patients. *Nephrology, Dialysis, Transplantation* **4**, 979–987.

Sunder-Plassmann, G. and Hörl, W. H. (1997). Erythropoietin and iron. *Clinical Nephrology* **47**, 141–157.

Taccone-Gallucci, M. *et al.* (1989). Platelet lipid peroxidation in hemodialysis patients: effects of vitamin E supplementation. *Nephrology, Dialysis, Transplantation* **4**, 975–978.

Takeuchi, M. *et al.* (1988). Comparative study of the asparagine-linked sugar chains of human erythropoietins purified from urine and the culture medium of recombinant Chinese hamster ovary cells. *Journal of Biological Chemistry* **263**, 3657–3663.

Tan, C. C., Eckardt, K.-U., and Ratcliffe, P. J. (1991). Organ distribution of erythropoietin messenger RNA in normal and uremic rats. *Kidney International* **40**, 69–76.

Tan, C. C., Eckardt, K.-U., and Ratcliffe, P. J. (1992). Feedback modulation of renal and hepatic erythropoietin messenger RNA in response to graded anemia and hypoxia. *American Journal of Physiology* **263**, F474–F481.

Tan, C. C., Tan, L. H., and Eckardt, K.-U. (1996). Erythropoietin production in rats with post-ischemic acute renal failure. *Kidney International* **50**, 1958–1964.

Tarng, D. C., Wen, C. T., Huang, T. P., Chen, C. L., Liu, T. Y., and Wei, Y. H. (2002). Increased oxidative damage to peripheral blood leucocyte DNA in chronic peritoneal dialysis patients. *Journal of the American Society of Nephrology* **13**, 1321–1330.

Taylor, J. E., McLaren, M., Henderson, I. S., Belch, J. J. F., and Stewart, W. K. (1992). Prothrombotic effect of erythropoietin in dialysis patients. *Nephrology, Dialysis, Transplantation* **7**, 235–239.

Teruel, J. L. *et al.* (1991). Hemodynamic changes in hemodialyzed patients during treatment with recombinant human erythropoietin. *Nephron* **58**, 135–137.

Thevenod, F., Radtke, H. W., Grützmacher, P., Vincent, E., Koch, K. M., and Fassbinder, W. (1983). Deficient feedback regulation of erythropoiesis in kidney transplant patients with polycythemia. *Kidney International* **24**, 227–232.

Tielemans, C. *et al.* (1985). Improvement of anemia with desferrioxamine in hemodialysis patients with aluminum-induced bone disease. *Clinical Nephrology* **24**, 237–241.

Touam, M. *et al.* (1983). Aluminium-induced, reversible microcytic anemia in chronic renal failure: clinical and experimental studies. *Clinical Nephrology* **19**, 295–298.

Tsuruoka, S. *et al.* (2002). Vitamin-E bonded hemodialyzer improves neutrophil function and oxidative stress in patients with end-stage renal failure. *American Journal of Kidney Diseases* **39**, 127–133.

Veys, N., Vanholder, R., and Ringoir, S. (1992). Correction of deficient phago-cytosis during erythropoietin treatment in maintenance hemodialysis patients. *American Journal of Kidney Diseases* **19**, 358–363.

Viganó, G., Benigni, A., Mendogni, D., Mingardi, G., Mecca, G., and Remuzzi, G. (1991). Recombinant human erythropoietin to correct uremic bleeding. *American Journal of Kidney Diseases* **18**, 44–49.

Wallner, S. F. and Vautrin, R. M. (1981). Evidence that inhibition of erythro-poiesis is important in the anemia of chronic renal failure. *Journal of Laboratory and Clinical Medicine* **97**, 170–178.

Wang, G. L. and Semenza, G. L. (1995). Verification and characterization of hypoxia-inducible factor 1. *Journal of Biological Chemistry* **270**, 1230–1237.

Wang, F. F., Kung, C. K.-H., and Goldwasser, E. (1985). Some chemical prop-erties of human erythropoietin. *Endocrinology* **116**, 2286–2292.

Wenger, R. (2002). Cellular adaptation to hypoxia: O_2-sensing protein hydr-oxylases, hypoxia-inducible transcription factors, and O_2-regulated gene expression. *FASEB Journal* **16**, 1151–1162.

Westenfelder, C., Biddle, D. L., and Baranowski, R. L. (1999). Human, rat and mouse kidney cells express functional erythropoietin receptors. *Kidney International* **55**, 808–820.

Wiesener, M. S., Jürgensen, J. S., Rosenberger, C., Scholze, C., Hörstrup, J. H., Warnecke, C., Mandriota, S., Frei, U., Pugh, C. W., Ratcliffe, P. J., Bachmann, S., Maxwell, P. M., and Eckardt, K.-U. (2003). Widespread, hypoxia-inducible expression of HIF-2 alpha in distinct cell populations of different organs. *FASEB Journal* **17**, 271–273.

Wiesener, M. S., Münchenhagen, P. M., Berger, I., Roigas, J., Schwiertz, A., Jürgensen, J. S., Gruber, G., Maxwell, P. H., Löning, S. A., Frei, U., Gröne, H. J., and Eckardt, K.-U. (2001). Constitutive activation of hypoxia-inducible genes related to overexpression of hypoxia-inducible factor-1α in clear cell renal carcinomas. *Cancer Research* **61**, 5215–5222.

Wiesener, M. S., Seyfarth, M., Warnecke, C., Jürgensen, J. S., Rosenberger, C., Morgan, N. V., Maher, E. R., Frei, U., and Eckardt, K.-U. (2002). Para-neoplastic erythrocytosis associated with an inactivating point-mutation of the von Hippel–Lindau gene in a renal cell carcinoma. *Blood* **99**, 3562–3565.

Wiesener, M. S., Turley, H., Allen, W. E., Willam, C., Eckardt, K.-U., Talks, K. L., Wood, S. M., Gatter, K. C., Harris, A. L., Pugh, C. W., Ratcliffe, P. J., and Maxwell, P. H. (1998). Induction of endothelial PAS domain protein-1 by hypoxia: characterization and comparison with hypoxia-inducible factor 1-α. *Blood* **92**, 2260–2268.

Wizemann, V., Kaufmann, J., and Kramer, W. (1992). Effect of erythropoietin on ischemia tolerance in anemic hemodialysis patients with confirmed coronary artery disease. *Nephron* **62**, 161–165.

Yoshimura, A. and Misawa, H. (1998). Physiology and function of the ery-thropoietin receptor. *Current Opinion in Hematology* **5**, 171–176.

Zappacosta, A. R., Caro, J., and Erslev, A. J. (1982). Normalization of hemat-ocrit in patients with end-stage renal disease on continuous ambulatory peritoneal dialysis. *American Journal of Medicine* **72**, 53–57.

Further reading

Eckardt, K.-U. (1994). Erythropoietin: oxygen-dependent control of erythro-poiesis and its failure in renal disease. *Nephron* **67**, 7–23.

Jelkmann, W., ed. *Erythropoietin: Molecular Biology and Clinical Use*. Johnson City, TN: F. P. Graham Publishing Co., 2003.

Macdougall, I. C. Erythropoietin therapy for renal anaemia. In *Advanced Renal Medicine* (ed. A. E. G. Raine), pp. 379–390. Oxford: Oxford University Press, 1992.

Ratcliffe, P. J. (1993). Nephrology forum: molecular biology of erythropoietin. *Kidney International* **44**, 887–904.

Valderrabano, F. (1996). Erythropoietin in chronic renal failure. *Kidney International* **50**, 1373–1391.

11.3.9 Skeletal disorders

Tilman B. Drüeke and Eberhard Ritz

Bony problems and extraosseous calcification may be a major obstacle to the rehabilitation of patients treated for endstage renal failure. Judi-cious management and preventive measures have helped to reduce the frequency of rapidly progressive secondary hyperparathyroidism. However, after prolonged haemodialysis, nephrologists are still plagued by persisting problems such as advanced hyperparathyroidism with nodular parathyroid hyperplasia, low bone turnover ('adynamic bone disease') often associated with soft tissue calcification, and finally, skeletal problems from β_2-microglobulin (β_2-m)-derived amyloidosis. In contrast, aluminium-related bone disease has become rare in recent years.

Current concepts concerning pathogenesis, clinical presentation, diagnosis, and management of bone disease in uraemia are summarized in this chapter. Particular emphasis is given to prophylactic measures.

Pathogenesis of disturbed calcium and phosphate metabolism and related issues leading to disturbances of bone metabolism in chronic renal failure

Early renal failure

Although present knowledge is incomplete, several mechanisms have been recognized by which hyperparathyroidism is initiated in early renal failure and maintained in advanced renal failure.

The development of secondary hyperparathyroidism in renal failure can be viewed as a disruption of the endocrine parathyroid hormone (PTH)–vitamin D axis. The hormonally active metabolite of vitamin D3 [1,25-dihydroxyvitamin D3, 1,25-(OH)2D3, or calcitriol] is synthesized from its precursor 25(OH)D3 by the rate-limiting enzyme 25-hydroxyvitamin D3-1α-hydroxylase in the renal epithelial cells, mainly of the proximal tubule. Calcitriol exerts negative feedback inhibition on the parathyroid by three mechanisms:

(1) possibly an increase in calcium sensitivity and a reduction in calcium-dependent secretion of preformed PTH from secretory granules;

(2) inhibition of PTH synthesis, that is, transcription of the pre-pro-PTH gene and translation of PTH mRNA;

(3) chronic inhibition of parathyroid cell proliferation, that is, devel-opment of hyperplasia (Naveh-Many *et al.* 1989; Szabo *et al.* 1989; Roussanne *et al.* 2001).

The effects of calcitriol on the parathyroid gland are mediated through a specific nuclear binding protein, that is, the vitamin D receptor (VDR), which is abnormally regulated in renal failure. In par-ticular, its expression is decreased (Fukuda *et al.* 1993) as is its trans-location from the cytoplasm to the nucleus (Patel *et al.* 1994a,b). In addition, the VDR also binds to the retinoic X receptor (RXR) which is part of another class of nuclear receptors. The RXR forms a stable heterodimer with VDR (RXR–VDR), thereby enhancing calcitriol-dependent transcription (Yu *et al.* 1991; Kliewer *et al.* 1992).

Reduced availability of calcitriol in renal failure will result in disinhibition of the parathyroid gland, that is, an interruption of chronic negative feedback inhibition. In this view, renal secondary hyperparathyroidism represents an adequate homeostatic response of the parathyroid gland to maintain the circulating calcitriol close to the normal range at the expense of elevated PTH concentrations.

Another potent control mechanism of PTH production which is disturbed in renal failure is the response of the parathyroid gland to the calcium ion (Ca^{2+}) via the calcium-sensing receptor localized in the parathyroid cell membrane (Brown *et al.* 1993). This calcium sensor mediates the known stimulatory effects of hypocalcaemia and the inhibitory effects of hypercalcaemia on PTH synthesis and secretion. The expression of calcium-sensing receptor mRNA and protein is decreased in chronic renal failure (Kifor *et al.* 1996; Gogusev *et al.* 1997).

Whether calcitriol upregulates the calcium-sensing receptor and calcitriol deficiency downregulates it remains a matter of debate (Rogerys *et al.* 1995; Brown *et al.* 1996). The probable importance of Ca^{2+} sensing in the genesis of secondary parathyroid hyperplasia is illustrated by the observation that activation of the calcium sensor by calcimimetic agents prevents parathyroid cell proliferation in experimental renal failure (Wada *et al.* 1997).

Finally, evidence has also been provided that an increased extracellular phosphate concentration, independent of low plasma calcium and calcitriol concentrations, not only stimulates PTH secretion in experimental animals (Lopez-Hilker *et al.* 1990) and human patients *in vivo* (Lafage *et al.* 1992; Fine *et al.* 1993; Combe and Aparicio 1994), but also *in vitro* under tissue culture conditions via a direct action independent of ionized Ca^{2+} or calcitriol (Almadén *et al.* 1996; Nielsen *et al.* 1996; Slatopolsky *et al.* 1996). In addition, phosphate also enhances parathyroid cell proliferation via a direct action on parathyroid cells (Roussanne *et al.* 2001).

Figure 1 summarizes these concepts and points, in addition to the possibility that unknown local factors (e.g. mitogens), as well as modifying enhancer and repressor genes, modulate parathyroid cell growth and activity.

Increased PTH concentrations are already found in some patients whose glomerular filtration rate ranges from 60 to 80 ml/min, as shown by increased intact PTH (Reichel *et al.* 1991). This is accompanied by the appearance of increased PTH action on bone, that is, increased osteoclast numbers and occurrence of woven osteoid and woven bone (Malluche *et al.* 1976) (Fig. 2). The signal triggering such early hyperparathyroidism has not been definitely elucidated. The 'trade-off' hypothesis of Bricker *et al.* (1969) emphasized an increase in serum phosphate as the initial event in the development of secondary hyperparathyroidism. However, fasting or postprandial serum phosphate is not elevated in early renal failure (Portale *et al.* 1984; Wilson *et al.* 1985). Thus, retention of phosphate, at least in the extracellular space, is presumably not sufficient to explain the initiation of secondary hyperparathyroidism in early renal failure. Undoubtedly, hyperphosphataemia plays an important role in the genesis of hyperparathyroidism of patients with advanced renal failure.

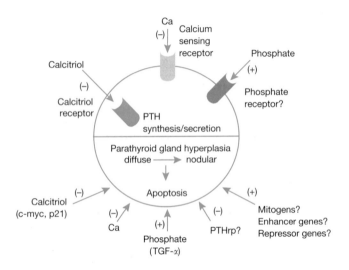

Fig. 1 A schematic summary of pathogenesis of secondary hyperparathyroidism in chronic renal failure: − inhibition; + stimulation of PTH secretion/synthesis and of parathyroid gland growth. Reproduced with permission from Drüeke and Zingraff (1994).

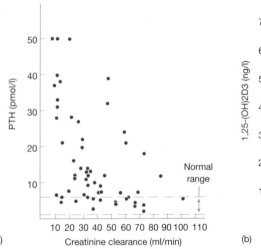

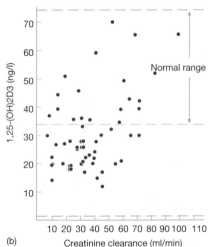

Fig. 2 (a) Intact plasma PTH values as a function of glomerular filtration rate in predialysis chronic renal failure; (b) serum 1,25-(OH)2D3 as a function of glomerular filtration rate in predialysis chronic renal failure. (Data from unselected consecutive patients presenting in a nephrology outpatients department.)

Llach and Massry (1985) found a trend towards a decrease in plasma ionized calcium in incipient renal failure, but hypocalcaemia is not demonstrable in all patients and no relation is found between total or ionized calcium and intact PTH (Reichel *et al.* 1991). Nevertheless, it is possible that continuous or intermittent hypocalcaemia triggers increased secretion of PTH in early renal failure through release of preformed hormone and an increase in synthesis of pre-pro-PTH mRNA (Yamamoto *et al.* 1989). However, secondary hyperparathyroidism occurred in subtotally nephrectomized dogs, even when the ionized calcium was increased above the normal range by the administration of calcium carbonate (Lopez-Hilker *et al.* 1986). The increase of plasma PTH in such hypercalcaemic dogs could be prevented by concomitant administration of calcitriol, demonstrating that hypocalcaemia is not an obligatory factor in the development of renal secondary hyperparathyroidism. These results suggest that reduced synthesis of calcitriol is involved in the hypersecretion of PTH.

More recent data document subtle disturbances of calcitriol biosynthesis in early renal failure (Table 1) which suggest an important role of calcitriol in the initiation of renal hyperparathyroidism. In early renal failure, serum calcitriol is usually within or slightly below the normal range (Wilson *et al.* 1985; Lucas *et al.* 1988). The relation between serum calcitriol and glomerular filtration rate in early renal failure is illustrated in Fig. 2. The relatively low serum calcitriol in early renal failure is clearly inappropriate, because one would expect increased concentrations in the presence of elevated PTH. As explained above, the most likely explanation is that calcitriol concentrations are maintained within or slightly below the normal range by increased parathyroid activity and the consecutive stimulation of renal 1α-hydroxylase activity.

This hypothesis is supported by the results of a study in which the reserve capacity of renal calcitriol biosynthesis in early renal failure was examined (Ritz *et al.* 1991). After infusion of synthetic human 1,38-PTH the increase in serum calcitriol in patients with early renal failure was clearly attenuated in proportion to the prevailing PTH concentration, suggesting a decrease in the reserve capacity of the renal 25-(OH)2D3-1α-hydroxylase as a result of continuous stimulation by PTH. This situation is similar to that of incipient adrenal insufficiency where plasma cortisol levels are still maintained in the normal range, despite diminished adrenal mass, through increased secretion of adrenocorticotropic hormone (ACTH). Further arguments in favour of an early impairment of vitamin D metabolism are provided by studies documenting decreased function of vitamin-D-dependent target organs, for example reduction of the active intestinal absorption of calcium in early renal failure (Malluche *et al.* 1978).

Finally, as shown in Table 2, the role of calcitriol deficiency is also supported by the results of a recent placebo-controlled prospective multicentre trial (Ritz *et al.* 1995). Daily administration of 0.125 μg calcitriol prevented a further increase of elevated baseline PTH concentrations without altering serum calcium or serum phosphate concentrations or the urinary calcium excretion rate.

Thus, absolute or relative calcitriol deficiency is probably involved in the initiation of hyperparathyroidism. Such a deficiency could be explained on anatomical or functional grounds. It appears unlikely that impaired calcitriol synthesis in early renal failure, that is, at a glomerular filtration rate of 60–70 ml/min, is merely the consequence of reduced renal mass. The impairment may at least in part be functional because serum calcitriol of patients with moderate renal failure is modulated appropriately by reducing the intake of dietary phosphate (Portale *et al.* 1984). Moreover, when healthy subjects undergo unilateral nephrectomy, serum calcitriol is reduced transiently but returns to the normal range in parallel with an increase in PTH concentration (Lucas *et al.* 1986; Friedlander *et al.* 1988). In order to explain the phosphate-dependent changes in early renal failure, it has been suggested that phosphate accumulates in a putative critical intracellular compartment of the tubular epithelial cells (Bonjour 1988). This would result in functional inhibition of 25-(OH)2D3-1α-hydroxylase and reduced calcitriol synthesis, as well as reduced tubular threshold for phosphate reabsorption and a tendency for hypophosphataemia. Against this proposal stands the observation that equilibration of patients with incipient renal failure on a low-phosphate diet fails to alter calcitriol or PTH concentrations (Seidel *et al.* 1991). Alternatively, it is possible that the activity of the renal 1α-hydroxylase is depressed by the retention of uraemic toxins such as purines (including guanidinosuccinic acid) (Hsu and Patel 1992).

Table 1 Disturbances of calcitriol biosynthesis in early renal failure

Inadequately low plasma calcitriol concentration in the presence of elevated plasma intact PTH (Reichel *et al.* 1991)

Diminished reserve capacity of the renal 25-(OH)$_2$ vitamin D3-1α-hydroxylase (Ritz *et al.* 1990)

Signs of decreased activity of calcitriol in its target organs, i.e. intestine (Malluche *et al.* 1978)

Abnormal substrate dependence of renal and extrarenal 1α-hydroxylases (Dusso *et al.* 1988; Lucas *et al.* 1988)

Table 2 Effect of low-dose calcitriol (0.125 μg/day for 12 months) on plasma intact PTH and plasma chemistry in predialysis patients with chronic renal failure

	Placebo (n = 24)		Calcitriol (n = 28)		Normal range
	Baseline[a]	Final[a]	Baseline[a]	Final[a]	
Intact PTH (pmol/l)	14.0 (6.7–63.3)	27.8[b] (4.2–68.5)	16.2 (6.85–82.0)	18.2 (4.45–75.5)	1.0–6.0
Calcium (mmol/l)	2.44 (2.0–2.6)	2.40 (2.01–2.64)	2.40 (2.13–24.0)	2.41 (2.0–2.6)	2.25–2.60
Phosphate (mmol/l)	1.20 (0.82–1.7)	1.32 (0.52–1.83)	1.19 (0.56–1.8)	1.18 (0.75–1.8)	0.870–1.7
Creatinine (mg/dl)	3.06 (1.57–6.76)	3.48 (1.01–9.58)	3.31 (1.47–5.46)	4.07 (1.53–10.2)	0.60–1.10

[a] Intention to treat analysis: median and range shown.

[b] $p < 0.05$ versus placebo.

Still another hypothesis is that calcidiol cannot penetrate into proximal tubular epithelium from the luminal side due to a decreased availability or functional impairment of megalin in renal failure. This multifunctional receptor protein, which is located in the brush border membrane, is required to allow the internalization of filtered calcidiol and its binding protein (DBP) into the tubular epithelium and to serve as substrate for the renal enzyme 1α-OH vitamin D hydroxylase (Nykjaer *et al.* 1999) (Fig. 3). This obligate entry pathway for calcidiol was actually discovered in mice by serependicity, namely after the knock-out of the *megalin* gene. However, the validity for the human situation of this mechanism established in the mouse has subsequently been questioned, since 1α-OH vitamin D hydroxylase expression was found not only in the proximal, but also in the distal tubular epithelium of human kidney, that is, in tubular areas in which megalin apparently is not expressed (Zehnder *et al.* 1999).

An altered rate of metabolic clearance of calcitriol does not appear to contribute to decreased plasma calcitriol, at least in early chronic renal failure. The metabolic clearance rate was measured in experimental renal failure, and was found to be unchanged in uraemic dogs (Dusso *et al.* 1989) and diminished in rats with advanced uraemia (Hsu *et al.* 1987). The decreased degradation could be related to the accumulation of ultrafiltrable substances, possibly oxidized purine derivatives (Hsu *et al.* 1991). This disturbance partially offsets the decreased synthetic capacity of the 1α-hydroxylase in chronic renal failure. Another possible explanation of the disruption of calcitriol metabolism arises from studies of its interaction with the VDR (Patel *et al.* 1994b). In the past, conflicting results have been published with respect to the specific binding of calcitriol (Korkor 1987; Szabo *et al.* 1991), but there is agreement that VDR regulation is abnormal in renal failure (Szabo *et al.* 1991; Koyama *et al.* 1994). Recently, covalent modification of the VDR, which blunts the action of calcitriol on its target organs, has been observed. The net result is presumably additive to diminished synthesis of calcitriol and leads to decreased stimulation of vitamin D target organs (see above). Resistance to the action of calcitriol is potentially an alternative or complementary explanation for the disruption of the feedback interaction of calcium-regulating hormones in early renal failure (Kurokawa 1993).

A decreased calcaemic response to the action of PTH may be a further factor involved in the stimulation of the parathyroid gland in uraemic patients. Massry *et al.* (1976) found a diminished calcaemic response to the infusion of PTH, suggesting that PTH oversecretion was necessary to maintain eucalcaemia. The subsequent cloning of the PTH/PTHrp receptor ('PTH1-R') (Jüppner *et al.* 1991) allowed

a better insight into the molecular mechanism of the resistance to PTH. The observation of a downregulation of the PTH1-R mRNA in kidney, heart, and cartilage of uraemic rats and of an impaired transmembranous signal transduction mechanism points to a reduced responsiveness at the cellular target level (Ureña *et al.* 1993, 1994; Smogorzewski *et al.* 1995). Whether such a reduction in PTH1-R expression also occurs in the bone of uraemic patients is still a matter of debate. Thus, Picton *et al.* (2001) observed a decrease, whereas Langub *et al.* (2001) actually found an increase, in the skeletal PTH1-R expression of chronic dialysis patients. Further studies showed the expression of several PTH1-R isoforms in various organs and tissues whose precise function, however, remains unknown. In summary, there is an impressive body of evidence suggesting that the initiation of secondary hyperparathyroidism in early renal failure is associated with disturbed calcitriol biosynthesis, and possibly also a reduced action of calcitriol and PTH on their respective target organs. Reduced biosynthesis of calcitriol can be corrected by administration of calcitriol. However, it is obvious that additional factors are also involved, and this requires further study.

Advanced renal failure

With progression of renal failure the spontaneous intake of calcium by uraemic patients tends to decrease to amounts of less than 500 mg of elemental calcium per day (Ritz *et al.* 1980). Together with a reduction in vitamin-D-dependent active intestinal transport of calcium, the diminished intake of calcium results in a tendency towards negative calcium balance and further stimulation of PTH synthesis and secretion. At earlier stages of renal failure, serum phosphate can still be maintained in the normal range through an increase in fractional phosphate clearance, that is, enhanced phosphate clearance per nephron. Despite this compensatory mechanism, the progressive reduction of nephron mass ultimately leads to retention of phosphate in the plasma, usually when the glomerular filtration rate decreases to less than 30 ml/min/1.73 m². Hyperphosphataemia may further enhance hypocalcaemia through formation of calcium–phosphate complexes, although this concept has been questioned by Adler *et al.* (1985). Definitively, hyperphosphataemia stimulates the parathyroid glands directly, independent of changes in circulating calcium or calcitriol concentrations (see above).

Serum calcium may be low, normal, or high in endstage renal disease. It has been shown that hyperparathyroidism may progress even in the presence of normocalcaemia or hypercalcaemia (Dunstan *et al.* 1985). This can be explained by additional factors that stimulate the parathyroids in advanced renal failure independently of serum calcium (Table 3). While normal parathyroid glands have an extremely low proliferative activity, uraemia leads to parathyroid tissue hyperplasia, that is, to recruitment of additional, hormonally active cells. Transition from diffuse hyperplasia to nodular hyperplasia is found in cases with severe hyperparathyroidism (Mendes *et al.* 1983). More recently, it has been shown that growth in parathyroid glands with nodular hyperplasia is predominantly mono- or multiclonal, based on the observation of clonal growth in the parathyroid glands of at least 60 per cent of dialysis patients who underwent parathyroidectomy (Arnold *et al.* 1995), as well as on the demonstration of allelic loss of proven or presumed tumour suppressor genes (Falchetti *et al.* 1993; Arnold *et al.* 1995; Chudek *et al.* 1998). Impaired growth control in such glands is also suggested by the observations of increased rates (approximately 30 per cent) of local recurrence after successful subtotal

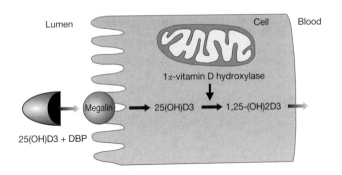

Fig. 3 Luminal uptake of calcidiol [25(OH)D3] and its binding protein (DBP) via a megalin-dependant mechanism.

Table 3 Pathogenesis of secondary renal hyperparathyroidism

Abnormal plasma biochemistry
    Low plasma calcium
    Low plasma calcitriol
    High plasma phosphate?

Excessive parathyroid tissue mass (hypertrophy/hyperplasia)

Resistance to PTH action
    Decreased PTH receptor expression
    Postreceptor events?

Autonomous PTH synthesis/secretion
    Abnormal parathyroid gland calcitriol receptors?
    Abnormal parathyroid gland calcium sensing protein?
    Altered Ca set point?
    Abnormal expression of growth-enhancing or
        growth-repressing genes?
    Nodular monoclonal growth of parathyroid tissue

parathyroidectomy (Gagné et al. 1992) and locally invasive growth of parathyroid autotransplants in the forearms of at least some patients (Frei et al. 1981; Korzets et al. 1987). In glands with nodular hyperplasia, focal areas of low VDR expression are frequently found (Fukuda et al. 1993). Low VDR expression and/or diminished transfer of the VDR—calcitriol complex from the cytoplasm to the nucleus of the parathyroid cell (Patel et al. 1994a) may explain why uraemic patients with advanced hyperparathyroidism often have a reduced response or even no response at all to treatment with calcitriol (Fischer and Harris 1993; Herrmann et al. 1994; Quarles et al. 1994). This is particularly the case in patients in whom plasma Ca and/or phosphorus increase under calcitriol therapy.

With respect to the stimulatory action of hypocalcaemia, it is important to define whether the calciostatic function of the parathyroid glands, that is, the rate of secretion of PTH in response to changes in ionized calcium, is altered in renal failure. Both in vitro (Brown et al. 1982) and in vivo (Delmez et al. 1989) studies suggested that there was an increase in the 'set point' of PTH secretion, that is, higher concentrations of ionized calcium were required to inhibit PTH secretion half-maximally. The set point decreased after intravenous calcitriol treatment. Dialysis patients with severe secondary hyperparathyroidism have a set point shift to the right (Felsenfeld et al. 1995; Goodman et al. 1996, 1998); in contrast, such a shift was not observed in uraemic patients with less severe hyperparathyroidism (Ramirez et al. 1993).

Abnormalities of the skeletal response to PTH (see discussion above) as well as alterations in the metabolism of PTH have also been implicated in the maintenance of renal hyperparathyroidism. Catabolism of PTH is disturbed in chronic renal failure. PTH is mostly degraded in the liver and in the kidney. Bio-inactive fragments of the PTH peptide are normally excreted by the kidney. In uraemia, these peptide fragments accumulate in the circulation (Freitag et al. 1978). However, it is unlikely that in a servocontrolled hormonal system decreased catabolism would cause alterations in the steady-state concentration of the hormone. In the past, bio-inactive fragments have interfered with PTH radioimmunoassays. Subsequently, it was held that this problem had been entirely solved with the modern two-site immunoradiometric assays of so-called 'intact PTH' which had indeed revolutionized the clinical diagnosis of hyperparathyroidism.

However, more recent findings showed that these 'intact PTH' assays actually recognized a considerable amount of amino-terminally truncated PTH fragments (~50 per cent of total PTH), in addition to intact PTH (Lepage et al. 1998). Therefore, a new radioimmunometric assay has been developed which has been claimed to measure intact PTH alone (see below) (John et al. 1999).

It would be wrong to assume that hyperparathyroidism is invariably present in advanced renal failure. Perhaps because of iatrogenic measures (positive calcium balance, administration of calcitriol), an increasing proportion of patients on dialysis (in our experience approximately 30–40 per cent) have PTH concentrations in the normal range. Because of the altered skeletal response to PTH in chronic renal failure (Cohen-Solal et al. 1991; Quarles et al. 1992), this may be a factor in the genesis of 'adynamic bone disease'. Plasma 'intact PTH' is elevated two- to tenfold in approximately 50–60 per cent of untreated patients and more than tenfold in approximately 5–10 per cent of them. Apart from iatrogenic interventions, namely, the administration of calcium, and/or active vitamin D metabolites, marked interpatient variability may also be related to the type of nephropathy, vitamin D status, aluminium overload status, and individual dietary habits with respect to the intake of calcium and phosphate. A more hypothetical possibility is interindividual differences in VDR or PTH receptor status. Excessive PTH concentrations may exert effects on a variety of non-classical target organs which are unrelated to hormonal control of calcium metabolism, for example the myocardium, arteries, several endocrine glands, the peripheral and central nervous system, and haematopoietic cells, for most of which PTH receptors have been demonstrated recently (Mannstadt et al. 1999). It has been claimed that excess PTH may have numerous, potentially serious clinical consequences unrelated to disturbed calcium metabolism (Massry et al. 1987).

Uraemic acidosis has also been implicated in the pathogenesis of impaired divalent ion metabolism in chronic renal failure. Metabolic, but not respiratory, acidosis promotes bone demineralization and a negative calcium balance (Kleeman 1994). This is due in part to direct effects of protons on bone cells, as found in bone cell culture models (Bushinsky 1993). It is also of interest that acidosis has been shown to inhibit renal 1α-hydroxylase activity by direct or indirect mechanisms. It has been suggested that correction of acidosis slows down progression of hyperparathyroidism in haemodialysis patients (Lefebvre et al. 1989). This observation could be explained by the fact that the correction of acidosis in haemodialysis patients increases the sensitivity of the parathyroid glands to calcium (Graham et al. 1997).

Vitamin D deficiency is common in renal patients, at least in Europe, where milk is not systematically supplemented with vitamin D. It is also true in Algerian patients with a theoretically high likelihood to have enough sunshine (Ghazali et al. 1999). The deficiency is diagnosed from low circulating 25(OH)D3 concentrations. It is important to take seasonal changes of 25(OH)D3 into consideration. During the summer, serum 25(OH)D3 ranges between 100 and 300 nmol/l but in winter it may be 50 per cent less. Vitamin D deficiency usually results from an altered lifestyle and reduced sun exposure (Ghazali et al. 1999), resulting in diminished actinic synthesis of vitamin D3 by the skin. In addition, increased UV irradiation may be required for vitamin D generation in the skin because of melanosis cutis. Furthermore, vitamin D metabolites bound to vitamin D binding protein may be lost to the urine in patients with nephrotic range proteinuria or to the peritoneal fluid in patients treated by CAPD (Schmidt-Gayk et al. 1977). Low 25(OH)D3 may be clinically important because more severe bone disease is found in vitamin-D-deficient uraemic patients (Bayard *et al.* 1973). Furthermore, in extrarenal tissues, synthesis of calcitriol is substrate dependent and thus is predictably diminished when 25(OH)D3 is reduced. Local calcitriol synthesis, for example by human bone cells (Puzas *et al.* 1987), may build up high local (paracrine) calcitriol concentrations which are not necessarily reflected by circulating (endocrine) concentrations. Because it is unknown to what extent hypothetically increased local calcitriol concentrations are restored by administration of calcitriol alone, it is wise to correct vitamin D deficiency, if present.

Disturbances related to dialysis procedure (see also Chapters 12.3 and 12.5)

Renal replacement therapy, together with dietary measures and drug treatment, is aimed at improving many of the perturbations of calcium and phosphate metabolism which are induced by the uraemic state. The degree of improvement may vary with the type of renal replacement modality. Unfortunately, however, iatrogenic perturbations may also be introduced.

Haemodialysis and haemodiafiltration techniques influence calcium balance via diffusive and convective loss of calcium during the dialysis procedures. To overcome these losses, in the past, a high dialysate calcium concentration (generally 1.75 mmol/l) was chosen to achieve a net positive balance of calcium during the dialysis session, taking also into consideration that the patients are in negative calcium balance during the interdialytic interval because of intestinal malabsorption of calcium, unless they receive high doses of calcium-containing phosphate binders or active vitamin D derivatives. The magnitude of net calcium uptake during the dialysis session is dependent on the transmembrane gradient of diffusible calcium (Argilés *et al.* 1993) and the amount of ultrafiltration (Memoli *et al.* 1991). Such net uptake is relatively small compared with what is achieved with high oral doses of calcium supplementation. Nevertheless, an inappropriately high dialysate calcium may cause hypercalcaemia and undesirably low PTH concentrations, particularly in patients on calcitriol treatment. This may render the management of hyperparathyroidism in dialysed patients difficult.

It has been claimed that CAPD allows for greater net removal of phosphate and greater net uptake of calcium than haemodialysis, but there is no conclusive evidence for this (Weinreich *et al.* 1992). It is highly probable, however, that the previous habit of using relatively high calcium concentrations for the preparation of peritoneal dialysis fluid was responsible for the much higher prevalence of adynamic bone disease in patients treated by CAPD than in those treated by intermittent haemodialysis (Sherrard *et al.* 1993; Torres *et al.* 1995). Serum 25-(OH)2D3 and calcitriol, bound to vitamin D binding protein, may be lost into the peritoneal dialysis fluid (Zucchelli *et al.* 1984) by a mechanism analogous to plasmapheresis, but vitamin D deficiency related to this mechanism is rare and can be relevant only in vitamin-D-deficient patients in whom the rate of peritoneal loss of vitamin D metabolites approximates the rate of vitamin D synthesis.

Extrarenal synthesis of calcitriol has been found in some dialysis patients (Dusso *et al.* 1991). One possible source of excess calcitriol synthesis is ectopic production of calcitriol by activated macrophages

(Adams *et al.* 1985; Reichel *et al.* 1987) and granulomatous tissue. This has been reported in dialysed patients with granulomatous disease, for example, sarcoidosis or tuberculosis. It is also of note that circulating monocytes from haemodialysis patients may synthesize calcitriol (Dusso *et al.* 1991), possibly mediated by contact of cells with dialysis membranes (Reichel *et al.* 1992). The 25(OH)D-1α-hydroxylase activity of extrarenal tissue is not hormonally controlled, and product inhibition by calcitriol does not occur (Reichel *et al.* 1987). Calcitriol synthesis by extrarenal 1α-hydroxylation is substrate dependent, and this may explain the finding that circulating calcitriol in uraemic patients increases under vitamin D or 25(OH)D3 therapy (Dusso *et al.* 1991), whereas in normal subjects calcitriol synthesis is not influenced by increasing serum 25(OH)D3.

The serum magnesium concentration is generally increased in chronic renal failure. The increase tends to be even more pronounced in patients who ingest magnesium-containing phosphate binders. Since elevated circulating magnesium could impair skeletal mineralization, some authors advocate drastic reduction of the magnesium concentration in the dialysate, or even its omission from the dialysis fluid, for patients who are receiving magnesium-containing drugs. In this case, close monitoring of plasma magnesium is necessary to avoid magnesium depletion (Kenny *et al.* 1987). A more reasonable approach seems to be to aim at the maintenance of near-normal serum magnesium.

Plasma β_2-m is increased in chronic renal failure and may reach very high concentrations in anuric patients. They cannot be normalized despite highly efficient dialysis or haemofiltration modalities and usually remain 10–20 times above normal levels. This could be partially responsible for non-PTH-related stimulation of osteoclastic bone resorption, since β_2-m is capable of stimulating calcium release from bone by an enhancement of osteoclast activity *in vitro* (Moe and Sprague 1992). Furthermore, plasma β_2-m correlates with the degree of bone turnover as reflected by biochemical determination of serum markers and histomorphometric measurements of bone cell numbers (Ferreira *et al.* 1995).

Bone disease secondary to severe aluminium intoxication, namely, osteomalacia or adynamic bone disease, became a major complication in dialysis patients during the 1970s and 1980s. However, owing to the recognition of its cause, the identification of effective treatments, and in particular the establishment of preventive measures, the prevalence of clinically relevant aluminium-associated osteopathy has become negligible during recent years, at least in Western Europe.

Aluminium can enter the body of the uraemic patient through two main routes, namely the dialytic and the gastrointestinal pathway. During the 1970s and 1980s, dramatic aluminium overload states had been observed in haemodialysis or CAPD patients whose dialysis fluid was heavily contaminated by the trace element. Before the introduction of systematic deionization and reverse osmosis of dialysis water, high aluminium concentrations of tap water in several geographical areas led to aluminium intoxication in an almost routine manner. This danger has now been overcome in general in most centres of the Western hemisphere. However, extremely high water contamination may still lead to an aluminium overload via that route, even in the presence of adequate technical equipment. Moreover, a transiently or permanently defective water purification system will allow the trace element to enter the body if its concentration is elevated in drinking water, as illustrated by the dramatic accidental aluminium intoxication which occurred in a dialysis centre in Portugal in 1994 (Simoes *et al.* 1994).

The other route by which aluminium overload can occur is excessive intestinal aluminium absorption, generally due to the oral intake of large amounts of the trace element in the form of aluminium-containing phosphate binders such as aluminium hydroxide or carbonate. Although the ingestion of small doses of such compounds (e.g. up to 3 g of aluminium hydroxide daily) does not usually lead to a clinically significant overload, it is no longer considered acceptable at present, even in patients with uncontrollable elevation of serum phosphorus, because of the availability of new, calcium- and aluminium-free phosphate binders (see below). The prescription of aluminium-containing phosphate binders is absolutely contraindicated in the presence of short bowel syndrome and in patients with concomitant administration of citrate which has been shown to enhance intestinal aluminium absorption markedly.

In plasma, aluminium is mainly bound to transferrin and albumin. It probably competes with iron for transferrin binding sites (VanLandeghem *et al.* 1997). Iron overload apparently protects the body against excessive entry of the trace element, whereas iron deficiency appears to enhance its entry into the organism and its distribution to targets tissues (Cannata *et al.* 1991; Smans *et al.* 1996). Heavy aluminium overload may induce two different types of skeletal disease, namely osteomalacia or 'adynamic' (also called 'aplastic') bone disease, but this is not an inexorable outcome. The clinical, laboratory, and radiological expression of aluminium-related osteomalacia is similar to that of vitamin D deficiency. Histologically, there are minor differences which may allow the two conditions to be differentiated. The hallmark of aluminium overload is the presence of aluminium deposits at the mineralization front (see below). The skeletal lesions induced by aluminium are probably due to both direct and indirect effects (Plachot *et al.* 1984; Lieberherr *et al.* 1987). The latter involve interactions with the metabolism and action of calcium-regulating hormones, that is, PTH and calcitriol (Fig. 4).

It is noteworthy that even marked aluminium overload may remain histologically silent in patients with pre-existing moderate to severe osteitis fibrosa. Therefore, the finding of osteitis fibrosa or mixed bone disease is not incompatible with the presence of even marked aluminium overload. Under such conditions, the deposition of aluminium may best be revealed by a positive desferrioxamine test (see below).

In cases of suspected aluminium toxicity, an assessment of plasma aluminium is indicated both in the basal state and after infusion of the chelating agent desferrioxamine. Basal plasma concentrations of aluminium are increased to greater than the normal range (<5 µg/l) in virtually all patients on maintenance haemodialysis.

Basal plasma aluminium is not a reliable indicator of the presence of aluminium-related bone disease. Therefore, a desferrioxamine infusion test may be required which generally gives more precise information. To avoid toxicity, we recommend infusion of 5 mg/kg body weight desferrioxamine over 1 h at the end of a dialysis session. Reliable criteria for defining a positive test have not been established. As a rule of thumb, aluminium intoxication can be assumed if aluminium increases threefold above the basal value, or if the absolute increment is more than 150 µg/l (5.6 µmol/l) 24–48 h later. The test may be paradoxically negative in patients with low bone turnover (adynamic bone disease), but in this case the pathogenetic implication of aluminium is unclear.

Diagnostic procedures

Diagnosis, clinical presentation, and management of hyperparathyroid bone disease and other bone problems are discussed in the following sections. The syndrome of dialysis-related β_2-m amyloidosis is described in detail in Chapter 4.2.

Laboratory tests

Table 4 provides a list of biochemical tests that are useful in the evaluation of uraemic patients with bone disease. The measurement of plasma total calcium, ionized calcium, and phosphorus is not helpful in recognizing the pattern of bone involvement, that is, in distinguishing osteitis fibrosa from other types of bone disease, particularly osteomalacia and low bone turnover with or without aluminium overload. Only when a patient presents with combined hypocalcaemia and hypophosphataemia can the diagnosis of vitamin D deficiency and osteomalacia be made with a certain degree of accuracy. Hypercalcaemia is common in both advanced osteitis fibrosa and low bone turnover including aluminium bone disease. Patients with low bone turnover are particularly prone to develop hypercalcaemia if they receive vitamin D metabolites or oral calcium supplements. Probably, calcium uptake and hence the calcium buffering capacity of uraemic bone are decreased (Kurz *et al.* 1994). The following aetiologies should be considered first in the dialysis patient with hypercalcaemia:

(1) advanced hyperparathyroidism;

(2) positive calcium balance (calcium-containing phosphate binders, high dialysate calcium, and active vitamin D metabolites, particularly in patients with low bone turnover/aluminium bone disease);

(3) overtreatment with vitamin D or its more active derivatives (exogenous vitamin D overload); or

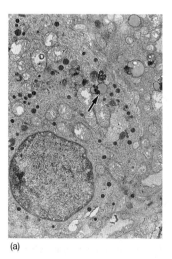
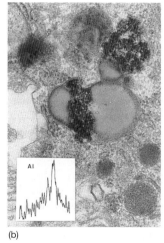

(a)   (b)

Fig. 4 Electron microscopy of parathyroid tissue in aluminium intoxication. (a) Ultrastructural aspect of a parathyroid gland chief cell from an aluminium-intoxicated haemodialysis patient. Note the numerous mitochondria, secretion granules, and folding of plasmalemma indicating active hormone synthesis (magnification 12,000×). (b) Dense deposits (arrow) which emit X-rays characteristic of aluminium are present within lipoid bodies (magnification 63,000×).

Table 4 Serum biochemistry in the evaluation of renal osteodystrophy

	Comments	Normal range
Calcium	Low, normal, or elevated (tendency for elevation in severe HPT, intoxication, vitamin D excess, therapy with Ca-containing phosphate binders)	2.2–2.6 mmol/l
Phosphate	Elevated in advanced renal failure (GFR < 30 ml/min)	0.8–1.4 mmol/l
PTH		
Intact 1-84 peptide	Elevated in HPT; can be normal or even low (mostly in cases of Al intoxication adynamic bone disease, overtreatment with calcitriol, prior parathyroidectomy)	1–6 pmol/l or 10–65 pg/ml
Fragment assays	Obsolete since PTH fragments accumulate in chronic renal failure	
25(OH)D3 (calcidiol)	Low or normal; seasonal variations; if increased, check for exogenous source	50–200 nmol/l
Calcitriol	Low (rarely low normal); if increased, check for calcitriol ingestion; rarely, endogenous overproduction	25–75 pg/ml
Total AP	Normal or increased, elevated in severe HPT (exclude concomitant liver disease by determination of γGT)	60–170 IU/l
Osseous AP isoenzyme	Normal or increased; elevated in HPT; measurement by monoclonal antibody technology has better sensitivity and specificity for HPT than total AP	3–22 μg/l (may depend on assay)
Osteocalcin	Changes similar to AP; fragments accumulate in chronic renal failure; probably no extra information in addition to intact PTH and osseous AP	ca. 3–8 μg/l* (may depend on assay)
Magnesium	Normal or elevated (decreased renal excretion)	0.8–1.3 mmol/l

* Range for normal renal function.

HPT, hyperparathyroidism; GFR, glomerular filtration rate; AP, alkaline phosphatase; γGT, γ-glutamyl transferase.

(4) endogenous calcitriol excess (granulomatous disease);

(5) increased bone resorption from immobilization or neoplasia (myeloma, metastasizing carcinoma).

The serum phosphate depends on dietary phosphate intake, vitamin D therapy, catabolic state, residual renal function, efficacy of dialysis, and other factors (Schaefer 1994); therefore, it is not a useful index of bone disease. The risk of soft tissue calcification parallels the degree of hyperphosphataemia and the Ca × P product (Ureña et al. 1999; Goodman et al. 2000), as well as the amount of oral calcium intake (Guerin et al. 2000).

Serum total alkaline phosphatases must be interpreted in relation to prevailing γ-glutamyl transferase to exclude cholestasis, with potential elevation of the hepatic isoenzyme of alkaline phosphatase. Measurement of the bone-specific isoenzyme of alkaline phosphatase provides a more sensitive index and has been proposed as a non-invasive probe to monitor the type of bone disease, in particular to assess the degree of bone formation (Ureña et al. 1995; Coutteyne et al. 1997). However, its value in distinguishing low from normal bone turnover in ESRD patients is not yet definitely established. Other non-invasive serum markers have been proposed for the assessment of bone formation such as intact osteocalcin (GLA protein) and procollagen type I C-terminal propeptide (PICP) (Ureña and deVernejoul 1999). For the evaluation of osteoclastic bone resorption, type I collagen cross-linked telopeptide (ICTP), the bone collagen derivatives pyridinoline (PYD) and deoxypyridinoline (DPD), and tartrate-resistant acid phosphatase (TRAP) have been reported to be useful, at least by some groups (Ureña et al. 1999). However, it remains uncertain at present whether they provide useful clinical information over and above that provided by a combination of serum calcium, phosphorus, PTH, aluminium and total alkaline phosphatases.

Table 5 Plasma intact PTH versus bone histology

	Bone histology	Plasma PTH (pmol/l)
Healthy subjects	Normal	1–6
Dialysis patients	Normal	6 (−12)–18
	Osteitis fibrosa	12–18
	'Adynamic bone disease'	0–9

Modified from Hutchinson et al. (1993).

Measurement of serum 25(OH)D3 is useful for assessing the vitamin D status. As discussed above, vitamin D deficiency is not uncommon in uraemic patients. It can also be used to monitor compliance of patients treated with cholecalciferol or 25(OH)D3. Monitoring of calcitriol treatment and measurement of serum calcitriol is not useful because of the short half-life of this compound. The finding of increased calcitriol (which is usually low in uraemic patients) may occasionally be useful as an indicator of sarcoidosis or other granulomatous diseases in dialysed patients with hypercalcaemia of unknown origin.

Plasma so-called 'intact PTH' generally exhibits a reasonably good, but not perfect, relation with bone histology parameters (Hutchison et al. 1993) (Table 5). In a more recent study ((Ureña et al. 1995), we found better correlations with bone histomorphometry parameters for serum bone-specific alkaline phosphatase isoenzyme and serum PYD than for intact PTH. In rare cases, however, elevation of 'intact PTH' by a factor of 2–8 may be associated with normal bone histology. The subsequent development of a radioimmunometric assay measuring full-length intact PTH only (John et al. 1999) is a further step in our attempt to assess the precise concentration of truly biologically active, inact PTH alone. However, the N-terminal PTH fragment, which is also

Table 6 Laboratory tests in renal osteodystrophy

	Osteitis fibrosa	Aluminium osteopathy/intoxication	β_2-m Amyloidosis
Calcium	Variable, high normal in advanced hyperparathyroidism	Tendency for hypercalcaemia	Non-specific
Phosphate	Rises in advanced hyperparathyroidism	Non-specific	Non-specific
Intact PTH	Elevated	Less elevated than in hyperparathyroidism or normal	Non-specific
Alkaline phosphatases	Usually elevated	Tends to be low	Non-specific
Aluminium	Variable, usually <100 μg/l	Mostly elevated (>60 μg/l)	Non-specific
Increase of aluminium after desferrioxamine	Variable, may be marked or nil	Marked increase, often >150 μg/dl or threefold above baseline	Non-specific

biologically active, is not measured by this assay. It remains to be seen whether the use of the new radioimmunometric assay provides a significant benefit over that of the so-called 'intact PTH' assays in clinical practice, in particular, with respect to a better distinction between mild osteitis fibrosa and adynamic bone disease. Recently, Faugere *et al.* (2001) have proposed that the use of the ratio of the concentration of true intact PTH to that of large PTH fragments (calculated from the difference between true PTH and so-called 'intact PTH') allowed a more reliable assessment of bone turnover than either assay alone. Several other research groups could however not confirm this observation.

In the last decade, a large number of new growth factors and cytokines, as well as their agonists, antagonists, and receptors, have been recognized and their respective roles in the fine tuning of bone activity defined. Here it would not be proper to present an exhaustive review of this rapidly evolving chapter of bone physiology and pathophysiology. Suffice to say that in the future we will have to take into account various bone formation regulatory systems such as the IGF and IGF-receptor protein family (Jehle *et al.* 2000), as well as bone resorption regulatory systems such as the osteoprotegerin, RANK, and RANK-L protein family (deVernejoul 2001) for a more precise evaluation of the disturbances of bone metabolism in chronic renal failure.

At any rate, preventive and therapeutic measures will have to be re-evaluated using novel serum markers for bone turnover. At present, the determination of such markers is only indicated if, in the presence of clinical problems, PTH concentrations are modestly elevated, and thus do not permit safe conclusions with respect to bone histology, or when there are discrepancies between PTH concentrations and other clinical findings (Table 5).

Table 6 summarizes the utility of laboratory tests to differentiate between osteitis fibrosa, low bone turnover ('aplastic bone disease'), aluminium osteopathy, and bone involvement unrelated to disturbed calcium metabolism, for example, β_2-m-related amyloidosis.

X-ray and other imaging techniques

Evaluation of the hand skeleton should be carried out using plain radiography or magnification techniques. A complete series of skeletal radiographs (Table 7) should be taken when a patient begins dialysis treatment. Follow-up radiography of the hand skeleton at yearly intervals is advisable and sufficient.

The radiographic findings in osteitis fibrosa are quite characteristic. The typical signs are summarized in Table 8. Typical lesions include

Table 7 Recommended skeletal X-ray series for assessment of secondary hyperparathyroidism

Hand, anteroposterior
Shoulder, lateral
Skull, lateral
Spine, lateral
Pelvis, anteroposterior

Table 8 Radiographic signs of renal osteodystrophy in patients with chronic renal failure

Hyperparathyroidism
Accelerated bone resorption
    Subperiosteal resorption, maximal at radial aspect of middle phalanx of index and midfinger, also at distal ends of clavicles, and in the skull (pepper-pot aspect); acro-osteoylsis of terminal phalanges; cortical bone thinning; cortical striation, fluffy trabecular structure, seldom pathological fractures
Enlarged syndesmoses
    Resorption of cortex of lateral clavicle, of symphysis, and of sacroiliac joints
Osteosclerosis
    Increased density of ground plates of vertebrae (rugger jersey spine), or of radial and tibial metaphyses, or osteosclerosis of diploe (ground glass)
Accelerated bone apposition
    Periosteal neostosis
Soft tissue calcification
    Periarticular and vascular radiodense deposits; less frequently deposits in viscera (lungs, myocardium) and skin

Aluminium-related bone disease
Generally no specific radiological signs; pseudofractures (Looser zones) at predilection sites; low mineral density

Differential diagnosis
β_2-Microglobulin-associated osteo-arthropathy
    Periarticular bone erosions, subchondral bone cysts, destructive arthropathy

resorptive defects on the external and internal surfaces of cortical bone, particularly resorption and new bone formation (periosteoneostosis) at the subperiosteal surface. Resorption within cortical bone enlarges the Haversian channels, resulting in longitudinal striation; resorption at the endosteal surface causes cortical thinning. These lesions are detected first and most easily in the hand skeleton (Fig. 5). Accelerated bone deposition at the periosteal surface (periosteal neostosis) can be seen on radiographs [Fig. 5(b)]. Another characteristic feature is resorptive loss of acral bone (acro-osteolysis), for example at the terminal phalanges [Fig. 5(a)], at the distal end of the clavicles, and 'punched out' resorptive lesions in the skull ('pepper-pot' aspect) (Fig. 6). Syndesmoses, that is, tight fibrous bone connections, may be enlarged by bone resorption, for example, at the acromioclavicular joint, the symphyses, or the sacroiliac joints. The mass (volume fraction) of spongy bone tends to be increased, particularly in the metaphyses. This phenomenon results in the characteristic sclerotic aspect of the upper and lower thirds of the vertebrae, contrasting with the rarefaction of the centre ('rugger jersey spine') (Fig. 7).

Osteosclerosis of the diploë leads to a 'ground glass' appearance of the skull radiograph. Osteosclerosis is also commonly seen in radiographs of the metaphyses of the radius and tibia. In addition to the skeletal lesions, radiographs often reveal various types of soft tissue calcification.

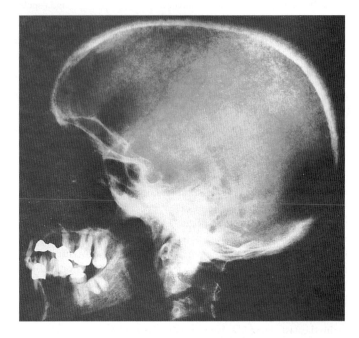

Fig. 6 Resorptive defects of diploë (pepper-pot aspect) in the skull of a haemodialysis patient with severe hyperparathyroidism.

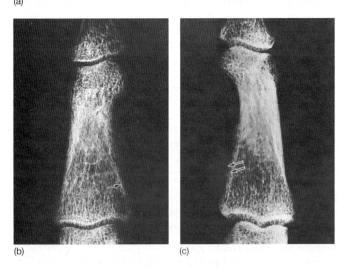

(a)

(b)   (c)

Fig. 5 Radiographic signs in hand skeletons of haemodialysis patients with severe secondary hyperparathyroidism: (a) subperiostal erosion (particularly pronounced in middle phalanges) and acro-osteolysis of the terminal phalanges; (b) periostal new bone formation (periostal neostosis) (arrow); (c) subperiostal resorption zones (arrow). Both (b) and (c) show cortical thinning, cortical striation, and fluffy trabecular structure.

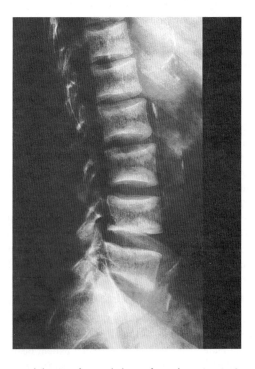

Fig. 7 Increased density of ground plates of vertebrae contrasting with radiolucency of the central vertebral slices (rugger jersey spine) in a haemodialysis patient with severe hyperparathyroidism. Note the severe aortic calcification.

These comprise vascular calcifications, that is, calcification of intimal plaques (aorta, iliac arteries), as well as diffuse calcification of the media (Mönckeberg type) of peripheral muscular arteries [Fig. 8(a)]. Finally, calcium deposits may be seen in periarticular tissue or bursas [Fig. 8(b) and (c)].

There are no specific radiographic signs that prove the presence of aluminium-related bone disease, but the demonstration of Looser zones in the predilection sites (Fig. 9) is suggestive of aluminium osteopathy. Looser zones are usually sharply delineated zones of radiolucency, corresponding to zones subjected to high mechanical stress where lamellar bone has been replaced by primitive, poorly mineralized woven bone. Looser zones at both ischiopubal branches of the pelvis in a haemodialysis patient with severe aluminium intoxication are shown in Fig. 10. Furthermore, aluminium intoxication favours the development of extraosseous calcifications [Fig. 8(b) and (c)]. In some

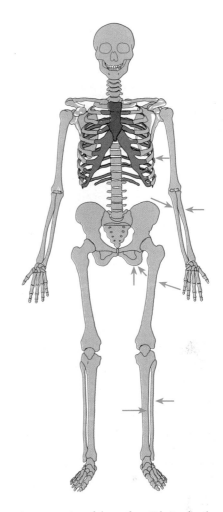

Fig. 9 Schematic presentation of the preferential sites for the occurrence of Looser zones in aluminium-intoxicated uraemic patients. Less frequent localizations (e.g. at the scapula) are not shown.

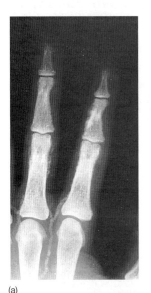

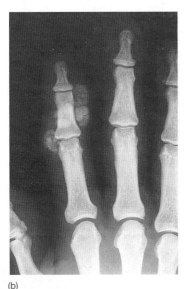

(a)

(b)

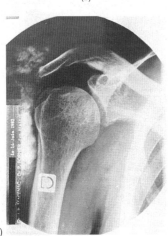

(c)

Fig. 8 Extraosseous calcifications in terminal renal failure: (a) calcifications of small peripheral (digital) arteries in a dialysis patient with severe osteitis fibrosa with concomitant existence of subperiostal erosions; (b) pseudotumoural calcinosis in a dialysis patient with severe aluminium intoxication in the absence of radiological evidence of hyperparathyroidism; (c) pseudotumoural calcinosis of the shoulder in a dialysis patient with severe aluminium intoxication in the absence of secondary hyperparathyroidism.

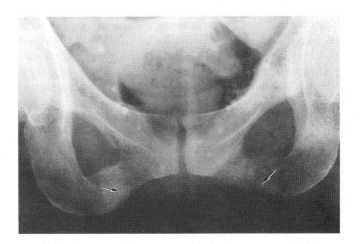

Fig. 10 Looser zones (arrows) at both pubic bones in a haemodialysis patient with severe aluminium intoxication.

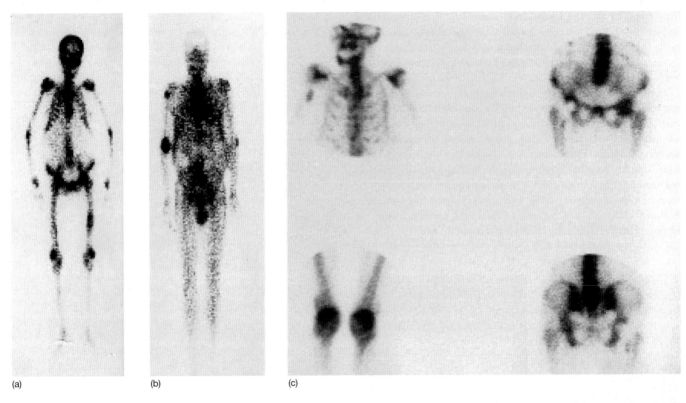

(a)   (b)   (c)

Fig. 11 Contrasting bone scintigrams in the major bony complications of uraemia (osteitis fibrosa, osteomalacia, and β_2-m-related amyloidosis) obtained using ^{99m}Tc-methylene diphosphonate as the bone-seeking marker substance: (a) markedly increased tracer uptake by skeletal areas consisting of spongy bone (skull, axial skeleton) in a haemodialysis patient with severe hyperparathyroidism; (b) decreased bone uptake with persistence of tracer in extraskeletal areas (presumably blood vessels and soft tissues) in a haemodialysis patient with severe osteomalacia; (c) localized increase of tracer uptake at the site of the shoulder, iliac, femoral, and knee joints in a haemodialysis patient with biopsy-proven β_2-m amyloid deposits.

cases, the use of complementary imaging techniques may be advisable. Technetium diphosphonate scans show characteristic patterns in osteitis fibrosa and aluminium bone disease: diffusely increased uptake, particularly in the skull, is typical of osteitis fibrosa, whereas aluminium osteopathy may result in reduced skeletal uptake of tracer with preferential uptake in soft tissue (but focal uptake at sites of Looser zones may occur). Characteristic scintigrams are shown in Fig. 11.

Specific imaging of β_2-m amyloid deposits using radio-iodinated human serum amyloid P-component (Nelson *et al.* 1991) or radio-iodinated β_2-m purified from human serum (Floege *et al.* 1990, 2001) has been described. These procedures have been used for investigative purposes only (Floege and Ketteler 2001). Areas of active amyloid deposition (e.g. bone cysts) can also be visualized by technetium diphosphonate scanning [Fig. 11(c)]. Although less specific for amyloid than the P-component or β_2-m scans, the technetium diphosphonate scan may be a useful procedure for distinguishing amyloidosis from other types of uraemic bone disease (Grateau *et al.* 1988; Sethi *et al.* 1990).

Computed tomography (CT) may be helpful in patients with complex vertebral problems in order to differentiate bacterial spondylitis, amyloid spondyloarthropathy, and chondrocalcinosis of intervertebral discs. Magnetic resonance imaging (MRI) may provide diagnostically useful, specific information in cases with suspected spondylitis, by showing soft tissue swelling (Fig. 12). It is also useful in visualizing active lesions in amyloid spondylarthropathy. After renal transplantation, osteonecrosis of the femoral head, and less frequently of the

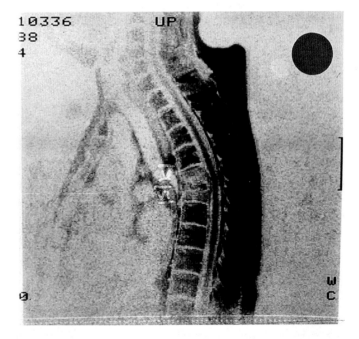

Fig. 12 MRI scan of the spine of a haemodialysis patient with spondylodiscitis C5/C6. Note the destruction of vertebral bodies and compression by soft tissue swelling of the spinal cord.

humerus, knee, or other joint regions, can be visualized by radiography (Fig. 13). Early diagnosis of osteonecrosis is possible with technetium diphosphonate scintigraphy and earliest with MRI.

Visualization of the parathyroid glands before a first parathyroidectomy is not mandatory because these glands are best localized by an experienced surgeon during the operation although some surgeons find it useful because of the 3–5 per cent prevalence of ectopic parathyroids, particularly of retrosternal location (Tominaga *et al.* 1997). However, before a planned second operation, parathyroid glands should always be visualized by imaging techniques. The methods available include ultrasonography or, in doubtful cases, magnetic resonance, tomography, and selective arteriography; the latter three may be particularly helpful in localizing retrosternal parathyroid tissue (Winzelberg 1987; Levin and Clark 1988). An enlarged parathyroid gland in a paratracheal site, detected by CT scan, is shown in Fig. 14. In our experience, and that

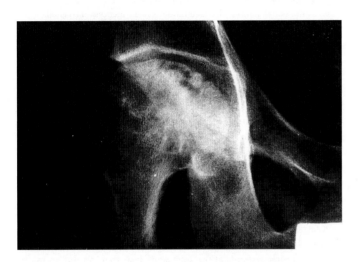

Fig. 13 Unilateral femoral head necrosis in a patient with a kidney transplant.

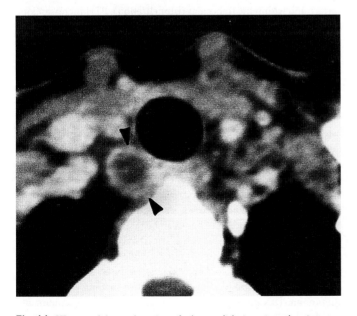

Fig. 14 CT scan of the neck region of a haemodialysis patient showing an enlarged parathyroid gland in paratracheal localization.

of others, technetium–thallium subtraction scintigraphy has not lived up to its promise. A promising more recent scintigraphic technique uses ^{99m}Tc-sestamibi in conjunction with subtraction ^{123}I-scanning in primary hyperparathyroidism (Casas *et al.* 1993). Its usefulness in secondary hyperparathyroidism has since been newly demonstrated.

If visualization of the parathyroid glands by imaging techniques is not possible, selective venous catheterization for measurements of PTH from the thyroid, jugular, subclavian, and innominate veins is indicated. This method may allow localization of enlarged parathyroid glands by demonstrating PTH gradients.

Bone mineral density can be determined by dual-energy X-ray absorptiometry (DEXA) and quantitative computerized tomography (qCT) in the spine, and by DEXA in the forearm. The usefulness of determining bone mineral density in patients with chronic kidney disease remains a matter of debate.

Patterns of bone involvement

Various patterns of bone involvement in addition to classical osteitis fibrosa (see later) have been identified (Table 9). Some characteristic features of osteomalacia, low bone turnover (adynamic bone disease), and osteopenia/osteoporosis are summarized in Tables 10, 11, and 12.

After medical control of hyperparathyroidism has been achieved in a substantial proportion of patients, a new pattern of bone involvement has emerged in the last decade, that is, a state of low bone turnover called 'adynamic bone disease' (Hercz *et al.* 1993; Sherrard *et al.* 1993). The cause of this type of osteopathy is multifactorial. It was initially thought to be a specific consequence of aluminium overload. However, it is mainly seen at present in patients who have been exposed either to small amounts of aluminium or not exposed to it at all. In most instances, plasma 'intact PTH' is at best slightly elevated, but usually normal or low. Hypercalcaemia develops more readily in patients with low bone turnover in response to oral calcium or vitamin D supplementation than in patients with osteitis fibrosa, and hyperphosphataemia is observed with similar frequency. The resulting elevation of the calcium × phosphorus product increases the risk of development or aggravation of soft tissue calcification.

Bone histology

Bone biopsies can be taken either with the Jamshidi needle or by using an electrical drill. The Jamshidi needle is completely satisfactory for

Table 9 Differential diagnosis of bone disease in uraemia

Osteitis fibrosa

Osteomalacia (aluminium overload, vitamin D deficiency)

Mixed lesions

Low bone turnover (adynamic bone disease)

Osteopenia/osteoporosis

Dialysis-related amyloidosis

Rare causes of bone disease
    Oxalosis (primary or secondary)
    Fluorosis
    Infection (e.g. osteomyelitis, spondylitis)
    Causes unrelated to uraemia (e.g. multiple myeloma, secondary
       metastases)

Table 10 Osteomalacia in uraemic patients

Cause	Aluminium overload or vitamin D deficiency
Clinical aspects	Bone and joint pain Skeletal deformities Proximal myopathy
Plasma chemistry	Elevated aluminium (>60 μg/l) or decreased 25(OH)D3
Radiographic	Low bone mineral density Woven spongiosal texture Looser zones
Bone histomorphometry	Decreased bone formation Increased osteoid seams Variable bone resorption (positive aluminium stain)

Table 11 Adynamic bone disease of dialysed patients

Cause	Unknown (aluminium? high calcium? low PTH? diminished response to PTH?)
Clinical findings	No symptoms Post-transplant osteonecrosis? Tendency to hypercalcaemia Tendency to extraosseous calcification
Bone histomorphometry	Decreased bone formation and resorption
Predisposing factors	Low PTH Diabetes mellitus Hypothyroidism Glucocorticoid treatment

Table 12 Osteopenia/osteoporosis in uraemic patients

Causes	Same as in general population Oestrogen deficiency? Glucocorticoids after renal transplant
Clinical aspects	Non-specific Loss of height
Plasma chemistry	Unremarkable (tendency to hypercalcaemia?)
Radiography	Diffuse demineralization Longitudinal striation of vertebral bodies Wedge deformity of vertebral bodies
Bone histomorphometry	Decreased bone mass

clinical diagnostic purposes, whereas drilling is preferable for scientific investigations because a larger sample with fewer microfractures is obtained. The biopsy is taken from the anterior iliac crest. Quantitative techniques are available which allow manual or automatic analysis of volumes and surfaces of mineralized bone or osteoid as well as assessment of cell numbers (micromorphometry). The full potential of bone biopsy can only be realized if undecalcified sections are examined. The Masson–Goldner stain, which differentiates mineralized from unmineralized tissue, and the von Kossa silver stain are the most useful.

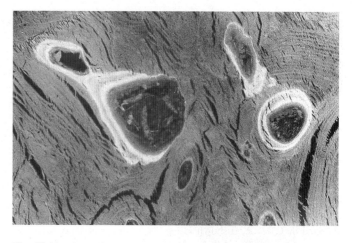

Fig. 15 Histology of normal bone. Two distinct tetracycline labels are found at the bone–osteoid interface (undecalcified sections, unstained, fluorescence light microscopy, 200×).

The von Kossa stain is suitable for assessing bone mineralization (mineralized tissue is stained black). The dynamics of bone remodelling can be examined by administering (prior to the bone biopsy) tetracycline, which locks firmly into the mineralization front. Currently, we use the following schedule: an oral dose of 500 mg tetracycline is given on days 20 and 19 before biopsy, and subsequently on days 6, 5, and 4 before biopsy. By using fluorescence microscopy the rate of bone mineralization can be precisely calculated from the distance between the tetracycline markers administered at different times, and thus the sites of ongoing mineralization in the bone section can be identified. Two distinct tetracycline labels in normal bone are illustrated in Fig. 15.

Histological evidence of increased PTH hormone activity in bone is found in most patients at the start of dialysis therapy and on maintenance dialysis. Typical lesions consist of focal or diffuse fibrosis of bone marrow (endosteal fibrosis) and increased sites of osteoclastic bone resorption. Erosive cavities are detected both on the trabecular surface and within the trabeculas (tunnelization). PTH increases bone turnover by activating sites of bone remodelling, that is, local bone resorption followed by apposition. Consequently, the proportion of the trabecular surface covered by apposition and resorption surfaces is increased. Histological changes of bone in osteitis fibrosa are shown in Fig. 16.

Bone tissue under the influence of excess PTH consists of immature bone in which the texture of the collagen fibres is irregular (woven osteoid and irregularly calcified woven bone). This pattern is usually found in the fetal skeleton, and mature bone normally has a regular lamellar texture (lamellar osteoid, lamellar bone). These two types of osteoid can be distinguished by the presence or absence (in woven bone) of birefringence under polarized light. The histological pattern of woven bone in osteitis fibrosa is shown in Fig. 16.

The aluminium burden of bone can be determined indirectly using an aluminium-specific stain with a tricarboxycyclic acid (Aluminon stain), which identifies aluminium in the mineralization front, that is, the interface between osteoid and mineralized bone. Acid solochrome azurine has been introduced as an alternative staining technique for aluminium. This agent gave more intense staining than Aluminon and correlated well with the biochemically analysed bone aluminium (Kaye *et al.* 1990). The most frequent histological type of aluminium

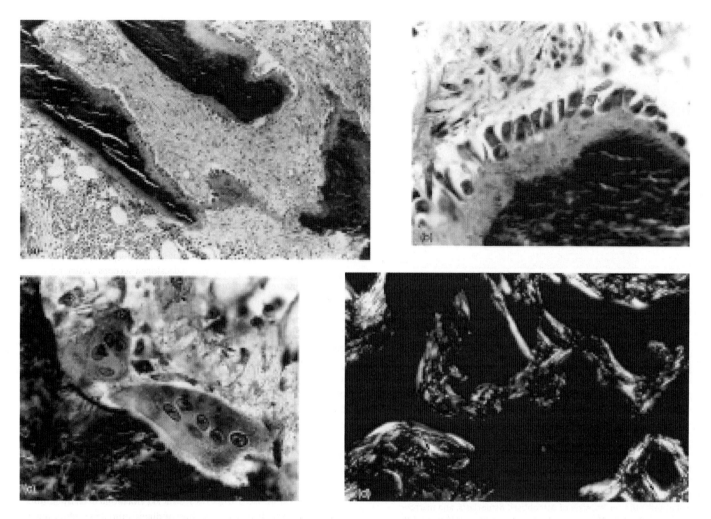

Fig. 16 Bone histology in osteitis fibrosa. (a) The mineralized trabeculas are covered by broad osteoid seams; osteoblasts are numerous and cellular fibrosis is seen in the marrow spaces (magnification 125×). (b) Active osteoblasts with irregular polygonal shapes along an osteoid seam (magnification 800×). (c) Multinucleated osteoclasts resorb the mineralized matrix; note cytoplasmic folding (brush border) in contact with bone tissue (undecalcified section) (toluidine blue stain; magnification 800×). (d) The main bone type observed is woven bone; at some sites (arrows) trabeculas are covered by thin layers of lamellar bone (undecalcified sections; polarized light microscopy; magnification 125×).

osteopathy is characterized by broad unmineralized seams of lamellar osteoid, decreased cancellous bone mass, and little cell activity on the trabecular surface (Fig. 17). The mineralization rate is reduced. Thus, aluminium-related osteopathy most frequently presents as generalized osteomalacia with low bone turnover. It must be stressed that the correlation between stainable and biochemically determined total bone aluminium is poor. Aluminium osteopathy should be thoroughly excluded in patients scheduled to undergo parathyroidectomy because the risk of developing low-turnover bone disease is increased after surgery. Osteomalacia unrelated to aluminium toxicity (Fig. 18) is rarely found in uraemic patients nowadays. This form of osteomalacia, which is due to vitamin D deficiency or hypophosphataemia, also presents with broad unmineralized osteoid seams. The interface between osteoid and mineralized bone is blurred, and cellular activity is usually greater than in aluminium-related osteomalacia. Adynamic (or aplastic) bone disease is a special form of osteopathy where the build-up of broad osteoid seams is presumably prevented by some impairment of osteoblast activity (Fig. 19). The disease results in low-turnover osteopenia. Aluminium was initially incriminated as the most important,

if not the sole, factor involved. However, an aluminium-negative form of adynamic bone disease without osteopenia has been described subsequently (Moriniere *et al.* 1989; Fournier *et al.* 1994) which is the predominant form. It has been proposed that high doses of calcitriol and/or calcium salts, when administered to uraemic patients for prolonged periods of time, cause relative or absolute hypoparathyroidism which is usually found in patients with this type of osteopathy (Hercz 1993; Goodman *et al.* 1994; Fournier 1995).

Further examples of bone histology are shown in Figs 20–24.

Clinical syndromes

Osteitis fibrosa

Excessive activity of PTH at the site of bone tissue results in fibro-osteoclasia, that is, focal or diffuse fibrosis of bone marrow and osteoclastic bone resorption. Even in asymptomatic patients, this may be evident at the macroscopic (radiology) and microscopic level

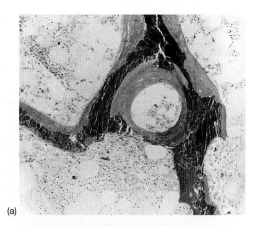

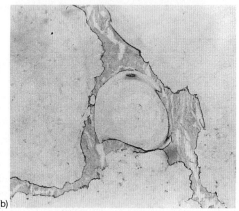

Fig. 17 Renal osteodystrophy: bone histology in aluminium-related low-turnover osteomalacia. (a) Osteoid tissue surrounds the mineralized trabeculas, and the interface between osteoid and mineral is sharply delineated; note the absence of osteoblasts, osteoclasts, and marrow fibrosis (undecalcified sections; toluidine blue stain; magnification 125×). (b) Aluminium deposits at the osteoid–bone interface (undecalcified sections; aurintricarboxylic stain for aluminium; magnification 125×).

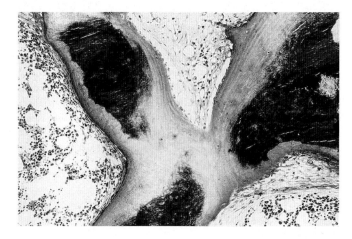

Fig. 18 Renal osteodystrophy: bone histology in non-aluminium-related osteomalacia. Broad lamellar osteoid seams cover the calcified tissue. The interface between osteoid and mineral is blurred. Marrow fibrosis is found along the trabeculas (undecalcified sections; toluidine blue stain; magnification 125×).

(histology). Clinical signs and symptoms are found only in advanced stages. It is unusual that bone disease is symptomatic before the start of maintenance dialysis. Exceptions occur in patients with a long pre-dialytic course (e.g. analgesic nephropathy) or with superimposed problems (e.g. severe vitamin D deficiency or intestinal malabsorption). When patients develop symptoms, they usually complain of pain on exertion in skeletal sites that are subjected to biomechanical stress. Pain in the lower back or foot may be experienced when walking downstairs or on uneven ground. Pain at rest and localized pain are rather unusual and suggest other problems, such as aluminium osteopathy, amyloid bone disease, or osteomyelitis. Patients may present with additional symptoms, for example, the red eye syndrome, pruritus, cutaneous calcification, and pseudogout. Pseudogout is a form of painful joint involvement of acute or subacute onset caused by intra-articular deposition of radio-opaque crystals of calcium pyrophosphate dihydrate. Diagnosis of pseudogout requires demonstration of typical pipe-shaped crystals with weak birefringence under polarized light. The red eye syndrome is a transient local irritation in the eye associated with visible inflammation and injected conjunctival vessels. It is due to deposition of calcium phosphate in the alkaline fluid covering the conjunctiva. Severe proximal myopathy is seen in some patients, even in the absence of vitamin D deficiency.

Unlike that which is seen in severe osteomalacia, bone deformities and pathological fractures are not common in osteitis fibrosa. Rupture of the patella or avulsion of tendons may be observed in advanced cases. Vertebral compression fractures may occur in patients who have epileptic seizures.

Vertebral height is commonly diminished in advanced osteitis fibrosa ('seated dwarf' or 'Sitzzwerg'). Disproportionate loss of height is typical in patients with severe bone lesions; the patient may be able to reach the popliteal region with the hand when standing in an upright position. Acro-osteolysis, that is, erosive loss of the ends of bone, is usually detected on radiographic examination. Occasionally this lesion may become clinically manifest as pseudoclubbing, that is, redundancy of soft tissue covering dissolved terminal phalanges of the fingers. Calciphylaxis, that is, cutaneous eschar formation ('calcific uraemic arteriolopathy', see below), may be encountered in patients with severe hyperparathyroidism (Gipstein *et al.* 1976), but this association has become infrequent in recent years, at least in Europe.

Patients with severe hyperparathyroidism and advanced bone lesions often appear severely ill. This may be related, amongst other causes, to multiple actions of PTH on non-classical target organs (e.g. skeletal muscle, heart, blood vessels, bone marrow, pancreas, sexual organs, and nervous system) by interaction with the PTH/PTHrP receptor. These findings have led to the suggestion that PTH is a 'uraemic toxin' (Massry 1987).

Aluminium-associated bone disease

The patient with aluminium osteopathy often presents with osteo-articular pain, both at rest and after exertion. In contrast with those suffering from osteitis fibrosa, these patients tend to have bone deformities and spontaneous fractures. Fractures are of both the fatigue fracture type (Looser zones) and true fractures.

Radiological evidence of osteitis fibrosa often appears before clinical symptoms are present. The opposite is true for aluminium-related bone disease in which patients may complain of osteoarticular pain without any bone lesions demonstrable on radiographic examination. Another

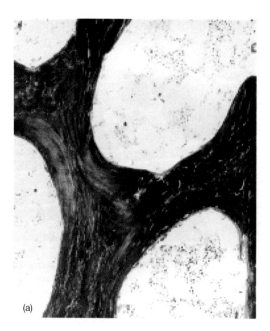
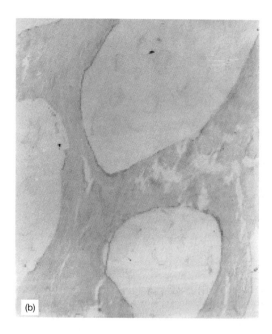

Fig. 19 Bone histology in aluminium-related adynamic bone disease (serial sections): (a) no osteoid tissue is observed. Osteoblasts, osteoclasts, and marrow fibrosis are absent (undecalcified sections; toluidine blue stain; magnification 125×); (b) aluminium deposits are present along the mineralized trabeculas (undecalcified sections; aurintricarboxylic stain for aluminium; magnification 125×).

Fig. 20 Photomicrograph of trabecular bone from a haemodialysis patient with aluminium-intoxication. Trabeculas (arrow) are surrounded by large osteoid seams (ost). Note the absence of bone marrow fibrosis (toluidine blue; magnification 120×) (Figures 19–23, courtesy Dr Giulia Cournot, CNRS URA 583, Hôpital Necker—Enfants Malades, Paris).

Fig. 21 Photomicrograph of trabecular bone from a haemodialysis patient with aluminium-intoxication. Trabeculas are surrounded by deep red lines corresponding to aluminium deposits (arrow). Similar deposits are observed along cement lines (arrow).

typical symptom is myopathy, presenting as asthenia of the proximal musculature. Patients have difficulty in getting up from a supine position or in raising their arms. Common features of aluminium-related bone disease are hypercalcaemia after oral calcium supplementation or low doses of vitamin D derivatives, and the presence of extensive soft tissue calcifications.

Aluminium intoxication may be accompanied by systemic manifestations, such as microcytic hypochromic anaemia (or simply normocytic anaemia) resulting from suppression of erythropoiesis, encephalopathy resulting from involvement of the central nervous system, and cachexia.

Aluminium osteopathy is particularly common after parathyroidectomy in patients with aluminium overload, with the consecutive state of low bone turnover.

Bone problems and calcium metabolism after renal transplantation (see also Chapter 13.5)

Successful renal transplantation is generally associated with a rapid decline in serum 'intact PTH' which parallels the decline in serum creatinine. Serum calcitriol usually normalizes within a few days of

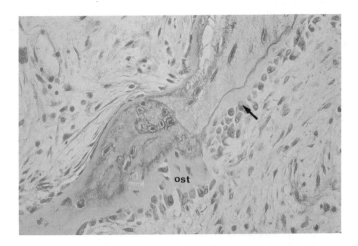

Fig. 22 Photomicrograph of trabecular bone from a haemodialysis patient with severe secondary hyperparathyroidism and osteitis fibrosa. The trabacula is surrounded by enlarged osteoid seams (ost). Numerous active osteoblasts (arrow) are aligned along the osteoid. Note the presence of extensive bone marrow fibrosis (toluidine blue, magnification 300×).

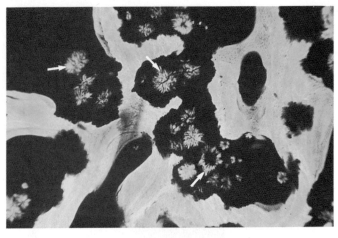

Fig. 24 Microradiograph of trabecular bone from a haemodialysis patient with primary hyperoxaluria and bone involvement. Numerous oxalate crystal clusters (arrows) are observed in the bone marrow between the eroded trabeculas (magnification 120×).

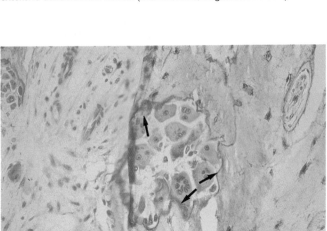

Fig. 23 Photomicrograph of trabecular bone from a haemodialysis patient with severe secondary hyperparathyroidism and osteitis fibrosa. A large resorption cavity has developed within the trabecula. Large multinucleated osteoclasts (arrow) are observed within Howship's lacunae. Note the presence of extensive bone marrow fibrosis (toluidine blue; magnification 300×).

Table 13 Disturbances of mineral metabolism after successful renal transplantation

Unrelated to glucocorticoid therapy
Persistent hyperparathyroidism*
Renal phosphate wasting
Abnormal regulation of 25(OH)D3-1-hydroxylase

Complications of glucocorticoid therapy
Osteonecrosis
Osteopenia
Negative calcium balance

Lesion of uncertain aetiology
Osteo-articular pain of lower limbs with metaphyseal impaction

* Glucocorticoids have been shown to enhance PTH secretion *in vitro* (Peraldi *et al.* 1990).

transplantation. Nevertheless, perturbations of mineral metabolism may persist even after successful transplantation. Common types of bony problems after transplantation are listed in Table 13. However, these perturbations do not have clinical consequences in most cases. Interstitial fibrosis and tubular damage as a result of chronic rejection are presumably the cause of renal loss of phosphate and disturbed feedback regulation of renal calcitriol biosynthesis. The rate of calcitriol production is no longer tightly feedback-regulated in transplanted patients, so that calcitriol does no longer inhibit its own production. Similar to what is seen in the patient with uraemia, the synthesis of calcitriol depends on the concentration of its precursor substance 25(OH)D3 (Lucas *et al.* 1988). Hypophosphataemia, which is found in a large proportion of transplanted patients, may arise from a primary PTH-independent renal loss of phosphate (Rosenbaum *et al.* 1981; Parfitt *et al.* 1986), but elevated plasma PTH and glucocorticoid administration also contribute to tubular wasting of phosphate.

Hyperparathyroidism is usually not completely reversible after successful renal transplantation. Detailed investigations have demonstrated persistently elevated basal serum levels of PTH in the majority of patients (Parfitt 1982), or at least abnormal PTH secretion in response to hypocalcaemia (Mitlak *et al.* 1991). The most likely explanation is persistent hyperplasia of parathyroid glands (Parfitt 1982) with persisting basal, non-suppressible secretion of PTH. Parfitt (1982) estimated that the size of enlarged parathyroid glands decreases by only 2–3 per cent per year; therefore, involution of hyperplastic parathyroid glands will require many years. Steroids may also contribute to elevated PTH synthesis and/or secretion by a direct effect on the parathyroid cell (Sugimoto *et al.* 1989; Peraldi *et al.* 1990), by impairment of intestinal absorption of calcium, and by increasing renal calcium excretion.

Despite persistently elevated serum PTH, the radiographic signs of osteitis fibrosa usually disappear after transplantation.

Hypercalcaemia is a relatively frequent complication after renal transplantation (Parfitt 1982). It may appear either soon or only several months after transplantation. Close monitoring of hypercalcaemic patients is necessary because hypercalcaemia potentially endangers the function of the graft and predisposes to renal stone formation.

The most important bone complication in transplanted patients is steroid-induced osteonecrosis. Osteonecrosis is a known complication of endogenous hypercortisolism and administration of steroids. Predisposing factors are the reduction of trabeculas in cancellous bone (due to steroid osteopenia), fatty transformation of bone marrow (resulting in impaired microcirculation), and reduced capacity to repair microfractures (due to low bone turnover).

In the distant past, osteonecrosis was observed in approximately 20 per cent of transplanted patients (Ibels *et al.* 1978), but the incidence has dramatically decreased in subsequent years (Ritz and Rieden 1985). This is probably due to the general reduction of steroid dose after introduction of cyclosporin, although it is agreed upon that osteonecrosis is not strictly related to the steroid dose. Osteonecrosis has been observed after administration of glucocorticoids at low doses for short duration (in our experience after 16 mg prednisone for 3 days), so that there is probably an individually variable threshold for its development. Cumulative, peak, or average steroid doses do not correlate with the incidence of osteonecrosis in individual cases (Ritz *et al.* 1982). Osteonecrosis may be a late complication of glucocorticoid therapy in patients with a history of immunosuppressive therapy for the nephrotic syndrome, vasculitis, or preceding renal transplantation.

Osteonecrosis develops most frequently in the femoral head. The onset is mostly bilateral but may be unilateral. The lesion may also develop in knee and elbow joints, the calcaneus, and the humeral head. Most frequently it develops in the first year after transplantation and is not clearly related to the type of underlying renal disease, the presence of pre-existing osteitis fibrosa, or plasma PTH, although this point is still controversial. No curative conservative treatment is available. Patients must be managed with weight reduction, if appropriate, and analgesics. As a prophylactic measure, the lowest possible steroid dose should be selected and additional measures may be tried, for example, vitamin D metabolites, thiazides, or bisphosphonates. Surgery is less urgent and more risky when the knee or the humerus are involved, but total hip endoprosthesis is highly successful in advanced forms of necrosis of the femoral head. Surgery should be carried out when patients complain of pain at rest, in the presence of advanced destructive lesions of the femoral head.

The occurrence of osteopenia in transplant recipients is primarily related to the known action of glucocorticosteroids on bone (Avioli 1984). Decreased bone mass, diminished bone formation, and decreased rates of apposition with unchanged rates of resorption have been found in transplanted patients with fractures (Nielsen *et al.* 1996). Today, with the use of lower doses of steroids, fractures in transplanted patients have become more infrequent. Mineral loss from the forearm was only modest (Neubauer *et al.* 1984), but loss of vertebral mineral density was more marked (Julian *et al.* 1991). Bone loss is much more dramatic in recipients of heart and liver transplants (Katz and Epstein 1992). Loss of bone mass could be prevented by prophylactic administration of bisphosphonates (Fan *et al.* 2000).

Some renal transplant patients complain of severe pain at rest and during exercise in the metaphyseal region of long bones. In at least part of them MRI revealed localized bone resorption, presumably as a result of sympathetic reflex osteodystrophy (Goffin *et al.* 1993).

Successful renal transplantation will result in the resolution of aluminium intoxication and removal of aluminium from bone surfaces (Nordal *et al.* 1992).

Alternative types of bone disease

The most common problem of differential diagnosis is β_2-m-related amyloidosis. Unfortunately, there is no specific laboratory test for β_2-m amyloidosis. The diagnosis must rely on clinical criteria, that is, demonstration of subchondral bone erosions and cysts in joint areas, with a characteristic pattern on radiography and other imaging techniques including ultrasound, CT scan, and MRI. Specific scintigraphic techniques have been developed but are not generally available at present (see above). Amyloid-related cysts are characterized by their articular location, the lack of a cellular reaction of the surrounding tissue, a tendency for osteosclerosis of surrounding bone, and complete radiolucency (for further details see Chapter 12.5).

Occasionally, rarer causes of bone disease must be considered. The radiological and clinical findings of oxalosis may mimic hyperparathyroid bone disease (Julian *et al.* 1987; Thompson and Weinman 1988) and result in pathological fractures, osteosclerosis, subperiosteal resorption, and extraskeletal calcifications (Fig. 25). The secondary oxalosis of chronic renal failure may result in extraskeletal deposition of calcium oxalate in the joint, myocardium, or peripheral vessels. The diagnosis of oxalosis can be made from bone biopsy or from biopsy of affected tissues by the demonstration of oxalate crystals under polarized light.

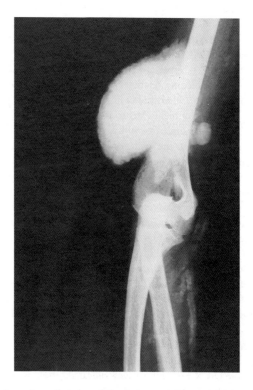

Fig. 25 Extensive soft tissue calcifications in a dialysis patient with primary hyperoxaluria. Diffuse calcium deposits are present in skin and blood vessels. A periarticular tumour-like calcium deposit is present in the elbow area.

Patients from areas where the drinking water has a high fluoride content or who ingest large quantities of fluoride-containing mineral water (e.g. from the Vichy Saint-Yorre spring) may exhibit fluorosis. This disease is characterized by osteosclerosis of the vertebral bodies, the formation of osteophytes, and a tendency to develop bone fractures.

Dialysis patients are prone to develop bacteraemia, generally related to vascular access infections. Therefore, spondylitis or osteomyelitis must always be considered in the differential diagnosis of localized, painful bone problems. In cases where the diagnosis remains doubtful, bone biopsy is indicated to rule out bone disease unrelated to uraemia, such as myeloma or metastatic bone disease.

Soft tissue calcification in uraemic patients

Patients with advanced renal failure may develop several types of soft tissue calcification. An exhaustive description is beyond the scope of this chapter, but we shall highlight some of them. For more detailed information, see recent reviews (Llach 1998; Drüeke et al. 2000; Rostand and Thornley-Brown 2001).

The first and most dramatic type is calciphylaxis, also called 'calcific uraemic arteriolopathy' at present. It is a clinical syndrome characterized by rapidly progressive, painful cutaneous necrosis and eschar formation at the extremities, the lower abdomen and the buttocks. Its precise pathogenesis is unknown. As mentioned above, it may be encountered in patients with severe hyperparathyroidism (Gipstein et al. 1976; Angelis et al. 1997; Coates et al. 1998), but this association has become infrequent in recent years (Mawad et al. 1999). Hyperphosphataemia and female gender, and possibly obesity and diabetes were found to be predisposing clinical conditions (Ahmed et al. 2001; Mazhar et al. 2001). High serum phosphorus, elevated serum alkaline phosphatases, and low serum albumin were also independent predictors. Iron overload is also thought to be associated with systemic calciphylaxis, at least in some cases (Rubinger et al. 1986; Zacharias et al. 1999), especially when high dose IV iron dextran is administered to overcome relative erythropoietin unresponsiveness due to iron depletion. Other studies implicated protein C or protein S deficiency in its development (Mehta et al. 1990; Perez-Mijares et al. 1996), because of the similarity with warfarin-induced skin necrosis (Comp et al. 1990), but the evidence is not completely convincing. It has been proposed that parathyroidectomy should be carried out whenever ischaemic skin lesions associated with peripheral vessel calcifications appear in uraemic patients. Unfortunately, however, only those patients appear to respond to this intervention who present with clearly elevated serum intact PTH levels (Mawad et al. 1999). Hyperbaric oxygen therapy may be another option.

Arterial calcification. Because of the increasing age and high prevalence of diabetes mellitus in dialysis patients, atherosclerosis is found with high frequency. At present, it is the most frequent cause of vascular calcification (Rostand et al. 2001). Calcification of atherosclerotic intimal plaques must not be confounded with typical vascular calcification of the media layer seen in uraemic patients. This Mönckeberg type of lesion is characterized by calcification of the tunica media and internal elastic lamina of medium and small resistance arteries. On X-ray, this variant of calcification is diffuse, in contrast to the patchy distribution of atheromatous calcium deposits (Fig. 26). In addition, atheromatous plaques of uraemic patients are much more frequently calcified than those of non-uraemic control subjects, as documented by light microscopy studies (Schwarz et al.

2000). Diffuse medial calcification is also a manifestation of ageing, and in this perspective uraemia can be considered premature and accelerated ageing. Aortic calcification and stiffening account for the reduced vascular distensibility and increased vascular resistance observed in patients with renal failure (London and Drüeke 1997; Guerin et al. 2000).

A role of secondary hyperparathyroidism in uraemic arterial calcification has long been demonstrated. Thus, clinical and experimental studies have shown that PTX could either reverse or prevent the development of arterial calcification (Ejerblad et al. 1979; Drüeke et al. 2000), although others were unable to observe a beneficial effect of the correction of uraemic hyperparathyroidism (DeFrancisco et al. 1985). Arterial distensibility has been found to be inversely associated with serum iPTH concentration, suggesting a role for iPTH in vascular compliance (Barenbrock 1998). A marked contribution of pharmacological doses of vitamin D and its active derivatives to vascular calcification has also been reported (Milliner et al. 1990).

In more recent years, a predominant role of hyperphosphataemia, hypercalcaemia, and the serum calcium × phosphate product in the pathogenesis of coronary and carotid artery calcification as well as cardiac valve calcification has become apparent, even in the absence of hyperparathyroidism (Ureña et al. 1999; Goodman et al. 2000; Raggi et al. 2002). Moreover, an association was found between vascular calcification and the dose of oral calcium supplements administered for the control of hyperphosphataemia (Goodman et al. 2000; Guerin et al. 2000). These noxious effects probably play a role in the recently reported association of an elevated serum phosphorus and a high calcium × phosphate product with increased relative mortality risk in dialysis patients (Block et al. 1998; Amann et al. 1999).

Novel mechanisms involved in arterial calcification. Until recently, vessel wall calcification was considered solely a passive process, especially in uraemic patients with an elevated calcium × phosphate product. According to this view, PTH and vitamin D would mainly contribute via an elevation in the calcium × phosphate product. However, there had

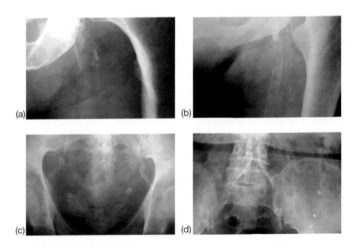

Fig. 26 Calcification of the femoral artery intima (a) and media (b), respectively. Calcification of the media of the m-pelvic arteries (c) and mixed calcifications of the iliac arteries (d). Assessment by posteroanterior fine-detail native, unenhanced X-ray of the pelvis and the thigh taken from chronic haemodialysis patients in recumbent position. Reproduced with permission from London, G. et al. (2003). *Nephrology, Dialysis, Transplantation* **18**, 1731–1740.

been some claims to the contrary. Thus, it was proposed, for instance, that local accumulation of vitamin K dependent proteins with high calcium affinity might play a role (Robert *et al.* 1985).

Recently, several lines of evidence have been provided in support of the 'active' intervention of several gene products and of cellular mechanisms in the pathogenesis of extraskeletal calcification (Parhami and Demer 1997; Shanahan *et al.* 1998; Schinke *et al.* 1999). The paradoxical osteoporotic loss of bone mineral together with the occurrence of vascular calcification, which is of the same composition as bone mineral hydroxyapatite, also suggests that neither process is attributable to simple systemic calcium excess or deficiency (Parhami and Demer 1997).

Several proteins with high calcium affinity have been isolated and characterized during the last decades, both during the progressive unravelling of the normal skeletal calcification process and during that of pathological renal, biliary, and pancreatic stone formation. The expression of these proteins, together with others involved in the physiological mineralization process of extracellular bone matrix (osteoid), has also been observed in various soft tissues, in particular, in the blood vessel wall (Table 14). They include collagen-I and several non-collagenous matrix proteins such as osteocalcin, osteopontin, and bone morphogenetic protein-2a (BMP-2a), which are normally involved in the formation of extracellular matrix and the deposition of hydroxyapatite in bone. In addition, matrix GLA protein (MGP), which is expressed in chondrocytes, but not osteoblasts, has also been found in vascular smooth muscle cells (Luo *et al.* 1997), in calcified plaques (Shanahan *et al.* 1994), and in tissue culture models of vascular calcification (Proudfoot *et al.* 1998; Tintut *et al.* 1998). The presence of matrix vesicles has also been reported in blood vessels, similar to the extracellular matrix vesicles of bone which secrete enzymes that modify inhibitory factors contained in the osteoid and provide a protective environment in which mineral ions can accumulate and transform into apatite crystals (Boskey *et al.* 1997). Recently, an enhanced expression of the bone matrix proteins osteopontin, type I collagen, bone sialoprotein, and alkaline phosphatase was observed in the arterial media of dialysis patients. The expression of these proteins was strongly correlated with the degree of arterial calcification (Moe *et al.* 2002).

Osteocalcin and MGP belong to a family of calcium-binding proteins, the GLA proteins, that also include coagulation factors II, VII, and IX as well as anticlotting factors, protein C and protein S. To attain functional status, certain glutamate residues on these proteins undergo carboxylation to form γ-carboxyglutamic acid (GLA). This process is vitamin K dependent. The GLA residues are responsible for the calcium binding properties of these proteins (Booth 1997; Luo *et al.* 1997).

Osteopontin belongs to a family of phosphorylated glycoproteins containing polyaspartic acid and polyglutamic acid sequences that are found often in mineral-binding proteins. It may inhibit or stimulate crystal formation depending on its concentration (Fitzpatrick *et al.* 1994). It is similarly found in normal vascular tissue and may inhibit calcification, perhaps by binding directly to crystal surfaces (Wada *et al.* 1999). Osteoprotegerin is a member of the TNF receptor superfamily and functions as an inhibitor of osteoclastogenesis. It is of interest, to note that it is not only expressed in bone but also in cartilage and arteries (Bucay *et al.* 1998).

The most compelling evidence suggesting that collagen-I and non-collagen matrix proteins may be involved in soft tissue calcification stems from recent gene knock-out studies. Thus, Luo *et al.* showed that the genetic induction of MGP deficiency in mice was associated with the presence of extracellular matrix vesicles and rapid calcification by apatite of elastic lamina and media of elastic and muscular arteries, including the coronary arteries, but not arterioles (Luo *et al.* 1997). It is interesting to note that these lesions are similar to those seen in renal failure. The findings suggest that MGP is normally expressed in vascular tissues in order to inhibit calcium deposition in soft tissues. Bucay *et al.* showed that gene deletion of osteoprotegerin in mice led to medial calcification of the aorta and renal arteries, together with the development of severe osteopenia (Bucay *et al.* 1998), conditions often seen in uraemia.

As a consequence of the above observations, Schinke *et al.* (1997) have suggested that ectopic calcification may result from reduced expression of extracellular matrix proteins, such as MGP and others, that normally protect arterial walls and cartilage from calcification, thus allowing these physiologically uncalcified tissues to ossify. Figure 27 shows a schematic presentation of the potential preventive

Table 14 Proteins potentially involved in soft tissue calcification

Vitamin K dependent proteins	Vitamin K independent proteins
Osteocalcin	Collagen-I
MGP	Osteopontin
	BMP-2a
	Osteoprotegerin
	Bone alkaline phosphatase
	Bone sialoprotein
	Fetuin

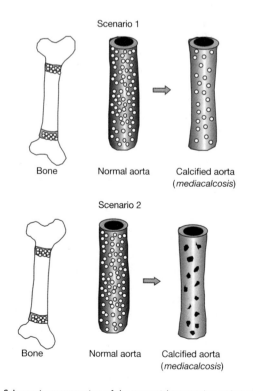

Fig. 27 Schematic presentation of the potential preventive action of MGP or similar proteins against abnormal calcium deposition.

action of MGP or similar proteins against abnormal calcium deposition. In bone, the presence of such proteins in the growth plate protects again premature calcification and thereby allows bone elongation to occur during growth. Accordingly, in the vessel wall, the normal expression of calcium-binding proteins would prevent calcium from precipitating. In contrast, a quantitative or a qualitative change in protein expression would lead to a reduced protection against calcification. The figure shows two different scenarios, namely a decrease of protein expression and altered protein structure or function, respectively.

Loss of the less potent inhibitor of calcification, osteoprotegerin, will lead to increased bone resorption, making calcium more available for deposition in soft tissues. Such a mechanism is another plausible explanation for vascular calcification in chronic renal failure.

According to recent studies, vascular smooth muscle cells do not represent a single cell type but rather are a mixture of cells derived from different lineages (Majesky et al. 1996). Among these cells are some that are felt to be pericytes having the capacity to differentiate into chondrocytes, adipocytes, fibroblasts, vascular smooth muscle cells, and osteoblasts (Doherty and Canfield 1999). Those that become osteoblast-like, calcifying cells are able to secrete osteopontin and other osteoblastic bone markers (Giachelli et al. 1991). Demer and her associates (Balica et al. 1997; Parhami and Demer 1997) have described and studied a subtype of vascular smooth muscle cells with fibroblast morphology that expresses several osteoblastic markers including osteopontin, bone morphogenic protein type 2 (BMP-2), osteocalcin, and MGP and is capable of inducing the formation of distinct, calcified nodules via the production of extracellular matrix. The main components of matrix secreted by vascular calcifying cells are type I collagen and fibronectin (Watson et al. 1998). Vascular calcification by apatite crystals was shown to be dependent on membrane-bound alkaline phosphatase (ALP) (Hui et al. 1997; Wada et al. 1999), and also on non-collagenous matrix proteins. A population of slowly mineralizing, bovine aortic cells developed the calcifying vascular cell phenotype when cultured on purified type I collagen or fibronectin. Treatment of such calcifying cells grown on fibronectin with an antibody to the integrin $\alpha 5$ subunit decreased ALP activity, suggesting that ALP expression is mediated at least in part through the interaction between the integrin $\alpha 5 \beta 1$ heterodimer and fibronectin (Watson et al. 1998).

The phenotypic modulation of vascular smooth muscle cells is influenced by a number of factors (Jacoby-IV and Semenkovich 2000). The importance for the genesis of vascular calcification in uraemic patients is currently unclear. Factors promoting transformation of vascular smooth muscle cells to osteoprogenitor-like cells include 25(OH) cholesterol, 17β estradiol, and calcitriol. Furthermore, TGF-β induces phenotypic changes of vascular smooth muscle cells, and it is therefore of interest that hyperglycaemia favours the expression of TGF-β. Advanced glycation end-products (AGEs) are found in atheromatous lesions (Vlassara 1996) and also promote osteoblastic differentiation into calcifying vascular cells (Yamagishi et al. 1999). These findings may be relevant to explain the propensity of diabetic patients to develop vascular calcifications. To explain calcification of lipid-laden plaques it is of interest that oxidized LDL also transform vascular smooth muscle cells into the above phenotype.

The applicability of cellular models of vascular calcification to calcium deposits in other tissues is uncertain but seems reasonable. For example, studies of the mechanism of heart valve calcification have been performed in native human heart valves and xenograft prostheses by Srivatsa et al. (1997) who found that zones of calcification within native heart valves were associated with the expression of non-collagen matrix proteins, osteopontin, and osteocalcin. These noncollagen matrix proteins are also found in injured myocardium, lung, and kidney (Srivatsa et al. 1997) and have also been observed in skin (Contri et al. 1996).

Management of the uraemic patient with disturbed calcium metabolism

Prophylaxis of secondary hyperparathyroidism

As outlined above, the abnormalities that ultimately lead to nodular hyperplasia of the parathyroid gland and symptomatic osteitis fibrosa evolve early in renal failure. Because parathyroid hyperplasia and skeletal lesions are not readily reversed by treatments available at present, a consensus has emerged that prophylactic interventions should be started in asymptomatic patients. This opinion is based on evidence that prophylactic calcitriol administration prevents an increase in parathyroid weight, that is, parathyroid hyperplasia, and inhibits parathyroid cell proliferation in experimental studies when administered immediately after subtotal nephrectomy. In contrast, once parathyroid hyperplasia has been established, calcitriol fails to reverse it, although it still suppresses parathyroid cell proliferation (Szabo et al. 1989). In other words, it is easier to prevent parathyroid cell proliferation than to cause involution of parathyroid cells by apoptosis. Clinical observations have shown that the weight of the parathyroids increases progressively with increasing duration of renal failure, and nodular hyperplasia develops in a substantial proportion of patients (Mendes et al. 1983). Monoclonal growth of parathyroid tissue (Arnold et al. 1995), resulting from various mutations of tumour-enhancing and tumour-suppressing genes, is found in nodular hyperplasia. This may explain why many patients with advanced hyperparathyroidism fail to respond to high doses of calcitriol, given either intravenously or orally (Fischer and Harris 1993; Herrman et al. 1994; Quarles et al. 1994). It is not an attractive option to wait until advanced hyperparathyroidism ('intact PTH' 10–20 times normal) and bony lesions (indicated by elevated bone alkaline phosphatase isoenzyme and radiography findings) necessitate administration of high doses of calcitriol. At that stage, it is uncertain whether parathyroid hyperplasia can be reversed and whether bone histology can be completely normalized. This leads to the question of which patients should be given prophylactic calcitriol and at what stage of renal dysfunction. We propose to monitor 'intact PTH' early on. In our view, once a consistent increase to values greater than 12–18 pmol/l, that is, two–three times the upper limit of the normal value, has been established, the organism has signalled the need for additional exogenous calcitriol to make up for defective endogenous calcitriol synthesis or impaired calcitriol action. We propose that calcitriol supplementation should be started at this point.

It has been suggested that, as an alternative to administration of exogenous calcitriol, attempts should be made to stimulate endogenous calcitriol synthesis via reduction of phosphate retention and increased phosphate levels in a hypothetical intracellular compartment of proximal tubular epithelial cells. This can be obtained by dietary phosphate restriction or the prescription of oral calcium supplements.

The two approaches are not mutually exclusive. Indeed, it may be necessary to administer calcitriol as well as calcium salts as phosphate binders although such an association favours the occurrence of hypercalcaemia and hyperphosphataemia. In this case, alternative phosphate binders are indicated. There is no doubt that hypocalcaemia (Yamamoto et al. 1989) activates the parathyroid gland independently of calcitriol. Hyperphosphataemia may also stimulate PTH synthesis/ secretion directly (Silver et al. 1994), in addition to its proven indirect effect. Therefore, both hypocalcaemia and hyperphosphataemia must be corrected.

Recommended prophylactic measures include: (a) the administration of calcitriol or other bioactive metabolites of vitamin D, (b) the reduction in the net intake of phosphate either by lower dietary intake or ingestion of phosphate binders, and (c) the administration of calcium salts. Points (b) and (c) are covered by administration of calcium carbonate or calcium acetate, for instance 2–3 g per day in addition to baseline dietary calcium intake, to counteract the tendency to hyperphosphataemia and hypocalcaemia.

Vitamin D metabolites

In several controlled trials, oral calcitriol at a dose of 0.25 μg/day or more (Coen et al. 1986; Nordal and Dahl 1988; Baker et al. 1989) or alfacalcidol at a dose of 0.5 μg/day (Hamdy et al. 1995) has been shown to reduce PTH concentrations, to slow down the development of hyperparathyroidism, and to ameliorate the skeletal lesions of osteitis fibrosa on bone biopsy. In the past, there was concern that calcitriol might cause deterioration in renal function unrelated to hypercalcaemia or hypercalciuria (Christiansen et al. 1978). This concern has been completely dispelled in controlled trials. In addition, Bertoli et al. (1990) demonstrated stable renal function by inulin clearance in predialysis uraemic patients who received 0.5 μg calcitriol daily over 4 months. In experimental studies, it has been demonstrated that calcitriol is renoprotective (Schwarz et al. 1998). While 0.25 μg calcitriol per day does not seem detrimental to residual renal function under controlled circumstances, administration of this compound is still fraught with the risks of hypercalciuria and hypercalcaemia in case of an overdose. Consequently, careful long-term monitoring of urinary and serum calcium, and of renal structure by ultrasonography for early recognition of nephrocalcinosis, is mandatory when conventional doses of active vitamin D metabolites are administered. The risk may be even greater with coadministration of thiazide diuretics, which promote tubular calcium reabsorption.

These risks can be circumvented by using lower doses of calcitriol, that is, 0.125 μg/day, which prevent the increase in PTH concentration (see Table 2) despite having no effect on serum calcium or phosphate and urinary excretion of calcium, thus increasing the safety of prophylaxis with calcitriol.

Baker et al. (1989) found that bone turnover decreased to less than the normal range after long-term calcitriol therapy. The clinical relevance of this finding is not clear, but 'overcorrection' of hyperparathyroidism and development of low bone turnover are matters of potential concern. It is recommended that intact PTH should be monitored periodically during long-term calcitriol therapy, and that treatment should be stopped as soon as concentrations are less than 12–18 pmol/l. In the future, monitoring of non-invasive indicators of bone metabolism may also be useful.

As already mentioned, classical vitamin D deficiency is by no means rare in renal patients; it can be diagnosed from low 25(OH) vitamin D3. Since vitamin D deficiency promotes secondary hyperparathyroidism (Bayard et al. 1973; Ghazali et al. 1999), depletion of vitamin D3 stores should be corrected by administration of physiological doses of vitamin D, that is, 500–1000 IU vitamin D3 (cholecalciferol) daily or 25(OH) vitamin D (calcidiol), for example, 10–20 μg daily.

One has to be aware of the fact that calcitriol also acts on non-classical target organs (Merke et al. 1987). Calcitriol decreases the number of mitoses and suppresses compensatory renal growth in uni-nephrectomized rats (Matthias et al. 1991). It also interferes with the development of glomerulosclerosis in uraemia, which is desirable (Schwarz et al. 1998). Calcitriol is also involved in the regulation of glucose-mediated insulin secretion (Cade and Norman 1987) and in the differentiation of haematopoietic cells (Reichel et al. 1989). Thus, treatment with calcitriol could improve some disturbances associated with the uraemic syndrome, for example, correction of the insulin secretion defect or amelioration of impaired immune function (Tabata et al. 1988). However, intake of vitamin D has been associated with the development of atherosclerotic lesions in animal models and vascular calcification in uraemic patients (Milliner et al. 1990), and calcitriol causes accumulation of triglycerides in monocytes in vitro (Roullet et al. 1989). These observations raise the possibility of increased atherogenesis, at least with high doses of calcitriol.

Prevention and treatment of hyperphosphataemia by calcium salts, aluminium-containing compounds, or calcium and aluminium-free phosphate binders

Disturbed phosphate metabolism and relative or absolute calcium deficiency play important roles in the genesis of secondary hyperparathyroidism. Hyperphosphataemia should be corrected to prevent: (a) suppression of renal 1α-hydroxylase, (b) reduction of ionized calcium through the formation of insoluble calcium–phosphate complexes (a concept which has remained controversial), (c) a direct stimulation of the parathyroid cell, and (d) extraskeletal calcification. Normalization of serum phosphate is obligatory before treatment with active vitamin D metabolites is started. Persistent hyperphosphataemia is an absolute contraindication to therapy with vitamin D metabolites. It is commonly recommended that treatment of hyperphosphataemia should start as soon as phosphate begins to exceed the normal range. While this usually occurs at a serum creatinine of 300–400 μmol/l, no strict relation with serum creatinine concentration is found because serum phosphate depends not only on residual renal clearance but also on confounding factors such as the amount of dietary phosphate and the degree of protein catabolism.

As phosphate is ubiquitous in food, reduction of dietary intake of phosphate is difficult to achieve. However, the patient should be advised to avoid dairy products (because of the high phosphate content of cow's milk) and food products with added phosphate (e.g. sausages and phosphate-rich soft drinks), but care should be taken to avoid the risk of malnutrition. One desirable side-effect of a low-protein diet is the concomitant reduction in phosphate intake. While usual phosphorus intake in Western Europe is approximately 1000–1200 mg/day, adherence to a low-protein diet of 0.8 g/kg daily is associated with a reduced daily phosphorus intake, that is approximately 800 mg/day. Correspondingly lower serum phosphate is found in patients who follow a protein-restricted diet.

Dietary modification is usually not sufficient to control hyperphosphataemia. The patients remain in positive phosphate balance unless oral phosphate binders are administered. These compounds sequester phosphate in the intestine by forming insoluble phosphate salts. Phosphate binders must be taken before or with meals, but not between meals (Schiller *et al.* 1989). The daily dose should be divided between meals according to their estimated phosphate content. Ingestion of calcium-containing phosphate binders between meals is potentially hazardous: enhanced uptake of calcium increases the risk of calcium overload and hypercalcaemia. Until recently, available phosphate binders included calcium carbonate or alternative calcium salts and aluminium-containing compounds, magnesium salts, α-ketoacids, and alginate in a calcium phase, as listed in Table 15. The use of some of these agents has become contraindicated (aluminium), and several of them have only a limited efficacy or tolerance. The use of calcium carbonate was first recommended by Makoff *et al.* (1969); subsequently, it was heavily promoted by others (Fournier *et al.* 1986; Slatopolsky *et al.* 1986, 1989; Renaud *et al.* 1988) to replace oral aluminium salts or gels which may be toxic when taken in large amounts. Calcium carbonate has at least four therapeutic advantages:

(1) it corrects hyperphosphataemia through binding of phosphate in the intestine (Makoff *et al.* 1969; Slatopolski *et al.* 1986; Hercz and Coburn 1987; Ghazali *et al.* 1993);

(2) it increases serum calcium as 25–30 per cent of inorganic calcium is absorbed (with large variations between individual patients) (Recker *et al.* 1988);

(3) it partially corrects metabolic acidosis (Makoff *et al.* 1969), although this has not been the experience of all investigators;

(4) it helps to establish a positive calcium balance as a result of increased passive intestinal absorption of calcium.

The latter is beneficial in the predialytic stage if low-dose calcium supplements are given, since spontaneous calcium intake tends to be low and, in addition, intestinal calcium absorption is reduced in uraemic patients (Ritz *et al.* 1980). This potential advantage becomes undesirable at high doses since hypercalcaemia and soft tissue calcifications develop, as discussed below. This is particularly common in dialysis patients.

The recommended daily dose of calcium carbonate is 2–5 g/day. Some authors have prescribed daily doses of up to 15 g calcium

carbonate which certainly is excessive. The dose should be divided in proportion to the phosphate content of meals (Locatelli *et al.* 2002).

The dose of calcium carbonate must be titrated individually since intestinal absorption of calcium varies widely between patients; one of the reasons for this is that the efficacy of calcium carbonate is reduced at neutral pH (e.g. in patients with atrophic gastritis). Hypercalcaemia, which is the main side-effect, is usually reversible after a reduction in dose. The risk of hypercalcaemia is increased in patients with concomitant calcitriol therapy, aluminium overload, low bone turnover (aplastic bone disease), and immobilization. Gastrointestinal side-effects (mostly constipation; rarely diarrhoea) have also been observed.

Calcium citrate has been recommended in the treatment of hyperphosphataemia (Cushner *et al.* 1988). It also carries the risk of inducing hypercalcaemia and, when taken together with aluminium salts, of stimulating intestinal aluminium absorption (Molitoris *et al.* 1989). Calcium citrate and aluminium must never be given together. Because there may be concealed sources of aluminium, we believe that the use of calcium citrate should be discouraged (Schaefer 1994).

Experiments *in vitro* have suggested that calcium acetate may also be a suitable agent for treatment of hyperphosphataemia. Calcium acetate is effective in binding phosphorus even at neutral pH, whereas calcium carbonate is less efficacious at alkaline than at acidic pH (Sheikh *et al.* 1989). On a weight basis, calcium acetate is more effective, but the risk of hypercalcaemia was almost the same when calcium carbonate and calcium acetate were compared at doses which lowered serum phosphate to an identical extent. Some calcium acetate preparations are less well tolerated because of their gastric side-effects. There is little overall difference between the two compounds (Benthamida *et al.* 1993; Schaefer 1994) and certainly calcium acetate is not the panacea, as had been hoped on the basis of the initial *in vitro* studies.

Recently, long-term follow-up of treatment with high doses of calcium supplements has become available. Although previously Renaud *et al.* (1988) and Clark *et al.* (1989) found no influence of calcium supplements on vascular calcification using relative insensitive methods such as plain X-ray or ^{99m}Tc-pyrophosphate scan, more recent studies provided definitive evidence, based on ultrasonographic techniques (Guerin *et al.* 2000) and electron-beam computerized tomography (Goodman *et al.* 2000). Thus, a positive calcium balance clearly is a matter of concern, even in the absence of hypercalcaemia.

Table 15 Oral phosphate binders in patients with advanced chronic renal failure

Agents	Daily recommended dose[a]	Side-effects and contraindications
Calcium-containing compounds		Hypercalcaemia, soft tissue calcification, gastrointestinal symptoms, constipation, diarrhoea
Calcium carbonate	3–6(–10) g, drug of first choice	
Calcium acetate	2–4(–6) g, drug of first choice	
Calcium citrate	Not recommended	Stimulation of intestinal aluminium-absorption
Calcium alginate	4–6 g	Variable efficacy
Aluminium-containing compounds[b]		Aluminium intoxication (osteopathy, central nervous system symptoms, etc.), constipation, ileus
Aluminium hydroxyde	Maximum 3–4 g	
Magnesium-containing compounds		Hypermagnesaemia, diarrhoea, abdominal pain
Magnesium hydroxyde	1.0–4.0 g	
Magnesium carbonate	0.5–1.5 g	
α-Ketoacids	8–500 mg N depending on body weight	Decreased muscle mass

[a] Fixed dosing schedules do not exist; the doses given are those above which, at least in the authors' experience, the frequency of side-effects increased.
[b] Owing to their side-effects, aluminium-containing phosphate binders should be avoided; if satisfactory control of serum phosphate by calcium carbonate or calcium acetate alone is not possible, aluminium-containing phosphate binders can be added in small doses.

Various aluminium salts, such as aluminium hydroxide and aluminium carbonate, are available as oral phosphate binders. The risk of inadvertent absorption of aluminium varies greatly between individuals. Unfortunately, it is unpredictable. Currently, there is consensus that aluminium-containing phosphate binders should be avoided (DeBroe et al. 1993).

What should be done in patients with uncontrollable hyperphosphataemia? Compliance should be monitored, phosphate release from the skeleton as a result of increased bone resorption should be looked for in patients with excessive PTH, and dialysis efficacy should be monitored and increased if possible (Schaefer 1994). In patients on dialysis, tolerance for calcium carbonate is improved, that is, the risk of hypercalcaemia is diminished, if the dialysate calcium concentration is reduced (see below). If all these measures fail, aluminium-containing phosphate binders may cautiously be considered, but this necessitates regular monitoring of serum aluminium concentrations.

Both magnesium carbonate and magnesium sulfate have been recommended for the control of serum phosphate (Oe et al. 1987). Because of the frequent occurrence of hypermagnesaemia in chronic renal failure, treatment of patients with magnesium compounds necessitates lowering of the concentration of magnesium in the dialysate. Magnesium salts are laxatives, and their efficacy in controlling serum phosphate, at least in our experience, is less than impressive.

The advent of novel oral phosphate binders, which are free of calcium, magnesium, and aluminium, can be considered as an important step forward in the control of hyperphosphataemia without causing major side effects. Extensive clinical experience is only available for sevelamer hydrochloride, a non-absorbable exchange resin, which has proved to be equivalent, although not superior, to calcium carbonate or calcium acetate in terms of its phosphate chelating capacity (Bleyer et al. 1999; Chertow et al. 1999). In addition, sevelamer also decreases LDL-cholesterol and increases HDL cholesterol. In a recent prospective, randomized, double blind, multicentre study performed in 200 haemodialysis patients, sevelamer was able to prevent the progression of coronary artery and aortic calcium calcification over a 1 year period, as evaluated by EBCT-assessed score, whereas patients receiving calcium carbonate or calcium acetate had significant lesion progression (Chertow et al. 2002).

Several other novel phosphate binders are presently under investigation, including iron citrate, polynuclear iron preparations and lanthanum carbonate (Hergesell and Ritz 2002; Yang et al. 2002). The latter does, however, undergo significant intestinal absorption, which at least theoretically constitutes a serious limitation because of potential long-term toxicity (Hergesell and Ritz 2002).

A final, safe, and non-toxic way of controlling hyperphosphataemia in terminal renal failure is to increase the efficiency of dialysis. The elimination kinetics of phosphate during dialysis are complex because phosphate is slowly mobilized from several intracellular pools (Hercz and Coburn 1987). The dialysis 'dose' (surface area, blood flow, duration, and schedule) should be selected according to the predialysis level of phosphate. The most efficient way to improve phosphate removal is to increase dialysis frequency. Thus, 'daily' nocturnal haemodialysis has been shown to be extremely effective (Mucsi et al. 1998); however, this strategy faces great logistic problems.

Choice of dialysate calcium concentration

As discussed above, long-term negative calcium balance will result in exacerbation of hyperparathyroidism. Several factors favour the development of a negative calcium balance in uraemia. First, experimental and clinical studies suggest that passive intestinal absorption of calcium (along a concentration gradient and not requiring thermodynamic work) is unchanged in uraemic patients, whereas active intestinal absorption of calcium (dependent on calcitriol and requiring thermodynamic work) is impaired (Sheikh et al. 1988). Therefore, dialysis patients cannot adapt to low-calcium diets; this is important since uraemic patients on self-selected diets tend to ingest amounts of calcium below the recommended dietary allowance. Second, convective loss of calcium during ultrafiltration in haemodialysis sessions and intestinal calcium loss further aggravate the tendency to negative calcium balance.

In the past, a calcium concentration of 7 mg/100 ml (1.75 mmol/l) in the dialysate has been selected to compensate for the negative calcium balance resulting from low calcium intake and reduced intestinal calcium absorption in the interdialytic interval (Drücke et al. 1977). This dialysate calcium concentration causes net calcium uptake during dialysis sessions and compensates not only for the negative intestinal calcium balance, but also for convective loss of calcium during dialysis sessions. If the calcium concentration in the dialysate is lowered, higher doses of calcium-containing phosphate binders and/or of vitamin D metabolites are tolerated without development of hypercalcaemia. It may be useful to lower dialysate calcium concentration to 6.0 mg/100 ml (1.5 mmol/l), or temporarily even 5.0 mg/100 ml (1.25 mmol/l), to avoid hypercalcaemia under such conditions. If this approach is chosen, it is essential to ensure the compliance of the patient, that is, adherence to treatment with calcium carbonate and/or vitamin D derivatives. Otherwise, negative calcium balance with exacerbation of secondary hyperparathyroidism may ensue. The long-term outcome of the strategy to lower dialysate calcium concentration has not been sufficiently documented, although several acute and subacute studies suggest that it is practicable (Sawyer et al. 1989; Slatopolsky et al. 1989; Argilés et al. 1993; Weinreich et al. 1995).

Treatment of manifest secondary hyperparathyroidism

Conservative management

The management of the patient with manifest secondary hyperparathyroidism, that is, markedly elevated intact PTH (more than approximately 50 pmol/l or eight times normal), elevated bone alkaline phosphatase isoenzyme, or radiographic signs of osteitis fibrosa, requires a different approach. Such patients require higher doses of calcitriol (or alternative vitamin D metabolites) than those used in the prophylaxis of asymptomatic patients. Treatment should start with relatively low doses of calcitriol (e.g. 0.5 μg/day). It is important to verify that such a dose is well tolerated, without developing hypercalcaemia or hyperphosphataemia. The dose can be increased in a stepwise fashion until a decrease of intact PTH without hypercalcaemia is noted. Recently, there have been discussions concerning the optimal mode of administration of calcitriol. Slatopolsky et al. (1984) noted that elevated PTH was effectively reduced by intravenous calcitriol administered in an intermittent fashion. PTH concentrations decreased even prior to a detectable increase in serum calcium. The efficacy of intravenous calcitriol has been confirmed in several prospective controlled trials (Gallieni et al. 1990).

The original rationale for using intravenous calcitriol was, among other reasons, to achieve high peak plasma concentrations of calcitriol, so that the parathyroid VDR was more completely saturated by the ligand. Intermittent oral calcitriol does not achieve similarly high peak plasma concentrations of calcitriol, but it is equally effective (Klaus et al. 1991; Tsukamoto et al. 1991; Kwan et al. 1992; Hermann et al. 1994). This observation argues against a crucial role of high peak plasma calcitriol, at least under clinical conditions. Calcitriol given orally in an intermittent fashion is able to lower PTH effectively (Klans et al. 1991; Tsukamoto et al. 1991; Kwan et al. 1992) even when given only once weekly. Indeed, recent head-on comparisons of intravenous and oral bolus calcitriol failed to detect significant differences between the two routes of administration (Fischer and Harris 1993; Quarles et al. 1994). However, it must be admitted that the beta error is considerable because of large interpatient variation. The marked efficacy of intermittent calcitriol is plausible in view of the finding that a single oral dose of calcitriol causes prolonged suppression of circulating PTH concentrations for more than 96 h (Seidel et al. 1993); the PTH concentration is still suppressed when serum calcitriol has returned to baseline. This finding is in line with experimental observations (Silver et al. 1985) that show prolonged suppression of pre-pro-PTH mRNA after one single dose of calcitriol.

Apparently, the response of the parathyroid to calcitriol is quantitatively different when it is administered in an intermittent fashion, at least in the experimental animal. This is suggested by a study in subtotally nephrectomized rats (Reichel et al. 1993). An identical dose of calcitriol was given by either osmotic minipump or intermittent intraperitoneal injection. Intermittent calcitriol caused a greater reduction of circulating PTH, less gain of parathyroid weight, and more effective suppression of pre-pro-PTH mRNA (Table 16). One would predict that intermittent schedules of calcitriol administration should also be more effective in uraemic patients. However, a recent controlled comparison of daily versus intermittent calcitriol in patients with moderate hyperparathyroidism failed to show significant differences in the proportion of patients responding and in the rate of decline of intact PTH (Hermann et al. 1994). One cannot exclude the possibility that the known considerable interpatient variability obscured an underlying difference; however, such a minor difference would not be of major clinical importance. Undoubtedly, intermittent administration offers the advantage that administration of calcitriol can be supervised as patient compliance is notoriously poor. In our own study, compliance for calcitriol, monitored with an electronic system, was less than 50 per cent.

1α-Cholecalciferol (alfacalcidol) is also widely used. This compound must be transformed in the liver to active calcitriol by a cytochrome-P-450-dependent enzyme system. The rate of this transformation may be variable and can be influenced by hepatic disease, cigarette smoking, and drugs that modulate the activity of cytochrome P-450. Barbiturates, diphenylhydantoin or other anticonvulsive drugs, and glucocorticoids decrease cytochrome P-450 activity, whereas oestrogens increase it. Doses of 1α-cholecalciferol need to be approximately twice those of calcitriol (in μg/day). 1α-cholecalciferol behaves identically to calcitriol after hepatic activation. The use of vitamin D3 (cholecalciferol) or 25(OH)D3 (calcidiol) in the treatment of manifest hyperparathyroidism should be discouraged because the management of patients is more difficult. The long half-lives of these compounds will result in prolonged hypercalcaemia if the dose administered is inadvertently too high.

In sum, in haemodialysis patients calcitriol or alfacalcidol can be given either orally or intravenously. The oral administration can be on a daily basis (e.g. 0.125–0.5 μg) or as intermittent bolus ingestions (e.g. 0.5–2.0 μg or more for each dose), whereas the IV administration is always intermittent (also 0.5–2.0 μg or more per injection). The route and mode of administration of calcitriol or alfacalcidol probably play only a minor role.

Since the highly active 1α-hydroxylated vitamin D derivatives can easily induce hypercalcaemia, intensive research has focused on the development of so-called non-hypercalcaemic analogues, including the natural vitamin D compound 24,25-(OH)2D3, 22-oxa-calcitriol, 19-nor-1,25-(OH)2D3, hexafluorocalcitriol, and 1α-(OH)D2. Despite numerous studies done in experimental animals (Brown et al. 1991; Finch et al. 1992; Kubrusly et al. 1993; Hirata et al. 1999; Monier-Fougere et al. 1999; GalMoscovici et al. 2000; Slatopolsky et al. 2000) and uraemic patients (Kurokawa et al. 1996; Llach et al. 1998; Frazao et al. 2000; Maung et al. 2001), none of these compounds has been shown to have entirely lost the capacity of inducing an increase in plasma calcium or phosphate in the clinical setting. In controlled trials, none has so far been demonstrated to be clearly superior to calcitriol or alfacalcidol in the long run.

The therapy described above must be monitored. Its efficacy can be assessed by measuring serum intact PTH, which usually decreases to approximately 50 per cent of the original value after 4–8 weeks in responders and to lower values after 6–12 months of therapy (Klaus et al. 1991). Alkaline phosphatase, bone-specific alkaline phosphatase, and, to a lesser degree, osteocalcin usually decrease in parallel (Cannella et al. 1994). A transitory increase of alkaline phosphatases and osteocalcin in the first few weeks is not unusual and indicates that

Table 16 Effect of continuous versus intermittent calcitriol on parathyroid function experimental uraemia

	Normal	Nx, vehicle treatment	Nx, continuous calcitriol	Nx, intermittent calcitriol
PTH/β-actin mRNA ratio (arbitrary units)	1.0	2.36	1.53	1.32[a]
Serum N-terminal PTH (pg/ml)	32 ± 3	52 ± 4	38 ± 4	46 ± 4[a]
Parathyroid gland weight (μg/g body weight)	0.70 ± 0.04	1.30 ± 0.18	1.15 ± 0.17	0.99 ± 0.20[b]

[a] $p < 0.05$ versus Nx, continuous calcitriol.
[b] $p < 0.05$ versus Nx, vehicle treatment.
Nx, subtotal nephrectomy.

osteoclastic resorption zones are repaired by osteoblastic apposition fronts. The risk of hypercalcaemia is particularly high when elevated intact PTH returns to the upper normal range and/or elevated alkaline phosphatase returns to the normal range. These findings indicate decrease or normalization of bone turnover and reduced capacity of the bone to take up calcium. Unfortunately, changes induced by calcitriol at the level of bone tissue are not necessarily reflected by plasma intact PTH in all circumstances, even though this can be accepted as a general rule. Thus, Goodman *et al.* (1994) showed in uraemic adolescents on CAPD that osteitis fibrosa healed under calcitriol treatment even though there was no decrease of plasma intact PTH. In contrast, plasma *N*-terminal or *C*-terminal PTH decreased even though osteoclast activity was increased, at least in some patients, during IV calcitriol treatment (Andress *et al.* 1989). Non-invasive markers of bone metabolism will have to be developed to recognize such discrepancies. This will be important to avoid excessive reduction of bone turnover (adynamic bone disease).

A new, promising class of CaR agonists ('calcimimetics') is presently under clinical evaluation for the medical treatment of hyperparathyroidism. For primary hyperparathyroidism, only short-term (3 weeks) experience is available in published form, showing that the calcimimetic drug cinacalcet is able to reduce serum PTH and Ca^{2+} concentrations in hyperparathyroid postmenopausal women (Shoback *et al.* 2003).

In uraemic patients with secondary hyperparathyroidism of moderate to severe degree, promising medium-term (26 weeks) experience is available with the calcimimetic drug cincalcot (Block *et al.* 2004). It shows that, on average, plasma PTH can be lowered by at least 30 per cent and the calcium × phosphate product can also be significantly reduced, in contrast to treatment strategies based on calcium and/or vitamin D derivatives. Of considerable potential siginificance is the experimental observation that calcimimetics prevent parathyroid hyperplasia in uraemia (Wada *et al.* 1997).

Surgical procedures

Surgical reduction of parathyroid glands should be considered in patients with advanced hyperparathyroidism, that is, intact PTH greater than 60–80 pmol/l (10–12 times normal) (Table 17). The following points may help in deciding whether to choose medical or surgical management.

With calcitriol or alfa-calcidol, irrespective of their mode of administration, medical management carries a considerable risk of

Table 17 Indications for parathyroidectomy in patients with chronic renal failure

Persistent refractory hypercalcaemia and/or hyperphosphataemia associated with high plasma intact PTH

Severe clinical osteitis fibrosa (e.g. biochemical problems), due to parathyroid overfunction i.e. not manageable by calcitriol

Marked enlargement of parathyroid glands, associated with high intact PTH values (8–10 times normal or higher), and unresponsiveness to an 8–12 week course of calcitriol therapy

Marked soft tissue calcification and high plasma intact PTH
Intractable pruritus and high plasma intact PTH

Note: It is imperative to exclude other causes of hypercalcaemia, soft tissue calcification, and, in particular, aluminium intoxication. If present, aluminium intoxication should be treated by desferrioxamine before parathyroidectomy.

hypercalcaemia and/or hyperphosphataemia. Furthermore, a high proportion of patients fail to respond, at least in terms of plasma intact PTH (Hermann *et al.* 1994; Quarles *et al.* 1994). One is often only buying time in those who do respond, so that ultimately it is still necessary to resort to parathyroidectomy. Consequently, one should not hesitate to consider parathyroidectomy if patients do not respond to a short (6–8 weeks) course of calcitriol by a reduction of at least 30 per cent in serum intact PTH, since virtually all patients who respond will do so within a few weeks (Klaus *et al.* 1991). This decision will be helped by the consideration that nodular hyperplasia with diminished focal expression of VDRs (Fukuda *et al.* 1993) and evidence of monoclonal growth (Falchetti *et al.* 1993; Arnold *et al.* 1995) is often present in patients with advanced long-standing hyperparathyroidism. This strategy will probably be revised in the near future, with the advent of calcimimetics. This class of drugs leads to a decrease of serum calcium and the calcium-phosphorous product.

It has been proposed that parathyroidectomy should be considered if the mass of parathyroid tissue estimated by imaging procedures exceeds approximately 0.5–1 g (Ritz *et al.* 1993; Fukagawa *et al.* 1996; Indridason *et al.* 1996). As shown in Table 16, further indications for parathyroidectomy include hypercalcaemia or hyperphosphataemia when they are resistant to conservative management. Calcitriol therapy is contraindicated in this setting. Furthermore, parathyroid surgery should be considered when biomechanical problems arise (e.g. fractures, tendon rupture), which necessitate rapid management, or when severe pruritus remains refractory to medical management in a patient with massively elevated PTH concentrations. Unfortunately, only a minority of patients with pruritus will respond to parathyroid surgery. Calciphylaxis in the context of increased intact PTH is a definite indication for parathyroidectomy.

The exclusion of aluminium bone disease and other bone pathologies is essential before parathyroidectomy. This may necessitate a bone biopsy and/or a desferrioxamine test. When the aluminium burden is high, the postoperative risk of symptomatic low-turnover aluminium bone disease is particularly high (Andress *et al.* 1985).

The surgical options are subtotal resection of all identifiable parathyroid tissue except a portion of the fourth gland, or total parathyroidectomy with immediate autotransplantation of several small fragments of parathyroid tissue into the musculature of the forearm or abdominal subcutaneous fat. Cryopreservation of excised parathyroid tissue is recommended to ensure that further tissue is available if the first graft fails. As the risk of recurrent disease appears to be greater with parathyroid nodules (Gagné *et al.* 1992), excision of these from the glands and implantation only of tissue portions with diffuse hyperplasia seems preferable (Wallfelt *et al.* 1988; Neyer *et al.* 2002). It has been claimed that invasive growth of parathyroid grafts points to a semimalignant character.

Kaye *et al.* (1989) proposed that total parathyroidectomy without reimplantation of parathyroid tissue should be the preferred technique. After total parathyroidectomy, low concentrations of plasma PTH can apparently be secreted from parathyroid remnant tissue in the thymus, at least in the experimental animal (Gunther *et al.* 2000). Nevertheless, finite amounts of PTH are required to maintain bone turnover within the normal range, and these amounts appear to be greater in patients with renal failure. The long-term consequences of low PTH levels with low bone turnover are not yet well known. An increased incidence of hip fractures (Coco and Rush 2000) and vertebral fractures has been reported (Atsumi *et al.* 1999). A definitive

Table 18 Algorithm for managing the hyperparathyroid patient

1. Monitor serum calcium, serum albumin, serum phosphate, serum 25(OH)D3, serum aluminium, plasma intact PTH

2. Prophylaxis

   If 25(OH)D3 is low (<20 nmol/l) administer vitamin D (500–1000 IU/day)

   If serum calcium low, serum phosphate high → administer CaCO₃ 0.5–1.5 g with each meal

   If plasma intact PTH still remains above 12–18 pmol/l (2–3 times normal) and serum calcium and serum phosphate are normal(ized) → administer 0.25 μg (−0.5 μg) calcitriol

3. Treatment (usually dialysed patients)

   If plasma intact PTH remains elevated above approximately 20 pmol/l normalize serum calcium and serum phosphate as follows

   (i) Administer oral calcium carbonate (or calcium acetate)

   (ii) Reduce phosphate intake

   (iii) Increase dialysis efficacy

   (iv) Adjust dialysate calcium (if hypercalcaemia persists, reduce to 6 mg/dl or 5 mg/dl)

   If serum calcium and serum phosphate have been normalized

   (i) Administer increasing doses of 0.5–3 μg calcitriol 1–2 (−3) times per week depending on plasma intact PTH

   (ii) Monitor serum calcium, serum phosphate, plasma intact PTH

   If plasma intact PTH falls below 20 pmol/l, stop calcitriol and monitor plasma intact PTH

   If plasma intact PTH does not decrease and uncontrollable hypercalcaemia or hyperphosphataemia develop, consider parathyroidectomy

disadvantage of total parathyroidectomy is that the patient will be dependent on vitamin D supplements, particularly after renal transplantation. On the other hand, an argument for total parathyroidectomy would be the semimalignant autonomous character of the growth of parathyroid glands with nodular hyperplasia. A dogmatic statement on total versus subtotal parathyroidectomy is not possible at present.

Subtotal parathyroidectomy or total parathyroidectomy with autotransplantation of parathyroid tissue to the forearm are roughly equivalent with respect to primary failures (rare), persistent hypoparathyroidism (approximately 30 per cent), and late recurrence (approximately 30 per cent) (Gagné *et al.* 1992). The selection of the procedure should be left to the surgeon.

If surgery is contraindicated or refused, some alternative procedures deserve consideration. These include coagulation of at least the large visible parathyroid glands by alcohol injection under sonographic guidance (Charboneau *et al.* 1988; Giangrande *et al.* 1992; Cintin *et al.* 1994; Kitakoa *et al.* 1994). The disadvantage is that instillation of alcohol causes scarring and renders subsequent neck surgery more difficult. Whether the direct injection of calcitriol into parathyroid glands leads to better results than ethanol injection, as claimed by some authors (Tanaka *et al.* 2003), remains uncertain since it could not be confirmed by others (Edevanilson de Barros Gueiros *et al.* 2004).

Table 18 summarizes our recommendations for the management of the hyperparathyroid patient.

References

Adams, J. S. *et al.* (1985). Isolation and structural identification of 1,25-dihydroxyvitamin D3 produced by cultured alveolar macrophages in sarcoidosis. *Journal of Clinical Endocrinology and Metabolism* **60**, 960–966.

Adler, A. J., Ferran, N., and Berlyne, G. M. (1985). Effect of inorganic phosphate on serum ionized calcium concentration *in vitro*; a reassessment of the 'trade-off hypothesis'. *Kidney International* **28**, 962–966.

Ahmed, S., O'Neill, K. D., Hood, A. F., Evan, A. P., and Moe, S. M. (2001). Calciphylaxis is associated with hyperphosphatemia and increased osteopontin expression by vascular smooth muscle cells. *American Journal of Kidney Diseases* **37**, 1267–1276.

Almadén, Y. *et al.* (1996). Direct effect of phosphorus on parathyroid hormone secretion from whole rat parathyroid glands *in vitro*. *Journal of Bone and Mineral Research* **11**, 970–976.

Amann, K., Gross, M. L., London, G. M., and Ritz, E. (1999). Hyperphosphataemia—a silent killer of patients with renal failure? *Nephrology, Dialysis, Transplantation* **14**, 2085–2087.

Andress, D. L., Ott, S. M., Maloney, N. A., and Sherrard, D. J. (1985). Effect of parathyroidectomy on bone aluminum accumulation in chronic renal failure. *New England Journal of Medicine* **312**, 468–473.

Andress, D. L., Norris, K. C., Coburn, J. W., Slatopolsky, E., and Sherrard, D. J. (1989). Intravenous calcitriol in the treatment of refractory osteitis fibrosa of chronic renal failure. *New England Journal of Medicine* **321**, 274–279.

Angelis, M., Wong, L. L., Myers, S. A., and Wong, L. M. (1997). Calciphylaxis in patients on hemodialysis: a prevalence study. *Surgery* **122**, 1083–1090.

Argilés, A., Kerr, P. G., Canaud, B., Flavier, J. L., and Mion, C. (1993). Calcium kinetics and the long-term effects of lowering dialysate calcium concentration. *Kidney International* **43**, 630–640.

Arnold, A., Brown, M. F., Ureña, P., Gaz, R. D., Sarfati, E., and Drüeke, T. B. (1995). Monoclonality of parathyroid tumors in chronic renal failure and in primary parathyroid hyperplasia. *Journal of Clinical Investigation* **95**, 2047–2054.

Atsumi, K., Kushida, K., Yamazaki, K., Shimizu, S., Ohmura, A., and Inoue, T. (1999). Risk factors for vertebral fractures in renal osteodystrophy. *American Journal of Kidney Diseases* **33**, 287–293.

Avioli, L. V. Effects of chronic corticosteroid therapy on mineral metabolism and calcium absorption. In *Glucocorticoid Effects and Their Biological Consequences* (ed. C. G. L. V. Avioli and B. Imbimbo). New York, NY: Plenum, 1984.

Baker, L. R. J. *et al.* (1989). 1,25(OH)₂ vitamin D3 administration in moderate renal failure: a prospective double blind trial. *Kidney International* **35**, 661–669.

Balica, M., Boström, K., Shin, V., Tillisch, K., and Demer, L. L. (1997). Calcifying subpopulation of bovine aortic smooth muscle cells is responsive to 17 beta-estradiol. *Circulation* **95**, 1954–1960.

Bayard, F., Bec, P., Ton That, H., and Louvet, J. P. (1973). Plasma 25-hydroxycholecalciferol in chronic renal failure. *European Journal of Clinical Investigation* **3**, 447–450.

BenHamida, F., ElEsper, I., Compagnon, M., Moriniere, P., and Fournier, A. (1993). Long-term (6 months) cross-over comparison of calcium acetate with calcium carbonate as phosphate binder. *Nephron* **63**, 258–262.

Bertoli, M., Luisetto, G., Ruffatti, A., Urso, M., and Romagnoli, G. (1990). Renal function during calcitriol therapy in chronic renal failure. *Clinical Nephrology* **33**, 161–163.

Bleyer, A. J. *et al.* (1999). A comparison of the calcium-free phosphate binder sevelamer hydrochloride with calcium acetate in the treatment of hyperphosphatemia in hemodialysis patients. *American Journal of Kidney Diseases* **33**, 694–701.

Block, G. A., Hulbert-Shearon, T. E., Levin, N. W., and Port, F. K. (1998). Association of serum phosphorus and calcium × phosphorus product with mortality risk in chronic hemodialysis patients: a national study. *American Journal of Kidney Diseases* **31**, 607–617.

Block, G. A. *et al.* (2004). The calcimimetic cinacalcet hydrochloride (AMG073) for the treatment of secondary hyperparathyroidism in hemodialysis patients. *New England Journal of Medicine* (in press).

Bonjour, J. P. 1,25-Dihydroxy vitamin D and phosphate homeostasis in early chronic renal failure—the 'trade-off hypothesis' revisited. In *Nephrology* (ed. A. M. Davison). London: Baillière Tindall, 1988.

Booth, S. L. (1997). Skeletal functions of vitamin K-dependent proteins: not just for clotting anymore. *Nutrition Review* **55**, 282–284.

Boskey, A. L., Boyan, B. D., and Schwartz, Z. (1997). Matrix vesicles promote mineralization in a gelatin gel. *Calcified Tissue International* **60**, 309–315.

Bricker, N. S., Slatopolsky, E., Reiss, E., and Avioli, L. V. (1969). Calcium, phosphorus, and bone in renal disease and transplantation. *Archives of Internal Medicine* **123**, 543–553.

Brown, A. J. *et al.* (1991). The noncalcemic analogue of vitamin D, 22-oxacalcitriol, suppresses parathyroid hormone synthesis and secretion. *Journal of Clinical Investigation* **84**, 728–732.

Brown, A. J. *et al.* (1996). Rat calcium-sensing receptor is regulated by vitamin D but not by calcium. *American Journal of Physiology* **270**, F454–F460.

Brown, E. M., Wilson, R. E., Eastman, R. C., Pallota, J., and Marynick, S. P. (1982). Abnormal regulation of parathyroid hormone release by calcium in secondary hyperparathyroidism due to renal chronic renal failure. *Journal of Clinical Endocrinology and Metabolism* **54**, 172–179.

Brown, E. M. *et al.* (1993). Cloning and characterization of an extracellular Ca^{2+}-sensing receptor from bovine parathyroid. *Nature* **366**, 575–580.

Bucay, N. *et al.* (1998). Osteoprotegerin-deficient mice develop early onset osteoporosis and arterial calcification. *Genes & Development* **12**, 1260–1268.

Bushinsky, D. A. (1993). Effect of metabolic and respiratory acidosis on bone. *Current Opinions in Nephrology and Hypertension* **2**, 588–596.

Cade, C. and Norman, A. W. (1987). Rapid normalization/stimulation by 1,25-dihydroxyvitamin D3 of insulin secretion and glucose tolerance in the vitamin D-deficient rat. *Endocrinology* **120**, 1490–1497.

Cannata, J. B. *et al.* (1991). Role of iron metabolism in absorption and cellular uptake of aluminium. *Kidney International* **39**, 799–803.

Cannella, G. *et al.* (1994). Evidence of healing of secondary hyperparathyroidism in chronically hemodialyzed uremic patients treated with long-term intravenous calcitriol. *Kidney International* **46**, 1124–1132.

Casas, A. T., Burke, G. J., Sathyanarayana, Mansberger, A. R., and Wei, J. P. (1993). Prospective comparison of technetium-99m-sestamibi/iodine-123 radionuclide scan versus high-resolution ultrasonography for the preoperative localization of abnormal parathyroid glands in patients with previously unoperated primary hyperparathyroidism. *American Journal of Surgery* **166**, 369–373.

Charboneau, J. W., Hay, I. D., and Heerden, J. Av. (1988). Persistent primary hyperparathyroidism: successful ultrasound-guided percutaneous ethanol ablation of an occult adenoma. *Mayo Clinic Proceedings* **63**, 913–991.

Chertow, G. M. *et al.* (1999). A randomized trial of sevelamer hydrochloride (RenaGel) with and without supplemental calcium. Strategies for the control of hyperphosphatemia and hyperparathyroidism in hemodialysis patients. *Clinical Nephrology* **51**, 18–26.

Chertow, G. M., Burke, S. K., Raggi, P., and Treat to Goal Working Group (2002). Sevelamer attenuates the progression of cardiovascular calcification in hemodialysis patients. *Kidney International* **62**, 245–252.

Christiansen, C., Rodbro, P., Christiansen, M. S., Hartnack, B., and Transbol, I. B. (1978). Deterioration of renal function during treatment of chronic renal failure with 1,25-dihydroxycholecalciferol. *Lancet* **2**, 700–708.

Chudek, J., Ritz, E., and Kovacs, G. (1998). Genetic abnormalities in parathyroid nodules of uremic patients. *Clinical Cancer Research* **4**, 211–214.

Cintin, C., Karstrup, S., Ladefoged, S. D., and Joffe, P. (1994). Tertiary hyperparathyroidism treated by ultrasonographically guided percutaneous fine-needle ethanol injection. *Nephron* **68**, 217–220.

Clark, A. G., Ward, G., Turner, C., and Chantler, C. (1989). Safety and efficacy of calcium carbonate in children with chronic renal failure. *Nephrology, Dialysis, Transplantation* **4**, 539–544.

Coates, T. *et al.* (1998). Cutaneous necrosis from calcific uremic arteriolopathy. *American Journal of Kidney Diseases* **32**, 384–391.

Coco, M. and Rush, H. (2000). Increased incidence of hip fractures in dialysis patients with low serum parathyroid hormone. *American Journal of Kidney Diseases* **36**, 1115–1121.

Coen, G., Mazzaferro, S., Bonucci, E., and Ballantini, P. (1986). Treatment of secondary hyperparathyroidism of predialysis chronic renal failure with low doses of $1,25(OH)_2D3$: humoral and histomorphometric results. *Mineral and Electrolyte Metabolism* **12**, 375–382.

Cohen-Solal, M. E., Boudailliez, B., Sebert, J. L., Westeel, P. F., Bouillon, R., and Fournier, A. (1991). Comparison of intact, mid region and carboxyterminal assays of parathyroid hormone for the diagnosis of bone disease in hemodialyzed patients. *Journal of Clinical Endocrinology and Metabolism* **73**, 516–524.

Combe, C. and Aparicio, M. (1994). Phosphorus and protein restriction and parathyroid function in chronic renal failure. *Kidney International* **46**, 1381–1386.

Comp, P. C., Elrod, J. P., and Karszenski, S. (1990). Warfarin induced skin necrosis. *Seminars in Thrombosis and Hemostasis* **16**, 293–298.

Contri, M. B., Boraldi, F., Taparelli, F., and Ronchetti, A. D. P. P. (1996). Matrix proteins with high affinity for calcium ions are associated with mineralization within the elastic fibers of pseudoxanthoma elasticum dermis. *American Journal of Pathology* **148**, 569–577.

Couttenye, M. M., D'Haese, P. C., Deng, J. T., Hoof, V. O. V., Verpooten, G. A., and Broe, M. E. D. (1997). High prevalence of adynamic bone disease diagnosed by biochemical markers in a wide sample of the European CAPD population. *Nephrology, Dialysis, Transplantation* **12**, 2144–2150.

Cushner, H. M., Copley, J. B., Lindberg, J. S., and Foulks, C. J. (1988). Calcium citrate, a nonaluminum-containing phosphate-binding agent for treatment of CRF. *Kidney International* **33**, 95–99.

DeBroe, M. E., Drüeke, T. B., and Ritz, E. (1993). Diagnosis and treatment of aluminium overload in end-stage renal failure patients. *Nephrology, Dialysis, Transplantation* **8** (Suppl. 1), 1–4.

DeFrancisco, A. M. *et al.* (1985). Parathyroidectomy in chronic renal failure. *Quarterly Journal of Medicine* **55**, 289–315.

Delmez, J. A., Tindra, C., Grooms, P., Dusso, A., Windus, D., and Slatopolsky, E. (1989). Parathyroid hormone suppression by intravenous $1,25(OH)_2$ vitamin D. A role for increased sensitivity to calcium. *Journal of Clinical Investigation* **83**, 1349–1355.

deVernejoul, M. C. and Marie, J. M. New aspects of bone biology. In *The Spectrum of Renal Osteodystrophy* (ed. T. B. A. S. Drueke). Oxford, UK: Oxford University Press, 2001.

Doherty, M. J. and Canfield, A. E. (1999). Gene expression during vascular pericyte differentiation. *Critical Reviews Eukaryotic Gene Expression* **9**, 1–17.

Drüeke, T., Bordier, P., Man, N. K., Jungers, P., and Marie, P. (1977). Long term effects of high dialysis calcium concentration on bone remodelling, serum biochemistry and parathyroid hormone of hemodialyzed patients with renal osteodystrophy. *Kidney International* **11**, 267–274.

Drüeke, T. and Zingraff, J. (1994). The dilemma of parathyroidectomy in chronic renal failure. *Current Opinions in Nephrology and Hypertension* **3**, 386–395.

Drüeke, T. B., Touam, M., Thornley-Brown, D., and Rostand, S. G. (2000). Extraskeletal calcification in patients with chronic kidney failure. *Advances in Nephrology from the Necker Hospital* **30**, 333–356.

Dunstan, C. R. *et al.* (1985). The pathogenesis of renal osteodystrophy: role of vitamin D, aluminium, parathyroid hormone, calcium and phosphorus. *The Quarterly Journal of Medicine* **55**, 127–44.

Dusso, A. *et al.* (1989). Metabolic clearance rate and production rate of calcitriol in uremia. *Kidney International* **35**, 860–864.

Dusso, A. S. *et al.* (1991). Extrarenal production of calcitriol in normal and uremic humans. *Journal of Clinical Endocrinology and Metabolism* **72**, 157–164.

Ejerblad, S., Eriksson, I., and Johansson, H. (1979). Uræmic arterial disease: an experimental study with special reference to the effect of parathyroidectomy. *Scandinavian Journal of Urology and Nephrology* **13**, 161–169.

Falchetti, A. *et al.* (1993). Progression of uremic hyperparathyroidism involves allelic loss on chromosome 11. *Journal of Clinical Endocrinology and Metabolism* **76**, 139–144.

Fan, S. L. S., Almond, M. K., Ball, E., Evans, K., and Cunningham, J. (2000). Pamidronate therapy as prevention of bone loss following renal transplantation. *Kidney International* **57**, 684–690.

Felsenfeld, A. J., Jara, A., Pahl, M., Bover, J., and Rodriguez, M. (1995). Differences in the dynamics of parathyroid hormone secretion in hemodialysis patients with marked secondary hyperparathyroidism. *Journal of the American Society of Nephrology* 6, 1371–1378.

Ferreira, A. *et al.* (1995). Relationship between serum β2-microglobulin, bone histology and dialysis membranes in uraemic patients. *Nephrology, Dialysis, Transplantation* 10, 1701–1707.

Finch, J. L., Brown, A. J., Mori, T., Nishi, Y., and Slatopolsky, E. (1992). Suppression of PTH and decreased action on bone are partially responsible for the low calcemic activity of 22-oxacalcitriol. *Journal of Bone and Mineral Research* 7, 835–839.

Fine, A., Cox, D., and Fontaine, B. (1993). Elevation of serum phosphate affects parathyroid hormone levels in only 50 per cent of hemodialysis patients, which is unrelated to changes in serum calcium. *Journal of the American Society of Nephrology* 3, 1947–1953.

Fischer, E. R. and Harris, D. C. H. (1993). Comparison of intermittent oral and intravenous calcitriol in hemodialysis patients with secondary hyperparathyroidism. *Clinical Nephrology* 40, 216–220.

Fitzpatrick, L. A., Severson, A., Edwards, W. D., and Ingram, R. T. (1994). Diffuse calcification in human coronary arteries: association of osteopontin with atherosclerosis. *Journal of Clinical Investigation* 94, 1597–1604.

Floege, J. and Ketteler, M. (2001). Beta(2)-microglobulin-derived amyloidosis: an update. *Kidney International* 59, S164–S171.

Floege, J. *et al.* (1990). Imaging of dialysis-related amyloid (AB-amyloid) deposits with ^{131}I-beta2-microglobulin. *Kidney International* 38, 1169–1176.

Fournier, A. (1995). Adynamic bone disease—is it actually a disease? *Nephrology, Dialysis, Transplantation* 10, 454–457.

Fournier, A., Moriniere, P., and Sebert, J. L. (1986). Calcium carbonate, an aluminum free agent for control of hyperphosphatemia, hypocalcemia and hyperparathyroidism in uremia. *Kidney International* 18, S114–S119.

Fournier, A. *et al.* (1994). Adynamic bone disease in patients with uremia. *Current Opinions in Nephrology and Hypertension* 3, 396–410.

Frazao, J. M. *et al.* (2000). Intermittent doxercalciferol [1alpha-hydroxyvitamin D(2)] therapy for secondary hyperparathyroidism. *American Journal of Kidney Diseases* 36, 550–561.

Frei, U., Klempa, I., Schneider, M., Scheuermann, E. H., and Koch, K. M. (1981). Tumour-like growth of parathyroid autografts in uraemic patients. *Proceedings of the European Dialysis and Transplantation Association* 18, 548–555.

Freitag, J. J., Martin, K. J., Hruska, K. A., and Slatopolsky, E. (1978). Impaired parathyroid hormone metabolism in patients with chronic renal failure. *New England Journal of Medicine* 298, 29–34.

Friedlander, M. A., Lemke, J. H., and Horst, R. L. (1988). The effect of uninephrectomy on mineral metabolism in normal human kidney donors. *American Journal of Kidney Diseases* 11, 393–401.

Fukagawa, M., Kitaoka, M., and Kurokawa, K. (1996). Ultrasonographic intervention of parathyroid hyperplasia in chronic dialysis patients: a theoretical approach. *Nephrology, Dialysis, Transplantation* 11, 125–129.

Fukuda, N., Tanaka, H., Tominaga, Y., Fukagawa, M., Kurokawa, K., and Seino, Y. (1993). Decreased 1,25-dihydroxyvitamin D3 receptor density is associated with a more severe form of parathyroid hyperplasia in chronic uremic patients. *Journal of Clinical Investigation* 92, 1436–1442.

Gagné, E. R. *et al.* (1992). Short and long-term efficacy of total parathyroidectomy with immediate autografting compared with subtotal parathyroidectomy in hemodialysis patients. *Journal of the American Society of Nephrology* 3, 1008–1017.

Gallieni, M., Brancaccio, O., Padovese, P., Roulla, D., and Tarolo, C. (1990). Clinical effects of low doses intravenous calcitriol in 83 hemodialysis patients with mild to severe hyperparathyroidism. *Symposium 'Renal Bone Disease, PTH and Vitamin D'*, Singapore.

GalMoscovici, A., Rubinger, D., and Popovtzer, M. M. (2000). 24,25-dihydroxyvitamin D-3 in combination with 1,25-dihydroxyvitamin D-3 ameliorates renal osteodystrophy in rats with chronic renal failure. *Clinical Nephrology* 53, 362–371.

Ghazali, A., Ben Hamida, F., Bouzernidj, M., el Esper, N., Wetseel, P. F., and Fournier, A. (1993). Management of hyperphosphatemia in patients with renal failure. *Current Opinion in Nephrology and Hypertension* 2, 566–579.

Ghazali, A. *et al.* (1999). Is low plasma 25-(OH)vitamin D a major risk factor for hyperparathyroidism and Looser's zones independent of calcitriol? *Kidney International* 55, 2169–2177.

Giachelli, C., Bae, N., Lombardi, D., Majesky, M., and Schwartz, S. (1991). Molecular cloning and characterization of 2B7, a rat mRNA which distinguishes smooth muscle cell phenotypes *in vitro* and is identical to osteopontin (secreted phosphoprotein I,2aR). *Biochemical and Biophysical Research Communication* 177, 867–873.

Giangrande, A., Castiglioni, A., Solbiati, L., and Allaria, P. (1992). US-guided percutaneous fine-needle ethanol injection into parathyroid glands in secondary hyperparathyroidism. *Nephrology, Dialysis, Transplantation* 7, 412–420.

Gipstein, R. M. *et al.* (1976). Calciphylaxis in man. *Archives of Internal Medicine* 136, 1273–1280.

Goffin, E., vande Berg, B., Pirson, Y., Malghem, J., Maldague, B., and van Ypersele de Strihou, C. (1993). Epiphyseal impaction as a cause of severe osteoarticular pain of lower limbs after renal transplantation. *Kidney International* 44, 98–106.

Gogusev, J., Duchambon, P., Hory, B., Giovannini, M., Sarfati, E., and Drüeke, T. B. (1997). Depressed expression of calcium receptor in parathyroid gland tissue of patients with primary or secondary uremic hyperparathyroidism. *Kidney International* 51, 328–336.

Goodman, W. G. *et al.* (1994). Development of adynamic bone in patients with secondary hyperparathyroidism after intermittent calcitriol therapy. *Kidney International* 46, 1160–1166.

Goodman, W. G., Belin, T. R., and Salusky, I. B. (1996). *In vivo* assessments of calcium-regulated parathyroid hormone release in secondary hyperparathyroidism. *Kidney International* 50, 1834–1844.

Goodman, W. G., Veldhuis, J. D., Belin, T. R., VanHerle, A. J., Juppner, H., and Salusky, I. B. (1998). Calcium-sensing by parathyroid glands in secondary hyperparathyroidism. *Journal of Clinical Endocrinology and Metabolism* 83, 2765–2772.

Goodman, W. G. *et al.* (2000). Coronary-artery calcification in young adults with end-stage renal disease who are undergoing dialysis. *New England Journal of Medicine* 342, 1478–1483.

Graham, K. A., Hoenich, N. A., Tarbit, M., Ward, M. K., and Goodship, T. H. J. (1997). Correction of acidosis in hemodialysis patients increases the sensitivity of the parathyroid glands to calcium. *Journal of the American Society of Nephrology* 8, 627–631.

Grateau, G. *et al.* (1988). Radionuclide exploration of dialysis amyloidosis. Preliminary experience. *American Journal of Kidney Diseases* 11, 231–237.

Guerin, A. P., London, G. M., Marchais, S. J., and Metivier, F. (2000). Arterial stiffening and vascular calcifications in end-stage renal disease. *Nephrology, Dialysis, Transplantation* 15, 1014–1021.

Gunther, T. *et al.* (2000). Genetic ablation of parathyroid glands reveals another source of parathyroid hormone. *Nature* 406, 199–203.

Hamdy, N. A. T. *et al.* (1995). Effect of alfacalcidol on natural course of renal bone disease in mild to moderate renal failure. *British Medical Journal* 310, 358–363.

Hercz, G. and Coburn, J. W. (1987). Prevention of phosphate retention and hyperphosphatemia in uremia. *Kidney International* 22 (Suppl.), S215–S220.

Hercz, G. *et al.* (1993). Aplastic osteodystrophy without aluminum: the role of 'suppressed' parathyroid function. *Kidney International* 44, 860–866.

Hergesell, O. and Ritz, E. (2002). Phosphate binders in uraemia: pharmacodynamics, pharmacoeconomics, pharmacoethics. *Nephrology, Dialysis, Transplantation* 17, 14–17.

Herrmann, P. *et al.* (1994). Comparison of intermittent and continuous oral administration of calcitriol in dialysis patients: a randomized prospective trial. *Nephron* 67, 48–53.

Hirata, M. *et al.* (1999). 22-Oxacalcitriol ameliorates high-turnover bone and marked osteitis fibrosa in rats with slowly progressive nephritis. *Kidney International* 56, 2040–2047.

Hsu, C. H. and Patel, S. (1992). Uremic plasma contains factors inhibiting 1 alpha-hydroxylase activity. *Journal of the American Society of Nephrology* **3**, 947–952.

Hsu, C. H., Patel, S., Young, E. W., and Simpson, R. U. (1987). Production and degradation of calcitriol in renal failure rats. *American Journal of Physiology* **253**, F1015–F1019.

Hsu, C. H., Vanholder, R., Patel, S., De Smet, R. R., Sandra, P., and Ringoir, S. M. (1991). Subfractions in uremic plasma ultrafiltrate inhibit calcitriol metabolism. *Kidney International* **40**, 868–873.

Hui, M., Li, S. Q., Holmyard, D., and Cheng, P. (1997). Stable transfection of nonosteogenic cell lines with tissue nonspecific alkaline phosphatase enhances mineral deposition in the presence and absence of beta-glycerophosphate: possible role for alkaline phosphatase in pathological mineralization. *Calcified Tissue International* **60**, 467–472.

Hutchison, A. J. et al. (1993). Correlation of bone histology with parathyroid hormone, vitamin D3, and radiology in end-stage renal disease. *Kidney International* **44**, 1071–1077.

Ibels, L. S., Alfrey, A. C., Huffer, W. E., and Weil, R. III (1978). Aseptic necrosis of bone following renal transplantation: experience in 194 transplant recipients and review of the literature. *Medicine (Baltimore)* **57**, 25–45.

Indridason, O. S., Heath, H., III, Khosla, S., Yohay, D. A., and Quarles, L. D. (1996). Non-suppressible parathyroid hormone secretion is related to gland size in uremic secondary hyperparathyroidism. *Kidney International* **50**, 1663–1671.

Jacoby-IV, M. G. and Semenkovich, C. F. (2000). The role of osteoprogenitors in vascular calcification. *Current Opinion in Nephrology and Hypertension* **9**, 11–15.

Jehle, P. M. et al. (2000). Insulin-like growth factor system components in hyperparathyroidism and renal osteodystrophy. *Kidney International* **57**, 423–436.

John, M. R., Goodman, W. G., Gao, P., Cantor, T. L., Salusky, I. B., and Juppner, H. (1999). A novel immunoradiometric assay detects full-length human PTH but not amino-terminally truncated fragments: implications for PTH measurements in renal failure. *Journal of Clinical Endocrinology and Metabolism* **84**, 4287–4290.

Julian, B. A., Faugere, M. C., and Malluche, H. H. (1987). Oxalosis in bone causing a radiographical mimicry of renal osteodystrophy. *American Journal of Kidney Diseases* **9**, 436–440.

Julian, B. A., Laskow, D. A., Dubovsky, J., Dubovsky, E. V., Curtis, J. J., and Quarles, L. D. (1991). Rapid loss of vertebral mineral density after renal transplantation. *New England Journal of Medicine* **325**, 544–550.

Jüppner, H. et al. (1991). A G protein-linked receptor for parathyroid hormone and parathyroid hormone-related peptide. *Science* **254**, 1024–1026.

Katz, I. A. and Epstein, S. (1992). Posttransplantation bone disease. *Journal of Bone and Mineral Research* **7**, 123–126.

Kaye, M., D'Amour, P., and Henderson, J. (1989). Elective total parathyroidectomy without autotransplantation in end-stage renal disease. *Kidney International* **35**, 1390–1399.

Kaye, M., Hodsman, A. B., and Malynowsky, L. (1990). Staining of bone for aluminum: use of acid solochrome azurine. *Kidney International* **37**, 1142–1147.

Kenny, M. A., Casillas, E., and Ahmad, S. (1987). Magnesium, calcium and PTH relationships in dialysis patients after magnesium repletion. *Nephron* **46**, 199–205.

Kifor, O. et al. (1996). Reduced immunostaining for the extracellular Ca2+-sensing receptor in primary and uremic secondary hyperparathyroidism. *Journal of Clinical Endocrinology and Metabolism* **81**, 1598–1606.

Kitakoa, M., Fukagawa, M., Ogata, E., and Kurokawa, K. (1994). Reduction of functioning parathyroid cell mass by ethanol injection in chronic dialysis patients. *Kidney International* **46**, 1110–1117.

Klaus, G., Mehls, O., Hinderer, E., and Ritz, E. (1991). Is intermittent oral calcitriol safe and effective in renal secondary hyperparathyroidism? (Letter). *Lancet* **i**, 800.

Kleeman, C. R. (1994). The role of chronic anion gap and/or nonanion gap acidosis in the osteodystrophy of chronic renal failure in the predialysis era: a minority report. *Mineral and Electrolyte Metabolism* **20**, 81–96.

Kliewer, S. A., Umesono, K., Mangelsdorf, D. J., and Evans, R. M. (1992). Retinoid X receptor interacts with nuclear receptors in retonoic acid, thyroid hormone, and vitamin D3 signalling. *Nature* **355**, 446–449.

Korkor, A. B. (1987). Reduced binding of 3H-1,25 dihydroxyvitamin D3 in the parathyroid glands of patients with renal failure. *New England Journal of Medicine* **316**, 1573–1577.

Korzets, Z., Magen, H., Kraus, L., and Bernheim, J. (1987). Total parathyroidectomy with autotransplantation in haemodialysed patients with secondary hyperparathyroidism—should it be abandoned? *Nephrology, Dialysis, Transplantation* **2**, 341–346.

Koyama, H. et al. (1994). Impaired homologous upregulation of vitamin D receptor in rats with chronic renal failure. *American Journal of Physiology* **266**, F706–F712.

Kubrusly, M. et al. (1993). Effect of 22-oxa-calcitriol on calcium metabolism in rats with severe secondary hyperparathyroidism. *Kidney International* **44**, 551–556.

Kurokawa, K. (1993). The kidney and calcium homeostasis. *Kidney International* **44**, S97–S105.

Kurokawa, K., Akizawa, T., Suzuki, M., Akiba, T., Ogata, E., and Slatopolsky, E. (1996). Effect of 22-oxacalcitriol on hyperparathyroidism of dialysis patients: results of a preliminary study. *Nephrology, Dialysis, Transplantation* **11**, 121–124.

Kurz, P. et al. (1994). Evidence for abnormal calcium homeostasis in patients with adynamic bone disease. *Kidney International* **46**, 855–861.

Kwan, J. T. C., Almond, M. K., Beer, J. C., Noonan, K., Evans, S. J. W., and Cunningham, J. (1992). Pulse oral calcitriol in uraemic patients: rapid modification of parathyroid response to calcium. *Nephrology, Dialysis, Transplantation* **7**, 829–834.

Lafage, M.-H., Combe, C., Fournier, A., and Aparicio., M. K. (1992). Physiological calcium intake and native vitamin D improve renal osteodystrophy. *Kidney International* **42**, 1217–1225.

Langub, M. C., MonierFaugere, M. C., Qi, Q. L., Geng, Z., Koszewski, N. J., and Malluche, H. H. (2001). Parathyroid hormone/parathyroid hormone-related peptide type 1 receptor in human bone. *Journal of Bone and Mineral Research* **16**, 448–456.

Lefebvre, A., Vernejoul, M. C. D., Gueris, J., Goldfarb, B., Graulet, A. M., and Morieux, C. (1989). Optimal correction of acidosis changes progression of dialysis osteodystrophy. *Kidney International* **36**, 1112–1118.

Lepage, R. et al. (1998). A non-(1–84) circulating parathyroid hormone (PTH) fragment interferes significantly with intact commercial PTH assay measurements in uremic samples. *Clinical Chemistry* **44**, 805–809.

Levin, K. E. and Clark, O. H. (1988). Localization of parathyroid glands. *Annual Review of Medicine* **39**, 29–40.

Lieberherr, M., Grosse, B., Cournot-Witmer, G., Hermann-Erlee, M. P., and Balsan, S. (1987). Aluminum action on mouse bone cell metabolism and response to PTH and 1,25(OH)$_2$D$_3$. *Kidney International* **31**, 736–743.

Llach, F. (1998). Calcific uremic arteriolopathy (calciphylaxis): an evolving entity? *American Journal of Kidney Diseases* **32**, 513–518.

Llach, F. and Massry, S. G. (1985). On the mechanism of secondary hyperparathyroidism in moderate renal insufficiency. *Journal of Clinical Endocrinology and Metabolism* **61**, 601–606.

Llach, F. et al. (1998). Suppression of parathyroid hormone secretion in hemodialysis patients by a novel vitamin D analogue: 19-nor-1,25-dihydroxyvitamin D2. *American Journal of Kidney Diseases* **32**, S48–S54.

Locatelli, F. et al. (2002). Management of disturbances of calcium and phosphate metabolism in chronic renal insufficiency, with emphasis on the control of hyperphosphataemia. *Nephrology, Dialysis, Transplantation* **17**, 723–731.

London, G. M. and Drüeke, T. B. (1997). Atherosclerosis and arteriosclerosis in chronic renal failure (editorial review). *Kidney International* **51**, 1678–1695.

Lopez-Hilker, S., Galceram, T., Chan, U. L., Rapp, N., and Martin, K. J. (1986). Hypocalcemia may not be essential for the development of secondary hyperparathyroidism in chronic renal failure. *Journal of Clinical Investigation* **78**, 1097–1102.

Lucas, P. A., Brown, R. C., and Woodhead, J. S. (1986). Acute responses of parathyroid hormone and 1,25 dihydroxyvitamin D3 to unilateral nephrectomy in healthy donors. *Nephrology, Dialysis, Transplantation* **1**, 199–203.

Lucas, P. A., Woodhead, J. S., and Brown, R. C. (1988). Vitamin D3 metabolites in chronic renal failure and after renal transplantation. *Nephrology, Dialysis, Transplantation* **3**, 70–76.

Luo, G. *et al.* (1997). Spontaneous calcification of arteries and cartilage in mice lacking matrix GLA protein. *Nature* **386**, 78–81.

Majesky, M. W., Dong, X. R., and Topouzis, S. (1996). Smooth muscle diversity and extracellular matrix in a rat model of restenosis. *Puerto Rico Health Sciences Journal* **15**, 187–191.

Makoff, D. L., Gordon, A., Franklin, S. S., Gerstein, A. R., and Maxwell, M. H. (1969). Chronic calcium carbonate therapy in uremia. *Archives of Internal Medicine* **123**, 15–21.

Malluche, H. H. *et al.* (1976). Bone histology in incipient and advanced renal failure. *Kidney International* **9**, 355–362.

Malluche, H., Werner, E., and Ritz, E. (1978). Intestinal absorption of calcium and whole-body calcium retention in incipient and advanced renal failure. *Mineral and Electrolyte Metabolism* **1**, 263–270.

Mannstadt, M., Juppner, H., and Gardella, T. J. (1999). Receptors for PTH and PTHrP: their biological importance and functional properties. *American Journal of Physiology. Renal Physiology* **277**, F665–F675.

Massry, S. G. (1987). Parathyroid hormone: a uremic toxin. *Advances in Experimental Medicine and Biology* **223**, 1–17.

Massry, S. G. *et al.* (1976). Skeletal resistance to the calcemic action of parathyroid hormone in uremia: role of 1,25(OH)$_2$D3. *Kidney International* **1**, 467–474.

Matthias, S., Busch, R., Merke, J., Mall, G., Thomasset, M., and Ritz, E. (1991). Effects of 1,25(OH)$_2$D3 on compensatory renal growth in the growing rat. *Kidney International* **40**, 212–218.

Maung, H. M. *et al.* (2001). Efficacy and side effects of intermittent intravenous and oral doxercalciferol [1alpha-hydroxyvitamin D(2)] in dialysis patients with secondary hyperparathyroidism: a sequential comparison. *American Journal of Kidney Diseases* **37**, 532–543.

Mawad, H. W., Sawaya, B. P., Sarin, R., and Malluche, H. H. (1999). Calcific uremic arteriolopathy in association with low turnover uremic bone disease. *Clinical Nephrology* **52**, 160–166.

Mazhar, A. R. *et al.* (2001). Risk factors and mortality associated with calciphylaxis in end-stage renal disease. *Kidney International* **60**, 324–332.

Mehta, R. L., Scott, G., Sloand, J. A., and Francis, C. W. (1990). Skin necrosis associated with acquired protein C deficiency in patients with renal failure and calciphylaxis. *American Journal of Medicine* **88**, 252–257.

Memoli, B., Gazzotti, R. M., Dello Russo, A., Libetta, C., and Andreucci, V. E. (1991). Bicarbonate and calcium kinetics in postdilutional hemodiafiltration. *Nephron* **58**, 174–179.

Mendes, V. *et al.* (1983). Secondary hyperparathyroidism in chronic haemodialysis patients: a clinico-pathologic study. *Proceedings of the European Dialysis Transplantation Association* **20**, 731–738.

Merke, J. *et al.* (1987). 1,25(OH)$_2$D3 Receptors and endorgan response in experimental aluminium intoxication. *Kidney International* **32**, 204–211.

Milliner, D. S., Zinsmeister, A. R., Lieberman, E., and Landing, B. (1990). Soft tissue calcification in pediatric patients with end-stage renal disease. *Kidney International* **38**, 931–936.

Mitlak, B. H., Alpert, M., Lo, C., Delmonico, F., and Neer, R. M. (1991). Parathyroid function in normocalcemic renal transplant recipients: evaluation by calcium infusion. *Journal of Clinical Endocrinology and Metabolism* **72**, 350–355.

Moe, S. H. and Sprague, S. M. (1992). β2-Microglobulin induces calcium efflux from cultured neonatal mouse calvariae. *American Journal of Physiology* **263**, F540–F545.

Moe, S. M. *et al.* (2002). Medial artery calcification in ESRD patients is associated with deposition of bone matrix proteins. *Kidney International* **61**, 638–647.

Molitoris, B. A., Froment, D. H., Mackenzie, T. A., Huffer, W. H., and Alfrey, A. C. (1989). Citrate: a major factor in the toxicity of orally administered aluminum compounds. *Kidney International* **36**, 949–953.

Monier-Faugere, M. C. *et al.* (1999). 22-Oxacalcitriol suppresses secondary hyperparathyroidism without inducing low bone turnover in dogs with renal failure. *Kidney International* **55**, 821–832.

MonierFaugere, M. C. *et al.* (2001). Improved assessment of bone turnover by the PTH-(1-84) large C-PTH fragments ratio in ESRD patients. *Kidney International* **60**, 1460–1468.

Moriniere, P. *et al.* (1989). Disappearance of aluminic bone disease in a long term asymptomatic dialysis population restricting Al(OH)$_3$ intake: emergence of an idiopathic adynamic bone disease not related to aluminum. *Nephron* **53**, 93–101.

Mucsi, I., Hercz, G., Uldall, R., Ouwendyk, M., Francoeur, R., and Pierratos, A. (1998). Control of serum phosphate without any phosphate binders in patients treated with nocturnal hemodialysis. *Kidney International* **53**, 1399–1404.

Naveh-Many, T., Friedlander, M., Mayer, H., and Silver, J. (1989). Calcium regulates PTH mRNA but not calcitonin mRNA *in vivo* in the rat. Dominant role of 1,25-(OH)$_2$D3. *Endocrinology* **125**, 275–280.

Nelson, S. R. *et al.* (1991). Imaging of haemodialysis-associated amyloidosis using 123-I-serum amyloid P component. *Lancet* **338**, 335–339.

Neubauer, E., Neubauer, N., Ritz, E., Dreikorn, K., and Krause, K. H. (1984). Bone mineral content after renal transplantation. Placebo-controlled prospective study with 1,25-dihydroxy vitamin D3. *Klinische Wochenschrift* **62**, 93–96.

Neyer, U., Hoerandner, H., Haid, A., Zimmermann, G., and Niederle, B. (2002). Total parathyroidectomy with autotransplantation in renal hyperparathyroidism: low recurrence after intra-operative tissue selection. *Nephrology, Dialysis, Transplantation* **17**, 625–629.

Nielsen, P. K., Feldt-Rasmussen, U., and Olgaard, K. (1996). A direct effect of phosphate on PTH release from bovine parathyroid tissue slices but not from dispersed parathyroid cells. *Nephrology, Dialysis, Transplantation* **11**, 1762–1768.

Nordal, K. P. and Dahl, E. (1988). Low dose calcitriol versus placebo in patients with predialysis renal failure. *Journal of Clinical Endocrinology and Metabolism* **67**, 937–941.

Nordal, K. P., Dahl, E., Halse, J., Aksnes, L., Thomassen, Y., and Flatmark, A. (1992). Aluminum metabolism and bone histology after kidney transplantation: a one-year follow-up study. *Journal of Clinical Endocrinology and Metabolism* **74**, 1140–1145.

Nykjaer, A. *et al.* (1999). An endocytic pathway essential for renal uptake and activation of the steroid 25-(OH) vitamin D3. *Cell* **96**, 507–515.

Oe, P. L., Lips, P., van der Meulen, J., de Vries, P. M., van Bronswijk, H., and Donker, A. J. (1987). Long-term use of magnesium hydroxide as a phosphate binder in patients on hemodialysis. *Clinical Nephrology* **28**, 180–185.

Parfitt, A. M. (1982). Hypercalcemic hyperparathyroidism following renal transplantation: differential diagnosis, management and implications for cell population control in the parathyroid gland. *Mineral and Electrolyte Metabolism* **8**, 92–112.

Parfitt, A. M., Kleerekoper, M., and Cruz, C. (1986). Reduced phosphate reabsorption unrelated to parathyroid hormone after renal transplantation: implications for the pathogenesis of hyperparathyroidism in chronic renal failure. *Mineral and Electrolyte Metabolism* **12**, 356–362.

Patel, S., Ke, H. Q., Vanholder, R., and Hsu, C. H. (1994a). Inhibition of nuclear uptake of calcitriol receptor by uremic ultrafiltrate. *Kidney International* **46**, 129–133.

Patel, S. R., Ke, H. Q., and Hsu, C. H. (1994b). Effect of vitamin D metabolites on calcitriol degradative enzymes in renal failure. *Kidney International* **45**, 509–514.

Parhami, F. and Demer, L. L. (1997). Arterial calcification in face of osteoporosis in ageing: can we blame oxidized lipids? *Current Opinion in Lipidology* **8**, 312–314.

Peraldi, M. N. *et al.* (1990). Dexamethasone increases preproparathyroid hormone messenger RNA in human hyperplastic parathyroid cells *in vitro*. *European Journal of Clinical Investigation* **20**, 392–397.

Perez-Mijares, R., Guzman-Zamudio, J. L., Payan-Lopez, J., Rodriguez-Fernandez, A., Gomez-Fernandez, P., and Alaraz-Jimenez, M. (1996). Calciphylaxis in a hæmodialysis patient: functional protein S deficiency. *Nephrology, Dialysis, Transplantation* **11**, 1856–1859.

Picton, M. L. *et al.* (2000). Down-regulation of human osteoblast PTH/PTHrP receptor mRNA in end-stage renal failure. *Kidney International* **58**, 1440–1449.

Plachot, J. J. *et al.* (1984). Bone ultrastructure and X-ray microanalysis of aluminum-intoxicated hemodialyzed patients. *Kidney International* **25**, 796–803.

Pogglitsch, H., Estelberger, W., Petek, W., Zitta, S., and Ziak, E. (1989). Relationship between generation and plasma concentration of anorganic phosphorus. *In vivo* studies on dialysis patients and *in vitro* studies on erythrocytes. *International Journal of Artificial Organs* **12**, 524–532.

Portale, A. A., Booth, B. E., Halloran, B. P., and Morris, R. C. (1984). Effect of dietary phosphorus on circulating concentrations of 1,25-dihydroxyvitamin D and immunoreactive parathyroid hormone in children with moderate renal insufficiency. *Journal of Clinical Investigation* **73**, 1580–1589.

Proudfoot, D., Skepper, J. N., Shanahan, C. M., and Weissberg, P. L. (1998). Calcification of human vascular cells *in vitro* is correlated with high levels of matrix gla protein and low levels of osteopontin expression. *Arteriosleros, Thrombosis and Vascular Biology* **18**, 379–388.

Puzas, J. E., Turner, R. T., Howard, G. A., Brand, J. S., and Baylink, D. J. (1987). Synthesis of 1,25-dihydroxycholecalciferol and 24,25-dihydroxycholecalciferol by calvarial cells. Characterization of the enzyme systems. *The Biochemical Journal* **245**, 333–338.

Quarles, L. D., Lobaugh, B., and Murphy, G. (1992). Intact parathyroid hormone overestimates the presence and severity of parathyroid-mediated osseous abnormalities in uremia. *Journal of Clinical Endocrinology and Metabolism* **75**, 145–150.

Quarles, L. D. *et al.* (1994). Prospective trial of pulse oral versus intravenous calcitriol treatment of hyperparathyroidism in ESRD. *Kidney International* **45**, 1710–1721.

Raggi, P. *et al.* (2002). Cardiac calcification in adult hemodialysis patients. A link between end-stage renal disease and cardiovascular disease? *Journal of the American College of Cardiology* **39**, 695–701.

Ramirez, J. A. *et al.* (1993). Direct *in vivo* comparison of calcium-regulated parathyroid hormone secretion in normal volunteers and patients with secondary hyperparathyroidism. *Journal of Clinical Endocrinology and Metabolism* **76**, 1489–1494.

Recker, R. R., Bammi, A., Barger-Lux, M. J., and Heaney, R. P. (1988). Calcium absorbability from milk products, an imitation milk, and calcium carbonate. *American Journal of Clinical Nutrition* **47**, 93–95.

Reichel, H., Koeffler, H. P., Barbers, R., and Norman, A. W. (1987). Regulation of 1,25-dihydroxyvitamin D3 production by cultured alveolar macrophages from normal human donors and from patients with pulmonary sarcoidosis. *Journal of Clinical Endocrinology and Metabolism* **65**, 1201–1209.

Reichel, H., Koeffler, H. P., and Norman, A. W. (1989). The role of the vitamin D endocrine system in health and disease. *New England Journal of Medicine* **320**, 980–991.

Reichel, H., Deibert, B., Schmidt-Gayk, H., and Ritz, E. (1991). Calcium metabolism in early chronic renal failure: implications for the pathogenesis of hyperparathyroidism. *Nephrology, Dialysis, Transplantation* **6**, 162–169.

Reichel, H., Recker, A., Deppisch, R., Stier, E., and Ritz, E. (1992). 25-Hydroxyvitamin D3 metabolism *in vitro* by mononuclear cells from hemodialysis patients. *Nephron* **62**, 404–412.

Reichel, H. *et al.* (1993). Intermittent versus continuous administration of 1,25-dihydroxyvitamin D3 in experimental renal hyperparathyroidism. *Kidney International* **44**, 1259–1265.

Renaud, H., Atik, A., Hervé, M., Morinière, P., Hocine, C., and Fournier, A. (1988). Evaluation of vascular calcinosis risk in patients on chronic hemodialysis. Lack of influence of $CaCO_3$ doses. *Nephron* **48**, 28–32.

Ritz, E. and Rieden, K. (1985). Prophylaxe und Therapie osteologischer Komplikationen nach Nierentransplantation. *Mitteil Klin Nephrol* **13**, 55–70.

Ritz, E., Dreikorn, K., Weisschedell, E., and Mehls, O. (1982). Aseptische Knochennekrosen nach Nierentransplantation. *Nieren Hochdruckkrankh* **11**, 240–245.

Ritz, E., Mehls, O., and Krempien, B. (1980). Calcium and phosphorus metabolism in maintenance hemodialysis. *Advances in Nephrology from the Necker Hospital* **9**, 71–108.

Ritz, E., Szabo, A., and Reichel, H. (1993). Parathyroidectomy in secondary (renal) hyperparathyroidism—whom, when, how? *International Journal of Artificial Organs* **16**, 7–10.

Ritz, E. *et al.* (1995). Low-dose calcitriol prevents the rise in 1,84 iPTH without affecting serum calcium and phosphate in patients with moderate renal failure (prospective placebo-controlled multicenter trial). *Nephrology, Dialysis, Transplantation* **10**, 2228–2234.

Robert, D. *et al.* (1985). Does vitamin K excess induce ectopic calcifications in hemodialysis patients? *Clinical Nephrology* **24**, 300–304.

Rogers, K. V., Fox, J., Dunn, C. K., Conklin, R. L., Lowe, H., and Petty, B. A. (1995). Parathyroid gland calcium receptor mRNA levels are unaffected by chronic renal insufficiency or low dietary calcium in rats. *Endocrine* **3**, 769–774.

Rosenbaum, R. W., Kruska, K. A., and al AKe. (1981). Decreased phosphate absorption after renal transplantation. Evidence for a mechanism independant of calcium and parathyroid hormone. *Kidney International* **19**, 568–578.

Rostand, S. G. and Thornley-Brown, D. Soft tissue calcification in chronic renal failure. In *The Spectrum of Renal Osteodystrophy* (ed. T. B. A. S. Drueke). Oxford, UK: Oxford University Press, 2001.

Roullet, J. B., Haluska, M., Morchoisne, O., and McCarron, D. A. (1989). 1,25-Dihydroxyvitamin D3-induced alterations of lipid metabolism in human monocyte-macrophages. *American Journal of Physiology* **257**, E290–E295.

Roussanne, M. C., Lieberherr, M., Souberbielle, J. C., Sarfati, E., Drueke, T., and Bourdeau, A. (2001). Human parathyroid cell proliferation in response to calcium, NPS R-467, calcitriol and phosphate. *European Journal of Clinical Investigation* **31**, 610–616.

Rubinger, D., Friedlaender, M. M., Silver, J., Kopolovic, Y., Czaczkes, W. J., and Popovtzer, M. M. (1986). Progressive vascular calcification with necrosis of extremities in hemodialysis patients: a possible role of iron overload. *American Journal of Kidney Diseases* **7**, 125–129.

Sawyer, N., Nooman, K., and Altman, P. (1989). High dose calcium carbonate with stepwise reduction in dialyse calcium concentration: effective phosphate control and aluminium avoidance in haemodialysis patients. *Nephrology, Dialysis, Transplantation* **4**, 105–109.

Schaefer, K. (1994). Unsatisfactory control of serum phosphate: why is it so common and what can be done? *Nephrology, Dialysis, Transplantation* **9**, 1366–1367.

Schiller, L. R., Ana, C. S., Sheikh, M. S., Emmett, M., and Fordtran, J. S. (1989). Effect of the time of administration of calcium acetate on phosphorus binding. *New England Journal of Medicine* **320**, 1110–1113.

Schinke, T., McKee, M. D., and Karsenty, G. (1999). Extracellular matrix calcification: where is the action? *Nature Genetics* **21**, 150–151.

Schmidt-Gayk, H. *et al.* (1977). 25-Hydroxy-vitamin-D in nephrotic syndrome. *Lancet* **2**, 105–108.

Schwarz, U., Amann, K., Orth, S. R., Simonaviciene, A., Wessels, S., and Ritz, E. (1998). Effect of 1,25(OH)$_2$ vitamin D3 on glomerulosclerosis in subtotally nephrectomized rats. *Kidney International* **53**, 1696–1705.

Schwarz, U. *et al.* (2000). Morphology of coronary atherosclerotic lesions in patients with end-stage renal failure. *Nephrology, Dialysis, Transplantation* **15**, 218–223.

Seidel, A., Herrmann, P., Klaus, G., Mehls, O., Schmidt-Gayk, H., and Ritz, E. (1993). Kinetics of serum 1,84 iPTH after high dose of calcitriol in uremic patients. *Clinical Nephrology* **39**, 210–213.

Seidel, A., Stein, G., Schneider, S., Schmidt-Gayk, H., and Ritz, E. (1991). Do limited changes in phosphate intake modulate 1,25(OH)$_2$D3 levels in early renal failure? *Clinical Nephrology* **36**, 274–280.

Sethi, D., Naunton Morgan, T. C., Brown, E. A., Jewkes, R. F., and Gower, P. E. (1990). Technetium-99-labelled methylene diphosphonate uptake scans in patients with dialysis arthropathy. *Nephron* **54**, 202–207.

Shanahan, C. M., Cary, N. R., Metcalfe, J. C., and Weissberg, P. L. (1994). High expression of genes for calcification-regulating proteins in human atherosclerotic and plaques. *Journal of Clinical Investigation* **93**, 2393–2402.

Shanahan, C. M., Proudfoot, D., Farzaneh-Far, A., and Weissberg, P. L. (1998). The role of Gla proteins in vascular calcification. *Critical Reviews in Eukaryotic Gene Expression* **8**, 357–375.

Sheikh, M. S., Ramirez, A., Emmett, M., Santa Ana, C., Schiller, L. R., and Fordtran, J. S. (1988). Role of vitamin D-dependent and vitamin D-independent mechanisms in absorption of food calcium. *Journal of Clinical Investigation* **81**, 126–132.

Sheikh, M. S., Maguire, J. A., Emmett, M., Ana, C. A. S., Schiller, L. R., and Fordtran, J. S. (1989). Reduction of dietary phosphorus by phosphate binders: a theoritical *in vitro* and *in vivo* study. *Journal of Clinical Investigation* **83**, 66–73.

Sherrard, D. J. *et al.* (1993). The spectrum of bone disease in end-stage renal failure—an evolving disorder. *Kidney International* **43**, 436–442.

Shoback, D. M., Bilezikian, J. P., Turner, S. A., McCary, L. C., Guo, M. D., and Peacock, M. (2003). The calcimimetic cinacalcet normalizes serum calcium in subjects with primary hyperparathyroidism. *Journal of Clinical Endocrinology and Metabolism* **88**, 5644–5649.

Silver, J., Russel, J., and Sherwood, M. L. (1985). Regulation by vitamin D metabolites of messenger ribonucleic acid for preproparathyroid hormone in isolated bovine parathyroid cells. *Proceedings of the National Academy of Sciences USA* **82**, 4270–4273.

Silver, J., Moallem, E., Epstein, E., Kilav, R., and Naveh-Many, T. (1994). New aspects in the control of parathyroid hormone secretion. *Current Opinion in Nephrology and Hypertension* **3**, 379–385.

Simoes, J., Barata, J. D., D'Haese, P. C., and De Broe, M. E. (1994). Cela n'arrive qu'aux autres (aluminium intoxication only happens in the other nephrologist's dialysis centre). *Nephrology, Dialysis, Transplantation* **9**, 67–68.

Slatopolsky, E., Weerts, C., Thielan, J., Horst, R., Harter, H., and Martin, K. J. (1984). Marked suppression of secondary hyperparathyroidism by intravenous administration of 1,25-dihydroxy-cholecalciferol in uremic patients. *Journal of Clinical Investigation* **74**, 2136–2143.

Slatopolsky, E. *et al.* (1986). Calcium carbonate as a phosphate binder in patients with chronic renal failure undergoing dialysis. *New England Journal of Medicine* **315**, 157–161.

Slatopolsky, E. *et al.* (1989). Long-term effects of calcium carbonate and 2.5 mEq/liter calcium dialysate on mineral metabolism. *Kidney International* **36**, 897–903.

Slatopolsky, E. *et al.* (1996). Phosphorus restriction prevents parathyroid gland growth: high phosphorus directly stimulates PTH secretion *in vitro*. *Journal of Clinical Investigation* **97**, 2534–2540.

Slatopolsky, E., Finch, J., Ritter, C., and Takahashi, F. (1998). Effects of 19-nor-1,25(OH)$_2$D2, a new analogue of calcitriol, on secondary hyperparathyroidism in uremic rats. *American Journal of Kidney Diseases* **32**, S40–S47.

Smans, K. A., Van Landeghem, F. G., D'Haese, P. C., Couttenye, M. M., and De Broe, M. E. (1996). Is there a link between erythropoietin therapy and adynamic bone disease? *Nephrology, Dialysis, Transplantation* **11**, 1248–1249.

Smogorzewski, M., Tian, J., and Massry, S. G. (1995). Down-regulation of PTH-PTHrP receptor of heart in CRF: role of [Ca^{2+}]i. *Kidney International* **47**, 1182–1186.

Srivatsa, S. S. *et al.* (1997). Increased cellular expression of matrix proteins that regulate mineralization is associated with calcification of native human and porcine xenograft bioprosthetic heart valves. *Journal of Clinical Investigation* **99**, 996–1009.

Sugimoto, T., Brown, A. J., Ritter, C., Morrissey, J., Slatopolsky, E., and Martin, K. J. (1989). Combined effects of dexamethasone and 1,25-dihydroxyvitamin D3 on parathyroid hormone secretion in cultured bovine parathyroid cells. *Endocrinology* **125**, 638–641.

Szabo, A., Merke, J., Beier, E., Mall, G., and Ritz, E. (1989). 1,25(OH)2 vitamin D3 inhibits parathyroid cell proliferation in experimental uremia. *Kidney International* **35**, 1045–1056.

Szabo, A., Merke, J., Thomasset, M., and Ritz, E. (1991). No decrease of 1,25(OH)2D3 receptors and duodenal calbindin-D9k in uraemic rats. *European Journal of Clinical Investigation* **321**, 521–526.

Tabata, T. *et al.* (1988). *In vivo* effect of 1 alpha-hydroxyvitamin D3 on interleukin-2 production in hemodialysis patients. *Nephron* **50**, 295–298.

Thompson, C. S. and Weinman, E. J. (1988). The secondary oxalosis of chronic renal failure. *Seminars in Dialysis* **1**, 94–99.

Tintut, Y., Parhami, F., Bostrom, K., Jackson, S. M., and Demer, L. L. (1998). cAMP stimulates osteoblast-like differentiation of calcifying vascular cells. Potential signaling pathway for vascular calcification. *Journal of Biological Chemistry* **273**, 7547–7553.

Tominaga, Y., Numano, M., Tanaka, Y., Uchida, K., and Takagi, H. (1997). Surgical treatment of renal hyperparathyroidism. *Seminars in Surgical Oncology* **13**, 87–96.

Torres, A. *et al.* (1995). Bone disease in predialysis, hemodialysis, and CAPD patients: evidence of a better bone response to PTH. *Kidney International* **47**, 1434–1442.

Tsukamoto, Y. *et al.* (1991). The oral 1,25-dihydroxyvitamin D3 pulse therapy in hemodialysis patients with severe secondary hyperparathyroidism. *Nephron* **57**, 23–28.

Ureña, P. and deVernejoul, M. C. (1999). Circulating biochemical markers of bone remodeling in uremic patients. *Kidney International* **55**, 2141–2156.

Ureña, P., Malergue, M. C., Goldfarb, B., Prieur, P., Guedon-Rapoud, C., and Petrover, M. (1999). Evolutive aortic stenosis in hemodialysis patients: analysis of risk factors. *Nephrologie* **20**, 217–225.

Ureña, P. *et al.* (1993). Parathyroid hormone (PTH)/PTH-related peptide receptor-messenger ribonucleic acids are widely distributed in rat tissues. *Endocrinology* **133**, 617–623.

Ureña, P. *et al.* (1994). The renal PTH/PTHrP receptor is down-regulated in rats with chronic renal failure. *Kidney International* **45**, 605–611.

Ureña, P. *et al.* (1995). Serum pyridinoline as a specific marker of collagen breakdown and bone metabolism in hemodialysis patients. *Journal of Bone and Mineral Research* **10**, 932–939.

VanLandeghem, G. F., D'Haese, P. C., Lamberts, L. V., and De Broe, M. E. (1997). Competition of iron and aluminum for transferrin: the molecular basis for aluminum deposition in iron-overloaded dialysis patients? *Experimental Nephrology* **5**, 239–245.

Vlassara, H. (1996). Advanced glycation end-products and atherosclerosis. *Annals of Medicine* **28**, 419–426.

Wada, M. *et al.* (1997). The calcimimetic compound NPS R-568 suppresses parathyroid cell proliferation in rats with renal insufficiency. Control of parathyroid cell growth via a calcium receptor. *Journal of Clinical Investigation* **100**, 2977–2983.

Wada, T., McKee, M. D., Steitz, S., and Giachelli, C. M. (1999). Calcification of vascular smooth muscle culture: inhibition by osteopontin. *Circulation Research* **84**, 166–178.

Wallfelt, C. H., Larsson, R., Gylfe, E., Ljunghall, S., Rastad, J., and Åkerström, G. (1988). Secretory disturbance in hyperplastic parathyroid nodules of uremic hyperparathyroidism: implications for parathyroid autotransplantation. *World Journal of Surgery* **12**, 431–438.

Warrell, R. P., Jr., Issacs, M., Alcock, N. W., and Bockman, R. S. (1987). Gallium nitrate for treatment of refractory hypercalcemia from parathyroid carcinoma. *Annals of Internal Medicine* **107**, 683–686.

Watson, K. E., Parhami, F., Shin, V., and Demer, L. L. (1998). Fibronectin and collagen I matrixes promote calcification of vascular cells *in vitro*, whereas collagen IV matrix is inhibitory. *Arteriosclerosis, Thrombosis and Vascular Biology* **18**, 1964–1971.

Weinreich, T., Rambausek, H., and Ritz, E. (1992). Is control of secondary hyperparathyroidism optimal with the currently used calcium concentration in the CAPD fluid? *Nephrology, Dialysis, Transplantation* **6**, 843–845.

Weinreich, T., Passlick-Deetjen, J., and Ritz, E. (1995). Low dialysate calcium in continuous ambulatory peritoneal dialysis: a randomized controlled multicenter study group. *American Journal of Kidney Diseases* **25**, 452–460.

Wilson, I., Felsenfeld, A., Drezner, M. K., and Llach, F. (1985). Altered divalent ion metabolism in early renal failure: role of 1,25(OH)$_2$D3. *Kidney International* **27**, 565–573.

Winzelberg, G. G. (1987). Parathyroid imaging. *Annals of Internal Medicine* **107**, 64–70.

Yamagishi, S., Fujimori, H., Yonekura, H., Tanaka, N., and Yamamoto, H. (1999). Advanced glycation endproducts accelerate calcification in microvascular pericytes. *Biochemical Biophysical Research Communication* **258**, 353–357.

Yamamoto, M., Igarashi, T., Muramatsu, M., Fukagawa, M., Motokura, T., and Ogata, E. (1989). Hypocalcemia increases and hypercalcemia decreases the steady-state level of parathyroid hormone messenger RNA in the rat. *Journal of Clinical Investigation* **83**, 1053–1056.

Yang, W. C., Yang, C. S., Hou, C. C., Wu, T. H., Young, E. W., and Hsu, C. H. (2002). An open-label, crossover study of a new phosphate-binding agent in haemodialysis patients: ferric citrate. *Nephrology, Dialysis, Transplantation* **17**, 265–270.

Yu, V. C. *et al.* (1991). RXR beta: a coregulator that enhances binding of retinoic acid, thyroid hormone, and vitamin D receptors to their cognate response elements. *Cell* **67**, 1251–1266.

Zacharias, J. M., Fontaine, B., and Fine, A. (1999). Calcium use increases risk of calciphylaxis: a case–control study. *Peritoneal Dialysis International* **19**, 248–252.

Zehnder, D. *et al.* (1999). Expression of 25-hydroxyvitamin D3-1 alpha-hydroxylase in the human kidney. *Journal of the American Society of Nephrology* **10**, 2465–2473.

Zingraff, J. *et al.* (1987). Hypocalcaemic effect of WR 2721, 5-2 63-aminopropylaminol ethyl-phosphorothioic acid in an anuric haemodialysis patient. *Nephrology, Dialysis, Transplantation* **2**, 48–52.

Zucchelli, P., Catizone, L., Casanova, S., Fusaroli, M., Fabbri, L., and Ferrari, G. (1984). Renal osteodystrophy in CAPD patients. *Mineral and Electrolyte Metabolism* **10**, 326–332.

11.3.10 β2M Amyloidosis

Michel Jadoul and Charles van Ypersele

Introduction

Dialysis-related amyloidosis has emerged as the price paid for the long-term survival of patients on renal replacement therapy (RRT). It results from the precipitation of β2-microglobulin (β2m) fibrils (Gejyo *et al.* 1985).

In the absence of renal failure, β2m amyloid is detected only occasionally in the prostate (Cross *et al.* 1992). Although it has been observed occasionally in patients with a long history of chronic renal failure but not receiving dialysis (Zingraff *et al.* 1990), it is seen mainly in patients on RRT (Miyata *et al.* 1998), whatever its modality, except renal transplantation. β2m amyloidosis, abbreviated as Aβ2m in accordance with World Health Organization (WHO) guidelines on the nomenclature of amyloidosis (Westermark *et al.* 2002), involves mainly the joints and bone but may also extend to various organs.

Pathology

The systematic study of joints harvested at autopsy in patients on RRT has revealed the various steps of Aβ2m deposition (Garbar *et al.* 1999) (Fig. 1). In peripheral joints, Aβ2m first deposits on the surface of the cartilage. It further extends into capsules and synovia and subsequently into adjacent bones where it generates typical cysts that may lead to pathological fractures. Eventually, Aβ2m deposits undergo advanced glycation (Miyata *et al.* 1993) and are invaded by macrophages. The first pathological evidence of Aβ2m was obtained in these late deposits and led to physiopathological considerations that are now revised.

Pathological evidence of Aβ2m joint deposits is observed in up to 20 per cent of patients within 24 months after the onset of dialysis (Jadoul *et al.* 1997a) and in virtually all patients examined after more than or equal to 7 years of dialysis. Interestingly, clinical symptoms such as arthralgias develop later and are probably associated with macrophage-dependent inflammation.

In the spine, Ohashi *et al.* (1992) detected Aβ2m as early as within 24 months of dialysis, in discs sustaining severe mechanical stress.

There is no pathological evidence that joint Aβ2m deposits regress significantly after transplantation (Jadoul *et al.* 1997b).

Aβ2m is observed much later, after more than 10 years of dialysis, in the tongue and various organs with a decreasing prevalence in heart (80 per cent), gastrointestinal tract (78 per cent), lung (59 per cent), liver (41 per cent), kidney (33 per cent), and spleen (5 per cent) (Jadoul and van Ypersele 1999). In these locations, Aβ2m precipitates first in the vascular endothelium to extend subsequently within the organ parenchyma where, occasionally, clinical symptoms become apparent.

Clinical manifestations

β2M amyloidosis usually manifests as the carpal tunnel syndrome (CTS). Later arthralgias together with periarticular bone cysts sometimes complicated by bone fractures, or signs of spondyloarthropathy, and usually asymptomatic visceral deposits develop (Fig. 2).

Carpal tunnel syndrome

Carpal tunnel syndrome may be observed within 3–5 years after the onset of dialysis. Paresthesiae of the palmar surface of the first three to four fingers are eventually followed by sensory and motor loss with wasting of the thenar muscles. The pain is typically worse at night and during dialysis sessions and sooner or later becomes bilateral (Bardin 1996). Other manifestations of Aβ2m may include paresthesias of the palmar surface of the fourth or fifth finger, the so-called Guyon syndrome, and a progressive impairment of hand function, reflecting not

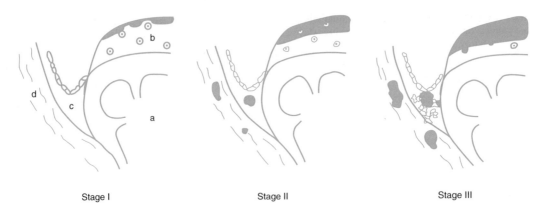

Fig. 1 Schematic representation of the three stages of Aβ2m deposition. Aβ2m is represented in black (a, bone; b, cartilage; c, synovium; d, capsule). Macrophages accumulate around synovial Aβ2m in stage III.

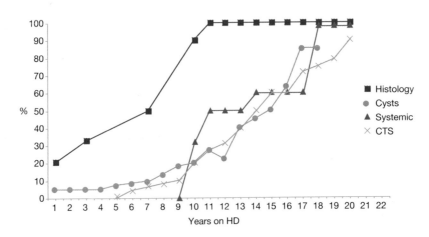

Fig. 2 Clinical manifestations of Aβ2m. (—■—) Histological articular Aβ2m (data from Jadoul et al. 1997a); (—●—) histological systemic Aβ2m (data from Miyata et al. 1998); (—▲—) operated carpal tunnel syndrome (data from Charra et al. 1988); (—✕—) radiological bone cysts (data from van Ypersele de Strihou et al. 1991).

only the CTS but also Aβ2m-induced tenosynovitis of the palmar tendons (Limaye et al. 2001). Results of electromyography help differentiate CTS from uraemic neuropathy and cervical root compression.

Aβ2m is not the only cause of CTS in dialysed patients. In particular, patients with diabetes mellitus, multiple myeloma with AL amyloidosis, and middle-aged women are known to be at risk of developing CTS not caused by Aβ2m. CTS of Aβ2m origin should be suspected in patients dialysed long-term (>5 years), especially when associated with chronic arthralgias.

Amyloid arthropathy: peripheral joints

Initially insidious arthralgia involves first the shoulders and subsequently hips, knees, and wrists (Charra et al. 1988). It worsens progressively, becomes bilateral and restricts joint mobility. Pain is worse at night and during dialysis sessions. Joint swelling or effusions may be present. The synovial fluid usually shows features of low-grade inflammation except when there is a haemarthrosis, observed in a minority of patients. It may occasionally contain Aβ2m fragments. Subsequently bone cysts develop in the adjacent bone and may lead to pathological fractures, especially of the femoral neck (Bardin 1996; Maldague et al. 1996). Subcutaneous

β2m amyloid tumours with a periarticular location (elbow, hip, knee) may also be observed occasionally.

Amyloid arthropathy: spine

Various forms of destructive spondyloarthropathy complicate long-term haemodialysis but the pain is usually moderate. Radiological signs include either cysts of the vertebral plates without significant osteophytes, or erosions of the intervertebral disc but with narrowing of the intervertebral space (Maldague et al. 1996). Although histological evidence of Aβ2m is sometimes available, this spondyloarthropathy is probably not specific of Aβ2m. Other contributing factors include severe hyperparathyroidism, aluminum overload and mechanical stress (Bardin 1996; Miyata et al. 1998).

Rarely, β2m amyloid masses develop in the epidural space and joints of the cervical spine and eventually result in nerve compression with quadriparesis or occipital nerve neuralgia (Bardin 1996).

Visceral manifestations

β2M amyloidosis deposits are found in various organs, usually in patients who have been on haemodialysis (HD) for 10 or more years.

They are usually small, located in blood vessel walls, and asymptomatic. They infrequently cause heart failure, pulmonary hypertension or various complications in the digestive tract (macroglossia or lingual nodules, bleeding, perforation, infarction or pseudo-obstruction, or diarrhoea) (Jadoul and van Ypersele 1999). Aβ2m may exceptionally present as visceral tumour-like lesions, for example, ovarian masses.

Diagnosis

Histology

The gold standard for the diagnosis of Aβ2m, as for all other types of amyloidosis, remains histological examination of the affected tissue. Unfortunately, biopsy of osteoarticular tissue is an invasive procedure and entails definite risks in dialysis patients. Occasionally, the punctured swollen joints yield synovial fluid containing Aβ2m in tissue fragments. This test proved positive in six of seven evaluated patients (Jadoul and van Ypersele 1999). In contrast to other types of amyloidosis, biopsies of subcutaneous fat and rectal submucosa are insensitive (Miyata *et al.* 1998).

Bone radiology

Periarticular bone cysts have long been recognized as a hallmark of Aβ2m. The radiological pattern of bone lesions is similar in Aβ2m and in AL amyloidosis (Maldague *et al.* 1996). Swelling of soft tissues, with a preserved or widened joint space is followed by the development of juxta-articular cystic bone defects located mainly in the wrist, shoulder, and hip. Bone cysts develop within 5–15 years of starting dialysis. They increase in size and number over time, together with displacement of fat pads (reflecting soft tissue swelling). Skeletal X-rays may allow a specific diagnosis of bone Aβ2m provided that strict criteria are applied. To be diagnostic, the cyst size should exceed 10 mm (hip, shoulder) or 5 mm (wrist) and should be located outside areas prone to synovial inclusions such as the femoral neck and outside the weight-bearing area of the acetabulum. A normal joint space adjacent to the bone defect allows the exclusion of osteoarthritic bone cysts. When cysts affect a weight-bearing area or sites of synovial inclusions, only defects whose diameter increases by more than 30 per cent per year are considered significant. Diagnosis of Aβ2m requires the involvement of at least two joints. When the two affected joints are the wrists, at least two significant bone defects must be detected in one of them (Fig. 3). In our experience, these criteria have proven very specific but not sensitive for Aβ2m (van Ypersele *et al.* 1991; Maldague *et al.* 1996).

Ultrasonography

Capsulosynovial ('soft tissue') swelling precedes the development of bone cysts in Aβ2m.

Advanced techniques of ultrasonography now permit an accurate assessment of capsule and tendon thickness and provide a more sensitive tool for Aβ2m diagnosis. Thickened supraspinatus shoulder tendons and femoral neck capsules have been documented in patients with Aβ2m (Jadoul *et al.* 1993).

Computed tomography–magnetic resonance imaging

Soft-tissue changes and early cystic Aβ2m bone lesions are more easily detected with computed tomography (CT) (Fig. 4) or magnetic resonance imaging (MRI) than with plain X-rays (Escobedo *et al.* 1996). MRI may also be helpful in the differential diagnosis of dialysis spondyloarthropathy with spondylodiscitis: infection is unlikely in the absence of high signal intensity on *T*2-weighted images (Maldague *et al.* 1996).

Serum amyloid P and β2m scintigraphy

Serum amyloid P scintigraphy

Serum amyloid P (SAP) component, a non-fibrillar plasma glycoprotein synthesized by the liver, undergoes non-covalent calcium-dependent binding to almost all types of amyloid fibrils. This avidity has been used in scintigraphic studies with ^{123}I-labelled SAP, first in a mouse model of systemic amyloidosis and then in various types of human amyloidosis (see Chapter 4.2.1).

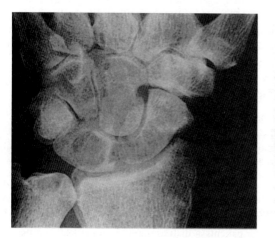 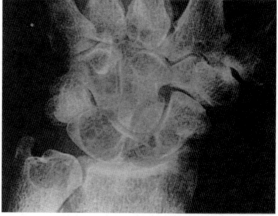

Fig. 3 Evolution of typical β2m bone defects of the wrist in a 52-year-old male, over a 5-year period of time. Left panel: after 11 years of dialysis, typical bone defects in the navicular, the lunate, the proximal angle of the hamate, and the distal end of the ulna. Right panel: 5 years later (16 years of dialysis), increase in size of each of the previous bone defects and development of new defects in the hamate, the capitatum, the distal radius, and the proximal end of metacarpals 3, 4, and 1.

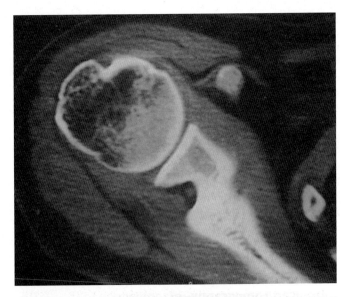

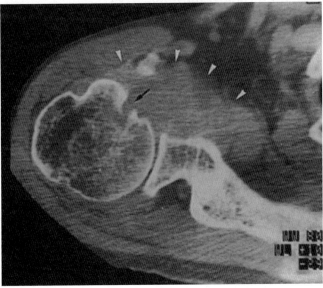

Fig. 4 Comparative CT of the shoulder in a normal subject (upper panel), and in a patient with β2m shoulder arthropathy (lower panel). Aβ2m deposits lead to thickening of the muscles ventral to the scapulohumeral joint (arrowheads) and to the presence of marginal defects of the ventral aspect of the humerus (arrow).

In a cross-sectional study of 38 long-term HD patients, ^{123}I-labelled SAP accumulated at all sites of histology proven Aβ2m and at many sites of clinically suspected Aβ2m. Wrist uptake was predominant. Surprisingly, however, splenic uptake was observed in 12 of 38 long-term HD patients, although histological Aβ2m is highly uncommon at that site and, when present, minimal. In contrast, hip uptake was infrequent and shoulder uptake was not detected in seven of 19 cases with clinical manifestations (Nelson et al. 1991). Splenic uptake is probably an artefact, whereas the lack of hip or shoulder uptake reflects methodological problems. Thus, both specificity and sensitivity of the method seem limited (Jadoul et al. 1997a,b).

The specificity of SAP scintigraphy is further limited by the fact that SAP binds to all types of amyloid and, thus, does not distinguish

Aβ2m from the other amyloidoses, including that associated with age, frequently present although in small amounts in dialysis patients (Garbar et al. 1999). The ability of SAP scintigraphy to quantify amyloid deposit is as yet not supported by convincing histologic evidence.

β2m Scintigraphy

β2-Microglobulin Labelled by ^{131}I has also been utilized in scintigraphic studies. Sensitivity and specificity were excellent for the detection of large Aβ2m deposits in 42 long-term HD patients but no information is available for small, incipient deposits (Floege et al. 1990). Unfortunately, β2m scintigraphy cannot be used in patients with a significant residual renal function, because β2m is readily excreted by the kidney. [111]Indium-labeled recombinant or natural human β2m scintigraphy has been recently developed, in order to reduce radiation exposure (Schäffer et al. 2000). Although sensitivity appears somewhat better, it remains suboptimal as some patients in whom predicted prevalence of histological Aβ2m reached 100 per cent, have proved negative. Histological validation of this new method has been limited to four involved sites, calling for further experience.

Risk factors for Aβ2m

A careful clinical, radiological, and postmortem evaluation of cohorts of patients on dialysis has unravelled several risk factors for the onset of Aβ2m.

Types of renal replacement therapy

With the exception of renal transplantation, Aβ2m development has been reported with all types of RRT: HD, peritoneal dialysis (PD), haemofiltration (HF), and also in a few patients with severe chronic renal failure prior to RRT (Zingraff et al. 1990). Histological Aβ2m prevalence at postmortem was slightly but not significantly less in patients on PD than in those on HD, matched for age and time on dialysis (Jadoul et al. 1998).

More recently, the prevalence of CTS as evaluated by the need for surgical decompression, was reported to be less in patients on convective (haemodiafiltration, HF) than on diffusive (HD) treatment modalities, again independently of age and time on RRT (Locatelli et al. 1999). This observation fits with the better clearance of β2m with convective than diffusive treatments. The prevalence of Aβ2m with newer treatment modalities such as daily short or nocturnal HD is as yet unknown.

Time on haemodialysis

The prevalence of Aβ2m, as judged by the need for CTS surgery, the presence of typical radiological signs or histological Aβ2m at postmortem, increases markedly with the time spent on dialysis (Fig. 2) (Charra et al. 1988; Chanard et al. 1989; van Ypersele et al. 1991; Jadoul et al. 1997a).

Age at dialysis onset

Older patients at dialysis onset are at markedly greater risk of clinical (CTS), radiological, and histological Aβ2m, independently of the time spent on dialysis (van Ypersele et al. 1991; Jadoul et al. 1997a). This consistent observation remains unexplained.

Haemodialysis membrane type

Many studies have used clinical (CTS) or radiological (bone) endpoints to investigate the potential contribution of HD membrane type to the development of Aβ2m. All are retrospective, due to the long time required for the development of clinical or radiological signs of Aβ2m. After appropriate statistical adjustments for other known risk factors for Aβ2m (age at HD onset, time on HD), high-flux biocompatible membranes such as polycrylonitrile (AN69) or polysulfone (PS) delayed onset of Aβ2m as compared with low-flux bioincompatible membranes such as cuprophane (Chanard *et al.* 1989; van Ypersele *et al.* 1991; Küchle *et al.* 1996; Koda *et al.* 1997).

Pathophysiology

Role of β2m retention

β2M amyloidosis has not been reported in the absence of elevated β2m serum concentration except in the prostate gland. β2m concentrations are influenced by several factors, none of which have a demonstrable effect on the prevalence of Aβ2m:

1. *β2m Production:* activation and proliferation of lymphoid cells, the presumed major synthesis site of β2m, stimulates β2m production. Thus, patients with clonal B cell disorders, rheumatoid arthritis, systemic lupus, Crohn's disease, various viral infections have increased serum β2m (Miyata *et al.* 1998). Treatment with interferon-α (IFN-α) for hepatitis C has recently also been shown to increase serum β2m in HD patients, an effect reversible upon IFN-α withdrawal (Espinosa *et al.* 2001).

2. *Residual glomerular filtration rate (GFR):* even a minimal residual GFR reduces serum β2m: serum β2m is twice as high in HD patients with a GFR less than 1 ml/min than in those with a GFR of 4–5 ml/min (Miyata *et al.* 1998).

3. *Age and time spent on dialysis:* older patients have lower β2m, independently of residual GFR, an observation in striking contrast with their known increased propensity to develop Aβ2m. When residual GFR and age are considered in a multivariate analysis, time spent on dialysis does not emerge as an independent determinant of serum β2m (Kabanda *et al.* 1994).

4. *Metabolic acidosis:* limited but consistent *in vitro* and *in vivo* data suggest that acidosis stimulates β2m production (Sonikian *et al.* 1996). This single observation is yet to be confirmed in a large group of patients.

5. *Dialysis modality:* serum β2m is some 30 per cent lower in patients on PD or high-flux HD than in those on low-flux HD; this reflects both the high-flux and peritoneal clearance of β2m as well as the higher residual GFR on PD. In a large randomized study using PS membranes, serum β2m was not lower with haemodiafiltration than with high-flux HD (Locatelli *et al.* 1999). Nocturnal daily high-flux dialysis is associated with a further 50 per cent decrease of serum β2m (Raj *et al.* 2000).

Many studies have been performed to elucidate the mechanism(s) of the membrane effect.

Some *in vitro* studies have suggested that complement-activating membranes such as cuprophane stimulate β2m production whereas the results of *in vivo* studies are discordant. The *in vivo* relevance of membrane-induced changes in β2m production is limited when compared with the β2m clearance of various dialysis modalities (van Ypersele *et al.* 1994).

Whatever the dialysis modality, β2m accumulates progressively as β2m removal fails to meet its production.

Role of β2m modification and of cells infiltrating Aβ2m deposits

By analogy with other amyloidogenic proteins, it has been suggested that β2m has to be modified to generate amyloid fibrils. The potential role of proteolytic cleavage of β2m fibrils has been controversial for years. Truncated β2m was initially isolated from Aβ2m deposits (Linke *et al.* 1989), an observation subsequently contradicted (Campistol *et al.* 1996; Garcia-Garcia *et al.* 1997). This discrepancy has been recently attributed to the origin of the amyloid deposits, and to the purification procedures which may favour self-aggregation and precipitation of truncated peptides (Stoppini *et al.* 2000).

A number of recent studies have identified conformational alterations or amyloidogenic characteristics of the β2m molecule (Heegard *et al.* 2002; McParland *et al.* 2002; Trinh *et al.* 2002; Verdone *et al.* 2002), but their relevance to Aβ2m formation remains to be proved.

An *in vitro* model has shown the positive effect of low pH (Naiki *et al.* 1997) on fibrillar extension as well as the inhibitory effect of apolipoprotein E (ApoE) on β2m depolymerization (Yamaguchi *et al.* 2001). These studies do not elucidate the initial steps of β2m fibrillar precipitation.

Large, late Aβ2m deposits undergo advanced glycoxidative (AGE) modification (Miyata *et al.* 1993). AGE-modified β2m binds *in vitro* to human synovial fibroblasts through the receptor for AGE (Hou *et al.* 2002). This interaction induces the release of chemoattractants for monocytes and stimulates them to secrete proinflammatory cytokines (Miyata *et al.* 1993, 1998). AGE modification of β2m may thus attract inflammatory cells and contribute to the overt, clinical phase of Aβ2m. However, it is still unlikely to initiate Aβ2m precipitation. Indeed, neither AGE-modified β2m nor cellular infiltrates are observed in the early stages of Aβ2m, involving only the cartilage (Garbar *et al.* 1999).

Role of dialysate purity

In contrast to a Japanese single centre study (Koda *et al.* 1997), a German single centre, retrospective study reported a conspicuous decline of clinical Aβ2m prevalence between 1988 and 1996 (Schwalbe *et al.* 1997). A significant, yet limited change in HD membrane type over this period was taken to be insufficient to account for the change in prevalence. A role for lower bacteriological and endotoxin concentrations in dialysate in recent years was therefore suggested.

An uncontrolled study by Baz *et al.* (1991) also claimed that CTS prevalence was lower when ultrapure dialysate rather than standard dialysate was used. Recent studies have shown that the shift to ultrapure dialysate reduces serum AGEs, an observation of interest if the latter are involved in Aβ2m formation. Moreover, ultrapure dialysate use has recently been associated with improved preservation of residual GFR (Schiffl *et al.* 2002) and thus potentially with lower serum β2m (see above).

Role of inhibitors of Ab2m degradation

Several other proteins are detected in Aβ2m deposits, for example: α2-macroglobulin (α2mG), ApoE, and SAP. Interestingly, they are also present in most other types of amyloid (e.g. AA, AL) deposits.

α2mG, a major serum antiprotease, has been claimed to prevent the proteolysis of deposited Aβ2m (Argiles *et al.* 1989). Similarly, ApoE inhibits the *in vitro* depolymerization of β2m amyloid fibrils at a neutral pH (Yamaguchi *et al.* 2001). SAP, a ubiquitous component of amyloid deposits, is highly resistant to proteolysis. It is thought that its high affinity binding to amyloid deposits protects them from proteolysis (Pepys *et al.* 2002). The relevance of these results to *in vivo* pathogenesis remains as yet unproven.

Factors accounting for the preferential osteoarticular involvement

The affinity of Aβ2m for osteoarticular tissues remains a mystery. It may be related to their high content in glycosaminoglycans such as heparan and keratan sulfate, which have a high affinity for β2m, as well as to their high content of some collagen subtypes (Ohashi *et al.* 2002).

β2m itself has been shown to exert *in vitro* various effects on osteoarticular tissues: it stimulates the expression of vascular cell adhesion molecule I and cyclooxygenase-2 (COX-2) by synovial fibroblasts, the synthesis of collagenases and cytokines, and the dissolution of bone mineral (Balint *et al.* 2000; Chen *et al.* 2002). Again, the relevance of *in vitro* data to the pathogenesis of Aβ2m in humans remains unclear.

Prevention and treatment of Aβ2m

Prevention

The best way to prevent Aβ2m is by successful renal transplantation. If this is not possible, prevention relies on the best possible removal of β2m by high-flux membranes (Jadoul and van Ypersele 1999). Whether the higher β2m removal rates provided by nocturnal daily haemodialysis or by sorbent therapy (Ameer *et al.* 2001; Winchester *et al.* 2002), will delay Aβ2m development remains to be demonstrated. The preventive role of drugs either inhibiting advanced glycoxidation such as aminoguanidine or producing pharmacological depletion of SAP (Pepys *et al.* 2002) has not been investigated.

Medical treatment

Chronic arthralgias are best treated by paracetamol/dextropropoxyphene/COX-2 inhibitors, to avoid the risk of gastric complications in high risk patients. Intra-articular corticosteroid injections are especially helpful when a single joint is very painful. Their effect is transient and carries a low but definite risk of infection. If these first-line therapies fail, oral prednisone (0.1 mg/kg/day) may be helpful (Bardin 1996).

In a few small uncontrolled and up to now unconfirmed studies, switching patients from cuprophane HD to PD or high-flux HD has been reported to improve arthralgias.

Surgical treatment

Symptomatic CTS is best treated by early surgery in order to prevent serious irreversible neuromuscular impairment. CTS cure may be achieved either classically or endoscopically although experience with the latter procedure in HD patients remains limited (Okutsu *et al.* 1993).

Recurrence should be rare with an experienced surgeon and systematic epineurotomy (Bardin 1996).

Severe shoulder arthralgias may benefit, at least transiently, from various endoscopic or surgical procedures: endoscopic resection of the coracoacromial ligament or arthroscopic synovectomy of the shoulder, open surgery with curettage of humeral cysts and ceramic implantation together with resection of hypertrophied synovium and masses. The long-term success rate of such interventions has not yet been proven (Miyata *et al.* 1998).

Pathological fractures or spinal cord compression usually require a joint prosthesis or laminectomy with vertebral fusion (Bardin 1996).

Renal transplantation

Renal transplantation should be urgently considered whenever possible in all patients with symptomatic Aβ2m. Successful transplantation results in a striking, almost immediate improvement of Aβ2m joint symptoms. In the short term, this effect has been ascribed to the high doses of steroids. It persists, however, in the long term despite the reduction and, sometimes, the interruption of steroid treatment. Progression of Aβ2m deposits is stopped as demonstrated by the lack of progression of typical amyloid bone cysts (Jadoul *et al.* 1997a,b).

Regression of Aβ2m deposits after transplantation remains a controversial issue. The reduction in labelled SAP uptake, within 3–5 years after a successful transplantation, has been taken to indicate significant Aβ2m regression (Tan *et al.* 1996). In contrast, radiological bone cysts do not regress up to 15 years after transplantation and histological evidence of Aβ2m persists up to 12 years after a successful transplantation. These findings taken together with the lack of specificity of SAP scintigraphy and its inability to quantitate amyloid deposits, strongly suggest that Aβ2m deposits remain largely unchanged after transplantation (Jadoul *et al.* 1997b).

References

Ameer, G. A. *et al.* (2001). A novel immunoadsorption device for removing beta2-microglobulin from whole blood. *Kidney International* **59**, 1544–1550.

Argiles, A. *et al.* (1989). High-molecular-mass proteins in haemodialysis-associated amyloidosis. *Clinical Science* **76**, 547–552.

Balint, E., Marshall, C. F., and Sprague, S. M. (2000). Role of interleukin-6 in beta2-microglobulin-induced bone mineral dissolution. *Kidney International* **57**, 1599–1607.

Bardin, T. Arthropathy and carpal tunnel syndrome of β2-microglobulin amyloidosis. In *Dialysis Amyloid* (ed. C. van Ypersele and T. B. Drüeke), pp. 71–97. Oxford: Oxford University Press, 1996.

Baz, M. *et al.* (1991). Using ultrapure water in hemodialysis delays carpal tunnel syndrome. *International Journal of Artificial Organs* **14**, 681–685.

Campistol, J. M. *et al.* (1996). Polymerization of normal and intact beta 2-microglobulin as the amyloidogenic protein in dialysis-amyloidosis. *Kidney International* **50**, 1262–1267.

Chanard, J. *et al.* (1989). Carpal tunnel syndrome and type of dialysis membrane. *British Medical Journal* **298**, 867–868.

Charra, B., Calemard, E., and Laurent, G. (1988). Chronic renal failure treatment duration and mode: their relevance to the late dialysis periarticular syndrome. *Blood Purification* **6**, 117–124.

Chen, N. X. *et al.* (2002). Signal transduction of beta2m-induced expression of VCAM-1 and COX-2 in synovial fibroblasts. *Kidney International* **61**, 414–424.

Cross, P. A., Bartley, C. J., and McClure, J. (1992). Amyloid in prostatic corpora amylacea. *Journal of Clinical Pathology* **45**, 894–897.

Escobedo, E. M. *et al.* (1996). Magnetic resonance imaging of dialysis-related amyloidosis of the shoulder and hip. *Skeletal Radiology* **25**, 41–48.

Espinosa, M. *et al.* (2001). Alpha-interferon therapy increases serum beta2-microglobulin levels in hemodialysis patients. *Clinical Nephrology* **56**, 378–381.

Floege, J. *et al.* (1990). Imaging of dialysis-related amyloid (AB-amyloid) deposits with 131I-beta 2-microglobulin. *Kidney International* **38**, 1169–1176.

Garbar, C. *et al.* (1999). Histological characteristics of sternoclavicular beta 2-microglobulin amyloidosis and clues for its histogenesis. *Kidney International* **55**, 1983–1990.

Garcia-Garcia, M. *et al.* (1997). Monometric and dimeric beta 2-microglobulin may be extracted from amyloid deposits in vitro. *Nephrology, Dialysis, Transplantation* **12**, 1192–1198.

Gejyo, F. *et al.* (1985). A new form of amyloid protein associated with chronic hemodialysis was identified as beta 2-microglobulin. *Biochemical and Biophysical Research Communications* **129**, 701–706.

Heegaard, N. H. *et al.* (2002). Cleaved beta 2-microglobulin partially attains a conformation that has amyloidogenic features. *Journal of Biological Chemistry* **277**, 11184–11189.

Hou, F. F. *et al.* (2002). Receptor for advanced glycation end products on human synovial fibroblasts: role in the pathogenesis of dialysis-related amyloidosis. *Journal of the American Society of Nephrology* **13**, 1296–1306.

Jadoul, M. and van Ypersele de Strihou, C. β2-Microglobulin amyloidosis. In *Complications of Long-term Dialysis* (ed. E. A. Brown and P. S. Parfrey), pp. 121–144. Oxford: Oxford University Press, 1999.

Jadoul, M. *et al.* (1993). Ultrasonographic detection of thickened joint capsules and tendons as marker of dialysis-related amyloidosis: a cross-sectional and longitudinal study. *Nephrology, Dialysis, Transplantation* **8**, 1104–1109.

Jadoul, M. *et al.* (1997a). Histological prevalence of β2-microglobulin amyloidosis in hemodialysis: a prospective post-mortem study. *Kidney International* **51**, 1928–1932.

Jadoul, M. *et al.* (1997b). Does dialysis-related amyloidosis regress after transplantation? *Nephrology, Dialysis, Transplantation* **12**, 655–657.

Jadoul, M. *et al.* (1998). Prevalence of histological beta2-microglobulin amyloidosis in CAPD patients compared with hemodialysis patients. *Kidney International* **54**, 956–959.

Kabanda, A. *et al.* (1994). Determinants of the serum concentrations of low molecular weight proteins in patients on maintenance hemodialysis. *Kidney International* **45**, 1689–1696.

Koda, Y. *et al.* (1997). Switch from conventional to high-flux membrane reduces the risk of carpal tunnel syndrome and mortality of hemodialysis patients. *Kidney International* **52**, 1096–1101.

Küchle, C. *et al.* (1996). High-flux hemodialysis postpones clinical manifestation of dialysis-related amyloidosis. *American Journal of Nephrology* **16**, 484–488.

Limaye, V. *et al.* (2001). Evaluation of hand function in patients undergoing long term haemodialysis. *Annals of Rheumatic Diseases* **60**, 278–280.

Linke, R. P. *et al.* (1989). Lysine-specific cleavage of beta 2-microglobulin in amyloid deposits associated with hemodialysis. *Kidney International* **36**, 675–681.

Locatelli, F. *et al.* (1999). Comparison of mortality in ESRD patients on convective and diffusive extracorporeal treatments. *Kidney International* **55**, 286–293.

Maldague, B., Malghem, J., and Van de Berg, B. Radiology of dialysis amyloidosis. In *Dialysis Amyloid* (ed. C. van Ypersele and T. B. Drüeke), pp. 98–135. Oxford: Oxford University Press, 1996.

McParland, V. J. *et al.* (2002). Structural properties of an amyloid precursor of beta(2)-microglobulin. *Nature Structural Biology* **9**, 326–331.

Miyata, T. *et al.* (1993). Beta 2-microglobulin modified with advanced glycation end products is a major component of hemodialysis-associated amyloidosis. *Journal of Clinical Investigation* **92**, 1243–1252.

Miyata, T. *et al.* (1998). Beta-2 microglobulin in renal disease. *Journal of the American Society of Nephrology* **9**, 1723–1735.

Naiki, H. *et al.* (1997). Establishment of a kinetic model of dialysis-related amyloid fibril extension in vitro. *Amyloid: International Journal of Experimental and Clinical Investigation* **4**, 223–232.

Nelson, S. R. *et al.* (1991). Imaging of haemodialysis-associated amyloidosis with 123I-serum amyloid P component. *Lancet* **338**, 335–339.

Ohashi, K., Kisilevsky, R., and Yanagishita, M. (2002). Affinity binding of glycosaminoglycans with beta(2)-microglobulin. *Nephron* **90**, 158–168.

Ohashi, K. *et al.* (1992). Cervical discs are most susceptible to beta 2-microglobulin amyloid deposition in the vertebral column. *Kidney International* **41**, 1646–1652.

Okutsu, I. *et al.* (1993). Results of endoscopic management of carpal-tunnel syndrome in long-term haemodialysis versus idiopathic patients. *Nephrology, Dialysis, Transplantation* **8**, 1110–1114.

Pepys, M. B. *et al.* (2002). Targeted pharmacological depletion of serum amyloid P component for treatment of human amyloidosis. *Nature* **417**, 231–233.

Raj, D. S. *et al.* (2000). Beta(2)-microglobulin kinetics in nocturnal haemodialysis. *Nephrology, Dialysis, Transplantation* **15**, 58–64.

Schäffer, J. *et al.* (2000). Recombinant versus natural human 111In-beta2-microglobulin for scintigraphic detection of Abeta2m amyloid in dialysis patients. *Kidney International* **58**, 873–880.

Schiffl, H., Lang, S. M., and Fischer, R. (2002). Ultrapure dialysis fluid slows loss of residual renal function in new dialysis patients. *Nephrology, Dialysis, Transplantation* **17**, 1814–1818.

Schwalbe, S. *et al.* (1997). Beta 2-microglobulin associated amyloidosis: a vanishing complication of long-term hemodialysis? *Kidney International* **52**, 1077–1083.

Sonikian, M. *et al.* (1996). Potential effect of metabolic acidosis on beta 2-microglobulin generation: in vivo and in vitro studies. *Journal of the American Society of Nephrology* **7**, 350–356.

Stoppini, M. S. *et al.* (2000). Detection of fragments of beta2-microglobulin in amyloid fibrils. *Kidney International* **57**, 349–350.

Tan, S. Y. *et al.* (1996). Long term effect of renal transplantation on dialysis-related amyloid deposits and symptomatology. *Kidney International* **50**, 282–289.

Trinh, C. H. *et al.* (2002). Crystal structure of monomeric human beta-2-microglobulin reveals clues to its amyloidogenic properties. *Proceedings of the National Academy of Sciences of the United States of America* **99**, 9771–9776.

van Ypersele de Strihou, C. *et al.* (1991). Effect of the dialysis membrane and patient's age on signs of dialysis related amyloidosis. *Kidney International* **39**, 1012–1019.

van Ypersele de Strihou, C. *et al.* (1994). Amyloidosis and its relationship to different dialysers. *Nephrology, Dialysis, Transplantation* **9** (Suppl. 2), 156–161.

Verdone, G. *et al.* (2002). The solution structure of human beta2-microglobulin reveals the prodromes of its amyloid transition. *Protein Science* **11**, 487–499.

Westermark, P. *et al.* (2002). Amyloid fibril protein nomenclature—2002. *Amyloid: Journal of Protein Folding Disorders* **9**, 197–200.

Winchester, J. F. *et al.* (2002). The next step from high-flux dialysis: application of sorbent technology. *Blood Purification* **20**, 81–86.

Yamaguchi, I. *et al.* (2001). Apolipoprotein E inhibits the depolymerization of beta 2-microglobulin-related amyloid fibrils at a neutral pH. *Biochemistry* **40**, 8499–8507.

Zingraff, J. J. *et al.* (1990). Beta 2-microglobulin amyloidosis in chronic renal failure. *New England Journal of Medicine* **323**, 1070–1071.

11.3.11 Effect on the immune response

Alessandro Amore and Rosanna Coppo

Introduction

Uraemia interferes with the immune response through complex modifications of molecular pathways with clinically relevant consequences.

Almost half a century ago, impairment of humoral immunity in uraemia was detected, accounting for enhanced susceptibility to bacterial infections (Dammin *et al.* 1957). Later effects on cell-mediated immunity with hyporesponsiveness to thymus-dependent vaccines and skin grafts were described (Smiddy *et al.* 1961). The immune deficiency of uraemia *is considered* secondary to interferences with immune system cell biological functions due to accumulation of uraemic toxins (Vanholder *et al.* 2001) with loss of essential components and functions.

Paradoxically, a large series of studies have shown that in uraemic patients phenotypic and functional signs of chronic immune activation exist, and the system is primed in a manner mimicking autoimmunity (reviewed in Amore and Coppo 2002).

Despite the great improvements in renal replacement therapy over time, no beneficial effect on the immune system abnormalities in uraemic patients has been achieved. It has also become evident that repeated use of synthetic extracorporeal circuits and unphysiological dialysate buffers challenge the immune system, resulting in a state of persistent microinflammation. The long-term systemic effects of this subtle condition are deleterious, since this relentless process promotes a vasculopathy which contributes to the morbidity and mortality of patients on dialysis.

The aim of this chapter is to summarize the physiological properties of the various cell lines of the immune system, and then to focus on their dysfunction in uraemia and their modulation by repeated dialysis treatments.

Physiological immune response

A precise and effective immune response depends upon an orchestration of different bone-marrow-derived cells, each of which has acquired specific functions during fetal and postnatal development.

Natural immunity is an ancestral process which precedes the exposure to infectious or foreign agents and does not show any modulation by contact with foreign substances. The players of the innate immunity are mostly phagocytic cells (polymorphonuclear leucocytes, mononuclear phagocytes, and natural killer T-cells), circulating molecules (as complement components), and soluble mediators which are active on other cells [such as interferon-α, interferon-β, tumour necrosis factor (TNF)-α, and macrophage-derived cytokines].

Acquired or specific immunity is a more complex system, finely regulated by the exposure to foreign substances. This system is exquisitely specific for distinct macromolecules and increases in magnitude and defensive efficiency with each subsequent exposure to antigens. Its complete activity is the result of a precise cooperation among 'T' (Thymus derived) lymphocytes deputed to cell-mediated immunity (delayed hypersensitivity and cytotoxic reactions) and 'B' (Bursa derived) lymphocytes specialized in the production of antibodies. The development, differentiation, and acquisition by these cells of the full activity depend upon the presence of accessory antigen presenting cells, mainly dendritic cells and monocyte/macrophages expressing HLA class II molecules.

T-cell function

T-lymphocytes play a pivotal role in the acquired immune response. Their precursors arise in the bone marrow and mature in the thymus.

Mature T-lymphocytes express CD2 and CD3 surface markers. They differentiate into functionally distinct populations, the best defined of which are helper T, suppressor T, and cytotoxic T-cells. The surface markers CD4 or CD8 allow their identification into CD4+CD8− T-helper lymphocytes and CD4−CD8+ T-suppressor lymphocytes.

CD4 and CD8 are involved in the recognition of the major histocompatibility complex (MHC) expressed on the antigen presenting cells (APCs).

The T-cell receptor (TCR) CD3 is required for recognition of the foreign nature of the antigen-derived peptides presented by the MHC. Its activation initiates the complex reactions required to provide the organism with defence against non-self antigens. However, the full T-lymphocyte activation requires the participation of accessory or costimulatory molecules expressed on T-cells and on APCs including B7 1 and B7 2 (CD86 and CD80) and their ligands CD28 and LFA3. The lack of expression of some of the costimulatory molecules results in a deficient T-cell activation and anergy.

Once allo-recognition is complete, the activation of intracellular signalling results in synthesis of specific cytokines with autocrine and paracrine activity [such as interleukin (IL)-2] leading to lymphoblast transformation and clonal expansion.

According to the pattern of lymphokines produced, two major subclasses of CD4+CD8− T-cells—Th1 and Th2 lymphocytes—have been identified. The former mainly secrete IL-2 and interferon-γ and are involved in cell-mediated reactions (such as rejection of grafted organs), the latter are mostly involved in humoral and allergic reactions and secrete IL-4, IL-5, IL-6, and IL-10. A mutual control exists between Th1 and Th2 T-lymphocytes as interferon-γ inhibits the Th2 response, while IL-10, being a controller of Th1 activity, is provided with anti-inflammatory activity.

B-cell function

Although B-cells are fundamentally different from T-cells, they share common aspects including several points of development, signalling, tolerogenic mechanisms, and receptor structure.

B-lymphocytes are destined to provide synthesis of immunoglobulins, products of specific genes belonging to a large series of 'immune' genes. Immunoglobulins are characteristic of humoral immunity and, after binding to the B-cell membrane, they form B-cell receptors (BCRs) for antigens, equivalent to TCRs.

Some of the progeny of antigen-stimulated B-cells do not differentiate into effector (plasma) cells, but become memory lymphocytes, which are capable of surviving for long periods, perhaps 20 years or more, in the absence of further antigenic stimulation. These lymphocytes are able to increase antibody production rapidly after further antigenic stimulation. Memory B-lymphocytes are, therefore, extremely important for providing long-lasting immunity against infections.

B-cells express on their surface other molecules involved in the interactions with immunocompetent T-cells, such as MHC class II molecules and receptors for complement factors (C3b and C3d).

The contact of the B-cells with a non-self antigen, directly or via T-cell mediation, induces lymphocyte activation with blast transformation, proliferation, and differentiation into a B-cell clone specific for the challenging antigen. The clonal expansion and the differentiation into plasma cells leads to production of IgM and thereafter successive switching to IgG, IgA, or IgE. The switching programme is regulated by cytokines produced by antigen-activated T-cells.

Mononuclear cell function

Mononuclear cells constitute the second major population of the immune system and consist of cells whose primary function is phagocytosis. They play a key role in both innate and acquired immunity. Macrophages phagocytose foreign particles, such as microbes, macromolecules, including antigens and even self-tissues that are injured or dead, such as senescent or apoptotic cells. The recognition involves receptors for phospholipids and carbohydrate residues, and the degradation is mediated by lysosomal enzymes. Mononuclear phagocytic cells are the principal 'scavenger system' of the body.

To exert their effector role fully in the innate immunity, mononuclear phagocytic cells produce a large variety of proinflammatory and 'killer' molecules including complement proteins, proteases, reactive oxygen species (ROS), nitric oxide, and metabolites of arachidonic acid (prostaglandins and leukotrienes).

In acquired immunity, mononuclear phagocytic cells function as accessory and effector cells playing an important role in recognition, activation, and effector phases. The expression of MHC class II molecules allows them to act as APCs, reacting with TCR expressed on T-cells, then initiating the recognition phase of non-self antigens. Moreover, by expressing costimulatory molecules they promote the full T-cell activation.

The synthesis and release of interferon-γ by antigen-stimulated T-cells activate mononuclear phagocytic cells and lead them to become cytotoxic effector cells. Such activated macrophages are more efficient in performing phagocytic, degradative, and cytocidal functions than are unstimulated cells.

In the effector phase of the humoral immune response, foreign antigens become coated or opsonized by antibody molecules and complement proteins. Mononuclear cells express surface receptors for the Fc portion of Ig (FcR) and complement proteins (CR1), and participate in antibody-mediated cellular toxicity.

Mononuclear cells produce cytokines such as interferon-γ, IL-1, TNF-α, IL-6, and metabolic products of arachidonic acid to exert their effector activities. Cytokines function in autocrine and paracrine pathways. Their activity is receptor-mediated and elicits a cascade of intracellular events inducing the nuclear translocation of transcriptional factors (NF-κB, AP-1, NFAT) leading to the final effects of the release of cytokines. These cytokines are not constitutively expressed, and gene transcription is enhanced by challenge by various stimuli such as infections, bacterial lipopolysaccharide (LPS), and other mediators of inflammation.

Cytokine activity is finely regulated in order to limit the cell and tissue damage. These mechanisms of control include transcriptional and post-transcriptional internal events, shedding of soluble receptors (e.g. the soluble TNF-α receptor), and self-induced synthesis of receptor antagonists which compete for receptor occupancy (e.g. IL-1 receptor antagonist, IL-1-Ra).

Polymorphonuclear cell function

Polymorphonuclear cells are often referred to as inflammatory cells, because they play important roles in inflammation and natural immunity and function to eliminate microbes and dead tissues. However, like macrophages, granulocytes are stimulated by T-cell-derived cytokines and are able to phagocytose opsonized particles, thereby serving important effector functions in the specific immune response as well. Besides a critical role in host defence against infections, granulocytes can damage normal cells and digest connective tissue by releasing a large variety of injurious agents including ROS and proteases.

These effects are finely orchestrated and consist of a series of events initiating with polymorphonuclear cell cytoskeletal rearrangement in response to chemotactic agents, adherence to vascular endothelium, trans-endothelial migration and full expression of injurious potential. All these activities are regulated by specific membrane receptors, soluble mediators, and extremely precise biochemical mechanisms of oxygen-dependent and oxygen-independent lytic pathways. The adherence of granulocytes to endothelial cells is favoured by upregulation of β2 integrins (CD11a/CD18 and CD11b/CD18) enhanced by TNF-α, the proinflammatory platelet activating factor (PAF), and leukotrienes, which also induce an upregulation on endothelial cells of the ligands β2 integrins, ICAM-1. The passage across the endothelial layer in the subintimal space is regulated by chemoattractant cytokines or chemokines such as IL-8 and monocyte chemoattractant protein-1 (MCP-1) or complement anaphylotoxins (C3a and C5a), whose gene expression and translation is induced by proinflammatory agents including IL-1β, TNF-α, and LPS.

Neutrophils also possess receptors for IgG and complement proteins (FcR and CR1), allowing them to migrate and accumulate at sites of complement activation, where they avidly phagocytose opsonized particles and function as effector cells of humoral immunity. Granulocytes are provided with two main pathways to exert their bactericidal activity: the first is oxygen-dependent and, following the activation of the NADPH oxidase, produces extremely reactive oxygen intermediates; the second is constituted by a patrimony of lytic enzymes stored in the characteristic granules that are released upon activation.

Immune dysregulation in uraemia and dialysis

Uraemia is a condition characterized by immunodepression paradoxically coexisting with both phenotypic and functional signs of immune cell activation. This condition is worsened rather than corrected by haemodialysis treatment.

In uraemic endstage renal failure (ESRF) and in dialysed patients, the total leucocyte number and CD4+/CD8+ ratio is normal (Chatenoud *et al.* 1986), with a relative lymphopenia sometimes associated with monocytosis.

A defect in *in vitro* lymphocyte proliferation with a significant reduction in synthesis and release of the activation-dependent cytokines interferon-γ and IL-2 has been reported (Meuer *et al.* 1987; Gerez *et al.* 1991). Since this defect is accentuated in the presence of uraemic serum, the involvement of circulating toxins has been advocated. Even though a dysregulated expression of CD3/TCR on T-cell surface has been described (Stachowski *et al.* 1991), the proliferative activity of T-cells in uraemia is completely restored by the coincubation of heterologous APCs or by the administration of CD28 ligands (Girndt *et al.* 1993, 2001). This finding suggests that the defect of lymphocyte proliferation is not the fault of T-cells but of the costimulatory mechanisms of the APCs. This hypothesis is supported by the observation that B-cells in uraemia proliferate normally and produce immunoglobulins *in vitro* when the activation is independent from APC or T-cell activity.

The defect in uraemic APCs does not involve class II antigens, but depends on the synthesis and expression of costimulatory molecules. The costimulatory molecule B7 2 (CD86), which binds to CD28 on T-cells, is significantly reduced in uraemia and in patients in haemodialysis (Girndt *et al.* 1993, 2000, 2001), while the expression of B7 1 (CD80) is not affected (reviewed in Girndt *et al.* 2001).

The defective expression of B7 2 limits the intracellular signals eliciting IL-2 synthesis (Williams *et al.* 1992). Conversely, IL-2 R (CD25) is upregulated on T-lymphocyte surface (Chatenoud *et al.* 1986) and increased numbers of cells expressing CD25 have been described (Stachowski *et al.* 1991), thus increasing the sensitivity of T-lymphocytes to the effect of IL-2. Plasma levels of soluble CD25 levels are increased from the onset of progressive reduction of renal function, and rise further with advancement of uraemia to a peak in haemodialysis patients (Descamps-Latscha *et al.* 1995).

Thus, in uraemia the opposite features of depression and chronic non-specific activation of T-cells coexist.

In uraemia, the process of differentiation of CD4+ T-cells into Th1 or Th2 subsets is reduced, possibly due to defective synthesis of IL-2, the cytokine that plays a pivotal role in T-lymphocyte expansion. In haemodialysis patients, a higher prevalence of Th1 CD4+ T-cells has been reported, suggesting a more heavily compromised Th2 subset. This bias in Th1 differentiation seems to be related to monocyte overexpression of IL-12 (Sester *et al.* 2000) (Fig. 1).

During the interdialytic interval, the production of monocyte-derived cytokines (IL-1β, IL-6, and TNF-α) is normal, but can be enhanced more than in healthy subjects under stimulation. This 'preactivation' state of monocytes suggests a condition of chronic intermittent inflammatory activation alongside the immune deficiency (Girndt *et al.* 1995). A key molecule in this dual phenomenon is the cytokine IL-10, produced by monocytes and providing a counter-regulatory action limiting the proinflammatory response (De Wall-Malefyt *et al.* 1991). Uraemia and haemodialysis with repeated complement activation induce the synthesis and release of IL-1 and IL-6, which have a physiological role in defence. However, in the absence of specific pathogens, this response results in immune failure as high levels of IL-1 and IL-6 upregulate the secretion of IL-10 in an attempt to limit the inflammatory response (Brunet *et al.* 1998). IL-10 gene polymorphisms, which discriminate high or low producers of IL-10, may modulate immune system function in uraemic patients through the above-mentioned feedback mechanism (Turner *et al.* 1997).

While specific defects in T-cell function in uraemia have been described by several authors, alterations in B-cell activity are still controversial. Even though immunoglobulin levels are in the normal range in uraemic patients (Descamps-Latscha *et al.* 1994), inadequate

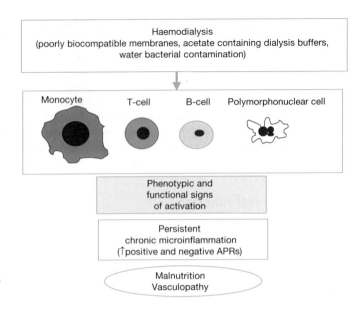

Fig. 1 Schematic of increased mononuclear production of cytokines during uraemia and haemodialysis.

B-cell responses with deficient specific antibody production as well as increased non-specific antibody production have been described. Observations of interest are: a high frequency of false-positive HIV antibodies in some cohorts of patients on dialysis (Vardinon *et al.* 1999); and spontaneous antibodies against ethylene oxide (Wass *et al.* 1988). Some studies indicate a high prevalence of non-specific antibodies against several autoantigens, phospholipids, and immunoglobulins (rheumatoid factor) in uraemia.

The altered B-cell response has been ascribed to increased level of soluble CD23, the low-affinity FcR of IgE, a marker of B-cell activation which acts as a functional cytokine (Descamps-Latscha *et al.* 1993). Since it is predominantly expressed on activated B-cells, this finding suggests an intrinsic B-cell activation state.

Actually, it is not certain whether the B-cell dysregulation in uraemia is intrinsic or due to an abnormal B–T-cell cooperation.

Vaccination response in uraemic and dialysed patients

A defective or absent response to vaccine antigens requiring T-cell-dependent mechanisms (such as hepatitis B and influenza) and the lower and time-limited responses against T-cell-independent vaccines, including tetanus, varicella, and diphtheria toxoid, has been one of the clinical observations that induced nephrologists to evaluate the function of the immune system in uraemia.

Beside non-specific factors, such as age, nutritional status, and the route of administration, particular attention has been devoted to the role of MHC genes. For instance, a particular HLA haplotype (A1 B8 DR3) and DR2 seem to modulate the responsiveness to HB vaccine (Alper *et al.* 1989; Pol *et al.* 1990).

In addition, defective expression of costimulatory molecules, alteration in CD3/TCR T-cell receptor (Stachowski *et al.* 1994), limited expression of adhesion molecules resulting in altered monocyte-dependent T-cell activation all play a role in regulating the immune response to vaccines in uraemic patients.

Monocyte-mediated responses in chronic uraemia and dialysis

Besides defective expression of costimulatory molecules on mononuclear cells leading to inappropriate T-cell function, an altered FcR-mediated internalization of opsonized particles is responsible in these patients for defective antigen presentation and phagocytosis in the effector phase of the immune response.

However, several lines of evidence suggest that uraemic mononuclear cells are actually in a continuous state of activation.

Mononuclear cells express receptors with specificity for molecules that accumulate during uraemia, including advanced glycosylated end products (AGE) (reviewed in Schimdt *et al.* 1996) and oxidized low-density lipoprotein (ox LDL) (Hamilton 1997). Activation of AGE receptor (RAGE) on mononuclear cells results in synthesis of proinflammatory cytokines (particularly IL-1β, IL-6, TNF-α), altered intracellular redox state, and activation of apoptotic pathways.

Oxidized LDL acts similarly by increasing the synthesis of IL-6 and adhesion molecules. Advanced oxidized protein products (AOPPs) levels increase with progression of renal failure and are closely related to monocyte activation, as indicated by serum levels of neopterin, TNF, and its soluble receptor (Descamps-Latscha and Witko-Sarsat 2001). Moreover, AOPPs can trigger monocyte activation and by altering intracellular redox state, promote apoptosis (Fig. 2).

Similar effects are elicited by carbonyl compounds. They are formed by auto-oxidation of carbohydrates and lipids, leading to the eventual formation of AGEs and advanced lipo-oxidation end products (ALEs) (Miata *et al.* 1994, 1999). AGEs, pentosidine and carboxymethyllysine (CML), and ALEs, malonyldialdehyde (MDA)-lysine, as well as precursor carbonyl compounds derived from carbohydrates and lipids are present in high levels in plasma and tissues of uraemic patients (Miata *et al.* 1994, 1999).

The increased levels of AGEs and ALEs are not a direct effect of glucose or loss of glomerular clearance. In uraemia, the increased levels of these molecules depend upon an accumulation of low molecular weight AGE or ALE precursor carbonyl compounds (such as glyoxal, methylglyoxal, 3-deoxyglucosone, MDA) (Miata *et al.* 1994, 1999, 2001) (Fig. 2).

The state of continuous oxidation in uraemia leads to red blood damage, platelet dysfunction, mononuclear cell activation. Clinical consequences of the oxidative stress are the appearance of amyloid arthropathy due to β2 microglobulin chemical modification and premature ageing- and apoptotis-related vasculopathy associated with long-term dialysis.

During haemodialysis, mononuclear cells are activated in other ways, including the direct contact with dialysis membranes, acetate-containing dialysis fluids, bacterial-derived material contaminating water, or dialysate. Cytokine transcription and/or production is enhanced in mononuclear cells leading to the acute and chronic inflammatory reactions dealing with the 'dialysis syndrome'. This reflects the 'interleukin hypothesis' proposed more than 20 years ago by Henderson (Henderson *et al.* 1983). This proposed the release by activated mononytes of IL-1β (Dinarello 1992; Schindler *et al.* 1993), required for IL-2 and IL-2R gene transcription, as responsible for the clinical syndrome following blood interaction with bioincompatible membranes. Recently, several other mediators have been detected, including TNF-α (Roccatello *et al.* 1993) and IL-6 (reviewed in Pertosa *et al.* 2000).

Both cuprophane membrane and acetate contained in the dialysis buffer, by activating the transcription of IL-1β and TNF-α in mononuclear cells, are responsible for inducible nitric oxide synthase (iNOS) gene transcription and translation in endothelial cells with release of toxic high amounts of NO (Amore *et al.* 1995, 1997; Amore and Coppo 2002).

The dialyser *per se* is a major factor, as the simple adherence of mononuclear cells to membrane surface stimulates mRNA expression of mediators such as IL-1β and IL-6 and oncogenes (Pertosa *et al.* 1993; reviewed in Pertosa *et al.* 2000).

The gene transcription is not always followed by mRNA translation and release of cytokines. For instance, recombinant C5a and cuprophane membrane stimulate IL-6 gene transcription rather than translation, and LPS or IL-1 are required for the translational signal (Schindler *et al.* 1990).

The literature on cytokines in haemodialysis is full of controversy. The issue is further complicated by high levels of circulating soluble receptors during dialysis making the understanding of the role of cytokines in the haemodialysis inflammation more complex. In fact, specific inhibitors of cytokines are concomitantly produced after immune system challenge. For instance, TNF-α soluble receptors (TNF-sRs) (TNF-sR55 and TNF-sR75) bind to TNF (Pereira and Dinarello 1994; Pereira *et al.* 1994; Descamps-Latscha *et al.* 1995; Ward *et al.* 1996) thus neutralizing its biological effects or, paradoxically, by stabilizing its tertiary structure, TNF-α soluble receptors prolong its effects. Conversely, IL-1-RAs competitively block IL-1 receptor, without activating any intracellular signalling. Parallel to the progressive loss of renal function, TNF-sR and IL-1-RA increase, but while TNF-sR is further increased during the course of the dialysis session, the levels of IL-1-RA decrease during haemodialysis (Pereira and Dinarello 1994; Descamps-Latscha *et al.* 1995).

TNF-sRs are considered not only as inhibitors of TNF-α function, but also as reservoirs of the cytokine. The low levels of IL-1-RA, in part

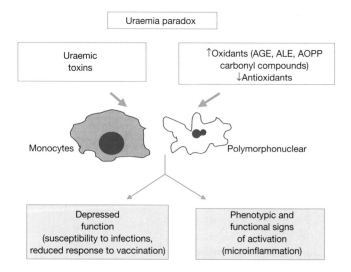

Fig. 2 Schematic of uraemic mononuclear cells in a continuous state of activation.

due to loss during haemodialysis, are not able to counteract IL-1β wasting activity, hence IL-1-RA is considered a specific marker of inflammation in chronic uraemia.

In any event, the increased mononuclear production of cytokines during uraemia and even more during haemodialysis is presently considered as the pathogenetic mechanism responsible for the microinflammatory state of long-term dialysed patients, characterized by an increase in the *so-called* acute phase reactants (APRs) including C reactive protein, amyloid, fibrinogen, and haptoglobin and a coincident decrease in albumin and transferrin (reviewed in Amore and Coppo 2002) (Fig. 3).

Polymorphonuclear dysfunction in uraemia and dialysis

Polymorphonuclear cell function is altered in uraemia rendering patients with chronic renal failure particularly susceptible to bacterial infections. Chemotaxis, phagocytosis, intracellular killing by proteolytic enzymes, and toxic oxygen radical production is partially inhibited in uraemia.

Causal factors are interdependent including iron overload, high intracellular calcium (related to PTH levels), hypophosphataemia, and various low and high molecular weight plasma circulating factors, apart from haemodialysis treatment *per se*.

Polymorphonuclear cell phagocytic ability is depressed by high intracellular iron and Ca^{2+} concentrations, which also alter calcium signal activation after stimulation of FcγRIII receptor. Erythropoietin, vitamin D, and calcium channel blockers are able to partially restore polymorphonuclear cell phagocytosis (reviewed in Massry and Smogorzewski 2001).

In the last few years, several small peptides that accumulate during uraemia have been isolated from haemodialysis ultrafiltrate or continuous ambulatory peritoneal dialysis (CAPD) effluent, and identified as molecules provided with inhibitory effects on different polymorphonuclear cell activities. Among those are the so-called granulocyte and degranulating inhibitory proteins GIP and DIP.

GIP I has high homology with free immunoglobulin light chains (IgLCs) that interfere with chemotaxis, oxidative metabolism, phagocytosis, and glucose uptake. In particular, GIP I inhibits chemotactic movements of polymorphonuclear cells induced by formyl-methionyl-leucyl-phenylalanine, a member of the *N*-formyl-peptides released by microorganisms (Horl *et al.* 1990).

GIP II has a strict homology with β2 microglobulin modified by advanced glycation and inhibits deoxyglucose uptake and polymorphonuclear cells' oxidative metabolism stimulated by phorbol-myristate-acetate, while it stimulates the synthesis of IL-1β, IL-6, and TNF from mononuclear cells (Haag-Weber *et al.* 1994; Miata *et al.* 1994).

Angiogenin, also known as DIP I, blocks the release of several polymorphonuclear enzymes such as collagenase, gelatinase, and lactoferrin, but does not modify the other polymorphonuclear functions (Tschesche *et al.* 1994).

By using a three-step chromatographic isolation procedure, another degranulating inhibitory protein has been isolated and identified as the complement Factor D (Balke *et al.* 1995). Similarly to DIP I, Factor D inhibits the release of lactoferrin in a dose-dependent manner, without affecting polymorphonuclear cells phagocytosis and chemotaxis. Unlike DIP I, Factor D or DIP II enhances oxygen radical production in resting cells.

IgLCs are present in normal conditions and their concentrations increase in uraemia and even more after repeated haemodialysis treatments. Free IgLCs inhibit polymorphonuclear cell chemotaxis, glucose uptake, and oxidative metabolism. Furthermore, free IgLCs influence

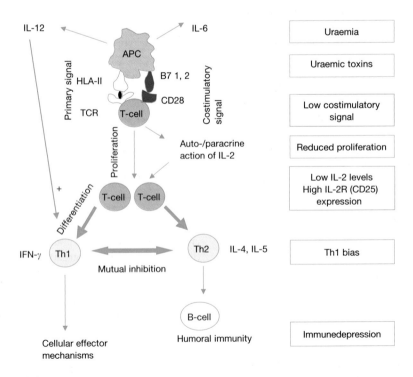

Fig. 3 Th1 differentiation in haemodialysis patients.

the percentage of viable cells by inhibiting spontaneous apoptotic death. These effects may contribute not only to the diminished immune function of the polymorphonuclear cell in the innate immunity against infectious agents, but also to the condition of preactivation of the polymorphonuclear cell responsible for chronic microinflammation in uraemic patients in dialysis (reviewed in Cohen *et al.* 1997).

A modified form of ubiquitin (Cohen *et al.* 1998) isolated from CAPD effluent is able to inhibit polymorphonuclear cell chemotaxis, while the uraemic toxin *p*-cresol (Vanholder *et al.* 1995), at the concentration found in uraemic patients, depresses the whole blood respiratory burst activity and the synthesis of PAF.

Altered CR1, FcγR, and desensitization to C5a receptors result in a defective chemotactic and oxidative response to opsonized zymosan (Lewis *et al.* 1986) interpreted as a consequence of repeated and chronic exposure to activated complement fragments.

Glycated products (either AGEs or ALEs) and carbonyl compounds present in uraemic sera influence polymorphonuclear cell function. Early glycated products, such as Amadori adducts, increase in the polymorphonuclear cell glucose uptake and accelerate apoptotic death, while late glycation products (AGEs or ALEs) increase polymorphonuclear cell chemotaxis (reviewed in Amore and Coppo 2002). This finding suggests an enhancement of the polymorphonuclear cell in the early phases of disease leading to functional impairment in a later phase.

Haemodialysis *per se* modifies polymorphonuclear cell function profoundly. Leucopenia in the initial phase of the treatment is a phenomenon related to the generation of complement components following contact of neutrophils with bioincompatible membranes. The simultaneous overexpression of surface molecules, such as Mac-1 (CD11b/CD18) and MoF11 (reviewed in Descamps-Latscha 1996) participate in the sequestration of neutrophils in the lungs and increased adhesiveness to endothelial cells. CD11b molecules remain elevated (Himmelfarb *et al.* 1992) during the whole dialysis session, despite the return to the baseline values of the neutrophil count. This phenomenon is strictly related to a decreased expression on endothelial cells of the counter-receptor for CD11b, L-selectin, involved in the rolling phase of polymorphonuclear cells on the vessel wall surface during inflammation, possibly due to dialysis-induced shedding of this molecule. This alteration could be responsible for the impairment of defence against infections in patients repeatedly treated by poorly biocompatible devices. Dialysis membrane bioincompatibility also enhances ROS production and release of granulocyte enzymes. Phagocytic polymorphonuclear cell function is depressed as a consequence of the relentless activation. A lower incidence of infections by using biocompatible membranes has been demonstrated in patients in acute and chronic renal failure.

Finally, uraemic polymorphonuclear cells are more prone to undergo apoptotic death. Uraemic toxins, particularly polyamines, carbamylated proteins, hydroxyurea, hyperhomocysteinaemia, glycated products, and carbonyl compounds (as other oxidants) act as proapoptotic agents. An enhancement of the apoptotic pathway could be also related to the complex network of cytokines produced during dialysis treatment. Dysregulation of apoptosis may play an important role in the pathogenesis of immune dysfunction in uraemia (reviewed in Jaber *et al.* 2001).

Conclusions

The progressive loss of renal function induces accumulation of several molecules that are extremely reactive with immunocompetent cells, with consequent depression or dysfunction of immunity in uraemic patients. Both innate and acquired immunity are involved. The reduced expression of costimulatory molecules on mononuclear cells together with the increased synthesis of IL-6, IL-10, and IL-12 seem to be the pivotal factors governing T- and B-cell dysfunctions in uraemia. Paradoxically, for almost each cell line phenotypic and functional signs of activation coexist and these effects parallel the progressive accumulation of uraemic toxins.

Conversely, haemodialysis acts as a repeated stimulus on mononuclear cells, which enhances a persistent microinflammatory status with clinical expression of malnutrition and vasculopathy in long-term dialysis patients.

Different therapeutic interventions can prevent or, at least, limit these events. Among these are: (a) adequate treatment with discrete Kt/V could in part restore the immune system function by removing the molecules that accumulate in uraemia and interfere with the function of the immune system; (b) the use of biocompatible membranes to limit complement activation and cytokine release; and (c) the use of sterile water. These approaches represent the basic principles to reduce the immune dysfunction in uraemia and particularly the chronic state of inflammation during long term haemodialysis.

References

Alper, C. A. *et al.* (1989). Genetic prediction of nonresponse to hepatitis B vaccine. *New England Journal of Medicine* **321**, 708–712.

Amore, A. and Coppo, R. (2002). Immunological basis of inflammation in dialysis. *Nephrology, Dialysis, Transplantation* **17**, 16–24.

Amore, A. *et al.* (1995). Enhanced production of nitric oxide by blood-dialysis membrane interaction. *Journal of the American Society of Nephrology* **6**, 1278–1283.

Amore, A. *et al.* (1997). Acetate intolerance is mediated by enhanced synthesis of nitric oxide by endothelial cells. *Journal of the American Society of Nephrology* **9**, 1431–1436.

Balke, N. *et al.* (1995). Inhibition of human polymorphonuclear leukocytes by complement factor D. *FEBS Letter* **371**, 300–302.

Brunet, P. *et al.* (1998). IL-10 synthesis and secretion by peripheral blood mononuclear cells in hemodialysed patients. *Nephrology, Dialysis, Transplantation* **13**, 1745–1751.

Chatenoud, L. *et al.* (1986). Presence of preactivated T-cells in hemodialyzed patients: their possible role in altered immunity. *Proceedings of the National Academy of Sciences USA* **83**, 7457–7461.

Cohen, G., Haag-Weber, M., and Horl, W. H. (1997). Immune dysfunction in uraemia. *Kidney International* **52**, 79–82.

Cohen, G., Rudnicki, M., and Horl, W. H. (1998). Isolation of modified ubiquitin as a neutrophil chemotaxis inhibitor from uraemic patients. *Journal of the American Society of Nephrology* **9** (3), 451–456.

Dammin, G. J., Couch, N. P., and Murray, J. E. (1957). Prolonged survival of skin homografts in uraemic patients. *Annals of the New York Academy of Sciences USA* **64**, 967–976.

Descamps-Latscha, B. and Witko-Sarsat, V. (2001). Importance of oxidatively modified proteins in chronic renal failure. *Kidney International* **78** (Suppl.), S108–S113.

Descamps-Latscha, B. *et al.* (1993). Soluble CD23 as an effector of immune dysregulation in chronic uraemia and dialysis. *Kidney International* **43**, 878–884.

Descamps-Latscha, B. *et al.* (1994). The immune system in end-stage renal disease. *Seminars in Nephrology* **14**, 253–260.

Descamps-Latscha, B. *et al.* (1995). Balance between IL-1β, TNF-α and their specific inhibitors in chronic renal failure and maintenance dialysis.

Relationships with activation markers of T-cells, B-cells and monocytes. *Journal of Immunology* 154, 882–892.

Descamps-Latscha, B. *et al.* (1996). New molecular aspects of chronic uraemia and dialysis related immunecompetent T-cell activation. *Nephrology, Dialysis, Transplantation* 11, 121–124.

De Wall-Malefyt, R., Abrams, J., and Bennet, B. (1991). Interleukin 10 (IL-10) inhibits cytokines synthesis by human monocytes: an autoregulatory role of IL-10 produced by monocytes. *Journal of Experimental Medicine* 174, 1209–1220.

Dinarello, C. A. (1992). Cytokines: agents provocateurs in haemodialysis? *Kidney International* 41, 683–694.

Gerez, L. *et al.* (1991). Regulation of interleukin-2 and interferon-gamma gene expression in renal failure. *Kidney International* 40, 266–272.

Girndt, M., Kohler, H., and SchiedhelmWeick, E. (1993). T-cell activation defect in haemodialysis patients: evidence for a role of B7/CD28 pathway. *Kidney International* 44, 359–365.

Girndt, M. *et al.* (1995). Production of interleukin 6, tumor necrosis factor and interleukin 10 *in vitro* correlates with the clinical immune defect in chronic haemodialysis patients. *Kidney International* 47, 559–565.

Girndt, M. *et al.* (2000). Molecular aspects of T- and B-cells in uraemia. *Kidney International* 59 (Suppl. 78), S206–S211.

Girndt, M. *et al.* (2001). Defective expression of B7-2 (CD86) on monocytes of dialysis patients correlates to the uraemia-associated immune defect. *Kidney International* 59 (4), 1382–1389.

Haag-Weber, M., Mai, B., and Horl, W. H. (1994). Isolation of a granulocyte inhibitory protein from uraemic patients with homology with beta2 microglobulin. *Nephrology, Dialysis, Transplantation* 9, 382–388.

Hamilton, C. A. (1997). Low-density lipoprotein and oxidised low-density lipoprotein: their role in the development of atherosclerosis. *Pharmacology & Therapeutics* 4 (1), 55–72.

Henderson, L. W. *et al.* (1983). Hemodialysis hypotension: the interleukin-1 hypothesis. *Blood Purification* 1, 3–8.

Himmelfarb, J., Zaoui, P., and Hakim, R. (1992). Modulation of granulocyte LAM-1 and MAC-1 during dialysis. A prospective, randomized controlled trial. *Kidney International* 41, 388–395.

Horl, W. H. *et al.* (1990). Physicochemical characterization of a polipeptide present in uraemic serum that inhibits the biological activity of polymorphonuclear cells. *Proceedings of the National Academy of Sciences USA* 87, 6353–6357.

Jaber, B. L. *et al.* (2001). Apoptosis of leukocytes: basic concepts and implications in uraemia. *Kidney International* 78 (Suppl.), S197–S205.

Lewis, S. L., Van Epps, D. E., and Chenoweth, D. E. (1986). C5a receptor modulation on neutrophils and monocytes from chronic haemodialysis and peritoneal dialysis patients. *Clinical Nephrology* 26, 37–44.

Massry, S. G. and Smogorzewski, M. (2001). Dysfunction of polymorphonuclear leukocytes in uraemia: role of parathyroid hormone. *Kidney International* 78 (Suppl.), 195–196.

Meuer, S. C. *et al.* (1987). Selective blockade of the antigen-receptor-mediated pathway of T-cell activation inpatients with impaired primary immune responses. *Journal of Clinical Investigation* 80, 743–749.

Miata, T. (2001). Reactive carbonyl compounds related uraemic toxicity ('carbonyl stress'). *Kidney International* 78, S25–S31.

Miata, T. *et al.* (1994). Involvement of beta2 microglobulin modified with advanced glycation end products in the pathogenesis of haemodialysis associated amyloidosis. Induction of monocyte chemotaxis and macrophage secretion of tumor necrosis factor alpha and interleukin 1. *Journal of Clinical Investigation* 93, 521–528.

Miata, T. *et al.* (1999). Alterations in nonenzymatic biochemistry in uremia: origin and significance of 'carbonyl stress' in long-term uremic complications. *Kidney International* 55, 389–399.

Pereira, B. J. G. and Dinarello, C. A. (1994). Production of cytokines and cytokine inhibitory proteins in patients on dialysis. *Nephrology, Dialysis, Transplantation* 9 (Suppl. 2), 60–70.

Pereira, B. J. G. *et al.* (1994). Plasma levels of IL-1β, TNFα and their specific inhibitors in undialyzed chronic renal failure, CAPD and haemodialysis patients. *Kidney International* 45, 1000.

Pertosa, G. *et al.* (1993). Influence of haemodialysis on interleukin-6 production and gene expression by peripheral blood mononuclear cells. *Kidney International* 39 (Suppl.), S149–S153.

Pertosa, G. *et al.* (2000). Clinical relevance of cytokines production in haemodialysis. *Kidney International* 58 (Suppl. 76), S104–S111.

Pol, S. *et al.* (1990). Genetic basis of non response to hepatitis B vaccine in hemodialyzed patients. *Journal of Hepatology* 11, 385–387.

Roccatello, D. *et al.* (1993). Induction of mRNA for tumor necrosis factor alpha in emodialysis. *Kidney International* 39 (Suppl.), S144–S148.

Schindler, R. *et al.* (1990). Transcription, not synthesis, of interleukin-1 and tumor necrosis factor by complement. *Kidney International* 37, 85–93.

Schindler, R. *et al.* (1993). Gene expression of interleukin-1 beta during haemodialysis. *Kidney International* 43, 712–721.

Schmidt, A. M. *et al.* (1996). RAGE: a novel cellular receptor for advanced glycation end products. *Diabetes* 45, S77–S80.

Sester, U. *et al.* (2000). T-cell activation follows Th1 rather than Th2 pattern in haemodialysis patients. *Nephrology, Dialysis, Transplantation* 15, 1217–1233.

Smiddy, F. G., Burwell, R. G., and Parsons, F. M. (1961). Influence of uraemia on the survival of skin homografts. *Nature* 190, 732.

Stachowski, J. *et al.* (1991). Immunodeficiency in ESRD-patients is linked to altered IL-2 receptor density on T-cell subsets. *Journal of Clinical and Laboratory Immunology* 4, 171–177.

Stachowski, J. *et al.* (1994). Non-responsiveness to hepatitis B vaccination in haemodialysis patients: association with impaired TCR/CD3 antigen receptor expression regulating costimulatory processes in antigen presentation and recognition. *Nephrology, Dialysis, Transplantation* 9, 144–152.

Tschesche, H. *et al.* (1994). Inhibition of degranulation of polymorphonuclear leukocytes by angiogenin and its tryptic fragment. *Journal of Biological Chemistry* 269, 30274–30280.

Turner, D. M. *et al.* (1997). An investigation of polymorphism in the interleukin-10 gene promoter. *European Journal of Immunogenetics* 24, 1–8.

Vanholder, R. *et al.* (1995). Mechanisms of uraemic inhibition of phagocyte reactive species production: characterization of the role of p-cresol. *Kidney International* 47, 510–517.

Vanholder, R. *et al.* (2001). Uraemic toxicity: present state of the art. *International Journal of Artificial Organs* 24 (10), 695–725.

Vardinon, N. *et al.* (1999). Anti-HIV indeterminate Western blot in dialysis patients: a long-term follow-up. *American Journal of Kidney Diseases* 34, 146–149.

Ward, R. and McLeish, K. R. (1996). Soluble TNF alpha receptors are increased in chronic renal insufficiency and haemodialysis and inhibit neutrophil priming by TNF alpha. *Artifical Organs* 20 (5), 390–395.

Wass, U., Belin, L. and Delin, K. (1988). Longitudinal study of specific IgE and IgG antibodies in a patient sensitized to ethylene oxide through dialysis. *The Journal of Allergy and Clinical Immunology* 82 (4), 679–685.

Williams, T. M. *et al.* (1992). CD-28 stimulated IL2 gene expression in Jurkatt T-cells occurs in part transcriptionally and it is cyclosporine A sensitive. *Journal of Immunology* 148, 2609–2616.

11.3.12 Coagulation disorders

*Paola Boccardo, Carla Zoja, and
Giuseppe Remuzzi*

Introduction

Bleeding in patients with renal failure was first recognized by Giovan Battista Morgagni in 1764, then by Richard Bright in 1827, and after that was often reported as one of the major complications of uraemia. Ecchymoses and epistaxis are the major bleeding manifestations seen today, with gastrointestinal bleeding, haemopericardium, or subdural haematoma occurring only occasionally. Modern dialysis techniques and the use of erythropoietin (EPO) to correct anaemia have reduced the frequency of uraemic bleeding, which, however, still limits surgery and invasive procedures, including biopsies, in these patients.

Pathogenesis

Research over the past 30 years has revealed a variety of abnormalities, but the exact nature of uraemic bleeding has not been fully clarified. The pathogenesis is considered multifactorial (Table 1) and the major defects involve platelet–platelet and platelet–vessel wall interactions (Remuzzi 1988). The impairment of primary haemostasis in uraemia has two constant abnormalities: reduced adhesiveness of platelets, and a prolonged bleeding time which is the best predictor of clinical bleeding (Mattix and Singh 1999): it depends on platelet number and function, vascular integrity, and the haematocrit, and thus gives an excellent overall assessment of primary haemostasis.

Platelet dysfunction

Thrombocytopenia is found in 16–55 per cent of uraemic patients, suggesting platelet overconsumption or inadequate production. However,

Table 1 Factors involved in the pathogenesis of uraemic bleeding

Platelet dysfunction
Subnormal dense granule content
Reduction in intracellular ADP and serotonin
Impaired release of the platelet α-granule protein and
  β-thromboglobulin
Increased intracellular cAMP
Abnormal mobilization of platelet Ca^{2+}
Reduced thromboxane A_2 generation
Defective platelet aggregation
Abnormal activation-dependent binding activity of $\alpha_{IIb}\beta_3$

Abnormal platelet–vessel wall interaction
Abnormal platelet adhesion
Increased synthesis of vascular PGI_2
Alterations in nitric oxide synthetic pathway

Anaemia
Altered blood rheology
Erythropoietin deficiency

platelet number is rarely less than 80,000/µl, a concentration generally considered adequate for normal haemostasis. On the other hand, complex abnormalities in platelet function have been described which may contribute to defective platelet aggregation and adhesion to injured vessels (Joist *et al.* 1994; Weigert and Schafer 1998). They include a reduction in platelet adenosine diphosphate (ADP) and serotonin content, a defect in the mechanisms of platelet secretion and release of the α-granule protein and β-thromboglobulin, increased platelet cyclic adenosine monophosphate, and reduced generation of thromboxane A_2. An increased platelet calcium content was described as well as an abnormal mobilization of calcium flux in response to stimulation.

Data on platelet aggregation in uraemia are conflicting. Defective platelet aggregation *in vitro* in response to stimuli such as ADP, epinephrine, collagen, and thrombin has been documented in a great number of studies. By contrast, in several other reports, platelet aggregation was found to be normal or increased. In a subpopulation of uraemic patients, irreversible platelet aggregation did not occur in response to platelet activating factor, a phospholipid able to induce aggregation and secretion in human platelets, playing a role in primary haemostasis (Macconi *et al.* 1992). This abnormality appeared as a result of the reduced capability to form thromboxane A_2 in response to platelet activating factor.

Platelet–vessel wall interaction

Normal platelet adhesion requires initial platelet contact followed by platelet spreading on the subendothelial matrix. Two adhesive proteins, fibrinogen and von Willebrand factor (vWF), and two platelet adhesion receptors, glycoprotein (GP)Ib and the $\alpha_{IIb}\beta_3$ (GPIIb/IIIa) complex, play a vital role in the formation of platelet thrombi at sites of injury. At high shear rates, such as those found in the capillary circulation, contact is dependent on the binding of vWF to the platelet GPIb. Binding of GPIb to vWF is normal in uraemic patients (Benigni *et al.* 1993), as is the surface expression of the receptor (Mezzano *et al.* 1996), whereas a decrease in the total content of platelet GPIb has been documented, accompanied by an increase in glycocalicin, a soluble proteolytic fragment of GPIb, probably due to proteolytic damage to membrane GPIb. The normal surface expression of this receptor and the total decrease in content account for a redistribution from the intraplatelet pool to the surface pool. The activation-dependent receptor function of the $\alpha_{IIb}\beta_3$ complex is defective in uraemia, as shown by decreased binding of both vWF and fibrinogen to stimulated platelets (Benigni *et al.* 1993; Gawaz and Mujais 1995). The number of $\alpha_{IIb}\beta_3$ receptors expressed on the platelet membrane is normal. Removal of substances present in uraemic plasma markedly improved the $\alpha_{IIb}\beta_3$ defect. Thus, a reversible abnormality of the activation-dependent binding activity of $\alpha_{IIb}\beta_3$ caused by a dialysable toxic substance or substances, or due to receptor occupancy by fibrinogen fragments present in uraemic plasma (Sreedhara *et al.* 1996), is probably a major component of the altered platelet function in uraemia. The impaired $\alpha_{IIb}\beta_3$ activation in uraemia may explain aggregation defect as well as reduced vWF-dependent adhesion and thrombus formation (Gawaz and Mujais 1995).

Plasma vWF has been found to be normal or elevated in uraemia, and conflicting data are available for qualitative abnormalities of vWF. That a functional defect in the vWF–platelet interaction may play a role in the abnormal haemostasis of uraemic patients rests on the findings that cryoprecipitate, a plasma derivative rich in factor VIII and vWF, and desmopressin, a synthetic derivative of antidiuretic hormone that releases autologous vWF from storage sites, both shortened the bleeding time of these patients (Mannucci *et al.* 1983).

An increased synthesis by the vascular endothelium of prostacyclin, a potent vasodilator and inhibitor of platelet function, was documented in uraemic patients as well as in experimental uraemia (Remuzzi *et al.* 1980; Zoja *et al.* 1988). Plasma of uraemic patients stimulated prostacyclin generation by cultured endothelial cells more than normal plasma (Defreyn *et al.* 1980). It was suggested that this could be due to parathormone (PTH), which is elevated in the uraemic circulation and which increased urinary excretion of 6-keto-prostaglandin F1α (Saglikes *et al.* 1985), a prostacyclin metabolite.

Experimental and clinical data are available to show that the bleeding tendency in uraemia is associated with an excessive formation of nitric oxide (NO), a potent vasoactive molecule. Rats made uraemic by extensive surgical ablation of renal mass had a prolonged bleeding time, and plasma concentrations of the stable NO metabolites, nitrites and nitrates, were higher than normal (Aiello *et al.* 1997). Moreover, administration of *N*-monomethyl-L-arginine (L-NMMA), a specific inhibitor of NO synthesis, returned the bleeding time of these rats to normal and increased *ex vivo* platelet adhesion. This effect was completely reversed by giving the animals the NO precursor L-arginine. Excessive formation of NO at systemic levels derives from vessels, as documented by the increased NO synthase (NOS) activity and high expression of both inducible NO synthase (iNOS) and endothelial NOS (eNOS) in the aorta of uraemic animals (Aiello *et al.* 1997). In the same model, the shortening effect on bleeding time of either conjugated oestrogen mixture or its active component, 17β-oestradiol, was also abolished by L-arginine, indicating that the effect of these drugs on haemostasis in uraemia could be mediated by changes in the NO synthetic pathway. In this context, in uraemic rats, 17β-oestradiol, at a dose that normalized the prolonged bleeding time, fully corrected the excessive formation of NO by markedly reducing the expression of both eNOS and iNOS in vascular endothelium (Noris *et al.* 2000). Besides its vasoactive properties, NO inhibits platelet aggregation *in vitro* and platelet adhesion to cultured endothelial cells. Patients with chronic renal failure had a defective platelet aggregation associated with higher than normal platelet NO synthesis (Noris *et al.* 1993). Uraemic plasma potently induced *in vitro* NO synthesis in cultured human umbilical vein endothelial cells as well as in human microvascular endothelial cells, suggesting that substances are accumulating in uraemic plasma that upregulate the NO synthetic pathway. Cytokines such as tumour necrosis factor-α and interleukin-1β are possible candidates since both are potent inducers of iNOS and circulate in increased amounts in the blood of patients with chronic renal failure either undialysed or on maintenance haemodialysis (Horl 2002).

Role of anaemia

Platelet adhesion and aggregation in flowing systems are markedly potentiated by red blood cells, which play an important role *per se* in platelet adhesion and thrombus formation: the red cell deformability influences the rheology of blood, modifying the transport mechanism in flowing blood. The role of anaemia in the bleeding tendency of uraemia has been investigated extensively in the past and a significant negative correlation was found between bleeding time and packed cell volume (PCV). Increasing PCV over 30 per cent by red cell transfusions or by recombinant human EPO (Livio *et al.* 1982; Viganò *et al.* 1991) in uraemic patients was associated with a significant shortening of bleeding time and with an improvement of platelet function.

Dialysis

Dialysis may contribute to the haemostatic abnormalities of uraemic patients because the interaction between blood and artificial surfaces may induce chronic activation of platelets. Moreover, heparin, used to obtain systemic anticoagulation, can occasionally induce platelet activation and thrombocytopenia. Monocytes can be activated during haemodialysis, due to adhesion to the dialysis membrane, resulting in interleukin-1 and tumour necrosis factor-α production. Increased production of cytokines may also be triggered by bacterial toxins that may cross the dialysis membrane. Because of massive release of cytokines during dialysis, there is an increase in NO synthesis by vascular endothelium, which further contributes to platelet dysfunction and possibly to other complications such as haemodialysis-associated hypotension. Uraemic patients may occasionally have an increase in plasma levels of NO metabolites during haemodialysis. Plasma collected after haemodialysis stimulated NO synthesis by cultured endothelial cells more than plasma from the same patients before dialysis (Noris *et al.* 1998). Thus, the capacity of the dialysis procedure to remove uraemic toxins is negatively counterbalanced by its effects on platelet activation and NO synthesis.

On the other hand, under optimal haemodialysis conditions that induce no or minimal cytokine activation, the exaggerated NO synthesis is corrected, possibly by removing from uraemic plasma some dialysable NO-releasing substances (Noris and Remuzzi 1999). Guanidinosuccinate (GSA), a guanidino compound related to arginine, that accumulates in uraemic plasma in micromolar concentrations, induced in endothelial cells an increase in NO release, abrogated by treating cells with specific NOS inhibitors. The effect of GSA of stimulating NO release provides a biological explanation for the data generated in the early 1970s showing that among uraemic toxins, GSA was the only one that consistently inhibited platelet function.

Coagulation and fibrinolysis disorders

Activated partial thromboplastin, prothrombin, and thrombin times are generally within the normal range in patients with endstage renal failure; fibrinogen and factor VIII procoagulant are usually increased. Low plasma concentrations of antithrombin III, protein C anticoagulant activity, and free protein S have been reported. Thrombin is continuously formed, as demonstrated by increased levels of thrombin–antithrombin III complex, D-dimer, and fibrinopeptide A (Sagripanti and Barsotti 1997). These alterations suggest that a hypercoagulable state exists in chronic uraemia that may result in thrombotic complications.

Data regarding fibrinolysis are conflicting. Total fibrinolytic activity is usually reduced in uraemia, in the face of hypercoagulation. Reduced release of tissue plasminogen activator from vascular endothelium and increased plasma of plasminogen activator inhibitor type I (PAI-I) has been measured in uraemic patients. Uraemic toxins are likely to be responsible for fibrinolytic impairment because uraemic serum stimulated endothelial PAI-I production, which was corrected by haemodialysis. By contrast, activation of fibrinolysis, with an increase of plasmin–antiplasmin complexes and fibrinogen and fibrin degradation products has also been described (Sagripanti and Barsotti 1997).

Clinical manifestations

The most common haemorrhagic complications of uraemia are ecchymoses, purpura, epistaxis, and bleeding from venepuncture sites. Bleeding from the gastrointestinal tract, although less frequent, is an important cause of morbidity and mortality. It is associated with peptic ulcers and telangiectasia. Dialysis patients suffering from human immunodeficiency virus (HIV) nephropathy may have specific lesions such as Kaposi's sarcoma, cytomegalovirus colitis, or non-Hodgkin's lymphoma that contribute to gastrointestinal bleeding. Retroperitoneal bleeding may complicate percutaneous femoral catheterization. Subcapsular haematoma of the liver has also been described. Subdural haematoma may also occur, primarily due to the degree of hypertension in these patients (reviewed by Lohr and Schwab 1991).

Treatment

Dialysis and systemic anticoagulation

An effective haemodialysis regimen shortens the prolonged bleeding time of uraemic patients and partially corrects platelet and platelet–endothelial dysfunctions. However, it may not completely avert the risk of bleeding. The role of haemodialysis in the correction of the uraemic haemostatic abnormalities remains controversial: the continuous platelet activation induced by the interaction between blood and artificial surface, and the release of platelet-derived proteins, can induce platelet 'exhaustion' and favour bleeding.

The risk of haemorrhage may be further increased by systemic anticoagulation with unfractionated heparin, used to inhibit clotting in the extracorporeal circuit. Regional and low-dose heparinization, use of prostacyclin, high-flow-rate haemodialysis without anticoagulation, and regional citrate anticoagulation have been shown to reduce bleeding complications (Lohr and Schwab 1991). Each of these methods, however, has its own technical difficulties, limitations, and complications (Ouseph and Ward 2000).

Antiplatelet agents, aspirin and dipyridamole analogues, and prostaglandin E_1 have also been used, but without obtaining any real advantage over heparin.

The infusion of dermatan sulfate has also been proposed as an anticoagulant agent during haemodialysis (Ryan et al. 1992), because it caused less bleeding than heparin in animal models. This was likely due to its reduced effect on platelet function. Dermatan sulfate also induced a moderate prolongation of activated partial thromboplastin time (APTT). A comparative short-term clinical study performed on 10 haemodialysed patients demonstrated that dermatan sulfate dose can be individually titrated to suppress clot formation during haemodialysis as efficiently as does individualized heparin (Boccardo et al. 1997).

Peritoneal dialysis, when applicable, avoids the risk of bleeding associated with heparin or anticoagulants. However, this procedure may cause platelet hyper-reactivity.

Recombinant human erythropoietin

The cloning of the human EPO gene and the production of recombinant human EPO have provided clinicians with a powerful tool to correct the anaemia associated to uraemia, allowing to eliminate red blood cell transfusion. Early studies showed that increasing doses of EPO, when given to haemodialysis patients with a history of bleeding,

severe anaemia (haematocrit < 23 per cent), and a long basal bleeding time (>19 min), induced a progressive increase in haematocrit accompanied by significant shortening of the bleeding time (Moia et al. 1987). No consistent changes were found in platelet number, platelet aggregation, or platelet thromboxane A_2 formation (Moia et al. 1987; Zwaginga et al. 1991). A randomized study established that in uraemic patients on EPO a threshold haematocrit between 27 and 32 per cent effectively normalized bleeding time (Viganò et al. 1991).

Although the efficacy of EPO is indisputable, the question of the target haematocrit or haemoglobin to be achieved remains unresolved. Current evidence-based recommendations suggest a target haematocrit range of 33–36 per cent. Whether patients may benefit from haematocrit greater than 36 per cent, and closer to the normal range of healthy persons, is a matter of controversy. Small studies suggest that normalization of haematocrit with EPO may benefit haemodialysis patients in terms of brain function, physical performance, quality of life, and prevention of progressive left ventricular dilatation (Murphy and Parfrey 1999). However, a randomized controlled clinical trial (the USA Normal Hematocrit Cardiac Study) of the effects of normal as compared with low haematocrit values in haemodialysis patients with symptomatic cardiac disease receiving EPO was terminated early because of an increase in both mortality and the rate of vascular access thrombosis in the group allocated to normalization of haematocrit (Besarab et al. 1998). Therefore, in patients with clinically evident congestive heart failure or ischaemic heart disease, administration of EPO to raise their haematocrit to 42 per cent is currently not recommended.

Cryoprecipitate and desmopressin

Cryoprecipitate is a plasma product enriched in vWF, fibrinogen, and fibronectin. The observation that cryoprecipitate shortened the bleeding time of patients with platelet storage-pool disease prompted Janson et al. (1980) to use it in uraemic patients with a bleeding time of greater than 15 min. This time was significantly shortened in all the patients as early as 1 h after the infusion, the effect being maximal between 4 and 12 h. However, because this therapy carries the risk of transmitting blood-borne diseases it was largely replaced by other approaches.

The possibility that the beneficial effect of cryoprecipitate may be related to the increase in vWF-related properties suggested that desmopressin—(1-deamino-8-D-arginine vasopressin, DDAVP), a synthetic derivative of the antidiuretic hormone that induces release of autologous vWF from storage sites—might be effective. In two randomized double-blind crossover trials (Mannucci et al. 1983; Viganò et al. 1989), DDAVP was effective in shortening the bleeding time of uraemic patients at a dose of 0.3 μg/kg given intravenously or subcutaneously. Peak responses were achieved after a 30–90 min delay when the subcutaneous route was employed. The shortening of the bleeding time lasted 6–8 h. DDAVP was also effective and well tolerated when administered intranasally. DDAVP loses its efficacy when administered repeatedly, probably due to a progressive depletion of vWF stores in endothelial cells. Although remarkably free of serious side-effects, DDAVP is reported to cause a mild to moderate decrease in platelet count, facial flushing, mild transient headache, nausea, abdominal cramps, mild tachycardia, water retention, and hyponatraemia. Rarely, thrombotic events followed DDAVP administration, particularly in patients with underlying advanced cardiovascular disease. The use of DDAVP was suggested for treating acute bleeding in uraemia and preventing abnormal bleeding in connection with surgery or invasive procedures (Mannucci 1997).

Conjugated oestrogens

Patients with gastrointestinal or intracranial bleeding, or those undergoing major surgery, require a lasting haemostatic effect. These patients may benefit from the use of conjugated oestrogens, first proposed for treatment of uraemic bleeding (Liu *et al.* 1984), because of the observation that abnormal bleeding in women with von Willebrand's disease improved during pregnancy, when blood oestrogens increase. A double-blind crossover trial (Livio *et al.* 1986) showed that infusions of conjugated oestrogen, in a cumulative dose of 3 mg/kg divided over five consecutive days, shortened bleeding time in uraemic patients. The effect manifested only after several hours but lasted 14 days. A subsequent dose–response study (Viganò *et al.* 1988) showed that the minimum dose of oestrogens that could reduce the bleeding time was 0.6 mg/kg, and that four or five infusions 24 h apart were needed to obtain at least a 50 per cent decrease in bleeding time. Recently, low-dose transdermal oestrogen (oestradiol 50–100 mg/24 h) applied as a patch twice weekly was found to reduce recurrent gastrointestinal bleeding with parallel improvement in bleeding time and no side-effects (Sloand and Schiff 1995).

Thrombotic complications

Paradoxically, haemodialysis may expose uraemic patients to the thrombotic complications of arteriovenous shunts (Joist *et al.* 1994; Sagripanti and Barsotti 1997). The thrombotic occlusion of vascular access accounts for a substantial percentage of hospital admissions in chronic haemodialysis patients and represents an ongoing contributor to their morbidity and mortality.

Because platelet aggregation plays a major role in thrombus formation, antiplatelet agents have been used with encouraging results. Aspirin, dipyridamole, ticlopidine, or sulfinpyrazone have proved useful in several studies. Fibrinolytic agents, such as streptokinase or urokinase, as well as recombinant tissue plasminogen activator have produced contrasting results.

The vast majority of uraemic patients has several risk factors for developing atherosclerotic cardiovascular disease, either pre-existing or caused by chronic renal failure, namely dyslipoproteinaemia, hypertension, glucose intolerance, and hyperparathyroidism.

References

Aiello, S. *et al.* (1997). Renal and systemic nitric oxide synthesis in rats with renal mass reduction. *Kidney International* **52**, 171–181.

Benigni, A. *et al.* (1993). Reversible activation defect of the platelet glycoprotein IIb–IIIa complex in patients with uremia. *American Journal of Kidney Diseases* **22**, 668–676.

Besarab, A. *et al.* (1998). The effects of normal as compared with low hematocrit values in patients with cardiac disease who are receiving hemodialysis and Epotin. *New England Journal of Medicine* **339**, 584–590.

Boccardo, P. *et al.* (1997). Individualized anticoagulation with dermatan sulphate for hemodialysis in chronic renal failure. *Nephrology, Dialysis, Transplantation* **12**, 2349–2354.

Defreyn, G. *et al.* (1980). A plasma factor in uraemia which stimulates prostacyclin release from cultured endothelial cells. *Thrombosis Research* **19**, 695–699.

Gawaz, M. P. and Mujais, S. K. (1995). Platelet membrane glycoprotein abnormalities in uremia. *Journal of Nephrology* **8**, 12–19.

Horl, W. H. (2002). Hemodialysis membranes: interleukins, biocompatibility, and middle molecules. *Journal of the American Society of Nephrology* **13**, S62–S71.

Janson, P. A. *et al.* (1980). Treatment of the bleeding tendency in uremia with cryoprecipitate. *New England Journal of Medicine* **303**, 1318–1322.

Joist, J. H., Remuzzi, G., and Mannucci, P. M. Abnormal bleeding and thrombosis in renal disease. In *Hemostasis and Thrombosis. Basic Principles and Clinical Practice* (ed. R. W. Colman, J. Hirsh, V. J. Marder, and E. W. Salzman), pp. 921–935. Philadelphia: J.B. Lippincott Company, 1994.

Liu, Y., Kosfeld, R., and Marcum, S. (1984). Treatment of uraemic bleeding with conjugated oestrogen. *Lancet* **ii**, 887–890.

Livio, M. *et al.* (1982). Uraemic bleeding: role of anaemia and beneficial effect of red cell transfusion. *Lancet* **ii**, 1013–1015.

Livio, M. *et al.* (1986). Conjugated estrogens for the management of bleeding associated with renal failure. *New England Journal of Medicine* **315**, 731–735.

Lohr, J. W. and Schwab, S. J. (1991). Minimizing hemorrhagic complications in dialysis patients. *Journal of the American Society of Nephrology* **2**, 961–975.

Macconi, D. *et al.* (1992). Defective platelet aggregation in response to platelet-activating factor in uremia associated with low platelet thromboxane A2 generation. *American Journal of Kidney Diseases* **19**, 318–325.

Mannucci, P. M. (1997). Desmopressin (DDAVP) in the treatment of bleeding disorders: the first 20 years. *The Journal of the American Society of Hematology* **90**, 2516–2521.

Mannucci, P. M. *et al.* (1983). Deamino-8-D-arginine vasopressin shortens the bleeding time in uremia. *New England Journal of Medicine* **308**, 8–12.

Mattix, H. and Singh, A. K. (1999). Is the bleeding time predictive of bleeding prior to a percutaneous renal biopsy. *Current Opinion in Nephrology and Hypertension* **8**, 715–718.

Mezzano, D. *et al.* (1996). Hemostatic disorders of uremia: the platelet defect, main determinant of the prolonged bleeding time, is correlated with indices of activation of coagulation and fibrinolysis. *Thrombosis Haemostasis* **76**, 312–321.

Moia, M. *et al.* (1987). Improvement in the haemostatic defect of uraemia after treatment with recombinant human erythropoietin. *Lancet* **i**, 1227–1229.

Murphy, S. T. and Parfrey, P. S. (1999). Erythropoietin therapy in chronic uremia: the impact of normalization of hematocrit. *Current Opinion in Nephrology and Hypertension* **8**, 573–578.

Noris, M. and Remuzzi, G. (1999). Uremic bleeding: closing the circle after 30 years of controversies? *Blood* **94**, 2569–2574.

Noris, M. *et al.* (1993). Enhanced nitric oxide synthesis in uremia: implications for platelet dysfunction and dialysis hypotension. *Kidney International* **44**, 445–450.

Noris, M. *et al.* (1998). Effect of acetate, bicarbonate dialysis and acetate-free biofiltration on nitric oxide synthesis: implications for dialysis hypotension. *American Journal of Kidney Diseases* **32**, 115–124.

Noris, M. *et al.* (2000). 17β-Estradiol corrects hemostasis in uremic rats by limiting vascular expression of nitric oxide synthases. *American Journal of Physiology. Renal Physiology* **279**, F626–F635.

Ouseph, R. and Ward, R. A. (2000). Anticoagulation for intermittent hemodialysis. *Seminars in Dialysis* **13**, 181–187.

Remuzzi, G. (1988). Bleeding in renal failure. *Lancet* **i**, 1205–1208.

Remuzzi, G. *et al.* Prostaglandins, plasma factors and haemostasis in uraemia. In *Hemostasis, Prostaglandins and Renal Disease* (ed. G. Remuzzi, G. Mecca, and G. De Gaetano), pp. 273–281. New York: Raven Press, 1980.

Ryan, K. E. *et al.* (1992). Antithrombotic properties of dermatan sulphate (MF 701) in haemodialysis for chronic renal failure. *Thrombosis and Haemostasis* **68**, 563–569.

Saglikes, Y. *et al.* (1985). Effect of PTH on blood pressure and response to vasoconstrictor agonists. *American Journal of Physiology* **248**, F674–F681.

Sagripanti, A. and Barsotti, G. (1997). Bleeding and thrombosis in chronic uremia. *Nephron* **75**, 125–139.

Sloand, J. A. and Schiff, M. J. (1995). Beneficial effect of low-dose transdermal estrogen on bleeding time and clinical bleeding in uremia. *American Journal of Kidney Diseases* **26**, 22–26.

Sreedhara, R., Itagaki, I., and Hachim, R. M. (1996). Uremic patients have decreased shear-induced platelet aggregation mediated by decreased availability of glycoprotein IIb–IIIa receptors. *American Journal of Kidney Diseases* **27**, 355–364.

Viganò, G. *et al.* (1988). Dose–effect and pharmacokinetics of estrogens given to correct bleeding time in uremia. *Kidney International* **34**, 853–858.

Viganò, G. *et al.* (1989). Subcutaneous desmopressin (DDAVP) shortens the bleeding time in uremia. *American Journal of Hematology* **31**, 32–35.

Viganò, G. *et al.* (1991). Recombinant human erythropoietin to correct uremic bleeding time. *American Journal of Kidney Diseases* **18**, 44–49.

Weigert, A. L. and Schafer, A. I. (1998). Uremic bleeding; pathogenesis and therapy. *American Journal of Medical Science* **316**, 94–104.

Zoja, C. *et al.* (1988). Prolonged bleeding time and increased vascular prostacyclin in rats with chronic renal failure: effects of conjugated estrogens. *Journal of Laboratory Clinical Medicine* **112**, 380–386.

Zwaginga, J. J. *et al.* (1991). Treatment of uraemic anemia with recombinant erythropoietin also reduces the defects in platelet adhesion and aggregation caused by uraemic plasma. *Thrombosis and Haemostasis* **66**, 638.

11.3.13 Dermatological disorders

Claudio Ponticelli, Angelo Valerio Marzano, and Ruggero Caputo

Skin problems are commonly seen in patients with renal failure. In the past, the most frequent findings were uraemic frost and 'erythema papulatum uremicum'. Uraemic roseola and uraemic erysipeloid were also seen in patients with advanced renal failure. More recently, with the advent of dialysis, these manifestations have become rare, but several other abnormalities of the skin and the appendages have emerged, their frequency increasing with the period of maintenance dialysis.

Cutaneous disorders

Abnormal pigmentation

Although alterations in the cutaneous pigmentation can be seen early in renal insufficiency, prevalence is greater in patients with longer duration of dialysis (Avermaete *et al.* 2001). Macular hyperpigmentation of the palms and soles, and brown diffuse hyperpigmentation, more evident in the areas exposed to sunlight, are seen in many dialysis patients (Pico *et al.* 1992).

Rare cases of diffuse bluish-grey discolouration of the skin and nails, referred to as 'argyria', have also been observed in patients on long-term haemodialysis (Sue *et al.* 2001). Acquired hair and skin fairness, a result perhaps of a disturbance of phenylalanine metabolism, may occasionally be found in dialysis patients (Ben Huida *et al.* 1996). A sudden deepening of pigmentation during haemodialysis can develop in patients with severe haemolysis (Seukeran *et al.* 1997).

Abnormal keratinization

Cutaneous dryness (xerosis) is the most frequent cutaneous abnormality in uraemic patients. It generally develops before the start of dialysis treatment and seems to be little influenced by it. The incidence is similar in patients whether treated with haemodialysis or peritoneal dialysis (Bencini *et al.* 1985).

When xerosis is associated with desquamation, it can cause an ichthyosis-like appearance with a picture of dry skin and fish-like scales mostly on the limbs and over the trunk (Fig. 1). The extensor surfaces of legs and arms are most severely affected, with large dark scales. The flexor surfaces, the axillae, and the antecubital and popliteal fossae are relatively spared. Over the abdomen, the scales are whitish to translucent and somewhat smaller and finer. The margins of the scale tend to turn up, which accounts for the rough feeling of the surface. The scalp is frequently involved, with pityriasic and, occasionally, lamellar desquamation.

Patients with dry skin may also show signs of abnormal keratinization or excessive production of keratin, such as follicular keratosis, onychodystrophy, and plantar hyperkeratosis, which is also an early and frequent finding in patients with diabetes mellitus. Sometimes, variable degrees of hyperkeratosis occur even without concomitant xerosis.

The pathogenesis of these abnormalities is still poorly understood. Uraemic xerosis may be caused, at least in part, by an impairment of the function of exocrine sweat glands (Park *et al.* 1995), but other mechanisms are also postulated. Since the hydration of the stratum corneum influences the appearance of the skin, lack of water might be one of the causes of xerosis. The water content of the stratum corneum has been reported to be reduced in dialysis patients (Kato *et al.* 2000). However, others found that the transepidermal water loss was normal in dialysis patients (Ostlere *et al.* 1994). Either hyper- or hypovitaminosis A may cause xerosis and skin desquamation. The plasma and skin content of vitamin A and its carrier, retinol-binding protein, are increased in uraemic patients (Vahlquist *et al.* 1985). These data suggested that xerosis and ichthyosiform dermatosis are due to a state of hypervitaminosis A, specific to uraemia. However, Stein *et al.* (1986) reported that, despite raised serum concentrations, the vitamin A stores are not increased in uraemia. Electron transmission microscopy studies of the skin of uraemic patients with xerosis revealed an

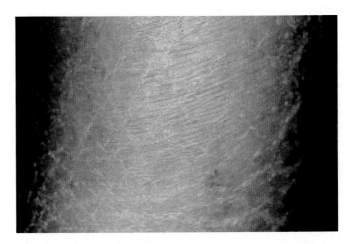

Fig. 1 Xerosis with ichthyosis-like appearance.

increased number of corneal cell layers with desmosomal junctions present up to the skin surface, and an increased number of keratinosomes (Bencini *et al.* 1994). Morphological abnormalities of keratinosomes, which are essential for desquamation, have also been described in other forms of inherited keratinization disorders, such as lamellar congenital ichthyosis, as a consequence of a disturbance in the metabolism of epidermal lipids. Similar pathogenetic mechanisms might also operate in uraemic patients. Alternatively, a disorder in vitamin D metabolism might account for these cutaneous disorders. In fact, keratinocytes contain receptors for $1,25(OH)_2$-vitamin D which induces terminal differentiation and inhibits proliferation of keratinocytes in culture. Elevated parathyroid hormone values with relatively low concentrations of $1,25(OH)_2$-vitamin D were found in non-uraemic patients with various disorders of keratinization, some of whom showed secondary hyperparathyroidism similar to uraemic patients (Milstone *et al.* 1992). Since elevated plasma parathyroid hormone and reduced $1,25(OH)_2$-vitamin D are common in patients with chronic renal failure, a role of these metabolic disorders in uraemic xerosis is not excluded.

There is no specific treatment for xerosis and ichthyosiform dermatosis. Emollients are of mild benefit for initial xerosis but are ineffective for more severe forms.

Pruritus

Chronic renal failure is probably the most common cause of persistent and long-lasting pruritus in clinical medicine. The frequency of pruritus tends to increase with the increasing severity of renal failure (Murphy and Carmichael 2000). Although pruritus sometimes improves with dialysis, in many instances it persists or even develops after it has been started (Balaskas *et al.* 1993). About 60–90 per cent of dialysis patients suffer from some degree of itching. No difference is found between haemodialysis and peritoneal dialysis (Ponticelli and Bencini 1992; Balaskas *et al.* 1993). Pruritus may be mild or severe, transient or continuous, generalized or localized. The axillae, scalp, nose, and ears are the most frequent areas of pruritus; however, it can frequently change its location. Pruritus often worsens at bedtime. For about 25 per cent of patients with pruritus, it occurs only during or soon after dialysis and it is most severe at these times for an additional 42 per cent of patients (Gilchrest *et al.* 1982). For some patients, pruritus can be severe enough to cause depression and even thoughts of suicide.

There is a degree of inverse correlation between the severity of itching and the efficacy of dialysis (Masi and Cohen 1992). Moreover, patients with pruritus have higher predialysis values of blood urea nitrogen and β_2-microglobulin and lower K_t/V_{urea} than patients without pruritus (Hiroshige *et al.* 1995). These data suggest that dialysis itching is related to the efficacy of dialysis.

The skin may appear normal or mildly xerotic. However, in some patients itching and scratching may lead to cutaneous lesions such as 'prurigo nodularis' or keratotic papules in generalized pruritus and lichen simplex in localized pruritus. Prurigo nodularis is characterized by typical multiple brown nodules often covered by scales, crusts, and abrasions. It is caused by inflammation secondary to continuous scratching and may be accompanied by infection and bleeding. Keratotic papules are red or violaceous with a typical central plug. They range in size from 3 to 12 mm and usually occur on the extensor surfaces of limbs, although they can also develop in other sites with the exception of the palms and

soles (Fig. 2). Histopathological findings show epidermal hyperplasia of the contiguous skin with areas of parakeratosis in laminated or columnar array, keratin, and basophilic debris. Perforation of the epithelium can occur with spillage of material into the dermis. Keratotic papules have been classified as a perforating folliculitis (Hurwitz 1985), as a variety of Kyrle's disease (Hood *et al.* 1982), or as uraemic follicular hyperkeratosis (Garcia-Bravo *et al.* 1985). In lichen simplex, there is hyperplasia of all components of the epidermis with hyperkeratosis and acanthosis. The dermis contains a chronic inflammatory infiltrate, forming a plaque-like structure. The skin appears thickened, hyperpigmented, and hyperkeratotic. Skin markings are accentuated.

The pathophysiology of pruritus in uraemia is still incompletely explained. The major difficulty is the fact that pruritus is a subjective sensation and is strongly influenced by the psychological status of the subject. A number of studies of uraemic patients have excluded any pathogenetic role of xerosis (Ostlere *et al.* 1994; Park *et al.* 1995; Kato *et al.* 2000) but some investigators found a strong association between the intensity of xerosis and pruritus (Szepietowski et al. 2004). Blood serotonin is increased in uraemic patients but does not correlate with pruritus (Kerr *et al.* 1992). It is possible that secondary hyperparathyroidism, abnormal mast cell proliferation, increased plasma histamine, and non-specific enolase-positive sensory nerve endings in the skin are implicated in the pathogenesis of itching (Murphy and Carmichael 2000).

Secondary hyperparathyroidism is frequently accompanied by intractable pruritus and parathyroidectomy is often, although not always, followed by dramatic relief of itching within a few hours Moreover, hyperparathyroidism can cause hypercalcaemia and skin calcifications and can stimulate skin mast cells with consequent release of histamine (Dimkovic *et al.* 1992). All these factors may contribute to pruritus. These observations assign an important role to parathyroid hormone in the genesis of uraemic pruritus. However, not all patients with secondary hyperparathyroidism of sufficient severity to warrant surgery have pruritus. Moreover, a correlation between the intensity of uraemic pruritus and parathyroid hormone concentrations has been ruled out (Cho *et al.* 1997). Finally, pruritus can recur after parathyroidectomy if patients have a high product calcium × phosphorus (Chou *et al.* 2000). Thus, it is unlikely that the elevated parathyroid hormone itself is a cause of pruritus. As the concentrations of calcium,

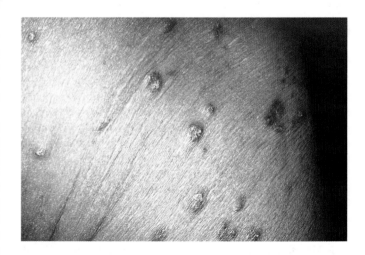

Fig. 2 Keratotic papules.

magnesium, and phosphorus in skin from patients with uraemic pruritus are greater than those in skin from either non-pruritic dialysis patients or healthy volunteers (Blachley *et al.* 1985), microprecipitation of divalent ions in the skin might be one of the causes of uraemic pruritus. Alternatively, pruritus may be due to an increase in dermal mast cells and increased plasma histamine. However, no relationship was found between plasma histamine, the number of skin mast cells, and the extent of pruritus in uraemic patients (Mettang *et al.* 1990). Finally, Stähle-Backdahl (1988) used indirect immunochemistry to evaluate neuron-specific enolase immunoreactive nerve fibres and terminals after skin biopsy. Sprouting of fibres through the epidermal layers was found in uraemic patients but not in controls. These data were not confirmed by Fantini *et al.* (1992) who found no difference between uraemic and normal subjects with respect to the distribution pattern of the enolase-positive nerve fibres. However, these investigators reported a reduction in the total number of skin nerve terminals in uraemic patients, possibly as a consequence of neuropathy. Actually, a relationship was found between pruritus and somatic neuropathy in uraemic patients (Zakrzewska-Pniewska and Jedras 2001). Finally, a possible role for 'substance P', a neurotransmitter widely distributed in the afferent sensory neurons, has been suggested (Cho *et al.* 1997). In summary, it is difficult to identify a single cause for uraemic pruritus. It is probable that in most patients it is caused by a combination of the factors described above and possibly by a circulating pruritogenic substance, the existence of which has been postulated but not yet demonstrated.

Before any therapeutic measures are initiated, it is necessary to perform a careful examination of the skin of a patient with pruritus to exclude other clinical causes. For example, scabies, which can mimic uraemic pruritus, is a potential complication in dialysis patients and can be easily treated. Since itching may also be a sign of inadequate dialysis, every effort should be made in order to ensure that efficient dialysis is being performed (Hiroshige *et al.* 1995; Ponticelli and Bencini 1995). When pruritus is associated with hypercalcaemia and hyperparathyroidism, it responds dramatically to parathyroidectomy. The relief from pruritus generally parallels the rapid decline in serum calcium concentration, suggesting a reduction of skin calcium concentration.

Several measures have been tried for patients without these problems. In a randomized trial, nicergoline 30 mg orally four times daily plus 5 mg intravenously at dialysis for 2 weeks, significantly improved the pruritus score (Bousquet *et al.* 1989). Prolonged phototherapy with ultraviolet B with total body exposure three times weekly can relieve pruritus in most patients (Twicrons *et al.* 2003). By a meta-analysis of the controlled trials published between 1966 and 1991 Tan *et al.* (1991) concluded that ultraviolet B phototherapy is the treatment of choice for moderate to severe uraemic pruritus. The mechanisms for the effect of ultraviolet B are unknown. It may inactivate a putative circulating pruritogenic substance; it may form a photoproduct which relieves pruritus (Fjellner 1981); it may alter the skin content of divalent ions (Blachley *et al.* 1985), or it may induce mast cell apoptosis (Szepietowski *et al.* 2002). In some patients, encouraging results have also been reported with electrical needle stimulation, a modified acupuncture technique (Duo 1987); with topical capsaicin 0.025 per cent, an irritant cream which depletes substance P in peripheral sensory neurons (Cho *et al.* 1997), and with the mast cell stabilizer ketotifen (1–2 mg twice daily) (Francos *et al.* 1991). It has been claimed that erythropoietin therapy relieves pruritus through a reduction of plasma histamine concentration (De Marchi *et al.* 1992), but these results were not confirmed in other studies (Balaskas and Uldall 1993). Naltrexone, an opioid

antagonist, was found to be effective in a controlled study of 1 week (Peer *et al.* 1996), but no benefit was reported by another randomized trial, in which the drug was administered for 4 weeks (Pauli-Magnus *et al.* 2000). Oral supplementation of primrose oil, 2 g per day, significantly improved the symptoms of pruritus in a randomized trial (Yoshimoto-Furuie *et al.* 1999).

Arteriovenous fistula dermopathies

About 8 per cent of patients on chronic haemodialysis suffer from arteriovenous fistula dermatitis (Goh and Phay 1988). This is characterized by irritant contact dermatitis from soaps, disinfectants, and alcohol used for skin cleansing during haemodialysis. This dermatitis is more common in patients with pruritus. About 50 per cent of patients may respond to treatment with mild topical steroids and substitution of normal saline for skin cleansing before haemodialysis. Dermopathy associated with venous hypertension of the hand caused by the fistula is much rarer. It is characterized by swelling, induration, hyperpigmentation, and even ulcer formation restricted to the thumb and index finger. This disorder may be related to pericapillary cuffs of fibrin due to venous hypertension (Brakman *et al.* 1994).

Pseudo-Kaposi's sarcoma

Pseudo-Kaposi's sarcoma is a term used to describe benign lesions clinically and histologically similar to those of Kaposi's sarcoma which occur in the vicinity of the arteriovenous fistula (Hwang *et al.* 1999). Clinical lesions consist of purplish nodules or papules, slowly evolving into scaly crusted violaceous patches. Histological features include vascular and fibroblast proliferation in the superficial dermis vascular slits, mitotic figures, and extravasated red blood cells. The lesions may improve if the shunt or arteriovenous fistula is tied off.

Pseudoporphyria cutanea

Pseudoporphyria cutanea tarda, a bullous disorder clinically and histopathologically indistinguishable from porphyria, was described by Gilchrest *et al.* (1975) who called it 'bullous dermatosis of haemodialysis'. In the same year, Korting (1975) also observed several uraemic patients with skin changes mimicking porphyria cutanea tarda and coined the term 'pseudoporphyria'. Whether bullous dermatosis and pseudoporphyria are two separate entities or reflect the same disorder is still controversial. The disorder usually occurs in patients on maintenance haemodialysis but may also develop in patients on peritoneal dialysis (Kelly and O'Rourke 2001). Lesions develop more frequently during the summer and are located in areas exposed to the sun, generally on the back of fingers and hands, and less frequently on the face and neck (Fig. 3). Some cases are very mild and can be detected only by careful examination. Lesions include vesiculae and/or bullae which may resolve in several weeks, leaving erosions with haemorrhagic crusts and atrophic scarring. Fragility of the skin is constant. Pseudomiliary cysts and mild hirsutism may also be observed.

Plasma porphyrins, which were reported to be normal in the first descriptions of uraemic pseudoporphyria, have now been found to be raised in several patients (Glynne *et al.* 1999). Since porphyrins circulate in high molecular weight protein-bound complexes, they are not removed by either haemodialysis or haemofiltration. The deficiency of uroporphyrinogen decarboxylase in uraemic patients (Mamet *et al.* 1995) coupled with the impaired renal and dialysis clearance of

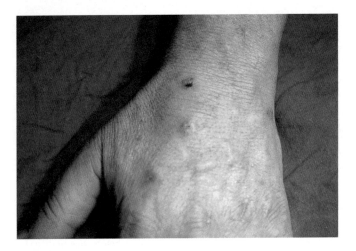

Fig. 3 Pseudoporphyria cutanea tarda.

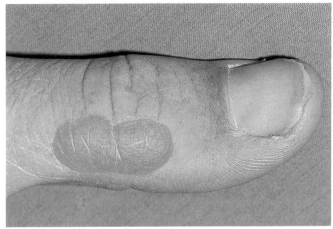

Fig. 4 Bullous lesion on the left thumb of a patient on haemodialysis.

porphyrins can lead to an accumulation of uroporphyrins, with increased passage into the tissues and an increase in photodynamic activity. Oxygen free radicals may be important pathogenetic mediators in dialysis-associated pseudoporphyria (Green and Manders 2001). The possibility that dialysis patients may suffer from a genuine hereditary porphyria cutanea tarda should also be kept in mind. In these cases, a course of intravenous iron (McKane *et al.* 2001) or hepatitis C reactivation after treatment with interferon alpha (Albalate *et al.* 2001) may precipitate the development of the disease.

Because uraemic pseudoporphyria is usually triggered or aggravated by exposure to sun, a trial of avoidance of such exposure is the first step. Protection from the sun can reduce the blister formation, but it may be months before any improvement appears. Plasma exchanges and chloroquine are of little, if any, benefit in uraemic pseudoporphyria. Phlebotomy has considerably improved the prognosis of idiopathic porphyria cutanea tarda. Its mechanism of action is related to reduction of iron stores in the body. Ferrous ions *in vitro* inhibit uroporphyrinogen decarboxylase activity, with possible enhanced production of uroporphyrin I (Sampietro *et al.* 1999). For dialysis patients without severe anaemia and with increased iron stores, small repeated phlebotomies may produce marked biochemical improvement and complete clinical remission (Glynne *et al.* 1999). In milder cases, low-dose erythropoietin can induce stable remission of pseudoporphyria cutanea tarda (Sarkell and Patterson 1993; Peces *et al.* 1994). In fact, the drug causes removal of large quantities of iron from stores owing to the enhanced production of red blood cells. In more severe, cases erythropoietin treatment allows the use of small phlebotomies (120–180 ml) with further reduction of ferritin and porphyrin levels. Good results with the antioxidant *N*-acetylcysteine have also been reported (Vadoud-Seyedi *et al.* 2000). Pseudoporphyria may spontaneously remit after renal transplantation which normalizes blood porphyrin concentrations (Stevens *et al.* 1993).

Drug-induced bullous dermatosis

This disorder is caused by exposure to photosensitizing drugs. It is clinically and histologically indistinguishable from both porphyria cutanea tarda and haemodialysis-related pseudoporphyria (Breier *et al.* 1998). A number of drugs can cause bullous dermatosis, including high-dose frusemide, tetracycline, piroxicam, vancomycin, ciprofloxacin, atorvastatin, and naproxen. The diagnosis is based on a positive history of

photosensitive drug ingestion. Resolution of bullous dermatosis usually occurs after the causative agent is discontinued, but in some cases photosensitivity may persist for several months after the drug is stopped (Fig. 4).

Cutaneous and subcutaneous calcifications

Soft tissue calcification is common in dialysis patients with a chronically raised calcium × phosphorus product in the blood. Deposits of calcium may occur between dermal collagen fibres or within epidermal appendages. They may appear as plaques or as intensely pruritic whitish papules. The papular lesions may occur in a linear pattern in skin previously excoriated due to pruritus. Exceptional cases of metastatic soft calcifications presenting as large tongue masses (Walker *et al.* 1993) or perforating papules (Enelow *et al.* 1998) have also been reported. Calcific arteriopathy may result in painful livedo reticularis, followed by progressive digital gangrene. Panniculitis of the legs may occur, with tenderness, induration, and necrosis of the overlying skin. Soft tissue calcification is closely related to hyperphosphataemia and secondary hyperparathyroidism. Control of these may prevent and sometimes even resolve cutaneous papules and arterial calcification.

Precancerous and cancerous lesions

Basal cell carcinoma is the most frequent skin cancer in uraemia, as it is in the general population. This tumour, which is painless and is not preceded by precancerous changes, appears as a non-inflamed smooth translucent or pearly nodule which can show numerous telangiectasia vessels near its surface and can have brown pigmentation. Nodules often ulcerate and form a crust. A variant presenting as a finely scaling, erythematosus patch is less common (Fig. 5). The tumour may rarely invade nearby structures such as bone, nerves, or brain, but it rarely, if ever, metastasizes.

Multiple actinic keratoses, which are more frequent in uraemic patients than in general population (Tercedor *et al.* 1995) may occur in skin exposed to sun and appear as scaly rough red plaques. These lesions may progress to squamous cell carcinoma, which is a painless red nodule or plaque with scales on its surface. Ulceration and crusting may occur, and the tumour sometimes metastasizes. Porokeratosis, a precancerous lesion characterized by crater-shaped keratosis, may develop on

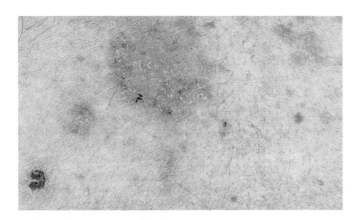

Fig. 5 Basal cell carcinomas on the back of a patient on peritoneal dialysis.

the access site for haemodialysis (Nakazawa *et al*. 1991). Rare cases of angiosarcoma occurring at the site of an arteriovenous fistula have been observed after renal transplantation (Bessis *et al*. 1998).

Vascular disorders

Microangiopathy

Severe microangiopathy has been detected in skin biopsies from 75 per cent of patients with chronic renal failure of various degrees (Gilchrest *et al*. 1980). The histological picture consists of endothelial cell activation and/or necrosis, basement membrane zone thickening, and reduplication of the basal lamina involving both venules and arterioles. The severity of the microangiopathy correlates with the duration of renal failure (Lundin *et al*. 1995). These lesions tend to regress after a successful renal transplantation.

Skin necrosis

Proximal skin necrosis and/or peripheral gangrene may occur in uraemic patients as a consequence of vascular disease, diabetes, or calciphylaxis. Proximal skin necrosis can involve the trunk, shoulders, buttocks, or thighs. The lesion usually spreads rapidly, covering large areas, and has an ominous prognosis (Fig. 6). Distal skin necrosis of the fingers and toes can lead to digital gangrene, but the disease is usually self-limiting. In patients with calciphylaxis the subcutaneous arteries and arterioles are narrowed or occluded by mural calcification, with or without intimal fibrosis. The pathogenesis involves abnormalities in calcium and phosphorus metabolism with acute deposition of calcium in the vessels of the subcutis and consequent skin necrosis. Many patients with calciphylaxis have elevated levels of serum parathyroid hormone (Llach and Velasquez Forero 2001).

Parathyroidectomy has been suggested for treatment of proximal skin necrosis even if the levels of parathyroid hormone are not very elevated (Garrigue *et al*. 2002). However, the results of parathyroidectomy are unpredictable. Frequent haemodialysis to normalize calcium and phosphorus levels and local debridement of skin lesions may be helpful in few cases (Kang *et al*. 2000). Hyperbaric oxygen may also improve the skin necrotic ulcers in some patients (Podimow *et al*. 2001).

Exceptional cases of skin necrosis induced by heparin and protein S deficiency have been reported (Denton *et al*. 2001).

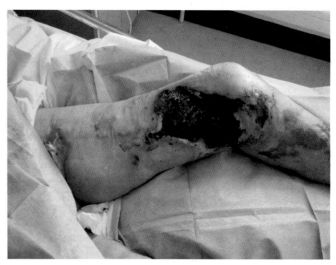

Fig. 6 Skin necrosis from calciphylaxis. Courtesy of Prof C. Winearls.

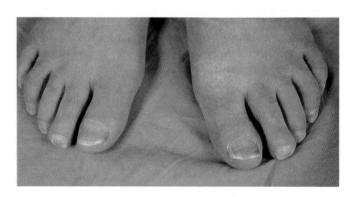

Fig. 7 Half-and-half nail.

Disorders of appendages

Nails

Several abnormalities of nail pigmentation can be seen in chronic renal failure. Double white transverse subungual bands, called Muercke's striae, and single transverse white strips, known as Mee's lines, have been reported in uraemic patients but have also been described in many other pathological conditions. Splinter haemorrhages have been observed in patients treated with either haemodialysis or peritoneal dialysis. Although non-specific, these haemorrhages are more common in dialysis patients than in the general population.

The so-called 'half-and-half nail' is typical of uraemia. The distal portion of each nail bed is red, pink, or brown, occupies 20–60 per cent of the total nail length, and always sharply demarcated; the proximal portion has a dull whitish ground-glass appearance (Lindsay 1967). When pressure is applied, the discoloration does not fade completely. This change can affect single nails, or all the nails of the hands, feet, or both (Fig. 7). Half-and-half nail often begins before dialysis. It occurs in 15–50 per cent of patients on regular dialysis (Kint *et al*. 1974; Lubach *et al*. 1982). The histology of the nail plate itself shows no change and it contains no melanin. The number of capillaries under the nail plate is increased, with remarkable thickening of the capillary walls. The increase in capillary density of the nail bed might account for the band of discoloration. The disorder is probably partially reversible. In some patients a lightening of the colour and a decrease in the width of the brown nail arc have been seen after months of observation (Kint et al. 1974).

Pincer nail deformity associated with pseudo-Kaposi's sarcoma may develop as a consequence of venous hypertension caused by arteriovenous fistula. There is over curvature of the nails, in which the lateral edge of the nail is pressed deeply into the lateral nail fold (Hwang et al. 1999).

Onychodystrophy

Some uraemic patients have nails similar to those of older subjects. The nail plate is thick, dull, and opaque, with a yellowish, whitish, or grey colour. Rarely, a severe onychodystrophy with spontaneous resolution may occur (Caputo et al. 1997).

Changes of pilosebaceous unit

About half of dialysis patients suffer from 'keratosis pilaris', an abnormal keratinization of the hair follicles which become raised giving a sensation of a grater. More rare is perforans folliculitis (Hurwitz 1985). Several hair changes have been observed in dialysis patients, including alopecia (Sarris et al. 2002), and hair discolouration. Electron microscopic studies showed that all dialysis patients investigated had some hair shaft abnormalities (irregular diameter, flattening, twisting) as well as a disordered disposition of the cuticular tiles (Bencini et al. 1992). The cause of these hair changes remains obscure. In a few patients, these abnormalities can result in hair break.

References

Albalate, M. et al. (2001). Development of porphyria cutanea tarda in a hemodialysis patient after reactivation of hepatitis C virus infection. Nephron 88, 170–173.

Avermaete, A., Altmeyer, P., and Bacharach-Buhles, M. (2001). Skin changes in dialysis patients: a review. Nephrology, Dialysis, Transplantation 16, 2293–2296.

Balaskas, E. V. and Uldall, R. P. (1993). Erythropoietin treatment does not improve uremic pruritus. Peritoneal Dialysis International 12, 330–331.

Balaskas, E. V., Chu, M., Uldall, R. P., Gupta, A., and Oreopulos, D. G. (1993). Pruritus in continuous ambulatory peritoneal dialysis and hemodialysis patients. Peritoneal Dialysis International 13, S527–S532.

Bencini, P. L., Brusasco, A., Graziani, G., Ponticelli, C., and Caputo, R. (1994). Acquired ichthyosis in uremic patients. European Journal of Dermatology 4, 310–312.

Bencini, P. L., Graziani, G., and Crosti, C. (1992). Hair shaft abnormalities in uremia, a SEM study. Preliminary report. European Journal of Dermatology 2, 119–121.

Bencini, P. L. et al. (1985). Cutaneous abnormalities in uremic patients. Nephron 40, 316–321.

Ben Huida, M. et al. (1996). Hypopigmentation in hemodialysis. Dermatology 192, 148–152.

Bessis, D. et al. (1998). Endothelin-secreting angiosarcoma occurring at the site of an arteriovenous fistula for haemodilaysis in a renal transplant recipient. British Journal of Dermatology 138, 361–363.

Blachley, J. D., Blankenship, M., Menter, A., Parker, T. F., III, and Knochel, J. P. (1985). Uremic pruritus: skin divalent ion content and response to ultra-violet phototherapy. American Journal of Kidney Diseases 5, 237–241.

Bousquet, J. et al. (1989). Double-blind, placebo-controlled study of nicergoline in the treatment of pruritus in patients receiving maintenance hemodialysis. Journal of Allergy and Clinical Immunology 83, 825–828.

Brakman, M., Faber, W. R., Zeegelaar, J. E., Bousema, M. T., van Proosdij, J. L., and Kerckhaert, J. A. M. (1994). Venous hypertension of the hand caused by hemodialysis shunt: immunofluorescence studies of pericapillary cuffs. Journal of the American Academy of Dermatology 31, 23–26.

Breier, F., Feldmann, R., Pelzl, M., and Gschnait, F. (1998). Pseudophorphyria cutanea tarda induced by furosemide in a patient undergoing peritoneal dialysis. Dermatology 197, 271–273.

Caputo, R., Gelmetti, C., and Cambiaghi, S. (1997). Severe self-healing nail distrophy in a patient on peritoneal dialysis. Dermatology 194, 274–275.

Cho, Y.-L., Liu, H.-N., Huang, T.-P., and Tarng, D.-C. (1997). Uremic pruritus: roles of parathyroid hormone and substance P. Journal of the American Academy of Dermatology 36, 538–543.

Chou, F. F., Ho, J. C., Huang, S. C., and Sheen-Chen, S. M. (2000). A study on pruritus after parathyroidectomy for secondary hyperparathyroidism. Journal of the American College of Surgeons 190, 65–70.

De Marchi, S., Cecchin, E., Villalta, D., Sepiacci, G., Santini, G., and Bartoli, E. (1992). Relief of pruritus and decreases in plasma histamine concentrations during erythropoietin therapy in patients with uremia. New England Journal of Medicine 326, 969–974.

Denton, M. D., Mauiyyedi, S., and Bazari, H. (2001). Heparin-induced skin necrosis in a patient with end-stage renal failure and functional protein S deficiency. American Journal of Nephrology 4, 289–293.

Dimkovic, N., Djukanovic, L., Radmilovic, A., Bojic, P., and Juloski, T. (1992). Uremic pruritus and skin mast cells. Nephron 61, 5–9.

Duo, L. J. (1987). Electrical needle therapy of uremic pruritus. Nephron 47, 179–183.

Enelow, T. J., Huang, W., and Williams, C. M. (1998). Perforating papules in chronic renalfailure. Archives of Dermatology 134, 98–99.

Fantini, F., Baraldi, A., Sevigliani, C., Spattini, A., Pincelli, C., and Giannetti, A. (1992). Cutaneous innervation in chronic renal failure patients. Acta Dermatoveneorologica (Stockholm) 72, 102–105.

Fjellner, B. (1981). Experimental and clinical pruritus. Acta Dermatovenereologica (Stockholm) 97 (Suppl.), 1–34.

Fjellner, B. and Hägermark, O. (1982). Influence of ultraviolet light on itch and flare reactions in human skin induced by histamine and histamine liberator compound 48/80. Acta Dermatovenereologica (Stockholm) 62, 137–140.

Francos, G. C. et al. (1991). Elevated plasma histamine in chronic uremia. Effects of ketotifen on pruritus. International Journal of Dermatology 30, 884–889.

Garcia-Bravo, R., Rodriguez-Pichardo, A., and Camacho, F. (1985). Uraemic follicular hyperkeratosis. Clinical and Experimental Dermatology 10, 448–454.

Garrigue, V. et al. (2002). Necrotic skin lesions in a dialysis patient: a multifactory entity. Clinical Nephrology 57, 163–166.

Gilchrest, B. A., Rowe, J. W., and Mihm, M. C., Jr. (1975). Bullous dermatosis of hemodialysis. Annals of Internal Medicine 83, 480–483.

Gilchrest, B. A., Rowe, J. W., and Mihm, M. L. (1980). Clinical and histological cutaneous findings in uremia: evidence for a dialysis-resistant transplant responsive microangiopathy. Lancet ii, 1271–1275.

Gilchrest, B. A. et al. (1982). Clinical features of pruritus among patients undergoing maintenance hemodialysis. Archives of Dermatology 118, 154–156.

Glynne, P. et al. (1999). Bullous dermatoses in end-stage renal failure: porphyria or pseudo porphyria. American Journal of Kidney Diseases 34, 155–160.

Goh, C. L. and Phay, K. L. (1988). Arterio-venous shunt dermatitis in chronic renal failure patients on maintenance haemodialysis. Clinical and Experimental Dermatology 13, 379–381.

Green, J. J. and Manders, S. M. (2001). Pseudophorphyria. Journal of the American Academy of Dermatology 44, 100–108.

Hiroshige, K., Kabashima, N., Takasugi, M., and Kuroiwa, A. (1995). Optimal dialysis improves uremic pruritus. American Journal of Kidney Diseases 25, 413–419.

Hood, A. F., Hardegen, G. L., Zarate, A. R., Nigra, T. P., and Gelfand, M. C. (1982). Kyrle's disease in patients with chronic renal failure. *Archives of Dermatology* 118, 85–88.

Hurwitz, R. M. (1985). The evolution of perforating folliculitis in patients with chronic renal failure. *American Journal of Dermatopathology* 7, 231–239.

Hwang, S. M., Lee, S. H., and Ahn, S. K. (1999). Pincer nail deformity and pseudo-Kaposi sarcoma: complications of an artificial arteriovenous fistula for haemodialysis. *British Journal of Dermatology* 141, 1129–1132.

Kang, A. S. *et al.* (2000). Is calciphylaxis best treated surgically or medically? *Surgery* 128, 967–971.

Kato, A. *et al.* (2000). Pruritus and hydration state of stratum corneum in hemodialysis patients. *American Journal of Nephrology* 20, 437–442.

Kelly, M. A. and O'Rourke, K. D. (2001). Treatment of porphyria cutanea tarda with phlebotomy in a patient on peritoneal dialysis. *Journal of the American Academy of Dermatology* 44, 336–338.

Kerr, G. P., Argiles, A., and Mion, C. (1992). Whole blood serotonin levels are markedly elevated in patients on dialytic therapy. *American Journal of Nephrology* 12, 14–18.

Kint, A., Bussels, L., Fernandes, M., and Ringoir, S. (1974). Skin and nail disorders in relation to chronic renal failure. *Acta Dermatovenereologica (Stockholm)* 54, 137–140.

Korting, G. W. (1975). Uber Porphyria-cutanea-tarda-artige hautveranderungen bei Langzeithalodialysepatienten. *Dermatologica* 150, 58–61.

Lindsay, P. G. (1967). The half-and-half nail. *Archives of Internal Medicine* 119, 583–587.

Llach, F. and Velasquez Forero, F. (2001). Secondary hyperparathyroidism in chronic renal failure: pathogenic and clinical aspects. *American Journal of Kidney Diseases* 38 (Suppl. 5), S20–S33.

Lubach, D., Strubbe, J., and Schmidt, J. (1982). The 'half and half nail' phenomenon in chronic hemodialysis patients. *Dermatologica* 164, 350–353.

Lundin, A. P., Fani, K., Berlyne, G. M., and Friedman, E. A. (1995). Dermal angiopathy in hemodialysis patients: the effect of time. *Kidney International* 47, 1775–1780.

Mamet, R. *et al.* (1995). Decreased uroporphyrinogen decarboxylase activity in patients with end-stage renal disease undergoing hemodialysis. *Nephron* 70, 202–206.

Masi, C. M. and Cohen, E. P. (1992). Dialysis efficacy and itching in renal failure. *Nephron* 62, 257–261.

McKane, W., Green, C. A., and Farrington, K. (2001). Porphyria cutanea tarda precipitated by intravenous iron in a haemodialysis patient. *Nephrology, Dialysis, Transplantation* 16, 1936–1938.

Mettang, T., Fritz, P., Weber, J., Machleidt, C., Hubel, E., and Kuhlmann, U. (1990). Uremic pruritus in patients on hemodialysis or continuous ambulatory peritoneal dialysis (CAPD): the role of plasma histamine and skin mast cells. *Clinical Nephrology* 34, 136–141.

Milstone, M. L., Ellison, A. F., and Insogna, K. L. (1992). Serum parathyroid hormone level is elevated in some patients with disorders of keratinization. *Archives of Dermatology* 128, 926–930.

Murphy, M. and Carmichael, A. J. (2000). Renal itch. *Clinical and Experimental Dermatology* 25, 103–106.

Nakazawa, A., Matsuo, I., and Ohkido, M. (1991). Porokeratosis localized to the access region for hemodialysis. *Journal of the Academy of Dermatolology* 25, 338–340.

Ostlere, L. S., Taylor, C., Baillod, R., and Wright, S. (1994). Relationship between pruritus, transepidermal water loss, and biochemical markers of renal itch in haemodialysis patients. *Nephrology, Dialysis, Transplantation* 9, 1302–1304.

Park, T. H. *et al.* (1995). Dry skin (verosis) in patients undergoing maintenance haemodialysis: the role of decreasing sweating of the eccrine swear gland. *Nephrology, Dialysis, Transplantation* 12, 2269–2273.

Pauli-Magnus, C. *et al.* (2000). Naltrexone does not relieve uremic pruritus. Results of a randomized, double-blind, placebo-controlled crossover study. *Journal of the American Society of Nephrology* 11, 514–519.

Peces, R. *et al.* (1994). Successful treatment of haemodialysis-related porphyria cutanea tarda with erythropoietin. *Nephrology, Dialysis, Transplantation* 9, 433–435.

Peer, G. *et al.* (1996). Randomised crossover trial of naltrexone in uraemic pruritus. *Lancet* 348, 1552–1554.

Pico, M. R., Lugo-Solinos, A., Sanchez, J. L., and Burgos-Calderon, R. (1992). Cutaneous alterations in patients with chronic renal failure. *International Journal of Dermatology* 31, 860–863.

Podimow, T., Wherrett, C., and Burns, K. D. (2001). Hyperbaric oxygen in the treatment of calciphylaxis: a case series. *Nephrology, Dialysis, Transplantation* 16, 2176–2180.

Ponticelli, C. and Bencini, P. L. (1992). Uremic pruritus. A review. *Nephron* 50, 1–5.

Ponticelli, C. and Bencini, P. L. (1995). Pruritus in dialysis patients: a neglected problem. *Nephrology, Dialysis, Transplantation* 10, 2174–2175.

Sampietro, M., Fiorelli, G., and Fargion, S. (1999). Iron overload in porphyria cutanea tarda. *Haematologica* 84, 248–253.

Sarkell, B. and Patterson, J. W. (1993). Treatment of porphyria cutanea tarda of end-stage renal disease with erythropoietin. *Journal of the American Academy of Dermatology* 29, 499–500.

Sarris, E. *et al.* (2003). Diffuse alopecia in a hemodialysis patient caused by a low-molecular-weight heparin, tinzapirin. *American Journal of Kidney Diseases* 41, E15.

Seukeran D., Flecher S., Sellars L., and Vestey J. P. (1997). Sudden deepening of pigmentation during haemodialysis due to severe haemolysis. *British Journal of Dermatology* 137, 997–999.

Stähle-Backdahl, M. (1988). Stratum corneum hydration in patients undergoing maintenance hemodialysis. *Acta Dermatoveneorologica (Stockholm)* 68, 531–544.

Stein, G. *et al.* (1986). No tissue level abnormality of vitamin A concentration despite elevated serum vitamin A of uremic patients. *Clinical Nephrology* 25, 87–93.

Stevens, B. R., Fleischer, A. B., Jr., Piering, F., and Crosby, D. L. (1993). Porphyria cutanea tarda in the setting of renal failure. Response to renal transplantation. *Archives of Dermatology* 129, 337–339.

Sue, Y. M. *et al.* (2001). Generalized argyria in two chronic hemodialysis patients. *American Journal of Kidney Diseases* 37, 1048–1051.

Szepietowski, J. C., Morita, A., and Tsuji, T. (2002). Ultraviolet B induces mast cell apoptosis: a hypothetical mechanism of ultraviolet B treatment of uraemic pruritus. *Med Hypotheses* 58,167–170.

Szepietowski, J. C. *et al.* (2003). Uremic pruritus: a clinical study of maintenance hemodialysis patients. *Journal of Dermatology* 29, 621–627.

Tan, J. K .L., Haberman, H. F., and Coldman, A. J. (1991). Identifying effective treatment for uremic pruritus. *Journal of the American Academy of Dermatology* 25, 811–818.

Tercedor, J. *et al.* (1995). Multivariate analysis of cutaneous markers of aging in chronic hemodialyzed patients. *International Journal of Dermatology* 34, 546–550.

Twicross, R. *et al.* (2003). Itch: scratching more than surface. *Q J Med* 96, 7–26.

Vadoud-Seyedi, J., de Dobbeleer, G., and Simonart, T. (2000). Treatment of hemodialysis-associated pseudoporphyria with *N*-acetylcysteine: report of two cases. *British Journal of Dermatology* 142, 580–581.

Vahlquist, A., Berne, B., Danielson, B. G., Grefberg, N., and Berne, C. (1985). Vitamin A losses during continuous ambulatory peritoneal dialysis. *Nephron* 41, 179–183.

Walker, R. P. *et al.* (1993). Metastatic soft calcification presenting as a tongue mass. *Otolaryngology and Head and Neck Surgery* 109, 540–542.

Yoshimoto-Furuie, K. *et al.* (1999). Effects of oral supplementation with evening primrose oil for six weeks on plasma essential fatty acids and uremic skin symptoms in hemodialysis patients. *Nephron* 81, 151–159.

Zakrewska-Priewska, B. and Jedras, M. (2001). Is pruritus in chronic uremic patient related to the peripheral somatic and autonomic neuropathy? Study by R.R. interval variation test (RRLV) and by sympathetic skin response (SSR). *Neurophysiologie Clinique—Clinical Neurophysiology* 31, 181–193.

11.3.14 Neuropsychiatric disorders

Andrew Davenport

Peripheral neuropathy

Introduction

Patients with chronic renal failure who have a generalized polyneuropathy usually have uraemic neuropathy, but other conditions should also be considered (Table 1). Similarly, dialysis patients may develop neuropathies as a result of the accumulation of toxins, alcohol abuse, vitamin deficiencies, and drugs including amiodarone, colchicine, cyclosporine, isoniazid, metronidazole, and nitrofurantoin. After recovery from acute renal failure some patients are found to have developed an intensive care neuromyopathy caused by ischaemia, typically resulting in a motor axonal polyneuropathy, ischaemic muscle changes with atrophic fibres, and thick filament loss (Sandler *et al.* 2002).

Clinical manifestations of uraemic neuropathy

In the early days of dialysis, about 50 per cent of patients starting treatment had clinical evidence of a peripheral neuropathy (Thomas 1978). Because of earlier initiation of dialysis today, neuropathy is usually asymptomatic. Classically, patients presented with a distal sensorimotor, predominantly axonal, neuropathy. Loss of ankle vibration sensation and the ankle jerk were often the first manifestations, progressing to a burning sensation in the feet, followed by motor deficit, such as weakness of ankle dorsiflexion (Schaumberg *et al.* 1992). This could then progress to a stocking neuropathy with weakness and wasting of the distal leg muscles. After regular dialysis treatment symptomatic distal parethesiae cleared rapidly, although in some, a peripheral neuropathy, usually sensory, rather than motor, persisted. Despite symptomatic clinical improvement, nerve conduction studies have shown that nerve function can deteriorate over time (Jurcic *et al.* 1998).

Uraemic neuropathy can be exacerbated by both nerve ischaemia and hypoxia. Muscle cramps can occur in other peripheral neuropathies, and motor neurone disease, but are more frequent in haemodialysis than continuous ambulatory peritoneal dialysis (CAPD) patients, typically during the last hour of haemodialysis, and may be due to a reduction in oxygen delivery to the distal nerves.

Pruritus

Pruritus in dialysis patients may be multifactorial due to a combination of dry skin, hyperparathyroidism (Chou *et al.* 2000), hypercalcaemia and/or hyperphosphataemia, hypermagnesaemia, retention of bile salts, and dialysis exposure to plastizers and other chemicals. Many treatments have been advocated for pruritus, but pruritus does improve symptomatically following the institution of better quality dialysis (Pierratos and Ouwendyk 1999). In some studies, it is only resolved after successful transplantation (Murphy and Carmichael 2000). Uraemic pruritus has been shown to be associated with altered sympathetic innervation of the skin (Robles *et al.* 1999), and this correlated with impaired peripheral somatosensory nerve conduction, suggesting that uraemic pruritus is a manifestation of uraemic neuropathy (Zakzewska-Pniewska and Jedras 2001).

Restless legs

'Restless legs' are another clinical manifestation of uraemic neuropathy in dialysis patients, and is usually worse at night. It is often present in association with pruritus and sleep disturbances (Winkelman *et al.* 1996). Many treatments have been tried including benzodiazepines, such as clonazepam, or the newer dopamine agonists, including pramipexole. The response is variable. As with pruritus, increasing the dose of dialysis, for example, by daily dialysis, and renal transplantation have been reported to cure this distressing condition (Winklemann *et al.* 2002).

Pathophysiology of uraemic neuropathy

Electrophysiological studies of severely uraemic patients showed extensive slowing in peripheral nerve conduction of both upper and low limb sensory and motor nerves, followed by a decline in the amplitude of the nerve action potential (Schaumburg *et al.* 1992). However, these electrophysiological abnormalities were markedly out of proportion to the clinical symptoms and findings on physical examination. Following successful renal transplantation, nerve conduction velocity improves rapidly (Oh *et al.* 1978).

Histological studies in uraemic neuropathy revealed nerve fibre degeneration, characterized by axonal degeneration, and demyelination of apparently normal looking axons (Forno and Alston 1967). Typically the large diameter axons in the distal nerve trunks supplying the legs were affected, with relative sparing of the unmyelinated and the small myelinated afferent neurons. The spinal roots and cervical dorsal columns are usually intact, as are the anterior horn cells, although they may show chromatolytic change (Schaumberg *et al.* 1992). Paranodal demyelination and separation of the axolemma sheath have also been reported, but probably reflect axonal damage. Those fibres with axonal degeneration have abnormal nerve tubules, due to defective assembly of tubulin proteins. Nerve biopsies also showed onion like structures due to several layers of Schwann cell processes around myelinated nerve fibres, suggesting repeated episodes of demyelination followed by remyelination (Dyan *et al.* 1970). Although there may well be a defect in Schwann cell function in uraemia, the predominant defect is one of axonal loss with secondary demyelination. Following renal transplantation, early remyelination accounts for the initial rapid improvement in nerve conduction, whereas nerve regeneration is a slow process taking many months (Oh *et al.* 1978). Similarly, there is no significant improvement in nerve conduction studies following a single haemodialysis treatment (Laaksonen *et al.* 2002). There may be an additional ischaemic component to uraemic neuropathy, as increasing the haematocrit with erythropoietin therapy improved nerve conduction times (Sobh *et al.* 1992).

The biochemical pathogenesis of uraemic neuropathy remains to be elucidated. It is certainly multifactorial, in that neuropathy is exacerbated by hypermagnesaemia and hypercalcaemia. Nerve function and muscle strength improve following parathyroidectomy (Chou *et al.* 2000). However, the most likely explanation is that retention of 'uraemic toxins' (Hörl 1998) leads to a reduction in energy dependent processes, and failure to transport and assemble tubulin within the cell correctly. The ouabain sensitive calcium ATPase pump activity has been shown to be decreased in uraemia, thereby affecting the sodium–calcium exchanger, and hence, reducing the normal calcium gradient of 10,000 : 1 (outside to inside) across these excitable cells (Shibahara *et al.* 1990). Various 'uraemic toxins' have been proposed, including

Table 1 Spinal cord and peripheral nerve involvement in renal patients with endstage renal failure treated by dialysis due to conditions which can lead to both chronic renal failure and cerebral damage, and complications associated with dialysis

Underlying condition	Spinal cord	Peripheral nerve
Fabry's disease		Burning painful peripheral neuropathy Autonomic neuropathy
Porphyria		Peripheral neuropathy
Sickle-cell disease	Cord ischaemia	Mononeuropathy
HIV	Transverse myelitis	Peripheral neuropathy Guillain–Barré syndrome Autonomic neuropathy
HTLV-1	Cord ischaemia	Ascending spastic paralysis
Polyarteritis nodosa		60% multifocal mononeuropathy—often painful
Churg–Strauss syndrome		75% multifocal mononeuropathy
Wegener's granulomatosis		Multifocal mononeuropathy and polyneuropathy
Rheumatoid arthritis	Atlantoaxial subluxation	Sensory neuropathy, rarely mononeuropathy Sensorimotor neuropathy
Systemic lupus erythematosus	Transverse myelitis	Distal sensory neuropathy Sensorimotor neuropathy
Sjögren's syndrome	Dorsal root gangliopathy	Peripheral neuropathy Autonomic neuropathy
Sarcoidosis		Peripheral neuropathy
Diabetes mellitus	Cord ischaemia	Distal sensory neuropathy—may be painful Motor mononeuropathy Autonomic neuropathy
Amyloid	Cord ischaemia	Peripheral neuropathy Autonomic neuropathy
Multiple myeloma	Cord compression	Peripheral neuropathy
POEMS	Cord ischaemia	50% motor neuropathy
Waldenström's		Sensory and motor neuropathy
Cryoglobulinaemia		Multiple mononeuropathy
Tuberculus osteomyelitis	Cord compression	Nerve root entrapment
Staphylococcus aureus osteomyelitis	Cord compression	Nerve root entrapment
Dialysis amyloid	Cord compression	Carpal tunnel syndrome
Lead toxicity		Motor neuropathy—wrist and foot drop
Mercury toxicity		Sensory neuropathy
Thallium toxicity		Painful motor and sensory neuropathy
Thiamine deficiency		Sensory neuropathy
Pyridoxine deficiency/toxicity		Peripheral neuropathy
Vitamin B_{12} deficiency	Dorsal column	Peripheral neuropathy
Coeliac disease		Peripheral neuropathy
Vascular steel due to arteriovenous fistula/graft		Carpal tunnel syndrome Ischaemic neuropathy
Complications of central venous access		Brachial nerve palsy Femoral nerve palsy
Postrenal transplantation		Femoral nerve palsy

guanidine compounds, particularly methylguanidine which can inhibit the sodium ATPase pump, polyamines, phenol metabolites, myoinositol, and 3-carboxy-4-methyl-5-propyl-2-fluranpropanoic acid, which inhibits organic acid transport. Other suggestions include toxin induced inhibition of other key enzymes, such as transketolase, and pyridoxal phosphate kinase (Pietrzak and Baczyk 2001).

Electrolyte abnormalities and peripheral nerve function

Hyperkalaemia may present in dialysis patients with generalized muscle weakness in association with a reduction in peripheral sensation, in a stocking distribution with loss of reflexes. Hypermagnesaemia can also cause muscle weakness and peripheral neuropathy (Davenport 1998). Profound hypocalcaemia following parathyroidectomy, can lead to tetany, with carpopedal spasm, as can severe hypomagnesaemia.

Carpal tunnel syndrome (see Chapter 11.3.10)

Carpal tunnel syndrome (CTS) is due to compression of the median nerve as it passes deep to the flexor retinaculum at the wrist, causing numbness, tingling, and burning sensations in the hand and fingers. Gentle percussion of the median nerve at the wrist may reproduce these symptoms (Tinel's sign). Occasionally, pain may radiate proximally up the arm, even as far as the elbow. Parathesiae may be restricted to the radial fingers, but often affect all digits. The pain is typically worse at night and during haemodialysis. Eventually weakness of thumb abduction occurs with wasting of the thenar eminence. CTS is more common in middle aged and older women, diabetics, patients with hypothyroidism, and patients who have dialysed for more than 7 years (Jadoul and De Broe 1999), and may well have a genetic predisposition (Omori et al. 2002). Although CTS usually starts on the same side as an arteriovenous fistula, most dialysis patients develop bilateral disease. It is usually caused by β2-microglobulin amyloid deposition in the median nerve tunnel. Although haemodialysis with a high flux polyacrylonitrile, or haemodiafiltration, have been reported to reduce the deposition of β2-microglobulin, other factors including dialysate water composition and microbacteriological quality are also important in determining the frequency of CTS (Floege and Kettler 2001).

The diagnosis of CTS can be confirmed by measuring a delay in median nerve conduction across the wrist, and also by ultrasound of the wrist demonstrating bone cysts and distortion of the flexor tendons (Beekman and Visser 2002).

β2 Amyloid deposition in the palm can lead to local ulnar nerve compression with pain and parathesiae over the fourth and fifth fingers (Jadoul and De Broe 1999). Late on, patients are left with very restricted movement in the hands, as β2 amyloid becomes deposited not only in the wrist compartment, but also in the palm and around tendon sheaths, causing flexion contractures. In addition deposition in the lower cervical and lumbar vertebrae can result in bony destruction, and collapse with cord compression.

Forearm nerve damage

Forearm arteriovenous fistula formation changes blood flow in the forearm. As more and more of the dialysis population are diabetic and elderly, then these patients may have pre-existing vascular disease, and are more likely to suffer from vascular steal and nerve ischaemia following fistula formation (Sessa et al. 2000).

Autonomic neuropathy

Autonomic dysfunction is more commonly found in diabetics and elderly patients. Early studies in dialysis patients suggested that the prevalence of autonomic dysfunction was greater than 50 per cent (Ewing and Winney 1975). More recent reports have shown similar prevalence to that of an age matched population (Jassal et al. 1998). Autonomic neuropathy improves after the institution of dialysis (Laaksonen et al. 2000), and resolves following successful transplantation. Secondary autonomic neuropathy has also been described in alcoholism, Wernicke's encephalopathy, and drugs, including phenothiazine tranquillizers, tricyclic antidepressants, α-blockers such as doxazosin and labetalol, and angiotensin-converting enzyme inhibitors.

Most centres test for autonomic neuropathy by power spectral analysis of heart rate variability in response to postural change, hyperventilation, the Valsalva manoeuvre, and breath holding. Blood pressure changes with posture and exercise (hand grip) can also be assessed (Savica et al. 2001). Other tests include measurement of plasma noradrenaline in response to posture and/or tilt test, sweat responses to heat, and pupillary responses to cocaine. In dialysis patients the most common defect is one of failure of the sensing baroreceptor in the afferent limb of the autonomic loop, whereas the efferent limb is usually found to be functioning normally (Dheenan et al. 1997).

Although the aetiology of hypotension during haemodialysis is multifactorial, some patients show a paradoxical bradycardia in response to hypotension—Bezold–Jarisch reflex. This is similar to withdrawal of sympathetic tone in carotid sinus hypersensitivity, and idiopathic orthostatic hypotension. Patients with autonomic dysfunction have been shown to have more cardiac arrhythmias during dialysis and are more prone to intradialytic hypotension (Calvo et al. 2002).

Management includes withdrawal of drugs, which block autonomic nerves and dialysing the patient in a bed rather than in a chair, and maintaining an adequate haematocrit, more than 30 per cent. Peritoneal dialysis patients with postural hypotension may benefit from surgical support stockings, and volume expansion, and fludrocortisone. Haemodialysis patients should be dialysed with cooled dialysate and may benefit from blood volume and reverse sodium profiling. Sertraline, a selective serotonin reuptake inhibitor, and venlafaxine, which additionally reduces nor-adrenaline reuptake, have been reported to reduce intradialytic hypotension (Dheenan and Henrich 2001). Midrodine, an oral sympathomimetic has also been advocated to improve intradialytic hypotension.

Myopathy

Introduction

Many dialysis patients complain of fatigue and muscle weakness. The weakness is predominantly proximal, and can be accompanied by muscle wasting. Bone and joint pain, due to underlying renal osteomalacia, osteoarthritis, intrajoint calcified foreign bodies, and periarticular soft tissue calcification, exacerbate the functional incapacity. Similarly, tendon weakness, due to hyperparathyroidism, or tendon calcification also impair effective muscle contraction. Many dialysis patients take little or no exercise, and this increases the risk of disuse atrophy (Johansen 1999). Elderly patients may have pre-existing major vascular disease, suffering claudication, or small vessel disease, thus some patients have a predisposition to ischaemic muscle damage

(Gambhir *et al.* 1995). More recently calcific arteriolopathy has been described in dialysis patients. This affects small arterioles supplying muscles, causing muscle ischaemia, reducing exercise ability and exacerbating intradialytic cramps.

Uraemic patients may develop myositis due to prescription of hydroxymethylglutaryl coenzyme A3 reductase inhibitors (statins), fibrates, and/or nicotinic acid, for secondary hyperlipidaemia. Myositis can also occur in acute renal failure, not only due to crush injury, but also secondary to drugs, including amphetamines and cocaine. Colchicine has also been reported to result in a proximal myopathy and myositis.

General causes of muscle weakness

Prior to the introduction of vitamin D analogues, patients with renal failure developed osteomalacia, characterized by proximal muscle weakness and underlying bone pathology (Ritz *et al.* 1980). $1,25(OH)_2D3$ is anabolic to muscle, accelerating protein muscle synthesis and increasing local ATP concentrations. It also increases muscle contractility by regulating calcium binding to the troponin complex. Hypophosphataemia, usually associated with malnutrition, can also lead to profound muscle weakness. Hyperparathyroidism is a well-recognized cause of proximal muscle weakness in dialysis patients (Ritz *et al.* 1980). Parathyroid hormone not only increases muscle proteolysis, but also impairs energy production, transfer, and utilization. This may be exacerbated by the development of an enthesiopathy, as tendon insertion into surface of the underlying bone can be affected by high bone turnover, and can result in tendon rupture.

Many patients starting dialysis have been protein restricted, either by protein restricted diets, or self-restriction caused by the effect of advancing uraemia on appetite. Even in dialysis patients, malnutrition remains the greatest predictor of muscle weakness (Fahal *et al.* 1997), and muscle biopsy studies showed that many dialysis patients have reduced muscle glycogen levels (Davenport *et al.* 1993).

Uraemic myopathy

Dialysis patients, whether treated by peritoneal or haemodialysis have been shown not only to be weaker than controls, but also to have reduced muscle relaxation rates (Fahal *et al.* 1996). Muscle biopsies from uraemic patients show predominantly type II fibre atrophy with abnormal variation in fibre diameter, and a variety of cytoarchetectural changes, including internal nuclei, fibre splitting, and the appearance of ring fibres (Davenport *et al.* 1993).

Biochemical studies have shown that skeletal muscle in anaemic dialysis patients contains increased levels of inorganic phosphate, with reduced oxidative capacity. During exercise these dialysis patients developed increased intracellular acidosis and phosphocreatine breakdown (Thompson *et al.* 1994). This would suggest a defect in mitochondrial oxidative capacity. Carnitine supplementation has been shown to improve skeletal muscle energetics, as assessed by magnetic resonance (MR) spectroscopy in anaemic dialysis patients. Several studies using L-carnitine supplementation reported improvement in muscle fatigue and cramps during haemodialysis (Sakurauchi *et al.* 1998). However, when MR spectroscopy studies were repeated after treatment with erythropoietin, baseline muscle energy kinetics improved, suggesting that the most important feature affecting uraemic muscle was oxygen delivery (Thompson *et al.* 1997). Under these circumstances carnitine supplementation, showed either a small, or no benefit.

Disorders of cerebral function in the dialysis patient

Cognitive and psychological dysfunction

Cognitive function can be depressed by comorbid conditions that result in cerebrovascular disease, which may have been present prior to the advent of dialysis, or developed either during, or as a consequence of dialysis (Lass *et al.* 1999) (Table 2). Similarly, psychological factors can depress cognitive function. Compared to patients with other chronic medical conditions, dialysis patients have been reported to have an increased hospitalization rate not only for depression and other affective disorders, but also organic disorders and dementias; alcohol and other drug disorders, schizophrenia and other psychoses; and anxiety and other personality disorders (Kimmel *et al.* 1998). Depression is the most common psychological disorder in the dialysis patients, with a prevalence of around 50 per cent of patients starting dialysis (Watnick *et al.* 2003), but even following transplantation psychological problems may persist (Griva *et al.* 2002).

It has been well documented that chronic haemodialysis patients under perform on psychometric testing, with delayed responses to visual or auditory stimuli, which improve somewhat following a haemodialysis session. However, normalization of haematocrit with erythropoietin therapy, was reported not only to improve cognitive function but also quality of life assessments, and reduce depression (Furuland *et al.* 2003).

Encephalopathy

Uraemic encephalopathy is an organic brain syndrome, which occurs both in patients with endstage renal failure, and those treated by dialysis. Following the move towards a policy of earlier initiation of dialysis, combined with quality initiatives to improve the adequacy of dialysis, this syndrome is now only rarely observed. Uraemic encephalopathy typically occurs following a rapid decline in residual renal function, precipitated and/or exacerbated by hypertension, electrolyte imbalances, sepsis, and/or drug toxicity. Initially symptoms are rather non-specific; fatigue, apathy and poor attention span, varying from day to day. Progressing through confusion, and occasionally delirium, to coma. Motor function is often abnormal, with intention tremor, leading to asterixis. Myoclonic jerks may develop and can progress to generalized tonic–clonic seizures (Lederman and Henry 1978). Tone is generally increased, with hyper-reflexia, and extensor plantar responses. In the very advanced stages of uraemic encephalopathy patients may exhibit signs of meningism.

EEG recordings of severely uraemic patients show an increased prevalence of delta and theta slow wave activity, typically over the frontal lobes, with a corresponding reduction in alpha and beta waves compared to normal healthy controls (Fig. 1). Treatment with peritoneal dialysis or haemodialysis reverses these changes. Similarly the response to visual or auditory stimuli is slowed in uraemia, and improves following dialysis (Davenport and Bramley 1993).

Cerebral imaging with computed tomography (CT) or magnetic resonance imaging (MRI) is not diagnostic in uraemic encephalopathy, although it will exclude other causes of confusion, such as a subdural haematoma, cerebral abscess, meningitis, or hydrocephalus. The pathophysiology of uraemic encephalopathy, as with uraemic neuropathy remains to be elucidated. Cerebral metabolic rate is reduced,

Table 2 Cerebral dysfunction in the patient with endstage renal failure treated by dialysis due to conditions which can lead to both chronic renal failure and cerebral damage

Underlying condition	Aetiology	Clinical manifestations
Alport's syndrome	Loss α-3(IV) α-4(IV) α-5(IV) Cochlear basement membrane	High tone sensorineural deafness
Fabry's disease	Endothelial damage ↓ α-Galactosidase	Multi-infarct dementia Cerebrovascular accident
Methyl malonic acidaemia	Endothelial damage ↓ Methylmalonyl CoA mutase	Cognitive impairment Cerebrovascular accident
Mitochondrial myopathy	Endothelial damage A3243G point mutation Leu gene	Encephalopathy Cerebrovascular accident
Cystinosis	Cystine crystal accumulation Defective lysosomal carrier	Small vessel brain disease Cortical atrophy, cystic necrosis
Hyperoxaluria	Endothelial deposition AGT deficiency; EC 2.6.1.44	Small vessel brain disease Cerebrovascular accident Seizures
Porphyria	Hypertension	Small vessel brain disease Cerebrovascular accident
Sickle-cell disease	Sickled erythrocytes	Small vessel brain disease
Haemoglobin S/S, S/C, S/D, S/E	Valine → glutamic acid (6 β chain)	Cerebrovascular accident
Von Hippel–Lindau disease	Hamartoma formation VHL gene 3p25–p26	Cognitive impairment Cerebrovascular haemorrhage Seizures
Tuberous sclerosis	Hamartoma formation Gene TSC2-GTPase activator	Cognitive impairment Cerebrovascular haemorrhage Seizures
Polycystic kidney disease	Hypertension, cerebral artery aneurysms (berry) Cardiac valve prolapse	Small vessel brain disease Cerebrovascular infarct Embolic stroke
Polyarteritis nodosa	Necrotizing vasculitis Secondary hypertension	Encephalopathy Focal infarction, haemorrhage Seizures
Churg–Strauss syndrome	Necrotizing vasculitis	Encephalopathy
Wegener's granulomatosis	Necrotizing vasculitis	Focal cerebral ischaemia Cranial diabetes insipidus
Systemic lupus erythematosus	Immune complex vasculitis Secondary hypertension	Encephalopathy Seizures Focal infarction
Anticardiolipin syndrome	Small vessel occlusion Secondary hypertension	Encephalopathy Seizures Focal infarction
Sjögren's disease	Anti-Ro and -La antibodies Inflammatory vasculitis	Psychiatric disorders Focal cerebral ischaemia
Behçet's syndrome	Lymphomonocytic vasculitis	Brain stem strokes Meningoencephalitis
Systemic sclerosis	Hypertension	Focal cerebral ischaemia
Malignant hypertension	Vasculopathy and ischaemia	Encephalopathy Cerebrovascular accident
Cholesterol emboli syndrome	Atheroma	Focal cerebral ischaemia Cerebrovascular accident

Table 2 Continued

Underlying condition	Aetiology	Clinical manifestations
Diabetes mellitus	Vasculopathy and ischaemia	Focal cerebral ischaemia Cerebrovascular accident
Amyloid	Vasculopathy	Focal cerebral ischaemia Cerebrovascular accident
Plasma cell dyscrasias	Hyperviscosity	Encephalopathy
Multiple myeloma, POEMS		Cerebrovascular accident
Waldenström's macroglobulinaemia		Subarachnoid haemorrhage
Cryoglobulinaemia Types I, II, and III	Hyperviscosity and secondary vasculitis	Cerebrovascular accident Transient ischaemic attack
Sarcoidosis	Inflammatory granulomata	Focal cerebral ischaemia Cerebrovascular accident Cranial diabetes insipidus

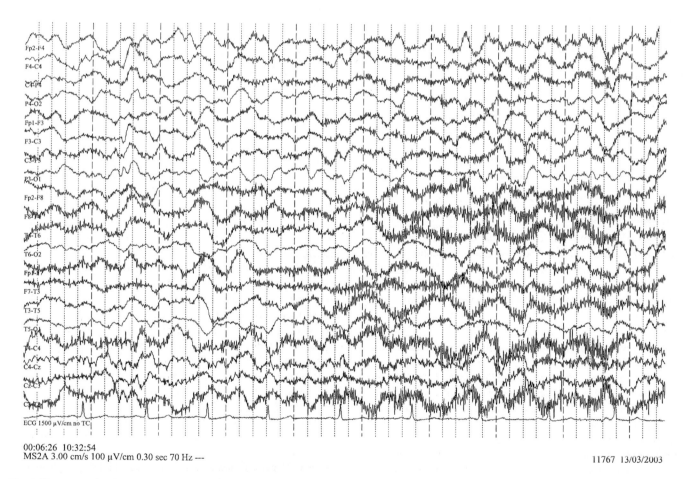

00:06:26 10:32:54
MS2A 3.00 cm/s 100 µV/cm 0.30 sec 70 Hz ---

11767 13/03/2003

Fig. 1 Electroencephalographic recording from a patient with uraemic encephalopathy. The recording is predominantly ν (4–8 Hz) and δ (<4 Hz) wave activity, with no normal α (8–13 Hz) or β (>13 Hz) waves.

as is cerebral oxygen uptake. It has been postulated that the ouabain sensitive calcium ATPase pump activity is decreased in uraemia (Fraser 1988), this would then affect the sodium–calcium exchanger, so increasing intracellular calcium. This could then effect electrophysiolgical gradients and the general release of neurotransmitters.

Studies on the brains and cerebrospinal fluid (CSF) of patients with uraemia, have shown major differences from subjects with normal renal function, with up to 30-fold increases in methylguanidine and 100-fold in guanidine reported. Methylguanidine can also inhibit the Na^+,K^+-ATPase pump. In addition, these guanidine compounds could affect cerebral neurotransmission, as *in vitro* studies have shown them as competitive receptor antagonists, blocking GABA$_A$ and glycine receptors, and potentiate *N*-methyl-D-aspartate receptor activation (De Deyn *et al.* 2001).

Electrolyte disturbances and drugs

Encephalopathy may occur in uraemic patients, usually as a result of major electrolyte derangements.

Sodium

Astrocytes and/or glial cells maintain local homeostasis, by taking up water, toxins and neurotransmitters. If hyponatraemia develops rapidly, this results in brain oedema. The patient presents with non-specific symptoms of headache, malaise, nausea, vomiting and then progressing from drowsiness through to confusion, possibly delirium, and then finally to coma (Strange 1992).

Hypernatraemia is unusual in dialysis patients, the resulting hyperosmolality causing shrinkage of the brain. As in non-ketotic hyperosmolar hyperglycaemia patients may become confused, possibly delirious, develop focal or generalized seizures, and hemipareses or other cerebrovascular like deficits before progressing to coma.

Calcium

Hypercalcaemia usually results from a combination of the use of high calcium dialysate, the prescription of calcium based phosphate binders and vitamin D analogues (Davenport 1998). Patients initially present with impaired cognitive function, lethargy, and constipation. Progression to confusion may occur, occasionally delirium, and finally coma. Myoclonic jerks and generalized seizures have also been reported.

Magnesium

Although most patients with chronic renal failure have an increased total body magnesium, this does not cause symptoms. However, symptomatic hypermagnesaemia can occur due to high magnesium dialysates and prescription of magnesium based phosphate binders. Patients become drowsy and develop peripheral neuropathy.

Drugs

Drug toxicity from accumulation is common in the uraemic patient resulting in confusion, occasionally fitting and even coma. The most common drugs are: cimetidine, penicillin and cephalosporin antibiotics, isoniazid, parenteral acyclovir and ganciclovir, and opiates.

Dialysis patients may also take recreational drugs, which affect cerebral function. Whereas heroin and marijuana often result in cerebral depression, 3,4-methylenedioxmethamhetamine and phencyclidine can lead to severe psychiatric or psychotic disturbances, and cocaine severe hypertension resulting in cerebrovascular accident, and seizure. Asian and South American patients have been reported to develop encephalopathy following ingestion of the star fruit (*Averrhoa carambola*).

Wernicke's encephalopathy

Thiamine is a water-soluble vitamin, but due to tight plasma protein binding, losses during peritoneal and/or standard haemodialysis are not increased. Even so, Wernicke's encephalopathy continues to be encountered in dialysis patients due to a combination of an underlying genetic predisposition, chronic malnourishment, anorexia, and the administration of glucose based fluids (Thara *et al.* 1999). The classic triad of ataxia, ophthalmoplegia, and confusion is often not always present in dialysis patients. Whereas Wernicke's encephalopathy is effectively cured by prompt treatment with thiamine, Korsakoff's psychosis does not respond so readily to thiamine.

Dialysis disequilibrium syndrome

Cerebral water content increases following a routine haemodialysis session, yet most chronic haemodialysis patients are unaware of this. However, when patients with cerebral oedema or following acute brain injury were haemodialysed, intracranial pressure (ICP) increased significantly during treatment (Davenport 1995). This is similar to the dialysis disequilibrium syndrome (DDS) (Rosen *et al.* 1964), first described when severely uraemic patients were dialysed infrequently for prolonged periods against a low sodium dialysate. The DDS has a spectrum of presentations ranging from mild symptoms of headache, nausea, progressing through to restlessness, confusion, or even generalized seizures.

Initially, the DDS was thought to be due to the rapid removal of urea from the vascular compartment with a smaller loss from the CSF and brain, which then led to water moving into the brain down an osmotic gradient. This theory was supported by animal experiments which showed that rapid haemodialysis, caused a more rapid change in osmotic gradients, which then resulted in greater cerebral water accumulation than slower haemodialysis (Silver *et al.* 1994), and that DDS could be prevented by adding urea to the dialysate.

One of the functions of dialysis treatment is to correct metabolic acidosis. During haemodialysis bicarbonate diffuses from the dialysate into the plasma, leading to an increase in plasma pH. Bicarbonate, being charged, is relatively impermeable to cells, and has to be converted through to CO_2 to allow passage across the blood brain barrier and into cells. Thus the rapid infusion of bicarbonate can lead to intracellular acidosis, due to the rapid movement of CO_2 and the slow exchange of HCO_3^-.

Intracellular acidosis leads to the breakdown of cell proteins and phosphate moieties with the generation of idiogenic osmoles, so creating an osmotic gradient for the passage of water into the brain (Arieff 1996). In addition, cerebral hypoxia/hypoperfusion results in increased lactate production, and the release of other locally active vasodilatators and increased flow through the hypoxic area, with a consequent rise in ICP (Davenport 2001).

Thus in daily clinical practice, patients with long standing uraemia undergoing their first haemodialysis treatment and those with underlying structural intracerebral lesions (acute stroke or subdural haemorrhage) are most at risk of the DDS. To minimize osmotic gradients developing across the blood brain barrier, dialysis duration is shortened to 2 h or less, and blood pump speeds slowed to 200 ml/min, in combination with a small surface area dialyser. In addition, a high sodium dialysate is typically used, with the dialysate bicarbonate reduced to 30 mmol/l, to limit the rate of increase in plasma pH. Prophylactic mannitol (15.5 g), or hypertonic saline (30 ml 3 N NaCl) may be given as a bolus after 60 min of dialysis to maintain the effective plasma volume and increase plasma osmolality. Similarly, cooling the dialysate to 35°C, also improves cardiovascular stability during haemodialysis. Daily dialysis minimizes urea gradients, and provided the patient remains stable then the duration and blood pump speed can be increased. After 4–5 days, alternate day dialysis can usually be introduced (Davenport 2001).

Fitting and other acute cerebral deterioration during dialysis may not always be due to DDS. Other conditions such as intracranial and/or subdural haemorrhage, acute cerebrovascular events, hypoglycaemia, hypertensive encephalopathy, epileptic seisure, intracerebral abscess, cardiac arrhythmia, air embolus, dialysate toxin, or microbacteriological contamination with cyanobacteria, and dialysate hyperthermia need to be excluded.

Cerebral cortical disorders

Cerebrovascular disease

Cerebral atrophy is the major abnormality found in CT and MRI brain scans of dialysis patients (Kamata *et al.* 2000), with hypertension proposed as the major cause. Transient ischaemic attacks (TIAs), by definition, last less than 24 h and are usually due to atheroembolic events. Although many TIAs result in loss of cortical function, lacunar infarcts typically affect the internal capsule, or basal ganglia, without affecting higher cortical function, and are usually due to pre-existing intracerebral vascular disease, and may result in form of Parkinson's disease (Fig. 2).

The causes of ischaemia and infarction are identical, as prolonged ischaemia leads to infarction, especially if the collateral supply is inadequate. Many patients who have been on long-term dialysis develop calcification of both the heart valve rings and the valves themselves, and these could act as possible sources of emboli. In addition, many dialysis patients have extensive vascular calcification, including the cerebral vessels. This may lead to small vessel ischaemia and infarction (Fig. 3). Other causes of TIAs or infarcts include a transient fall in blood pressure, which may occur during both haemo- and peritoneal dialysis, and can result in catastrophic blindness due to optic nerve ischaemia (Abe *et al.* 2002). After excluding a source of emboli, patients with TIAs should be treated with aspirin, and if appropriate antihypertensive and/or cholesterol lowering agents. Those who present with a stroke, are at risk of the DDS during dialysis as cerebral oedema develops around the infarct.

Haemodialysis patients are at greater risk of haemorrhagic stroke (Kawamura *et al.* 1998), and subdural haemorrhage than the general population. Some studies have suggested that haemorrhagic stroke is more severe in the haemodialysis patient because of the use of heparin during dialysis, and other anticoagulants such as warfarin and antiplatelet agents.

Dementia

Although hypertension and small vessel vascular disease can lead to multi-infarct dementia, aluminium accumulation in the brain was once the significant cause of dementia in haemodialysis patients (D'Haese and De Broe 1999). The main source was the dialysate prepared from domestic water, which had been treated with alum. However, aluminium intoxication has been reported in CAPD patients due to ingestion of aluminium-containing phosphate binders. Plasma aluminium concentrations do not necessarily reflect total body burden, as aluminium is mainly intracellular (Davenport *et al.* 1991). Thus monitoring the response to a test dose of 5 mg/kg desferrioxamine given during the last hour of dialysis may be helpful in assessing the aluminium burden, as a rise in plasma aluminium prior to the subsequent dialysis session of not less than 50 μg/l is suggestive of aluminium accumulation, and warrants a three month trial of desferrioxamine chelation therapy (D'Haese and De Broe 1999).

Clinically, patients developed stuttering speech, difficulty performing complex tasks, a Parkinsonian like gait and micrographia, disorientation, and dementia. EEG abnormalities, characterized by bursts of high voltage slowing and spike and wave activity in the frontal leads, could precede the onset of symptoms by up to 6 months (Fraser and Arieff 1994).

Aluminium is not the only metal contaminant that can result in central nervous system dysfunction. Manganese has also been reported to cause dementia in dialysis patients, and the trace elements cadmium, mercury, lead, copper, nickel, thallium, boron, and tin can also cause nervous system damage (Fraser and Arieff 1994).

Sleep disorders

Although sleep disorders are common in uraemic patients who have not been dialysed, the initiation of dialysis does not necessarily improve the symptoms (Hanly *et al.* 2003). Up to one-third of haemodialysis patients have significant daytime sleepiness, and this correlates negatively with quality of life health scores (Iliescu *et al.* 2003). Correction of anaemia with erythropoietin has been reported to improve the quality of sleep, in

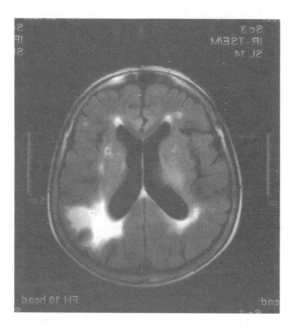

Fig. 2 MRI scan from a dialysis patient showing multiple small vessel ischaemic disease and extensive intracerebral arterial calcification.

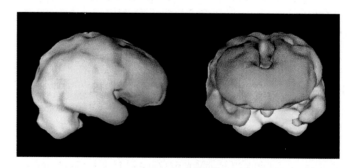

Fig. 3 Isotope brain scan of a normotensive haemodialysis patient showing multiple cerebral cortical infarcts using 473 MBq Tc-99m Bicisate neurolite.

terms of sleep fragmentation, arousal from sleep, and reduce periodic limb movements during sleep, with improved day time alertness (Benz *et al.* 1999). As there is a correlation between restless legs syndrome and sleep disturbances, it has been suggested that there is a uraemic component to the pathogenesis of these sleep disturbances. This is supported by improvements in sleep patterns and day time alertness when patients were switched to daily nocturnal haemodialysis (Hanly *et al.* 2003).

References

Abe, M., Chutorian, M. D., Winterkorn, J. M. S., and Geffer, M. (2002). Anterior ischemic optic neuropathy in children: case reports and review of the literature. *Pediatric Neurology* **26**, 358–364.

Arieff, A. I. (1994). Dialysis disequilibrium syndrome: current concepts on pathogenesis and prevention. *Kidney International* **45**, 629–635.

Beekman, R. and Visser, L. H. (2002). Sonography in the diagnosis of carpal tunnel syndrome: critical review of the literature. *Muscle & Nerve* **27**, 26–33.

Benz, R. L., Pressman, M. R., Hovick, E. T., and Peterson, D. D. (1999). A preliminary study of the effects of correction of anemia with recombinant human erythropoietin therapy on sleep, sleep disorders, and day time sleepiness in hemodialysis patients (The SLEEPO study). *American Journal of Kidney Diseases* **34**, 1089–1095.

Calvo, C., Maule, S., Mecca, F., Quadri, R., Martia, G., and Cavallo Perin, P. (2002). The influence of autonomic neuropathy on hypotension during hemodialysis. *Clinical Autonomic Research* **12**, 84–87.

Chou, F. F., Ho, J. C., Huang, S. C., and Sheen-Chen, S. M. (2000). A study on pruritus after parathyroidectomy for secondary hyperparathyroidism. *Journal of the American College of Surgeons* **190**, 65–70.

Davenport, A. (1995). Renal replacement therapy in patients at risk of cerebral edema/hypoxia. *New Horizons* **3**, 717–727.

Davenport, A. Neurological disorders in patients with acute renal failure. In *Critical Care Nephrology* (ed. C. Ronco and R. Bellomo), pp. 1081–1104. London: Kluwer Academic Publishers, 1998.

Davenport, A. (2001). Renal replacement therapy in the patient with acute brain injury. *American Journal of Kidney Diseases* **37**, 457–466.

Davenport, A. and Bramley, P. N. (1993). Cerebral function analysing monitor and visual evoked potentials as a non-invasive method of detecting cerebral dysfunction in patients with acute hepatic and renal failure treated with intermittent hemofiltration. *Renal Failure* **15**, 515–522.

Davenport, A., Davison, A. M., Will, E. J., Newton, K. E., and Toothill, C. (1991). Aluminium mobilisation following renal transplantation and the possible effect on susceptibility to bacterial sepsis. *Quarterly Journal of Medicine* **289**, 407–423.

Davenport, A., King, R. F. G. J., Ironside, J. W., Will, E. J., and Davison, A. M. (1993). The effect of treatment with recombinant human erythropoietin on the histological appearance and glycogen content of skeletal muscle in patients with chronic renal failure treated by regular hospital hemodialysis. *Nephron* **64**, 89–94.

De Deyn, P. P., D'Hooge, R., Van Bogaert, P. P., and Marescau, B. (2001). Endogenous guanidine compounds as uremic toxins. *Kidney International* **59** (Suppl. 78), S77–S83.

D'Haese, P. C. and De Broe, M. E. Aluminium, silicon, and strontium accumulation/intoxication as a complication of long-term dialysis. In *Complications of Long Term Dialysis* (ed. E. A. Brown and P. S. Parfrey), pp. 104–120. Oxford: Oxford University Press, 1999.

Dheenan, S. and Henrich, W. L. (2001). Preventing dialysis hypotension: a comparison of usual protective maneuvers. *Kidney International* **59** (3), 1175–1181.

Dheenan, S., Venkatesan, J., Grubb, B. P., and Henrich, W. L. (1997). Effect of setraline hydrochloride on dialysis hypotension. *American Journal of Kidney Diseases* **31**, 624–630.

Dyan, A. D., Gardner-Thorpe, C., Down, P. F., and Gleadle, R. I. (1970). Peripheral neuropathy in uremia. *Neurology* **20**, 649–652.

Ewing, D. J. and Winney, R. (1975). Autonomic function in patients with chronic renal failure on intermittent hemodialysis. *Nephron* **15**, 424–429.

Fahal, I. H., Ahmad, R., and Edwards, R. H. T. (1996). Muscle weakness in continuous ambulatory peritoneal dialysis patients. *Peritoneal Dialysis International* **16** (Suppl. 1), S419–S423.

Fahal, I. H., Bell, G. M., Bone, M. J., and Edwards, R. H. T. (1997). Physiological abnormalities of skeletal muscle in dialysis patients. *Nephrology, Dialysis, Transplantation* **12**, 119–127.

Floege, J. and Ketteler, M. (2001). β_2 Microglobulin-derived amyloidosis: an update. *Kidney International* **59** (Suppl. 78), S164–S171.

Forno, L. and Alston, W. (1967). Uremic polyneuropathy. *Acta Neurologica Scandinavica* **43**, 640–646.

Fraser, C. L. Neurological manifestations of the uremic state. In *Metabolic Brain Dysfunction in Systemic Disorders* (ed. A. I. Arieff and R. C. Griggs), **139**, pp. 66–76. Little Brown: Boston, 1988.

Fraser, C. L. and Arieff, A. I. (1994). Metabolic encephalopathy as a complication of renal failure: mechanisms and mediators. *New Horizons* **2**, 518–526.

Furuland, H., Linde, T., Ahlmen, J., Christensson, A., Strömbom, U., and Danielson, B. G. (2003). A randomized controlled trial of hemoglobin normalization with epoetin alfa in pre-dialysis and dialysis patients. *Nephrology, Dialysis, Transplantation* **18**, 353–361.

Gambhir, I. S., Bayen, P. K., Singh, R. G., Usha, R., and Katiyar, B. C. (1995). Neuromuscular changes in acute renal failure. *The Journal of the Association of Physicians of India* **43**, 263–264.

Griva, K., Ziegelmann, J. P., Thompson, D., Jayasena, D., Davenport, A., Harrison, M., and Newman, S. P. (2002). *Nephrology, Dialysis, Transplantation* **17**, 22,044–22,211.

Hanly, P. J., Gabor, J. Y., Chan, C., and Pierratos, A. (2003). Daytime sleepiness in patients with chronic renal failure: impact of nocturnal hemodialysis. *American Journal of Kidney Diseases* **41**, 403–410.

Hörl, W. H. The patient with uremia. In *Oxford Textbook of Clinical Nephrology* 2nd edn. (ed. A. M. Davison, J. S. Cameron, J. P. Grünfeld, D. N. S. Kerr, E. Ritz, and C. G. Winearls), pp. 1822–1836. Oxford: Oxford University Press, 1988.

Iliescu, E. A., Coo, H., McMurray, M. H., Meers, C. L., Quinn, M. M., Siger, M. A., and Hopman, W. M. (2003). Quality of sleep and health-related quality of life in hemodialysis patients. *Nephrology, Dialysis, Transplantation* **18**, 126–132.

Jadoul, M. and De Broe, M. E. β_2-Microglobulin amyloidosis. In *Complications of Long Term Dialysis* (ed. E. A. Brown and P. S. Parfrey), pp. 121–144. Oxford: Oxford University Press, 1999.

Jassal, S. V., Douglas, J. F., and Stout, R. W. (1998). Prevalence of central autonomic neuropathy in elderly dialysis patients. *Nephrology, Dialysis, Transplantation* **13**, 1702–1708.

Johansen, K. L. (1999). Physical functioning and exercise capacity in patients on dialysis. *Advanced Renal Replacement Therapy* **6**, 141–148.

Jurcic, D., Bago, J., Eljuga, D., Milutinovic, S., Bobinac, A., Bakula, V., and Bilic, C. (1988). Features of uremic neuropathy in long term dialysis. *Collegium Antropologicum* **22**, 119–125.

Kawamura, M., Fijimoto, S., Hisanga, S., Yamamoto, Y., and Eto, T. (1998). Incidence, outcome, and risk factors of cerebrovascular events in patients undergoing maintenance hemodialysis. *American Journal of Kidney Diseases* **31**, 991–996.

Kamata, T., Hishida, A., Takita, T., Sawada, K., Ikegaya, N., Maruyama, Y., Miyajima, H., and Kaneko, E. (2000). Morphological abnormalities in the brain of chronically hemodialysed patients without cerebrovascular disease. *American Journal of Nephrology* **20**, 27–31.

Kimmel, P. L., Thamer, M., Richard, C. M., and Ray, N. F. (1998). Psychiatric illness in patients with end-stage renal disease. *American Journal of Medicine* **105**, 214–221.

Laaksonen, S., Metsärinne, K., and Viopio-Pulkki, L. M. (2002). Neurophysiological parameters and symptoms in chronic renal failure. *Muscle & Nerve* **25**, 884–890.

Laaksonen, S., Viopio-Pulkki, L. M., Erkinjutti, M., Asola, M., and Falck, B. (2000). Does dialysis therapy improve autonomic and peripheral nervous system abnormalities in chronic uremia? *Journal of Internal Medicine* **248**, 21–26.

Lass, P., Buscombe, J. R., Harber, M., Davenport, A., and Hilson, A. J. (1999). Cognitive impairment in patients with renal failure is associated with multi-infarct dementia. *Clinical Nuclear Medicine* **24**, 561–565.

Lederman, R. J. and Henry, C. E. (1978). Progressive dialysis encephalopathy. *Annals of Neurology* **4**, 199–204.

Murphy, M. and Carmichael, A. J. (2000). Renal itch. *Clinical and Experimental Dermatology* **25**, 103–106.

Oh, S. J., Clements, R. S., Lee, Y. W., and Diethelm, A. G. (1978). Rapid improvement in nerve conduction velocity following renal transplantation. *Annals of Neurology* **4**, 369–372.

Omori, K., Kazama, J. J., Song, J., Goto, S., Takada, T., Saito, N., Sakatsume, M., Narita, I., and Gejyo, F. (2002). *Amyloid* **3**, 175–182.

Pierratos, A. and Ouwendyk, M. (1999). Nocturnal hemodialysis: five years later. *Seminars in Dialysis* **12**, 419–423.

Pietrzak, I. and Baczyk, K. (2001). Erythrocyte transketolase activity and guanidine compounds in hemodialysis patients. *Kidney International* **59** (Suppl. 78), S97–S101.

Ritz, R., Boland, R., and Kreusser, W. (1980). Effects of vitamin D and parathyroid hormone on muscle: potential role in uremia. *American Journal of Nutrition* **33**, 1522–1529.

Robles, N. R., Solis, M., Albarran, L., Esparrago, J. F., and Roncero, F. (1999). Sympathetic skin response in hemodialysis patients: correlation with nerve conduction studies and adequacy of dialysis. *Nephron* **82**, 12–16.

Rosen, S. M., O'Connor, K., and Shaldon, S. (1964). Hemodialysis disequilibrium syndrome. *British Medical Journal* **2**, 672–675.

Sakurauchi, Y., Matsumoto, Y., Shinzato, T., Takai, I., Nakamura, Y., Sato, M., Nakai, S., Miwa, M., Morita, H., Miwa, T., Amano, I., and Maeda, K. (1999). Effects of L-carnitine supplementation on muscular symptoms in hemodialyzed patients. *American Journal of Kidney Diseases* **32**, 258–264.

Sandler, H. W., Golden, M., and Danon, M. J. (2002). Quadriplegic areflexic ICU illness: selective thick filament loss and normal nerve histology. *Muscle & Nerve* **26**, 499–505.

Savica, V., Musolino, R., Di Leo, R., Santoro, D., Vita, G., and Bellinghieri, G. (2001). Autonomic dysfunction in uremia. *American Journal of Kidney Diseases* **38** (Suppl. 1), S118–S121.

Schaumburg, H. H., Berger, A. R., and Thomas, P. K. Uremic neuropathy. In *Disorders of Peripheral Nerves* 2nd edn. (ed. R. A. Davis), pp. 156–163. Philadelphia: WB Saunders Co, 1992.

Sessa, C., Pecher, M., Maurizi-Balzan, J., Pichot, O., Tonti, F., Farah, I., Magne, J. L., and Guidicelli, H. (2000). Critical hand ischemia after angio-access surgery: diagnosis and treatment. *Annals of Vascular Surgery* **14**, 583–593.

Shibahara, N., Okada, S., Onishi, S., Hamada, K., Takasaki, N., Miyazaki, S., Nakagaki, I., and Sasaki, S. (1990). Axoplasmic electrolyte contents measured by X-ray microanalysis in experimental uremic neuropathy. *Nippon Jinzo Gakkai Shi* **32**, 885–892.

Silver, S. M., Sterns, R. H., and Halperin, M. L. (1996). Brain swelling after dialysis: old urea or new osmoles? *American Journal of Kidney Diseases* **28**, 1–13.

Sobh, M. A., El-Tantawy, A. H., Said, E., Atta, M. G., Refaie, A., Nagati, M., and Ghoneim, M. (1992). Effect of treatment of anemia with erythropoietin on neuromuscular function in patients on long term dialysis. *Scandinavian Journal of Urology and Nephrology* **26**, 65–69.

Strange, K. (1992). Regulation of solute and water balance and cell volume in the central nervous system. *Journal of the American Society of Nephrology* **3**, 12–27.

Thara, M., Ito, T., Yanagihara, C., and Nishimura, Y. (1999). Wernicke's encephalopathy associated with hemodialysis: report of two cases and review of the literature. *Clinical Neurology and Neurosurgery* **101**, 118–121.

Thomas, P. K. (1978). Screening for peripheral neuropathy in patients treated by chronic hemodialysis. *Muscle & Nerve* **1**, 396–399.

Thompson, C. H., Irish, A. B., Kemp, G. J., Taylor, D. J., and Radda, G. K. (1997). The effect of propionyl L-carnitine on skeletal muscle metabolism in renal failure. *Clinical Nephrology* **47**, 372–378.

Thompson, C. H., Kemp, G. J., Barnes, P. R. J., Rajagopalan, B., Styles, P., Taylor, D. J., and Radda, G. K. (1994). Uremic muscle metabolism at rest and during exercise. *Nephrology, Dialysis, Transplantation* **9**, 1600–1605.

Watnick, S., Kirwi, P., Mahnensmith, R., and Concato, J. (2003). The prevalence and treatment of depression among patients starting dialysis. *American Journal of Kidney Diseases* **41**, 105–110.

Winkelman, J. W., Chertow, G. M., and Lazarus, J. M. (1966). Restless legs syndrome in end-stage renal disease. *American Journal of Kidney Diseases* **28**, 372–378.

Winklemann, J., Stautner, A., Samtleben, W., and Trenkwalder, C. (2002). Long term course of restless legs syndrome in dialysis patients after kidney transplantation. *Movement Disorders* **17**, 1072–1076.

Zakzewska-Pniewska, B. and Jedras, M. (2001). Is pruritus in chronic uremic patients related to peripheral somatic and autonomic neuropathy? *Neurophysiologie Clinique* **31**, 181–193.

12

The patient on dialysis

12.1 Dialysis strategies

Vincenzo Cambi, Salvatore David, and Dante Tagliavini

Introduction

Dialysis provides incomplete replacement of lost renal excretory function and is generally considered as a compromise between an acceptable outcome for the patient and an acceptable cost and inconvenience. The idea of a treatment able to substitute fully the functions of the failed kidney is misleading, because of the complexity of the kidney and the metabolic and endocrine functions which are not reproducible by any device. Only a continuous highly efficient treatment could restore the '*milieu interieur*' but technical problems of a 'wearable device' remain unsolved. Moreover, it has never been shown that an uninterrupted treatment provides the best clinical outcome, nor has the detoxification threshold below which no further advantage is gained, been identified.

Hitherto, although different dialysis strategies are available, the great majority of the patients are still treated in a standard way—which is a compromise, but not necessarily the best treatment. Alternative methods tailored to the individual patient's need, are available for particular clinical problems.

Although dialysis adequacy links clinical outcomes to a given dialysis dose, measured as small solute clearance, it is now agreed that other treatment-related factors affect patient outcome. The type of dialysis membrane, the method of solute removal (by convection or by diffusion), treatment-dependent factors of tolerance to ultrafiltration, the dialysis interval, are examples of relevant factors that may affect outcome of dialysis independently of its dose, particularly in high-risk patients. The gold standard for dialysis therapy has not been certainly identified yet and the aim of standard dialysis strategy is to reach an acceptable level of survival and rehabilitation for the majority of patients. Unfortunately, this level is far from being reached, as can be seen from the persistent high mortality rate in the dialysis population (USRDS 2001).

When to initiate dialysis in chronic renal failure

The appearance of symptoms of uraemia is an absolute indication to initiate dialysis (Table 1). However, it is a good clinical practice to prevent severe metabolic derangement by starting therapy before any symptoms appear (Hakim and Lazarus 1995).

The slow progression of renal failure allows adaptation of the patient to changes in metabolic state and the feeling of well-being is often maintained in spite of very low residual renal function. Appropriate pharmacological therapy may further delay the appearance of uraemic symptoms, for example, recombinant erythropoietin

Table 1 Absolute indications for initiating dialysis

Hyperkalaemia, not related to drug intake (i.e. RAS antagonists)
Bleeding
Fluid overload or pulmonary oedema
Hypertension, resistant to drug therapy
Pericarditis
Anorexia, nausea, vomiting
Uraemic neuropathy

for the improvement of anaemia or bicarbonate for the correction of acidosis. On the other hand, symptoms caused by adverse effects of drug therapy (e.g. antihypertensive drugs) may be inappropriately attributed to uraemia. The decision to start dialysis is reached, therefore, from a comprehensive clinical evaluation of the patient—a real challenge for the nephrologist's expertise. Indeed, patients free of symptoms are generally unwilling to start dialysis. There is also a tendency to delay the start for as long as possible because of limitations of dialysis resources. Objective measures to inform a correct decision have been identified, but should be considered only a guide and cannot substitute the clinical evaluation of the patient. Residual renal function is considered a crucial parameter in the patient follow-up. It is a widely held opinion that a glomerular filtration rate (GFR) less than 8–10 ml/min (Hakim and Lazarus 1995) is usually insufficient to maintain a stable clinical condition, but it has not been identified as an exact criterion for initiating dialysis. In fact, in some patients, without overt comorbidity and closely observing dietary prescription, dialysis may be further delayed, provided fluid balance, blood pressure, and phosphate concentration are controlled by pharmacological therapy.

On the contrary, significant comorbidities, such as diabetes mellitus or cardiovascular disease (CVD), or early signs of malnutrition suggest dialysis should be started despite higher values of residual renal clearance. Laboratory indexes may be misleading, unless linked to clinical evaluation of the patient. Increases in urea and creatinine may underestimate the real degree of insufficiency (Shemesh *et al.* 1985), since a spontaneous reduction of protein and energy intake may cause loss of lean body mass and a lower generation of both solutes, which may appear stable in time, hiding progressive malnutrition. Incipient malnutrition may be identified by the evaluation of body weight changes. Interference of fluid accumulation on body weight may be calculated by bioimpedance, a fast, non-invasive test of body composition. Malnutrition may also be detected with the help of laboratory parameters, such as albumin, prealbumin, serum transferrin, cholesterol (Hakim 1993), and creatinine itself, an expression of muscle mass. USRDS data suggest that a plasma creatinine concentration less than 10 mg/dl (880 μmol/l) at the start of dialysis is associated with an increased mortality rate (USRDS 1992).

Accurate measurement of GFR requires the use of other markers (Levey 1990), such as inulin or ^{125}I-iothalamate, since creatinine clearance overestimates residual renal function, due to tubular secretion, and urea clearance underestimates it, with an error of about 30–35 per cent in both cases. However, mean value of urea and creatinine clearance may provide an acceptable estimate of GFR because the errors balance out. The suggestion that dialysis be started when GFR values are less than 10 ml/min also arises from DOQI guidelines for peritoneal dialysis initiation (NKF-DOQI Clinical Practice Guidelines for Peritoneal Dialysis Adequacy). Indeed, a GFR of 10.5 ml/min per 1.73 m^2 corresponds to a urea clearance of about 7 ml/min and provides a weekly urea Kt/V of 2, the dose of continuous ambulatory peritoneal dialysis (CAPD) considered to be adequate.

Early initiation of dialysis, according to DOQI guidelines, could have some beneficial effect on patient survival, although clinical observations have provided conflicting results (Bonomini et al. 1985; Korevaar et al. 2001). Timely initiation of dialysis can prevent malnutrition, not always reversed following dialysis therapy, and improves patient rehabilitation. Furthermore, early dialysis may allow better control of hypertension and hyperphosphataemia, by means of the removal of fluid overload and phosphate excess, factors responsible for left ventricle hypertrophy and coronary vessel calcifications, respectively.

Patients with chronic renal failure should be prepared for dialysis when creatinine clearance is in the range of 15–20 ml/min and dialysis should be started if malnutrition is detected or, control of hypertension or hyperphosphataemia is unsatisfactory, irrespective of the clearance value. The strong working recommendation is not to delay starting dialysis when residual GFR is less than 10 ml/min.

Historical background

A review of the development of dialysis shows that the characteristics of standard dialysis have completely changed from the pioneering era of the artificial kidney, leading to a dramatic improvement in patient outcome.

In the early 1960s, when dialysis became a maintenance treatment for chronic renal failure, very long sessions lasting 10–12 h were necessary for a minimum acceptable control of uraemia, because of the low efficiency of the devices. Technical complications such as blood leaks in extracorporeal circulation, bacterial contamination of dialysate, unstable composition of dialysis solutions, and limited and fluctuating ultrafiltration rates were common problems causing unpredictable and often unsatisfactory results. Dialysis adequacy was empirically evaluated on the basis of the lack of uraemic symptoms. The advantage of a thrice weekly schedule in comparison to twice weekly dialysis was identified early on clinical grounds. When more efficient dialysers and A-V fistulae with high blood flows became available, the length of dialysis session could be reduced and short dialysis (4 h thrice weekly or 3 h every 2 days) became the standard dialysis strategy (Cambi et al. 1975).

The square metre/hour hypothesis (proposed by Scribner in 1971) to quantify dialysis prescription, was based on the concept that the volume of large solutes removed per week, with a given surface area, rather than the blood urea and creatinine, were important to prevent uraemic neuropathy, a troublesome and frequent complication of uraemia in that era. Later the middle molecule hypothesis stressed the important contribution of high molecular weight solutes in the uraemic toxicity.

In the late 1970s, the application of pharmacokinetic derived models to dialysis provided a more accurate guide to dialysis quantification, resulting in the 1980s in the formulation of the dialysis index Kt/V. Since the analysis of National Cooperative Dialysis Study, published in 1985, outcome of dialysis therapy was related to a combination of adequate protein-energy intake and a quantified amount of small solute clearance. Attention shifted from urea concentration to urea clearance, since concentration is not a constant parameter, depending on both dialysis removal and protein intake and so the Kt/V has now become the most popular parameter for dialysis dose quantification.

Although clinical evidence suggested the pivotal role of small solutes in the uraemic toxicity, the prospect of a better outcome of dialysis with the removal of larger toxic solutes was not invalidated and the availability of high flux membranes lead to introduction of haemofiltration in the 1970s. This treatment allowing removal of high molecular weight solutes by convection, mimics the performance of the kidney, although small solute clearances are limited by relatively low ultrafiltration rates, in comparison to diffusive clearance. Mixed convective and diffusive treatment, called haemodiafiltration, balances the low convective clearance. An improvement of the vascular stability was also observed with these treatments, offering a way to prevent dialysis hypotension.

In the middle 1980s, when dialysis amyloidosis was identified, these methods appeared as a possible means to remove β_2-microglobulin, a solute of 11.800 Da molecular weight that accumulates to cause amyloid deposits. Convection-based treatments provided an important contribution to the improvement of the quality of dialysis solution, and the importance of good microbiological water quality was also recognized for haemodialysis treatment. The production of dialysis membranes less prone to activating the complement cascade contributed to treatment biocompatibility especially when used with near sterile dialysis solutions.

In the late 1970s, CAPD was introduced as an alternative treatment of endstage renal failure (Popovich et al. 1976). Previously peritoneal dialysis was limited to the treatment of acute renal failure. Improvement in technology has made peritoneal dialysis today a valid alternative therapeutic modality, providing facility for home treatment allowing an increase in the numbers of treated patients.

Peritoneal dialysis (see also Chapter 12.4)

Technical improvement in peritoneal catheter manufacture and connection systems allows longer preservation of peritoneal integrity and longer survival of this dialysis modality in comparison to the pioneering era of its application, largely a result of a lower incidence of peritonitis. The clinical success of CAPD is confirmed by patient survival being no different from that of patients on haemodialysis (Collins et al. 1999).

The lower dialysis efficiency is balanced by the continuity of the treatment and/or better removal of higher molecular weight solutes. Abnormally high concentration of toxic solutes persist due to the low urea Kt/V achieved with the commonly exchanged dialysis solution volumes (2 l four times daily), but toxic solute concentration peaking as in extracorporeal intermittent treatments is prevented. This effect, with a more physiological fluid excess withdrawal, contributes to the success of modality. However, a relationship between the efficiency of the dialysis and nutritional status to mortality, morbidity, and technique failure has been demonstrated (CANUSA Study 1996). A Kt/V urea of 2.1 and a weekly creatinine clearance of 70 l/1.73 m^2 body surface area were both associated with a 78 per cent expected two-year survival rate and a minimum total weekly Kt/V urea of 2.0 and a creatinine clearance of 60 l/1.73 m^2 is now recommended (NKF-DOQI Guidelines 2001), since both parameters are independent predictors of treatment success. To the prospect of improved outcome by use of larger exchange volumes have been recently negated by the results of a multicentre study demonstrating no difference in survival and complications in a group of patients treated with higher than recommended clearance values (Paniagua et al. 2002).

Beside CAPD, other types of intermittent peritoneal dialysis are available. The intermittent regimens typically utilize multiple short dwells and automated technology regulating inflow and outflow of dialysate. Automated peritoneal dialysis (APD) includes nightly intermittent peritoneal dialysis (NIPD), consisting in multiple overnight dwell with the abdominal cavity drained of dialysate daytime, and tidal peritoneal dialysis (TPD), performed with the peritoneal cavity always containing some dialysate (usually one-half full). TPD improves comfort and facilitates drainage in some patients, but it requires a larger volume of dialysate and is more difficult to perform (Juergensen et al. 1999). Continuous cyclic peritoneal dialysis (CCPD) is an automated form of therapy in which a cycler delivers three to six overnight exchanges with a 12–15 h daytime dwell. More dialysate fluid is generally required each day and this increases the cost of the technique.

The choice of the type of dialysis is made according to peritoneal permeability characteristics of the individual patient with the goal of maximizing solute transport and allowing adequate fluid withdrawal. Urea and creatinine diffuse easily into the dialysate and are rapidly removed in the first few hours of a dwell. Larger solutes do not equilibrate as rapidly and they continue to be removed throughout the dwelling time, although removal of β2-microglobulin is very low. The rate of small solute transport is however variable and it may be measured by the peritoneal equilibration test (Twardowski 1990). Patients are classified as rapid or slow transporters, with the possibility of intermediate categories. Rapid transporters achieve almost total equilibration between plasma and dialysate urea and creatinine in a few hours. They also absorb the glucose contained in the dialysate rapidly, thereby removing the osmotic drive to ultrafiltration. Eventually, solute removal is also impaired, since the solutes that have diffused into the dialysate are also absorbed back into the systemic circulation In this setting prolonged dwell times, as in CAPD, will not produce sufficient fluid or solute removal. This would require the more frequent use of hypertonic dialysate (2.5 or 4.25 per cent dextrose), potentially inducing hyperglycaemia, hypertriglyceridaemia, and obesity. An alternative in such cases is to perform frequent short dwells in order to prevent glucose absorption with NIPD. On the contrary, slow transporters need longer dwell times to remove small solutes but the glucose gradient is not dissipated, allowing ultrafiltration. Such individuals are good candidates for CAPD. Most patients may start peritoneal dialysis with CAPD or CCPD. The choice depends on patient's preference, since CCPD allows more time for daytime activities,

but requires the presence of a partner. It is a good choice for elderly dependent patients, allowing a family member to participate in patient care without interfering with their own lifestyle.

Treatment failure may occur over time when total solute clearance as measured by weekly Kt/V urea and creatinine clearance declines to less than a minimal allowed value because of loss of residual renal function (Burkart et al. 1996). A compensatory increase of peritoneal clearance is thus necessary to maintain dialysis efficiency, although it is not clear that peritoneal clearance is equivalent to renal clearance in terms of long-time results. A higher peritoneal clearance is not easy to obtain while maintaining an acceptable peritoneal integrity because of the patient discomfort of larger or more frequent volume exchanges. In this setting, it is sometime possible to improve peritoneal clearances by shifting the patient from CAPD to APD, with rapid and more frequent dwells in a limited part of the day. This modality also allows the maintenance of a good ultrafiltration rate, in spite of the high glucose reabsorption rate of the peritoneal membrane (Heimburger et al. 1990). APD, however, is a less continuous treatment than CAPD and higher clearances are necessary to maintain efficiency equivalent to that of CAPD. A 10–20 per cent increase in Kt/V and a 5–10 per cent increase in weekly urea clearance are recommended in CCPD and NIPD, respectively (NKF-DOQI 2001). These problems can explain the frequent treatment failure, and reinforce the need to assess the peritoneum efficiency regularly over time (at least every six months), for timely intervention to maintain adequate total clearances. When it is impossible, a switch to extracorporeal treatments is necessary, despite the reluctance of the patient to change.

Standard haemodialysis

Standard haemodialysis is performed thrice-weekly, for 4–5 h each session, with low-flux membranes. There has, since the 1960s, been a general technical improvement in dialysis machines, dialysers, and dialysis solutions. Dialyser performance has improved, thanks to better assembling of the fibres, more efficient fluid geometry, and higher membrane permeability per surface area unit. Improved haemodynamic stability is assured by accurate control of the ultrafiltration rate by new dialysis machines and more precise control of electrolyte dialysate composition. Reverse osmosis systems producing good quality water for dialysate generation are in common use and some dialysis machine are supplied with an additional ultrafiltration facility producing ultrapure dialysate. The substitution of acetate as dialysate buffer with bicarbonate has improved vascular stability. Cuprophan membranes have been replaced by more biocompatible cellulose-modified or synthetic membranes, sterilized with agents safer than ethylene oxide.

The dialyser

The choice of the dialyser is not straightforward. Dialyser efficiency is indicated by its permeability to solutes (KoA) and is proportional to the surface area, for the same membrane. This parameter allows one to calculate the expected solute diffusive clearance for each value of blood and dialysate flow (Salem and Mujais 1993). For standard dialysis, a urea KoA of 600 is generally adequate, since it provides a clearance of about 210 ml/min at 300 ml blood flow of the pump, when the Hct is 35 per cent, plasma protein 60 g/l and dialysate flow 500 ml/min. In this setting, a Kt/V of 1.2 may be reached in 240 min in a patient weighing 70 kg body weight. When higher clearances are required, for example, in larger patients, a dialyser with greater KoA will provide only small advantage, unless blood flow is increased. As an example, an increase of KoA to 800 will correspond to a urea clearance of 227 ml/min, when blood flow is set at 300 ml/min. An increase of blood flow up to 400 ml/min will provide a clearance of 240 and 266 ml/min when dialysers with 600 and 800 KoA, respectively, are used. The current trend is to choose more efficient dialysers, in the belief that 'more is better', but a very high KoA is no better for solute removal unless blood flow is also high.

Dialysers with KoA greater than 600 may be suitable for smaller patients. There is no need to use less efficient dialysers to prevent dialysis disequilibrium syndrome in the first dialysis sessions. This risk can be reduced by reversing the connection of dialysate lines with the dialyser (co-current) and reducing blood flow. As an example, when using a dialyser with 600 KoA in co-current flow at 200 ml/min blood flow, the clearance of urea is about 127 ml/min, low enough to prevent disequilibrium. In contrast, a reduction of blood flow to 200 ml/min, while maintaining a *counter*-current flow, corresponds to a high clearance of approximately 160 ml/min. Too low blood flow may increase the risk of clotting in the extracorporeal circuit.

Substitution of Cuprophan membranes with cellulose-modified or synthetic membranes is believed to improve the biocompatibility of the treatment (Hakim 1993). However, all components of dialysis apparatus contribute to biocompatibility including line composition and water and dialysate quality. *In vitro* and *in vivo* tests demonstrate lower complement activation and cytokine induction with biocompatible membrane. Clear evidence of prolonged survival or reduced morbidity with more biocompatible membrane is still lacking.

Synthetic and some cellulose-modified, but not Cuprophan membranes reduce plasma levels of β2-microglobulin and may thus delay the appearance of dialysis amyloidosis (Hakim *et al.* 1996). It is still debated whether better removal, lower generation, or both contribute to this effect. The use of Cuprophan membranes should therefore be avoided, or limited to patients likely to be on haemodialysis short term, for example, those with a high probability of early transplantation or elderly uncomplicated patient with short lifespan expectancy.

Dialysis with high-flux membranes

High-flux dialysis membranes are characterized by higher solute permeability, allowing better removal of larger solutes not usually affected by cellulose membranes. Solute and water permeability are necessarily related, thus high-flux membranes have a higher ultrafiltration coefficient. At spontaneous transmembrane pressure, due to inner filter resistance and venous line resistance, ultrafiltration may exceed the patient's need for balancing interdialysis weight gain. Dialysis machines equipped with ultrafiltration control automatically create a positive hydraulic pressure, preventing excessive weight loss, but causing backfiltration of dialysate. When a higher transmembrane pressure is applied, a higher ultrafiltration rate is achieved and the excessive fluid loss must be replaced by sterile solutions, infused into the extracorporeal circulation, as in haemofiltration and haemodiafiltration.

The improved microbiological quality of the water produced by sophisticated water-treatment systems and the possibility of producing ultrapure dialysate with a filter added in the dialysate circuit avoid the risk of blood contamination by dialysate backfiltration and allow the use of the same dialysis solution as on line produced reinfusion solutions. Indeed, larger volumes of reinfusion solution are needed, in particular for haemofiltration, since the high haematocrits obtained in patients on erythropoietin lower the real plasma water blood flow and the filtration fraction in the filter, thus limiting the solute clearance. In the majority of the patients, therefore, only the predilution modality is practicable, especially for haemofiltration, and a large reinfusion volume about 1.5 times the volume of total body water (i.e. about 65 l for 70 kg body weight.) is necessary to achieve an adequate Kt/V value. Only on line production keeps the cost of such treatment acceptable.

New dialysis membranes with high adsorption properties are able to capture endotoxin fragments crossing the filter because of their low molecular weight, and improve the safety of high-flux dialysis while maintaining larger solute clearances as high as those of convection-based modalities, without the need of reinfusion solution. High quality of the water is still recommended also for this modality of dialysis.

High-flux dialysis, which requires more complicated dialysis machines and a highly efficient water-treatment system, has not produced convincing clinical benefit. Controlled long-term studies comparing high- and low-flux treatments with clear-cut endpoints, such as mortality and morbidity are still lacking. The advantage of the observed reduction, albeit not to normal values, of the concentration of some identified high molecular weight toxic solutes, is still theoretical. A controlled randomized trial (Locatelli *et al.* 1996) failed to observe any advantages in terms of tolerance and improvement of nutritional parameters, while a marginal reduction of β2-microglobulin was observed. Further effects of these treatments on single solutes removal and cardiovascular stability are discussed below.

Limits of standard dialysis (see also Chapter 12.5)

Although CVD remains the main cause of death (USRDS 2001) in dialysis patients, several risks factors for increased morbidity and mortality have been identified. Apart from the usual CVD risk factors, specific risk factors related to uraemia or dialysis treatment *per se* have been identified (Cheung *et al.* 2000) namely anaemia, malnutrition, persistent fluid overload, accelerated atherosclerosis, calcium-phosphate imbalance, and chronic inflammation (Kaysen 2001). An optimal dialysis strategy should limit these factors, but despite four decades of uninterrupted advances of engineering, biophysical, microbiological research, and these have not radically changed mortality, morbidity, and quality of life of dialysis patients.

The real challenge for dialysis therapy is to modify current dialysis prescription to improve dialysis dose, further improving solute removal and uraemia-related complications, to enhance haemodynamic stability, by improving ultrafiltration and preventing biocompatibility-related reactions.

The problem of the effective dialysis dose

Dialysis dose is quantified by the Kt/V index, corresponding to body water fractional clearance, given by the product of urea clearance (K) and dialysis time (t), divided by the volume of body water (V). Survival data for dialysis patients shows the relationship between dialysis dose and the risk of death. This risk progressively declines with the increase of Kt/V and reaches a plateau beyond values of Kt/V

of 1.2–1.4, that is, 3.6 per week in a standard thrice weekly dialysis schedule, corresponding to the current treatment modality for the majority of patients. The Kt/V provided by normal kidney (weekly urea clearance per litre of body water) is about four times greater than that provided by dialysis therapy, so it is surprising that no advantage of higher dialysis doses is apparent.

Dialysis dose and urea removal

Thrice-weekly dialysis schedule is an asymmetric treatment, because there are two short interdialysis intervals and a long interval at the end of the week. In a hypothetical symmetric dialysis cycle with constant interdialysis interval, stable urea generation rate and constant Kt/V, pre- and postdialysis urea concentrations are the same in any dialysis session when a steady state has been achieved. The amount of urea removed by each dialysis is also the same as is the weekly removal if a weekly asymmetric dialysis cycle is considered. When Kt/V is modified (e.g. by increasing the clearance), a new steady state is reached after some dialysis sessions with reduced pre- and post-dialysis concentrations, but ultimately urea removal does not change. In fact, in a steady state condition, the stability requires removal of exactly the amount of urea generated. Since generation is constant, removal must also be constant—a paradox of constant removal in spite of different efficiency. Thus removal does not depend on dialysis efficiency so a Kt/V increase by means of higher clearance, while keeping dialysis duration unchanged, will not lead to an increased removal, but to a reduction of both pre- and postdialysis concentrations. However, this effect is limited and tends to plateau for very high Kt/V values, as it is shown in Fig. 1.

An increase of the dose beyond a Kt/V of 4–4.5, obtained by increasing the clearance in standard thrice weekly dialysis schedule does not increase urea removal, has a marginal effect on predialysis

urea concentration and will not affect the fluctuation of post- versus predialysis urea concentrations.

Dialysis interval as a parameter of dialysis efficiency

Independently of the level of postdialysis concentration, the interdialysis increase of urea concentration is constant for a given patient since urea generation rate is constant. Therefore, the only way to reduce urea accumulation and the consequent increase of urea concentration is to reduce the length of interdialysis interval. Change of interdialysis interval will have significant effects on the urea profile, independent of weekly Kt/V, and interdialysis interval behaves as a parameter of dialysis efficiency no less important than dialysis dose. Indeed, weekly dialysis dose apparently corresponds to the sum of Kt/V of the single dialysis sessions and in theory it should be possible to reach the same weekly dose independently of the number of dialyses, provided the Kt/V value of single session is appropriately modified. However, the effect on urea concentration of the same weekly dialysis dose is different if the length of interdialysis interval changes, as illustrated in Fig. 2.

The increase in dialysis frequency and the consequent reduction of the intervals progressively reduces fluctuation of pre- to postconcentration and this can in theory have same clinical advantage for the patient, since it improves the stability of body composition with favourable effects on dialysis-induced symptoms. Also predialysis concentration can be eventually lowered.

Removal of other toxic solute by dialysis

The morbidity and mortality of dialysis patients has been related to urea kinetics, independently of the low toxicity of this solute. Indeed, urea is only a marker of low molecular weight solutes, and uraemic toxicity is mainly related to this class of toxins. Clinical evidence confirms, however, that higher molecular weight solutes contribute to

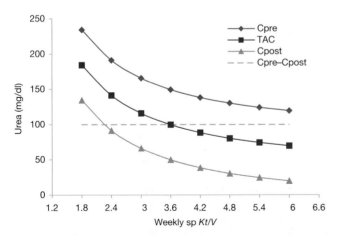

Fig. 1 Urea concentration change as function of weekly Kt/V, calculated with the single pool urea model (sp), in a thrice-weekly 4-h dialysis and variable clearance. A 50% increase of weekly Kt/V above the standard value (i.e. from 3.6 to 5.4) lowers predialysis concentration by only 17% (from 149 to 124 mg/dl) since the curve representing the concentration as a function Kt/V progressively flattens out with the increase in the dialysis efficiency. Time-averaged concentration (TAC) of urea features in a similar way. The difference of pre–post dialysis concentration is constant, in spite of increasing Kt/V values, since the generation is constant and removal is also constant. (Parameters: urea distribution volume = 35 l; generation = 11.2 mg/min; renal clearance = 0.)

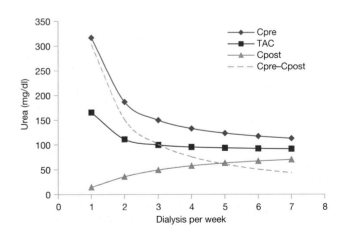

Fig. 2 Single pool (sp) urea kinetic model. Urea concentration change as function of the number of dialysis per week. Weekly sp Kt/V = 3.6, constant. Shortening dialysis interval causes lower fluctuation of pre- to postdialysis concentration. (Parameters: urea distribution volume = 35 l; generation rate = 11.2 mg/min; clearance = 200 ml/min; renal function = 0.)

uraemic toxicity so alternative dialysis strategies are needed to improve their removal.

β2-Microglobulin (see Chapter 11.3.10)

β2-Microglobulin is a 11.8 kDa-protein responsible of dialysis amyloidosis. Several factors contribute to the clinical manifestations of amyloidosis such as the dialysate composition and its microbiological quality. Such factors, which have changed over the last years as part of general improvements in dialysis care, may explain why the prevalence of the amyloidosis appears to be decreasing. Prevention or delay of the disease may be possible using high-flux synthetic membranes for haemodialysis or haemodiafiltration, since only in patients dialysed with more permeable synthetic high-flux membranes is a significant reduction of the plasma level described (Floege and Ketteler 2001). With these dialysis strategies, it is difficult to distinguish the effect of a better biocompatibility from that of an increased removal.

To improve the removal of such a large solute, the slow equilibration of its distribution volume with the plasma must be taken into account. Otherwise, the high postdialysis rebound will cancel the dialysis-induced reduction of plasma concentration. Therefore, high-flux membranes should be combined with prolonged dialysis sessions to allow intercompartmental solute shift to occur.

The simple reduction of dialysis interval, as in short daily haemodialysis, has little effect on reduction of plasma β2-microglobulin, nor has daily haemofiltration lowered the concentration to normal. Only frequent long treatments such as nocturnal haemodialysis, performed with high-flux membranes might return β2-microglobulin concentration towards normal.

Homocysteine

Hyperhomocysteinaemia is an independent risk factor for cardiovascular disease in chronic haemodialysis patients and treatment with folic acid normalizes total homocysteine (tHcy) in only a minority.

New dialysers with very high permeability may lead to significant reduction, but not normalization, of predialysis tHcy concentration, while normal high-flux membrane fail to show any effect on this solute (Van Tellingen 2001). The clinical advantages of this effect remains theoretical. Furthermore, it is possible that increased loss of water-soluble vitamins, such as folate, with high-flux membrane may have detrimental effects on homocysteine metabolism. The same is true for increased protein loss through highly permeable membranes in high-flux treatment, when up to 20 g of protein per session could be lost. The loss of protein may of course increase the removal of protein-bound toxic solutes, but the effect on nutrition of such a loss cannot be ignored.

Complement

The complement system can be activated in the extracorporeal circulation even if biocompatible membranes are used. Complement is an important candidate in the genesis of microinflammation and accelerated atherogenesis in ESRD and some authors have stressed the potential advantage, even still theoretical, of removing factor D with high-flux dialysis (Deppish 2001).

Leptin

Leptin is a protein produced by fat cells and involved in body weight regulation. Plasma leptin is significantly greater in some haemodialysis patients than in normal controls. In patients on haemodiafiltration with high-flux dialysers, a reduction of initial serum-free leptin values was observed, whereas bound leptin remained unaffected. Other studies have demonstrated that dialysis with high-flux dialysers and haemodiafiltration led to a substantial reduction of leptin concentration, while the cellulose membrane dialyser did not (Widjaja et al. 2000).

Advanced glycated endproducts

Advanced glycate endproduct (AGE) peptides, involved in the genesis of atherosclerosis, can be removed with highly permeable membranes. The removal is limited to compounds with a molecular mass less than 12 kDa. A significant reduction of plasma pentosidine during high-flux dialysis in non-diabetic patients has been described but protein associated compounds as the Amadori product fructoselysine are not removed (Henle et al. 1999). Once more, clinical advantages of these results have not been demonstrated.

Phosphate

Phosphate kinetics are those of a large solute. There is a high postdialysis rebound, reflecting a slow intercompartmental equilibration and the amount removed by dialysis is always insufficient to balance the phosphate intake when the protein content of the diet is appropriate. The use of high-flux membranes for haemodialysis or haemodiafiltration and increasing the surface area of the dialyser membrane can remove phosphate more efficiently, although no improvement is seen in the predialysis phosphate levels (Man et al. 1991). This contrasts with slow continuous treatments, as continuous venovenous dialysis (CVVH), which lead to subnormal phosphate levels and the need of phosphate supplementation during dialysis.

Daily dialysis does seem to be able to establish phosphate balance, and a reduction of the need for phosphate binders, in spite of an increase of protein intake, has been described. Long daily dialysis, for example, nocturnal dialysis, is effective for patients with phosphate imbalance, but a risk of adynamic bone disease has been described. In same cases, phosphate has been added to dialysate in order to prevent excessive mineral depletion.

It is interesting to note that longer dialysis treatments remove a higher mass of phosphate, but also may result in significantly higher postdialysis phosphate concentrations. This is explained by phosphate being mobilized to a greater extent in long dialysis, probably from pathological stores in bone. When plasma phosphate is very low, new phosphate synthesis occurs. This synthesis in a fourth pool located in the intracellular space must be taken into account for kinetic calculation. It probably corresponds to glycophosphate compounds as described in some in vitro studies (Spalding et al. 2002). This phenomenon, aimed to prevent life-threatening hypophosphataemia, could lead in the long term to phosphate depletion in some patients, since the newly generated phosphate compounds can also be eliminated by long-term treatment.

Effect of dialysis on special clinical problems

Anaemia

The most efficient therapy for uraemia-related anaemia is the administration of epoietin or darbepoietin and adequate iron supplementation.

Dialysis improves the effect of epoietin and some patients may achieve an adequate Hb without it. Low dialysis dose is associated with anaemia and an improvement in Hb may be obtained when Kt/V is increased to values greater than 1. There is some evidence of a further improvement of Hb with high efficiency dialysis and high flux membranes, however, controlled studies have failed to confirm these results (Locatelli et al. 2000). An increase in dialysis frequency, in particular daily dialysis, seems to improve Hb.

Membrane biocompatibility could impair erythrocyte survival by enhancing the so-called oxidant stress (i.e. production of ROS, lipid oxidation etc.), due to the leucocyte activation after membrane contact. Erythrocyte membrane changes may follow reducing red cell survival. Vitamin E coated membranes seems to reduce dialysis-related oxidant stress, but similar results could be obtained with the administration of the vitamin. Preventing leucocyte activation with the use of more biocompatible membrane and ultrapure dialysate should also reduce oxidant stress. Leucocyte activation may also contribute to the persistence of a chronic inflammatory status, identified through abnormal plasma acute phase proteins, such as SAA and C-reactive protein, as evidenced in several dialysis patients. In these conditions, the response to EPO administration is blunted.

Malnutrition

Malnutrition is a common problem in chronic renal failure manifesting as early as at a GFR of 50 (Ikizler et al. 1995). A variable proportion of chronic dialysis patients, ranging from 20 to 70 per cent in different countries, are malnourished.

The causes of malnutrition are the dialysis procedure itself, for example, loss of nutrients through the dialysate; the hypercatabolic effect of the bioincompatible dialysis membranes; metabolic acidosis; but the most important factor is chronic inflammation. A further important role is played by therapeutic measures: drugs, phosphate binders, and nutritional restrictions.

Inadequate dialysis may contribute to malnutrition, but the positive effects of increased dialysis dose beyond the recommended value is not obvious. It is possible that an increase of effective dialysis dose, obtained by changing dialysis schedule and reducing dialysis interval, may improve nutritional status. Recently, Galland et al. (2001) studied nutritional parameters in eight patients treated six times per week. Total weekly time and dialysis modalities were not changed. The weekly Kt/V only increased from 4.1 to 4.5. Each patient served as his own control. The increase in appetite and food intake was impressive. Several authors describing experience of either short daily dialysis (Kooistra and Vos 1999; Williams et al. 1999; Woods et al. 1999); long nocturnal daily dialysis (Pierratos and Ouwendyk 1999; Williams et al. 1999) or long thrice weekly treatment (Charra et al. 1992), confirm an improvement in appetite, protein intake, nutritional parameters, though not always statistically significant. The impressive clinical improvement in these patients especially the nutritional status is unequivocal and a contribution of the higher dialysis dose is a likely explanation.

The advantages of the treatment protocols in Tassin (Charra et al. 1992) may depend not only on the increase of the dose of each dialysis session, but also on the reduction, albeit small, of interdialysis interval, a consequence of the prolonged dialysis time (40 instead of 44 h, as in standard dialysis). Indeed, predialyis concentrations of markers are lesser than that reached by standard dialysis or short daily dialysis. How can the exceptional impact on nutrition obtained by short daily dialysis be explained? Dialysis strategies dealing with sessions of very long duration and daily frequency, share a better vascular stability and less postdialysis fatigue; moreover pre- and postdialysis swinging of solutes is less

than in standard dialysis. It is possible that this much reduced fluid and solute disequilibrium maintains a better homeostatic environment.

There is no doubt that increasing the effective dialysis dose is the key requirement to improve or even normalize the nutritional status in most dialysis patients and a real increase in dialysis dose can only be obtained by an increase in dialysis duration and/or dialysis frequency. Whereas in progressive renal failure the signs of uraemic toxicity appear with a spontaneous reduction of protein intake when the GFR is less than 50 ml/min, daily dialysis seems to correct most of the nutritional derangements in spite of a very limited correction of the retention of traditional uraemic toxins and a very limited increase in the effective clearance.

It can be postulated that the 'milieu interieur' of the dialysis patient responds with a physiological correction of malnutrition, as a consequence of the significant reduction of post- versus predialysis fluctuations.

Cardiovascular stability and tolerance to ultrafiltration

The role of the membrane and dialysis modality

Convection-based treatments such as haemofiltration and haemodiafiltration improve tolerance to fluid loss in comparison to haemodialysis, thanks to a more effective activation of physiological compensatory mechanisms to hypovolaemia. The explanation has not been identified, but several lines of evidence suggest that dialysis-induced hypotension is multifactorial. Sodium balance, temperature change, and treatment biocompatibility are probably the major factors accounting for the lower incidence of hypotensive episodes during convection-based treatments.

In spite of experimental evidence supporting the role of single factors, it is difficult to identify their relative contribution from results of clinical studies. However, it was possible to reproduce at least in part the good results of haemo(dia)filtration in haemodialysis, by manipulating both sodium balance and by cooling the dialysate.

Van der Sande et al. (2001) demonstrated that different thermal balance is achieved in haemodialysis and haemodiafiltration. Cooling dialysate probably makes haemodialysis as good as haemodiafiltration in respect of vascular stability. Moreover, when the infusion rate of solution at room temperature increases in haemodiafiltration, vascular stability increases, suggesting the pivotal role of thermal balance in preventing ultrafiltration-induced hypotension.

The importance of sodium balance is confirmed by the favourable results obtained by profiling the sodium concentration of dialysate, to combine high ultrafiltration rate with high sodium concentration in the first part of the session, when the increased plasma osmolality allows fluid removal without symptoms (Oliver et al. 2001). The sodium concentration, and the ultrafiltration rate, are thus progressively reduced during the session, to prevent positive sodium balance.

The role of biocompatibility in haemodynamic instability is a matter of debate. The lower incidence of intradialytic hypotension observed in haemofiltration and haemodiafiltration could be attributed to better biocompatibility of the synthetic membranes commonly used. On the other hand, high-flux synthetic membranes are more permeable to dialysate contaminants and dialysate contamination by pyrogen is considered as an important bio-incompatibility factor. Endotoxins derived from dialysate are able to cross most dialysis membranes by both backdiffusion and backfiltration transport mechanisms. The positive effects of membrane biocompatibility are therefore cancelled out by the endotoxin-dependent activation of white cells. The results of clinical studies aimed to compare different dialysis modalities are often both conflicting or inconclusive. No difference in the incidence of dialysis hypotension was in fact observed when polysulfone membranes were compared to Cuprophan membrane (Bergamo Study Group 1991).

Locatelli compared Cuprophan dialysis, low-flux polysulfone dialysis, high-flux polysulfone dialysis and high-flux polysulfone HDF in a prospective randomized study (Locatelli *et al.* 1996). Treatment tolerance, in terms of hypotension, was not different between the four dialysis methods, however, the incidence of hypotension in the population as a whole was low, which could have hidden any difference. Conflicting or inconclusive results of the other less controlled studies, comparing synthetic and cellulosic membrane reflect the difficulty of performing controlled clinical studies, in which all factors contributing to vascular instability are taken into account.

Recently, a relationship between inflammation and dialysis-induced hypotension, based on an increase in markers of inflammation in hypotension-prone patients has been proposed. It has also been suggested that convection-based treatments could reduce the risk of inflammation thanks to better biocompatibility and a lower risk of pyrogen transfer to the patient. This may depend on the fact that patient-related factors such as diastolic dysfunction or reduced vascular compliance may affect the tolerance to ultrafiltration more than treatment-related factors do.

The role of dialysis frequency and duration

Independently of the dialysis modality, the increase of the frequency and the length of the treatment improve the tolerance of ultrafiltration. Haemodynamic stability is a common benefit of both daily dialysis (Kooistra and Vos 1999; Williams *et al.* 1999; Woods *et al.* 1999; Galland *et al.* 2001) and traditional long dialysis sessions performed with smoother changes of fluid overload (Charra *et al.* 1992).

The correction or normalization of systolic and diastolic blood pressure, the reduction or complete withdrawal of antihypertensive therapy was a common achievement in all these studies. These results were always associated with an immediate reduction of postdialysis body weight, lower fluctuations of intradialytic weight, and disappearance of cramps or acute intradialysis hypotension.

When daily dialysis was prolonged up to 1 year, a significant reduction of left ventricular mass index was also observed (Galland *et al.* 2001). The almost immediate haemodynamic response confirms that volume overload is the main cause or, at least, the most important factor contributing to hypertension in almost all hypertensive dialysis patients. However, the total duration of the presently published trials of the new haemodialysis strategies especially daily dialysis, is limited and a long-term adaptation of the patients to the newly achieved fluid balance cannot be excluded. The only trial examining the haemodynamic results of daily dialysis is the long-term experience of Tassin but the limits of the haemodynamic parameters of this study have been emphasized (Gotch *et al.* 1997).

Choosing a dialysis strategy

Different dialysis modalities may be offered to patients starting dialysis therapy, but most guarantee clinical success. There being no gold standard treatment, practical considerations mean the best compromise between patient's need and therapeutic options should be sought.

Practice varies from country to country, depending on a number of factors, such as the economic state of the country, allocation of resources for health care, reliance on transplantation and not least, the local expertise. Moreover, some patient-related factors independent of clinical aspects, may determine the choice of the therapy. The distance of the patient from the hospital, availability of family support, patient's compliance and willingness to cooperate actively in his/her own care, employment, are some examples of factors affecting the choice of dialysis option. In some countries, economic reimbursement is offered to the patient's family to encourage home treatments.

The prospective of early transplantation may justify a suboptimal choice, although within the limits of adequacy, because the duration of time spent on dialysis will be short. It is, nevertheless, mandatory to ensure even in the short term, that effective control of anaemia, hypertension and Ca–P metabolism be achieved because of the future effects of these abnormalities on transplant survival and clinical complications. Moreover, the possibility of returning to dialysis therapy after transplant rejection means vascular access and peritoneal integrity of the patient must be preserved.

A good dialysis policy should offer not only a treatment tailored to the patient's need, but also the option to shift the patient to an alternative treatment in case of complication. When a complete range of therapeutic options is available, it is possible to encourage home dialysis as first-choice treatment, with the option to treat the patient with limited care or in-centre dialysis, not only during intercurrent illness, but also to relieve the patient or the family of the burden of clinical care. Early referral to a nephrologist allows the choice of the most suitable dialysis option, without the need for emergency vascular access.

There are few limitations to treatment choices, so the choice of the first treatment is often driven by patient preference. CAPD is not appropriate in cases of obesity, multiple abdominal surgical procedures, or abdominal herniae. Moreover, the patient's likely compliance and ability to perform the procedure safely must be taken into account. A clean environment at the patient's home or work is required. Obviously haemodialysis cannot be performed without vascular access. A severe coagulopathy is a relative contraindication, since treatment can be performed without anticoagulation of the extracorporeal circuit.

In patients with highly compromised vascular stability, CAPD may improve tolerance to fluid loss, although extracorporeal treatments may be acceptable with the help of cooling dialysate, sodium and ultrafiltration profiling, or the use of convection treatment.

Independently of the long-term effects on survival and morbidity, increasing dialysis frequency is a powerful tool to improve vascular stability. Our experience since mid-1970s (Cambi *et al.* 1975) confirms the good and sometimes unexpected results of every other day dialysis instead of classical thrice weekly schedule for a close control of fluid balance and prevention of dialysis-induced hypotension. The apparently high cost in terms of organization of such a policy should be accurately evaluated in the light of these favourable results. On the contrary, the application of sequential ultrafiltration–dialysis or sodium profile of dialysate not associated with ultrafiltration profile seems to be less effective for the prevention of dialysis hypotension (Oliver *et al.* 2001).

Specific circumstances may limit the choice of selected treatments, often because of difficulties in performing them, related to greater patient discomfort and logistic problem of dialysis unit. Difficulty in phosphate control, for instance, means the need for longer and more frequent extracorporeal treatments, such as nocturnal daily dialysis.

The feasibility of these options cannot be excluded *a priori* and should be evaluated taking account of saving days of hospitalization for dialysis complications.

In order to plan a correct dialysis strategy in an anuric dialysis patient, some important kinetic principles should be considered.

1. Urea kinetic model derived by the comparison between continuous treatment (CAPD) and intermittent dialysis has been proposed to evaluate the effect of different frequencies on the whole dialysis dose. It can be shown that in the absence of residual renal function, a dialysis frequency of two sessions per week does not reach even the minimum weekly standard required for peritoneal dialysis (stKt/V per week: 2) (Depner 1999).

2. The belief that an extreme increase of the dialyser clearance and short dialysis session is insufficient to obtain an effective correction of the uraemic environment is presently shared by most authorities. The exceptionally low mortality rate of the patients treated in Tassin by Charra, who is operating with a dialysis schedule of 8 h thrice weekly and a spKt/V of 1.6, can be explained not only by the more effective dialysis dose, but by a better control of hypertension. However, Gotch *et al.*, who analysed the results of the Tassin population, underlined the difficulties in relating the impact of survival to the Kt/V due to the wide distribution of the Kt/V values in these unselected population (Gotch *et al.* 1997).

3. Prolonged, more frequent treatment as the slow nocturnal haemodialysis combines the advantages of high frequency with the possibility of removing large or slowly diffusible solutes (including phosphate and β_2-microglobulin).

For almost three decades, technology has been oriented to maximize the value of the dialyser clearance and membrane geometry and just accepting a schedule of three times a week for 3–4 h per session. The logical endpoint was the development of hardware (dialysers, membranes, electronic sensors) very helpful in limiting the side-effect of extremely high clearance and ultrafiltration, but ignoring the fundamental need to correct the unphysiological internal environment.

The proper way to deal with daily constant solute generation, is to reduce the interdialysis interval and utilize the dialysis efficiency of the first part of the session properly. The endless debate on the nature of the uraemic toxins has been re-opened in the light of the preliminary results of daily dialysis. The most important achievement of the daily treatment is neither an extreme reduction of predialysis concentration of several solutes (small and especially larger solutes) nor a significant increase of the treatment time in comparison to the uninterrupted activity of the normal human kidney.

The improvement of the clinical status of the patients seems to be mainly related to a better management and reduced fluctuations of water, electrolytes, and acid–base homeostasis. The improvement of the subjective symptoms and quality of life outweighs the correction of small molecules retention. The control of fluid, electrolyte, and acid–base homeostasis is of paramount importance.

While anaemia and metabolic acidosis are completely controlled with epoetin and by an accurate choice of the dialysate composition, the recovery of protein intake is multifactorial but is certainly more influenced by the improvement of fluid homeostasis, including the control of postdialysis fatigue, acute and/or prolonged postdialysis hypotension, correction of metabolic acidosis, and hidden or manifest heart failure.

A very intriguing observation regarding clinical outcome of daily dialysis was made from Buoncristiani, the world's longest pioneer of daily dialysis (Buoncristiani 1998). In the early 1980s, they used to treat a limited patient population with low-efficiency daily dialysis with a session length of 90 min and a frequency of six to seven treatments per week. The average post- versus predialysis urea concentration was respectively 149 versus 182 mg/dl with a reduction of 19 per cent and the weekly Kt/V was approximately 1.9. In spite of this very modest dialysis dose, they describe in this pioneer paper a reduction of uraemia-related symptoms (thirst, lack of appetite, insomnia, fatigue), improvement of anaemia, peripheral neuropathy, physical strength and blood pressure control.

The discrepancy between the almost marginal correction of traditional uraemic markers and the general improvement of the clinical condition is intruiging. More recently, Kooistra and Vos (1999) moved 13 patients from thrice weekly to daily dialysis for a period of 6 months, without changing Kt/V. In this limited period, they did not observe a significant improvement of several nutritional parameters described by others. However, he stresses the improvement or disappearance of the same subjective uraemia-related symptoms described by Buoncristiani.

If the above observation is correct, it follows that the concept of replacing native kidney function completely with the artificial kidney is, in some sense, misguided. It is probably sufficient and more realistic, as suggested by daily dialysis and in part by peritoneal dialysis success, to limit fluctuations around the steady state and to maintain toxic solute concentrations below a certain threshold value not necessarily in the normal range.

In this sense, the artificial kidney is 'ideal' when, independently of any inappropriate comparison with the human kidney, it is capable of offering the patient the feeling of an appropriate physical and intellectual quality of life. This can be obtained with the present dialysis strategies, which guarantee a superior effective dialysis dose.

Dialysis treatment should always be appropriately tailored to each individual patient taking account of clinical state and residual renal function.

References

Bergamo Collaborative Dialysis Study Group (1991). Acute intradialytic well being: result of a clinical trial comparing polysulfone with Cuprophan. *Kidney International* **40**, 714–719.

Bonomini, V. *et al.* (1985). Benefits of early initiation of dialysis. *Kidney International* **17** (Suppl.), S57–S60.

Buoncristiani, U. (1998). Fifteen years of clinical experience with daily haemodialysis. *Nephrology, Dialysis, Transplantation* **13** (Suppl. 6), 148–151.

Burkart, J. M. *et al.* (1996). Solute clearance approach to adequacy of peritoneal dialysis. *Peritoneal Dialysis International* **16**, 457–470.

Cambi, V. *et al.* (1975). Short dialysis schedules (SDS)—finally ready to become routine? *Proceedings European Dialysis Transplantation Association* **11**, 112–120.

Canada-USA (CANUSA) Peritoneal Dialysis Study Group (1996). Adequacy of dialysis and nutrition in continuous peritoneal dialysis: association with clinical outcomes. *Journal of the American Society of Nephrology* **7**, 198–207.

Charra, B. *et al.* (1992). Survival as an index of adequacy of dialysis. *Kidney International* **41**, 1286–1291.

Cheung, A. K. *et al.* (2000). Atherosclerotic cardiovascular disease risks in chronic hemodialysis patients. *Kidney International* **58**, 353–362.

Collins, A. J. *et al.* (1999). Mortality risks of peritoneal dialysis and hemodialysis. *American Journal of Kidney Diseases* **34**, 1065–1069.

Depner, T. A. (1999). Why daily dialysis is better. *Seminars in Dialysis* **12**, 462–471.

Deppisch, R. M. (2001). Complement components as uremic toxins and their potential role as mediators of microinflammation. *Kidney International Supplement* **S78**, S271–S277.

Floege, J. and Ketteler, M. (2001). β_2-Microglobulin-derived amyloidosis: an update. *Kidney International* **59** (Suppl. 78), 164–168.

Galland, R. *et al.* (2001). Short daily hemodialysis rapidly improves nutritional status in hemodialysis patients. *Kidney International* **60**, 1555–1560.

Gotch, F. A. *et al.* (1997). Clinical outcome relative to the dose of dialysis is not what you think: the fallacy of the mean. *American Journal of Kidney Diseases* **30**, 1–15.

Hakim, R. M. (1993). Clinical implications of hemodialysis biocompatibility. *Kidney International* **44**, 484–490.

Hakim, R. M. *et al.* (1996). The effect of membrane biocompatibility on plasma β2-microglobulin levels in chronic hemodialysis patients. *Journal of American Society of Nephrology* **7**, 472–476.

Hakim, R. M. and Lazarus, J. M. (1995). Initiation of dialysis. *Journal of American Society of Nephrology* **6**, 1319–1322.

Hakim, R. M. and Levin, N. (1993). Malnutrition in hemodialysis patients. *American Journal of Kidney Diseases* **21**, 125–130.

Heimburger, O. *et al.* (1990). Peritoneal transport in CAPD patients and permanent loss of ultrafiltration capacity. *Kidney International* **38**, 495–499.

Henle, T. *et al.* (1999). Advanced glycated end-products (AGE) during haemodialysis treatment: discrepant results with different methodologies reflecting the heterogeneity of AGE compounds. *Nephrology, Dialysis, Transplantation* **14**, 1968–1975.

Ikizler, T. A. *et al.* (1995). Spontaneous dietary protein intake during progression of chronic renal failure. *Journal of the American Society of Nephrology* **6**, 1386–1391.

Juergensen, P. H. *et al.* (1999). Tidal peritoneal dialysis to achieve comfort in chronic peritoneal dialysis patients. *Advances in Peritoneal Dialysis* **15**, 125–130.

Kaysen, G. A. (2001).The microinflammatory state in uremia: causes and potential consequences. *Journal of the American Society of Nephrology* **12**, 1549–1557.

Kooistra, M. P. and Vos, P. F. (1999). Daily home hemodialysis: towards a more physiological treatment of patients with ESRD. *Seminars in Dialysis* **12**, 424–430.

Korevaar, J. C. *et al.* (2001). When to initiate dialysis: effect of proposed US guidelines on survival. *Lancet* **358**, 1046–1048.

Levey, A. S. (1990). Measurement of renal function in chronic renal disease. *Kidney International* **38**, 167–171.

Locatelli, F. *et al.* (2000) Effect of high-flux dialysis on the anaemia of haemodialysis patients. *Nephrology, Dialysis, Transplantation* **15**, 1399–1409.

Locatelli, F. *et al.* (1996). Effects of different membranes and dialysis technologies on patient treatment tolerance and nutritional parameters. The Italian Cooperative Dialysis Study Group. *Kidney International* **50**, 1293–1302.

Man, N. K. *et al.* (1991). Phosphate removal during hemodialysis, hemodiafiltration and hemofiltration. A reappraisal. *ASAIO Transactions* **36**, 463–465.

NKF-DOQI Clinical Practice Guidelines for Peritoneal Dialysis Adequacy (2001). Guidelines 1 and 2. *American Journal of Kidney Diseases* **37** (Suppl. 1), S70–S75.

Oliver, M. J., Edwards, L. J., and Churchill, D. N. (2001). Impact of sodium and ultrafiltration profiling on hemodialysis-related symptoms. *Journal of the American Society of Nephrology* **12**, 151–156.

Paniagua, R. *et al.* (2002). Effects of increased peritoneal clearances on mortality rates in peritoneal dialysis: ADEMEX, a prospective, randomized, controlled trial. *Journal of the American Society of Nephrology* **13**, 1307–1320.

Pierratos, A. and Ouwendyk, M. (1999). Nocturnal hemodialysis: five years later. *Seminars in Dialysis* **12**, 419–423.

Popovich, R. P. *et al.* (1976). The definition of a novel portable/wearable equilibrium dialysis technique. *Transactions American Society of Artificial Internal Organs* **5**, 64–66.

Salem, M. and Mujais, S. K. Dialyzers. In *Dialysis Therapy* (ed. A. R. Nissenson and R. N. Fine), pp. 65–72. Philadelphia: Hanley and Belfus Inc., 1993.

Shemesh, O. *et al.* (1985). Limitation of creatinine as a filtration marker in glomerulopathic patients. *Kidney International* **28**, 830–834.

Spalding, E. M., Chamney, P. W., and Farrington, K. (2002). Phosphate kinetics during hemodialysis: evidence for biphasic regulation. *Kidney International* **61**, 655–658.

Twardowski, Z. J. PET—A simpler approach. In *Advances in Peritoneal Dialysis* Vol. 7 (ed. R. Khanna *et al.*), pp. 186–191. Nashville: Peritoneal Dialysis Bulletin, 1990.

US Renal Data System (1992). Comorbid conditions and correlations with mortality risk among 3,399 incident hemodialysis patients. *American Journal of Kidney Diseases* **20**, 32–35.

US Renal Data System (2001). USRDS 2001 Annual Data Report. The National Institutes of Health, National Institute of Diabetes and Digestive and Kidney Diseases, Bethesda, MD, 2001 (http://www.usrds.org/).

van der Sande, F. M. *et al.* (2001). Thermal effects and blood pressure response during postdilution hemodiafiltration and hemodialysis: the effect of amount of replacement fluid and dialysate temperature. *Journal of the American Society of Nephrology* **12**, 1916–1920.

Van Tellingen, A. (2001). Long-term reduction of plasma homocysteine levels by super-flux dialyzers in hemodialysis patients. *Kidney International* **59**, 342–347.

Widjaja, A. *et al.* (2000). Free serum leptin but not bound leptin concentrations are elevated in patients with end-stage renal disease. *Nephrology, Dialysis, Transplantation* **15**, 846–850.

Williams, A. W., O'sullivan, D. A., and McCarthy, J. T. (1999). Slow nocturnal and short daily hemodialysis: a comparison. *Seminars in Dialysis* **12**, 431–435.

Woods, J. D. *et al.* (1999). Clinical and biochemical correlates of starting 'daily' hemodialysis. *Kidney International* **55**, 2467–2476.

12.2 Vascular access

Kazuo Ota

Introduction

For the patient on chronic dialysis, long-term maintenance of reliable fully functioning vascular access is vital. Quinton *et al.* (1960) described a cannula made of a silastic tube with a Teflon vessel tip at one end. Using this cannula inserted in the forearm, as vascular access for haemodialysis, they succeeded for the first time in sustaining the life of a patient with endstage renal disease. Later, several modified cannulae were designed including the Thomas shunt (Thomas 1969), which has a vascular graft attached at one end to suture the cannula end-to-side to the vessels. The development of these cannulae made long-term haemodialysis possible for patients with terminal renal failure. However, the high incidence of clotting and infection provided continual problems.

The introduction of the arteriovenous fistula by Brescia *et al.* (1966) made a significant contribution to overcoming these difficulties. This vascular access is now in use worldwide and has become the lifeline of haemodialysis patients. In 1969, the use of vascular grafts to create arteriovenous fistulae in patients whose limb vessels had been lost by repeated vascular access operations was reported. Others described the use of bovine grafts (Chinitz *et al.* 1972) or expanded polytetrafluoroethylene (E-PTFE) (Volder *et al.* 1973). Mehigan and McAlexander (1982) described a new site, well known as the anatomical snuff box or *tabatière*, as an alternative to the creation of a radial arteriovenous fistula. This increased the number of potential sites for creating vascular access.

A different approach, introduced by Shaldon *et al.* (1961), is the direct insertion of catheters into blood vessels. This type of vascular access has regained favour in recent years and is used predominantly in patients with acute renal failure as well as in patients with endstage renal disease without peripheral arteriovenous vascular access.

Vascular access devices introduced by Golding *et al.* (1980), Collins *et al.* (1981), Levin *et al.* (1998), and Beathard and Posen (2000) are the later innovations in the field and these will be described in the text.

Types of vascular access

The different types of vascular access in current clinical use are shown in Table 1. They can be divided into two fundamental categories; those with shunting of the bloodstream and those without.

Timing of formation and selection of method

Many factors must be considered when creating vascular access for haemodialysis depending on the general clinical status of the patient and on whether the renal failure is acute or chronic. The essential factors to be considered are: (a) age of the patient; (b) original disease; (c) degree of renal failure and possibility of recovery; (d) blood pressure and hydration; (e) presence of other complications; (f) status of limb blood vessels; and (g) degree of emergency for commencing dialysis.

Timing of formation

In patients with acute renal failure and in those with chronic renal failure accompanied by serious problems such as hyperkalaemia and overhydration, dialysis is usually started as an emergency treatment,

Table 1 Classification of vascular access

Classification of vascular access			Names of accesses in practice and sites of formation
With shunt			
External shunts	Cannula type		Quinton-Scribner, Allen-Braun, Thomas, Buseimeier
Arteriovenous	Button type (plug type)		Hemasite
fistulas	Simple anastomosis		Brescia-Cimino arteriovenous fistula and other variations
		Synthetic	Dacron, E-PTFE, and Sparks mandril grafts
	Grafts	Biological	Saphenous vein, bovine, swine, and umbilical cord vein graft
		Hybrid	Biograft, Omniflow
Without shunt			Direct puncture of artery and vein
Simple puncture	Temporary		Shaldon, Uldall, catheter
Catheter method	Tunneled-cuffed		Tesio catheter
	With subcutaneous device		Life Site, Dialock
Superficialized artery			Superficialization of the femoral, brachial, and radial artery
Jump grafts			Implantations of grafts to the femoral and brachial artery

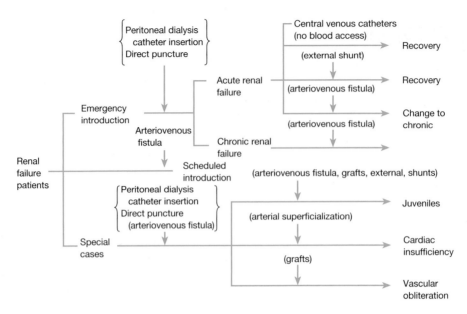

Fig. 1 Selection of access for dialysis.

most commonly by use of a percutaneous catheter. In this setting, there is little room for debate about when to create a permanent vascular access which in chronic patients should be undertaken as soon as the acute clinical status is stabilized. However, in patients with chronic renal failure without life-threatening complications, the correct timing for the formation of a vascular access is important. From my experience, an arteriovenous fistula should be created at least 4 weeks, or preferably earlier, before starting regular dialysis.

The age of the patient is as important as the underlying disease. Vascular access must be made relatively early in paediatric patients and also in patients with diabetic nephropathy, as the need for dialysis may arise relatively quickly. In contrast, as the progression of renal failure is slow in polycystic renal disease, it is best to avoid the early creation of vascular access in such patients. Thus, the creation of vascular access must be carefully timed, but is generally undertaken when the plasma creatinine of the patient is consistently in excess of 600 μmol/l or glomerular filtration rate (GFR) is less than 20 ml/min.

Selection of type

In adults requiring haemodialysis for chronic renal failure, an arteriovenous fistula is normally fashioned in the non-dominant forearm, usually the left. The fistula is made in the right forearm in patients who are left-handed or in patients whose blood vessels in the left forearm are unsuitable. In the case of paediatric patients whose distal vessels may be very small, a fistula may be made in the region of the elbow, or some other access may be formed such as the use of a graft or a Thomas external shunt (Thomas 1969). In patients with heart failure which a shunt might exacerbate, it is advisable to make use of arterial superficialization (Brittinger *et al.* 1970; Capodicasa *et al.* 1971) or a jump graft. For those patients without vascular access who require dialysis as an emergency, it was previously the practice to make an external shunt in the left forearm. However, such an external shunt damages important vessels in the forearm which may subsequently be required for an arteriovenous fistula. In view of this, it has been suggested that if an

external shunt is required, it should be inserted in the lower limb using the posterior tibial artery and the long saphenous vein just proximal to the ankle. However, in some instances when external shunts have been made in the forearm, they can be subsequently converted to arteriovenous fistulae by anastomosing the artery and the vein on removal of the cannulae (Siminian *et al.* 1977). Recently, the use of the catheter originally developed by Shaldon *et al.* (1961) has been re-evaluated, and since improved products are now commercially available (Perini *et al.* 2000), it has become the fashion to insert a catheter into the subclavian or internal jugular vein to provide vascular access while the arteriovenous fistula matures. Once this occurs, particularly when the subclavian vein has been used, the catheter is removed and dialysis is continued using the fistula. As the catheter may cause thrombosis and/or stenosis in the vein used (Vanherweghem *et al.* 1986), it is advisable to remove the catheter as early as possible.

In patients for whom the creation of vascular access presents special problems, and if there is no contraindication, peritoneal dialysis is often useful (Fig. 1).

Constructing an external shunt

Insertion of cannulae and installation of vascular access devices, such as Hemasite, are two ways of constructing external shunts.

Insertion of cannula

It has become less common to use cannulae for haemodialysis. Currently their use is confined to patients with acute renal failure or for short-term relief from vascular access problems.

The most appropriate region for the insertion of cannulae is a distal part of the forearm, using the radial artery and cephalic vein approximately 10 cm proximal to the wrist. Straight-type cannulae are more commonly used to avoid the formation of postoperative haematoma which frequently accompanies immediate postoperative systemic

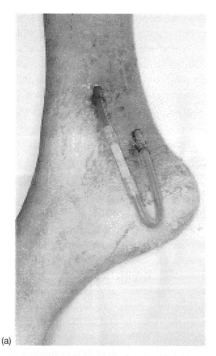

(a)

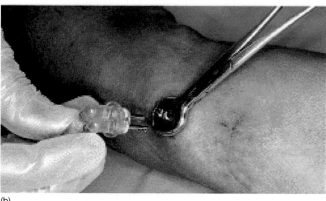

(b)

Fig. 2 (a) Appearance of straight-type external shunt at the ankle. (b) Implanted Hemasite being connected to blood lines.

heparinization. A straight-type cannula installed in the forearm is shown as an example in Fig. 2(a).

Installation of a vascular access device

Hemasite (Collins *et al.* 1981), a button-type vascular access device, is inserted in a fashion similar to that used for vascular grafts except for the positioning of the device for connection which is usually located at the centre of the graft [Fig. 2(b)]. Dialock (Levin *et al.* 1998) and Life Site (Beathard *et al.* 2000) are newly developed access devices, designed under the same concept. They consist of a catheter and a puncturable device. The catheter is introduced to the superior vena cava or to the right atrium through the internal jugular vein, and the opposite side of the catheter is connected to the device installed subcutaneously. The former needs two devices, for arterial and venous sides, while in the latter two devices are joined together into one.

Creating an arteriovenous fistula

Selection of the anastomotic site

The forearm is usually chosen for establishing an arteriovenous anastomosis. The standard location for anastomosis is 3–5 cm proximal to the wrist as the radial artery and cephalic vein come close together at this site. However, as there is a considerable individual variation in the venous system, a thorough examination of the veins should be undertaken before the operation.

Another suitable site, whose use was introduced by Harder *et al.* (1977), is the anatomical snuff box where the dorsal branch of the radial artery and cephalic vein are closely apposed. The advantages of creating an arteriovenous fistula at this site are: (a) to provide an extra site for the creation of an arteriovenous fistula; (b) to allow development of the artery and vein in the forearm to make subsequent operations easier.

Technique of anastomosis

The operation is usually carried out under local anaesthesia, using 10–20 ml of 0.5–1.0 per cent procaine hydrochloride or lidocaine. A skin incision of approximately 4 cm is placed transversely 3–5 cm proximal to the wrist and the radial artery and the cephalic vein are exposed. Branches of the artery and the vein are ligated and severed, leaving both vessels isolated.

There are four types of vascular anastomoses available in this setting; end-to-end, side(artery)-to-end(vein), end(artery)-to-side(vein), and side-to-side anastomosis. Most surgeons favour the use of side-to-side anastomoses.

The vein is ligated peripherally and is severed without proximal ligation. A 19-gauge Teflon cannula is inserted into the lumen from the severed end and heparinized saline is injected. If the solution passes into the lumen freely, this vein can be expected to remain open. After the vein has been occluded by small vascular forceps (bulldog clamps) applied as proximally as possible, a Teflon cannula is inserted and held in place by a single-bound suture, and the cannula is removed while gently injecting further heparinized saline. At this time, the previously single-bound ligated suture is ligated for a second time so that the vessel is bound as soon as the cannula is removed. This causes the isolated vein to swell like a long balloon, making surgical manipulation easier, and as the entire drainage vein is dilated, there is increased patency rate.

After the preparation of the venous side is completed, the radial artery is clamped using bulldog forceps and a longitudinal incision of 7 mm is made. To accommodate this, an incision of a similar size is performed on the prepared vein.

Anastomosis is started by placing stay sutures at the proximal and distal ends and two traction sutures are set at the centre of the anterior walls of the artery and vein. Suturing is started from the posterior wall using the suture previously set distally. When a continuous suture is started from this position, it turns back from the proximal posterior wall to the proximal anterior wall. In this way, the inflow and outflow tract, the most vital region of the anastomosis, can be sutured under direct vision. The two traction sutures are removed when the suture on the anterior wall reaches their position; when the suture reaches the distal end of the anastomosis, it is tied to the stay suture and the anastomosis is completed (Figs 3 and 4). Recently, small vascular clips are used instead of suturing to shorten the time of anastomosis.

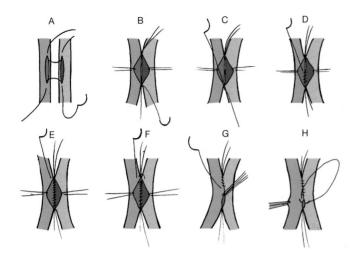

Fig. 3 Procedures for a side-to-side anastomosis. In the illustrations, the distal portion faces downward. If right-handed, the operator is situated to the left of each figure. It makes no difference whether the artery or vein locates to the right or left side.

Management of insufficient blood flow and prevention of occlusion

By lightly compressing the anastomotic site with a finger, any bleeding is usually controlled within 2–3 min. If there is complete haemostasis and the blood flow is satisfactory, the dilated vein distal to the anastomosis is ligated at a site as close as possible to the anastomosis and the blood in the lumen removed by a small incision. The remaining venous segment is not divided but is retained, since it may be required as access for possible postoperative declotting. Where there is complete haemostasis and either a thrill felt or a considerably strong murmur heard, skin closure is undertaken. However, in some cases after resumption of blood flow there is pulsation without a thrill and difficulty in stopping haemorrhage from the suture line. These are manifestations of stenosis, occlusion, and/or spasm in the drainage vein. In such cases, thrombi will develop eventually in the anastomotic region. If the state of blood flow is uncertain, it is advisable to auscultate with a sterilized stethoscope. If there is still no audible murmur, vascular dilation or removal of thrombi should be undertaken. It is at this time that the leftover venous segment becomes useful.

A 17-gauge Teflon needle or a No. 3 or 4 Fogarty catheter is inserted into the vascular lumen through the small incision placed previously in the distal portion of the leftover venous segment. As the blood vessel is dilated, thrombi are removed simultaneously. Manipulations are first performed on the venous side and then on the arterial. After the catheter is removed, the blood flow is stopped by clamping and ligating the distal venous segment and the operation is completed. Using these procedures and when a definite thrill has been felt, the remainder of the vein is ligated as close to the anastomotic region as possible to prevent the formation of a blind sac. The remaining blood is drained and the venous segment is left to be used in case of further occlusion. In cases where there is insufficient flow despite the absence of stenosis or thrombosis, arterial or venous spasm is frequently observed. This finding can be explained by considering the physiology of the vessel wall. In this case, the velocity of blood flowing in the artery becomes accelerated by being shunted to a dilated vein with a low resistance. The resultant increase in the velocity is perceived by the artery as haemorrhage and spasm of the wall takes place to minimize bleeding. Spasm of the vein is also a frequent occurrence and can be considered as a reaction to the sudden increase in blood flow and pressure. For these reasons, even after the clamps are released and a very strong thrill palpated, it does not mean that the operation is successful. Before, during, and after skin suturing, the presence of the thrill should be checked repeatedly (Fig. 5).

Factors influencing patency

There are five factors which influence the patency rate of the anastomosis. High blood pressure and the use of anticoagulant and/or antiplatelet drugs are two factors which increase patency rate.

Arterial and venous vasospasm and enhanced systemic as well as local coagulability are the three factors which decrease the patency rate, that is the patency rate of the anastomosis is decided by the balance of these antagonistic factors. Consequently, prevention of hypotension, avoidance of vasospasm, and local activation of coagulation factors are important for success. For better results, meticulous surgical technique for the isolation and anastomosis of small vessels is indispensable. However, it is also necessary to check the fluid status of the patient before operation; if dehydration is suspected, preoperative or intraoperative rehydration with saline should be administered. Immediate postoperative administration of hypertensive drugs such as carnigen and/or anticoagulants such as low molecular weight heparin are recommended in cases with poor blood flow. In patients without a bleeding risk, an intravenous bolus of low molecular weight heparin of 20 anti-Xa units/kg is given followed by a continuous infusion of 10 anti-Xa units/kg/h. In patients with a bleeding risk, the bolus dose is reduced to 10 anti-Xa units/kg with a maintenance infusion of 7.5 anti-Xa units/kg/h. The latter should be used only after complete haemostasis of the surgical field has been achieved.

Vascular access using a vascular graft
Varieties and characteristics of vascular grafts

Vascular grafts for vascular access must satisfy several specific criteria in addition to those required for conventional vascular grafts. They must be easy to puncture, prompt in haemostasis, durable to repeated puncture, and resistant to infection. Several vascular grafts listed in Table 1 were selected by those criteria and have been examined and used clinically. Among them, the E-PTFE graft (Volder *et al.* 1973) (Fig. 6) and the bovine graft (Chinitz *et al.* 1972) have been widely used; the umbilical cord vein graft (Mindich *et al.* 1975) and the polyurethane graft (Ota *et al.* 1987; Allen *et al.* 1996; Glickman *et al.* 2001) are being evaluated for their suitability for vascular access. The use of the autogenous saphenous vein graft, which was introduced by May *et al.* (1969), has decreased because of its short functional survival and its potential for use in coronary artery bypass surgery.

Indication and mode of implantation

Vascular graft implantation should be limited to those patients whose limb blood vessels have been destroyed by repeated access procedures or venous thromboses. The modes of implantation are divided into two categories: straight and looped. In addition, there are several modifications according to the localization of arteries and veins. Since

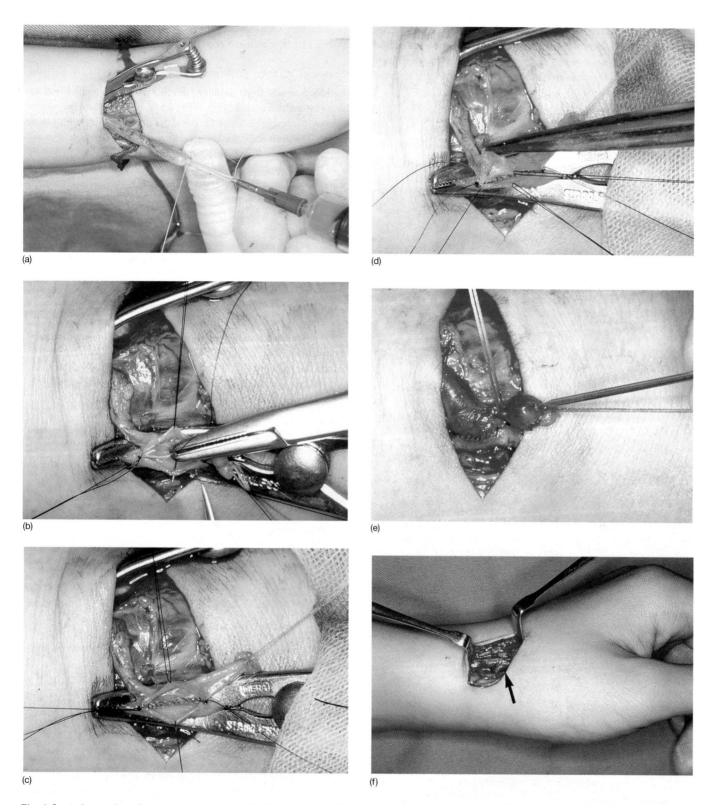

Fig. 4 Surgical procedures for arteriovenous fistula. (a) Saline is infused in the vein to check patency and bulldog forceps are applied to dilate the vessel wall. (b) Longitudinal incision of approximately 7 mm is made by a cutter in the artery. Four stay stutures are placed to fix the anastomotic site. (c) The anastomosis is started at the peripheral side of the posterior wall. (d) Using the same running suture the anterior wall is sutured from outside. (e) After declamping the left-over venous segment is ligated and blood is drained by a small incision. (f) An arteriovenous fistula anastomosing the dorsal branch of the radial artery and the cephalic vein at the tabatière is shown as a modification of the standard fistula.

limb joints between the arterial and venous anastomotic site decreases the patency rate of such grafts, insertion in such a manner should be avoided whenever possible. In situations in which it is unavoidable, it is advisable to pass the graft either to the radial or ulnar side to avoid severe kinking with joint movement. If no suitable site is found in the upper limbs, the thigh and popliteal regions may be used (Ota 1982a).

Method of vascular graft implantation

The blood vessels to be anastomosed to the vascular graft are determined by detailed examination of the arm. The techniques for surgical exposure of the vessels are similar to those described for arteriovenous fistulae. The graft to be used is selected according to the size of vessels to be anastomosed. Grafts with similar internal dimensions to the vessel to be anastomosed are easy to suture. However, in addition to the difficulties in cannulation, grafts with small diameters are prone to thrombosis. It is therefore recommended that a 6-mm graft for upper limbs and 6–8 mm for the lower limbs be used for adult patients.

After clamping the vessels to be anastomosed, a longitudinal incision of 1.0–1.5 cm is made in the venous wall, and three or four stay sutures are placed to fix the venous anastomotic opening to that of the graft which was created by bevelling the wall to an appropriate angle. The venous anastomosis is usually carried cut end(vein)-to-side, similar to the method used in the creation of an arteriovenous fistula. After completion of the anastomosis, a subcutaneous tunnel is created using a Hegar dilator or specially designed tunneller, through which the graft is passed. In the case of a loop graft, one to three small skin incisions are necessary to turn the graft back to the arterial anastomotic site. The use of the Hegar dilator and the completion of anastomosis are shown in Fig. 7.

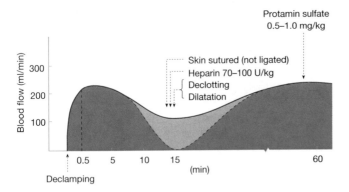

Fig. 5 Blood flow with time after declamping.

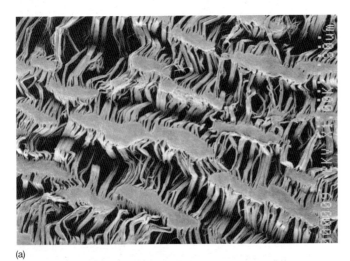

(a)

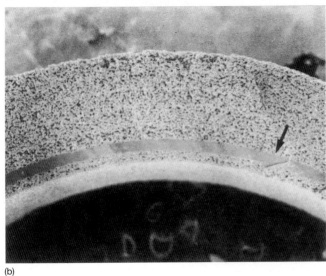

(b)

Fig. 6 Sectional view of polyurethane graft. An arrow indicates the dense layer: (a) E-PTFE graft; (b) polyurethane graft.

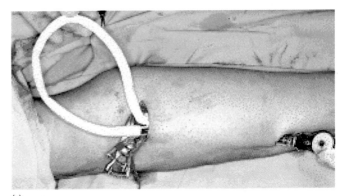

(a)

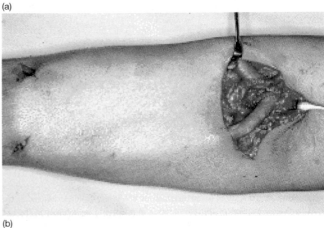

(b)

Fig. 7 Implantation of vascular graft. A subcutaneous tunnel is constructed using a specially designed tunneller or Hegar dilator which is also used to pull the graft through as seen in panel (a). Completion of implantation is demonstrated in panel (b).

Superficialization of arteries

Arterial superficialization, introduced by Brittinger *et al.* (1970) and Capodicasa *et al.* (1971), is the subcutaneous placement of an artery, without the creation of an arteriovenous fistula, to make arterial puncture easier and to avoid the formation of subfascial haematoma which often results from arterial puncture. The advantage of this vascular access is avoidance of cardiac overload which sometimes becomes a serious problem in elderly patients, in those with diabetes mellitus, and in patients with cardiovascular diseases. The sites used are the cubital fossa and upper arm and the thigh. The brachial artery is superficialized in the former and the superficial femoral artery is used for the latter. In cases of vascular access problems in patients without cardiac dysfunction, superficialization combined with venous anastomosis, using saphenous, basilic, or brachial vein, has also been utilized (Fig. 8).

Catheters and method of insertion

Catheters have been used for vascular access since 1961 when Shaldon *et al.* (1961) described the use of femoral catheters for haemodialysis. Uldall *et al.* (1980) used catheters with double lumens to make single-puncture placement possible. The subclavian vein and femoral vein are the vessels most commonly used at first, followed by the internal jugular vein. The Tesio system requires placement of two single lumen catheters (Fig. 9). At the time of insertion the Seldinger technique using a guidewire is used.

The advantages of vascular access using a catheter are: (a) avoidance of cardiac overload by blood shunting; (b) the ability to start dialysis without blood access surgery, either in an emergency or in patients without appropriate blood vessels to create vascular access. However, apart from catheter occlusion, a common complication is irritation inducing stenosis or occlusion of the subclavian vein making subsequent arteriovenous fistula formation in the upper limb of the affected side extremely difficult. The details of this complication will be described separately.

Needles for puncture, usage, and care of vascular access

Needles

There are three types of needles designed for use in haemodialysis; metal needles with a connecting tube, metal needles with a plastic sheath, and Y-shaped needles for single-needle dialysis. The last type has two forms: those with a single lumen and those with a double lumen (Fig. 10). The size of the needle most commonly used is 13–18 gauge. There are several advantages and disadvantages of each type.

Usage

To facilitate healing of the wound and dilatation of the vein, it is recommended that there should be at the very minimum a 2–3-week interval between surgery and starting puncture. The most important prerequisite in selecting the puncture site is to avoid intravascular

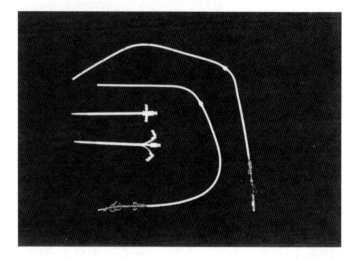

Fig. 9 Tesio catheters and two peel-away sheathes, lower one is being peeled.

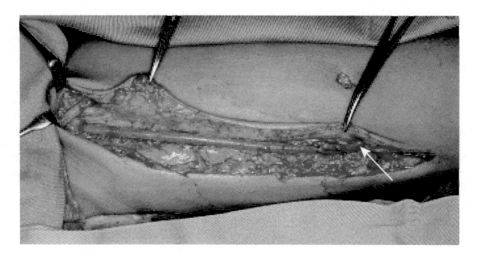

Fig. 8 Superficialization of femoral artery. The saphenous vein is anastomosed to a distal part of the superficialized artery as indicated by the arrow on the right. The vein passes subcutaneously and reappears as indicated by the arrow on the left.

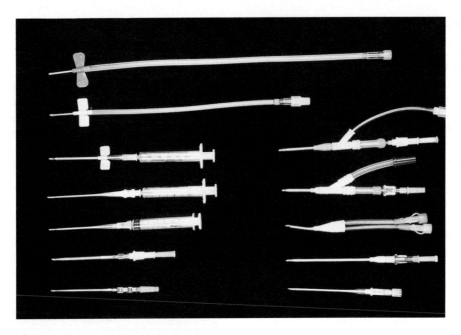

Fig. 10 Varieties of puncture needles.

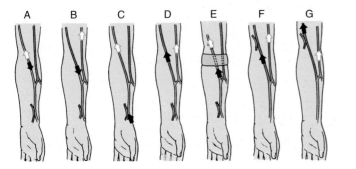

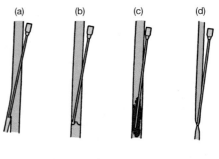

Fig. 11 The puncture sites of an arteriovenous fistula. A and B are the sites commonly employed; however, when the arterial sites shown in A and B have been mispunctured, it is better to apply model C. Model D is entirely suitable for use although the penetration direction of the arterial side is reversed. In model E, since the same vessel is used in the same direction, a tourniquet is applied between the sites. Models F and G demonstrate employment of the brachial artery with an anastomosed median cubital vein. Black arrows indicate the arterial side and white arrows the venous side; direction of the arrows indicates the direction of puncturing.

Fig. 12 Insufficient blood flow of an arteriovenous fistula occurs: (a) when the end of the needle has entered a small tributary; (b) when the end has been positioned near a venous valve; (c) when occlusion has resulted from thrombus. Pumping with a heparinized saline solution is carried out; (d) when the vascular walls have been drawn together by negative pressure to occlude the end. In this case, as shown in (e), a tourniquet is applied between the arterial and venous sides.

mixing of immediate postdialysed blood with predialysed blood. To satisfy this requirement, the puncture site for the arterial needle (inlet to the dialyser) should be upstream to that of the venous side. Several choices for puncture sites are shown in Fig. 11.

When using single-needle dialysis, the needle should be inserted in the same direction as the bloodstream to avoid mixing of dialysed and undialysed blood.

Problems encountered during dialysis

The major problems of vascular access encountered during dialysis can be attributed to insufficient blood flow from the arterial side and

elevation of pressure in the venous side. Possible causes of the problems are shown in Fig. 12. Situation (a) occurs when a needle tip enters a thin tributary. Situation (b) occurs when the tip has been situated near a venous valve. In situation (c), there is occlusion caused by a newly formed thrombus. Situation (d) occurs when the vein is narrow and the vessel walls have been sucked in, thereby occluding the needle tip. To counteract situations (a) and (b), it is advisable to draw the needle back slightly to find a more suitable site for withdrawing blood. In situation (c), it is necessary to inject heparinized saline solution until an adequate flow of blood can be achieved; if unsuccessful, resting is necessary. In situations such as (d), a tourniquet or a band must be applied between the arterial and venous sides to avoid mixing the blood. In situation (e), a tourniquet is applied in the same fashion as in situation (d) to obstruct passage of blood; the vein will then dilate, and this will prevent the walls from being drawn into the needle tip.

High venous pressure may arise in situations (a)–(c) in Fig. 12. In addition, when the blood vessel is narrow, as in situation (d), or when stenosis has occurred proximally, and the volume of blood withdrawn from the arterial side is greater than the drainage capacity of the venous side, there will be an increase in pressure.

It is important to take measures similar to those taken in situations (a)–(c) on the arterial side to obtain adequate blood flow. However, if a decrease in pressure is not obtained, there are no options other than to reduce the speed of the blood pump until the excessive pressure in the dialyser falls to an acceptable level or to find a new puncture site. There are numerous problems involved with newly constructed fistulae, but in general after 1 or 2 months, the blood vessels will dilate, and almost all the previous problems will resolve.

Daily care

The day to day care of an arteriovenous fistula is clearly easier than that of an external shunt. After use, pressure is applied to the punctured region for about 10–15 min. After haemostasis has been achieved, a gauze folded to approximately 3 cm^2 is applied to the puncture site and held by tapes or bandages. On the following day, the gauze may be removed and replaced by sterilized adhesive tape to cover the puncture site. Baths and showers should be avoided for 24 h after dialysis, but if the wound has healed sufficiently they may be permitted on the following day. The daily care of a superficialized artery is similar to that of an arteriovenous fistula.

Evaluation and examination of vascular access

Angiography, measurement of blood flow through the shunt, and cardiac output are the three methods used for long-term follow-up of vascular access.

Angiography

Conventional and digital subtraction angiography (Orofino *et al.* 1987) using contrast media have been most commonly used while sonography has become popular. Both are useful for morphological evaluation of the vascular access. The advantage of the former is that the total vasculature with functional blood flow may be visualized. The disadvantage is the necessity for contrast media which may cause side-effects. Sonographic examination causes no discomfort and there are no harmful side-effects. It can be performed at the bedside easily and repeatedly. Beside the easy availability, it visualizes blood flow pattern and velocity with the use of Doppler imaging which can be ulilized to calculate blood flow through the fistula (Dousset *et al.* 1991; Finlay *et al.* 1993; Kirschbaum and Compton 1995). Three angiograms of arteriovenous fistulae and two angiosonograms are shown in Figs 13 and 14.

Measurement of blood flow through an arteriovenous fistula

In external shunts it is possible to determine blood flow by introducing an electromagnetic flowmeter to the circuit. However, compared with the external shunt, measurement of blood flow in an arteriovenous

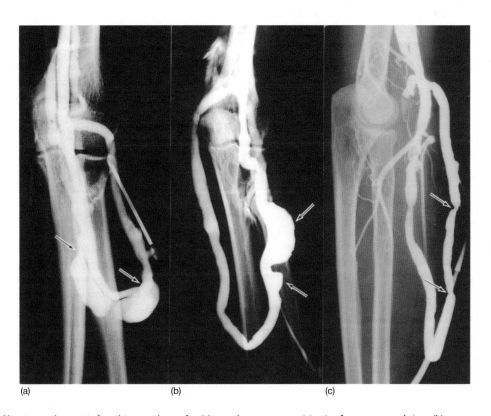

(a) (b) (c)

Fig. 13 Aneurysmal dilatation and stenosis found in vascular grafts: (a) pseudoaneurysms originating from punctured sites; (b) aneurysms of the graft originating from wall cleavage; (c) stenoses found in the graft.

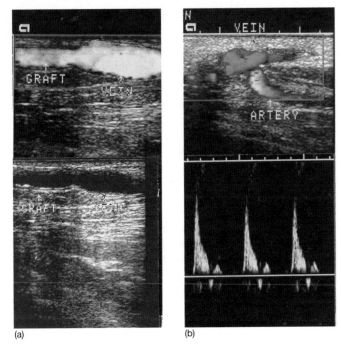

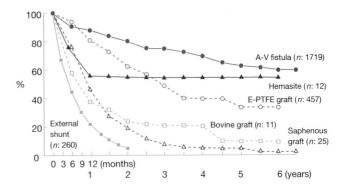

Fig. 15 Functional survival of the vascular access (by courtesy of S. Sakai, Shinrakuen Hospital).

Fig. 14 (a) Anastomotic site and flow pattern of a stenosed fistula. The anastomotic site of the fistula is visualized with colour imaging; artery in red and vein in blue. The Doppler image in the lower figure indicates the flow pattern of the artery adjacent to the anastomotic site. The sharp systolic peak with reverse flow suggests an increased peripheral pressure, presumably caused by severe stenosis in the outflow vein. (Apparatus used: ACUSON 128XP System, linear 7.0 MHz, a. CDE mode, b. CDI mode.) (b) An anastomotic site of a E-PTFE graft to vein. The wall of the graft is demonstrated as two layers. Postanastomotic dilation is observed in the venous segment on the right. Colour Doppler energy mode is useful to obtain a longitudinal section of the vessels at one shot. The lower panel shows the same vessel.

Factors influencing long-term patency

There are many factors associated with the long-term patency of the vascular access including age, gender, original disease, blood coagulability, blood pressure, development, and/or pre-existing damage of blood vessels in the limbs. In addition, the site of the anastomosis and size of the blood vessels used, local conditions of blood flow turbulence, and infections are also important. Turbulence in the vicinity of the anastomosis, especially on the venous side of the graft, enhances thickening of the intima, leading eventually to thrombosis. In addition, there is a tendency to kink at the site of venous branches due to stretching of the blood vessel, and this may also cause thrombosis. Infections of the punctured site and subsequent rupture and/or narrowing of the drainage vein are also important factors in determining the functional survival of the vascular access.

Other than these, long-term functional maintenance of vascular access is influenced by factors peculiar to the individual and other unforeseen problems. It is necessary to correct these conditions as much as possible to secure long-term patency, and maximum efforts must be made to guard against mispuncture and haematoma formation as well as maintenance of personal hygiene in order to prevent infection.

Complications of vascular access

Systemic complications

Systemic complications of vascular access are mainly caused by cardiac overload. The blood flow rate through an arteriovenous fistula constructed in the wrist region immediately after operation is 291 ± 187 ml/min (Anderson *et al.* 1977). However, after a period of time following the construction of the fistula, the anastomosed arterial as well as the venous lumen will gradually enlarge, and the entire anastomotic area will become fully functional. If the anastomotic opening is too large, the blood flow which is approximately 5–10 per cent of the cardiac output at the time of formation, may increase to between 15 and 20 per cent, causing cardiac overload which sometimes leads to cardiac failure (Ahearn and Maher 1972; Fee *et al.* 1976). Concomitant anaemia is a contributing factor which will aggravate the problem.

High-output cardiac failure brought on by excessive shunt flow can be treated by closing the shunt and constructing another arteriovenous fistula with a smaller blood flow, or by narrowing the inflow artery or outflow vein of the fistula with a metal clip or Teflon tape. This is known as the banding method and is also available to treat steal syndrome (Fig. 16).

fistula, especially using non-surgical methods, is extremely difficult. Various methods have been proposed but none is completely satisfactory. Table 2 summarizes these together with the results obtained. Measurement of cardiac output is also utilized to calculate shunt blood flow.

Long-term results and factors influencing outcome

With the extension of life expectancy among dialysis patients, the long-term maintenance of satisfactory vascular access has become a prime concern.

Comparison of patency rates for various types of vascular access

It has been demonstrated that the best results are obtained by conventional arteriovenous fistulae and the poorest with external shunts (Fig. 15). The results obtained from arteriovenous fistulae using various grafts fall between the two. Among these, patients implanted with E-PTFE grafts have the best patency rate and those with autogenous saphenous vein grafts the poorest.

Table 2 Blood flow of vascular access

Method of measurement	Flow (ml/min)	Problems
Electromagnetic flow meter	242 ± 89 (radial) 599 ± 163 (brachial) 592 ± 134 (graft) (Anderson et al. 1977)	Since surgical intervention is necessary, it can be carried out only under special circumstances Direct measurement cannot be carried out The blood flow changes due to vasospasms

Doppler	728 ± 53 (radial)
	778 ± 152 (brachial)
	1195 ± 125 (graft)
	(Bouthier et al. 1983)
	806.2
	(Moran et al. 1985)
		In conventional arteriovenous fistula, since the
		   direction of the blood flow is not uniform and
		   there are many branches, exact values cannot
		   easily be obtained

Local thermal	>400 (forearm)
	65% of the cases examined
	(Greenwood et al. 1985)
		This method works well for determining the blood
		   flow in grafts but not in arteriovenous fistula
		   because of the existence of many branches

Plethysmography	242 (Hurwich 1969)	Blocking of the vein is (Hurwich 1969) unreliable;
		   when a high pressure is induced, the inflow from
		   the artery is reduced. Also, the blood flow
		   distribution can change due to an increase in
		   peripheral resistance at the time pressure is
		   increased

Cardiac output	1000 ± 80
	(Dongradi et al. 1979)
	(Thermodilution)
	640
	(Johnson and Blythe 1970)
	(Dye dilution)
	710 ± 17
	(Von Bibra et al. 1978)
	(Echocardiography)
		If done before and after the formation of the
		   fistula, the fistula is still in an underdeveloped
		   condition and with the beginning of dialysis, the
		   body fluids are variable
		Since the measured values are large, the error
		   margin is also large
		The Graham effect may appear

Indicator dilution technique combined with optical transcutaneous haematocrit sensor	153–2042 (Steuer et al. 2001)	
Miscellaneous	180–4000 (mean 1200) (Langescheid et al. 1977)	

Local complications

Stenosis and occlusion

Occlusion is the most frequent cause of failure of vascular access. The contributing factors which should be avoided and dealt with early are: hypotension caused by excessive removal of fluid; infection; hypercoagulability; turbulence at, or adjacent to, anastomoses or branches, and metastatic calcification of the vessel wall. Declotting can be undertaken using a Fogarty catheter followed by intravenous administration of heparin (5000 U) and urokinase (30,000–60,000 U). However, in arteriovenous fistulae, pre-existing stenosis of the draining vein is usually one of the contributing factors to occlusion. In such circumstances, surgical repair or percutaneous transluminal angioplasty (PTA) (Glanz et al. 1987; Beathard et al. 1992) of the stenotic portion in combination with declotting and/or stenting (Haage et al. 1999) is recommended (Figs 17 and 18).

If a stenosis is found at the anastomotic site and repair is considered difficult, it is advisable to create a new arteriovenous fistula 2–5 cm proximal to the original anastomosis. If there is a patent vein and pulsating artery in the anatomical snuff box, this can be used as an alternative. In vascular graft occlusion, a stenosis is often found at the venous anastomotic site. Surgical enlargement by endarterectomy with patch grafting or the formation of a new anastomosis at the proximal side of the vein by applying a new graft 3–5 cm long to reach a new anastomotic opening is recommended. Stenosis at the outflow vein often causes venous hypertension which will be described separately.

Infection

Infection is frequently encountered in patients with central catheters and cannulae but is rare in arteriovenous fistulae, puncture sites being the usual sites affected. In some patients the anastomotic site itself may become infected as a result of bacteraemia or septicaemia. The organisms responsible are usually *Staphylococcus aureus* and *Staphylococcus epidermidis*, followed by *Escherichia coli* (Nsouli et al. 1979). The incidence of bacteraemia is reported to be 0.15 episodes per patient dialysis year (Dobkin et al. 1978).

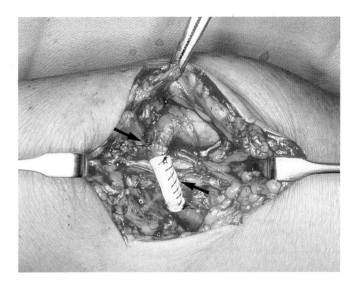

Fig. 16 Radial artery and cephalic vein were reanastomosed after removing dilated anastomotic site. A piece of E-PTFE sheet was used to wrap the radial artery to prevent further enlargement of the vessel. Arrows indicate the anastomotic site (left) and E-PTFE graft (right).

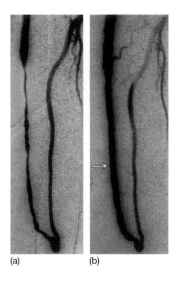

(a)   (b)

Fig. 17 Treatment of stenosis using a balloon catheter: (a) before treatment; (b) after treatment. The arrow indicates enlarged segment.

The causes of infection are: (a) inadequate disinfection of the skin; (b) contamination of the puncture needle; (c) manipulations of the needle during haemodialysis; (d) scratching of the puncture site due to pruritus; and (e) contamination at the time of bathing. Since *S. aureus* and *S. epidermidis* are the most frequently found causative organisms, cephalosporins and β-lactamase resistant penicillins are the first-choice antibiotics unless there is a high chance of methicillin resistant *S. aureus* being responsible. Vancomycin would then be used. Incision and drainage often become necessary in cases where a localized abscess is formed. The site of incision should be selected so as not to injure dilated draining veins, thereby avoiding massive haemorrhage. An abscess which is not drained often results in spontaneous rupture causing massive bleeding, or if occurring within the vessel, bacteraemia, which may lead to endocarditis (Cross and Steigbigel 1976).

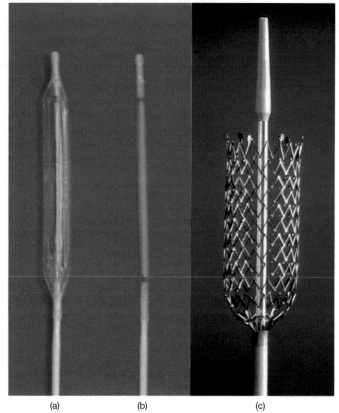

(a)   (b)   (c)

Fig. 18 Balloon catheter and self-expandable stent: (a) inflated; (b) deflated; (c) expanding self-expandable stent.

To stop bleeding, firm pressure with the fingers on the anastomotic site to limit arterial inflow and then application of a pneumatic tourniquet is recommended. The feeding artery and draining vein can then be ligated at the anastomotic site. If the 'side' of the artery has been used for the anastomosis, the distal part of the artery should be ligated at the same time, since a considerable amount of blood flow may come from the palmar arch. If haemostasis is not complete, ligation of the vein proximal and distal to the ruptured site or local application of gauze with compression may be indicated.

Infection occurring in heterologous or synthetic vascular grafts is very difficult to treat. Since vascular grafts (except autografts) are foreign materials with no self-defence mechanisms they are vulnerable to infection, which is difficult to eradicate. In addition to that, silent infection in non-functional clotted prosthetic grafts has been recognized as a frequent cause of bacteraemia (Nassar and Ayus 2001). Fungal infection may be a complicating factor (Onorato 1979). Skin necrosis and subsequent exposure of the graft ultimately lead to abandonment and removal (Fig. 19). To avoid such an unfavourable course, partial replacement of the graft is recommended.

Steal syndrome

The name 'steal syndrome' is derived from the stealing of blood which would normally flow to the palmar arch. In the case of arteriovenous fistulae constructed in the forearm, blood flow comes to the fistula from the radial artery both proximally and distally. For the latter, blood flows from the ulnar artery by the deep and superficial palmar arch, which may result in the blood supply to the palmar digital arteries becoming markedly decreased.

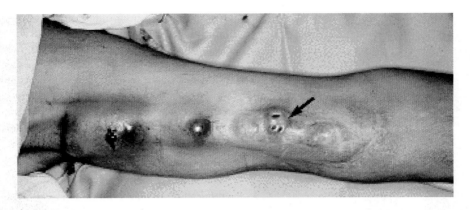

Fig. 19 Infection in the vascular graft. The original infection is indicated by the arrow on the right. Two others at the centre and left are disseminations.

The symptoms of the steal syndrome are a cold sensation and pallor of the fingers frequently accompanied by ischaemic pain. In severe cases, necrosis develops at the tips of the fingers which may be complicated by infection. Theoretically, it is most likely to occur following the creation of a fistula with high blood flow employing large vessels and in cases with vascular occlusive processes such as thromboangiitis obliterans, SLE, or diabetes mellitus. The incidence is about 1.6 per cent in various fistulae, but it increases to 33.3 per cent in brachial fistulae and 14 per cent in graft implantation (Haimov *et al.* 1975).

Basically, treatment of the steal syndrome is to decrease the blood flow through the fistula, thereby ensuring enough blood supply to the peripheral tissues. The following methods can be considered: (a) if the side of the artery is used, the distal arterial limb should be ligated (Bussell *et al.* 1971); (b) banding of the inflow artery or the outflow vein (Langescheid 1977); (c) the original large anastomosis is closed and a new fistula with a smaller blood flow is created either on the same or contralateral side. Wixon has proposed a new concept and strategies for the treatment of this problem (Wixon *et al.* 2000).

Venous hypertension

Venous hypertension is caused by an inflow of the arterial blood to the distal venous system. Clinical findings range from asymptomatic dilatation of veins to severe pain, swelling, and subsequent necrosis of the thumb and forefinger. The symptoms are enhanced particularly when there is narrowing or obstruction of the drainage vein. The most common clinical manifestation is the so-called 'sore-thumb syndrome'. This syndrome is prone to develop in standard arteriovenous fistulae when the radial artery and cephalic vein have been anastomosed side to side. In such a case, if the proximal side of the vein is occluded near the anastomotic site, blood is forced to flow distally and thus the veins of the hand become engorged with blood from the fistula disturbing the natural venous drainage with subsequent stasis.

Recently, with increased use of subclavian vein catheterization, stenosis or occlusion of this vein has become an important factor in causing venous hypertension. In addition to the effect of insertion of catheters, it has become clear that turbulence caused by inflow from the cephalic vein to the subclavian vein sometimes induces intimal thickening leading to stenosis and/or occlusion. In such cases, the upper limb becomes oedematous with varicose dilatation of the superficial veins. This is managed by reducing blood flow, either by narrowing the anastomotic site or by closing the anastomosis and forming a new one on the other side. It is therefore recommended that venography of

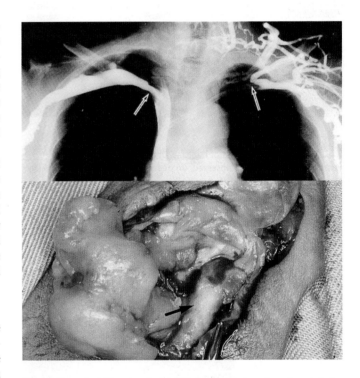

Fig. 20 Stenosis (left) and occlusion (right) caused by insertion of a subclavian catheter. The affected sites are indicated by arrows. A catheter remains inserted on the right-hand side.

the contralateral side should be undertaken to examine the patency of the subclavian vein and superior vena cava (Fig. 20).

In occlusion of the proximal draining vein, there are also two choices. One is to close the anastomosis and create a new one at some proximal part. The other is to create a bypass by anastomosing the dilated vein distal to the anastomosis to the basilic vein through a subcutaneous tunnel created either on the palmar side or dorsal side of the forearm near the wrist (Ota 1982b) (Fig. 21).

Aneurysmal or varicose dilatation of the vein

Aneurysmal and/or varicose dilatation occurring in the vascular access is often observed in patients on long-term maintenance dialysis. These

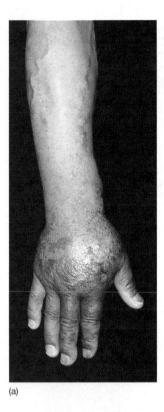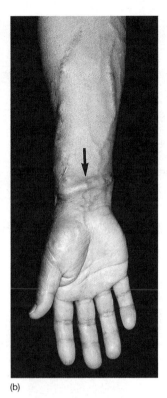

(a)   (b)

Fig. 21 Venous hypertension of the hand and its treatment: (a) hand oedema and ulceration are observed; (b) oedema has disappeared by means of a cephalobasilic anastomosis (arrow).

present few problems for function, but surgery is often necessary not only because of the danger of rupture but also for cosmetic reasons.

Aneurysmal dilatation in vascular access can be divided into four categories: (a) aneurysmal dilatation at the anastomotic site; (b) partial venous dilatation; (c) aneurysmal dilatation of the vascular graft; and (d) aneurysm of a superficialized artery.

Aneurysmal dilatation at the anastomotic site

In this condition, a stenotic segment is often found in the draining vein 1–3 cm proximal to the anastomotic site. A high internal pressure resulting from the stenosis is presumably the cause of the dilation. Surgical intervention is indicated when the aneurysmal dilatation is greater than 2 cm, and either pulsatile pain has developed in the aneurysm or glossy discolouration of the overlying skin is observed. Removal of the dilated anastomotic site followed by end-to-end anastomosis of the remaining end of the artery and vein is the solution of choice.

Partial venous dilatation

This manifests as venous dilatation up to 10 cm long. Blood flow can be obtained by puncturing the dilated site, but is difficult to obtain from elsewhere. Haemostasis after removal of the needles from the dilated segment is usually delayed. This phenomenon is seen in thrombosis of the cephalic vein at a site other than the anastomosis and where there is no suitable branch between the anastomosis and thrombosed segment to drain the inflowing blood. In such cases, the internal pressure is usually lower than that found in aneurysmal dilatation at the anastomotic site, and the risk of spontaneous rupture is small. However, surgical intervention is usually needed due to pain and difficulty in haemostasis following dialysis.

There are two ways to treat this complication. One is to dilate the stenotic portion immediately proximal to the dilated segment using

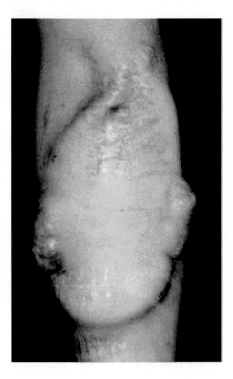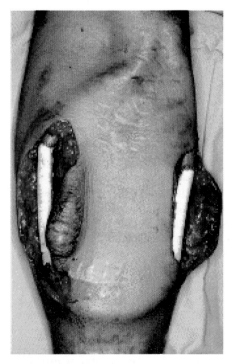

Fig. 22 Aneurysms from a vascular graft. Aneurysms are resected and replaced by two E-PTFE grafts.

thromboendarterectomy with patch grafting or an interposition graft. PTA has also been undertaken with both favourable (Dapunt *et al.* 1987; Glanz *et al.* 1987) and unfavourable (Tortolani *et al.* 1984) results.

Aneurysm of the vascular graft

Aneurysmal dilatation is one of the major complications of vascular access using grafts. As with aneurysms of native vessels they can be divided (in theory) into 'true' and 'false' aneurysms depending on the mechanism of development.

The true aneurysm develops subsequent to cleavage of the graft wall by repeated puncture of the same or a closely located site. The incidence depends on the type of graft used. Owens *et al.* (1978) reported that, when using Impra (E-PTFE) grafts, the incidence was 5 of 25 grafts over an average observation period of 8.25 months. The incidence increased with the duration of usage, repeated puncture at the same or a nearby site, and increased intraluminal pressure of the graft (Fig. 22). Surgical intervention is indicated where there is expansive growth with a diameter greater than 2 cm and rupture or impending rupture. Removal of the graft including the aneurysm and subsequent interposition of a new graft to preserve blood flow is the method of choice.

Aneurysm of a superficialized artery

As with vascular grafts, aneurysms develop in superficialized arteries after repeated puncture. It is, therefore, not advisable to puncture the same spot repeatedly. For this reason, the superficialized arterial segment should be long enough to allow an adequate selection of sites for puncture.

Indications for surgical treatment are similar to those of vascular grafts. Aneurysmorrhaphy is indicated for small aneurysms with a diameter of less than 2 cm, although excision followed by interposition of vascular graft is often required for larger ones.

Seroma

A seroma is a tumour arising from the accumulation of serum oozing from the wall of the implanted graft (Blumenberg *et al.* 1985). E-PTFE grafts are most prone to, and polyurethane grafts are almost free from, this complication. It develops adjacent to the arterial anastomotic site (Bolton *et al.* 1981) as an elastic hard hemispherical mass. The overlying skin surface becomes thin and glossy, and ultimately serum leaks through the ruptured skin.

Diagnosis is usually made by finding a hard hemispherical tumour at the anastomotic site of a E-PTFE graft. Differentiation from an aneurysm is by compressing the artery; if it is an aneurysm the 'tumour' collapses, but if a seroma no change is observed in its appearance. Surgery is indicated for aneurysms larger than 2 cm in diameter and showing continuous growth. This is an easy procedure which leaves the graft secreting serum continuously from its surface. The secretion can be stopped by electric or infrared cauterization. If it is difficult to stop secretion replacement of the affected segment by a new graft is indicated (Fig. 23).

Strategies for long-term maintenance of the vascular access

There are several important factors or conditions to consider in maintaining long-term function of the vascular access. From a systemic point of view, it is important to maintain a normal volume status. It is well known that hypotension from dehydration is one of the most common

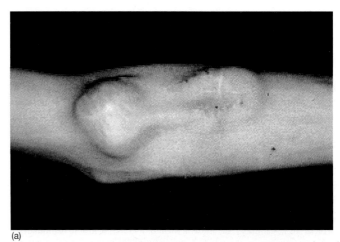

(a)

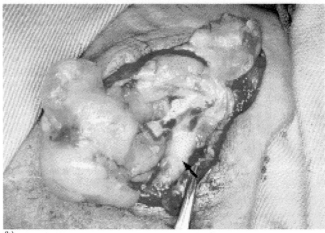

(b)

Fig. 23 Appearance (a) and findings of seroma at surgery (b). Contents of the tumour in (b) resembles a mass of fibrin; the arrow indicates an E-PTFE graft secreting serum.

causes of thrombosis of arteriovenous fistulae. Several local factors also contribute to thrombosis of the vascular access, including mispuncturing and formation of haematomas. Among these, the chain of events which results from mispuncture plays an important role. Repuncturing using the same needle causes contamination, leads to a high rate of infection, and should not be done. Compression by haematoma is an additional factor contributing to thrombosis. Another factor is turbulence of the bloodstream adjacent to the anastomosis. The resultant thickening of the intima often leads to occlusion of the draining vein. Antiplatelet drugs such as dipyridamole, ticlopidine, and prostaglandins may be used to prevent the process. The secret of success with vascular access is meticulous attention to detail, both when forming the access and in its subsequent use.

References

Ahearn, D. J. and Maher, J. F. (1972). Heart failure as a complication of hemodialysis arteriovenous fistula. *Annals of Internal Medicine* **77**, 201–204.

Allen, R. D. M., Yuill, E., Nankjvell, B. J., and Francis, D. M. A. (1996). Australian multicenter evaluation of a new polyurethane vascular access graft. *The Australian and New Zealand Journal of Surgery* **66**, 738–742.

Anderson, C. B., Etheredge, E. E., Harter, H. R., Codd, J. E., Graff, R. J., and Newton, W. T. (1977). Blood flow measurements in arteriovenous dialysis fistulae. *Surgery* **81**, 459–461.

Beathard, G. A. (1992). Percutaneous transvenous angioplasty in the treatment of vascular access stenosis. *Kidney International* **42**, 1390–1397.

Beathard, G. A. and Posen, G. A. (2000). Initial clinical results with the LifeSite® hemodialysis access system. *Kindey International* **58**, 2221–2227.

Blumenberg, R. M., Gelfand, M. L., and Dale, W. A. (1985). Perigraft seromas complicating arterial grafts. *Surgery* **97**, 194–204.

Bolton, W. *et al.* (1981). Seroma formation associated with PTFE vascular grafts used as arteriovenous fistulae. *Dialysis Transplantation* **10**, 60–66.

Bouthier, J. D., Levenson, J. A., Simon, A. C., Bariety, J. M., Bourquelot, P. E., and Safar, M. E. (1983). A noninvasive determination of fistula blood flow in dialysis patients. *Artificial Organs* **7**, 404–409.

Brescia, M. J., Cimino, J. E., and Hurwich, B. J. (1966). Chronic hemodialysis using vein puncture and a surgically created arteriovenous fistula. *New England Journal of Medicine* **275**, 1089.

Brittinger, W. D. *et al.* (1970). 16 months' experience with the subcutaneously fixed superficial femoral artery for chronic haemodialysis. *Proceedings of the European Dialysis and Transplant Association* **7**, 408.

Bussell, J. A., Abbott, J. A., and Lim, R. C. (1971). A radial steal syndrome with arteriovenous fistula for hemodialysis. *Annals of Internal Medicine* **75**, 387–394.

Capodicasa, G., Perna, N., and Giordano, C. (1971). Is a shunt an indispensable requirement for repeated haemodialysis? *Proceedings of the European Dialysis and Transplant Association* **8**, 517.

Chinitz, J. L., Yokoyama, T., Bower, R., and Swartz, C. (1972). Self-sealing prosthesis for arteriovenous fistula in man. *Transactions of the American Society for Artificial Internal Organs* **18**, 452–455.

Collins, A. J. *et al.* (1981). Blood access without skin puncture. *Transactions of the American Society for Artificial Internal Organs* **27**, 308–313.

Cross, A. S. and Steigbigel, R. T. (1976). Infective endocarditis and access site infections in patients on hemodialysis. *Medicine* **55**, 453–466.

Dapunt, O., Feurstein, M., Rendl, K. H., and Prenner, K. (1987). Transluminal angioplasty versus conventional operation in the treatment of haemodialysis fistula stenosis: results from a 5-year study. *British Journal of Surgery* **74**, 1004–1005.

Dobkin, J. F., Miller, M. H., and Steigbigel, N. H. (1978). Septicemia in patients on chronic hemodialysis. *Annals of Internal Medicine* **88**, 28–33.

Dongradi, G., Rocha, P., Kahn, J. C., Baron, B., Marichez., P., and Fendler, J. P. (1979). Arteriovenous fistula (AVF) blood flow in chronic haemodialysis patients (CHP): comparison of results obtained by the dye-dilution method (QAVF) and by variations in cardiac output during temporary occlusion of the AVF (OC). *Proceedings of the European Dialysis and Transplant Association* **16**, 690–691.

Dousset, V. *et al.* (1991). Hemodialysis grafts: color Doppler flow imaging correlated with digital subtraction angiography and functional status. *Radiology* **181**, 89–94.

Fee, H. J., Levisman, J., Doud, R. B., and Golding, A. L. (1976). High-output congestive failure from femoral arteriovenous shunts for vascular access. *Annals of Surgery* **183**, 321–323.

Finlay, D. E., Longley, D. G., Foshager, M. C., and Letourneau, J. G. (1993). Duplex and color Doppler sonography of hemodialysis arteriovenous fistulae and grafts. *RadioGraphics* **13**, 983–999.

Glanz, S., Gordon, D. H., Butt, K. M. H., Hong, J., and Lipkowitz, G. (1987). The role of percutaneous angioplasty in the management of chronic hemodialysis fistulae. *Annals of Surgery* **206**, 777–781.

Glickman, M. H., Gordon, K. S., Ross, J. R., Schuman, E. D., Sternbergh, W. C., III, Lindberg, J. S., Money, S. M., and Lorber, M. (2001). Multicenter evaluation of a polyurethaneurea vascular access graft as compared with the expanded polytetrafluoroethylene vascular access graft in hemodialysis application. *Journal of Vascular Surgery* **34**, 465–473.

Golding, A. L., Nissenson, A. R., Higgins, R., and Raible, D. (1980). Carbon transcutaneous access device (CTAD). *Transactions of the American Society for Artificial Internal Organs* **26**, 105–110.

Greenwood, P. N., Aldridge, C., Goldstein, L., Baker, L. R. I., and Cattell, W. R. (1985). Assessment of arteriovenous fistulae from pressure and thermal dilution studies: clinical experience in forearm fistulae. *Clinical Nephrology* **23**, 189–197.

Haage, P., Vorwerk, D., Piroth, W., Schuermann, K., and Guenther, R. W. (1999). Treatment of hemodialysis-related central venous stenosis or occlusion: results of primary wallstent placement and follow-up in 50 patients. *Radiology* **212**, 175–180.

Haimov, M., Baez, A., Neff, M., and Slifkin, R. (1975). Complications of arteriovenous fistulae for hemodialysis. *Archives of Surgery* **110**, 708–712.

Harder, F., Tondelli, P., and Haenel, A. F. (1977). Hamodialyse die arteriovenose Fistel distal des Handgelenkes. *Chirurgie* **48**, 719.

Hurwich, B. J. (1969). Plethysmographic forearm blood flow studies in maintenance haemodialysis patients with radial arteriovenous fistula. *Nephron* **6**, 673.

Johnson, G. and Blythe, W. (1970). Hemodynamic effects of arteriovenous shunts used for haemodialysis. *Annals of Surgery* **171**, 715.

Kirschbaum, B. and Compton, A. (1995). Study of vascular access blood flow by angiodynography. *American Journal of Kidney Diseases* **25**, 22–25.

Langescheid, C., Kramer, P., and Schelter, F. (1977). Use of a silver clip to reduce exaggerated A-V fistula blood flow rates. *Dialysis Transplantation* **6**, 56.

Levin, N. W., Yang, P. M., Hatch, D. A., Dubrow, A. J., Caraiani, N. S., Todd, S., Gandhi, V. C., Alto, A., Davila, S. M., Prost, F. R., Polaschegg, H. D., and Megerman, J. (1998). Initial results of a new access device for hemodialysis—technical note. *Kidney International* **54**, 1739–1745.

May, J. *et al.* (1969). Saphenous vein arteriovenous fistula in regular dialysis treatment. *New England Journal of Medicine* **280**, 770.

Mehigan, J. T. and McAlexander, R. A. (1982). Snuffbox arteriovenous fistula for hemodialysis. *American Journal of Surgery* **143**, 252–253.

Mindich, B. P., Silverman, M. J., Elguezabel, A., and Levowitz, B. S. (1975). Umbilical cord vein fistula for vascular access in hemodialysis. *Transactions of the American Society for Artificial Internal Organs* **21**, 273.

Moran, M. R., Rodriguez, J. M., Boyero, M. R., Enriquez, A. A., and Morin, A. I. (1985). Flow of dialysis fistulae. *Nephron* **40**, 63–66.

Nassar, G. M. and Ayus, J. C. (2001). Infectious complications of the hemodialysis access. *Kidney International* **60**, 1–13.

Nsouli, K. A., Lazarus, J. M., Schoenbaum, S. C., Gottlib, M. N., Lowrie, E. G., and Shocair, M. (1979). Bacteremic infection in haemodialysis. *Archives of Internal Medicine* **139**, 1255–1258.

Onorato, I. M., Axelrod, J. L., Lorch, J. A., Brensilver, J. M., and Bokkenheuser, V. (1979). Fungal infections of dialysis fistulae. *Annals of Internal Medicine* **91**, 50–52.

Orofino, L., Marcen, R., Ouereda, C., Castano, C., and Ortuno, J. (1987). Digital angiography and haemodialysis vascular access. *Nephron* **46**, 394.

Ota, K., Sasaki, Y., Nakagawa, Y., and Teraoka, S. (1987). A completely new poly(ether-urethane) graft ideal for hemodialysis blood access. *Transactions of the American Society for Artificial Internal Organs* **33**, 129–135.

Ota, K., Takahashi, K., Ara, R., and Agishi, T. Popliteal region—a new site for vascular graft implantation. In *Access Surgery* (ed. G. Kootstra and P. J. G. Jorning), p. 3038. Boston: MTP, 1982a.

Ota, K., Takahashi, K., Ara, R., and Agishi, T. Cephalobasilic anastomosis for venous hypertension. In *Access Surgery* (ed. G. Kootstra and P. J. G. Jorning), p. 153. Boston: MTP, 1982b.

Owens, M. L., Shinaberger, J. H., Wilson, S. E., and Wang, S. M. S. (1978). Aneurysmal enlargement of E-PTFE AV fistulae. *Dialysis Transplantation* **7**, 692.

Perini, S., LaBerge, J. M., Pearl, J. M., Santiestiban, H. L., Ives, H. E., Omachi, R. S., Graber, M., Wilson, M. W., Marder, S. R., Don, B. R., Kerlan Jr., R. K., and Gordon, R. L. (2000). Tesio catheter: radiological guided placement, mechanical performance, and adequacy of delivered dialysis. *Radiology* **215**, 129–137.

Quinton, W. E., Dillard, D., and Scribner, B. H. (1960). Cannulation of blood vessels for prolonged hemodialysis. *Transactions of the American Society for Artificial Internal Organs* **6**, 104.

Shaldon, S., Chiandussi, L., and Higgs, B. (1961). Haemodialysis by percutaneous catheterization of the femoral artery and vein with regional heparinization. *Lancet* **ii**, 857.

Siminian, S. J. *et al.* (1977). Conversion of a Scribner shunt to an arteriovenous fistula for chronic dialysis. *Surgery* **82**, 448–451.

Steuer, R. R., Miller, D. R., Zhang, S., Bell, D. A., and Leypoldt, J. K. (2001). Noninvasive transcutaneous determination of access blood low rate. *Kidney International* **60**, 284–291.

Thomas, G. I. (1969). A large-vessel appliqué A-V shunt for hemodialysis. *Transactions of the American Society for Artificial Internal Organs* **15**, 288.

Tortolani, E. C., Tanm, A. H. S., and Butchart, S. (1984). Percutaneous transluminal angioplasty. *Archives of Surgery* **119**, 221–223.

Uldall, P. R. *et al.* (1980). A double-lumen subclavian cannula (DLSC) for temporary hemodialysis access. *Transactions of the American Society for Artificial Internal Organs* **26**, 93.

Vanherweghem, J. L. *et al.* (1986). Subclavian vein thrombosis: a frequent complication of subclavian vein cannulation for haemodialysis. *Clinical Nephrology* **26**, 235–238.

Volder, J. G. R., Kirkham, R. L., and Kolff, W. J. (1973). A-V shunts created in new ways. *Transactions of the American Society for Artificial Internal Organs* **19**, 38–48.

Von Bibra, H. *et al.* (1978). The effects of arteriovenous shunts on cardiac function in renal dialysis patients—an echocardiographic evaluation. *Clinical Nephrology* **9**, 205.

Wixon, C. L., Hughes, J. D., and Milles, J. L. (2000), Understanding strategies for the treatment of ischemic steal syndrome after hemdialysis access. *Jounal of the American College of Surgeons* **191**, 301–310.

12.3 Haemodialysis, haemofiltration, and complications of technique

Christopher Olbricht, Gerhard Lonnemann, and Karl-Martin Koch

The principle of haemodialysis

The principle of haemodialysis is relatively simple, as illustrated in Fig. 1. Blood flows on one side of a semipermeable membrane, and dialysis fluid, an osmotically balanced solution of electrolytes, buffer, and glucose in water, flows on the other. The pores of the semipermeable membrane allow water molecules and small molecular weight solutes to pass through into the dialysate, but larger solutes such as proteins and blood cells are retained in the blood. Solute transport across the membrane can occur by diffusion or ultrafiltration-based convection: in haemodialysis, diffusion is the main transport mechanism, whereas in haemofiltration convection predominates. The net rate of passage of a given solute across the membrane depends on the magnitude and direction of its concentration gradient between blood and dialysate. To maintain a maximal concentration gradient during haemodialysis, blood and dialysis fluid flow through the compartments in opposite directions (Fig. 1). The rate of diffusion of a molecule across the semipermeable membrane depends also on its molecular weight and on the membrane resistance to diffusion, decreasing with increasing molecular weight and increasing membrane resistance. The resistance will be high if the membrane is thick and if there are few pores which are small in size. Additional factors affecting the diffusion rate are the size, shape, and charge of the molecules.

Ultrafiltration is applied in haemodialysis to remove excess water from the patient. If, for instance, the hydrostatic pressure is greater in the blood compartment than in the dialysate compartment, the small water molecules are forced through the membrane from blood to dialysate. In a process called solvent drag, solutes with low molecular weights that can pass through the membrane pores are swept along with the water.

The history of haemodialysis

The idea of removing solutes from body fluids by dialysis dates back to the beginning of the century. The first experimental haemodialysis in dogs was performed by at the Johns Hopkins Medical School in Baltimore. The first human dialysis was performed by Georg Haas from Gießen, Germany. He dialysed four patients with terminal renal failure between 1924 and 1928, using large celloidin tubes mounted in glass containers. Technical and anticoagulation problems limited the treatment and the patients died after temporary improvement of their uraemic conditions (Haas 1925). Willem Kolff at the Groningen University Hospital in The Netherlands introduced the first dialyser suitable for use in man in 1943. The first patient whose life was saved by treatment with the artificial kidney was a women with acute renal failure. However, problems of vascular access limited the use of dialysis to patients with acute renal failure who only needed renal replacement therapy for a short time (Kolff 1964). In 1960, the arteriovenous cannula system was introduced as vascular access for haemodialysis by Belding H. Scribner in Seattle in the United States, and 6 years later the surgically created arteriovenous fistula was introduced by Brescia and coworkers (Quinton *et al.* 1960; Brescia *et al.* 1966). These new techniques for creating permanent vascular access made it possible to perform an unlimited number of dialysis in patients with chronic, irreversible renal failure.

Technical aspects of renal replacement therapy

The major components of a haemodialysis system include the blood circuit (Fig. 2) and the dialysate circuit (Fig. 3). The central part of both circuits is the dialyser where waste products, excess electrolytes and water are removed from the patient's blood. Dialysis fluid and blood are pumped through the dialyser in a countercurrent direction, separated by the semipermeable membrane. The blood compartment is monitored to control the pressures, flow, and accidental entry of air into the blood circuit. In the dialysis-fluid compartment, the composition of the dialysis fluid, flow, pressure, temperature and accidental entry of blood into the dialysate due to rupture of the dialyser membrane need to be monitored.

The extracorporeal blood circuit

Blood is pumped from the patient's vascular-access cannula through the dialyser and back to the patient. The portion of the circuit from the patient to the dialyser is commonly referred to as the arterial segment and that from the dialyser back to the patient as the venous segment. Pressures in the blood circuit are usually measured between the arterial access and the blood pump, optionally at an arterial air trap between

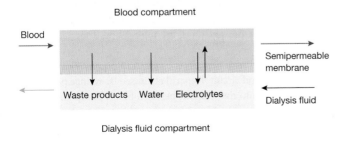

Fig. 1 Schematic representation of the haemodialysis principle.

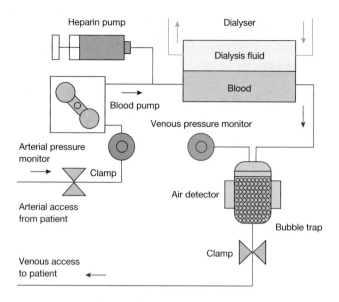

Fig. 2 The haemodialysis blood circuit.

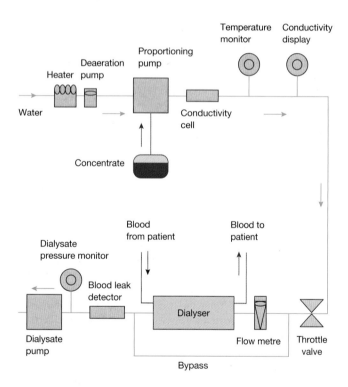

Fig. 3 The dialysis fluid circuit.

pump and dialyser, and at the venous air trap between the dialyser and the venous access. The air detector is usually located on the venous air trap. A clamp positioned just below the air trap is activated when air enters it. Heparin for anticoagulation is typically infused between the blood pump and the dialyser. When any of the alarms is activated the blood pump stops and the arterial and venous blood lines are clamped to protect the patient.

Access needles and blood tubing

The vascular-access cannulas constitute the major resistances to blood outflow and inflow. They should be large enough to allow flows of approximately 300 ml/min, but small enough to allow a smooth puncture without severe pain. Taking into account the large number of punctures per year per patient, smaller cannulas may be less detrimental for the arteriovenous fistula than larger needles. In our experience 16-gauge (1.6 mm diameter) needles of 2 cm length are sufficient to achieve blood flows in the region of 300 ml/min, with suitable arterial and venous pressures. If greater blood flows are needed, larger needles are preferable. For the arterial needle, a back eye at the tip is advantageous to prevent suction of the vessel wall into the needle tip. The connection between the access cannulas and tubing should be of the Luer-lock type to prevent disconnection. Blood tubing is mainly made of polyvinylchloride and less commonly of silicone.

Blood pump and heparin pump

The use of the arteriovenous fistula necessitates the use of a pump to ensure circulation through the blood circuit, since the pressure gradient between the fistula needles is not sufficient to achieve adequate blood flow. The flow rate at which blood perfuses the dialyser is important because it influences the efficiency of solute transport across the membrane. A peristaltic roller pump, usually integrated into the dialysis machine, is most commonly used. A special compressible segment of the arterial blood line is inserted into a curved roller track in the blood pump. The rotation of the rollers compresses the tubing, forcing blood out of the pump segment. After passage of the roller, blood is drawn in as the tubing resumes its original shape. Most pumps have two rollers. The occlusion of the pump segment between the rollers and the roller track must be adjustable: inadequate occlusion causes back flow, foaming, and haemolysis, while overocclusion may lead to damage of the tubing resulting in spallation of silicone particles (see below, section on biocompatibility), rupture with blood loss, as well as increased haemolysis. In well-adjusted blood pumps at standard flows, haemolysis is insignificant and of no clinical relevance (Hyde and Sadler 1969). Blood pumps are usually provided with a handle for manual operation in the event of power failure. The output of the blood pump is the product of stroke volume and pump speed. Blood pumps have a meter that supposedly indicates blood flow, but the value displayed is pump speed. If the stroke volume varies, even precise measurement of pump speed will not indicate flow rates accurately. Changes of stroke volume depend on variations in the internal diameter of the pump segment, the inlet suction pressure, and the elasticity of the pump segment. These variables may cause flow errors as great as 25 per cent in comparison to the displayed values, making regular calibration of the blood pump advisable.

Blood flow in the extracorporeal circuit can be determined by injecting an air bubble into the tubing and measuring the transit time through a 2 m length. The method is accurate only if the injected bubble fills the entire cross-section of the tubing, and if the blood line is horizontal.

Anticoagulation with heparin is essential to prevent clotting in the extracorporeal blood circuit. Heparin is infused by syringe pump or by peristaltic pump into the segment between blood pump and dialyser. Infusion upstream of the blood pump would increase the risk of air embolism because of the subatmospheric pressure in this segment. The infusion site should be before the dialyser to achieve adequate anticoagulation before the blood comes in contact with the large surface of the dialyser. The optimal location for other infusions and injections is the venous air trap: most blood-line systems have a short connecting tube at the air trap for that purpose. The infusion pump should be capable of accurate delivery against the pressure typically generated downstream of the blood pump.

Pressure and air-leak monitoring

The typical pressure profile of the blood circuit is illustrated in Fig. 4. The pressure before the blood pump is negative due to the resistances of the access needle and the tubing, and this carries the risk of air entry at poor connections. The pressure between the blood pump and the dialyser is always positive. The 'venous' pressure after the dialyser is measured in the air trap. The monitoring of pressures in the blood circuit allows tubing disconnections and obstructions caused by clots, kinks, or clamps to be detected, and also allows control of the fluid removal. The main determinant of fluid removal by ultrafiltration is the transmembrane pressure (TMP), which may be generated by applying positive blood-compartment pressure, negative dialysate pressure, or a combination of both. The blood-compartment pressure is estimated by averaging the pressures at inlet and outlet of the dialyser. In routine clinical practice, the venous pressure is a reasonable approximation of blood-compartment pressure. An increase in resistance downstream from the air trap will cause an increase in 'venous' pressure that may rupture the dialyser. A reduction in blood flow as well as disruption of the tubing between the air trap and venous needle will reduce the pressure and activate the low-pressure alarm.

Pressure can be monitored with mechanical manometers, electronic manometers, and—less desirable—the collapsible 'pillow' pressure monitor, which is a crude method and susceptible to frequent false alarms. All manometers and pressure transducers are protected from blood by disposable, elastic, non-permeable membranes or bellows to prevent the transmission of infections by blood. Pressure monitors should have an accuracy of ±10 mmHg at pressures of less than 50 mmHg and ±10 per cent at pressures greater than 50 mmHg. The maximum spread of pressure alarm limits should be set by the machine, with operator adjustment only within these limits. The low limit of the venous pressure should be above atmospheric pressure and close to the displayed value to enable early detection of disconnections in the venous blood line.

Any leak in the part of blood circuit with subatmospheric pressure (see Fig. 4) may lead to entry of air into the blood circuit. Causes include leaks around tubing connections and accidental removal of the arterial needle. Air may also enter from empty intravenous-fluid containers connected to the blood circuit before the blood pump: this risk should be reduced by the use of intravenous solutions in collapsible plastic bags rather than glass bottles, and their placement downstream from the blood pump. Air detectors are essential components of the dialysis blood circuit for prevention of air embolism. The ideal air detector will respond to foam as well as to air and not to saline; if there is an alarm it stops the blood pump and activates a tubing clamp immediately downstream of the air trap (see Fig. 2). Many different physical principles have been employed: probably the most reliable air detectors are ultrasonic devices. Ultrasonic waves pass through the bubble trap and are recorded at the opposite side. Since blood and other fluids transmit sound more efficiently than air, the presence of foam or air will therefore decrease the recorded intensity of the ultrasonic waves.

Dialysers

The transport of molecules across dialyser membranes is mainly diffusive, and the ratio of membrane surface to blood volume should be high for optimum efficacy. This implies that there will be thin blood films between the membranes and short diffusion distances. The two designs of haemodialyser most widely used to accomplish this goal are the parallel plate (Fig. 5) and the hollow fibre (Fig. 6). The use of disposable parallel-plate dialysers decreased over the last years reaching less than 10 per cent of all European dialysis patients; the majority of patients (90 per cent) dialyses with capillary hollow-fibre dialysers and this proportion is increasing.

The parallel-plate dialysers contain multiple layers of membranes separated by flat supports. The membrane surface area may range from 0.8 to 1.5 m^2; the average dialyser has a surface of around 1.1 m^2, and an average blood-compartment volume of approximately 100 ml. This volume increases with increasing pressure in the blood compartment. This characteristic is called the compliance of the dialyser. The hollow-fibre dialysers consist of a bundle of capillaries encased in a plastic tubular housing and potted at both ends in tightly sealing material. Blood enters and leaves the device via manifolds, and the dialysate flows in a countercurrent direction around the fibre bundles. Surface areas commonly in use are approximately 1.2 m^2. Hollow-fibre dialysers have almost no compliance and the blood-compartment volume rarely exceeds 90 ml. Ethylene oxide gas is still most widely used to sterilize dialysers but

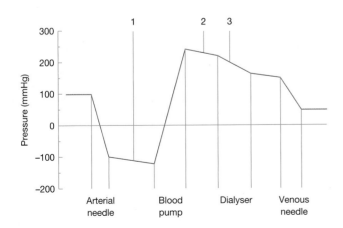

Fig. 4 Pressure profile in the blood circuit. 1, 2, and 3 indicate pressure monitors.

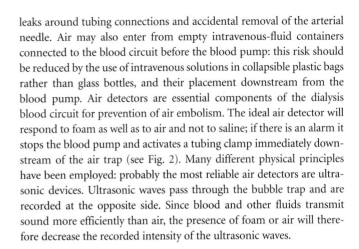
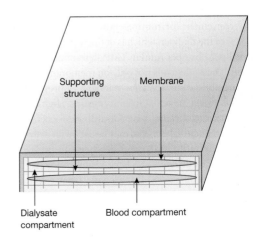

Fig. 5 Schematic representation of a parallel-plate dialyser.

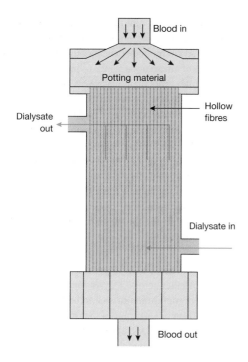

Fig. 6 Hollow-fibre dialyser.

steam and γ-radiation are more frequently applied in the past 10 years. One important reason to avoid ethylene oxide is that this gas may cause allergic reactions (see below).

Membranes

There are two types of dialyser membrane: cellulose-based and synthetic. The former include Cuprophan®, the most widely used dialyser membrane in the 1990s, which is made of reconstituted cellulose. Examples of synthetic membranes are polysulfone, polycarbonate, polyamide, and polyacrylonitrile. The membranes differ in their solute permeability, hydraulic permeability, and interaction with blood. In general, synthetic membranes provoke less interaction with blood cells and plasma proteins than membranes made of reconstituted cellulose. However, membranes made of modified cellulose exhibit only low-grade interactions with blood.

The solute permeability of a membrane is high if it is thin and the pores are numerous and of large diameter. A measure of the hydraulic permeability convenient for routine clinical use is the ultrafiltration coefficient (K_f) of the dialyser, which is defined as the volume of ultra-filtrate formed per hour per mmHg TMP, determined at a blood flow of 200 ml/min. The K_f depends not only on membrane characteristics, but also on membrane surface area: standard Cuprophan® dialysers have K_f values between 3.5 and 7 ml/min/mmHg. High-flux dialysers, made of synthetic membranes, have ultrafiltration coefficients up to 60 ml/min/mmHg. Such dialysers can only be used with dialysis machines that have reliable ultrafiltration control systems to prevent excessive volume loss. High-flux dialysers also have greater convective permeability to molecules of 5000–25,000 Da, allowing faster removal of larger solutes from the blood.

Clearance

The solute transport characteristics of a dialyser may be expressed as clearance, analogous to the use of this term in renal physiology. This is

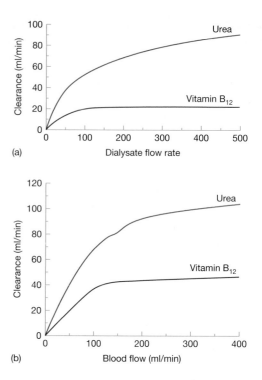

Fig. 7 (a) Relationship between dialysate flow rate and clearance, blood flow rate 200 ml/min. (b) Relationship between blood flow rate and clearance, dialysate flow rate 500 ml/min.

a clinically meaningful measure since it describes the dialyser as a part of the patient's circulatory system. Clearance is defined as the amount of solute removed from the blood per unit of time, divided by the incoming blood concentration. The clearances of solutes depend on membrane permeability and the flow rate at which blood perfuses the dialyser (Q_B). The removal of small solutes such as urea and creatinine is influenced to a greater extent by the flow rates of blood and dialysis fluid than by the diffusive resistance of the dialyser membrane (Fig. 7). The removal of large solutes such as vitamin B_{12} (1355 Da) is, however, mainly influenced by the diffusive resistance of the membrane and to a much smaller extent by blood and dialysate flow rates. High-flux membranes have a comparatively low diffusive resistance, and greater clearances of larger solutes are achieved by such dialysers. Clearance data for dialysers are specified for a blood-flow rate of 200 ml/min. The urea clearance of commonly used dialysers is approximately 160 ml/min.

Reuse of dialysers

It is estimated that dialysers are reused in over 80 per cent of patients on haemodialysis in the United States, but only in approximately 10 per cent of patients on dialysis in Europe (Fassbinder *et al.* 1991; Tokars *et al.* 2000). To minimize side-effects, it is essential to adhere to the recommended standards for all steps of reuse (AAMI—Association for the Advancement of Medical Instrumentation 1993). Immediately after disconnection of the patient, both compartments of the dialyser are extensively rinsed with dialysis water. The procedures for rinsing often include reverse ultrafiltration in which the dialysate compartment is pressurized relative to the blood compartment to remove blood from the capillaries of the dialyser more effectively. Rinsing is followed by cleaning of the blood compartment. A mixture of peroxyacetic acid and hydrogen peroxide (PAM, Renalin™) is the most common agent used to clean dialysers. Sodium hypochlorite (bleach) can also be used but this agent has several disadvantages (Dumler 1994). It may damage the membrane, reducing its burst strength and increasing the ultrafiltration coefficient (Deane and Bemis 1982; Pizziconi 1990). Hypochlorite-processed polysulfone dialysers may leak substantial quantities of protein; the degree of protein loss increases with each reuse (Kaplan *et al.* 1995). The dialyser is tested after cleaning, usually by a fibre-bundle volume test combined with measurement of the ultrafiltration coefficient and pressure testing to detect leaking (Krivitski *et al.* 1998).

For consecutive disinfection the dialysate and blood compartments are filled with germicides. The most commonly used germicide is PAM (4.5 per cent peroxyacetic acid, 28 per cent hydrogen peroxide), but 4 per cent formaldehyde or 0.8 per cent glutaraldehyde can also be used. Before subsequent use of the dialyser the sterilants must be removed and the amount of residual disinfectant in each dialyser has to be determined. The AAMI recommends formaldehyde concentrations of less than 5 mg/l.

Heat disinfection is an alternative to chemical sterilization. The dialyser is filled with dialysis-quality water and placed in a 105°C convection oven for 20 h. Heat may damage the casing and the potting material of the dialyser and substantially reduce the number of reuses (Kaufman *et al.* 1992). To reduce thermal stress on dialysers, the heat disinfection process has been modified by addition of 1.5 per cent citric acid and using lower temperatures (95°C). Heat sterilization has thus far been tested only in polysulfone dialysers with heat-resistant polycarbonate casings and polyurethane resin (Levin *et al.* 1995).

The number of reuses from a single dialyser varies widely among patients and dialysis units. In the United States, a median number of 14 reuses nationally and a maximum number of 30 reuses in single dialysis units have been reported (Tokars *et al.* 2000).

The main argument in favour of reuse is to reduce the cost of treatments. The clinical benefit attributed to reuse was a lower incidence of first-use reactions. However, a controlled prospective cross-over study found no difference in the incidence of symptoms after the reuse or single use of regenerated cellulosic dialysers (Cheung *et al.* 1991). Reuse may be associated with several undesirable effects. Infections with *Mycobacterium chelonei* and common water pathogens, such as *Pseudomonas aeruginosa* and *Pseudomonas maltophilia*, were reported in patients treated with reused dialysers (Lowry *et al.* 1990; Vanholder *et al.* 1992). However, either deficient disinfectant mixing or lower than currently recommended concentrations of the disinfectant have been applied in these cases. A doubled incidence of febrile reactions due to retained endotoxins in patients on reused high-flux dialysers has been reported by some (Petersen *et al.* 1981; Gordon *et al.* 1988), but comparative randomized clinical trials have not shown an increased risk of pyrogenic reactions with dialyser reuse (Kant *et al.* 1981; Churchill *et al.* 1988; Fleming *et al.* 1991). There is an increased loss of albumin through the dialyser when bleach has been used in the cleansing (Kaplan *et al.* 1995).

A loss of dialyser performance is of concern. Although negligible effects on urea, creatinine, and phosphorus removal have been found with cellulose derived membranes (Fleming *et al.* 1991), the delivered dialysis dose *Kt/V* may decrease with an increased number of reuses (Sherman *et al.* 1994). The removal of β_2-microglobulin is enhanced, impaired or remains unaffected, depending on the combination of membranes and cleaning agents (Petersen *et al.* 1991; Westhuyzen *et al.* 1992; Cheung *et al.* 1999). Ultrafiltration may fall slightly after reuse with PAM and increase after reuse with bleach and formaldehyde (Fleming *et al.* 1991). In a recent retrospective study, the relative risk of death was increased in patients treated with reused low-flux dialysers

disinfected with glutaraldehyde or PAM, but treatment with reused formaldehyde-disinfected low-flux dialysers was not associated with greater risk ($p = 0.088$) than in the non-reuse group. The results were quite different with high-flux dialysers.

Mortality was somewhat lower in units reusing high-flux dialysers with PAM or glutaraldehyde and similar with formaldehyde when compared to units using non-reprocessed low-flux dialysers (Held *et al.* 1994). Studies showing mortality risks associated with some reuse practices (Collins *et al.* 1998; Kimmel and Miskin 1998) may be unreliable because of multiple problems, including selection bias, global interference drawn from unit-level data, and poorly characterized or unknown centre effects (Kimmel and Miskin 1998). Two well designed consecutive studies showed no effect on mortality and confirmed the general safety of reuse with high-flux dialysers (Ebben *et al.* 2000; Port *et al.* 2001). These results are almost certainly due to the improved quality control of reuse practices as well as a significant increase in use of synthetic membranes.

Although adequately performed cleaning of high-flux dialysers for reuse appears to be safe, potential for side-effects exist and there seems to be no clinical benefit. It should be recognized that the driving force behind dialyser reuse is cost-savings. Even in the United States, the National Kidney Foundation took no position concerning whether dialysers should or should not be reused (National Kidney Foundation 1997).

Single-needle haemodialysis

In patients with limited puncture sites on the arteriovenous fistula, allowing insertion of one needle only, and in acute dialysis where vascular access is achieved by percutaneous cannulation of major veins, the so-called single-needle dialysis can be applied (Fig. 8). The basic principle involves alternating the direction of blood flow through a single access needle joined to a Y-junction that connects the arterial and the

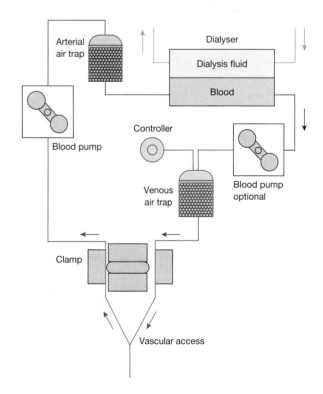

Fig. 8 Single-needle dialysis system.

venous ends of the standard blood circuit. The alternation of flow can be achieved in different ways. One system uses two clamps situated on the arterial and venous lines as close as possible to the Y-connection. When the arterial clamp is opened, the pump draws blood into the circuit against the closed venous clamp. The pressure in the blood compartment increases to an upper limit, at which the arterial clamp closes, stopping the blood pump and opening the venous clamp. Blood flows back into the patient due to the high pressure in the blood compartment. When the pressure reaches a lower limit, the low-pressure alarm closes the venous clamp, opens the arterial clamp, and starts the blood pump. The system can be optimized by using two separate pumps for arterial withdrawal and venous return. In single-needle dialysis, the compliance of the blood circuit must be enhanced by an arterial bubble trap between pump and dialyser, serving as an expansion chamber. Recirculation of blood in the Y-connection does occur and amounts to 20 per cent of the blood flow, reducing the solute clearance. To achieve effectiveness comparable to that of a standard, 4 h two-needle dialysis a blood flow greater than 400 ml/min and a 10–20 per cent increase in the duration of dialysis are mandatory (Vanholder *et al.* 1989).

The dialysis-fluid circuit

The dialysate circuit most commonly used today is the single-pass system (Fig. 3). Dialysate is continuously produced by a proportioning device that mixes purified water and a concentrated salt solution in a ratio of 1 : 35–1 : 45. The concentrate may be delivered from a central supply system or from bedside containers. Water is heated and de-aerated before being mixed with concentrate: since a considerable amount of air is usually dissolved in water, dialysis solutions prepared from water that is not de-aerated tend to 'degas' under conditions of negative pressure and heating. This may lead to maldistribution of the flow and a decrease in the performance of the dialyser. The temperature of the dialysate must be kept close to 37°C to keep the temperature of the blood in the extracorporeal circuit within physiological limits. Monitoring, which is essential to ensure the composition of the dialysate is adequate, depends on the specific conductivity of the total ionic strength of the dialysate [expressed in milliSiemens (mS)]. The conductivity of the dialysate depends mainly on sodium and chloride (see Table 2): at standard sodium concentrations of between 135 and 150 mmol/l the conductivity is between 13.5 and 15.0 mS. Conductivity cells ensure that if the quality of the dialysate is outside the desired limits, it bypasses the dialyser. The flow rate and the pressure within the dialysate circuit are set by a dialysate pump downstream and a throttle valve upstream of the dialyser. The negative pressure so generated in the dialysate compartment of the dialyser increases the TMP required for fluid transfer from blood to dialysate. The dialysate flow meter is located before the dialyser, and the dialysate pressure monitor is between the dialyser and the dialysate pump.

The presence of red blood cells in the dialysate, due to membrane rupture, is monitored by a blood-leak detector downstream of the dialyser, which measures the change in optical transmission caused by haemoglobin. The detection threshold is between 0.25 and 0.35 ml of blood per litre of dialysate.

Preparation of tap water for dialysis

Tap water needs to be purified for the purposes of dialysis. Drinking water regulations are based on a weekly exposure of about 14 l, whereas the patient on dialysis is exposed to between 300 and 500 l a week. These patients have severely impaired renal function and, hence, compromised urinary excretion of toxic substances ingested with drinking water. Unlike gastrointestinal absorption, diffusion across the dialysis membrane is unselective. The requirements of dialysis water are therefore more stringent than those for drinking water, and additional purification is essential. Contaminants of tap water with documented toxicity include aluminium sulfate, chloramines, copper and other trace metals, fluoride, nitrates, and other organic materials. In areas where water is hard due to excess calcium, the 'hard water syndrome' (see below) may occur, and calcium must be removed from tap water.

A standard water-treatment system device consists of a water softener, an activated carbon filter, a sediment filter, and a reverse osmosis module (Fig. 9). Activated carbon filters remove chlorine, chloramines, and dissolved organics, but, because of their microporous structure, these filters tend to release carbon particles and a sediment filter has to be placed downstream. This filter also removes particulate matter from the water, protecting water-purification equipment downstream of the filter from obstruction by particles. Water softeners are ion exchangers containing a cationic resin that exchanges sodium ions for calcium, magnesium, and other polyvalent ions. The effectiveness of softening is monitored by measuring the hardness of the effluent water. Water softening not only prevents the hard water syndrome, but also protects the reverse-osmosis membrane, used in the final step of water treatment, from a build-up of scale and subsequent failure. In reverse osmosis, the water is forced through a highly semipermeable polyamide or cellulose membrane under high pressure. This removes 90–100 per cent of inorganic and organic substances, pyrogens, bacteria and particulate matter, and water thus treated meets the standards for dialysis water (Table 1). Water is pumped from the reverse-osmosis module to the patient's individual stations in a recirculating loop which delivers the water produced in excess of that actually required for dialysis back to the reverse-osmosis module, preventing wastage of high-quality water. Continuous circulation of water may reduce microbial growth and the formation of biofilm on the inner surface of the tubing (see below). The ring type of distribution system is considered as standard for dialysis units.

The limit for microbiological contamination has been set at a maximum total viable count of 100 cfu/ml for the water used to prepare the dialysis fluid and 1000 cfu/ml for effluent dialysate at the end of the dialysis procedure (Association for the Advancement of Medical Instrumentation 1993; Baldamus *et al.* 1999). The endotoxin contamination of dialysis water measured in the Limulus amebocyte lysate assay should be less than 0.25 endotoxin units (EU)/ml and less than 0.50 EU/ml in dialysate (Baldamus *et al.* 1999). Water-treatment devices are susceptible to microbial proliferation: sediment filters and

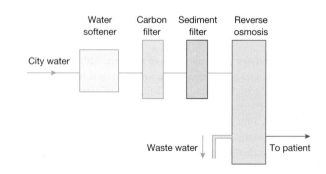

Fig. 9 Schematic representation of a water treatment device for haemodialysis.

Table 1 Water quality standards of haemodialysis according to the Association for the Advancement of Medical Instrumentation (AAMI)

Substance	Maximum concentration (mg/l)
Aluminium	0.01
Chloramine	0.10
Copper	0.10
Zinc	0.10
Fluoride	0.20
Nitrate	2.00
Sulfate	100.00
Calcium	2.0 (0.1 mEq/l)
Magnesium	4.0 (0.3 mEq/l)
Potassium	8.0 (0.2 mEq/l)
Sodium	70.0 (3.0 mEq/l)

Table 2 Composition of extracellular fluid and a standard dialysis fluid

	Serum water (mmol/l)	Dialysis fluid (mmol/l)
Sodium	152	140–145
Potassium	4.5	1–3
Calcium	1.5	1.5
Magnesium	0.5	0.5
Chloride	109	100–110
Acetate or	0	30–35
Bicarbonate	30	32–38
Glucose	5	0–10

carbon filters should be regularly replaced, and water-softening devices need regular bacteriological surveillance and disinfection. Although reverse osmosis is effective for removal of bacteria, viruses, and pyrogens, microbial growth can occur on the module, which may cause small defects in the membrane allowing bacteria and pyrogens to penetrate it and contaminate the water produced. The reverse-osmosis module must therefore be disinfected regularly. To avoid bacterial growth in stagnant water, water-treatment devices are put into operation intermittently by automated control systems during the night and at weekends when dialysis does not normally take place. Stagnant water in the connecting tubes between the recirculating water supply loop and the dialysis monitors is the most important cause of bacterial growth in the water distribution system. Microorganisms stick to the inner surface of water and dialysate tubing and grow in an organic matrix of bacterial origin called biofilm (Man *et al.* 1998). Discharge of bacteria and bacterial products from biofilm may lead to intermittent or continuous contamination of dialysis water. In order to reduce biofilm formation phases with stagnant water in the system should be reduced to a minimum and disinfection of the water distribution loop including the connecting tubes on a regular basis is recommended.

Composition of the dialysate

The composition of dialysis fluid should be similar to that of normal interstitial body fluid appropriately corrected for protein content (Table 2). A sodium dialysate concentration of 138–140 mmol/l is appropriate for most patients (Redaelli *et al.* 1979), but some may need greater concentrations of sodium in the dialysate to prevent muscle cramps during and after the dialysis session. Sodium concentrations exceeding 145 mmol/l are associated with increased thirst, fluid intake between dialyses, and hypertension. Sodium concentrations less than 138 mmol/l may be accompanied by an increased incidence of hypotension and muscle cramps during treatment.

At an average ultrafiltration of 2 l of plasma water (sodium concentration 135–145 mmol/l) during one dialysis session, about 280 mmol (16 g)

of sodium will be removed, an amount approximately equal to that ingested by the average patient over 2 or 3 days. In patients with treatment resistant hypertension, it may be necessary to further reduce salt intake and, in the same time, to use low dialysate sodium concentrations (below plasma sodium concentration) to remove also sodium by diffusive transport in order to control blood pressure (Krautzig *et al.* 1998).

In patients with hypotension or muscle cramps during haemodialysis 'sodium profiling' or 'sodium ramping' has been applied to prevent these side effects. The initial dialysate sodium may be for instance 148 mmol/l and is decreased during dialysis to 138 mmol/l (see section describing acute complication during dialysis).

The standard dialysate potassium concentration is usually 2 mmol/l: this can be changed by using different concentrates. Zero potassium is desirable in patients with severe hyperkalaemia; in those with a normal predialysis potassium and a tendency to cardiac arrhythmias a dialysate potassium of 3 or even 4 mmol/l should be used.

The routine dialysate calcium concentration should be 1.5 mmol/l unless there is substantial hyper- or hypocalcaemia: this concentration allows a zero calcium balance to be achieved (Wing 1968). The administration of calcium salts as phosphate binders and/or of calcitriol may induce hypercalcaemia; in response the dialysate calcium should be reduced temporarily to 1.25 mmol/l (Sawyer *et al.* 1988; Slatopolsky *et al.* 1989). The serum calcium should be measured regularly to avoid unphysiological concentrations. When a positive calcium balance is desired, the dialysate calcium concentration may be increased to 1.75 mmol/l.

Most dialysis centres use 0.5–0.75 mmol magnesium per litre in dialysate to maintain normal serum magnesium concentrations (Markell *et al.* 1993). Hypomagnesaemia can be detrimental as it may play a part in the development of dialysis-related cramps and cardiac arrhythmias in susceptible patients (Kenny *et al.* 1987). The clinical impact of hypermagnesaemia is controversial (Catto *et al.* 1974): it may protect against soft tissue calcification (Meema *et al.* 1987), but others have claimed it may be involved in the development of polyneuropathy (Ahmad 1984), pruritus (Graf *et al.* 1979), and renal osteodystrophy (Drüeke 1984), and have recommended a dialysate magnesium of less than 0.5 mmol/l.

Dialysate buffer: bicarbonate haemodialysis

Although not a physiological buffer, acetate has been used for a long time as buffer in dialysis fluid: it is readily metabolized in the liver, resulting in the generation of bicarbonate from carbon dioxide (Mion *et al.* 1964). The introduction of acetate instead of the physiological bicarbonate was necessary with the advent of single-pass, on-line preparation of dialysate from concentrated dialysis fluids. The presence of bicarbonate in calcium- and magnesium-containing concentrates may lead to the precipitation of calcium and magnesium carbonates and the deposition of these insoluble salts in the dialysate pathway. With the use of high-efficiency dialysers, the influx of acetate will substantially increase and may exceed the metabolic capacity of the liver and the muscles, resulting in an elevated serum acetate accompanied by cardiovascular instability, nausea, and vomiting (Graefe *et al.* 1978; Vreman *et al.* 1980). It is now recognized that vascular stability during dialysis is improved with bicarbonate rather than acetate haemodialysis. Several studies have demonstrated that the compensatory vasoconstrictive response to hypovolaemia is inhibited when acetate is used as buffer (Keshaviah 1982). Further dialysis-induced complications attributed to the use of acetate include hypoxaemia, incomplete correction of acidosis, and an increased release of cytokines (Dolan *et al.* 1981; Kaiser *et al.* 1981; Bingel *et al.* 1987). These acetate-related problems stimulated development of the equipment necessary for safe, on-line delivery of bicarbonate dialysate and subsequently the use of bicarbonate dialysis has increased in many European countries from 55 to 97 per cent of all haemodialyses (Geerlings *et al.* 1994).

To prevent precipitation of calcium and magnesium carbonates, two concentrates are required for bicarbonate dialysis: a bicarbonate concentrate containing sodium bicarbonate and sodium chloride, and an acidified concentrate containing sodium, potassium, calcium, magnesium, chloride, glucose, and acetic acid. Acetic acid is included in the calcium- and magnesium-containing concentrate to achieve a slightly acidic pH when the two concentrates are mixed, thereby preventing precipitation of calcium and magnesium carbonates. Two proportioning pumps are necessary for bicarbonate dialysis, one for the acidic and one for the bicarbonate concentrate. The conductance is measured after each mixture. In most modules, controlling the speed of the concentrate pump is used as an extra safeguard. Both conductance and motor speed must be regulated between narrow limits to avoid errors in the composition of the dialysate. Control of the pH of the ultimate dialysate is advocated as an additional safeguard (von Breitenfelder 1986b). Most modules are capable of varying the bicarbonate concentration of the dialysate. In clinical practice in many centres, acetate and bicarbonate dialyses may be going on simultaneously. These procedures are done with dialysis machines equipped for the optional use of acetate and bicarbonate buffers. Hence, there is an increasing chance of mistakenly using the wrong concentrate. This can result in a dangerous composition of the dialysate, with a pH of 3–4, when only acid concentrate is used erroneously for both concentrates. To reduce this risk, the storage containers and the machine input tubes should be colour-coded, and there should be a selective mechanical interlock between the containers and the connection of the tubing to the module. Furthermore, the pH of the ultimate dialysate should be controlled.

Bicarbonate dialysis will lead to the precipitation of calcium and magnesium salts in the dialysis system, possibly associated with unreliable measurements of conductance and ultrafiltration volume. Therefore, besides careful disinfection, it is of great importance to decalcify the dialysate system daily after dialysis, for instance with citric acid.

The use of liquid bicarbonate dialysate concentrate is associated with two problems: a decrease in the bicarbonate concentration due to loss of CO_2 and microbial contamination since it is an excellent growth medium (Mion *et al.* 1987). To avoid substantial bicarbonate loss and

significant bacterial growth, the concentrate should be used within 7–8 h once the container has been opened (von Breitenfelder 1986a,b). To prevent bacterial contamination, pure, dry sodium bicarbonate powder in a plastic cartridge or bag has been introduced. The stored powder does not permit bacterial growth, so there is only minimal contamination. By passing warm, degassed water through the cartridge, a saturated bicarbonate solution is produced, which is then proportioned as described for the liquid bicarbonate concentrate (Delin *et al.* 1988). Another system to avoid the problems related to liquid bicarbonate concentrate is termed 'acetate-free biofiltration', where the dialysate is buffer-free and an appropriate volume of 1 M bicarbonate is infused into the venous bubble trap to substitute for the loss of buffer base (Zucchelli *et al.* 1990).

Because of the considerable variation in the requirements for bicarbonate from patient to patient, the dialysis machine must be able to provide dialysates with variable concentrations of bicarbonate (Gennari 1985). The therapeutic goal is to achieve postdialysis bicarbonate concentrations of from 26 to 28 mmol/l (Gennari 1985), and the bicarbonate concentration in the dialysate should be selected accordingly. For most patients on dialysis an initial dialysate bicarbonate of between 30 and 32 mmol/l is appropriate. Bicarbonate concentrations at or greater than 35 mmol/l should be used with caution, since several dialysis-associated complications may be aggravated by these larger concentrations. The serum ionized calcium is lower in comparison to dialysate containing 30 mmol/l of bicarbonate, leading to decreases in vascular tone and cardiac contractility (Leunissen *et al.* 1989). A faster increase in pH may be associated with the rapid development of hypokalaemia, probably with associated cardiac arrhythmias (Wiegand *et al.* 1979). Furthermore, a substantial post-dialysis alkalosis with clinical symptoms is conceivable in haemodialysis using dialysate with a very high bicarbonate concentration.

Regeneration of dialysate

Conventional haemodialysis with single pass of dialysate requires approximately 150 l of pretreated water per session. In an attempt to reduce this volume and thereby to meet the requirements for a portable artificial kidney, several methods of regenerating the dialysate have been developed. The only system with wide application is named REcirculating DialYsis (REDY) (Drukker and Van Doorn 1989), and it incorporates a dialysate reservoir containing 6 l of dialysate which is continuously recirculated at a flow rate of 250 ml/min through a disposable regeneration cartridge. The REDY is similar to the standard dialysis machine and is provided with the usual monitors and alarm systems.

The regeneration cartridge is in five layers. The first layer consists of activated carbon and zirconium oxide, and binds trace metals and oxidizing agents such as chlorine, chloramine, sodium hypochloride, and others that may be present after disinfection and rinsing of the system or in the water used to prepare the dialysis fluid. The second layer contains urease, which catalyses the decomposition of urea to ammonium ions and bicarbonate ions. The third layer consists of zirconium phosphate and acts as a cation exchanger loaded with hydrogen ions and sodium ions in a ratio of 1 : 8, which are exchanged for ammonium, calcium, magnesium, and potassium ions. The complete removal of calcium, magnesium, and potassium means that these anions must be added continuously as acetate salts to the regenerated dialysate by a separate infusate system. In the fourth layer of cartridge, containing zirconium oxide, anions such as phosphate and fluoride are exchanged for acetate. The fifth layer consists of activated carbon and adsorbs creatinine, uric acid, and other waste products of nitrogen metabolism.

Haemodialysis using the REDY system has some peculiar features. The process of regeneration limits the dialysate flow to a maximum of 250 ml/min, and clearance of small molecular-weight solutes are therefore less than in standard haemodialysis with a dialysate flow of 500 ml/min. The ability of the REDY system to remove urea is limited by the capacity of the third zirconium phosphate layer to exchange ammonium ions. Cartridges with a capacity to remove approximately 43 and 60 g of urea are available: this may be insufficient in patients with a high rate of protein catabolism. If the capacity of the cartridge for ammonium is exceeded, the patient will be exposed to increasing concentrations of ammonium present in the effluent of the cartridge. The generation of bicarbonate by the cartridge is an important source of buffer base: minor sources are the acetate in the initial dialysis solution, the infused acetate salts of calcium, magnesium, and potassium, and the acetate generation in the fourth layer. These sources of buffer base have been structured to deliver an amount of base sufficient to correct moderate predialysis acidosis. However, in patients with a low predialysis urea and on short-time dialysis, the amount of urea adsorbed by the cartridge is reduced and an insufficient amount of bicarbonate may be generated. Additional bicarbonate must be added.

The bicarbonate generated by the conversion of urea and the bicarbonate originating from the patient's blood react with the protons delivered from the zirconium phosphate, and decompose into water and carbon dioxide when the pH is less than 7. For this reason, the P_{CO_2} in the dialysate will increase, sometimes up to 300 mmHg, CO_2 will be transferred to the blood, and the P_{CO_2} of the blood leaving the dialyser will be high. However, the total amount of carbon dioxide delivered to the patient is small in comparison to the amount generated by the patient's metabolism, and the arterial P_{CO_2} will not increase in patients with normal ventilatory function.

Due to the exchange of ammonium, calcium, magnesium, and potassium for sodium and hydrogen ions in the third layer, the sodium concentration in the fluid leaving the cartridge will be greater than that in the incoming dialysate. During a 4 h dialysis the dialysate sodium may increase by some 30–35 mmol/l; an initial dialysis fluid sodium concentration of 105–115 mmol/l is recommended.

Despite these complicated and specific properties, there is evidence that the blood chemistry and clinical features in long-term REDY-treated patients are similar to those of patients on chronic dialysis treated by conventional, single-pass haemodialysis (Mansell and Wing 1977). However, REDY is more expensive than conventional dialysis and continuous ambulatory peritoneal dialysis, owing to the high cost of disposable cartridge. The independence from a water supply achieved by the REDY system offers the chance for dialysis patients to travel without major limitations, but chronic ambulatory peritoneal dialysis, which is less expensive and easier to operate, has superseded REDY in this respect. REDY has also been recommended for where moving the dialysis machine to the patient is preferable to moving the patient, for instance in intensive-care units and in hospitals without facilities for dialysis, but small, portable, reverse-osmosis modules connected to the conventional dialysis machine are now available and continuously deliver water of dialysis quality. Haemodialysis with portable, reverse-osmosis modules needs only tap water, and is cheaper and less complicated than REDY. In our opinion, chronic ambulatory peritoneal dialysis and dialysis with portable, reverse-osmosis modules are the better alternatives to the REDY system.

Single-pass batch haemodialysis system

A batch dialysis system such as the REDY system has the disadvantage of accumulation of urea and other uraemic toxins in the dialysate tank. Consequently, the diffusion gradient across the dialyser membrane and the efficiency of dialysis decreases progressively with time. Recirculation of dialysate promotes growth of microorganisms and release of pyrogens causing pyrogenic reactions such as shivering attacks which were common in the early days of haemodialysis using batch systems.

Tersteegen designed a batch type machine combining the advantages of a batch system with those of a modern single-pass dialysis system (Fassbinder 1998). The advantages of this system are simplicity of design and preserved flexibility regarding dialysate composition. The dialysate for one treatment session is stored in an air-free 75 l glass container which is completely filled with dialysate as shown in Fig. 10. The acetate-free bicarbonate-buffered dialysis fluid is prepared from sterile reverse osmosis water and prepacked salts (NaCl, KCl, $CaCl_2$, $MgCl_2$, $NaHCO_3$). The dialysis fluid is heated to a temperature of 38–40°C during the filling process of the 75 l tank of the dialysis system. The composition of the dialysis fluid (Na^+ 135–145 mmol/l, HCO_3^- 25–45 mmol/l, K^+ 1–4 mmol/l, Ca^{2+} 1.0–2.0 mmol/l, Mg^{2+} 0.3–1.2 mmol/l, Glucose 0–11 mmol/l) can be adapted to the needs of the individual patient by varying the prepacked salts. The glass walls of the container provide thermal isolation so that heating of the dialysate during a 5-h treatment session is not necessary. Special two-lumen quartz glass tubes in the axis of the tank allow separate access to the top and the bottom of fluid compartment of the tank. Fresh dialysis fluid is pumped from the top of the tank into the dialysate compartment of the dialyser. In the closed dialysate loop, used dialysate is pumped from the dialyser through the central tube to the bottom of the tank. Because of a small difference in temperature, the slightly cooler (−1°C) used dialysate entering the bottom of the tank does not mix with fresh dialysis fluid on top. Only one roller pump with two pump-segments is present in the extracorporeal system circulating blood and dialysate with the same speed of 250 ml/min each in a countercurrent manner. With this pump speed the 75 l tank lasts for

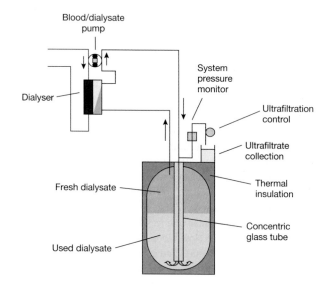

Fig. 10 Single-pass batch haemodialysis system.

a treatment session of 5 h. An ultrafiltrate line with adjustable pump is connected to the closed, completely filled dialysate compartment allowing ultrafiltration rates between 20 and 1000 ml/h and providing a simple and exact method of volumetric ultrafiltration control: fluid removed from the dialysate compartment under the control of the ultrafiltration monitor has to be generated by ultrafiltration from the patients blood.

The single-pass batch haemodialysis system (trade name: Genius® system) provides ultra-pure quality of dialysis fluid because the design combines the following factors: (a) ultra-pure reverse osmosis water which is UV irradiated to suppress bacterial growth; (b) dry salt concentrates reducing the risk of bacterial contamination are used to mix dialysis fluid; (c) the whole blood and dialysate tubing is single use material, there are no multiple-use connectors in the system which are known sites of bacterial growth; and (d) the material of the machine is mostly glass and dead spaces are avoided to prevent accumulation of micro-organisms.

Due to the flexibility of the system with respect to dialysis fluid composition, and independency of water supply during treatment, it is suitable for use in the treatment of chronic renal failure as well as for extended daily veno-venous haemodialysis in the treatment of acute renal failure in intensive care (Lonnemann et al. 2000).

The control of ultrafiltration

One essential goal of haemodialysis is the removal of fluid from the patient by ultrafiltration. The driving force for ultrafiltration is the TMP, which is determined by the mean hydrostatic pressures in the dialysate (P_d) and blood compartment (P_b), and the oncotic pressure (P_o) in the blood compartment, according to the equation:

$$\text{TMP} = P_b - (P_o + P_d)$$

The volume of ultrafiltrate is determined by the TMP and by the ultra-filtration coefficient (K_f) of the dialyser. Theoretically, it would be possible to control ultrafiltration through TMP. The mean pressure in the blood compartment of the dialyser can be derived from the blood inlet and outlet pressures [(2) and (3) in Fig. 4]. The dialysate pressure can be derived from dialysate inlet and outlet pressures of the dialyser. However, the control of ultrafiltration by controlling and adjusting TMP is accompanied by many uncertainties. It assumes accurate measurements of four pressures as well as knowledge of the accurate K_f of the dialyser in vivo. In the clinical setting only two pressures are monitored, at the blood outlet and dialysate outlet. The K_f of dialysers is usually specified with a standard deviation of ±10–20 per cent and it is subject to changes during dialysis due to membrane-protein interactions. In the light of these problems, the control of ultrafiltration by TMP is unreliable. Corrections of TMP are necessary during dialysis to achieve the desired volume removal. Consequently, the patient may be subject to varying rates of ultrafiltration with the potential of hypovolaemic hypotension or inadequate fluid removal.

Recently, systems that measure and directly control the rate of ultra-filtration have been developed. These systems, which assure the uniform, accurate, and predictable removal of fluid during haemodialysis, include the flow sensor, the closed loop, and the volumetric balancing. The flow-sensor system measures and compares the inflow and outflow of the dialysate (Fig. 10): the difference between these values corresponds to the ultrafiltrate volume and is automatically adjusted to the desired volume by changing the TMP. In the closed-loop system, the dialysate

circulates in a closed loop (Fig. 11). An additional pump removes a volume of fluid from the closed circuit, equal to the ultrafiltration rate. The circulating dialysate is replaced at intervals by fresh dialysate. The volumetric-balancing system is similar to the closed loop (Fig. 12). Matched pumps keep the dialysate inflow exactly equal to the dialysate outflow, creating a 'semiclosed' loop. Ultrafiltration is governed by an additional pump removing fluid from this loop.

Dialysers with high-flux membranes need to be used in dialysis machines with reliable volume control of ultrafiltration to prevent excessive fluid loss. The use of high-flux dialysers may result in filtration from dialysate to blood in the efferent part of the dialyser due to a reverse TMP gradient: this effect is called 'back filtration' (Stiller et al. 1986). Only a slightly negative dialysate pressure is necessary to achieve a sufficient net ultrafiltration rate in dialysis with high-flux dialysers. At the dialysate inlet (blood outlet) of the dialyser the dialysate pressure is close to zero. The hydrostatic pressure in the blood compartment

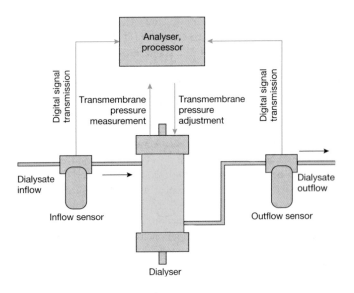

Fig. 11 The flow-sensor system of ultrafiltration control.

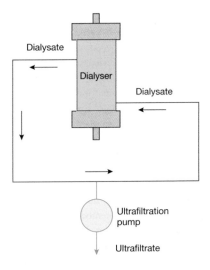

Fig. 12 The closed-loop system of ultrafiltration control.

decreases from blood inlet to blood outlet, while the oncotic pressure remains almost constant along the blood pathway. At the blood-outlet part of the dialyser, therefore, the effective filtration pressure (hydrostatic pressure – oncotic pressure) within the blood compartment forcing fluid from the blood into the dialysate compartment may be lower than the hydrostatic pressure in the dialysate compartment, and back filtration may occur. Back filtration may cause convective transfer of pyrogenic substances derived from bacteria from the dialysate to the blood. If a membrane leak occurs at the efferent part of the dialyser, dialysate will enter the blood and the leakage may not be detected. The possible clinical consequences are described below.

Haemofiltration

Haemofiltration is an alternative form of renal replacement therapy where solute removal is achieved only by convection, rather than diffusion, as in haemodialysis (Henderson *et al.* 1973). Instead of a dialyser, a haemofilter is incorporated into the blood circuit. The highly permeable membranes of the haemofilter, made of polysulfone, polyamide, and polyacrylonitrile, allow ultrafiltration rates of between 120 and 180 ml/min under appropriate conditions of blood flow and TMP. The ultrafiltrate containing urea, creatinine, uric acid, and other waste products is substituted with an equal volume of lactate-, acetate-, or bicarbonate-buffered Ringer's solution introduced into either the arterial line (predilution) or the venous line (postdilution). The filtration rate is measured gravimetrically, and the infusion of substitution fluid is adjusted automatically to the filtration rate. Adequate removal of urea and other small molecular waste products requires the exchange volume per treatment to be around 40 per cent of the body weight; three treatments are required per week. To maintain the high filtration rates of between 120 and 180 ml/min necessary for adequate treatment in an appropriate time, blood-flow rates of from 350 to 500 ml/min are required, making a vascular access with a high flow rate a prerequisite. Clinical advantages of haemofiltration over haemodialysis include better haemodynamic stability during treatment, less hypotension after treatment, and no exposure to dialysate fluid, which may contain pyrogens (Baldamus *et al.* 1982). In spite of these advantages only 3 per cent of all patients on renal replacement therapy in Europe are treated by haemofiltration: a major reason for this is certainly the greater cost, since haemofilters cost twice as much as low-flux dialysers, and sterile and pyrogen-free substitution solution costs more than dialysate. In most patients, the clinical benefit of haemofiltration may be absent or to small to justify the greater expense. Where there is pronounced vascular instability, however, haemofiltration may be applied with major advantages for the patient. The advantage of haemodialysis of high removal of small solutes has been combined with the improved cardiovascular stability of haemofiltration in hybrid systems that include both convection and diffusion (Schmidt 1986): this has been termed 'haemodiafiltration'. Three per cent of all patients on renal replacement therapy in Europe are treated by haemodiafiltration. This low acceptance rate may be explained in part by the complex machinery necessary for haemodiafiltration and by higher costs in comparison to haemodialysis.

Online haemodiafiltration

The preparation of substitution fluid for haemofiltration and haemodiafiltration by the haemodialysis proportioning system (on-line preparation) became popular during the last decade for several reasons. First of all, high-flux treatment modalities with a high degree of convective transmembrane transport to improve middle molecule

clearances require large volumes of substitution fluid. In conventional haemofiltration and haemodiafiltration, the volume ultrafiltered from the patient is replaced by intravenous infusion of replacement fluid which is provided prefabricated in plastic bags. In particular when high volume haemofiltration and haemodiafiltration with ultrafiltration volumes as high as 50 l per treatment are performed and bicarbonate- instead of lactate-buffer is used, expenses for replacement fluid increase tremendously. Alternatively, the online preparation of substitution fluid, in other words the use of fluid produced by the dialysis machine for intravenous infusion, provides the opportunity of cost-effective convective high-flux therapies. The problem of on-line preparation of infusion fluid is to ensure its sterility.

For on-line production of infusion fluid, minimal contamination of reverse osmosis water provided by the central water supply system is a precondition. The water quality should be controlled on a regular basis and has to fulfil recommended standards (bacterial growth < 100 cfu/ml; endotoxin content < 0.25 EU/ml). Single-step ultrafiltration through pyrogen-adsorbing filters made of polysulfone or polyamide ensures ultra-pure quality of dialysis fluid (bacterial growth: <0.1 cfu/ml; endotoxin: <0.03 EU/ml). In order to further improve safety and sterility, double filtration of dialysis fluid through two synthetic high-flux filters in series has been introduced (Canaud *et al.* 2000). Today, there are several modifications of on-line haemodiafiltration machines available. All systems use two ultrafilters in series to filter the dialysis fluid prepared from ultra-pure water, acid, and bicarbonate concentrates (Fig. 13). One ultrafilter (UF 1) is installed in the

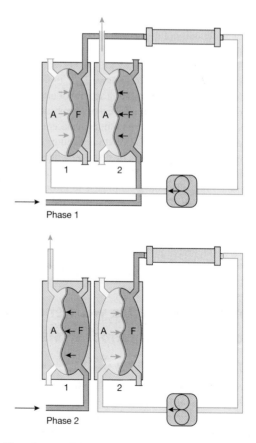

Fig. 13 The volumetric-balancing system using diaphragm pumps for ultrafiltration control. A, spent dialysate; F, fresh dialysate.

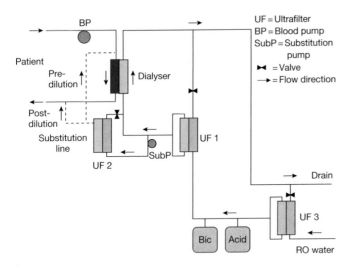

Fig. 14 Preparation of ultra-pure substitution fluid for online haemodiafiltration from dialysis fluid.

dialysis fluid circuit and is included in the rinsing and disinfection program of the dialysis machine. The second ultrafilter (UF 2) is also integrated in the dialysis fluid circuit and replaced together with UF 1 every 100 treatments, or is a disposable filter for single use. In all systems, single-filtered fluid is used as dialysate and double-filtered fluid is used for intravenous substitution in on-line haemofiltration or haemodiafiltration. To ensure ultra-pure quality of reverse osmosis water before mixing of dialysis fluid, one on-line system employs an additional ultrafilter (UF 3) at the water entry of the dialysis monitor (Fig. 14).

All modifications of on-line systems have been used for high volume haemodiafiltration and the bacteriological quality as well as the endotoxin concentration (using a very sensitive LAL-assay, detection limit 0.005 EU/ml) and the cytokine-inducing activity of ultrafiltered dialysis fluid were repeatedly tested in samples from the substitution line. Over study periods of up to 12 months and routine replacement of ultrafilters every 100 sessions, neither bacterial growth nor endotoxin nor cytokine-induction were detected in samples of single-step filtered dialysis fluid and two-step filtered infusion fluid (Ward *et al.* 2000; Canaud *et al.* 2001; Lin *et al.* 2001). Comparing these parameters to those in commercially available sterile infusion solutions, on-line prepared substitution fluid can be referred to as sterile and pyrogen-free (Ledebo and Nystrand 1999; Vaslaki *et al.* 2000). Today, double filtration through pyrogen-adsorbing synthetic membranes is a practical, safe and cost effective approach to produce pyrogen-free substitution fluid on-line.

Treatment of patients with endstage renal disease by haemodialysis

The number of patients on dialysis

The number of patients on dialysis varies largely from country to country. In Europe, the number of patients per million population (pmp) treated by regular dialysis ranges from 157 (Estonia) to 891 (Belgium) (Frei *et al.* 2001). A higher prevalence of renal replacement therapy has been reported from the United States (1209 pmp) and Japan (1629 pmp). The large differences may be partly due to differences in the rates of

kidney transplantation, but the major reason is certainly economic. In general, there is a correlation between gross national product and the number of patients on dialysis in a given country. About 50 per cent of the world population have no access to renal replacement, owing to the lack of financial resources.

Organization of haemodialysis

In most Western European countries, haemodialysis mostly takes place in a specialized centre, which may be integrated into a hospital or in a private practice. The centre provides a full medical service and close monitoring during and between treatments. Such treatment is expensive, mainly because of the high staff: patient ratio, and therefore programmes have been developed to teach patients to haemodialyse themselves.

Selected patients at low medical risk can be trained for home haemodialysis as long as the constant support of a family member and adequate space are available. Home haemodialysis may place substantial stress on domestic relationships, and this may be one reason why its popularity has declined steadily. Other reasons are the increasing number or patients being treated by continuous ambulatory peritoneal dialysis and the increased number of dialysis centres. In addition, patients starting haemodialysis during the last decade are older and have significant comorbidity necessitating regular medical care in a dialysis centre. Four per cent of all patients on haemodialysis are treated in the home in Europe (Geerlings *et al.* 1994). In Germany, the percentage of home-haemodialysis patients decreased to 0.9 per cent in 2000 (Frei *et al.* 2001). A form of dialysis between in-centre and home haemodialysis is the so-called limited-care dialysis, in which patients at comparatively low medical risk are trained to dialyse themselves without major assistance and supervision in a dialysis centre. The staffing required for these centres is less than in full-service centres. The increasing age and morbidity of the dialysis population have also led to a decline in this form of dialysis provision.

Patient selection

The selection of patients for haemodialysis may be influenced by restricted facilities for renal replacement or may be based purely on medical grounds. In countries where dialysis facilities are restricted, the number of patients on dialysis as well as the number of new patients admitted to dialysis per year are much lower than in countries with unrestricted facilities. Between 53 and 175 new patients pmp per year were accepted for renal replacement therapy during 1998 in Europe. The respective numbers for the United States and Japan were 313 and 253 new patients pmp per year (Frei *et al.* 2001). Since it seems reasonable to assume that there is no significant difference between European countries in the incidence of endstage renal disease, a selection process has to be assumed to be taking place with the consequence that a considerable number of patients are excluded from renal replacement therapy. The most common discriminant for selection is age. Other selection criteria include the expected quality of life, anticipated compliance, quality of vascular access, ability to self-dialyse, and the acceptability for transplantation. Criteria used by the Seattle Medical Advisory Board in the 1960s can be used as a historical example. These criteria selected stable patients under 45 years of age with no irreversible cardiovascular disease who were expected to cooperate well (Murray *et al.* 1962). However, some physicians felt that, if selection is necessary, a 'first come-first serve' policy is the one most ethically acceptable (Abrams 1976). In countries with limited facilities, one regulatory factor is the phenomenon of 'under-referral' from primary care physicians, as reported from the United Kingdom (Challah *et al.* 1984).

Withholding of dialysis is also not uncommon under circumstances where dialysis facilities are not a restricting factor (Singer 1992; Hirsch *et al.* 1994; Sekkarie and Moss 1998). For instance, American nephrologists consider withholding dialysis in the following situations: patients with severe and irreversible dementia; patients who are in the vegetative state; patients with endstage lung, liver, or heart disease without the prospect of organ transplantation; patients with severe, continuous and uncontrollable pain. Dialysis should not be used merely to prolong the dying process (Lowance 1993; Moss 1995). However, it is extremely difficult to assess the quality of life, as perceived from the patients view point and as long as the patient does not refuse dialysis, it should be initiated and continued. Since many patients may not have their full decision-making capacity when dialysis is necessary, it is important to discuss dialysis as early as possible in the course of renal failure. Every patient should have the chance to prepare proper advance directives about initiation of dialysis. In patients who are incompetent to decide the nephrologist should search for previously given written directives and should ask family members about explicit oral advance directives or strongly held beliefs that would be inconsistent with dialysis. When there is doubt about chances of recovery from a severe underlying disease, a trial of dialysis may be offered. Withdrawal of dialysis at a later time is preferable to withholding it from the beginning.

Age, *per se*, is not a sufficient reason to withhold dialysis. Five-year survival rates of patients aged 65 or more are 20–40 per cent, the median life expectancy is approximately 3–4 years, which is lower than that of patients without endstage renal disease (Held *et al.* 1990; Ismail *et al.* 1993). Survival among patients greater than 80 years of age is between 26 and 29 months with a tendency to increase during the last decade. In these very old patients on haemodialysis life expectancy was not shorter in comparison to octogenarians without dialysis (Peri *et al.* 2001). Dialysis improves the condition of most elderly patients considerably and many patients have a high quality of life on dialysis (Ahmed *et al.* 1999). Thus, dialysis should not be denied to elderly patients, even the very old, if there is hope for prolongation of enjoyable additional years of life.

Once the decision to start dialysis is made, the optimal form of renal replacement for the individual patient should be considered. Either peritoneal dialysis and haemodialysis should be offered to the patient whenever possible, and the selection should be based on the patients preference. Although haemodialysis is an adequate renal replacement therapy for most patients, peritoneal dialysis may be obligatory for some patients (see Chapter 10.6) including those with major vascular access problems and with severe diabetic retinopathy, since anticoagulation during haemodialysis may cause deterioration of vision due to retinal bleeding. In patients with severe cardiac insufficiency, continuous fluid removal by chronic ambulatory peritoneal dialysis is better tolerated than intermittent fluid removal by haemodialysis and better blood pressure control is achieved.

Start of maintenance haemodialysis

The preparation of patients with endstage renal disease for renal replacement therapy should begin with providing vascular access well in advance of its need. The Cimino–Brescia arteriovenous fistula in the forearm is the access of choice for most patients. A new fistula takes between 2 weeks and 4 months to mature into an access with sufficient blood flow and puncture sites, depending on the vascular status of the patient. In general, vascular access surgery should be performed when the clearance is between 10 and 15 ml/min. Patients with rapid progression of renal failure and with anticipated 'slow access maturation' should undergo access surgery earlier. If patients present with far advanced uraemia, requiring immediate dialysis, acute vascular access through percutaneous cannulation of large veins is necessary until the arteriovenous fistula matures.

Initiation of haemodialysis is mandatory in patients with severe uraemic symptoms, such as pericarditis, volume overload with pulmonary oedema refractory to diuretics, severe hyperkalaemia, progressive uraemic encephalopathy, and persistent nausea and vomiting. In asymptomatic patients with deteriorating renal function, there is no general rule about when to begin dialysis: although initiation of dialysis at a clearance greater than 10 ml/min may be associated with longer survival and lower morbidity on dialysis (Bonomini *et al.* 1985), this view is not shared by others (Korevaar *et al.* 2001). Clinical experience indicates that for most patients maintenance dialysis is best initiated when the creatinine clearance is approximately 5 ml/min (Maher 1976; Ratcliffe *et al.* 1983). It should be emphasized, however, that the patient's clinical condition is more important than laboratory values. Occasional patients survive in excellent condition without dialysis for as long as 3 years after reaching a creatinine value of 900 μmol/l (Maher 1976). Other patients may have uraemic symptoms with a creatinine clearance greater than 10 ml/min. An important consideration to start dialysis may be malnutrition. A direct correlation exists between creatinine clearance and dietary protein intake (Ikizler *et al.* 1995). For instance, patients without dietary intervention with a creatinine clearance greater than 50 ml/min consumed 1.1 g/kg per day of protein, while those with a creatinine clearance less than 10 ml/min had a protein intake of 0.54 g/kg per day. Plasma albumin is decreased in patients with decreased protein intake and the risk of death in patients starting haemodialysis with hypoalbuminaemia is substantially greater than in patients with a normal albumin concentration (USRDS 1992). Therefore, low protein intake and hypoalbuminaemia in patients with a creatinine clearance less than 15–20 ml/min may be an indication to start dialysis after exclusion of other causes of anorexia (NKF-DOQI 2001). Protein intake can be estimated from daily urinary urea nitrogen excretion by using the following formula (Maroni *et al.* 1985):

$$\text{Estimated protein intake} = 6.25(\text{urine urea nitrogen} + 0.03 \\ \times \text{body weight in kg})$$

The standard dialysis schedule is 4–5 h three times per week, depending on residual renal function, age, body weight, and fluid volume status (see also in section 'adequacy of dialysis'). The initial four to five dialysis treatments should be considerably shorter (2–3 h) to prevent the development of the so called dialysis disequilibrium (described below).

Patients treated by home haemodialysis usually have longer treatment hours, probably responsible for the better outcome associated with home haemodialysis (Mailloux *et al.* 1996; Oberley and Schatell 1996; Woods *et al.* 1996; McGregor *et al.* 2000). First experiences with six to seven nocturnal haemodialysis sessions per week indicate a better control of blood pressure, phosphate metabolism and fluid balance leading to a significant better rehabilitation in comparison to standard haemodialysis (Galland *et al.* 2001; Mohr *et al.* 2001). Long-term prospective studies comparing daily haemodialysis with standard haemodialysis concerning health benefits, survival and costs are yet not available. It seems to be premature to recommend daily home haemodialysis before such studies are available.

Anticoagulation during haemodialysis

Interaction between the extracorporeal blood circuit and the clotting system

The flow of blood through the extracorporeal circuit activates the intrinsic coagulation pathway, leading to the formation of thrombin and fibrin. Circulating platelets adhere to the artificial surface of the dialyser and undergo a series of changes that include spreading, and release of ADP, thromboxane A2, and other highly reactive products from their granules (Salzman 1987). Platelet adhesion also interacts with the activated clotting system: thrombin stimulates the release of factors which enhance platelet adhesion and aggregation, and aggregated platelets activate prothrombin at their cell surface. The final result of these interactions is thrombus formation.

Heparin

Heparin is the anticoagulant most widely used to prevent clotting in the extracorporeal blood circuit in haemodialysis patients. Heparin is a highly anionic charged sulfated glycosaminoglycan that accelerates the formation of a molecular complex between antithrombin III, a constituent of normal plasma, and coagulation factors of the intrinsic coagulation system. In concert with heparin, antithrombin III inhibits the activated clotting factors IX, X, XI, XII, and thrombin. Heparin preparations presently in use are a heterogeneous mixture of molecules that vary in molecular weight from about 2000–40,000, averaging around 15,000–18,000. The anticoagulant activity of heparin is a function of its molecular size. With decreasing molecular weight there is an increase in factor Xa (activated) inhibition and a reduction in thrombin inhibition. Low molecular weight heparin has a high affinity for antithrombin III and strongly inhibits factor Xa and XIIa, but only weakly inhibits thrombin and factors IX and XI. In contrast to normal unfractionated heparin, low molecular weight heparin causes only a slight increase in partial thromboplastin and thrombin time. The size of heparin molecules also influences its interaction with platelets, and the interaction of platelets with dialyser membranes (Hirsch et al. 1985). Unfractionated heparin enhances the adhesion of platelets at dialyser membranes and may significantly reduce platelet count over the course of haemodialysis (Lindsay et al. 1977). Low molecular weight heparin appears to have a lower potential to induce thrombocytopenia during haemodialysis (Huisse et al. 1982): the undesirable side-effects of heparin attributable to higher molecular weight fractions led to the introduction of heparin preparations with lower molecular weights (average 4000–5000 Da).

The effect of low molecular weight heparin is monitored using the chromogenically determined anti-factor Xa activity (Bratt et al. 1983). Such monitoring is laborious, and costs are greater than those for standard heparin. A comparison of standard and low molecular weight heparin showed equivalent antithrombotic effectiveness in haemodialysis. The number of blood transfusions given during the study period was slightly lower in the patients given low molecular weight heparin: this was interpreted as indicating reduced occult blood loss (Schrader et al. 1988). Long-term treatment with low molecular heparin may cause a decrease in triglycerides and cholesterol in haemodialysis patients unlike long-term treatment with conventional heparin (Deuber and Schulz 1991). Whether low molecular weight heparin reduces the risk of atherosclerotic complications in patients on maintenance haemodialysis

remains to be determined. Low molecular weight heparin is associated with a considerably lower rate of heparin-induced thrombocytopenia (Warkentin et al. 1995). There is no doubt that safe and effective haemodialysis can be performed using low molecular weight heparin. Whether the slight advantages justify the routine use of low molecular weight heparin for anticoagulation in all haemodialysis patients remains debatable. Until further data are available, it is important to recognize that low molecular weight heparin is much more expensive than conventional heparin and it may therefore be preferable to standard heparin only in patients with severe hyperlipidaemia.

Under-anticoagulation with the risk of clotting in the extracorporeal blood circuit; overheparinization with the potential of overt and occult bleeding may result in blood loss. The narrow therapeutic limits mean that precise control of heparin anticoagulation is necessary (Farrell et al. 1978). Determination of the standard partial thromboplastin time as a control needs a coagulation laboratory, and is therefore also time consuming. Adequate tests for bedside monitoring of anticoagulation during haemodialysis are the whole blood activated clotting time and the whole blood activated partial thromboplastin time. The whole blood activated clotting time differs from the whole blood clotting time in that an activator of surface contact factors, such as kaolin, is added to speed up the initial stages of the coagulation cascade. Thus, the normal whole blood activated clotting time ranges from 90 to 140 s. The whole blood activated partial thromboplastin time is based on the same principle, except that the activator contains a platelet lipid surrogate as well as surface contact activators. The normal value for this test is between 50 and 80 s. During haemodialysis the optimal whole blood activated clotting time lies between 200 and 240 s, and the whole blood activated partial thromboplastin time is between 120 and 160 s (Farrell et al. 1978).

The standard heparinization procedure includes administration of an initial bolus of heparin prior to the connection of the patient to the extracorporeal circuit and continuous infusion of heparin during haemodialysis. Since the dose of heparin required may vary widely within the dialysis population and may change with time on dialysis in the individual patient, heparin requirements should be assessed by the above tests during the first three haemodialyses the patient undergoes. An example of an assessment of the heparin dose is given in the final section of this chapter. The heparin dose should be reassessed if there is untoward clotting or bleeding. If clotting occurs in spite of adequate heparinization, enhanced interaction of platelets with the dialyser membrane may be suspected, and it is reasonable to treat the patient with an antiplatelet drug such as low dose of acetylsalicylic acid (Lindsay et al. 1972).

Heparin-induced thrombocytopenia (HIT)

Heparin may induce thrombocytopenia by two different pathways associated with different clinical syndromes (Warkentin et al. 2001). HIT I usually occurs within 4 days after heparin treatment has started, the platelet count seldom declines to less than 100,000, there are no haemorrhagic or thromboembolic sequelea, and the platelet count often returns to normal with continued heparin administration. The mechanism of the thrombocytopenia appears to be due to a direct effect of heparin on platelet activation, as described above for higher molecular heparin fractions. HIT II is an immune-mediated disorder, characterized by formation of antibodies against the heparin–platelet factor IV complex. The platelet count usually decreases to 30,000–55,000, haemorrhagic sequelae rarely occur, but thromboembolic events including arterial and a v-shunt thrombosis occur in 30–80 per cent. The frequency of HIT II in patients receiving unfractionated heparin is between 1 and 3 per cent, while low molecular weight heparin is associated with a lower incidence of HIT II (Warkentin *et al.* 1995; Yamamoto *et al.* 1996; O'Shea *et al.* 2002). The appearance of otherwise unexplained thrombocytopenia, thrombosis associated with thrombocytopenia, or even a normal platelet count which has fallen 50 per cent or more from prior value should raise the possibility of HIT II in patients undergoing haemodialysis with heparin. The diagnosis of HIT is initially made on clinical grounds and heparin should be stopped immediately. The confirmatory laboratory tests for HIT II include the serotonin release assay, the heparin-induced platelet aggregation test, and a solid phase immunoassay of the heparin–platelet factor IV complexes.

Avoidance of low molecular weight heparin is recommended in HIT II patients since it may crossreact with heparin induced antibodies and may induce heparin-dependent IgG antibody formation. In addition, thrombocytopenia and the hypercoagulable state may persist when low molecular weight heparin is substituted for unfractionated heparin (Warkentin 2001). The options for patients who have developed HIT II include regional citrate haemodialysis (see below), a change to peritoneal dialysis, or the administration of one of the three drugs that appear to be effective in patients with HIT II: danaparoid, recombinant hirudin, and argatroban. Danaparoid is a heparinoid which includes predominantly dermatan sulfate and heparan sulfate. The anticoagulant effect of danaparoid is monitored by measuring anti-factor Xa levels. There is substantial experience in HIT II but only limited experience in haemodialysis patients using this agent (Magnani *et al.* 1993). There is a 10 per cent crossreactivity between danaparoid and the antibody responsible for HIT II *in vitro* (Magnani *et al.* 1993). The persistence or recurrence of thrombocytopenia without thrombosis was noted in 6.5 per cent of non-dialysis patients with HIT II who were switched from heparin to danaparoid (Tardy-Poncet *et al.* 1999). Further disadvantages of danaparoid include its long half-life of 25 ± 100 h, and the absence of an antidote. Hence, danaparoid may not be the anticoagulant of choice for haemodialysis patients with HIT II.

Recombinant hirudin effectively prevents thromboembolic events in HIT II (Greinacher *et al.* 2000). Caution should be used in patients with renal insufficiency, since the drug is cleared by the kidney and its anticoagulant effect is not easily reversed. There is substantial experience with hirudin in haemodialysis (Vanholder *et al.* 1994; Van Wyck *et al.* 1995; Nowak *et al.* 1997; Vanholder *et al.* 1997; Bucha *et al.* 1999; Dager and White 2001). Most authors recommend a single bolus injection of 0.08–0.15 mg/kg body weight of hirudin immediately prior to start of haemodialysis. Adequate anticoagulant levels are monitored by measuring the activated partial thromboplastin time, which should be 1.5–2 times the base line value. There are substantial variations in the necessary dosage and in the elimination half-life of hirudin (2–107 h, median 9 h) in haemodialysis patients, probably related to residual renal function. These large variations require that the dosage be individually adjusted when repeated treatments are given (Vanholder *et al.* 1994; Van Wyck *et al.* 1995; Vanholder *et al.* 1997; Bucha *et al.* 1999; Dager and White 2001).

Argatroban is a small molecule that inhibits thrombin directly. It is metabolized by the liver, has a half-life of only 24 min, and dose adjustment is apparently not required in the presence of renal failure. To achieve an activated PTT of 1.5–2 times baseline a continuous infusion of 2 μg/kg/min is necessary; patients with hepatic dysfunction may start with 0.5 μg/kg/min (Lewis *et al.* 2001). Experience with haemodialysis is very limited (Matsuo *et al.* 1988).

Anticoagulation in patients with high bleeding risk

Dialysis is often required in patients with an intercurrent haemorrhagic problem such as gastrointestinal or retinal bleeding, or when a situation exists where over-heparinization may be dangerous, such as in those with pericarditis or following surgery. The bleeding risk associated with haemodialysis can be reduced by 'minimal heparinization'; this is administration of 50 per cent of the heparin dose as evaluated by the above methods. Another method is 'regional heparinization' in which heparin is neutralized by constant infusion of protamine before the blood returns to the patient. A heparin rebound may occur between 2 and 10 h after cessation of dialysis, potentially causing haemorrhage when the heparin–protamine complex is broken down in the reticuloendothelial system and heparin re-enters the circulation. In a clinical trial comparing minimal heparinization with regional heparinization, bleeding frequency was considerably greater with the latter (Swartz and Port 1979), and regional heparinization is therefore not recommended. In patients at high risk of bleeding, dialysis may be accomplished without any anticoagulation (Schwab *et al.* 1987). Heparin-free haemodialysis requires pretreating both the dialyser and blood lines with 2000–5000 units of heparin contained in a litre of normal saline. The heparinized saline is flushed from the extracorporeal lines prior to the start of dialysis treatment so that heparin is not administered to the patient. Extracorporeal blood flow should by as high as possible and the haemodialyser must be flushed with 100–200 ml isotonic saline every 15–30 min. A high ultrafiltration rate is required to remove the large fluid volume given to the patient. Heparin-free haemodialysis is the most common method of providing dialysis to patients at high bleeding risk and can be accomplished in approximately 90 per cent of cases (Schwab *et al.* 1987).

Prostacyclin prevents platelet aggregation and has also been applied as antithrombotic agent in dialysis patients with high bleeding risk (Zusman *et al.* 1981). In a prospective trial comparing prostacyclin and heparin for anticoagulation, a 50 per cent reduction in the frequency of bleeding was observed in the prostacyclin-treated patients (Swartz *et al.* 1988). Side-effects such as hypotension and clotting in the extracorporeal circuit have been reported repeatedly. Prostacyclin should be considered as a substitute for heparin in haemodialysis patients with high bleeding risk, but whether there is an advantage of prostacyclin over heparin free dialysis remains to be determined. In patients with acute renal failure undergoing continuous arteriovenous haemofiltration which often cannot be performed without heparin, prostacyclin is certainly an effective antithrombotic agent which may considerably reduce bleeding (Davenport *et al.* 1988).

Regional citrate anticoagulation involves the continuous infusion of isosmotic trisodium citrate solution (102 mmol/litre) into the arterial line. The fall in the free plasma calcium concentration induced by binding to citrate is responsible for the anticoagulant effect. The citrate–calcium complex is removed across the dialyser membrane. The citrate infusion is adapted to maintain the activated clotting time above 200 s in the arterial limb. Regional anticoagulation is achieved by the infusion of 5 per cent calcium chloride into the venous return line at a rate of 0.5 ml/min. The rate is constantly adjusted according to frequent measurements of plasma calcium concentrations to prevent hypocalcaemia or hypercalcaemia. Several modifications of this technique have been described. The major problems are hypocalcaemia or hypercalcaemia, hypernatraemia due to hypertonic trisodium citrate, and metabolic alkalosis due to bicarbonate generated during citrate metabolism. Therefore, close monitoring is essential (Janssen *et al.* 1996).

Acute complications of haemodialysis

In the early years of haemodialysis, complications due to technical failure of the equipment were very common. Substantial technical improvements have made such events rare, and haemodialysis has become a safe therapeutic procedure. If technical complications occur at all, they are mostly caused by inappropriate use and not by primary technical faults. Today, acute complications during haemodialysis are mainly related to medical problems of the patients and to factors and mechanisms inherent to the intermittent dialytic procedure itself. An acute event accompanying haemodialysis is frequently the consequence of a synergy between patient's pathology and a dialysis-induced process.

Complications due to technical faults or inappropriate application of haemodialysis equipment

Incorrect proportions of water and dialysate concentrate leading to major deviations in sodium concentration and osmolality of the dialysate are unlikely to occur due to reliable on-line control of the ionic strength by conductivity meters. If, however, the patient is accidentally exposed to hypotonic dialysate, haemolysis, hyperkalaemia, and cerebral oedema may occur with the early symptoms of lumbar and abdominal pain. Once the failure is recognized the patient should immediately be disconnected from the extracorporeal circuit. The haemolysed blood should be rinsed from the dialyser and dialysis should be reinstituted using a dialysate of correct composition. If indicated, oxygen, blood, and anti-convulsant drugs should be administered.

The increasing use of bicarbonate-buffered dialysate has created the risk of severe hyperchloraemic acidosis (Brueggemeyer *et al.* 1987). To prepare bicarbonate buffered dialysate on-line, an acidic and a basic concentrate have to be mixed with water. Mixture of only the acidic component with water may not be detected by the conductivity meter and, unless a pH meter is included in dialysate monitoring, an acidic dialysate will be delivered, inducing hyperchloraemic acidosis. Intravenous administration of bicarbonate and haemodialysis with bicarbonate dialysate of correct composition are the appropriate therapeutic measures.

Unlike sodium, the dialysate calcium concentration cannot be monitored by conductivity. The occurrence of acute hypercalcaemia during haemodialysis is in virtually all cases a consequence of inadequate preparation of tap water (Freeman *et al.* 1967). Untreated drinking water contains variable concentrations of calcium; failure of the water treatment devices to remove calcium may increase the dialysate calcium concentration, resulting in hypercalcaemia, the so called 'hard water syndrome'. The symptoms include nausea, vomiting, abdominal pain, headache, disorientation, confusion, and seizures. Some patients may develop pancreatitis. Acute treatment consists of correcting the hypercalcaemia by replacing the faulty dialysate by a low calcium dialysate and in continuing dialysis treatment.

Air embolism is one of the most serious complications of haemodialysis. Aspiration of air into the extracorporeal blood circuit is facilitated by the subatmospheric pressure between arterial vascular access and blood pump (Fig. 4). Safety measures include the air detector and the air trap, described above, and if air embolism occurs, it is almost always due to human error. The consequences of air embolism depend on the volume of air entering the patients vasculature, on the size of the air bubbles, and the position of the patient. If the patient is in an upright position central nervous symptoms predominate due to obstruction of cerebral veins; in a recumbent position air forms foam inside the heart and impairs cardiac performance with a subsequent decrease in cardiac output. If the air passes into the pulmonary artery the pulmonary pressure will increase. Further passage into the left ventricle may cause arrhythmias and cerebral symptoms induced by arterial air embolism. Symptoms which may be related to air embolism include sudden dyspnoea, cough, cyanosis, followed by unconsciousness. The venous return of blood must be stopped immediately by placing the patient head and chest down, and turned on the left side. Oxygen should be administered, and artificial ventilation should be initiated if necessary. In severe cases, it may be necessary to aspirate foam from the right ventricle by transthoracic puncture. In some cases, treatment in a compression chamber was of value. Air embolism is a life-threatening complication, and the mortality is in the range of 25 per cent in spite of adequate and intensive therapy.

The disequilibrium syndrome

When haemodialysis treatment is started in severely uraemic patients, neurological disturbances may occur, particularly when there is a fast solute removal from the extracellular space. The symptoms develop during or immediately after haemodialysis and include nausea, headache, blurred vision, disorientation, and increased blood pressure. More severely affected patients progress to confusion, seizures, coma and even death. Predisposing factors include markedly increased blood urea nitrogen (above 175 mg/dl), older age, paediatric patients, severe metabolic acidosis, and the presence of other central nervous system disease (Arieff 1994). With the preventive measures described below severe dialysis disequilibrium syndrome is rare in adults. Children remain at increased risk since up to 7 per cent may have dialysis-associated seizures (Glen *et al.* 1992). Cerebral oedema due to increased brain osmolality is considered to be the major cause for this symptoms, for which—in reference to the assumed pathogenesis—the term disequilibrium syndrome was introduced (Petersen 1964). Three concepts have been proposed to explain why cerebral oedema occurs: a reverse osmotic shift induced by urea removal, accumulation of intracellular osmolytes, and a fall in cerebral intracellular pH (Arieff 1994). It was assumed that clearance of urea would be more rapid from plasma than from brain tissue when high concentrations of urea are rapidly decreased by effective dialysis. The higher concentration of urea in brain tissue would lead to cerebral oedema. Such an assumption stemmed from the observed slower clearance of urea from cerebrospinal fluid than from plasma in patients undergoing rapid haemodialysis associated with higher urea concentrations in the cerebrospinal fluid following haemodialysis (Kennedy *et al.* 1962). The pathogenetic importance of urea has been demonstrated by experiments in uraemic rats where rapid dialysis was associated with a 6–8 per cent increase in brain water and with cerebral oedema. Rats dialysed against a bath containing urea did not develop cerebral oedema (Silver *et al.* 1992; Galons *et al.* 1996). The accumulation of osmolytes, including sugars, amino acids, polyols, and methylamine, within the brain cells during the hyperosmolar uraemic condition preceding terminal renal failure has also been discussed as a cause of the disequilibrium syndrome. When extracellular solutes are removed rapidly by haemodialysis these osmolytes may cause dissociation between intra- and extracellular osmolality, thereby causing cerebral oedema (Arieff *et al.* 1994). Another mechanism contributing to dialysis disequilibrium may be the decrease in cerebrospinal and brain pH observed during haemodialysis (Arieff 1994). The biochemical sequence leading to increases in brain H^+ ions is not known, but changes in CO_2 are certainly not the cause since cerebrospinal P_{CO_2} remains unchanged during haemodialysis. The increased H^+ ion activity in brain is accompanied by an increase of brain osmole content due to displacement of intracellularly bound Na^+ and K^+ ions from protein and due to the increased quantities of organic acids *per se* (Arieff 1994). However, not all reports have confirmed an increase in brain osmolytes and the reverse urea effect appears sufficient to explain most of the dialysis disequilibrium syndrome (Silver 1995; Galons *et al.* 1996). The risk of disequilibrium syndrome can be minimized if haemodialysis is initiated as frequent (daily) short (2–3 h) sessions of limited efficacy. To prevent critical reduction of extracellular osmolality the dialysate sodium concentration should be kept between 140 and 145 mmol/l. Symptoms of dialysis disequilibrium syndrome are self-limited and usually dissipate within several hours. Severe symptoms can be reversed more rapidly by raising the plasma osmolality with either hypertonic saline or mannitol.

Bleeding

Patients with uraemia have an increased incidence of bleeding episodes, caused by platelet dysfunction (Di Minnio *et al.* 1985). The risk of haemorrhage is further increased during haemodialysis due to the administration of heparin, and due to thrombocytopenia induced by heparin and/or platelet–membrane interactions. Petechial haemorrhages, blood blisters in the skin and bruising around fistula puncture sites are common. Serious bleeding during haemodialysis is rare, but may take the form of intracerebral haemorrhage, subdural haematoma, subarachnoid haemorrhage in patients with polycystic renal disease, subcapsular liver haematoma, and retroperitoneal and gastrointestinal bleeding. The possibility of internal blood loss must always be considered in any instance of unexplained hypotension during and after haemodialysis. In the presence of pericarditis which is not infrequent in uraemic patients (see also Chapter 9.6.2), and haemodialysis with heparin anticoagulation may cause haemopericardium with subsequent pericardial tamponade. Patients with pericarditis should therefore be dialysed without heparin, as described in the previous section. If tamponade occurs, it has to be treated immediately by pericardiocentesis.

Dialysis hypotension

Symptomatic hypotension is a very common complication during haemodialysis. It may be accompanied by nausea, vomiting, and muscle cramps, and may proceed to circulatory collapse. Inappropriate volume removal by ultrafiltration is the leading mechanism causing hypotension. The plasma water that is removed from the intravascular compartment by ultrafiltration is substituted by refilling from the interstitial fluid compartment. If the ultrafiltration rate exceeds the refilling rate, intravascular volume contraction will result. Another mechanism contributing to intravascular volume contraction is the reduction of the extracellular osmolality achieved by haemodialysis. There is a time lag in equilibration between intracellular and extracellular fluid causing a shift of fluid into cells. This will aggravate the extracellular fluid loss. Both mechanisms occur more often in short haemodialysis where the volume and the solutes accumulated between dialysis sessions have to be removed in 3 h or less. Another very common cause of plasma volume contraction is an underestimation of the so called dry weight to be achieved at the end of the dialysis session. As long as the circulatory system is able to respond by compensatory vasoconstriction, the plasma volume

contraction induced by haemodialysis does not result in symptomatic hypotension. Very often, however, the haemodynamic response is inadequate to prevent hypotension, even after removal of a low fluid volume. The major causes for this failure are impaired sympathetic response to volume removal (Henderson 1980), diminished cardiac reserve (Poldermans *et al.* 1999), and the vasodilatory action of acetate when applied as dialysate buffer (Schon *et al.* 1981). The impaired sympathetic response to volume loss may be due to uraemia induced defects in the autonomic nervous system (Heidbreder *et al.* 1985).

The acute management of low blood pressure associated with haemodialysis includes the following measures. Ultrafiltration should either be stopped or the rate decreased. The patient should be placed in the Trendelenburg position and the blood flow rate should be reduced. The intravascular volume should be replaced with isotonic saline or mannitol solutions. The use of 7.5 per cent hypertonic saline (approximately 30 ml) appears to be particularly effective since the rapid increase in plasma osmolality may have a positive effect on cardiac performance (Emili *et al.* 1999). Further treatment depends upon the cause of the hypotension. The prompt recognition of life-threatening causes of low blood pressure is essential. In particular, occult sepsis, cardiac or pericardial disease, and bleeding should be considered (Letteri 1998).

General measures to prevent repeated episodes of hypotension during haemodialysis include increase of the patients dry weight when appropriate, prolongation of dialysis time to reduce the rate of ultrafiltration per hour, use of a dialysis machine with controlled ultrafiltration, and application of bicarbonate buffered dialysate instead of acetate buffered dialysis fluid. Initial high volume ultrafiltration for approximately one hour followed by isovolaemic haemodialysis with little or no further volume removal may be an effective strategy to prevent hypotension. This manoeuvre requires prolongation of the time of dialysis to achieve an adequate Kt/V. An increase in the dialysate sodium concentration up to 145 mmol/l has been among the most efficacious and best tolerated therapies to prevent dialysis-associated hypotension (Stiller *et al.* 2001). Dialysate sodium profiling with an initial sodium concentration of 155 mmol/l continuously decreasing during haemodialysis to 140 mmol/l may be even more effective. However, both measures carry the risk of sodium accumulation associated with increased thirst with subsequent enhanced interdialytic weight gain and the development of hypertension. Sodium accumulation may, in fact, explain the reduced intradialytic morbidity reported in some short-term profiling studies. Sodium profiling, when performed appropriately, may have a lower risk of sodium accumulation as compared to a continuously elevated dialysate sodium concentration (Stiller *et al.* 2001). However, the long-term benefits and risks are unknown since randomized long-term studies have not been published. The frequency of dialysis-associated hypotension is increased in patients with a prior history of congestive heart failure, cardiomegaly, or ischaemic heart disease. These conditions lead to a diminished cardiac reserve in the case of a haemodynamic challenge (Poldermans *et al.* 1999). Cardiovascular performance can be enhanced in many dialysis patients by increasing the dialysate calcium concentration (Alappan *et al.* 2001) and/or by decreasing the temperature of the dialysate by approximately 2°C (Jost *et al.* 1993). Food ingestion during dialysis should be avoided, since it leads to a significant decline in systemic vascular resistance and may contribute to dialysis induced hypotension (Barakat *et al.* 1993). Patients on antihypertensive therapy suffering hypotension during haemodialysis may benefit from missing the medication prior to dialysis therapy. Among patients with autonomic neuropathy and perhaps others with severe haemodialysis induced hypotension not responsive to other measures, the selective alpha-1 adrenergic agonist midodrine may be effective and well tolerated (Flynn *et al.* 1996).

Biocompatibility of haemodialysis

Blood cells and proteins interact with dialyser membranes and blood tubing. The term 'biocompatibility' was introduced to characterize the extent of these interactions: materials that exhibit comparatively little interaction are said to be biocompatible. While many biological reactions within the extracorporeal circuit have been analysed and quantitated, their acute and chronic clinical consequences are not always clear. The term biocompatibility should not be restricted to blood–membrane interactions, but should also include such processes as the spallation of particles and the leaching of toxic substances from blood tubing.

Biological reactions induced by the extracorporeal circuit

Activation of complement

Contact between blood and the dialyser activates the alternative pathway of complement. Plasma concentrations of activated factors C3a and C5a increase during the first 15 min of haemodialysis and this reaction is most pronounced with regenerated cellulosic membranes such as Cuprophan. These concentrations subsequently decrease, but still remain significantly greater than before dialysis. Normal values are found within 30 min of completion of dialysis (Craddock *et al.* 1977). The use of dialysers with synthetic membranes as well as some modified cellulosic membranes is associated with a much lower increase in the concentrations of activated complement than is seen with membranes made of regenerated cellulose (Bingel *et al.* 1989). This is due to less activation of the alternative pathway in most membranes and/or greater adsorption of C3a and C5a to the membrane, for instance to polyacrylonitrile membranes (Cheung *et al.* 1990). C5a, also called anaphylatoxin, induces smooth-muscle contraction, increases vascular permeability, releases histamine from mast cells, enhances the adherence and autoaggregation of leukocytes and the degranulation of granulocytes, and increases the release of proteases and oxygen radicals from granulocytes, and the transcription of cytokines in mononuclear cells (Schindler *et al.* 1990). In view of these multiple biological effects, it is conceivable that many of the clinical reactions observed during haemodialysis, including anaphylactoid reactions, the trapping of neutrophils in the lung, and hypoxaemia may be related to complement activation.

Contact activation system

The contact system of plasma, which includes the proteins Hageman factor (factor XII), high molecular weight kininogen, and prekallikrein, can be activated by the negatively charged surfaces of biomaterials. Activation leads to the cleavage of high molecular weight kininogen by kallikrein and the release of bradykinin into the circulation, where it is normally inactivated within seconds by kininase I and II, the latter being identical with angiotensin-converting enzyme. Only the degradation products of kininase II are completely inactive. The activities of bradykinin include vasodilatation with a consequent reduction in blood pressure, the stimulation of vascular permeability, and the induction of inflammatory hyperaemia, oedema, and pain. The dose of bradykinin needed to decrease blood pressure by approximately 20 per cent can be reduced by two orders of magnitude in the presence of an angiotensin-converting enzyme inhibitor (Cochrane and Griffin 1982). The negatively charged AN69 polyacrylonitrile membrane *in vitro* generates low amounts of bradykinin in the absence of angiotensin-converting enzyme inhibitor, but generation is enhanced by the inhibitor in a concentration-dependent manner (Lemke and Fink 1992). In clinical dialysis, plasma bradykinin concentrations increased when dialysers with AN69 membranes were used while this reaction was rarely observed with other synthetic membranes such as polysulfone and only after reuse (Pegues *et al.* 1992). An increase in bradykinin concentrations has also been reported in low-density lipoprotein apheresis with negatively charged dextran sulfate columns.

Induction of cytokines

Cytokines such as interleukin-1 and tumour necrosis factor-α are potent mediators of the acute-phase inflammatory response (Dinarello 1994). Activated circulating mononuclear cells are the major source of cytokines and it has been shown that such cells are stimulated during haemodialysis to produce and release interleukin-1 and tumour necrosis factor-α (Herbelin *et al.* 1990; Lonnemann *et al.* 1990; Schindler *et al.* 1993a). The degree of cytokine induction appears to be dependent on the dialyser membrane used (Bingel *et al.* 1988; Herbelin *et al.* 1990; Schindler *et al.* 1993a). Recent *in vitro* and *in vivo* studies suggest that activated complement components and bacterial substances derived from contaminated dialysate are the most important inducers of cytokine production during haemodialysis. Under the conditions of *in vitro* dialysis with pyrogen-free dialysate, complement-activating cellulosic dialyser membranes induce transcription of mRNA coding for interleukin-1 and tumour necrosis factor-α in activated circulating mononuclear cells without causing translation and increased protein synthesis of these cytokines (Schindler *et al.* 1990). However, when a second stimulus—for example, bacterial endotoxin—is provided, activated circulating mononuclear cells, pre-stimulated ('primed') by C5a, produce more interleukin-1 and tumour necrosis factor-α than 'unprimed' cells (Schindler *et al.* 1990). Thus, haemodialysis with complement-activating dialyser membranes in the presence of contaminated dialysate may result in significant cytokine production *in vivo*, provided that the dialyser membrane is permeable for cytokine-inducing bacterial products derived from contaminated dialysate (Lonnemann 2000).

Routine dialysate is contaminated by Gram-negative microorganisms and *Pseudomonas* spp. such as *P. aeruginosa* and *P. maltophilia* are very common (Klein *et al.* 1990). These micro-organisms release cytokine-inducing substances such as endotoxins (lipopolysaccharides), other cell-wall components such as peptidoglycans, as well as exotoxins such as exotoxin A from *P. aeruginosa*, which is actively secreted from bacteria growing in contaminated dialysate. Lipopolysaccharide ($>$100,000 Da) and exotoxin A (66,000 Da) are large molecules and are not able to penetrate low- or high-flux dialyser membranes. However, *Pseudomonas* spp. grown in dialysate produce and release small molecular-weight pyrogens, which have been shown to penetrate standard, low-flux cellulosic as well as high-flux cellulosic and synthetic dialyser membranes (Schindler *et al.* 1996). It is likely that small molecular-weight fragments derived from bacteria in contaminated dialysate induce the production of proinflammatory cytokines in the activated circulating mononuclear cells of patients in endstage renal failure.

In general, it has to be concluded from all *in vitro* studies on pyrogen permeability that every dialyser membrane can be shown to be permeable for small, cytokine-inducing substances of bacterial origin. Several studies comparing low- and high-flux dialyser membranes have demonstrated that high-flux membranes are equally or even less permeable to pyrogenic bacterial fragments than low-flux cellulosic membranes (Lonnemann *et al.* 1992). Therefore, the pore size of the dialyser membrane seems not to be a crucial factor limiting pyrogen permeability. Quantitative differences in the pyrogen permeability of dialyser membranes depend on other factors such as the types of microorganism-derived pyrogens in the dialysate, the ability of the dialyser membranes to adsorb pyrogens (Lonnemann *et al.* 1988a,b), and the formation of a protein layer on the dialyser membrane (Lonnemann *et al.* 1995) as well as the presence of blood components, such as lipopolysaccharide-binding protein, bactericidal/permeability-increasing protein which influence the responsiveness of activated circulating mononuclear cells to bacterial substances (Schindler *et al.* 1993b). Synthetic high-flux membranes such as polysulfone and polyamide have greater adsorptive capacity for small molecular pyrogens than cellulosic membranes, and have been used successfully as ultrafilters to remove cytokine-inducing substances from highly contaminated fluids such as bicarbonate dialysate (Dinarello *et al.* 1987).

As the induction of cytokines in mononuclear cells is probably the most sensitive system for detecting pyrogens *in vitro* as well as *in vivo*, the activation of circulating mononuclear cells was studied in patients with endstage renal failure on low-flux haemodialysis with regenerated cellulosic membranes and either non-filtered or ultrafiltered bicarbonate dialysate. Whereas in non-filtered dialysate the median of the bacterial count was 148 cfu/ml (range 61–400), there were no cfu/ml detectable in polysulfone-ultrafiltered dialysate. Even in comparison to this very moderate contamination of dialysate, the use of sterile dialysate reduced significantly the cytokine content in activated circulating mononuclear cells from patients with endstage renal failure (Schindler *et al.* 1994). Similar results were obtained when ultra-pure dialysate and routine dialysate (385 cfu/ml) were compared in low-flux haemodialysis using haemophan membranes (modified cellulose) (Lonnemann 2000). These data indicate that pyrogens derived from contaminated dialysate are able to penetrate low-flux dialyser membranes *in vivo* and induce cytokine production in activated circulating mononuclear cells. The use of ultrafiltered dialysate in combination with non-complement activating dialyser membranes may be most effective in reducing or even in preventing haemodialysis-associated cytokine induction.

The clinical correlates of cytokine induction during haemodialysis may be classified as definitive, probable, and speculative. Definitive clinical indicators are fever and chills, which commonly occur during haemodialysis with bacteria-contaminated dialysate, since interleukin-1 and tumour necrosis factor-α are potent endogenous pyrogens. The headache felt by some patients after haemodialysis, frequent sleeping during haemodialysis, and the abnormal sleep patterns of patients on dialysis are rather speculatively correlated with cytokine induction. However, interleukin-1 and tumour necrosis factor-α induce the production of prostaglandin E_1 in the cerebrum, which could produce headache, and cytokines have been shown to induce slow-wave sleep. In addition to these acute symptoms, chronic pathological changes in patients on dialysis may be related to the repeated induction of cytokines by regular intermittent haemodialysis. For example, interleukin-1 has a systemic catabolic effect on muscle and connective tissue in experimental animals, and this may account, in part, for the wasting and negative nitrogen balance of patients on haemodialysis. In cell cultures, interleukin-1 and tumour necrosis factor-α increase bone resorption by osteoclasts, and the osteopenia described in patients on long-term dialysis may be contributed to by these cytokines (Schindler and Dinarello 1990).

Acute clinical correlates of biocompatibility

Acute adverse effects of dialysers ('hypersensitivity reactions', 'first-use syndrome')

Life-threatening acute reactions occur in a few susceptible patients during the initial 20 min of haemodialysis. Symptoms include urticaria, pruritus, dyspnoea, chest tightness, angioedema, or laryngeal oedema, swelling or fullness in mouth and throat, numbness of fingers, toes, lips, or tongue, anxiety, hypotension, and collapse. The reactions can be severe, leading to respiratory arrest and death (Daugirdas and Ing 1988). At first, these reactions were associated primarily with new dialysers, and the term 'first-use syndrome' was applied (Ing *et al.* 1983). Subsequently it became apparent that clinically identical symptoms occurred with reused dialysers (see below), and the more general terms 'hypersensitivity reactions' or 'dialyser reactions' were introduced. To distinguish these early reactions from usually milder symptoms occurring later during haemodialysis the former were termed type A and the latter type B reactions by some authors (Daugirdas and Ing 1988).

Pathogenic mechanisms

Ethylene oxide The underlying pathogenetic mechanism of the majority of acute reactions is hypersensitivity to ethylene oxide (Lemke *et al.* 1990; Salem *et al.* 1994). Ethylene oxide is commonly used to sterilize dialysers and blood tubing. Although the sterilization of these materials is usually followed by degassing, traces of ethylene oxide may remain in dialyser materials, especially if polyurethane is used as potting substance for the capillaries in hollow-fibre dialysers. Proper rinsing of the blood compartment with at least 2 l of saline solution and of the dialysate compartment by perfusion with 500 ml/min of dialysate for 30 min before the dialysis session is important to reduce residual ethylene oxide to a minimum (Ansorge *et al.* 1987; Bommer and Ritz 1987). Antibodies against ethylene oxide have been detected in 10–40 per cent of patients on haemodialysis, depending on the method of investigation. Ethylene oxide is also widely used for the sterilization of a large variety of foods, thus sensitization preceding the start of haemodialysis is not uncommon. However, the incidence of allergic reactions is certainly much less than the prevalence of ethylene oxide antibodies (Rumpf *et al.* 1985). Other substances used in the manufacture of dialysers, including isopropyl myristate, phthalates, and isocyanates, are extracted from the dialyser during rinsing and have been suspected to cause hypersensitivity reactions without definite proof (Salem *et al.* 1994). In order to avoid hypersensitivity reactions caused by gas or chemical sterilization, steam as well as gamma- and beta irradiation are increasingly being used.

Activation of complement factors

The generation of C5a and C3a were held responsible for hypersensitivity reactions, since reused cellulosic membranes did not show complement activation and were associated with a lower rate of such reactions. Patients dialysed with new cellulosic membranes and experiencing symptoms had higher levels of complement factors than patients without symptoms dialysed with new cellulosic membranes (Hakim *et al.* 1984). Recent controlled prospective studies, however, found no difference in the incidence of intradialytic symptoms between patients dialysed with complement-raising Cuprophan® dialysers and patients treated with non-complement-raising polysulfone or polyacrilonitrile membranes

(Bergamo Collaborative Dialysis Study Group 1991; Collins *et al.* 1993). Hypersensitivity reactions have been described with reused, non-complement activating membranes as well (Pegues *et al.* 1992). These observations raise doubt that the generation of C3a and C5a during dialysis is a common cause of hypersensitivity reactions. However, the possibility remains that complement activation may, by enhancing the release of histamine, thromboxane, or some other mediators, amplify hypersensitivity reactions due primarily to ethylene oxide or some other cause (Salem *et al.* 1994).

Bradykinin, AN69, and angiotensin-converting enzyme inhibitors In 1990, a series of acute reactions were described in patients receiving angiotensin-converting enzyme inhibitors combined with the use of an AN69 polyacrylonitrile-membrane dialyser (Tielemans *et al.* 1990; Verresen *et al.* 1990). Antibodies of the IgE Type and specifically against ethylene oxide could not be found, thereby excluding the possibility of an IgE-mediated reaction. There was no increase observed in C3a or histamine across the dialyser. Symptoms did not occur when the AN69 polyacrylonitrile dialyser was changed to another membrane or when the intake of angiotensin-converting enzyme inhibitors was discontinued (Verresen *et al.* 1994). Originally, two explanations were postulated for the reactions—contamination of dialysate with microbial products (Verresen *et al.* 1990) and the bradykinin hypothesis (Tielemans *et al.* 1990). The first explanation has been discarded since endotoxins are not known to induce hypersensitivity reactions of the immediate type (Dinarello 1991) and since reactions were not only observed during haemodialysis but also during haemofiltration, when no dialysate is in contact with the membrane (Petrie *et al.* 1991). The bradykinin hypothesis involves contact activation at the negatively charged AN69 poly-acrylonitrile-membrane surface leading to the release and accumulation of bradykinin in the presence of an angiotensin-converting enzyme inhibitor. Several lines of evidence support this hypothesis. *In vitro* AN69 generates low amounts of bradykinin in the absence of an angiotensin-converting enzyme inhibitor, but generation is enhanced by the inhibitor in a concentration-dependent manner (Lemke and Fink 1992). In clinical dialysis with AN69 polyacrylonitrile-membrane, plasma bradykinin concentrations were greater than in patients dialysed with other membranes (Verresen *et al.* 1994). Acute reactions were also observed in patients treated with an AN69 dialyser without angiotensin-converting enzyme inhibition and high concentrations of plasma bradykinin were measured (Verresen *et al.* 1994). Similar reactions have been reported, incriminating bradykinin as a mediator involved in reactions on low-density lipoprotein apheresis with negatively charged dextrane sulfate columns (Olbricht *et al.* 1992).

Dialysate There are reports that the use of acetate dialysate itself might cause acute reactions (Papadakis *et al.* 1991). The mechanism of such reactions is not clear. Metabolism of acetate generates adenosine, and adenosine can function as a bronchoconstrictor. Some believe that the effects of acetate on the pulmonary vasculature might contribute to acute reactions on haemodialysis (Salem *et al.* 1994).

Reuse Acute reactions also occurred with a variety of dialyser membranes, including polysulfone, when bleach, hydrogen peroxide, and peracetic acid were used to clean and sterilize the dialyser for reuse. Some of the patients were taking angiotensin-converting enzyme inhibitors, but not all. The reactions ceased once the reuse was discontinued, despite continued use of the inhibitors (Pegues *et al.* 1992). The pathogenesis of these acute dialyser reactions in reuse is unknown and may

be multifactorial. The possibility exists that the interaction of certain oxidative disinfectants with certain dialyser membranes generates bradykinin or some other mediators.

Treatment

The treatment of acute adverse effects of dialysers consists of immediate disconnection of the patient from the extracorporeal circuit without return of extracorporeal blood, and the administration of antihistamines, corticosteroids, adrenaline, oxygen, and respiratory support if needed. All further dialyses should be done with disposables, which are not ethylene oxide sterilized if ethylene oxide is the suspected cause. The dialyser should be thoroughly rinsed immediately before use to remove other compounds that may leach from dialyser materials. Treatment with angiotensin-converting enzyme inhibitors should be stopped and a change of AN69 membrane is indicated if these are suspected causes. Other measures include switching to a dialyser with a different membrane or changing from acetate- to bicarbonate-buffered dialysate.

Dialysis-induced hypoxaemia

Haemodialysis using acetate-buffered dialysate is accompanied by the development of hypoxaemia. Arterial oxygen tension begins to decrease after the onset of dialysis and persists for as long as dialysis is continued (De Broe 1994). The decrease in Po_2 may be up to 25 per cent, and this is relevant in patients with severely compromised cardiac or pulmonary function. Hypoxaemia is mainly due to hypoventilation caused by loss of CO_2 via the dialyser since Pco_2 in acetate dialysate is almost zero and the diffusion of CO_2 across the dialyser membrane occurs along the concentration gradient (Dolan *et al.* 1981). An aggravation of dialysis-induced hypoxaemia has been described in patients dialysed with complement-activating membranes. Therefore, as a second mechanism possibly involved in dialysis-induced hypoxaemia, complement-induced sequestration of white blood cells in the lung with a consequent decrease in diffusion capacity has been postulated (De Backer *et al.* 1983). Hypoxaemia of a milder degree may be present in haemodialysis using bicarbonate-buffered dialysate (Hunt *et al.* 1984). Since Pco_2 in bicarbonate dialysate exceeds the carbon dioxide tension in blood, loss of CO_2 via the dialyser is excluded as a cause of hypoventilation. Conceivable mechanisms contributing to hypoxaemia in bicarbonate-buffered haemodialysis include the complement-induced sequestration of white blood cells in the lung with a consequent decrease in diffusion capacity, and the suppression of respiratory drive resulting from a gain of bicarbonate from the dialysate (De Backer *et al.* 1983; Hunt *et al.* 1984).

Chronic clinical correlates of bioincompatibility

Effect of dialyser membranes on protein catabolism

Protein malnutrition is an important risk factor for morbidity and mortality in haemodialysis (Lowrie and Lew 1990). The dietary requirements for protein are increased in comparison to those of non-dialysed uraemic patients and to patients on continuous ambulatory peritoneal dialysis, suggesting that haemodialysis itself may enhance the net protein catabolism and/or impair the utilization of dietary protein (Bergström *et al.* 1990). Suggested pathogenic factors for increased net protein catabolism include a reduced protein intake induced by underdialysis, the inhibition of protein synthesis possibly induced by loss of amino acids in dialysis fluid (Lim *et al.* 1993), and the induction of protein breakdown by cytokines generated during haemodialysis (see cytokines above). Whether a complement-induced and prostaglandin-mediated mechanism plays a part in dialysis-associated malnutrition remains to be determined. The activation of C5 in normal individuals exposed to a cuprophane dialyser membrane without dialysate was accompanied by significantly greater protein catabolism in leg muscle than with a polyacrylonitrile membrane. This catabolic response could be abolished by giving indomethacin before and during the procedure, suggesting that the catabolic effect was mediated by prostaglandins (Gutierrez et al. 1992). However, these experiments were done on healthy volunteers and not patients on dialysis.

Bioincompatibility and infection

Between 15 and 20 per cent of all deaths in haemodialysis are due to infection (Vanherweghem et al. 1991). Causes include the repeated puncture of the vascular access, which provides an entry for bacteria, immunodeficiency due to uraemia and/or long-term dialysis (Descamps-Latscha and Herbelin 1993), and iron overload. Numerous studies have documented alterations in the function of neutrophils, B and T lymphocytes, and monocytes in patients on chronic haemodialysis, although it is difficult to form firm conclusions from the wide variety of findings (Descamps-Latscha and Herbelin 1993). Defects were found in chemotaxis, the adherence of leucocytes, the production of reactive oxygen species, and phagocytosis. It is uncertain whether and how these membrane-triggered events are related to death on haemodialysis due to infection. Phagocytic cell function and the production of reactive oxygen species by granulocytes were less impaired in patients dialysed with synthetic than with cuprophane membranes (Vanholder et al. 1991; Descamps-Latscha and Herbelin 1993; Himmelfarb and Hakim 1994). Conclusive clinical studies to support the hypothesis that haemodialysis with synthetic membranes is associated with a lower rate of infection are not available and further prospective studies are, therefore, needed to draw a clear-cut conclusion (Himmelfarb and Hakim 1994).

Effect of dialyser membranes on β_2-amyloidosis (see Chapter 11.3.10)

In patients on long-term dialysis, a specific amyloidosis preferentially involving bones and joints occurs. The precursor of this amyloid is β_2-microglobulin, a middle-sized molecule in the range of 11,800 Da that is retained in renal insufficiency, and its concentration is elevated up to 60-fold in patients on dialysis. Although the retention of β_2-microglobulin can induce amyloidosis in the absence of contact between blood and artificial membranes, that is, in patients on peritoneal dialysis (Maioraca et al. 1993) and also in rare, non-dialysed patients with chronic uraemia (Linke et al. 1986; Morinière et al. 1991), retrospective studies suggest that the characteristics of the dialysis membrane may influence the deposition of β_2-amyloid. For instance, the incidence of operated carpal-tunnel syndrome and amyloid bone cysts, both clinical consequences of β_2-amyloidosis, in patients treated with cuprophane or AN69 over longer periods was significantly greater in the cuprophane group (Chanard et al. 1989; Van Ypersele de Strihou et al. 1991; Miura et al. 1992). There are three conceivable mechanisms that might relate membrane characteristics to β_2-amyloid deposition: the influence of those characteristics on the production and/or release of β_2-microglobulin, the ability of membranes to activate or release proteases and reactive oxygen species from granulocytes, and the capacity of the membrane to clear β_2-microglobulin. The in vitro and in vivo data currently available do not demonstrate conclusively that the rate of synthesis of β_2-microglobulin is significantly influenced by the

characteristics of the dialysis membrane (Floege et al. 1991; Van Ypersele de Strihou et al. 1994). Proteases that are released from granulocytes during haemodialysis (Hörl et al. 1987) may modify β_2-microglobulins and increase amyloid deposition, since incomplete or atypical proteolysis could possibly enhance the amyloidogenicity of β_2-microglobulins (Linke et al. 1989). The release of proteases is greater in haemodialysis with cuprophane than with AN69 (Hörl et al. 1987). Likewise, the production of reactive oxygen species by granulocytes is increased during haemodialysis with cuprophane but not with AN69 (Nguyen et al. 1985), and it is conceivable that the deposition of β_2-amyloid is enhanced locally by the presence of reactive oxygen species (Capeillère-Blandin et al. 1991). Finally, the rates of removal of β_2-microglobulin during haemodialysis through diffusion and/or convection, and through adsorption, are greater with synthetic, high-flux membranes than with cuprophane and other low-flux membranes (Floege et al. 1988; Drüeke et al. 1989; Wizemann et al. 2000; Lonnemann and Koch 2002). Although the rate of removal of β_2-microglobulin by high-flux membranes remains less than the rate of its generation, the increased elimination of the precursor may delay the development of dialysis-related amyloidosis (Van Ypersele de Strihou et al. 1994).

Effect of dialyser membranes on mortality

There are several non-randomized, retrospective trials either published or reported in abstract form in which the annual mortality rate decreased from about 15–20 to 9–11 per cent concomitant with a switch from low-flux, complement-activating membranes to high-flux membranes with little complement activation. In a more recent study, a retrospective analysis of 715 patients treated by intermittent haemodialysis for up to 5 years was undertaken. Low-flux polysulfone dialysers were used exclusively for 252 patients and 463 patients were dialysed for at least 3 months with high-flux polysulfone. Patients treated with high-flux dialysis had a lower mortality (21 versus 36 per 1000 years) and significantly lower standardized mortality ratio. For non-diabetic patients, the 5-year probability of survival was significantly greater for patients treated with high-flux dialysers (Kaplan-Meier: 92 versus 69 per cent; $p = 0.036$) (Woods and Nandakumar 2000). It is not clear whether this decrease in mortality represents a membrane effect, since in all of these retrospective studies multiple differences existed between study populations, including dose, use of erythropoietin, dialysate composition and buffer, and volumetric control. A large randomized and prospective trial showed no effect of dialyser membranes on morbidity, further suggesting that results from retrospective studies should be interpreted with caution (Martin-Malo and Castillo 1993). Ongoing prospective multicentre studies such as the American haemodialysis outcome (HEMO) study and the European membrane permeability outcome (MPO) study will have the statistical power to answer reliably the question whether the use of synthetic high-flux membranes is associated with improved survival in patients on haemodialysis (Locatelli et al. 2001).

The best, long-term survival data in the world for haemodialysis were achieved when exclusively the complement-activating, bioincompatible Cuprophan membrane was used. The survival rate was 87 per cent at 5 years, 75 per cent at 10 years, 55 per cent at 15 years, and 43 per cent at 20 years (Charra et al. 1992). These outstanding survival rates were attributed to long hours of dialysis with excellent control of blood pressure without the use of antihypertensive drugs. This suggests that membrane biocompatibility may be less important than the dose of dialysis, which includes the capacity to remove urea, sufficient removal of salt and water to control blood pressure, and the time of dialysis.

Spallation of particles and leaching of toxins from blood tubing

The most widely used materials for blood lines are polyvinyl chloride and silicone, both of which are subject to spallation of particles shed by the shearing stress of the roller pumps. Trapped silicone particles may initiate granulomas in the liver, lung spleen, bone marrow, and skin of patients on dialysis (Leong *et al.* 1982; Bommer *et al.* 1983). However, clinical symptoms attributable to silicone storage, consisting of an enlarged liver and spleen with increased levels of liver enzymes, and pancytopenia due to hypersplenism, are uncommon. Although spallation has been demonstrated *in vitro* for both silicone and polyvinyl chloride materials, polyvinyl chloride granulomas have not so far been found in patients on dialysis (Bommer *et al.* 1983).

To ensure that polyvinyl chloride is flexible and elastic, plasticizers such as diethyl hexyl phthalate must be added: these chemicals can be released from the blood tubing into the circulation (Lewis *et al.* 1977; Ono *et al.* 1980), and substantial amounts have been found in the liver tissue of patients on dialysis (Bommer *et al.* 1983). The toxicity of plasticizers for liver has been demonstrated in experimental animals (Kevy and Jacobson 1983), and a hepatitis-like syndrome and cases of necrotizing dermatitis have been observed in patients on dialysis. Although these are likely to be related to the leaching of plasticizers from polyvinyl chloride blood tubing, this has not been proved (Neergard *et al.* 1971; Bommer *et al.* 1979). Whether this problem can be mitigated by plasticizers with a lower rate of release from blood tubing remains to be determined.

Haemodialysis in children

According to the European Dialysis and Transplantation Association report on regular dialysis and transplantation for 1992, approximately 2000 children (age < 15 years) were on renal replacement therapy in Europe; 25 per cent of these children were treated by haemodialysis, 57 per cent were transplanted, and 18 per cent were treated by peritoneal dialysis (Loirat *et al.* 1994). The basic principles, procedures, and complications of haemodialysis are the same as in adults.

However, several modifications in equipment and techniques are required for haemodialysis in children. Vascular access is a major problem in young patients. For acute access, venous cannulas of appropriate calibre can be inserted into the vena cava using the subclavian, internal jugular, or femoral approach. Silicone rubber catheters with an internal diameter of 1.6–2.6 mm may be used for chronic vascular access in infants. These catheters are inserted via the subclavian vein, fixed subcutaneously with a Dacron cuff, and may be left in place for prolonged periods. In infants weighing between 5 and 10 kg, a saphenous-loop fistula between the distal end of the saphenous vein and the side of the femoral artery can be constructed; in older children the Cimino–Brescia arteriovenous fistula is the common mode of vascular access. Fistula needles of gauge 18 to 14 are required for adequate blood flow. Single-needle dialysis is adequate, even in children with only a short area of vessel available for fistula puncture. Since the extracorporeal blood volume should never exceed 8 ml/kg body weight (approximately 10 per cent of total blood volume), special paediatric blood lines with a volume varying between 20 and 60 ml and a surface area of 0.25–0.8 m^2, are used.

Blood-flow rates must be individually determined for each patient and should be sufficient to obtain a dialyser urea clearance of 3.0 ml/min per kg body weight: this is calculated using the blood flow-urea clearance correlation of the dialyser (Fig. 7). Special pump heads that precisely deliver blood-flow rates of from 10 to 200 ml/min are necessary. The dialysate flow rate should be 500 ml/min and bicarbonate-buffered dialysate is preferred as it maintains better haemodynamic stability. The ultrafiltration rate must be carefully controlled since children are especially prone to develop hypotension because of their small blood volume. Fluid removal per haemodialysis session should not usually exceed 5 per cent of body weight. Dialysis machines with volumetric control of ultrafiltration are recommended since they allow safe withdrawal of fluid.

Children have a greater requirement for calories, protein, and fluid relative to body weight than adults, and since the metabolic rate is proportional to the intake of nutrients, and the requirement for dialysis is proportional to the metabolic rate, child patients need more dialysis in relation to body weight than adults. Dialysis treatment is usually given three times per week: adequate dialysis time can be assessed by using Kt/V concept as demonstrated in the section on adequacy of haemodialysis. K is the urea clearance in litres per hour, t is the session time in hours, and V is the urea space. The target value for Kt/V is approximately 1.2; $K = 3$ ml/min/kg $= 0.18$ l/h/kg; $V =$ approximately $0.6 \times$ body weight. The equation can be solved for the required session length, and in the present example is 4 h. The usual length of session for child patients is 3–4 h.

Heparinization should follow the guidelines given for adults. The initial heparin dose should be 30–50 u/kg body weight. If there is a risk of bleeding the patient can be dialysed with minimal or no heparin.

Acute complications of haemodialysis are similar in children and adults. Children are, however, especially prone to develop the disequilibrium syndrome, and this can be prevented if the initial dialysis sessions do not exceed 2 h, with a maximum blood-flow rate of 3 ml/min per kg body weight. Other preventive measures include prophylactic infusion of mannitol before haemodialysis and the maintenance of the dialysate sodium at or slightly above the plasma concentration.

Guidelines for heparin administration in haemodialysis

The target whole-blood activated partial thromboplastin time (WBAPTT) during haemodialysis may be 140 s.

1. Do a baseline WBAPTT. Normal values are between 40 and 80 s.

2. Administer a loading dose of 1500 u heparin, which is based on the average patient's heparin sensitivity of 0.04 s increase in WBAPTT per unit of heparin, amounting to a total increase of 60 s.

3. Allow 3 min to pass and do a second WBAPTT. This will give the patient's response to heparin ($=$WBAPTT$_2$ $-$ WBAPTT$_1$). The heparin sensitivity can be calculated by dividing the response by the heparin bolus dose. The correlation between response measured by WBAPTT and heparin dose is linear, and the response can be used to calculate the appropriate heparin dose for a given target WBAPTT.

4. Adjust the WBAPTT to the desired value by giving additional heparin or by decreasing the loading dose before the next dialysis.

5. Attach the patient to the extracorporeal blood circuit and set infusion rate to 1000 u heparin per hour.

6. Do a WBAPTT 30–60 min later to check appropriate infusion rate. For every 5 s below 140 s, change infusion rate by 250 u/h. Give a bolus dose according to the calculated response if the WBAPTT is less than 200 per cent of initial value.

7. Repeat procedure at hourly intervals.

8. Stop infusion 0.5 h before the end of haemodialysis. From the information so obtained the heparin loading dose and the rate of infusion required during dialysis will be ascertained.

References

AAMI (Association for the Advancement of Medical Instrumentation) (1993). Recommended practice for reuse of hemodialyzers. Arlington, Virginia, USA.

Abrams, H. S. Psychiatry and prolongation of life. In *Proceedings of the Conference on Emerging Medical, Moral and Legal Concerns* (ed. S. Siemsen and I. Greifer), pp. 63–68. Honululu: St. Francis Hospital, 1976.

Ahmad, R. (1984). Magnesium induced neuropathy in patients undergoing haemodialysis. *British Medical Journal* 288, 1654–1657.

Ahmed, S. *et al.* (1999). Opinions of elderly people on treatment for end stage renal disease. *Gerontology* 45, 156–165.

Alappan, R. *et al.* (2001). Treatment of severe intradialytic hypotension with the addition of high dialysate calcium concentration to midodrine and/or cool dialysate. *American Journal of Kidney Diseases* 37, 294–298.

Ansorge, W., Pelger, M., Dietrich, W., and Baurmeister, F. (1987). Ethylene oxide in dialyzer rinsing fluid: effect of rinsing technique, dialyzer storage time, and potting compound. *Artificial Organs* 11, 118–122.

Arieff, A. I. (1994). Dialysis disequilibrium syndrome: current concepts on pathogenesis and prevention. *Kidney International* 45, 629–635.

Baldamus, C. A., Ernst, W., Frei, U., and Koch, K. M. (1982). Sympathetic and hemodynamic response to volume removal during different forms of renal replacement therapy. *Nephron* 31, 324–332.

Baldamus, C., Bommer, J., Fiegel, P., Graefe, U., Kopp, F. K., Mann, H., and Meins, K. (1999). Anforderungen und Überprüfung der mikrobiologischen Wasserqualität für die Hämodialyse. *Mitteilungen der Deutschen Arbeitsgemeinschaft für klinische Nephrologie*, 111–113.

Barakat, M. M. *et al.* (1993). Hemodynamic effects of intradialytic food ingestion and the effects of caffeine. *Journal of the American Society of Nephrology* 3, 1813–1817.

Bergamo Collaborative Dialysis Study Group (1991). Acute intradialytic well-being: results of a clinical trial comparing polysulfone with cuprophan. *Kidney International* 40, 714–719.

Bergström, J., Alvestrand, A., Lindhold, B., and Tranaeus, A. (1990). Relationship between Kt/V and protein catabolic rate is different in continuous peritoneal dialysis and haemodialysis patients. *Journal of the American Society of Nephrology* 2, 358.

Bingel, M., Lonnemann, G., Koch, K. M., Dinarello, C. A., and Shaldon, S. (1987). Enhancement of *in vitro* human interleukin I production by sodium acetate. *Lancet* i, 14–16.

Bingel, M., Lonnemann, G., Koch, K. M., Dinarello, C. A., and Shaldon, S. (1988). Plasma interleukin-1 activity during hemodialysis: the influence of dialysis membranes. *Nephron* 50, 273–276.

Bingel, M., Arndt, W., Schulze, M., Floege, J., Shaldon, S., Koch, K. M., and Götze, O. (1989). Comparative study of C5a plasma levles with different hemodialysis membranes using an enzyme-linked immunosorbent assay. *Nephron* 51, 320–324.

Bommer, J. and Ritz, E. (1987). Ethylene oxide (ETO) as a major cause of anaphylactoide reactions in dialysis (a review). *Artificial Organs* 11, 111–117.

Bommer, J., Ritz, E., and Andrassy, K. (1979). Necrotizing dermatitis resulting from hemodialysis with polyvinylchloride tubing. *Annals of Internal Medicine* 91, 869–870.

Bommer, J., Waldherr, R., and Ritz, E. (1983). Silicon storage disease in long-term hemodialysis patients. *Contributions to Nephrology* 36, 115–125.

Bonomini, V., Feletti, C., Scolari, M. P., and Stefoni, S. (1985). Benefits of early initiation of dialysis. *Kidney International* 17, S57–S59.

Boulton-Jones, M. (1994). Dialysis membranes: clinical effects. *The Lancet* 344, 559.

Bratt, G., Törnebohm, E., Lockner, D., and Bergström, K. (1983). Pharmacokinetics of low molecular weight heparin as compared with conventional heparin in humans. *Thrombosis Haemostasis* 50, 184–189.

Brescia, M. J., Cimino, J. E., Appel, K., and Hurwich, B. J. (1966). Chronic hemodialysis using venipuncture and a surgically created arteriovenous fistula. *New England Journal of Medicine* 275, 1089–1093.

Brueggemeyer, C. D. and Ramirez, G. (1987). Dialysate concentrate: a potential source of lethal complications. *Nephron* 46, 397–401.

Brunet, P., Jaber, K., Serland, Y., and Baz, M. (1992). Anaphylactoid reactions during hemodialysis and hemofiltration: role of associating AN69 membrane and angiotensin I converting enzyme inhibitors. *American Journal of Kidney Diseases* 9, 444–447.

Bucha, E., Nowak, G., Czerwinski, R., and Thieler, H. (1999). R-hirudin as anticoagulant in regular hemodialysis therapy: finding of therapeutic R-hirudin blood/plasma concentrations and respective dosages. *Clinical Applied Thrombosis and Hemostasis* 5, 164–170.

Canaud, B., Bosc, J. Y., Leray-Moragues, H., Stec, F., Argiles, A., Leblanc, M., and Mion, C. (2000). On-line haemodiafiltration. Safety and efficacy in long-term clinical practice. *Nephrology, Dialysis, Transplantation* 15 (Suppl. 1), 60–67.

Canaud, B., Wizemann, V., Pizzarelli, F., Greenwood, R., Schultze, G., Weber, C., and Falkenhagen, D. (2001). Cellular interleukin-1 receptor antagonist production in patients receiving on-line haemodiafiltration therapy. *Nephrology, Dialysis, Transplantation* 16, 2181–2187.

Capeillère-Blandin, C., Delaveau, T., and Descamps-Latscha, B. (1991). Structural modifications of human beta-2-microglobulin treated with oxygen-derived radicals. *Biochemical Journal* 277, 175–182.

Catto, G. R. D., Reid, I. W., and MacLeod, M. (1974). The effect of low magnesium dialysate on plasma, ultrafiltrable, erythrocyte and bone magnesium concentrations from patiens on maintenance haemodialysis. *Nephron* 13, 372–378.

Challah, S., Wing, A. J., Bauer, R., Morris, R. W., and Schroeder, S. A. (1984). Negative selection of patients for dialysis and transplantation in the United Kingdom. *British Medical Journal* 288, 1119–1121.

Chanard, J., Bindi, P., and Lavaud, S. (1989). Carpal tunnel syndrome and type of dialysis membrane. *British Medical Journal* 298, 867–868.

Charra, B., Calemard, E., Ruffet, M., Chazot, C., Terrat, J. C., Vanel, T., and Laurent, G. (1992). Survival as an index of adequacy of dialysis. *Kidney International* 41, 1286–1291.

Cheung, A. K., Parker, C. J., Wilcox, L. A., and Janatova, J. (1990). Activation of complement by hemodialysis membranes: polyacrilonitrile binds more C3a than cuprophan. *Kidney International* 37, 1055–1059.

Cheung, A. K., Dalpias, D., Emmerson, R., and Leypolt, J. K. (1991). A prospective study on intradialytic symptoms associated with reuse of hemodialysers. *American Journal of Nephrology* 11, 397–401.

Cheung, A. K. *et al.* and the Hemodialysis (HEMO) Study Group (1999). Effects of hemodialyzer reuse on clearances of urea and Beta-2-microglobulin. *Journal of the American Society of Nephrology* 10, 117–

Churchill, D. N., Taylor, D. W., Shimizu, A. G., Beecroft, M. L., Singer, J., Barnes, C. C., Ludwin, D., Wright, N., Sackett, D. L., and Smith, E. K. (1988). Dialyzer re-use—a multiple crossover study with random allocation to order of treatment. *Nephron* 50, 325–331.

Cochrane, C. G. and Griffin, J. H. (1982). The biochemistry and pathophysiology of the contact system of plasma. *Advances in Immunology* 33, 241–306.

Collins, D. M., Lambert, M. B., Tannenbaum, J. S., Oliverio, M., and Schwab, S. J. (1993). Tolerance of hemodialysis: a randomized prospective trial of high-flux versus conventional high-efficiency hemodialysis. *Journal of the American Society of Nephrology* **4**, 148–154.

Collins, A. J., Ma, J. Z., Constantini, E. G., and Everson, S. E. (1998). Dialysis and patient characteristics associated with reuse practices and mortality: 1989–1993. *Journal of the American Society of Nephrology* **2**, 2108.

Craddock, P. R., Fehr, J., Dalmasso, A. P., Brigham, K. L., and Jacob, H. S. (1977). Hemodialysis leukopenia: pulmonary vascular leukostasis resulting from complement activation by dialyzer cellophane membrane. *Journal of Clinical Investigation* **59**, 879–888.

Dager, W. E. and White, R. H. (2001). Use of lepirudin in patients with heparin-induced thrombocytopenia and renal failure requiring hemodialysis. *Annals of Pharmacotherapeutics* **35**, 885–890.

Davenport, A., Davison, A. M., and Will, E. J. (1988). Anticoagulation with prostacyclin in patients treated by continuous haemofiltration (abstract). *XXVth Congress of the European Dialysis and Transplant Association.* Madrid, Spain, Abstract Book, 160.

Daugirdas, J. T. and Ing, T. S. (1988). First use reactions during hemodialysis: a definition of subtypes. *Kidney International* **24**, S37–S43.

Deane, N. and Bemis, J. A. (1982). Multiple use of hemodialyzers. New York, Manhattan Kidney Center, National Nephrology Foundation, pp. 64–82.

De Backer, W. A., Verpooten, G. A., Borgonjon, D. J., Vermeire, P. A., Lins, R. L., and De Broe, M. E. (1983). Hypoxemia during hemodialysis: effects of different membranes and dialysate composition. *Kidney International* **23**, 738–743.

De Broe, M. E. (1994). Hemodialysis-induced hypoxemia. *Nephrology, Dialysis, Transplantation* **9** (Suppl. 2), 173–175.

Delin, K., Attman, P. O., Dahlberg, M., and Awell, M. (1988). A clinical test of a new device for on-line preparation of dialysis fluid from bicarbonate powder: the Gambro BiCart. *Nephrology, Dialysis, Transplantation* **17**, 468–469.

Descamps-Latscha, B. and Herbelin, A. (1993). Long-term dialysis and cellular immunity: a critical survey. *Kidney International* (Suppl. 41), S135–S142.

Deuber, H. J. and Schulz, W. (1991). Reduced lipid concentrations during four years of dialysis with low molecular weight heparin. *Kidney International* **40**, 496–500.

Di Minno, G., Martinez, J., McKean, M., De La Rosa, J., Burke, J. F., and Murphy, S. (1985). Platelet dysfunction in uremia. Multifaceted defect partially corrected by dialysis. *American Journal of Medicine* **79**, 552–557.

Dinarello, C. A. (1991). ACE inhibitors and anaphylactoid reactions to high-flux membrane dialysis. *Lancet* **337**, 370.

Dinarello, C. A. (1994). The interleukin-1 family: 10 years of discovery. *FASEB Journal* **8**, 1314–1325.

Dinarello, C. A., Lonnemann, G., Maxwell, R., and Shaldon, S. (1987). Ultrafiltration to reject human interleukin-1-inducing substances derived from bacterial cultures. *Journal of Clinical Microbiology* **25**, 1233–1238.

Dolan, M. G., Whipp, B. J., Davidson, W. D., Weitzman, R. E., and Wassermann, K. (1981). Hypopnea associated with acetate hemodialysis: carbon dioxide-flow-dependent ventilation. *New England Journal of Medicine* **305**, 72–75.

Drüeke, T. (1984). Does Mg excess play a role in renal osteodystrophy. *Contributions to Nephrology* **38**, 195–201.

Drüeke, T., Urena, P., Man, N. K., and Zingraff, J. (1989). Membrane transfer, membrane adsorption and possible membrane-induced generation of beta-2-microglobulin. *Contributions to Nephrology* **74**, 113–119.

Drukker, W. and Van Dorn, A. W. J. Dialysis regeneration. In *Replacement of Renal Function by Dialysis* (ed. J. F. Maher), pp. 417–438. Dordrecht: Kluwer Academic Publishers, 1989.

Dumler, F. (1994). Reuse of hemodialyzers. *Seminars in Dialysis* **7**, 257.

Ebben, J. P. *et al.* (2000). Impact of disease severity and hematocrit level on reuse-associated mortality. *American Journal of Kidney Diseases* **35**, 244.

Emili, S., Black, N. A., and Paul, R. V. (1999). A protocol-based treatment for intradialytic hypotension in hospitalized patients. *American Journal of Kidney Diseases* **33**, 1107–1112.

Farrell, P. C., Ward, R. A., Schindhelm, K., and Gotch, F. A. (1978). Precise anticoagulation for routine hemodialysis. *Journal of Laboratory and Clinical Medicine* **92**, 164–176.

Fassbinder, W. (1998). Renaissance of the batch method? *Nephrology, Dialysis, Transplantation* **13** (12), 3010–3012.

Fassbinder, W. *et al.* (1991). Combined report on regular dialysis and transplantation in Europe, XX, 1989. *Nephrology, Dialysis, Transplantation* **6** (Suppl. 1), 5–12.

Fleming, S. J., Foreman, K., Shanley, K., Mihrshahi, R., and Siskind, V. (1991). Dialyser reprocessing with Renalin. *American Journal of Nephrology* **11**, 27–31.

Floege, J., Granolleras, C., Shaldon, S., and Koch, K. M. (1988). Which membrane? Should beta-2-microglobulin decide on the choice of todays hemodialysis membrane? *Nephron* **50**, 177–181.

Floege, J., Bartsch, A., Schulze, M., Shaldon, S., Koch, K. M., and Smeby, L. C. (1991). Turnover of beta-2-microglobulin in hemodialyzed patients. *Journal of Laboratory and Clinical Medicine* **118**, 153–165.

Flynn, J. J., Mitchell, M. C., Caruso, F. S., and McElligot, M. A. (1996). Mododrine treatment for patients with hemodialysis hypotension. *Clinical Nephrology* **45**, 261–264.

Freeman, R. M., Lawton, R. L., and Chamberlain, M. A. (1967). Hard-water syndrome. *New England Journal of Medicine* **276**, 1113–1116.

Frei, U. and Schober-Halstenberg, H.-J. *Nierenersatztherapie in Deutschland: Bericht über Dialysebehandlung und Nierentransplantation in Deutschland 2000*, Berlin: QuaSi-Niere GmbH, 2001, ISBN 3-00-008745-1.

Galland, R. *et al.* (2001). Short daily hemodialysis rapidly improves nutritional status in hemodialysis patients. *Kidney International* **60**, 1555–1562.

Galons, J. P., Trouard, T., Gmitro, A. F., and Lien, Y. H. (1996). Hemodialysis increases apparent diffusion coefficient of brain water in nephrectomized rats measured by isotropic diffusion-weighted magnetic resonance imaging. *Journal of Clinical Investigation* **98**, 750–758.

Geerlings, W., Tufveson, G., Ehrich, J. H. H., Jones, E. H. P., Landais, P., Loirat, C., Mallick, N. P., Margreiter, R., Raine, A. E. G., Salmela, K., Selwood, N. H., and Valderrabano, F. (1994). Report on management of renal failure in Europe, XXIII. *Nephrology, Dialysis, Transplantation* **9** (Suppl. 1), 6–25.

Gennari, F. J. (1985). Acid–base balance in dialysis patients. *Kidney International* **28**, 678–688.

Glenn, C. M., Astley, S. J., and Watkins, S. L. (1992). Dialysis associated seizures in children and adolescents. *Pediatric Nephrology* **6**, 182–186.

Gordon, S. M., Tipple, M., Bland, L. A., and Jarvis, W. R. (1988). Pyrogenic reactions associated with the reuse of disposable hollow fibre dialysers. *Journal of the American Medical Association* **260**, 2077–2081.

Graefe, U., Milutinovich, J., Folette, W. C., Vizzo, J. E., Babb, A. C., and Scribner, B. H. (1978). Less dialysis induced morbidity and vascular instability with bicarbonate in dialysate. *Annals of Internal Medicine* **88**, 332–336.

Graf, H., Kovarik, J., Stummvoll, H. K., and Wolf, A. (1979). Disappearance of uraemic pruritus after lowering dialysate magnesium concentration. *British Medical Journal* **2**, 1478–1481.

Greinacher, A. *et al.* (2000). Heparin-induced thrombocytopenia with thromboembolic complications: meta-analysis of 2 prospective trials to assess the value of parenteral treatment with lepirudinand its therapeutic aPTT range. *Blood* **96**, 846.

Gutierrez, A., Bergstöm, J., and Alvestrand, A. (1992). Protein catabolism in sham-hemodialysis: the effect of different membranes. *Clinical Nephrology* **38**, 20–29.

Haas, G. (1925). Versuche der Blutauswaschung am Lebenden (Experiments on cleansing of blood *in vivo* by means of dialysis). *Klinische Wochenschrift* **4**, 13–19.

Hakim, R. M., Breillatt, J., Lazarus, J. M., and Port, F. K. (1984). Complement activation and hypersensitivity reactions to dialysis membranes. *New England Journal of Medicine* **311**, 878–882.

Heidbreder, E., Schafferhans, K., and Heidland, A. (1985). Autonomic neuropathy in chronic renal insufficiency: comparative analysis of diabetic and nondiabetic patients. *Nephron* **41**, 50–56.

Held, P. J. *et al.* (1990). Five-year survival for end-stage renal disease patients in the United States, Europe and Japan 1982 to 1987. *American Journal of Kidney Diseases* 15, 451–466.

Held, P. J., Wolfe, R. A., Gaylin, D. S., Port, F. K., Levin, N. W., and Turenne, M. N. (1994). Analysis of the association of dialyzer reuse practices and patient outcomes. *American Journal of Kidney Diseases* 23, 692–708.

Henderson, L. W. (1980). Symptomatic hypotension during hemodialysis. *Kidney International* 17, 571–577.

Henderson, L. W., Livoti, L. G., Ford, C. A., Kelly, A. B., and Lysaght, M. J. (1973). Clinical experience with intermittent hemofiltration. *Transactions of the American Society of Artificial Internal Organs* 19, 119–121.

Herbelin, A., Nguyen, A. T., Zingraff, J., Urena, P., and Descamps-Latscha, B. (1990). Influence of uremia and hemodialysis on circulatory interleukin-1 and tumor necrosis factor alpha. *Kidney International* 37, 116–125.

Himmelfarb, J. and Hakim, R. M. (1994). Biocompatibility and risk of infection in haemodialysis patients. *Nephrology, Dialysis, Transplantation* 9 (Suppl. 2), 138–144.

Hirsch, D. J. *et al.* (1994). Experience with not offering dialysis to patients with a poor prognosis. *American Journal of Kidney Diseases* 23, 463.

Hirsch, J., Ofosu, F., and Buchanan, M. (1985). The rational behind the development of low molecular weight heparin derivatives. *Seminars in Thrombosis and Hemostasis* 11, 13–16.

Hörl, W. H., Riegel, W., Steinhauer, H. B., Wanner, C., Schollmeyer, P., Schaefer, R., and Heidland, A. (1987). Plasma levels of main granulocytic components during hemodialysis. *Contributions to Nephrology* 59, 35–43.

Huisse, M. G., Guillin, M. C., and Bezeaud, A. (1982). Heparin associated thrombocytopenia. *In vitro* effects of different molecular weight heparin fractions. *Thrombosis Research* 27, 485–490.

Hunt, J. M., Chappell, T. R., Henrich, W. L., and Rubin, L. J. (1984). Gas exchange during dialysis. Contrasting mechanisms contributing to comparable alterations with acetate and bicarbonate buffers. *American Journal of Medicine* 77, 255–260.

Hyde, S. E. III and Sadler, J. H. (1969). Red blood cell destruction in haemodialysis. *Transactions of the American Society of Artificial Internal Organs* 15, 50–52.

Ikizler, T. A., Greene, J. H., and Wingard, R. L. (1995). Spontaneous dietary protein intake during progression of chronic renal failure. *Journal of the American Society of Nephrology* 6, 1386–1391.

Ing, T. S., Daugirdas, J. T., Popli, S., and Gandhi, V. C. (1983). First-use syndrome with cuprammonium cellulose dialyzers. *International Journal of Artificial Internal Organs* 6, 235–239.

Ismail, N., Hakim, R. M., Oreopolus, D. G., and Patrikarea, A. (1993). Renal replacement in the elderly: part 1. Hemodialysis and chronic peritoneal dialysis. *American Journal of Kidney Diseases* 22, 759–782.

Janatova, J., Cheung, A. K., and Parker, C. J. (1991). Biomedical polymers differ in their capacity to activate complement. *Complement Inflammation* 8, 61–69.

Janssen, M. J. *et al.* (1996). Citrate compared to low molecular weight heparin anticoagulation in chronic hemodialysis patients. *Kidney International* 49, 806–813.

Jost, C. M., Agarwal, R., Khair-el-Din, T., Grayburn, P. A., Victor, R. G., and Henrich, W. L. (1993). Effects of cooler temperature dialysate on hemodynamic stability in problem dialysis patients. *Kidney International* 44, 606–612.

Kaiser, B. A., Potter, D. E., Bryant, R. E., Vreman, H. J., and Weiner, M. V. (1981). Acid–base changes and acetate metabolism during routine and high efficiency hemodialysis in children. *Kidney International* 19, 70–79.

Kant, K. S., Pollak, V. E., Cathey, M., Goetz, D., and Berlin, R. (1981). Multiple use of dialyzers: safety and efficacy. *Kidney International* 19, 728–738.

Kaplan, A. A., Hallay, S. E., Lapkin, R. A., and Graeber, C. W. (1995). Dialysate protein losses with bleach processed polysulphone dialysers. *Kidney International* 47, 573–581.

Kaufman, A. M. *et al.* (1992). Clinical experience with heat sterilization for processing dialyzers. *ASAIO Journal* 38, M338.

Kennedy, A. C., Linton, A. L., and Eaton, J. C. (1962). Urea levels in cerebrospinal fluid after heamodialysis. *Lancet* 1, 410–411.

Kenny, M. A., Casillas, E., and Ahmad, S. (1987). Magnesium, calcium and PTH relationships in dialysis patients after magnesium repletion. *Nephron* 46, 199–203.

Keshaviah, P. (1982). The role of acetate in the etiology of symptomatic hypotension. *Artificial Organs* 6, 378–382.

Kevy, S. and Jacobson, M. (1983). Hepatic effects of the leaching of phthalate ester plasticizers and silicon. *Contribution to Nephrology* 36, 82–89.

Kimmel, P. L. and Miskin, G. J. (1998). Dialyzer reuse and the treatment of patients with end-stage renal disease by hemodialysis. *Journal of the American Society of Nephrology* 9, 2153.

Klein, E., Pass, T., Harding, G. B., Wright, R., and Million, C. (1990). Microbial and endotoxin contamination in water and dialysate in the central United States. *Artificial Organs* 14, 85–94.

Kolff, W. J. (1964). De kunstmatige Nier (The artificial kidney). MD Thesis, University of Groningen, The Netherlands, Kampen JH Kok NV.

Korevaar, J. C., Jansen, M. A. M., and Dekker, F. W. (2001). When to initiate dialysis: effect of proposed US guidelines on survival. *Lancet* 358, 1046–1050.

Krautzig, S., Janssen, U., Koch, K. M., Granolleras, C., and Shaldon, S. (1998). Dietary salt restriction and reduction of dialysate sodium to control hypertension in maintenance haemodialysis patients. *Nephrology, Dialysis, Transplantation* 13, 552–553.

Krivitsky, N. M., Kislukhin, V. V., and Snyder, J. W. (1998). *In vivo* measurement of hemodialyzer fiber bundle volume: theory and validation. *Kidney International* 54, 1751.

Ledebo, I. and Nystrand, R. (1999). Defining the microbiological quality of dialysis fluid. *Artificial Organs* 23, 37–43.

Lemke, H. D. and Fink, E. (1992). Accumulation of bradykinin formed by the AN69- or PAN DX-membrane is due to the presence of an ACE inhibitor *in vitro*. *Journal of the American Society of Nephrology* 3, 376 (abstract).

Lemke, H. D., Heidland, A., and Schaefer, R. M. (1990). Hypersensitivity reactions during hemodialysis: role of complement fragments and ethylene oxide antibodies. *Nephrology, Dialysis, Transplantation* 5, 264–269.

Leong, A. S. Y., Disney, A. P. S., and Gove, D. W. (1982). Spallation and migration of silicone from blood-pump tubing in patients on hemodialysis. *New England Journal of Medicine* 306, 135–136.

Letteri, J. M. (1998). Symptomatic hypotension during hemodialysis. *Seminars in Dialysis* 11, 253–262.

Leunissen, K. M. L., van den Berg, B. W., and van Hooff, J. P. (1989). Ionized calcium plays a pivotal role in controlling blood pressure during hemodialysis. *Blood Purification* 7, 233–239.

Levin, N. W. *et al.* (1995). The use of citric acid for dialyser reprocessing. *Journal of the American Society of Nephrology* 6, 1578–1582.

Lewis, B. E. *et al.* (2001). Argatroban anticoagulant therapy in patients with heparin-induced thrombocytopenia. *Circulation* 103, 1838–1890.

Lewis, L. M., Flechtner, T. W., Kerkay, J., Pearson, K. H., Chen, W. T., Popowniak, K. L., and Nakamoto, K. M. (1977). Determination of plasticizer levles in serum of hemodialysis patients. *Transactions of the American Society of Artificial Internal Organs* 23, 566–568.

Lim, V. S., Bier, D. M., Flanigan, J. M., and Sum-Ping, S. T. (1993). The effect of hemodialysis on protein metabolism: a leucine kinetic study. *Journal of Clinical Investigation* 91, 2429–2436.

Lin, C. L., Yang, C. W., Chiang, C. C., Chang, C. T., and Huang, C. C. (2001). Long-term on-line hemodiafiltration reduces predialysis beta-2-microglobulin levels in chronic hemodialysis patients. *Blood Purification* 19, 301–307.

Lindsay, R. M., Ferguson, D., Prentice, C. R. M., Burton, J. A., and McNicol, G. P. (1972). Reduction of thrombus formation on dialyzer membranes by aspirin and RA 233. *Lancet* 2, 1287–1290.

Lindsay, R. M., Rourke, J. T. B., Reid, B. D., Linton, A. L., Gilchrist, T., Courtney, J., and Edwards, R. O. (1977). The role of heparin on platelet retention by acrylonitrile co-polymer dialysis membranes. *Journal of Laboratory and Clinical Medicine* **89**, 724–734.

Linke, R. P., Bommer, J., Ritz, E., Waldherr, R., and Eulitz (1986). Amyloid kidney stones of uremic patients consist of beta-2-microglobulin fragments. *Biochemical and Biophysical Research Communications* **136**, 665–671.

Locatelli, F., Andrulli, S., and D'Amico, M. (2001). Evaluation of dialysis outcomes: experimental versus observational evidence. *Journal of Nephrology* **148** (Suppl. 4), S101–S108.

Loirat, C., Ehrich, J. H. H., Geerlings, W., Jones, E. H. P., Landais, P., Mallick, N. P., Margreiter, R., Raine, A. E. G., Salmela, K., Selwood, N. H., Tufveson, G., and Valderrabano, F. (1994). Report on management of renal failure in children in Europe, XXIII. *Nephrology, Dialysis, Transplantation* **9** (Suppl. 1), 26–40.

Lonnemann, G. (2000). Should ultra-pure dialysate be mandatory? *Nephrology, Dialysis, Transplantation* **15** (Suppl. 1), 55–59.

Lonnemann, G. and Koch, K. M. (2002). Online predilution HDF versus low-flux HD with ultrafiltered dialysate: longterm influence on mediators of inflammation. *Blood Purification* **20**, 202 (abstract).

Lonnemann, G., Koch, K. M., Shaldon, S., and Dinarello, C. A. (1988a). Studies on the ability of hemodialysis membranes to induce, bind, and clear human interleukin-I. *Journal of Laboratory and Clinical Medicine* **112**, 76–86.

Lonnemann, G., Bingel, M., Floege, J., Koch, K. M., Shaldon, S., and Dinarello, C. A. (1988b). Detection of endotoxin-like interleukin-1-inducing activity during *in vitro* dialysis. *Kidney International* **3**, 29–35.

Lonnemann, G., Haubitz, M., and Schindler, R. (1990). Hemodialysis-associated induction of cytokines. *Blood Purification* **8**, 214–222.

Lonnemann, G., Behme, T. C., Lenzner, B., Floege, J., Schulze, M., Colton, C. K., Koch, K. M., and Shaldon, S. (1992). Permeability of dialyzer membranes to TNF alpha-inducing substances derived from water bacteria. *Kidney International* **42**, 61–68.

Lonnemann, G., Schindler, R., Lufft, V., Mahiout, A., Shaldon, S., and Koch, K. M. (1995). The role of plasma coating on the permeation of cytokine-inducing substances through dialyser membranes. *Nephrology, Dialysis, Transplantation* **10**.

Lonnemann, G., Floege, J., Kliem, V., Brunkhorst, R., and Koch, K. M. (2000). Extended daily veno-venous high-flux haemodialysis in patients with acute renal failure and multiple organ dysfunction syndrome using a single path batch dialysis system. *Nephrology, Dialysis, Transplantation* **15** (8), 1189–1193.

Lowance, D. C. (1993). Factors and guidelines to be considered in offering treatment to patients with end-stage renal failure: a personal opinion. *American Journal of Kidney Diseases* **21**, 679.

Lowrie, E. and Lew, N. (1990). Death risk in hemodialysis patients: the predictive value of commonly measured variables and an evaluation of death rate differences between facilities. *American Journal of Kidney Diseases* **5**, 458–482.

Lowry, P. W., Beck-Sague, C. M., Bland, L. A., and Aguero, S. M. (1990). Mycobacterium chelonei infection among patients receiving high-flux dialysis in a hemodialysis clinic in California. *Journal of Infectious Diseases* **161**, 85–90.

Magnani, H. N. (1993). Heparin-induced thrombocytopenia (HIT): an overview of 230 patients treated with Orgaran. *Thrombosis and Haemostasis* **70**, 554–561.

Maher, J. F. (1976). When should maintenance dialysis be initiated? *Nephron* **16**, 83–85.

Mailloux, L. U. *et al.* (1996). Home hemodialysis: patient outcomes during a 24-year period of time from 1970 through 1993. *Advances in Renal Replacement Therapy* **3**, 112–121.

Maioraca, R., Cancarini, G. C., Brunori, G., Camerini, C., and Manili (1993). Morbidity and mortality of CAPD and hemodialysis. *Kidney International Supplement* **40**, S4–S15.

Man, N. K., Degremont, A., Darbord, J. C., Collet, M., and Vaillant, P. (1998). Evidence of bacterial biofilm in tubing from hydraulic pathway of hemodialysis system. *Artificial Organs* **22** (7), 596–600.

Mansell, M. A. and Wing, A. J. (1977). Long term experience of home dialysis with sorbent regeneration of dialysate. *Proceedings of the European Dialysis and Transplant Association* **13**, 275–279.

Markell, M. S., Altura, B. T., Sarn, Y., Delano, B. G., Ifudu, O., Friedman, E. A., and Altura, B. M. (1993). Deficiency of serum ionized magnesium in patients receiving hemodialysis or peritoneal dialysis. *Transactions of the American Society of Artificial Internal Organs* **39**, 801–804.

Maroni, B. J., Steinman, T. I., and Mitch, W. E. (1985). A method for estimating nitrogen intake of patients with chronic renal failure. *Kidney International* **27**, 58–64.

Martin-Malo, A. and Castillo, D. (1993). Adequacy of dialysis: is it really determined by the type of membrane and buffer? *Proceedings of the European Dialysis and Transplant Association* **147** (abstract).

Matsuo, T., Chikahira, Y., Yamada, T., Nakao, K., Ueshima, S., and Matsuo, O. (1988). Effect of synthetic thrombin inhibitor (MD805) as an alternative drug on heparin induced thrombocytopenia during hemodialysis. *Thrombosis Research* **52**, 165–171.

McGregor, D. O., Buttimore, A. L., and Lynn, K. L. (2000). Home hemodialysis: excellent survival at less cost, but still underutilized. *Kidney International* **57**, 2654–

Meema, H. E., Oreopoulos, D. G., and Rapoport, A. (1987). Serum magnesium level and arterial calcification in end stage renal disease. *Kidney International* **32**, 388–394.

Mion, C. M., Hegstrom, R. M., Boen, S. I., and Scribner, B. H. (1964). Substitution of sodium acetate for sodium bicarbonate in the bath fluid for hemodialysis. *Transactions of the American Society of Artificial Internal Organs* **10**, 110–114.

Mion, C. M., Canaud, B., Francesqui, M. P., Ortiz, J. P., N'Guyen, Q. V., Armynot, A. M., Simeon, M., and Athisso, M. (1987). Bicarbonate concentrate: a hidden source of microbial contamination of dialysis fluid. *Blood Purification* **7**, 32–38.

Miura, Y., Ishiyama, T., Inomata, A., Takeda, T., Senma, S., Okuyama, K., and Suzuki, Y. (1992). Radiolucent bone cysts and the type of dialysis membrane used in patients undergoing longterm hemodialysis. *Nephron* **60**, 268–273.

Mohr, P. E. *et al.* (2001). The case or daily dialysis: its impact on costs and quality of life. *American Journal of Kidney Diseases* **37**, 777–782.

Moriniére, P., Marie, A., El Esper, N., Fardellone, P., Deramond, H., Remond, A., Sebert, J. L., and Fournier, A. (1991). Destructive spondylarthropathy with beta-2-microglobulin amyloid deposits in an uremic patient before chronic hemodialysis. *Nephron* **59**, 654–657.

Moss, A. H. (1995). To use dialysis appropriately: the emerging consensus on patients selection guidelines. *Advance in Renal Replacement Therapy* **2**, 175.

Murray, J. S., Tu, W. H., Alberts, J. B., Burnell, J. H., and Scribner, B. H. (1962). A community hemodialysis center for the treatment of chronic uremics. *Transactions of the American Society of Artificial Internal Organs* **10**, 110–114.

National Kidney Foundation Report on Dialyzer Reuse (1997). Task Force on Reuse of Dialyzers, Council on Dialysis, National Kidney Foundation. *American Journal of Kidney Diseases* **30**, 859.

National Kidney Foundation-DOQI (2001). Clinical Practice Guidelines for Peritoneal Dialysis Adequacy. Guidelines 1 and 2. *American Journal of Kidney Diseases* **37** (Suppl. 1), S70–

Neergard, J., Nielsen, B., Faurby, V., Christensen, D. H., and Nielsen, O. F. (1971). Plasticizers in PVC and the occurrence of hepatitis in a haemodialysis unit: a preliminary communication. *Scandinavian Journal of Urology and Nephrology* **5**, 141–145.

Nguyen, A. T., Lethias, C., Zingraff, J., Herbelin, A., Naret, C., and Descamps-Latscha, B. (1985). Hemodialysis membrane-induced activation of phagocyte oxidative metabolism detected in vivo and in vitro within microamounts of whole blood. *Kidney International* **28**, 158–167.

Nowak, G., Bucha, E., Brauns, I., and Czerwinski, R. (1997). Anticoagulation with r-hirudin in regular haemodialysis with heparin-induced thrombocytopenia (HIT II). The first long-term application of r-hirudin in a haemodialysis patient. *Wiener Klinische Wochenschrift* **109**, 343–345.

Oberley, E. and Schattell, D. (1996). Home hemodialysis: survival, quality of life and rehabilitation. *Advances in Renal Replacement Therapy* **3**, 147–153.

Olbricht, C. J., Schaumann, D., and Fischer, D. (1992). Anaphylactoid reactions, LDL apheresis with dextrane sulfate, and ACE inhibitors. *Lancet* **340**, 908–909.

Ono, K., Ikeda, T., Fukumitsu, T., Tatsukawa, R., and Wakimoto, T. (1980). Migration of plasticizers from haemodialysis blood tubing. *Proceedings of the European Dialysis and Transplant Association* **12**, 571–573.

O'Shea, S. I., Sands, J. J., Nudo, S. A., and Ortel, T. L. (2002). Frequency of anti-heparin-platelet factor 4 antibodies in hemodialysis patients and correlation with recurrent vascular access thrombosis. *American Journal of Hematology* **69**, 72–73.

Papadakis, J. T., Patrikarea, A., Saradi, S., Papakostas, K., Leondi, A., Kravaritis, A., and Vafiadis, S. (1991). Hypersensitivity reactions during hemodialysis related to the use of acetate dialysate. *Clinical Nephrology* **35**, 224–226.

Pappius, H. M. and Dossetor, J. B. (1967). The effects of rapid hemodialysis on brain tissues and cerebrospinal fluid of dogs. *Canadian Journal of Physiology and Pharmacology* **45**, 129–147.

Pegues, D. A., Beck-Sague, C. M., and Woollen, S. W. (1992). Anaphylactoid reactions associated with reuse of hollow-fiber hemodialyzers and ACE-inhibitors. *Kidney International* **42**, 1232–1237.

Peri, U. N., Fenves, A. Z., and Middleton, J. P. (2001). Improving survival of octogenerian patients selected for haemodialysis. *Nephrology, Dialysis, Transplantation* **11**, 2201–2206.

Peterson, H. D. (1964). Acute encephalopathy occurring during hemodialysis. *Archives of Internal Medicine* **113**, 8777–8800.

Petersen, J. *et al.* (1991). The effects of reprocessing cuprophane and polysulfone dialyzers on beta-2-microglobuline removal from hemodialysis patients. *American Journal of Kidney Diseases* **17**, 174–178.

Petersen, N. J., Carson, A., and Favero, M. S. (1981). Bacterial endotoxin in new and reused dialysers: a potential cause of endotoxemia. *Transactions of the American Society of Artificial Internal Organs* **27**, 155–160.

Petrie, J. J. B., Campbell, Y., Hawley, C. M., and Hogan, P. G. (1991). Anaphylactoid reactions in patients on hemofiltration with AN69 membrane whilst receiving ACE inhibitors. *Clinical Nephrology* **36**, 264–265.

Pizziconi, V. B. (1990). Performance and integrity testing in reprocessed dialysers: a QC update. *AAMI, Standards and Recommended Practices* Vol. 3, Dialysis, Arlington: Association for the Advancement of Medical Instrumentation, 1990.

Poldermans, D. *et al.* (1999). Cardiac evaluation in hypotension-prone and hypotension-resistant hemodialysis patients. *Kidney International* **56**, 1905–1909.

Port, F. K. *et al.* (2001). Mortality risk by hemodialyzer reuse practice and dialyzer membrane characteristics. *American Journal of Kidney Diseases* **37**, 276–286.

Quinton, W. E., Dillard, D., and Scribner, B. E. (1960). Cannulation of blood vessels for prolonged hemodialysis. *Transactions of the American Society of Artificial Internal Organs* **6**, 103–106.

Ratcliffe, P. J., Phillips, R. E., and Oliver, D. V. (1983). Late referal for maintenance dialysis. *British Medical Journal* **288**, 441–445.

Redaelli, B., Sforzini, S., Bondoldi, G., Dadone, C., DiFillipo, S., Filoramo, F., Limido, D., Pincella, G., and Vigano, M. R. (1979). Hemodialysis with adequate sodium concentration in dialysate. *International Journal of Artificial Organs* **2**, 133–140.

Rumpf, K. W., Seubert, S., Seubert, A., Lowitz, H. D., Valentin, R., Rippe, H., Ippen, H., and Scheler, F. (1985). Association of ethylene oxide induced IgE antibodies with symptoms in dialysis patients. *Lancet* **2**, 1385–1387.

Salem, M., Ivanovich, P. T., Ing, T. S., and Daugirdas, J. T. (1994). Adverse effects of dialyzers manifesting during the dialysis session. *Nephrology, Dialysis, Transplantation* **9** (Suppl. 2), 127–137.

Salzman, E. W. Interaction of blood with artificial surfaces. In *Hemostasis and Thrombosis* (ed. R. W. Colman, J. Hirsh, V. J. Marder, and E. W. Salzman), pp. 1335–1354. New York: Lippincott, 1987.

Sawyer, N., Noonan, K., Altman, P., Marsh, F., and Cunningham, J. (1988). High dose calcium carbonate with stepwise reduction in dialysate calcium concentration: effective phosphate control and aluminum avoidance in haemodialysis patients. *Nephrology, Dialysis, Transplantation* **3**, 1–5.

Schindler, R. and Dinarello, C. A. Interleukin 1. In *Growth Factors, Differentiation Factors, and Cytokines* (ed. A. Habenicht), pp. 85–102. Berlin: Heidelberg, Springer Verlag, 1990.

Schindler, R., Lonnemann, G., Shaldon, S., Koch, K. M., and Dinarello, C. A. (1990). Transcription, not synthesis, of interleukin-1 and tumor necrosis factor by complement. *Kidney International* **37**, 85–93.

Schindler, R., Linnenweber, S., Schulze, M., Oppermann, M., Dinarello, C. A., Shaldon, S., and Koch, K. M. (1993a). Gene expression of interleukin-1 beta during hemodialysis. *Kidney International* **43**, 712–721.

Schindler, R., Marra, N. M., McKelligon, B. M., Lonnemann, G., Schulzeck, P., Schulze, M., Oppermann, M., and Shaldon, S. (1993b). Plasma levels of bactericidal/permeability-increasing protein (BPI) and lipopolysaccharide-binding protein (LBP) during hemodialysis. *Clinical Nephrology* **40**, 346–351.

Schindler, R., Lonnemann, G., Schäffer, J., Shaldon, S., Koch, K. M., and Krautzig, S. (1994). The effect of ultrafiltered dialysate on the cellular content of interleukin-1 receptor antagonist in patients on chronic hemodialysis. *Nephron* **68**, 229–233.

Schindler, R., Krautzig, S., Lufft, V., Lonnemann, G., Mahiout, G., Marra, M. N., Shaldon, S., and Koch, K. M. (1996). Induction of interleukin-1 and interleukin-1 receptor antagonist during contaminated *in-vitro* dialysis with whole blood. *Nephrology, Dialysis, Transplantation* **11** (1), 101–108.

Schmidt, M. Hemodiafiltration. In *Hemofiltration* (ed. L. W. Henderson, E. Quellhorst, C. A. Baldamus, and M. J. Lysaght), pp. 265–271. Berlin, Heidelberg, New York, Tokyo: Springer Verlag, 1986.

Schon, D. C., Klein, S., Mitshuishi, Y. H., and Jahn, H. A. (1981). Correlation between plasma sodium acetate concentration and systemic vascular resistance. *Proceedings of the European Dialysis and Transplant Association* **18**, 160–166.

Schrader, J., Stibbe, W., Armstrong, V. W., Kandt, M., Muche, R., Köstering, H., Seidel, D., and Scheler, F. (1988). Comparison of low molecular weight heparin to standard heparin in hemodialysis/hemofiltration. *Kidney International* **33**, 890–896.

Schwab, S. J., Onorato, J. J., Sharar, L. R., and Dennis, P. A. (1987). Hemodialysis without anticoagulation: 1 year prospective trial in hospitalized patients at risk for bleeding. *American Journal of Medicine* **83**, 405–410.

Sekkarie, M. A. and Moss, A. H. (1998). Withholding and withdrawing dialysis: the role of physician specialty and education and patients functional status. *American Journal of Kidney Diseases* **31**, 464.

Sherman, R. A., Cody, R. P., Rogers, M. E., and Solanchick, J. C. (1994). The effect of dialyzer reuse on dialysis delivery. *American Journal of Kidney Diseases* **24**, 924–928.

Silver, S. M. (1995). Cerebral edema after rapid dialysis is not caused by an increase in brain organic osmolytes. *Journal of the American Society of Nephrology* **6**, 1600.

Silver, S. M., DeSimone, J. A., Smith, D. A., and Sterns, R. H. (1992). Dialysis disequilibrium in the rat: role of the reverse urea effect. *Kidney International* **42**, 161–165.

Singer, P. A. (1992). Nephrologists experience with and attitudes towards decisions to forego dialysis. *Journal of the American Society of Nephrology* **2**, 1235.

Slatopolsky, E., Weerts, C., Norwood, K., Giles, K., Fryer, P., and Finch, L. L. (1989). Long-term effects of calcium carbonate and 2.5 mEq/liter calcium dialysate on mineral metabolism. *Kidney International* **36**, 897–903.

Stiller, S., Mann, H., and Brunner, H. (1986). Backfiltration in haemodialysis with highly permeable membranes. *Contributions to Nephrology* **46**, 23–32.

Stiller, S., Bonnie-Schorn, E., Grassmann, A., Uhlenbusch-Körwer, I., and Mann, H. (2001). A critical review of sodium profiling for hemodialysis. *Seminars in Dialysis* **14**, 337–347.

Swartz, R. D. and Port, F. K. (1979). Preventing hemorrhage in high-risk hemodilaysis: regional versus low-dose heparin. *Kidney International* **16**, 513–518.

Swartz, R. D., Flamenbaum, W., Dubrow, A., Hall, J. C., Crow, J. W., and Cato, A. (1988). Epoprostol (PGI2, prostacyclin) during high-risk hemodialysis: preventing further bleeding complications. *Journal of Clinical Pharmacology* **28**, 818–825.

Tardy-Poncet, B., Tardy, B., and Reynaud, J. (1999). Efficacy and safety of danaparoid sodium in critically ill patients with heparin-associated thrombocytopenia. *Chest* **115**, 1616–1620.

Tielemans, C., Madhoun, P., Lenaers, M., Schandene, L., Goldman, M., and Vanherweghem, J. L. (1990). Anaphylactoid reactions during hemodialysis on AN69 membranes in patients receiving ACE inhibitors. *Kidney International* **38**, 982–984.

Tokars, J. I., Miller, E. R., Alter, M. J., and Arduino, M. J. (2000). National surveillance of dialysis associated diseases in the United States, 1997. *Seminars in Dialysis* **13**, 75–85.

US Renal Data System (1992). Comorbid conditions and correlations with mortality risk among 3399 incident hemodialysis patients. *American Journal of Kidney Diseases* **20** (5 Suppl. 2), 32–38.

Vanherweghem, J. L., Tielemans, C., Goldman, M., and Boelaert, J. (1991). Infections in chronic haemodialysis patients. *Seminars in Dialysis* **4**, 240–244.

Vanholder, R., Hoenich, N. A., and Ringoir, S. Single needle haemodialysis. In *Replacement of Renal Function by Dialysis* (ed. J. F. Maher), pp. 382–399. Dordrecht: Kluwer Academic Publishers, 1989.

Vanholder, R., Ringoir, S., Dhondt, A., and Hakim, R. M. (1991). Phagocytosis in uremic and hemodialysis patients: a prospective and cross sectional study. *Kidney International* **39**, 320–327.

Vanholder, R., Vanhaecke, E., and Ringoir, S. (1992). Pseudomonas septicaemia due to deficient disinfectant mixing during reuse. *International Journal of Artificial Organs* **15**, 19–24.

Vanholder, R. C., Camez, A. A., Veys, N. M., Soria, J., Mirshahi, M., Soria, C., and Ringoir, S. (1994). Recombinant hirudin: a specific thrombin inhibiting anticoagulant for hemodialysis. *Kidney International* **45**, 1754–1759.

Vanholder, R. C., Camez, A. A., Veys, N. M., Van Loo, A., Dhondt, A. M., and Ringoir, S. (1997). Pharmacocinetics of recombinant hirudin in hemodialyzed end-stage renal failure patients. *Thrombosis and Haemostasis* **77**, 650–655.

Van Wyk, V., Badenhorst, P. N., Luus, H. G., and Kotzé, H. F. (1995). A comparison between the use of recombinant hirudin and heparin during hemodialysis. *Kidney International* **48**, 1338–1342.

Van Ypersele de Strihou Ch., Jadoul, M., Malghem, J., Maldague, J., and Jamart, J. (1991). Effect of dialysis membrane and patients age on signs of dialysis-related amyloidosis. *Kidney International* **39**, 1012–1019.

Van Ypersele de Strihou Ch., Floege, J., Jadoul, M., and Koch K. M. (1994). Amyloidosis and its relationship to different dialysers. *Nephrology, Dialysis, Transplantation* **9** (Suppl. 2), 156–161.

Vaslaki, L., Karatson, A., Vörös, P., Major, L., Pethö, F., Ladanyi, E., Weber, C., Mitteregger, R., and Falkenhagen, D. (2000). Can sterile and pyrogen-free on-line substitution fluid be routinely delivered? A multicentric study on the microbiological safety of on-line haemodiafiltration. *Nephrology, Dialysis, Transplantation* **15** (Suppl. 1), 74–78.

Verresen, L., Waer, M., Vanrentergem, Y., and Michielsen, P. (1990). Angiotensin-converting-enzyme inhibitors and anaphylactoid reactions to high-flux membrane dialysis. *Lancet* **336**, 1360–1362.

Verresen, L., Fink, E., Lemke, H. D., and Vanrenterghem, Y. (1994). Bradykinin is a mediator of anaphylactoid reactions during hemodialysis with AN69 membranes. *Kidney International* **45**, 1497–1503.

von Breitenfelder, W. (1986a). Technische Aspekte der Bikarbonat-Hämodialyse, part 1. *Medizintechnik* **106**, 84–87.

von Breitenfelder, W. (1986b). Technische Aspekte der Bikarbonat-Hämodialyse, part 2. *Medizintechnik* **106**, 121–125.

Vreman, H. J., Assomul, V. M., Kaiser, B. A., Blaschke, T. F., and Weiner, M. W. (1980). Acetate metabolism and acid–base homeostasis during hemodialysis: influence of dialyzer efficiency and metabolic capacity of acetate metabolism. *Kidney International* **18**, S62–S74.

Ward, R. A., Schmidt, B., Hullin, J., Hillebrand, G. F., and Samtleben, W. (2000). A comparison of on-line hemodiafiltration and high-flux hemodialysis: a prospective clinical study. *Journal of the American Society of Nephrology* **11**, 2344–2350.

Warkentin, T. E. (2001). Heparin-induced thrombocytopenia (HIT): yet another treatment paradox? *Thrombosis and Haemostasis* **85**, 947–952.

Warkentin, T. E., Levine, M. N., Hirsh, J., Horsewood, P., Roberts, R. S., Gent, M., and Kelton, J. G. (1995). Heparin-induced thrombocytopenia in patients treated with low-molecular-weight heparin or unfractionated heparin. *New England Journal of Medicine* **332**, 1330–1335.

Westhuyzen, J., Foreman, K., Battistutta, D., Saltissi, D., and Fleming, S. J. (1992). Effect of dialyzer reprocessing with Renalin on serum beta-2-microglobulin and complement activation in hemodialysis patients. *American Journal of Nephrology* **12**, 29–36.

Wiegand, C., Dvin, T., Raji, L., and Kjellstrand, C. (1979). Life threatening hypokalemia during hemodialysis. *Transactions of the American Society of Artificial Internal Organs* **25**, 416–418.

Wing, A. J. (1968). Optimum calcium concentration of dialysis fluid for maintenance haemodialysis. *British Medical Journal* **4**, 145–149.

Wizemann, V., Lotz, C., Techert, F., and Uthoff, S. (2000). On-line haemodiafiltration versus low-flux haemodialysis. A prospective randomized study. *Nephrology, Dialysis, Transplantation* **15** (Suppl. 1), 43–48.

Woods, H. F. and Nandakumar, M. (2000). Improved outcome for haemodialysis patients treated with high-flux membranes. *Nephrology, Dialysis, Transplantation* **15** (Suppl. 1), 36–42.

Woods, J. D. *et al.* (1996). Comparison of mortality with home hemodialysis and center hemodialysis: a national study. *Kidney International* **49**, 1464–1471.

Yamamoto, S., Koide, M., Matsuo, M., Suzuki, S., Ahtaka, M., Saika, S., and Matsuo, T. (1996). Heparin-induced thrombocytopenia in hemodialysis patients. *American Journal of Kidney Diseases* **28**, 82–85.

Zucchelli, P., Santoro, A., Ferrari, G., and Spongano, M. (1990). Acetate-free biofiltration: hemodiafiltration with base-free dialysate. *Blood Purification* **8**, 14–22.

Zusman, R. M., Rubin, R. H., Cato, A. E., Cocchetto, D. M., Crow, J. W., and Tolkoff-Rubin, N. (1981). Hemodialysis using prostacyclin instead of heparin as the sole antithrombotic agent. *New England Journal of Medicine* **304**, 934–939.

12.4 Peritoneal dialysis and complications of technique

Ram Gokal

History

Peritoneal dialysis (PD) is now a well-established treatment of endstage renal failure but its development and refinement has taken time. Ganter's (1923) animal and human studies provided many of the principles that are still true today. The hundred patients with uraemia who had had PD between 1923 and 1948 were reviewed by (Odel *et al.* 1950). The results were poor because of technical problems with catheters, peritonitis, and dialysis fluid composition. Despite subsequent changes and improvement, use of PD was not satisfactory as a long-term treatment.

The modern era of PD started in 1959 with the introduction of a simplified method based on intermittent irrigation of the peritoneal cavity using a single, disposable catheter and commercially prepared dialysis solutions (Maxwell *et al.* 1959). However, repeated abdominal puncture, peritonitis, and the lower efficacy than haemodialysis (HD) limited its use in patients with terminal renal failure. A major advance came in the late 1960s when Tenckhoff and Schechter (1968) described the use of a permanent, indwelling, silicone-rubber catheter with two Dacron cuffs but this 'periodic' intermittent PD (IPD) was regarded as having little place in the treatment of patients in endstage renal failure (Tenckhoff *et al.* 1973). The situation changed dramatically after 1976 when Popovich *et al.* (1976) introduced the concept of a 'portable/wearable equilibration' PD technique. This new approach, resulting in steady-state, low blood concentrations of uraemic metabolites, was later developed into continuous ambulatory peritoneal dialysis (CAPD). This technique gained rapid and widespread acceptance. At the end of 2001 approximately 1,30,000 patients worldwide were on PD, that is, 13 per cent of the total world dialysis population. This rapid increase over the last 25 years has stimulated attempts to refine the treatment.

Peritoneal anatomy and physiology

Peritoneal dialysis requires solute and fluid exchange between peritoneal capillary blood and a dialysis solution in the peritoneal cavity across the peritoneal 'membrane', which consists of a vascular wall, the interstitium, the mesothelium, and adjacent fluid films. Solute movements follow physical laws of diffusion and convective transport, whilst fluid shifts relate to osmosis. The crucial components of the PD system are, therefore, peritoneal blood flow, the membrane, and the 'flow rate' of the PD fluids. The various techniques and regimens are designed to exploit these transport characteristics.

Morphology and ultrastructure

The peritoneal surface area of the adult ranges between 1.7 and 2.0 m^2, similar to the surface area of the skin. The membrane itself consists of three layers: the capillary endothelium, the interstitium, and the mesothelium, but peritoneal thickness varies according to the area examined (Di Paolo and Sacchi 2000).

Mesothelium

The resting normal mesothelium appears as a continuous layer formed by flattened, polygonal, mononuclear cells. The luminal aspect has numerous projecting microvilli, which not only increase the surface area of the mesothelium by a factor of 20, but, by possessing anionic fixed charges, may play a significant part in the transperitoneal transfer of anionic macromolecules such as proteins (Gotloib and Shustack 1987). Microvilli are extremely sensitive to minor injury and loss of microvilli represents an early sign of impending apoptosis (Kondo *et al.* 1997). Several groups have demonstrated a surface-active material made up of phospholipids in the dialysate effluent (di Paolo *et al.* 1986). Dobbie and Lloyd (1989) have shown onion-layered organelles or lamellar bodies at the surface of the mesothelium, protruding by exocytosis from the surface and appearing as blebs and blisters (podocytosis). This has been linked to the secretory function (release of phospholipids and phosphatidylcholine) of the mesothelial cells, providing a lubricating surface with water-repellent properties. Mesothelial cells also release cytokines [interleukin (IL)-1 and IL-6], factors for fibrinolysis (PAI-1 and -2), transforming growth factor-β (TGF-β), fibronectin and growth factors important in peritoneal transport (vascular endothelial growth factor, VEGF). Recently, aquaporin channels (aquaporin-1 and -3) have been demonstrated in the mesothelial cells, the expression of which can be modulated by both osmotic and non-osmotic stimuli (Pannakeet *et al.* 1996; Lai *et al.* 2002). Their relevance to peritoneal permeability is unknown.

Interstitium

The submesothelial connective tissue consists of fibroblasts, mast cells, macrophages, and lymphatic vessels. Occasionally, fibroblasts are found near bundles of collagen. Proteoglycans make up the major component of the colloid-rich ground substance. These are also negatively charged, as are fibroblasts and collagen fibres, thus influencing solute transport. Wayland and Silverberg (1978) believe that the interstitium represents a network of aqueous channels of collagenous gels. Flessner and Schwab (1996) has shown that transfer of small solutes through the tortuous interstitial pathway is primarily by diffusion, with zero hydrostatic pressure under normal conditions but during clinical PD, the raised intra-abdominal pressure (4–10 cm water) drives fluid as well as solutes to the interstitium.

Blood microvessels

In the human parietal and visceral peritoneum microvessels have been classically described as of the continuous type but the fenestrated type has also been found, representing less than 2 per cent of the vessels (Gotloib and Shustack 1987). The endothelial-cell glycocalyx is a regular, well-organized polymeric carpet with an electronegative charge. The cells are linked by tight junctions. The microvascular endothelial cell is considered a highly active structure serving not only as a permeability barrier and an effective thromboresistant surface, but also as the location of important synthetic and other metabolic activities (Thorgeirsson and Robertson 1998). Recent identification of aquaporin-1 channels in the endothelium provides a molecular explanation of the water permeability of the peritoneal capillaries, where about 50 per cent of the transperitoneal water flow occurs (Pannekeet et al. 1996). The small pores in the three-pore model of solute and fluid transport (see later) are represented by the capillary clefts.

Mesothelial mass or turnover

Recently, Koomen et al. (1994) have shown that the cancertumour antigen (CA125) in the dialysate released by mesothelial cells can be regarded as a reflection of mesothelial mass or cell turnover in stable CAPD patients. This group has shown an inverse correlation of CA125 with the duration of CAPD, indicating a loss of cell mass with time (Ho-dac-Pannekeet et al. 1997a). However, there are conflicting results regarding the relationship of CA125 and time on PD (Ho-dac-Pannekeet et al. 1997a; Lai et al. 1997a,b), and longitudinal studies are needed.

Effect of peritoneal dialysis on morphology (Fig. 1)

The introduction of dialysis fluid into the peritoneal cavity has profound effects on the ultrastructure (Table 1). Early effects include the development of mesothelial intracellular oedema, destruction of organelles, interstitial oedema, diminished numbers of microvilli, and

submesothelial deposition of collagen and filamentous inclusion bodies, and some of the vascular changes similar to those seen in diabetic patients (Dobbie 1992; Dobbie et al. 1994; di Paolo and Sacchi 2000). These changes are reversible as shown by the fact that the peritoneum, if allowed to rest, completely regenerates within 10–30 days (Gotloib and Shustack 1987).

After an attack of acute bacterial peritonitis the ultrastructural changes are dramatic. The mesothelium is completely devoid of microvilli or completely denuded, and in severe episodes there may be accompanying layers of surface fibrin, all leading to obvious changes in permeability and ultrafiltration (UF). Recovery from peritonitis can take several paths. After cure of infection, there is remesothelialization but this may lead to membrane opacification and basement membrane reduplication. Prolonged and severe episodes may lead to a failure of regeneration of mesothelial tissue (tanned peritoneum), with increased and hyalinized collagen, widespread insudation of fibrin into the underlying interstitium, and, eventually, new membrane formation or mural fibrosis (Dobbie et al. 1994).

The situation is completely different for long-term patients, where loss of peritoneal function is a major cause of treatment failure (Davies et al. 1998). It is widely assumed that alterations in peritoneal function are related to structural changes in the peritoneal membrane. There is accumulating evidence that continuous exposure to the unphysiological dialysis solutions and repeated episodes of peritonitis could have a major influence on the membrane characteristics (Fuholler et al. 2002).

A recent study from the International Peritoneal Biopsy Study Group, which examined the morphological features of parietal peritoneal membranes in 130 PD patients and compared them with normal individuals, uraemic predialysis patients, and patients undergoing HD, has provided important data (Williams et al. 2002). The median thickness of the submesothelial compact collagenous zone was 50 μm for normal subjects, 140 μm for uraemic patients, 150 μm for HD patients, and 270 μm for patients on PD ($p = 0.001$ for all versus normals). Compact zone increased significantly with duration of PD therapy (Fig. 2). Vascular changes included progressive subendothelial hyalinization, with luminal narrowing or obliteration and prevalence of vasculopathy also increased with duration of PD therapy (Fig. 3). This study provides a comprehensive cross-sectional analysis of morphological changes associated with PD. The important findings include: some of the changes predate dialysis; those patients who do not develop problems with PD in the first 5 years are those who do not develop increased thickening of the submesothelial layer or significant vasculopathy. In addition, fibrosis did not occur without a degree of vasculopathy, suggesting that the latter predisposed to the

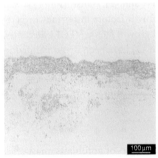
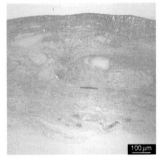

Normal parietal peritoneum   Parietal peritoneum >5 years PD

Fig. 1 Morphological features of parietal peritoneum from normal individual and a patient who has undergone long-term PD. Two zones can be observed. A compact submesothelial collagenous band and a deeper loose adipose connective tissue. The compact zone is markedly thickened in the sample from the PD patient, with markedly increased collagen fibres, mononuclear cells, and blood vessels (reproduced with permission from Williams et al. 2002).

Table 1 Various changes in the peritoneal membrane morphology described with long-term PD

Mesothelial denudation
Reduplication of capillary and mesothelial cell basement membrane
Submesothelial expansion: interstitial fibrosis and extracellular matrix deposition
Neoangiogenesis and vasculopathy
Changes in cytokine/growth factor expression

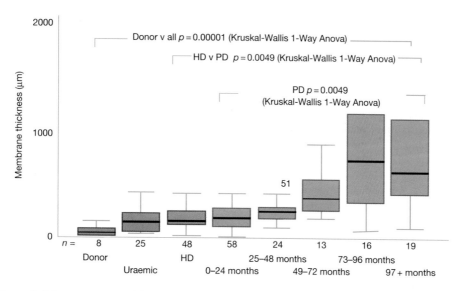

Fig. 2 Changes in the submesothelial compact zone with biopsy origin and with PD duration in the various groups of patients. Data are presented as box plots, with the boxes representing interquartile range. Lines extend from the box to the highest and lowest values and the median value is represented by the thick line across the box (reproduced with permission from Williams *et al.* 2002).

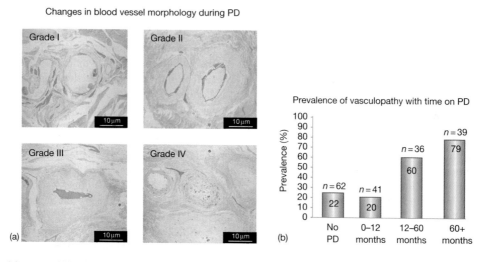

Fig. 3 (a) Morphological features of blood vessels in the parietal peritoneum. The subendothelial hyaline layer is slender (up to 7 μm), corresponding to grade 1. The subendothelial zone is greater than 7 μm but the lumen is not distorted or narrowed, corresponding to grade 2. The lumen is distorted or narrowed corresponding to grade 3. The lumen is occluded by connective tissue, corresponding to grade 4. (b) The prevalence of vasculopathy according to the duration of PD is represented in comparison to biopsies from predialysis patients (reproduced with permission from Williams *et al.* 2002).

development of the former. Functional correlates to these morphological findings were not studied.

Pathogenesis of peritoneal membrane derangements with long-term peritoneal dialysis

With PD, morphological changes do take place and with it, functional derangement. These morphological–functional relationships are, therefore, vitally important. The use of unphysiological PD solutions as well as episodes of infection and inflammation lead to changes in the peritoneal membrane described above. This tendency to 'fibrosis' has been reported in long-term dialysis patients (Dobbie *et al.* 1994; Hendriks *et al.* 1997) and it is partly related to advanced glycation endproducts (AGE) in the peritoneum from glucose–protein reactions

in the peritoneum (Nakayama *et al.* 1997). This process (a direct chemical reaction between sugars and primary amino groups in the protein forming irreversible Amadori products) gives rise to AGE, a process directly related to levels of glucose degradation products (GDPs) in the PD fluids (Devuyst 2002). This process may be accelerated by peritonitis when the submesothelium is exposed to a very high glucose concentration from the dialysate (Papanastasion *et al.* 1994; Park *et al.* 2000). This complex process involves interactions between released growth factors (VEGF and TGF-β), cytokines (IL-1–6) (Devuyst 2002; Miyata *et al.* 2002).

The end result of the changes is encapsulating peritoneal sclerosis (EPS), which is fortunately infrequent (Kawaguchi *et al.* 2000). The Australia and New Zealand Renal Registry Data (ANZ DATA) reported that 1.9–4.2 per cent of patients develop this syndrome (Rigby and Hawley 1998). The incidence is lower in Japan, 0.9–1.7 per cent (Nakamoto *et al.* 2002).

Loss of UF is the commonest peritoneal transport abnormality in long-term PD (Honda *et al.* 1996; Ho-dac-Pannekeet *et al.* 1997b). The major causes of UF failure are the presence of a large vascular peritoneal surface area and decrease in osmotic conductance to glucose—perhaps related to decreased aquaporin function or a decrease in the UF coefficient of the peritoneum. The diabetiform peritoneal neoangiogenesis appears to be an important, but not the only, cause of UF failure (Krediet *et al.* 2000).

There are several pathogenic factors responsible for changes in the peritoneal membrane, predominantly related to bioincompatibility of current PD solutions. These appear to be as follows:

1. Continuous exposure to bioincompatible dialysis fluids [shown to be toxic *in vitro* (Martis *et al.* 2000)]. The important factors are a combination of low pH and lactate and glucose itself, through its metabolism via the polyol pathway (Kaur *et al.* 1997), and molecular mechanisms—cytokines, growth factors, and nitric oxide synthase activity (Combet *et al.* 2000; Devuyst 2002).

2. Glucose exposure leading to vascular changes of neovascularization and deposition of type IV collagen in the interstitium (Mateijsen *et al.* 1999).

3. Formation of AGE in peritoneal tissue (Honda *et al.* 1999).

4. The presence of GDPs generated during steam sterilization, are directly cytotoxic and accelerate the process of AGE formation (Martis *et al.* 2000; An *et al.* 2001).

5. Patient related factors such as inflammation, peritonitis, oxidative stress, and diabetes (Devuyst 2002).

Glucose exposure is now regarded as the significant pathogenetic factor in peritoneal membrane alteration and the development of increased peritoneal permeability (or high transporter status on the standard peritoneal equilibration test, PET) (Davies *et al.* 2001). The goal for the clinician is to identify how to reduce patient exposure to glucose, minimize the total amount of glucose absorbed, and avoid the hyperosmolar stress and high glucose and GDP exposure to the peritoneum. Fortunately, non-glucose based PD solutions and lower GDP containing solutions are becoming available.

Peritoneal lymphatics

The lymphatic drainage from the peritoneal cavity is primarily by specialized end-lymphatic openings (stomata) located in the subdiaphragmatic peritoneum. From the stomata, the capillaries coalesce to form a plexus of collecting lymphatics within the diaphragm. The lacunae of the terminal lymphatics are separated from the peritoneal cavity by interdigitating mesothelium, a loose network of connective tissue and lymphatic endothelium (Tsilibary and Wissig 1987). The stomata are formed by the separation of adjacent mesothelial cells and permit absorption of intraperitoneal particles, cells, colloids, and fluid. Two indirect methods are available for estimating lymphatic absorption. Both apply the same physiological functions of the lymphatics. By assuming that intraperitoneal marker colloids are returned to the systemic circulation exclusively by the lymphatics without any alteration in the concentration of the index colloids, the lymphatic absorption rate may be estimated either from the mass

transfer rate of marker colloids from the peritoneal cavity to the blood or from the rate of disappearance from the peritoneal cavity (Mactier and Khanna 2000).

Effective lymphatic absorption rates (back-filtration) estimated from the disappearance of intraperitoneal colloids exceed 1 ml/min in most adult CAPD patients (Heimburger *et al.* 1995), and have a major influence on the kinetics of UF in long-dwell exchanges. On average, back-filtration reduces net UF volumes each day by 40–50 per cent.

Peritoneal physiology

Solute and fluid transport

The kinetics of solute and fluid transport across the peritoneal membrane during PD remain incompletely understood.

Solutes

The transfer of solutes across the peritoneal membrane occurs through two major mechanisms, diffusion and convection. The rate of solute transport by diffusion is proportional to the concentration difference between blood in the peritoneal capillaries and the PD fluid. The proportionality factor, which accounts for the extent of contact area between the peritoneum and the dialysis fluid, defines the permeability of the peritoneal membrane. Solute transport also occurs by convection or 'solvent drag' and is relatively more important for substances in the range of 50–500 Da. Whether diffusion or convection is the most important transport mechanism of a solute is dependent on the transcapillary UF rate, the diffusability of the solute, and its sieving coefficient (this is the convective proportionality factor; a value of 1 indicates no rejection of solute by the peritoneal membrane whereas a value of 0 indicates total hindrance to solutes relative to fluid movement. The sieving coefficient is one minus the reflection coefficient) (Staverman 1951). Solute and fluid removal are reduced during PD by direct absorption into peritoneal tissues and transport into lymphatics (back-filtration). Solutes passing from the blood in the peritoneal capillaries to the dialysate-filled peritoneal cavity have to pass at least three structures that can offer resistance: the capillary wall (probably the most important), the interstitial tissue, and mesothelial cell layer. Diffusion and transcapillary UF occur in two directions across these resistances.

Several mathematical models have been defined to describe the transport phenomena: the three most plausible are the homogeneous or membrane model (Kallen 1966), the capillary distributed theories (Flessner *et al.* 1984), and the three-pore model (Rippe and Krediet 1994).

It is now recognized that there are effectively 'three pores' that explain the capillary transport. This three-pore theory recognizes:

1. Ultrasmall pores (3–5 Å; aquaporin-1; the aquaporin chip is a 28-kDa, channel-forming, integral membrane protein which acts as an osmotically driven, water-selective pore), allowing the transport of water but not solutes. These have been identified in the mesothelium and the capillary endothelium. Glucose is effective as a crystalloid osmotic agent inspite of its small size of 2–3 Å, as it predominantly acts at this level. About 50 per cent of transcapillary UF occurs through these pores, inspite of the surface area being only 1–2 per cent.

2. Small pores (40–50 Å; interendothelial clefts have been considered the equivalent of small pores)—colloid osmosis occurs at this level.

3. Large pores (>150 Å; probably less than 0.1 per cent of total pore count), which are involved in macromolecular transport.

Because of the very complex structure of the various barriers to the peritoneal transport of solutes and fluid, it is simpler to regard this system as one membrane. The three-pore model of capillary permeability envisages at least two different exchange pathways across the capillary wall: one transcellular through the ultrasmall pore and the other through the dominant transcapillary pathway for small solutes and water (Fig. 4).

Another development of importance in solute transport has been the concept of quantification of solute removal and characterization of individual differences in peritoneal transport characteristics, which led to the development of the PET by Twardowski et al. (1987). The basis of this was the recognition that peritoneal permeability and peritoneal surface area were both important and that the solute transport rates can be influenced by both. The term describing this link is the mass transfer area coefficient (MTAC) or permeability area product, and is a fundamental measure of the rate of diffusive transport across the peritoneal membrane. This can be influenced by the contact area between the peritoneum and PD fluid, permeability of the capillaries, diffusivity within the peritoneal interstitium, and perfusion of peritoneal tissues.

There are two processes of solute transport—diffusive, which is more 'open', and convective transport, which is regarded as 'tight', akin to two separate barriers in series. The barrier proximal to the blood was postulated to be thin and tight (or restrictive) and this was thought to be the capillary endothelium. The distal barrier was postulated to be thick but open—the interstitium of the peritoneal membrane (Leypoldt 2002). Subsequent work by Rippe and Stelin (1989) provided a theory based on capillary physiology for understanding solute sieving by the peritoneum and proposed a two-pore model of capillary transport. This theory was, however, unable to explain the low sieving coefficient for the peritoneum. These investigators proposed water-only pathways giving rise to the three-pore theory, which has become the paradigm for describing the kinetics of fluid and solute transport during PD.

The peritoneal equilibration test
The PET is a simple, practical technique from which the dialysate to plasma concentration ratio ($D:P$) can be obtained in a standardized

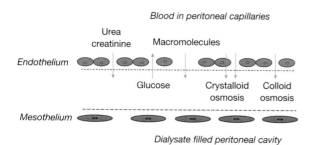

Blood in peritoneal capillaries

Urea
creatinine   Macromolecules

Endothelium

Glucose   Crystalloid   Colloid
osmosis   osmosis

Mesothelium

Dialysate filled peritoneal cavity

• Loss through lymphatics

Fig. 4 Diagramatic representation of the various pathways for the peritoneal transport of fluid and solutes on the three-pore model. Crystalloid osmosis (usually glucose based in CAPD) influence transport through small and ultrasmall pores, while colloid osmosis (icodextrin as an colloid osmotic agent is an example in PD) act predominantly at the small pores.

way, as can a ratio between dialysate glucose at the end of the dwell and after inflow ($D:D_0$) and compared to the drained volume after 4 h (Twardwoski et al. 1987). It is useful as a prognostic tool and as a means of assessing loss of UF, depending on the permeability of the membrane; high or high-average transporters have low UF, whilst low transporters have poor solute clearance. There are limitations in using PET to prescribe dialysis (Harty et al. 1995b); it tends to exaggerate clearances and is no substitute for 24 h dialysis collection.

Solute transport in long-term peritoneal dialysis
A number of studies have shown an increase in transport of low-molecular-weight solutes with time on PD (Krediet 1999). In the study by Davies et al. (2001), those patients with low and low-average transport characteristic progressively developed the membrane characterics of high and high-average transporter, probably related to glucose and bioincompatible fluid exposure as well as peritonitis. In another study, high transporters tended to become less 'permeable' with time on PD (Lo et al. 1994). More recently, increase in peritoneal transport rates were not found to be related to the PD modality or peritonitis rates, but led to lower UF in long-term PD patients (Fuholler et al. 2002).

Fluid transport (ultrafiltration)
The removal of excess fluid is critical to any form of dialysis; in PD this has traditionally been achieved by adding to the solutions various concentrations of glucose, which act as the driving force (osmotic agent). The transperitoneal UF rate is governed primarily by a complex interplay between the peritoneal membrane and physiological (osmotic and oncotic) forces across it. As the peritoneal membrane is a partially permeable membrane, a correction factor is required for each solute concentration difference to adjust for the degree of membrane leakiness. This factor is called the Staverman reflection coefficient (σ) and is dependent on the properties of solute and membrane as described before (Staverman 1951). The driving force across the peritoneum is made up of the hydrostatic capillary-pressure gradient (which probably remains fairly constant during PD) and the osmotic/oncotic-pressure gradient, which is the major component.

The flow of fluid (Q_f) is dependent on the peritoneal membrane factor (L_p is the permeability or proportionality coefficient, and A is the area) and the difference on either side of the membrane of the sum of the product of reflection coefficient (σ) and osmolalities (or molar concentration) of the solutes.

$$Q_f = L_p A \left[P - \sum_{j-1}^{n} (\sigma 1 C) \right]$$

where P is the hydrostatic pressure and $\sum_{j-1}^{n}(\sigma 1 C)$ is the sum of reflection coefficients of solvents and their differences in molar concentration (C) across the membrane.

Osmotic fluid flow between two isosmotic solutions can occur if they are separated by a permeable membrane and contain solute components with differing reflection coefficients (Mistry et al. 1987). This is the basis of colloid osmosis, similar to that induced by albumin across the capillary wall. During PD, water may be transferred across the peritoneal capillary in either direction depending on hydrostatic, oncotic, and crystalloid osmotic pressure. The intraperitoneal reabsorption of dialysate during PD involves at least two pathways—lymphatic and transcapillary (venular) fluid absorption in response to Starling forces.

Continuous ambulatory peritoneal dialysis

The concepts

The concept of CAPD described by Popovich *et al.* (1976) utilizes the smallest volume of dialysate to prevent uraemia. Using a double-pool model, they demonstrated that the accumulation of a metabolite in the body would be equal to the generation rate minus the combined effect of the residual renal function and overall dialysate clearance. Using this, they proposed that a patient would maintain a steady blood urea of about 30 mmol/l if 12 l of PD fluid (5 × 2 l plus 2 l of ultra-filtrate) were allowed to equilibrate with body fluids. This theoretical model was adapted to the current CAPD technique of four daily exchanges of 2 l, to produce, with UF, a total dialysate of 10 l daily.

If 2 l of fluid were allowed to dwell in the peritoneal cavity until equilibration had been achieved, then the drained volume would equal the urea clearance. They showed that varying the number of exchanges would have an impact on urea clearance (and hence fractional urea clearances). For the same dwell time, high-molecular-weight substances, such as creatinine or middle molecules, are dialysed continuously because the concentration gradient between the blood and dialysate is maintained for an extended period, much longer than in CAPD. Further, theoretical analysis by Teehan *et al.* (1985) showed that the maintenance of a steady level of urea on CAPD is dependent on the daily volume of fluid exchanged, the size of the patient, and the residual renal function (Fig. 5).

Technique and systems

CAPD entails a 'closed system', whereby fluid is initially instilled by gravity into the peritoneal cavity and drained out after a dwell period of several hours. The basic CAPD system remains unchanged and consists of the plastic bag containing 0.5–3.0 l of PD fluid, a transfer set, and a permanent, indwelling, silastic dialysis catheter. The connection between the bag and the transfer set is broken three to four times a day and the procedure must be performed using a strict, sterile, non-touch technique (about 1500 exchanges/year). The introduction of the Y-system

(Buoncristiani *et al.* 1980; Maiorca *et al.* 1983) was a major advance in the prevention of contamination related peritonitis compared to the spike systems. This method entails drainage of the effluent after the connection is made with a new bag, thereby enabling any touch contamination to be 'flushed' out before new fluid is drained into the peritoneal cavity (Fig. 6). Disconnect systems, which incorporate this principle, also allow total disconnection from the bags.

Night exchange device

This system was designed to provide a single extra exchange for CAPD patients, which is delivered automatically at a predetermined time, most often while the patient is asleep at night. It is set up before the patient goes to bed, just like a cycler but uses standard CAPD tubing. The patient performs a routine exchange in the morning upon awakening. The night exchange device (NXD) allows CAPD patients one or more night-time exchanges while reducing patient involvement and improving clearances. Though some patients on four or fewer exchanges may opt for this device as a life-style choice, the NXD is extremely helpful for patients needing five exchanges.

There are physiological and kinetic advantages to using the NXD. The long night dwell is 'divided', thus increasing small solute clearance but also allowing an increase in dwell volume, thus maximizing mass transfer without an increase in intraperitoneal pressure. The major advantage of NXD is to improve solute clearance, as well as to avoid positive fluid balance in patients retaining fluid overnight (those with high transporter status).

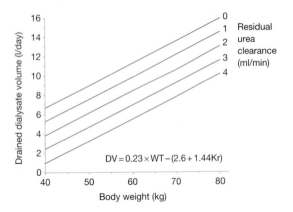

Fig. 5 Theoretical analysis of volume of totally equilibrated exchange of PD fluid over 24 h needed to maintain a steady-state blood urea of 25 mmol/l with a dietary protein intake of 1.2 g/kg body weight per 24 h. This volume of exchange is dependent on the weight of the patient and the residual renal function [adapted from Teehan *et al.* (1985) with permission].

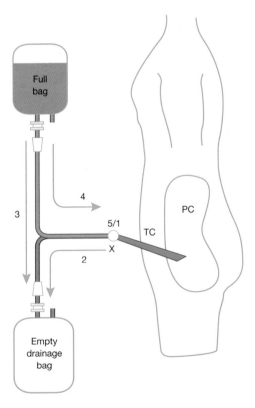

Fig. 6 The concept of 'flush before fill' utilized in the various disconnection systems or Y-sets as outlined by the steps (1–5) during the exchange procedure. PC, peritoneal cavity; TC, Tenckhoff catheter.

Automated peritoneal dialysis

Automated peritoneal dialysis (APD) is a broad term that is used to refer to all forms of PD employing a mechanical device to assist in the delivery and drainage of the dialysate. The various therapeutic regimens encompassed by APD are continuous cyclic PD (CCPD), IPD, nightly intermittent PD (NIPD), and tidal PD (TPD). The most obvious advantage of APD is that it eliminates the need for intensive manual involvement, reducing the work to two procedures daily—setting up the dialysis machine, and connecting and disconnecting the patient and dismantling the machine. It not only provides more solute clearance and UF than its CAPD counterpart, but also a more convenient life-style (Enoch et al. 2002). Daytime exchanges may also be necessary to improve total clearance. This complicates the procedures and intrudes into daytime routines. It is a home-based therapy carried out by the patient or by a helper overnight, which allows simultaneous rest and treatment and frees all parties from all procedures during the day.

Types of automated peritoneal dialysis (Fig. 7; Table 2)

The various APD regimens now in routine practice have evolved gradually. The traditional IPD is now seldom practised as a routine long-term therapy. Originally this technique was called periodic PD (Boen et al. 1962). IPD is only used in special circumstances, viz (a) temporarily, following catheter implantation, (b) during severe peritonitis in CAPD patients, and (c) at home in a patient requiring help with high peritoneal permeability and loss of UF. Its low efficiency results in inadequate solute and sodium clearance, poorly controlled blood pressure, and fluctuating concentrations of uraemic solutes. It also requires long periods of confinement.

Continuous cyclic peritoneal dialysis

This is based on the concept of continuous-equilibrium dialysis as proposed by Popovich et al. (1976) but incorporates a cycler. It was developed as an alternative to CAPD for patients who were not able to perform manual exchanges or were unwilling to interrupt their daily routine (Diaz-Buxo and Suki 1994). Technically, CCPD is a reversal of CAPD, where the shorter exchanges are automatically provided at night while the longer exchange is made during the day. A typical adult prescription consists of three to five nocturnal cycles with a final fill of hypertonic dialysis fluid. The catheter is then disconnected (Diaz-Buxo 1989). The provision of a day cycle is imperative to maintain the relatively steady physiological state and the targets for small-solute clearance. There is a linear relation between intraperitoneal pressure and intraperitoneal dialysate volume, which is least in a supine position. This diminishes any respiratory problems that might arise at night. CCPD is particularly suitable for children and those with high

Table 2 Various regimens used in PD[a]

Type of dialysis	Number of daytime exchanges	Number of nighttime exchanges	Volume of exchanges (l)
CAPD	2–3	1–2	1.0–3.0
CCPD	1	3–4	1.0–3.0
NIPD	0	3–5	2.0–3.0
NIPD 'wet day'	1–2	3–5	2.0–3.0
TPD	0	20	1.0–1.5

[a] CCPD here represents the original regimen; subsequent developments are here termed NIPD 'wet day' or high dose CCPD (incorporates the PD Plus and the Optimized Continuous PD concepts).

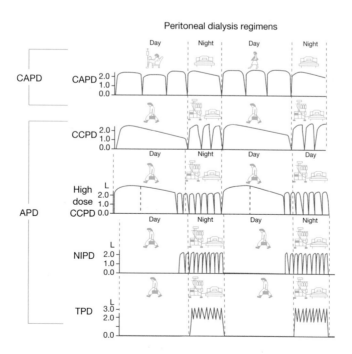

Fig. 7 Diagrammatic representation of various PD regimens (see text for explanations).

peritoneal permeability. Although no more effective than CAPD there are advantages such as reduced risk of peritonitis, abdominal and inguinal hernia, and pericatheter fluid leaks.

Nightly intermittent peritoneal dialysis

NIPD is done every night without a long-dwell daytime exchange. It has been advocated for use in patients with recurrent abdominal hernias, bladder prolapse, rapid glucose absorption resulting in poor UF, abdominal discomfort, and during fluid leaks. The main problem with NIPD is its low efficiency; 10–20 l need to be exchanged overnight.

High-dose CCPD or NIPD with a 'wet' day

To compensate for inadequate solute removal the patient may need to perform one or two exchanges in the daytime. This is usually referred to as high-dose CCPD or NIPD with a 'wet' day. Most APD regimens now entail a 'wet day' to improve solute and fluid removal. With icodextrin, the entire daytime exchange can be undertaken by a single bag of this solution, because it is able to achieve sustained UF with prolonged (8–16 h) dwell times (Mistry et al. 1987). This is of particular advantage to high transporters who need short dwells with glucose exchanges.

Tidal peritoneal dialysis

TPD can lead to an increase in clearance by 10–40 per cent. This is achieved by a portion of the dialysate being drained and then replaced with fresh PD fluid. The majority of the dialysate is in constant contact with the peritoneal membrane until the end of the dialysis. This is an expensive treatment as 20–30 l of fluid need to be exchanged overnight.

Choice of peritoneal dialysis regimen (Table 3)

The selection of a PD regime is mostly influenced by the patient's preference, the physicians advice and predictions, the availability of equipment and supplies, and the patient's clinical state, for example, a hyperpermeable peritoneal membrane. The most important consideration in the selection of APD other than patient preference is the individual's peritoneal-solute transport rate. Patients with high solute transport rates require more frequent cycles of short duration in order to accomplish adequate UF. NIPD is the therapy of choice in these instances. Large patients and those with greater dietary protein intake require greater clearance of small solutes; high-flow APD is recommended in their treatment. Unless fast peritoneal-solute transport dictates otherwise, continuous PD is preferable. NIPD with high PD fluid at night and with additional, manual, diurnal exchanges are available choices.

Peritoneal dialysis prescription (Table 4)

To decide on a prescription for a patient one needs to take into account the fixed variables, namely residual renal function (RRF), peritoneal membrane permeability, and size of the patient and then vary the dialysate volume, dwell times, the number of exchanges, and glucose (or icodextrin) concentration (Fig. 8). Table 4 lists some of the pitfalls in APD prescribing and how this therapy can be optimized.

A number of other factors must be considered when selecting PD prescription, for example, the patient's life-style.

Peritoneal dialysis solutions

As PD developed, it was soon realized that fluids needed to be similar to interstitial fluid, and hypertonic to plasma in order to achieve fluid

Table 3 Factors that need to be taken into account in choosing CAPD or APD

CAPD	APD
Easy technique	More difficult
Daytime exchange can be difficult if working or carer doing exchanges	None (with icodextrin) or only 1 daytime exchange
Poor UF if high transporter requiring use of higher concentration glucose exchanges	Easier to achieve good UF independent of transporter status
Some difficulty to increase adequacy by increasing number or volume of exchanges	Easier to increase adequacy by increasing number of exchanges overnight/daytime
Increasing exchange volume leads to increased intra-abdominal pressure when patient ambulant. Increased risk of hernia	Intra-abdominal pressure lower when supine. Decreased risk of hernia; better management of patient with hernias, leaks
Ease of travel	Can travel with machine or revert to CAPD
Peritonitis rate 1 episode/20–30 months	Peritonitis rate 1 episode/30–40 months

Table 4 APD prescribing

Common pitfalls in prescribing APD
1. Too many nighttime exchanges
2. Inappropriate nightly dwell times
3. Inappropriate 'day' time during the day
4. Failure to maximize instilled volume
5. Inappropriately long-dwell time

Ways to optimize clearances in APD (Fig. 11)
1. Increase nighttime instilled volume
2. Minimize drain time
3. Optimize nightly dwell times
4. Utilize entire 24-h period
5. Increase daytime instilled volume
6. Consider adding a daytime exchange

More fluid usage does not always lead to an increase in clearances; often an increase in number of exchanges, without optimizing dwell times, leads to a decrease in solute clearance

removal. Several osmotic agents were evaluated but glucose was found to be the safest and most effective (Odel et al. 1950).

Current solutions and problems with their use

The composition of the PD solutions currently available is shown in Table 5. The problems with the 'older' standard solutions are shown in Fig. 8. Newer solutions, however, focus on improving outcomes and the long-term viability of the peritoneal membrane by improving the biocompatibilty of the solutions. These centre around the pH, osmolarity, concentrations of glucose, use of lactate as a base, and the presence of GDP from the sterilization procedure.

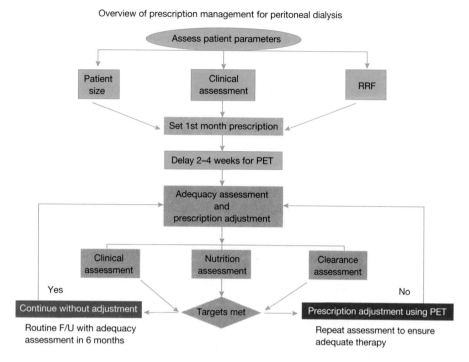

Fig. 8 Algorithm for managing prescription in PD patients from commencement of PD. Initially an arbitrary prescription is applied until a PET is evaluated 2–4 weeks after CAPD commencement. It takes that time for the PET to stabilize (Rocco *et al.* 1995). Thereafter, based on PET and small solute adequacy targets, the prescription is adjusted.

Table 5 Composition of standard PD fluids[a]

Sodium (mmol/l)	132–134
Potassium (mmol/l)	0–2
Calcium (mmol/l)	0–1.75
Magnesium (mmol/l)	0.25–0.75
Chloride (mmol/l)	95–106
Lactate (mmol/l)	35–40
Glucose (g/dl)	1.36–3.86 (dextrose anhydrous)
	1.5–4.25 (dextrose monohydrate)
Amino acids	1%
pH	5.2–5.5
Osmolality (mOsm)	358–511

[a] The ionic composition of the newer solutions do not differ much from standard solutions—differences relate to osmotic agents, higher pH, lower osmolality, and varying mixture of bicarbonate/lactate as a buffer.

Dextrose (D-glucose)

Glucose has several deficiencies which make it an unsuitable agent for standard, long-dwell PD, for example, metabolic side-effects and the impact on the integrity of the peritoneal membrane. The metabolic side-effects include obesity, glucose intolerance, hyperinsulinaemia, reduced peripheral sensitivity to insulin, and hyperlipidaemia. The bioincompatibility is related to hyperosmolality, but the high glucose concentration affects peritoneal cell metabolism adversely.

There is accumulating evidence that glucose is involved in the alteration of peritoneal tissues in long-term PD (Davies *et al.* 2001). The goal is to reduce patient exposure to glucose, minimize the total amount of glucose absorbed, avoid the hyperosmolar stress, and high glucose and GDP exposure to the peritoneum. Fortunately, non-glucose-based PD solutions as well as lower GDP-containing solutions are becoming available.

Glucose polymers (icodextrin)

Icodextrin is a glucose polymer, with mainly 1–4 glucosidic linkages between glucose molecules. It has a mean molecular weight of 16,500 and the 7.5 per cent solution has an osmolality of only 285 mOsm/kg of water (Mistry *et al.* 1987). Absorption is limited to 10–20 per cent of the instilled quantity during prolonged dwells (8–12 h). It exerts a colloidal rather than crystalline osmotic pressure to effect a sustained UF profile that is beneficial for long dwells in CAPD and APD (Fig. 9). A 7.5 per cent icodextrin solution exerts an osmotic pressure of only 282 mOsm compared to glucose 1.36, 2.27, and 3.86 per cent PD solutions which exert osmotic pressures of 358, 401, and 511 mOsm, respectively. The GDP content of icodextrin is very low compared to that of glucose containing solutions, with a resulting significant reduction in *in vitro* cell cytotoxicity, glycation of proteins, amadori adduct formation, and AGE formation (Dawney and Millar 1997; Ueda *et al.* 2000).

Studies done in the late 1980s showed the efficacy of icodextrin in producing prolonged UF over a 12-h dwell (Mistry and Gokal 1994). In a randomized multicentre study, the 7.5 per cent icodextrin solution was shown to be safe for overnight use, and three to five times more effective than the 1.36 per cent glucose solution for UF and equivalent to the 3.86 per cent glucose over long dwells (Mistry *et al.* 1994). More recent studies have shown that UF can be improved by icodextrin in patients who have lost UF. Wilkie *et al.* (1997) have shown improved technique survival with a median of 22 months in patients who would

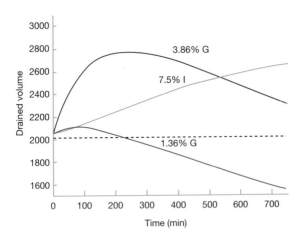

Fig. 9 Simulated intraperitoneal volume profile for glucose (G) 1.36 and 3.86% compared to icodextrin (I) 7.5% over long dwells of up to 12 h. The usual instillation volume for a PD exchange is 2000 ml.

Table 6 Indications for the use of icodextrin-based PD solutions

Long-dwell dialysis—overnight to replace 3.86% glucose
- daytime dwell in APD

Loss of UF—hyperpermeability (high transporter on PET)
- presence of large vascular surface area
- loss of aquaporins

During peritonitis

Glucose sparing; minimize metabolic side-effects

have otherwise needed transfer to HD. Icodextrin has been shown to produce sustained UF for up to 16 h when used in APD during the daytime long dwell (Posthuma *et al.* 1997; Woodrow *et al.* 1999; Plum *et al.* 2002). In patients with a hyperpermeable membrane who are particularly suitable to APD, icodextrin can be used during the long daytime dwell to enhance UF and solute clearance (Krediet and Mujais 2002). In a recent double blind randomized study in hypertensive PD patients using all 2.27 per cent glucose solutions the use of icodextrin improved the fluid status (Davies *et al.* 2003). In another pivotal study (The European APD outcome study—EAPOS) in anuric APD patients, UF at the start of the study predicted outcome; half the patients were on icodextrin for their long, daytime dwell to achieve adequate fluid removal (Brown *et al.* 2003).

Various studies suggest that icodextrin-based solutions are especially effective not only during long dwells, but also in UF failure due to a large effective peritoneal vascular surface area (Ho-dac-Pannekeet *et al.* 1996). With a high vascular surface area (associated with a high-transporter status) there are more perfused peritoneal capillaries. This makes a large number of capillaries available for transport and, therefore, a high UF rate. The only reason that this is not seen with glucose is that its absorption is also very high leading to a rapid disappearance of the osmotic gradient. When comparing the transcapillary UF rate with glucose and icodextrin, patients with high MTACs or high transporters have the lowest transcapillary UF rates with glucose, but the highest with icodextrin (Wang *et al.* 1998a). Peritonits is associated with UF failure due to a large vascular surface area; so in this situation, icodextrin achieves more UF (Gokal *et al.* 1995). Icodextrin solutions can only be administered once a day and, therefore, cannot replace glucose. No accumulation of the glucose polymers occurs with the once daily usage; plasma levels of maltose (end-product of icodextrin metabolism with amylase) and polymers remain in steady-state but come down rapidly within 7–10 days of stopping icodextrin (Mistry *et al.* 1994). There are potential advantages in minimizing the glucose load with the use of icodextrin, thereby improving the metabolic profile of PD patients (Gokal *et al.* 2002). The only other reported side-effects are allergic skin reactions in a few patients (Wolfson *et al.* 2002) and really cloudy effluents from a contaminant produced during fluid production. This has been eliminated (Gokal 2002). The indications for use of icodextrin are shown in Table 6.

Amino acids

Amino acid dialysis solutions have been studied for over 20 years but interest in them has been increased by the possibility that they may also alleviate malnutrition in PD patients, and reduce reliance on glucose-based solutions. The osmotic and dialysis efficacy is similar to glucose, and there are no adverse effects on peritoneal permeability, or lipids (Misra *et al.* 1997).

The effects of amino acid solutions on nutritional state have been widely investigated. Most, but not all, studies showed a benefit when they were used in malnourished patients (Kopple *et al.* 1995; Jones *et al.* 1998, 1999). Their use is associated with a rise in plasma urea and a mild metabolic acidosis, especially with two exchanges a day so this is the limit of their use. Indications for their use are to provide a protein source in individuals whose intake is limited; in hypercatabolic states, for example, peritonitis; and to minimize glucose exposure. There is no evidence that their use prevents the development of malnutrition.

Modified dialysis solutions

Two modifications make dialysis solutions more biocompatible. The first is reduction of the content of cytotoxic GDP, produced during heat sterilization (Wieslander *et al.* 1995). Although non-glucose-based PD solutions avoid systemic and local glucotoxicity, they cannot be used for all exchanges. The recent development of two-/three-chambered bags permits separation of glucose from other solution components, allowing glucose to be sterilized at a lower pH than is possible in single chamber bags (Rippe *et al.* 2001; Passlick-Deetjen *et al.* 2002). Mixing of the compartments results in a rise in the pH, which in the case of bicarbonate-containing formulations, is near neutral. The solution has a pH of 6.3 and is less cytotoxic. For bicarbonate-/lactate-buffered two-chamber systems, sterilization of glucose at lower pH reduces most of the identified GDPs. The second modification is the replacement of lactate buffer with bicarbonate.

Peritoneal dialysis fluid buffers

Because of the problem of calcium carbonate precipitation during sterilization, bicarbonate was replaced by lactate or acetate. A low pH and lactate are regarded to be deleterious to the peritoneum (Coles 1999). The introduction of bicarbonate solutions into clinical practice seemed the way forward and was made possible by advances in sterilization methods and delivery systems.

Several studies have reported clinical experience with these solutions, either as bicarbonate alone (Schmitt *et al.* 2002) or as a combination of bicarbonate and lactate (Coles *et al.* 1997). In a clinical study, this solution was found to be equivalent to 40 mmol/l lactate or 38 mmol/l bicarbonate solution (Coles *et al.* 1998).

There is no evidence that bicarbonate solutions benefit patients in terms of peritoneal transport and preservation of peritoneal membrane integrity. However, those patients who experience pain on infusion of PD fluid related to pH and lactate, have been shown, in a randomized trial, not to experience pain with bicarbonate and bicarbonate/lactate solutions (Mactier *et al.* 1998).

Outcomes in patients treated with peritoneal dialysis

Because CAPD is a continuous therapy, it provides stable blood concentrations of electrolytes and nitrogenous waste products. The actual blood concentrations depend upon the RRF, the daily dialysate volume, and the rate of generation of the waste products. In addition, the signs and symptoms of dysequilibrium associated with high-efficiency, intermittent procedures such as HD are infrequent in CAPD patients. With judicious use of hypertonic dialysis fluid, adequate amounts of sodium and water can be removed. Most patients have normal serum potassium concentrations even with an intake of 70–80 mmol/day and control of acidosis is achieved with dialysate lactate concentration of 40 mmol/l. Some patients become alkalotic, especially with concurrent consumption of calcium carbonate as a phosphate binder. Anaemia is better controlled with less need for erythropoietin as compared to HD patients.

Calcium–phosphate homeostasis (see Chapter 11.3.9)

Calcium–phosphate homeostasis is achieved on CAPD and there appears to be better control of hyperparathyroidism but a greater tendency to develop adynamic bone disease (Hutchison 2000). Once CAPD has begun, gastrointestinal absorption and peritoneal flux of calcium are the two major determinants of the overall calcium mass balance. The transfer of calcium to the patient from the fluid is dependent on both the serum ionized calcium and the UF rate. The mass balance is positive when 1.75 mmol/l calcium solutions are used (Hutchison *et al.* 1992), but neutral on lower calcium concentrations of 1.00–1.25 mmol/l. The use of calcium-containing binders often leads to hypercalcaemia unless a reduced-calcium PD solution (0.6–1.25 mmol/l) is used. These allow a greater use of oral calcium carbonate (Cunningham *et al.* 1992; Hutchison *et al.* 1992). Maintenance of a high serum ionized calcium and strict control of serum phosphate decreases the plasma parathyroid hormone (PTH) without the addition of vitamin D analogue (Hutchison *et al.* 1993). However, oversuppression (PTH < 50 pg/ml) is associated with adynamic bone histology, which is itself linked to metastatic and vascular calcification.

Nutritional aspects of peritoneal dialysis

Chronic renal failure is associated with derangements in carbohydrate, lipid, and protein metabolism in uraemia with a high incidence of malnutrition, all of which may be aggravated by dialysis (Pollock *et al.* 2000). Initially, patients on PD appear to be in an anabolic state over the first 2 years (Jager *et al.* 2001a). However, with long-term treatment, several harmful metabolic effects emerge, raising questions about the long-term safety of CAPD (Harty and Gokal 1995). The continuous peritoneal absorption of 100–200 g/day of glucose (20 per cent of total calorie intake) aggravates glucose intolerance and peripheral resistance to the action of insulin. Uraemic hypertriglyceridaemia and dyslipoproteinaemia persist during CAPD. These abnormalities are worse in the initial months and the changes correlate with the peritoneal glucose load (Pollock *et al.* 2000). With the raised triglycerides there is a concomitant decrease in high-density lipoprotein (HDL) cholesterol, altered apolipoprotein metabolism (low apo A-1 to apo B ratios), and abnormal accumulation of cholesterol in very low-density

lipoprotein (VLDL) and low-density lipoprotein (LDL) remnants, and raised lipoprotein (a) (Anwar *et al.* 1993), all thought to be atherogenic. This lipid profile appears to be more atherogenic than that seen in HD patients. Treatment of lipid abnormalities is difficult and the value of lowering cholesterol not substantiated. The substantial losses of protein in the dialysate contributes to the negative nitrogen balance in these patients. However, Kaysen and Schoenfield (1984) have reported that plasma albumin mass, total albumin mass, and the distribution of albumin are normal in CAPD. If this is so, then the lower values may well reflect either the dilutional effect of overhydration that most patients on CAPD display (Harty and Gokal 1995), or an inflammatory state (Stenvinkel *et al.* 2001).

Protein–energy malnutrition

During the first 6–12 months of CAPD, patients are in neutral or even positive nitrogen balance. Blumenkrantz *et al.* (1982) showed the relationship between intake and balance to be curvilinear: nitrogen balance increased as protein intake increased up to 1.1 g/kg per day but there was no additional increase in nitrogen balance with further increases in dietary protein. There is a gradual decrease in nutritional intake with time and a decrease in nitrogen balance after 2–5 years of CAPD (Sombolis *et al.* 1986). The reduced intake reflects decreased appetite, abdominal distension, delayed gastric emptying, and glucose absorption. Mild to moderate malnutrition is prevalent in 30–35 per cent and severe malnutrition in 8–10 per cent of CAPD patients (Young *et al.* 1991; Jones 1994).

Malnutrition and inflammation

Peritoneal dialysis is associated with a high cardiovascular mortality. Chronic inflammation, as evidenced by increased levels of proinflammatory cytokines and C-reactive protein, is common in PD patients and may mediate both malnutrition and accelerated atherosclerotic cardiovascular disease—the so called MIA syndrome—malnutrition, inflammation, atherosclerosis (Stenvinkel *et al.* 2001). Patients showing an increase in peritoneal permeability, often suffer the MIA syndrome which may partly explain the higher mortality in these patients.

The inflammation theory has led to the suggestion that there are two types of malnutrition. Type 1 (usually without comorbidity) is characterized by the absence of inflammation, low/normal serum albumin, decreased protein catabolism, low food intake, normal resting energy expenditure, and increased oxidative stress. Type 2 (associated with comorbidity) is characterized by inflammation and being 'cytokine driven' is characterized by low serum albumin, increased protein catabolism, low/normal food intake, elevated resting energy expenditure, and resistance to increased dialysis and nutritional support (Stenvinkel *et al.* 2000). If the inflammatory stimulus is removed there is an improvement in well being (Aguilera *et al.* 2001).

Although the assessment of nutritional state is difficult, it can be defined from body composition, serum proteins, dietary intake, and muscle function (Harty and Gokal 1995). A number of nutritional indices have been devised to encapsulate these variables into a single scoring system (Harty *et al.* 1994). Certain measures are suitable for screening during routine clinical practice: anthropometry, lean body mass from creatinine kinetics, subjective global assessment, and serum albumin. Muscle biopsies, neutron activation, dual energy X-ray absorptiometry, and isotope dilution methods are research methods.

Management of protein–calorie malnutrition (Table 7)

The recommended intake of protein, energy, and minerals is outlined in Table 8 (NKF : K/DOQI 2000). Dietary intake should be individualized,

Table 7 Prevention and treatment of malnutrition in CAPD[a]

1. *Identification of 'at risk' group*
   Elderly
   Diabetes mellitus
   Recurrent peritonitis
   Active comorbidity including depression
   Loss of RRF

	Method	Malnutrition risk
2. *Screening and monitoring*		
Dietary protein and calorie	3-day diet history	<0.8 g/kg IBW/day
	24-h urine + PD Protein Nitrogen Appearance	<30 kcal/kg IBW/day
Anthropometrics	MUAC, skinfold thickness AMA, dry weight	<15th percentile = mild to moderate malnutrition
		<5th = severe malnutrition
		<80% IBW (NHANES)
Serum albumin	Blood test	<30 g/l
SGA	GI symptoms	A—well nourished
	Loss of subcutaneous fat	B—moderate malnutrition
		C—severe malnutrition

3. *Possible interventions*
   Exclude possible GI disease
   Increase intake
   Correction of acidosis
   Modification of dialysis dose (if loss of RRF)
   Eradicate occult infection/inflammation
   Intraperitoneal aminoacids
   Parenteral nutrition

[a] IBW, ideal body weight; PNA, protein nitrogen appearance; MUAC, mid-upper arm circumference; AMA, arm muscle area; GI, gastrointestinal; NHANES, National Health and Nutritional Examination Surveys; SGA, subjective global assessment.

Table 8 Dietary nutritional requirements in PD[a]

Energy	30–50 kcal/kg IBW per day (including calories from glucose)
Protein	1.1–1.3 g/kg IBW per day
Sodium	About 100 mmol/day
Potassium	Usually no restriction
Phosphorus	0.7–1.2 g/day
Calcium	Individualized (usually no less than 1 g/day)
Iron	Individualized and dependent on erythropoietin use
Zinc	15 mg/day
Vitamins	
B_1	1.5 mg/day
B_2	1.7 mg/day
B_6	10 mg/day
C	60 mg/day
Niacin	20 mg/day
Folic acid	1 mg/day
D	Individualized

[a] IBW, ideal body weight.

but there should be a low threshold for the use of enteral supplementation. Parenteral nutrition has been shown to be of benefit and should be considered in catabolic illnesses requiring admission to hospital, for example, during severe peritonitis, especially in malnourished patients (Rubin 1990).

The use of amino acids as an alternative osmotic agent offers the potential additional advantage of providing 3–4 g of amino acids (8–10 g of protein) daily if one to two bags/day are used. Studies using a 1.1 per cent amino acid solution containing an increased amount of lactate (40 mmol/l) have demonstrated an improvement in nitrogen balance and an increase in creatinine and serum transferrin (Kopple *et al.* 1995). Side-effects include metabolic acidosis, an increase in serum urea, and nausea. Inadequate dialysis may result in a reduction in protein and calorie intake but the evidence that increasing dialysis solute removal improves nutritional state is controversial (Harty *et al.* 1995a, 1997; Davies *et al.* 2000). Certainly nutritional status is linked with residual renal function (Harty *et al.* 1996a,b; Wang *et al.* 2001). To maintain solute clearance any reduction in residual function should be offset by increasing PD dose.

Peritoneal dialysis adequacy—solute removal

Adequacy of PD is judged by both clinical assessment, solute-clearance measurements, and fluid removal. The well-dialysed patient has a good appetite, no nausea, minimal fatigue, and feels well. In contrast, the uraemic patient is anorectic with dysgeusia, nausea, and complains of fatigue. Broadbase adequacy refers also to appropriate control of blood pressure and fluid status, calcium and phosphate levels, acid–base status, nutrition, and anaemia. 'Adequacy' has, however, come to be equated with small-solute removal.

Measurement of dialysis adequacy

The clearances of urea and creatinine are used as markers of dialysis dose based on the urea kinetic-modelling concept of HD arising from the National Cooperative Dialysis Study.

1. The fractional clearance of urea: This is expressed as Kt/V, which is urea clearance (K) per unit time (t) related to total body water (V). Kt is obtained by multiplying the effluent: blood urea nitrogen concentration ratio (D/P urea) by the 24 h effluent drain volume. Renal urea nitrogen clearance is added to this. The daily value is multiplied by 7 to provide a weekly value. To compare clearance values between patients they are normalized to a function of patient size: for urea, the volume of urea distribution (v) calculated from the Watson normogram, or can be estimated as 60 per cent of weight in males and 55 per cent of weight in females. These various methods were assessed by Wong *et al.* (1995), who found that bioelectrical impedance was not sufficiently accurate for measurement of total body water whilst 58 per cent of body-weight methods consistently overestimated total body water. They recommended that the effect of body composition on the estimation of V needs to be evaluated by validated techniques such as deuterium oxide. Clearly this is not possible in routine practice.

2. Creatinine clearance (both peritoneal and residual renal): this is also obtained from a 24-h collection of dialysate, to which is added the average of the renal creatinine and urea nitrogen clearance (since creatinine clearance overestimates glomerular filtration rate due to tubular secretion of creatinine). An adjustment for body surface area (BSA) is also required. Creatinine clearance is normalized to BSA or ($K \times 1.73/BSA$).

Other techniques to estimate clearances include the dialysis index of Teehan *et al.* (1985) and the efficacy number (Brandes *et al.* 1992). In addition, when clearance values are compared between haemodialysis and CAPD the latter gives much lower values. This has given rise to the peak concentration hypothesis (Keshaviah *et al.* 1989), which explains this discrepancy in the intermittent nature of HD as compared to the continuous form of CAPD.

Residual renal function

A residual renal clearance of 1 ml/min equates to 10 l of dialysate per week, a not inconsequential amount given that values for creatinine clearance in peritoneal dialysate range from 30 to 50 l/week only. Residual renal urea clearance has been shown to contribute 17 per cent to the total Kt/V value, with residual creatinine clearance contributing 35 per cent to the total normalized creatinine (Harty *et al.* 1993). In addition, residual renal clearance accounts for the majority of the variation in the total clearance value. RRF declines with time with little remaining after 3–4 years of dialysis. The importance of RRF cannot be over emphasized in PD patients (Van Biesen *et al.* 2002). Several studies have shown its relation to outcome (Diaz-Buxo *et al.* 1999; Bargman *et al.* 2001; Rocco *et al.* 2002) and an interesting analysis showing an increase in left ventricular hypertrophy with declining RRF (Wang *et al.* 2002).

Targets for dialysis adequacy

The increasing number of studies which have demonstrated a relation between small-solute clearance and survival, emphasize the importance of assessing dialysis adequacy in CAPD patients. There is, however, controversy over the ideal target urea and creatinine clearances. Not only is there debate over minimal solute-clearance target (or threshold below which prescription has to be adjusted to increase solute clearance), but little is known about the optimal level beyond which there is no further clinical gain. Until recently there was no consensus as to whether dialysis dose was related to clinical outcome. Results of clinical studies have been contradictory. Teehan *et al.* (1990) and Rocco *et al.* (1993) using multivariate analyses found that low serum albumin and lower Kt/V predicted worse survival. Other univariate analytical studies (Blake *et al.* 1991; Brandes *et al.* 1992; DeAlvaro *et al.* 1992; Teehan *et al.* 1992) gave conflicting results when relating various targets of solute clearance with outcomes. Two key studies have been instrumental in broadening the debate.

The first was the CAN-USA study (Churchill *et al.* 1996), a 2-year longitudinal, cohort study of 680 new CAPD patients, the results of which suggested that both Kt/V and creatinine clearance were independent predictors of mortality but only so if the initial clearance values were maintained throughout the study. For every 0.1 increase in Kt/V and 5 l per week increase in creatinine clearance the relative risk of death was 5 per cent lower. Because the study was observational and not interventional, there was a decline in the total solute clearance over time, explained by a decline in RRF. A subsequent analysis of the CAN-USA study revealed that the mortality risk was entirely related to RRF (Bargman *et al.* 2001). This study cannot be used as evidence for setting targets as it did not answer the question of whether modifying dialysis clearance alone would be sufficient to compensate for the adverse impact of loss of RRF.

In the second study (Maiorca *et al.* 1995), the survival of 68 patients who had been on PD for about 35 months was followed and related to their Kt/V. Patients with values greater than 1.96 had the better survival. Somewhere between 1.7 and 1.96, there is a 'knuckle', where a steep decline changes to a more level relationship to survival. RRF affected outcome in this study too.

Target setting—guidelines

The debate about what solute clearance in PD patients should be, gained momentum with the publication of the National Kidney Foundation's (NKF) Dialysis Outcomes Quality Initiative (DOQI) (NKF : K/DOQI 1997). An 'evidence based' approach was supposed to have been used. Attempts to pick targets that would be consistent over time regardless of RRF were made. The guidelines advocated minimal Kt/V of 2.0 and creatinine clearance of 60 l/week/1.73 m^2 for CAPD patients (Table 9). Targets for APD were somewhat higher to compensate for the intermittent nature of the treatment.

Subsequently various studies have pointed out that the minimum Kt/V is less than 2.0. These also related the outcomes to RRF rather than peritoneal clearance (Diaz-Buxo *et al.* 1999; Szeto *et al.* 2000; Bargman *et al.* 2001) and furthermore the evidence in anuric patients was contradictory (Bhaskaran *et al.* 2000; Szeto *et al.* 2001). There was strong circumstantial evidence from a Chinese study in which patients undergoing 3×2 l exchanges—(Kt/V 1.6–1.8), had excellent survival, and that solute clearance was over emphasized in the DOQI guidelines (Lo *et al.* 1996). Inspite of attempts to reconcile the differences (Chatoth *et al.* 1999), there is no consensus. Randomized, controlled studies were needed and two have provided a clear way forward.

1. The ADEMEX Study (Paniagua *et al.* 2002). This was an active controlled, randomized, prospective study in 1968 on new and prevalent CAPD patients with a minimum follow-up of 2 years. Patients were randomized to control (standard 4×2 l regime to achieve a Kt/V 1.6–1.8 and creatinine clearance 45–50 l/week) or an intervention group (4×2.3–3.0 l regime to achieve a $Kt/V \geq 2.0$ and creatinine clearance 55–60 l/week). There was no difference

Table 9 The guidelines to solute clearance in CAPD and APD patients as advocated by the various international and national bodies[a]

	Kt/V	CCr/1.73 m^2 (l)
CAPD patients		
NKF : K/DOQI (1997)	2.0	60
NKF : K/DOQI (2000a)		
L and LA	2.0	50
HA and H	2.0	60
Canadian guidelines		
(Churchill *et al.* 1999)		
L and LA	2.0	50
HA and H	2.0	60
RARCPL (2002)	1.7	50
EDTA-ERA (2004)	1.7 (Peritoneal)	
APD patients		
NKF-DOQI CCPD	2.1	63
NIPD	2.2	66

[a] The NKF-DOQI guidelines were revised in 2000 to lower the creatinine clearance in low (L) and low average (LA) transporters as they have a better survival than high (H) and high average (HA) transporters. These transporter statuses are obtained on the PET.

in survival between the two groups (Fig. 10). Albumin (< or >30 g/l), diabetes, protein intake (normalized protein nitrogen appearance < or >0.8 g/kg/day), anuria, transport profile, and body size had no impact on survival either. In addition there was no difference in hospitalization or peritonitis rates between the treatment and control groups. ADEMEX was a well-controlled, randomized clinical trial designed to assess the effect of small-solute clearance on mortality in CAPD patients. The results were obtained in the context of a rigorous experimental design that assured proper randomization at baseline. The clinical study design was successful in achieving the intended separation in peritoneal creatinine and urea clearances throughout the course of the study. This study provides evidence that there is no difference in patient survival with variations in peritoneal small-solute clearance within ranges achievable in current clinical practice.

2. The second is the Hong Kong randomized prospective study on 331 new CAPD patients with a renal Kt/V less than 1.0, randomized to one of three arms of Kt/V: 1.5–1.7, 1.7–2.0, and greater than 2.0 with a mean follow-up of 2 years (Lo *et al.* 2003). There was no difference in survival between the three groups. There were more patients in the 1.5–1.7 group with complications requiring withdrawal from study (higher demand for erythropoietin and slightly higher hospitalization rate), but no difference in nutritional status. There was no significant difference between the two higher Kt/V arms.

Both these studies indicate that the minimum small-solute clearance for Kt/V is 1.7 and creatinine clearance 50 l/week. Solute clearance is important and more clearance desirable, especially if the patient is faring badly and showing features of uraemia despite these targets, which are a guide. Adjusting the prescription as RRF declines is essential. The debate about the equivalence of RRF and peritoneal clearance is not resolved but renal clearance provides more than just solute removal, so attempts to preserve it by avoiding nephrotoxic agents, fluid depletion and, in relevant cases, use of angiotensin-converting enzyme inhibitors should be strenuous. Whether to use Kt/V or creatinine clearance to assess solute removal is not resolved either. The latter is more influenced by RRF and targets are more difficult to achieve in anuric patients (Table 9).

Management of inadequate dialysis and prescription setting

Conventional CAPD offers some flexibility allowing increases in small-solute clearance by varying the volume and number of exchanges. Increasing the volume of exchange is resented by some patients who are intolerant of abdominal fullness and pain (Tattersall *et al.* 1994). There is undoubtedly a psychosomatic element to this perception as studies have shown that patients are unable to distinguish the difference in instilled volumes when administered blindly (Sarkar *et al.* 1999). Maximizing infusion volume should be attempted first, then with the availability of NXDs some patients can increase to five exchanges a day. An important way to increase dialysis dose is by APD which can be used to achieve solute-clearance targets even in anuric patients (Brown *et al.* 2001).

It is also important to vary the dwell times and volumes to maximize solute and fluid removal. Various computer programs are available to model the prescription based on the PET estimation of transporter status, weight, and RRF. Examples of these are given for APD (Fig. 11).

Peritoneal dialysis adequacy—fluid removal

The poor fluid balance in PD populations is widely reported (Gokal 1999a). Tzamaloukas *et al.* (1995) observed a 25 per cent prevalence of symptomatic fluid overload manifested by peripheral oedema, pulmonary venous congestion, pleural effusions, and hypertension which led to a higher hospitalization rate. Non-compliance with dietary and fluid restriction was the major predictor of fluid retention. Patients with high or high-average transporter status were most likely to experience UF failure. There is also a high prevalence of hypertension in this population, over 50 per cent of whom lose the nocturnal dip (Cocchi *et al.* 1999).

The impact of inadequate fluid and sodium removal was recently analysed by Ates *et al.* (2001). Both fluid and sodium overload were independent predictors of death in the 125 patients monitored for 3 years. Elevated systolic blood pressure was also associated with increased mortality. Moist *et al.* (2000) examined a variety of factors relevant to the decline of RRF. Here, a history of congestive heart failure was a strong predictor of decline in RRF. It seems, therefore, that the decline in RRF is accelerated in the presence of fluid overload.

There are two therapeutic goals: patients should be both oedema free and normotensive (Abu-Alfa *et al.* 2002). Hypertension in dialysis

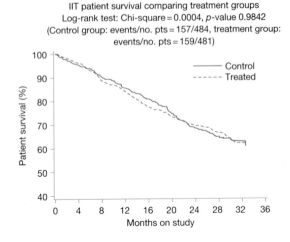

IIT patient survival comparing treatment groups
Log-rank test: Chi-square = 0.0004, *p*-value 0.9842
(Control group: events/no. pts = 157/484, treatment group: events/no. pts = 159/481)

Fig. 10 The ADEMEX Study showing patient survival in the control and treatment groups in the intention to treat life-table analysis (reproduced with permission from Paniagua *et al.* 2002).

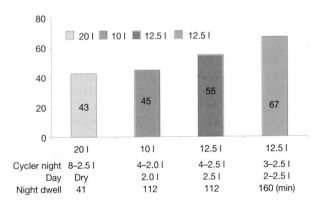

Fig. 11 Creatinine clearance value (l/week) with various regimes, volumes, and dwell period. A smaller volume (12.5 l) utilized as 5 × 2.5 l dwells gives a much higher clearance (purple bar) than 20 l cycled overnight (blue bar).

patients is predominantly volume dependent and salt sensitive (Bianchi 2000), and can be corrected by fluid and sodium restriction (Gunal *et al.* 2001). In this study, strict salt and fluid control allowed 44 out of 47 hypertensive patients to come off all antihypertensive drugs, a reduction in the cardiothoracic index, and a mean weight reduction of 2.8 kg. The only exception to this was in patients with autonomic insufficiency and cardiomyopathy where a degree of volume expansion is required to support the blood pressure (Kara and Somers 2002).

Therapeutic approach

If oedema is absent then blood pressure control and the degree of dependence on antihypertensive agents is examined. A series of interventions are available if there are deviations in either of these (Table 10).

Non-compliance is a major issue in PD patients and can alter fluid balance by affecting fluid and salt intake, adherence to diuretic regimens, and changes in PD prescription. These can be hard to implement as they require education and life-style changes (Bernardini *et al.* 2000). Non-compliance may be large in absolute terms but is usually intermittent, occurring in about 26 per cent of patients overall. Only ~2 per cent are consistently non-compliant in terms of dialysis exchanges (Bernardini *et al.* 2000).

Loss of ultrafiltration

There is now a considerable body of evidence to show that patients with increased low-molecular-weight solute transport (hyperpermeability) have a worse outcome (Churchill *et al.* 1998; Wang *et al.* 1998b; Chung *et al.* 2000). These patients experience difficulty in managing fluid balance and achieving dry-weight targets as their UF capacity is limited by their inability to maintain an osmotic gradient during long dwells, as practiced in the standard CAPD regime. This is almost certainly related to various morphological changes of the peritoneum.

Net UF failure is the most important transport abnormality in long-term CAPD (Selgas *et al.* 1994; Davies *et al.* 1996, 1998). The prevalence of UF failure increases from 3 per cent after 1 year on CAPD to 31 per cent after 6 years (Heimburger *et al.* 1990). This UF loss is mainly associated with increased transport of low-molecular-weight solutes implying both a large effective peritoneal vascular surface area and impaired transcellular water transport (Ho-dac-Pannekeet *et al.* 1997b).

Definition of ultrafiltration failure

There are various definitions of the level of UF failure. Excessive (three or more) 3.86 per cent dextrose exchanges per day points to UF failure but is not diagnostic. A more scientific definition proposed by Heimberger *et al.* (1990) is: 5.5 ml of UF/g of glucose absorbed. The more accepted definition is based on the modified PET (standard peritoneal permeability analysis, SPA), where less than 2400 ml drain volume is obtained after a 4 h dwell with 2 l 3.86 per cent glucose (Ho-dac-Pannekeet *et al.* 1997b). This is a deviation from the standard PET protocol which utilizes a 2.27 per cent dextrose. In the standard PET, UF failure is diagnosed if the drain volume is less than 2200 ml after a 4-h dwell.

Evaluation of ultrafiltration failure

The International Society of Peritoneal Dialysis (ISPD) recently published its guidelines on management of fluid problems and set out helpful algorithms (Mujais *et al.* 2000). When faced with a problem of fluid overload, one has to exclude reversible causes (dietary indiscretion and non-compliance with prescription, inappropriate prescription, mechanical problems—leaks and catheter malfunction), before diagnosing true UF failure that necessitates evaluation of peritoneal membrane function, using the SPA (Fig. 12a–c).

Management of ultrafiltration failure

Patients with a low drain volume and high-transport status (D/P creatinine > 0.8) represent the largest group with inadequate UF. About 10 per cent of patients starting PD have an inherent high-transport status, as do those with peritonitis. The group of most concern is the long-term PD patients. These have good solute clearance but poor UF on long-dwell PD regimes. If dwell times are mismatched for their membrane transport characteristic then they will have loss of UF. Icodextrin is ideal for the long dwell in these patients.

Encapsulating peritoneal sclerosis

This was formerly called sclerosing encapsulating peritonitis, a term that has been abandoned because of its morphological inaccuracy. It is a rare entity with an overall incidence between 0.5 and 4.4 per cent (Kawaguchi *et al.* 2000). The ANZ DATA report gave a figure of 1.9–4.2 per cent of patients suffering from this syndrome (Rigby and Hawley 1998), whereas the Japanese study reports a lower incidence of 0.9–1.7 per cent (Kawaguchi *et al.* 1999).

It comprises clinical syndromes of bowel obstruction, bloodstained effluent, UF failure, and abdominal mass. Distinct radiological features included peritoneal thickening and encapsulation, obstruction, cocooning identified by ultrasonography, contrast studies, and computed tomography (CT). The pathological derangements include loss of mesothelium, gross interstitial thickening within the membrane, which can be cellular or acellular, and variable amount of inflammatory cells.

The treatment approach is to stop PD, transfer to HD, and institute hyperalimentation if necessary. Stopping PD does not always halt or reverse progression. Subsequent treatment strategies vary, the experience being limited to case reports. These include corticosteroids,

---

Table 10 Areas for intervention in fluid overloaded

Dietary evaluation
Salt intake (<100 mmol/day)
Fluid intake (achieve negative balance)

RRF
Use of loop diuretics (e.g. frusemide 250–500 mg/day)
Monitor trends in urine volume and glomerular filtration rate
Avoid nephrotoxic agents (e.g. aminoglycoside, non-steroidal anti-inflammatory agents, contrast agents)
Use ACE inhibitors to preserve RRF

Compliance
Quality of life issues
Delivered dose and inventory control

Catheter function
Outflow obstruction
Leaks and hernias

Peritoneal UF profile
PET estimation
Modify dwell time, tonicity of glucose, use alternative osmotic agents
Evaluate both long and short dwells during CAPD and APD

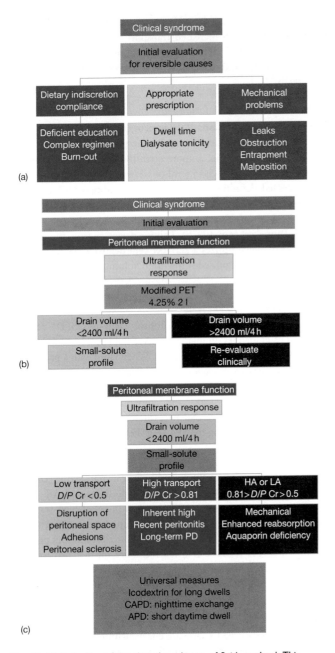

Fig. 12 (a) Evaluation of the clinical syndrome of fluid overload. This initially entails the evaluation and search of reversible causes. (b) When reversible causes are excluded then it is appropriate to evaluate peritoneal membrane function using the modified PET with 2 l of 3.86/4.25% glucose (SPA test). (c) Algorithm for further evaluation and treatment based on small-solute profile. For high-transport patients the therapy is outlined. For low-transport patients, PD may not be possible and serious consideration needs to be taken to exclude peritoneal sclerosis, especially of the encapsulating variety (EPS).

immmunosuppression, transplantation, peritoneal rest, long-term parenteral hyperalimentation, antifibrotic agents (tamoxifen), and surgical viscerolysis. The mortality of EPS is extremely high, varying between 20 and 93 per cent (Nomoto *et al.* 1996; Afthentopoulos *et al.* 1998; Rigby *et al.* 1998) death occuring in 60 per cent within 4 months of diagnosis.

Peritonitis

Since the introduction of CAPD, peritonitis remains the most serious complication, accounting for considerable morbidity and modality failure (Golper *et al.* 1996; Woodrow *et al.* 1997; Gokal 2000). The incidence of peritonitis has fallen since the early days when bottled fluid was used. The development of better delivery systems and connectors, and the widespread use of disconnect systems, have all contributed to the fall in incidence.

Definition and clinical diagnosis

The repeated drainage of the PD effluent offers a unique opportunity for the early detection of peritoneal inflammation. For both patient and doctor the turbidity of the effluent still remains the earliest sign of infection. The generally accepted definition of peritonitis in CAPD entails any two of the three features: signs or symptoms, cloudy dialysate with more than 100 cells/mm^3, and micro-organisms in the effluent.

Relapse is defined as the occurrence of peritonitis, with the same organisms, within 2 weeks of stopping antibiotics. The differentiation between relapsing peritonitis and reinfection is important as frequently relapsing peritonitis is an indication for catheter removal. A study based on biotyping and 'fingerprinting' by Western blotting has been able to distinguish reinfection from relapse in patients with multiple episodes of coagulase-negative staphylococcal peritonitis (Brown *et al.* 1989).

Cloudy effluent is not necessarily diagnostic of infective peritonitis. It can be due to blood, fibrin, intra-abdominal pathology, diarrhoea, and eosinophilic peritonitis. The latter is a syndrome including cloudy effluent in an asymptomatic patient with persistently negative cultures. It occurs during the early stages of CAPD and resolves spontaneously within weeks. The explanation appears to be an 'allergy' to constituents of the CAPD system (Gokal *et al.* 1981).

Routes of infection in cyclic ambulatory peritoneal dialysis peritonitis

The main pathway for infection of the peritoneal cavity (30–40 per cent of all episodes) is through the lumen of the catheter, followed by periluminal (20–30 per cent; around the outside of the catheter—the catheter exit-site) (Golper *et al.* 1996). There is a close link between these and the skin and nasal carriage of *Staphylococcus aureus* (Luzar *et al.* 1990). The other less common routes are transcolonic (20–25 per cent), haematogenous (5 per cent), and ascending from the female genital tract (2–5 per cent).

Microbial aetiology

The variety and frequency with which different organisms are isolated are given in Fig. 13. Gram-positive organisms cause up to 75 per cent of all episodes of peritonitis; of these, *Staphylococcus epidermidis* infections are usually mild and cure is readily obtained with appropriate antibiotic therapy. *S. aureus* is associated with a much more severe picture, with a tendency to abscess formation and a significant risk of death. Of the Gram-negative organisms *Pseudomonas* infections are similarly dangerous. They are difficult to eradicate and lead to loss of the peritoneal cavity. Fungal peritonitis is uncommon, is generally caused by *Candida* species and requires catheter removal. With the introduction of the disconnect systems there has been a reduction in *S. epidermidis*, polymicrobial, and sterile peritonitis but the rates for *S. aureus* and *Pseudomonas* are not different (Holley *et al.* 1994).

Culture-negative peritonitis accounts for 8–30 per cent of all episodes (Bunke *et al.* 1994). There are genuine causes for this, the most frequent being inadvertent use of antibiotics by the patient before culture, whilst peritoneal 'irritants' (chemicals, dialysis fluid components, endotoxins, and antiseptics) may also be important. Culture-negative peritonitis should not exceed 10 per cent of episodes. If it does, microbiological techniques should be reviewed (Keane *et al.* 1987).

Pathogenesis of peritonitis

Coagulase-negative Staphylococci are the major causative organisms in CAPD peritonitis, as they are of infections associated with other prosthetic devices and intravascular catheters. They tend to adhere to and grow on polymer surfaces, producing an extracellular, slimy substance resulting in a thick matrix with embedded organisms. Tenckhoff catheters examined using scanning electron microscopy of the external and internal surfaces (Dasgupta *et al.* 1987) also show this phenomenon. The slime or biofilm is thought to inhibit the chemotactic response of neutrophils, the proliferative response of lymphocytes, and opsonization of bacteria. Colonization of the external surface of the catheter reaches the external cuff 3 days after implantation, with the film reaching the peritoneal portion within 3 weeks (Read *et al.* 1989). This protected biofilm comprises an inherently antibiotic-resistant reservoir of bacteria that can cause repeated episodes of peritonitis. This subgroup could be identified by comparing the antibiotic sensitivities of a biofilm culture and a routine microbiological culture of the same PD effluent (Dasgupta and Larabie 2001). More recently Finkelstein *et al.* (2002) studied this problem in long-term PD patients. Of 90 pateints who had more than four episodes, 65 per cent had at least half or more of these caused by the same organism. Of 67 patients with catheter change, only 15 per cent developed repeat infection. This supports the hypothesis that bacterial biofilm is a cause of recurrent peritonitis in long-term patients on PD.

Clinical course

The incubation period of peritonitis is not known but it is estimated from touch contamination incidents, as well as prospective studies, to be 24–48 h. The timing has been cleverly studied by Zemel *et al.* (1995). CAPD patients stored the overnight PD effluent at 4°C for 2 days. If an episode of peritonitis occurred, two overnight bags were brought in. In this way nine episodes of peritonitis were assessed. The study found that at least 24 h prior to clinical peritonitis (and at times up to 48 h previously), bacteria were present in most of the PD effluents. There was also an increase in the number of peritoneal macrophages, a moderate increase in neutrophils, and a relative phagocytic malfunction of the macrophages. It seems, therefore, that in any bacterial invasion, the host defence mechanisms need to be overwhelmed before clinical peritonitis ensues.

In most cases of peritonitis the symptoms decrease rapidly after the initiation of treatment and disappear within 2–3 days. During this period the cell counts decrease and the bacterial cultures become negative. In the majority of the cases, positive peritoneal cultures are present for only 3–4 days. Persistence of symptoms is indicative of a complicated cause or a possible resistant organism, which is not responding well to antibiotics used; these require further investigation and often catheter removal.

Management of peritonitis

When peritonitis occurs, treatment should be started immediately after appropriate microbiological samples have been obtained (Keane *et al.* 1993). Many protocols of antibiotic treatment have been proposed. They differ in dose, duration, and route of administration. The management of CAPD peritonitis remains empirical (Fig. 14). There is an increasing consensus supporting a standardized approach combining continuation of CAPD, intraperitoneal antibiotics, and management of patients at home if possible. The latest ISPD Working Party report (Keane *et al.* 2000) provides recommendations for management.

Antibiotic regimens

The intraperitoneal administration of a single, broad-spectrum agent or a combination of antibiotics to give the widest possible cover against the major potential organisms is favoured. The initial first-line regimen should cure about 80 per cent of episodes without catheter removal, and a further 10 per cent should respond to changes in antibiotics. The treatment should provide broad coverage of all organisms without disturbing the patient's normal flora, should not encourage the development of resistant organisms, and should be convenient and cheap to administer (Van Biesen *et al.* 2002). Such a perfect regimen does not exist.

In their 1993 recommendations (Keane *et al.* 1993), The AdHoc Committee advocated the use of vancomycin as the mainstay against Gram-positive infections with ceftazidine or aminoglycoside to cover the Gram-negative organism as first line, blind therapy in the absence of an organism being identified on Gram stain at presentation. Since publication of that report, there has been a dramatic increase in the prevalence of vancomycin-resistant micro-organisms, especially entercocci (VRE), from approximately 0.5 per cent to nearly 14 per cent; especially in larger hospitals. Vancomycin resistance has been associated with resistance to penicillins and aminoglycosides creating a therapeutic challenge. This

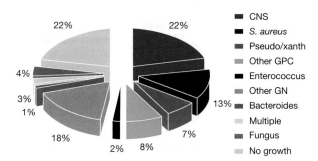

Fig. 13 Micro-organisms causing peritonitis. CNS, coagulase-negative staphylococcus; GPC, Gram-positive organisms.

	Urine output <100 ml/day	Urine output >100 ml/day
Cefazolin or Cephalothin	1 g/bag daily or 15 mg/kg BW/bag	20 mg/kg BW/bag daily
Ceftazidime	1 g daily in long dwell	20 mg/kg BW/bag once a day
Gentamicin Tobramycin Netilmycin	0.6 mg/kg BW/bag once a day	Not recommended

Fig. 14 Initial empirical treatment of PD peritonitis (modified with permission from Keane *et al.* 2000).

has prompted a number of agencies (Centres for Disease Control 1997) to discourage routine use of vancomycin for prophylaxis, for routine use, and for oral use against Clostridium difficile enterocolitis. The major concern is that the vancomycin resistance is transmitted to staphylococcal strains. The use of vancomycin as a first-line therapy is being reduced and the peritonitis sub-committee reverted to recommended first-generation cephalosporins in large doses. The latest ad hoc committee guidelines (Keane *et al.* 2000) have continued with the recommendations of 1996 with a few modifications. There is now evidence that aminoglycoside usage for PD peritonitis does lead to a decline in RRF (Shemin *et al.* 1999), which is also recognized to be an important marker of outcome of PD patients (Bargman *et al.* 2001). The Ad Hoc Peritonitis Committee has, therefore, recommended a change in the regime to replace the aminoglycoside with ceftazidime, given once daily as an initial empirical therapy, when the residual urine output is greater than 100 ml/day. Recent accumulating evidence points against any impact of aminoglycoside antibiotics on residual renal function in peritoneal dialysis (Baker *et al.* 2003). As a result the new ISPD guidelines on peritonitis management, due out in late 2004 will not recommend a regime based on residual renal function.

Initial empirical therapy for peritonitis

A first-generation cephalosporin antibiotic for Gram-positive and an aminoglycoside or ceftazidime for Gram-negative cover is recommended. Account is taken of urine output. This is to prevent automatic exposure to vancomycin and the emergence of resistant organisms. The antibiotic can be given as a single dose overnight (Lai *et al.* 1997a,b). Acceptance of this regimen is not universal because there is a relatively high failure rate especially if infection is caused by methicillin-resistant strains of *S. aureus* (MRSA). Goldberg *et al.* (2001) described an initial cure rate of 78 per cent (55 per cent Gram-positive infections and only 2 per cent methicillin-resistant); De Fijter *et al.* (2001) had only a 50 per cent cure rate with cephradine. Vas *et al.* (1997) had reasonable results but five out of nine methicillin-resistant strains did not respond. The findings of Sandoe *et al.* (1997) suggested that 50 per cent of coagulase-negative staphylococcus resistant to methicillin do not respond to cephalosporin. Local patterns and prevalence of organisms should be taken into account when choosing a regime. Many units, therefore, continue to use vancomycin.

Modification of treatment once culture and sensitivity results are available

Gram-positive bacteria

The management of patients with Gram-positive bacterial infection depends on the culture and sensitivity (Fig. 15). If the organism is *S. aureus*, its sensitivity to methicillin will dictate the choice of antibiotic. If it is sensitive to methicillin the aminoglycoside or ceftazidime should be discontinued and if the clinical response is unsatisfactory, rifampicin (600 mg/day by mouth) should be prescribed in addition to the intraperitoneal, first-generation cephalosporin. The use of rifampicin in areas with a high prevalence of tuberculosis is not recommended. If the *S. aureus* is methicillin resistant, rifampicin should be added and the first-generation cephalosporin should be switched to clindamycin or vancomycin.

Culture-negative peritonitis

In 10–20 per cent of cases cultures may be negative. If the patient is improving clinically after 4–5 days, and no suggestion of Gram-negative

organisms are seen on direct microscopy, only the cephalosporin should be continued for 2 weeks.

Gram-negative bacteria (Fig. 16)

A decision to discontinue the aminoglycoside or ceftazidime and continue with a first-generation cephalosporin will be guided by *in vitro* sensitivity testing. If the culture reveals multiple Gram-negative organisms (as occurs in 3–6 per cent of episodes) the possibility of intra-abdominal pathology necessitating surgical exploration must be excluded. Should the isolate be a *Pseudomonas* sp. (e.g. *Pseudomonas aeruginosa*), ceftazidime should be continued. An agent to which the isolated organism is sensitive should be added. Piperacillin, ciprofloxacin, aztreonam, an aminoglycoside, or sulfamethoxazole/trimethoprim are candidates for continued use with the ceftazidime. Evidence of catheter infection with pseudomonas (which is sometimes subtle) should be sought and if present removal of catheter is mandatory.

Fungal infection

Fungal peritonitis occurs in PD patients at rates of between 0.01/year and 0.11/year. The patients are usually acutely ill with severe abdominal pain and may deteriorate rapidly to die if catheter removal is delayed.

Enterococcus	S. aureus	Other (CNS)
• Stop cephalosporins Start ampicillin 125 mg/l each bag Consider adding aminoglycoside	• Stop ceftazidime or aminoglycoside Continue cefazolin Add rifampin 600 mg/d p.o.	• Stop ceftazidime or aminoglycoside Continue cefazolin
• If ampicillin resistant start vancomycin or clindamycin If VRE consider Synercid (Linezolid)	• If MRSA start vancomycin or clindamycin	• If MRSE and clinically not responding start vancomycin or clindamycin
Treat for 2 weeks	Treat for 3 weeks	Treat for 2 weeks

Fig. 15 Antibiotic treatment for Gram-positive organisms (modified with permission from Keane *et al.* 2000).

Single Gram-negative organism	Pseudomonas Stenotrophomonas	Multiple Gram-negatives and/or anaerobes
Adjust antibiotics to sensitivity >100 ml urine Ceftazidime <100 ml urine Aminoglycoside	Continue Ceftazidime and add: <100 ml urine Aminoglycoside >100 ml urine Ciprofloxacin: 500 mg bd oral or Piperacillin: 4 g IV 12 hourly Aztreonam: Load 1 g/l Maint 250 mg/l IP each bag	Continue cefazolin and ceftazidime Add Metronidazole 500 mg 8 hourly oral, IV or rectally If no change in clinical status consider surgery
Treat for 2 weeks	Treat for 3 weeks	Treat for 3 weeks

Fig. 16 Antibiotic treatment for Gram-negative organisms (modified with permission from Keane *et al.* 2000).

Few reports suggest that cure can be obtained with prolonged courses of antifungal agents (Lee *et al.* 1995). Prior antibiotic therapy is the predisposing cause of ~75 per cent of cases of *Candida peritonitis*.

Antifungal treatment should be continued after catheter removal for at least an additional 10 days.

Prophylaxis with oral nystatin during antibiotic therapy is reported to be effective in preventing fungal peritonitis in both children and adults (Robitaille *et al.* 1995), but this is not a universal finding (Williams *et al.* 2000). Patients requiring frequent or prolonged antibiotic therapy are a group likely to benefit.

Relapsing peritonitis

Peritonitis relapses after 10–20 per cent of episodes and is an indication for catheter removal, especially if rifampicin has been prescribed. The usual causes are tunnel infection and catheter colonization. The use of urokinase used to be advocated but in a randomized study of recurrent peritonitis comparing one-stage, Tenckhoff catheter replacement therapy with intraperitoneal urokinase, the results with urokinase were poor (Williams *et al.* 1989). The hypothesis was that the urokinase would lyse the fibrin, allowing antibiotic access to the source of reinfection.

Treatment of peritonitis in patients undergoing automated Peritoneal dialysis (Keane *et al.* 2000)

The cycler regimen should be adjusted to around the clock exchanges of 3–4 h until the fluid clears, which usually takes 24–72 h. During this time the patient must remain connected to the cycler or may disconnect for one dwell per 24 h as long as the full exchange is maintained. This may not be possible at home so admission to hospital may be required. An alternative is to place the antibiotics in the long day dwell (that is giving the antibiotic once daily). The patient may be switched to CAPD, with the addition of antibiotics to all exchanges. Diaz-Buxo *et al.* (2001) have outlined an antibiotic dose regimen based on pharmacokinetic studies for piperacillin, cefazolin, vancomycin, and tobramycin. Fielding *et al.* (2002) showed that once a day cefazolin with gentamicin is an effective treatment in APD peritonitis with 78 per cent treatment success. Warady *et al.* (2000) have produced guidelines for the treatment of peritonitis in paediatric patients. They advocate that for patients who receive nocturnal APD, the initial (24–48 h) treatment should include a prolongation of the dialysate dwell time to 3–6 h until there is clearing of the fluid.

Course and outcome of peritonitis

Complete cure is achieved in ~80 per cent of cases without recourse to catheter removal. Persistent symptoms beyond 96 h occur in about 13–39 per cent of episodes. Relapsing peritonitis is a feature in 8–16 per cent of episodes and catheter removal to effect a cure is necessary in upto 15 per cent of cases. Death is reported in 1–3 per cent of cases (Gokal 2000). Peritonitis and peritoneal catheter infections remain the cause of significant morbidity, including catheter loss, transfer to HD either permanently or temporarily and hospitalization (Woodrow *et al.* 1997).

Peritonitis results in a marked increase in effluent protein losses, which contributes to malnutrition already prevalent in PD patients, a transient decrease in UF and, over time, an increase in solute transport and loss of UF. This process has been shown to be exacerbated and accelerated by peritonitis and is related to the degree of inflammation and the number of infections especially if in quick succession (Davies *et al.* 1996).

The ability to resume PD after Tenckhoff catheter removal following severe peritonitis was studied by Szeto *et al.* (2002). One hundred patients with severe peritonitis had had their catheters removed. In half it was possible to resume PD, but failed in the remainder. In the group that continued PD, there was a rise in *D/P* creatinine with the need to use additional exchanges or hypertonic dialysis. The optimum time gap between the removal of catheter and reinsertion is not known but 3–4 weeks is usually allowed. Recent experience suggests that short intervals may be acceptable. Indeed some clinicians perform the removal of the old catheter and the insertion of the new one at the same operation (Mayo *et al.* 1995; Posthuma *et al.* 1998). This of course decreases hospitalization, and minimizes the need for back-up HD.

Peritonitis rates have hitherto been expressed as episodes per patient year of treatment or an episode per number of months. Schaefer *et al.* (2002) proposed using a median value of individual patient peritonitis rates. The median values give important information as some centres may have many patients with little or no peritonitis and a small subset with a very high rate of peritonitis.

Prevention of peritonitis

The incidence of peritonitis caused by *S. epidermidis*, most often due to touch contamination at the time of the exchange, has decreased following improvements in connection technology, especially the disconnect systems (Maiorca *et al.* 1983). Careful selection of patients and meticulous training also reduce this cause of peritonitis. The incidence of *S. aureus* infections may be reduced by applying mupirocin at the exit-site and eradication of nasal carriage (see later). Prophylactic daily cephalexin or trimethoprim 160 mg/sulfamethoxazole 800 mg was ineffective in reducing the risk of peritonitis, although the effect of the prophylaxis on the rates of individual organisms was not reported (Churchill *et al.* 1988). Although there is no means of reducing the incidence of peritonitis from gut organisms, constipation should be avoided. Prophylactic antibiotic therapy prior to invasive procedures such as colonoscopy, gynaecological, cholecystectomy, is recommended (Keane *et al.* 2000).

It is axiomatic that the good organization of a CAPD programme with appropriate staff and infrastructure will reduce infection rates (Uttley and Prowant 2000). Enhancing of heat-stable opsonic activity by intraperitoneal IgG given every 3 weeks (Lamperi *et al.* 1986) has been shown to be ineffective, as has vaccination against staphylococci (Poole-Warren *et al.* 1991). Prevention depends on good training and using connector systems that minimize contamination.

Peritoneal catheter related infections

Colonization of the exit-site with micro-organisms may lead to infection of the exit-site, which may spread along the subcutaneous pathway of the catheter to the inner cuff and subsequently to the peritoneum. Catheter infections, a term which includes both exit-site and tunnel infections, occur at a rate of 0.6/year although reported figures vary depending on the definitions used. *S. aureus* and *P. aeruginosa* are the most common and serious causes of catheter infections because they are difficult to eradicate and frequently result in peritonitis, leading to catheter loss.

Exit-site infection

This is defined as a purulent drainage at the peritoneal catheter exit-site, with or without erythema. The presence of induration and tenderness suggest a worse prognosis. Twardowski and Prowant (1996) have further classified the catheter related infections. This provides the basis of management—a regimen adopted by the recent report of the ISPD Committee on catheter and exit-site practices (Gokal et al. 1998). They divide exit-site infections into: (a) acute (purulent and/or bloody drainage from the exit-site which may be associated with erythema, tenderness, exuberant granulation tissue, and oedema), (b) chronic (the result of an untreated or inadequately treated acute infection), and (c) equivocal (purulent and/or bloody drainage only in the sinus, but cannot be expressed, accompanied by the regression of the epithelium, and occurrence of slightly exuberant granulation tissue in the sinus). The equivocal infected exit-site represents low-grade infection. These sometimes improve spontaneously, but most progress to overt infection if untreated.

Tunnel infection

This is diagnosed when there is pain, tenderness, erythema, induration, or any combination of these over the subcutaneous pathway of the catheter. However, many tunnel infections are occult, detected only by sonography of the subcutaneous catheter pathway (Plum et al. 1994). Using clinical criteria the infection rate was 0.13 episodes per patient year, but this almost trebled with ultrasound imaging.

If the ultrasound was negative there was no catheter loss, but 50 per cent when it was positive. Tunnel infections are present in approximately one-half of all exit-site infections, but occasionally occur in the absence of an exit-site infection. The infection can involve the outer cuff, intercuff segment, and/or inner cuff of the catheter. As the infection spreads along the tunnel towards the peritoneum, the risk of peritonitis greatly increases (Plum et al. 1994).

Pathogens

S. aureus is responsible for the majority of exit-site and tunnel infections. P. aeruginosa is much less common, but like S. aureus, is difficult to eradicate and frequently leads to peritonitis if catheter removal is delayed. S. epidermidis is a relatively infrequent cause of tunnel infection in contrast to peritonitis. Other Gram-positive organisms, Gram-negative bacilli, and rarely fungi account for the remaining infections.

Peritoneal infections and nasal carriage

S. aureus peritonitis occurs predominantly in patients who either have or have had a history of S. aureus catheter infections and in patients with S. aureus colonization either in the nares (Luzar et al. 1990; Turner et al. 1998), the skin (Pignatari et al. 1990), or at the peritoneal catheter exit-site (Swartz et al. 1991). Nasal carriage of S. aureus has been shown to be of particular importance in diabetics, immunosuppressed patients, and in whom prophylaxis is recommended (Vychytil et al. 1998). Almost one-half of patients carry S. aureus in their nares at the initiation of PD and these are the patients most likely to develop S. aureus exit-site, and tunnel infections (Turner et al. 1998). In a 3-year study of pericatheter and nasal colonization, Perez-Fontan et al. (2002) found that Gram-negative organisms were responsible for chronic carriage in 7 per cent of patients and partners, but was not associated with an increased risk of peritonitis.

Treatment of peritoneal dialysis catheter infections

Treatment of exit-site infections includes local care, systemic antibiotics, and revision of the tunnel surgically, and as a last resort, replacement of the catheter.

Exit-site, tunnel, and cuff infections require antibiotic therapy which should be started immediately before culture results are available (Gokal et al. 1998). For Gram-positive infections, oral penicillinase-resistant penicillins, oral trimethoprim/sulfamethoxazole, or cephalexin are convenient and cost-effective options. Vancomycin should be avoided in view of the emergence of VRE. In slowly resolving or particularly severe S. aureus exit-site infections, rifampicin can be added. Quinolones are generally used for P. aeruginosa catheter infections but ceftazidime may be added if necessary.

For chronic exit-site infections a combination of synergistic antibiotics is preferred to avoid emergence of resistant organisms during a prolonged treatment. The response to therapy is slow and the features of chronic infection change gradually to an 'equivocal exit' and then eventually to a 'good exit site'. Treatment should be continued until the exit-site appears completely normal. Topical treatment can be used as an adjunct to systemic antibiotics in treatment of exit infections or as initial therapy for low-grade infection (equivocally infected exit). Topical antibiotic therapy is not appropriate for acute and chronic exit infections. The latter may need external cuff exteriorization.

Prevention of exit-site and tunnel infections

Antibiotics given at the time of catheter insertion have been shown to decrease catheter related peritonitis in animal studies (Pecoits-Filho et al. 1998) but evidence in patients is lacking. Catheter immobilization, proper location of the exit-site, sterile wound care immediately after placement of the catheter, and avoidance of trauma are all recommended (Turner et al. 1992). The Network 9 study found that directing the subcutaneous portion of the catheter downwards decreased the risk of peritonitis associated with exit-site and/or tunnel infection by 38 per cent, while an upward-directed catheter had a 50 per cent increased risk of catheter related peritonitis, compared to horizontally directed tunnels (Golper et al. 1996).

S. aureus nasal carriage is a risk factor for S. aureus infection. Without prophylaxis the rates of S. aureus exit-site infections are about 0.34–0.41/year and reduced by 50 per cent with mupirocin prophylaxis. There have been four randomized studies (Zimmerman et al. 1991; Perez-Fontan et al. 1993; Bernardini et al. 1996; Mupirocin Study Group 1996) that have demonstrated mupirocin effectiveness in reducing S. aureus catheter infections and peritonitis (Fig. 17). The mupirocin must be repeated either monthly or when the nasal culture becomes positive for S. aureus. The disadvantages of the intranasal approach are expense and the need for repeated nose cultures (if therapy is based on positive cultures only). Zimmerman et al. (1991) reported the successful use of cyclical rifampicin but its use is not advocated because of side-effects and development of resistance. An alternative approach to decreasing S. aureus infections is to apply mupirocin to the exit-site as part of routine daily care (Bernardini et al. 1996). Routine use in clinical practice in all patients has been shown to reduce significantly not only staphylococcal exit-site infections and peritonitis, but also non-staphylococcal pathogens (Thodis et al. 1998; Casey et al. 2000; Prakashan et al. 2001). It is cost-effective (Davey et al. 1999).

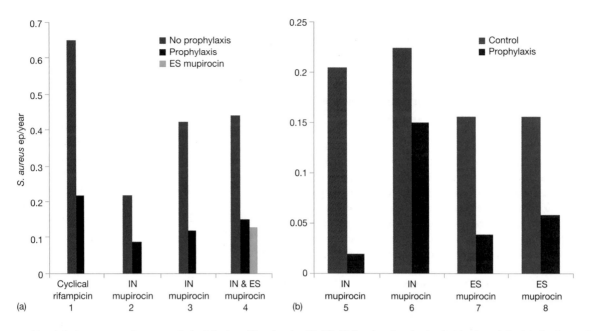

Fig. 17 Impact of prophylaxis to prevent *S. aureus* exit-site infections (a) and peritonitis (b). (a) Results of randomized trials of prophylaxis with rifampicin (1—Zimmerman *et al.* 1991), intranasal (IN) mupirocin (2—Perez-Fontan *et al.* 1993), IN mupirocin (3—Mupirocin Study Group 1996), and IN and exit-site (ES) mupirocin (4—Bernardini *et al.* 1996). (b) Impact of the prophylaxis on *S. aureus* peritonitis (episodes per patient year; ep/year) with IN mupirocin (5—Perez-Fontan *et al.* 1993), IN mupirocin (6—Mupirocin study group 1996), ES mupirocin (7—Bernardini *et al.* 1996), and ES mupirocin (8—Thodis *et al.* 1998).

Application of mupirocin to the exit-site as part of the daily routine is advocated as a means to prevent exit-site infection and does appear to result in development of bacterial resistance (Annigeri *et al.* 2001; Perez-Fontan *et al.* 2002).

Peritoneal catheters and exit-site practices

The key to successful PD is a permanent and safe access to the peritoneal cavity. Despite improvements in catheter survival over the last few years, catheter-related complications still occur, causing significant morbidity and requiring catheter removal and a permanent switch of the patient to HD.

Types of catheter

Several catheters have been designed to minimize the various complications of peritoneal access. Catheters for chronic PD have a variety of intraperitoneal designs, physically combined with a number of extraperitoneal designs (Ash 1990) (Fig. 18). Intraperitoneal designs of chronic catheters include a straight or coiled Tenckhoff catheter, the double-disc Toronto-Western catheter, the column-disc catheter, or the T-fluted catheter (Ash *et al.* 2002). The latter is a T-shaped catheter, which contains long flutes rather than holes. Extraperitoneal designs of chronic catheters include either a single or double Dacron cuff, disc-bubble two cuffs, arcuate (swan-neck—two cuffs with a preformed 150° bend in the inner cuff tubing to provide a caudally directed exit-site without strain on the cuffs; Twardowski *et al.* 1992), and Cruz (pail-handle—similar to the arcuate catheter but with two 90° bends; Cruz 1994). The double-cuff, straight Tenckhoff catheter is still the most widely used because it seems to satisfy the needs of most patients. The swan-neck catheter has become the second most popular catheter, with promising survival times for the device when compared to other types (Twardowski *et al.* 1992). The Cruz pail-handle

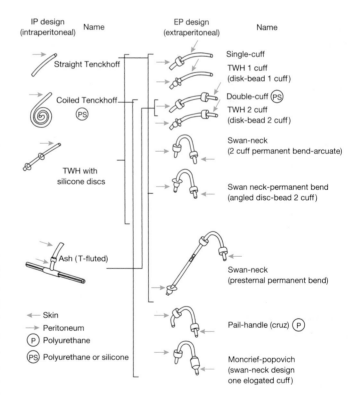

Fig. 18 Various types of PD catheters divided up into intra- and extraperitoneal portions (reproduced with permission Gokal *et al.* 1998).

catheter utilizes polyurethane, which, being a strong and smooth material, allows thinner walls, a greater internal diameter, and therefore a more rapid flow of dialysate. The coil catheter causes less discomfort by minimizing the 'jet effect' of the high flow of dialysis solutions and is potentially less prone to migration. This is also true of the Toronto-Western catheters, which have two discs perpendicular to the tubing axis.

Catheter choice and outcome

The minimum acceptable rate of catheter survival at 12 months is 50–60 per cent. At best, a 3-year catheter survival rate of 80 per cent should be expected. Results worse than the former percentages should lead to a review of the procedures used. Audit of results at regular intervals is vital. Two-cuff catheters are felt to be superior to single-cuff. Even though a survey of the current literature suggests that the most popular catheters are the two-cuff standard Tenckhoff and the swan-neck Missouri catheters, there have been no controlled studies to suggest the superiority of one over the other. The complication rates of peritoneal catheters by type and placement technique show improved results for the swan-neck, which require a surgical approach for insertion, but equally good results are reported for the peritoneoscopic approach to catheter implantation. It is important to stress that while these studies demonstrate varied outcomes, there is no hard evidence available to recommend discarding the use of any type of catheter. In support of this are two prospective randomized studies of different catheters (straight Tenckhoff, curled Tenckhoff, and Toronto-Western; Scott *et al.* 1994; straight Tenckhoff and swan-neck; Eklund *et al.* 1994), which showed no difference in complication rates. Recent studies by Nielsen *et al.* (1995) show superior survival of curled catheters over straight ones.

Implantation method

Implantation must be performed by a competent and experienced team. Although there are now six techniques of catheter implantation there are several areas of general agreement about technique (Gokal *et al.* 1998).

1. The insertion site should be paramedian.

2. The deep cuff should be in the musculature of the anterior abdominal wall.

3. The subcutaneous cuff should be near the skin surface and not less than 2 cm from the exit-site.

4. The exit-site should be facing downwards or directed laterally.

5. The intra-abdominal portion of the catheter should be placed between the visceral and parietal peritoneum.

    The various implantation techniques are as follows.

Surgical insertion (placement by dissection)

Dissective placement is essential for catheters with stabilizing devices (e.g. swan-neck, Toronto-Western, column-disc), but all catheters can be inserted this way.

Blind catheter insertion

This procedure, using a trocar, should not be used in patients who are extremely obese or who have had previous abdominal surgery.

Seldinger (guidewire) and peel-away sheath (Zappacosta et al. 1991)

This technique is similar to the split sheath used for the insertion of subclavian and internal jugular venous catheters. It can be used for straight Tenckhoff catheters as well as swan-neck, straight, and coiled catheters. Preparation of the patient is similar to that described for rigid catheters.

Peritoneoscopic insertion

The use of peritoneoscopy for peritoneal catheter placement was developed by Ash (1993). Tenckhoff and swan-neck, straight, and coiled catheters may be implanted. It is done through a single abdominal puncture and utilizes a Y-tec peritoneoscope.

The swan-neck presternal catheter

The catheter has the same intraperitoneal portion but the extraperitoneal portion is long and brought up externally at the sternum (Twardowski 2002). The rationale for this approach is that it provides greater catheter stability at the exit-site and good tunnel-wound healing, easy exit-site care, and some psychosocial advantages. Up to 2001 nearly a thousand such catheters had been implanted. Experience suggests that this catheter is particularly useful in obese patients (body mass index > 35), patients with 'ostomies', young patients requiring diapers, and those with faecal incontinence.

Moncrief and Popovich technique (Moncrief and Popovich 1994)

The distal external segment of the catheter is completely buried and remains in the subcutaneous tunnel until exteriorization 4 weeks after insertion. This is a new technique that allows tissue to grow into the cuff material without exposure to the skin surface. This necessitates insertion at least 4 weeks before use, at which time the catheter tip is brought out through a tiny exit in the skin. In a prospective randomized study this method of insertion did not reduce the risk of peritonitis or exit-site infections (Danielsson *et al.* 2002).

Catheter complications (Table 11)

Early soft-catheter complications

Early postinsertion complications are similar to those after implantation of a rigid catheter, but the frequency is lower, particularly with surgical and peritoneoscopic insertion. Blood-tinged dialysate is common but severe bleeding is very rare. Dialysate leaks are less likely to occur if PD delayed for at least 2 weeks after implantation.

Poor dialysate return is usually due to catheter obstruction, the most common causes of which are migration of the catheter tip, occlusion

Table 11 Complications of peritoneal catheters

Complication	Action
Operative and early postoperative complications	
Pain in perineal area	Analgesia
Leakage of PD fluid	Stop PD; antibiotic cover. If recurrence catheter replacement
Bleeding exit-site	Pressure bandage
Intraperitoneal bleeding	Lavage PD fluid
Severe haemorrhage	Surgery
Perforation of hollow viscus	Laparotomy
Exit-site infection	Antibiotics
Catheter tip migration	Treat constipation, catheter manipulation, surgery
Long-term complications	
Exit-site infections	Antibiotics, cuff exteriorization
Catheter cuff-erosion	Exteriorization
Catheter tip migration	As above
Leakage of PD fluid	As above

of the tip by bowel or bladder, and intraluminal clot formation. Emptying the bladder and using laxatives may restore catheter function. Clots can be prevented by using heparin or the catheter can be filled with urokinase (5000 units diluted in normal saline). These measures will relieve the obstruction in 10–15 per cent of cases. If the catheter is not kinked but does not function for 2 weeks, omental wrapping or multiple adhesions are likely to occur and omentectomy or adhesiolysis through a laparoscopy may be required.

Catheter migration and obstruction

The best position for the catheter tip is in the true pelvis. If the exit is directed caudally and the tunnel points cephalad, however, the catheter will then have an intraperitoneal bend. In this circumstance, the tip will migrate out of the true pelvis, owing to the 'shape memory' and resilience of the silastic.

Migration of the catheter out of the pelvis is frequently observed on abdominal radiographs taken for various reasons in patients with a functioning catheter. While about 20 per cent of catheters translocate to the upper abdomen, only one-fifth of these translocated catheters become obstructed. However, a catheter with its tip in the upper abdomen is about six times more likely to be obstructed than a normally positioned catheter.

Migration of the catheter tip may be the result of obstruction rather than its cause. Relocation of the catheter is best done surgically or laparoscopically.

Capture of the catheter by an active omentum causes outflow obstruction. This is usually an immediate postoperative event but can occur later, and when it does, it is usually associated with peritonitis. Late catheter migration is unusual unless associated with omental capture.

Slow drainage due to catheter translocation, or to occlusion of the tip by bowel or a fibrin clot, occurs from time to time in some patients. Constipation is a common cause of this complication, and laxatives and regular bowel emptying help to avoid the problem. For fibrin clots the addition of heparin, 500 units/l of dialysis solution, is usually successful in restoring good catheter function.

Another reason for obstruction is adherence of the catheter to the peritoneum. This complication, more commonly found in children, can be avoided by performing a partial omentectomy at the time of the insertion. Laparoscopic omentectomy can also be done to salvage malfunctioning catheters, with catheter fixation to the anterior pelvic wall (Lee and Donovan 2002). Relocation of such catheters may be attempted with a so-called whiplash technique. This entails insertion of a blunted steel trocar into the catheter. Using the cuff as a pivot and with short and rapid whiplash motions, the catheter is freed from the adherence site (Dobrashian et al. 1999). The outcome is generally poor, with a success rate of only 25 per cent (Nielsen et al. 1995).

Image-guided techniques in managing peritoneal access and managing complications have evolved over the decade (Taylor 2002). Fluoroscopy-guided wire manipulation combined with laparoscopic surgery has produced better results. In one small series, the overall success rate of repeated manipulation was 71 per cent (Kim et al. 2002). Laparoscopic manipulation has salvaged many catheters and in a small series, all patients were able to return to PD after this procedure (Ogunc 2002).

Catheter dialysate leaks

Dialysate leakage is a tiresome complication of PD which can develop at any time after catheter implantation. Its development is related to

technique of PD catheter insertion, the way PD is initiated, and/or weaknesses of the abdominal wall but not the type of catheter.

Early leakage is from the exit-site. There is an association between early leaks (<30 days) and immediate initiation of PD and midline catheter insertion. Leaks can be from the peritoneal cavity via the catheter. Abdominal weakness predisposes to late leaks (>30 days), which are usually subcutaneous. It can also present more subtly as subcutaneous swelling, weight gain, peripheral and genital oedema, and apparent UF failure. Dyspnoea is the first sign of a pleural leak, which is usually right sided. Such a leak may be difficult to prove but the best method is to do a CT scan after intraperitoneal contrast instillation (Letherland et al. 1992). Peritoneal scintigraphy has also been used in ascertaining the site of fluid leakage (Mellor et al. 2002).

Hernias and genital oedema

The presence of 2–3 l of fluid in the peritoneal cavity increases the intra-abdominal pressure significantly. Coughing and straining further increase the pressure and abdominal-wall tension which can lead to hernia formation in patients with congenital or acquired defects in or around the abdominal wall. A variety of hernias have been described in patients on PD (Bargman 2000); the most common are incisional, inguinal, or umbilical. Up to 11 per cent of patients developed hernias during a 5-year follow-up (O'Connor et al. 1986). The mean time for development of a hernia is 1 year and the risk increases by about 20 per cent for each year thereafter. The risk of hernias is not increased by the fill volume (Hussain et al. 1998).

Using a paramedian incision through the rectus muscle will reduce hernia risk and early fluid leakage. However, an important site for herniation is the processus vaginalis especially in children. The pressure of the fluid may convert this weakness into an indirect inguinal hernia.

Oedema of the labia or scrotum and penis is a distressing complication which occurs in ~10 per cent of CAPD patients (Tzamaloukas et al. 1992). Dialysate can track through the soft-tissue planes from the catheter insertion site, from a hernia, or from peritoneofascial defects and be associated with abdominal oedema (Letherland et al. 1992). CT, abdominal ultrasonography, and isotopic methods have been used to detect the site of the leak (Scanziani et al. 1992; Taylor 2002). The most worrisome complication is incarceration, and bowel and umbilical hernias are at particular risk of strangulation (Suh et al. 1994). Bowel incarceration can occasionally mimic peritonitis (Steiner et al. 1990).

The treatment of hernias is surgical, after which PD may need to be interrupted to allow healing. The hernia repair can be reinforced by using an overlying polypropylene mesh, allowing a quicker return to full-volume dialysis (Lewis et al. 1998). Treatment of genital oedema includes bed rest, scrotal elevation, and surgery for a hernia or patent processus vaginalis.

Hydrothorax is a rare but potentially life-threatening complication. It occurs predominantly on the right. The mechanism is unknown but defects in the diaphragm are not uncommon. Management options include: stopping PD, attempting pleurodesis, and low-volume PD.

Patient selection

The availability of PD allows a renal centre to be more flexible in managing patients in endstage renal failure (Table 12). In spite of over 25 years experience with CAPD there is as yet no 'profile' of a perfect PD patient (Table 13).

Table 12 Factors favouring PD as an initial dialysis therapy for ESRD patients, as compared to HD

Improving outcomes: equal or better survival in first 2–3 years
Better preservation of RRF versus HD
Higher haemoglobin levels; less erythropoietin use
Preservation of vascular access for HD
Provides continuous UF for improved blood pressure and volume control
Better outcomes post-transplant
Less risk of acquiring blood borne virus (hepatitis C)
Patient benefits including more flexible holidays and travel and higher employment rates; better quality of life than maintenance HD
Ability to expand patient numbers in a dialysis centre with limited need for resources and major capital investments
Lower staff to patient ratio than maintenance HD
Less costly than maintenance HD

Table 13 Factors that need to be taken into account in choosing between dialytic therapies in patients starting dialysis

Medical factors	Psychosocial factors
Age	Patient preference
Cardiovascular disease	Motivation
Diabetes mellitus	Compliance
Ease of transplantation	Family support
Extensive abdominal surgery	Distance from centre
Blindness	Occupation
Severe pulmonary disease	Concern with body image
Peripheral vascular disease	Travel
Extensive diverticulitis	
Extensive vascular disease—vascular access	

For new patients the essential factors are: motivation, physical and mental capability of carrying out the procedure, an insight into symptoms, and overall management of uraemia. A wish to be independent and be treated at home are useful pointers. Certain patients will have major difficulties with other types of dialysis. These are the 'high-risk' patient population, for example, diabetics and those with severe cerebro- and cardiovascular disease, in whom there may be few options other than PD (Wuerth *et al.* 2002).

For patients already on HD, a switch to PD is indicated in those with problems with vascular access, excessive weight gain between dialyses, severe hypertension, postdialysis disequilibration, and severe anaemia. Patients expecting a kidney transplant can be safely maintained on PD. This is especially so for children in whom PD is the preferred dialysis treatment prior to transplantation.

The peritoneal cavity may be unsuitable for PD because of adhesions, secondary to previous operations or systemic inflammatory disease. This is the only absolute contraindication to PD. Other relative contraindications are abdominal hernias (which can be repaired before PD), 'ostomies' (increase the risk of infection), progressive neurological diseases, movement disorders and severe arthritis which make PD impossible to perform (but a spouse or relative may be able to carry out the exchanges); severe psychological and social problems, chronic obstructive airways disease patients, and severe diverticular disease of the colon (risk of Gram-negative peritonitis or perforation).

Outcomes in peritoneal dialysis

Survival

PD and HD do not seem to differ in respect of mortality over the initial 4–5 years (Gokal 2002). The comparison is difficult to make as there has never been a randomized study comparing the two modalities. A number of factors impact on outcomes, not least of which is comorbidity and differences in patient characteristics at start (Nissenson *et al.* 1997; Xue *et al.* 2002). These need to be taken into account when making comparisons (Van Manen *et al.* 2002).

There are a number of useful published comparisons of PD and HD. Nolph (1996) analysed the relative risk of death on PD as compared to HD and found that the mortality risk was equal for HD and PD. The report of Bloembergen *et al.* (1995) based on the United States Renal Data Systems (USRDS) data on prevalent patients (1987, 1988, and 1989) showed that PD patients had a 19 per cent higher risk of mortality than those on HD. This caused considerable consternation in the United States and probably did the therapy a major disservice. Recent analyses from the Canadian Organ Replacement Registry (CORR) on patients starting RRT between 1990 and 1994, showed that for incident patients, the survival on PD was better in the first 2 years of treatment compared to HD and there was no difference at 4 years (Fenton *et al.* 1997). It also showed that there was a significantly lower risk of death in PD patients across all ages with diabetes. For ages 0–64 years the relative risk of death was 0.54 for non-diabetic PD patients (HD being 1) and 0.73 for diabetics. A further analysis from 11 Canadian centres showed that the apparent survival advantage of PD patients was due to lower comorbidity and a lower likelihood of dialysis being started acutely (Murphy *et al.* 2000). More recently the analysis of the Medicare patients in the United States (cohort of patients 1994–1997) by Collins *et al.* (1999) concluded that in the first 2 years of therapy short-term PD is associated with superior outcomes compared with HD at all ages except in elderly female diabetics. A more recent analysis from the USRDS database shows that after adjustment for comorbidity and other related factors, patients in the United States above the age of 67 years on PD had a higher risk of death, and this was greater for the diabetic population (Collins *et al.* 2002). A Danish registry reported results similar to the CORR database. This study corrected for comorbidity and transplant status and found that the relative risk of death was lower on PD compared to HD over the first 18 months, but the risk was the same thereafter (Heaf *et al.* 2002). The Netherlands Cooperative Study on the Adequacy of Dialysis (NECOSAD) prospective cohort study shows no difference in survival at 2 years (76 per cent for both HD and PD) (Jager *et al.* 2001b). Long-term survival from single-centre analysis shows no difference at 15 years between PD and HD patients (Maiorca and Cancarini 2000).

The overall conclusion from these data is that mortality is the same for HD and PD when comparing similar patients, at least for the first 3–4 years of RRT. Patient survival statistics from long-term studies in PD patients starting treatment during the 1990s show a 35–70 per cent 5-year survival (Davies *et al.* 1998) (see Table 14).

Technique survival

To achieve wider acceptance, several outstanding problems of PD currently need to be overcome. The two major issues are: the higher technique failure in PD compared to HD (still related in a third of drop-outs to HD to peritoneal infections) and the low rate of maintaining the treatment long-term. The latter problem is to a large extent a consequence of changes in peritoneal membrane structure and function. In the analysis

Table 14 Outcome studies in the 1990s showing patient and technique survival in cohorts of patients on PD

Source	Year	Mean age (years)	Proportion diabetics (%)	Proportion cardiovascular disease (%)	Patient survival at 5 years (%)	Technique survival at 5 years (%)
Maiorca et al.	1991	56.2	20.2	20–25	50	70
Rotellar et al.	1991	47	18	n/a	60	64
Lupo et al.	1994	58.4	13	31	48	59
Maiorca et al.	1996	62	13	22–25	60a	72
Kawaguchi et al.	1996	47.6	13.8	43.4	50	55
Fenton et al.	1997	63	32	43.4	35	n/a
Davies et al.	1998	58.8	14.8	32	55	70

by Davies *et al.* (1998) technique survival in the seven studies in the 1990s was 55–70 per cent at five years (Table 14). The major causes of discontinuation are shown in Fig. 19. A very small percentage of those that start PD (Gokal and Oreopoulos 1996) remain on it for greater than or equal to 10 years. A single-centre analysis show that technique survival is at best 20 per cent at 10 years (Maiorca and Cancarini 2000). The major cause of failure in long-term studies are UF failure, inadequate solute clearance, and peritonitis (Kawaguchi 1999a). In Japan, median survival of a cohort of 242 patients was 5.8 years (Kawaguchi 1999b). Failure of the technique was related to membrane problems. PD patients have a greater need for admissions to hospital, mainly due to peritonitis, comorbidity, and also to lack of experience (Habach *et al.* 1995).

Health-related quality of life in peritoneal dialysis

Several analyses have shown that quality of life is marginally better in PD patients than those on maintenance HD and this view is supported by two meta-analyses (Gokal *et al.* 1999; Cameron *et al.* 2000). The former meta-analysis includes 49 comparative studies of HRQL (well-being, emotional distress) in transplanted patients compared to HD (home, hospital) and CAPD, using sensitivity analyses and taking into account case mix, methodological rigour, and research design. Notwithstanding bias due to differences in case mix and publication bias, the transplant population had a higher well being and lower distress than hospital HD and CAPD patients. Hospital HD had lower HRQL than CAPD. In the second analysis, HRQL was linked with survival in 14 studies. The analysis showed that home dialysis (home HD and CAPD) treatment was associated with better outcomes than hospital HD but only a few reached statistical difference.

In the elderly, HRQL and outcomes are similar for PD and HD (Harris *et al.* 2002). That HRQL deteriorates on dialysis is well recognized. A recent longitudinal study in the United Kingdom reported on 88 PD patients over 24 months and showed that HRQL declined over the 24 months, with higher comorbidity (especially diabetes) being associated with worse scores (Bakewell *et al.* 2002).

Role of peritoneal dialysis in an integrated renal replacement therapy programme (Fig. 20)

Because survival results on PD are better than on HD in the initial years of therapy and technique survival on long-term PD is improving (Davies *et al.* 1998), it is tempting to advocate PD as an initial therapy (Coles and Williams 1998; Van Biesen *et al.* 2000a). If PD therapy fails

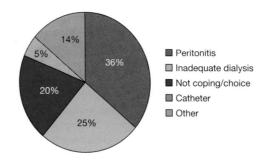

Fig. 19 Reasons for therapy change to HD in long-term PD patients in the 1990s. These are the averaged percentages of studies in Table 12 (reproduced with permission from Gokal *et al.* 2002).

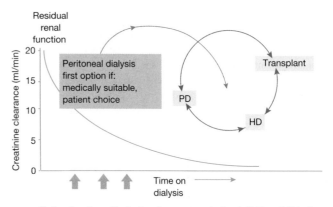

Early referral + patient education program before initiation of dialysis

Fig. 20 Schematic representation of the role of PD in an integrated/RRT programme, where patients are referred early, receive full education and therapy choice, and on the basis of medical and social conditions, and patient choice, are perhaps managed initially by PD (reproduced with permission from Gokal 1999b).

for whatever reason (usually peritonitis, inadequate dialysis, or patient related factors) then a switch from PD to HD can be made. In a Belgian study (Van Biesen *et al.* 2000b) of this approach, there was better survival in patients starting with PD than those starting with HD. It showed that patient outcome is not jeopardized by starting patients on PD, provided they are switched to HD in a timely manner when PD-related problems, especially loss of UF, arise. There are several advantages to using PD as the initial RRT (Table 12). RRF is better preserved (Moist *et al.* 2000), the risk of hepatitis C is decreased (Pereira and Levey 1997), vascular access sites are preserved (Van Biesen *et al.* 2000b), blood pressure control is better, and there is less cardiac dysfunction (Foley *et al.* 1998). Results of transplantation may be better too (Bleyer *et al.* 1999; Van Biesen *et al.* 2000c). It must be stressed that switching to HD at an appropriate time improves outcome. Failure to do so will lead to poorer results (Woodrow *et al.* 1997; Davies *et al.* 1998).

Non-medical factors and economics of dialysis therapy

It is not clear why PD is not more widely used. Medical factors suggest that about 18 per cent of patients would be suited to either HD or PD only (Little *et al.* 2001). The rest could be treated equally well by HD or PD. Figure 21 shows that the utilization of PD in various countries ranges from less than 5 to over 80 per cent. Such a discrepancy cannot be entirely linked to medical, social, and patient-related factors. In a study by Nissenson *et al.* (1997), five non-medical factors were listed—the most important reason for selecting a particular mode of dialysis proved to be financial and reimbursement policies. In countries with fixed annual allocations, the use of PD was high, reflecting the lower cost. In countries where financial aspects had less influence, factors such as physician bias and social mores were more important. There is greater use of PD in countries in which public health care systems dominate RRT provision. In mixed health economies the PD penetration is less and least in private provider dominated systems (Horl *et al.* 1999).

Another important factor is patient education before the need for dialysis. Several studies have shown that, when this is deficient there is bias towards HD. The USRDS in 1997 reviewed the patient-reported process of modality choice (USRDS 1997). In this analysis, Dialysis Mortality and Morbidity Study (Wave 2), only 25 per cent of patients starting HD were aware of the PD option. However, when patients were made aware of all the options, the proportion starting PD was higher. Of 1174 HD patients assessed, 17 per cent chose this dialysis modality when the decision was patient led, 53 per cent when it was medical team led, and 30 per cent when it was joint patient/medical team decision. Of 1049 PD patients, the percentages in the three categories were

35 per cent, 16 per cent, and 49 per cent respectively. Schreiber *et al.* (2000) assessed the impact of providing thorough dialysis treatment options education on modality choice in a US patient population of 5065 pre-ESRD patients over the time period 1997–1999. In this cohort, the patient choice was 55 per cent HD to 45 per cent PD. The patients actually starting RRT modality were 70 : 30 in favour of HD. Patients are frequently not given the choice and the physician makes the choice for them (Wuerth *et al.* 2002). In the United Kingdom, the initial choice of therapy was 55 : 45 HD versus PD when patients were given free choice of therapy and completely informed (Little *et al.* 2001). A recent United States multivariate analysis in 4025 patients (1996–1997) showed that selection of PD over HD was associated with lower age, white race, and fewer comorbid conditions. There was greater use of PD in employed, married subjects and those who are independent and educated. Earlier referral (>4 months) led to greater use of PD (Stack 2002).

Time of referral is another important determinant of modality use. Patients who are referred late are more likely to start HD immediately and remain on it (Lameire *et al.* 1997).

PD is a cheaper dialysis option than maintenance HD (Peeters *et al.* 2000). Dialysis programmes should encourage this home therapy (De Vecchi *et al.* 1999; Peeters *et al.* 2000; Lee *et al.* 2002; Sennfalt *et al.* 2002). In a cost–utility analysis, the cost per quality-adjusted life year was lower for PD as compared to HD by a factor of 12–31 per cent (age dependent) even though there was no difference in survival or transplantation rates (Sennfalt *et al.* 2002). In the developing world, the picture is different. Here the socioeconomic circumstances vary, as do government reimbursement policies for RRT (Correa-Rotter 2001). Treatment rates correlate with the gross national product and the choice of modality is highly influenced by factors other than the medical needs of the patient, especially the availability of staff and resources.

Current usage of peritoneal dialysis

The number of patients on dialysis worldwide at the end of 2002 is over a million. Of these, 13 per cent are managed by PD, the growth of which is steady but declining in some Western countries. Use in Asian countries is variable and heavily dependent on economic and non-medical factors (Wang *et al.* 2002) and survival figures are good despite the lower clearance achieved (Lo *et al.* 1996). The decline in the use of PD in some developed countries (Oreopoulos and Tzamaloukas 2000) is

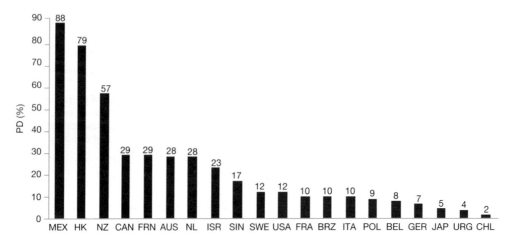

Fig. 21 PD utilization in various countries worldwide (from USRDS data 1999).

explained by physician bias, financial incentives, and late referral. In the United States, studies have shown that training of nephrologists in PD is inadequate, so they are less likely to suggest this option when in clinical practice (Mehrotra *et al.* 2002).

Future strategies

Existing PD solutions were formulated simply for the maintenance of fluid and electrolyte balance, removal of metabolic waste, and correction of acidosis. Recent emphasis has been on improving their biocompatibility to maintain peritoneal membrane integrity and, thereby, improve long-term outcomes (Holmes and Shockley 2000). Additives (procysteine, sulodexide) may help to maintain peritoneal function and enhance adequacy (hyaluron, atrial naturetic peptide) (Gokal 2002). Automation will increase with dialysate regeneration and the use of on-line systems to create mixed PD solutions prescribed to provide not only toxin and fluid removal but also nutritional and other clinical support (Roberts *et al.* 1999).

Molecular genetic approaches, by which the use of genetically modified mesothelium will be used to deliver potentially therapeutic recombinant proteins that might serve to preserve or improve the performance of the peritoneal membrane in long-term PD are possible (Nagy and Jackman 2000). The ability to genetically modify the peritoneal mesothelium by *ex vivo* and *in vivo* strategies demonstrates that the peritoneum is a modifiable membrane. This suggests that it may be possible to preserve or enhance the performance and integrity of the membrane for long-term use.

References

Abu-Alfa, A. K. *et al.* (2002). Approach to fluid management in peritoneal dialysis: a practical algorithm. *Kidney International* **62** (Suppl. 81), S8–S16.

Afthentopoulos, I. E. *et al.* (1998). Sclerosing peritonitis in CAPD patients: one centre's experience and review of the literature. *Advances in Renal Replacement Therapy* **5**, 157–167.

Aguilera, A. *et al.* (2001). *Helicobacter pylori* infection: a new cause of anorexia in peritoneal dialysis patients. *Peritoneal Dialysis International* **20** (Suppl. 3), S152–S156.

An, S. *et al.* (2001). Glucotoxicity of the peritoneal membrane: the case for VEGF. *Nephrology, Dialysis, Transplantation* **16**, 2299–2302.

Annigeri, R. *et al.* (2001). Emergence of mupirocin-resistant *Staphylococcus aureus* in chronic peritoneal dialysis patients using mupirocin prophylaxis to prevent exit-site infections. *Peritoneal Dialysis International* **21**, 554–559.

Anwar, N. *et al.* (1993). Serum liopoprotein (a) concentrations in patients undergoing CAPD. *Nephrology, Dialysis, Transplantation* **8**, 71–74.

Ash, S. Peritoneal access devices and placement techniques. In *Dialysis Therapy* (ed. A. M. Nissenson and R. N. Fine), pp. 23–30. New York: Hanely and Belfus, 1993.

Ash, S. R. (1990). Chronic peritoneal dialysis catheters: effects of catheter design, materials and location. *Seminars in Dialysis* **3**, 39–46.

Ash, S. R. *et al.* (2002). Clinical trials of the T-fluted (Ash Advantage) peritoneal dialysis catheter. *Seminars in Dialysis* **9**, 133–143.

Ates, K. *et al.* (2001). Effect of fluid and sodium removal on mortality in peritoneal dialysis patients. *Kidney International* **60**, 767–776.

Baker, R. J. *et al.* (2003). Emperical aminoglycosides for peritonitis do not affect residual renal function. *American Journal of Kidney Diseases* **41**, 670–675.

Bakewell, A. R. *et al.* (2002). Quality of life in peritoneal dialysis patients: decline over time and association with clinical outcomes. *Kidney International* **61**, 239–248.

Bargman, J. Non-infectious complications of peritoneal dialysis. In *Textbook of Peritoneal Dialysis* (ed. R. Gokal *et al.*), pp. 609–646. Dordrecht: Kluwer Academic, 2000.

Bargman, J. *et al.* (2001). Relative contribution of residual renal function and peritoneal clearance on adequacy of dialysis: a reanalysis of the CANUSA Study. *Journal of the American Society of Nephrology* **12**, 2158–2162.

Bernardini, J., Nagy, M., and Piraino, B. (2000). Pattern of non-compliance with dialysis exchanges in peritoneal dialysis patients. *American Journal of Kidney Diseases* **35**, 1104–1110.

Bernardini, J. *et al.* (1996). Randomised trial of *Staph. aureus* prophylaxis in PD patients: mupirocin calcium ointment 2% applied to the exit site versus oral rifampin. *American Journal of Kidney Diseases* **26**, 695–700.

Bhaskaran, S. *et al.* (2000). The effect of small solute clearances on survival of anuric peritoneal dialysis patients. *Peritoneal Dialysis International* **20**, 181–187.

Bianchi, G. (2000). Hypertension in chronic renal failure and end stage renal disease patients treated with haemodialysis and peritoneal dialysis. *Nephrology, Dialysis, Transplantation* **15** (Suppl. 5), 105–110.

Blake, P. *et al.* (1991). Lack of correlation between urea kinetic indices and clinical outcomes in CAPD patients. *Kidney International* **39**, 700–706.

Bleyer, A. *et al.* (1999). Dialysis modality and delayed graft function after cadaveric renal transplantation. *Journal of the American Society of Nephrology* **10**, 154–159.

Bloembergen, W. *et al.* (1995). Comparison of mortality in prevalent HD and PD treated dialysis patients. *Journal of the American Society of Nephrology* **6**, 177–183.

Blumenkrantz, M. *et al.* (1982). Metabolic balance studies and dietary protein requirements in CAPD. *Kidney International* **21**, 849–858.

Boen, S. T., Mulinari, A. S., Dillard, D. N., and Scribner, B. N. (1962). Periodic peritoneal dialysis in the management of chronic uraemia. *Transactions of the American Society of Artificial Internal Organs* **8**, 256–258.

Brandes, J. E., Piering, W. F., and Beres, J. A. (1992). Clinical outcome of CAPD by urea and creatinine kinetics. *Journal of the American Society of Nephrology* **2**, 1430–1435.

Brown, A. L. *et al.* (1989). Multiple episodes of coagulase-negative staphylococcal CAPD peritonitis—reinfection or relapse. *Nephrology, Dialysis, Transplantation* **4**, 493–496.

Brown, E. A. *et al.* (2001). Adequacy targets can be met in anuric patients by automated peritoneal dialysis: baseline data from EAPOS. *Peritoneal Dialysis International* **21** (Suppl. 3), S133–S137.

Brown, E. A. *et al.* (2003). Survival of functionally anuric patients on APD: the European APD Outcome Study. *Journal of the American Society of Nephrology* **14**, 2948–2957.

Bunke, M. *et al.* (1994). Culture negative CAPD peritonitis: the Network 9 study. *Advances in Peritoneal Dialysis* **10**, 174–178.

Buoncristiani, C. *et al.* (1980). A new safe simple connection system for CAPD. *International Journal of Urology and Nephrology* **1**, 45–50.

Cameron, J. L. *et al.* (2000). Differences in quality of life across renal replacement therapies: a meta-analytic comparison. *American Journal of Kidney Diseases* **35**, 629–637.

Casey, M. *et al.* (2000). Application of mupirocin cream at the catheter exit site reduces exit-site infections and peritonitis in peritoneal dialysis patients. *Peritoneal Dialysis International* **20**, 566–568.

Centres for Disease Control (1997). *Staphylococcus aureus* with reduced susceptibility to vancomycin: United States. *Morbidity and Mortality Weekly Report* **46**, 765–766.

Chatoth, D. K., Golper, T. A., and Gokal, R. (1999). Morbidity and mortality in redefining adequacy of peritoneal dialysis: a step beyond NKF-DOQI. *American Journal of Kidney Diseases* **33**, 617–632.

Chung, S. H. *et al.* (2000). Peritoneal transport characteristics, comorbid diseases and survival in CAPD patients. *Peritoneal Dialysis International* **20**, 541–547.

Churchill, D. N. *et al.* (1988). Peritonitis in CAPD patients: a randomised trial of cotrimoxazole prophylaxis. *Peritoneal Dialysis International* **8**, 125–128.

Churchill, D. N. *et al.* (1996). Adequacy of dialysis and nutrition in CAPD: association with clinical outcomes. *Journal of the American Society of Nephrology* 7, 198–207.

Churchill, D. N. *et al.* (1998). Increased peritoneal membrane transport is associated with decreased patient and technique survival for continuous peritoneal dialysis patients. *Journal of the American Society of Nephrology* 9, 1285–1293.

Churchill, D. N. *et al.* (1999). Clinical practice guidelines for dialysis. Canadian Society of nephrology. *Journal of the American Society of Nephrology* 13 (Suppl. 10), S289–S291.

Cocchi, R. *et al.* (1999). Prevalence of hypertension in patients on peritoneal dialysis: results of an Italian multicentre study. *Nephrology, Dialysis, Transplantation* 14, 1536–1540.

Coles, G. (1999). Biocompatibility and new fluids. *Peritoneal Dialysis International* 19 (Suppl. 2), S267–S270.

Coles, G. and Williams, J. (1998). What is the place of peritoneal dialysis in the integrated treatment of renal failure? *Kidney International* 54, 2234–2240.

Coles, G. A. *et al.* (1997). A randomised controlled trial of a bicarbonate- and bicarbonate/lactate-containing peritoneal dialysis solution. *Peritoneal Dialysis International* 17, 48–51.

Coles, G. A. *et al.* (1998). A controlled trial of two bicarbonate-containing fluids for CAPD—final report. *Nephrology, Dialysis, Transplantation* 13, 3165–3171.

Collins, A. J. *et al.* (1999). Mortality risks of peritoneal and hemodialysis. *American Journal of Kidney Diseases* 34, 1065–1074.

Collins, A. J. *et al.* (2002). Comparison and survival of hemodialysis and peritoneal dialysis in the elderly. *Seminars in Dialysis* 15, 98–102.

Combet, S., Miyata, T., Moulin, P., Pouthier, D., Goffin, E., and Devuyst, O. (2000). Vascular proliferation and enhanced expression of endothelial nitric oxide synthase in human peritoneum exposed to long-term peritoneal dialysis. *Journal of the American Society of Nephrology* 11, 717–728.

Correa-Rotter, R. (2001). The cost barrier to renal replacement therapy and peritoneal dialysis in the developing world. *Peritoneal Dialysis International* 21 (Suppl. 3), S314–S317.

Cruz, C. (1994). Cruz catheters: implantation technique and clinical results. *Peritoneal Dialysis International* 14 (Suppl. 3), S59–S62.

Cunningham, J. *et al.* (1992). Dialysate calcium reduction in CAPD patients treated with calcium carbonate and alfacalcidol. *Nephrology, Dialysis, Transplantation* 7, 63–68.

Danielsson, A. *et al.* (2002). A prospective randomised study of the effect of a subcutaneously 'buried' peritoneal dialysis catheter technique versus standard technique on the incidence of peritonitis and exit-site infections. *Peritoneal Dialysis International* 22, 211–219.

Dasgupta, M. K. and Larabie, M. (2001). Biofilms in peritoneal dialysis. *Peritoneal Dialysis International* 21 (Suppl. 3), S213–217.

Dasgupta, M. K. *et al.* (1987). Relationship of adherent bacterial bio films to peritonitis in CAPD. *Peritoneal Dialysis Bulletin* 7, 168–173.

Davey, P. *et al.* (1999). Cost-effectiveness of prophylactic nasal mupirocin in patients undergoing peritoneal dialysis based on a randomised, placebo-controlled trial. *Journal of Antimicrobial Chemotherapy* 43, 105–112.

Davies, S. J. (2000). Peritoneal solute transport—we know it is important, but what is it? *Nephrology, Dialysis, Transplantation* 15, 1120–1123.

Davies, S. J., Bryan, J., Phillips, L., and Russell, G. I. (1996). Longitudinal changes in peritoneal kinetics: the effects of peritoneal dialysis and peritonitis. *Nephrology, Dialysis, Transplantation* 11, 495–506.

Davies, S. J., Phillips, L., Naish, P. F., and Russell, G. I. (2001). Peritoneal glucose exposure and change in membrane transport with time on peritoneal dialysis. *Journal of the American Society of Nephrology* 12, 1046–1051.

Davies, S. J. *et al.* (1998). What really happens to people on long-term peritoneal dialysis? *Kidney International* 54, 2207–2217.

Davies, S. J. *et al.* (2000). Analysis of the effect of increasing delivered dialysis treatment to malnourished peritoneal dialysis patients. *Kidney International* 57, 1743–1754.

Davies, S. J. *et al.* (2003). Icodextrin improves the fluid status of peritoneal dialysis patients: result of a randomized double blind controlled trial. *Journal of the American Society of Nephrology* 14, 2338–2344.

Dawney, A. and Millar, D. (1997). Glycation and advanced glycation end-product formation with icodextrin and dextrose. *Peritoneal Dialysis International* 17, 52–58.

DeAlvaro, F. *et al.* (1992). Adequacy of peritoneal dialysis: does KKT/V have the same predictor value as in HD? Multicentre study. *Advances in Peritoneal Dialysis* 8, 93–97.

De Fijter, C. W. *et al.* (2001). Intraperitoneal ciprofloxacin and rifampicin versus cephradine as initial treatment of (C)APD-related peritonitis: a prospective randomized multicenter comparison (CIPPER trial). *Peritoneal Dialysis International* 21, 480–486.

De Vecchi, A. F., Dratwa, M., and Wiedermann, M. E. (1999). Healthcare systems and end-stage renal disease (ESRD therapies—an international review: costs and reimbursement/funding of ESRD therapies. *Nephrology, Dialysis, Transplantation* 14 (Suppl. 6), 31–41.

Devuyst, O. (2002). New insights in the molecular mechanisms regulating peritoneal permeability. *Nephrology, Dialysis, Transplantation* 17, 548–551.

Diaz-Buxo, J. A. (1989). Current status of continuous cyclic peritoneal dialysis (CCPD). 9, 9–14.

Diaz-Buxo, J. A. and Suki, W. N. Automated peritoneal dialysis. In *Textbook of Peritoneal Dialysis* (ed. R. Gokal and K. D. Nolph), pp. 399–418. Dordrecht: Kluwer Academic, 1994.

Diaz-Buxo, J. A., Crawford, T. L., and Bailie, J. R. (2001). Peritonitis in automated peritoneal dialysis: antibiotic therapy and pharmakokinetics. *Peritoneal Dialysis International* 21 (Suppl. 3), S197–S201.

Diaz-Buxo, J. A. *et al.* (1999). Peritoneal dialysis adequacy: a model to assess feasibility with various modalities. *Kidney International* 55, 2493–2501.

di Paolo, N. and Sacchi, G. (2000). Atlas of peritoneal histology in normal conditions and during peritoneal dialysis. *Peritoneal Dialysis International* 20 (Suppl. 3), S3–S100.

di Paolo, N. *et al.* (1986). Phosphatidylcholine and peritoneal transport during peritoneal dialysis. *Nephron* 44, 365–370.

Dobbie, J. W. (1992). Pathogenesis of pertioneal fibrosing syndrome (sclerosing peritonitis) in peritoneal dialysis. *Peritoneal Dialysis International* 12, 14–27.

Dobbie, J. W. and Lloyd, J. K. (1989). Mesothelium secretes lamellar bodies in a similar manner to type II pneumocytes secretion of surfactant. *Peritoneal Dialysis International* 9, 215–219.

Dobbie, J. W., Anderson, J. D., and Hind, C. (1994). Long-term effects of peritoneal dialysis on peritoneal morphology. *Peritoneal Dialysis International* 14 (Suppl. 3), 16–20.

Dobbie, J. W., Pavlina, T., Lloyd, J., and Johnson, R. C. (1988). Phosphatidylcholine synthesis by peritoneal mesothelium: its implications for peritoneal dialysis. *American Journal of Kidney Diseases* 12, 31–36.

Dobrashian, R. D. *et al.* (1999). The repositioning of migrated Tenchkoff CAPD catheters under fluoroscopic control. *British Journal of Radiology* 72, 452–456.

EDTA-ERA (2004). European Practice Guidelines on peritoneal dialysis. *Nephrology, Dialysis, Transplantation* (in press).

Eklund, B. H., Honkanes, E. O., Kala, A., and Kyllonen, L. (1994). Catheter configuration and outcome in patients on CAPD: a prospective comparison of two catheters. *Peritoneal Dialysis International* 14, 70–74.

Enoch, R., Aslam, N., and Piraino, B. (2002). Intra-abdominal pressure, peritoneal dialysis exchange volume and tolerance in APD. *Seminars in Dialysis* 15, 403–406.

Fenton, S. S. A. *et al.* (1997). Hemodialysis versus peritoneal dialysis: a comparison of adjusted mortality rates. *American Journal of Kidney Diseases* 30, 334–342.

Fielding, R. E. *et al.* (2002). Treatment and outcome of peritonitis in automated peritoneal dialysis, using a once-daily cefazolin-based regimen. *Peritoneal Dialysis International* 22, 345–349.

Finkelstein, E. S. *et al.* (2002). Patterns of infection in patients maintained on long-term peritoneal dialysis therapy with multiple episodes of peritonitis. *American Journal of Kidney Diseases* 39, 1278–1286.

Flessner, M. F. and Schwab, A. (1996). Pressure threshold for fluid loss from the peritoneal cavity. *American Journal of Physiology* **270**, F377–F390.

Flessner, M. F., Dedrick, R. L., and Schulz, J. S. (1984). A distributed model of peritoneal plasma transport: theoretical considerations. *American Journal of Physiology* **246**, 597–607.

Foley, R. *et al.* (1998). Mode of dialysis therapy and mortality in end stage renal disease. *Journal of the American Society of Nephrology* **9**, 267–276.

Fuholler, A., Nieden, S. R., Grabensee, B., and Plum, J. (2002). Peritoneal fluid and solute transport: influence of treatment time, peritoneal dialysis modality and peritonitis incidence. *Journal of the American Society of Nephrology* **13**, 1055–1060.

Ganter, G. (1923). Uber die Beseitigung giftiger Stoffeausdem Blute Durch Dialyse. *Muenchener Medizinische Wochenschrift* **70**, 1478–1480.

Gokal, R. (1999a). Fluid management and cardiovascular outcome in peritoneal dialysis patients. *Seminars in Dialysis* **12**, 126–132.

Gokal, R. (1999b). Taking peritoneal dialysis beyond the year 2000. *Peritoneal Dialysis International* **19** (Suppl. 3), S35–S42.

Gokal, R. (2000). Peritoneal dialysis: prevention and control of infection. *Drugs and Ageing* **17**, 269–282.

Gokal, R. (2002). Icodextrin associated sterile peritonitis. *Peritoneal Dialysis International* **22**, 445–448.

Gokal, R. and Oreopoulos, D. G. (1996). Is long-term technique survival on CAPD possible? *Peritoneal Dialysis International* **16**, 553–555.

Gokal, R., Ramos, J., Ward, M. K., and Kerr, D. N. S. (1981). Eosinophilic peritonitis in CAPD. *Clinical Nephrology* **15**, 328–330.

Gokal, R. *et al.* (1995). Peritonitis occurrence in a multicentre study of icodextrin and glucose in CAPD. *Peritoneal Dialysis International* **15**, 226–230.

Gokal, R. *et al.* (1998). Peritoneal catheters and exit-site practices towards optimum peritoneal access: 1998 update. *Peritoneal Dialysis International* **18**, 11–33.

Gokal, R. *et al.* (1999). Outcomes in peritoneal dialysis and haemodialysis—a comparative assessment of survival and quality of life. *Nephrology, Dialysis, Transplantation* **14** (Suppl. 6), 24–30.

Gokal, R. *et al.* (2002). Metabolic and laboratory effects of icodextrin. *Kidney International* **62** (Suppl. 81), S62–S71.

Goldberg, L. *et al.* (2001). Initial treatment of peritoneal dialysis peritonitis without vancomycin with a once daily cefazolin-based regimen. *American Journal of Kidney Diseases* **37**, 49–55.

Golper, T. A. *et al.* (1996). Risk factors for peritonitis in long-term peritoneal dialysis: the Network 9 peritonitis and catheter survival studies. *American Journal of Kidney Diseases* **28**, 428–436.

Gotloib, L. and Shustack, A. (1987). Ultrastructural morphology of the peritoneum: new findings and speculations on transfer of solutes and water during peritoneal dialysis. *Peritoneal Dialysis Bulletin* **7**, 119–129.

Gunal, A. I. *et al.* (2001). Strict volume control normalises hypertension in peritoneal dialysis pateints. *American Journal of Kidney Diseases* **37**, 588–593.

Habach, G., Bloembergen, W., Manger, E., Wolfe, R., and Port, F. (1995). Hospitalisation among United States dialysis patients: haemodialysis versus peritoneal dialysis. *Journal of the American Society of Nephrology* **5**, 1940–1948.

Harris, S. A. *et al.* (2002). Clinical outcomes and quality of life in elderly patients on peritoneal dialysis versus hemodialysis. *Peritoneal Dialysis International* **22**, 463–470.

Harty, J. and Gokal, R. (1995). Nutritional status in peritoneal dialysis. *Journal of Renal Nutrition* **5**, 2–10.

Harty, J., Venning, M., and Gokal, R. (1995a). Dialysis adequacy and nutritional status in CAPD—is there a link? *Seminars in Dialysis* **8**, 62–67.

Harty, J. *et al.* (1995b). Limitations of the peritoneal equilibration test in prescribing and monitoring dialysis therapy. *Nephrology, Dialysis, Transplantation* **10**, 252–257.

Harty, J. *et al.* (1996a). The influence of small solute clearance on dietary protein intake in CAPD patients: a methodological analysis based on cross-sectional and prospective studies. *American Journal of Kidney Diseases* **28**, 553–560.

Harty, J. *et al.* (1996b). Is peritoneal permeability an adverse risk factor for malnutrition in CAPD patients? *Mineral Electrolyte Metabolism* **22**, 97–101.

Harty, J. *et al.* (1997). Impact of increasing dialysis volume on adequacy targets: a prospective study. *Journal of the American Society of Nephrology* **8**, 1304–1310.

Harty, J. C. *et al.* (1993). Limitations of kinetic models as predictors of nutritional and dialysis adequacy in CAPD. *American Journal of Nephrology* **13**, 454–463.

Harty, J. C. *et al.* (1994). The normalised protein catabolic rate is a flawed marker of nutrition in CAPD patients. *Kidney International* **45**, 103–109.

Heaf, J. G. *et al.* (2002). Initial survival advantage of peritoneal dialysis relative to haemodialysis. *Nephrology, Dialysis, Transplantation* **17**, 112–117.

Heimburger, O., Wanewski, J., Wereynsha, A., Traenus, A., and Lindholm, B. (1990). Peritoneal transport in CAPD patients with permanent loss of ultrafiltration capacity. *Kidney International* **38**, 495–506.

Heimburger, O. *et al.* (1995). Lymphatic absorption in CAPD patients with loss of ultrafiltration capacity. *Blood Purification* **13**, 327–339.

Hendriks, P. M. *et al.* (1997). Peritoneal sclerosis in chronic peritoneal dialysis patients: analysis of clinical presentation, risk factors, and peritoneal transport kinetics. *Peritoneal Dialysis International* **17**, 136–143.

Ho-dac-Pannekeet, M. M., Hiralall, J. K., Sruijk, D. G., and Krediet, R. T. (1997a). Longitudinal follow-up of CA125 in peritoneal effluent. *Kidney International* **51**, 888–893.

Ho-dac-Pannekeet, M. M., Atasever, B., Struik, D., and Krediet, R. T. (1997b). Analysis of ultrafiltration failure in peritoneal dialysis patients by means of standard peritoneal permeability analysis. *Peritoneal Dialysis International* **17**, 144–150.

Ho-dac-Pannekett, M. M. *et al.* (1996). Peritoneal transport characteristic with glucose polymer based dialysate. *Kidney International* **50**, 974–986.

Holley, J. L. *et al.* (1994). Infecting organisms in CAPD patients on the Y set. *American Journal of Kidney Diseases* **23**, 569–573.

Holmes, C. J. and Shockley, T. R. (2000). Strategies to reduce glucose exposure in peritoneal dialysis patients. *Peritoneal Dialysis International* **20** (Suppl. 2), S37–S41.

Honda, K., Nitta, K., Yamara, S., and Nikei, W. (1996). Morphological changes in the peritoneal vasculature of patients on CAPD with ultrafiltration failure. *Nephron* **72**, 171–176.

Honda, K. *et al.* (1999). Accumulation of advanced glycation end products in the vasculature of CAPD patients with low ultra-filtration. *Nephrology, Dialysis, Transplantation* **14**, 1541–1549.

Horl, W. H., de Alvaro, F., and Williams, P. F. (1999). Healthcare systems and end-stage renal disease (ESRD) therapies—an international review: access to ESRD treatments. *Nephrology, Dialysis, Transplantation* **14** (Suppl. 6), 10–15.

Hussain, S. I., Bernardini, J., and Piraino, B. (1998). The risk of hernia with large exchange volumes. *Advances in Peritoneal Dialysis* **14**, 105–107.

Hutchison, A. Calcium, phosphate and renal osteodystrophy. In *Textbook of Peritoneal Dialysis* (ed. R. Gokal *et al.*), pp. 585–608. Dordrecht: Kluwer Academic, 2000.

Hutchison, A. J., Freemont, A. J., Boulton, H. F., and Gokal, R. (1992). Low calcium dialysis fluid and oral calcium carbonate in CAPD. A method of controlling hypophosphataemia whilst minimising aluminium exposure and hypercalcaemia. *Nephrology, Dialysis, Transplantation* **7**, 1219–1225.

Hutchison, A. *et al.* (1993). Correlation of bone histology with PTH, vitamin D and radiology in endstage renal disease. *Kidney International* **44**, 1071–1077.

Jager, K. J. *et al.* (2001a). Nutritional status over time in hemodialysis and peritoneal dialysis. *Journal of the American Society of Nephrology* **12**, 1272–1279.

Jager, K. J. *et al.* (2001b). What happens to patients starting dialysis in the Netherlands? *Netherland Journal of Medicine* **58**, 163–173.

Jones, C. H. *et al.* (1999). Fasting plasma amino acids are not normalised by 12-month amino-acid-based dialysate in CAPD patients. *Peritoneal Dialysis International* **19**, 174–177.

Jones, M. R. (1994). Etiology of severe malnutrition: results of an international cross sectional study in CAPD patients. *American Journal of Kidney Diseases* **23**, 412–420.

Jones, M. R. et al. (1998). Treatment of malnutrition with 1.1 per cent aminoacid peritoneal dialysis solution: results of a multicentre outpatient study. American Journal of Kidney Diseases 32, 761–769.

Kallen, R. J. (1966). A method for approximating the efficacy of peritoneal dialysis for uraemia. American Journal of Disease in Childhood 3, 156–160.

Kara, T. and Somers, V. K. (2002). Therapeutic strategies for orthostatic intolerance: mechanisms, observations, and making patients feel better. American Journal of Medicine 112, 419–421.

Kaur, D., Williams, J. D., Phillips, A. O., and Topley, N. (1997). Improved cell function in pyruvate-buffered peritoneal dialysis fluids is related to specific antagonism of the polyol pathway. Journal of the American Society of Nephrology 8, 266A.

Kawaguchi, Y. (1999a). Peritoneal dialysis as long-term treatment: comparison of technique survival between Asian and Western populations. Peritoneal Dialysis International 19 (Suppl. 2), S327–S328.

Kawaguchi, Y. (1999b). National comparisons: optimal peritoneal dialysis outcomes among Japanese patients. Peritoneal Dialysis International 19 (Suppl. 2), S9–S16.

Kawaguchi, Y. et al. (2000). Encapsulating peritoneal sclerosis: definition, etiology, diagnosis, and treatment. Peritoneal Dialysis International 20 (Suppl. 4), S43–S55.

Keane, W. F., Everett, E. D., Fine, R. N., Golper, T. A., Vas, S. I., and Peterson, P. K. (1987). CAPD related peritonitis management and antibiotic therapy recommendations. Peritoneal Dialysis Bulletin 7, 55–68.

Keane, W. F. et al. (1993). CAPD peritonitis treatment recommendations 1993 update. Peritoneal Dialysis International 13, 247–256.

Keane, W. F. et al. (2000). Adult peritoneal dialysis-related peritonitis treatment recommendations. Peritoneal Dialysis International 20, 396–411.

Keshaviah, P. R., Nolph, K. D., and Ban Stone, J. C. (1989). The peak concentrations hypothesis: a urea kinetic approach to comparing the adequacy of CAPD and haemodialysis. Peritoneal Dialysis International 9, 257–266.

Kim, H. J. et al. (2002). Use of fluoroscopy-guided wire manipulation and/or laparoscopic surgery in the repair of malfunctioning peritoneal dialysis catheters. American Journal of Nephrology 22, 532–538.

Kondo, T. et al. (1997). ERM-based molecular mechanism of microvillar breakdown at an early stage of apoptosis. Journal of Cell Biology 139, 749–758.

Koomen, G. C. M. et al. (1994). Dialysate cancer antigen (CA) 125 is a reflection of the peritoneal mesothelial mass in CAPD patients. Peritoneal Dialysis International 14, 132–136.

Kopple, J. D. et al. (1995). Treatment of malnourished CAPD patients with an amino acid based dialysate. Kidney International 47, 1148–1157.

Krediet, R. (1999). The peritoneal membrane in chronic peritoneal dialysis. Kidney International 55, 341–356.

Krediet, R. and Mujais, S. (2002). Use of icodextrin in high transport ultrafiltration failure. Kidney International 62 (Suppl. 81), S53–S61.

Krediet, R., Lindholm, B., and Rippe, B. (2000). Pathophysiology of peritoneal membrane failure. Peritoneal Dialysis International 20 (Suppl. 4), S22–S42.

Lai, K. N. et al. (1997a). Dialysate cell population and cancer antigen 125 in stable CAPD patients: their relationship with transport parameters. American Journal of Kidney Diseases 29, 699–705.

Lai, K. N. et al. (1997b). Intraperitoneal once-daily dose of cefazolin and gentamicin for treating CAPD peritonits. Peritoneal Dialysis International 17, 87–89.

Lai, K. N. et al. (2002). Expression of aquaporin 3 in human peritoneal mesothelial cells and its up-regulation by glucose in vitro. Kidney International 62, 1431–1439.

Lamiere, N. et al. (1997). The referral pattern of patients with ESRD is a determinant in the choice of dialysis modality. Peritoneal Dialysis International 17 (Suppl. 2), S161–S166.

Lamperi, S., Carozzi, S., and Nasilni, M. G. Intraperitoneal immunoglobulin treatment in prophylaxis of bacterial peritonitis in CAPD. In Advances in

CAPD 1986 (ed. R. Khanna et al.), pp. 110–113. Toronto: Peritoneal Dialysis Bulletin, Inc., 1986.

Lee, H. et al. (2002). Cost analysis of ongoing care of patients with end-stage renal disease: the impact of dialysis modality and dialysis access. American Journal of Kidney Diseases 40, 611–622.

Lee, M. and Donovan, J. F. (2002). Laparoscopic omentectomy for salvage of peritoneal dialysis catheters. Journal of Endourology 16, 241–244.

Lee, S. et al. (1995). Successful treatment of fungal peritonitis with intracatheter anti-fungal retention. Advances in Peritoneal Dialysis 11, 172–175.

Letherland, J., Gibson, M., and Banbrook, P. (1992). Investigations and treatment of poor drains of dialysate fluid associated with anterior abdominal leaks in CAPD patients. Nephrology, Dialysis, Transplantation 7, 1030–1034.

Lewis, D. M. et al. (1998). Polypropylene mesh hernia repair—an alternative permitting rapid return to peritoneal dialysis. Nephrology, Dialysis, Transplantation 13, 2488–2489.

Leypoldt, J. K. (2002). Solute transport across the peritoneal membrane. Journal of the American Society of Nephrology 13 (Suppl. 1), S84–S91.

Little, J. et al. (2001). Predicting a patient's choice of dialysis modality: experience in a UK renal department. American Journal of Kidney Diseases 37, 981–986.

Lo, W. K. et al. (1994). Changes in the peritoneal equilibration test in selected chronic peritoneal dialysis patients. Journal of the American Society of Nephrology 4, 1466–1474.

Lo, W. K. et al. (1996). Survival of CAPD patients in a center using 3 two-litre exchanges as standard regime. Peritoneal Dialysis International 16 (Suppl. 1), S163–S166.

Lo, W. K. et al. (2003). Effect of Kt/V on survival and clinical outcome in CAPD patients in a randomised prospective study. Kidney International 64, 649–656.

Lupo, A. et al. (1994). Longterm outcome in CAPD: a 10 year survey by the Italian Co-operative PD Study Group. American Journal of Kidney Diseases 24, 826–837.

Luzar, M. A. et al. (1990). Staphylococcus aureus nasal carriage and infection in patients on CAPD. New England Journal of Medicine 322, 505–509.

Mactier, R. A. and Khanna, R. Peritoneal lymphatics. In Textbook of Peritoneal Dialysis (ed. R. Gokal et al.), pp. 173–192. Dordrecht: Kluwer Academic, 2000.

Mactier, R. et al. (1998). Treatment of infusion pain by bicarbonate and bicarbonate/lactate containing PD solutions. Kidney International 53, 1061–1067.

Maiorca, R. and Cancarini, G. C. Outcome with peritoneal dialysis compared to haemodialysis. In The Textbook of Peritoneal Dialysis (ed. R. Gokal et al.), pp. 755–783. Dordrecht: Kluwer Academic, 2000.

Maiorca, R. et al. (1983). Prospective controlled trial of Y connector and disinfectant in CAPD. Lancet ii, 642–645.

Maiorca, R. et al. (1991). A multi-centre selection adjusted comparison of patient and technique survival on CAPD and hemodialysis. Peritoneal Dialysis International 11, 118–127.

Maiorca, R. et al. (1995). Predictive value of dialysis adequacy and nutritional indices for mortality and morbidity in CAPD and HD patients: a longitudinal study. Nephrology, Dialysis, Transplantation 10, 2255–2305.

Maiorca, R. et al. (1996). CAPD viability: a long-term comparison with hemodialysis. Peritoneal Dialysis International 16, 276–287.

Martis. L., Topley, N., and Holmes, C. J. Conventional and newer peritoneal dialysis solutions. In Dialysis and Transplantation: a Companion to Brenner and Rector's The Kidney (ed. W. F. Owen, J. G. Pereira, and M. H. Sayegh), pp. 179–198. Philadelphia, PA: W.B. Saunders, 2000.

Mateijsen, M. A. M. et al. (1999). Vascular and interstitial changes in the peritoneum of CAPD patients with peritoneal sclerosis. Peritoneal Dialysis International 19, 517–525.

Maxwell, M. N., Rockney, R. E., Kleeman, C. R., and Twiss, M. R. (1959). Peritoneal dialysis. 1. Technique and application. Journal of the American Medical Association 170, 917–924.

Mayo, R. R. *et al.* (1995). Pseudomonas peritonitis treated with simultaneous catéter replacement and removal. *Peritoneal Dialysis International* 15, 389–390.

Mehrotra, R. *et al.* (2002). An analysis of dialysis training in the United States and Canada. *American Journal of Kidney Diseases* 40, 152–160.

Mellor, J., Sahlmann, C. O., and Becker, W. (2002). Nuclear medicine studies in the dialysis patient. *Seminars in Dialysis* 15, 269–276.

Misra, M. *et al.* (1997). Six-month prospective cross-over study to determine the effects of 1.1% amino acid dialysate on lipid metabolism in patients on CAPD. *Peritoneal Dialysis International* 17, 279–286.

Mistry, C. D. and Gokal, R. (1994). Icodextrin in peritoneal dialysis. *Peritoneal Dialysis International* 14 (Suppl. 2), S13–S21.

Mistry, C. D., Mallick, N. P., and Gokal, R. (1987). Ultrafiltration with an isosmotic solution during long peritoneal dialysis exchanges. *Lancet* ii, 178–182.

Mistry, C. D., Gokal, R., peers, and the MIDAS Study Group (1994). A randomised mutlicentre clinical trial comparing isosmolar Icodextrin with hyperosmolar glucose solutions in CAPD. *Kidney International* 46, 496–503.

Miyata, T. *et al.* (2002). Towards better dialysis compatibility: advances in the biochemistry and pathophysiology of the peritoneal membranes. *Kidney International* 61, 375–386.

Moist, L. M. *et al.* (2000). Predictors of loss of residual renal function among new dialysis patients. *Journal of the American Society of Nephrology* 11, 556–564.

Moncrief, J. W. and Popovich, P. P. (1994). Moncrief/Popovich catheter: implantation techniques and clinical results. *Peritoneal Dialysis International* 14 (Suppl. 3), S56–S58.

Mujais, S. *et al.* (2000). Evaluation and management of ultrafiltration problems in peritoneal dialysis. *Peritoneal Dialysis International* 20 (Suppl. 4), S5–S21.

Mupirocin Study Group (1996). Nasal mupirocin prevents *S. aureus* exit site infection during peritoneal dialysis. *Journal of the American Society of Nephrology* 7, 2403–2408.

Murphy, S. W. *et al.* (2000). Comparative mortality of hemodialysis and peritoneal dialysis in Canada. *Kidney International* 57, 1720–1726.

Nagy, J. A. and Jackman, R. W. Peritoneal membrane biology. In *Dialysis and Transplantation* (ed. W. F. Owen, B. Pereira, and M. H. Sayegh), pp. 109–128. Philadelphia, PA: W.B. Saunders, 2000.

Nakamoto, H. *et al.* (2002). Encapsulating peritoneal sclerosis in patients undergoing continuous ambulatory peritoneal dialysis in Japan. *Advances in Peritoneal Dialysis* 18, 119–123.

Nakayama, M. *et al.* (1997). Immunohistochemical detection of advanced glycosylation end-products in the peritoneum and its possible pathophysiological role in CAPD. *Kidney International* 51, 182–186.

NKF : K/DOQI (1997). Clinical practice guidelines for peritoneal dialysis adequacy. *American Journal of Kidney Diseases* 30 (Suppl. 2), S67–S136.

NKF : K/DOQI (2000a). Clinical practice guidelines for peritoneal dialysis adequacy: update 2002. *American Journal of Kidney Diseases* 37 (Suppl. 1), S65–S136.

NKF : K/DOQI (2000b). Clinical practice guidelines for nutrition in chronic renal failure. *American Journal of Kidney Diseases* 35 (Suppl. 2), S1–S140.

Nielsen, P. K., Hemmingsen, C., Friis, J., Ladefoged, J., and Glgaard, K. (1995). Comparison of straight and curled Tenckhoff peritoneal dialysis catheters implanted by percutaneous technique: a prospective randomised study. *Peritoneal Dialysis International* 15, 18–21.

Nissenson, A. *et al.* (1997). ESRD modality selection into 21st century: the importance of non-medical factors. *ASAIO Journal* 43, 143–150.

Nolph, K. D. (1996). Why are reported relative mortality risks for CAPD and HD so variable? *Peritoneal Dialysis International* 16, 15–18.

Nomoto, Y. *et al.* (1996). Sclerosing peritonitis in patients undergoing CAPD: a report of the Japanese Sclerosing Encapsulating Peritonits Study Group. *American Journal of Kidney Diseases* 28, 420–427.

O'Connor, J., Rigby, R., and Handee, I. (1986). Abdominal hernias complicating CAPD. *American Journal of Nephrology* 6, 271–274.

Odel, H. M., Ferns, D. O., and Power, H. (1950). Peritoneal lavage as an effective means of extra renal excretion. *American Journal of Medicine* 9, 63–77.

Ogunc, G. (2002). Malfunctioning peritoneal dialysis catheter and accompanying surgical pathology repaired by laparoscopic surgery. *Peritoneal Dialysis International* 22, 454–462.

Oreopoulos, D. G. and Tzamaloukas, A. H. (2000). Peritoneal dialysis in the next millenium. *Advances in Renal Replacement Therapy* 7, 338–346.

Paniagua, R. *et al.* (2002). Effects of increased peritoneal clearances on mortality rates in peritoneal dialysis: ADEMEX, aprospective, randomised, controlled trial. *Journal of the American Society of Nephrology* 13, 1307–1320.

Pannekeet, M. M. *et al.* (1996). Demonstration of aquaporin-chip in peritoneal tissue of uraemic and CAPD patients. *Peritoneal Dialysis International* 16 (Suppl. 1), S54–S57.

Papanastasion, P. *et al.* (1994). Immunological quantification of advanced glycosulation end products in the serum of patients on haemodialysis or CAPD. *Kidney International* 46, 216–222.

Park, M. S. *et al.* (2000). Peritoneal accumulation of AGE and peritoneal membrane permeability. *Peritoneal Dialysis International* 20, 452–460.

Passlick-Deetjen, J., Schaub, T. P., and Schilling, H. (2002). Solutions for APD: special considerations. *Seminars in Dialysis* 15, 414–417.

Pecoits-Filho, R. *et al.* (1998). The effect of antibiotic prophylaxis on the healing of exit sites of peritoneal dialysis catheters in rats. *Peritoneal Dialysis International* 18, 60–63.

Peeters, P. *et al.* (2000). Analysis and interpretation of cost data in dialysis: review of Western European literature. *Health Policy* 54, 209–227.

Pereira, B. and Levey, A. (1997). Hepatitis C virus infection in dialysis and renal transplantation. *Kidney International* 51, 981–999.

Perez-Fontan, M. *et al.* (1993). Treatment of *Staph. aureus* nasal carriages in CAPD with Mupirocin: long term results. *American Journal of Kidney Diseases* 22, 708–712.

Perez-Fontan, M. *et al.* (2002). Incidence and clinical significance of nasal and pericatheter colonization by Gram-negative bacteria among patients undergoing chronic peritoneal dialysis. *Nephrology, Dialysis, Transplantation* 17, 118–122.

Pignatari, A. *et al.* (1990). *Staphylococcal aureus* colonisation and infection in patients on CAPD. *Journal of Clinical Microbiology* 28, 1898–1902.

Plum, J. *et al.* (1994). Result of ultrasound assisted diagnosis of tunnel infections in CAPD. *American Journal of Kidney Diseases* 23, 99–104.

Plum, J. *et al.* (2002). Efficacy and safety of a 7.5 per cent icodextrin solution in patients treated with automated peritoneal dialysis. *American Journal of Kidney Diseases* 39, 862–871.

Pollock, C. A. *et al.* Nutritional aspects of peritoneal dialysis. In *Textbook of Peritoneal Dialysis* (ed. R. Gokal *et al.*), pp. 515–543. Dordrecht: Kluwer Academic, 2000.

Poole-Warren, L. A. *et al.* (1991). Vaccination for prevention of CAPD associated staph infections. Results of a prospective multicentre clinical trial. *Clinical Nephrology* 35, 198–206.

Popovich, R. P., Moncrief, J. W., Dechard, J. F., Bomar, J. B., and Pyle, W. K. (1976). The definition of a novel portable/wearable equilibrium dialysis technique. *Transactions of the American Society of Artificial Internal Organs* 5, 64 (abstract).

Posthuma, N. *et al.* (1997). Icodextrin instead of glucose during the long day time dwell in CCPD patients increases ultrafiltration and 24-h dialysate creatinine clearance. *Nephrology, Dialysis, Transplantation* 12, 550–553.

Posthuma, N. *et al.* (1998). Simultaneous peritoneal dialysis catheter insertion and removal in catheter related infections without interruption of peritoneal dialysis. *Nephrology, Dialysis, Transplantation* 13, 700–703.

Prakashan, K. P. *et al.* (2001). Local application of mupirocin at the peritoneal catheter exit-site prevents early post-operative infections and should become standard practice. *Peritoneal Dialysis International* 21, 526–527.

Read, R. *et al.* (1989). Peritonitis in peritoneal dialysis: bacterial colonisation by biofilm spreading along the catheter surface. *Kidney International* **35**, 614–621.

RARCPL (Renal Association and Royal College of Physicians of London). *Treatment of Patients with Renal Failure: Recommended Standards and Audit Measures.* London: Royal College of Physicians, 2002.

Rigby, R. J. and Hawley, C. M. (1998). Sclerosing peritonitis: the experience in Australia. *Nephrology, Dialysis, Transplantion* **13**, 154–159.

Rippe, B. (1993). A three pore model of peritoneal transport. *Peritoneal Dialysis International* **13** (Suppl. 2), S35–S38.

Rippe, B. and Stelin, G. (1989). Simulations of peritoneal solute transport during CAPD. Application of two-pore formalism. *Kidney International* **35**, 1234–1244.

Rippe, B. *et al.* (2001). Long term clinical effects of a peritoneal dialysis fluid with less glucose degradation products. *Kidney International* **59**, 348–357.

Roberts, M., Ash, S. R., and Lee, D. B. N. (1999). Innovative peritoneal dialysis: flow-thru and dialysate regeneration. *ASAIO Journal* **45**, 372–378.

Robitaille, P. *et al.* (1995). Successful anti-fungal prophylaxis in chronic peritoneal dialysis: a pediatric experience. *Peritoneal Dialysis International* **15**, 77–78.

Rocco, M. V., Jordan, J. R., and Burkart, J. M. (1993). The efficacy number as a predictor of morbidity and mortality in peritoneal dialysis patients. *Journal of the American Society of Nephrology* **4**, 1184–1191.

Rocco, M. V., Jordan, J. R., and Burkart, J. M. (1995). Changes in peritoneal transport during first month of peritoneal dialysis. *Peritoneal Dialysis International* **15**, 12–17.

Rocco, M. V. *et al.* (2002). Risk factors for early mortality in US peritoneal dialysis patients: impact of residual renal function. *Peritoneal Dialysis International* **22**, 371–379.

Rotellar, C. *et al.* (1991). Ten years' experience with CAPD. *American Journal of Kidney Diseases* **17**, 158–164.

Rubin, J. (1990). Nutritional support during peritoneal dialysis related peritonitis. *American Journal of Kidney Diseases* **15**, 551–555.

Sandoe, J. A. T., Gokal, R., and Struthers, J. K. (1997). Vancomycin-resistant *Enterococci* and emperical Vancomycin for CAPD peritonitis. *Peritoneal Dialysis International* **17**, 617–618.

Sarkar, S. *et al.* (1999). Tolerance of large exchange volume by peritoneal dialysis patients. *American Journal of Kidney Diseases* **33**, 1136–1141.

Scanziani, R. *et al.* (1992). Peritoneography and peritoneal computerised tomography: a new approach to non-infectious complication of CAPD. *Nephrology, Dialysis, Transplantation* **7**, 1035–1038.

Schaefer, F. *et al.* (2002). Methodological issues in assessing the incidence of peritoneal dialysis-associated peritonitis in children. *Peritoneal Dialysis International* **22**, 234–238.

Schmitt, C. P. *et al.* (2002). Effects of pH-neutral, bicarbonate buffered dialysis fluid on peritoneal transport knietics in children. *Kidney International* **61**, 1527–1536.

Schreiber, M. *et al.* (2000). Preliminary findings from the national pre-ESRD education initiative. *Nephrology News Issues* **14**, 44–46.

Scott, P. *et al.* (1994). Peritoneal dialysis access. Randomised trial of three different peritoneal catheters—preliminary report. *Peritoneal Dialysis International* **14**, 289–290.

Selgas, R. *et al.* (1994). Functional longivity of the human peritoneum: how long is continuous peritoneal dialysis possible. *American Journal of Kidney Diseases* **23**, 64–73.

Sennfalt, K., Magnusson, M., and Carlsson, P. (2002). Comparison of hemodialysis and peritoneal dialysis—a cost–utility analysis. *Peritoneal Dialysis International* **22**, 39–47.

Shemin, D. *et al.* (1999). Effect of aminoglycoside use on residual renal function in peritoneal dialysis. *American Journal of Kidney Diseases* **34**, 14–20.

Sombolis, K., Berkelhammer, C., Baker, J., Wu, G., McNamee, P., and Oreopoulos, D. (1986). Nutritional assessment and skeletal muscle function in patients on CAPD. *Peritoneal Dialysis Bulletin* **6**, 53–58.

Stack, A. G. (2002). Determinants of modality selection among incident US dialysis patients: results from a national study. *Journal of the American Society of Nephrology* **13**, 1279–1287.

Staverman, A. J. (1951). The theory of measurement of osmotic pressure. *Recueil des Travaux Chemiques des Pays-Bas* **70**, 344–352.

Steiner, R. W. *et al.* (1990). Abdominal catastrophes and other unusual events in CAPD patients. *American Journal of Kidney Diseases* **15**, 1–7.

Stenvinkel, P. *et al.* (2000). Are there two types of malnutrition in chronic renal failure? Evidence for relationships between malnutrition, inflammation and atherosclerosis (MIA syndrome). *Nephrology, Dialysis, Transplantation* **15**, 953–960.

Stenvinkel, P. *et al.* (2001). Malnutrition, inflammation and atherosclerosis in peritoneal dialysis. *Peritoneal Dialysis International* **20** (Suppl. 3), S157–S162.

Suh, H. *et al.* (1994). Abdominal wall hernias in ESRD patients receiving peritoneal dialysis. *Advances in Peritoneal Dialysis* **10**, 85–88.

Swartz, R. *et al.* (1991). Preventing Staphylococcal infection during chronic peritoneal dialysis. *Journal of the American Society of Nephrology* **2**, 1085–1091.

Szeto, C. C. *et al.* (2000). Importance of dialysis adequacy in mortality and morbidity of Chinese CAPD patients. *Kidney International* **58**, 400–407.

Szeto, C. C. *et al.* (2001). Impact of dialysis adequacy on on the mortality and morbidity of anuric Chinese CAPD patients. *Journal of the American Society of Nephrology* **12**, 355–360.

Szeto, C. C. *et al.* (2002). Feasibility of resuming peritoneal dialysis after severe peritonitis and Tenckhoff catheter removal. *Journal of the American Society of Nephrology* **13**, 1040–1045.

Tattersall, J. G., Doyle, S., Greenwood, R. N., and Farrington, K. (1994). Maintaining adequacy in CAPD by individualising the dialysis prescription. *Nephrology, Dialysis, Transplantation* **9**, 749–752.

Taylor, P. M. (2002). Image-guided peritoneal access and management of complications in peritoneal dialysis. *Seminars in Dialysis* **15**, 250–258.

Teehan, B. P., Schleifer, S. R., Sigler, M. H., and Belgor, G. S. (1985). A quantitative approach to CAPD prescription. *Peritoneal Dialysis Bulletin* **5**, 152–156.

Teehan, B. P. *et al.* (1990). Urea kinetic analysis and clinical outcomes on CAPD: a few year longitudinal study. *Advances in Peritoneal Dialysis* **6**, 181–185.

Teehan, B. P., Schleifer, S. R., and Brown, J. (1992). Urea kinetic modelling is an appropriate assessment of adequacy. *Seminars in Dialysis* **5**, 189–192.

Tenckhoff, H. and Schechter, H. (1968). A bacteriologically safe peritoneal access device for repeated peritoneal dialysis. *Transactions of the American Society of Artificial Internal Organs* **14**, 181–186.

Tenckhoff, H., Blagg, C. R., Curtis, K. F., and Hickman, R. D. (1973). Chronic peritoneal dialysis. *Proceedings of the European Dialysis and Transplant Association* **10**, 363–370.

Thodis, E. *et al.* (1998). Decrease in *Staphylococcus aureus* exit-site infections and peritonitis in CAPD patients by local application of mupirocin ointment at the catheter exit-site. *Peritoneal Dialysis International* **18**, 261–270.

Thorgeirsson, G. and Robertson, A. L., Jr. (1998). The vascular endothelium: pathobiologic significance. *American Journal of Pathology* **95**, 801–848.

Tsilibary, E. C. and Wissig, S. L. (1987). Light and electron microscopic observations of the lymphatic drainage units of the peritoneal cavity of rodents. *American Journal of Anatomy* **180**, 195–207.

Turner, K. *et al.* (1992). Does catheter immobilization reduce exit-site infections in CAPD patients? *Advances in Peritoneal Dialysis* **8**, 265–268.

Turner, K. *et al.* (1998). Natural history of *Staphylococcal aureus* nasal carriage and its relationship to exit-site infections. *Peritoneal Dialysis International* **18**, 271–275.

Twardowski, Z. (2002). Presternal peritoneal catheters. *Seminars in Dialysis* **9**, 125–132.

Twardowski, Z. J. and Prowant, B. F. (1996). Classification of normal and diseased exit sites. *Peritoneal Dialysis International* **16** (Suppl. 3), S32–S50.

Twardowski, Z. J. *et al.* (1987). Peritoneal equilibration test. *Peritoneal Dialysis Bulletin* **7**, 138–147.

Twardowski, Z. J., Prowant, B. F., Nichols, K., Nolph, K. D., and Khanna, R. (1992). Six years experience with a swan neck catheter. *Peritoneal Dialysis International* **12**, 384–389.

Tzamaloukas, A. H. *et al.* (1992). Scrotal oedema in CAPD patients: causes, differential diagnosis and management. *Dialysis and Transplantation* **21**, 581–590.

Tzamaloukas, A. H. *et al.* (1995). Symptomatic fluid retention on patients on continuous peritoneal dialysis. *Journal of the American Society of Nephrology* **6**, 198–206.

Ueda, Y. *et al.* (2000). Effects of dwell time on carbonyl stress using icodextrin and amino acid PD fluids. *Kidney International* **58**, 2518–2524.

Uttley, L. and Prowant, B. Organisation of a PD programme: the nurse's role. In *Textbook of Peritoneal Dialysis* (ed. R. Gokal *et al.*), pp. 363–386, Dordrecht: Kluwer Academic, 2000.

USRDS (United States Renal Data Systems). *Annual Data Report*. The National Institutes of Health, National Institute of Diabetes and Digestive and Kidney Diseases, Bethesda, MD, 1997.

Van Biesen, W. *et al.* (2000a). The role of peritoneal dialysis as the first-line renal replacement modality. *Peritoneal Dialysis International* **20**, 375–383.

Van Biesen, W. *et al.* (2000b). Evaluation of an integrative care for ESRD patients. *Journal of the American Society of Nephrology* **11**, 116–125.

Van Biesen, W. *et al.* (2000c). Peritoneal dialysis favourably influences recovery of renal function after transplantation. *Transplantation* **69**, 508–514.

Van Biesen, W. *et al.* (2002). Peritoneal dialysis in anuric patients: concerns and cautions. *Seminars in Dialysis* **15**, 305–310.

Van Manen, J. *et al.* (2002). How to adjust for comorbidity in survival studies in ESRD patients: a comparison of different indices. *American Journal of Kidney Diseases* **40**, 82–89.

Vas, S., Bargman, J., and Oreopoulos, D. G. (1997). Treatment of PD patients peritonitis caused by Gram-positive organisms with single daily dose of antibiotics. *Peritoneal Dialysis International* **17**, 91–94.

Vychytil, A. *et al.* (1998). New strategies to prevent *Staphylococcal aureus* infections in peritoneal dialysis patients. *Journal of the American Society of Nephrology* **9**, 669–676.

Wang, A. Y. *et al.* (2001). Independent effects of residual renal function and dialysis adequacy on actual dietary proetein, calorie and other nutrient intake in patients on CAPD. *Journal of the American Society of Nephrology* **12**, 2450–2457.

Wang, A. Y. *et al.* (2002). A novel association between residual renal function and left ventricular hypertrophy in peritoneal dialysis patients. *Kidney International* **62**, 639–647.

Wang, T. *et al.* (1998a). Peritoneal fluid and solute transport with different polyglucose formulations. *Peritoneal Dialysis International* **18**, 193–203.

Wang, T. *et al.* (1998b). Increased peritoneal permeability is associated with decreased fluid and small solute removal and higher mortality in CAPD patients. *Nephrology, Dialysis, Transplantation* **13**, 1242–1249.

Wang, T. *et al.* (2002). Peritoneal dialysis in Asia in the 21st century: perspectives on and obstacles to peritoneal dialysis therapies in Asian countries. *Peritoneal Dialysis International* **22**, 243–248.

Warady, B. A. *et al.* (2000). Consensus guidelines for the treatment of peritonitis in pediatric patients receiving peritoneal dialysis. *Peritoneal Dialysis International* **20**, 610–624.

Wayland, N. and Silverberg, A. (1978). Blood to lymph transport. *Microvascular Research* **15**, 367–374.

Wieslander, A. P. *et al.* (1995). Are aldehydes in heat sterilised peritoneal dialysis fluids toxic *in vitro*? *Peritoneal Dialysis International* **15**, 348–352.

Wilkie, M. *et al.* (1997). Icodextrin 7.5 per cent dialysate solution (glucose polymer) in patients with ultrafiltration failure: extension of CAPD technique survival. *Peritoneal Dialysis International* **17**, 84–87.

Williams, A. J. *et al.* (1989). Tenckhoff catheter replacement or IP urokinase: a randomised trial in the management or recurrent CAPD-peritonitis. *Peritoneal Dialysis International* **9**, 65–67.

Williams, J. D. *et al.* (2002). Morphological changes in the peritoneal membrane of patients with renal disease. *Journal of the American Society of Nephrology* **13**, 470–479.

Williams, P. F., Moncrief, N., and Marriot, J. (2000). No benefit in using nysattin prophylaxis against fungal peritonitis in peritoneal dialysis patients. *Peritoneal Dialysis International* **20**, 352–353.

Wolfson, M. *et al.* (2002). Efficacy and long term safety of icodextrin in peritoneal dialysis. *American Journal of Kidney Diseases* **40**, 1055–1065.

Wong, V. K. *et al.* (1995). *KT/V* in CAPD by different estimations of *V*. *Kidney International* **48**, 563–569.

Woodrow, G. *et al.* (1997). Technique failure in peritoneal dialysis and its impact on patient survival. *Peritoneal Dialysis International* **17**, 360–364.

Woodrow, G. *et al.* (1999). Comparison of icodextrin and glucose solutions for the daytime dwell in automated peritoneal dialysis. *Nephrology, Dialysis, Transplantation* **14**, 1530–1535.

Wuerth, D. B. *et al.* (2002). Patients' description of specific factors leading to modality selection of chronic peritoneal dialysis or hemodialysis. *Peritoneal Dialysis International* **22**, 184–190.

Xue, J. L. *et al.* (2002). Peritoneal and hemodialysis. Differences in patients characteristics at initiation. *Kidney International* **61**, 734–740.

Young, G. *et al.* (1991). Nutritional assessment of CAPD: an international study. *American Journal of Kidney Diseases* **17**, 462–471.

Zappacosta, A. R., Perras, S. T., and Closkey, G. N. (1991). Seldinger technique for Tenckhoff catheter placement. *ASAIO Transactions* **37**, 13–15.

Zemel, D. *et al.* (1995). Analysis of inflammatory mediators and peritoneal permeability to macromolecules shortly before the onset of overt peritonitis in patients treated with CAPD. *Peritoneal Dialysis International* **15**, 134–141.

Zimmerman, S. W. *et al.* (1991). Randomised controlled trial of prophylactic rifampin for PD related infections. *American Journal of Kidney Diseases* **18**, 225–231.

12.5 Adequacy of dialysis

James Tattersall

Introduction

Current dialysis techniques provide, at most, 15 per cent of the urea clearance of normal renal function. This fraction is much lower for higher molecular weight solutes. Dialysis patients have mortality rates, which are 5–20 times higher than normal individuals of a similar age (Collins *et al.* 2001).

Numerous studies have demonstrated a link between mortality in dialysis patients and measures to quantify the efficacy of dialysis. These measures include blood pressure (Mazzuchi *et al.* 2000), serum phosphate (Block *et al.* 1998), serum bicarbonate (Lowrie and Lew 1990) and the clearance of urea and creatinine [Gotch and Sargent 1985; Canada–USA (CANUSA) Peritoneal Dialysis Study Group 1996]. There is now data available to define an 'adequate' level of dialysis, below which outcome is measurably worse. On the other hand, evidence for an optimal level of dialysis (which may be closer to normal renal function) has been elusive. The concept of dialysis adequacy combines principles of dialysis and human physiology with measurements of dialysis efficacy and data from dialysis outcome studies. It aims to define the minimum acceptable level of dialysis efficacy and to provide evidence-based, cost–benefit analysis to guide the dialysis prescription. A concept of dialysis adequacy is required in order to;

1. Ensure that the dialysis patient receives the minimum amount of dialysis for acceptable survival.

2. Prescribe the optimum amount of dialysis for the individual patient.

3. Plan a cost-effective and evidence-based dialysis programme.

The urea kinetic model

In the 1970s, Gotch and Sargent proposed the urea kinetic model as a tool for quantifying and predicting dialysis dose (Gotch 2001). The parameter Kt/V, derived from the model was shown to predict outcome in a re-analysis of the National Cooperative Dialysis Study (NCDS) (Gotch and Sargent 1985).

The urea kinetic model describes and predicts changes in urea mass balance in the patient. It accounts for urea clearance by dialysis and by the kidneys, urea generation by the patient, and the urea distribution volume of the patient. In intermittent treatments, the model also incorporates changes in body fluid content and the intermittent urea clearance by dialysis.

Why urea?

Urea is easy to measure and is present in high concentrations in the blood of uraemic patients. Of all of the waste products produced by the body, urea is produced in the greatest amount (2–3 mol/week).

Although high blood urea levels do not seem to be harmful, at least up to 40 mM/l (Depner 2001), numerous studies have linked the parameters calculated from urea clearance to outcome. Urea clearance can be considered as a marker for the clearance of other, more toxic solutes. Due to its low molecular weight, it is much easier to predict the clearance rate and changes in blood concentration of urea compared to other solutes.

Clearance

Measurement of the concentrations of urea and creatinine in blood alone are useless in quantifying dialysis, since the level is as much a function of generation rate as of clearance. The urea generation rate is dependent on protein intake and the creatinine generation rate is dependent on muscle mass (Keshaviah *et al.* 1994). A low blood urea or creatinine level could indicate a high clearance rate or malnutrition and reduced muscle mass. Similarly, measuring the mass of solute removed provides limited information on its own since, in steady state, the mass removed is always equal to the generation rate, independent of the dialysis dose.

The clearance concept is established as a means of quantifying renal function, independent of solute generation rate or blood level. Clearance is defined as the rate at which solute is removed from the body, divided by the concentration of the solute in the body. All methods of quantifying low molecular weight clearance in dialysis use this principle.

The single-pool model

The original urea kinetic model assumed that urea was evenly distributed throughout a single pool of body water quantified as the urea distribution volume (V). During intermittent haemodialysis, urea mass is cleared from the body at a rate quantified by the dialyser urea clearance (K) multiplied by the instantaneous urea concentration in blood at the dialyser inlet (C_t), representing urea concentration throughout the body water volume (Sargent and Gosch 1980).

As C_t falls during dialysis, the rate of fall also decreases, so that the fall becomes exponential. C_t can be predicted from the predialysis concentration (C_0), K, the duration of dialysis (t), and V; so that concentration can be described by an exponential equation:

$$C_t = C_0 \times e^{-(Kt/V)}.$$

In the period between dialyses, urea is generated in the liver and the urea concentration rises as described by the equation; $BUr = (G/V) \times t$.

More complex equations exist which allow for inclusion of the effects of urea generation, ultrafiltration and residual renal function.

The single-pool Kt/V (SpKt/V) may be predicted from the dialysis prescription where K is estimated from dialyser data, blood and dialysate flow rate, V is estimated from prediction equations and t is the prescribed dialysis time.

A dialysis time may be calculated to achieve a given SpKt/V using the estimated values of V and K and the equation $t = SpKt/V \times V/K$.

The SpKt/V delivered by dialysis may be independently calculated from pre- and postdialysis urea concentrations by a rearrangement of the equation describing the exponential fall in urea;

$$SpKt/V = \ln\left(\frac{C_0}{C_t}\right).$$

This calculation of delivered dose of dialysis does not require precise values for K or V.

The two-pool model

Sargent and Gotch (1980) have also described a two-pool model, which is more realistic. Urea is distributed in two compartments, central and peripheral, which were originally considered to represent intra- and extracellular fluid volumes. The two compartments could equally represent areas of the body with low and high rates of perfusion (Schneditz 1993). The model considers urea to be cleared from, and generated into, the central compartment. During dialysis, urea transfers from the peripheral to central compartment at a rate defined by the concentration difference between compartments multiplied by the intercompartment clearance rate.

The intercompartment clearance rate is either the product of diffusive permeability and area of the cell membranes or blood flow rate between compartments, depending on the mechanism of transfer.

The two-pool model was originally considered to be impractical as it is more complex and requires values for the relative volumes of the two compartments and the intercompartment clearance rate, which are hard to measure.

Measurements of blood urea during and immediately after dialysis are predicted accurately by the two-pool model, but not by the single-pool model. The single-pool model predicts only the pre- and immediate postdialysis urea concentrations, fails to predict the postdialysis rebound and always overestimates the dialysis dose, particularly in short dialysis treatments (Fig. 1).

More recent work has demonstrated that intercompartment urea transfer may be accurately predicted and that the two-pool model may be simplified and used routinely (Smye et al. 1999). The two-pool model is also appropriate for creatinine and, potentially to other solutes. Therefore, the single-pool model should be considered obsolete for quantifying haemodialysis dose.

The patient clearance time (t_p)

During dialysis, there is a time lag between the urea concentration in the fistula and the average urea concentration throughout the body. After the fist few minutes of dialysis, this lag is relatively constant and has been measured at around 35 min (Fig. 1) (Tattersall et al. 1996).

This time lag has been termed the patient clearance time (t_p). It is independent of dialysis dose or duration and can be used to predict

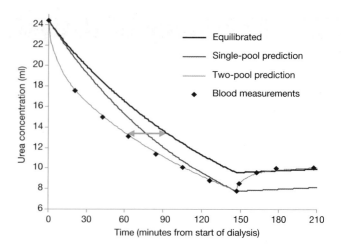

Fig. 1 Measured blood levels match closely to a two-pool model but not the single-pool model. A short, intensive dialysis is shown to emphasize the difference. There is a time-lag of approximately 35 min between blood levels and the equilibrated or mean concentrations (arrow).

the postdialysis rebound for urea, creatinine and, potentially, other solutes. A related approach has been validated in over 600 patients enrolled in the HEMO study and has been shown to predict the effect of the rebound on EqKt/V so that it may be calculated accurately from pre- and immediate postdialysis concentrations (Daugindas et al. 1997).

The urea kinetic model in peritoneal dialysis

In peritoneal dialysis, the urea kinetic model can also be used to quantify and predict dialysis dose (Gotch et al. 1993). The urea concentration in blood (BUr) can be predicted from the urea generation rate (G) equation and the sum of renal and dialysis urea clearance (K) using the equation; $BUr = G/K$.

K can be predicted from the dialysis prescription and the peritoneal mass transfer area coefficient (MTAC). K can also be calculated from the urea concentration in blood, the mass of urea measured in dialysate and urine collections. The osmotic removal of fluid can also be predicted using a three-pore model, accounting for the transfer of water and different sized solutes (Rippe 1993).

V is predicted from anthropometric data. A weekly Kt/V in continuous treatments is calculated using the duration of a week as t.

Measures of dialysis adequacy

Fluid and blood pressure homeostasis

Heart disease is the reported cause of over 65 per cent of the deaths in dialysis patients. The dialysis patients tend to have left ventricular hypertrophy (Foley et al. 1996; Prichard et al. 1996) considered to be caused by failure to control sodium and fluid overload and hypertension.

Hypertension in dialysis patients is often the only sign of fluid overload and should be excluded as the cause of raised blood pressure especially if this is proving resistant to antihypertensive drugs.

In peritoneal dialysis, the ability to remove fluid is crucial (Davies et al. 1999) and should be quantified as part of the adequacy quantification. This can be achieved using tools such as the standard peritoneal permeability analysis (SPA), peritoneal equilibration test (PET) or personal dialysis capacity (PDC) test (Davies 2001).

Low molecular weight solute clearance

Glomerular filtration rate

Renal function is normally quantified as glomerular filtration rate (GFR) in ml/min and corrected to a body surface area of 1.73 m^2. It can be estimated from the mean of urea and creatinine clearance (CCr), calculated from the urea and creatinine concentrations in blood and a 24-h urine collection and surface area calculated from height and weight.

Urea reduction ratio

The urea reduction ratio (URR) is a simple measure of small solute clearance achieved over a single haemodialysis session. It is calculated as the ratio of the fall in blood urea divided by the predialysis blood urea. It is easy to calculate, but fails to take urea generation, ultrafiltration, the postdialysis rebound, frequency, or duration of dialysis into account. It underestimates clearance in long dialysis (when urea generation becomes significant) and cannot be used to quantify renal function or continuous treatments. The URR can only be used to compare treatments, which are of similar duration and frequency.

Single-pool *Kt/V* (haemodialysis)

The single-pool *Kt/V* (Sp*Kt/V*) is the ratio of dialyser clearance (*K*) multiplied by dialysis duration (*t*) divided by urea distribution volume (*V*). It is a measure of urea clearance for a single dialysis treatment and does not take frequency of dialysis or the postdialysis rebound into account. Sp*Kt/V* can be estimated from the dialysis prescription when *K* is read from the dialyser data sheet, and *V* is estimated as 0.5 times the body weight. Sp*Kt/V* can be calculated directly from pre- and postdialysis blood samples without needing exact values for *K* or *V*. Sp*Kt/V* can take urea generation and ultrafiltration into account, but the mathematics is complex and requires a computer. It is difficult to include renal function into Sp*Kt/V* and it cannot be calculated for continuous treatments. Sp*Kt/V* can only be used to compare treatments of similar duration and frequency.

Equilibrated *Kt/V* (haemodialysis)

The equilibrated *Kt/V* (Eq*Kt/V*) is based on a more realistic model of dialysis where urea is cleared from the fistula blood, but the effect on the body depends also on the rate at which urea transfers from other areas of the body into the blood entering the fistula. Eq*Kt/V* is calculated directly from a predialysis blood sample and either a postdialysis sample taken 30–60 min postdialysis or from dialysate samples. Eq*Kt/V* may be estimated from Sp*Kt/V* but corrected using a time constant representing urea transfer from all parts of the body into the fistula.

Eq*Kt/V* can be used to compare treatments of differing duration but not frequency and should be used in preference to Sp*Kt/V*, which is now obsolete.

Kt/V (continuous treatment)

Kt/V as quoted for patients on continuous treatment (e.g. continuous ambulatory peritoneal dialysis or CAPD) is calculated in a different way and has a different meaning to the *Kt/V* used in intermittent treatments (e.g. haemodialysis). The continuous *Kt/V* is calculated from the mass of urea removed from the patient (e.g. measured in the 24-h dialysate drain) divided by the mass of urea in the patient (blood urea concentration multiplied by *V*). The *Kt/V* is normally quoted as a weekly value, in which case the 24-h value is multiplied by seven. In this way, *K* is the urea clearance, *t* is 1 week and *V* is the urea distribution volume. *Kt/V* (continuous treatment) may be calculated also for renal function and added to the dialysis component. For renal function, *Kt/V* is calculated from *K* as the renal urea clearance.

Solute removal index

Solute removal index (SRI) is numerically equivalent to *Kt/V* (continuous treatment) described above, but is also applicable to intermittent treatments (Keshaviah 1995). SRI is the mass of urea removed per week divided by the peak mass of urea in the patient.

In intermittent treatments, SRI is approximately equal to the URR multiplied by the number of dialyses per week and can be calculated from the same data as used for Eq*Kt/V*. A theoretical advantage of SRI in intermittent treatments is that it has the same relationship between concentration and generation rate as does the continuous clearance in renal function and continuous dialysis modalities. Any given SRI will result in the same peak urea concentration regardless of the dialysis type, duration and frequency. SRI can incorporate residual renal function and a combination of different dialysis types by calculating each component separately and adding together.

The SRI equivalence between dialysis modalities assumes that uraemic toxicity is related to the peak concentrations (rather than average concentrations), that the urea distribution volume is the same as the body water volume and that urea is a valid marker for uraemic toxins.

Standard *Kt/V* (Std*Kt/V*) is equivalent to SRI but specifically includes the effect of urea generation, postdialysis rebound, ultrafiltration and dialysis schedules which are not evenly spaced throughout the week (Gotch 2002). Peak mass is defined as the midweek peak (i.e. the second dialysis after the long interdialytic interval for three times weekly haemodialysis).

To prevent confusion with other types of *Kt/V*, the term SRI is used here in preference to Std*Kt/V* or *Kt/V* (continuous treatment), which are equivalent.

Weekly creatinine clearance

Since creatinine has a molecular weight around twice that of urea, it could be a more realistic marker for a uraemic toxin.

In peritoneal dialysis, CCr in (l/week/1.73 m^2) is calculated from dialysate and urine collections. Software for calculating CCr may calculate the renal component as the mean of urea and creatinine clearance.

CCr may also be calculated for haemodialysis using pre- and postrebound creatinine concentrations.

Equivalent renal urea clearance

The equivalent renal urea clearance (EkrU) has been proposed as a standardized method for reporting urea clearance for all dialysis modalities (Casino and Lopez 1996). EkrU is the urea generation rate divided by the time-averaged urea concentration and normalized to 1.73 m^2 surface area. The units of EkrU are the same as normally used to quantify renal function (ml/min/1.73 m^2). The difference between EkrU and SRI are that the normalizing factor is surface area rather than urea distribution volume and that any given EkrU results in the same time averaged urea concentration rather than peak concentration.

The EkrU has the advantage of using familiar units, readily under-standable by non-nephrologists. However, it is harder to calculate than SRI since it requires time-averaged concentration rather than the directly measurable peak concentration. In this chapter, the terms SRI and, where appropriate, $EqKt/V$ are used in preference. This is in the interests of simplicity rather than a recommendation of these terms. Figure 2 and Table 1 gives equivalences between the different adequacy measures.

Bicarbonate

Survival of dialysis patients has been shown to relate to their serum bicarbonate concentration (Lowrie and Lew 1990). Bicarbonate has a similar molecular weight as urea, so the relative mass of bicarbonate

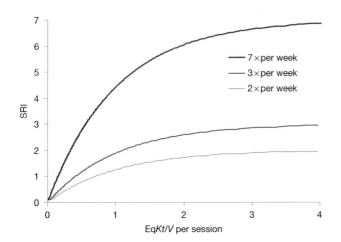

Fig. 2 Equivalent doses for different frequencies of intermittent dialysis.

Table 1 Equivalent adequacy measures for SRI = 2 per week, approximately the minimum dose recommended for all dialysis treatments

Weekly dialysis frequency	Dialysis time per session	SpKt/V	EqKt/V	URR
2 with renal function	4:00	1.37	1.20	0.70
2 with renal function	6:00	1.31	1.20	0.68
3	3:00	1.31	1.10	0.67
3	4:00	1.26	1.10	0.65
6	2:00	0.52	0.41	0.38
6	8:00	0.44	0.41	0.33
7	8:00	0.36	0.34	0.28

The patient is assumed to have V = 35 l, SA = 1.73 ml/min/m^2 and to be in fluid balance.

The two times weekly haemodialysis treatments assume 500 ml/day urine output, GFR 3 ml/min and 3.5 l of fluid removed during dialysis per week. It is not possible to achieve SRI = 2 without renal function by two times weekly dialysis.

All other treatments assume that the patient is anuric and 7 l of fluid are removed by dialysis per week.

transferred into the blood will be approximately proportional to the $EqKt/V$ and the bicarbonate concentration gradient across the mem-brane. A dialysate bicarbonate concentration of 40 mM will keep the patients bicarbonate concentration in the normal range (22–28 mM) in virtually all dialysis patients if SRI is 1.7. If the SRI is increased, a proportional reduction in concentration gradient is required so that for a SRI of 2.6, the dialysate bicarbonate concentration should be reduced to 35 mM. Individual variations in the dialysate bicarbonate concentration may be required to cope with differing metabolic rates, diets and oral base intake (e.g. calcium carbonate).

Phosphate

The kidneys normally excrete 30–50 mmol phosphate per day. Most of the filtered phosphate is reabsorbed in the tubules. As the kidneys fail, phosphate excretion is relatively well maintained as tubular phosphate reabsorption is decreased as filtration falls. Dialysis patients with residual renal function tend therefore to have better phosphate control than those without (Morduchowicz et al. 1994).

The clearance of phosphate by dialysis is approximately the same as the clearance of creatinine; around 60 l/week which would maintain serum phosphate at around 4 mM (i.e. four times higher than normal) with normal phosphate intake in the absence of renal function. The levels can be reduced to 1.5–3 times normal in dialysis patients by a combination of reduced intake, phosphate binders, and abnormal deposition of phosphate in the tissues.

The abnormal phosphate kinetics in dialysis patients have been linked to vascular calcification and mortality.

While phosphate clearance can be quantified and predicted, changes in phosphate concentration during dialysis are governed by active transfer of phosphate between intra- and extracellular compart-ments and into and out of bones. This has proved very difficult to pre-dict. The serum phosphate concentration may even rise during the final hour of dialysis and there is always a large postdialysis phosphate rebound. Therefore, the mass of phosphate removed by haemodialysis cannot yet be predicted from measurements of pre- and postdialysis concentration as it can for urea and creatinine (Spalding et al. 2002).

If we were to rely on dialysis alone to control phosphate, the dose would have to be much higher than currently achieved to normalize serum phosphate. This is currently only possible in overnight daily haemodialysis (Vanholder et al. 2002).

High molecular weight solute clearance

β-2-Microglobulin is a well-recognized large molecular weight uraemic toxin. Accumulation in dialysis patients has resulted in death (Kawano et al. 1998). It is now practical to measure the concentration of β-2-microglobulin in a predialysis blood sample. Although serum β-2-microglobulin levels have not been linked to overall survival β-2-microglobulin clearance is considered to be a valid marker for the clearance of uraemic toxins (Vincent et al. 1978).

Protein-bound solutes

The normal kidney clears small quantities of albumin. This may be a method for clearing albumin-bound uraemic toxins. Haemodialysis and haemofiltration techniques do not clear bound toxins. In this respect, CAPD is superior as it does clear some albumin. Methods for quantifying and clearing protein-bound solutes are still in the experimental stage (Vanholder *et al.* 2001).

Nutrition and adequacy

Malnutrition is common in dialysis patients and is associated with a high mortality and morbidity. Malnutrition may be caused by underdialysis (Lindsay and Spanner 1989) or inflammation (Kaysen *et al.* 2002). The early signs of malnutrition are easy to miss in dialysis patients, particularly if there is no weight loss due to fluid accumulation.

The patient's protein intake is related to the appearance of urea in urine and dialysate and can be measured as the protein equivalent of the nitrogen appearance rate (PNA). The PNA can be calculated from the same samples as used for the adequacy measurements and is normalized to ideal body weight as nPNA. Adequate values for nPNA are considered to be at least 0.8 g/kg/day.

Artefactual link between adequacy and nPNA

nPNA has been shown to correlate with urea-based adequacy in patients treated by both haemodialysis and CAPD. While it is generally accepted that adequacy should be inversely proportional to the concentration of an appetite-suppressing uraemic toxin in blood, the observed link between nPNA and adequacy could be entirely or partly artefactual (Harty *et al.* 1994).

If both nPNA and adequacy are calculated from the same 24-h collection in CAPD or from the same pre- and posthaemodialysis urea concentrations then any random variation in dose of dialysis delivered or measurement error will affect both nPNA and adequacy. This artefactual component may be minimized by ensuring that the dialysis dose delivered is stable and by averaging multiple values. It can be eliminated altogether by calculating nPNA independently from adequacy by using samples before and after the dialysis interval.

Interpretation of nPNA

Although the nPNA reflects the generation rate of urea, and has fixed adjustments for non-urea nitrogen losses to resemble the dietary protein intake (DPI), it is only indirectly related to DPI. The nPNA only reflects the DPI if the patient is in stable nitrogen balance and if the non-urea nitrogen losses are predictable. The malnourished patient may well be in negative nitrogen balance and relatively catabolic. In this case, the nPNA will be relatively high as urea is generated from muscle catabolism (Flanigan *et al.* 1995).

Other dietary assessment tools may be appropriate. These include measurement of skinfold thickness, assessment of muscle mass from creatinine generation rate, lean body mass from bioimpedance measurement, and assessment of dietary intake by food weighing or diaries.

What is adequate?

The minimum acceptable dose of dialysis

Numerous studies have demonstrated that survival is significantly reduced when dialysis fails to deliver more than an SRI of 1.7 (Eq$Kt/V \approx$ 0.9, URR $\approx$ 0.6 for 3 times per week haemodialysis and no renal function). The NCDS was the original landmark study demonstrating a link between haemodialysis dose and clinical outcome (as probability of death or hospitalization in a 6-month period). The NCDS was interpreted as evidence for an adequacy 'threshold' equivalent to SRI of 1.7 (Gotch and Sargent 1985). Patients whose doses were lower than this value fared badly. There were relatively few patients with SRI greater than 2, but there appeared to be no benefit to increasing dose above the 'threshold' level.

Analysis of the Japanese Data Registry suggested a more progressive relationship between haemodialysis dose and gross mortality rate but the increase in mortality rate became significant only when SRI fell below 1.7 (Eq$Kt/V \approx$ 0.85) (Fig. 3) (Teraoka *et al.* 1995).

The optimal dose of dialysis

The Canada–USA (CANUSA) study demonstrated a progressive relationship between SRI and survival in peritoneal dialysis [Canada–USA (CANUSA) Peritoneal Dialysis Study Group 1996]. Six hundred and eighty patients were studied for 2 years after dialysis was initiated. The SRI was 2.38 at initiation declining to 1.99 after 2 years due to loss of renal function. The dialysis component of SRI was relatively constant around 1.7 and that almost all of the variability in SRI was due to differences in renal function. The study was initially interpreted as suggesting that SRI should be pushed as high as possible, at least to 2, for optimal survival.

An alternative interpretation of the CANUSA study could be that only renal function influenced survival and the hypothesis that increasing dialysis dose would impact on survival was not tested (Bargman *et al.* 2001).

The ADEMEX study prospectively studied 965 prevalent patients who were being treated by CAPD. Patients were randomized to standard treatment (SRI $\approx$ 1.7) or intensive treatment (SRI $\approx$ 2.1). The study showed no significant survival advantage in the intensively treated group.

The HEMO study was set up to test the hypothesis that more intensive dialysis could increase survival in haemodialysis. Patients were randomized to conventional (SRI = 2, EqKt/V = 1.1) and intensively treated (SRI = 2.4, EqKt/V = 1.4). The dose of dialysis in the conventionally treated group was high enough to ensure that they were adequately or well dialysed by conventional criteria. The study failed to demonstrate a clear-cut benefit to intensive dialysis.

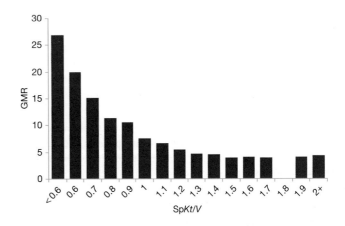

Fig. 3 Results from the Japanese Data Registry. Patients are grouped by SpKt/V, gross annual mortality rate (GMR) is shown for each group.

Practical limitations in increasing dialysis dose

It is hard to increase dialysis dose above an SRI of 2.5 using dialysis treatment in common use. With three times weekly haemodialysis it is impossible to increase SRI above 3, even if EqKt/V could be increased to infinity and postdialysis urea concentrations are zero. This is because the removal of solute is driven by its concentration in blood and its rate falls progressively during dialysis as concentration falls. With EqKt/V above 1.4, the peak or time-averaged concentrations in blood are dependent mostly on the accumulation of urea due to generation during the time between dialysis sessions.

In order to reduce the average or peak blood solute concentrations significantly lower than currently achieved with standard dialysis, it is necessary to reduce the time between sessions by increasing frequency of dialysis.

In peritoneal dialysis, clearance is limited by the MTAC of the peritoneal membrane and time in which the dialysate is in contact with the membrane. These factors are effectively limited. Conventional CAPD delivers an SRI of around 1.7. By using high fill volumes (up to 3 l) and increased exchange frequency (up to 20 l/day using automated equipment) SRI may be increased up to 2.2.

Potential side-effects of increasing dialysis dose

Considering that SRI in normal renal function is 25–30, common sense suggests that dialysis dose should optimally be far higher than an SRI of around 2 as delivered by current dialysis. However, no study has so far demonstrated any clear-cut advantage of an SRI greater than around 2. This raises the possibility that any advantage to the patient in clearing more solute is counteracted by some side-effect of the more intensive dialysis. Adverse factors of dialysis, which potentially increase in proportion to dialysis dose include inflammation due to endotoxin transfer from dialysis fluid to blood and bioincompatibility due to contact with the extracorporeal blood circuit or peritoneal dialysate (Chung et al. 2000; Kaysen et al. 2000).

Current adequacy guidelines

Current guidelines recommend a minimal level of dialysis dose of SRI = 1.9 in haemodialysis (EqKt/V = 1.0, SpKt/V = 1.2, URR = 0.65). In CAPD, the recommended minimum SRI level varies between 1.7 (UK and European guidelines) and 2.0 (US DOQI guidelines).

At present the guidelines do not recommend more intensive dialysis since there is no evidence to support it. Current opinion expects the recommended optimal level of dialysis to be increased significantly as dialysis efficacy, biocompatibility and safety improves, particularly with increasing use of daily haemodialysis.

Confounding effects of urea distribution volume on survival

The urea distribution volume (V) has been shown to be an independent predictor of survival in dialysis patients; patients with higher V have a better chance of survival compared to patients with a lower V. This is thought to be because V is a marker for muscle mass, nutritional status, and activity (Owen et al. 2000).

Since V is used as a normalizing factor in the calculation of the adequacy measures EqKt/V and SRI, it tends to blunt the association between survival and adequacy. Patients with a low V will tend to have a high EqKt/V yet have poor survival, presumably due to malnutrition.

It has been advocated that EqKt/V and SRI be multiplied by V to combine both the predictive effects of adequacy and V on survival (Lowrie et al. 1999). This combined parameter (Kt) has been shown to predict survival better than V or adequacy alone. However, the evaluation and interpretation of V separately from adequacy is likely to be more useful in the care of the individual patient.

Urea distribution volume

All measures of dialysis adequacy include an assessment of urea distribution volume (V). This is generally taken to be the body water volume. There are no practical methods for measuring this volume directly and a variety of indirect methods or estimations are used.

The simplest method of estimation of the urea distribution volume is to use a fixed fraction of the body weight. Traditionally, a value of 55 per cent for females and 58 per cent for males has been used although the originating evidence for these values is obscure. Recent evidence suggests that, for dialysis patients, body water volume is, on average 50 per cent of body weight for both males and females.

Estimating body water from demographic and anthropomorphic data

Since fat contains little water, and muscle has a relatively high water content, a more precise prediction may be obtained by including an estimate of fat and muscle mass using anthropomorphic and demographic data. The Watson equation is the most commonly used (Watson et al. 1980). The equation was derived from regression analysis of demographic and anthropomorphic data and measurements of body water by radioisotope dilution studies in normal volunteers. V (in litres) is calculated from weight (Wt in Kg), height (Ht in cm), and age (in years):

For men: $V = 2.447 + 0.3362 \times \text{Wt} + 0.1074 \times \text{Ht} - 0.09516 \times \text{age}$

For women: $V = -2.097 + 0.2466 \times \text{Wt} + 0.1069 \times \text{Ht}$.

Urea distribution volume from bioelectrical impedance

Bioelectrical impedance is currently the most precise method for estimating urea distribution volume (V) available in routine practice (Kushner and Roxe 2002). The method exploits the differing electrical impedance of muscle, fat, and extracellular water at differing frequencies.

Urea distribution volume from measurements of urea in intermittent dialysis

In intermittent dialysis, the urea distribution volume (V) may be calculated from measurements of pre- and postdialysis blood urea concentration and an estimation of the change in urea mass over the dialysis session. This requires values for the postrebound urea concentration, the urea generation rate, and mass of urea removed during dialysis.

The mass removed may be calculated from partial or total dialysate collections. The accuracy of the urea measurements in dialysate may be reduced by growth of urea-metabolizing bacteria in the dialysate, and calibration differences between measurements of urea in blood and dialysate.

Alternatively, the mass removed is calculated from the integration of urea clearance rate and blood urea concentration over the entire dialysis session. This requires either a realistic estimation of clearance over the entire dialysis session or semicontinuous clearance measurements.

Similarly, the blood urea concentration throughout dialysis may be estimated using the pre- and postdialysis blood samples and a urea kinetic model.

The single-pool urea kinetic model can be used to estimate V from pre- and immediate postdialysis blood samples and the dialyser datasheet to estimate clearance. By chance, the 15–20 per cent error introduced by ignoring the postdialysis rebound is almost exactly cancelled out by an error introduced by using a single-pool model rather than a more realistic double-pool model. These errors only cancel out when EqKt/V is close to one. The urea distribution volume will be underestimated at lower EqKt/V and overestimated at higher EqKt/V if this method is used.

A precise value for V or K is not required for the adequacy calculations in intermittent treatment if based on pre- and postdialysis blood samples. Values for EqKt/V, SRI, and urea generation rate depend mainly on the ratio of the pre- and postdialysate concentrations. Only the relatively small contribution of ultrafiltration is subject to errors in urea distribution volume.

The adequacy assessments of continuous treatments and the contribution of residual renal function depend on a value of urea distribution volume, which is most commonly calculated using the Watson equations.

Surface area

GFR and CCr are normalized to a surface area (SA) of 1.73 m². An estimate of surface area is obtained using one of the prediction equations listed in Table 2. The Gehan and George method is preferred as it has been validated in over 400 patients (Gehan and George 1970).

$$SA = 0.0235 \times Wt^{0.51456} \times Ht^{0.42246}.$$

The Du Bois and Du Bois method (Du Bois and Du Bois 1916) is widely used but was validated in 1916—in only nine patients!

Renal function

The kidneys are far more efficient at removing solute than any current dialysis technique. Of the techniques in current use, only daily dialysis has the potential to approach even 20 per cent of the urea clearance of the normal kidney. A typical CAPD or haemodialysis has an SRI of less than 10 per cent of normal renal function. When larger solutes are considered, this fraction falls even lower. Dialysis lacks the ability to match certain functions of the kidney altogether, these include the selective excretion of toxins by the renal tubule, certain homeostatic functions and the ability to clear protein-bound solute.

Control of certain key solutes including phosphate (Morduchowitz *et al.* 1994) and β-2-microglobulin (Amici *et al.* 1993) have been shown to be critically dependent on the presence of residual renal function in dialysis patients. Phosphate is removed by haemodialysis so that its level is low or low–normal at the end of dialysis. However, unless dialysis is performed daily, or there is significant renal function, phosphate accumulation in the period between dialysis sessions generally caused clinical problems for the patient.

The CANUSA study has shown that optimal survival in CAPD is critically dependant on residual renal function (Bergman *et al.* 2001).

All current guidelines recommend that renal function measurements are made as part of the assessment of peritoneal dialysis adequacy. Recent study has shown that renal function is also significant in haemodialysis patients (McKane *et al.* 2002) and the European

Best Practice Guidelines now recommend that renal function is measured as part of the assessment of haemodialysis adequacy also.

When to start dialysis

European guidelines now recommend starting at or above a GFR of 6 ml/min/1.73 m² regardless of symptoms or nutritional state.

A GFR of 6 ml/min equates to an SRI of around 1.2. This value is low compared to the minimum level for dialysis adequacy. However, in the failing kidney, the clearance rates of almost all solutes is at least 30 per cent higher than the urea clearance, in contrast to dialysis, which clears urea best. Therefore, the urea-based SRI underestimates the power of the kidneys compared to dialysis. When taking a range of solutes into account, a renal SRI of 1.2 is probably equivalent to current minimum levels for dialysis adequacy.

Incremental dialysis

Unless renal function stops suddenly, there is significant renal function at the time dialysis is started. Some useful renal function persists for some years after starting dialysis (Fig. 4). For a more rational prescription of dialysis, it has been advocated to start dialysis with a minimum dose (e.g. to top up the SRI to 2) and increase the dialysis dose progressively to match the decline in renal function (Fig. 5) (Golper 1998).

The haemodialysis prescription

Frequency of dialysis

In intermittent dialysis, the overall efficacy is reduced as the dialysis becomes less frequent, despite maintaining a constant weekly EqKt/V. This is because the mass of solute removed and the peak urea concentration are not linear functions of EqKt/V and very little extra urea can be cleared as EqKt/V is increased beyond 1.4. The maximum SRI achievable

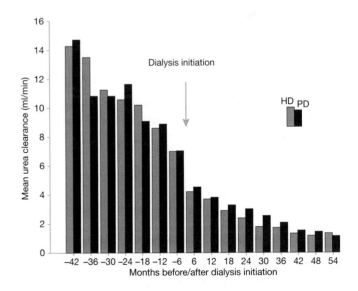

Fig. 4 The decline in renal function before and after dialysis is started. This study suggested that the rate of decline in renal function is similar in patients treated by haemodialysis and CAPD. Other papers suggest a more rapid decline in patients treated by haemodialysis.

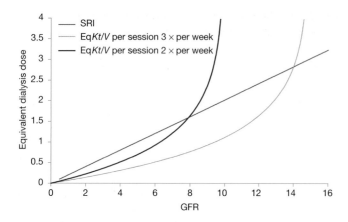

Fig. 5 The relationship between renal function (expressed as GFR) and an equivalent dialysis dose. The relationship considers only urea and assumes that urea clearance is 0.7 times GFR, which is approximately true at low GFR. Note that the relationship between EqKt/V and GFR is non-linear and would have to be infinite to be equivalent to GFR = 15 in three times weekly haemodialysis.

with intermittent dialysis is equal to the times the number of dialysis sessions per week and even this would require an infinite EqKt/V.

Daily or six times per week haemodialysis has proven to allow much better control of fluid overload, hypertension, and phosphate than three times per week haemodialysis.

The urea clearance (K)

A value for K for the chosen blood flow rate may be read off a graph on the dialyser data sheet.

Alternatively, K may be predicted from the overall dialyser mass transfer coefficient (KoA), blood flow rate (Q_b), and dialysate flow rate (Q_d) using Renkin's equation below. KoA is the theoretical maximum K for a given dialyser at infinite blood and dialysate flow rates and depends mainly on membrane area and permeability. KoA is also inversely related to the molecular weight of the solute.

$$K = \left[\frac{1 - e^{KoA \times (Q_b - Q_d)/(Q_b - Q_d)}}{(1/Q_b) - (1/Q_d) \times e^{KoA \times (Q_b - Q_d)/(Q_b - Q_d)}} \right].$$

If a value for KoA is not available, it can be calculated from clearance values in the data-sheets or (more satisfactorily) from clearance measurements. The equation for calculating KoA from dialyser clearance values is shown below.

$$KoA = \left[\frac{Q_b}{1 - (Q_b/Q_d)} \right] \times \ln \left[\frac{1 - (K/Q_d)}{1 - (K/Q_b)} \right].$$

The renal component of EqKt/V

The renal component of EqKt/V is calculated from the renal component of SRI and subtracted from the desired EqKt/V to return the target dialysis component EqKt/V as shown below where n is the number of dialyses per week. The renal component of SRI is measured from urine collections as described in the section on measuring renal function. If the renal component of SRI is more than n, the EqKt/V

cannot be calculated since it will be more than the maximum possible for haemodialysis.

$$EqKt/V = \ln \left[\frac{1}{1 - (SRI/n)} \right].$$

Calculating dialysis time (t)

The dialysis time (t in minutes) required to achieve a given target dialysis component of EqKt/V is given by

$$t = \left(\frac{V}{K} + 35 \right) \times EqKt/V.$$

The value 35 is needed to correct for the effect of the postdialysis rebound described later.

Optimizing EqKt/V in haemodialysis

K may be increased by increasing blood flow rate or dialyser surface area. However, the relationship between K and either blood flow rate or surface area are non-linear. Increasing either may well result in only modest increases in K. Only if there is a proportional increase in both flow rates and surface area, will a proportional increase in K result.

If high blood flows are chosen to increase clearance, there is a tendency for the pressure in the blood pump segment to fall. This may result in blood pump inaccuracy due to partial collapse of the pump segment. Also stoppages due to pressure alarms may increase. These pressure problems can be avoided by reducing the hydraulic resistance of the fistula needles in proportion to the increase in blood flow. This can be achieved by reducing needle length (e.g. from 15 to 10 mm) and/or increasing needle internal diameter (e.g. from 15 to 14 g).

Optimizing fluid removal by haemodialysis

Haemodialysis removes fluid from the vascular compartment, potentially causing hypotension and hypovolaemia at the end of dialysis even if there is excess fluid elsewhere in the body. Therefore, any physical assessment of fluid balance should not be performed immediately after dialysis.

The rate at which fluid can be removed safely is limited to the rate at which fluid transfers into the circulation. This varies from 2–3 l/h in overloaded patients to near zero as the patient approaches dry weight. The rate also depends on the function of the capillaries and may be reduced by vascular disease, diabetic neuropathy, and antihypertensive drugs.

Fluid removal can be optimized by longer or more frequent dialysis, which allows a lower ultrafiltration rate. Reducing the dialysate temperature has been shown to reduce hypotension during dialysis by preventing the reflex vasodilatation caused by a temperature rise. Ultrafiltration profiling, where the ultrafiltration rate is highest at the start of dialysis, when the patient is fluid overloaded, and progressively reduces towards the end of dialysis as dry weight is approached.

Optimizing higher molecular weight solute clearance in haemodialysis

While it may be possible to increase K by choosing high blood flow rates, the clearance of higher molecular weight solutes may not increase in proportion unless the dialyser membrane surface area is also increased. For this reason, blood flow should be prescribed in proportion to dialyser surface area so that around 1 m^2 of surface is available for each 250 ml/min of blood flow.

Other measures to increase high molecular weight clearance include using convection (haemofiltration or haemodiafiltration) (Ledebo 1998) and more porous dialyser membranes.

Finally, residual renal function is important in clearing high molecular weight solute. It makes sense to take measures designed to protect or maintain residual renal function for as long as possible.

Recirculation

During haemodialysis, some of the blood entering the dialyser inlet has flowed from the dialyser outlet without passing through the peripheral circulation. This flow of dialysed blood from dialyser outlet to inlet is termed recirculation and is quantified as the flow rate of recirculated blood entering the dialyser, expressed as a fraction of the extracorporeal blood flow rate.

Access recirculation

Access recirculation occurs when a proportion of the blood returning to the patient in the venous line is immediately drawn into the arterial needle and dialysed again without leaving the fistula. This occurs when the arterial needle is placed downstream of the venous needle or when the extracorporeal blood flow rate exceeds the blood flow rate in the fistula due to a critical stenosis.

The effect of access recirculation is included in the measurement of delivered EqKt/V, by ensuring that the postdialysis sample is taken after 15–30 seconds of low blood flow. Access recirculation should be suspected if EqKt/V falls below 80 per cent of the value predicted by the prescription.

Cardiopulmonary recirculation

Due to the configuration of the circulation, 5–10 per cent of the blood in the fistula will have recirculated through the heart and lungs without passing through the systemic circulation. The effect of cardiopulmonary recirculation is included in the 35-min rebound correction—contributing about 5 min.

Prescribing adequate peritoneal dialysis

The peritoneal mass transfer area coefficient

The clearance of a specific solute is limited by its peritoneal MTAC. This is the maximum possible clearance rate when the concentration in the dialysate is zero. MTAC is inversely related to the molecular weight of the solute and directly proportional to the peritoneal membrane surface area. The clearance rate dialysis approaches MTAC for a short time after the start of an exchange when the concentration in dialysate is low.

To aid interpretation of MTAC, peritoneal function is commonly reported relative to a population mean as the *transport type* (Table 2).

In patients with a high transport type, the SRI approaches the weekly exchange volume divided by the V, provided that dwell times are at least 4 h, so that the dialysate urea concentration is close to the blood urea concentration by the time the exchange is drained.

Table 2 Peritoneal transport types and approximate MTAC range

Transport type	MTAC urea	MTAC creatinine
High	25–40	20–35
High average	20–25	12–20
Low average	15–20	6–12
Low	12–15	3–6

In practice, the urea concentration in the dialysate is between 0.7 and 0.9 times the plasma urea concentration due to limitations imposed by MTAC and dwell time. This will reduce the SRI by the same amount. On the other hand, the mass of urea removed by dialysis is increased by about the same amount due to osmotic removal of fluid, increasing the drain volume.

As a rule of thumb, for CAPD with all dwell times at least 4 h, the weekly exchange volume (drained in) required to achieve a given SRI can be predicted by:

$$\text{PDvol/week} = V \times \text{SRI}.$$

The effect of dwell time and MTAC can be predicted for each exchange, where PDvol is the volume of the individual exchange and n is the number of times the exchange is performed per week;

$$\text{SRI} = \frac{\text{PDvol}}{V} \times (1 - e^{(\text{MTAC} \times \text{dwell})/\text{PDvol}}) \times n.$$

The influence of osmotic removal of fluid on SRI is harder to predict and requires a sophisticated three-pore model and a computer.

The total SRI will be the sum of the SRIs for each exchange and the renal SRI.

Maximizing small solute clearance in peritoneal dialysis

Small solute clearance depends on the weekly exchange volume, which should be as high as is practical. Dwell time should always be maximized by avoiding periods when the peritoneal cavity is 'dry'. Increasing dwell volume, which distends the peritoneal cavity and increases its surface area, may increase MTAC. High dwell volume (up to 3 l) is better tolerated at night when the patient is lying down.

Maximizing the clearance of larger solutes

In peritoneal dialysis, large solute clearance is limited by MTAC and overall dwell time. Increasing the number of exchanges makes little difference to large solute clearance. Increasing MTAC by increasing dwell volume, increasing dwell time by avoiding 'dry' periods and maximizing osmotic fluid removal will help to increase large-solute clearance.

Maximizing osmotic fluid removal

Osmotic fluid removal carries small and large solutes with it and has been shown to predict survival.

Fluid is removed by osmosis as long as the dialysis fluid has a higher osmotic pressure than the blood. Traditionally, glucose is used as the osmotic agent as it is relatively cheap and biocompatible. However, is rapidly absorbed, particularly if the MTAC is high so that its effect is short-lived. Furthermore, the high concentration of glucose and associated glucose degradation products and advanced glycation end products have been shown to cause clinical problems.

For maximum osmotic effect and minimum toxicity, hypertonic glucose dwells should be of short duration, typically, 2–4 h.

Alternatively, a glucose polymer should be used as the osmotic agent. The polymer is not absorbed. In contrast to glucose, the polymer is more effective when the dwell time is long as urea diffusing out of the blood adds to the osmotic effect. Typically, exchanges containing a glucose polymer would be used overnight in CAPD or the long day dwell in automated peritoneal dialysis (APD).

Measurement of dialysis adequacy

Measurement of renal function

Renal function is calculated from the volume (UVol), urea and creatinine concentrations (UUr, UCr), and duration (t in minutes) of a urine collection. The peak concentrations of urea and creatinine in blood (BUr, BCr) during the collection, the urea distribution volume (V), and the surface area (SA in m^2) are also required. Apart from SA and t, the units do not matter but must be consistent.

$$SRI = \frac{UVol \times UUr \times 10{,}080}{BUr \times V \times t}$$

$$CCr = \frac{UVol \times UCr \times 1.73 \times 10{,}080}{BCr \times SA \times t}.$$

In patients who are not yet on dialysis or who are treated by continuous dialysis, the urine is usually collected over 24 h ($t = 1440$) and the concentrations in blood are estimated from a single blood sample at the end of the collection period.

In patients treated by intermittent dialysis, renal function may be lower immediately after a dialysis session, compared to immediately before. Therefore, the urine is collected over the entire interdialytic interval. In intermittent treatments, according to the peak equivalence hypothesis, BUr and BCr are the peak or predialysis levels.

CCr is an overestimation of GFR by 10–100 per cent due to tubular secretion of creatinine. The difference between GFR and urea and CCr is greater at lower GFR. By chance, the urea clearance underestimates GFR by approximately the same amount due to tubular reabsorption of filtered urea. Therefore, GFR may be estimated by the mean of urea and CCr:

$$GFR = \frac{UVol \times 1.73}{t \times SA \times 2} \times \left(\frac{UUr}{BUr} + \frac{UCr}{BCr}\right).$$

In some software for calculating peritoneal dialysis adequacy, the renal component of CCr is calculated as the mean of urea and creatinine clearance.

Measuring haemodialysis adequacy

Predialysis sampling method

The sample is taken from a fistula needle just after it has been inserted, preferably without having been prefilled with any fluid. If the needle has been prefilled or if the patient is dialysing via an indwelling catheter, an adequate quantity of blood (usually 10 ml) is withdrawn and discarded before sampling.

Since adequacy measurements depend on the ratio of pre- to postdialysis urea, precision can be greatly improved by ensuring that the

pre- and postdialysis samples are analysed consecutively in the same analytical run. Therefore, the predialysis sample should be kept until the end of the dialysis and sent to the laboratory together with the postdialysis sample.

Postdialysis sample method

At the end of dialysis and for a further 30–60 s, the blood urea level is relatively stable. After this, the concentration varies rapidly and unpredictably due to the postdialysis rebound and the washback until a new relatively stable level is reached 30–45 min after the end of dialysis.

For reproducible quantification of dialysis, the postdialysis sample should be taken directly from the arterial needle at the end of dialysis after a the blood pump has been slowed to 50 ml/min for 5–10 s to allow any recirculated blood to clear.

If the sample is taken from a port in the arterial line, 15–30 s are required to allow the recirculated blood to clear.

Alternatively, the postdialysis sample can be measured after the rebound is complete, 30–45 m after the end of dialysis.

Another option to obtain a more accurate measurement of renal function and nPNA, a third (pre2) blood sample can be taken immediately before the following dialysis.

Calculating the urea reduction ratio

URR is calculated from pre- and immediate postdialysis blood urea concentrations.

$$URR = 1 - \frac{post}{pre}.$$

Calculating the postrebound concentration

The postrebound concentration (reb) can be calculated from the pre- and immediate postdialysis concentrations using the equation below. The value t in the equation is the time difference between the pre- and postdialysis sample times.

$$reb = pre \times \left(\frac{post}{pre}\right)^{t/(t+35)}.$$

The value 35 in the equation is the same value as used to correct for rebound effects when prescribing dialysis and is the patient clearance time (t_p). The postrebound creatinine can also be predicted using value of 70 instead of 35.

Calculating adequacy from pre- and postrebound concentrations

Since the generation rate of urea (G) during dialysis competes with the clearance, it must be accounted for in the calculations. It can be measured using the following equation:

$$G = \frac{pre2 \times V2 - reb \times (V - ufV) + UVol \times UUr}{tin}.$$

The values UVol and UUr are the volume and urea concentrations in the interdialytic urine collection, tin is the time (in minutes) between the dialyses and also the duration of the urine collection period. The values pre2 and V2 are the urea concentration and V just before the dialysis following the usual pre- and postsample. The value ufV, is the difference between the pre- and postdialysis weight in kilogram. V is calculated from the Watson equation described previously using the predialysis weight.

If pre2 and V2 are not available, G may approximated by

$$G = \frac{(\text{pre} - \text{reb}) \times V \times n}{10{,}080 - n \times t}.$$

The value n is the number of dialyses per week and 10,080 is the number of minutes in the week. This approximation assumes that the dialyses are evenly spaced and that the rise of urea concentration between dialyses is linear. The approximate method will underestimate G if there is significant renal function and after a short interdialytic interval. G will be overestimated after an atypically long interdialytic interval. G calculated by the approximate method is not precise enough to calculate nutritional parameters but, since G has a relatively small influence on the adequacy calculations, it will result in errors of less than 4 per cent.

$$\text{Eq}Kt/V = \ln\left[\frac{\text{pre} \times V}{\text{reb} \times (V - \text{uf}V) - G \times t}\right]$$

$$\text{SRI} = \frac{\text{pre} \times V - \text{reb} \times (V - \text{uf}V) + G \times t}{\text{pre} \times V} \times n.$$

Weekly CCr can be calculated using creatinine concentrations.

$$\text{CCr} = \frac{\text{pre} \times V - \text{reb} \times (V - \text{uf}V) + G \times t}{\text{pre} \times \text{SA}} \times 1.73 \times n.$$

V largely cancels out in the equations and errors in V have relatively little impact.

The Daugirdas rate equation for correcting Sp*Kt*/*V*

As an alternative to calculating or measuring the postrebound concentration, the Daugirdas rate equation may be used to correct the Sp*Kt*/*V* (Daugirdas et al. 1997). The Sp*Kt*/*V* is first calculated using the equations above but using the immediate postdialysis concentration instead of the postrebound concentration. The Eq*Kt*/*V* is then calculated from Sp*Kt*/*V* using the Daugirdas rate equation;

$$\text{Eq}Kt/V = \text{Sp}Kt/V - \left(\frac{36 \times \text{Sp}Kt/V}{t}\right) + 0.03.$$

This approach is mathematically similar to the calculation of the postrebound method. The value 36 is equivalent to the patient clearance time used to predict the rebound.

Calculating delivered adequacy from a dialysate collection

The dialysate collection method has the advantage of avoiding the need for a postdialysis or postrebound blood sample or an estimate of urea generation rate (Argiles et al. 1997). However, unlike the blood concentration method, the dialysate method requires an accurate value for V.

Special measures are required to avoid growth of urea-metabolizing bacteria in the dialysate during collection. Some dialysis machines can use the partial dialysate collection method to avoid these problems. The dialysate output volume is automatically measured on line and a proportion continuously diverted for the concentration measurement.

In the dialysate method, the total mass of solute removed by dialysis including ultrafiltration is calculated from the total dialysate

output volume (dV) multiplied by the average solute concentration in the dialysate (dC). In this way, the dialysis is quantified in exactly the same way as is renal function and CAPD.

$$\text{Eq}Kt/V = \ln\left[\frac{1}{1 - (\text{dV} \times \text{dC})/(V \times \text{pre})}\right]$$

$$\text{SRI} = \frac{\text{dV} \times \text{dC} \times n}{V \times \text{pre}}$$

$$\text{CCr} = \frac{\text{dV} \times \text{dC} \times 1.73 \times n}{\text{pre} \times \text{SA}}.$$

Calculating t_p

The values of 35 and 70 min used to quantify the urea and creatinine rebound represent mean values for the patient clearance time (t_p). These values may not predict the rebound precisely in some patients. In particular, patients with ascites or heart failure may need higher values to predict the rebound. The patient clearance time may be calculated from the dialysis duration (t, min), predialysis, postdialysis, and postrebound (pre, post, reb) concentrations in blood. This post-rebound sample should be taken at least 30 min and preferably 45 min after the end of dialysis.

The postdialysis and postrebound samples should be corrected for the effect of urea generation by subtracting $t \times G/V$ where t is the time between the sample time and the start of dialysis (Tattersall et al. 1996).

$$t_p = t \times \frac{\ln(\text{reb}/\text{post})}{\ln(\text{pre}/\text{reb})}.$$

Validating Eq*Kt*/*V* and trouble-shooting

The delivered Eq*Kt*/*V* calculated from the pre- and postdialysis urea measurements can be crosschecked with the prescribed Eq*Kt*/*V* predicted from the dialysis prescription. The prescribed Eq*Kt*/*V* can be calculated from the urea clearance (K calculated from KoA as described previously), dialysis time (t) and the urea distribution volume (V, calculated from anthropometric data) using the equation:

$$\text{Eq}Kt/V = \frac{K \times t}{V + 35 \times K}.$$

The value 35 corrects for the rebound.

The prescribed Eq*Kt*/*V* should be within 20 per cent of the delivered Eq*Kt*/*V*. Delivered values less than 80 per cent of the prescribed values suggest problems with the dialysis delivery, for example, access recirculation, interrupted dialysis due to alarms or failure to achieve the prescribed blood flow throughout dialysis. Delivered Eq*Kt*/*V* more than 120 per cent of the prescribed value suggests that the postdialysis sample was taken incorrectly (e.g. after the washback or without an adequate period of slow flow in the presence of recirculation).

On average, delivered Eq*Kt*/*V* values tend to be slightly higher than the prescribed values, at least when V is estimated using the Watson equations. This indicates that the true urea distribution volume in haemodialysis patients is less than the body water volume estimated by the Watson equations. Since the Watson equations are not believed to overestimate body water, this raises the possibility that the urea distribution volume may be less than the body water.

Measuring peritoneal dialysis adequacy

Batch UKM

In batch UKM, all the dialysate effluent and urine output is collected from the patient over a 24-h period. A blood sample is drawn at the end of the collection period. The total volume of the dialysate is measured and a single sample of the total mixed dialysate volume is taken. This may be achieved either by mixing all of the dialysate before sampling and measuring or by measuring the volume in each dialysate bag and taking a sample of proportional volume from each bag and mixing the samples.

Batch UKM allows calculation of SRI, CCr, glucose absorption, fluid removal, and nPNA but not MTAC.

Peritoneal function test

In the peritoneal function test (PFT), the urine and dialysate effluent in each drain bag is measured and sampled separately over a 24-h period. A blood sample is also taken, ideally at the end of the collection period (Gotch 1993). In CAPD, each of the four or five effluent bags are sampled. In APD, samples are taken from the effluent of the overnight exchanges, day dwell and any additional exchanges and the volumes of each component are either measured or read from the APD machine record.

The peritoneal function test allows calculation of all the adequacy parameters including MTAC. The test requires more samples but avoids the need for a PET.

The peritoneal equilibration test

The peritoneal equilibration test (PET) is used to quantify MTAC and residual fluid volume (Twardowski 1990). Measurements are made on the overnight dwell bag and from a standard test exchange, performed in the clinic. A blood sample is taken at the start of the test. The test bag is sampled soon after it has been drained in and mixed by rolling the patient from side to side. The bag is drained out after 4 h and an additional sample is taken at 2 h.

PET cannot be used to quantify clearance or nutrition.

Standard permeability analysis

The Standard permeability analysis (SPA) tests the ability of the peritoneum to remove fluid under standard conditions (Ho-dac-Pannekeet *et al.* 1997). The 'ultrafiltration' volume removed by a 2 l, 3.86 per cent glucose, 4-h dwell is measured. Ultrafiltration failure is defined as less than 400 ml.

SPA cannot be used to quantify clearance or nutrition.

Personal dialysis capacity

The personal dialysis capacity (PDC) analyses peritoneal function using a three-pore model (Rippe 1993). The model accounts for peritoneal transport of albumin, water, urea, glucose, sodium, and creatinine.

The PDC is performed using a standardized five-exchange CAPD prescription.

The PDC predicts SRI, CCr, glucose absorption, and ultrafiltration for any prescription. Adequacy is not calculated directly by the PDC, but can be estimated for the patient's usual prescription using the three-pore model and the peritoneal function parameters.

Since the PDC is not performed under the patient's normal dialysis prescriptions, the patient cannot be assumed to be in steady state and nutrition cannot be quantified.

Calculating peritoneal dialysis small-solute clearance

The dialysis components of adequacy in CAPD are calculated from the volume the urea and creatinine concentrations (UUr, UCr) and drain volumes (DVol) of the dialysate collections and number of time each component is performed per week (n).

$$\text{SRI} = \frac{\text{PDvol} \times \text{PDUr}}{\text{BUr} \times V} \times n$$

$$\text{CCr} = \frac{\text{PDvol} \times \text{PDcr} \times 1.73}{\text{BCr} \times \text{SA}} \times n.$$

For batch UKM there is only one component and $n = 7$. For peritoneal function tests, adequacy is calculated as the sum of each component. An iterative computer simulation may be used to predict the peak blood concentration from the measured blood concentration. This peak concentration is used as BUr and BCr.

Commonly used software for calculating CCr calculates the renal component of CCr as GFR multiplied by 10.08 to convert from ml/min/1.73 m^2 to l/week/1.73 m^2. GFR (calculated as the mean of urea and CCr) is used in this software rather than CCr to prevent overestimation of the renal component.

Peritoneal mass transfer area coefficient

MTAC is calculated from PD dwell volume (PDvol), dwell time (t), Blood concentration (BC), and PD effluent concentration (PDC);

$$\text{MTAC} = \frac{\text{PDvol}}{t} \times \ln\left[\frac{1}{1 - (\text{PDC/BC})}\right].$$

MTAC may be calculated for urea, creatinine, and glucose from data collected using the PET or PFT.

Residual fluid volume

Residual fluid volume (RV) may be calculated from the volume of the test exchange (PDvol) and urea concentrations in dialysate drained out immediately before the PET and in the $t = 0$ sample (PDur$_{\text{pre}}$, PDur$_0$).

$$\text{RV} = \text{PDvol} \times \frac{\text{PDur}_0}{\text{PDur}_{\text{pre}}}.$$

Calculation of nPNA

All methods to calculate nPNA rely on the principle that urea generation in the body is entirely a result the metabolism of protein. Nitrogen accounts for around 14 per cent of the mass of protein and a mole of urea contains 28 g of nitrogen.

The nPNA can be calculated from the urea nitrogen appearance (UNA in g/24 h), ideal body weight (IBW in kilograms) and the protein loss in dialysate and urine (Ploss in g/24 h) using the Bergstrom equation (Lindholm and Bergstrom 1992)

$$nPNA = \frac{15.1 + (6.95 \times UNA) + Ploss}{IBW}.$$

The constant 15.1 represents obligatory nitrogen losses in skin and faeces (in g/day). In haemodialysis, the dialysate protein loss is negligible and can be ignored.

The urine and peritoneal dialysate protein losses can be calculated from measurements of volume (Vol in l), protein concentration (Prot in g/l) and collection time (t in minutes);

$$Ploss = \frac{Vol \times Prot \times 1440}{t}.$$

Ideal body weight can be calculated from $V/0.58$.

In continuous treatments, or when a dialysate collection is available, UNA is calculated from the volumes (UVol, DVol in l) and urea concentrations (UUr, DUr in mM) in 24-h urine and dialysate collections.

$$UNA = (UVol \times UUr + DVol \times DUr) \times 0.028.$$

The value 0.028 converts the urea from mM to urea nitrogen in g/l. If urea is measured as urea nitrogen in mg/dl, then the conversion factor should be 0.01 instead of 0.028.

In intermittent treatments, urea generation can be quantified from appearance of urea in the urine and the rise in urea concentration between dialysis sessions. Taking ultrafiltration volume (ufV), fluid accumulation between dialysis, changes in nitrogen balance, and renal function into account the following equation is used;

$$UNA = [(BUr_{pre2} \times V_{pre2} - BUr_{post1} \times (V_{pre2} - ufV)$$
$$+ UVol \times UUr) \times 0.028 \times 1440]/tin.$$

The equation calculates the UNA from measurements over the interdialytic interval. Blood urea is measured postdialysis (and corrected for rebound) and immediately before the following dialysis (BUr_{post1}, BUr_{pre2}). V is estimated immediately before both dialyses (V_{pre1}, V_{pre2}). The urine is collected over the entire interdialytic period (between post1 and pre2). The time between the post1 and pre2 samples (tin in min) is measured.

The pre2 sample may be estimated from pre1 and post1 but this requires an iterative computer programme. If pre2 is estimated rather than measured, nPNA will be artefactually linked to adequacy.

References

Amici, G. *et al.* (1993). Serum beta-2-microglobulin level and residual renal function in peritoneal dialysis. *Nephron* **65**, 469–471.

Argiles, A. *et al.* (1997). Precise quantification of dialysis using continuous sampling of spent dialysate and total dialysate volume measurement. *Kidney International* **52**, 530–537.

Bargman, J. M., Thorpe, K. E., and Churchill, D. N. (2001). Relative contribution of residual renal function and peritoneal clearance to adequacy of dialysis: a reanalysis of the CANUSA study. *Journal of the American Society of Nephrology* **12**, 2158–2162.

Block, G. A., Hulbert-Shearon, T. E., Levin, N. W., and Port, F. K. (1998). Association of serum phosphorus and calcium × phosphate product with mortality risk in chronic hemodialysis patients: a national study. *American Journal of Kidney Diseases* **31**, 607–617.

Canada–USA (CANUSA) Peritoneal Dialysis Study Group (1996). Adequacy of dialysis and nutrition in continuous peritoneal dialysis: association with clinical outcomes. *Journal of the American Society of Nephrology* **7**, 198–207.

Casino, F. G. and Lopez, T. (1996). The equivalent renal urea clearance: a new parameter to assess dialysis dose. *Nephrology, Dialysis, Transplantation* **11**, 1574–1581.

Chung, S. H., Stenvinkel, P., Bergstrom, J., and Lindholm, B. (2000). Biocompatibility of new peritoneal dialysis solutions: what can we hope to achieve? *Peritoneal Dialysis International* **20** (Suppl. 5), S57–S67.

Collins, A. J., Li, S., Ma, J. Z., and Herzog, C. (2001). Cardiovascular disease in end-stage renal disease patients. *American Journal and Kidney Diseases* **38**, S26–S29.

Daugirdas, J. T. *et al.* (1997). Comparison of methods to predict equilibrated Kt/V in the HEMO Pilot Study. *Kidney International* **52**, 1395–1405.

Davies, S. J. (2001). Monitoring of long-term peritoneal membrane function. *Peritoneal Dialysis International* **21**, 225–230.

Davies, S. J. *et al.* (1999). Impact of peritoneal membrane function on long-term clinical outcome in peritoneal dialysis patients. *Peritoneal Dialysis International* **19** (Suppl. 2), S91–S94.

Du Bois, D. and Du Bois, E. F. (1916). A formula to estimate the approximate surface area if height and weight be known. *Archives of Internal Medicine* **17**, 863–971.

Depner, T. A. (2001). Uremic toxicity: urea and beyond. *Seminars in Dialysis* **14**, 246–251.

Flanigan, M. J., Lim, V. S., and Redlin, J. (1995). The significance of protein intake and catabolism. *Advances in Renal Replacement Therapy* **2**, 330–340.

Foley, R. N. *et al.* (1996). Impact of hypertension on cardiomyopathy, morbidity and mortality in end-stage renal disease. *Kidney International* **49**, 1379–1385.

Gehan, E. and George, S. L. (1970). Estimation of human body surface area from height and weight. *Cancer Chemotherapy Reports* **54**, 225–235.

Golper, T. A. (1998). Incremental dialysis. *Journal of the American Society of Nephrology* **9**, S107–S111.

Gotch, F. A. (1993). Adequacy of peritoneal dialysis. *American Journal of Kidney Diseases* **21**, 96–98.

Gotch, F. A. (2001). Evolution of the single-pool urea kinetic model. *Seminars in Dialysis* **14**, 252–256.

Gotch, F. A. and Sargent, J. A. (1985). A mechanistic analysis of the National Cooperative Dialysis Study (NCDS). *Kidney International* **28**, 526–534.

Gotch, F., Gentile, D. E., and Schoenfeld, P. Y. (1993). CAPD prescription in current clinical practice. *Advance is Peritoneal Dialysis* **9**, 69–72.

Harty, J. C. *et al.* (1994). The normalized protein catabolic rate is a flawed marker of nutrition in CAPD patients. *Kidney International* **45**, 103–109.

Ho-dac-Pannekeet, M. M., Atasever, B., Struijk, D. G., and Krediet, R. T. (1997). Analysis of ultrafiltration failure in peritoneal dialysis patients by means of standard peritoneal permeability analysis. *Peritoneal Dialysis International* **17**, 144–150.

Kawano, M. *et al.* (1998). Fatal cardiac beta2-microglobulin amyloidosis in patients on long-term hemodialysis. *American Journal of Kidney Diseases* **31**, E4.

Kaysen, G. A., Dubin, J. A., Muller H. G., Rosales, L. M., and Levin, N. W. (2000). The acute-phase response varies with time and predicts serum albumin levels in hemodialysis patients. The HEMO Study Group. *Kidney International* **58**, 346–352.

Kaysen, G. A. *et al.* (2002). Relationships among inflammation nutrition and physiologic mechanisms establishing albumin levels in hemodialysis patients. *Kidney International* **61**, 2240–2249.

Keshaviah, P. (1995). The solute removal index—a unified basis for comparing disparate therapies. *Peritoneal Dialysis International* **15**, 101–104.

Keshaviah, P. R., Nolph, K. D., and Van Stone, J. C. (1989). The peak concentration hypothesis: a urea kinetic approach to comparing the adequacy of continuous ambulatory peritoneal dialysis (CAPD) and hemodialysis. *Peritoneal Dialysis International* **9**, 257–260.

Keshaviah, P. R. *et al.* (1994). Lean body mass estimation by creatinine kinetics. *Journal of the American Society of Nephrology* **4**, 1475–1485.

Kushner, R. F. and Roxe, D. M. (2002). Bipedal bioelectrical impedance analysis reproducibly estimates total body water in hemodialysis patients. *American Journal of Kidney Diseases* **39**, 154–158.

Ledebo, I. (1998). Principles and practice of hemofiltration and hemodiafiltration. *Artificial Organs* **22**, 20–25.

Lindholm, B. and Bergstrom, J. (1992). Nutritional aspects on peritoneal dialysis. *Kidney International* **38** (Suppl.), S165–S171.

Lindsay, R. M. and Spanner, E. (1989). A hypothesis: the protein catabolic rate is dependent upon the type and amount of treatment in dialyzed uremic patients. *American Journal of Kidney Diseases* **13**, 382–389.

Lowrie, E. G. and Lew, N. L. (1990). Death risk in hemodialysis patients: the predictive value of commonly measured variables and an evaluation of death rate differences between facilities. *American Journal of Kidney Diseases* **15**, 458–482.

Lowrie, E. G., Chertow, G. M., Lew, N. L., Lazarus, J. M., and Owen, W. F. (1999). The urea (clearance × dialysis time) product (Kt) as an outcome-based measure of hemodialysis dose. **56**, 729–737.

Mazzuchi, N., Carbonell, E., and Fernandez-Cean, J. (2000). Importance of blood pressure control in hemodialysis patient survival. *Kidney International* **58**, 2147–2154.

McKane, W., Chandna, S. M., Tattersall, J. E., Greenwood, R. N., and Farrington, K. (2002). Identical decline of residual renal function in high-flux biocompatible hemodialysis and CAPD. *Kidney International* **61**, 256–265.

Morduchowicz, G. Winkler, J., Zabludowski, J.R., and Boner, G. (1994). Effects of residual renal function in haemodialysis patients. *International Urology and Nephrol* **26**, 125–131.

Owen, W. F., Jr., Coladonato, J., Szczech, L., and Reddan, D. (2001). Explaining counter-intuitive clinical outcomes predicted by Kt/V. *Seminars in Dialysis* **14**, 268–270.

Paniagua, R. *et al.* (2002). Effects of increased peritoneal clearances on mortality rates in peritoneal dialysis: ADEMEX, a prospective, randomized, controlled trial. *Journal of the American Society of Nephrology* **13**, 1307–1320.

Prichard, S., Sniderman, A., Cianflone, K., and Marpole, D. (1996). Cardiovascular disease in peritoneal dialysis. *Peritoneal Dialysis International* **16** (Suppl. 1), S19–S22.

Rippe, B. (1993). A three-pore model of peritoneal transport. *Peritoneal Dialysis International* **13** (Suppl. 2), S35–S38.

Sargent, J. A. and Gotch, F. A. (1980). Mathematic modeling of dialysis therapy. *Kidney International* (Suppl. 10), S2–S10.

Schneditz, D., Van Stone, J. C., and Daugirdas, J. T. (1993). A regional blood circulation alternative to in-series two compartment urea kinetic modeling. *ASAIO Journal* **39**, M573–M577.

Smye, S. W., Tattersall, J. E., and Will, E. J. (1999). Modeling the postdialysis rebound: the reconciliation of current formulas. *ASAIO Journal* **45**, 562–567.

Spalding, E. M. Chamney P. W., and Farrington, K. (2002). Phosphate kinetics during hemodialysis: evidence for biphasic regulation. *Kidney International* **61**, 655–667.

Tattersall, J. E., DeTakats, D., Chamney, P., Greenwood, R. N., and Farrington, K. (1996). The post-hemodialysis rebound: predicting and quantifying its effect on Kt/V. *Kidney International* **50**, 2094–2102.

Teraoka, S. *et al.* Current status of renal replacement therapy in Japan. *American Journal of Kidney Diseases* **25**, 151–164.

Twardowski, Z. J. (1990). PET—a simpler approach for determining prescriptions for adequate dialysis therapy. *Advances in Peritoneal Dialysis* **6**, 186–191.

Vanholder, R., De Smet, R., and Lameire, N. (2001). Protein-bound uremic solutes: the forgotten toxins. *Kidney International* **78** (Suppl.), S266–S270.

Vanholder, R., Veys, N., Van Biesen, W., and Lameire, N. (2002). Alternative timeframes for hemodialysis. *Artificial Organs* **26**, 160–162.

Vincent, C., Revillard, J. P., Galland, M., and Traeger, J. (1978). Serum beta2-microglobulin in hemodialyzed patients. *Nephron* **21**, 260–268.

Watson, P. E., Watson, I. D., and Batt, R. D. (1980). Total body water volumes for adult males and females estimated from simple anthropometric measurements. *American Journal of Clinical Nutrition* **33**, 27–39.

12.6 Medical management of the dialysis patient

Claude Jacobs

Introduction

Patients relying on long-term renal replacement therapy (RRT) either haemodialysis (HD) or peritoneal dialysis (PD) remain uraemic because the clinical, biological, immunological, and other disturbances are only partly corrected by dialysis. The removal of 'uraemic toxins' by dialysis methods depends on their physicochemical characteristics, mainly their degree of binding to plasma proteins (Dhondt *et al.* 2000). The overall medical management of HD and PD patients has many features in common, but some differences specific to the actual technique. The four main objectives of the long-term treatment of endstage renal failure (ESRF) are: (a) minimizing morbidity and mortality; (b) imitating the normal clinical and metabolic status as best as one can; and (c) striving for the best possible quality of life. A detailed description of the uraemic syndrome and the effects on organ system is covered in Chapter 11.3.1.

Main causes of mortality and morbidity in dialysis patients

Less than 50 years ago ESRF was invariably lethal. Over the last three decades maintenance dialysis methods have successfully prolonged the life of patients with terminal uraemia. In 1996 more than one million ESRF patients were alive on various modes of RRT worldwide, some of whom had been treated for more than 20 years (Schena 2000).

Despite this impressive achievement the annual mortality rates reported for patients on long-term dialysis in 1999 in the United States were 247 and 231 per thousand patient-years (ptpy) at risk in HD and PD patients, respectively. Mortality rates are highly dependent on the patients' age and underlying renal disease. In 1999, the annual mortality rate of prevalent patients on HD in the United States was 87.4 ptpy among those aged 30–39 years, but rose to 359.8 ptpy in those aged 70–79 years. In the same year, the mortality rate of prevalent HD patients aged 60–64 years with primary glomerulonephritis and of those with diabetes was 166.8 and 246.9 ptpy, respectively (USRDS 2001). Overall the expected lifetime of dialysis patients evaluated in the 1996 prevalent patient cohort was estimated to be between 17 and 39 per cent of that of the sex-, age-, and race-matched US population (USRDS 1998). It is, however, noteworthy that in several major countries of the developed world the death rates of dialysis patients decreased markedly in the last decade of the twentieth century compared with that recorded in the 1970s and 1980s. This trend is well documented in recent surveys conducted in six Western European Countries (Van Dijk *et al.* 2001), the United States (USRDS 2000;

Meier-Kriesche 2001), Canada (Schaubel *et al.* 2000), and Japan (Iseki *et al.* 2002a,b).

The improvement in survival observed in dialysis patients over the past 15 years is all the more remarkable as the mean age of incident patients has steadily increased during this time period. In six European Countries recently surveyed by the European Renal Association and European Dialysis and Transplant Association (ERA-EDTA) Registry (Austria, Finland, French Belgium, The Netherlands, Norway, and Scotland), the mean age of incident dialysis patients has increased by 14 years over a period of 20 years (Van Dijk *et al.* 2001). In the 1040 adult patients, first taken onto dialysis treatment in 1998 in the greater Paris-Ile-de-France area (10.7 million inhabitants), the mean age at the start of RRT was 59.8 years, and the incidence was about six times higher in males aged greater than or equal to 75 years than in those aged 18–39 years (Jungers *et al.* 2000). In the Japanese Island of Okinawa, the average age of patients starting dialysis increased from 46.4 to 53.8 years in the period 1991–2000 (Iseki *et al.* 2002a). During this period the comorbidity of many of the incident patients has increased, for example, the much higher proportion of diabetics who accounted in 1999 for 43 per cent of incident patients in the United States, 23 per cent in the six previously cited European Countries, 20 per cent in the French-Ile-de-France region, and 30 per cent in Okinawa.

Data collected in most of the large national/international registries show unequivocally that the mortality in dialysis patients is largely due to cardiac and vascular causes (which is also true for the general populations of the developed countries). Thus, among the dialysis patients who died in the United States during the 1997–1999 period (239 ptpy, all ages combined), 41 per cent had a cardiac cause (cardiac arrest 21 per cent, acute myocardial infarction 8.8 per cent, arrhythmias 5.4 per cent), followed by septicaemia (11.3 per cent) and cerebrovascular accidents (CVA 5.7 per cent). A similar distribution of the causes of death is reported for dialysis patients who died during the 1991–1999 period in the six European countries, cardiac deaths accounting for 36 per cent of all deaths, followed by infections and strokes.

Besides fatal complications, dialysis patients often suffer a wide array of more or less distressing and disabling complications. Some are directly related to the dialysis technique such as dysfunction of the vascular or peritoneal access. Others interefere with the patients' quality of life (QOL) and social/vocational rehabilitation such as chronic fatigue frequently associated with depression and/or sexual dysfunction (see Chapter 11.3.3).

Numerous studies of the factors which most influence the morbidity and mortality of dialysis patients show them to be in two categories:

1. Pre-existing factors (many that cannot be changed) which will have significant effects during the course of RRT, for example, age,

gender, underlying disease responsible for renal dysfunction (e.g. diabetes mellitus, systemic lupus, myeloma), or the consequences of comorbid conditions that result from either inadequate pre-dialysis care, poor compliance, or late referral to a specialized nephrological team (Jungers 2002).

2. Factors which result from inadequate dialysis or care or non-compliance with dialysis, dietary, or drug regimens.

The factors that contribute most to mortality and morbidity in dialysis patients are: a previous history of (non-skin) malignant disease, coronary heart disease, congestive heart failure, cerebrovascular or peripheral vascular disease, chronic obstructive pulmonary disease, and malnutrition (suggested by low serum albumin, prealbumin), parathyroid hormone (PTH) and creatinine concentrations (Foley and Parfrey 1998; Avram et al. 2001; Combe et al. 2001). Most of the established risk factors involved in the development of atherosclerotic cardiovascular disease are already present in (too) many patients at the time of starting RRT, for example, uncontrolled hypertension, dyslipidaemias, and heavy smoking. Although dialysis and associated medical treatments may be effective in improving many of the clinical and metabolic complications of uraemia, they cannot reverse the detrimental consequences of ageing or the extrarenal established complications of systemic diseases (e.g. diabetic retinopathy or neuropathy) or the disastrous consequences of poor medical care.

Main components of the medical management of dialysis patients

The dismal results reported on the outcome of patients in the United States at the end of the 1980s, with an annual mortality rate above 20 per cent (Eggers et al. 1990) was a 'wake-up' call for the nephrological community. It became clear that dialysis had to move from an empirical procedure applied according to individual physician's experience (and prejudices) to be more standardized and evidence-based. This cultural revolution gave rise to 'Clinical Practice Guidelines' elaborated by several groups of experts who had reviewed the available literature on the major issues in various areas of dialysis. Clinical practice guidelines for dialysis patients were thus first published in September–October 1997 in the United States as the National Kidney Foundation Dialysis Outcome Quality Initiative (NKF/DOQI 1997). They were extended and updated in 2000 (NKF/DOQI 2000) and 2001 (NKF/DOQI 2001). There were similar initiatives in the United Kingdom (The Renal Association 1997) and in Canada (Churchill et al. 1999). The guidelines were soon widely circulated among the nephrological community and have become a reference point. The guidelines are, however, no more than recommendations and should not be considered binding. Nevertheless, these clinical practice guidelines assist in the aim of providing more standardized and best practice care.

The case for 'timely initiation of dialysis' (see Chapter 12.1)

The rationale for timely initiation of dialysis is to: (a) *avoid* the debilitating and sometimes life-threatening complications of advanced uraemia; (b) *maintain* reasonable health and quality of life; and (c) *prevent* morbidity–mortality late in the course of RRT. Dialysis should be initiated to maintain well being and not to rescue from illness

(Burkart 1998; Golper 1999). At present the main causes for less than optimal initiation of dialysis remain: late referral of severely uraemic patients to nephrologists (Levin 2000; Jungers 2002); underestimating the true severity of renal failure (Rahn et al. 1999), poor patient compliance or refusal to start dialysis and, unfortunately, the persisting shortage of dialysis facilities. The debate is sometimes obscured by conceptual and academic conflicts around dietary means for delaying the initiation of dialysis treatment (Walser et al. 1999; Mehrotra et al. 2000).

'Timely initiation of dialysis' is based primarily on a small set of measurements. Serum creatinine (Scr) and creatinine clearance (Ccr) have been found to be unreliable markers of residual renal function (RRF) in ESRF patients (Walser et al. 1999), which is better estimated by the formula [Ccr + urea clearance (ml/min/1.73 m^2)/2] (Burkart 1998). The accuracy of another indicator of RRF (as well as of adequacy of dialysis): Kt/V urea, suffers from errors made in the evaluation of the urea distribution volume, that is, total body water (TBW). The use of sophisticated formulae based on anthropometric data (Watson et al. 1980) or recent biophysical methods such as bioelectrical impedance (Plum et al. 2001; Kushner et al. 2002) yield more accurate results, but are not widely available. In the year 2000, update of the NKF/DOQI guidelines (National Kidney Foundation 2001) the criteria for 'initiating some form of dialysis' for ESRF patients have not been altered. The working group supported the contention that once the RRF expressed as weekly Kt/V urea falls below 2.0, patients are at increased risk of malnutrition and uraemic complications. Hence, dialysis should be implemented at a weekly K_RT/V urea (R for residual) of 2.0, which approximates a kidney urea clearance of 7 ml/min (normalized to TBW) and a kidney Ccr between 9 and 14 ml/min/1.73 m^2, the glomerular filtration rate (GFR) estimated by the arithmetic mean of the urea clearance and Ccr being then at about 10.5 ml/min/1.73 m^2. Dialysis should also be started when there is a deterioration in the nutritional indicators such as a greater than 6 per cent involuntary reduction in oedema-free usual body weight or a reduction of serum albumin by greater than or equal to 0.3 g/dl and to less than 4.0 g/dl in the absence of acute infection or inflammation, confirmed by repeat laboratory testing. Recent data on the level of renal function at the initiation of dialysis in the United States clearly show that these targets are far from being achieved (Obrador et al. 1999) with 63 per cent among 90,897 patients starting dialysis between April 1995 and September 1997 having a 'predicted' GFR between 5 and 10 ml/min/1.73 m^2 and 25 per cent lower than 5 ml/min/1.73 m^2. The current and future constraints on the facilities for RRT in many countries raise serious questions as to whether the guidelines for initiation of RRT will be applicable to the majority of the ESRF populations.

The lively debate sustained by the advocates and opponents of a protein restricted diet for delaying the initiation of some form of RRT should actually be clarified with more precise definitions of 'early dialysis'. It should be acknowledged that a standard 'protein restricted diet' providing patients with a residual GFR less than 25 ml/min, 0.6 g/kg/day of protein including greater than or equal to 35 kcal/kg and less than or equal to 10 mg/kg of phosphate, should not delay a 'timely initiation of dialysis' as defined by the DOQI guidelines (residual GFR ~ 10 ml/min). On the other hand, carefully prescribed and monitored dietary prescriptions on the above basis should be preferred to an 'early initiation of dialysis', that is, when the residual GFR is still between 15 and 25 ml/min (Maroni 1998).

Another approach developed for more customized care of patients with advanced ESRF is that of 'Incremental dialysis'. The concept is based on the principle that patients with advanced chronic renal failure (CRF) should maintain a constant weekly global Kt/V urea of 2.0 by adding to their RRF an adequately titrated dose of dialysis. This dose of dialysis has to be increased over time according to the progressive fall of the RRF. Furthermore, the qualitative and quantitative nature of waste removal performed by any dialysis method cannot be considered as strictly equivalent to that achieved by RRF and thus cannot really be added arithmetically. The dose of dialysis that needs to be added to RRF to provide a total weekly therapy equivalence of Kt/V urea of 2.0 varies according to whether a continuous or intermittent technique of dialysis is used (Golper 1998). The main reasons for using incremental dialysis include either patient-specific psycho-social situations, or local economic restrictions, for example, a shortage in facilities precluding full-scale conventional dialysis therapy.

Whatever the mode of follow-up applied for patients with advanced CRF, its efficacy and safety is analogous to that operating for a smooth landing of an aircraft at a 'dialysis initiation airport'. The universally available navigation instruments for meeting this goal are listed in Table 1.

Adequate/optimal dialysis prescription and delivery (see Chapters 12.4 and 12.5)

On the basis of the results of the National Cooperative Dialysis Study, Gotch and Sargent (1985) coined the concept of 'dialysis dose', equating the prescription of dialysis for a uraemic patient to that of a pharmacological treatment.

'Adequate dialysis' has thus been defined as the dose of dialysis below which one observes a 'significant worsening of mortality–morbidity'. Optimal dialysis would be the dose of dialysis above which no further improvement in the patients' morbidity–mortality could be expected (Hakim et al. 1992). Numerous outcome studies have demonstrated a correlation between the delivered dose of dialysis and patient morbidity and mortality (Hakim et al. 1994; Held et al. 1996). The Haemodialysis Adequacy Working Group of the NKF/DOQI has extensively reviewed the key issues of adequate/optimal dialysis prescription, measurement, and delivery in the update of the 1997 guidelines published in 2001 (Haemodialysis Adequacy Working Group 2001). The dialysis care team should deliver a Kt/V of at least 1.2 (single pool) for both adult and paediatric patients. For those using the 'urea reduction ratio' (URR) the delivered dose should be equivalent to a Kt/V of 1.2, that is, an average URR of 65 per cent. However, URR can vary substantially as a function of fluid removal. These are absolute minimum values and to prevent the Kt/V or URR for any patient from declining to below the minimum delivered dose the working group suggested that the prescribed minimum Kt/V be 1.3 and the URR targeted at 70 per cent for patients dialysing three times per week. When a double pool model is used for calculating Kt/V, the minimum prescribed dose should be 1.05 for patients dialyzing three times per week. In order to avoid misleading results of measurements of Kt/V and URR, careful attention should be taken to blood sampling procedures, particularly for postdialysis blood samples, which may be polluted by postdialysis urea rebound secondary to angioaccess and cardiopulmonary recirculation. The technical requirements required for meeting the currently accepted criteria for delivery of adequate dialysis are listed in Table 2.

Just providing a recommended minimum value of Kt/V or URR for the patients is not a sufficiently adequate dialysis protocol. The main clinical and biological criteria to be met for HD patients are listed in Table 3.

Table 1 Clinical and biological requirements for a safe 'touch down' of patients with chronic renal failure at the time of initiation of dialysis

GFR ([Ccr + Cl urea]/2): 10 ml/min/1.73 m^2
Residual weekly Kt/V urea: 2
Absence of fluid overload
Blood pressure: ≤140/90 mmHg
Serum bicarbonate: ≥22 mmol/l
Serum potassium: <5.0 mmol/l
Serum calcium: 2.3–2.5 mmol/l
Serum phosphate: <1.6 mmol/l
Serum iPTH (1–84) 130–250 pg/ml
Serum albumin: >35 g/l
Hb concentration: >11.5 g/dl
MNCV (lower limb[a]): >40 m/s

[a] Motor nerve conduction velocity.

Table 2 Technical requirements for delivery of adequate dialysis (adult patients)

Conventional haemodialysis
Vascular access: blood flow ≥ 300 ml/min
Dialysis fluid: bicarbonate buffered, sterile, pyrogen-free QD: ≥500 ml/min
Volumetric ultrafiltration control
Dialyser:
    Highly permeable, biocompatible membrane
    Surface area: ≥1 m^2
Dose of dialysis:
    Minimum Kt/V urea: 1.2–1.3 (single pool)
    Minimum urea reduction rate: 65–70%
    Measurement of dialysis dose: once monthly
Weekly dialysis time: ≥12 h (4–4.5 h × 3)

Peritoneal dialysis
CAPD: minimum weekly Kt/V urea: 2 minimum total creatinine
    clearance: 60 l/1.73 m^2
CCPD: minimum weekly Kt/V urea: 2.1
APD: minimum total creatinine clearance: 63 l/1.73 m^2

Table 3 Basic criteria to be met by adequate dialysis

Fluid removal permitting return to correctly evaluated 'dry weight' at end of dialysis

Predialysis blood pressure < 140/90 mmHg with or without antihypertensive drugs

Predialysis plasma concentrations
    Potassium: ≤5.5 mmol/l without absorption of ion exchange resins
    Bicarbonate: ≥24 mmol/l
    Inorganic phosphate: ≤1.6 mmol/l without oral binding agents
    Urea: <35 mmol/l with daily protein-intake 1.2 g/kg/BW
    Albumin: ≥40 g/l
    Haemoglobin: 11.5–13 g/100 ml with or without rHu-EPO
    Motor nerve conduction velocity (common peroneal nerve): ≥45 m/s

Not included are, however, the very important issues pertaining to the patients' comfort, tolerance, and impact on their QOL.

The clinical practice guidelines for PD adequacy have also been updated in detail in 2000 by the NKF/DOQI PD working group (2001). For patients treated with continuous ambulatory peritoneal dialysis (CAPD), the delivered PD dose should be a total Kt/V urea of at least 2.0 per week and a total Ccr of at least 60 l/week/1.73 m^2 for high and high-average transporters and 50 l/week/1.73 m^2 in low and low-average transporters (NKF/DOQI 2001). The dose requirements for other PD techniques (continuous cyclic PD, nocturnal intermittent PD, automated PD) are deemed to be slightly higher (Kt/V urea of at least 2.2 and total weekly Ccr around 65 l/1.73 m^2). Providing an 'adequate' dose of PD calculated according to the above criteria and frequent monitoring of the persistance of PD adequacy over time is critical for achieving an optimal patient and technique survival. The results of the Canada–United States (CANUSA) study reporting on 680 incident CAPD patients showed a 5 per cent decrease in patient survival for every 0.1 decrease in total weekly Kt/V urea for Kt/V urea between 1.5 and 2.3. The risk of technique failure increased by 5 per cent for every 5 l/week decrease in Ccr (Churchill *et al.* 1996).

Control of fluid, electrolyte, and acid–base balance

Maintaining the volume and composition of body fluids as close as possible to normal is a key aim of dialysis care.

Control of fluid volume

Most dialysis patients are chronically fluid overloaded (their daily urinary output being frequently less than 500 ml) explaining the development of oedema, hypertension, left ventricular hypertrophy (LVH), and acute and chronic left ventricular dysfunction. The dialysis prescription aims for removal of the accumulated interdialytic fluid restoring the patient's 'dry weight', defined as the lowest weight at the end of a dialysis session (or during the steady state of a PD patient) that a patient can tolerate without symptomatic hypotension in the absence of oedema. The clinical assessment of a true dry weight is fraught with errors. Overestimation of dry weight and chronic hypervolaemia is the main cause of persistent hypertension (and 'pseudoresistant' hypertension) in dialysis patients, whereas underestimation of dry weight manifests as symptomatic intra- and/or inter dialytic hypotensive episodes, which respond favourably to diminution of fluid removal and carefully controlled dry weight gain (Jaeger and Mehta 1999). New techniques to determine the dry weight through a more accurate evaluation of the extra- and intracellular fluid volume status of the patients and their respective variations during the dialytic procedure have been developed. Examples include pre- and postdialysis plasma levels of cyclic guanosine monophosphate (cGMP), atrial natriuretic peptide (ANP), *N*-terminal proANP (Metry *et al.* 2001; Plum *et al.* 2001), ultrasound measurement of the inferior vena cava diameter (Katzarski *et al.* 1997; Yanagiba *et al.* 2001) bioimpedance spectroscopy (Cox-Reijen *et al.* 2001), bipedal bioimpedance analysis (Kushner *et al.* 2002). Despite their technological sophistication, none of these methods has proved superior to careful clinical assessment and some yield conflicting results. Their use remains limited to research oriented dialysis facilities. Because fluid removal is only from the patients' blood compartment, intradialytic ultrafiltration, by inducing a sharp decrease in blood volume, is the major determinant of hypovolaemia-related symptoms, primarily symptomatic hypotension. Recent technological advances

allow non-invasive monitoring of blood volume changes by measuring haematocrit (Hct), using optical or impedance methods, or total protein concentration by ultrasonic evaluation (Locatelli *et al.* 1998b; Santoro *et al.* 1998; Shulman *et al.* 2001). However, the reduction in blood volume during HD is subject to considerable intra- and interindividual variations and thus routine blood-volume monitoring remains currently of limited interest in the prevention of dialysis-related hypotension (Locatelli 1998b; Leypoldt *et al.* 2002).

Maintaining adequate hydration status in a steady-state dialysis patient requires a restriction of the interdialytic daily fluid intake to a volume not exceeding 500 ml more than the residual urinary output and a reduction of the daily dietary sodium intake to approximately 80–100 mmol of sodium chloride, that is, no more than 6 g of salt. Such a regimen would require an intradialytic fluid removal of about 2.5 kg with a modest ultrafiltration rate and a dialysis-fluid sodium concentration no greater than 140 mmol/l (see Chapter 12.3). Unfortunately, interdialytic weight gains are usually two- or threefold greater, requiring intense fluid removal within a short period of time provoking clinical manifestations of dialysis intolerance, such as headache, cramps, vomiting, hypotensive episodes, arrhythmias, and interdialytic exhaustion. This intradialytic symptomatology can be alleviated by prolonging the dialysis time, slowing the ultrafiltration rate, close monitoring of fluid loss by volumetric ultrafiltration control, and by optimizing the dialysate sodium concentration. The optimal value of dialysate sodium concentration is that, which restores the physiological value of the exchange sodium pool at the end of dialysis. Specially designed software, based on biofeedback techniques using on-line sensors and kinetic modelling, have been recently developed aiming at a fully automated determination of the optimal dialysate sodium concentration according to the patients' predialytic hydration status and sodium concentration (Locatelli *et al.* 1998a; Bosetto *et al.* 1999; Petitclerc *et al.* 1999).

The use of sodium profiling, time-dependent profile of the sodium concentration in the dialysis fluid over the course of a HD session, aims at keeping the plasma osmolality in a physiological range despite the loss of urea and other solutes across the dialyser, thus preventing dialysis intolerance symptoms and improving vascular stability. Careful monitoring of sodium balance is required with this technique, to prevent inappropriate sodium accumulation that may cause increased interdialytic thirst, weight gain, and the development or aggravation of hypertension (Oliver *et al.* 2001; Stiller *et al.* 2001). Oral administration of frusemide at doses ranging from 500 to 1000 mg daily may be helpful for improving the hydration status of dialysis patients, since at these doses the loop diuretic significantly increases, at least for a while, the patients' urinary sodium excretion. Patients should, however, be checked regularly for toxic effects of these high doses of frusemide.

Potassium

Hyperkalaemia is an ever-present lethal threat to patients with ESRF and accounted for 4.0 and 2.6 deaths ptpy in HD and PD patients, respectively, in the United States during the year 1999 (USRDS 2001).

On the other hand, hypokalaemia (<2.5 mmol/l) may develop in malnourished patients or in case of acute or chronic potassium loss via the digestive tract (vomiting or diarrhoea) creating a risk of cardiac arrhythmias. Although the usual concentration of potassium in dialysate is 2 mmol/l, ensuring adequate removal of interdialytic potassium accumulation, it may have to be lowered to 1 mmol/l (at least temporarily) in chronically hyperkalaemic patients. Conversely, it has to be increased to 3–3.5 mmol/l in patients with low predialysis potassium serum concentrations, especially for those on digitalis treatment.

Hyperkalaemia is enhanced by any associated metabolic or respiratory acidosis and hypoaldosteronism and should be sought in diabetic patients (Ahmed and Weisberg 2001). Dialysis patients need to be reminded, which are the dangerous potassium-rich foods which must be severely restricted. This is best done by regular dietary advice.

Acute hyperkalaemia (>6.5 mmol/l) requires emergency dialysis. Prior to the start of dialysis electrocardiogram (ECG) monitoring is mandatory, whilst symptomatic treatment is provided through intravenous (IV) infusion of calcium chloride or gluconate, or of hypertonic glucose solution with insulin or infusion/inhalation of salbutamol (Allon 1993), a β-2 adrenergic agonist, which stimulates the potassium flux into the cells. IV administration of salbutamol is reported as appropriate in patients with life-threatening hyperkalaemia (Kemper et al. 1996). The efficacy of IV infusion of bicarbonate is unpredictable in its capacity to correct significant elevations of serum potassium. Sodium polystyrene cation exchange resin (Kayexalate®) by mouth or enema is useful when less rapid correction of hyperkalaemia is needed. The chronic administration of Kayexalate® as prevention of hyperkalaemia is ill-advised because of the high sodium content and because such a prescription leads to a false sense of security encouraging patients to relax the restriction of potassium-rich foods in their diets.

Acid–base balance

All patients with ESRF are prone to metabolic acidosis. A total of 70–80 mmol of H^+ are retained daily in anuric, non-hypertacabolic adult subjects ingesting ~70 g of protein. Besides increasing the risk of hyperkalaemia, uncontrolled acidosis has many detrimental effects, including the stimulation of protein catabolism leading to protein malnutrition (Franch and Mitch 1998), depression of myocardial contractility predisposing to arrhythmias. Metabolic acidosis plays an important role in the development of bone disease in uraemic patients, leading to depletion of alkaline bone-calcium salts as compensation for the negative H^+ ion balance. Metabolic acidosis is worsened in dialysis patients by an excessive exogenous H^+ intake (high protein diet) or endogenous production (ketosis, lactic acidosis) or by additional bicarbonate loss via the digestive tract (acute or chronic diarrhoea).

Metabolic acidosis has to be corrected during dialysis by the buffer contained in the dialysate, described in detail in Chapter 12.2, or by direct infusion as in the acetate-free biofiltration (AFB) technique (Zucchelli et al. 1994). Technical advances have led to the universal replacement of acetate-buffered dialysate by bicarbonate buffered dialysis fluids used for all extracorporal dialysis techniques (Mercadal et al. 1999). The main advantages attributed to bicarbonate dialysis are the avoidance of the symptoms and adverse effects of acetate intolerance observed in patients with limited or impaired capacity for acetate metabolism and its beneficial effects on vascular stability during the dialysis sessions particularly in patients treated with short (<4 h) treatments. Adequate correction of metabolic acidosis in dialysis patients is indicated by a postdialysis plasma bicarbonate concentration of 26–28 mmol/l, which should not decline to less than 22 mmol/l by the time of the next dialysis session.

In addition to the buffer provided during dialysis, the calcium carbonate prescribed to many dialysis patients as calcium supplementation and a phosphate-binding agent also contributes significantly to the correction of metabolic acidosis. Whilst correction of metabolic acidosis and maintenance of a normal pH are one of the principal aims and criteria of dialysis, it has to be remembered that excessive postdialytic alkalosis enhances postdialytic hypokalaemia, increasing the risk of cardiac arrhythmias.

Calcium

Calcium transfer from the dialysis fluid into the patient, oral supplementation with calcium salts, and oral or IV administration of calcitriol $1,25 (OH)_2D_3$ or other vitamin D sterols such as paracalcitol, doxercalciferol, or alfacalcidol (Steddon et al. 2001) are the three ways of compensating for the long-term negative calcium balance observed in dialysis patients. This results from a reduction of dietary intake of both calcium and phosphate with impaired intestinal absorption of calcium caused by a deficient renal biosynthesis of calcitriol. Normalization of calcium balance is essential at all stages of renal failure and particularly in dialysis patients to reduce the manifestations of osteodystrophy by controlling secondary hyperparathyroidism (HPT).

Calcium fluxes in dialysis patients depend on the calcium concentration in the dialysate, the volume of ultrafiltration that removes the non-protein bound diffusible calcium, and the plasma calcium and phosphate concentrations at start of dialysis. The optimal calcium concentration in the dialysate for achieving a zero or slightly positive calcium balance cannot be the same for every dialysis patient. Given the widespread use of calcium salts administered to the patients as phosphate binders, any adjustment of the calcium concentration in the dialysate has to take account of the risk of being either too low (such as 1.25 mmol/l) leading to a negative calcium balance and enhanced secretion of PTH, or too high (such as 1.75 mmol/l leading to hypercalcaemia, which carries the risk of vascular and tissue deposition of calcium. Since it is not easy to 'customize' the calcium concentration of the dialysis fluid to meet the specific requirements of each individual patient, an 'intermediate' calcium concentration of 1.50–1.60 mmol/l is generally accepted for most HD patients. The goal is to reach a predialysis total calcium serum concentration of 2.40–2.50 mmol/l (1.25–1.30 mmol/l of ionized calcium), that is, at the upper limit of the normal range by adjusting the prescriptions of the doses of oral calcium and vitamin D analogues according to the results of frequent pre- and postdialysis measurements of plasma calcium, phosphate, alkaline phosphatase, and intact PTH (i-PTH) concentrations. Hypercalcaemia (>2.70 mmol/l) requires temporary withdrawal of calcium-containing phosphate binders and of vitamin D analogues and if necessary a temporary decrease of the dialysate calcium concentration to 1.25 mmol/l.

Phosphate (see Chapter 11.3.9)

Phosphate retention and hyperphosphataemia are present in all the patients with ESRF and play a key role in the development of secondary HPT, renal bone disease (osteitis fibrosa), and extra osseous (particularly vascular) calcium deposition. Since hyperphosphataemia per se is a potent stimulus for PTH secretion (Almaden et al. 1998) close control of plasma phosphate concentration is critical for preventing and treating secondary HPT. The means available for achieving this goal are threefold: (a) decrease of the dietary phosphate intake; (b) enhanced removal of phosphate by dialysis; and (c) use of compounds/drugs that inhibit the intestinal absorption of phosphate (Malluche et al. 1999).

The average daily amount of phosphate contained in an 'ordinary' Western daily diet ranges between 1000–1800 mg of which 60–70 per cent is absorbed in the duodenum and jejunum. The main sources of phosphate are milk and all dairy products, other protein-rich foodstuffs such as eggs, liver, baked/dried beans or peas, lentils, wholegrain or cornbread, and soft drinks such as 'colas' that all have to be carefully rationed in hyperphosphataemic patients, the daily intake not to exceed 800 mg.

This rationing is necessary since no currently used conventional dialysis technique is able to remove all the excess phosphate contained in a free diet. This is due in part to the intercompartmental transfer resistance for phosphate between the intra- and extracellular spaces. Recent studies have revealed the complexity of phosphate kinetics during haemodialysis involving up to four phosphate pools. Postdialysis plasma phosphate concentrations have been found to be higher after long than after short dialysis sessions despite removal of a greater mass of phosphate (Spalding *et al.* 2002). Recent studies showed that the postdialytic rebound of serum phosphate was more rapid and of a greater extent after a haemodiafiltration (HDF) session than after a conventional HD session, whilst the serum phosphate levels immediately after the end of each of these two treatments did not differ. In a group of patients receiving HDF for 3 months the predialysis serum phosphate concentration diminished significantly, whereas those recorded in a control group treated during the same period with conventional HD remained unchanged. Utilization of convective treatment methods thus amplifies the mobilization of phosphate from intracellular compartments (Minutolo *et al.* 2002).

Enhancing phosphate removal thus requires either the use of large surface area dialysers or prolonging dialysis time or ensuring high blood flows. The best results are currently achieved with long slow nocturnal HD. The phosphate-removal performance is so good that addition of phosphate to the dialysate may be necessary to maintain normal phosphate levels (Mucsi *et al.* 1998; Pierratos 1999). A 75 per cent reduction of the prescription of phosphate binders, despite a big increase in phosphate intake has also been achieved without further elevation of serum phosphate in a series of patients treated with short daily dialysis sessions, 2.5 h six times per week (Galland *et al.* 2001). In patients treated with PD, peritoneal phosphate clearance has been found to be higher with ambulatory peritoneal dialysis than with conventional CAPD, depending on plasma phosphate levels, daily volume of dialysis prescribed and peritoneal membrane transport characteristics (Gallar *et al.* 2000). Whatever dialysis technique is employed, the goal of maintaining a pre-HD (or permanent level in PD patients) plasma phosphate concentration less than or equal to 1.60 mmol/l and a calcium × phosphate product lesser than 4 requires the regular intake of phosphate-binding agents by the majority of dialysis patients.

Aluminium-containing phosphate binders have been abandoned for the long-term prevention of hyperphosphataemia since they have been directly incriminated in the development of the severe complications related to aluminium toxicity, including encephalopathy, myopathy, osteomalacia or adynamic bone disease, microcytic anaemia, and resistance to the action of erythropoietin (EPO) (Drüeke 1993).

Calcium-containing compounds (mainly carbonate and acetate) have been the most widely used phosphate binders in recent years. Daily doses range from 1 to 3 g of elemental calcium. The greater efficacy found in some studies of calcium acetate is attributed to the lesser efficacy of calcium carbonate in the presence of gastric anacidity (Pflanz *et al.* 1994). Calcium citrate has also been shown to be an effective, although not superior, phosphate binder, but enhances the intestinal absorption of aluminium, exposing the patients to the risks of aluminium toxicity. This is especially important when aluminium compounds are still prescribed to patients with advanced chronic renal failure (Coburn *et al.* 1991). Calcium salts should be taken with meals, the daily dosage being distributed in order to match the amount of phosphate ingested with each meal. Careful attention to the early detection of (even mild) hypercalcaemia is essential as this may favour the development of extraskeletal calcification, particularly in central and peripheral arteries, coronary arteries and cardiac valves, which have been

demonstrated with modern vascular imaging techniques and are currently considered as high morbidity and mortality risks (Goodman *et al.* 2000; Salusky and Goodman 2002). For the prevention of the consequences of extraskeletal (cardiovascular) calcification it has been suggested that the upper-limit target serum levels should be revised to 2.4 mmol/l for calcium, 1.7 mmol/l for phosphate, less than 4 for Ca × P product and 100–200 pg/ml for i-PTH (Block *et al.* 2000). Meeting such objectives has stimulated the interest of using novel, calcium- and aluminium-free phosphate binders such as sevelamer hydrochloride (Slatopolsky *et al.* 1999) polynuclear iron preparations such as ferric citrate (Chang-Yang *et al.* 2002) or lanthanum (Hutchinson 1999). The latter two compounds are still under clinical trials, whereas the efficacy of sevelamer hydrochloride is already proven (Amin 2002). It also has a beneficial effect in lowering serum lipids in HD patients (Chertow *et al.* 1999). At the present recommended dosage of about 4800 mg per day, sevelamer hydrochloride significantly reduces serum phosphate and Ca × P product with a potency equivalent to that seen with calcium acetate therapy, but with considerably less risk of elevation of serum calcium levels (Amin 2002). Such a modification of the patients' calcium–phosphate equilibrium should have a beneficial effect by reducing the development of coronary and aortic calcification. Further studies are needed before advocating broader use of sevelamer. Improved palatability that would ensure greater patient acceptance, a reduction of the gastrointestinal side-effects (constipation or diarrhoea, flatulence, vomiting) and also a decrease in the currently high cost of the drug would be welcome (Hergesell and Ritz 2002). A reasonable compromise would include the prescription of relatively low dosages of calcium carbonate in patients whose serum calcium concentration remains in the normal range and with no evidence of soft tissue/vascular calcifications. If with such a regimen the serum phosphate concentration remains greater than 1.8 mmol/l, and after having carefully checked compliance to the calcium salt prescription, the introducion of sevelamer is a reasonable option.

Hypophosphataemia can develop in dialysis patients either through marked protein deficiency, excessive phosphate binder dosage or during parenteral nutrition. Sustained hypophosphataemia may provoke serious cardiac or muscular complications. Phosphate supplementation should then be provided either orally or through the dialysis fluid (Pierratos 1999).

Magnesium

At a dialysis fluid magnesium (Mg) concentration of 0.5 mmol/l, the Mg serum concentration of the dialysis patient is usually maintained within the normal range (1–1.30 mmol/l). Hypermagnesaemia may develop in patients taking large quantities of Mg salts for digestive symptoms which then would require a lowering or withdrawal of magnesium from the dialysis fluid.

Control of blood pressure (see Chapters 11.3.4 and 11.3.5)

Hypertension is the single most important risk factor for the development of cardio- and cerebrovascular complications, the leading causes of morbidity and mortality in dialysis patients. This has been repeatedly demonstrated in all survival statitics published worldwide over the past 40 years. The founding father of maintenance dialysis, B.H. Scribner reinforced the notion that 'adequate control of blood pressure (BP) must become a part of the definition of dialysis adequacy along with an adequate dose of dialysis and adequate intake of protein' (Charra et al. 1992). Long-term uncontrolled hypertension causes LVH (Canella et al. 2000), is an independent risk factor for cardiomyopathy, cardiac failure, ischaemic heart disease (IHD), and death (Foley et al. 1996). Despite the universally recognized detrimental effect of hypertension in dialysis patients, 60–70 per cent of patients reported on in clinical studies performed in Europe as well as in North America remain hypertensive while undergoing HD (Canella et al. 2000; Rahman et al. 2000; Grekas et al. 2001) or PD treatment (Menon et al. 2001; Rocco et al. 2001; Wang et al. 2001).

Manual home BP monitoring and ambulatory blood pressure monitoring (ABPM) both provide more precise and useful information of the patients' true BP profile than the routine pre- and postHD BP measurements. Several recent studies have clearly documented the persisting inadequate control of BP in a vast majority of patients during more than half of the interdialytic periods despite antihypertensive (AH) therapy (Canella et al. 2000; Grekas et al. 2000). A satisfactory estimation of the BP load can, however, be approached by using the average value of 12 predialysis BP measurements over a 1-month period (Zoccali et al. 1999). Monitoring of the circadian variations of BP reveals that the normal nocturnal reduction of systolic and diastolic BP (-15 and -20 per cent, respectively) is blunted or absent in 60–80 per cent of dialysis patients (Canella et al. 2000; Narita et al. 2001) a factor with a strongly negative impact on the cardiovascular prognosis of ESRF patients. The decrease in nocturnal fall of BP has been found to be associated with an increase of extracellular volume, even in patients without overt clinical fluid overload, and with insufficient delivery of dialysis (Narita et al. 2001).

The lack of understanding of the pathophysiology of hypertension in dialysis patients accounts in part for the poor control of BP in this population. Certainly, extracellular fluid expansion is the most consistent factor (Bianchi 2000; Hörl and Hörl 2002; Leypoldt et al. 2002). Actually, BP can be maintained within a normal range in the vast majority of dialysis patients by strict control of an extracellular volume excess, as has been clearly demonstrated by the results obtained with the Tassin-long-slow HD technique (Chazot et al. 1995) or more recently with nocturnal home HD (Pierratos 1999), or short-daily dialysis regimens (Traeger et al. 1998). In most of the patients who benefited from such HD modalities, AH drugs could be withdrawn and a significant reduction of LVH demonstrated after 6 months of treatment (Faguali et al. 2001; Galland et al. 2001).

The more stable fluid status provided by PD does not consistently provide better control of BP. A large proportion of patients remain chronically overtly or covertly fluid overloaded, which worsens as residual renal function declines (Menon et al. 2001). Significant LVH and increased left ventricular mass index have been documented in CAPD as well as in continuous cycling peritoneal dialysis patients, particularly after more than 5 years of treatment (Takeda et al. 1998; Wang et al. 2001).

An excessive expansion of extracellular volume cannot account exclusively for persistent (or resistant) hypertension in dialysis patients, a significant proportion of whom remain hypertensive despite having reached their 'dry weight' (see above). Several studies failed to demonstrate a relation between interdialytic weight gain and rise of BP (Luik et al. 1997a,b). Other factors which have been investigated and may play a role in the persistence of hypertension in dialysis patients (Luik et al. 1997a,b) include an inappropriate activation of the renin–angiotensin system, which would cause an inappropriate increase in systemic vascular resistance, but this is an inconsistent finding in hypertensive dialysis patients. The role of increased concentrations of endothelin-1, a result of decreased renal clearance or endothelial cell damage is also a matter of controversy as are accumulation of endogenous inhibitors of the vascular endothelium-generated vasoactive compound nitric oxide such as asymmetric-dimethyl arginine (1-ADMA).

Increased activity of the sympathetic system has also been demonstrated in HD patients. This should originate in the diseased kidneys, since it is not seen in bilaterally nephrectomized patients (Augustyniac et al. 2002). In contrast, recent clinical studies based on pre- and post-dialysis adrenaline and noradrenaline plasma levels failed to show an association of sympathetic activity with hypertension in dialysis patients (Grekas et al. 2001).

Administration of exogenous EPO (epoetin) may cause exacerbation or new hypertension in about 20 per cent of dialysis patients. Many factors are involved (Hörl and Horl 2002) and are not completely understood. Careful and frequent assessment of dry body weight with appropriate reduction in blood volume and slow titration of the epoetin dose are recommended. Correction of anaemia to normal levels of Hct (42 ± 3 per cent) with epoetin can actually be achieved without an increase of BP (Conlon et al. 2000).

Dietary sodium restriction, maintaining an optimal dry weight and prescription of appropriate AH drugs are the three means of controlling BP satisfactorily in dialysis patients. Optimal levels for systolic and diastolic pressures are a matter of debate (Hörl and Hörl 2002). There is no reason why the target BP in hypertensive dialysis patients should differ from that recommended for the age-matched general population. The mortality risk is 'U-shaped' being higher among patients with predialysis systolic BP higher than 180 mmHg or lower than 110 mmHg or markedly hypotensive after dialysis. Predialysis BP levels of 140–150/90 mmHg are desirable targets. The overriding necessity for dietary sodium restriction is often overlooked given the high amount of sodium removal possible by many currently used extracorporeal dialysis techniques. Removal of high sodium loads is more difficult to achieve with standard PD fluids. A return to normal BP with a significant reduction of body weight can be obtained in 80 per cent of PD patients without recourse to AH drugs, by adherence to rigid dietary salt restriction and enhanced ultrafiltration using hypertonic dialysis fluid solutions (Gunal et al. 2001). The disadvantage of this is the reduction in the daily residual urinary volume. In HD patients, with a daily sodium chloride intake not exceeding 6 g and careful ultrafiltration, interdialytic weight gain, and BP decrease progressively, reflected in a reduction of the left ventricular wall thickness (Ozkahya et al. 1999). A significant reduction of BP allowing withdrawal of AH drugs may occur only after a 'lag period' of several weeks or months, as the peripheral vascular resistance decreases. Setting the individual hourly fluid removal profile and end-of-dialysis 'dry weight' remains a challenge. Poor haemodynamic tolerance to aggressive ultrafiltration performed during short-duration (3–4 h) dialysis sessions may trigger symptomatic hypotensive episodes and initiate a vicious circle if fluid and/or sodium supplementation are needed to relieve acute symptoms. Postdialysis residual fluid overload and interdialytic hypertension will require AH medication which will give rise to intradialytic hypotension during the next dialysis session (Fig. 1).

Sudden and profound falls of BP during dialysis are particularly dangerous in patients with vascular instability, for example, the elderly or diabetics, in whom they can precipitate angina, myocardial infarction or CVA. Long, slow, volumetrically controlled HD sessions, an isolated ultrafiltration period during a HD session, use of cooled dialysate

(Hoeben *et al.* 2002), dialysate sodium modelling, or a daily dialysis regimen are options for reducing intradialytic vascular instability. For patients who still develop hypotensive episodes despite optimally tailored dialysis sessions, particularly those with severe autonomic dysfunction, the prescription of a pharmacological treatment such as the α-adrenergic agonist midodrine or of the selective serotonin re-uptake inhibitor sertraline is then indicated (Perazella 2001).

Prescription of AH drugs is needed for patients who do not achieve BP levels less than or equal to 150/90 mmHg with a salt-restricted diet and intensive dialysis–ultrafiltration. The choice between the type and dose depends on their efficacy, patients' tolerance (which governs compliance) and their intra- and interdialytic side-effects (Table 4).

The occurrence and mechanisms of acute anaphylactoid reactions, which occur in some patients treated with AN69 (polyacronitrile) membranes and receiving angiotensin-I converting enzyme inhibitors (ACE-I) have been extensively documented and investigated (Tielemans 1990). These reactions occur at the start of dialysis and comprise acute hypotension, most frequently with flushing, abdominal pain, swelling of the throat, and nausea leading to immediate interruption of dialysis. These symptoms occur with first-use or reused AN69 dialysers, in conventional HD, haemofiltration, or HDF. Bradykinin has been clearly identified as the principal mediator of these reactions. The excessive accumulation of bradykinin results both from an increase of generation and release caused by the contact of blood with the negatively charged AN69 membrane and from its reduced breakdown due to the inhibition of kininase II (identical to Angiotensin Converting Enzyme) by the ACE-I. However, anaphylactoid reactions with elevated bradykinin concentrations have also been reported in patients dialysed on AN69 membranes and who had not received ACE-I (Verresen *et al.* 1994; EBPG 2000).

Angiotensin (AT)I–AT II receptor antagonists are increasingly popular for the treatment of hypertension in the dialysis population. They are very effective, and do not accumulate in endstage renal disease (ESRD) patients with repeated dosing (Sica *et al.* 1997). Anaphylactoid reactions similar to those reported with ACE-I are extremely rare, since their metabolism does not interfere with that of bradykinin (John *et al.* 2001).

A stepwise protocol for the use of AH drugs in dialysis patients is suggested in Table 5. 'Resistant hypertension' may turn out to be

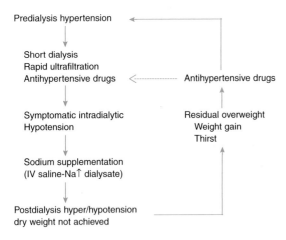

Fig. 1 The vicious circle of dialysis hypertension.

Table 5 Stepwise protocol for prescription of antihypertensive drugs in haemo/peritoneal dialysis patients

Indication: Blood pressure > 140/90 mmHg despite dietary sodium restriction (≤6 g/day) and true dry weight achieved with ultrafiltration
Step 1: Monotherapy: ACE-inhibitor; AT1-angiotensin II receptor antagonist; β-blocker
Step 2: Add loop diuretic, if daily urinary output > 600 ml: oral frusemide 500–1000 mg/day
Step 3: Two/three drug combination: with drugs used in steps 1 and 2 + calcium channel blocker
Step 4: If all of the above ineffective: (rare event!) bilateral nephrectomy??

Table 4 Use of antihypertensive drugs in haemodialysis patients

Drugs	Preferred indication	Specific side-effects in HD patients	Special precautions
ACE inhibitors	LV heart failure, diabetes	Anaphylactoid reactions with AN69 membrane	Reactions unpredictable Select other AHT drug or dialysis membrane
ATI angiotensin II receptor antagonist	Idem	—	Avoid excessive dehydration
Calcium channel blockers	Associated coronary heart disease		Avoid association with β-blockers
β-Blockers	Associated coronary heart disease	Excessive bradycardia with liposoluble compounds	Avoid association with Ca-channel blockers
Centrally acting anti-adrenergic drugs	None	Post-HD hypertensive rebound with clonidine	Avoid
Alpha-adrenergic receptor blockers	None	—	Beware of severe hypotension
Direct vasodilators (diazoxide, nitroprusside)	Emergency treatment of hypertensive crisis	—	Use only in well-equipped hospital setting

'pseudoresistant' hypertension when modest and clinically inapparent fluid overload is corrected by a further small decrease in body weight. Bilateral nephrectomy for 'malignant' or 'intractable' hypertension has become very rare, but remains a 'rescue' measure applicable for the small subset of dialysis patients with repeated hypertensive crises and cerebrovascular complications who do not respond to the full range of AH treatments (Zazgornik *et al.* 1998).

Acute hypertensive episodes with neurological or ocular symptoms, or pulmonary oedema may require an emergency lowering of BP. This goal may be achieved by IV administration of calcium-channel blockers (nicardipine), clonidine, labetabol, nitroprusside, or diazoxide. All these drugs need to be administered with care and continuous monitoring of BP, heart rate, and ECG recording, to prevent too abrupt a reduction in BP and to detect any cardiac ischaemia. Less acute hypertensive emergencies may respond quickly to an oral administration of a fast-acting ACE-I (captopril). Sublingual nifedipine is also very effective, but is considered as dangerous since ischaemic S-T changes, angina pectoris, and acute myocardial infarctions have been reported even in patients who had no relevant history. A sublingual low dose of captopril (25 mg) is safe and more effective for lowering BP in patients with hypertensive emergencies (Angeli *et al.* 1991).

Correction of anaemia (Chapter 11.3.8)

The introduction of recombinant human EPO (Rhu-EPO) for the treatment of uraemic anaemia is probably the single most important advance in the management of chronic renal failure in the last 20 years (Eschbach *et al.* 1989). For the steadily increasing number of patients who benefit from epoetin, the risks associated with repeated blood transfusions such as immunization against HLA antigens, transmission of infectious agents (mainly hepatitis B and C and HIV), haemochromatosis due to iron overload, and erythroid bone marrow suppression have been almost completely eliminated. The beneficial effects of an even incomplete correction of anaemia are multifold (Winearls 1998) and well beyond the well-documented improvement of overall well being, exercise performance, and cognitive function (Moreno *et al.* 2000; Valderrabano *et al.* 2001). Several studies have shown a reduction of prevalence of LVH with increase of haemoglobin (Hb) even with incomplete correction of anaemia (reviewed in Sünder-Plassmann and Hörl 2001). Raising the Hb level to approximately 12 g/dl has a highly beneficial effect on the risk of congestive heart failure (Silverberg 2000), and a Hct of 33–36 per cent has been found associated with a 10 per cent reduction in the risk of death as compared with patients maintained in a Hct range of 30–33 per cent (Ma *et al.* 1999).

After close to 15 years of clinical use the most important factor which prevents a generalized unrestricted prescription of epoetin for all renal failure patients remains its high cost! The side/adverse effects of the drug are few and in most cases easily preventable and curable. Actually, as demonstrated in large multinational studies the most frequent problems encountered are related to undetected or underestimated causes of hyporesponsiveness or 'resistance'.

In the first 5 years after its introduction, the mode of use and evaluation was largely empiric. Recently, a panel of experts in the United States produced the first NKF/DOQI Clinical Practice Guidelines for Anemia of Chronic Kidney Disease, which were updated in 2000

(NKF/DOQI 2001). In 1999, a European Working Party completed a set of European Best Practice Guidelines (EBPG) for the management of anaemia in patients with chronic renal failure (Working Party 1999). Both groups based their guidelines on extensive literature review according to the principles of evidence-based medicine.

The management of anaemia in dialysis patients is thus currently well codified (Eschbach 2000) and its main features are shown in Table 6. The rationalization effort for the improvement of prescription, follow-up, prevention, and treatment of adverse effects of epoetin therapy provided by the guidelines has not yet solved all of the issues pertaining to the utilization of the drug. The main controversies that remain unresolved are listed in Table 7.

It is uncertain whether the benefits of raising Hb concentrations to normal values are significant enough to justify an increase in dose,

Table 6 Main guidelines for the management of renal anaemia with erythropoietin (EPO)

1. *Rule out other possible causes of anaemia*
   (blood loss, haemolysis, nutritional deficiencies, comorbidities . . .)

2. *Start EPO if Hb concentration* (Hb) consistently <11 g/dl
   (haematocrit < 33%)

3. *Target Hb concentration*
   Patients with standard causes of CRF: 85% of the patient population
   should have Hb > 11 g/dl. Mean or median Hb thus ~12–12.5 g/dl
   Patients with cardiovascular diseases, diabetics: not exceed
   Hb 11.5–12 g/dl
   Patients with sickle-cell disease: maintain Hb: 7–9 g/dl

4. *Ensure and monitor adequate iron availability*
   Serum ferritin: 200–500 μmol/l
   TSAT: 30–40%
   Hypochromic red cells: <10%
   Reticulocyte Hb content: ~29 pg
   Monitor iron stores at least every 3 months
   Carefully assess origin of iron deficiency (Table 10)
   Withhold iron supplementation if serum ferritin > 800 μmol/l

5. *Increase dose of EPO gradually* during the initial correction-phase to
   reach target Hb in about 3 months. Usual maintenance dose will then
   be around 100 U/kg/week, range 50–300 U/kg/week

6. *If blunted/non-response to above doses, check for cause* (Table 9)

7. *Detect early and treat adverse effects*: hypertension, vascular access
   problems, development of anti-EPO antibodies

Adapted from: *Nephrology, Dialysis, Transplantation* (14 Suppl. 5), 1999.

Table 7 Main unsolved issues on the use of epoetin in uraemic/dialysis patients

1. Which optimal target haemoglobin concentration?

2. Which more appropriate route and frequency of administration?

3. Which factors involved in the optimization of results of epoetin therapy?

4. Diagnosis and management of hyporesponsiveness/resistance to epoetin therapy

5. Prevention and management of adverse effects related to epoetin therapy

which would entail a 50–100 per cent increase in cost. This debate was fuelled by the results of a US multicentre study documenting a more frequent occurrence of myocardial infarction and higher mortality after 2 years in HD patients who had a previous history of ischaemic heart disease or congestive heart failure and in whom the mean Hct had been increased to 42 per cent versus a control group of patients whose Hct had been maintained around 30 per cent (Besarab *et al.* 1998). This study has however been widely and strongly criticized for its methodology and interpretation. On the other hand, several studies conducted in Europe and in the United States have shown that high (but not normal) Hct or Hb levels were associated with lower morbidity and mortality rates (Locatelli *et al.* 1998b; Ma *et al.* 1999; Moreno *et al.* 2000).

The shared US and European consensus is that a reasonable target range for correction of anaemia in dialysis patients should be Hct 33–39 per cent (i.e. 11–13 g Hb/dl), but that attempts to reach normal values should not be made for patients with cardiac disease, congestive heart failure, or ischaemic cardiopathy (Collins 2002; Lopez-Gomez and Carrera 2002).

The advantages and shortcomings of IV versus subcutaneous (SC) administration of epoetin remain debated for HD patients, but the SC route is of course essential in PD patients. The issue remains focused on attempts to use the lowest possible dose of epoetin to achieve the Hb concentration target. Whereas several studies favoured the SC route for meeting this objective (Kaufmann *et al.* 1998) it has also been shown that there may be no advantage of SC over IV route of administration of epoetin in HD patients if optimal care is taken to correct any iron deficiency in the IV treated patients (Sünder–Plassmann and Hörl 1995).

The issue of optimal frequency of administration of epoetin has become a live issue since the recent introduction of darbepoetin alfa (also known as 'novel erythropoiesis stimulating protein' or NESP). This molecule stimulates erythropoiesis by the same mechanism as both native and recombinant epoetin. The modification of the latter compound by addition of extra sialic acid residues results in a two- to threefold longer elimination half-life (Macdougall *et al.* 1999). Darbepoetin given weekly or fortnightly is as effective as epoetin given more frequently (Locatelli *et al.* 2001; Macdougall 2001a,b). The recommended starting dose for NESP is about 0.45 µg/kg once weekly either SC or IV (1 µg of NESP is equivalent to 200 IU of epoetin). Initiation and maintenance procedures, monitoring for efficacy, and detection of side-effects are identical with darbepoetin and epoetin. (NESP Usage Guidelines Group 2001). There are no reports of antibodies to darbepoetin. The main advantage of darbepoetin lies in the reduction of frequency of injections. However, it has been shown that a similar objective could be reached in using epoetin beta (Weiss *et al.* 2000; Locatelli *et al.* 2002a).

Despite more than a decade of clinical experience the data collected by early 1999 in the European Survey on Anaemia Management (ESAM) study (Valderrabano *et al.* 2000) revealed that only 53.6 per cent of a 12,540 dialysis patient cohort investigated in 14 European countries achieved the EBPG guideline of a greater than 11 g/dl Hb concentration at the end of the 6 month study.

Several factors account for the still largely unsatisfactory results obtained with epoetin therapy, the majority of which are readily reversible (Table 8).

Iron deficiency is the most important reason for a suboptimal response to epoetin therapy. The first step is to establish whether a patient has absolute or functional iron deficiency. Absolute iron deficiency

Table 8 Main causes of hyporesponsiveness/resistance to epoetin therapy

Absolute or functional iron deficiency
Acute/chronic inflammatory/infectious states
Malignant disease
Aluminium overload
Vitamin B_6, B_9 (folate), B_{12} deficiencies
Chronic haemolysis (sickle-cell disease)
Anti-epoetin antibodies
ACE-inhibitors interaction?

results mostly from overt or occult blood loss, usually from the gastrointestinal tract. Functional iron deficiency is caused by inadequate mobilization of normal or even elevated iron stores to the bone marrow by transferrin. The tests assessing iron status used for establishing the accurate cause of iron deficiency are listed in Table 9. The sensitivity of serum ferritin and of transferrin saturation (TSAT) for assessing iron deficiency is poor. A raised serum ferritin concentration due to inflammation, infection, malignancy, or liver disease may mask true iron deficiency. A low TSAT value may indeed reflect iron deficiency or result from an intense erythropoeisis with a disequilibrium between iron storage, circulation, and the bone marrow. The percentage of hypochromic red cells measurable with currently available automated haematology analysers provides a much better estimation of the availability of iron for production of red cells by the bone marrow. More recently it has been shown that the reticulocyte Hb content (CH_R) is an even more reliable marker for detecting iron deficiency, providing 'on-line information' on iron status, whereas the percentage of hypochromic red cells, dealing with mature erythrocytes gives more 'delayed' readout on the iron availability to the bone marrow. CH_R can also be performed during routine blood testing for Hb and Hct on modern automated haematology analysers. The use of CH_R for monitoring iron status showed much less variability than any other test, led to less IV epoetin administration compared to reliance on other indices with similar results for target Hb and epoetin dose requirements (Fishbane *et al.* 2001). Simultaneous measurements of CH_R and C-reactive protein, a sensitive marker of inflammation, are helpful for avoiding useless and potentially harmful administration of iron. A low CH_R associated with a high C-reactive protein concentration suggests this inflammation or infection should be ruled out before increasing iron supplementation.

There is a large literature on the modes of administration of iron to dialysis patients. Severe adverse reactions and even fatalities have been reported with the use of IV iron dextran. Iron sucrose or gluconate are therefore the most widely prescribed compounds. A test dose need not be performed with the use of one of the two latter iron preparations (Macdougall 2000). IV administration may be performed in various ways: short (5–10 min) or slow 60–120 min infusions, depending on the amount of iron to be injected. There are multiple infusion regimens, either small doses (20–40 mg) delivered at each dialysis sessions, or larger doses infused at monthly–bimonthly time intervals (Macdougall 2000; Kosch *et al* 2001). 200–300 mg doses of iron sucrose diluted in 250 ml of normal saline and administered as an IV infusion over 2 h through an infusion pmp is considered as a safe and

Table 9 Iron deficiency in uraemic/dialysis patients

Type	Mechanism	Cause	Indices
Absolute	Insufficient iron stores	Blood loss (digestive tract, gynaecology, etc.)	Hypochromic red cells $\geq 10\%$ Reticulocyte Hb content $< 29\ \mu g$ Serum ferritin $< 100\ \mu g/l$ TSAT: $<20\%$
Functional	Inadequate mobilization or transport from iron stores to bone marrow	Inflammation Infection Malignancy	Serum ferritin > 100 to $> 1000\ \mu g/l$ TSAT $\leq 20\%$ C-reactive protein $> 15\ mg/l$

efficacious means of iron supplementation in HD, PD, and predialysis patients (Chandler *et al.* 2001).

The efficacy of oral iron supplementation is reduced because of the poor intestinal absorption of iron preparations and their dislike by the patients. They are unpleasant to taste and there is a high frequency of (mostly digestive) side-effects at their required daily dosages: 200–400 mg iron fumarate, ascorbate, or sulfate. Nevertheless, exclusive oral iron supplementation was reported in 43.7 per cent of the 945 PD patients, but in only 3.8 per cent of the 10,964 HD patients who participated in the ESAM study (Valderrabano *et al.* 2000). IV infusions delivered to PD patients in an outpatient setting on a once or bimonthly schedule have been shown to be more effective than continuous oral iron supplementation (Johnson *et al.* 2001). Intraperitoneal instillation of iron dextran (500 mg) repeated at a mean interval of 14 days has also been found effective, well tolerated and without negative impact on peritoneal performances, but the study was short term (Mars *et al.* 2001).

It is essential to assess the iron status in patients receiving epoetin therapy regularly; at least every 4–6 weeks during the initial 'correction' phase of epoetin treatment and at least once every 3 months for patients in the 'maintenance' phase. TSAT should not exceed 50 per cent or serum ferritin 800 $\mu g/l$ if iron toxicity is to be avoided.

Apart from adequate iron supplementation and availability, other measures improve the response to epoetin therapy. A significant sparing effect on epoietin requirements for reaching a given target Hct has been shown in patients receiving a higher dialysis dose ($Kt/V \geq 1.4$) versus that observed in a control group in whom Kt/V was lesser than or equal to 1.2 (Movilli *et al.* 2001). Despite the fact that putative medium–large on higher molecular weight erythropoiesis inhibitors may be better removed by high permeability membranes, the use of a high flux polymethylmetacrylate did not result in a significant difference in Hct increase compared with the results obtained in patients dialysed with a conventional cellulose membrane (Locatelli *et al.* 2000). Increasing the duration of HD sessions has a beneficial effect on Hct, eliminating almost all transfusion requirements. This was clearly shown in the patients treated with the long–slow HD technique in Tassin (Charra *et al.* 1992). Finally, a significant rise in Hct values associated with a 20–50 per cent reduction in epoetin requirements were reported in several series of patients treated with daily or nocturnal dialysis schedules (Lacson and Diaz-Buxo 2001). 'Good dialysis' undoubtedly has a beneficial effect on the Hb status and for reducing exogenous epoetin requirements.

Optimizing the quality of the water used for the preparation of the dialysis fluid also contributes to reducing the degree of anaemia and the requirements of exogenous epoetin for its correction. Various chemical contaminants (aluminium, copper, lead, chlorine) and bacterial contamination of the dialysis fluid, which trigger the generation of cytokines

and enhance an inflammatory state in the patients, act as inhibitors of erythropoiesis. The use of pyrogen free, 'ultrapure', dialysate results in a decrease of interleukin (IL)-6 and C-reactive protein levels together with a significant and sustained reduction of epoetin dosage for maintaining a preset Hb concentration (Sitter *et al.* 2000).

Supplementation of several vitamins may have a beneficial effect on the responsiveness to epoetin therapy. Recent studies have revealed depletion of the active moiety of pyridoxine and a significant loss of folate accross the dialyser during high-efficiency dialysis in patients not supplemented with water soluble vitamins (Leblanc *et al.* 2000). It is therefore recommended that dialysis patients be supplemented with 100–150 mg vitamin B_6, 2–3 mg folic acid per week, and 0.25 mg vitamin B_{12} per month (Sünder-Plassman and Hörl 2001). Subclinical vitamin C deficiency is also encountered in some patients, a result of insufficient dietary intake or loss during dialysis sessions. It has been shown that IV administration of vitamin C (300 mg thrice weekly) corrected epoetin-resistant anaemia in patients with functional iron deficiency, even in the presence of iron overload. Ascorbic acid acts by mobilizing the iron from the reticuloendothelial system, promotes iron release to transferrin, and facilitating its incorporation into protoporphyrin (Tarng *et al.* 2001). However, the safety of long-term administration of high doses of ascorbic acid to HD patients has not been established, the anxiety being the development of secondary oxalosis resulting from the metabolism of ascorbic acid. When vitamin C depletion is suspected on clinical grounds it seems reasonable to restrict its supplementation to 1 g orally per day for 4 weeks. It is not proven whether IV supplementation of vitamin C is a benefit to patients who have a normal response to epoetin therapy.

Several studies have shown that administration of L-carnitine (usually 1 g IV at the end of each dialysis session) results in a significant decrease of epoetin requirements for reaching or even exceeding a target Hb (Bommer 1999; Hurot *et al.* 2002). However, no significant differences were found in free or total carnitine plasma concentrations between responders and non responders to L-carnitine supplementation. The mechanisms by which carnitine may reduce epoetin requirements have not been explained. The recommendation issued by a Consensus Group some years ago, was that L-carnitine supplementation should be reserved for patients with an unexplained poor response to epoetin therapy (Consensus Group 1994).

Secondary HPT also interferes with the action of epoetin by causing marrow fibrosis. Patients with marked elevation of i-PTH require greater doses of EPO to reach and maintain a target Hb than patients with lower levels of PTH. Active treatment of HPT either with vitamin D derivatives or parathyroidectomy (PTX) improves the action of EPO in uraemic patients, entailing a simultaneous increase in Hb and reduction of EPO doses in patients whose moderate to severe secondary HPT was controlled (Goicoechea *et al.* 1998).

Whether ACE-I significantly inhibit the response to epoetin therapy remains a matter of controversy. Data from the ESAM study show no differences in epoetin doses in HD patients between those receiving or not ACE-Is, whereas epoetin requirements were significantly higher in ACE-I treated PD patients (Vaderrabano *et al.* 2000). No negative effect on the correction of anaemia in HD patients was recently reported with the use of eight different ACE-Is prescribed in moderate doses (Hayashi *et al.* 2001). Several factors have been proposed to explain the blunting effect. Recently, a spectacular increase in the plasma concentration of *N*-acetyl-seryl-aspartyl-lysyl-proline (AcSDKP), a physiological inhibitor of erythropoiesis in patients treated with ACE-I, has been described (Macdougall 2001b).

An inhibitory effect of ACE-I on epoetin response appears more likely to develop in patients receiving both high doses of ACE-I and low doses of epoetin. The blunting effect of ACE-I on epoetin effectiveness can be overcome by increasing the epoetin dose. There are conflicting results among the few available studies examining the effects of AT II blockers on epoetin responsiveness. The higher dose requirement of epoetin to maintain a target Hct level in patients receiving captopril versus patients treated with Losartan may have been related to increased levels of AcSDKP in patients receiving the ACE-I (Schiffl and Lang 1999).

Patients with either acute or chronic, inflammatory diseases or malignancy are also frequently poorly responsive to epoetin. This is explained by failure of iron release from its storage sites in the reticuloendothelial system and also several cytokines such as IL-1, TNFα, which are generated in excess during inflammatory states and have an inhibitory action on erythropoiesis.

Plasma fibrinogen and/or C-reactive protein plasma concentrations are useful diagnostic tools for evaluation of inflammatory diseases. The response to epoetin in these situations can be improved by increasing the dose and restored by eliminating the cause of inflammation.

Aluminium overload is now uncommon, and usually causes a normo- or microcytic anaemia. Significant aluminium overload may cause a decreased response to epoetin which can often be overcome by increasing the dose, but the essential action is to detect and eliminate the cause(s) of aluminium overload. Aluminium overload is best diagnosed by the IV desferrioxamine test or bone biopsy and requires withdrawal of aluminium-containing phosphate binders, with or without desferrioxamine chelation therapy, and review of the dialysis-water purification system.

The aggravation of pre-existing hypertension or the development of hypertension in previously normotensive patients with ESRD (whether or not treated with dialysis methods) is the most frequently reported adverse effect in clinical practice. This effect is recorded in about 20–25 per cent of HD or PD patients who require the institution or increase of AH drugs, whereas this problem has not been reported in patients with non-uraemic anaemia treated with epoetin. The mechanisms of epoetin-induced hypertension have been extensively studied and include an increase in peripheral vascular resistance along with a reduction in cardiac index. Several factors are involved in the increase of peripheral vascular resistance, including the increase in blood viscosity due to the increased red cell mass, a reduction of the vasodilatation due to the hypoxia linked to anaemia, direct vasopressor effects attributed to increased calcium uptake and augmentation of endothelin-I synthesis and release by endothelial vascular cells. An increase in thromboxane A2 generation and reduction of prostacyclin synthesis by the endothelium might lead to an enhanced response of peripheral vascular tone to endogenous vasoconstrictors. All these factors suggest a possible link between endothelial damage or dysfunction and the development of hypertension (see Chapter 11.3.4).

The elevation of BP usually develops during the early ('correction') phase of epoetin treatment, occurs more commonly in patients with preexisting hypertension and is frequently correlated with the rapidity of the increase of Hct. The control of epoetin induced hypertension is easily achieved in most cases, by reducing excessive extracellular volume through more intensive dialysis–ultrafiltration. If necessary, AH drugs should be prescribed, at least temporarily, until appropriate reduction of dry weight is obtained. No single class of AH drugs is particularly indicated for treating epoetin induced hypertension. A high incidence of seizures caused great concern when epoetin therapy was first used but the problem has been resolved by careful control of BP and insisting on slow increase in Hct.

Well functioning native arteriovenous (AV) fistulae do not appear to be at risk (De Marchi *et al.* 1997), but thrombosis is more common in patients with synthetic vascular access. During the 5 months of the ESAM study an episode of vascular access thrombosis occured in 4.4 per cent of the patients with an AV fistula, compared to 14.5 per cent of those with a synthetic graft. Curiously, the risk of access thrombosis was highest in those who had a Hb level lower than 9 g/dl and lowest in the group with Hb levels between 11.0 and 11.9 g/dl (Valderrabano *et al.* 2000). The haemostatic alterations resulting from platelet activation during dialysis raise the issue of whether to prescribe prophylactic antiplatelet therapy to patients with synthetic vascular grafts but the efficacy of antiplatelet drugs for prevention of vascular access thrombosis in dialysis patients is unproven. Moreover, it has to be remembered that the reversal of the inhibition of platelet aggregation entailed by aspirin, ticlopidine, or clopidogrel may take up to 7 days after discontinuation of the medication (Kaufman *et al.* 2000) which creates risks for patients needing emergency surgery or undergoing renal transplantation. It has also been shown that higher epoetin dose, more blood transfusions, and large doses of iron supplements were required in patients receiving antiplatelet medications, a consequence of increased bleeding from access sites in patients with synthetic grafts and (probably) also gastrointestinal blood loss (Goiecochea *et al.* 2000).

The increase in Hct following epoetin administration may result in a slight reduction of some solute clearances in patients treated with HD particularly for substances that have a slow coefficient of transfer from the red cells to the serum and are dependent on serum water clearance such as creatinine and phosphate. It has thus been shown that an increase of Hct from 20 up to 40 per cent would reduce HD creatinine and phosphate removal by 8 and 13 per cent, respectively (Lim *et al.* 1990). On the other hand, the improved feeling of well being and appetite in patients with increased Hct often led to a (beneficial) greater protein and caloric intake with an increased protein catabolic rate. It may be necessary in some patients to increase the dialysis dose by 15–20 per cent using *Kt/V* urea as the dose indicator (Paganini 1995).

Pure red cell aplasia

There has been a recent disturbing increase in the number of patients developing pure red cell aplasia (PRCA), leading to transfusion dependence while being treated with recombinant EPO. This has, in most cases, been shown to be a complication of the development of a neutralizing antibody to the conformational protein moiety of EPO, native and recombinant (Casadevall *et al.* 2002). This rare complication, which occurs in 50/100,000 patient-years of exposure should be suspected if a profound anaemia with reticulocytes less than $10,000 \times 10^{12}$/mm without a fall in leucocyte and platelet counts develops. The bone marrow appearances are diagnostic. Antibody testing should be performed in laboratories with appropriate expertise. Other marrow disorders, such as myelofibrosis and myeloma, will cause epoetin-resistant anaemia, but the marrow appearances are quite different. Parvo virus infection can cause transient red cell aplasia. In these rare cases there is no point in switching to alternative epoetin products or darbepoetin. Patients do recover, and antibody titres fall after discontinuation of epoetin therapy. Some have been treated with immunosuppression and renal transplantation and IV γ-globulin. The numbers are too small to recommend a particular treatment strategy. This side-effect is most frequently seen in patients receiving epoetin-α subcutaneously.

Skeletal disorders

Renal osteodystrophy (see also Chapter 11.3.9)

Skeletal disorders in renal failure are the result of complex metabolic and hormonal disturbances, which start early in its course and are aggravated by metabolic toxic or iatrogenic factors such as aluminium overload or β2-microglobulin (β2-M) accumulation in more advanced stages.

The complex spectrum of the bone disorders of ESRF is best characterized by static and dynamic histomorphometric analyses of bone biopsy specimens. An abridged classification and some of the main features of the bone disorders in dialysis patients is given in Table 10. Whilst osteitis fibrosa of variable intensity and mixed bone disease remain the more prevalent disorder, the spectrum of the other bone disorders has changed: true oesteomalacia is rare (at least in the developed countries); the frequency of aluminium-related osteomalacia has considerably decreased with the lesser use of aluminium-containing phosphate binders. In contrast, aplastic (or adynamic) bone disease without aluminium deposits has been documented in close to 50 per cent of biopsies in dialysis patients, particularly those with diabetes mellitus and those on CAPD (Sherrard et al. 1996). Bone biopsy remains, however, mainly indicated for research purposes or for a limited number of dialysis patients in whom the value of biochemical markers or radiological data needs to be confirmed by a sound histological proof to substantiate a specific diagnosis or therapeutic procedure, for instance PTX (Malluche et al. 1999). For the majority of dialysis patients the interpretation of laboratory and imaging data provides sufficient information to decide on appropriate therapeutic interventions. Laboratory investigations should thus include at least monthly determinations of serum total (and if possible ionized) calcium, inorganic phosphate, and alkaline phosphatase, and quarterly measurements of serum intact PTH and aluminium (Ferreira 2000). In patients exposed to aluminium, basal serum concentration of aluminium may not be sufficient. A desferrioxamine (DFO) stimulation test is then necessary (D'Haese et al. 1996; Fournier et al. 1998). The radiographical features of secondary HPT are increased bone resorption particularly on the phalanges of the hands, clavicles and skull, osteosclerotic lesions giving the characteristic 'Rugger Jersey' spine and soft tissue calcification seen in periarticular spaces and as vascular deposits. Osteomalacic lesions are suggested by Looser zones in their preferential sites (ischiopubal rami of the pelvis, the femoral neck, or pseudofractures of the ribs).

At the time of initiation of dialysis secondary HPT will be the prominent, although not exclusive, feature of renal osteodystrophy. The main objectives are to prevent the aggravation, and if possible, reverse the symptoms and signs of HPT and to avoid superimposed toxic or iatrogenic complications such as overcorrection of HPT, or aluminium deposition (Martin and Gonzalez 2001b).

Effective control of secondary HPTH can be achieved by various measures that include: (a) limitation of dietary phosphate intake; (b) administration of calcium salts, which simultaneously improve calcium balance, act as phosphate binders in the intestine and contribute to the correction of acidosis; (c) administration of non-calcium, non-aluminium-containing phosphate binders such as sevelamer; (d) appropriate adjustment of calcium concentration in the dialysate; (e) adequate dialysis delivery, including optimal correction of metabolic acidosis (Lefebvre et al. 1989); and (f) careful administration of vitamin D analogues (Table 11).

Comprehensive algorithms and reviews detailing the management of HPT have been published recently by several authorative groups (Medical Expert Group 2000a,b; Locatelli et al. 2002b). The administration of 1,25 $(OH)_2D_3$ (calcitriol) or 1α $(OH)D_3$ is highly effective for reducing the severity of adverse effects of secondary HPTH in dialysis patients, but requires careful clinical and biochemical surveillance to

Table 10 Bone lesions in endstage renal disease

Type of bone disorder	Bone formation	Main features	Main causes
High turnover Mild/severe HPT[a]	High	Osteoid surface ↑ Osteoblasts/clasts ↑ Eroded bone surface ↑ Marrow fibrosis ↑	Secondary HPT (1)
Low turnover Osteomalacia	Low	Osteoblasts/clasts ↓ Unmineralized osteoid ↑ (a) Bone surface Al. staining +	Calcium deficiency (2) Aluminium overload (3)
Aplastic bone disease		(b) No Al. osteoid vol. normal	Over correction of HPT (4)
Mixed uraemic osteodystrophy	Low/high	'Mixed'	(1) + (2)
β2-Microglobulin amyloidosis	Variable	Cystic β2-microglobulin deposits	Undetermined

[a] HPT: hyperparathyroidism.

Table 11 Management of secondary hyperparathyroidism in
dialysis patients

Aim
Control excess secretion of PTH
Maintain serum concentration of 1-84 i-PTH at 130–250 pg/ml

Methods
1. Prevention of phosphate retention and hyperphosphataemia: dietary
   measures, increase dialysis dose, Al or Ca phosphate binders,
   Sevelamer HCl

2. Maintenance of normal serum calcium concentration
   Adjustment of calcium concentration in dialysate
   Oral calcium supplementation
   Calcitriol (oral, IV)
3. Novel vitamin D derivatives: 22-oxacalcitriol, paricalcitol, alfacalcitol . . .
4. Calcimimetic agents: clinical use currently under investigation (2002)
5. If medical armamentorium falls: surgery: subtotal or total PTX

avoid the complications of overdosage. The targets include maintaining
the serum concentrations of total calcium, phosphate, and i-PTH no
greater than 2.6 mmol/l, 1.7 mmol/l, and 250 pg/ml, respectively. In
particular, serum concentration of intact 1-84 PTH should range
between 130 and 250 pg/ml, that is 2–3 times the upper normal level
(65 pg/ml) (Torres *et al.* 1995). Prescription of calcitriol (at a dosage of
0.25–0.50 μg/day) should be considered if calcium salts supplementation, dietary phosphate restriction, and adequate dialysis are insufficient
to meet these objectives. Marked hyperphosphataemia is a contraindication to calcitriol use because of the risk of development of extraskeletal
calcification. Numerous studies have been conducted to evaluate the possible advantages of intermittent IV or oral boluses of calcitriol over the
conventional daily intake of the drug (Andress *et al.* 1989). IV pulses
are given twice or thrice weekly at the end of dialysis sessions. Doses are
usually in the range of 1–2 μg per IV pulse, but depend on the effects on
serum calcium, phosphate, and PTH.

The advantages of more recently introduced vitamin D analogues lie
in their capacity for suppressing the pre-pro PTH gene transcription
and PTH secretion without generating increases in intestinal calcium
and phosphate absorption (Martin and Gonzalez 2001a). Several compounds have been tested in recent years such as 22-oxacalcitriol, paracalcitol, 1α-hydroxy-vitamin D$_2$ (doxercalciferol). The uniform result
obtained with these compounds is a marked fall (up to 75 per cent) of
serum PTH concentrations without a substantial rise of calcium and
phosphate serum levels (Goodman 2002; Slatopolsky *et al.* 2002). The
doses of each of these drugs vary according to their route and frequency of administration, namely oral or IV, and daily or thrice weekly
(Steddon 2001). For example, it has been shown that intermittent
(thrice weekly) oral and IV doxercalciferol reduced i-PTH levels effectively and similarly compared with baseline values (43–50 per cent after
10–12 weeks of treatment). Episodes of hypercalcaemia and hyperphosphataemia were less pronounced with the IV route (Maung *et al.*
2001). Discontinuation of vitamin D sterols administration is followed
by a rapid return of serum PTH levels to their pretreatment values, as
has been documented in a clinical trial with doxercalciferol (Frazao *et al.*
2000). However, clinical trials comparing the efficacy of intermittent,
either IV or oral, with continuous administration of active vitamin D
derivatives have not proved conclusive (Locatelli *et al.* 2002b).

Calcimimetic agents may prove useful for the treatment of secondary HPT in dialysis patients (Frazao *et al.* 2002). These small organic
molecules increase the activation by calcium of the calcium-sensing
receptor (CaSR) in the parathyroid glands and reduce PTH release
from the parathyroid cells. The changes in PTH secretion that are mediated through the CaSR occur within seconds or minutes, in contrast
with that induced by other PTH-lowering agents whose action is
delayed over hours or days. The action of the calcimimetics is also transient with a return to predosing levels after 18–24 h. The reduction in
PTH release occurs without being triggered by a rise in extracellular calcium concentration, which actually decreases to a significant extent after
administration of calcimimetic compounds. The mechanisms of this phenomenon remains to be elucidated. Calcimimetic agents will therefore
be prescribed for lowering PTH serum concentrations in patients with
hypercalcaemia in whom calcitriol or other vitamin D derivatives are
contraindicated (Goodman *et al.* 2002). Several calcimimetic drugs are
being tested at present in clinic trials (R-568, AM 073). The impact of
daily large and rapid variations of serum PTH concentrations on the
biochemical markers of mineral metabolism and skeletal modifications
remain to be established before extensive use of calcimimetic agents in
uraemic patients is promoted (Goodman *et al.* 2002).

Despite the introduction of new medical means for treating
secondary HPT, PTX remains necessary for some dialysis patients.
Clinical symptoms and signs of HPT such as soft tissue or vascular
calcification, intractable pruritus, spontaneous tendon ruptures, and
calciphylaxis may be greatly ameliorated only after subtotal or total
PTX. Surgery should be preceded by imaging of the parathyroid glands.
Ultrasonography, computed tomography (CT) scan, magnetic resonance imaging (MRI), colour Doppler sonography, and scintigraphic
methods such as ^{99m}Tc Sestamibi (Mibi) are techniques used for displaying the number, size, volume, and structure of the parathyroid glands,
but remain neither available nor affordable everywhere (Ambrosoni
et al. 2000).

The use of sestamibi scintigraphy has become popular for identifying
the presence of hyperfunctioning nodular or autonomous parathyroid
glands, for example, in tertiary HPT following renal transplantation, or
in cases of recurrent HPT originating from autotransplanted parathyroid
tissue after total PTX (Olaizola *et al.* 2000; Torregrosa *et al.* 2000).
Among 21 patients who underwent surgical PTX, the overall sensitivity
of the sestamibi scan in correctly locating parathyroid glands was only
50 per cent, although its specificity was 100 per cent. Of note, sensitivity
was 100 per cent in a subgroup of patients with recurrent secondary HPT
(Olaizola *et al.* 2000). This method is thus less useful for identifying
diffuse parathyroid hyperplasia than for localizing ectopic glands or
remaining parathyroid tissue after PTX.

Total PTX with autotransplantation of parathyroid tissue (most
frequently into the brachioradialis muscle in the non-fistula bearing
forearm) is successful provided that the hyperplastic or nodular
parathyroid tissue has effectively been removed, that sufficient functional parathyroid tissue has been autografted to avoid subsequent
development of hypoparathyroidism and that no overactivity will
develop in the autografted fragments (De Francisco *et al.* 2000). In a
series of 1053 total PTXs reported on by a Japanese group over a 20-year
period, per/postoperative complications were less than 2 per cent, no
patient required retransplantation of cryopreserved parathyroid
tissue, 1.4 per cent of the patients had to be reoperated because of persistent HPT originating in supernumerary parathyroid glands and the
incidence of graft-dependent recurrent HPT was 8.1 per cent, with an

incidence increasing over time after grafting, being 30 per cent in the seventh year after PTX (Tominaga *et al.* 2001).

A recently described technique consisting in an intraoperative selection of parathyroid tissue for transplantation using a stereomagnifier is of interest for minimizing the recurrence of HPT originating in the autotransplanted grafted fragments (Neyer *et al.* 2002).

Subtotal PTX (meaning a total resection of three glands and 75 per cent of the fourth) carries the risk of great surgical difficulties if reoperation(s) become(s) necessary. High doses of calcium, administered IV in the immediate postoperative period and orally thereafter, sometimes for several months, together with calcitriol are usually mandatory after successful PTX as bone resorption rapidly decreases and bone formation becomes very active with large quantities of calcium reentering into the skeleton ('hungry bone syndrome').

Percutaneous fine-needle injection of ethanol into enlarged hyperplastic or nodular parathyroid glands under ultrasonic Doppler flow guidance is an alternative treatment for severe refractory HPT. Results obtained with this technique are conflicting. In a series of 46 patients treated by a Japanese group, parathyroid function was maintained within the fixed target-range in 80.4 per cent of the patients at 1 year after injection with no subsequent surgical PTX required in any patient (Kakuka *et al.* 1999). British experience involving 22 patients was much less successful, with 11 (50 per cent) of them requiring subsequent PTX for clinically persistent HPT.

Aluminium overload should be carefully excluded by DFO testing before PTX and, if necessary, bone biopsy. DFO treatment to remove aluminium overload is mandatory prior to PTX. PTX patients are particularly susceptible to aluminium-induced osteomalacia by redistribution of the aluminium previously deposited on the bone surface into the osteoid/calcified bone interface.

The widespread use of deionizers and reverse osmosis filters in dialysis systems along with the decreasing use of aluminium-containing phosphate binders explain the reduction of aluminium-related bone diseases observed in recent years. However, great caution should continue to be exerted to prevent the multiple complications related to aluminium overload, which impairs skeletal mineralization and alters bone cell formation and/or proliferation. Accumulation of aluminium leads to the decline of osteoblastic activity and collagenase synthesis and thus ends up in reduced bone formation. Histologically, aluminium bone disease may be either of the osteomalacic type with an excess accumulation of unmineralized osteoid and large aluminium deposits on the bone surface, or of the aplastic type with normal or small amounts of osteoid and aluminium. Both types share an abnormally small number of osteoclasts and a decreased rate of bone formation. Overall, aluminium can be recognized as 'bone toxin' (Malluche 2002).

Bone biopsy remains the gold standard for diagnosis of aluminium bone disease. Histologically stainable bone aluminium content at the mineralization front does correlate with the known changes of aluminium bone disease, whereas there is no correlation between bone aluminium content and histological abnormalities (Faugère and Malluche 1986). Bone biopsy remains an invasive and costly procedure and requires a great expertise for an accurate interpretation. Hence, regular monitoring of serum aluminium concentration two to three times per year remains the routine surveillance procedure applied for the majority of dialysis patients without characterized or heavily suspected skeletal problems. Baseline serum aluminium levels reflect recent exposure and as such offers greatest value for detection of incipient aluminium loading. The patients' iron status has to be taken into

account for correctly interpreting the results of serum aluminium determinations, since patients with functional iron depletion may exhibit spuriously increased serum aluminium levels in the presence of only a low aluminium body burden when evaluated with a DFO test. While the normal range of serum aluminium concentration in healthy persons is less than 5 μg/l, levels up to 20–30 μg/l are acceptable in dialysis patients (Ferreira 2000). Aluminium overload should be suspected when aluminium serum concentrations are greater than 50–60 μg/l. In a recent series of 258 patients who underwent a bone biopsy and measurement of serum aluminium level, only 50 per cent of the patients with a serum aluminium equal to or greater than 40 μg/l had biopsy-proven aluminium bone disease, but this diagnosis was made in 14.2 per cent of patients who were below this threshold. Thus, the serum aluminium level alone is not a very reliable predictor of the presence of aluminium bone disease (Kausz *et al.* 1999). A low dose (5 mg/kg) DFO test is a useful tool for assessing more precisely the risk of aluminium overload in patients with elevated baseline serum aluminium levels. A clearly positive test (>50 per cent increase in serum aluminium) used in combination with the results of i-PTH measurements provides useful information on the presence of aluminium-related bone disease. Patients with a serum aluminium concentration greater than 50 μg/l and a serum i-PTH greater than 650 pg/ml have aluminium overload, but are not prone to develop aluminium bone disease, whereas patients with the same increase in serum aluminium but a serum i-PTH less than 650 pg/ml are at risk of developing aluminium bone lesions. The patients at highest risk are those with i-PTH levels less than 150 pg/ml (D'Haese *et al.* 1996). Patients with documented aluminium-related bone disease require aluminium-chelation therapy with DFO. The objective is to decrease the stainable bone surface aluminium and to increase bone formation rate. DFO therapy is not devoid of side-effects. It is administered usually once weekly in low doses under close surveillance (D'Haese *et al.* 1996). The removal of the aluminoxamine complex is optimized with the use of high-flux (polysulfone) dialysis membranes or with the addition of a charcoal haemoperfusion column ahead of the dialyser. The duration of DFO treatment is based on the results of two successive DFO tests performed each at 1-month interval after a 3 month course followed by 1-month of wash-out. If the serum aluminium concentration after DFO test is less than 50 μg/l greater than baseline, it can be concluded that the aluminum overload has been adequately removed. Six to 12 months of DFO therapy may be necessary to reach this goal in severely aluminium-intoxicated patients.

Even with preventive measures, positive aluminium balance may still occur, even with low aluminium concentration in the dialysate (to be kept at <5 μg/l). Prescription of aluminium-containing phosphate binders should be abandoned.

Osteomalacia due to nutritional calcium or phosphate deficiency is rarely seen nowadays in well-nourished and vitamin D replete patients. Osteomalacic lesions can, however, develop as a result of a combination of several contributing factors such as: (a) a negative calcium balance if the calcium content of the dialysate is too low (<1.50 mmol/l) and not compensated for by oral calcium supplementation; (b) a sustained acidosis due to inadequate buffering of the dialysate; or (c) vitamin D deficiency related for instance to lack of solar exposure in sun deprived countries. Osteomalacia is usually encountered when serum concentrations of 25-hydroxy-vitamin D are below 20 nmol/l. It has been shown that 25-hydroxy-vitamin D may be more effective in promoting bone formation than 1α $(OH)_2D_3$ (Fournier 1979). Supplementation of 1000 units per day or a once weekly dose of 10,000 units of cholecalciferol aiming at raising the plasma 25-hydroxy-vitamin D concentrations above 50 nmol/l under close supervision to avoid vitamin D intoxication and hypercalcaemia has therefore been recommended (Schäuming and Ritz 2000).

The pathophysiology of non-aluminium related aplastic bone disease is not understood. An oversuppression of PTH activity is currently the most popular explanation (Fournier 1995). Adynamic bone disease has usually been regarded as asymptomatic, that is it does not cause fractures, but this view has been challenged recently, since it could be shown that dialysis patients with low serum PTH levels had an increased incidence of hip fractures (Coco and Rush 2000). Moreover, and maybe more importantly, it is associated with the risk of development of extraskeletal calcification due to excessive elevation of the Ca × P product. An elevated serum calcium concentration together with a normal (or low) i-PTH level and the absence of aluminum overload (by DFO test if necessary) are sufficient to confirm the diagnosis, avoiding the need for bone biopsy. This combination should lead to discontinuing any administration of vitamin D metabolites, restricting or even entirely avoiding oral calcium supplementation to control serum phosphate and, if required, decrease the calcium concentration of the dialysate to about 1.25 mmol/l. A non-calcium, non-aluminium-containing phosphate binder is a valuable alternative in this condition. PTH levels should be permitted to fluctuate between 100 and 200 pg/ml in HD patients and 100 and 300 pg/ml in PD patients (Fournier 1995).

Management of osteoarticular complications of β2-microglobulin amyloidosis (see Chapter 11.3.10)

Carpal tunnel syndrome, arthropathy, bone disease, and much less frequently visceral deposits are the principal manifestations of dialysis-related β2-microglobulin amyloidosis (β2-MA). Arthropathy with joint effusion usually affects the shoulders, knees, hips, or wrists. The spondyloarthropathies result in destructive changes of intervertebral disks or radiolucent cysts located in the cervical spine. Cystic lesions are frequently located at the site of tendon insertions. They are filled with amyloid deposits and can cause pathological fractures, particularly when close to a weight-bearing joint (Floege and Ketteler 2001). The prevalence of β2-MA increases progressively with the duration of RRT. Lesions are rarely present less than 5 years after start of dialysis, but affect more than 80 per cent of patients dialysed for 15 years or more. A high frequency of β2-MA has also been demonstrated in elderly patients, independent of the duration of RRT. There is a considerable discrepancy between clinical and radiological signs (i.e. carpal tunnel syndrome and bone radiolucencies), which are present in 2 and 4 per cent, respectively in a series of patients compared to histological evidence of β2-MA in 48 per cent (Jadoul et al. 1997). An unequivocal diagnosis of β2-MA still relies on histology of the affected area or the synovial fluid from an affected joint. Ultrasonography is helpful in selected joints. CT and MRI may help differentiate amyloid cystic lesions from lucent lesions of a different origin but have a low specificity. Among several scintigraphic methods investigated in recent years, scanning with ^{111}In-labelled β2-M or ^{111}In-labelled recombinant human β2-M are currently considered as the most useful and safe (Ketteler et al. 2001).

The management of dialysis-related amyloidosis is largely that of pain-relief, while prevention is based on optimal reduction of the plasma concentration of β2-M. Non-steroidal anti-inflammatory drugs may relieve joint-pain, but intra- or periarticular steroid injections have only transient effects and carry the risk of infection. Reports of substantial improvement of amyloid arthropathy following kidney transplantation prompted trials of low-dose oral prednisone (0.1 mg/kg/day) for patients suffering from joint pain. Patients remain steroid-dependent for a long term, because pain reoccurs after discontinuation of treatment. Carpal tunnel associated symptoms require early surgical intervention to relieve pain and also to preserve median nerve function.

The most effective prevention of β2-MA is not to allow time for it to develop by expediting renal transplantation. β2-M plasma levels return to normal values rapidly after successful renal transplantation, with a relief of pain at the osteoarticular sites. This is, however, due at least in part, to the effect of steroid therapy. Amyloid cysts, seen on X-ray, may persist 10 years or more after transplantation.

The only alternative for delaying deposition of amyloid fibrils in dialysis patients is to maximize the removal of β2-M by the dialysis filtration methods, the absence of an unequivocally proven close relationship between the plasma concentration of β2-M and the development of amyloid deposits not withstanding. Given the molecular weight of β2-M (11,800 Da), its removal can be enhanced by increasing its convective versus diffusive transmembrane transport by haemofiltration or HDF. A high rebound of plasma β2-M levels occurs after high-efficiency filtration sessions, and none of the available techniques are able to maintain the concentration in the normal range (David et al. 1998). Whether the use of biocompatible versus bioincompatible (cellulosic) dialysis membranes has advantages for delaying the development of β2-M-related lesions and symptoms remains a long-standing controversy. The current consensus is that a biocompatible dialysis/ filtration membrane is preferred for all the patients who are at increased risk for developing β2-M related complications, that is, all patients who, for any reason have only a small chance of receiving a renal transplant, or for elderly patients (>60 years) independently or not of whether they are transplant candidates (Floege and Ketteler 2001; Jaradat and Moe 2001). Recent studies with the long nocturnal (8 h) dialysis strategy show that the mass of β-M removed using a small-area dialyser (0.7 m^2 polysulfone) and moderate blood and dialyser flows (281 and 99 ml/min, respectively) was significantly greater than that achieved with a conventional thrice weekly dialysis regimen using a 1.80 m^2 polysulfone dialyser, with a close to 50 per cent sustained clearance of baseline β2-M serum concentration, down to 13.7 ± 4.4 mg/dl at 9 months (Raj et al. 2000). Haemoperfusion methods using selective β-M adsorption columns have also been shown as effective for improving clinical symptoms in patients with documented periarticular amyloid lesions, but their high cost and unproven safety have thus far limited their utilization (Kazama et al. 2001). Finally, the dialysis/filtration devices are not the sole factor to be taken into account for the prevention of β2-M amyloid. The use of ultrapure, pyrogen-free dialysate in minimizing the inflammatory reactions provoked by dialysate endotoxins crossing the filter membrane is also believed to be important (Schwalbe et al. 1997).

CAPD can remove only a small amount of β2-M per day because the peritoneal membrane clearance is very low. The lower serum concentration of β2-M that has been reported in some series of PD patients compared with HD patients can in fact be attributed to a better and longer preservation of residual renal function in patients treated with PD. The daily peritoneal dialytic clearance of β2-M has been found to be lower with nocturnal PD than with conventional CAPD (Brophy et al. 1999). The overall poor performance of PD for removal of β2-M explains why the prevalence of amyloid deposits is not significantly different from that observed in HD patients matched for age and duration of dialysis (Jadoul 1998b).

Management of nutritional status

Prevention of protein–energy malnutrition

A close association between protein–energy malnutrition and morbidity–mortality rates in chronic dialysis populations has been documented in numerous retrospective and prospective studies conducted over the past 20 years (Hakim and Levin 1993; Bergström 1995). This holds true in recently published single-centre or nationwide surveys: prealbumin serum concentration, a validated nutritional marker, has been shown to be the best biochemical predictor of mortality in a series of 130 HD and 128 PD patients monitored prospectively for 10 years (Mittman et al. 2001). Data collected between 1996 and 1998 in 1610 patients treated with HD in 20 French centres showed that serum concentrations of albumin and prealbumin and not indicators of dialysis adequacy (Kt/V urea or urea reduction ratio) were significant predictors of survival (Combe et al. 2001). Although malnutrition is widely documented as a major contributing factor to the high mortality rates in dialysis patients, it is quite disappointing to observe its current persistence in a large proportion of dialysis populations. 'Life-threatening denutrition' was recorded (according to nutritional parameters) in 20–36 per cent of 7123 HD patients treated in France (Aparicio et al. 1999). Among the first 1000 patients randomized in the HEMO study in the United States, a daily energy intake and protein intake below the values recommended by the NKF/DOQI guidelines were recorded in 76 and 62 per cent of the patients, respectively (Rocco et al. 2002).

Substantial advances in the understanding of protein metabolism and the pathogenesis of protein–energy malnutrition have been made in recent years, which allow the best way to improve the nutritional status of the individual patient (Lim and Kopple 2000; Kaysen et al. 2002). The main causes of protein malnutrition in dialysis patients are listed in Table 12. Anorexia is the major contributor and is of multifactorial origin (Bergström 1996). It can be corrected somewhat by improvements in medical care (adequate dietary supervision; increased and customized dialysis regimens) and/or psychosocial or economic support. Correction of metabolic acidosis improves negative nitrogen balance and the consequent reduction of muscle mass (Franch and Mitch 1998). Reduction of peritonitis episodes minimizes the loss of albumin in PD patients. A specific link between malnutrition,

inflammation and atherosclerosis has in recent years been identified in ESRD patients as shown by a significant elevation of serum concentrations of biological markers of inflammation, such as C-reactive protein and proinflammatory cytokines (Bergström and Lindholm 1998; Stenvinkel et al. 1999). Malnutrition in dialysis patients is thought to be of at least two different types: one related to low protein–energy intake, which may be amenable to adequate dialysis and dietary support, the other being associated with inflammation and atherosclerotic cardiovascular disease which can only be reversed if the acute or chronic infectious or inflammatory state can be cured. The contribution of some components of dialysis itself, such as bioincompatible dialysis membranes and/or bacteria/toxin contaminated dialysate to a perpetual systemic inflammatory state remains a matter of debate (Lindholm et al. 1998; Schiffl et al. 2001; Memoli et al. 2002).

The clinical practice guidelines for nutrition in chronic renal failure proposed by the NKF/DOQI™ working group and a recent European Consensus on nutritional status in dialysis patients have described in great detail the methods for assessment and management of nutritional deficiencies encountered in dialysis patients (NKF/DOQI 2000; Locatelli et al. 2002c). The tools for evaluating the nutritional status of dialysis patients are listed in Table 13. The key role of a qualified renal dietician and of a careful overall medical supervision cannot be overemphasized. Among the routinely available biochemical markers a low serum albumin level and body mass index (BMI) have been identified as the most informative markers of malnutrition. Elevation of serum C-reactive protein level reflecting the presence of infection or inflammation is associated with hypoalbuminaemia (Qureschi et al. 1998). In other studies the prealbumin concentrations were found to be the best predictor of mortality in a long-term survey of dialysis patients (Mittmann et al. 1001). For a more sophisticated determination of body composition, dual-energy-X-ray absorptiometry (DEXA) is considered the most reliable, but is not universally available (Locatelli 2002c).

The widely accepted recommendations for the management of energy–protein malnutrition are listed in Table 14. At least half of the recommended daily protein intake should include protein of high biological value from animal origin (fish, meat, or dairy products). Anorexia and financial constraints may represent major obstacles for adequate protein intake or supply. Several types of protein–energy supplementation have been introduced in clinical practice: oral supplementation of

Table 12 Main causes of protein–energy malnutrition in dialysis patients

	Low protein intake	Hypercatabolism and protein waste
	Absence/inadequate dietary counselling	Metabolic acidosis
	Uraemic toxicity (underdialysis)	Dialysis loss of amino acids and/or albumin (PD)
	Comorbid illness(es)	Endocrine disturbances
Anorexia	Psychosocial factors (Depression–low income)	Chronic systemic inflammation (bioincompatibilities of dialysis coexisting
	Intolerance to dialysis techniques	infections, heart failure and atherosclerosis (?)

Table 13 Assessment of nutritional status in dialysis patients

Routine clinical practice	More detailed information
1. Frequent dietary counselling	1. Subjective Global Assessment (SGA) Questionnaire
2. Follow-up of dry weight (% of standard BW)	2. Investigations on fat mass and lean body mass
3. Anthropometric measurements (Body mass index—four sites-skinfold thickness mid-arm muscle circonference)	Dual energy-X-ray-absorptiometry (DEXA) Bioimpedance analysis (?)
4. Biochemical markers: albumin, prealbumin, creatinine, bicarbonate, transferrin, cholesterol	Exchangeable sodium/potassium ratios—total body water (isotopic methods)
5. Determination of protein catabolic rate	3. Measurement of serum levels of proinflammatory cytokines: IL-1, IL-6, TNFα
6. Markers of inflammation: C-reactive protein	

Table 14 Main recommendations for the management of the energy–protein nutritional status in dialysis patients

1. Provide optimal energy and protein intake
    35 kcal/kg standard BW/day in patients <60 years;
      30 kcal/kg/day in those >60 years
  At least
    1.2 g/kg/day in HD patients
    1.2–1.3 g/kg/day in PD patients
    (50% protein of animal origin)
  If required: oral, parenteral, intraperitoneal
    amino acid supplementation
2. Provide sustained dietary supervision by
  qualified renal dietician
	3. Reduce/suppress hypercatabolic factors
	  Provide 'adequate' dialysis dose
	  HD: Kt/V urea: 1.2–1.3
	  PD: total weekly Kt/V urea: 2.0–2.2
	  Correct metabolic acidosis: predialysis
	    bicarbonate $\geq$ 22 mmol/l
	  Diagnose and treat comorbid conditions:
	    infections—cardiovascular complications
	  Reduce dialysis-induced inflammation
	    Use ultra-pure pyrogen-free dialysate
	    Use biocompatible membranes (?)
	  Increase dialysis efficiency $\rightarrow$ daily dialysis

branched-chain amino acids (Hiroshige *et al.* 2001), use of amino acid based dialysate in malnourished PD patients (Kopple *et al.* 1995), parenteral nutrition during acute surgical or infectious complications. Injections of recombinant human insulin growth factor-1 (rH IGF-1) are effective for inducing a strong and sustained anabolic effect in protein-deficient CAPD patients (Fouque *et al.* 2000). Finally, a spectacular improvement of nutritional status has been documented in patients treated with long nocturnal HD as well as with short daily HD strategies. Both allow freedom from dietary restrictions and reduction or avoidance of phosphate binders. Patients experience a rapid increase in body weight and a significant rise of serum albumin and prealbumin concentrations (Pierratos 1999; Galland *et al.* 2001). On the basis of these recent reports a temporary shift to a daily dialysis technique can be recommended for improving the nutritional status of severely malnourished dialysis patients who have a persistently insufficient spontaneous oral protein–energy intake.

Management of lipid abnormalities (see Chapter 11.3.5)

Numerous studies have demonstrated cardiovascular complications as the leading cause of death in dialysis patients. Several plasma lipid abnormalities have been shown to be closely associated with markers of atherosclerosis such as carotid–intima media thickness and aortic stiffness, whilst, for example, the genetically determined apo(a) phenotype of lipoprotein(a) has been found to be a strong and independent risk predictor for coronary events in dialysis patients (Kronenberg 1999). The main dyslipidemic abnormalities present in patients with ESRD include elevated triglyceride levels, low high-density lipoprotein-cholesterol (HDL-C), frequently normal or low low-density lipoprotein-cholesterol (LDL-C) concentrations, a profile which may result in either low, normal, or elevated total-cholesterol levels. The most characteristic feature of uraemia-associated dyslipidamia is currently described as the accumulation of apolipoprotein-B containing triglyceride-rich particles in the very-low-density (VLDL) and intermediate-density lipoprotein (IDL) range (Wanner 2000). It has been recently suggested that IDL-C is the lipoprotein that should be most closely controlled in the management of dyslipidaemia. Determination of IDL-C levels show that they account for approximately 15 per cent of the LDL-C level measured with the Friedewald formula, with a normal range lower than 15 mg/dl corresponding to an LDL-C level below 100 mg/dl (Shoji *et al.* 2002). The recommended level for LDL-C in dialysis patients is thus in

accordance with those proposed for the general population (Kasiske 1998). Screening of the lipoprotein profile is at present not recommended for the routine follow-up of the total dialysis population. It should be reserved for selected high-risk subgroups of patients, for example, diabetics and those with atherosclerotic complications. For all patients, a quarterly determination of plasma triglycerides, total-cholesterol, HDL-C, LDL-C (calculated with the Friedewald formula) is recommended (Medical Expert Group 2000a).

The therapeutic guidelines are to maintain a plasma LDL-C concentration at or less than 100 mg/dl (2.6 mmol/dl), which would keep the most detrimental IDL-C fraction within the normal range. Dietary restriction of saturated fat products (dairy products, meat) is of limited efficacy and may worsen an already impaired nutritional status. The patients' lipid profile may be improved by the use of highly permeable dialysis membranes (Biankenstijn *et al.* 1995) and also by the replacement of unfractioned heparin by low molecular weight heparin (Schmitt and Schneider 1993). The phosphate binder sevelamer hydrochloride has been shown to have a beneficial effect on lipid profiles of HD patients, with a 30 per cent decrease of LDL-C and an 18 per cent increase of HDL-C concentrations over baseline values, respectively (Chertow *et al.* 1999).

Fibric acid analogues, among which gemfibrozil is the drug of choice, are effective for lowering serum triglycerides and raising HDL-C levels, but with no effect on LDL-C. Low dosage and close monitoring of creatine–phosphokinase levels (CPK) are recommended to detect rhabdomyolysis. (HMG-CoA) reductase inhibitors (statins) are very effective, reducing the level of LDL-C and other non-LDL-C fractions in HD and PD patients by up to 30 per cent (Harris *et al.* 2002; Saltissi *et al.* 2002; Shoji *et al.* 2002). Statins are well tolerated and safe, side/adverse effects are generally limited to a dose-related increase of hepatic enzymes in a small percentage of patients. An increase of the frequency of monitoring CPK will be required with stopping of the agent if they rise. The combination of a fibric acid derivative and a statin is contraindicated because of the increased risk of rhabdomyolysis. An independent association between the use of statins and a reduction of cardiovascular-specific (-37 per cent) and a total mortality (-32 per cent) in dialysis patients has been recently published. No such effect was found with the use of fibrates (Seliger *et al.* 2002). However, the design of the study did not reveal whether the lower mortality observed in statin users was related to changes in lipid levels, nor whether the association between statin use and reduced mortality differed among patients with or without hyperlipidaemia. Studies currently under way are investigating the degree of relationship between the lipid-lowering effects of statins and reduction of mortality in dialysis patients.

Nutritional supplementations

Vitamins

Dialysis patients may suffer from water-soluble vitamin deficiencies either because of impaired dietary intake and intestinal malabsorption or dialysis losses. To compensate for ascorbic acid (vitamin C) losses during dialysis, particularly if convective techniques are used (Morena et al. 2002) a routine daily supplementation of 50 mg of vitamin C is recommended (Locatelli et al. 2002c). Higher doses are not required and carry the risk of development of hyperoxalaemia and subsequent calcium oxalate deposits in blood vessels and solid organs, particularly the heart. Thiamine deficiency with neurological manifestation may develop during acute, severe, medical, or surgical complications requring large quantities of glucose infusions. It can be prevented with an oral supplementation of 1–2 mg daily supplementation of vitamin B_1. Folic acid (vitamin B_9) and pyridoxine (vitamin B_6) are useful adjuncts for optimizing the action of exogenous epoetin at a daily dosage of 1 and 5–10 mg, respectively (Hörl 1999).

Hyperhomocysteinaemia (tHcy) has been identified in several series of patients as an independent risk factor for the occurrence of atherosclerotic complications in uraemic patients. A clear association has recently been shown in a prospective study involving a cohort of 175 HD patients between tHcy levels, incident cardiovascular mortality and atherosclerotic events (Mallamacci et al. 2002). Raised tHcy concentrations have been documented in up to 90 per cent of patients on HD and in 67 per cent of PD patients (Mallamacci et al. 2002). The level of tHcy was inversely related to plasma folate concentration. Daily administration of 10–15 mg of folic acid results in a significant decrease of tHcy (Billion et al. 2002). A beneficial impact of concomitant vitamin B_{12} supplementation is debatable, being dependent on the daily dosage of folic acid administered. The results of a recent, prospective, randomized trial show a comparable reduction of tHcy levels obtained with IV folinic acid, oral folinic acid, and oral folic acid in patients already receiving IV vitamin B_6 and oral vitamin B_{12} (Ducloux et al. 2002). The question as to whether higher doses of folic acid (>10–15 mg per day) should become a routine prescription for preventing or delaying the incidence of cardiovascular complications in dialysis patients requires further confirmation. It is worth noting that the use of 'super-flux' dialysers has been shown to have a greater effect on tHcy levels than conventional high-flux dialysers, presumably due to a maximization of convective transport and removal of large (protein-bound) uraemic toxins which may interfere with tHcy metabolism (Van Tellingen 2001). Finally, frequent nocturnal HD (six/seven nights per week) has been found to have a greater effect in lowering tHcy levels than standard HD in two groups of patients otherwise submitted to identical therapeutic regimens within the same dialysis unit (Friedman 2002).

Prevention of communicable diseases

Hepatitis B virus infection

Despite the reduction in the need of blood transfusions for dialysis patients following the availability of epoetin, hepatitis B virus (HBV) infection remains a serious risk for ESRD populations, medical and nursing staff and their families. Patients may become infected through failure to screen blood products, or nosocomial transmission caused by failure to observe proper precautions. All patients and staff members who are hepatitis B surface antigen (HBs Ag) negative or have a low antibody (Ab) titre should be immunized. The likelihood of developing a protective Ab titre decreases with the severity of renal failure and associated impairment of the immune responses. Vaccination against HBV should therefore be started early in the course of renal insufficiency.

Several vaccination protocols have been developed for non-immune dialysis patients aiming at maximizing the seroconversion rate and duration of immunity. The comparative results of intradermal (ID) and intramuscular (IM) vaccination protocols have been found similar in a recent randomized prospective study—conversion rates of 97.6 per cent for ID versus 90.5 per cent for IM, $p = 0.16$, time required for seroconversion, peak Ab titre reached, proportion of patients with a peak Ab titre of 1000 U/l or greater, and duration of immunity post vaccination (Charest et al. 2000). A low dose repeated ID vaccination protocol has been shown as particularly effective for obtaining a secondary seroconversion in HD patients who had failed to respond to a standard IM vaccination scheme (Fabrizi et al. 1997). A regular follow-up of Ab titres should be performed after a successful vaccination (defined as a minimum titre of 100 U/l and an optimum titre of 1000 U/l), the frequency being adjusted to the rate of the fall of Ab titre.

Administration of a booster dose (40 μg IM) is recommended when the Ab titre falls to less than 20 U/l (Charest et al. 2000). The use of an immunomodulator (AM3 Immunoferon®) has been shown recently to prolong the duration of the protective antibody titre in a population of HD patients vaccinated with an IM protocol (Perez-Garcia et al. 2002).

To provide isolation in a separate area and the use of individually dedicated dialysis machines and instruments remain mandatory measures for HBV positive patients to prevent transmission of the disease to other patients or staff.

Hepatitis C virus infection

As in the general population, hepatitis C virus (HCV) infection is currently much more common than HBV among dialysis patients in developed countries. Patient testing for HCV includes enzyme-linked immunosorbent assay (ELISA 3rd generation), polymerase chain reaction (PCR) and reverse transcription (RT), which provide evidence of viral replication, identify the genotype, and quantify the viral load (Barrera 2000). Nosocomial transmission of HCV within the dialysis facilities is the main cause of patient seroconversion, certainly more common than transmission by blood products or IV drug abuse, the latter cause being common in some countries. Nosocomial transmission is most frequently the result of cross infection from an HCV-infected patient to other patients through contaminated hands of staff members, or from sharing of instruments (e.g. clamps, scissors) than internal contamination of dialysis machines or reuse of dialysers. Long-term longitudinal studies have clearly shown that, in contrast to what is imperative for HBV+ patients, isolation in separate rooms or use of separate monitors is not necessary to reduce to zero the incidence of HCV seroconversion in HD patients, as long as the 'Universal precautions for prevention of transmission of bloodborne pathogens' set out by the Centre of Disease Control are rigidly implemented and enforced (MMWR 1988; Jadoul et al. 1998a). These measures include careful cleaning and disinfection of instruments, and surfaces, widespread use of disposable instruments, and tissues, prohibition of sharing objects (razors, toothbrushes, scissors, knives) between patients, and for staff members frequent hand washing, wearing of gloves, gowns, face-masks, and goggles (Jadoul et al. 2000). Sterilization of the dialysis machine after each dialysis session has become mandatory by law in some countries.

All these measures also apply for human-immunodeficiency virus (HIV) positive patients who represent quite a substantial proportion of dialysis patients in some countries. Great care should be taken for disposal of drained PD bags, which represent a source of contamination.

References

Ahmed, J. and Weisberg, L. S. (2001). Hyperkalemia in dialysis patients. *Seminars in Dialysis* **14**, 348–356.

Allon, M. (1993). Treatment and prevention of hyperkalemia in end-stage renal disease. *Kidney International* **43**, 1197–1209.

Almaden, Y. *et al.* (1998). High phosphate level directly stimulates parathyroid hormone secretion and synthesis by human parathyroid tissue *in vitro*. *Journal of the American Society of Nephrology* **9**, 1845–1852.

Ambrosoni, P. *et al.* (2000). The role of imaging techniques in the study of renal osteodystrophy. *American Journal of Medical Sciences* **320**, 90–95.

Amin, N. (2002). The impact of improved phosphorus control: use of sevelamer hydrochloride in patients with chronic renal failure. *Nephrology, Dialysis, Transplantation* **17**, 340–345.

Andress, D. L. *et al.* (1989). Intravenous calcitriol in the treatment of refractory osteitis fibrosa of chronic renal failure. *New England Journal of Medicine* **321**, 274–279.

Angeli, P. *et al.* (1991). Comparison of sublingual Captopril and Nifedipine in immediate treatment of hypertensive emergencies. A randomized, single blind clinical trial. *Archives of Internal Medicine* **151**, 678–682.

Aparicio, M. *et al.* (1999). Nutritional status of haemodialysis patients: a French National Cooperative Study. French Study Group for Nutrition in Dialysis. *Nephrology, Dialysis, Transplantation* **14**, 1679–1686.

Augustyniac, R. A. *et al.* (2002). Sympathetic overactivity as a cause of hypertension in chronic renal failure. *Journal of Hypertension* **20**, 3–9.

Avram, M. M. *et al.* (2001). Survival on hemodialysis and peritoneal dialysis over 12 years with emphasis on nutritional parameters. *American Journal of Kidney Diseases* **37** (Suppl. 2), S77–S80.

Barrera, J. M. (2000). Diagnostic tests for hepatitis-C virus infection. *Nephrology, Dialysis, Transplantation* **15** (Suppl. 8), 15–18.

Bergström, J. (1995). Nutrition and mortality in hemodialysis. *Journal of the American Society of Nephrology* **6**, 1329–1341.

Bergström, J. and Lindholm, B. (1998). Malnutrition, cardiac disease and mortality, an integrated point of view. *American Journal of Kidney Diseases* **32**, 834–841.

Besarab, A. *et al.* (1998). The effect of normal as compared with low hematocrit values in patients with cardiac diseases who are receiving hemodialysis and erythropoeitin. *New England Journal of Medicine* **339**, 584–590.

Bianchi, G. (2000). Hypertension in chronic renal failure and end-stage renal disease patients treated with hemodialysis on peritoneal dialysis. *Nephrology, Dialysis, Transplantation* **15** (Suppl. 5), 105–110.

Biankestijn, P. J. *et al.* (1995). High-flux dialysis membranes improve lipid profile in chronic hemodialysis patients. *Journal of the American Society of Nephrology* **5**, 1703–1708.

Billion, S. *et al.* (2002). Hyperhomocysteinaemia: folate and vitamin B_{12} in unsupplemented dialysis patients: effect of oral therapy with folic acid and vitamin B_{12}. *Nephrology, Dialysis, Transplantation* **17**, 455–461.

Block, G. A. and Port, F. K. (2000). Re-evaluation of risks associated with hyperphosphatemia and hyperparathyroidism in dialysis patients. Recommendations for a change in management. *American Journal of Kidney Diseases* **37**, 1331–1333.

Bommer, J. (1999). Saving erythropoietin by administering L-carnitine? *Nephrology, Dialysis, Transplantation* **14**, 2819–2821.

Bosetto, A., Bene, B., and Petitclerc, T. (1999). Sodium management in dialysis by conductivity. *Advances in Renal Replacement Therapy* **6**, 243–254.

Brophy, D. F. *et al.* (1999). Small and middle molecular weight solute clearance in nocturnal intermittent peritoneal dialysis. *Peritoneal Dialysis International* **19**, 534–539.

Burkart, J. M. (1998). Clinical experience: how much earlier should patients really start renal replacement therapy? *Journal of the American Society of Nephrology* **9** (Suppl.), S118–S123.

Canella, G. *et al.* (2000). Inadequate diagnosis and therapy of arterial hypertension as causes of left ventricular hypertrophy in uremic dialysis patients. *Kidney International* **58**, 260–268.

Casadevall, N. *et al.* (2002). Pure red-cell aplasia and anti-erythropoietin antibodies in patients treated with recombinant erythropoietin. *New England Journal of Medicine* **346**, 469–475.

Chandler, G., Marchowal, J., and MacDougall, I. C. (2001). Intravenous iron sucrose: establishing a safe dose. *American Journal of Kidney Diseases* **38**, 988–991.

Chang-Yang, W. *et al.* (2002). An open-label, cross-over study of a new phosphate-binding agent in hemodialysis patients: ferric citrate. *Nephrology, Dialysis, Transplantation* **17**, 265–270.

Charest, A. F., McDougall, J., and Goldstein, M. B. (2000). A randomized comparison of intra-dermal and intra-muscular vaccination against hepatitis B virus in incident chronic hemodialysis patients. *American Journal of Kidney Diseases* **36**, 976–982.

Charra, B. *et al.* (1992). Survival as index of adequacy of dialysis. *Kidney International* **41**, 1286–1291.

Chazot, C. *et al.* (1995). Interdialytic blood pressure control by long haemodialysis sessions. *Nephrology, Dialysis, Transplantation* **10**, 831–837.

Chertow, G. M. *et al.* (1999). Long-term effects of sevelamer hydrochoride on the calcium $\times$ phosphorus product and lipid profile of haemodialysis patients. *Nephrology, Dialysis, Transplantation* **14**, 2907–2914.

Churchill, D. N. *et al.* (1996). Adequacy of dialysis and nutrition in continuous peritoneal dialysis: association with clinical outcomes. *Journal of the American Society of Nephrology* **7**, 198–207.

Churchill, D. N. *et al.* (1999). Clinical practice guidelines of the Canadian Society of Nephrology for treatment of patients with chronic renal failure. *Journal of the American Society of Nephrology* **10** (Suppl. 13), S287–S310.

Coburn, J. W. *et al.* (1991). Calcium citrate markedly enhances aluminium absorption from aluminium hydroxide. *American Journal of Kidney Diseases* **17**, 708–711.

Coco, M. and Rush, H. (2000). Increased incidence of hip fractures in dialysis patients with low serum parathyroïd hormone. *American Journal of Kidney Diseases* **36**, 1115–1121.

Collins, A. (2002). Influence of target hemoglobin in dialysis patients on morbidity and mortality. *Kidney International* **61** (Suppl. 80), S44–S48.

Combe, C. *et al.* (2001). Influence of nutritional factors and hemodialysis adequacy on the survival of 1610 French patients. *American Journal of Kidney Diseases* **37** (Suppl. 2), S81–S88.

Consensus Group Statement (1994). The role of L-carnitine in treating renal dialysis patients. *Dialysis and Transplantation* **23**, 177–181.

Conlon, P. J. *et al.* (2000). Normalization of hematocrit in hemodialysis patients with cardiac disease does not increase blood pressure. *Renal Failure* **22**, 435–444.

Cox-Reijven, P. L. *et al.* (2001). Role of impedance spectroscopy in assessment of body water compartments in hemodialysis patients. *American Journal of Kidney Diseases* **38**, 832–838.

David, S. *et al.* (1998). Behaviour of β_2-microglobulin removal with different dialysis schedules. *Nephrology, Dialysis, Transplantation* **13** (Suppl. 6), 49–54.

De Francisco, A. L. M. *et al.* (2002). Parathyroidectomy in dialysis patients. *Kidney International* **61** (Suppl. 80), S161–S166.

De Marchi, S. *et al.* (1997). Long-term effects of erythropoietin therapy on fistula stenosis and plasma concentrations of PDGF and MCP-1 in hemodialysis patients. *Journal of the American Society of Nephrology* **8**, 1147–1156.

D'Haese, P. C., Couttenye, M. M., and De Broe, M. E. (1996). Diagnosis and treatment of aluminium bone disease. *Nephrology, Dialysis, Transplantation* **11** (Suppl. 3), 74–79.

Dhondt, A. *et al.* (2000). The removal of uremic toxins. *Kidney International* **58** (Suppl. 76), S47–S59.

Drüeke, T. B. (1993). Adynamic bone disease, anaemia, resistance to erythropoietin and iron-aluminium interaction. In Consensus Conference: Diagnosis and treatment of aluminium overload in end-stage renal failure. *Nephrology, Dialysis, Transplantation* **8** (Suppl. 1), 12–27.

Ducloux, D. *et al.* (2002). Hyperhomocysteinaemia therapy in dialysis patients: folinic versus folic acid in combination with vitamin B_6 and B_{12}. *Nephrology, Dialysis, Transplantation* **17**, 865–870.

Eggers, P. W. (1990). Mortality rates among dialysis patients in Medicare's End-Stage Renal Disease Program. *American Journal of Kidney Diseases* **15**, 414–421.

Eschbach, J. W. (2000). Current concepts of anaemia management in chronic renal failure: impact of NKF-DOQI. *Seminars in Nephrology* **20**, 320–329.

Eschbach, J. W. *et al.* (1989). Treatment of anaemia of progressive renal failure with recombinant human erythropoietin. *New England Journal of Medicine* **321**, 158–163.

European Best Practice Guidelines Expert Group on Renal Transplantation (2000). Evaluation, selection and preparation of the potential transplant recipient. *Nephrology, Dialysis, Transplantation* **15** (Suppl. 7), 3–37.

Fabrizi, F. *et al.* (1997). Intradermal versus intra-muscular revaccination in non-responsive chronic dialysis patients: a prospective randomized study with cost-effectiveness evaluation. *Nephrology, Dialysis, Transplantation* **12**, 1204–1211.

Fagugli, R. M. *et al.* (2001). Short-daily hemodialysis: blood pressure control and left ventricular mass reduction in hypertensive hemodialysis patients. *American Journal of Kidney Diseases* **38**, 371–376.

Faugere, M. C. and Malluche, H. H. (1986). Stainable aluminium and not aluminium bone content reflects bone histology in dialyzed patients. *Kidney International* **30**, 717–722.

Ferreira, M. A. *et al.* (2000). Diagnosis of renal osteodystrophy: when and how to use biochemical markers and non-invasive methods; when bone biopsy is needed. *Nephrology, Dialysis, Transplantation* **15** (Suppl. 5), 8–14.

Fishbane, S. *et al.* (2001). A randomized trial of iron deficiency testing strategies in hemodialysis patients. *Kidney International* **60**, 2406–2411.

Floege, J. and Ketteler, M. (2001). Beta-microglobulin-derived amyloidosis: an update. *Kidney International* **59** (Suppl. 78), 164–171.

Foley, R. N. and Parfrey P. S. (1998). Cardiovascular disease and mortality in ESRD. *Journal of Nephrology* **11**, 239–245.

Foley, R. N. *et al.* (1996). Impact of hypertension on cardiomyopathy, morbidity and mortality in end-stage renal disease. *Kidney International* **49**, 1379–1385.

Fouque, D. *et al.* (2000). Recombinant human insulin-like growth factor-1 induces an anabolic response in malnourished CAPD patients. *Kidney International* **57**, 646–654.

Fournier, A., Moriniere, Ph., and Marie, A. (1995). Adynamic bone disease: is it actually a disease? *Nephrology, Dialysis, Transplantation* **10**, 457–457.

Fournier, A. *et al.* (1979). Comparison of 1 α-hydroxycholecalciferol and 25 hydroxycholecalciferol in the treatment of renal osteodystrophy: greater effect of 25 hydroxycholecalciferol on bone mineralization. *Kidney International* **15**, 196–204.

Fournier, A. *et al.* (1998). Renal osteodystrophy in dialysis patients: diagnosis and treatment. *Artificial Organs* **22**, 530–557.

Franch, H. A. and Mitch W. E. (1998). Catabolism in uremia: the impact of metabolic acidosis. *Journal of the American Society of Nephrology* **9** (Suppl. 12), S78–S81.

Frazao, J. M. *et al.* (2000). One-alpha-hydroxy-vitamin D2 (Doxercalciferol) effectively and safely suppresses intact parathyroid hormone levels in hemodialysis patients with moderate to severe hyperparathyroidism. Results of a multi-center, double blinded, placebo controlled study. *American Journal of Kidney Diseases* **36**, 562–565.

Frazao, J. M., Martins, P., and Coburn, J. W. (2002). The calcimimetic agents: perspectives for treatment. *Kidney International* **61** (Suppl. 80), S149–S154.

Friedman, A. N. (2002). Plasma total homocysteine levels among patients undergoing nocturnal vs standard hemodialysis. *Journal of the American Society of Nephrology* **13**, 265–268.

Galland, R. *et al.* (2001). Short daily hemodialysis rapidly improves nutritional status in hemodialysis patients. *Kidney International* **60**, 1555–1560.

Gallar, P. *et al.* (2000). Influencing factors in the control of phosphorus in peritoneal dialysis. Therapeutic options. *Nefrologia* **20**, 355–361.

Goicoechea, M. *et al.* (1998). Intravenous calcitriol improves anaemia and reduces the need for erythropoietin in hemodialysis patients. *Nephron* **78**, 23–27.

Goicoechea, M. *et al.* (2000). Antiplatelet therapy alters iron requirements in hemodialysis patients. *American Journal of Kidney Diseases* **36**, 80–87.

Golper, Th. A. (1998). Incremental dialysis. *Journal of the American Society of Nephrology* **32** (Suppl. 4), S107–S111.

Golper, Th. A. (1999). The rationale for healthy start of dialysis. *Blood Purification* **17**, 1–9.

Goodman, W. G. (2002). Calcimimetic agents and secondary hyperparathyroidism: treatment and prevention. *Nephrology, Dialysis, Transplantation* **17**, 204–207.

Goodman, W. G. *et al.* (2000). Coronary-artery calcification in young adults with end-stage renal disease who are undergoing dialysis. *New England Journal of Medicine* **342**, 1478–1483.

Goodman, W. G. *et al.* (2002). The calcimimetric agent AMG073 lowers parathyroid hormone levels in hemodialysis patients with secondary hyperparathyroidism. *Journal of the American Society of Nephrology* **13**, 1017–1024.

Gotch, F. A. and Sargent, J. A. (1985). A mechanistic analysis of the National Cooperative Dialysis Study. *Kidney International* **28**, 526–534.

Grekas, D. *et al.* (2000). Hypertension in chronic hemodialysis patients: current view on pathophysiology and treatment. *Clinical Nephrology* **53**, 164–168.

Grekas, D. *et al.* (2001). Effect of sympathetic and plasma renin activity on hemodialysis hypertension. *Clinical Nephrology* **55**, 115–120.

Gunal, A. I. *et al.* (2001). Strict volume control normalizes hypertension in peritoneal dialysis patients. *American Journal of Kidney Diseases* **37**, 588–593.

Hakim, R. M. and Levin, N. (1993). Malnutrition in hemodialysis patients. *American Journal of Kidney Diseases* **21**, 125–137.

Hakim, R. M. *et al.* (1992). Adequacy of dialysis. *American Journal of Kidney Diseases* **20**, 107–23.

Hakim, R. M. *et al.* (1994). Effects of dose of dialysis on morbidity and mortality. *American Journal of Kidney Diseases* **23**, 661–669.

Harris, K. P. G. *et al.* (2002). A placebo-controlled trial examining atorvastatin in dyslipidemic patients undergoing CAPD. *Kidney International* **61**, 1469–1474.

Hayashi, K., Hasegawa, K., and Kobayashi, S. (2001). Effects of angiotensin converting enzyme inhibitors on the treatment of anemia with erythropoietin. *Kidney International* **60**, 1110–1116.

Held, P. J. *et al.* (1996). The dose of hemodialysis and patient mortality. *Kidney International* **50**, 550–556.

Hergesell, O. and Ritz, E. (2002). Phosphate binders in uraemia: pharmacodynamics, pharmacoeconomics, pharmacoethics. *Nephrology, Dialysis, Transplantation* **17**, 14–17.

Hiroshige, K. *et al.* (2001). Oral supplementation of branched-chain amino acids improves nutritional status in elderly patients on chronic haemodialysis. *Nephrology, Dialysis, Transplantation* **16**, 1856–1862.

Hoeben, H. *et al.* (2002). Hemodynamics in patients with intradialytic hypotension treated with cool dialyzate or Midodrine. *American Journal of Kidney Diseases* **39**, 102–107.

Hörl, W. H. (1999). Is there a role for adjuvant therapy in patients being treated with epoetin. *Nephrology, Dialysis, Transplantation* **14**, 2819–2821.

Hörl, M. P. and Hörl, W. H. (2002). Hemodialysis associated hypertension. Pathophysiology and therapy. *American Journal of Kidney Diseases* **39**, 227–244.

Hurot, J. M. *et al.* (2002). Effects of L-carnitine supplementation in maintenance hemodialysis patients: a systematic review. *Journal of the American Society of Nephrology* **13**, 708–714.

Hutchinson, A. J. (1999). Calcitriol, lanthanum carbonate and other new phosphate binders in the management of renal osteodystrophy. *Peritoneal Dialysis International* **19** (Suppl. 2), S408–S412.

Iseki, K. *et al.* (2002a). Demographic trends in the Okinawa Dialysis Study Registry (1971–2000). *Kidney International* **61**, 668–675.

Iseki, K. *et al.* (2002b). Hypocholesterolemia is a significant predictor of death in a cohort of chronic hemodialysis patients. *Kidney International* **61**, 1887–1893.

Jadoul, M. (2000). Epidemiology and mechanisms of transmission of the hepatitis C virus in haemodialysis. *Nephrology, Dialysis, Transplantation* **15** (Suppl. 8), 39–41.

Jadoul, M. *et al.* (1997). Histological prevalence of beta$_2$-microglobulin amyloidosis in hemodialysis: a prospective post-mortem study. *Kidney International* **51**, 1928–1932.

Jadoul, M. *et al.* (1998a). Universal precautions prevent hepatitis C virus transmission: a 54-months follow-up of the Belgian Multicenter study. *Kidney International* **53**, 1022–1025.

Jadoul, M. *et al.* (1998b). Prevalence of histological beta$_2$-microglobulin amyloidosis in CAPD patients compared with hemodialysis patients. *Kidney International* **54**, 956–959.

Jaeger, J. Q. and Mehta, R. L. (1999). Assessment of dry weight in hemodialysis: an overview. *Journal of the American Society of Nephrology* **10**, 392–403.

Jaradat, M. I. and Moe, S. M. (2001). Effect of hemodialysis membranes on beta2-microglobulin amyloidosis. *Seminars in Dialysis* **14**, 107–112.

John, B., Anijeet, H. K., and Ahmad, R. (2001). Anaphylactic reaction during hemodialysis on AN69 membrane in a patient receiving angiotensin II receptor antagonist. *Nephrology, Dialysis, Transplantation* **16**, 1955–1956.

Johnson, D. W. *et al.* (2001). A prospective cross over trial comparing intravenous and continuous oral iron supplements in peritoneal dialysis patients. *Nephrology, Dialysis, Transplantation* **16**, 1879–1884.

Jungers, P. (2002). Late referral: loss of chance for the patient, loss of money for society. *Nephrology, Dialysis, Transplantation* **17**, 373–375.

Jungers, P. *et al.* (2000). Epidemiology of end-stage renal disease in the Ile de France area: a prospective study in 1998. *Nephrology, Dialysis, Transplantation* **15**, 2000–2006.

K/DOQI™ (2000). Clinical practice guidelines for nutrition in renal failure. *American Journal of Kidney Diseases* **35** (Suppl. 2), S1–S54.

Kasiske, B. L. (1998). Hyperlipidemia in patients with chronic renal disease. *American Journal of Kidney Diseases* **32** (Suppl. 3), S142–S156.

Katuka, T. *et al.* (1999). Prognosis of parathyroid function after successful percutaneous ethanol injection therapy guided by color doppler flow mapping in chronic dialysis patients. *American Journal of Kidney Diseases* **33**, 1091–1099.

Katzarski, K. S. *et al.* (1997). A critical evaluation of ultrasound measurement of inferior vena cava diameter for assessing dry weight in normotensive and hypertensive hemodialysis patients. *American Journal of Kidney Diseases* **30**, 459–465.

Kaufman, J. S. *et al.* (1998). Subcutaneous compared with intravenous epoetin in patients receiving hemodialysis. *New England Journal of Medicine* **339**, 678–683.

Kaufman, J. S. *et al.* (2000). A pharmacodynamic study of clopidogrel in chronic hemodialysis patients. *Journal of Thrombosis and Thrombolysis* **10**, 127–131.

Kausz, A. T. *et al.* (1999). Screeming plasma aluminium levels in relation to aluminium bone disease among asymptomatic dialysis patients. *American Journal of Kidney Diseases* **34**, 688–693.

Kaysen, G. A. *et al.* (2002). Relationships between inflammation nutrition and physiologic mechanisms establishing albumin levels in hemodialysis patients. *Kidney International* **61**, 2240–2249.

Kazama, J. J., Maruyama, H., and Gejyo, F. (2001). Reduction of circulating beta2-microglobulin level for treatment of dialysis related amyloidosis. *Nephrology, Dialysis, Transplantation* **16** (Suppl. 4), 31–35.

Kemper, M. J., Harps, E., and Müller-Wiefel, D. E. (1996). Hyperkalemia: therapeutic options in acute and chronic renal failure. *Clinical Nephrology* **46**, 67–69.

Ketteler, M., Koch, K. M., and Floege, J. (2001). Imaging techniques in the diagnosis of dialysis related amyloidosis. *Seminars in Dialysis* **14**, 90–93.

Kopple, J. D. *et al.* (1995). Treatment of malnourished CAPD patients with an amino-acid based dialysate. *Kidney International* **47**, 1148–1157.

Kosch, M. *et al.* (2001). A randomized, controlled parallel group trial on efficacy and safety of iron sucrose (Venofer^R) vs iron gluconate (Ferrlecit^R) in hemodialysis patients treated with Rhu-EPO. *Nephrology, Dialysis, Transplantation* **16**, 1239–1239.

Kronenberg, F. (1999). The low molecular weight apo(a) phenotype is an independent predictor for coronary artery disease in hemodialysis patients: a prospective follow-up. *Journal of the American Society of Nephrology* **10**, 1027–1036.

Kushner, R. F. and Roxe, D. M. (2002). Bipedal bioelectrical impedance analysis reproducibly estimates total body water in hemodialysis patients. *American Journal of Kidney Diseases* **39**, 154–158.

Lacson, E. and Diaz-Buxo, J. A. (2001). Daily and nocturnal hemodialysis: how do they stock-up? *American Journal of Kidney Diseases* **38**, 225–239.

Leblanc, M. *et al.* (2000). Folic acid and pyridoxal-5′-phosphate losses during high efficiency hemodialysis in patients without hydrosoluble vitamin supplementation. *Journal of Renal Nutrition* **10**, 196–201.

Lefebvre, A. *et al.* (1989). Optimal correction of acidosis changes progression of dialysis osteodystrophy. *Kidney International* **36**, 1112–1118.

Levin, A. (2000). Consequences of late referral on patient outcomes. *Nephrology, Dialysis, Transplantation* **15** (Suppl. 3), 8–13.

Levin, A. (2002). Anemia and left ventricular hypertrophy in chronic kidney disease populations: a review of the current state of knowledge. *Kidney International* **61** (Suppl. 80), S44–S48.

Leypoldt, J. K. *et al.* (2002). Relationship between volume status and blood pressure during chronic hemodialysis. *Kidney International* **61**, 266–275.

Lim, V. S. and Kopple, J. D. (2000). Protein metabolism in patients with chronic renal failure: role of uremia and dialysis. *Kidney International* **58**, 1–10.

Lim, V. S. *et al.* (1990). Effect of hematocrit on solute removal during high-efficiency hemodialysis. *Kidney International* **37**, 1557–1562.

Lindholm, B. *et al.* (1998). Influence of different treatments and schedules on the factors conditioning the nutritional status in dialysis patients. *Nephrology, Dialysis, Transplantation* **13**, 66–73.

Locatelli, F., Baldamus, C. A., Villa, G., Ganea, A., and Martín de Francisco, A. L. (2002a). Once weekly compared with three-times-weekly subcutaneous epoetin β: results from a randomised, multi-centre, therapeutic study. *American Journal of Kidney Diseases* **40**, 119–125.

Locatelli, F., Cannata-Andía, J. B., Drüeke, T. B., Hörl, W. H., Fouque, D., Heimburger, O., and Ritz, E. (2002b). Management of disturbances of calcium and phosphate metabolism in chronic renal insufficiency, with emphasis on the control of hyperphosphataemia. *Nephrology, Dialysis, Transplantation* **17**, 723–731.

Locatelli, F., Fouque, D., Heimburger, O., Drüeke, T. B., Cannata-Andía, J. B., Hörl, W. H., and Ritz, E. (2002c). Nutritional status in dialysis patients: a European consensus. *Nephrology, Dialysis, Transplantation* **17**, 563–572.

Locatelli, F. *et al.* (1998a). Effect of on-line conductivity plasma ultra-filtrate kinetic modeling on cardiovascular stability of hemodialysis patients. *Kidney International* **53**, 1052–1060.

Locatelli, F., Conte, F., and Marcelli, D. (1998b). The impact of haematocrit levels and erythropoeitin treatment on overall and cardiovascular mortality. The experience of the Lombardy Dialysis Registry. *Nephrology, Dialysis, Transplantation* **13**, 1642–1644.

Locatelli, F. *et al.* (2000). Effect of high-flux dialysis on the anaemia of haemodialysis patients. *Nephrology, Dialysis, Transplantation* **15**, 1399–1409.

Locatelli, F. *et al.* (2001). Novel erythropoiesis stimulating protein for treatment of anemia in chronic renal insufficiency. *Kidney International* **60**, 41–47.

Lopez–Gomez, J. M. and Carrera, F. (2002). What should optimal target hemoglobin be? *Kidney International* **61** (Suppl. 80), S39–S43.

Luik, A. J., Kooman, J. P., and Leunissen, K. M. L. (1997a). Hypertension in hemodialysis patients: is it only hypervolaemia? *Nephrology, Dialysis, Transplantation* **12**, 1557–1560.

Luik, A. J. *et al.* (1997b). Effects of hypervolaemia on interdialytic hemodynamics and blood pressure control in hemodialysis patients. *American Journal of Kidney Diseases* **30**, 466–474.

Ma, J. Z. *et al.* (1999). Hematocrit level and associated mortality in hemodialysis patients. *Journal of the American Society of Nephrology* **10**, 610–619.

Macdougall, I. C. (2000). Intravenous administration of iron in epoetin-treated haemodialysis patients: Which drugs? Which regimen? *Nephrology, Dialysis, Transplantation* **15**, 1743–1745.

Macdougall, I. C. (2001a). An overview of the efficacy and safety of novel erythropoeisis stimulatin protein (NESP). *Nephrology, Dialysis, Transplantation* **16** (Suppl. 3), 14–21.

Macdougall, I. C. (2001b). ACE inhibitors and erythropoeitin responsiveness. *Ameican Journal of Kidney Diseases* **38**, 649–651.

Macdougall, I. C., Gray, S. J., Elston, O., Breen, C., Jenkins, B., Browne, J., and Egrie, J. (1999). Pharmacokinetics of novel erythropoiesis stimulating protein compared with epoetin alfa in dialysis patients. *Journal of the American Society of Nephrology* **10**, 2392–2395.

Mallamaci, F. *et al.* (2002). Hyperhomocysteinaemia predicts cardio-vascular outcomes in haemodialysis patients. *Kidney International* **61**, 609–614.

Malluche, H. H. (2002). Aluminium and bone disease in chronic renal failure. *Nephrology, Dialysis, Transplantation* **17** (Suppl. 2), 21–24.

Malluche, H. H. *et al.* (1999). The role of bone biopsy in clinical practice and research. *Kidney International* **56** (Suppl. 73), 520–525.

Maroni, B. J. (1998). Protein restriction in the pre-end-stage renal disease patient: who, when, how and the effect on the subsequent ESRD outcome. *Journal of the American Society of Nephrology* **32** (Suppl. 4), S100–S506.

Mars, R. L. *et al.* (1999). Use of bolus intraperitoneal iron dextran in continuous ambulatory peritoneal dialysis or cyclic peritoneal dialysis patients receiving recombinant human erythropoietin. *Advances in Peritoneal Dialysis* **15**, 60–64.

Martin, K. J. and Gonzalez, A. (2001a). Vitamin D analogues for the management of secondary hyperparathyroidism. *American Journal of Kidney Diseases* **38** (Suppl. 5), S34–S40.

Martin, K. J. and Gonzalez, A. (2001b). Strategies to minimize bone disease in renal failure. *American Journal of Kidney Diseases* **38**, 1430–1436.

Maung, H. M. (2001). Efficacy and side effects of intermittent intravenous and oral Doxercalciferol (1α-hydroxy vitamin D2) in dialysis patients with secondary hyperparathyroidism: a sequential comparison. *American Journal of Kidney Diseases* **37**, S32–S43.

Medical Expert Group (2000a). Clinical algorithms on renal osteodystrophy. *Nephrology, Dialysis, Transplantation* **15** (Suppl. 5), 40–57.

Medical Expert group (2000b). Clinical algorithm on cardiovascular risk factors: antihypertensive management in PD and HD patients. *Nephrology, Dialysis, Transplantation* **15** (Suppl. 5), 126–135.

Mehrotra, R. and Nolph, K. D. (2000). Treatment of advanced renal failure: low-protein diets or timely initiation of dialysis (?). *Kidney International* **58**, 1381–1388.

Meier-Kriesche, H. U. *et al.* (2001). Survival improvement among patients with end-stage renal disease: trends over time for transplant recipients and wait-list patients. *Journal of the American Society of Nephrology* **22**, 1293–1296.

Memoli, B. *et al.* (2002). Changes of serum albumin and C-reactive protein are related to changes of interleukin-6 release by peripheral mononuclear cells in hemodialysis patients treated with different membranes. *American Journal of Kidney Diseases* **39**, 266–273.

Menon, M. K. *et al.* (2001). Long-term blood pressure control in a cohort of peritoneal dialysis patients and its association with residual renal function. *Nephrology, Dialysis, Transplantation* **16**, 2207–2213.

Mercadal, L. *et al.* (1999). Duocart biofiltration: a new method of hemodialysis. *ASAIO Journal* **45**, 151–156.

Metry, G. *et al.* (2001). Fluid balance in patients with chronic renal failure assessed with *N*-terminal pro-atrial natriuretic peptide, atrial natriuretic peptide and ultrasonography. *Acta Physiologia Scandinavica* **171**, 117–122.

MMWR update (1988). Universal precautions for prevention of transmission of human immuno-deficiency virus, hepatitis B virus and other blood borne pathogens in health-care settings. *Journal of the American Medical Association* **260**, 462–465.

Minutolo, R. *et al.* (2002). Post-dialytic rebound of serum phosphorus: pathogenetic and clinical insights. *Journal of the American Society of Nephrology* **13**, 1054–2002.

Mittman, N. *et al.* (2001). Serum prealbumin predicts survival in hemodialysis and peritoneal dialysis 10 years of prospective observation. *American Journal of Kidney Diseases* **38**, 1358–1364.

Morena, F. *et al.* (2002). Convective and diffusive losses of vitamin C during haemodiafiltration session: a contributive factor to oxydative stress in haemodialysis patients. *Nephrology, Dialysis, Transplantation* **17**, 422–427.

Moreno, F. *et al.* (2000). Increasing the hematocrit has a beneficial effect on quality of life and is safe in selected hemodialysis patients. Spanish Cooperative Renal Patients Quality of Life Study Group of the Spanish Society of Nephrology. *Journal of the American Society of Nephrology* **11**, 335–342.

Movilli, E. *et al.* (2001). Adequacy of dialysis reduces the doses of recombinant erythropoietin independently from the use of biocompatible membranes in hemodialysis patients. *Nephrology, Dialysis, Transplantation* **16**, 111–114.

Mucsi, I. *et al.* (1998). Control of serum phosphate without any phosphate binders in patients treated with nocturnal hemodialysis. *Kidney International* **53**, 1399–1404.

Narita, I. *et al.* (2001). The circadian blood pressure rythm in non-diabetic hemodialysis patients. *Hypertension Research* **24**, 111–117.

National Kidney Foundation NKF/DOQI (1997). Clinical practice guidelines for hemodialysis adequacy and peritoneal dialysis adequacy. *American Journal of Kidney Diseases* **30** (Suppl. 2), S1–S138.

National Kidney Foundation NKF/DOQI (2000). K/DOQI clinical pratice guidelines for nutrition in chronic renal failure. *American Journal of Kidney Diseases* **35** (Suppl. 2), S1–S140.

National Kidney Foundation K/DOQI (2001). Clinical practice guidelines for hemodialysis and peritoneal adequacy, vascular access and anemia of chronic diseases. *American Journal of Kidney Diseases* **37** (Suppl. 1), S1–S238.

NESP Usage Guidelines Group (2001). Practical guidelines for the use of NESP in treating renal anaemia. *Nephrology, Dialysis, Transplantation* **16** (Suppl. 3), 22–28.

Neyer, U. *et al.* (2002). Total parathyroïdectomy with autotransplantation in renal hyperparathyroïdism: low recurrence after intra-operative tissue selection. *Nephrology, Dialysis, Transplantatis* **17**, 625–629.

Obrador, G. *et al.* (1999). Level of renal function at the initiation of dialysis in the U.S. end-stage renal disease population. *Kidney International* **56**, 227–235.

Olaizola, I. *et al.* (2000). [(99 m)Tc]. Sestamibi parathyroid scintigraphy in chronic haemodialysis patients: static and dynamic explorations. *Nephrology, Dialysis, Transplantation* **15**, 1201–1206.

Oliver, M. J., Edwards, L. J., and Churchill, D. N. (2001). Impact of sodium and ultrafiltration profiling on hemodialysis related symptoms. *Journal of the American Society of Nephrology* **12**, 151–156.

Ozkahya, M. *et al.* (1999). Treatment of hypertension in dialysis patients by ultrafiltration: role of cardiac dilatation and time factor. *American Journal of Kidney Diseases* **34**, 218–221.

Paganini, E. P. (1995). Adapting the dialysis unit to increased hematocrit levels. *American Journal of Kidney Diseases* **25** (Suppl. 4), S12–S17.

Perazella, M. A. (2001). Pharmacologic options to treat symptomatic intradialytic hypotension. *American Journal of Kidney Diseases* **38** (Suppl. 4), S26–S36.

Perez-Garcia, R. *et al.* (2002). AM3 (Immunoferon^R) as an adjuvant to hepatitis B vaccination in dialysis patients. *Kidney International* **61**, 1845–1852.

Petitclerc, Th. (1999). Recent developments in conductivity monitoring of haemodialysis session. *Nephrology, Dialysis, Transplantation* **14**, 2607–2613.

Pflanz, S. *et al.* (1994). Calcium acetate versus calcium carbonate as phosphate-binding agents in chronic haemodialysis. *Nephrology, Dialysis, Transplantation* **9**, 1121–1124.

Pierratos, A. (1999). Nocturnal home haemodialysis: an update on a 5 year experience. *Nephrology, Dialysis, Transplantation* **14**, 2835–2840.

Plum, J. *et al.* (2001). Comparison of body fluid distribution between chronic haemodialysis and peritoneal dialysis patients as assessed by biophysical and biochemical methods. *Nephrology, Dialysis, Transplantation* **16**, 2378–2385.

Qureshi, A. R. *et al.* (1998). Factors predicting malnutrition in hemodialysis patients. *Kidney International* **53**, 773–782.

Rahman, M. *et al.* (2000). Interdialytic weight gain, compliance with dialysis regimen and age are independent predictors of blood pressure in dialysis patients. *American Journal of Kidney Diseases* **35**, 257–265.

Rahn, K. M., Heidenreich, S., and Bruckner, D. (1999). How to assess glomerular function and damage in humans. *Journal of Hypertension* **17**, 309–317.

Raj, D. S. C. *et al.* (2000). β2-Microglobulin kinetics in nocturnal dialysis. *Nephrology, Dialysis, Transplantation* **15**, 58–64.

Rocco, M. V. *et al.* (2001). Risk factors for hypertension in chronic hemodialysis patients: baseline data from the HEMO study. *American Journal of Nephrology* **21**, 280–288.

Rocco, M. V. *et al.* (2002). Nutritional status in the HEMO study cohort at baseline. *American Journal of Kidney Diseases* **39**, 245–256.

Saltissi, D. *et al.* (2002). Safety and efficacy of simvastatin in hypercholesterolemic patients undergoing chronic renal dialysis. *American Journal of Kidney Diseases* **39**, 283–290.

Salusky, I. B. and Goodman, W. G. (2002). Cardiovascular calcification in end-stage renal disease. *Nephrology, Dialysis, Transplantation* **17**, 336–339.

Santoro, A. *et al.* (1998). Blood volume regulation during hemodialysis. *American Journal of Kidney Diseases* **32**, 739–748.

Schaubel, D. E. *et al.* (2000). Trends in mortality on peritoneal dialysis: Canada (1991–1997). *Journal of the American Society of Nephrology* **11**, 126–133.

Schena, F. P. (2000). Epidemiology of end-stage renal disease: international comparisons of renal replacement therapy. *Kidney International* **57** (Suppl. 74), S39–S45.

Schiffl, H. and Lang, S. M. (1999). Angiotensin-converting enzyme inhibitors but not Angiotensin II AT1 receptor antagonists affect erythropoiesis in patients with anemia of end-stage renal disease. *Nephron* **81**, 106–108.

Schiffl, H. *et al.* (2001). Effect of ultra pure dialysis fluid on nutritional status and inflammatory parameters. *Nephrology, Dialysis, Transplantation* **16**, 1863–1869.

Schmitt, Y. and Schneider, H. (1993). Low-molecular-weight heparin: influence on blood lipids in patients on chronic hemodialysis. *Nephrology, Dialysis, Transplantation* **8**, 438–442.

Schöming, M. and Ritz, E. (2000). Management of disturbed calcium metabolism in uraemic patients. Use of vitamin D metabolites. *Nephrology, Dialysis, Transplantation* **15** (Suppl. 5), 18–24.

Schwalbe, S. *et al.* (1997). Beta2-microglobulin associated amyloidosis: a vanishing complication of long-term haemodialysis. *Kidney International* **52**, 1077–1083.

Seliger, S. L. *et al.* (2002). HMG-COA reductase inhibitors are associated with reduced mortality in ESRD patients. *Kidney International* **61**, 297–304.

Sherrard, D. J. *et al.* (1996). The aplastic form of renal osteodystrophy. *Nephrology, Dialysis, Transplantation* **11** (Suppl. 3), 29–31.

Shoji, T. *et al.* (2002). Atherogenic lipoproteins in end-stage renal disease. *American Journal of Kidney Diseases* **38** (Suppl. 1), S30–S33.

Shulman, T. *et al.* (2001). Preserving central blood volume: changes in body fluid compartments during hemodialysis. *ASAIO Journal* **47**, 615–618.

Sica, D. A. *et al.* (1997). The pharmacokinetics of irbesartan in renal failure and maintenance hemodialysis. *Clinical Pharmacology and Therapeutics* **62**, 610–618.

Silverberg, D. S. *et al.* (2000). The use of subcutaneous erythropoietin and intravenous iron for the treatment of the anemia of severe, resistant congestive heart failure improves cardiac and renal function and functional cardiac class and markedly reduces hospitalizations. *Journal of the American College of Cardiology* **35**, 1737–1744.

Sitter, T., Bergner, A., and Schiffl, H. (2000). Dialysate related cytokine induction and response to recombinant erythropoietin in haemodialysis patients. *Nephrology, Dialysis, Transplantation* **15**, 1207–1211.

Slatopolsky, E., Dusso, A., and Brown, A. J. (2002). Control of uremic bone disease: role of vitamin D analogs. *Kidney International* **61** (Suppl. 80), S143–S148.

Slatopolsky, E. A. *et al.* (1999). Renagel, a non-absorbed calcium and aluminium-free phosphate binder lowers serum phosphorus and parathyroid hormone. *American Journal of Kidney Diseases* **33**, 694–701.

Spalding, E. M., Chamney, P. W., and Farrington, K. (2002). Phosphate kinetics during hemodialysis. Evidence for biphasic regulation. *Kidney International* **61**, 655–667.

Steddon, S. J., Schroeder, N. J., and Cunningham, J. (2001). Vitamin D analogues: how do they differ and what is their clinical role? *Nephrology, Dialysis, Transplantation* **16**, 1915–1967.

Stenvinkel, P. *et al.* (1999). Strong association between malnutrition, inflammation and atherosclerosis in chronic renal failure. *Kidney International* **55**, 1899–1911.

Stiller, S. *et al.* (2001). A critical review of sodium profiling for hemodialysis. *Seminars in Dialysis* **14**, 337–347.

Sünder-Plassmann, G. and Hörl, W. H. (1995). Importance of iron supply for erythropoietin therapy. *Nephrology, Dialysis, Transplantation* **10**, 2070–2076.

Sunder-Plassmann, G. and Hörl, W. H. (2001). Effect of erythropoietin on cardiovascular diseases. *American Journal of Kidney Diseases* **38** (Suppl. 1), S20–S25.

Takeda, K. *et al.* (1998). Disadvantage of long-term CAPD for preserving cardiac performance: an echocardiographie study. *American Journal of Kidney Diseases* **32**, 482–487.

Tarng, D. C., Huang, T. P., and Wei, Y. H. (2001). Erythropoietin and iron: the role of ascorbic acid. *Nephrology, Dialysis, Transplantation* **16**, 35–39.

The Renal Association. *Treatment of Adult Patients with Renal Failure: Recommended Standards and Audit Measures*, pp. 1–126. London: Publication Unit of the Royal College of Physicians of London, 1997.

Tominaga, Y. *et al.* (2001). More than 1000 cases of total parathyridectomy with forearm autograft for renal hyperparathyroidism. *American Journal of Kidney Diseases* **38** (Suppl. 4), S168–S171.

Torregrosa, J. V. *et al.* (2000). [(99m)-Tc]Sestamibi scintigraphy and cell cycle in parathyroid glands of secondary hyperparathyroidism. *World Journal of Surgery* **24**, 1386–1390.

Torres *et al.* (1995). Bone disease in pre-dialysis, hemodialysis and CAPD patients: evidence of a better bone response to PTH. *Kidney International* **47**, 1434–1442.

Traeger, J. *et al.* (1998). Daily versus standard hemodialysis: one year experience. *Artificial Organs* **22**, 558–563.

United States Renal Data System USRDS. *Annual Data Report*. Bethesda, MD: National Institutes of Health, Institute of Diabetes and Digestive and Kidney Diseases, 1998.

United States Renal Data System USRDS. *Annual Data Report*. Bethesda, MD: National Institutes of Health, Institute of Diabetes and Digestive and Kidney Diseases, 2000.

United States Renal Data System USRDS. *Annual Data Report: Atlas of End-Stage Renal Disease in the United States*. Bethesda, MD: National Institutes of Health, National Institute of Diabetes and Digestive and Kidney Diseases, 2001.

Valderrabano, F., Jofre, R., and Lopez-Gomez, J. M. (2001). Quality of life in end-stage renal disease patients. *American Journal of Kidney Diseases* **38**, 443–464.

Valderrabano, F. *et al.* (2000). European survey on anaemia management (ESAM Study). *Nephrology, Dialysis, Transplantation* **15** (Suppl. 4), 1–56.

Van Dijk, P. C. W. *et al.* (2001). Renal replacement therapy in Europe: the results of a collaborative effort by the ERA–EDTA registry and six national or regional registries. *Nephrology, Dialysis, Transplantation* **16**, 1121–1129.

Van Tellingen, A. *et al.* (2001). Long-term reduction of plasma homocysteine levels by super-flux dialysers in hemodialysis patients. *Kidney International* **59**, 342–347.

Verresen, L. *et al.* (1994). Bradykinin is a mediator of anaphylactoid reactions during hemodialysis with AN69 membranes. *Kidney International* **45**, 1497–1503.

Walser, M. and Hill, S. (1999). Can renal replacement therapy be deffered by a supplemented very-low protein diet? *Journal of the American Society of Nephrology* **10**, 110–116.

Wang, M. C. *et al.* (2001). Blood pressure and left ventricular hypertrophy in patients on different peritoneal dialysis regimens. *Peritoneal Dialysis International* **21**, 36–42.

Wanner, C. (2000). Importance of hyperlipidaemia and therapy in renal patients. *Nephrology, Dialysis, Transplantation* **15** (Suppl. 5), 92–96.

Watson, P. E., Watson, I. D., and Batt, R. D. (1980). Total body water volumes for males and females estimated from simple anthropometric measurements. *American Journal of Clinical Nutrition* **33**, 27–29.

Weiss, L. G. *et al.* (2000). The efficacy of once weekly compared with two or three times weekly subcutaneous epoetin β: results from a randomized controlled multicentre trial. *Nephrology, Dialysis, Transplantation* **15**, 2014–2019.

Winearls, C. G. (1998). Recombinant human erythropoietin: 10 years of clinical experience. *Nephrology, Dialysis, Transplantation* **13** (Suppl. 2), 3–8.

Working Party for European Best Practice Guidelines for the management of anaemia in patients with chronic renal failure (1999). European Best Practice Guidelines for the management of anaemia in patients with chronic renal failure. *Nephrology, Dialysis, Transplantation* **14** (Suppl. 5), 1–50.

Yanagiba, S. *et al.* (2001). Utility of the inferior vena cava diameter as a marker of dry weight in non oliguric hemodialyzed patients. *ASAIO Journal* **47**, 528–532.

Zazgornik, J. *et al.* (1998). Bilateral nephrectomy: the best, but often overlooked treatment for refractory hypertension in hemodialysis patients. *American Journal of Hypertension* **11**, 1364–1370.

Zoccali, C. *et al.* (1999). Prediction of left ventricular geometry by clinic, pre-dialysis and 24-h-ambulatory BP monitoring in haemodialysis patients. *Journal of Hypertension* **17**, 1751–1758.

Zucchelli, P., Santoro, A., and Spongano, M. (1994). Acetate-free biofiltration: acidosis correction and cardiovascular stability. *Contributions to Nephrology* **108**, 105–113.

12.7 Psychological aspects of treatment for renal failure

Richard B. Weiner

Adapting to endstage renal disease

Psychological reactions

In the early years of haemodialysis, patients with endstage renal disease (ESRD) who were accepted for dialysis therapy were in many respects ideally suited to adapt to this dramatic change in lifestyle. Since maintenance haemodialysis was very expensive and funds to pay for it were severely limited, the patients selected were under 50 years of age, employed, and with supportive family relationships. How long a patient could survive was unknown, and the first decade of haemodialysis was one of experimentation. While the pioneering dialysis units provided an environment which was exciting for the medical staff, the situation was more uncertain and anxiety provoking for the patients. Nevertheless, many were grateful and, for the most part, willing to be 'guinea pigs'.

Patients presenting for treatment of renal failure are often viewed as angry, anxious, uncertain (about what the future holds), afraid, depressed, and very often denying the reality of the nature and demands of their illness (Dingwall 1997). Along with trying to cope with a loss of renal function, these patients may also have to cope with a loss of sexual function, a loss of personal freedom, a reduced life expectancy, and a possible loss of their position in the family and in society (i.e. economic loss). A high incidence of suicide, withdrawal from treatment, and fatal non-compliance were also noted (Abram *et al.* 1971).

Kaplan De-Nour (1982) concluded that denial can be usefully adaptive when one does not ignore the existence of severe problems by rejecting needed treatments and assistance while refusing to accept that these problems must necessarily have a detrimental impact on oneself. Examples of such adaptation are individuals who overcome blindness, deafness, and paralysis. To a well-adapted dialysis patient, these would seem much more severe handicaps. Today, dialysis patients are said to use denial of an uncertain future constructively by focusing on and living in the present (Hoothay and Leary 1990). This is possible where medical and psychosocial complications do not interfere. However, denial can be harmful when it interferes with compliance and adaptation to a necessary medical regimen.

From the early- to mid-1970s and into the 1980s, the number of patients on haemodialysis has grown as government financial support for their treatment has become available. Therapeutic advances were similarly remarkable.

By the end of the twentieth century, the following statistical data on ESRD were noted for the United States (USRDS 2001).

In 1999, the period prevalence of patients with ESRD was approximately 425,000, of whom 243,000 were on dialysis, 85 per cent receiving in-centre haemodialysis; 90,000 new patients started renal replacement and 13,500 kidney transplants were performed, 65 per cent from cadaver donors.

Patient selection criteria became increasingly less rigid, and patients with psychological and additional life-limiting medical problems were offered treatment. Depression began to be seen as a normal step on the path to adaptation, resolving with stable health and longer time on haemodialysis (Kutner *et al.* 1985). In some patients depression did not begin with renal failure but was present before (Craven *et al.* 1987). It was treatable with psychotherapy (Kaplan De-Nour 1970) or antidepressants (Kennedy *et al.* 1989). Resolution of depression came to be viewed as successful adaptation.

Adaptation to dialysis

Problems with coping

Having avoided death, the dialysis patient has to then cope with a less than normal existence. A necessary dependence on a machine for life struggles with the independence needed to maintain a 'normal' life. A study by Hagren *et al.* (2001) indicated that patients on haemodialysis experienced areas of suffering that related to a loss of freedom because of dependence on the machine as a lifeline, and dependence on the dialysis staff. The lifestyle of dependency was seen to affect the nature and quality of marital, family, and social relationships. Prolonged stress due to unresolved physiological and psychosocial problems reduces the ability to cope. Physiological stresses were seen as being more troublesome than psychosocial ones, and were felt by patients to be harder to control. Devins *et al.* (1993) have studied the role of illness intrusiveness in determining patient adaptation. An illness is intrusive when it substantially interferes with one's desired lifestyle. As measured by 13 important life domains, ESRD is not more intrusive than rheumatoid arthritis and is less so than multiple sclerosis. Results of a study of 75 patients aged 18–65 years, on maintenance haemodialysis for at least 1 year (Cristovao 1999) showed that patients identified high levels of stress, and that psychosocial stressors were as challenging as physiological ones.

Not surprisingly, individuals who have difficulty dealing with the normal stresses of life will have problems with dialysis. Personalities marked by low frustration tolerance, acting out, non-therapeutic denial, gains from assuming the sick role, and obsessive–compulsive traits do not adapt well in terms of either compliance or rehabilitation (Kaplan De-Nour 1978). Poll and Kaplan De-Nour (1980) analysed a patient's locus of control as a way of judging adaptation to dialysis. Locus of control is a method of looking at how patients view their ability to control their lives. From the perspective of this construct, patients can be divided into three groups: the internally controlled, the externally controlled, and (possibly constituting a majority) those with mixed locus of control depending on the situation. Patients with an internal locus of control (independent) adjust and adapt better than those with an external locus (dependent). They have better compliance with diet, greater vocational rehabilitation, and more readily accept their limitations. They also have a greater tendency to seek information and to adopt an active, problem-solving, and intellectual approach to cope with their situation (Weng 1984). They tend to believe that their actions can affect what happens to them, whereas those who are externally oriented believe that their behaviour has little or no impact upon life events.

Levels of expectation of dialysis staff seem to be more often too low than too high and, because of their unique dependence on the dialysis staff, patients are likely to make these staff expectations part of their behaviour. The often stated inability of dialysis to rehabilitate can become a self-fulfilling prophecy where staff expectations are low, dialysis therapy is inadequate, and other medical problems are neither treated nor prevented. Poor or inattentive medical care from the physician can cause or contribute to a symptomatic uraemic state due to inadequate dialysis treatment. In situations where the nurses and physicians give most of their attention to the technical aspects of their work and avoid meaningful personal interactions with patients, patient adaptation will lag.

Promoting adaptation

For ESRD, patient acceptance is the adaptation to a new lifestyle and a life without cure. At best, it can be a life with minimal interference from physiological and psychosocial stresses. At worst, it can be an existence full of sickness and uncertainty. However, almost everyone must make compromises in life, and adaptation to a life dependent on a machine is certainly within human ability.

Factors found to be predictive of coping were family relationships, predialysis functioning in terms of coping styles, and personality (Olsen 1983). Patients with good family support, adequate premorbid stress defences, and agreeable personalities should adapt well to the limitations and difficulties of dialysis. The caring support of loved ones is a great advantage to one who is attempting to cope with a loss. The influence of the family and friends on psychological adjustment of ESRD patients is well supported in the literature (Burton *et al.* 1983; Siegal *et al.* 1987). Understanding how families adapt to chronic illness may be important to caregivers in providing support for healthy family members stressed in trying to deal with another member's illness. Flaherty and O'Brien (1992), in explaining how families try to cope, conceptualize five different styles:

Remote: illness of one member leaves other family members unaffected in their lives and activities.

Enfolded: family members band together to work as a unit in dealing with problems and issues of the illness.

Altered: the illness itself causes significant changes for and between family members both within and outside the home.

Distressed: family members become anguished and grieve over the effects of illness on both the patients and themselves.

Receptive: family members accept the illness and begin to make adjustments. Such groupings may prove useful in promoting family well-being.

Within the family, particular attention should be paid to the partners of dialysis patients who reflect the anxieties of the patients as well as harbouring fears of their own. Their stability is necessary for ultimate patient adaptation. A potent influence on patient and family acceptance of dialysis is knowing about other people in the same situation who are doing well. This awareness helps alleviate feelings of isolation and gives patients and family hope that their burden can be overcome. Meeting with other patients, singly or in groups, can be very beneficial in aiding adjustment. Patients can share experiences, problems, and solutions with those who 'have been there'. Such meetings can be facilitated by patient-run organizations such as the American Association of Kidney Patients in the United States or the National Federation of Kidney Patient Associations in the United Kingdom. Most countries which offer access to dialysis probably have similar organizations.

The importance of internally localized control for coping with and survival on dialysis should inspire care-giving staff members, without feeling threatened, to allow such patients to take as much responsibility as possible for their own dialysis regimens. A useful strategy for the large mixed locus group is to encourage greater participation in the treatment regimen. Patients incapable of taking any responsibility for their own care require considerable attention, providing more than enough work for dialysis professionals. Active involvement in their own treatment as well as outside activities through education, with staff support, promotes compliance, decreases perceived illness intrusiveness, and helps to integrate therapy into a patient's lifestyle (Devins 1994). Rittman *et al.* (1993) suggest that the potentially dehumanizing experience of the technical aspects of dialysis can be offset by a caring staff. Psychiatrists and psychologists have roles to play in identifying maladaptive defences, diagnosing personality disorders, and recommending appropriate treatment.

Compliance

In medical terms, compliance means faithfully adhering to a prescribed regimen. For many patients, feeling forced to give in to a restrictive treatment or to bend to a severely limiting prescription is an invitation to rebellion.

Non-compliance with dialysis treatment remains a problem. By strict definition, most patients on dialysis are non-compliant in some aspect of their treatment. The most commonly used measures of compliance are blood urea, serum creatinine, plasma potassium, and phosphate, together with interdialytic weight gain. A patient can be labelled as compliant or non-compliant depending on how closely he or she adheres to levels of blood values or weight gain established by a facility. However, such limits should reflect both common sense and ranges appropriate for dialysed patients. For example, the upper limit of 'normal' for potassium may be 5.5 mmol/l on a chemistry profile, yet a stable dialysis patient can expect few difficulties with a predialysis potassium level of approximately 7 mmol/l drawn just before the treatment following a weekend. Insisting to a patient that a Monday morning potassium level of 6.0 mmol/l represents a case of non-compliance will uselessly reduce staff authority. Likewise, fluid intake that does not cause an increase in blood pressure even if one goes above an arbitrary weight-gain cut-off is unlikely to be harmful. A greater problem is the failure of unit personnel to assist the patient in achieving a true dry weight where moderate fluid intake will not increase the blood pressure. Non-compliance may be viewed more meaningfully by a measure which relates to good health for the dialysis patient. In this regard percentage of prescribed dialysis time achieved may be more useful since it relates to dialysis adequacy (Kobrin *et al.* 1991). Further examination of early sign-offs and missed dialysis treatments reveals plausible reasons for many such episodes (Rocco and Burkart 1993). Various discomforts occurring during dialysis accounted for 55 per cent of 2108 early sign-offs, while personal reasons such as other appointments, family responsibilities, or transportation problems explained another 36 per cent. In this study a substantial proportion of non-compliance with prescribed length of therapy was correctable by delivering more comfortable dialysis treatments and offering greater flexibility in scheduling.

Insisting upon compliance with a treatment regimen is often justified by the assumption, frequently in the absence of proof, that the required therapy has a positive impact on survival. Kaplan De-Nour and Czaczkes (1972) reported that eight out of 10 deaths in an Israeli dialysis unit were due to dietary non-compliance. Severe hyperkalaemia does kill and is seen more often in the patient inclined to suicide or ignorant of the proper diet. Repetitive bouts of excessive fluid gain and removal should not be very good for the heart. However, Ruggiero *et al.* (1992), in a study of 110 haemodialysis patients, failed to find support for the validity of dietary compliance variables as good predictors of survival. These results would indicate that at least moderate dietary non-compliance, by currently defined parameters, is of minimal risk.

Wolcott *et al.* (1986) described the determinants for compliance in ESRD patients as being due to the following:

1. situational factors (e.g. being out of or forgetting medications);
2. nature of illness or treatment (e.g. requirement for strict dietary restrictions);
3. sociodemographic events (e.g. adolescence, living alone);
4. family relationships (e.g. support, communication);
5. physician–patient interactions (e.g. trust, persuasion).

Personalities and interpersonal relationships underlie all these determinants. Theories of compliance behaviour, such as learning, cognitive, and health belief, rely on patients having some insight into and concern about health matters as well as a willingness to learn. Compliant patients are more likely to see the personal risks of non-compliance as well as the benefits accruing from adherence to a regimen (Hartman and Becker 1978).

Non-compliance with the prescribed routines of dialysis (including such things as diet, pharmacotherapy, and the treatment protocols themselves) can have a significant effect on both the success of treatment and patient care.

A study by Kutner *et al.* (2002) observed that a younger patient age was predictive of missed treatments. Perceived (negative) effects of kidney disease on daily life, and (decreased) perceived control over future health outcomes also predicted shortened treatments. No significant association was found between the type of dialysis treatment (haemodialysis versus peritoneal dialysis) and non-compliance.

Another study (Frazier *et al.* 1994) recognized factors that were associated with non-compliance among adult renal transplant recipients. This study found that recipients who were younger, female, unmarried, retransplanted, and with lower incomes tended to be non-compliant with medications. Those who were unmarried, low income, not insulin-dependent and with a longer time post-transplant tended to be non-compliant with their follow-up regimens. Those who reported higher stress and more depression, who coped with stress by using avoidance strategies, and who believed that health outcomes were beyond their control tended to be less compliant with both medication and follow-up.

Patient education and/or individualized attention, supervision, encouragement and support are commonly promoted as strategies to improve patient compliance with dialysis (Kutner 2001).

Probably, the most important causes of non-compliance are personality traits and socio-cultural factors unrelated to dialysis. The immature impulsive patient with an adolescent personality is unlikely to cooperate with the necessary restrictions of dialysis. Kaplan De-Nour and Czaczkes (1972) found that low frustration tolerance and primary and secondary gains from assuming a sick role were the most frequent causes for non-compliance. Inability to resolve depression, anger, and hostility, whether due to ingrained personality traits or to arbitrarily imposed conditions within a dialysis facility, may prevent a patient from coming to an acceptance of the necessity for dialysis. Not surprisingly, young males with an external locus of control may have the most trouble in limiting intradialytic fluid weight gains (Everett *et al.* 1993). O'Brien (1990) believes that episodes of extreme non-compliance should be understood either as simply an expression of the patient's frustration with the strict renal dietary restrictions, or as some (maladaptive) use of denial of the illness. Whatever the reason, since ongoing non-compliance with the dietary regimen or other aspects of the treatment can foreshadow serious physiological consequences, such patients warrant continuing evaluation and assessment.

Socio-cultural influences must be taken into account. For example some ethnic diets rely heavily on foods high in salt and potassium. In diverse societies such as that of the United States, influences of different cultures may be at work within a single facility. Mistrust of those in charge or a reliance on different authority figures (e.g. folk healers) may also play a role.

Placing responsibility for the outcome of their care back in the patients' hands as they are ready to receive it usually wins compliance. Winning successful compliance may require different approaches and take years. Failures must never be answered with anger, however understandable that response may appear to be. True compliance is best won by reason and calm persuasion; it is less easily compelled.

Quality of life and withdrawal of therapy

Definitions of quality of life (QOL) include a number of variables or domains such as physical health, social and psychological functioning, family life, financial well-being, and happiness with one's job. Satisfaction with ESRD therapy seems to be more *related* to fulfilment of needs and avoidance of problems than to the mode of therapy itself (Fox *et al.* 1991; Gokal 1993). Sensky (1993) concludes that, in terms of rehabilitation, adjustment, or QOL, some patients simply do better than others, regardless of the method of renal replacement therapy. Ferrans and Powers (1993) noted that haemodialysis patients were generally satisfied with the areas of their lives that they felt most important to them, and, for the most part, enjoyed a high QOL.

QOL has been increasingly viewed as a useful measure of the outcome of treatment. QOL of patients with ESRD is influenced by the disease itself and by the type of replacement therapy (Valderrabano *et al.* 2001). Among the various replacement therapies, renal transplantation seems to show the best improvements in the QOL. With this, recent trends have shown that patients' greatest concerns are about their anxieties about long-term renal function and overall health and they have fewer concerns about short-term issues, such as kidney rejection (Keown 2001).

Newer immunosuppressive agents used in the transplant patient, with improved side effect profiles, may also contribute to the improved QOL of these patients.

One study (Bakewell *et al.* 2002) noted a decline over the 2-year study period of the quality of life QOL of peritoneal dialysis patients. The most significant changes were observed for these items: general health symptoms/problems, burden of kidney disease, emotional well-being and patient satisfaction. QOL was also found to vary inversely with the number of hospital admissions.

Withdrawing treatment after it has been started, usually because of a poor QOL, is a topic of increasing interest. Between 9 and 18 per cent of dialysis patients may have their treatment stopped either by their own choice if competent or by a surrogate if not (Neu and Kjellstrand 1986; Mailloux *et al.* 1993). Most patients were older and in deteriorating mental or physical condition. Attitudes of dialysis medical directors about withholding and withdrawing treatment vary (Moss *et al.* 1993). Most (92 per cent) would honour a competent patient's wish. In patients with dementia, however, 32 per cent would stop dialysis but 68 per cent would continue.

Psychosocial problems with endstage renal disease in special cases

Diabetes mellitus

To the diabetic patient with ESRD, treatments such as haemodialysis and peritoneal dialysis, although life-prolonging, may seem more like the proverbial 'straw that breaks the camel's back'. Many of these patients are already dealing with major losses such as impaired or absent vision and loss of peripheral sensation in addition to problems with their cardiac, vascular, and autonomic systems. New limitations imposed on an already restricted diet are particularly discouraging.

Compliance with the dialysis regimen is a particularly difficult problem (Ruff 1983). Several factors are found to be influential.

1. *Complexity of the regimen.* The more complex the treatment, the more difficult it is to understand and the harder it is to implement successfully. When dealing with children or adolescents, the regimen should be carefully explained, bearing in mind the developmental level of the child.

2. *Family support.* Deterioration of a loved one may induce withdrawal of family or friends as part of the normal separation process, adding to the psychosocial stress of the patient. With families of patients, this process has been ongoing as the patient has been experiencing failure of other body functions. At the time of renal failure, when the diabetic patient is often angry, depressed, or in denial, the family may be emotionally exhausted. Reinvolving family to win their support for the patient is essential if health-restoring or preserving measures are to have any chance of success. Their love for the patient, while often strained by the circumstances can be sustaining during the darkest times.

3. *Support of medical staff.* With the onset of ESRD, the doctor or nurse may be ready to give up on the patient. However, this is the time when they need to be most actively involved. The empathetic care and support of medical and nursing staff is essential to the patient. Whether aggressive management can alter the otherwise grim prognosis for medically compromised diabetic patients with dialysis as treatment for ESRD is still to be proven.

Seeing themselves at the end of the road, diabetic patients with ESRD are usually eager to try a kidney transplant. Typically, however, they experience more problems with psychosocial adaptation following transplant than do non-diabetics (Gulledge *et al.* 1983). Although they show increased self-esteem and independence after the transplant, with decreased feelings of depression and anxiety, diabetic patients do not return to work or school or take up leisure activities to the same degree as their non-diabetic peers. Although renal function has been restored, diabetes has not been cured. In some cases, immunosuppressive drugs may make control of glucose more difficult and, in addition, exacerbate cardiovascular complications.

Because of their multiple health care needs which require frequent intervention, diabetics with renal failure, perhaps to an even greater extent than other chronically ill patients must take an active role in their own care, including diet and medication. Lower weight gains may lead to better blood pressure control, while greater adherence to diet and more precise use of diabetic medications may result in better glucose control. As with other patients, good outcomes for diabetic patients depends on compliance and knowledge.

Children

The United States Renal Data System (USRDS 2001) provides statistics for children on ESRD. The incident rates of ESRD in children have risen 2–3 per cent over the past 10 years. In these patients, the primary causes of the disease include glomerulonephritis and cystic/congenital/hereditary diseases. Boys have a higher likelihood of renal failure.

Most young children who receive a first renal transplant receive it from a living donor, in contrast to the pattern in adults. Second transplants are more likely to be from a cadaver donor.

Children under the age of five have a survival rate of 93 per cent after a kidney transplant, compared with 62 per cent for children in this age group on dialysis. Other paediatric age groups (5–9, 10–14, and 15–19 years) show five-year survivals on dialysis treatment that exceeds 81 per cent.

Over the past few decades, newer and more effective methods for the care and treatment of children with ESRD have been devised. These include better nutrition, continuous ambulatory peritoneal dialysis (CAPD), and transplantation with lower steroid dosages and newer immunosuppressants.

How the child reacts to an illness is a function of several factors (Lewis 1982):

1. *Developmental stage.* Children can adapt remarkably well to illness. The earlier in life that *restrictions* and modifications imposed by renal disease are learned, the better the adjustment is (Reynolds *et al.* 1986).

2. *Nature of relationship with parents.* The normal parent–child relationship changes when a child is chronically or fatally ill. Parents suffering feelings of guilt, may become overprotective, ignoring the emotional needs of other siblings. Even after parents have realized that their child does not necessarily have an immediately fatal illness and, with dialysis and transplantation, can have a long life, the abnormal relationship can be hard to reverse. The child may remain emotionally immature, complicating separation from parents as he or she passes through adolescence. These 'spoilt brats' do not endear themselves to adult nephrologists who eventually assume their care.

3. *Effects of the illness and its treatments.* An illness with frequent ups and downs, few prolonged plateaus, and uncomfortable procedures will impede the child's physical, emotional, and social development.

Parents and siblings share the stresses of children with ESRD, which come as a result of marked changes in diet, activity levels, school attendance, and activities of daily living (Fielding *et al.* 1985). Marital discord, as well as an increased incidence of behavioural dysfunction in siblings, have been observed in some families. Parents of sick children may be anxious and depressed, and manifest somatic symptoms. Others have the ability, despite a child's illness, to mobilize their resources and strengthen rather than weaken their marriage (Reynolds *et al.* 1988). In children with a more complicated illness, instances of family disruption are more noticeable. Parents who do not deal well with stress will have an adverse effect on the development of the healthy siblings as well as that of the sick child.

The importance of the family environment in predicting outcomes in different forms of kidney disease was found in one study (Soliday *et al.* 2001). Families with increased conflicts were predictive of more externalizing behavioural symptoms and the need for an increased number of prescribed medications. When there was a strong degree of family cohesion, fewer hospitalizations were needed.

An earlier study by the same group (Soliday *et al.* 2000) also concluded that a closely knit and supportive family structure might buffer the stresses caused by illness with kidney disease.

Psychological functioning and adjustment to dialysis were assessed in the families of 60 children and adolescents undergoing chronic dialysis (Fielding and Brownbridge 1999). Important factors found to be associated with poor adjustment to the treatment and/or anxiety and depression in children and adolescents included: parents in lower socioeconomic status homes; parents with large families; parents with limited support; parents of young children; and greater functional impairment as a result of the disease.

A number of researchers have written about the psychological aspects of adaptation to ESRD from the perspective of the developmental level of a child (Topor 1981; Frauman 1983). Very young (preschool), children are usually on dialysis only while awaiting a transplant. They are observed to become less depressed and increasingly more capable and playful within a few weeks of beginning dialysis. Nevertheless, serious dietary management problems remain since they are not able to understand the need for regulation of protein, sodium, potassium, and fluid intake. The children lag behind in personality development and growth, but this improves following successful transplantation.

When school-age children begin dialysis, behavioural and attitude problems improve as uraemic symptoms are ameliorated. These children are particularly open to peers and staff when revealing their fears and anxieties. As they are still developmentally dependent, family influence and support remain very important. Emotional deterioration may be reversed through the fostering of new interests and challenges. School-age children usually respond quite well to uncomplicated dialysis and transplantation.

Adolescents face greater emotional risks than any other group because of the many behavioural tasks that need to be accomplished. These include struggles with issues of dependence/independence, establishment of satisfactory peer and social relationships, dealing with sexuality, and planning the goals of life (education and career). They are frequently alienated from their peer group because of impaired growth, surgical scars, and the side-effects of medications. They are concerned about their body image, and their sense of self-esteem is weakened at a time when it needs to be strengthened. The consequence may be social isolation and withdrawal. Depression is common. In the future, they may have problems in forming normal sexual relationships. Adolescents are also poorly compliant with dietary modifications, and this is seen as defiant acting-out in the struggle to achieve independence.

Solutions to the problems of adolescents with ESRD are not easily found. Being in a struggle for control and mastery and independence from adults, they have a need to be considered partners in their overall treatment. Adolescents can help each other with shared feelings and experiences in support groups, enhancing self-worth and calming fears about altered body image. Such obviously beneficial associations do not develop easily, indicating the need for active encouragement by parents and staff. Cognitive coping strategies such as positive self-talk, relaxation, talking to someone, and problem-solving activity are better developed in children with chronic illnesses when compared with their healthy younger adolescent peers (Olson *et al.* 1993). Such strategies can help children and adolescents adapt to unfavourable and disturbing events. Whatever the developmental stage, fear of death underlies all anxieties. Defences include denial or projection. Dealing with this fear is an important issue in the psychotherapeutic management of children with ESRD.

Children on CAPD, which has enabled many paediatric patients to undergo dialysis at home, require special consideration. An improvement in psychological and social functioning of both patients and families has been noted (LePontois *et al.* 1987). Although families may remain stressed, children on CAPD are noted to experience an increased sense of self-worth and accomplishment as they begin to accept increasing responsibility for their own care. They experience fewer interruptions to their school schedules and activities when compared with children on haemodialysis.

Caregivers need to be aware that CAPD affects patients and family members in different ways at different developmental stages. Infants and toddlers must depend on their mothers for dialysis treatments. Mothers may feel guilt, anxiety, and depression because of the added life-supporting responsibility, particularly if there are complications. A sense of growing competence in management skills may ease the burden.

School-age children need to be encouraged to participate in all the normal social and educational activities. A sense of lowered self-esteem and poor self-image brought about by growth impairment can be aggravated by the presence of a peritoneal catheter. Some compensation can be made by encouraging the child's mastery of the techniques required by the dialysis process. A sense of pride and accomplishment may then lead to other achievements in school.

CAPD represents something of a contradictory task for adolescents. Developmentally, normal adolescents are testing the boundaries between dependence on and independence of parental authority. Conflict is heightened in situations such as CAPD or home haemodialysis where parents have been required to supervise the child's care very closely. The adolescent may respond to the parents' intense concern with rebellious non-compliance. Clearly, it is a time that requires much mutual respect and understanding between parents and children.

The elderly

The ESRD population grows steadily older as patients previously excluded by age are accepted for dialysis treatment and even transplantation. A paper by Luke and Beck (1999) provides these statistics about the elderly receiving treatment for ESRD: the average age for patients beginning dialysis for ESRD in the United States is 62 years and continues to increase. Twenty per cent of all ESRD-treated patients in the United States are older than 75 years, and about 50 per cent of all haemodialysis patients are over the age of 65 years. The annual incidence rates of new ESRD patients are highest in the age group 65–74 years, at approximately 1 per 1000.

For elderly patients on dialysis, comorbidity increases with age; over the age of 70 years, there are, on average, five comorbid conditions compared with 2–5 in those under 70 years. Compliance with therapy falls off rapidly and adverse side effects increase exponentially once more than five different medications are being taken.

A number of studies have compared older (>65 years of age) with younger patients in terms of psychosocial issues. Most found that the healthy elderly viewed life on dialysis with less stress and greater accommodation (Schultz and Powers 1987). One reason may be that selection of the elderly for dialysis is more health dependent. Another explanation may be that events such as serious illness, which are traumatic for a younger individual, may be developmentally on time for the elderly and thus less psychologically disturbing (Zarit and Kahn 1975). As a mark of their adaptation, hospital admissions for complications arising from failure to comply with the regimen are seldom required (Walker *et al.* 1976).

Results of a study of elderly dialysis patients and their dialysis nurses (Hines *et al.* 2001) indicated that these patients seek information that will enable them to cope with debilitating dialysis treatments rather than information nurses believe is necessary for them to make informed choices about whether to undergo such treatment. A key reason why communication about end-of-life issues is frequently confusing is the conflict between the information patients want to cope successfully with life and the information they need to decide intelligently about treatments that stave off death.

Older patients are more likely to have other complications that lead to shorter life expectancy. Husebye *et al.* (1987) studied the influence of 29 demographic, social, psychological, and somatic factors on survival of 78 dialysis patients aged over 70 years. Only four factors, all psychological, were prognostically important. The surviving patients rated higher on an activities scale, gained less weight between treatments, underwent home dialysis more often, and wished for transplantation less often. These results suggested that surviving patients were more in control of their treatment and had satisfactorily adapted to dialysis. Consistent with the importance of health status in the elderly, functional activity predicts survival (Kutner *et al.* 1994).

Optimum care of the elderly ESRD patient demands an interdisciplinary team approach in which the primary care physician in the early stages of disease is the leader, with the geriatrician or nephrologist becoming the leader as more complex disease interactions develop (Luke and Beck 1999).

Bia (1999) summarizes some important geriatric issues in renal transplantation: (a) a tremendous increase in the numbers of geriatric patients with ESRD, along with data showing survival after transplant in the elderly is, as in all adult age groups, better than for patients on dialysis, necessitates more skillful transplant surgeons for patients over the age of 60 years; (b) the chronic shortage of cadaveric donor organs has led to consideration of expanding the donor pool with older kidneys whose long-term survival may be shorter than those from younger donors; (c) the shortage of donors, together with data showing improved survival of living related and unrelated donor transplants has yielded an increased number of older donors (those over 60 years of age) who want to donate to a spouse, relative, or friend.

Although renal transplantation remains the most successful form of renal replacement therapy, only a small fraction of elderly ESRD patients are transplanted. The substantial mortality and comorbidity experienced by this population makes their management a difficult and ongoing challenge (Stack and Messana 2000).

Renal transplantation

In restoring a more normal life, a successful kidney transplant can markedly improve a patient's perspective. The psychological experiences that one faces following transplantation are grouped by Chambers (1982–1983) into the following stages: pretransplant, and immediate, early, middle, and late transplant. Before transplantation, patients have usually been on dialysis for some time, often growing unhappy with their lot. However, a sense of optimism begins to grow as the time to receive the kidney grows closer. In the immediate postoperative period, the patient anxiously finds himself or herself immobile, surrounded by a variety of machines, medicines, nurses, and medical staff. Painful activities are demanded of patients who would prefer to be left alone to sleep.

During the first few postoperative days, patients may respond with a sense of euphoria or hypomania when they realize that the kidney is beginning to function. Some of this effect may be the effect of corticosteroids which can produce strong, even psychotic, symptoms in a few patients. For some patients, the euphoria may dissolve to marked feelings of anxiety as they realize that the graft may not work. In this early stage, it is important that positive emotional ties are developed with the treating staff. Greater compliance with medications and diet may be a later benefit.

There is a period early after surgery (between 5 and 14 days if the kidney is working) when anxiety markedly diminishes, and the patient experiences a calm and comfortable sense of well-being. The patient has begun to accept the transplanted kidney as a functioning part. If the kidney continues to work successfully, by the middle postoperative stage (2–6 weeks), the patient will begin to focus on the future, formulating plans for a life of greater freedom and independence.

After leaving the hospital with a functioning kidney, most patients adjust satisfactorily. In one study, however, psychiatric morbidity indicating a need for therapy occurred in 25 per cent of patients with a transplant for more than 5 years (Kalman *et al.* 1983). Sensky (1989) found that previous psychiatric history was the main predictor of problems during follow-up.

In some patients, concerns relating to possibilities of graft failure, side-effects, and costs of medications, and donor fantasies may begin to emerge. Fearful of rejection, patients of all ages as well as their families employ a variety of coping defences and strategies to deal with the stress (Hudson and Hiott 1986). This fear can lead to any or all of the following emotional responses: anxiety, denial, anger, depression, guilt, frustration, diminished sense of self-worth and self-esteem, and a grief reaction.

When kidney failure cannot be reversed, a return to dialysis is indicated. When confronted with this harsh reality, patients may use denial maladaptively. If not supported, the patient could become pessimistic and feel abandoned by the staff. Over time, most will adjust to the new reality. Patients need support from family and professionals in the period of graft loss to enable a resolution of conflicts, providing for a more normal return and readjustment to life on dialysis. Staff attitudes and how they should handle the patient with irreversible rejection are important: many patients undergoing graft rejection will feel a sense of relief if they are given the opportunity to discuss their feelings about the loss of the transplant. In this way, they are not different from the dialysis patient with failed vascular access. Both patients may view the event as a risk to their life. If the staff members justifiably see the loss of a transplant or an access as only a temporary setback to the patient, they should have little difficulty in offering welcome encouragement and support. However, staff members who are deeply involved in a successful transplant outcome or who have difficulty in dealing with failure or patient depression will tend to withdraw.

Illness behaviour may become manifest through abnormal feelings in relation to both donor and kidney. This important topic has not been much explored. Not surprisingly, with living related donors, pre-existing family conflicts may be exacerbated after the transplant (Bisch 1973). Fantasies about the donor can affect recipients of cadaveric kidneys, causing serious difficulties for some in integrating the new organ into their body image. For these reasons, thorough psychological screening before the transplant can be helpful.

The importance of having a full life supported by family and friends apart from the treatment environment is important for a patient to function well after a transplant. Involvement in a transplant support group can help patients who live alone or in very poor social circumstances. Such a group can provide a forum to discuss problems, encouraging patients to verbalize and explore feelings about the whole transplant process. Others in similar circumstances can help through times of crisis with successful solutions for meeting the demands and responsibilities of the medical condition. Transplant groups can improve feelings of self-worth and self-image by allowing patients to see others with similar problems doing well.

References

Abram, H. S., Moore, G. L., and Westervelt, F. B. (1971). Suicidal behavior in chronic dialysis. *American Journal of Psychiatry* 127, 1199–1204.

Bakewell, A. B., Higgins, R. M., and Edmunds, M. E. (2002). Quality of life in peritoneal dialysis patients and association with clinical outcomes. *Kidney International* 61 (1), 239–248.

Bia, M. J. (1999). Geriatric issues in renal transplantation. *Geriatric Nephrology Urology* 9 (2), 109–113.

Bisch, S. H. (1973). The intrapsychic integration of a new organ—some observations of recipients and donors. *Psychoanalysis Quarterly* 41, 364–384.

Burton, H. J., Lindsay, R. M., and Kline, S. A. (1983). Social support as a mediator of psychological dysfunctioning and a determinant of renal failure outcomes. *Clinical and Experimental Dialysis and Apheresis* 7, 371–389.

Chambers, M. (1982–1983). Psychological aspects of renal transplantation. *International Journal of Psychiatry in Medicine* 12, 229–236.

Craven, J. L., Rodin, G. M., Johnson, L., and Kennedy, S. H. (1987). The diagnosis of major depression in renal dialysis patients. *Psychosomatic Medicine* 49, 482–492.

Cristovao, F. (1999). Stress, coping and quality of life among chronic haemodialysis patients. *EDTNA ERCA Journal* 25 (4), 35–38.

Devins, G. M. (1994). Illness intrusiveness and the psychosocial impact of lifestyle disruptions in chronic life-threatening disease. *Advances in Renal Replacement Therapy* 1, 251–263.

Devins, G. M., Edworthy, S. M., Seland, T. P., Klein, G. M., Paul, L. C., and Mandin, H. (1993). Differences in illness intrusiveness across rheumatoid arthritis, end-stage renal disease, and multiple sclerosis. *Journal of Nervous and Mental Diseases* 181, 377–ß381.

Dingwall, R. R. (1997). Living with renal failure: the psychological issues. *EDTNA ERCA Journal* 23 (4), 28–30, 35.

Everett, K. D., Sletten, C., Carmack, C., Brantley, P. J., Jones, G. N., and McKnight, T. (1993). Predicting noncompliance to fluid restrictions in haemodialysis patients. *Dialysis and Transplantation* 22, 614–620.

Ferrans, C. E. and Powers, M. J. (1993). Quality of life of haemodialysis patients. *American Nephrology Nurses Association Journal* 20, 575–581.

Fielding, D. and Brownbridge, G. (1999). Factors related to psychosocial adjustment in children with end-stage renal disease. *Journal of Pediatric Nephrology* 13 (9), 766–770.

Fielding, D., Moore, B., Dewey, M., Ashley, R., McKendrick, T., and Pinkerton, P. (1985). Children with end-stage renal failure: psychological effects on patients, siblings, and parents. *Journal of Psychosomatic Research* 29, 457–465.

Flaherty, M. J. and O'Brien, M. E. (1992). Family styles of coping in end stage renal disease. *American Nephrology Nurses Association Journal* 19, 345–349.

Fox, E., Peace, K., Neale, T. J., Morrison, R. B. I., Hatfield, R. T., and Mellsop, G. (1991). Quality of life for patients with end-stage renal failure. *Renal Failure* 13, 31–35.

Frauman, A. C. Habilitation of the child with chronic renal failure. In *Psychonephrology 2* (ed. N. B. Levy), pp. 207–212. New York: Plenum, 1983.

Frazier, P. A., Davis-Ali, S. H., and Dahl, K. E. (1994). Correlates of noncompliance among renal transplant recipients. *Clinical Transplant* 8 (6), 550–557.

Gokal, R. (1993). Quality of life in patients undergoing renal replacement therapy. *Kidney International* 43 (Suppl. 40), S23–S27.

Gulledge, A. D., Buszta, C., and Montague, D. K. (1983). Psychosocial aspects of renal transplantation. *Urologic Clinics of North America* 10, 327–335.

Hagren, B., Pettersen, I. M., Severinsson, F., Lutzen, K., and Clyne, N. (2001). The haemodialysis machine as a lifeline: experiences of suffering from end-stage renal disease. *Journal of Advanced Nursing* 34 (2), 196–202.

Hartman, P. E. and Becker, M. N. (1978). Noncompliance with prescribed regimen among chronic hemodialysis patients: a method of prediction and education diagnosis. *Dialysis and Transplantation* 7, 978–986.

Hines, S. C., Babrow, A. S., Badzek, L., and Moss, A. (2001). From coping with life to coping with death: problematic integration for the seriously ill elderly. *Health Communication* 13 (3), 327–342.

Hoothay, F. and Leary, E. M. (1990). Life satisfaction and coping of diabetic haemodialysis patients. *American Nephrology Nurses Association Journal* 17, 361–365.

Hudson, K. and Hiott, K. (1986). Coping with pediatric renal transplant rejection. *American Nephrology Nurses Association Journal* 13, 261–263.

Husebye, D. G., Westlie, L., Styn-oky, T. J., and Kjellstrand, C. M. (1987). Psychological, social, and somatic prognostic indicators in old patients undergoing long-term dialysis. *Archives of Internal Medicine* 147, 1921–1924.

Kalman, T. P., Wilson, P. G., Concetta, M., and Kalman, R. N. (1983). Psychiatric morbidity in long-term renal transplant recipients and patients undergoing haemodialysis. *Journal of the American Medical Association* 250, 55–58.

Kaplan De-Nour, A. (1970). Psychotherapy with patients on chronic haemodialysis. *British Journal of Psychiatry* 116, 207–215.

Kaplan De-Nour, A. Prediction of adjustment to chronic haemodialysis. In *Psychonephrology 1* (ed. N. B. Levy), pp. 117–232. New York: Plenum, 1978.

Kaplan De-Nour, A. (1982). Psychosocial adjustment to illness scale (PAIS): a study of chronic haemodialysis patients. *Journal of Psychosomatic Research* 26, 11–22.

Kaplan De-Nour, A. and Czaczkes, J. W. (1972). Personality factors in chronic haemodialysis patients causing noncompliance with medical regimen. *Psychosomatic Medicine* 34, 333–344.

Kennedy, S. H., Craven, J. L., and Rodin, G. M. (1989). Major depression in renal dialysis patients: an open trial of antidepressant therapy. *Journal of Clinical Psychiatry* 50, 60–63.

Keown, P. (2001). Improving quality of life—the new target for transplantation. *Transplantation* 72 (Suppl. 12), S67–S74.

Kobrin, S. M., Kimmel, P. L., Simmens, S. J., and Reiss, D. (1991). Behavioral and biochemical indices of compliance in haemodialysis patients.

Transactions of the American Society of Artificial Internal Organs **37**, M378–M380.

Kutner, N. G. (2001). Improving compliance in dialysis patients: does anything work? *Seminars in Dialysis* **14** (5), 324–327.

Kutner, N. G., Fair, P. L., and Kutner, M. H. (1985). Assessing depression and anxiety in chronic dialysis patients. *Journal of Psychosomatic Research* **29**, 23–31.

Kutner, N. G., Linn, L. S., Fielding, B., Brogan, D., and Hall, W. D. (1994). Continued survival of older haemodialysis patients: investigation of psychological predictors. *American Journal of Kidney Diseases* **24**, 42–49.

Kutner, N. G., Zhang, R., McClellan, W. M., and Cole, S. A. (2002). Psychosocial predictors of non-compliance in haemodialysis and peritoneal dialysis patients. *Nephrology, Dialysis, Transplantation* **17** (1), 93–99.

LePontois, J., Moel, D. I., and Cohn, R. A. (1987). Family adjustment to pediatric ambulatory dialysis. *American Journal of Orthopsychiatry* **57**, 78–83.

Lewis, M. Psychological reactions to illness and hospitalization. In *Clinical Aspects of Child Development* (ed. M. Lewis), pp. 307–323. Philadelphia, PA: Lea and Febiger, 1982.

Luke, R. G. and Beck, L. H. (1999). Gerontologizing nephrology. *Journal of the American Society of Nephrology* **10**, 1824–1827.

Mailloux, L. U., Bellucci, A. G., Napolitano, B., Mossey, R. T., Wilkes, B. M., and Bluestone, P. (1993). Death by withdrawal from dialysis: a 20-year clinical experience. *Journal of the American Society of Nephrology* **3**, 1631–1637.

Moss, A. H., Stocking, C. B., Sachs, G. A., and Siegler M. (1993). Variation in the attitudes of dialysis unit medical directors toward decisions to withhold and withdraw dialysis. *Journal of the American Society of Nephrology* **4**, 229–234.

Neu, S. and Kjellstrand, C. M. (1986). Stopping long-term dialysis: an empirical study of withdrawal of life-supporting treatment. *New England Journal of Medicine* **314**, 14–20.

O'Brien, M. E. (1990). Compliance behavior and long-term maintenance dialysis. *American Journal of Kidney Diseases* **15**, 209–214.

Olsen, C. A. (1983). A statistical review of variables predictive of adjustment in haemodialysis: patients. *Nephrology Nurse* **5**, 16–27.

Olson, A.-L., Johansen, S. G., Powers, L. E., Pope, J. B., and Klein, R. B. (1993). Cognitive coping strategies of children with chronic illness. *Journal of Developmental and Behavioral Pediatrics* **14**, 217–223.

Poll, I. B. and Kaplan De-Nour, A. (1980). Locus of control adjustment to chronic haemodialysis. *Psychological Medicine* **10**, 153–157.

Reynolds, J. M., Garralda, M. E., Jameson, R. A., and Postlethwaite, R. J. (1986). Living with chronic renal failure. *Child: Care, Health and Development* **12**, 401–407.

Reynolds, J. H., Garralda, M. E., Jameson, R. A., and Postlethwaite, R. J. (1988). How parents and families cope with chronic renal failure. *Archives of Disease in Childhood* **63**, 821–826.

Rittman, M., Northsea, C., Hausauer, H., Green, C., and Swenson, L. (1993). Living with renal failure. *American Nephrology Nurses Association Journal* **20**, 327–331.

Rocco, M. V. and Burkart J. M. (1993). Prevalence of missed treatments and early sign-offs in haemodialysis patients. *Journal of the American Society of Nephrology* **4**, 1178–1183.

Ruff, S. E. (1983). Measurement of compliance in patients with diabetes mellitus on hemodialysis. *Nephrology Nurse* **5**, 8–12.

Ruggiero, L., Brantley, P. J., Bruce, B. K., McKnight, G. T., and Cocke, T. B. (1992). The role of dietary compliance in survival of haemodialysis patients. *Dialysis and Transplantation* **21**, 14–17.

Schultz, K. O. and Powers, M. J. (1987). Adjustment of older patients to haemodialysis. *Dialysis and Transplantation* **16**, 234–242.

Sensky, T. (1989). Psychiatric morbidity in renal transplantation. *Psychotherapeutics and Psychosomatics* **52**, 41–46.

Sensky, T. (1993). Psychosomatic aspects of end-stage renal failure. *Psychotherapeutics and Psychosomatics* **59**, 56–68.

Siegal, B. A., Calsyn, R. J., and Cuddihee, R. M. (1987). The relationship of social support to psychological adjustment in end-stage renal disease. *Journal of Chronic Disease* **40**, 337–344.

Soliday, E., Kool, E., and Lande, E. (2000). Psychosocial adjustment in children with kidney disease. *Journal of Pediatrics and Psychology* **25** (2), 93–103.

Soliday, E., Kool, E., and Lande, E. (2001). Family environment, child behavior, and medical indicators in children with kidney disease. *Child Psychiatry and Human Development* **31** (4), 279–295.

Stack, A. G. and Messana, J. M. (2000). Renal replacement therapy in the elderly: medical, ethical and psychosocial considerations. *Advances in Renal Replacement Therapy* **7** (1), 52–62.

Topor, M. (1981). Chronic renal disease in children. *Nursing Clinics of North America* **16**, 587–597.

U.S. Renal Data System, USRDS (2001). Annual Data Report: Atlas of End-Stage Renal Disease in the United States, National Institutes of Health, National Institute of Diabetes and Digestive and Kidney Diseases, Bethesda, MD.

Valderrabano, F., Jofre, R., and Lopez-Gomez, J. M. (2001). Quality of life in end stage renal patients. *American Journal of Kidney Diseases* **38** (3), 443–464.

Walker, P. J. *et al.* (1976). Long-term haemodialysis for patients 50. *Geriatrics* **31** (9), 55–61.

Weng, B. K. (1984). Locus of control and reaction to illness: a study of patients with chronic renal failure. *Medical Journal of Malaysia* **39**, 275–278.

Wolcott, D. L., Maida, C. A., Diamond, R., and Nissenson, A. R. (1986). Treatment compliance in end-stage renal disease patients on dialysis. *American Journal of Nephrology* **6**, 329–338.

Zarit, S. H. and Kahn, R. L. (1975). Aging and adaptation to illness. *Journal of Gerontology* **30**, 67–72.

Zetin, M., Plummer, M. J., Vaziri, N. D., and Cramer, M. (1981). Locus of control and adjustment to chronic haemodialysis. *Clinical and Experimental Dialysis and Apheresis* **5**, 319–334.

13

The transplant patient

13.1 Selection and preparation of the recipient

Andries J. Hoitsma and Lukas B. Hilbrands

Introduction

In the early days of renal transplantation, the selection of patients for this procedure was relatively easy. The high mortality rate necessitated the use of stringent criteria with regard to age and general condition of the patient. With improvements in surgical techniques, and the introduction of highly effective, less hazardous modes of immunosuppression, both very young and elderly patients, and those with complicating diseases, have become potential candidates for a kidney graft. In these patients, however, it may be very difficult to weigh the advantages of renal transplantation against the risks. This is reflected in the great variability in acceptance criteria emerging from a survey conducted in the United States. University-based and large centres accepted more medically complicated patients; heterogeneity in the evaluation was especially apparent in the areas of viral hepatitis, cardiovascular disease, and non-compliance (Ramos *et al.* 1994). In a more recent European survey, heterogeneity was found with respect to oxalosis, gastric ulcers, and lack of compliance (Fritsche *et al.* 2000). Careful screening of the recipient is required and this can best be done by using a standardized check-list. On the other hand, the patient should not undergo too many unnecessary investigations in an attempt to exclude all possible operative risks. In the first part of this chapter we will give a summary of the routine investigations that are minimally required before the patient can be placed on a waiting-list. In the following sections, special patient groups, complicating diseases, and specific preparatory measures are discussed.

Routine assessment of the patient before transplantation

A complete medical interview, including history taking and a general physical examination, should be conducted at the transplantation centre. If the patient is being treated in a centre outside the transplantation centre, the referring centre can do most of the additional routine investigations. All information must be available when the patient presents to the transplantation centre for preoperative assessment. Table 1 gives a check-list of necessary procedures. Detailed guidelines to screen a recipient for renal transplantation have recently been published (European Best Practice Guidelines for Renal Transplantation 2000).

History

General

It is important, wherever possible, to establish the nature of the underlying renal disease causing the renal failure. If possible, the pathologist should be asked to re-examine the previous renal biopsies, since this

Table 1 Assessment of the patient before transplantation

History and physical examination
General
    Cause of renal failure, duration of disease, duration of hypertension
    Infections (especially urinary tract, viral, tuberculosis)
    Previous transplantations
Other diseases
    Cardiovascular, previous or current malignancies, respiratory, gastrointestinal
    Diabetes mellitus
Previous operations
    Nephrectomy, splenectomy, parathyroidectomy, appendectomy, other
Family history

Current clinical data and treatment
Mode and duration of dialysis
Blood pressure
Urine production
Signs or symptoms of neuropathy
Previous blood transfusions, pregnancies
Diet, drugs

Laboratory examinations
Haematocrit
Leucocyte count and differential, thrombocyte count
Calcium, phosphorus, alkaline phosphatase, parathormone
Liver function tests
CMV antibodies, HBs antigen, HBs antibodies, HCV antibodies, EBV antibodies, HIV antibodies
Urine culture

Radiological examinations
Chest radiograph, abdominal ultrasound

Miscellaneous investigations
Electrocardiogram
Fundoscopy
Urological examination

Immunologic investigations
Blood-group typing
Tissue typing, family typing
Antibody screening

CMV, cytomegalovirus; HBs, hepatitis B (surface); HCV, hepatitis C virus; EBV, Epstein–Barr virus; HIV, human immunodeficiency virus.

may help to estimate the risk of recurrence of the original renal disease. Information on the cause of the disease may also lead to additional preparatory measures, such as urological investigations or pretransplant nephrectomy of native kidneys. If there is a history of thrombotic microangiopathy, one should be cautious about prescribing calcineurin inhibitors after transplantation since these drugs may induce a similar syndrome in the graft.

The duration of the original renal disease and of the frequently accompanying hypertension can often indicate which complications are likely to be already present, or can be expected to develop in the near future. For example, patients with polycystic disease often show extensive signs of vascular atherosclerotic disease. This is probably caused by the relatively slow progression of renal failure in these patients, while hypertension often develops at an early stage.

Active urinary tract infection is generally considered a contraindication for renal transplantation. The infection should first be eradicated with appropriate antibiotic treatment. If this fails and one or both kidneys appear to be the source of the infection, unilateral or bilateral nephrectomy should follow. In some patients with asymptomatic urinary tract infections, a focus cannot be identified: if the lower urinary tract is found to be normal, the renal transplantation should be done under short-term antibiotic cover, with maintenance therapy being instituted when infection repeatedly recurs after transplantation.

The residual urine volume of dialysis patients can vary widely depending on the underlying cause of the renal disease, time on dialysis, and volume status. The residual urine volume must be accounted for when estimating graft function after transplantation. It is therefore important to collect precise information on daily urine production when the patient is interviewed before transplantation.

One should also examine the patient for the presence of other infectious foci, but in the absence of obvious signs or symptoms, an extensive search is not necessary. Although some centres perform routine radiological examination of the paranasal sinuses and a complete dental screening, this is of questionable benefit, since infections originating from these sites are, in our experience, not more frequent or harmful than in normal individuals.

If the patient has lost a previous transplant, it is important to assess whether the failure was due to technical or immunological problems. Rapid rejection (within 6 months) increases the risk of failure of a subsequent transplant (Arndorfer *et al.* 2001).

Patients should preferably have a body mass index below 30, because the outcome of renal transplantation in obese patients is worse than that in non-obese patients (Meier-Kriesche *et al.* 2002).

Other diseases

Patients with cardiovascular disease, diabetes mellitus, and a few rare conditions leading to renal failure form special risk groups that will be dealt with separately. For patients with diseases that are unrelated to the cause of the renal failure, general guidelines cannot be given. The risks of the procedure must be weighed against the consequences of life-long dialysis for each individual. Lung function tests may be indicated in patients with a history of respiratory disease.

Family history

Since almost 10 per cent of the primary causes of renal failure are hereditary or familial, a carefully taken family history can provide important information. It can also serve as a starting point for approaching relatives who might be considering kidney donation.

Previous operations

The patient's surgical history should be established. This is especially important, since previous abdominal operations raise the question of the possible presence of adhesions. The history may also play a part in deciding on which side the donor kidney can best be placed.

Psychological aspects

Most transplant candidates are well aware of the benefits of transplantation as compared to chronic dialysis treatment. They should also carefully be informed about the possible risks both in the short and in the long term. The importance of compliance with the immunosuppressive treatment must be stressed, but also an explanation of the potential side-effects and dangers of these drugs, including the increased risk for malignancy in the long term, is necessary. Patients should also be aware that there is at least a 50 per cent chance that they will have to take antihypertensive drugs after transplantation to control blood pressure.

The risk of recurrent disease should be mentioned during the interview, if applicable. This is especially important if live donor transplantation is planned. In this case, the prospective donor must also be informed of this additional risk. If, in a high-risk patient, it has been decided that there is no absolute contraindication to transplantation, the patient should be given ample opportunity to weigh the advantages and disadvantages of current dialysis treatment against the pros and cons of renal transplantation.

Laboratory examinations

Data on calcium and phosphorus metabolism help to predict potential hypercalcaemia due to secondary hyperparathyroidism, developing as a result of a reduction in serum phosphorus and a return to normal vitamin D metabolism after renal transplantation. Since disturbances of liver function frequently occur after renal transplantation, either due to cytomegalovirus infection or as a consequence of drug toxicity (cyclosporin, azathioprine, tacrolimus), results of routine liver enzyme assays must be available before transplantation. The determination of antibodies against cytomegalovirus, hepatitis B virus, hepatitis C virus, Epstein–Barr virus (EBV), and human immunodeficiency virus is important. Cytomegalovirus infection occurs frequently after renal transplantation, and is usually benign in those previously infected who have antibodies against the virus. Vaccination of seronegative transplant candidates with live, attenuated cytomegalovirus can possibly decrease the infection rate in these patients after transplantation of a kidney from a seropositive donor (Gonczol and plotkin 2001). However, since prophylactic treatment with ganciclovir after transplantation is very effective, this is now the treatment of choice in seronegative recipients receiving a kidney from a seropositive donor. The chance that a transplant candidate is seronegative for EBV declines with age and is less than 5 per cent at adulthood. Nevertheless, seronegative recipients that acquire a primary EBV infection during immunosuppressive treatment have an increased risk to develop post-transplant lymphoproliferative disease. Patients with human immunodeficiency virus infection are generally not eligible for renal transplantation because immunosuppressive treatment seems to hasten the unrelenting course of the disease considerably (Lang *et al.* 1991). With the availability of highly active antiretroviral therapy, this policy may be reconsidered in individual cases. However, the toxicity and potential interaction of immunosuppressive and antiviral drugs hinder safe transplantation in HIV-infected patients.

Radiological examinations

Only a few routine radiographic examinations are necessary; more extensive examinations need only be done on specific indications.

Chest radiographs will usually have been made at regular intervals in patients with renal failure. If a reasonably recent film shows no abnormalities and the patient has no signs or symptoms of pulmonary or heart disease, it is not necessary to repeat this investigation before transplantation. If arterial obstruction of the iliac vessels is clinically suspected, additional Doppler ultrasonography and arteriography may be indicated to help establish the best surgical approach.

A urological examination need not be made in every patient. Some centres require a micturition cystourethrogram in all patients before transplantation. However, in patients with primary renal involvement, such as biopsy-proven glomerulonephritis, and in the absence of problems with micturition, this investigation is not necessary. If voiding cystourethrography is indicated, it should be done via suprapubic puncture whenever possible, to avoid possible infection of the urinary tract caused by retrograde catheterization of the bladder. Great care should be taken to make exposures during micturition and after voiding in order to visualize the urethra and to check for complete emptying of the bladder.

Immunological investigations

There is ample evidence that matching for HLA-DR antigens, and probably also for HLA-A and -B antigens, between donor and recipient improves patient and graft survival. Therefore, tissue typing, including family typing when homozygosity is suspected, is now generally accepted as a necessary routine procedure before renal transplantation. In addition, there must be routine screening for HLA antibodies at 3-monthly intervals.

Living related transplantation

Recipient

Graft survival in recipients of a living donor kidney has proven to be superior to that achieved in cadaveric donor transplantation, irrespective of the number of HLA mismatches (Terasaki *et al.* 1995). The superior quality of a living donor kidney seems therefore to be more important than HLA-matching. In light of the shortage of cadaveric donors, these results justify the use of kidneys from living donors for transplantation. Kidneys from non-related living donors are currently only acceptable when a spouse or a person with a long-lasting relationship with the recipient, the so-called emotionally involved donor, wants to donate.

Donor

For the donor the acute mortality risk related to surgery is very low. Estimates vary from 1 in 1600 to 1 in 3000 kidney donations (0.03 per cent) (Johnson *et al.* 1997). Bay and Hebert (1987) compared this risk with other daily risks. Using the rate of mortality from traffic accidents in Ohio, they calculated that a kidney donor incurs as much risk from the transplant procedure as the average Ohio citizen does of dying in a traffic accident for each 2–4 years of residence in Ohio. Such comparisons may be helpful in explaining the acute mortality risk of surgery to a prospective donor. Nephrectomy can be performed by open surgery or by a laparoscopic procedure. Major complications (bleeding, pneumothorax requiring a chest tube, wound infection, pneumonia) occur in 3 per cent of the open procedures. Estimates of minor

complications (asymptomatic pneumothorax, urinary retention, urinary tract infection) amount to 17 per cent (Shaffer *et al.* 1998). With the use of laparoscopic removal of kidneys, the number of hospitalization days and overall morbidity are reduced. However, in a systematic review comparing the open procedure with the laparoscopic procedure, Merlin *et al.* (2000) concluded that the evidence base for laparoscopic live donor nephrectomy was inadequate to make safety and efficacy recommendations. Although the complications from any type of donor nephrectomy are relatively low and in general treatable, the donor should be carefully informed about these potential problems.

Concern about the possible development of renal failure by glomerular hyperfiltration in the single remaining kidney of the donor has not been borne out by clinical studies. A 45-year follow-up after uninephrectomy in young adults showed that this procedure has few, if any, adverse effects (Narkun-Burgess *et al.* 1993). Quality of life in Norwegian kidney donors was even better than in the general population (Westlie *et al.* 1993).

The donor should be healthy and free from complicating diseases. A definite age limit for donation cannot be given, but the donor must have reached the age of legal majority. Also at older age, the clinical condition and renal function are the decisive criteria for acceptance as a kidney donor. The donor must be completely free in his or her decision, and not under any pressure from the recipient or the relatives. Women of childbearing age can also serve as kidney donors. The course of subsequent pregnancies is similar to that in the general population and changes in renal function have not been noted. Complete blood-group and HLA typing of donor and recipient are required. The presence of antibodies against the donor HLA antigens in the recipient must be excluded, and this test must be repeated shortly before transplantation. The topics that deserve special attention in the assessment of a living donor are given in Table 2. Preoperative visualization of the renal arteries is mandatory in each living donor procedure. Computed tomography or magnetic resonance angiography are nowadays first choice, because of the potentially lower morbidity, improved donor convenience, and reduced cost. With these techniques an IVU is made simultaneously. In case of ambiguity, renal angiography is still the gold standard.

Table 2 Important factors in the assessment of a prospective living donor

History
Exclude hereditary renal diseases
Exclude congenital abnormalities of the urinary tract
Exclude recurrent urinary tract infections
Physical examination
Careful measurement of blood pressure
Laboratory tests
Blood group and HLA typing
Urinalysis (protein, glucose)
Urine culture
Careful examination of the urinary sediment
Serum creatinine
Screening for HIV, hepatitis B and C, cytomegalovirus, Epstein–Barr virus
Electrocardiogram
Radiological examination
Computed tomographic angiography

Pre-emptive transplantation

Transplantation before the endstage of renal failure has been reached, for instance as soon as the creatinine clearance has declined to less than 15 ml/min, would be the preferred approach for every patient since it has the potential to avoid dialysis related morbidity and is cost-saving. Especially when living donor kidneys are used, pre-emptive transplantation results in longer allograft survival than transplantation performed after the initiation of dialysis (Mange *et al.* 2001). Therefore, pre-emptive transplantation should be encouraged for all patients whenever a living donor is available. Several patient categories can particularly benefit from pre-emptive transplantation, such as children, diabetics, and patients with primary hyperoxaluria type I (see below). Transplantation with a cadaveric donor kidney before the endstage of renal failure has been reached is not generally applicable as long as there is a waiting list of patients on dialysis.

Special patient groups

Children

Although there are conflicting results in the literature, the success rate of renal transplantation in children younger than 2 years seems to be less than in older children. In children, vascular thrombosis is an important cause of graft loss. In children younger than 2 years, the risk of thrombosis in a cadaveric graft may be as high as 9 per cent, decreasing to 5.5 and 4.4 per cent in children aged 2–5 and 6–12 years, respectively (Singh *et al.* 1997). At our institution, we have set the minimal body-weight for a pediatric recipient at 11 kg, which usually correlates with an age of 18–24 months. In most of these children, it is technically feasible to transplant a kidney from an adult, particularly from a female donor.

In addition to the age of the recipient, the age of the donor also affects the success rate in paediatric transplantation. Lower graft survival rates with transplantation of kidneys from infant donors is mainly due to an increased risk of graft thrombosis. The best results in children can be achieved with kidneys from young adult donors, especially when there is no acute tubular necrosis (Sarwal *et al.* 2000).

If these restrictions are taken into account, the results of paediatric renal transplantation (with kidneys from either a cadaveric or a living donor) are comparable with those obtained in adults. As in adults, the results for living donor transplantations are superior to those obtained with cadaveric kidneys. A live-related, parental donor kidney is, therefore, often preferred.

Elderly patients

In the past, elderly patients (>60 years) with endstage renal disease (ESRD) were often not offered the possibility of transplantation because of the increased risk of mortality and morbidity. However, with newer treatment modalities the results of renal transplantation in older recipients have improved and nowadays the survival of transplant recipients 60–74 years of age is superior compared to waiting-list patients of the same age (Wolfe *et al.* 1999). The loss of grafts from rejection is even less than in younger patients (Tesi *et al.* 1994). This is most likely explained by the decrease of immune responsiveness with ageing. However, the loss of functioning grafts as a result of the death of the recipient is higher, resulting in an overall result comparable to that in other age groups. Thus, age by itself is not a contraindication for renal transplantation and there is no definite upper age limit for renal transplantation. Transplantation in patients older than 70 years is not frequently performed, but is certainly possible when their physical condition is good. Careful examination for the existence of comorbidity, especially cardiovascular diseases, in these patients may prevent early mortality after renal transplantation and may further improve graft survival results.

With the growing number of older patients receiving a transplant, an increase of the donor shortage can be expected. A solution for this problem might be the expansion of the donor pool by including older donors. Registry data show that kidney grafts from old donors have a shorter graft survival (Cecka 2000). This may not be a problem for older recipients because they will require a functioning graft for a shorter period than younger patients.

Patients with urological problems

In patients with anatomical or functional abnormalities of the lower urinary tract, urological examination, including ultrasound, voiding cystourethrography, urodynamic studies, and cystoscopy, is necessary (Glazier *et al.* 1996). The presence of vesicoureteric reflux is only an indication for nephroureterectomy if there is a hydroureter or if it is the cause of recurrent infections. In patients with abnormalities of the bladder, every attempt should be made at surgical correction. Patients with long-standing anuria on dialysis may have very small bladder capacities, but the bladder rather quickly regains its original size after a successful transplantation. Infravesical obstruction by urethral valves or prostatic hypertrophy, should be corrected only if there is still diuresis, otherwise the correction should be delayed until after a successful transplantation.

In patients with a neurogenic bladder without urinary incontinence, but with an inability to void spontaneously, self-catheterization after transplantation is a feasible policy. If the patient's own bladder cannot be used, kidney transplantation can be performed with implantation of the ureter into a urinary diversion. Ileal or colonic conduits are used for this purpose and excellent results have been reported (Warholm *et al.* 1999). The conduit must be constructed at least 6 weeks before transplantation.

Patients with hepatitis

Carriers of the hepatitis B virus surface (HBs) antigen must be identified, mainly because they constitute an infection risk to the surgical team. Graft loss due to rejection is probably not different from that in HBs-negative patients. Some centres have reported poor long-term survival, but this has not been confirmed in more recent publications. Patients with markers of active viral replication (HBe antigen or HBV-DNA) have an increased probability of death from liver disease (Hiesse *et al.* 1992). In addition, patients who are HBe antigen negative but have increased transaminase levels are at risk for chronic active hepatitis. In all these cases, a liver biopsy should be performed. If the biopsy shows signs of active infection, interferon (IFN-α) and lamivudine treatment should be considered before registration on the transplant waiting list (IFN-α is contraindicated after renal transplantation). In patients with cirrhosis, renal transplantation is contraindicated and continuation on dialysis or a combined liver and kidney transplantation should be discussed. Vaccination of all HB-negative dialysis patients is advisable, since it affords effective protection in the great majority. In HBs antigen-negative patients, hepatitis C virus (HCV) infection is the main cause of unexplained liver dysfunction after transplantation. The clinical course of HCV infection in transplanted patients appears to be similar to that in dialysis patients, but this observation is based on studies with a relatively short follow-up (Pereira *et al.* 1998). The pretransplant serum alanine aminotransferase has no predictive value for the course of liver disease after transplantation in HCV infection, and as a consequence many centres recommend liver biopsy in these patients. In patients with signs of chronic active hepatitis or cirrhosis on biopsy, the risk for progressive liver disease after renal transplantation is increased. Patients with chronic hepatitis may be candidates for IFN-α therapy during the dialysis period, although there are no data showing that this interferon therapy improves survival after transplantation (Morales *et al.* 2000).

Patients with a history of malignancy

The decision to perform a renal transplantation in a patient who has previously been treated for a malignancy is not an easy one. Penn (1993) has provided helpful guidelines based on data collected in an international transplant tumour registry. Overall, 22 per cent of 823 patients with a pretransplant malignancy developed a recurrence of the malignancy after transplantation. Of the recurrences, 53, 34, and 13 per cent occurred in patients transplanted at 0–24 months, 24–60 months, and more than 60 months, respectively, after treatment for the malignancy. There is also substantial variability among the rates of recurrence of different tumours (Table 3). An unsuspected renal carcinoma is sometimes found in a patient who undergoes pretransplant nephrectomy for other reasons: this is not surprising since the frequency of renal carcinoma is increased in patients with long-standing endstage renal failure and acquired renal cysts. The subsequent course in these patients is favourable as recurrent or metastatic disease has not been reported after transplantation.

Based on these data, a waiting period of 2 years seems justified for most neoplasms. No waiting time is necessary in incidentally discovered renal carcinoma, *in situ* carcinomas, focal neoplasms, low-grade bladder cancers, and basal-cell skin cancers. A waiting time of more than 2 years is required in malignant melanoma, breast carcinoma, colorectal carcinoma, and uterine carcinoma.

High-risk patients

Diabetic nephropathy

Patients with diabetic nephropathy form a special category of transplant recipients because, apart from the nephropathy, other complications almost invariably occur. The most important causes of death in patients with diabetic nephropathy and a renal transplant are myocardial infarction and congestive heart failure. Although the risk for atherosclerosis is greater in diabetics over the age of 45 years and in those with a history of smoking, neither clinical symptoms nor the cardiovascular risk profiles are sufficiently reliable to document or exclude the presence of coronary artery disease (Koch *et al.* 1997). Therefore, non-invasive screening tests (see below) should be carried out in all diabetic transplant candidates before transplantation. If abnormalities are found, a coronary angiography is indicated before a renal transplantation can be performed. In addition, special attention should be directed to urinary bladder emptying and the presence of foot ulcers.

Since patient survival and quality of life are substantially better after renal transplantation than with haemodialysis, diabetic patients should already be considered for transplantation when the creatinine clearance declines to less than 15–20 ml/min. The availability of a living donor graft may provide the opportunity to circumvent the need for dialysis. Early renal transplantation can prevent the progression of uraemic neuropathy, although the extrarenal complications of the diabetes mellitus are not halted. Peripheral vascular insufficiency, frequently necessitating limb amputations remains a common and frustrating problem after renal transplantation in diabetics.

Combined kidney–pancreas transplantation improves quality of life still further due to the freedom of insulin. Moreover, normoglycaemia prevents the development of diabetic glomerulosclerosis in the graft and there is stabilization, and in some cases improvement, of peripheral and autonomic diabetic neuropathy. The beneficial effects on the course of retinopathy and vascular disease are less clear. Recent data indicate that after simultaneous kidney–pancreas transplantation the annual mortality risk is reduced with more than 50 per cent as compared with renal transplantation alone (Becker *et al.* 2000; Smets *et al.* 2000). In patients who have the option to receive a kidney from a living donor, pancreas-after-kidney transplantation may be a preferable alternative. Since there is an excess risk of perioperative morbidity and mortality associated with combined kidney–pancreas transplantation, this procedure is usually offered only to young patients (<50 years) without overt cardiovascular disease.

Cardiovascular disease

Cardiovascular disease is the most important cause of death after renal transplantation. Major risk factors are: age more than 50 years, diabetes mellitus, history of angina pectoris, congestive heart failure, and an abnormal electrocardiogram (ECG). The cardiac mortality after renal transplantation in patients with one or more risk factors was found to be as high as 17 per cent at a mean follow-up of 2 years,

Table 3 Recurrence rates for different tumours

Recurrence rate	Type of tumour
Low (0–10%)	Incidentally discovered renal carcinoma Testicular tumours Uterine cervical carcinoma Thyroid carcinoma Lymphoma
Intermediate (11–25%)	Uterine body carcinoma Wilms' tumour Colorectal carcinoma Prostate carcinoma Breast carcinoma
High (≥26%)	Bladder carcinoma Sarcoma Malignant melanoma Symptomatic renal carcinoma Non-melanoma skin carcinoma Myeloma

From Penn (1993).

whereas it was 1 per cent in the low-risk group (Le *et al.* 1994). In the high-risk group, the cardiac prognosis is determined by the extent of coronary artery disease and by left ventricular function. We consider preoperative work-up by a cardiologist warranted in all patients older than 70 years or in the presence of other aforementioned risk factors. Resting echocardiography is a valuable tool to detect valvular diseases and to evaluate (residual) left ventricular function. Non-invasive methods to screen for the presence of coronary artery disease are hampered by the fact that uraemic patients (and especially those with diabetes) frequently have a poor exercise tolerance and can have aspecific basal ECG abnormalities. Combined dipyridamole and exercise thallium imaging as well as dobutamine stress echocardiography probably have the highest sensitivity and specificity in these circumstances (Dahan *et al.* 1998; Herzog *et al.* 1999). We advocate to repeat the screening for coronary artery disease every two years in high risk patients who are on the waiting list. Patients with a positive screening test should undergo coronary arteriography. If there is significant narrowing of the major coronary vessels, revascularization before transplantation is recommended. Several studies suggest that in dialysis patients bypass surgery leads to a better long-term outcome as compared to percutaneous transluminal coronary angioplasty (Szczech *et al.* 2001), although the results of the latter procedure may be improved by stenting and use of antiplatelet therapy. Nevertheless, in uraemic patients all kinds of revascularization procedures are associated with an increased mortality risk. Therefore, especially in older dialysis patients with subclinical coronary heart disease, one should always consider whether continued treatment by dialysis is not a better choice than transplantation preceded by coronary revascularization.

Routine examination of the iliac vessels is not necessary. If there is a history of claudication or when physical examination reveals signs of arterial insufficiency, non-invasive vascular studies can help to select patients in whom angiography is indicated. If an aortoiliac reconstruction is necessary, it should preferably be performed prior to transplantation as a scheduled procedure.

In patients with a history of transient ischemic attacks or cerebrovascular accident, carotid Doppler studies should be performed to screen for the presence of vascular disease.

Oxalosis (see also Chapter 16.5.2)

Patients with primary hyperoxaluria type I form another group with increased risks after transplantation. This disease is caused by a deficiency of the enzyme alanine glyoxalate aminotransferase and it leads to nephrolithiasis and nephrocalcinosis. ESRD usually occurs in these patients before the age of 20. As a consequence, oxalate excretion is completely interrupted and oxalate deposition throughout the body proceeds at an increased rate. This may account for the disappointing results of dialysis treatment in these patients, and emphasizes the need for early transplantation. After renal transplantation, there is an increased risk of graft destruction by massive deposition of oxalate, especially in patients with primary nonfunction. Strategies to reduce oxalate deposition in the kidney include aggressive preoperative dialysis, forced diuresis, and administration of pyridoxine, orthophosphates, and thiazide diuretics after transplantation. Since the enzyme defect can be reconstituted by liver transplantation, combined liver and renal transplantation has currently become the treatment of choice (Cochat 1999). It should be preferably carried out when the glomerular filtration rate drops below 25 ml/min. Isolated kidney transplantation,

preferably with a living donor kidney to avoid delayed graft function, can be considered in adults with a late-onset form of the disease.

Risk of recurrent disease after transplantation (see also Chapter 13.3.3)

Certain types of glomerulonephritis may recur following renal transplantation (see Chapter 13.3.3). In many of the diseases, such as systemic lupus and vasculitis, the likelihood of recurrence may be greater if the disease was fulminant and if the period on dialysis was short (<3 months). However, neither extrarenal manifestations nor markers of disease activity, such as titers of antineutrophil cytoplasmic antibody (ANCA) or antinuclear antibody, always correlate with disease recurrence. In contrast, the continued presence of circulating antibodies against the glomerular basement membrane (GBM) (detected by either enzyme immunoassay or indirect immunofluorescence) is generally considered a contraindication to renal transplantation because of the increased risk for disease recurrence. Focal–segmental glomerulosclerosis (FSGS) is also a disease with a high recurrence in transplants. In children with FSGS, a living donor allograft does not have a survival advantage compared to a cadaveric graft (Baum *et al.* 2001). One should therefore be more cautious to use a living donor kidney in patients with FSGS, particularly when a previous graft was lost to recurrent FSGS. Since a remission of recurrent FSGS can be induced with plasmapheresis, it has been proposed to start plasmapheresis prior to a planned transplantation to prevent recurrence (Ohta *et al.* 2000).

Special therapeutic or preparatory measures

Nephrectomy

The earlier practice of performing bilateral nephrectomy in patients before transplantation has been abandoned. The fears that, in patients with glomerulonephritis, the presence of the native kidneys would lead to recurrence of the original disease in the graft have proved to be completely unjustified. Nowadays, the patient's own kidneys are only removed on special indications. Large renal stones or gross abnormalities of the urinary tract, with persistent infection, are absolute indications for removal of one or both kidneys. If the ureters are abnormal, they should also be removed. Otherwise, they should be left intact, because they may be of use at later stages to construct a new anastomosis with the renal pelvis of the graft if urological complications involve the donor ureter. Recurrent asymptomatic urinary-tract infections are not an indication for nephrectomy.

Polycystic kidney disease by itself is not an indication for bilateral nephrectomy, since it does not affect the incidence of sepsis after renal transplantation (Sanfilippo *et al.* 1983). Only persistent infection or very large kidneys, which will hinder the placement of the graft, are an indication for nephrectomy. In the latter case, the removal of only one kidney will suffice.

In patients with endstage renal failure, fluid overload is the most common cause of hypertension. If, after the exclusion of this factor, the hypertension remains drug-resistant, bilateral nephrectomy is indicated. With the new, potent antihypertensive drugs this procedure is now very seldom necessary. Although the prevalence of post-transplant hypertension is clearly less in patients in whom the native kidneys have been removed, this is in itself no reason to subject them to pretransplant nephrectomy. The incidence of complications associated with this procedure in patients with endstage renal disease is relatively high. Moreover, most transplant patients respond well to antihypertensive treatment, and the blood pressure tends to show a spontaneous and gradual decrease in patients with stable graft function (Huysmans et al. 1987).

If bilateral nephrectomy cannot be avoided, it should preferably be performed in a separate session before transplantation.

In patients who undergo a second transplantation, removal of the first graft is only necessary when there are signs of active rejection or if placement of the subsequent graft is otherwise not possible.

Blood transfusion

Pretransplant blood transfusions can cause sensitization, with the formation of potentially destructive HLA antibodies. Broad sensitization against HLA antigens makes it difficult to find a suitable donor kidney (see below). On the other hand, it was shown in the past that pretransplant blood transfusions can also afford graft protection. Ample discussions have been devoted to this problem. Some have claimed that the graft-protecting effect can be induced by a single transfusion, which minimizes the risk of broad sensitization (Persijn et al. 1979). Others have maintained that graft survival rates improve further with increased numbers of transfusions (Opelz and Terasaki 1978). This controversy has never been solved. Subsequent evidence that a single blood transfusion is only protective if there is sharing of one HLA-DR antigen (or one HLA-B and one HLA-DR antigen) between donor and recipient has remained unconfirmed. However, there is general agreement that perioperative transfusions do not have a protective effect. The controversial reports on the effect of transfusion and the fact that the mechanism by which the transfusion has its effect has never been clarified have led many centers to abandon pretransplant transfusions. Moreover, with the introduction of recombinant erythropoietin (epoetin), the need for transfusions to treat the anaemia of chronic renal failure has vanished. With the current immunosuppressive possibilities, the 1-year graft survival is about 90 per cent in non-transfused patients, thus equivalent or even better than the results in transfused patients in previous studies. As transfusions still carry a small risk of alloimmunization and transmission of infectious diseases, there are no indications at present to systematically give pretransplant blood transfusions to all transplant candidates.

In living donor transplantation, excellent results have been reported in recipients who received three blood transfusions from their related kidney donors with one or two haplotype mismatches. Unfortunately, this procedure also induced the production of donor-specific cytotoxic T cell antibodies in about 20 per cent of the recipients, thus precluding transplantation of a kidney from that particular donor. Attempts to prevent the sensitization under an umbrella of immunosuppressive therapy have only been partly successful. As a consequence, this approach has not found wide acceptance in renal transplantation. Procedures such as infusion of stem cells or bone marrow cells seemed a promising procedure (De Pauw et al. 1998), but until now there are no new studies to support this strategy.

Highly sensitized patients

10–20 per cent of patients on waiting-lists for renal transplantation have developed broadly reactive cytotoxic antibodies against HLA. Sensitization against HLA may occur as a consequence of pregnancy, blood transfusion, graft rejection, or a combination of these factors. These highly immunized patients have antibodies against almost all HLA antigens and it is therefore very difficult to find a donor with a negative cross-match. Of course, transplantation of an HLA-identical kidney could circumvent the problem, but such kidneys are not easily found. Another attempt to solve this problem has been to screen for negative cross-matches by testing the sera of these patients against each available donor in a large donor pool (Opelz 1991). One can also screen the sera before transplantation against special donor panels to identify so-called acceptable mismatches, that is, foreign HLA antigens against which the recipient has no antibodies (Claas and van Rood 1988). Graft survival rates of patients transplanted within these programmes have been quite satisfactory.

A completely different approach is the active removal of the circulating antibodies by plasma exchange or by extracorporeal immunoadsorption, with prevention of resynthesis of antibodies by concomitant immunosuppression (Palmer et al. 1989). The basic idea of this procedure is that the broad reactivity against HLA in the serum of about 60 per cent of highly immunized patients is caused by cross-reactivity due to the high titres of the antibodies. When the titre is reduced by plasma exchange or immunoadsorption, the cross-reactivity disappears and the sera prove to be reactive against only one or two HLA specificities. It is then much easier to find a suitable donor with a negative cross-match. Since the first report, only a few studies have been published, all comprising a small number of patients and giving variable results (Reisaeter et al. 1995; Higgins et al. 1996). To establish if the procedure indeed removed antibodies against the HLA antigens of the kidney, donor cross-matches with sera before and after immunoadsorption have to be compared. In many instances the cross-matches with the pretreatment sera have not been done. This makes it difficult to interpret the results. More, carefully planned trials are required before this approach can be implemented into clinical practice.

A somewhat similar method has been recommended to enable the use of ABO-incompatible kidneys from living donors, when an ABO-compatible donor is not available (Alexandre et al. 1987). More recent results are described by Shishido et al. (2001). Before transplantation, natural anti-A or anti-B antibodies are removed in the recipient by plasma exchange. Splenectomy done before or at the time of transplantation is necessary to prevent hyperacute, antibody-mediated rejection. This is a serious disadvantage since splenectomy carries a considerable risk in these patients, as will be discussed in a separate section. Therefore, the procedure should be reserved for patients for whom there is no satisfactory alternative. An exemption can possibly be made for the transplantation of kidneys of blood group A_2 into non-A recipients. A graft from a donor carrying this antigen does not appear to be very immunogenic, probably because the A_2 antigen is only weakly expressed on the endothelial cells of the donor. Successful transplants have been reported in patients in whom preparative measures, such as plasma exchange and splenectomy, had not been taken. A high titre in the recipient serum of IgG antibodies against A red blood cells before transplantation seems to predict low graft survival. Therefore, transplantation of A_2 kidneys into O or B recipients is only recommended if the pretransplant anti-A antibody titre is less than 1 : 8 (Nelson *et al.* 1992).

Other surgical procedures

Splenectomy

Pretransplant removal of the spleen has been proposed as a means of decreasing the immune responsiveness of the host. Indeed, early results showed that graft survival rates 2 years after transplantation were significantly better in splenectomized recipients. However, in a follow-up study, this difference appeared to have gradually disappeared during the subsequent years, and there were more late deaths from sepsis in the splenectomized group (Sutherland *et al.* 1984). It is now generally agreed that there is no place for routine splenectomy before renal transplantation.

Parathyroidectomy

Severe secondary hyperparathyroidism can most often be prevented in patients with chronic renal failure by treatment with phosphate-binding agents and active vitamin D_3. If there is uncontrolled hyperparathyroidism, one should consider subtotal or total parathyroidectomy. Effective medical treatment of hyperparathyroidism to avoid surgery before transplantation is of great importance because the need for parathyroidectomy decreases markedly after successful transplantation (Malberti *et al.* 2001).

Pretransplant vascular surgery and urological operations have already been dealt with in previous sections.

Immediate preoperative preparation

Cross-match

Analogous to the common practice in blood transfusion, a cross-match of the lymphocytes of the donor with the recipient's serum is performed before transplantation to avoid hyperacute rejection. A cross-match is not necessary for patients who never had any PRA in previous screenings, because in these cases the cross-match will always be negative (Matas and Sutherland 1998). With this policy, it is possible to reduce cold ischemia time with at least 6 h. In sensitized patients, more sensitive cross-matches using separated T and B cells are necessary. Both, a recent serum and the historical sera, in which PRA have been demonstrated earlier, should be included in the test. The class I (HLA-A and HLA-B) antibodies of the IgG class are almost always detrimental. Most IgM antibodies against lymphocytes are probably harmless. If they do not show a definite HLA specificity, their presence can be disregarded. In many patients, they are broadly reactive and react also with the recipient's own lymphocytes (autoantibodies). Since they can cause false-positive cross-matches they should be removed from the serum by adding dithiothreitol (DTT). A positive DTT cross-match with donor T cells in one or more of the sera is generally considered to be an absolute contraindication for transplantation. Tests with isolated B cells are necessary to identify antibodies against HLA-DR with sufficient sensitivity. Antibodies against HLA-DR, nonspecific antibodies, or autoantibodies can cause a positive B cell cross-match, in the presence of a negative T cell cross-match. Only HLA-DR antibodies of the IgG class are potentially destructive. By performing all tests also in the presence of DTT, most false-positive cross-matches can be eliminated.

Antibiotics

In most transplant centers, antibiotic prophylaxis is given before transplantation, although controlled trials demonstrating the effectiveness of this strategy are lacking. The most frequently used regimen is a single dose of a third-generation cephalosporin (sometimes together with an aminopenicillin).

Tuberculosis reactivates more frequently in patients under immunosuppression, particularly when the tuberculin test is positive and there is radiologic evidence of inactive tuberculosis. Tuberculosis prophylaxis is indicated in patients at risk, but the difficulty lies in the identification of such patients. A negative tuberculin test, for instance, is unreliable because in patients with chronic renal failure the test can be a false negative as a consequence of a decreased cellular immune responsiveness. Moreover, the prophylactic treatment with isoniazid (drug of choice) is potentially hepatotoxic, especially if used together with azathioprine. It may also interfere with immunosuppressive drugs that are metabolized by the cytochrome P450 system (Wen *et al.* 2002). Patients who have received adequate treatment in the past do not need prophylactic treatment. If this is not the case and radiologic evidence of an inactive tuberculosis infection exists, prophylactic treatment with isoniazid (300 mg daily) during the first 9 months after transplantation is recommended. If possible, this treatment course should be given during the dialysis period because this will avoid the undesirable interference with immunosuppressive drugs after transplantation.

Anticoagulation

There are no studies demonstrating convincingly that anticoagulation during or after the transplantation procedure will decrease the incidence of thrombotic complications. The risk associated with anticoagulation therapy after the renal transplant operation is, of course, increased blood loss, particularly because of the already existing uremic bleeding tendency. Despite this, it is now common to treat renal transplant recipients with low-molecular-weight heparin after operation (Alkhunaizi 1998). More intensive anticoagulation is probably advisable in patients with a history of thrombosis or an increased risk for thrombosis, recipients of young age, or if a donor kidney of a child aged less than 2 years is used.

Dialysis

Dialysis immediately preceding transplantation should only be carried out if hyperkalaemia or an unacceptable fluid overload occurs. In all other situations, dialysis should be avoided because of an increased risk of bleeding complications after transplantation. If pretransplant dialysis must be performed, it is important to keep the patient well hydrated, since this improves the chances of immediate graft function.

Patients on peritoneal dialysis should continue dialysis until the time of the transplantation. The peritoneal cavity should be drained immediately before surgery. In case of a transplantation with a living donor kidney, the chance of postoperative need for dialysis is small enough to justify removal of the catheter during the transplantation operation.

Immunosuppression

Immunosuppressive therapy should generally be started before the kidney is implanted. Corticosteroids and anti-T cell antibodies can be given by intravenous injection before or during surgery. The strategies for cyclosporine and tacrolimus treatment differ between centres. Some administer a first dose before transplantation to ensure therapeutic blood values as early as possible, while at other centres the start of treatment is delayed until after transplantation to circumvent the acute nephrotoxic effects of these drugs during the early period when the graft is recovering from the ischaemic insult. Mycophenolate mofetil and azathioprine are usually started postoperatively.

Measures to reduce acute renal failure

Hydration protocol

Acute renal failure due to acute tubular necrosis is a major postoperative complication after cadaveric kidney transplantation. The age and haemodynamic condition of the donor before nephrectomy and the length of the cold ischaemia time of the donor kidney are the main determinants in the development of acute tubular necrosis after surgery. However, the haemodynamic condition of the recipient during the transplantation procedure is important as well. Several studies showed that optimal hydration of the recipient could substantially reduce the incidence of acute renal failure after transplantation. Since this approach requires invasive haemodynamic monitoring and prolonged mechanical ventilation, simpler hydration protocols have been sought. One effective option is to infuse 250 ml mannitol 20 per cent during the last 10 min before revascularization, combined with a moderate hydration protocol (van Valenberg *et al.* 1987).

Renal vasodilatory agents

Treatment of the recipient with several renal vasodilatory agents has been attempted with variable outcome. Atrial natriuretic factor or dopamine appear to be ineffective. Calcium-channel blockers reduced the rate of delayed graft function in open studies, but not in the few placebo-controlled trials (Ladefoged and Andersen 1994).

References

Alexandre, G. P. J. *et al.* (1987). Present experiences in a series of 26 ABO-incompatible living donor renal allografts. *Transplantation Proceedings* **19**, 4538–4542.

Alkhunaizi, A. M. *et al.* (1998). Efficacy and safety of low molecular weight heparin in renal transplantation. *Transplantation* **66**, 533–534.

Arndorfer, J. A. *et al.* (2001). Time to first graft loss as a risk factor for second renal allograft loss. *Transplantation Proceedings* **33**, 1188–1189.

Baum, M. A. *et al.* (2001). Loss of living donor renal allograft survival advantage in children with focal segmental glomerulosclerosis. *Kidney International* **59**, 328–333.

Bay, W. H. and Hebert, L. A. (1987). The living donor in kidney transplantation. *Annals of Internal Medicine* **106**, 719–727.

Becker, B. N. *et al.* (2000). Simultaneous pancreas–kidney transplantation reduces excess mortality in type 1 diabetic patients with end-stage renal disease. *Kidney International* **57**, 2129–2135.

Cecka, J. M. (2000). The UNOS Scientific Renal Transplant Registry—2000. *Clinical Transplantation* 1–18.

Claas, F. H. J. and van Rood, J. J. (1988). The hyperimmunized patient: from sensitization to transplantation. *Transplant International* **1**, 53–57.

Cochat, P. (1999). Primary hyperoxaluria type 1. *Kidney International* **55**, 2533–2547.

Dahan, M. *et al.* (1998). Diagnostic accuracy and prognostic value of combined dipyridamole–exercise thallium imaging in hemodialysis patients. *Kidney International* **54**, 255–262.

De Pauw, L. *et al.* (1998). Isolation and infusion of donor CD34+ bone marrow cells in cadaver kidney transplantation. *Nephrology, Dialysis, Transplantation* **13**, 34–36.

European Best Practice Guidelines for Renal Transplantation (Part 1) (2000). *Nephrology, Dialysis, Transplantation* **15** (Suppl. 7), 1–85.

Fritsche, L. *et al.* (2000). Practice variations in the evaluation of adult candidates for cadaveric kidney transplantation: a survey of the European transplant centers. *Transplantation* **70**, 1492–1497.

Glazier, D. B. *et al.* (1996). Evaluation of voiding cystourethrography prior to renal transplantation. *Transplantation* **62**, 1762–1765.

Gonczol, E. and Plotkin, S. (2001). Development of a cytomegalovirus vaccine: lessons from recent clinical trials. *Expert Opinion on Biological Therapy* **1**, 401–412.

Herzog, C. A. *et al.* (1999). Dobutamine stress echocardiography for the detection of significant coronary artery disease in renal transplant candidates. *American Journal of Kidney Diseases* **33**, 1080–1090.

Hiesse, C. *et al.* (1992). Impact of HBs antigenemia on long-term patient survival and causes of death after transplantation. *Clinical Transplantation* **46**, 461–467.

Higgins, R. M. *et al.* (1996). Prevention of hyperacute rejection by removal of antibodies to HLA immediately before renal transplantation. *Lancet* **348**, 1208–1211.

Huysmans, F. T. M., Hoitsma, A. J., and Koene, R. A. P. (1987). Factors determining the prevalence of hypertension after renal transplantation. *Nephrology, Dialysis, Transplantation* **2**, 34–38.

Johnson, E. *et al.* (1997). Complications and risks of living donor nephrectomy. *Transplantation* **64**, 1124–1128.

Koch, M. *et al.* (1997). Relevance of conventional cardiovascular risk factors for the prediction of coronary artery disease in diabetic patients on renal replacement therapy. *Nephrology, Dialysis, Transplantation* **12**, 1187–1191.

Ladefoged, S. D. and Andersen, S. B. (1994). Calcium channel blockers in kidney transplantation. *Clinical Transplantation* **8**, 128–133.

Lang, P. *et al.* (1991). Update and outcome of renal transplant patients with human immunodeficiency virus. *Transplantation Proceedings* **23**, 1352–1353.

Le, A. *et al.* (1994). Prospective risk stratification in renal transplant candidates for cardiac death. *American Journal of Kidney Diseases* **24**, 65–71.

Malberti, F. *et al.* (2001). Parathyroidectomy in patients on renal replacement therapy: an epidemiologic study. *Journal of the American Society of Nephrology* **12**, 1242–1248.

Mange, K. C., Joffe, M. M., and Feldman, H. I. (2001). Effect of the use or nonuse of long-term dialysis on the subsequent survival of renal transplants from living donors. *New England Journal of Medicine* **344**, 726–731.

Matas, A. J. and Sutherland, D. E. (1998). Kidney transplantation without a final crossmatch. *Transplantation* **66**, 1835–1836.

Meier-Kriesche, H. U., Arndorfer, J. A., and Kaplan, B. (2002). The impact of body mass index on renal transplant outcomes: a significant independent risk factor for graft failure and patient death. *Transplantation* **73**, 70–74.

Merlin, T. L. *et al.* (2000). The safety and efficacy of laparoscopic live donor nephrectomy: a systematic review. *Transplantation* **70**, 1659–1666.

Morales, J. M. and Campistol, J. M. (2000). Transplantation in the patient with hepatitis C. *Journal of the American Society of Nephrology* **11**, 1343–1353.

Narkun-Burgess, D. M. *et al.* (1993). Forty-five year follow-up after uninephrectomy. *Kidney International* **43**, 1110–1115.

Nelson, P. W. *et al.* (1992). Current experience with renal transplantation across the ABO barrier. *American Journal of Surgery* **164**, 541–545.

Ohta, T. *et al.* (2001). Effect of pre- and postoperative plasmapheresis on post-transplant recurrence of focal segmental glomerulosclerosis in children. *Transplantation* **71**, 628–633.

Opelz, G. and Terasaki, P. I. (1978). Improvement of kidney-graft survival with increased numbers of blood transfusions. *New England Journal of Medicine* **299**, 799–803.

Opelz, G. (1991). Collaborative transplant study kidney exchange trial for highly sensitized recipients. *Clinical Transplantation* **5**, 61–64.

Palmer, A. *et al.* (1989). Removal of anti-HLA antibodies by extracorporeal immunoadsorption to enable renal transplantation. *Lancet* **i**, 10–12.

Penn, I. (1993). The effect of immunosuppression on pre-existing cancers. *Transplantation* **55**, 742–747.

Pereira, B. J. *et al.* (1998). Effect of hepatitis C infection and renal transplantation on survival in end-stage renal disease. *Kidney International* **53**, 1374–1381.

Persijn, G. G. *et al.* (1979). Retrospective and prospective studies on the effect of blood transfusions in renal transplantation in the Netherlands. *Transplantation* **28**, 396–401.

Ramos, E. L. *et al.* (1994). The evaluation of candidates for renal transplantation. The current practice of U.S. transplant centers. *Transplantation* **57**, 490–497.

Reisaeter, A. V. *et al.* (1995). Pretransplant plasma exchange or immunoadsorption facilitates renal transplantation in immunized patients. *Transplantation* **60**, 242–248.

Sanfilippo, F. P. *et al.* (1983). Transplantation for polycystic disease. *Transplantation* **36**, 54–59.

Sarwal, M. M. *et al.* (2000). Adult-size kidneys without acute tubular necrosis provide exceedingly superior long-term graft outcomes for infants and small children: a single center and UNOS analysis. United Network for Organ Sharing. *Transplantation* **70**, 1728–1736.

Shaffer, D. *et al.* (1998). Two hundred one consecutive living-donor nephrectomies. *Archives of Surgery* **133**, 426–431.

Shishido, S. *et al.* (2001). ABO-incompatible living-donor kidney transplantation in children. *Transplantation* **72**, 1037–1042.

Singh, A., Stablein, D., and Tejani, A. (1997). Risk factors for vascular thrombosis in pediatric renal transplantation: a special report of the North American Pediatric Renal Transplant Cooperative Study. *Transplantation* **63**, 1263–1267.

Smets, Y. F. *et al.* (2000). Insulin secretion and sensitivity after simultaneous pancreas-kidney transplantation estimated by continuous infusion of glucose with model assessment. *Transplantation* **69**, 1322–1327.

Sutherland, D. E. R. *et al.* (1984). Long-term effect of splenectomy versus no splenectomy in renal transplant patients. *Transplantation* **38**, 619–624.

Szczech, L. A. *et al.* (2001). Differential survival after coronary revascularization procedures among patients with renal insufficiency. *Kidney International* **60**, 292–299.

Terasaki, P. I. *et al.* (1995). High survival rates of kidney transplants from spousal and living unrelated donors. *New England Journal of Medicine* **333**, 333–336.

Tesi, R. J. *et al.* (1994). Renal transplantation in older people. *Lancet* **343**, 461–464.

van Valenberg, P. L. J. *et al.* (1987). Mannitol as an indispensable constituent of an intraoperative protocol for the prevention of acute renal failure after renal cadaveric transplantation. *Transplantation* **44**, 784–788.

Warholm, C. *et al.* (1999). Renal transplantation in patients with urinary diversion: a case-control study. *Nephrology, Dialysis, Transplantation* **14**, 2937–2940.

Wen, X. *et al.* (2002). Isoniazid is a mechanism-based inhibitor of cytochrome P450 1A2, 2A6, 2C19 and 3A4 isoforms in human liver microsomes. *European Journal of Clinical Pharmacology* **57**, 799–804.

Westlie, L. *et al.* (1993). Quality of life in Norwegian kidney donors. *Nephrology, Dialysis, Transplantation* **8**, 1146–1150.

Wolfe, R.A. *et al.* (1999) Comparison of mortality in all patients on dialysis, patients on dialysis awaiting transplantation, and recipients of a first cadaveric transplant. *New England Journal of Medicine* **341**, 1725–1730.

13.2 Transplant immunology

13.2.1 The immunology of transplantation

Manikkam Suthanthiran and Terry B. Strom

Allograft rejection is a complex process and multiple cell types contribute to and participate in the rejection of histoincompatible allografts (Suthanthiran and Strom 1994). Cell to cell interactions proceed via physical contacts between alloreactive T cells and antigen-presenting cells (APCs) and a variety of soluble factors, cytokines, and chemokines, are important components of the anti-allograft repertoire. A vibrant assortment of cells including CD4+ T cells, CD8+ cytotoxic T cells, antibody-forming B cells, and other proinflammatory leucocytes participate in the antiallograft response (Fig. 1 and Table 1).

Transmembrane signalling of T cells: the immune synapse

The immunological synapse comprises multiple T cell surface proteins that form clusters thereby creating a platform for antigen recognition and generation of various crucial T cell activation related signals (Dustin and Cooper 2000). The synapse begins to form when the initial adhesions between certain T cell (e.g. CD2, LFA-1) and APC cell-surface proteins (e.g. CD58, ICAM-1) are formed (Table 2). These adhesions create intimate contact between T-cells and APCs and thereby provide an opportunity for T cells to recognize antigen. Antigen-driven T-cell activation, a tightly regulated, preprogrammed process, begins when T cells recognize intracellularly processed fragments of foreign proteins (approximately 8–16 amino acids) embedded within the groove of the major histocompatibility complex (MHC) proteins expressed on the surface of APCs (Unanue and Cerottini 1989; Germain 1994; Acuto and Cantrell 2000). Some recipient T cells directly recognize the allograft, that is, donor antigen(s) presented on the surface of donor APCs, while other T cells recognize the donor antigen after it is processed and presented by self APCs (Shoskes and Wood 1994) (Fig. 1).

The T-cell antigen receptor (TCR)/CD3 complex is composed of clonally distinct TCR-α and -β peptide chains that recognize the antigenic peptide in the context of MHC proteins and clonally invariant CD3 chains that propagate intracellular signals originating from antigenic recognition (Suthanthiran 1990; Jorgensen et al. 1992; Dustin and Cooper 2000) (Fig. 2). The TCR variable, diversity, junctional, and constant region genes, that is, genes for regions of the clone-specific antigen receptors, are spliced together in a cassette-like fashion during T-cell maturation (Jorgensen et al. 1992). A small population of T cells express TCR-γ and δ chains instead of the TCR-α and β chains.

CD4 and CD8 proteins, expressed on reciprocal T-cell subsets, bind to non-polymorphic domains of human leucocyte antigen (HLA) class II (DR, DP, DQ) and class I (A, B, C) molecules, respectively (Jorgenson et al. 1992; Dustin and Cooper 2000) (Fig. 1 and Table 2). A threshold of TCR to MHC–peptide engagements is necessary to stabilize the immunological synapse stimulating a redistribution of cell surface proteins and co-clustering of the TCR/CD3 complex with the T-cell surface proteins (Brown et al. 1989; Suthanthiran 1990; Beyers et al. 1992). CD5 proteins (Brown et al. 1989; Beyers et al. 1992) join the synapse. The TCR cluster already includes integrins (e.g. LFA-1) and non-integrins for example, CD2 (Brown et al. 1989; Suthanthiran 1990; Dustin and Cooper 2000) that have created T-cell–APCs adhesions. Hence, antigen recognition stimulates a redistribution of cell-surface proteins and co-clustering of the TCR/CD3 complex with the T-cell surface proteins (Brown et al. 1989; Suthanthiran 1990; Jorgensen et al. 1992; Dustin and Copper 2000) and signalling molecules. This multimeric complex functions as a unit in initiating T-cell activation.

Following activation by antigen, the TCR/CD3 complex and co-clustered CD4 and CD8 proteins are physically associated with intracellular protein–tyrosine kinases (PTKs) of two different families, the src (including p59^{fyn} and p56^{lck}) and ZAP 70 families (Dustin and Copper 2000). The CD45 protein, a tyrosine phosphatase, contributes to the activation process by dephosphorylating an autoinhibitory site on the p56^{lck} PTK. Intracellular domains of several TCR/CD3 proteins contain activation motifs that are crucial for antigen-stimulated signalling. Certain tyrosine residues within these motifs serve as targets for the catalytic activity of src family PTKs. Subsequently, these phosphorylated tyrosines serve as docking stations for the SH2 domains (recognition structures for select phosphotyrosine-containing motifs) of the ZAP-70 PTK. Following antigenic engagement of the TCR/CD3 complex, select serine residues of the TCR and CD3 chains are also phosphorylated (Acuto and Cantrell 2000; Dustin and Cooper 2000).

The wave of tyrosine phosphorylation triggered by antigen recognition encompasses other intracellular proteins and is a critical event in initiating T-cell activation. Tyrosine phosphorylation of the phospholipase Cg$_1$ activates this coenzyme and triggers a cascade of events that lead to full expression of T-cell programmes: hydrolysis of phosphatidylinositol 4,5-biphosphate (PIP$_2$) and generation of two intracellular messengers, inositol 1,4,5-triphosphate (IP$_3$) and diacylglycerol (Nishizuka 1992); IP$_3$, in turn, mobilizes ionized calcium from

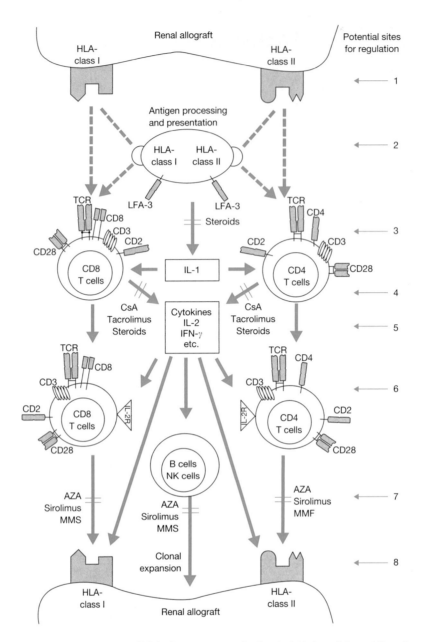

Fig. 1 The antiallograft response. Schematic representation of HLA, the primary stimulus for the initiation of the antiallograft response; cell surface proteins participating in antigenic recognition and signal transduction; contribution of the cytokines and multiple cell types to the immune response; and the potential sites for the regulation of the antiallograft response. Site 1: minimizing histoincompatibility between the recipients and the donor (e.g. HLA matching). Site 2: prevention of monokine production by APCs (e.g. corticosteroids). Site 3: blockade of antigen recognition (e.g. OKT3 mAbs). Site 4: inhibition of T-cell cytokine production [e.g. cyclosporin (CsA)]. Site 5: inhibition of cytokine activity [e.g. anti-interleukin-2 (IL-2) antibody]. Site 6: inhibition of cell cycle progression (e.g. anti-IL-2 receptor antibody). Site 7: inhibition of clonal expansion [e.g. azathioprine (AZA)]. Site 8: prevention of allograft damage by masking target antigen molecules (e.g. antibodies directed at adhesion molecules). HLA class I: HLA-A, B, and C antigens; HLA class II: HLA-DR, DP, and DQ antigens. IFN-γ, interferon-gamma; NK cells, natural killer cells; MMF, mycopenolate mofetil; AZA, azathioprine.

intracellular stores, while diacylglycerol, in the presence of increased cytosolic free Ca^{2+}, binds to and translocates protein kinase C (PKC)— a phospholipid/Ca^{2+}-sensitive protein serine/threonine kinase—to the membrane in its enzymatically active form (Nishizuka 1992; Acuto and Cantrell 2000). Sustained activation of PKC is dependent on diacylglycerol generation from hydrolysis of additional lipids such as phosphatidylcholine.

The increase in intracellular free Ca^{2+} and sustained PKC activation promote the expression of several nuclear regulatory proteins [e.g. nuclear factor of activated T cells (NF-AT), nuclear factor kappa B (NF-κB), activator protein 1 (AP-1)] and the transcriptional activation, and expression of genes central to T-cell growth [e.g. interleukin-2 (IL-2) and receptors for IL-2 and IL-15] (Waldman *et al.* 1998; Actuo and Cantrell 2000; Dustin and Cooper 2000). Calcineurin, a Ca^{2+}- and calmodulin-dependent serine/threonine phosphatase, is crucial to Ca^{2+}-dependent, TCR-initiated signal transduction (Clipstone and Crabtree 1992; O'keefe *et al.* 1992). Inhibition by cyclosporin and tacrolimus (FK-506) of the phosphatase activity of calcineurin

Table 1 Cellular elements contributing to the antiallograft response

Cell type	Functional attributes
T cells	The CD4+ T cells and the CD8+ T cells participate in the antiallograft response. CD4+ T cells recognize antigens presented by HLA-class II proteins, and CD8+ T cells recognize antigens presented by HLA-class I proteins. The CD3/TCR complex is responsible for recognition of antigen and generates and transduces the antigenic signal
CD4+ T cells	CD4+ T cells function mostly as helper T cells and secrete cytokines such as IL-2, a T-cell growth/death factor, and IFN-γ, a proinflammatory polypeptide that can up-regulate the expression of HLA-proteins as well as augment cytotoxic activity of T cells and NK cells. Recently, two main types of CD4+ T cells have been recognized: CD4+ TH1 and CD4+ TH2. IL-2 and IFN-γ are produced by CD4+ TH1 type cells, and IL-4 and IL-5 are secreted by CD4+ TH2 type cells. Each cell type regulates the secretion of the other, and the regulated secretion is important in the expression of host immunity
CD8+ T cells	CD8+ T cells function mainly as cytotoxic T cells. A subset of CD8+ T cells expresses suppressor cell function. CD8+ T cells can secrete cytokines such as IL-2, IFN-γ, and can express molecules such as perforin, granzymes that function as effectors of cytotoxicity
APC	Monocytes/macrophages and dendritic cells function as potent APCs. Donor's APCs can process and present donor antigens to recipient's T cells (direct recognition) or recipient's APCs can process and present donor antigens to recipient's T cells (indirect recognition). The relative contribution of direct recognition and indirect recognition to the antiallograft response has not been resolved. Direct recognition and indirect recognition might also have differential susceptibility to inhibition by immunosuppressive drugs
B cells	B cells require T cell help for the differentiation and production of antibodies directed at donor antigens. The alloantibodies can damage the graft by binding and activating complement components (complement dependent cytotoxicity) and/or by binding the Fc receptor of cells capable of mediating cytotoxicity (antibody dependent cell mediated cytotoxicity)
NK cells	The precise role of NK cells in the antiallograft response is not known. Increased NK cell activity has been correlated with rejection. NK cell function might also be important in immune surveillance mechanisms pertinent to the prevention of infection and malignancy

Reproduced from Suthanthiran, M., Morris, R. E., and Strom, T. B. Transplantation immunobiology, Chapter 13. In *Campbell's Urology* 7th edn. (ed. P. C. Walsh, A. B. Retik, E. D. Vaughan Jr., and A. J. Wein), pp. 491–504. Philadelphia, PA: W.B. Saunders Co., 1997.

Table 2 Cell-surface proteins important for T-cell activation

T cell surface	APC surface	Functional response	Consequence of blockade
LFA-1 (CD11a, CD18) ICAM1 (CD54)	ICAM1 (CD54) LFA-1 (CD11a, CD18)	Adhesion	Immunosuppression
CD8, TCR, CD3 CD4, TCR, CD3	MHCI MHCII	Antigen recognition	Immunosuppression
CD2 CD40L (CD154) CD5	LFA3 (CD58) CD40 CD72	Co-stimulation	Immunosuppression
CD28 CD28	B7-1 (CD80) B7-2 (CD86)	Co-stimulation	Anergy
CTLA4 (CD152) CTLA4 (CD152)	B7-1 (CD80) B7-2 (CD86)	Inhibition	Immunostimulation

Receptor counter-receptor pairs that mediate interactions between T cells and APCs are shown in this table. Inhibition of each protein-to-protein interaction, except the CTLA4–B7.1/B7.2 interaction, results in an abortive *in vitro* immune response. Initial contact between T cells and APCs requires an antigen-independent adhesive interaction. Next, the T cell antigen receptor complex engages processed antigen presented within the antigen-presenting groove of MHC molecules. Finally, co-stimulatory signals are required for full T-cell activation. An especially important signal is generated by B7-mediated activation of CD28 on T cells. Activation of CD28 by B7.2 may provide a more potent signal than activation by B7.1. CTLA4, present on activated but not resting T cells, imparts a negative signal.

Reproduced from Suthanthiran, M., Morris, R. E., and Strom, T. B. Transplantation immunobiology, Chapter 13. In *Campbell's Urology* 7th edn. (ed. P. C. Walsh, A. B. Retik, E. D. Vaughan, Jr., and A. J. Wein), pp. 491–504. Philadelphia, PA: W.B. Saunders Co., 1997.

is considered central to their immunosuppressive activity (Liu *et al.* 1991).

Signalling of T cells via the TCR/CD3 complex (antigenic signal) is necessary, but insufficient, in itself to induce maximal T-cell proliferation; plenary activation is dependent on both the antigenic signals and the co-stimulatory signals engendered by the contactual interactions between cell surface proteins expressed on antigen-specific T cells and the APCs (Schwarz 1993; Suthanthiran 1993) (Fig. 2 and Table 2). Interaction of the CD2 protein on the T-cell surface with the CD58 [leucocyte function-associated antigen 3 (LFA-3)] protein on the APCs, of the CD11a/CD18 (LFA-1) proteins with the CD54 [intercellular adhesion molecule 1 (ICAM-1)] (Dustin and Springer 1989)

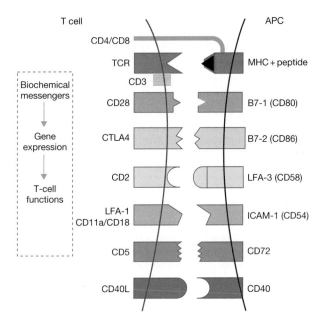

Fig. 2 *T-cell/antigen-presenting cell contact sites.* In this schema of T-cell activation, the antigenic signal is initiated by the physical interaction between the clonally variant TCR, heterodimer and the antigenic peptide displayed by MHC on APCs. The antigenic signal is transduced into the cell by the CD3 proteins. The CD4 and the CD8 antigens function as associative recognition structures, and restrict TCR recognition to class II and class I antigens of MHC, respectively. Additional T-cell surface receptors generate the obligatory co-stimulatory signals by interacting with their counter receptors expressed on the surface of the APCs. The simultaneous delivery to the T cells of the antigenic signal and the co-stimulatory signal results in the optimum generation of second messengers (such as calcium) expression of transcription factors (such as nuclear factor of activated T cells) and T-cell growth promoting genes (such as IL-2). The CD28 antigen as well as the CTLA4 antigen can interact with both the B7-1 and B7-2 antigens. The CD28 antigen generates a stimulatory signal, and the recent studies of CTLA4-deficient mice suggest that CTLA4, unlike CD28, generates a negative signal. CD, cluster designation; MHC, major histocompatibility complex; LFA-1, leucocyte function associated antigen-1; ICAM-1, intercellular adhesion molecule-1. (Reproduced from Suthanthiran, M. (1996). Transplantation tolerance: fooling mother nature. *Proceedings of the National Academy of Sciences USA* **93**, 12072–12075.) Copyright (1996), National Academy of Sciences, USA (Suthanthiran 1996).

proteins, and/or the CD5 with the CD72 proteins (Beyers *et al.* 1992) contribute to the generation of the obligatory co-stimulatory signal.

Recognition of the B7-1 (CD80) and B7-2 (CD86) proteins expressed upon CD4+ T cells generates a very powerful T-cell co-stimulus (Lenschow *et al.* 1996). Monocytes and dendritic cells constitutively express CD86. Cytokines, for example, granulocyte-macrophage colony stimulating factor (GM-CSF) or interferon-γ (IFN-γ), stimulate expression of CD80 on monocytes, B cells, and dendritic cells (Lenschow *et al.* 1996). Many T cells express B7 binding proteins, that is, CD28 proteins that are constitutively expressed on the surface of CD4+ T cells and CTLA-4 (CD152), a protein whose ectodomain is closely related to that of CD28, is expressed following activation of CD4+ and CD8+ T cells. CD28 binding of B7 molecules stimulates a Ca^{2+}-independent activation pathway that leads to stable transcription of the IL-2, IL-2 receptors, and other activation genes resulting in vigorous T-cell proliferation (Lenschow *et al.* 1996). CD28 is an important co-stimulatory receptors but other T-cell surface proteins

function as co-stimulatory receptors since robust T-cell activation occurs in CD28-deficient mice (Shahinian *et al.* 1993). For example, the interaction between CD40 expressed upon APCs and the CD40 ligand (CD154) expressed on T cells (Noelle 1996) results in the generation of a powerful co-stimulatory signal. The delivery of the antigenic signal and the co-stimulatory signal leads to stable transcription of the IL-2, several T-cell growth factor receptors, and other pivotal T-cell activation genes (Table 2). The Ca^{2+}-independent co-stimulatory CD28 pathway has a greater resistance to inhibition by cyclosporin or FK-506 as compared to the calcium-dependent pathway of T-cell activation. In contrast to positive co-stimulation resulting from CD28/B7 proteins, recognition of B7 proteins by CTLA-4, a protein primarily expressed on activated T-cells, generates a negative signal to T-cells. The CTLA-4 derived signal is important for the induction of peripheral T-cell tolerance (Ooesterwegel *et al.* 1999).

The formulation that full T-cell activation is dependent on the co-stimulatory signal as well as the antigenic signal is significant, as the T-cell molecules responsible for co-stimulation and their cognate receptors on the surface of APC then represent target molecules for the regulation of the antiallograft response. Indeed, transplantation tolerance has been induced in experimental models by targeting cell-surface molecules that contribute to the generation of co-stimulatory signals.

Interleukin-2/interleukin-15 stimulated T-cell proliferation

Autocrine and paracrine type of T-cell proliferation occurs as a consequence of the T-cell activation-dependent production of IL-2 and the T-cell expression of multimeric high affinity IL-2 receptors formed by the non-covalent association of three IL-2 binding α, β, and γ chains (Smith 1988; Waldman 1991; Takeshita *et al.* 1992; Waldmann *et al.* 1998). IL-15 is a paracrine-type T-cell growth factor family member with very similar overall structural and identical T-cell stimulatory qualities to IL-2 (Waldman *et al.* 1998). The IL-2 and IL-15 receptor complexes share β and γ chains that are expressed in low abundance upon resting T-cells; expression of these genes is amplified in activated T-cells. The α chain receptor components of the IL-2 and IL-15 receptor complexes are distinct and expressed upon activated, but not resting, T-cells. The intracytoplasmic domains of the IL-2 receptor β and γ chains are required for intracellular signal transduction. The ligand-activated, but not resting, IL-2/IL-15 receptors are associated with intracellular PTKs (Fung *et al.* 1991; Hatakeyama *et al.* 1991; Remillard *et al.* 1991; Waldman *et al.* 1998). Raf-1, a protein serine/threonine kinase that is a prerequisite for IL-2/IL-15 triggered cell proliferation, associates with the intracellular domain of the shared β chain (Maslinski *et al.* 1992). Translocation of IL-2 receptor bound Raf-1 serine/threonine kinase into the cytosol requires IL-2/IL-15-stimulated PTK activity. The ligand activated common γ chain recruits a member of the Janus kinase family, Jak 3, to the receptor complex that leads to activation of a member of the STAT family. Activation of this particular Jak-STAT pathway is a prerequisite for proliferation of antigen-activated T cells. The subsequent events leading to IL-2/IL-15 dependent proliferation are not fully resolved; however, IL-2/IL-15 stimulated expression of several DNA binding proteins including bcl-2, c-jun, c-fos, and c-myc contributes to cell cycle progression (Shibuya *et al.* 1992; Taniguchi 1995). It is interesting and probably significant that IL-2, but not IL-15, triggers apoptosis of many antigen-activated

T cells. In this way, IL-15 triggered events are more detrimental to the allograft response than IL-2. As IL-15 is not produced by T cells, IL-15 expression is not regulated by cyclosporin or FK-506.

Immunobiology of rejection

The net consequence of cytokine production and acquisition of cell-surface receptors for these transcellular molecules is the emergence of antigen specific and graft destructive T cells (Fig. 1). Cytokines also facilitate the humoral arm of immunity by promoting the production of cytopathic antibodies. Moreover, IFN-γ and tumour necrosis factor-α (TNF-α) can amplify the ongoing immune response by upregulating the expression of HLA molecules as well as co-stimulatory molecules (e.g. B7) on graft parenchymal cells and APCs (Fig. 1). We and others have demonstrated the presence of antigen-specific cytotoxic T lymphocytes (CTL) and anti-HLA antibodies during or preceding a clinical rejection episode (Strom et al. 1975; Suthanthiran and Garovoy 1983). We have detected messenger RNA (mRNA) encoding the CTL selective serine protease (granzyme B) perforin, and Fas ligand attack molecules and immunoregulatory cytokines, such as IL-10 and IL-15, in human renal allografts undergoing acute rejection (reviewed in Strom and Suthanthiran 2000). Indeed these gene expression events can anticipate clinically apparent rejection. More recent efforts to develop a non-invasive method for the molecular diagnosis of rejection have proved rewarding. Using either peripheral blood (Vasconcellos et al. 1998) or urinary leucocytes Li et al. (2001), rejection-related gene expression events evident in renal biopsy specimens are also detected in peripheral blood or urinary sediment specimens. We suspect that a non-invasive molecular diagnostic approach to rejection may prove pivotal in the detection of insidious, clinically silent rejection episodes that are steroid sensitive but capable of leading to chronic rejection if left untreated Li et al. (2001).

Immunopharmacology of allograft rejection

The calcineurin inhibitors: cyclosporin and tacrolimus (FK-506)

Cyclosporin, a small cyclic fungal peptide, and FK-506, a macrolide antibiotic, block the Ca^{2+}-dependent antigen triggered T-cell activation (the antigenic signal) (Schreiber 1992). The immunosuppressive effects of cyclosporin and FK-506 are dependent on the formation of a heterodimeric complex that consists of the native compound (cyclosporin or FK-506) and its respective cytoplasmic receptor 'immunophilin' proteins, cyclophilin, and FK binding protein (FKBP). Cyclosporin–cyclophilin and FK-506/FKBP complexes bind to calcineurin and inhibit its phosphatase activity (Table 3). The inhibition of the enzymatic activity of calcineurin is considered central to the immunosuppressive effects of cyclosporin and FK-506.

The phosphorylation status of a number of transcription factors alter their intracellular localization. Cyclosporin/FK-506 inhibition of phosphatase activity of calcineurin interferes with the dephosphorylation of cytoplasmic NF-AT and unmasking of its nuclear localization signal and importation into the nucleus. The phosphorylation status of transcription factors can also affect their DNA binding ability and

Table 3 Mechanisms of action of immunosuppressants

Immunosuppressant	Subcellular site(s) of action
Azathioprine	Inhibits purine synthesis
Corticosteroids	Blocks cytokine gene expression
CsA/Tacrolimus	Blocks Ca^{2+}-dependent T-cell activation pathway via binding to calcineurin
Mycophenolate Mofetil	Inhibits inosine monophosphate dehydrogenase and prevents de novo guanosine and deoxyguanosine synthesis in lymphocytes
Sirolimus	Blocks IL-2 and other growth factor signal transduction; blocks CD28-mediated co-stimulatory signals

interaction with the rest of the transcriptional machinery. For example, the DNA binding activities of c-jun increases on dephosphorylation. Also, cyclosporin inhibits the expression of not only NF-AT but other DNA binding proteins such as NF-κB and AP-1 Li et al. (1991).

Blockade of cytokine gene activation does not fully account for the antiproliferative effect of cyclosporin and FK-506. It is significant that cyclosporin, in striking contrast to its inhibitory activity on the induced expression of IL-2, enhances the expression of transforming growth factor-β (TGF-β) (Sehajpal et al. 1993). Because TGF-β_1 is a potent inhibitor of T-cell proliferation and generation of antigen-specific CTL (Kehrl et al. 1986), heightened expression of TGF-β_1 may contribute to the antiproliferative/immunosuppressive activity of cyclosporin. This novel effect of cyclosporin also suggests a mechanism for some of the complications (e.g. renal fibrosis and tumour metastasis) of therapy with cyclosporin because TGF-β_1 is a fibrogenic and angiogenic cytokine.

Glucocorticosteroids

Glucocorticosteroids inhibit T-cell proliferation, T-cell-dependent immunity, and cytokine gene transcription (including IL-1, IL-2, IL-6, IFN-γ, and TNF-α genes) (Arya et al. 1984; Knudsen et al. 1987; Zanker et al. 1990). While no single cytokine can reverse the inhibitory effects of corticosteroids on mitogen-stimulated T-cell proliferation, a combination of cytokines is effective (Almawi et al. 1991). The glucocorticoid and glucocorticoid receptor bimolecular complex block IL-2 gene transcription via impairment of the cooperative effect of several DNA binding proteins (Vacca et al. 1992). Corticosteroids also inhibit the formation of free NF-κB, a DNA binding protein required for cytokine and other T-cell activation gene expression events (Auphan et al. 1995) (Fig. 1 and Table 3).

Azathioprine

A thioguanine derivative of 6-mercaptopurine (Elion 1967), azathioprine is a purine analogue that acts as a purine antagonist and functions as an effective antiproliferative agent (Elion 1967; Bach and Strom 1986) (Fig. 1 and Table 3).

Mycophenolate Mofetil

Mycophenolate Mofetil (MMF) is the semisynthetic derivative of mycophenolic acid, and it diminishes proliferation of T and B lymphocytes, decreases generation of cytotoxic T-cells, and suppresses antibody formation (Sweeney 1972; Morris and Wang 1991; Lui and Halloran 1996). MMF inhibits inosine monophosphate dehydrogenase (IMPDH), an enzyme in the *de novo* pathway of purine synthesis. Lymphocytes are dependent upon this biosynthetic pathway to satisfy their guanosine requirements (Table 3) [reviewed in Lui and Halloran 1996]. Clinical trials have utilized MMF to replace azathioprine in the cyclosporin and steroid-based immunosuppressive regimen. These controlled, prospective trials have shown a diminished incidence of early acute rejection episodes (US Renal Transplant Mycophenolate Mofetil Study Group and Sollinger 1995; Lui and Halloran 1996; European Mycophenolate Mofetil Cooperative Study Group 1999). Follow-up studies have indicated an advantage for MMF over azathioprine after 3 years of follow-up (European Mycophenolate Mofetil Cooperative Study Group 1999).

Sirolimus (Rapamycin)

Rapamycin (Chung *et al.* 1992; Kuo *et al.* 1992; Morris 1992) is a macrocyclic lactone isolated from *Streptomyces hygroscopicus* that, like FK-506, binds to FKBP. Yet, rapamycin and FK-506 affect different and distinctive sites in the signal transduction pathway (Table 3). Whereas rapamycin blocks IL-2 and other growth factor-mediated proliferative response, FK-506 (or cyclosporin) has no such capacity. Also, the rapamycin/FKBP complex, unlike the FK-506/FKBP complex, does not bind calcineurin. The antiproliferative activity of the rapamycin/FKBP complex is linked to blockade of the activation of the 70 kDa S6 protein kinases and blockade of expression of the bcl-2 proto-oncogene. Rapamycin also blocks the Ca^{2+}-independent CD28-induced co-stimulatory pathway. Substitution of rapamycin for azathioprine in a triple therapy regimen reduced the frequency and severity of acute rejection (Kahan 2000).

Immunosuppressive regimens

The management of the transplant recipient, including anti-rejection therapy, is organized around a few general principles. The first consideration is careful patient preparation and, in the circumstance of living donor renal transplantation, selection of the best available ABO-compatible HLA match in the event that several potential living related donors are available for organ donation. The second is a multi-tiered approach to immunosuppressive therapy similar in principle to that used in chemotherapy; several agents are used simultaneously, each of which is directed at a different molecular target within the allograft response (Fig. 1 and Table 3). Additive/synergistic effects are achieved through application of each agent at a relatively low dose, thereby limiting the toxicity of each individual agent while increasing the total immunosuppressive effect. The third is the principle that higher immunosuppressive drug doses and/or more individual immunosuppressive drugs are required to gain early engraftment and to treat established rejection than are needed to maintain immunosuppression in the long term. Hence, intensive induction and lower dose maintenance drug protocols are used. The fourth is careful investigation of each episode of post-transplant graft dysfunction, with the realization that most of the common causes of graft dysfunction, including rejection, can (and frequently do) coexist. Successful therapy, therefore, often involves several simultaneous therapeutic manoeuvres. The fifth is the appropriate reduction or withdrawal of an immunosuppressive drug when that drug's toxicity exceeds its therapeutic benefit.

The basic immunosuppressive protocol used in most transplant centres involves the use of at least two and often three drugs, each directed at a discrete site in the T-cell activation cascade (Fig. 1) and each with distinct side effects. Whereas CsA + MMF + glucocorticoids is the most widely used regimen, there are a number of variations of the basic calcineurin inhibitor based triple drug protocol. A calcineurin-free non-nephrotoxic regimen consisting of rapamycin, MMF, and glucocorticosteroids has been developed and may have merit for use in recipients at high risk for delayed graft function (Kreis *et al.* 2000).

Many centres employ a sequential immunosuppressive protocol. Monoclonal anti-T cell (e.g. OKT3) or polyclonal antilymphocyte antibodies (e.g. thymoglobulin), are used as induction therapy for 5–14 days in the immediate post-transplant period, thereby establishing an immunosuppressive umbrella that enables early engraftment without immediate use of calcineurin inhibitors during the early post-transplant period. During this critical period, the graft is particularly vulnerable to CsA/FK-506-induced nephrotoxic effects. The incidence of early rejection episodes is reduced by the prophylactic use of anti-lymphocyte antibodies. This protocol is particularly beneficial for patients at high risk for immunological graft failure (e.g. broadly pre-sensitized or retransplant patients). The efficacy of the polyclonal anti-lymphocyte antibody preparation or mAbs in preventing rejection is impressive, but profound lymphopenia and an increase in the incidence of opportunistic infections and lymphoma results. Because of selective targeting of IL-2R+ T-cells, anti-CD25 mAb treatment might be safer than treatment with thymoglobulin or anti-T cell mAbs. Insofar as activated but not resting T cells express the IL-2 receptor α chain, anti-CD25 mAbs are employed as humanized (Vincenti *et al.* 1998; Ekberg *et al.* 2000) or chimeric (Hong and Kahan 1999; Kahan *et al.* 1999) mAbs to selectively target and destroy alloreactive T cells. These efforts are based on successful exploration and application of IL-2 receptor targeted therapy in preclinical models (Strom *et al.* 1993). Human anti-IL-2 receptor α mAbs are being explored as replacement for OKT3 (which targets both resting and activated T-cells) or polyclonal antilymphocyte antibodies in a sequential immunosuppressive protocol. Preliminary results with a low dose tacrolimus and sirolimus protocol (McAlister *et al.* 2000) may prove to rival the current sequential immune therapy regimens for use in patients at high risk to reject an allograft.

HLA and renal transplantation

The genes that code for the HLA antigens are lodged within the short arm of chromosome 6 (Klein and Sato 2000a,b). The class I proteins, HLA-A, B, and C antigens, are composed of a 41-kDa polymorphic chain linked non-covalently to a 12-kDa β_2-microglobulin chain that is encoded in chromosome 15. The class I molecules are expressed by all nucleated cells and platelets. The class II molecules, HLA-DR, DP, and DQ, are composed of an α chain of 34 kDa and a β chain of 29 kDa. MHC class II molecules are constitutively expressed on the surface of B cells, monocytes/macrophages, and dendritic cells. Additional lymphoid cells such as T cells and many non-lymphoid cells such as renal tubular epithelial cells express class II proteins only on stimulation with cytokines.

The clinical benefits of HLA matching are readily appreciable in the recipients of renal grafts from living related donors. An analysis of the

United Network for Organ Sharing (UNOS) scientific renal transplant registry data has revealed that the 1 year graft survival rate is 94 per cent in recipients of two-haplotype-matched, HLA-identical kidneys and 89 per cent and 90 per cent, respectively, when a one-haplotype-matched parent or sibling is the donor (Cecka and Terasaki 1992). The Collaborative Transplant Study, an international study that draws on 305 transplant centres located in 47 countries for data, has also demonstrated that the survival rate of HLA-identical transplants is superior to that of one-haplotype-matched grafts, even in the cyclosporin era (Opelz *et al.* 1999).

The advantage of HLA-matching is maintained beyond the first year of transplantation. UNOS registry data (Cecka and Terasaki 1992) show estimated half-lives (the time needed for 50 per cent of the grafts functioning at 1 year post-transplantation to fail) of 26.9 years for HLA-identical grafts and 12.2 years and 10.8 years for one-haplotype-matched sibling grafts and parental grafts, respectively. Data from the Collaborative Transplant Study, comprising 22,414 living related grafts, have also revealed a substantial long-term benefit (Opelz *et al.* 1999) of HLA matching in recipients of living related grafts.

The effect of matching for HLA in cadaveric graft recipients has been examined in a prospective US study (Takemoto *et al.* 1992) in which kidneys were shared nationally on the basis of matching for HLA-A, B, and DR antigens. All transplantation centres in the United States participated in this study. The 1 year graft survival rate was 88 per cent for HLA-matched kidneys and 79 per cent for HLA-mismatched kidneys. Moreover, the benefit of HLA matching persisted beyond the first year of post-transplantation; the estimated half-life of the HLA-matched renal graft was 17.3 years and that of HLA-mismatched renal allografts, 7.8 years.

Since the inception of the US national kidney sharing programme in 1987, more than 7500 cadaveric kidneys have been distributed to transplantation centres located in 48 states, and a recent analysis confirmed and extended the observation that HLA-matched transplants have a superior outcome compared to HLA-mismatched transplants (Takemoto *et al.* 2000). The estimated 10-year rate of cadaveric graft survival was 52 per cent for HLA-matched transplants and was 37 per cent for HLA-mismatched transplants. Furthermore, the incidence of rejection was lower in HLA-matched transplants compared to mismatched ones. Interestingly, the mean duration of cold-ischaemia time of nationally shared kidneys was not that different from locally transplanted kidneys, and was 23 h as compared to 22 h for non-shared kidneys (Takemoto *et al.* 2000).

A stepwise increase in the survival rate of cadaveric renal allografts has also been documented with increasing levels of HLA-A, B, and DR antigen matching. The improvement in the graft survival rate following HLA matching is more apparent when matching is based on better-resolved HLA antigens (HLA split antigens) than when based on broad HLA antigens, and the improvement in the graft survival rate between the best-matched and the worst-matched grafts increases with time (Cicciarelli and Cho 1992). In the UNOS registry data, the difference in the graft survival rate between the best-matched and worst-matched recipient was 10 per cent at 1 year post-transplantation, and this difference increased to 18 per cent by 3 years post-transplantation. The Collaborative Transplant Study of more than 67,000 primary cadaver grafts has also demonstrated a significant correlation between the number of HLA mismatches and graft loss (Opelz *et al.* 1999).

A threshold level of HLA matching might exist: allografts that are matched for four or more HLA antigens (or two or less HLA mismatches) have a superior short- as well as long-term outcome compared to less than four HLA antigen matches (or greater than two antigen mismatches) (Cicciarelli and Cho 1992). It is noteworthy that the beneficial effect of different degrees of matching/mismatching for the HLA-A, B, and DR antigens (Terasaki *et al.* 1992), with the exception of phenotypically identical HLA transplants, is more evident in white recipients as compared to black recipients of cadaveric renal allografts (Cecka and Terasaki 1992; Cicciarelli and Cho 1992).

The impact of each of the HLA loci, HLA-A locus, HLA-B locus, and HAL-DR locus, on renal allograft outcome has been investigated. Each locus impacts graft outcome. In the Collaborative Transplant Study, the influence of HLA-DR mismatch was greater than that of HLA-A or HLA-B mismatches in the first year of transplantation; with increased post-transplantation time, mismatches at any of the three loci impacted adversely on graft survival rates (Opelz *et al.* 1999).

Molecular techniques for the finer resolution of the HLA system hold considerable promise (Opelz *et al.* 1993). Existing molecular methodologies have already helped resolve the discrepancies associated with the serological identification of the HLA-DR antigens. The clinical advantage of molecular matching is suggested by the observation that the 1 year cadaveric renal graft survival rate is 87 per cent in patients who received kidneys that are HLA-DR identical not only by the serological methods but also by molecular methods (DNA-RFLP method), but only 69 per cent in patients who received kidneys that are not HLA-DR identical by the molecular methodology (Opelz *et al.* 1991). Application of molecular techniques for the identification of HLA-DR antigens has also resulted in the appreciation of a stepwise increase in the survival of cadaveric renal allografts matched for zero, one, or two HLA-DR antigens (Opelz *et al.* 1993, 1999). Molecular typing has also been used to detect mismatches at the HLA-A or HLA-B locus. Mismatches that were missed by conventional serological techniques but identified by molecular techniques were found to adversely impact graft survival (Opelz *et al.* 1999).

Current data suggest minimal impact of matching for HLA-C locus antigens. Matching for the HLA-DP antigen, on the other hand, appears to be important in repeat but not primary grafts (Opelz *et al.* 1999).

Crossmatch

Crossmatches, testing of recipient's serum for antibodies reacting with the donor's HLA antigens, must be performed prior to renal transplantation. The standard crossmatch test consists of incubating the serum from the recipient with the donor's lymphocytes in the presence of rabbit serum as a source of complement.

The presence in the recipient's serum of cytotoxic antibodies directed at the donor's class I antigen (positive T-cell crossmatch) is an absolute contraindication to transplantation because 80–90 per cent of transplants performed in the presence of a positive crossmatch are subject to hyperacute rejection (Cicciarelli and Cho 1992). The sensitivity of the standard crossmatch test has been increased by the addition of sublytic concentrations of antihuman globulin (AHG) to the test system. The graft survival rate is about 5 per cent lower in recipients with a positive AHG test compared to recipients with a negative AHG test (Williams *et al.* 1968).

The significance of antibodies reacting with the donor's class II antigens (positive B-cell crossmatch) is not fully resolved. A survival disadvantage, 7 per cent in primary transplants and 15 per cent in repeat transplants, has however been noted in recipients with a positive B-cell crossmatch (Ogura 1993).

A number of centres are currently evaluating the usefulness of flow cytometry based methodology to detect donor-specific antibodies. Flow cytometry cross-matches permit detection of low, sublytic concentrations of complement fixing as well as no complement fixing antibodies. The clinical impact of a positive flow cytometry cross-match is being analysed by the transplantation community. In the UNOS kidney transplant registry data (Cook *et al.* 1999), a positive flow cytometry crossmatch was associated with an increased incidence of early graft dysfunction requiring dialytic support, primary non-function of the allograft, prolonged hospitalization and a greater incidence of allograft rejection. The negative impact of a flow cytometry crossmatch was greater in repeat transplants compared to primary transplants. Whereas a positive flow crossmatch was associated with a 5 per cent decrease in the 3 year survival rate of primary grafts, a 19 per cent decrease was observed in the 3 year survival of repeat grafts. In primary transplants, a T+B+ flow cytometry crossmatch and a T−B+ cross-match had a similar outcome (76 per cent 3 year graft survival rate versus 74 per cent), and in repeat transplants a T+B+ flow cytometry crossmatch has a much inferior outcome compared to a T−B+crossmatch (60 per cent 3 year graft survival rate versus 73 per cent).

Transplantation tolerance

Transplantation tolerance can be defined as an inability of the organ graft recipient to express a graft destructive immune response in the absence of exogenous immunosuppressive therapy. While this statement does not restrict either the mechanistic basis or the quantitative aspects of immune unresponsiveness of the host, true tolerance is antigen-specific, induced as a consequence of prior exposure to the specific antigen, and is not dependent on the continuous administration of exogenous non-specific immunosuppressants.

A classification of tolerance on the basis of the mechanisms involved, site of induction, extent of tolerance, and the cell primarily tolerized is provided in Table 4. Induction strategies for the creation of peripheral tolerance are listed in Table 5.

Table 4 Classification of tolerance

A. Based on the major mechanism involved
1. Clonal deletion
2. Clonal anergy
3. Suppression

B. Based on the period of induction
1. Fetal
2. Neonatal
3. Adult

C. Based on the cell tolerized
1. T cell
2. B cell

D. Based on the extent of tolerance
1. Complete
2. Partial, including split

E. Based on the main site of induction
1. Central
2. Peripheral

Several hypotheses, not necessarily mutually exclusive and at times even complementary, have been proposed for the cellular basis of tolerance. Data from several laboratories support the following mechanistic possibilities for the creation of a tolerant state: clonal deletion, clonal anergy, and immunoregulation.

Clonal deletion

Clonal deletion is a process by which self-antigen-reactive cells, especially those with high affinity for the self antigens, are eliminated from the organism's immune repertoire. This process is called central tolerance. In the case of T cells, this process takes place in the thymus, and the death of immature T cells is considered to be the ultimate result of high-affinity interactions between a T cell with productively rearranged TCR and the thymic non-lymphoid cells, including dendritic cells that express the self-MHC antigen. This purging of the immune repertoire of self-reactive T cells is termed negative selection and is distinguished from the positive selection process responsible for the generation of the T-cell repertoire involved in the recognition of foreign antigens in the context of self-MHC molecules. Clonal deletion or at least marked depletion of mature T cells as a consequence of apoptosis can also occur in the periphery (reviewed in Van Parijs and Abbas 1998). The form of graft tolerance occurring as a consequence of mixed haematopoietic chimerism entails massive deletion of alloreactive clones (Werkerle *et al.* 1998). Tolerance to renal allografts has been achieved in patients who have accepted a bone marrow graft from the same donor (Sayegh *et al.* 1991; Spitzer *et al.* 1999). It is interesting that IL-2, the only T-cell growth factor that triggers

Table 5 Potential approaches for the creation of tolerance

A. Cell depletion protocols
1. Whole body irradiation
2. Total lymphoid irradiation
3. Panel of monoclonal antibodies

B. Reconstitution protocols
1. Allogeneic bone marrow cells with or without T-cell depletion
2. Syngeneric bone marrow cells

C. Combination of strategies A and B

D. Cell surface molecule targeted therapy
1. Anti-CD4 mAbs
2. Anti-ICAM-1 + anti-LFA-1 mAbs
3. Anti-CD3 mAbs
4. Anti-CD2 mAbs
5. Anti-IL-2 receptor α (CD25) mAbs
6. CTLA4Ig fusion protein
7. Anti-CD40L mAbs
8. Campain-1H

E. Drugs
1. Azathioprine
2. Cyclosporin
3. Rapamycin

F. Additional approaches
1. Donor-specific blood transfusions with concomitant mAb or drug therapy
2. Intrathymic inoculation of cells/antigens
3. Oral administration of cells/antigens

T-cell proliferation as well as apoptosis, is an absolute prerequisite for the acquisition of organ graft tolerance through the use of non-lymphoablative treatment regimens (Dai *et al.* 1998; Li *et al.* 1999). Tolerance achieved under these circumstances also involves additional mechanisms, including clonal anergy and suppressor mechanisms (Suthanthiran 1996; Waldmann 1999; Li *et al.* 2000).

Clonal anergy

Clonal anergy refers to a process in which the antigen-reactive cells are functionally silenced. The cellular basis for the hyporesponsiveness resides in the anergic cell itself, and the current data suggests that the anergic T cells fail to express the T-cell growth factor, IL-2, and other crucial T-cell activation genes because of defects in the antigen stimulated signalling pathway.

T-cell clonal anergy can result from suboptimal antigen-driven signalling of T cells, as mentioned earlier. The full activation of T cells requires at least two signals, one signal generated via the TCR/CD3 complex, and the second (co-stimulatory) signal initiated/delivered by the APCs. Stimulation of T cells via the TCR/CD3 complex alone—provision of signal 1 without signal 2—can result in T-cell anergy/paralysis (Fig. 3 and Table 2).

B-cell activation, in a fashion analogous to T-cell activation, requires at least two signals. One signal is initiated via the B-cell antigen receptor immunoglobulin, and a co-stimulatory signal is provided by cytokines or cell surface proteins of T-cell origin. Thus, delivery of the antigenic signal alone to the B cells without the instructive cytokines or T-cell help can lead to B-cell anergy and tolerance.

Immunoregulatory (suppressor) mechanisms

Antigen-specific T or B cells are physically present and are functionally competent in tolerant states resulting from suppressor mechanisms. The cytopathic and antigen-specific cells are restrained by the suppressor cells or factors or express non-cytopathic cellular programmes. Each of the major subsets of T cells, the CD4+ T cells and the CD8+ T cells, has been implicated in mediating suppression. Indeed, a cascade involving MHC antigen-restricted T cells, MHC antigen-unrestricted T cells, and their secretory products have been reported to collaborate to mediate suppression. At least four distinct mechanisms have been advanced to explain the cellular basis for suppression: (a) an anti-idiotypic regulatory mechanism in which the idiotype of the TCR of the original antigen-responsive T cells functions as an immunogen and elicits an anti-idiotypic response; the elicited anti-idiotypic regulatory cells, in turn, prevent the further responses of the idiotype-bearing cells to the original sensitizing stimulus; (b) the veto process by which recognition by alloreactive T cells of alloantigen-expressing veto cells results in the targeted killing (veto process) of the original alloreactive T cells by the veto cells; (c) immune deviation, a shift in CD4+ T-cell programmes away from Th1-type (IL-2, IFN-γ expressing) toward the Th2 type (IL-4, IL-10 expressing) programme; and (d) the production of suppressor factors or cytokines. For example, the production of TGF-β by myelin basic protein-specific CD8+ T cells or other cytokines with antiproliferative properties. The process leading to full tolerance is infectious. Tolerant T cells recruit non-tolerant T cells into the tolerant state (Waldmann 1999). The tolerant state also establishes a condition in which foreign tissues housed in the same micro-environment as the specific antigen to which the host has been tolerized are protected from rejection (Waldmann 1999). Tolerance is a multi-step process (Suthanthiran 1996; Waldmann 1999; Li *et al.* 2000).

Clearly more than one mechanism is o erative in the induction of tolerance (Fig. 3). The tolerant state is not an all-or-nothing phenomenon but is one that has several gradations. Of the mechanisms proposed for tolerance, clonal deletion might be of greater importance in the creation of self-tolerance, and clonal anergy and immunoregulatory mechanisms might be more applicable to transplantation tolerance. More recent data suggest that both clonal depletion and immunoregulatory mechanisms are needed to create and sustain central or peripheral tolerance. From a practical viewpoint, a non-immunogenic allograft (e.g. located in an immunologically privileged site or physically isolated from the immune system) might also be 'tolerated' by an immunocompetent organ graft recipient.

Authentic tolerance has been difficult to identify in human renal allograft recipients. Nevertheless, the clinical examples, albeit infrequent, of grafts functioning without any exogenous immunosuppressive drugs (either due to non-compliance of the patient or due to discontinuation of drugs for other medical reasons) do suggest that some long-term recipients of allografts develop tolerance to the transplanted organ and accept the allografts. The recent progress in our understanding of the immunobiology of graft rejection and tolerance and the potential to apply molecular approaches to the bedside hold significant promise for the creation of a clinically relevant tolerant state and transplantation without exogenous immunosuppressants.

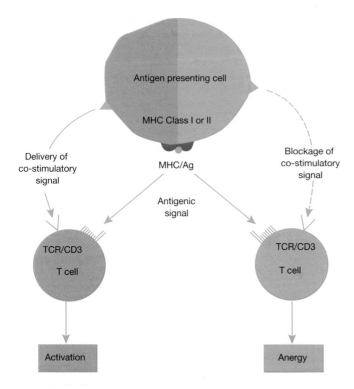

Fig. 3 *T-cell activation/anergy decision points.* Several potential sites for the regulation of T-cell signalling are shown. The antigenic peptide displayed by MHC (site 1), co-stimulatory signals (site 2), TCR (site 3), and cytokine signalling (site 4) can influence the eventual outcome. Altered peptide ligands, blockade of co-stimulatory signals, down regulation of TCR, and IL-10 favour anergy induction, whereas fully immunogenic peptides, delivery of co-stimulatory signals, appropriate number of TCR, and IL-12 prevent anergy induction and facilitate full activation of T cells. (Reproduced from Suthanthiran, M. (1996). Transplantation tolerance: fooling mother nature. *Proceedings of the National Academy of Sciences USA* **93**, 12072–12075.) Copyright (1996), National Academy of Sciences, USA (Suthanthiran 1996).

Acknowledgements

The authors are grateful to Ms Linda Stackhouse and Ms Frances Pechenick for their meticulous help in the preparation of this chapter.

References

Acuto, O. and Cantrell, D. (2000). T cell activation and the cytoskeleton. *Annual Review of Immunology* **18**, 165–184.

Almawi, W. Y. *et al.* (1991). Abrogation of glucocorticosteroid-mediated inhibition of T cell proliferation by the synergistic action of IL-1, IL-6 and IFN-gamma. *Journal of Immunology* **146**, 3523–3527.

Arya, S. K., Won-Staal, J., and Gallo, R. C. (1984). Dexamethason-mediated inhibition of human T cell growth factor and gamma-interferon messenger RNA. *Journal of Immunology* **133**, 273–276.

Auphan, N. *et al.* (1995). Immunosuppression by glucocorticoids: inhibition of NF-kappaB activity through induction of I-kappaB synthesis. *Science* **270**, 286–290.

Bach, J. F. and Strom, T. B. The mode of action of immunosuppressive agents. In *Research Monographs in Immunology* (ed. J. F. Bach and T. B. Strom), pp. 105–158. Amsterdam: Elsevier, 1986.

Beyers, A. D., Spruyt, L. L., and Williams, A. F. (1992). Molecular associations between the T-lymphocyte antigen receptor complex and the surface antigens CD2, CD4, or CD8 and CD5. *Proceedings of the National Academy of Sciences USA* **89**, 2945–2949.

Brown, M. H. *et al.* (1989). The CD2 antigen associates with the T-cell antigen receptor CD3 antigen complex on the surface of human T lymphocytes. *Nature* **339**, 551–553.

Cecka, J. M. and Terasaki, P. I. The UNOS Scientific Renal Transplant Registry—1991. In *Clinical Transplants 1991* (ed. P. I. Terasaki and J. M. Cecka), pp. 1–11. Los Angeles: UCLA Tissue Typing Laboratory, 1992.

Chung, J. *et al.* (1992). Rapamycin-FKBP specifically blocks growth-dependent activation of and signaling by the 70 kd 56 protein kinases. *Cell* **69**, 1227–1236.

Cicciarelli, J. and Cho, Y. HLA matching: univariate and multivariate analyses of UNOS registry data. In *Clinical Transplants 1991* (ed. P. I. Terasaki and J. M. Cecka), pp. 325–333. Los Angeles: UCLA Tissue Typing Laboratory, 1992.

Clipstone, N. A. and Crabtree, G. R. (1992). Identification of calcineurin as a key signalling enzyme in T-lymphocyte activation. *Nature* **357**, 695–697.

Cook, D. J. *et al.* Flow cytometry crossmatching (FXCM) in the UNOS kidney transplant registry. In *Clinical Transplants 1998* (ed. J. M. Cecka and P. I. Terasaki), pp. 413–419. Los Angeles: UCLA Tissue Typing Laboratory, 1999.

Dai, Z. *et al.* (1998). Impaired alloantigen-mediated T cell apoptosis and failure to induce long-term allograft survival in IL-2-deficient mice. *Journal of Immunology* **161**, 1659–1663.

Dustin, M. L. and Cooper, J. A. (2000). The immunological synapse and the actin cytoskeleton: molecular hardware for T cell signaling. *Nature Immunology* **1**, 23–29.

Dustin, M. L. and Springer, T. A. (1989). T-cell receptor cross-linking transiently stimulates adhesiveness through LFA-1. *Nature* **341**, 619–624.

Ekbergh, H. *et al.* (2000). Daclizumab prevents acute rejection and improves patient survival post transplantation: 1 year polled analysis. *Transplantation International* **13**, 151–159.

Elion, G. B. (1967). Biochemistry and pharmacology of purine analogues. *Federal Proceedings* **26**, 898–904.

European Mycophenolate Mofetil Cooperative Study Group (1999). Mycophenolate Mofetil in renal transplantation: 3-year results from the placebo-controlled trial. *Transplantation* **68**, 391–396.

Fung, M. R. *et al.* (1991). A tyrosine kinase physically associates with the alpha-subunit of the human IL-2 receptor. *Journal of Immunology* **147**, 1253–1258.

Germain, R. N. (1994). MHC-dependent antigen processing and peptide presentation: providing ligands for T lymphocyte activation. *Cell* **76**, 287–299.

Hatakeyama, M. *et al.* (1991). Interaction of the IL-2 receptor with the src-family kinase p56^lck: identification of novel intermolecular association. *Science* **252**, 1523–1528.

Hong, J. C. and Kahan, B. D. (1999). Use of anti-CD25 monoclonal antibody in combination with rapamycin to eliminate cyclosporine treatment during the induction phase of immunosuppression. *Transplantation* **68**, 701–704.

Jorgensen, J. L. *et al.* (1992). Molecular components of T-cell recognition. *Annual Review of Immunology* **10**, 835–873.

Kahan, B. D. (2000). Efficacy of sirolimus compared with azathioprine for reduction of acute allograft rejection: a randomized multicentre study. *Lancet* **356**, 194–202.

Kahan, B. D., Rajagopalan, P. R., and Hall, M. (1999). Reduction of the occurrence of acute cellular rejection among renal allograft recipients treated with basiliximab, a chimeric anti-interleukin-2-receptor monoclonal antibody. United States Simulect Renal Study Group. *Transplantation* **67**, 276–284.

Kehrl, J. H. *et al.* (1986). Production of transforming growth factor beta by human T lymphocytes and its potential role in the regulation of T cell growth. *Journal of Experimental Medicine* **163**, 1037–1050.

Klein, J. and Sato, A. (2000a). The HLA system. First of two parts. *New England Journal of Medicine* **343**, 702–709.

Klein, J. and Sato, A. (2000b). The HLA system. Second of two parts. *New England Journal of Medicine* **343**, 782–786.

Knudsen, P. J., Dinarello, C. A., and Strom, T. B. (1987). Glucocorticoids inhibit transcriptional and post-transcriptional expression of interleukin-1 in U937 cells. *Journal of Immunology* **139**, 4129–4134.

Kreis, H. *et al.* (2000). Sirolimus in association with mycophenolate mofetil induction for the prevention of acute graft rejection in renal allograft recipients. *Transplantation* **69**, 1252–1260.

Kuo, C. J. *et al.* (1992). Rapamycin selectively inhibits interleukin-2 activation of p70 56 kinase. *Nature* **358**, 70–73.

Lenschow, D. J., Walunas, T. L., and Bluestone, J. A. (1996). CD28/B7 system of T cell costimulation. *Annual Review of Immunology* **14**, 233–258.

Li, B. *et al.* (1991). Differential regulation of transforming growth factor beta and interleukin-2 genes in human T cells: demonstration by usage of novel competitor DNA constructs in the quantitative polymerase chain reaction. *Journal of Experimental Medicine* **174**, 1259–1262.

Li, Y. *et al.* (1999). Blocking both signal 1 and signal 2 of T-cell activation prevents apoptosis of alloreactive T cells and induction of peripheral allograft tolerance. *Nature Medicine* **5**, 1298–1302.

Li, S. C. *et al.* (2000). The role of T cell apoptosis in transplantation tolerance. *Current Opinion in Immunology* **12**, 522–527.

Li, B. *et al.* (2001). Non-invasive diagnosis of renal allograft rejection by quantification of cytotoxic genes in urinary cells. *New England Journal of Medicine* **344**, 947–954.

Liu, J. *et al.* (1991). Calcineurin is a common target of cyclophilin-cyclosporin A and FKBP-FK506 complexes. *Cell* **66**, 807–815.

Lui, S. L. and Halloran, P. F. (1996). Mycophenolate mofetil in kidney transplantation. *Current Opinion in Nephrology and Hypertension* **5**, 508–513.

Maslinski, W. *et al.* (1992). Interleukin-2 (IL-2) induces tyrosine kinase-dependent translocation of active Raf-1 from the Il-2 receptor into the cytosol. *Journal of Biological Chemistry* **267**, 15281–15284.

McAlister, V. C. *et al.* (2000). Sirolimus tacrolimus combination immunosuppression. *Lancet* **355**, 376–377.

Morris, R. E. (1992). Rapamycins: antifungal, antitumor, antiproliferative, and immunosuppressive macrolides. *Transplantation Reviews* **6**, 39–48.

Morris, R. E. and Wang, J. (1991). Comparison of the immunosuppressive effects of mycophenolic acid and the morpholinoethyl ester of mycophenolic acid (RS-61433) in recipients of heart allografts. *Transplantation Proceedings* **23**, 493–496.

Nishizuka, Y. (1992). Intracellular signaling by hydrolysis of phospholipids and activation of protein kinase C. *Science* **258**, 607–614.

Noelle, R. J. (1996). CD40 and its ligand in host defense. *Immunity* **4**, 415–419.

O'Keefe, S. J. *et al.* (1992). FK506- and CsA-sensitive activation of the IL-2 promoter by calcineurin. *Nature* **357**, 692–694.

Ogura, K. Clinical Transplants 1992. In *Clinical Transplants 1992* (ed. P. I. Terasaki and J. M. Cecka), pp. 357–369. Los Angeles: UCLA Tissue Typing Laboratory, 1993.

Oosterwegel, M. A. *et al.* (1999). CTLA-4 and T cell activation. *Current Opinions in Immunology* **11**, 294–300.

Opelz, G. *et al.* (1991). Survival of DNA HLA-DR typed and matched cadaver kidney transplants. *Lancet* **338**, 461–463.

Opelz, G. *et al.* (1993). Revisiting HLA matching for kidney transplants. *Transplantation Proceedings* **25**, 173–175.

Opelz, G. *et al.* (1999). HLA compatibility and organ transplant survival. *Reviews of Immunogenetics* **1**, 334–342.

Remillard, B. *et al.* (1991). Interleukin-2 receptor regulates activation of phosphatidylinositol 3-kinase. *Journal of Biological Chemistry* **266**, 14167–14170.

Rush, D. *et al.* (1998). Beneficial effects of treatment of early subclinical rejection: a randomized study. *Journal of the American Society of Nephrology* **9**, 2129–2134.

Sayegh, M. H. *et al.* (1991). Immunologic tolerance to renal allografts after bone marrow transplants from the same donors. *Annals of Internal Medicine* **114**, 954–955.

Schreiber, S. L. (1992). Immunophilin-sensitive protein phosphatase action in cell signaling pathways. *Cell* **70**, 365–368.

Schwartz, R. H. (1993). T cell anergy. *Scientific American* **269**, 62–63, 66–71.

Sehajpal, P. K. *et al.* (1993). Synergism between the CD3 antigen- and CD2 antigen-derived signals: exploration at the level of induction of DNA-binding proteins and characterization of the inhibitory activity of cyclosporine. *Transplantation* **55**, 1118–1124.

Shahinian, A. *et al.* (1993). Differential T cell co-stimulatory requirements in CD28-deficient mice. *Science* **261**, 609–612.

Shibuya, H. *et al.* (1992). IL-2 and EGF receptors stimulate the hematopoietic cell cycle via different signaling pathways: demonstration of a novel role for c-myc. *Cell* **70**, 57–67.

Shoskes, D. A. and Wood, K. J. (1994). Indirect presentation of MHC antigens in transplantation. *Immunology Today* **15**, 32–38.

Smith, K. A. (1988). Interleukin-2: inception, impact, and implications. *Science* **240**, 1169–1176.

Spitzer, T. R. *et al.* (1999). Combined histocompatibility leukocyte antigen-matched donor bone marrow and renal transplantation for multiple myeloma with end stage renal disease: the induction of allograft tolerance through mixed lymphohematopoietic chimerism. *Transplantation* **68**, 480–484.

Strom, T. B. and Suthanthiran, M. (2000). Prospects and applicability of molecular diagnosis of allograft rejection. *Seminars in Nephrology* **20**, 103–107.

Strom, T. B. *et al.* (1975). Identity and cytotoxic capacity of cells infiltrating renal allografts. *New England Journal of Medicine* **292**, 1257–1263.

Strom, T. B. *et al.* (1993). Interleukin-2 receptor-directed therapies: antibody- or cytokine-based targeting molecules. *Annual Review of Medicine* **44**, 343–353.

Suthanthiran, M. (1990). A novel model for the antigen-dependent activation of normal human T cells: transmembrane signaling by crosslinkage of the CD3/T cell receptor-alpha/beta complex with the cluster determinant 2 antigen. *Journal of Experimental Medicine* **171**, 1965–1979.

Suthanthiran, M. (1993). Signaling features of T cells: implication for the regulation of the anti-allograft response. *Kidney International* **43** (Suppl.), S3–S11.

Suthanthiran, M. (1996). Transplantation tolerance: fooling mother nature. *Proceedings of the National Academy of Sciences USA* **93**, 12072–12075.

Suthanthiran, M. and Garovoy, M. R. (1983). Immunologic monitoring of the renal transplant recipient. *Urological Clinics of North America* **10**, 315–325.

Suthanthiran, M. and Strom, T. B. (1994). Renal transplantation. *New England Journal of Medicine* **334**, 365–376.

Sweeney, M. J. (1972). Metabolism and biochemistry of mycophenolic acid. *Cancer Research* **32**, 1803–1809.

Takemoto, S. *et al.* (1992). Survival of nationally shared, HLA-matched kidney transplants from cadaveric donors. *New England Journal of Medicine* **327**, 834–839.

Takemoto, S. K. *et al.* (2000). Twelve years' experience with national sharing of HLA-matched cadaveric kidneys for transplantation. *New England Journal of Medicine* **343**, 1078–1084.

Takeshita, T., Asao, H., and Ohtani, K. (1992). Cloning of the gamma chain of the human IL-2 receptor. *Science* **257**, 379–382.

Taniguchi, T. (1995). Cytokine signalling through non-receptor protein tyrosine kinases. *Science* **260**, 251–255.

Terasaki, P. I. *et al.* UCLA and UNOS registries: overview. In *Clinical Transplants 1992* (ed. P. I. Terasaki and J. M. Cecka), pp. 409–430. Los Angeles: UCLA Tissue Typing Laboratory 1992.

Unanue, E. R. and Cerottini, J. C. (1989). Antigen presentation. *FASEB Journal* **3**, 2496–2502.

US Renal Transplant Mycophenolate Mofetil Study Group, Sollinger, H. W. (1995). Mycophenolate mofetil for the prevention of acute rejection in primary cadaveric renal allograft recipients. *Transplantation* **60**, 225–232.

Vacca, A. *et al.* (1992). Glucocorticoid receptor-mediated suppression of the interleukin-2 gene expression through impairment of the cooperativity between nuclear factor of activated T cells and AP-1 enhancer elements. *Journal of Experimental Medicine* **175**, 637–646.

Van Parijs, L. and Abbas, A. K. (1998). Homeostasis and self-tolerance in the immune system: turning lymphocytes off. *Science* **280**, 243–248.

Vasconcellos, L. M. *et al.* (1998). Cytotoxic lymphocyte gene expression in peripheral blood leukocytes correlates with rejecting renal allografts. *Transplantation* **66**, 562–566.

Vincenti, F. *et al.* (1998). Interleukin-2 receptor blockade with daclizumab to prevent acute rejection in renal transplantation. Daclizumab Triple Therapy Study Group. *New England Journal of Medicine* **338**, 161–165.

Waldman, T. A. (1991). The interleukin-2 receptor. *Journal of Biological Chemistry* **266**, 2681–2684.

Waldmann, H. (1999). Transplantation tolerance—where do we stand? *Nature Medicine* **5**, 1245–1248.

Waldmann, T., Tagaya, Y., and Bamford, R. (1998). Interleukin-2, interleukin-15, and their receptors. *International Review of Immunology* **16**, 205–226.

Wekerle, T. *et al.* (1998). Extrathymic T cell deletion and allogeneic stem cell engraftment induced with co-stimulatory blockade is followed by central T cell tolerance. *Journal of Experimental Medicine* **187**, 2037–2044.

Williams, G. M. *et al.* (1968). 'Hyperacute' renal-homograft rejection in man. *New England Journal of Medicine* **279**, 611–618.

Zanker, B. *et al.* (1990). Evidence that glucocorticosteroids block expression of the human interleukin-6 gene by accessory cells. *Transplantation* **49**, 183–185.

13.2.2 Immunosuppression for renal transplantation

Daniel Abramowicz, K. Martin Wissing, and Nilufer Broeders

Introduction

The two major goals after renal transplantation are to avoid acute rejection episodes and to limit the numerous side effects of immuno-suppressive drugs (Table 1).

It has been repeatedly shown that the occurrence of an acute rejection episode represents an important risk factor for renal graft loss either by uncontrollable rejection or by chronic rejection (Vereerstraeten *et al.* 1997). The risk of acute rejection is greatest during the first three months after transplantation and peaks during the first month, as inflammation caused by graft ischaemia increases transplant immunogenicity. Therefore, the most intense immunosuppression is required during this period.

Several new immunosuppressive drugs appeared in the clinical arena during the 1990s (Table 1): tacrolimus, which like cyclosporine A (CsA) is a calcineurin inhibitor (CNI); mycophenolate mofetil (MMF), which like azathioprine (AZA) inhibits lymphocyte proliferation; sirolimus (rapamycin) and everolimus (RAD for rapamycine-derivative), which both inhibit cell proliferation induced by cytokines and growth factors, and anti-interleukin-2 (IL-2) receptor antibodies, which block IL-2-induced lymphocyte proliferation. These new drugs have been combined with those already available in a number of clinical studies that focused on the reduction of rejection rates and the feasibility of dose reduction or withdrawal of CNI or steroids.

This chapter outlines the different strategies of immunosuppression that are used today after renal transplantation.

Prevention of acute rejection

Calcineurin inhibitors: CsA and tacrolimus

Calcineurin inhibitor has been the mainstay of immunosuppressive treatment for the last 20 years (Table 2). Two drugs are currently available: CsA and tacrolimus. These two molecules, upon entry into the cells, bind with cytoplasmic proteins named immunophilins. The immunophilin–CsA or –tacrolimus complexes bind to and inhibit calcineurin. Calcineurin is a phosphatase that when active dephosphorylates the nuclear factor of activated T cells (NFAT). This facilitates the entry of NFAT into the nucleus, where it activates the transcription of various cytokines such as IL-2, IL-3, IL-4, IL-5, interferon-γ, and tumour necrosis factor-α. Inhibition of calcineurin prevents the transcription of these cytokines, and thus inhibits T-cell activation. In addition, CsA and tacrolimus enhance the expression of transforming growth factor-β (TGF-β), which displays potent immunosuppressive effects as it inhibits IL-2-stimulated T-cell proliferation and generation of cytotoxic T lymphocytes, but also has a pro-fibrotic action, which can culminate in chronic nephrotoxicity.

The introduction of CsA in the mid-1980s in combination with steroids allowed for a 10–20 per cent improvement in graft survival after 1–3 years as compared to the AZA–steroid regimen. Nevertheless, the improvements in short-term graft survival did not translate into improved long-term survival, probably because CsA nephrotoxicity

Table 1 Main characteristics of immunosuppressive agents

Agent	Mechanism of action	Side effects
ATG	Binds to several antigens on lymphoid cells; depletes circulating lymphocytes	Cytokine release syndrome; leucopenia, thrombopenia; serum sickness
OKT3	Binds CD3 present on T lymphocytes; depletes circulating lymphocytes	Cytokine release syndrome; pro-coagulant effect; possible sensitization with loss of efficacy
Daclizumab	Binds the α chain of interleukin-2 receptor; blocks IL-2-induced proliferation	Unreported
Basiliximab	Binds the α chain of interleukin-2 receptor; blocks IL-2-induced proliferation	Anaphylaxis (rare)
Cyclosporine	Binds cyclophylin; inhibits calcineurin; inhibits cytokine gene transcription	Nephrotoxicity; hypertension; hypercholesterolaemia; hypertrichosis; gingival hypertrophy
Tacrolimus	Binds FKBP-12; inhibits calcineurin; inhibits cytokine gene transcription	Nephrotoxicity; neurotoxicity; hypertension; diabetes mellitus
Azathioprine	Inhibits purine biosynthesis and lymphocyte proliferation	Leucopenia
Mycophenolate mofetil	Inhibits purine biosynthesis and lymphocyte proliferation	Diarrhoea; leucopenia; anaemia
Sirolimus/ everolimus	Binds FKBP-12; inhibits the proliferative response to cytokines and growth factors	Hyperlipaemia; arthralgia; pneumonitis; impaired wound healing

Table 2 Main immunosuppressive regimens for the first transplant year

Immunosuppressive regimen	Rejection rates (1 year) in (%)	Main features
CNI + MMF + steroids	15–20	Most popular regimen; withdrawal of CNI, steroids or MMF can be undertaken after 3–6 months in low-risk patients
Tacrolimus + AZA + steroids	20–25	Reasonable efficacy; AZA less costly than MMF
CsA + sirolimus + steroids	15–20	CsA or sirolimus must be stopped after 3 months because of nephrotoxicity; excellent 1 year renal function under sirolimus + steroids
Tacrolimus + sirolimus + steroids	10–15	Validation ongoing, but already popular. Apparently not nephrotoxic like the CsA-sirolimus combination
Anti-IL-2R mAb + CNI + MMF + steroids	10	Very low rejection rates; appropriate for patients with immunological risk factors. Allows for the use of low-dose/withdrawal of CNI and/or steroids
ATG/OKT3 + CNI + MMF + steroids	5–10	Very potent combination; appropriate for high-risk patients

and cardiovascular toxicity has resulted in graft and patient loss. Tacrolimus is the second CNI that has been developed and has since been extensively compared to CsA. Before we describe the main trials where CsA and tacrolimus have been compared, it is important to appreciate that the formulation of CsA has evolved over time.

From CsA–Sandimmun to CsA–microemulsion (Neoral®)

Cyclosporine A is a highly lipophilic molecule, and was initially delivered as an olive-oil-based formulation (Sandimmun). Its absorption was bile-dependent with high inter and intra-patient variability, sometimes resulting in insufficient CsA exposure and thus inadequate immunosuppression. A water-miscible micro-emulsion formulation of CsA (Neoral) with improved absorption was introduced in 1996. This formulation resulted in an area under the concentration time curve (AUC) that was 30–50 per cent more than with Sandimmun despite similar 12-h CsA trough concentrations.

Do improved pharmacokinetics translate into fewer rejections? A meta-analysis of nine studies in *de novo* renal transplantation indeed showed that rejection rates decreased from 50 per cent with Sandimmun to 35 per cent with Neoral-based immunosuppression (Shah *et al.* 1999).

Tacrolimus versus CsA–Sandimmun with AZA and steroids

Tacrolimus was initially compared to CsA–Sandimmun in two large, prospective, randomized studies, one performed in the United States and one in Europe (Mayer *et al.* 1997; Pirsch *et al.* 1997). Concomitant immunosuppression consisted of AZA and steroids. Mean blood tacrolimus concentrations in both studies were approximately 15 ng/ml during the first 3 months. Results were similar in the two trials: the proportion of patients who experienced a biopsy-proven rejection episode was close to 45 per cent with CsA–Sandimmun, and 25–30 per cent with tacrolimus ($P < 0.01$). In addition, the incidence of the most severe rejections—those that required rescue therapy with lymphocyte antibodies—was 20 to 25 per cent with CsA–Sandimmun, versus 10 per cent with tacrolimus ($P < 0.01$). Nevertheless, at 1 year, renal function was similar across both arms in the two studies. There were no significant differences in 1-year patient or graft survival, which were approximately 95 per cent and 85–90 per cent respectively.

At the 5-year follow-up, both the US and European trials again showed equivalent patient and graft survival between CsA- and tacrolimus-treated patients (Mayer 2002; Vincenti *et al.* 2002). The lack of improvement in 5-year graft survival in tacrolimus-treated patients in spite of a large reduction in both acute and corticosteroid resistant rejection rates might seem puzzling at first sight. One explanation might be that in both the US and the European trials, as many as 12 per cent of CsA patients crossed over to tacrolimus because of resistant rejection. As discussed below, conversion to tacrolimus has been shown to improve the outcome of grafts suffering from severe rejections.

Tacrolimus versus CsA–Neoral with AZA and steroids

Tacrolimus was directly compared to CsA–Neoral in a large, prospective trial that evaluated as primary endpoint the proportion of patients with biopsy-proven rejection at 6 months (Margreiter 2002). Mean tacrolimus and CsA blood concentrations at 1 month were roughly 12 and 250 ng/ml, thus corresponding to standard guidelines. Concomitant immunosuppression consisted of AZA for 3 months and steroids. While patient and graft survival were similar, the rate of biopsy-proven rejection was significantly less with tacrolimus than with CsA (20 versus 37 per cent, $P < 0.0001$), as was the rate of corticosteroid-resistant rejection episodes (9 per cent with tacrolimus versus 21 per cent with CsA–Neoral, $P < 0.0001$).

Thus, when combined with AZA, there is evidence that tacrolimus when given at a sufficient dose prevents renal graft rejection better than CsA–Neoral.

Tacrolimus versus CsA–Neoral with MMF and steroids

In early studies, tacrolimus and CsA were combined with AZA. Since then, it appeared that combining CsA with MMF and steroids resulted in incidences of biopsy-proven acute and cortico-resistant rejection rates of 20 and 10 per cent, respectively. These incidences are similar to those reported with the tacrolimus–AZA–steroid combination.

How does tacrolimus compare to CsA–Neoral when combined with MMF rather than AZA? One multi-centre trial directly compared three groups of recipients of first cadaveric renal grafts, who were randomized to receive tacrolimus + AZA (1.5–2 mg/kg/day) + steroids, tacrolimus + MMF (2 g/day) + steroids, or CsA–Neoral + MMF (2 g/day) + steroids (Johnson *et al.* 2000). The incidence of rejection was not different across the three groups (15–20 per cent). Cortico-resistant rejections were numerically, but not significantly, less in the tacrolimus–MMF group as compared to the CsA–MMF group (4 versus 11 per cent). These findings were corroborated by two single-centre trials, where the incidence of 1-year AR was ±15 per cent in patients who received either tacrolimus or CsA with MMF and steroids, with no significant difference between both CNI.

Thus, when combined with MMF, there is no convincing evidence for the superiority of tacrolimus over CsA in the prevention of acute or cortico-resistant rejection episodes.

A comparison of efficacy between tacrolimus and CsA: summary

Tacrolimus was more potent than CsA at preventing AR when combined with azathioprine, but this does not translate into superior graft or patient survival at 5 years. The efficacy of both drugs is similar when combined with MMF. It seems likely that some further improvement in CsA–Neoral efficacy will take place with C2 monitoring. Therefore, the choice between these two molecules should be based on their side effects rather than on efficacy.

Side effects of CsA and tacrolimus

The two CNIs differ with respect to cosmetic inconveniences: up to 10 per cent of patients complain of alopecia with tacrolimus, or alternatively of hirsutism and gingival hypertrophy with CsA (Pirsch *et al.* 1997). Neurological side effects such as tremor and paresthesia are distinctly more common under tacrolimus (Mayer *et al.* 1997; Pirsch *et al.* 1997). Several trials have reported higher incidences of deep venous thrombosis with tacrolimus than with CsA (Pirsch *et al.* 1997; Margreiter 2002).

Unfortunately, both drugs are associated with the development of chronic nephrotoxicity. As an example, patients included in the US trial that compared CsA and tacrolimus underwent a renal graft biopsy after 2 years (Solez *et al.* 1998). Histological evidence of CNI nephrotoxicity, such as arterial hyalinosis, was evident in 24 per cent and 17 per cent of patients treated with tacrolimus and CsA, respectively. Along the same line, heart-transplant recipients experience similar primary renal function impairment whether they received tacrolimus or CsA. Therefore, reducing the dose or avoiding CNI may ultimately improve graft and patient survival, and these strategies are actively studied in renal transplantation.

Another major concern is that both CsA and tacrolimus display significant cardiovascular side effects. Tacrolimus can cause diabetes, and CsA is associated with hyperlipidaemia and hypertension.

In early studies, the incidence of *de novo* post-transplant diabetes mellitus (PTDM), which was defined as the requirement of insulin administration for at least 1 month, was higher with tacrolimus (10–20 per cent) than with CsA (2–5 per cent) (Mayer *et al.* 1997; Pirsch *et al.* 1997). The risk factors for developing PTDM include older age, a family history of diabetes, black race, and high doses of tacrolimus or steroids. Although a reduction in tacrolimus and steroid doses frequently makes it possible to stop insulin therapy, up to 50 per cent of patients with *de novo* diabetes require insulin indefinitely, suggesting that this complication is sometimes irreversible. With the use of lower tacrolimus concentrations (10–15 ng/ml), the incidence of PTDM has

been reduced to around 5 per cent, which is numerically, but not significantly, above the figures reported for CsA (Margreiter 2002).

In summary, tacrolimus is diabetogenic mainly among patients exposed to high blood concentrations. Careful monitoring of glucose abnormalities, reduction of tacrolimus and steroid doses, and if necessary withdrawal of tacrolimus should help in limiting the incidence of PTDM.

Patients treated with CsA experience an increase in both total cholesterol and triglycerides of approximately 30 mg/dl, and an increase in LDL cholesterol of approximately 20 mg/dl (Wissing *et al.* 2000). Unlike CsA, tacrolimus does not influence lipid metabolism. Thus, total cholesterol was approximately 30 mg/dl higher among CsA patients as compared to those receiving tacrolimus in several large-scale randomized comparative trials (Pirsch *et al.* 1997; Margreiter 2002). Switching patients from CsA to tacrolimus results in significant reductions in total cholesterol, LDL cholesterol, and triglycerides, with no change in HDL cholesterol (McCune *et al.* 1998).

CsA causes arterial hypertension, with up to 80 per cent of CsA-treated patients requiring antihypertensive therapy. Mechanisms are multiple and may involve renal and systemic vasoconstriction, volume expansion, sympathetic activation, and endothelial dysfunction with increased production of endothelin and decreased generation of NO. While it was initially thought that tacrolimus induced hypertension as much as CsA (Mayer *et al.* 1997; Pirsch *et al.* 1997), it was later observed that conversion from CsA to tacrolimus resulted in a significant reduction of mean arterial pressure of approximately 10 mmHg (Ligtenberg *et al.* 2001).

How should cardiovascular side effects of CNI influence clinical practice? To date, there are no data indicating that one CNI prevents death from cardiovascular events better than the other, so that the ultimate choice may depend on the individual patient risk profile. For instance, patients with definite risk factors for diabetes should probably not receive tacrolimus, while it may be preferable to avoid CsA in those with poorly controlled hypertension or hyperlipaemia.

Monitoring of CsA therapy

Like many other immunosuppressive drugs, CsA has a low therapeutic index and requires individualized monitoring to secure optimal efficacy and reduced toxicity. In addition, there is a substantial between-subject variability in absorption efficiency. Low oral bioavailability has been recognized as an important risk factor for AR. CsA dosages have traditionally been adapted according to the 12 h trough level (C_{min} or C0), a time point initially observed to strongly correlate with 12 h AUC. Since then, however, multiple studies have shown that C0 is poorly correlated with CsA exposure in the early stages of transplantation (Levy *et al.* 2002). Recent work has identified blood CsA measured 2 h after administration (C2) as the best single time-point predictor of CsA exposure (Levy *et al.* 2002). On clinical grounds, results from retrospective trials consistently showed that C2 levels are significantly and positively correlated with the probability of freedom from rejection (Levy *et al.* 2002). The use of C2 monitoring has been strongly encouraged for adult *de novo* renal transplant patients, and tentative target values for C2 according to the time interval from transplantation have been proposed (Levy *et al.* 2002).

It must be stressed, however, that no prospective, randomized trial has yet tested whether adjustment of CsA doses according to C2 results in decreased rejection rates and improved outcomes as compared to C0 monitoring. Of note, as many as 30–50 per cent of patients do not reach target C2 concentrations at days 3–5 (International Neoral Renal

Transplantation Study Group 2002), and will require rapid and sometimes massive CsA dose escalation. The safety of this strategy remains to be established. Obviously, more data are needed to ascertain that the improved accuracy of C2 with respect to CsA exposure translates into improved outcome.

Monitoring of tacrolimus therapy

Tacrolimus, like CsA, displays a variable absorption within and between patients, a narrow therapeutic window, and significant systemic side effects, justifying the use of therapeutic drug monitoring (TDM). C0 levels are widely used in TDM of tacrolimus, and indeed most studies have reported a good correlation ($r^2 > 0.75$) between the 12 h trough and the AUC (0–12) (Kahan et al. 2002).

As observed for CsA, achieving adequate target tacrolimus blood levels during the very first days after transplantation is critical to avoid rejection (Undre et al. 1999).

Mycophenolate mofetil

Mycophenolate mofetil has been extensively studied in association with CNIs and steroids with the aim of reducing the approximately 50 per cent incidence of rejection seen with CsA and steroid dual therapy.

MMF is the semi-synthetic morpholinoethyl ester of mycophenolic acid (MPA), which is the active compound. After oral administration, the ester linkage is cleaved by ubiquitous esterases to yield MPA. The bioavailability of MPA from oral MMF is above 90 per cent. MPA undergoes glucuronidation in the liver to form mycophenolic acid glucuronide (MPAG), which is excreted in urine. MPAG is also secreted into the bile, where it is converted to MPA and undergoes entero-hepatic recirculation. MPA prevents T and B lymphocyte proliferation by inhibiting the enzyme inosine monophosphate dehydrogenase (IMPDH), the rate-limiting enzyme in the de novo pathway for purine synthesis (Allison and Eugui 2000).

Efficacy studies

Three large randomized, prospective, double-blind, controlled trials of high quality compared AZA or placebo to MMF 2 g/day or MMF 3 g/day, in combination with CsA (Sandimmun) and steroids, for the prevention of renal allograft rejection (European Mycophenolate Mofetil Cooperative Study Group 1995; Sollinger for the US Renal Transplant Mycophenolate Mofetil Study Group 1996; The Tricontinental Mycophenolate Mofetil Renal Transplantation Study Group 1996). Altogether, nearly 1500 patients were enrolled. At 1 year, in a pooled efficacy analysis of the three trials, the incidence of biopsy-proven rejection episodes in the AZA/placebo group was 41 per cent, which was significantly greater than the 20 per cent and 17 per cent incidence recorded among patients who received 2 and 3 g of MMF, respectively (Halloran et al. 1997). The incidence of cortico-resistant rejections requiring rescue therapy with antilymphocyte antibodies was significantly less in patients treated with MMF (5 per cent for MMF 3 g; 9 per cent for MMF 2 g; and 20 per cent for AZA/placebo) (Halloran et al. 1997). The incidence of first-semester rejections was only slightly lower with 3 g than with 2 g, and it is widely accepted that the 2 g/day dose represents the best compromise between efficacy and toxicity when MMF is used with CsA. The 3 g/day dose is probably appropriate for high-risk patients. In spite of reduced rejection rates, graft survival was similar (~90 per cent) at 1 year in the MMF 2 g, MMF 3 g, and the AZA/placebo groups (Halloran et al. 1997).

What about long-term outcomes? A simple meta-analysis of the 3 year follow-up reports from the three pivotal studies (Mele and Halloran 2000) indicates that both graft (81 versus 75 per cent, $P = 0.03$) and patient survival (91.4 versus 89.7 per cent, $P = $ NS) were higher for MMF as compared to AZA patients. These numbers are amazingly similar to those reported by the UNOS scientific registry that compared patients taking a CNI with either AZA or MMF at discharge after the transplant hospitalization (Ojo et al. 2000). Indeed, at 4 years, both patient survival (MMF: 91.4 versus AZA: 89.8 per cent, $P = 0.002$) and death-censored graft survival (MMF: 85.6 per cent versus AZA: 81.9 per cent) were higher under MMF (Ojo et al. 2000). A better prevention of both acute and chronic rejection seems to explain the improved outcomes seen with MMF therapy.

Does this mean that MMF should be continued indefinitely? Several studies have documented that discontinuation of MMF after 3 months from a CNI + steroid combination among low-risk patients with stable graft function is associated with no risk (Wuthrich et al. 2000) or only a minor (Sadek et al. 2002) (<5 per cent) risk of AR, with no penalty with respect to graft function or proteinuria in the short term. In the absence of definite data, it may be wise to continue MMF therapy in patients considered to be at higher immunological risk.

Although used initially with CsA, MMF has since been widely prescribed together with tacrolimus, with similar efficacy. However, as many as 30–50 per cent of patients who received 2 g/day of MMF together with tacrolimus discontinued MMF within months because of gastrointestinal intolerance or leucopenia. This withdrawal rate was much higher than when the same dose of MMF was used together with CsA. It was then recognized that the trough levels and the AUC for MPA are 30–50 per cent higher when the same dose of MMF is given with tacrolimus as compared to CsA (Zucker et al. 1997). The reason is that CsA, but not tacrolimus, impedes the entero-hepatic recirculation of MPA.

With these pharmacokinetic data in mind, two dose-finding studies were performed, one in the United States and one in Europe, in order to determine whether the optimal dose of MMF given together with tacrolimus was 1 or 2 g/day. With respect to rejection rates, MMF 2 g/day was found to be superior in the US trial, whereas MMF 1 g/day appeared equivalent to 2 g/day in Europe. This discrepancy is probably due to the fact that patients in the US trial were on average at greater immunological risk than European patients. As for CsA, the dose of MMF should thus take the individual immunological risk into account. Furthermore, the full benefit from the high 2 g/day dose may probably be achieved if given only for the initial post-transplant weeks. In clinical practice, most European centres give MMF at the dose of 1 g/day when combined with tacrolimus, and 2 g/day when given with CsA.

Side effects of MMF

The main side effects of MMF are leucopenia, anaemia, and gastrointestinal intolerance. When given with CsA, the dose of MMF had to be reduced in close to 25 per cent of patients because of leucopenia (The Tricontinental Mycophenolate Mofetil Renal Transplantation Study Group 1996). This figure was not different than with AZA. Diarrhoea was distinctly more frequent with MMF than with AZA. It affects between 10 and 20 per cent of MMF-treated patients and responds most frequently either to splitting the dose into several administrations or reducing the dose (The Tricontinental Mycophenolate Mofetil Renal Transplantation Study Group 1996). Gastrointestinal complications such as oesophagitis, gastritis, and gastro-intestinal haemorrhage were also more frequent in the MMF versus the AZA group (Mele and Halloran 2000). Importantly, and in contrast to other immunosuppressive drugs, MMF does not cause hypertension, hyperlipaemia, diabetes, nephrotoxicity, or osteoporosis. For this reason, MMF has been used in the majority of recent trials that tried to limit the use of CNI and steroids.

Monitoring of MMF therapy

There are at least two reasons that would justify the therapeutic drug monitoring of MMF. First, like other immunosuppressants, a fixed dose of MMF results in a more than 10-fold inter-individual variation in MPA exposure. Second, both retrospective and prospective studies have shown a positive correlation between MPA exposure, as measured by full AUC (0–12) or trough levels, with the incidence of rejection episodes (van Gelder *et al.* 1999).

These observations stimulated the evaluation of limited sampling strategies for the determination of MPA AUC. The correlation between MPA trough levels (C0) and the AUC (0–12) was found to be present but moderate ($r^2 \sim$ 0.5–0.6) (Pawinski *et al.* 2002). A model using three samples (C0, C30min and C2h) gave a better correlation ($r^2 \sim$ 0.8) (Pawinski *et al.* 2002), and seems appropriate for clinical use.

What are the present indications for MMF monitoring? Given the relatively low toxicity of MMF as compared to CsA or tacrolimus, there is no need to monitor MMF therapy in every patient. Furthermore, dose reductions should be dictated by adverse events as they are not significantly correlated to total MPA exposure. Therefore, it seems reasonable to ensure that the patients with the highest immunological risk—young, poor HLA compatibility, immunized, etc.—display sufficient MMF exposure during the early stages of transplantation. In addition, monitoring is also likely to be useful when the discontinuation of CNI or steroids is contemplated in order to secure sufficient immunosuppression by MMF. The tentative target values are approximately 30–40 μg h/ml for MPA AUC (0–12), and above 2 μg/ml for the 12 h trough levels (Shaw *et al.* 2001).

Sirolimus

Sirolimus has a molecular structure similar to tacrolimus, and binds to the same FKBP12 intracellular immunophilin. However, the sirolimus–FKBP12 complex does not bind to calcineurin but to the mammalian target of rapamycin (mTOR), a protein kinase involved in signal transmission through receptors of growth-promoting cytokines such as IL-2. Sirolimus inactivates the kinase activity of mTOR and inhibits cytokine-induced mRNA translation of numerous proteins critical for cell growth. This interrupts cell cycle progression from the G1 to the S phase. Everolimus (RAD) is a second mTOR inhibitor that has been derived from sirolimus through alkylation at position 40. Everolimus is more hydrophilic than sirolimus, has a shorter half-life and greater bioavailability but displays the same immunosuppressive mechanism and adverse effect profile. Like MMF, sirolimus has been associated with CNIs and steroids with the aim of lowering rejection rates.

Efficacy studies

Sirolimus has been compared to AZA (Kahan 2000) or placebo (Macdonald 2001) in two prospective phase III trials in *de novo* renal transplant patients receiving CsA and corticosteroids. In the first study, 719 patients were randomized to AZA 2–3 mg/kg/day ($N = 161$),

sirolimus 2 mg/day ($N = 284$), or sirolimus 5 mg/day ($N = 274$) (Kahan 2000). The incidence of biopsy-proven AR at 12 months was 31 per cent in AZA-treated patients versus 22 per cent in the sirolimus 2 mg/day group ($P < 0.05$) and 15 per cent in the sirolimus 5 mg/day group ($P < 0.001$). The histological severity of ARs was significantly less in both sirolimus groups, as was the proportion of patients requiring antibody therapy for rejection. Unexpectedly, and in spite of the reduced incidence and severity of AR episodes, patients treated with sirolimus displayed a significantly poorer graft function. Creatinine clearance was 67.5 ml/min among AZA-treated patients, 62 ml/min in the sirolimus 2 mg/day group ($P < 0.01$) and 55.5 ml/min in the sirolimus 5 mg/day group ($P < 0.001$).

A similar design was used in a second randomized trial, except that the control group received placebo instead of AZA (Macdonald 2001). The incidence of biopsy proven ARs at 6 months was reduced by about half in patients receiving sirolimus 2 mg/day (24.7 per cent, $P < 0.01$) and 5 mg/day (19.2 per cent, $P < 0.001$) as compared to the placebo group (41.5 per cent). Fewer AR episodes required antibody therapy. Graft survival was above 94 per cent in all three groups ($P = NS$) and there were no significant differences in patient survival. Again graft function was lower in the 5 mg/day group (55.4 ml/min) as compared to the placebo group (62.6 ml/min).

In two large-scale randomized prospective trials, RAD (everolimus) 1.5 and 3 mg/day have been compared to MMF 2 g/day in patients treated with Neoral and steroids. Rejection rates were similar across the three groups (RAD, 17–22 per cent; MMF, 23.5 per cent). Graft survival did not differ between groups in either study and patient survival was consistently greater than 95 per cent. Similar to the CsA–sirolimus combination, graft function was lower in RAD-treated patients than in the MMF group.

The availability of intracellular FKBP12 is sufficient to permit co-administration of tacrolimus and sirolimus without competitive inhibition of drug binding. A large scale ($N = 361$) randomized prospective study compared sirolimus 2 mg/day to MMF 2 g/day in patients receiving tacrolimus and corticosteroids. The incidence of AR at 6 months was 11 per cent in the sirolimus group versus 13 per cent in the MMF group ($P = NS$). Graft function at 6 months was significantly better in patients receiving the tacrolimus–MMF combination (Pcreat 1.44 mg/dl) as compared to the group treated with tacrolimus and sirolimus (Pcreat 1.77 mg/dl) (Gonwa *et al.* 2003).

In conclusion, the combination of CNIs with sirolimus provides potent immunosuppression with an incidence of AR comparable to the CNI–MMF combination. The CNI–sirolimus combination is hampered by nephrotoxicity, for reasons unclear to date. As a result, the CsA–sirolimus combination has received regulatory approval in Europe only for the initial three post-transplantation months, after which either CsA or sirolimus must be discontinued.

Side effects

Sirolimus causes a dose-dependent increase in plasma cholesterol and triglycerides that requires lipid-lowering therapy in approximately two-thirds of patients (Kahan 2000; Johnson *et al.* 2001; Macdonald 2001; Gonwa *et al.* 2002). Despite therapy, mean total cholesterol at 12 months is 230–240 mg/dl with CsA–sirolimus–Pred, and 240–260 mg/dl with sirolimus–Pred dual therapy. Mean triglyceride ranged between 200 and 270 mg/dl in various studies (Johnson *et al.* 2001; Gonwa *et al.* 2002). Sirolimus has myelosuppressive properties resulting in leucopenia, thrombopenia, and anaemia. Although rarely a severe problem when sirolimus is combined with CNIs, thrombopenia and anaemia have been reported as adverse events in nearly half of the patients receiving sirolimus in association with AZA or MMF (Groth *et al.* 1999; Kreis *et al.* 2000). The antiproliferative and antifibrotic properties of sirolimus probably account for an increased incidence of delayed wound healing and formation of lymphoceles. In the pivotal US study, lymphoceles were observed in 12–15 per cent of patients receiving sirolimus versus 3 per cent of patients receiving AZA (Kahan 2000).

Early experience with sirolimus was complicated by a high incidence of *Pneumocystis carinii* pneumonia that can be prevented by trimethoprim–sulfamethoxazole prophylaxis (Kahan 2000; Johnson *et al.* 2001; Macdonald 2001; Gonwa *et al.* 2002). Sirolimus is a rare cause of drug-induced interstitial pneumonitis, which responds favourably to dose reduction or withdrawal of the drug (Morelon *et al.* 2001).

Sirolimus also triggers miscellaneous adverse events that can cause significant patient discomfort such as arthralgia and bone pain (20 per cent) (Groth *et al.* 1999; Macdonald 2001), painful aphtous mouth ulcers (up to 20 per cent) and epistaxis (up to 10 per cent).

In initial experience, everolimus shares the same adverse event profile as sirolimus.

Monitoring of sirolimus and everolimus therapy

Similar to tacrolimus, sirolimus has a relatively poor oral bioavailability (average 14 per cent) and a T_{max} of 1–2 h. The drug has a large volume of distribution and a long terminal half-life of approximately 60 h. The large inter-subject and intra-subject variability of drug exposure and the narrow therapeutic window mandates therapeutic drug monitoring. There is a very good correlation between 24 h trough levels and full AUC ($r^2 \sim 0.8$). In association with CsA, sirolimus trough levels of less than 6 ng/ml have been associated with an increased incidence of AR while levels greater than 15 ng/ml were associated with more frequent adverse events. Similar to sirolimus, everolimus also requires therapeutic drug monitoring by liquid chromatography. An increased incidence of AR has been observed in patients with trough levels less than 3.5 ng/ml (Kovarik *et al.* 2002).

The use of MMF or sirolimus as adjunct to CNIs: summary

Today, most centres have moved away from dual CsA + steroids or triple CsA + AZA + steroids therapy, and combine either MMF or sirolimus to a CNI and steroids. Both MMF and sirolimus/everolimus decrease rejection rate from approximately 50 per cent to 15–20 per cent when added to CNI and steroids. What are the main pros and cons for the use of either drug? At 4 years, the CNI + MMF regimen resulted in improved graft and patient survival; such data are not available yet for the CNI/sirolimus combination. Because of nephrotoxicity, the CsA + sirolimus combination must be discontinued after 3 months; nevertheless, discontinuation of CsA in this setting is safe, and patients maintained with sirolimus + steroids had excellent renal function at 1 year. The combination of sirolimus with tacrolimus shows promise, both in terms of efficacy and safety, but definite results are pending. Therefore, there is no strong argument in favour of one or another strategy, and the choice should probably be tailored to individual patient's conditions. For instance, a renal transplant candidate with serious digestive problems or leucopenia should probably not receive MMF, while a recipient with severe hyperlipaemia should probably be spared sirolimus/everolimus.

Antilymphocyte preparations

Interleukin-2 receptor antibodies

Upon activation, T cells up-regulate the third chain of the IL-2R, the IL-2Rα chain [CD25, T-activation (Tac) antigen]. IL-2 binds with high affinity to the trimeric IL-2$\alpha\beta\gamma$ complex, and triggers T-cell division. Two monoclonal antibodies (mAbs) targetting the α-chain of the IL-2 receptor have recently been made available in clinical transplantation: basiliximab (Simulect®) and daclizumab (Zenapax®). Their main mechanism of action is the inhibition of IL-2-induced T-cell proliferation. Basiliximab is a chimeric mAb that was engineered by grafting the entire Fab variable regions of the parental mouse Ab on the constant regions of a human IgG$_1$ molecule. Daclizumab is a humanized IgG$_1$ mAb that retains from its murine anti-Tac parent only the mouse hypervariable antigen-binding sequences.

The anti-IL-2R mAbs exhibit several features that make them more specific and less toxic than OKT3 and ATG. First, in contrast to OKT3 and ATG that target all T cells, the anti-IL-2R mAbs bind only to activated T cells that have up-regulated the α chain of the IL-2 receptor. Therefore, only T cells involved in the rejection process are blocked, while the bulk of other naive and memory T cells are not affected. Second, chimeric and humanized antibodies have a much longer half-life than rodent antibodies—of in the order of weeks rather than days. Third, the disappearance of the largest part of xenogeneic epitopes considerably reduces the immunogenicity of chimeric and humanized mAbs. Although anti-idiotypic antibodies may still arise, sensitization rates have been consistently below 2 per cent, as compared to 20–50 per cent among patients treated with the murine mAb OKT3. Finally, since the α chain of the IL-2 receptor is unable to give rise to an activation signal, antibodies against the IL-2R do not trigger the cytokine release syndrome that occurs with OKT3 or ATG, and are, therefore, very well tolerated.

Anti-IL-2R mAbs with CsA and steroids

Three large, prospective, randomized, double-blind, placebo-controlled studies have compared the anti-IL-2R mAbs to placebo in patients receiving CsA (Neoral) and steroids (Nashan *et al.* 1997, 1999; Kahan *et al.* 1999). The results were remarkably consistent across the trials: there was a significant 30–40 per cent reduction in the incidence of biopsy-proven AR at 6 months (controls: 45–50 versus 28–35 per cent with anti-IL-2R). Likewise, the incidence of resistant rejection treated with antilymphocyte antibodies was lowered by approximately 50 per cent. Nevertheless, overall, a third of the patients experienced a rejection episode during effective IL-2R blockade, suggesting that T cells might be activated by cytokines distinct from IL2, such as IL15. The remarkable observation was that both basiliximab and daclizumab were perfectly tolerated, with adverse event profiles comparable to that of the placebo. No patient discontinued the study drug because of side effects. There was no increase in cancer or infections, and in fact, the incidence of CMV infection was consistently lower in the anti-IL-2R groups.

Anti-IL-2R mAbs with CsA, AZA, and steroids

The efficacy and safety of basiliximab and daclizumab in patients receiving immunosuppressive triple therapy with CsA, AZA, and steroids was examined in two prospective, randomized, double-blind, placebo-controlled studies (Vincenti *et al.* 1998; Ponticelli *et al.* 2001). In the control groups, biopsy-proven rejection occurred in 35 per cent (Vincenti *et al.* 1998) and 29 per cent of patients. Again, daclizumab and basiliximab significantly reduced rejection rates with similar efficacy (reduction in rejection rates: 37 per cent for daclizumab and 36 per cent for basiliximab). The incidence of antibody-treated rejection was reduced by 43 per cent with daclizumab, and by 46 per cent with basiliximab. Safety and tolerance were similar to placebo.

Is there any evidence that anti-IL-2R mAbs improved patient or graft survival? While none of the five trials mentioned above was powered to do so, a simple meta-analysis indicates a trend in favour of anti-IL-2R treatment at 1 year. Longer follow-up and registry data with large numbers of patients should help to clarify this issue.

Anti-IL-2R mAbs with a CNI, MMF, and steroids

No sufficiently powered efficacy trial compared an anti-IL-2R to placebo in patients receiving a CNI, MMF, and steroids with a reduction in rejection rates as primary outcome. Nevertheless, a meta-analysis of published data reporting on 703 patients at low-immunological risk showed that rejection incidence was 9.2 per cent, graft survival 95 per cent, and patient survival 98 per cent at 6–12 months (Ciancio *et al.* 2002; Lebranchu *et al.* 2002; Lawen *et al.* 2003), indicating that this regimen allows for very low rejection rates and excellent safety.

In summary, anti-IL-2R antibodies demonstrate an excellent efficacy/toxicity ratio in renal transplantation. They reduce rejection rates by 30–40 per cent whatever the associated immunosuppression with no apparent toxicity. Although daclizumab and basiliximab have not been compared head to head, evidence to date suggests they are equally immunosuppressive. The very low rejection rate observed with the regimen combining an anti-IL-2R mAb with a CNI, MMF, and steroids has been a starting point for several studies that evaluated the reduction/avoidance of CNI, steroids, or both.

OKT3 and ATG

OKT3 is a monoclonal mouse antibody directed against the CD3 complex, a series of proteins associated with the lymphocyte T antigen receptor. Polyclonal ATG (for antithymocyte globulins) formulations are obtained by immunizing rabbits or horses by means of human lymphocytes. They contain antibodies targeting numerous membrane antigens, some of which are solely present on T cells, such as CD3, CD4, or CD8, whereas others, like the adhesion molecules CD11b and CD18, are also found on other circulating cells. This probably explains the leucopenia and thrombopenia that may develop during ATG treatment. The principal mechanism of action of OKT3 and ATG consists of T lymphocyte depletion from blood. OKT3 and ATG trigger a cytokine release syndrome caused by transient T-cell activation after the first dose (Abramowicz *et al.* 1989). Both OKT3 and ATG can induce sensitization, resulting in neutralization and loss of efficacy due to anti-idiotypic antibodies in patients receiving OKT3 (Abramowicz *et al.* 1999) and serum sickness due to immune complexes in patients receiving ATG.

The efficacy of OKT3 and ATG in treating AR has led to their use for 1–2 weeks during the early post-operative period. This strategy was called 'induction therapy'. Meta-analysis of prospective, randomized studies (Szczech *et al.* 1997) as well as data from scientific registries (Opelz 1995) indicate that ATG and OKT3 induction not only considerably reduced the incidence of rejection, but also increased long-term

graft survival by approximately 5 per cent among low-risk patients receiving CsA (Sandimmun) + AZA + steroids. OKT3/ATG induction was most beneficial in high-immunological risk patients, as improvements of long-term renal graft survival reached 15 per cent and even more among blacks, immunized, and retransplanted patients, in those with two HLA-DR mismatches or receiving kidneys with long cold ischaemia times (Abramowicz *et al.* 1999).

Only few studies provide data of OKT3/ATG induction in patients receiving the combination of CNI, MMF, and steroids. Aggregated results show a 1 year rejection rate of 10–15 per cent with this type of quadruple therapy, with no particular safety concern (Lebranchu *et al.* 2002).

Antilymphocyte preparations: summary

Quadruple therapy with an anti-IL-2R mAb or OKT3/ATG and a CNI, MMF, and steroids allows for very low rejection rates. In low-risk patients, anti-IL-2R mAbs are probably the best choice because of their favourable toxicity profile. Nevertheless, it is must be appreciated that patients with high immunological risk, such as those who have previously lost one or more grafts or those who are highly sensitized to HLA antigens, were not included in the above-mentioned clinical trials. Prospective studies are ongoing to compare anti-IL-2R mAbs with OKT3 or ATG in high-risk patients. Until then, ATG or OKT3 induction with a CNI, MMF, and steroids is the preferred strategy in this indication, because of the definite survival benefit observed in high-risk groups in the era of sandimmun and AZA.

Calcineurin inhibitors withdrawal and avoidance

Increasing evidence indicates that the toxic effects of CNIs contribute to kidney graft loss by cardiovascular death and chronic allograft nephropathy. In fact, these are currently the two major causes of late graft loss. Restricting the use of CNIs to the first months after transplantation, when rejection is more prevalent, would take advantage of adequate early immunosuppression while avoiding long-term vascular and renal toxicity. Attempts to discontinue CsA have been actively pursued, first by switching to AZA, and later to MMF and sirolimus.

CNI withdrawal

CNI withdrawal under AZA

Several groups have studied the impact of CsA withdrawal in stable renal transplant patients on maintenance therapy with AZA and corticosteroids. These results have been recently pooled in a meta-analysis (Kasiske *et al.* 2000). Patients withdrawn from CsA experienced a significant, 11 per cent higher incidence in ARs as compared to patients who remained on CsA. However, there was no difference in the incidence of graft loss. Two large, prospective randomized studies have followed patients for up to 10 years (Hollander *et al.* 1995; MacPhee *et al.* 1998). Patient survival and death-censored graft survival tended to be better after CsA withdrawal. Patients in both studies also had significantly improved graft function, less requirement for antihypertensive medication, and a reduction in cardiovascular mortality by about half (Hollander *et al.* 1995; MacPhee *et al.* 1998).

Despite these favourable reports, systematic switching to AZA has not become routine practice, mainly because of the fear of an AR in an otherwise stable patient. The availability of more potent drugs such as MMF and sirolimus has rekindled the interest in CsA discontinuation.

CNI withdrawal under MMF

Several prospective randomized studies have been conducted to investigate whether MMF had the potential to further increase the safety and feasibility of CNI withdrawal (Abramowicz *et al.* 2002; Schnuelle *et al.* 2002; Smak Gregoor *et al.* 2002). Smak Gregoor *et al.* (2002) randomized 212 patients under CsA–MMF–Pred triple therapy and stable graft function at 6 months to CsA withdrawal ($N = 63$), steroid withdrawal ($N = 76$), or continuous triple therapy ($N = 73$). CsA withdrawal was rapid with a 50 per cent reduction at randomization and complete withdrawal 2 weeks later. Prednisone was increased to 0.15 mg/kg in the withdrawal groups. Fourteen patients (22 per cent) rejected after CsA withdrawal compared to only one on triple therapy ($P = 0.0001$). Furthermore, nine out of 14 AR episodes were histologically moderate or severe (BANFF $\geq$ II) and six required treatment with antilymphocyte antibodies. CsA withdrawal did not result in improved graft function as compared to triple therapy.

Schnuelle *et al.* (2002) adopted a more cautious approach in their CsA withdrawal protocol. Low-risk patients with stable graft function 3 months after transplantation on CsA–MMF–Pred were randomized to either CsA ($N = 44$) or MMF ($N = 40$) withdrawal. CsA withdrawal was progressive over 9 weeks and oral steroids were increased to 25 mg/day during taper. The incidence of AR was low after withdrawal of either CsA (11.3 per cent) or MMF (5 per cent) ($P = NS$). Graft function was significantly improved in the CsA withdrawal group (GFR 72 ml/min versus 61 ml/min, $P < 0.05$). CsA withdrawal was also associated with a significantly lower arterial blood pressure and significantly reduced use of lipid lowering agents.

A similar protocol was used in a large multicentre CsA withdrawal study (Abramowicz *et al.* 2002). Patients transplanted between 12 and 30 months and having stable graft function under CsA-based immunosuppression were randomized to either CsA withdrawal ($N = 85$) or continuing triple therapy ($N = 85$). CsA dose was tapered by one-third every 6 weeks. Prednisolone could be increased at the discretion of the investigator to up to 25 mg/day during the withdrawal phase. Rejection incidence was 10.6 per cent in the withdrawal group versus 2.4 per cent in the triple therapy group ($P < 0.05$). All AR episodes occurred late in the taper period or early after CsA withdrawal. Interestingly, the majority of patients who rejected received less than 2 g/day of MMF and/or less than 10 mg/day of prednisone at the time of rejection, suggesting that some might have been under-immunosuppressed after CsA withdrawal. Graft function was significantly improved in the withdrawal group when analysis was restricted to per-protocol patients who had not experienced episodes of rejection and remained on a CsA-free regimen. There was no difference in graft function when the intent-to-treat populations were compared.

It is noteworthy that MPA exposure has not been assessed in any of these trials. One may speculate that proceeding with complete CsA discontinuation only in those patients who showed sufficient MPA exposure might have further reduced the incidence of rejection. Furthermore, a slow discontinuation of CsA and a transient increase of steroid dose might help to successfully discontinue CsA under MMF therapy.

CNI withdrawal under sirolimus

A large-scale randomized prospective trial has investigated whether CsA could be withdrawn after 3 months in patients treated with CsA,

sirolimus, and steroids, leaving patients on dual therapy with sirolimus and steroids (Johnson *et al.* 2001). Patients were randomized to either continuing triple therapy ($N = 215$) or CsA withdrawal ($N = 215$). In the withdrawal group, the daily sirolimus dose was increased in order to attain trough levels between 20 and 30 ng/ml, and CsA was progressively withdrawn in 4–6 weeks. Between 3 months and 1 year, 10 per cent of patients experienced AR in the withdrawal group versus 4 per cent in the triple therapy group ($P < 0.05$). All AR episodes in the withdrawal group were mild or moderate. CsA withdrawal was associated with a significant increase in GFR (63 ml/min at 12 months versus 57 ml/min in the triple therapy group; $P < 0.001$). Similar to other trials, CsA withdrawal was followed by a significant reduction in the requirement for antihypertensive medications. In spite of the low incidence of AR and excellent graft function, the proportion of patients that discontinued sirolimus was significantly higher in the withdrawal group (27 versus 18 per cent, $P < 0.05$). It must be kept in mind that CsA interferes with sirolimus metabolism, so that CsA withdrawal reduces sirolimus exposure (Johnson *et al.* 2001). As a matter of fact, a significant proportion of patients who rejected during CsA withdrawal had sirolimus trough levels less than 12 ng/ml and CsA trough levels less than 50 ng/ml (Johnson *et al.* 2001). Therefore, close monitoring of sirolimus levels and rapid dose adjustments are needed in this setting. A second trial of smaller size has confirmed that CsA withdrawal during the third month is safe among patients receiving sirolimus (Gonwa *et al.* 2002). Among black patients, who are at increased immunological risk, CsA withdrawal did not increase the incidence of acute rejection but caused a marked improvement in graft function (Pcreat 1.6 mg/dl versus 2.7 mg/dl among black patients on triple therapy; $P = 0.01$) (Gonwa *et al.* 2002).

CNI avoidance

MMF + steroids, with ATG or anti-IL-2R induction

Besides small-scale trials showing satisfactory results with the association of ATG induction with MMF and steroids without CNI, the main trial exploring this strategy involved the combination of the anti-IL-2R daclizumab with MMF (3 g/day) and steroids, which has been evaluated in 98 low-risk recipients (Vincenti *et al.* 2001b). Biopsy-proven rejection had developed in 48 per cent of patients at 6 months. A CNI had to be given to two-thirds of the patients, predominantly because of rejection. In spite of excellent 1 year patient and graft survival (>95 per cent) and adequate graft function at 1 year, the widespread use of this regimen is not feasible because of the high incidence of AR and the difficult tolerability of the 3 g/day MMF dose.

Sirolimus + AZA or MMF + steroids

Sirolimus, in association with AZA and steroids, has been compared to CsA in a prospective, randomized study (Groth *et al.* 1999). The incidence of rejection proved to be similar: nearly 40 per cent in the two arms. The serum creatinine was lower in the sirolimus group at 4 months (1.4 mg/dl versus 1.7 mg/dl in the CsA arm) and at 1 year (1.3 versus 1.5 in the CsA arm). These encouraging results led to a second clinical trial in which sirolimus was once again compared to CsA, but this time in association with MMF and steroids (Kreis *et al.* 2000). Both clinical rejections (sirolimus, 50 per cent; CsA, 29 per cent) and biopsy-proven rejections (sirolimus, 27 per cent; CsA, 18 per cent) were more frequent among sirolimus patients. In spite of this, at 1 year, renal function was slightly better among patients receiving sirolimus (serum creatinine: 1.4 mg/dl, versus 1.6 mg/dl with CsA). However, when administered at doses required to maintain trough levels of 20–30 ng/ml, the toxicity profile of sirolimus is substantial. Forty-three per cent of patients receiving sirolimus discontinued from the protocol (Kreis *et al.* 2000). Therefore, it is unlikely that the use of the sirolimus + MMF + steroids association during the early post-transplant period will become widespread.

Sirolimus + MMF + steroids, with IL-2R antibodies induction therapy

In order to further reduce the incidence of AR and the dosage of sirolimus, basiliximab anti-IL-R mAb has been added to sirolimus and MMF in a small prospective study (Flechner *et al.* 2002). Sixty-one patients were randomized to sirolimus (trough levels 10–12 ng/ml, $N = 30$) or Neoral (trough levels 200–250 ng/ml, $N = 31$). All patients received basiliximab, MMF 2 g/day and steroids. The incidence of biopsy-confirmed AR at 1 year was 6.4 per cent in sirolimus-treated and 16.6 per cent in CsA-treated patients. Creatinine clearance at 1 year was significantly better in sirolimus-treated patients (81 versus 61 ml/min; $P < 0.001$). Adverse events were few and comparable in both groups. The results of this study need confirmation in larger trials but combining anti-IL-2R induction with sirolimus and MMF seems a very promising immunosuppressive therapy.

CNI withdrawal and avoidance: summary

CNI withdrawal/avoidance is a highly valuable goal in renal transplantation, but to date long-term follow-up figures are available only for AZA-based regimen and show essentially equivalent, but not superior, graft survival. It is likely that what is gained with respect to graft failure from CNI nephrotoxicity is lost from increased rates of chronic rejection in AZA-treated patients. AR rates after CNI withdrawal appear to be lower in patients switched to MMF or sirolimus, but obviously the possible benefits of this strategy will only be fully appreciated in a decade. The same is true for CNI avoidance regimens where antibody induction is given together with sirolimus + MMF. In the meantime, it seems premature to propose systematic CsA withdrawal/avoidance to all patients. Rather, this strategy is likely to be of particular benefit in low-risk recipients who receive poorly functioning kidneys, or who develop severe CNI toxicities.

Steroid withdrawal and avoidance

In the early days of transplantation, steroids, besides AZA, were the only immunosuppressive drugs available, and they were given in rather high doses. Steroids, like CsA, adversely impact cardiovascular risk factors such as diabetes, hypertension, and hyperlipaemia. In addition, steroids cause osteoporosis, amyotrophy, cataracts, impaired wound healing, and cosmetic changes. Steroids are, therefore, considered to reduce both the quantity and the quality of life after renal transplantation. This has prompted many investigators, as soon as CsA became available, to study the withdrawal of steroids, or to try to avoid them completely after renal transplantation.

Steroid withdrawal

A recent meta-analysis examined 10 randomized, controlled studies that compared prednisone withdrawal with prednisone maintenance in patients receiving CsA-based immunosuppression (Kasiske *et al.* 2000).

AR was increased by 14 per cent ($P < 0.001$) and there were 40 per cent more graft failures after steroid withdrawal ($P = 0.012$). Besides typical AR, some patients may also have developed insidious increases in plasma creatinine and proteinuria after steroid discontinuation, probably as correlates of chronic rejection. Concerns about steroid withdrawal have been largely influenced by the Canadian multicentre trial, the largest study on steroid withdrawal so far. While graft survival was similar after 2 years, a significant decrease in allograft survival became apparent in the steroid withdrawal group at 5 years, underscoring the need for long-term follow-up in this setting (Sinclair 1992).

Nevertheless, these somewhat disappointing results by no means prove that steroids represent an essential ingredient of a successful immunosuppressive regimen. An alternative explanation is that in most of the former trials, patients were left under-immunosuppressed after steroid withdrawal, for reasons such as immunosuppression with Sandimmun instead of Neoral, low CsA target levels (~100 ng/ml), or the use of only low doses of AZA. The fact that classical immunological risk factors such as HLA-B and DR mismatches, black race, previous rejection, and previous transplantation were found to be predictors of AR and/or graft loss after steroid withdrawal in various trials lend support to the hypothesis that many patients were left under-immunosuppressed after steroid withdrawal. What about withdrawal trials in patients receiving MMF and/or tacrolimus? A recent European multi-centre trial has shown that, in association with CsA and MMF, the use of reduced steroid doses for 3 months followed by complete steroid withdrawal was associated with only a modest increase in the incidence of biopsy-proven ARs (25 per cent with reduced doses/withdrawal, versus 15 per cent in controls at 1 year) (Vanrenterghem *et al.* 2000). Most of the increase in rejection in the reduced-dose steroid group took place during the first 15 days. One-year serum creatinine was the same in both groups, and patients who received reduced steroid doses enjoyed lower blood pressure, lower lipid levels, and better preservation of bone density. Nevertheless, a similar study performed in the United States revealed that black patients on CsA and MMF (2 g/day) still experienced high rates of AR (~45 per cent) after steroid withdrawal (Ahsan *et al.* 1999), confirming that higher MMF doses may be necessary to prevent rejection in this group of patients.

Steroid avoidance

Two uncontrolled studies used ATG induction together with MMF and CsA (Cantarovich *et al.* 2000; Birkeland 2001). One group reported poor tolerance to ATG, with serum sickness involving the kidney in some patients (Cantarovich *et al.* 2000). In the other study, the incidence of rejection was quite low (15 per cent), but median serum creatinine reached 2.8 mg/dl at 3 years, probably reflecting the high doses of CsA used throughout the study. In two small-scale trials, one controlled (Vincenti *et al.* 2001a) and the other not (Cole *et al.* 2001), anti-IL-2R mAbs were administered together with CsA and MMF. Rejection rates were between 20 and 25 per cent, with serum creatinine at 1 year being 1.5 (Vincenti *et al.* 2001a) to 1.8 mg/dl (Cole *et al.* 2001). These preliminary results are encouraging and call for further controlled trials with long-term follow-up.

Steroid withdrawal and avoidance: summary

With present immunosuppressive drugs, steroid withdrawal/avoidance can be performed with no obvious penalty with regard to AR in low immunological risk patients, provided they receive sufficient immunosuppression. Withdrawal of corticosteroids has short-term beneficial effects on clinical and metabolic parameters, but long-term follow-up of graft survival is essential for validation of this strategy. In practice, steroid withdrawal/avoidance is likely to benefit mainly low-risk patients with co-morbidities such as diabetes, obesity, or osteoporosis. Furthermore, this approach should probably not be attempted in patients with proteinuria, unsatisfactory graft function, or those who required steroids for their primary kidney disease.

Treatment of acute allograft rejection

The widely validated Banff scheme of renal allograft pathology defines three types of AR (Racusen et al. 1999). Type I consists in infiltration of the interstitium and tubuli by mononuclear cells, without arteritis. Type II rejections are characterized by mild to moderate arteritis, while type III rejections show transmural arteritis and/or arterial fibrinoid change and necrosis of medial smooth muscle cells.

The initial treatment of an AR episode should involve methylprednisolone boluses (250, 500, or 1000 mg) for 3–5 days. This treatment is expected to reverse most episodes, and is given as first-line therapy to the vast majority of patients. The most important advantages of corticosteroids are their ease of administration and low cost. Successful responses are more common in recipients experiencing a Banff grade I or II rejection (92 versus 75 per cent for Banff grade III, $P = 0.009$) (Gaber et al. 1998). Success of steroid treatment is identifiable as early as day 2 or 3 of therapy by the fact that serum creatinine will increase only minimally or already decrease, and will return to rejection value or less by day 5. It may also be of interest to switch patients to MMF and/or tacrolimus at the time of rejection, as both drugs significantly reduced the need for antilymphocyte agents to treat refractory rejection as well as the incidence of recurrent rejection (The Mycophenolate Mofetil Acute Renal Rejection Study Group 1998; Dudley 2001).

Although the use of ATG/ALG or OKT3 as first-line therapy results in rejection reversal rates higher than with steroids (Ortho Multicentre Transplant Study Group 1985; Kamath et al. 1997), their adverse events and cost have led many centres to reserve these agents for initially severe (Banff IIB or III) or steroid-resistant rejections. A rejection can be considered resistant to steroids when serum creatinine continues to increase by day 3 of methylprednisolone boluses, and continues to rise unless treated with a different antirejection therapy.

The polyclonal rabbit ATG preparations (Sangstat® and Fresenius®) and OKT3 reverse corticosteroid-resistant AR episodes in more than 60 per cent of patients, and are considered of equivalent potency.

Besides antilymphocyte agents, limited experience has shown that both tacrolimus and MMF can be of value as therapy of refractory rejection.

Finally, intravenous immunoglobulin therapy can be successful in steroid and antilymphocyte antibody resistant rejections as suggested by preliminary evidence from small-scale trials (Casadei et al. 2001; Luke et al. 2001).

In summary, AR of histologically mild (Banff I) or moderate (Banff II) severity should be treated by steroid boluses, and a switch to tacrolimus and/or MMF might be considered. Histologically severe (Banff III), cortico-resistant, and recurrent rejections should be treated with rabbit ATG or OKT3.

Treatment of chronic allograft nephropathy

Chronic allograft nephropathy (CAN) is a clinico-pathological entity characterized by progressive loss of graft function and chronic histological lesions such as tubular atrophy, interstitial fibrosis, glomerular sclerosis, and graft vessels arteriosclerosis. The development of CAN is the common final pathway of numerous types of graft injury that can be either immune-mediated such as chronic rejection, or alloantigen-independent such as advanced donor age, brain death, reperfusion injury, and CNI toxicity. The relative contribution of non-immune and immune mechanisms to graft damage varies in individual patients, a fact that is important for clinical decision making and is not appropriately reflected by the single diagnostic entity of 'CAN' (Halloran 2002). A predominant immune mechanism is often attested by the presence of circulating antidonor antibodies while histology, in addition to the non-specific CAN lesions described above, may show characteristic features such as obliterative endarteritis and transplant glomerulopathy. This diagnosis is further supported by the presence of the C4d component of complement in the peritubular capillaries as a marker for antibody-mediated injury (Regele et al. 2002) and a history of multiple or vascular rejection. The lesions typical of CNI nephrotoxicity are hyalinosis of the glomerular afferent arteriole and band fibrosis (Bennett et al. 1996).

A first therapeutic approach in CAN is to reduce or even completely withdraw calcineurin inhibitors with the rationale that CNI nephrotoxicity exceeds the benefit of immunosuppression. One trial was restricted to patients with CNI toxicity, excluding those with histological evidence of either acute or chronic rejection (Mourad et al. 1998). Among patients who received CsA, AZA, and steroids, a 50 per cent reduction of CsA maintenance dose was associated with an increase of GFR from 40 to 47 ml/min ($P < 0.05$). Only one in 23 patients had an episode of AR during the 2 year follow-up. Weir et al. (2001) conducted an uncontrolled study with a mean follow-up of 2 years of CNI reduction ($N = 100$) or withdrawal ($N = 18$) among patients with deteriorating graft function and biopsy-proven CAN. The proportion of patients with obliterative endarteritis and transplant glomerulopathy was not specified. Overall, CNI reduction and withdrawal were associated with stabilization or improvement of graft function in approximately 50 per cent of patients. Complete withdrawal of CNI was followed by stabilization or improvement of graft function among 91 per cent of patients. There was a 15 per cent incidence of mostly mild or borderline AR (Weir et al. 2001). In the 'MMF Creeping Creatinine Study Group', patients with a history of progressively increasing creatinine were randomized to MMF treatment and CsA withdrawal or maintenance CsA. Preliminary results show that after CsA withdrawal ($N = 73$), 58 per cent had stable or improving graft function versus 30 per cent in the CsA group ($N = 70$) ($P = 0.002$). Furthermore, mean GFR increased from 37 to 43 ml/min in the CsA withdrawal group but decreased from 36.9 to 34.4 ml/min in the CsA group (Tedesco 2002).

In practice, CNIs should probably be withdrawn or strongly reduced when the medical history and graft biopsy suggests that the immune component in graft dysfunction is minimal. MMF should be maintained at 2 g/day and prednisolone not decreased to less than

0.1 mg/kg/day. Furthermore, the subpopulation of patients who do not show improved graft function after CsA withdrawal should be closely monitored and considered for a control biopsy to exclude rejection.

In addition to modification of the immunosuppressive regimen, patients with CAN should receive aggressive treatment of cardiovascular risk factors such as hypertension and hyperlipidaemia, which may contribute to graft loss from CAN, particularly among patients who have experienced previous AR episodes (Wissing *et al.* 2000). Proteinuria is a major predictor of both graft loss and patient death (Roodnat *et al.* 2001). The ability of inhibitors of the renin–angiotensin system to reduce proteinuria and to slow progression of chronic renal failure in primary kidney disease emphasizes the need for controlled prospective trials of ACE-inhibitors or sartans in patients with CAN. Preliminary evidence suggests that ACE-inhibitors or sartans might help to prevent both allograft failure and patient death in patients with CAN. With regard to lipid lowering therapy, a large prospective placebo-controlled study has shown that fluvastatin use by renal transplant patients was associated with a statistically significant reduction in cardiac death and myocardial infarction (Holdaas *et al.* 2003). While there is currently no definite evidence that statin therapy slows the progression of CAN, their use should be encouraged in this patient population.

Conclusions

Newly introduced immunosuppressive drugs have markedly changed our perspectives in renal transplantation. AR that was in the past plaguing the field has now become an oddity. The expansion of choices in the immunosuppressive agent armamentarium has provided kidney transplant professionals with the ability to tailor therapy to match individual risks. The initial post-transplantation immunosuppressive regimen should be selected first according to immunological risk. Once the AR period is over, the immunosuppressive regimen should be tailored according to the individual tolerability and cardiovascular safety. For instance, if renal graft function is suboptimal, the obvious move is to reduce or discontinue the calcineurin inhibitor and keep the patient on a combination of MMF or sirolimus and steroids. If the patients develops hyperlipidaemia, drugs such as cyclosporin and sirolimus should be avoided if possible. A history or the development of diabetes or glucose intolerance speaks against the introduction or maintenance of tacrolimus and steroids in the regimen.

It remains true, however, that as long as patients take immunosuppressive drugs, they will continue to face potentially fatal opportunistic infections, cancers, and cardiovascular events. Understandably, much effort is currently being devoted to tolerance-inducing protocols, which should allow a recipient to tolerate the graft antigens while still recognizing and eliminating other pathogenic environmental antigens. It is not unrealistic to expect that within 5–10 years, transplant patients will, following a period of tolerance induction, be able to live without or with only minimal immunosuppressants.

References

Abramowicz, D., Wissing, K. M., and Broeders, N. (1999). Induction therapy with anti-CD3 antibodies. *Current Opinion in Organ Transplantation* **4**, 312–317.

Abramowicz, D. *et al.* (1989). Release of tumor necrosis factor, interleukin-2, and gamma-interferon in serum after injection of OKT3 monoclonal antibody in kidney transplant recipients. *Transplantation* **47**, 606–608.

Abramowicz, D. *et al.* (2002). Cyclosporine withdrawal from a mycophenolate mofetil-containing immunosuppressive regimen in stable kidney transplant recipients: a randomized, controlled study. *Transplantation* **74**, 1725–1734.

Ahsan, N. *et al.* (1999). Prednisone withdrawal in kidney transplant recipients on cyclosporine and mycophenolate mofetil—a prospective randomized study. Steroid Withdrawal Study Group. *Transplantation* **68**, 1865–1874.

Allison, A. C. and Eugui, E. M. (2000). Mycophenolate mofetil and its mechanisms of action. *Immunopharmacology* **47**, 85–118.

Bennett, W. M. *et al.* (1996). Chronic cyclosporine nephropathy: the Achilles' heel of immunosuppressive therapy. *Kidney International* **50**, 1089–1100.

Birkeland, S. A. (2001). Steroid-free immunosuppression in renal transplantation: a long-term follow-up of 100 consecutive patients. *Transplantation* **71**, 1089–1090.

Cantarovich, D. *et al.* (2000). Prevention of acute rejection with antithymocyte globulin, avoiding corticosteroids, and delaying cyclosporin after renal transplantation. *Nephrology, Dialysis, Transplantation* **15**, 1673–1676.

Casadei, D. H. *et al.* (2001). A randomized and prospective study comparing treatment with high-dose intravenous immunoglobulin with monoclonal antibodies for rescue of kidney grafts with steroid-resistant rejection. *Transplantation* **71**, 53–58.

Ciancio, G. *et al.* (2002). Daclizumab induction, tacrolimus, mycophenolate mofetil and steroids as an immunosuppression regimen for primary kidney transplant recipients. *Transplantation* **73**, 1100–1106.

Cole, E. *et al.* (2001). A pilot study of steroid-free immunosuppression in the prevention of acute rejection in renal allograft recipients. *Transplantation* **72**, 845–850.

Dudley, C. R. (2001). Conversion at first rejection: a prospective trial comparing cyclosporine microemulsion with tacrolimus in renal transplant recipients. *Transplantation Proceedings* **33**, 1034–1035.

European Mycophenolate Mofetil Cooperative Study Group (1995). Placebo-controlled study of mycophenolate mofetil combined with cyclosporin and corticosteroids for prevention of acute rejection. *Lancet* **345**, 1321–1325.

Flechner, S. M. *et al.* (2002). Kidney transplantation without calcineurin inhibitor drugs: a prospective, randomized trial of sirolimus versus cyclosporine. *Transplantation* **74**, 1070–1076.

Gaber, A. O., Moore, L. W., and Schroeder, T. J. (1998). Observations on recovery of renal function following treatment for acute rejection. *American Journal of Kidney Diseases* **31**, S47–S59.

Gonwa, T. A. *et al.* (2002). Improved renal function in sirolimus-treated renal transplant patients after early cyclosporine elimination. *Transplantation* **74**, 1560–1567.

Gonwa, T. *et al.* (2003). Randomized trial of tacrolimus in combination with sirolimus or mycophenolate mofetil in kidney transplantation: results at 6 months. *Transplantation* **75**, 1213–1220.

Groth, C. G. *et al.* (1999). Sirolimus (rapamycin)-based therapy in human renal transplantation: similar efficacy and different toxicity compared with cyclosporine. Sirolimus European Renal Transplant Study Group [see comments]. *Transplantation* **67**, 1036–1042.

Halloran, P. F. (2002). Call for revolution: a new approach to describing allograft deterioration. *American Journal of Transplantation* **2**, 195–200.

Halloran, P. *et al.* (1997). Mycophenolate mofetil in renal allograft recipients: a pooled efficacy analysis of three randomized, double-blind, clinical studies in prevention of rejection. The International Mycophenolate Mofetil Renal Transplant Study Groups [published erratum appears in Transplantation 1997 **63** (4), 618]. *Transplantation* **63**, 39–47.

Holdaas, H. *et al.* (2003). Effect of fluvastatin on cardiac outcomes in renal transplant recipients: a multicentre, randomised, placebo-controlled trial. *Lancet* **361**, 2024–2031.

Hollander, A. A. *et al.* (1995). Beneficial effects of conversion from cyclosporin to azathioprine after kidney transplantation. *Lancet* **345**, 610–614.

International Neoral Renal Transplantation Study Group (2002). Randomized, international study of cyclosporine microemulsion absorption profiling in renal transplantation with basiliximab immunoprophylaxis. *American Journal of Transplantation* **2**, 157–166.

Johnson, C. *et al.* (2000). Randomized trial of tacrolimus (Prograf) in combination with azathioprine or mycophenolate mofetil versus cyclosporine (Neoral) with mycophenolate mofetil after cadaveric kidney transplantation. *Transplantation* **69**, 834–841.

Johnson, R. W. *et al.* (2001). Sirolimus allows early cyclosporine withdrawal in renal transplantation resulting in improved renal function and lower blood pressure. *Transplantation* **72**, 777–786.

Kahan, B. D. (2000). Efficacy of sirolimus compared with azathioprine for reduction of acute renal allograft rejection: a randomised multicentre study. The Rapamune US Study Group. *Lancet* **356**, 194–202.

Kahan, B. D., Rajagopalan, P. R., and Hall, M. (1999). Reduction of the occurrence of acute cellular rejection among renal allograft recipients treated with basiliximab, a chimeric anti-interleukin-2-receptor monoclonal antibody. United States Simulect Renal Study Group. *Transplantation* **67**, 276–284.

Kahan, B. D. *et al.* (2002). Therapeutic drug monitoring of immunosuppressant drugs in clinical practice. *Clinical Therapy* **24**, 330–350.

Kamath, S. *et al.* (1997). Efficacy of OKT3 as primary therapy for histologically confirmed acute renal allograft rejection. *Transplantation* **64**, 1428–1432.

Kasiske, B. L. *et al.* (2000). A meta-analysis of immunosuppression withdrawal trials in renal transplantation. *Journal of the American Society of Nephrology* **11**, 1910–1917.

Kovarik, J. M. *et al.* (2002). Exposure-response relationships for everolimus in *de novo* kidney transplantation: defining a therapeutic range. *Transplantation* **73**, 920–925.

Kreis, H. *et al.* (2000). Sirolimus in association with mycophenolate mofetil induction for the prevention of acute graft rejection in renal allograft recipients. *Transplantation* **69** (7), 1252–1260.

Lawen, J. G. *et al.* (2003). Randomized double-blind study of immunoprophylaxis with basiliximab, a chimeric anti-interleukin-2 receptor monoclonal antibody, in combination with mycophenolate mofetil-containing triple therapy in renal transplantation. *Transplantation* **75**, 37–43.

Lebranchu, Y. *et al.* (2002). Immunoprophylaxis with basiliximab compared with antithymocyte globulin in renal transplant patients receiving MMF-containing triple therapy. *American Journal of Transplantation* **2**, 48–56.

Levy, G. *et al.* (2002). Patient management by Neoral C(2) monitoring: an international consensus statement. *Transplantation* **73**, S12–S18.

Ligtenberg, G. *et al.* (2001). Cardiovascular risk factors in renal transplant patients: cyclosporin A versus tacrolimus. *Journal of the American Society of Nephrology* **12**, 368–373.

Luke, P. P. *et al.* (2001). Reversal of steroid- and anti-lymphocyte antibody-resistant rejection using intravenous immunoglobulin (IVIG) in renal transplant recipients. *Transplantation* **72**, 419–422.

Macdonald, A. S. (2001). A worldwide, phase III, randomized, controlled, safety and efficacy study of a sirolimus/cyclosporine regimen for prevention of acute rejection in recipients of primary mismatched renal allografts. *Transplantation* **71**, 271–280.

MacPhee, I. A. *et al.* (1998). Long-term outcome of a prospective randomized trial of conversion from cyclosporine to azathioprine treatment one year after renal transplantation. *Transplantation* **66**, 1186–1192.

Margreiter, R. (2002). Efficacy and safety of tacrolimus compared with cyclosporin microemulsion in renal transplantation: a randomised multicentre study. *Lancet* **359**, 741–746.

Mayer, A. D. (2002). Chronic rejection and graft half-life: five-year follow-up of the European Tacrolimus Multicenter Renal Study. *Transplantation Proceedings* **34**, 1491–1492.

Mayer, A. D. *et al.* (1997). Multicenter randomized trial comparing tacrolimus (FK506) and cyclosporine in the prevention of renal allograft rejection: a report of the European Tacrolimus Multicenter Renal Study Group. *Transplantation* **64**, 436–443.

McCune, T. R. *et al.* (1998). Effects of tacrolimus on hyperlipidemia after successful renal transplantation: a Southeastern Organ Procurement Foundation multicenter clinical study. *Transplantation* **65**, 87–92.

Mele, T. S. and Halloran, P. F. (2000). The use of mycophenolate mofetil in transplant recipients. *Immunopharmacology* **47**, 215–245.

Morelon, E. *et al.* (2001). Characteristics of sirolimus-associated interstitial pneumonitis in renal transplant patients. *Transplantation* **72**, 787–790.

Mourad, G. *et al.* (1998). Long-term improvement in renal function after cyclosporine reduction in renal transplant recipients with histologically proven chronic cyclosporine nephropathy. *Transplantation* **65**, 661–667.

Nashan, B. *et al.* (1997). Randomised trial of basiliximab versus placebo for control of acute cellular rejection in renal allograft recipients. CHIB 201 International Study Group [published erratum appears in *Lancet* (1997) **350** (9089), 1484]. *Lancet* **350**, 1193–1198.

Nashan, B. *et al.* (1999). Reduction of acute renal allograft rejection by daclizumab. Daclizumab Double Therapy Study Group. *Transplantation* **67**, 110–115.

Ojo, A. O. *et al.* (2000). Mycophenolate mofetil reduces late renal allograft loss independent of acute rejection. *Transplantation* **69**, 2405–2409.

Opelz, G. (1995). Efficacy of rejection prophylaxis with OKT3 in renal transplantation. Collaborative Transplant Study [see comments]. *Transplantation* **60**, 1220–1224.

Ortho Multicentre Transplant Study Group (1985). A randomized clinical trial of OKT3 monoclonal antibody for acute rejection of cadaveric renal transplants. *New England Journal of Medicine* **313**, 337–342.

Pawinski, T. *et al.* (2002). Limited sampling strategy for the estimation of mycophenolic acid area under the curve in adult renal transplant patients treated with concomitant tacrolimus. *Clinical Chemistry* **48**, 1497–1504.

Pirsch, J. D. *et al.* (1997). A comparison of tacrolimus (FK506) and cyclosporine for immunosuppression after cadaveric renal transplantation. FK506 Kidney Transplant Study Group. *Transplantation* **63**, 977–983.

Ponticelli, C. *et al.* (2001). A randomized, double-blind trial of basiliximab immunoprophylaxis plus triple therapy in kidney transplant recipients. *Transplantation* **72**, 1261–1267.

Racusen, L. C. *et al.* (1999). The Banff 97 working classification of renal allograft pathology. *Kidney International* **55**, 713–723.

Regele, H. *et al.* (2002). Capillary deposition of complement split product C4d in renal allografts is associated with basement membrane injury in peritubular and glomerular capillaries: a contribution of humoral immunity to chronic allograft rejection. *Journal of the American Society of Nephrology* **13**, 2371–2380.

Roodnat, J. I. *et al.* (2001). Proteinuria after renal transplantation affects not only graft survival but also patient survival. *Transplantation* **72**, 438–444.

Sadek, S. *et al.* (2002). Short-term combination of mycophenolate mofetil with cyclosporine as a therapeutic option for renal transplant recipients: a prospective, multicenter, randomized study. *Transplantation* **74**, 511–517.

Schnuelle, P. *et al.* (2002). Open randomized trial comparing early withdrawal of either cyclosporine or mycophenolate mofetil in stable renal transplant recipients initially treated with a triple drug regimen. *Journal of the American Society of Nephrology* **13**, 536–543.

Shah, M. B. *et al.* (1999). The evaluation of the safety and tolerability of two formulations of cyclosporine: neoral and sandimmune. A meta-analysis. *Transplantation* **67**, 1411–1417.

Shaw, L. M. *et al.* (2001). Pharmacokinetic, pharmacodynamic, and outcome investigations as the basis for mycophenolic acid therapeutic drug monitoring in renal and heart transplant patients. *Clinical Biochemistry* **34**, 17–22.

Sinclair, N. R. (1992). Low-dose steroid therapy in cyclosporine-treated renal transplant recipients with well-functioning grafts. The Canadian Multicentre Transplant Study Group [see comments]. *Canadian Medical Association Journal* **147**, 645–657.

Smak Gregoor, P. J. *et al.* (2002). Withdrawal of cyclosporine or prednisone six months after kidney transplantation in patients on triple drug therapy: a randomized, prospective, multicenter study. *Journal of the American Society of Nephrology* **13**, 1365–1373.

Solez, K., Vincenti, F., and Filo, R. S. (1998). Histopathologic findings from 2-year protocol biopsies from a U.S. multicenter kidney transplant trial comparing tarolimus versus cyclosporine: a report of the FK506 Kidney Transplant Study Group. *Transplantation* **66**, 1736–1740.

Sollinger, H. W. for the U.S. Renal Transplant Mycophenolate Mofetil Study Group (1996). Mycophenolate Mofetil for the prevention of acute rejection in primary cadaveric renal allograft recipients. *Transplantation* **60**, 225–232.

Szczech, L. A. *et al.* (1997). Effect of anti-lymphocyte induction therapy on renal allograft survival: a meta-analysis. *Journal of the American Society of Nephrology* **8**, 1771–1777.

The Mycophenolate Mofetil Acute Renal Rejection Study Group (1998). Mycophenolate mofetil for the treatment of a first acute renal allograft rejection. *Transplantation* **65**, 235–241.

The Tricontinental Mycophenolate Mofetil Renal Transplantation Study Group (1996). A blinded, randomized clinical trial of mycophenolate mofetil for the prevention of acute rejection in cadaveric renal transplantation. *Transplantation* **61**, 1029–1037.

Undre, N. A. *et al.* (1999). Low systemic exposure to tacrolimus correlates with acute rejection. *Transplantation Proceedings* **31**, 296–298.

van Gelder, T. *et al.* (1999). A randomized double-blind, multicenter plasma concentration controlled study of the safety and efficacy of oral mycophenolate mofetil for the prevention of acute rejection after kidney transplantation. *Transplantation* **68**, 261–266.

Vanrenterghem, Y. *et al.* (2000). Double-blind comparison of two corticosteroid regimens plus mycophenolate mofetil and cyclosporine for prevention of acute renal allograft rejection. *Transplantation* **70**, 1352–1359.

Vereerstraeten, P. *et al.* (1997). Absence of deleterious effect on long-term kidney graft survival of rejection episodes with complete functional recovery. *Transplantation* **63**, 1739–1743.

Vincenti, F. *et al.* (1998). Interleukin-2-receptor blockade with daclizumab to prevent acute rejection in renal transplantation. Daclizumab Triple Therapy Study Group [see comments]. *New England Journal of Medicine* **338**, 161–165.

Vincenti, F. *et al.* (2001a). Rapid steroid withdrawal versus standard steroid therapy in patients treated with basiliximab, cyclosporine, and mycophenolate mofetil for the prevention of acute rejection in renal transplantation. *Transplantation Proceedings* **33**, 1011–1012.

Vincenti, F. *et al.* (2001b). Multicenter trial exploring calcineurin inhibitors avoidance in renal transplantation. *Transplantation* **71**, 1282–1287.

Vincenti, F. *et al.* (2002). A long-term comparison of tacrolimus (FK506) and cyclosporine in kidney transplantation: evidence for improved allograft survival at five years. *Transplantation* **73**, 775–782.

Weir, M. R. *et al.* (2001). Long-term impact of discontinued or reduced calcineurin inhibitor in patients with chronic allograft nephropathy. *Kidney International* **59**, 1567–1573.

Wissing, K. M. *et al.* (2000). Hypercholesterolemia is associated with increased kidney graft loss caused by chronic rejection in male patients with previous acute rejection. *Transplantation* **70**, 464–472.

Wuthrich, R. P. *et al.* (2000). Randomized trial of conversion from mycophenolate mofetil to azathioprine 6 months after renal allograft transplantation. *Nephrology, Dialysis, Transplantation* **15**, 1228–1231.

Zucker, K. *et al.* (1997). Unexpected augmentation of mycophenolic acid pharmacokinetics in renal transplant patients receiving tacrolimus and mycophenolate mofetil in combination therapy, and analogous *in vitro* findings. *Transplantation Immunology* **5**, 225–232.

13.3 Management of the renal transplant recipient

13.3.1 Surgery and surgical complications

Michael Nicholson

Introduction

Successful human renal transplantation has been a clinical reality for nearly 50 years. In many ways, the principles of the technical aspects of renal transplantation have changed very little in this period. There have, nonetheless, been very significant improvements in surgical instrumentation and the fine details of surgical techniques. Indeed, very high rates of technical success and very low surgical complication rates are now expected throughout the world.

Procurement of kidneys for transplantation

The kidney is a relatively difficult organ to remove because of its retroperitoneal position. This has been confirmed by a recent analysis of the UK National Transplant Database, which reported a 19 per cent incidence of kidney damage at the time of retrieval. If a kidney is removed without damaging its blood vessels and ureter, then the subsequent transplant operation will be easier to perform and the associated technical complication rate reduced. The temptation to delegate organ retrieval surgery to junior surgical staff must therefore be resisted.

The most important principle of organ retrieval from heart beating cadaveric donors is that warm ischaemia must be minimized. This is achieved by cannulating the circulation to the kidneys and other organs whilst the heart is still beating and then perfusing the organs with cold preservation fluid, immediately prior to cardiac arrest (Rosenthal *et al.* 1983). The kidneys are most commonly removed as part of a multiple organ donation procedure in which the order of removing organs is as follows: the heart and lungs first, followed by the liver and pancreas and, finally, the kidneys. Multiple organ retrieval operations are performed through a long midline thoracoabdominal incision running from the sternal notch to the pubis. The superior and inferior vena cava are isolated and controlled with slings and a cannula is placed in the ascending aorta for administration of a cardioplegic preservation fluid. The abdominal organs are perfused *in situ* to reduce the warm ischaemic interval to a minimum. There are three important effects of flushing organs with cold preservation fluid: blood is washed out thus preventing local thrombosis; the organs are cooled so that their metabolic demand is reduced; and the normal interstitial fluid is replaced with preservation fluid. Perfusion fluids are designed to prevent cell death by inhibiting cellular swelling. Local cooling can be augmented by the liberal use of crushed ice; this surface cooling is very efficient. There are two main approaches for the dissection of the abdominal organs: the standard operation and the rapid flush technique. In the standard operation, most of the dissection of the vascular supply of the organs is performed with the heart beating. This facilitates identification of the vascular anatomy, but this method tends to be time-consuming and the extensive dissection required may lead to significant blood loss. In the rapid flush technique, the abdominal aorta and portal vein are cannulated early in the operation and very little, if any, preliminary dissection of the organs is performed at this stage. The organs are then flushed with preservation fluid and the vascular dissection takes place in a bloodless field. This is a quicker procedure, which is particularly useful in haemodynamically unstable donors. Its disadvantage is that asanguinous structures are more difficult to identify and, therefore, more easily damaged.

The hepatic hilum is dissected first to identify the hepatic artery, the portal vein, and the bile duct. A portal venous catheter is placed via the inferior mesenteric vein. Once the hepatic and pancreatic dissections have been completed, attention is turned to the kidneys. The intestines must first be mobilized to gain access to the retroperitoneal space. This involves division of the peritoneal reflections of the ascending and descending colon from their hepatic and splenic flexures to the pelvis. The root of the small bowel mesentery is also mobilized so that the small and large bowel can be reflected upwards and out of the way. The aorta is identified at the level of the diaphragm and at its bifurcation. It is controlled with vascular slings and cannulated using a large bore perfusion catheter introduced through the right common iliac artery. The vena cava is similarly identified and slung above the renal veins and at its bifurcation. The ureters are then mobilized from the pelvic brim to the renal hilum taking care to preserve a generous amount of periureteric connective tissue. The superior, lateral, and inferior attachments of the kidneys can then be divided, the safest technique being to stay outside the layer of Gerota's fascia. The organs are then perfused with an appropriate organ preservation fluid, such as hyperosmolar citrate or University of Wisconsin solution. The final step is to remove the kidneys from the abdomen with intact blood vessels and ureters. This may be done *en bloc* or the kidneys can be removed separately (Ackermann and Snell 1968; Linke *et al.* 1975).

As the liver and pancreas are removed first, the aorta and vena cava will have been transected above the renal vessels. In the *en bloc* technique, the kidneys are lifted forward and the aorta and vena cava are freed by dividing their posterior attachments in the prevertebral plane. This dissection is carried to the level of the bifurcation of the great vessels where they are transected. The kidneys are then transferred to a bowl containing iced preservation solution. The vessels are separated at this stage by dividing the left renal vein where it joins the vena cava. The rest of the vena cava should stay with the right kidney in order to allow subsequent lengthening of the right renal vein by fashioning a caval tube (Fig. 1). The aorta is next divided in the midline posteriorly (between the paired lumbar arteries) and anteriorly taking care to identify and preserve the renal arteries. Once the kidneys have been separated, no further dissection of the perinephric fat should be performed as overpreparation at this stage may easily cause serious damage to the vasculature. The kidneys are placed in sterile plastic bags with a small amount of preservation fluid and are transported in crushed ice. The alternative method involves the division of the aorta and vena cava within the abdomen. Many surgeons prefer this approach as the kidneys and vessels are easier to separate as they lie fixed in their usual anatomical positions.

The technique of organ procurement is modified slightly when the kidneys are being retrieved alone. The abdomen is opened through a full midline incision and the right colon and small bowel mesentery are mobilized to demonstrate the vena cava and aorta. These are slung with tapes or rubber slings at the level of their bifurcations. The infrahepatic vena cava is similarly controlled with a sling. The anterior aspect of the aorta is then dissected to identify and ligate the inferior and superior mesenteric arteries. The latter is found immediately above the left renal vein, where it crosses the anterior aortic wall. The infracoeliac aorta can now be slung and controlled. Once the vessels have been secured in this way, the ureters can be mobilized from the pelvic brim to the renal hilum and the lateral attachments of the kidneys dissected free. Alternatively, this step can be performed after *in situ* perfusion. A large-bore perfusion cannula is placed in the aorta and the *in situ* perfusion commenced. The effluent blood is drained either by placing a cannula in the vena cava at the level of its bifurcation or by simply incising the vein at this point and placing a sucker directly into the lumen. Slush ice can also be placed around the kidneys to aid rapid cooling. The aim is to reduce the renal core temperature below 10°C as quickly as possible; oxygen consumption decreases exponentially with falling temperature and is 10 per cent of normal at 10°C.

Non-heart-beating kidney donation

Kidneys are removed from non-heart-beating donors (NHBDs) after a variable period of cardiac arrest, and hence, warm ischaemia. The main requirement of organ procurement from NHBDs is to achieve rapid *in situ* perfusion of the kidneys in order to limit the duration of warm ischaemia. This requires a rapid response team consisting of surgeons and transplant coordinators. NHBDs may be either uncontrolled (Maastricht categories I and II) or controlled (Maastricht categories III and IV). In controlled donors, the cardiac arrest is planned and it is therefore possible to reduce the warm time to only a few minutes. In the uncontrolled donor, cardiac arrest occurs suddenly and this may result in prolonged warm times of up to 40–60 min. Some NHBD protocols include continuation of external cardiac massage and ventilation with 100 per cent oxygen after death (Booster *et al.* 1993; Dunlop *et al.* 1995). This is best achieved by the use of a mechanical resuscitator (Szostek *et al.* 1995). The aim is to provide continuing renal perfusion with oxygenated blood, but the effectiveness of this intervention has never been proven.

In situ cooling of the kidneys can be achieved in a number of different ways. The simplest and most popular method is intravascular cooling using a double balloon triple lumen intra-aortic catheter (Garcia-Rinaldi *et al.* 1975). The femoral artery and vein are exposed via a cut-down in the groin and the perfusion catheter is introduced into the aorta via an arteriotomy in the common femoral artery (Fig. 2). The lower (abdominal) balloon is inflated with dilute radiographic contrast media and the catheter is gently withdrawn until the abdominal balloon jams at the aortic bifurcation. The upper (thoracic) balloon is now inflated, again using dilute contrast media. Cold preservation fluid, for example, hyperosmolar citrate held at 4°C, is infused through the main lumen of the aortic catheter. This washes blood out of the kidneys, cools them and replaces their interstitial fluid with preservation fluid. In an attempt to reduce intravascular thrombosis and intrarenal vasospasm, heparin (10,000 AU) and an α blocker, such as phentolamine (10 mg), can be added to the first bag of perfusion fluid. The system is vented by placing a return

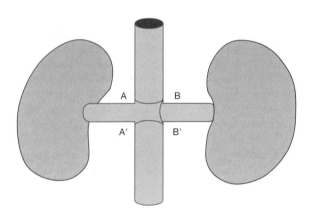

Fig. 1 Kidneys showing lengthened right renal vein by fashioning of a caval tube.

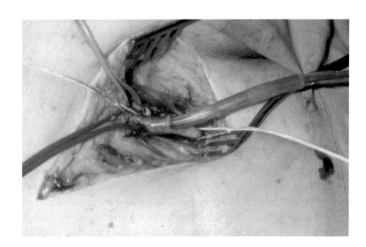

Fig. 2 Perfusion catheter introduced into the aorta via an arteriotomy in the common femoral artery.

catheter in the common femoral vein or the inferior vena cava. The success of this technique depends on effective isolation of the arterial blood supply to both kidneys. Correct positioning of the catheter balloons is vital and this can be checked by performing an urgent abdominal X-ray (Fig. 3). If this is available quickly, it is possible to reposition an incorrectly placed catheter. A common error is to pull the abdominal balloon too far so that it lies in the iliac system rather than the aorta. This leaves the thoracic balloon placed below the renal arteries (Fig. 4). In these circumstances, the perfusion fluid is lost to the contralateral leg, and this may be suspected clinically by comparing the surface temperature of the legs by palpation. The efficiency of organ perfusion can be assessed by inspection of the venous effluent and by monitoring the perfusion flow rate. Initially, the effluent fluid is heavily blood-stained, but this gradually clears until it is virtually blood-free. A flow rate of 100–200 ml/min, with the perfusate reservoir held 1 m above the kidneys, suggests that the system is working well. The size of the venous return catheter is an important flow-limiting factor, but this can be overcome by using a large-bore (>24 G), incompressible venous cannula. The flow of perfusion fluid must be maintained until the point of organ retrieval and this may require the use of 15–20 l of perfusate.

Two other techniques are in use: intraperitoneal cooling (Orloff *et al.* 1994) and extracorporeal total-body cooling (Gomez *et al.* 1993). Intraperitoneal cooling can be performed alone or in combination with intravascular cooling. A small midline abdominal incision is made to allow insertion of a 32Fr chest drain into the pelvis. A Foley catheter with a 30 ml balloon is introduced through the same incision to occlude the fascial defect. Surface cooling is achieved by running Ringer's lactate solution at 4°C into the abdomen through the chest tube and draining this via the Foley catheter. A more sophisticated modification of this technique employs the use of an ice–alcohol cooling coil that reaches subzero temperatures (Light *et al.* 1996). This allows an intraperitoneal temperature of 10°C to be reached in a few minutes. Once this level of cooling has been achieved, an emergency laparotomy is performed for kidney retrieval.

Extracorporeal total-body cooling can be performed using a simple cardiopulmonary bypass circuit. Large bore cannulas placed in the femoral artery and vein are connected to a circuit consisting of a roller pump, oxygenator and heat exchanger. Initial bypass is performed at normothermic temperature for a period of 15–20 min. The heat exchanger temperature is then rapidly decreased to 4°C until the core body temperature falls to 15°C, at which point organ retrieval is performed. The advantage of this method is the ability to maintain extracorporeal circulation for many hours. This may be especially useful in situations where the consent for organ donation is delayed. The requirement for expensive equipment and the relative complexity of this method are disadvantages.

NHBD kidneys are procured at laparotomy using the surgical techniques that have already been described for cadaveric donors. As the kidneys have already been cooled and are the only abdominal organs to be removed, the operation can be completed in around 45 min.

Live donor nephrectomy

Several different operative approaches have been used for live-donor nephrectomy, the most recent advance being the introduction of laparoscopically assisted operations. The options for traditional open

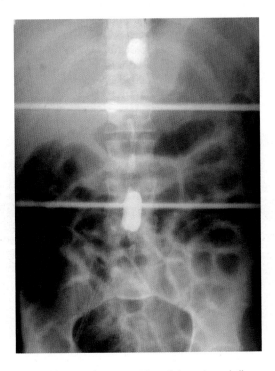

Fig. 3 Abdominal X-ray indicating position of the catheter balloon.

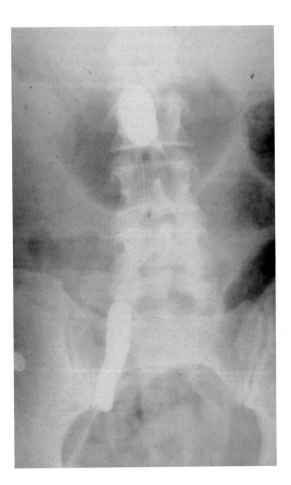

Fig. 4 Thoracic balloon placed incorrectly below the renal arteries.

operations include extra- and intraperitoneal approaches to the kidney made through a variety of anterior or loin incisions. The main alternative to this is to employ a retroperitoneal approach without rib resection. Some surgeons still use anterior intraperitoneal access to remove live donor kidneys. This has the disadvantage of breaching the peritoneal cavity, which may lead to adhesion formation. Such operations are associated with a 2 per cent risk of adhesive bowel obstruction in the long-term.

Open retroperitoneal nephrectomy with or without rib resection

The left kidney is used most commonly as the renal vein tends to be much longer than that of the right kidney and this facilitates implantation in the recipient. The right kidney is chosen in cases where it has a single artery and the left kidney has multiple arteries. The patient is placed on their side with the operating table broken to open up the space between the ribs and the pelvis. The incision is made along the line of the twelfth rib and carried forward into the abdomen towards the umbilicus. Division of the skin, superficial fat and muscles exposes the twelfth rib which is cleared of its periosteal attachments and then divided posteriorly and removed (Fig. 5). Care needs to be taken in order to avoid damage to the associated neurovascular bundle. At the anterior end of the wound, the oblique abdominal muscles are divided down to the peritoneum, which must be carefully preserved. The fascia of Gerota and the perinephric fat are divided to demonstrate the kidney, which can then be delivered into the wound to allow dissection of the hilar structures. The ureter is dissected free from its bed by sweeping away the anteriorly placed peritoneum and gonadal vessels. The ureter should be ligated and divided at the level of the pelvic brim to give a length of at least 10 cm for anastomosis in the recipient. The renal vein is dissected from the hilum towards the inferior vena cava with ligation and division of its gonadal, adrenal, and posterior lumbar tributaries. The renal artery is dissected free to its origin from the abdominal aorta. The surgeon must always look for previously unidentified accessory renal arteries, which tend to be small and polar in distribution. This is particularly important in the case of the lower polar arteries, as these may provide the important ureteric arterial supply. After removal of the kidney, the vessel stumps are oversewn

with vascular suture material and a suction or tube drain placed in the renal bed. The wound is closed by opposing the divided muscle layers using non-absorbable nylon sutures. If a right nephrectomy is required, the operation proceeds according to the same general plan. The right renal vein is often rather short and in order to obtain the maximum length possible, a side-biting vascular clamp is placed on the inferior vena cava at the level of the renal vein.

A similar approach can be used to remove the kidney without resecting the rib. This is made possible by the use of modern fixed retractor systems that allow nephrectomy to be performed through a smaller loin incision running from the tip of the twelfth rib towards the umbilicus.

Laparoscopy-assisted live donor nephrectomy

The traditional open donor nephrectomy operations leave a significant wound and the recovery period after surgery tends to be relatively prolonged. There is no doubt that this is a considerable disincentive to potential donors, particularly those in employment or with a young family to bring up. Many donors, especially young females, also have concerns about the cosmetic outcome of nephrectomy incisions (Fig. 6). Recent developments in minimal access surgery have made it possible to perform live donor nephrectomy using laparoscopy-assisted techniques. These newer operations have the potential to remove some of the disincentives to donors, but there is still a need to obtain high quality evidence in order to define their role.

The laparoscopic operation

Preoperative imaging by spiral computed tomography (CT) angiography greatly facilitates the laparoscopic operation as it can be used to create computerized three-dimensional (3D) reconstructions of the kidney and its vascular anatomy (Fig. 7). This technique provides definition of the renal arterial anatomy that is at least as good as that from conventional intra-arterial digital subtraction angiography (Shaffer et al. 1998). Its advantage lies in the superior quality of the information provided about the renal venous anatomy. This is invaluable in planning the operation and in particular avoiding damage to difficult venous tributaries such as short posterior lumbar veins arising from the posterior aspect of the renal vein. In open surgery, an avulsion injury to such a vessel is easily controlled by direct pressure and then

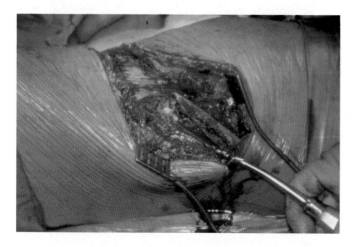

Fig. 5 Incision made along the line of the twelfth rib and carried forward into the abdomen.

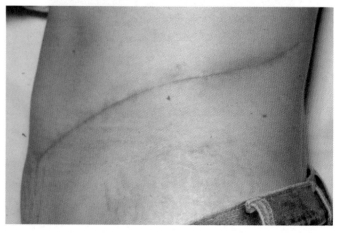

Fig. 6 Cosmetic outcome of nephrectomy incision in a young female donor.

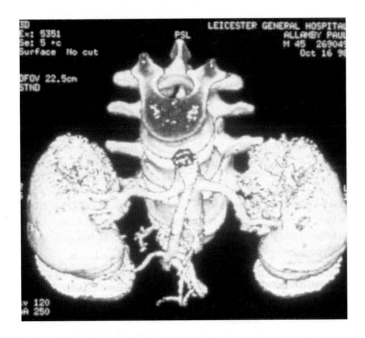

Fig. 7 Preoperative imaging by spiral computed tomography (CT).

repaired using a fine vascular suture. A similar injury during laparoscopic surgery is far more difficult to control as the surgeon does not have direct access to the vessels. The donor should be prehydrated on the night before the nephrectomy by the administration of 2 l of intravenous crystalloid solution. There are important differences in the operative approaches to the right and left kidneys and the more commonly performed left nephrectomy will be described first.

Laparoscopy-assisted donor nephrectomy is performed under general anaesthesia, usually using a transperitoneal approach although the retroperitoneum is gaining in popularity. The donor is placed in a modified lateral position and the operation begins with the creation of a pneumoperitoneum by needle insufflations of carbon dioxide into the abdominal cavity. Three 12 mm incisions are made for the insertion of the main laparoscopic operating ports. A video laparoscope and various dissection instruments are introduced through these ports. The operation begins with mobilization of the colon to demonstrate the kidney within Gerota's fascia. After the colon has been reflected medially, the kidney is exposed and the ureter dissected. It is very important to avoid stripping the ureter of its rather tenuous blood supply and one good way of doing this is to dissect the ureter and gonadal vessels together so that there is a wide margin of surrounding meso-ureteric tissue. The gonadal vein is then followed superiorly to its junction with the renal vein. This is mobilized and its gonadal, adrenal, and lumbar tributaries are secured between metal clips and divided. Attention is then turned to the renal artery, which is dissected back to its origin from the abdominal aorta. The ureter is clipped and divided at the pelvic brim and all the fascial attachments of the kidney are divided. The kidney is now only attached by its vascular pedicle, and at this stage a 6–8 cm retrieval incision is made in the abdominal wall. A short suprapubic Pfannenstiel incision gives the best cosmetic result but a midline incision around the umbilicus is favoured by some surgeons. A plastic kidney retrieval bag is now placed into the abdominal cavity through the retrieval incision. The

renal artery and then the renal vein are divided using an endovascular stapling device. This places several rows of metal staples across the vessel and then divides it, leaving the stump of the vessel safely secured. The kidney is then transferred to the plastic retrieval bag, which is pulled out through the retrieval incision. The kidney is immediately placed in a bowl of iced preservation fluid and following excision of the arterial and venous staple lines the kidney is flushed with approximately 500 ml of an appropriate preservation fluid held at 4°C. The Pfannenstiel incision is closed with a non-absorbable suture and the pneumoperitoneum is then re-established so that the stumps of the renal vessels and the renal bed itself can be inspected for haemostasis.

Considerable modification of the technique is required for a right-sided laparoscopic nephrectomy. The dissection proceeds in the same way but the vessels are dealt with differently and the kidney is removed through a 6–8 cm transverse muscle cutting incision in the right upper quadrant. This allows direct control of the inferior vena cava with a side-biting vascular clamp so that the full length of the relatively short right renal vein can be obtained. The right renal artery is clamped behind the vena cava and after division of the renal artery and vein, the kidney is removed directly through the right upper quadrant incision without the need for a retrieval bag.

Intraoperative fluid management is very important during laparoscopic donor nephrectomy. The pneumoperitoneum is maintained at a pressure of 12–16 mmHg and this can cause considerable compromise of renal perfusion over a 3-h operation. A central venous catheter is mandatory and the CVP should be maintained in the high normal range. The adequacy of renal perfusion can be directly observed during laparoscopy by viewing the renal vein, which should remain well filled throughout the procedure. This often requires the administration of large volumes of crystalloid solutions (up to 6–8 l). A diuresis should also be stimulated immediately prior to division of the renal vessels by the administration of intravenous mannitol (0.5 g/1 kg) and/or frusemide (80 mg intravenous). All donors should receive prophylactic subcutaneous heparin preoperatively, but systemic anticoagulation is not absolutely necessary prior to clamping the renal vessels.

Alternative minimally invasive techniques

The first laparoscopic donor nephrectomy was performed in Baltimore, United States in 1995 (Ratner *et al.* 1995). Since then, many centres in the United States and Europe have adopted this technique. The operation does require a high level of advanced laparoscopic skills and this may limit its wide application as it is unusual for surgeons to be trained in both transplant and laparoscopic surgery. 'Handoscopic' methods are an innovation which may broaden the application of laparoscopically assisted live donor nephrectomy. In this technique, a pneumoperitoneum is established as before, then the surgeon introduces one hand into the abdominal cavity through an airtight sleeve, but uses laparoscopic instruments to dissect the kidney. This combined method improves the tactile sense of the surgeon and this may facilitate the dissection of important structures such as the renal vessels and possibly reduces the total operating time (Slakey *et al.* 1999). This technique adds an element of safety to the operation as inadvertent damage to the renal vessels can easily be controlled by direct pressure whilst further measures are taken to secure the haemorrhage. Retroperitoneal handoscopic techniques have also been introduced recently and have the added advantage of not breaching the peritoneal cavity and thus avoiding the formation of intra-abdominal adhesions (Suzuki *et al.* 1997).

13 THE TRANSPLANT PATIENT

Comparative results of open and laparoscopic live donor nephrectomy

A number of studies have compared the outcome of the newer laparoscopic techniques with historical control data from traditional open operations (Flowers *et al.* 1997; Ratner *et al.* 1997; Philosophe *et al.* 1999). Each of these studies has suggested that compared with traditional open nephrectomy, the laparoscopic technique is associated with a shorter hospital stay, less requirement for postoperative analgesia and improved donor recovery times. In general, laparoscopic donors drove their cars after only 2 weeks, resumed exercise and felt able to return to work after 3 weeks and actually returned to work after 4–6 weeks. These recuperation times are between one-third and two-thirds shorter than recovery rates from open operations. The cosmetic results of laparoscopic donor nephrectomy are also better than those from open operations, especially if the kidney is removed through a Pfannensteil incision hidden under the pubic hairline.

Potential problems with laparoscopic donor nephrectomy

Despite the advantages to the donor claimed by the proponents of laparoscopic donor nephrectomy, the outcome in the recipient must also be considered. There is a legitimate concern that laparoscopic surgery could lead to the kidney being damaged during retrieval, with the result that morbidity is transferred from the donor to the recipient. It has also been noted that transplant kidneys removed laparoscopically are associated with a slower reduction in serum creatinine over the first 2 weeks post-transplant (Nogueira *et al.* 1999; Ratner *et al.* 1999). This is likely to be a consequence of the pneumoperitoneum exposing the kidney to a relatively prolonged period of elevated intra-abdominal pressure, leading to a reduction in renal blood flow and urine output (Kirsch *et al.* 1994). There have also been reports of a higher incidence of ureteric complications following the early experience of the laparoscopic operation (Philosophe *et al.* 1999). The ureteric blood supply of a transplanted kidney is provided exclusively by a small branch of the renal artery which runs a variable course downwards from the hilum of the kidney. This vessel may be damaged during any donor nephrectomy operation but this may happen more often during blunt laparoscopic dissection. Ureteric ischaemia may also occur at a lower level if the ureteric blood supply is accidentally stripped away. One way of avoiding this is to dissect the ureter and gonadal vessels to ensure the preservation of a good margin of periureteric areolar tissue. The ureteric complication rate has also been shown to fall with increasing experience (Philosophe *et al.* 1999; Sasaki *et al.* 1999).

Two groups in Baltimore have recorded a significant increase in the number of live donations since the introduction of the laparoscopic operation and have attributed this to the perceived advantages of the technique (Flowers *et al.* 1997; Ratner *et al.* 1997). However, it is common in the United States for patients to travel thousands of miles to undergo surgery in specialist centres, and some of the local increases in living donation described may to some extent reflect a redistribution of activity.

Laparoscopy-assisted live donor nephrectomy has the potential to become a major advance in renal transplantation. Enthusiasm for laparoscopic nephrectomy is increasing around the world, but there is currently insufficient evidence to support its widespread introduction. It is timely therefore to consider performing large multicentre prospective randomised trials comparing laparoscopic and open donor nephrectomy operations.

Renal transplantation

Successful human kidney transplantation has now been performed for nearly half a century and the fundamentals of the procedure have changed little during this time. The transplant kidney is placed heterotopically in one or other iliac fossa. This requires a curved muscle cutting incision running from just medial to the anterior superior iliac spine to the midline above the pubis. The inferior epigastric vessels are ligated as is the round ligament of the uterus in female patients. In males, the spermatic cord should be carefully mobilized and preserved. The peritoneum should not be breached and is swept superiorly to reveal the extraperitoneal bed into which the transplant kidney will be placed to lie on the iliacus and psoas muscles. The iliac blood vessels are then mobilized taking care to meticulously ligate all the associated lymphatic channels in order to reduce the risk of developing a post-transplant lymphocele.

Vascular anatomosis

The renal vein is anatomized end to side to the external iliac vein using a continuous fine monofilament vascular suture. In cases where the renal vein is very short, division of the internal iliac vein is a very useful manoeuvre as this frees the external iliac vein, bringing it into a more superficial position in the wound; this makes the venous anastomosis much easier to perform. The arterial anastomosis can be performed either end to side to the external iliac artery or end to end to the divided internal iliac artery (Fig. 8). The end to side anastomosis is technically easier and is the usual method employed in cadaveric transplantation where it is possible to include a funnel shaped cuff of aorta with the renal artery (a Carrell patch). The external iliac artery is controlled by vascular clamps and then opened as a longitudinal arteriotomy. The size of this is tailored to the length of the Carrell patch and although this is quite variable depending on the age and size of the donor, it is usually possible to create a relatively large (15–25 mm) anastomosis and this makes suture placement easier, so reducing the risk of technical errors. Again, a fine continuous monofilament vascular suture such as 5/0 or 6/0 polypropylene is used for the anastomosis.

In the case of a live donor kidney it is not possible to include a Carrell aortic patch and here it is preferable to anastomose the renal artery end to end to the divided internal iliac artery. If the renal artery is larger than the main trunk of the internal iliac artery (this can arise

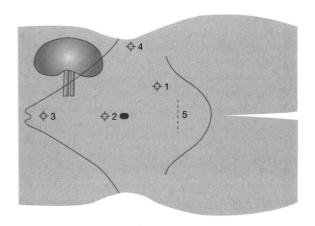

Fig. 8 Optional locations for performing arterial anastomosis.

if the donor is larger than the recipient, e.g. in a male to female live transplant) then a funnel shaped end to the internal vessel can be fashioned by dividing the bridge of tissue between it two main branches. If the renal artery is smaller than the main trunk of the internal iliac artery (donor smaller than recipient e.g. female to male transplant), then a suitably sized branch of the internal iliac artery is chosen for the anastomosis. As this type of end to end anastomosis is smaller and more technically demanding than the end to side variety, it is usual to use fine interrupted vascular sutures such as 6/0 or 7/0 polypropylene. Anastomosis to the internal iliac artery can also be chosen for cadaveric renal transplants where the Carrell patch has been inadvertently (or sometimes deliberately) excised. Difficult circumstances sometimes arise when there is no Carrell patch and the internal iliac artery is not available for anastomosis because of severe atheroma, or the fact that it has been used for a previous transplant. In such a case it is possible to anastomose the renal artery directly to the external iliac artery without a patch. This should be avoided if possible as the external iliac artery tends to have a much thicker wall than the renal vessel and this increases the likelihood of technical errors, in particular narrowing the anastomosis.

Correct positioning of the graft after completion of the vascular anastomoses is an important and under-appreciated technical aspect of renal transplantation. The kidney must sit in such a position that the renal vessels are not kinked. This is more likely to affect the thin walled low pressure renal venous drainage than the arterial supply. With left kidneys, the renal vein is usually significantly longer than the artery and this may lead to twisting or kinking of the vein if the kidney is not positioned correctly. On the other hand, as the right renal artery is longer than the vein, right kidneys are more susceptible to kinking of the renal artery. The transplant kidney can be placed laterally in the iliac fossa or may be placed in a subrectus pouch fashioned specifically for the purpose. In the latter case, the renal vessels run laterally from the kidney and this needs to be noted when performing a needle-core biopsy. An operative diagram of the disposition of the kidney and its vessels is therefore a worthwhile addition to the clinical notes.

Multiple vessels

There are a number of strategies for dealing with multiple renal vessels. As a general principle, it is best to reduce the number of anastomoses as far as possible and this can usually be achieved by careful bench surgery prior to implantation. Two or more arteries arising from the aorta close together are simply dealt with by taking a large Carrell patch and using a single large iliac arteriotomy. If double arteries are widely spaced on the aorta then a large strip of aorta needs to be taken and the central portion of this can then be excised and the two smaller patches then sutured together so that only a single anastomosis is required. Occasionally small polar arteries will only be recognized after a kidney has been retrieved, and such vessels may well have been excised without an aortic patch. In this case, bench surgery is performed to anastomose the cut polar artery to the side of the main renal artery. It is particularly important to reanastomose lower polar arteries accurately, as these may provide all the ureteric blood supply.

In the case of double renal veins, the most common course of action is simply to ligate the smaller vein as the larger one is usually sufficient to drain the whole kidney. If there are two equally sized veins, then it is usually also safe to ligate one of these and anastomose the other.

A more cautious approach is to place a bulldog or other suitable clamp on the lower of the two veins and then anastomose the upper vein to the external iliac vein. On clamp release, if there are no signs of venous congestion, then the lower vein can be ligated, but if there is any doubt about the situation, the second lower renal vein can then be anastomosed to the external iliac vein at a lower level. This can be achieved without interrupting the drainage of the upper renal vein by reclamping the external iliac vein below this first venous anastomosis.

Urinary drainage

If possible this should be performed by implanting the transplant ureter into the recipient bladder by creating a ureteroneocystostomy. The traditional method for doing this is the technique described by Politano and Leadbetter in 1958 but many surgeons now prefer the simpler onlay extravesical ureteroneocystostomy described by Gregoir (1977).

The Politano–Leadbetter (PL) technique involves the formation of a transvesical ureteroneocystostomy with creation of a submucosal antireflux tunnel (Fig. 9). The bladder is opened via a midline anteriorly placed incision. Scissors or a right angle forceps are used to develop a submucosal tunnel over a distance of 2–3 cm. The muscular layers of the bladder wall are then incised from outside down to the tip of an instrument placed in the submucosal tunnel. This allows the end of the ureter to be drawn through the submucosal tunnel from outside to inside the bladder. The end of the ureter is then spatulated and sutured to the bladder mucosa using four interrupted absorbable sutures. The anterior cystotomy should be closed using two layers of an absorbable suture material.

The Gregoir–Lich (GL) technique involves the creation of an onlay or external ureteroneocystostomy (Fig. 10). Two stay sutures are placed in the bladder after it has been distended with irrigation fluid. The bladder muscles of the anterolateral wall of the bladder are then incised down to the mucosa over a distance of 3 cm. The bulging mucosa is then incised over a distance of 1 cm at the distal end of the muscle incision. Following drainage of the irrigation fluid, the spatulated end of

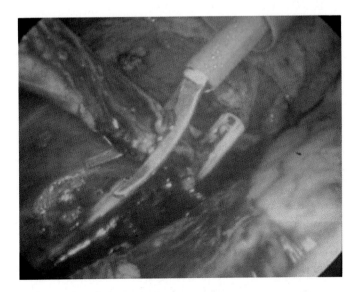

Fig. 9 Formation of ureteroneocystostomy with creation of submucosal antireflux tunnel (Politano–Leadbetter technique).

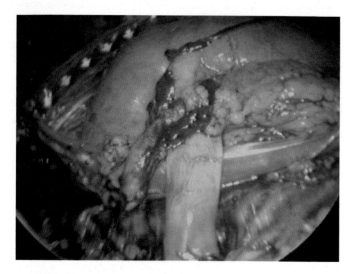

Fig. 10 Creation of onlay or external ureteroneocystostomy (Gregoir–Lich technique).

the ureter is anastomosed to the cystostomy with careful apposition of mucosa to mucosa. The divided muscle layer is then resutured over the ureter to create a short antireflux muscle tunnel. This technique is simpler than the PL method because an initial anterior cystostomy is not required. The onlay method also has the advantage of being possible with only a short length of ureter. This is important as the ureter is maintained only by its blood supply from the renal artery, the more distal aortic, iliac and vesical arterial supply having been divided during kidney retrieval. The shorter the ureter, the less likely there will be an inadequate blood supply to the distal end thereby reducing the risks of ischaemic ureteral leaks or stenosis. The potential disadvantage of the onlay method is that the antireflux mechanism may be less effective than that associated with the PL technique, although there is no definite evidence for this.

Ureteric stents

In both the PL and the GL techniques of ureteroneocystostomy, the surgeon has a choice of placing a ureteric stent or not. Stents have the advantage of reducing the incidence of technical errors leading to ureteric stenosis, but on the other hand they are a potential source of urinary infection, can become encrusted or blocked by debris, and they do have to be removed. They are usually removed 4–6 weeks post-transplant and this can be performed under local anaesthetic using a flexible cystoscope. A large randomized trial comparing the PL and the GP techniques with or without stenting showed an incidence of urinary complications (ureteric leaks or obstruction) of 13 and 21 per cent for the PL and GL operations, respectively, when a stent was not used. In distinct contrast, there were no urinary leaks following either the PL or the GL techniques when the ureter was stented (Pleass *et al.* 1995). PL with stenting was, however, associated with a higher incidence of clot retention compared to GL with stenting (12 versus 0 per cent, respectively).

Alternative techniques of urinary reconstruction

Pyeloureteral anastomosis and ureteroureteral anastomoses have been used in the past but have largely fallen out of favour. The problem with

these methods is that a native nephrectomy is required and the native urinary tract must be normal without evidence of reflux. These methods are therefore more complicated than the formation of a ureteroneocystostomy and may be associated with higher rates of urinary fistula.

Renal transplantation is now quite commonly performed in patients who have abnormal bladders. In many cases, it is possible to anastomose the transplant ureter to the abnormal bladder in the hope that this can be rehabilitated. Alternatively, patients can perform intermittent self-catheterization after the transplant. Nonetheless, a number of cases require urinary diversion using an ileal conduit. The conduit should be fashioned at least 6 weeks prior to transplantation, but in some cases will have been present for many years. In this case, a contrast study (a conduitogram) should be performed to exclude the development of conduit stenosis. The transplant kidney is best placed in the ipsilateral iliac fossa to avoid tension in the ureter and it may be preferable to deliberately place the transplant kidney upside down so that the ureter runs cranially and has a more direct route to the conduit. After revascularization, the peritoneum is opened and the distal blind end of the conduit identified by passing a suitable dilator through the urinary stoma. The spatulated end of the ureter is then anastomosed to the conduit using interrupted absorbable sutures and ensuring mucosa to mucosa continuity. It is possible to place a double-J stent through this anastomosis and to hold this in place by suturing it to the edge of the abdominal urinary stoma. Excellent long-term results have been achieved using this technique (Nguyen *et al.* 1990; Abusin *et al.* 1998).

Drainage and closure of the wound

It is essential to drain both the transplant bed and the subcutaneous tissues using a closed suction drainage system. This prevents the accumulation of serosanguinous fluid or lymph around the transplant kidney. The muscles are closed by a mass technique using a continuous large gauge non-absorbable monofilament suture material. The skin is best closed using a subcuticular suture and then dressed with a clear adhesive dressing so that ultrasound scanning can be performed early without disturbing the wound.

Vascular, lymphatic, and urological complications of renal transplantation

All transplant series have a small but significant incidence of technical complications. One of the keys to reducing the technical complication rate is to avoid damage to the kidneys at the time of the retrieval operation. Nonetheless, the presence of multiple renal vessels and donor atherosclerotic disease does increase the incidence of problems. Recipient obesity, atherosclerosis, and previous transplantation also increase the risk of technical problems.

Anastomotic haemorrhage

This should occur only rarely and is usually an early event due to a technical surgical error. It can also occur some weeks after a transplant due to the development of a mycotic aneurysm of the renal artery, but this is very rare indeed. The patient may complain of pain over the graft and this symptom should always be taken very seriously. There may also be pain in the back or the rectum caused by a tension haematoma in the retroperitoneum or pelvis. Significant haemorrhage will be attended by circulatory collapse with tachycardia and hypotension and a fall in the haemoglobin and haematocrit, sometimes to alarmingly low levels. In these circumstances, the patient must be returned to the operating theatre immediately and the transplant re-explored. The anastomosis can then be repaired by the placement of additional sutures. In the rare case of a ruptured mycotic aneurysm, an immediate graft nephrectomy is required but the mortality of this condition is high.

Renal arterial thrombosis

This is rare and should occur in only 1 per cent of all kidney transplants. The usual outcome is loss of the allografted kidney. Acute arterial thrombosis may occur immediately on table or during the first few days or weeks post-transplant. Whilst there are a number of potential causes including hyperacute rejection and the presence of a procoagulant state, in most cases the cause is a technical error made during the anastomosis of small or atheromatous vessels (Nerstrom et al. 1972). The vessels must not be under tension and the edges must be averted so that there is a smooth transition between the two intimal surfaces. This is critical, as vascular adventitia is thrombogenic and must not finds its way into the lumen of the anastomosis. Fine monofilament vascular sutures are used and these must be carefully placed through all layers of the vessel walls so that an intimal flap is avoided (Fig. 11).

Renal arterial thrombosis presents with sudden anuria, the differential diagnoses being a blocked urinary catheter, dehydration, or a urological complication. A high index of suspicion is required to make this diagnosis, particularly in the immediate postoperative period where anuria can be ascribed to the development of acute tubular necrosis. The only worthwhile investigation is an urgent duplex ultrasound scan (Reuther et al. 1989), but if the diagnosis is seriously entertained, then the only hope of saving the transplant is to re-explore it immediately in the hope that a correctable cause can be found. The reality is that unless

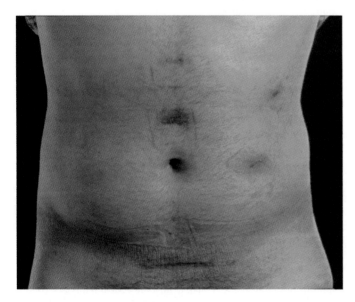

Fig. 11 Fine monofilament vascular sutures.

the acute arterial thrombosis occurs on-table, there is virtually no chance of saving the transplant kidney. Acutely thrombosed grafts must nevertheless be explored and removed to avoid the development of sepsis in a necrotic graft, as this could prove fatal.

Renal vein thrombosis

This is more common than arterial thrombosis occurring in 1–6 per cent of renal transplants (Jones et al. 1988). Whilst it may result from a technical error at the time of surgery, its aetiology is usually less certain. The renal vein can certainly be twisted or kinked if it is not correctly placed after completion of the vascular and ureteric anastomoses. It is worthwhile spending some time placing the kidney in different positions to find the optimal orientation. This can be confirmed by palpating the renal vein to exclude any obvious venous congestion. There is a possible link between renal vein thrombosis and the introduction of cyclosporin therapy, which has been shown to have an appreciable effect on platelet adhesion (Vanrenterghem et al. 1985). The apparent increased incidence of renal vein thrombosis with the introduction of cyclosporin (Richardson et al. 1990) may simply relate to more accurate diagnosis with early graft losses in the azathioprine era being attributed to rejection rather than thrombosis.

The peak incidence of renal vein thrombosis occurs 3–9 days posttransplant (Nerstrom et al. 1972) and the clinical features may be striking. A transplant with good initial graft function will have a sudden loss of urine output associated with severe pain arising from swelling and even rupture of the allograft with the formation of a perigraft haematoma. The ipsilateral leg may also swell if there is involvement of the iliac venous system. In contrast, renal vein thrombosis may also be occult and is one of the differential diagnoses of delayed graft function. Colour Doppler duplex ultrasound scanning is the best investigation. In an established renal vein thrombosis, this may show an obviously swollen allograft with surrounding haematoma and an absence of renal perfusion. Lesser degrees of thrombosis, or indeed incipient thrombosis, may be highlighted by an absence of arterial flow in diastole. An even later development is a reversal of flow in diastole. An isotope renogram is an alternative test that will show a nonperfused graft, but ultrasound is usually more readily available.

As with arterial thrombosis, if this diagnosis is entertained, then the best course of action is to re-explore the transplant as an emergency. After applying vascular clamps to the iliac venous system, the renal vein anastomosis can be opened along the whole length of one side of the vein to allow clot to be extracted. The venotomy can then be closed and the kidney observed for improvement. A more radical alternative would be to immediately explant the kidney by taking down the arterial, venous, and ureteric anastomoses. The kidney can then be reflushed with cold perfusion fluid on the back-table and held in preservation fluid at 4°C. This allows much more time to assess the cause of the venous thrombosis and if the kidney remains viable, then the transplant operation can then be repeated. If the transplant is already infarcted or cannot be adequately flushed with preservation fluid, then the organ will need to be discarded anyway and nothing is lost by immediate explanation. Successful emergency surgical exploration with subsequent long-term function will be rare.

Interventional radiological techniques offer an alternative to surgery. The renal vein can be selectively catheterized via the ipsilateral femoral vein and graft thrombolysis may then be attempted.

Transplant renal artery stenosis

To a certain extent, the rate of renal artery stenosis depends on how carefully it is looked for. The reported rates of 1–23 per cent also reflect the differing diagnostic criteria used (Margules et al. 1973; Lacombe 1975; Halimi et al. 1999). Furthermore, not all stenoses are of functional or clinical significance as shown by studies in which all functioning transplants have undergone arteriography (Lacombe 1975). Aetiological factors include donor vascular disease, early arterial damage and severe acute rejection. More and more elderly and marginal donors are being used as a source of transplant organs, and there is a high incidence of significant atherosclerosis in the renal arteries of these kidneys. Direct arterial damage may occur both at the time of organ retrieval and implantation. The intima may be damaged by traction or during cannulation for perfusion and it is likely that such damage can be the precursor of stenotic disease many months or even years later. Technical errors due to poor vascular technique, such as excessive handling of the intima during arterial anastomosis, may also be responsible for the later development of renal artery stenosis. The role of acute or chronic rejection in the pathogenesis of renal artery stenosis is unknown. The renal artery obviously contains the same mismatched HLA antigens as the renal parenchyma and as such is susceptible to ongoing immune attack. Nonetheless, the localized nature of renal artery stenotic disease suggests that alloimmunity is not a particularly important factor.

There are three different patterns of renal artery stenosis. The first type, an anastomotic stenosis, is likely to be due to errors of technique, especially when the renal artery is small and the more technically demanding end to end anastomosis is used. The second pattern is a postanastomotic stenosis usually situated about 1 cm distal to the original suture line. This type is more common and has a multifactorial aetiology including intimal damage, turbulent postanastomotic blood flow, and external compression by the fibrous reaction to surgery. This is seen more commonly in transplanted right kidneys, suggesting that poor positioning and kinking of the somewhat longer right renal artery may play a role. The third pattern involves multiple stenoses in the smaller branches of the renal artery within the renal substance itself. These are associated with the development of chronic allograft nephropathy and angiography shows a beaded appearance.

Renal artery stenosis presents with new or increasingly severe hypertension that may need treatment with three or more antihypertensive agents. Simultaneous allograft dysfunction is common, the pattern being a gradually increasing serum creatinine. Even mild renal artery stenosis may be dramatically unmasked by the introduction of an angiotensin-converting enzyme (ACE) inhibitor with a sudden marked elevation of serum creatinine and even anuria (Curtis et al. 1983). In view of this, it is advisable to perform a Duplex ultrasound scan of the renal allograft prior to initiating treatment with ACE inhibitors. Even if this does not show any evidence of renal artery stenosis, ACE inhibitors must be introduced at a low dose initially and the serum creatinine should be carefully monitored for several days. Bruits are commonly heard over renal allografts and are most commonly due to small arteriovenous fistulae as a result of needle-core biopsy. Nonetheless, the detection of a new bruit in association with worsening hypertension is a significant finding that should be investigated.

Duplex Doppler ultrasound scanning is a sensible investigation of any renal allograft recipient with deteriorating renal function. As with all ultrasound techniques, this examination is very operator dependent and some series show poor predictive values for the diagnosis of renal artery stenosis. The current gold standard investigation for obtaining a definitive diagnosis is an intra-arterial digital subtraction angiography with selective catheterization of the transplant arterial system (Arlart 1985). More modern techniques such as magnetic resonance angiography may prove to be just as good in the future but as yet there is not enough experience of this method to suggest that it can supercede intra-arterial DSA (Bakker et al. 1998).

Management

This depends on the site and the severity of the stenotic disease. A needle-core biopsy may be helpful in decision-making. If this shows severe chronic allograft nephropathy with significant interstitial fibrosis, glomerulosclerosis, and concentric narrowing of the arterioles, then there may be little to be gained in treating any concomitant renal artery stenosis. On the other hand, changes such as tubular atrophy and glomerular crowding are consistent with prerenal ischaemia suggesting that an attempt to improve graft perfusion should be made.

Stenoses of less than 50 per cent are probably not significant and should be treated conservatively. For stenoses of greater than 50 per cent, the treatment options are percutaneous transluminal angioplasty (PTA) and surgery. Re-operations on long-standing renal transplants are technically demanding because most transplants excite a severe perigraft fibrotic reaction. This factor taken together with the fact that the results of PTA are as good as surgery in terms of blood pressure control (Ruggenenti et al. 2001), make PTA the first choice treatment in most cases. The disadvantage of PTA is that it is attended by a high rate of restenosis, although this may occur less if the lesion is stented as part of the angioplasty procedure.

Lymphocele

Incidence and aetiology

Small, clinically insignificant lymphatic collections can be demonstrated by ultrasound scanning in up to 50 per cent of renal transplants (Pollak et al. 1988). Larger lymphoceles that cause complications or require treatment occur in 2–10 per cent of cases (Zinke et al. 1975; Morris et al. 1978). It has been convincingly demonstrated that the source of peritransplant lymph leaks is the lymphatic channels around the iliac arterial system rather than the lymphatics of the transplant kidney itself (Ward et al. 1978). In view of this during the dissection of the iliac arterial system, all the surrounding lymphatic channels must be meticulously secured with non-absorbable ligatures, such as silk, or by the application of metals clips. The lymphatics cannot be simply sealed by surgical diathermy or even left unligated because lymph does not contain any clotting factors and so a divided lymphatic would never seal spontaneously.

Presentation and diagnosis

Only large lymphatic collections (probably of the order of >100 ml) produce clinical symptoms. Compression of the transplant ureter leading to renal dysfunction is only produced by very large lymphoceles with a volume greater than 300 ml. The peak incidence is 6 weeks post-transplant but a lymphatic collection may present between 2 weeks and 6 months post-transplant (Pollak et al. 1988). Most lymphatic collections are found anterior to the iliac vessels and lying between the transplant kidney and the bladder. The most common presenting features are the development of wound or ipsilateral thigh swelling in association with suprapubic discomfort and urinary frequency due to bladder compression. Other presentations include pain over the transplant kidney sometimes associated with a fever, frank ureteric obstruction with renal dysfunction, and ipsilateral thrombophlebitis. However, the vast majority are asymptomatic and present as an incidental finding during an ultrasound scan being performed for another reason. It is important to aspirate all peritransplant fluid collections under ultrasound control in order to aid diagnosis. Macroscopic findings are usually sufficient to differentiate infected from non-infected lymph and biochemical analysis of the fluid allows a urine leak to be excluded. A CT or magnetic resonance imaging (MRI) scan is an essential investigation if surgery is being contemplated, particularly if a laparoscopic procedure is planned (Fig. 12). These allow accurate definition of the relationship between the lymphocele and the transplant ureter.

Treatment

Meticulous technique during surgery will reduce the incidence of lymphoceles. In addition, great attention should be paid to the timing of suction drain removal in the post-transplant period. These should not be removed until less than 20 ml of fluid is produced on two consecutive days. It is safe to leave drains in place for several weeks post-transplant to allow a low volume lymphatic leak to seal by gradual fibrosis. Despite the theoretical risk of infection, this does not seem to be a problem in practice.

Many lymphoceles do not require any treatment because they are small and asymptomatic. They will resolve spontaneously given enough time. If action is deemed to be necessary then the first line treatment is aspiration under ultrasound control. If recurrence occurs, further aspirations can be performed or an external drain can be placed under ultrasound guidance. These drainage procedures can be combined with the use of sclerosants such as povidone-iodine. If these simple measures fail then internal surgical drainage may be required.

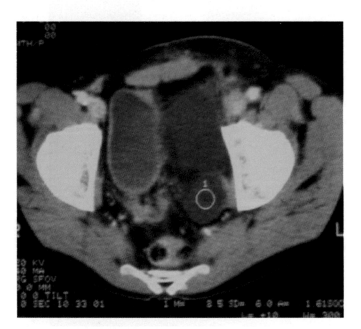

Fig. 12 CT scan taken for planning laparoscopy.

The procedure involves the removal of a 5 cm diameter disc of the lymphocele wall to create a large opening into the peritoneal cavity to allow reabsorption through the abdominal lymphatic drainage system. The peritoneal window has a tendency to heal before the lymphocele is completely reabsorbed, leading to early recurrence. The fenestration can be stented open with a plug of omentum (Bry *et al.* 1990) or a continuous ambulatory peritoneal dialysis (CAPD) tube in an attempt to avoid this. A laparoscopic procedure offers shorter hospitalization and quick postoperative recovery. Identification of the boundaries of the lymphocele is improved by the preoperative injection of methylene blue. The early experience suggests that laparoscopic treatment of lymphoceles can be achieved with a high level of success and no complications.

Urological complications

Urinary tract complications are relatively common after renal transplantation, having an incidence of approximately 5–14 per cent (Mundy *et al.* 1981; Loughlin *et al.* 1984). Whilst urological complications can be serious and difficult to manage, they only rarely cause graft loss or mortality. The relatively high incidence of urological problems is a consequence of the rather tenuous blood supply of the transplant ureter. After kidney retrieval, the only ureteric blood supply that is preserved is derived from the renal artery near the hilum of the kidney. This ureteric branch can be easily damaged where it passes through a 'golden triangle' of fatty connective tissue around and below the kidney. On the left side, this triangle is bounded by the renal hilum, the lower pole of the kidney and the junction of the gonadal and renal veins. On the right side, the triangle is formed by the renal hilum, the lower pole of the kidney and the junction of the vena cava and renal vein. The preservation of the tissue in this triangle is one of the fundamental requirements of donor nephrectomy in both cadaveric and the living donors.

Urinary leaks

These most commonly occur as a result of ischaemic necrosis in any part of the transplant urinary collecting system. The distal ureter has the poorest blood supply and is therefore the most common site of urinary leak. Leaks can also occur from the renal pelvis or the midportion of the ureter, but these are less usual sites, which may be due to unrecognized direct damage to the ureter during organ retrieval. Urinary leaks tend to occur in the first few days after transplantation but can also happen much later. The usual presentation is with straw coloured fluid leaking directly from the transplant wound or accumulating in the drains, in association with oliguria. Alternatively, the extravasating urine may accumulate as a peritransplant fluid collection. This presents as a painful swelling of the wound and the patient may also have a fever. In either case, the extravasated fluid must be differentiated from lymph. The simplest screening test is to dipstick the fluid for glucose, the presence of which would tend to exclude a urine leak. A sample of the undiagnosed fluid, and if possible a known urine specimen, should also be sent for formal biochemical analysis. Urine will have greater urea and creatinine compared to the patient's serum, whereas lymph will have a similar biochemical profile to serum.

Investigation

The presence of a urinary fistula should be confirmed by appropriate radiology. Radioisotope scanning using ^{99m}Tc DTPA can demonstrate the site of a leak but will not show the anatomy with any great accuracy. This is better delineated by either an antegrade or a retrograde pyelogram. Both of these techniques present difficulties in this situation. Antegrade puncture of a non-dilated pelvicalyceal system is a technical challenge for the radiologist, but is usually possible. Retrograde cannulation of the transplant ureteric orifice can be attempted using a flexible cystoscope. This is usually a difficult manouevre due to the fact that the transplant ureter is implanted into the dome of the bladder rather than at its base. Ultrasound scanning is the best initial investigation if the urine leak is contained as a urinoma. This will demonstrate a fluid collection between the transplant kidney and the bladder, which can be sampled by simple needling or drained by the placement of a suitable percutaneous catheter. Contrast-enhanced CT scanning may also be of help in the investigation of undiagnosed peritransplant fluid collections.

Management

The management of urinary leaks has changed significantly in recent years. The former practice of early re-exploration and surgical reconstruction (Palmer and Chatterjee 1978) is no longer always necessary. These operations are usually difficult as the transplant kidney, its blood supply and the ureter are encased in dense fibrous tissue. Percutaneous interventional radiological techniques offer an alternative, at least for initial treatment. The aim is to place a double-J ureteral stent across the region of damage to allow time for the urinary fistula to heal (Nicholson et al. 1991). The first step is to perform a percutaneous nephrostomy, following which the track into the renal substance is dilated. A guide wire is fed through the transplant ureter and into the bladder, and a double-J stent may then be introduced so that the self-retaining pigtail ends are placed in the renal pelvis and the bladder.

Urine leaks can also be managed by endoscopic placement of a double-J stent. A retrograde pyelogram may be possible using a flexible cystoscope, following which a double-J stent can be fed into the ureter over a guide wire. The technical difficulty of this procedure should not be underestimated. The transplant ureteral opening is difficult to cannulate and it is common to encounter significant oedema of the ureteral orifice in the early transplant period.

These techniques are unlikely to be successful in the presence of a significant amount of ischaemic necrosis of the ureter. In view of this surgery still has a role to play. Re-exploration of kidney transplants is straightforward in the early postoperative procedure but may be a considerable challenge later because of the development of an intense peritransplant fibrotic reaction. The choice of operative procedure for a necrotic distal ureter depends on the length of remaining viable ureter. If there is sufficient length after excision of the necrotic distal end, then the transplant ureter may be simply re-implanted into the bladder. In cases where this is not possible, the urinary tract should be reconstructed using the patients' native ureter. Here, there is a choice between anastomosing the native ureter to the transplant ureter proximal to the ischaemic segment or anastomosing the native ureter to the transplant renal depending to a certain extent on the amount of remaining viable transplant ureter. Whichever technique is chosen, it is advisable to protect the new anastomosis with a double-J stent. Although these techniques require the native ureter to be ligated proximally, there is no need to perform an ipsilateral nephrectomy (Lord et al. 1991). Postoperatively, the antegrade nephrostomy can be left in situ so that a contrast study can be performed after 7–10 days to confirm healing of the new anastomosis. Double-J stents are a potential source of sepsis in the immunosuppressed patient and should be removed after 4–6 weeks. In some cases, the transplant recipient will have undergone an ipsilateral nephrectomy in the past or the native ureter is present but too diseased to be used for reconstruction. In these rare cases, a Boari bladder flap can be used to reconstruct the urinary tract.

Ureteric obstruction

Obstruction of the transplant ureter may occur at anytime after transplantation. Its presentation as deterioration in transplant function, associated with hydronephrosis dictates that the investigation of all episodes of transplant dysfunction must include an ultrasound scan.

Causes

Early obstruction is uncommon and is suggestive of a technical error. The most common error during the PL technique is to create a submucosal bladder tunnel that is too tight. There may also be other mistakes such as kinking of a redundant length of ureter, or incorrect suture placement during anastomosis. Each of these problems should occur less frequently when the ureter has been stented and this is an argument for using double-J stents routinely. The urinary tract may also be obstructed early in the post-transplant course by blood clot in the ureter, bladder, or catheter. Bleeding may occur from the ureterovescical anastomosis, the cystotomy (in the PL technique) or as a result of a needle-core transplant biopsy (see Fig. 13). It is now common practice to drain the urinary bladder using relatively small diameter one-way Foley catheters and these may easily be blocked by blood clot. If haematuria is present in the immediate post-transplant hours then it is sensible to replace a standard Foley catheter with a two-way irrigation catheter of the type used routinely by urologists

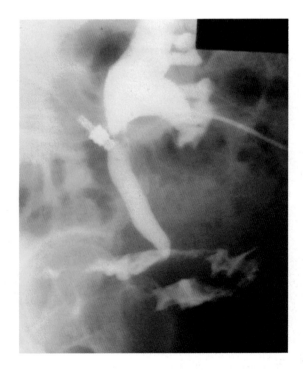

Fig. 13 Bleeding as a result of needle core biopsy.

after transurethral resection operations. The transplant ureter may also be obstructed by a large lymphocele.

Late ureteric obstruction may occur at the ureterovesical or pelvi-ureteric junctions. Ischaemia that is not severe enough to cause necrosis is presumed to be the cause of most ureterovesical obstructions. Renal transplants invariably excite a pronounced perigraft fibrotic response and this is more likely to be the cause of an obstruction at the level of the pelviureteric junction. It is difficult to be sure of the role played by acute rejection episodes. As pointed out previously, the urinary drainage system of the kidney expresses the same HLA antigens as the renal parenchyma and so must be susceptible to acute rejection episodes and the subsequent development of fibrosis. This mechanism could certainly be the cause of rare cases where the whole of the transplant pelvis and ureter become stenosed (Fig. 14).

Investigation

An ultrasound scan will demonstrate a dilated pelvicalyceal system. There is however an important difficulty here: longstanding kidney transplants may have quite marked pelvicalyceal dilatation without being obstructed. This may cause confusion when the apparent hydronephrosis occurs in a long-standing transplant with biopsy proven chronic allograft nephropathy. Further investigation will be required in order to confirm or refute the presence of obstruction and to define its anatomy.

Contrast studies and radioisotope scans are of limited benefit in this situation. Intravenous pyelography usually produces poor images due to a failure of the transplant kidney to concentrate the radiographic contrast media sufficiently. Indeed, an intravenous urography is only successful if the renal function is relatively good with a creatinine less than 250 μmol/l. Retrograde pyelography is an alternative, but has a low success rate because of the difficulty of catheterizing the transplant ureteric orifice at cystoscopy. Isotope scans can be used to confirm the

diagnosis of obstruction. An F-15 renogram may be especially useful in equivocal cases. A diuresis is stimulated by the administration of frusemide 15 min before injection of the isotope. The limitation of isotope scans is that they do not provide good anatomical localization of the problem. In view of these considerations, percutaneous nephrostomy followed by antegrade pyelography is the investigation of choice in suspected transplant ureteric obstruction. The nephrostomy is performed under antibiotic cover using ultrasound control to define an appropriate transplant calyx. The nephrostomy tube should be left in place for a few days. If the serum creatinine falls during this period, then obstruction is confirmed. If there is no improvement in renal function, significant obstruction can be confidently excluded. This simple observation avoids the need to use urodynamic investigations such as the Whittaker test, which tend to be difficult to interpret in transplant kidneys. Following external decompression of the transplant kidney for a few days, an antegrade pyelogram is performed to accurately define the anatomy of the obstructing lesion.

Treatment

Non-operative approaches for the treatment of transplant ureteric obstruction have been used for some time now (Goldstein et al. 1981). The key innovation was the introduction of double-J ureteric stents. These are made of soft silicone rubber that has a memory for its shape. The pigtail configuration at either end may be straightened by the introduction of a guide-wire during insertion and will reform when the guide-wire is removed. The simplest treatment of a transplant ureteric stricture is to place a double-J stent across the lesion via a percutaneous nephrostomy. This may require initial percutaneous balloon dilatation of the ureteral stricture via the nephrostomy (Streem et al. 1988). The stent can be removed after 6 weeks but the re-stenosis rate is high. An alternative is to leave a stent in place in the long-term. Stents left in this way can be changed at cystoscopy on a 6 monthly basis. The clear disadvantage of this method is a high incidence of urinary tract infection and long-term antibiotic prophylaxis is a sensible precaution.

Open surgical management still has its place in the management of ureteral obstruction. The operation performed depends on the site of obstruction and the remaining length of healthy transplant ureter proximal to the obstruction. In cases of obstruction at the ureterovesical, it may be possible to excise the strictured segment and to reimplant the transplant ureter into the bladder as a new ureteroneocystostomy. If there is insufficient transplant ureter to allow this, or the stricture is placed proximally, then the urinary tract is best reconstructed using the ipsilateral native ureter. This may be as a native to transplant uretero-ureterostomy or ureteropyelostomy, depending on the specific anatomy of the lesion. The native ureter may be difficult to identify in the dense peritransplant fibrotic reaction. The operation is therefore facilitated by catheterizing the native ureter at an initial cystoscopy and by the use of an intraperitoneal approach through virgin tissue. The native ureter can be divided and ligated proximally without the need for nephrectomy as long as the native kidney is non-functioning and has not been a source of previous infection. If the native ureter is absent or diseased then it is possible to reconstruct the drainage system by fashioning a tube from the bladder (a Boari flap).

Finally, it is worth stating that not all cases of obstruction require treatment. The overall status of the kidney, the degree of renal impairment and complicating factors such as urinary tract infection need to be taken into account. Where there is a mild degree of obstruction, not associated with any urinary tract infection and in

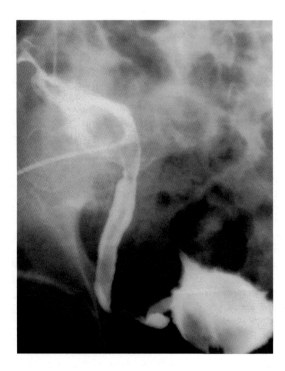

Fig. 14 Stenosed whole pelvis and ureter.

a long-standing kidney that is affected by chronic allograft nephropathy, then it may be better to simply monitor the situation and only intervene if the obstruction worsens.

Complications in the transplant bed

A number of nerves may be encountered in the retroperitoneal dissection required for kidney transplantation. These include the lateral femoral cutaneous nerve and the femoral, obturator, and sacral nerves. Each of these may be damaged by a traction injury, particularly when modern fixed wound retraction systems are used as these can exert a great deal of pressure on the surrounding tissues. As these injuries are neuropraxias, they should recover completely but this may take some months and they can be very disabling. In male transplant recipients the spermatic cord must be mobilized during the dissection to gain access to the retroperitoneal space. This may lead to postoperative scrotal complications such as an acute hydrocele, epididymoorchitis and testicular atrophy.

References

Abusin, K. *et al.* (1998). Long term adult renal graft outcome after ureteric drainage into an augmented bladder or ileal conduit. *Transplant International* 11 (Suppl. 1), S147–S149.

Ackerman, J. R. and Snell, M. E. (1968). Cadaveric renal transplantation: a technique for donor kidney removal. *British Journal of Urology* 40, 515–521.

Arlart, I. P. (1985). Digital subtraction angiography (DSA) in renal and renovascular hypertension: diagnostic value and application in follow-up studies after PTA. *Uremia Investigation* 9, 217.

Bakker, J. *et al.* (1998). Renal artery stenosis and accessory renal arteries: accuracy of detection and visualisation with gadolinium-enhanced breath-hold MR angiography. *Radiology* 207, 497.

Booster, M. H. *et al.* (1993). *In situ* preservation of kidneys from non-heartbeating donors: a proposal for a standardised protocol. *Transplantation* 56, 613.

Bry, J. *et al.* (1990). Treatment of recurrent lymphoceles following renal transplantation: remarsupialization with omentoplasty. *Transplantation* 49, 477.

Curtis, J. J. *et al.* (1983). Inhibition of angiotensin-converting enzyme in renal transplant recipients with hypertension. *New England Journal of Medicine* 308, 377–380.

Dunlop, P. *et al.* (1995). Non-heart-beating donors: the Leicester experience. *Transplantation Proceedings* 27, 2940.

Flowers, J. L. *et al.* (1997). Comparison of open and laparoscopic live donor nephrectomy. *Annals of Surgery* 226, 483.

Garcia-Rinaldi, R. *et al.* (1975). *In situ* preservation of cadaver kidneys for transplantation: laboratory observations and clinical application. *Annals of Surgery* 182, 576.

Goldstein, I. *et al.* (1981). Nephrostomy drainage for renal transplant complications. *Journal of Urology* 126, 159.

Gomez, M. *et al.* (1993). Cardiopulmonary bypass and profound hypothermia as a means for obtaining kidney grafts from irreversible cardiac arrest donors: cooling technique. *Transplantation Proceedings* 25, 1501.

Gregoir, W. Lich–Gregoir operation. In *Surgical Pediatric Urology* (ed. H. B. Epstein, R. Hohenfellner, and D. I. Williams), pp. 265. Stuttgart: Thieme, 1977.

Halimi, J. M. *et al.* (1999). Transplant renal artery stenosis: potential role of ischemia/reperfusion injury and long term outcome following angioplasty. *Journal of Urology* 161 (1), 28–32.

Jones, R. M. *et al.* (1988). Renal vascular thrombosis of cadaveric renal allografts in patients receiving cyclosporine, azathioprine and prednisolone triple therapy. *Clinical Transplantation* 2, 122–127.

Kirsch, A. J. *et al.* (1994). Renal effects of CO_2 insufflation oliguria and acute renal dysfunction in a rat pneumoperitoneum model. *Urology* 43, 453–459.

Lacombe, M. (1975). Arterial stenosis complicating renal allotranplantation in man. *Annals of Surgery* 181, 293–296.

Light, J. A. *et al.* (1996). New profile of cadaveric donors: what are the kidney donor limits? *Transplantation Proceedings* 28, 17.

Linke, C. A. *et al.* (1975). Cadaver donor nephrectomy. *Urology* 6, 133–138.

Lord, R. H. *et al.* (1991). Ureteroureterostomy and pyeloureterostomy without native nephrectomy in renal transplantation. *British Journal of Urology* 67, 349.

Loughlin, K. R. *et al.* (1984). Urologic complications in 718 renal transplant patients. *Surgery* 95, 297.

Margules, R. M. *et al.* (1973). Surgical correction of renovascular hypertension following renal allotransplantation. *Archives of Surgery* 106, 13–16.

Morris, P. J. *et al.* (1978). Results from a new renal transplantation unit. *Lancet* 2, 1353.

Mundy, A. R. *et al.* (1981). The urological complications of 1,000 renal transplants. *British Journal of Urology* 53, 397.

Nerstrom, B. *et al.* (1972). Vascular complications in 155 consecutive kidney transplantations. *Scandinavian Journal of Urology and Nephrology* 6 (Suppl. 15), 64.

Nguyen, D. H. *et al.* (1990). Outcome of renal transplantation after urinary diversion and enterocystoplasty: a retrospective, controlled study. *Journal of Urology* 144, 1349.

Nicholson, M. L. *et al.* (1991). Urological complications of renal transplantation: the impact of double J ureteric stents. *Annals of the Royal College of Surgeons of England* 73, 316–321.

Nogueira, J. M. *et al.* (1999). A comparison of recipient renal outcomes with laparoscopic versus open live donor nephrectomy. *Transplantation* 67, 722–728.

Orloff, M. S. *et al.* (1994). Non-heart-beating cadaveric organ donation. *Annals of Surgery* 220, 578.

Palmer, J. M. and Chatterjee, S. M. (1978). Urologic complications in renal transplantation. *The Surgical Clinics of North America* 58, 305.

Philosophe, B. *et al.* (1999). Laparoscopic versus open donor nephrectomy: comparing ureteral complications in the recipients and improving the laparoscopic technique. *Transplantation* 68, 497.

Pleass, H. C. *et al.* (1995). Orologic complications after renal transplantation: a prospective randomised trial comparing different techniques of ureteric anastomosis and the use of prophylactic ureteric stents. *Transplantation Proceedings* 27, 1091.

Politano, V. A. and Leadbetter, W. F. (1958). An operative technique the correction of vesicoureteral reflux. *Journal of Urology* 79, 932–941.

Pollak, R. *et al.* (1988). The natural history of and therapy for perirenal fluid collections following renal transplantation. *Journal of Urology* 140, 716.

Ratner, L. E. *et al.* (1995). Laparoscopic live donor nephrectomy. *Transplantation* 60, 1047.

Ratner, L. E. *et al.* (1997). Laparoscopic assisted live donor nephrectomy—a comparison with the open approach. *Transplantation* 63, 229.

Ratner, L. E. *et al.* (1999). Technical considerations in the delivery of the kidney during laparoscopic live donor nephrectomy. *Journal of the American College of Surgeons* 189, 427.

Reuther, G. *et al.* (1989). Acute renal vein thrombosis in renal allografts detection with duplex Doppler US. *Radiology* 170, 557–558.

Richardson, A. J. *et al.* (1990). Spontaneous rupture of renal allografts: the importance of renal vein thrombosis in the cyclosporin era. *British Journal of Surgery* 77, 558–564.

Rosenthal, J. T. *et al.* (1983). Principles of multiple organ procurement. *Annals of Surgery* 198, 617–621.

Ruggenenti, P. *et al.* (2001). Post transplant renal artery stenosis: the hemodynamic response to revascularization. *Kidney International* 60, 309–318.

Sasaki, T. *et al.* (1999). Is laparoscopic donor nephrectomy here to stay? *American Journal of Surgery* 177, 368–370.

Shaffer, D. *et al.* (1998). Two hundred consecutive living donor nephrectomies. *Archives of Surgery* **133**, 426–431.

Slakey, D. P. *et al.* (1999). Laparoscopic living donor nephrectomy: advantages of the hand-assisted method. *Transplantation* **68**, 581.

Streem, S. B. *et al.* (1988). Long-term efficacy of ureteral dilation for transplant ureteral stenosis. *Journal of Urology* **140**, 32.

Suzuki, K. *et al.* (1997). Retroperitoneoscopy assisted live donor nephrectomy: the initial 2 cases. *Journal of Urology* **158**, 1353–1356.

Szostek, M. *et al.* (1995). Successful transplantation of kidneys harvested from cadaver donors at 71 to 259 minutes following cardiac arrest. *Transplantation Proceedings* **27**, 2901.

Vanrenterghem, Y. *et al.* (1985). Thromboembolic complications and haemostatic changes in cyclosporine-treated cadaveric kidney allograft recipients. *Lancet* **1**, 999–1000.

Ward, K. *et al.* (1978). The origin of lymphoceles following renal transplantation. *Transplantation* **25**, 346.

Zinke, H. *et al.* (1975). Experience with lymphoceles after renal transplantation. *Surgery* **77**, 444.

13.3.2 The early management of the recipient

Phuong-Thu T. Pham, Phuong-Chi T. Pham, and Alan H. Wilkinson

Early post-transplant factors including delayed graft function (DGF), acute rejection episodes, nephrotoxic agents, post-transplant hypertension, dyslipidaemia, and/or diabetes mellitus among others have been implicated in both short- and long-term causes of morbidity and mortality after renal transplantation. Optimal management of the transplant recipient begins in the immediate postoperative period. This chapter provides a stepwise approach to the medical management of the transplant recipient in the first 6 months after transplantation. Surgical and urological complications are discussed elsewhere. Although postoperative recovery may differ among patients, management of the transplant recipient can be divided into three periods: the immediate postoperative period, the first week post-transplant, and the first 6 months post-transplant. Immunosuppressive therapy is discussed in Chapter 13.2.2.

Immediate postoperative period

Patients should be evaluated immediately upon arrival in the recovery room, preferably by a combined medical surgical team. The initial assessment is similar to that following any major surgical procedure and attention should be paid to cardiovascular and respiratory stability. Most patients are successfully extubated and awake, and pain control should be administered. Further evaluation should include a full electrolyte panel including sodium, potassium, creatinine, glucose, calcium, phosphorus, magnesium, complete blood count with platelets, chest X-ray, and electrocardiography (ECG). Intraoperative blood loss

Table 1 Maintenance and replacement fluids

Maintenance fluid: D5 1/2 NS
Replacement fluid
For urine output ≤200 ml/h, replace cc per cc with 1/2 NS
For urine output >200 ml/h, give 200 cc plus half of remainder of urine output
For urine output >300 ml for four consecutive hours, hold replacement fluid and reassess in 2 h
For urine output >500 ml/h for two consecutive hours, hold replacement fluid and reassess in 2 h
For urine output <50 ml/h, check for Foley catheter patency, reassess haemodynamic status. Volume challenge and/or high dose diuretics as clinically indicated. Imaging studies if no response

and volume replacement should be assessed and operative report reviewed.

In general, it is possible to anticipate early graft function based on preoperative and postoperative characteristics of the donor and the recipient as well as the intraoperative perfusion characteristics of the kidney allograft. In patients with minimal residual urine output, an immediate postoperative increase in urine output may serve as an indicator of early graft function. A brisk large volume diuresis following graft revascularization may be due to preoperative volume overload, osmotic diuresis in previously uraemic patients, intraoperative use of mannitol and/or frusemide, and/or excessive intraoperative intravenous crystalloid or colloid fluid administration. Total fluid intake and output should be monitored on an hourly basis. The intraoperative use of dopamine can be promptly discontinued in polyuric patients. Suggested maintenance and urine replacement fluids are given in Table 1.

An abrupt cessation or significant reduction in urine output should prompt immediate investigation. Irrigation of the Foley catheter to check for patency should be performed. In a persistently anuric patient, Doppler ultrasound or radioisotope flow scan to ensure ongoing blood flow to the allograft and to exclude surgical complications should be done in the recovery room. The absence of blood flow to the allograft requires urgent evaluation by the surgical team for possible re-exploration. The length of time a patient remains in the recovery room may vary. A stable patient may typically be transferred to the general transplant care unit within 1–2 h. Intensive care unit observation is usually not required except under special circumstances such as in patients with postoperative ECG changes or in patients with known cardiomyopathy and a low preoperative ejection fraction (EF of 40 per cent or less) who are at risk for congestive heart failure in the perioperative period. In these patients, intraoperative Swan–Ganz placement for continuous monitoring of cardiovascular and volume status is recommended.

The first postoperative week

In general, stable patients should be encouraged to ambulate within 24–48 h. Liquid diet may be started when bowel function returns, usually on the first postoperative day. Intravenous fluid can usually be discontinued when the patient is able to tolerate solid food diet. Electrolyte abnormalities are not uncommon in the early postoperative period and laboratory evaluation should initially be performed every 6 h, then daily. Suggested postoperative orders on transfer to the transplant care unit are shown in Table 2.

Specific management of patients in the first postoperative week depends on the immediate functional status of the graft, which may be categorized as immediate graft function, slow recovery of graft function, and DGF.

Patients with immediate graft function

For patients who have immediate graft function, the first postoperative week is generally characterized by gradual improvement in the patient's general sense of well being. Serum creatinine commonly decreases by 88.40 to greater than or equal to 354 μmol/l daily. Patients with immediate graft function can usually be discharged on postoperative day 4 or 5 following successful Foley catheter removal and voiding trial.

Patients with slow recovery of graft function

Patients who have slow recovery of graft function are generally non-oliguric and experience a slow decline in serum creatinine. The level typically decreases by 17.70 to 79.56 μmol/l daily. These patients usually do not require dialysis support. However, great care must be given to fluid management. Volume depletion must be avoided to prevent precipitation of acute tubular necrosis. An initial reduction in urine output may be challenged with administration of intravenous fluid and/or frusemide after a careful assessment of the patient's volume status. If there is no response to these manoeuvres, Doppler ultrasound or nuclear imaging studies should be obtained to assess renal blood flow and to rule out obstruction or urine leak. The serum creatinine of patients with slow graft function generally does not normalize within the first postoperative week. Nevertheless, most patients can be discharged on postoperative day 5–10 with close outpatient follow-up. In patients who are at high risk for obstruction such as diabetics with neurogenic bladder or male patients with benign prostatic hypertrophy and a high postvoid residual ($\geq$125–150 ml) it is advisable to leave the Foley catheter in place or to instruct the patient to perform self-catheterization prior to discharge. In addition, these patients may

benefit from an α-2-blocker (terazosin or doxazosin) and/or a prostate relaxant (tamsulosin). In recipients at risk for developing a urine leak or rupture at the ureterovesical junction in the presence of a high urine volume such as those with a small contracted bladder (bladder capacity $\leq$ 100 ml), it is also wise to leave the Foley catheter in place for a more prolonged period (7–14 days).

Patients with delayed graft function

The incidence of DGF may range from 10 to 50 per cent in some centres (Lehtonen *et al.* 1997; Ojo *et al.* 1997; Shokes and Cecka 1997; Marcen *et al.* 1998; Paff *et al.* 1998) and can often be anticipated based on both recipient and donor factors (Table 3). Unless these patients have adequate residual urine output from the native kidneys, most will require temporary dialysis support for volume, hyperkalaemia, or uraemia. Although peritoneal dialysis may be performed in patients with a functioning Tenckhoff catheter in place, haemodialysis may be more effective in the early postoperative period when severe hyperkalaemia is present or prolonged absence of bowel function is a problem. Peritoneal dialysis should be avoided when there is evidence of a peritoneal leak or infection. The differential diagnoses of DGF are shown in Table 3. A systematic approach to the evaluation of DGF may be divided into prerenal (or preglomerular type), intrinsic, and postrenal. Although uncommon, vascular causes of DGF must be excluded, particularly in the early postoperative period.

Prerenal causes of DGF

Intravascular volume depletion and nephrotoxic drugs
Severe intravascular volume depletion is usually suggested by a careful review of the patient's preoperative history and intraoperative report. If haemodialysis is performed preoperatively, it is preferable to keep the patient slightly above his or her estimated dry weight (approximately 1 k above their dry weight) to facilitate diuresis following graft revascularization. Both calcineurin inhibitors (CNIs) cyclosporin and, to a lesser extent, tacrolimus have been shown to cause a dose-related reversible afferent arteriolar vasoconstriction and 'preglomerular type'

Table 2 Postrenal transplant orders

Nursing care
Vital signs q 1 h × 12 h, q 2 h × 8 h, then q 4 h
Fluid input and output q 1 h
Daily weight
Turn, cough, and deep breathe q 1 h, encourage incentive spirometry q 1 h
  while awake
Out of bed first postoperative day, ambulate q.i.d. thereafter
Elevate head of bed 30°
Change dressing q.d. and p.r.n.
Check dialysis access for function q 4 h and record
No blood pressure checks or venipunctures in extremity with dialysis access
Foley catheter to drainage, irrigate gently with 30 ml normal saline p.r.n. for
  clots or no urine flow
Catheter care q 8 h
N.P.O. until diet is changed by surgical team

Laboratory orders
Complete blood count with platelets, electrolytes, creatinine, glucose
  q 6 h × 3, then daily
Alkaline phosphatase, total bilirubin, calcium, phosphorus, SGOT, SGPT,
  LDH, urine culture, and sensitivity twice a week
Cyclosporin or tacrolimus level every morning

Table 3 Differential diagnosis of DGF

Prerenal (or preglomerular type)
Volume contraction
Nephrotoxic drugs (see text)
Vascular complications
    Arterial or venous thrombosis
    Renal artery stenosis

Intrinsic renal
Acute tubular necrosis
Accelerated acute or acute rejection
Thrombotic microangiopathy
Recurrence of primary glomerular disease (particularly FSGS)

Postrenal
Catheter obstruction
Perinephric fluid collection (lymphocele, urine leak, haematoma)
Ureteral obstruction
    Intrinsic (blood clots, poor re-implantation, ureteral slough)
    Extrinsic (ureteral kinking)
Neurogenic bladder
Benign prostatic hypertrophy

allograft dysfunction that manifests clinically as delayed recovery of allograft function. Intraoperative direct injection of the calcium channel blocker verapamil into the renal artery has been suggested to reduce capillary spasm and improve renal blood flow (Dawidson et al. 1991, 1994; Gritsch and Rosenthal 2001). Most centres have advocated the use of non-dihydropyridine calcium channel blockers (i.e. diltiazem) to counteract the vasoconstrictive effect of CNIs in addition to the allowance for CNI dose reduction. Their use may permit a reduction in the cyclosporin dose of up to 40 per cent. Other commonly used drugs that may potentially precipitate acute 'preglomerular type' allograft dysfunction include angiotensin-converting enzyme inhibitors (ACEIs), Amphotericin B, non-steroidal anti-inflammatory drugs, and contrast dye.

Vascular complications/renal artery stenosis

Arterial or venous thrombosis generally occurs within the first 2–3 postoperative days but may occur as long as 2 months post-transplant. In most series reported, the incidence of arterial/venous thrombosis ranges from 0.5 per cent to as great as 8 per cent with arterial accounting for one-third and venous thrombosis for two-third of cases.

Thombosis occurring early after transplantation is most often due to technical surgical complications while the later onset is generally due to acute rejection (Fotiadis et al. 2001; Gritsch and Rosenthal 2001). Diagnostic studies and management of surgical complications are discussed elsewhere. In patients with initial good allograft function, thombosis is generally heralded by the acute onset of oliguria or anuria associated with deterioration of allograft function. Clinically, the patient may present with graft swelling or tenderness, and/or gross haematuria. In patients with DGF and good residual urine output from the native kidneys, there may be no overt signs or symptoms and the diagnosis rests on clinical suspicion and prompt imaging studies. Confirmed arterial or venous thrombosis typically necessitates allograft nephrectomy. Suggested predisposing factors for vascular thrombosis include arteriosclerotic involvement of the donor or recipient vessels, intimal injury of graft vessels, kidney with multiple arteries, younger recipient and/or younger donor age, history of recurrent thrombosis, the presence of antiphospholipid antibodies (anticardiolipin antibody and/or lupus anticoagulant antibody), and thrombocytosis. In a series of 96 consecutive renal transplant recipients, renal artery or renal vein thrombosis has been reported to occur in up to 16 per cent of patients with systemic lupus erythematosus who were positive for antiphospholipid antibody (Stone et al. 1999).

There has been no consensus on the optimal management of recipients with abnormal hypercoagulability profile such as abnormal activated protein C resistance ratio or factor V Leiden mutation, antiphospholipid antibody positivity, protein C or protein S deficiency, or antithrombin III deficiency. However, unless contraindicated, perioperative and/or postoperative prophylactic anticoagulation should be considered particularly in patients with a prior history of recurrent thrombotic events. Transplant of paediatric *en bloc* kidneys into adult recipient with a history of thrombosis should probably be avoided. The duration of anticoagulation has not been well defined but lifelong anticoagulation should be considered in high-risk candidates.

Transplant renal artery stenosis

Transplant renal artery stenosis may occur as early as the first week but is usually a late complication and is discussed under allograft dysfunction in the first 6 months.

Intrinsic renal causes of DGF

Intrinsic renal causes of DGF typically include acute tubular necrosis, acute rejection, thrombotic microangiopathy (TMA), or recurrence of glomerular disease affecting the native kidneys.

Acute tubular necrosis

Post-transplant acute tubular necrosis (ATN) is the most common cause of DGF. The two terms are often used interchangeably although not all cases of DGF are caused by ATN. Its incidence varies widely among centres and has been reported to occur in 20–25 per cent of patients (range 6–50 per cent) (Troppmann et al. 1996; Lehtonen et al. 1997; Ojo et al. 1997; Shokes and Cecka 1997; Marcen et al. 1998; Paff et al. 1998). The difference in the incidence reported may, in part, be due to the more liberal use of organs from marginal donors by some centres but not by others and/or the difference in the criteria used to define DGF. Unless an allograft biopsy was performed, post-transplant ATN should be a diagnosis of exclusion. In the absence of superimposed hyperacute or acute rejection, ATN typically resolves over several days and occasionally over several weeks (4–6 weeks), particularly in recipients of older donor kidneys. Recovery of ATN is usually heralded by a steady increase in urine output associated with a decrease in interdialytic increase in serum creatinine and eventual dialysis independence. Prolonged DGF should prompt a diagnostic allograft biopsy. Some centres perform serial biopsies in patients with prolonged DGF to exclude covert acute rejection or other intrinsic causes of allograft dysfunction. Both donor and/or recipient factors are important determinant(s) of early allograft function (Table 4). ATN is exceptional in living donor renal transplants while it may occur in 20–50 per cent of cadaveric renal transplants.

Risk factors

Prolonged cold ischaemia time (CIT) and older donor age have been regarded as major risk factors for DGF secondary to ATN. In a retrospective review of 383 cadaveric renal allograft transplants performed at 44 European centres, DGF has been reported to occur in 44 per cent of patients. Univariate analysis revealed that the rate of DGF in grafts with a CIT of more than 24 h was 20 per cent higher than in grafts with shorter CIT (60 versus 39 per cent, $P = 0.001$) (Hetzel et al. 2002). Data from the UNOS Scientific Renal Transplant Registry revealed that the incidence of DGF increased from 17 per cent when the CIT was less than 12 h to 39 per cent when the kidneys have been in cold storage for 49–72 h. The incidence of DGF has also been shown to increase with increasing donor age. The need for dialysis within the first postoperative week was 17 per cent when the donors were 15–20 years of age while more than 40 per cent required dialysis when the donors were more than 65 years of age (Cecka 1998). Data from the United States Renal Data System showed that every 6 h of CIT increases the risk of DGF by 23 per cent (Ojo et al. 1997). Other potential risk factors for DGF are shown in Table 4.

Potential mechanisms of post-transplant ATN

Post-transplant ATN is primarily an ischaemic injury that may be exacerbated by both immunological and non-immunological insults. The former is suggested by the observation that DGF is more prevalent in recipients of re-allograft transplants compared to those of primary transplants irrespective of donor source (i.e. living-related or cadaveric donor kidney) and the latter by the observation that the

Table 4 Risk factors for DGF due to ATN in cadaveric renal transplantation

Donor factors	Recipient factors
Premorbid factors	*Premorbid factors*
Age (<10 or >50)	African American
Donor hypertension	(compared to caucasians)
Donor macro- or microvascular	Peripheral vascular disease
disease	Presensitization (PRA > 50)
Cause of death (cerebrovascular	Re-allograft transplantation
versus traumatic)	
Preoperative donor characteristics	*Peri- and postoperative factors*
Brain-death stress	Recipient volume contraction
Hypotension, shock	Early high dose calcineurin inhibitors
Prolonged use of vasopressors	± Early use of OKT3
Preprocurement ATN	
Non-heart beating donor	
Nephrotoxic agents	
Organ procurement surgery	
Hypotension prior to	
cross-clamping of aorta	
Traction on renal vasculatures	
Cold storage flushing solutions	
Kidney preservation	
Prolonged warm ischaemia time	
(± contraindication to	
donation)	
Prolonged cold ischaemia time	
Cold storage versus machine	
perfusion	
Intraoperative factors	
Intraoperative haemodynamic	
instability	
Prolonged rewarm time	
(anastomotic time)	

incidence of DGF was significantly higher among recipients of cadaveric donor kidneys than for living-donor transplants (Shokes and Cecka 1997). Indeed, the cadaveric kidney is vulnerable to ischaemic injury at various time points starting at the diagnosis of donor brain death, maintenance of circulatory and respiratory stability following brain death, procurement surgery and cold storage, and ending at the time of renal arterial anastomosis or rewarming time.

In a rat study, explosive brain death has been shown to be associated with upregulation of macrophage [interleukin (IL)-1, IL-6, and tumour necrosis factor (TNF)-α] and T-cell-associated products [IL-2 and interferon (IFN)-α] in the peripheral organs, rendering them more susceptible to subsequent host inflammatory and immunological responses (Takada *et al.* 1998). Following brain death, maintenance of cardiovascular stability becomes increasingly difficult as time elapses. Persistent hypotension, the use of pressors, hypothermia, metabolic and electrolyte disturbances may all contribute to multiorgan failure. Intense sympathetic stimulation either from direct neurosympathetic activity, or from endogenous release of cathecholamines may further result in markedly decrease organ perfusion and consequently in donor ATN. In addition to donor factors, the overall medical condition of the recipient at the time of transplant and any adverse intraoperative or early postoperative events may also predispose the kidney allograft to ATN.

Following revascularization, the kidney allograft may be further exposed to ischaemia–reperfusion injury, particularly, in donor organs with a long CIT. During prolonged ischaemia, depletion of ATP results in anaerobic metabolism of the nucleotide adenosine. After reperfusion, the reintroduction of oxygen into tissues results in a profound increase in oxygen free radicals, superoxide anion, and hydrogen peroxide production leading to peroxidation of membrane lipids, glutathione depletion, and eventual cellular destruction. Recently, St Peter *et al.* (2002) have identified a genetic allele that is protective against reperfusion injury. Under the stress of reperfusion, inducible enzymes such as glutathione-S-transferase (GST) are believed to play an important role in attenuating the deleterious effects of reactive oxygen species. GSTs are encoded by two supergene families including a family of soluble GSTs, currently known to comprise at least 16 genes, and a separate family of microsomal GST enzymes comprising of at least six genes (Hayes and Strange 2000). It has been suggested that polymorphisms of the enzymes within each gene family may confer differential protection against oxidative stress. GSTP1, GSTM1, and GSTT1 are three polymorphic enzymes that have been extensively studied. St Peter *et al.* have shown that the presence of a donor GSTM1 *B allele was associated with a reduced risk of DGF in kidneys transplanted after a CIT of more than 24 h. In their studies, only three of 19 individuals who carried the GSTM1 *B allele required haemodialysis in the first week after transplantation, compared to 40 of 84 who received a kidney from a donor who lacked this allele ($P < 0.05$). No association was found between any enzyme polymorphism in the recipients and the development of DGF.

Effect of DGF/ATN on graft survival and function

Studies on the impact of DGF on long-term graft survival have yielded conflicting results (Troppmann *et al.* 1996; Lehtonen *et al.* 1997; Ojo *et al.* 1997; Shokes and Cecka 1997; Marcen *et al.* 1998). Data from the UNOS Scientific Renal Transplant Registry revealed that DGF reduced 1-year graft survival from 91 to 75 per cent ($P < 0.0001$) and graft half-life from 12.9 to 8.0 years, independent of early acute rejection. In the presence of early acute rejection occurring before hospital discharge, DGF reduced 1-year graft survival from 81 to 66 per cent ($P < 0.001$) and graft half-life from 9.5 to 7.7 years. When any episode of acute rejection occurring within the first 6 months was considered, DGF reduced 3-year graft survival from 77 to 60 per cent and graft half-life from 9.4 to 6.2 years ($P < 0.001$). The deleterious effect of DGF with or without acute rejection on graft half-life remained significant after adjusting for discharge serum creatinine of less than 2.5 mg/dl ($P < 0.001$). Interestingly, in the presence of DGF with or without acute rejection, the survival advantage of well-matched kidneys (0–1 mismatch) over those of poorly matched kidneys (5–6 mismatches) was no longer seen. In fact, the graft half-life of five to six HLA mismatch kidneys without DGF or early acute rejection was found to be superior to that of 0–1 HLA-mismatch kidney with DGF and/or acute rejection (Shokes and Cecka 1998). In contrast to the results obtained from the UNOS Scientific Renal Transplant Registry, a number of studies have shown that in the absence of acute rejection, DGF does not affect long-term graft survival. Other investigators suggested that DGF is deleterious to graft outcome only when associated with reduced renal mass and hyperfiltration injury (Barrientos *et al.* 1994). In a retrospective study of a single-centre cohort of primary cadaveric kidney recipients with good allograft function at 1 year (defined as serum creatinine ≤176.80 μmol/l at 1 year after transplantation), Troppmann *et al.*

showed that DGF *per se* was not a significant risk factor for decreased graft survival while the worst outcome was seen in a subgroup of recipients with both DGF and rejection. In contrast, rejection significantly increased the risk of graft loss irrespective of their DGF status. The authors speculated that for recipients with both DGF and rejection, a chronic ongoing process may have led to late graft failure (Troppmann *et al.* 1996). Similar results were obtained by Marcen *et al.* The authors showed that in the absence of rejection, graft survival rates at 1 and 6 years (censored for death with functioning grafts) were similar in patients with immediate graft function compared to those with DGF (96 and 81 per cent versus 95 and 83 per cent, respectively). In contrast, rejection adversely affected graft survival rates at 1 and 6 years, both in patients with immediate graft function ($P < 0.05$ versus no DGF/no rejection) and more deeply in those with DGF ($P < 0.001$ versus no DGF/no rejection). DGF, when combined with rejection, had an additive adverse effect on allograft survival (Marcen *et al.* 1998).

Regardless of the true impact of DGF (independent of other factors) on long-term graft survival, DGF may undoubtedly prolong hospitalization and complicate patient management in the early postoperative period. Hence, efforts should be made to modify risk factors including minimizing CIT, avoidance of intraoperative and perioperative volume contraction, and/or use of CNI sparing protocol. Some centres have advocated the use of sequential antibody induction therapy in the presence of anticipated or established DGF. In these cases, CNI is introduced when the serum creatinine reaches 221–265.20 µmol/l or less. The antibody can be discontinued once adequate CNI level has been achieved.

Acute rejection

While hyperacute or accelerated acute rejection due to presensitization may occur immediately after transplantation or a delay of several days, classic cell mediated acute rejection is typically seen after the first post-transplant week. Accumulating evidence suggests that there is an interactive effect between ATN and acute rejection. Ischaemia–reperfusion injury has been shown to cause upregulation of multiple cytokines and growth factors within the allograft including IL-1, IL-2, IL-6, TNF, IFN-α, and transforming growth factor β among others. The proinflammatory cytokine response may, in turn, trigger acute allograft rejection through upregulation of various costimulatory and adhesion molecules as well as through increased expression of major histocompatibility complex class I and class II antigen (Shokes *et al.* 1990; Bryan 2001). It is, therefore, prudent to perform a diagnostic allograft biopsy in the face of prolonged ATN.

Thrombotic microangiopathy

Thrombotic microangiopathy is a well-recognized complication after renal allograft transplantation. In most cases, CNI is believed to play a role in the development of this disorder. In a large series consisting of 188 recipients of kidney alone, simultaneous kidney–pancreas or pancreas after kidney transplantation, TMA has been reported to occur in up to 14 per cent of those cases treated with cyclosporin- or tacrolimus-based immunosuppression. It may develop as early as 4 days postoperative to as late as 6 years post-transplantation (Zarifian *et al.* 1998). In recipients of renal allograft, renal dysfunction is the most common manifestation. Thrombocytopenia and microangiopathic haemolysis are often mild or absent. Indeed, the diagnosis of post-transplant TMA is often made on graft biopsies performed to determine the cause of

DGF or to rule out acute rejection (Pham *et al.* 2000). Although there have been no controlled trials comparing the different treatment modalities of this condition, dose reduction or discontinuation of the offending agent appears to be pivotal to management. Adjunctive plasmapheresis with fresh frozen plasma replacement may offer survival advantages. In transplant recipients with cyclosporin-associated TMA, successful use of tacrolimus immunosuppression has been reported (McCauley *et al.* 1989; Pham *et al.* 2002). However, recurrence of TMA in renal transplant recipients treated sequentially with cyclosporin and tacrolimus has been described and clinicians must remain vigilant for signs and symptoms of recurrence of TMA in patients who are switched from cyclosporin to tacrolimus or vice versa (Pham *et al.* 2000). There have been anecdotal reports of the successful use of sirolimus and/or mycophenolate mofetil in transplant recipients with CNI-associated TMA (Lecornu-Heuze *et al.* 1998; Heering *et al.* 2000). However, recently, sirolimus has also been suspected to cause TMA in recipients of renal allografts (unpublished observation). The use of the monoclonal antibody muromonab-CD3 OKT3 has also been associated with the development of post-transplant TMA, although infrequently (Ruggenenti 2002).

Other potential causative factors of post-transplant-associated TMA include the presence of lupus anticoagulant and/or anticardiolipin antibody, cytomegalovirus (CMV) infection, and, less frequently systemic viral infection with parvovirus B19 or influenza A virus (Asaka *et al.* 2000; Luisa *et al.* 2000). An increased incidence of TMA has also been described in a subset of renal allograft recipients with concurrent hepatitis C virus (HCV) infection and anticardiolipin antibody positivity (Baid *et al.* 1999).

Recurrence of glomerular disease of the native kidneys

Recurrence of glomerular disease of the native kidneys is discussed in Chapter 13.3.3.

Postrenal causes of DGF

Postrenal DGF is generally due to obstruction and may occur anywhere from the intrarenal collecting system to the level of the bladder–catheter drainage system. The latter is generally due to blood clots and can often be managed by flushing the catheter with saline solution. Nursing care orders should routinely include irrigation of the Foley catheter as needed for clots or no urine flow. In patients with persistent gross haematuria, continuous bladder irrigation may be helpful. However, potential serious complications such as bleeding from vascular anastomoses or graft thrombosis should first be excluded. Table 3 summarizes the possible causative factors of postrenal causes of DGF. Obstruction secondary to urological complications is discussed under surgical complications.

The first 6 post-transplant months

The first post-transplant month involves the transition from inpatient to outpatient care. The frequency of clinic visits may vary between centres. However, patients should be seen two to three times a week for the first 2 weeks, twice a week for the next 2 weeks, and weekly for the next month. After the first 2 months, the frequency of outpatient visits largely depends on the complexity of the patient's early postoperative course. Most patients with stable graft function and an uneventful postoperative course can return to work and/or their regular daily activities 2–3 months post-transplant. Laboratory assessment during the first 1–2 months should include a complete blood count with platelets, urinalysis, serum creatinine, immunosuppressive drug concentration, electrolyte, and metabolic panel including potassium, calcium, phosphorus, and glucose. Liver enzymes and cholesterol should also be monitored regularly.

Acute allograft dysfunction

An increase of 10–20 per cent in serum creatinine from baseline commonly represents laboratory variability and can be rechecked within 48–72 h at the clinicians' discretion. However, a 25 per cent or greater increase in serum creatinine should prompt further evaluation. Prerenal azotaemia is usually evident through obtaining a medical history and/or physical exam. The presence of fever, graft tenderness, and/or pyuria suggest pyelonephritis. In the era of potent immunosuppression, fever and graft tenderness are usually absent during acute allograft rejection episodes. Accurate diagnosis necessitates an allograft biopsy. All medications must be reviewed to exclude any drug-induced nephrotoxicity. Deteriorating allograft function associated with markedly elevated cyclosporin or tacrolimus concentrations may be managed expectantly by dose reduction. Acute CNI typically improves within 24–48 h after dosage adjustment. Hence, a persistently elevated serum creatinine warrants further evaluation.

In contrast, acute allograft dysfunction in the face of persistently low cyclosporin or tacrolimus concentrations, high pretransplant panel reactive antibody (PRA), and/or in re-transplantation raises the possibility of acute rejection and requires more aggressive diagnostic and/or therapeutic intervention. Initial evaluation with Doppler ultrasound to exclude vascular complications and to rule out hydronephrosis, or perinephric fluid collection (due to lymphocele, haematoma, or urine leak) is appropriate. If perirenal drains are still in place or if there is copious drainage through the incision, the fluid should be sent urgently for measurement of creatinine. Elevated fluid creatinine concentration to more than one and a half times over that of plasma suggests urine leak and appropriate steps should be taken. Diagnostic imaging studies and management of surgical and urological complications are discussed elsewhere. A diagnostic allograft biopsy can be performed after vascular and urological causes of graft dysfunction have been excluded. In patients with high risks for complications (those who are anticoagulated, or those in whom an allograft biopsy may difficult due to overlying bowels or obesity), it may be appropriate to proceed with pulse corticosteroids without biopsy confirmation particularly when there is a high clinical suspicion for acute rejection.

Allograft rejection

Allograft rejection can be classified as hyperacute, accelerated acute, acute, and chronic rejection. Chronic rejection is discussed under long-term management and complications.

Hyperacute rejection

Hyperacute rejection can be recognized by the surgeon immediately following completion of vascular anastomosis or it can occur within minutes to hours after graft revascularization. Grossly, the kidney allograft may appear flaccid or cyanotic and hard, and graft rupture may occur within minutes after revascularization (Helderman and Goral 2001).

Histomorphological examination reveals widespread vascular thrombosis affecting arteries, arterioles, and glomeruli. Polymorphonuclear leucocytes are typically and regularly incorporated in the thrombi (Nast and Cohen 2001). Hyperacute rejection is mediated by preformed, cytotoxic IgG anti-HLA class I antibody that are produced in response to previous exposure to alloantigen through multiple pregnancies, blood transfusions, and/or prior transplants. These antibodies bind to the graft vascular endothelium, activate complement leading to severe vascular injury including thrombosis and obliteration of the graft vasculature (Helderman and Goral 2001). Hyperacute rejection almost uniformly leads to graft loss and prevention with meticulous cross-match is the mainstay of management. Hyperacute rejection can also occur as a result of ABO blood group incompatibility due to preformed anti-ABO blood group antibodies of the IgM isotype. With the current pretransplant cytotoxic cross-match as well as ABO-matching policy, hyperacute rejection has virtually been non-existent.

Accelerated acute rejection

Accelerated acute rejection occurs after the first 24 h to 7 days after transplantation and has been suggested to be mediated by both humoural and cellular mechanisms. However, histomorphological examination may reveal less intense tubulointerstitial infiltrates compared to that of classic acute cellular rejection. Accelerated acute rejection probably represents a delayed amnestic response to prior sensitization. It may be seen after donor-specific transfusions in recipients of living-related donor transplant due to a primed T-cell response (Helderman and Goral 2001). Treatment of accelerated acute rejection generally requires aggressive treatment with antibody therapy (OKT3 or antithymocyte antibody), intravenous immunoglobulin (IVIG) with or without adjunctive plasmapheresis. Anecdotal reports in small series of patients have shown that pre-emptive pretransplant combination therapy with plasma exchange and IVIG have allowed living donor kidneys to be successfully transplanted into cross-match positive recipients (Montgomery et al. 2000). Despite aggressive treatment, accelerated acute rejection commonly results in early graft loss. The T-cell flow cytometry cross-match (FCXM) may be useful in the pretransplant evaluation of sensitized or re-allograft transplant candidates whose antibody levels may have declined but who can mount a rapid amnestic response upon rechallenge. Transplant across a positive T-cell FCXM have been reported to be associated with a higher rate of early acute rejection episodes (Lazda et al. 1988; Bryan et al. 1998; Kimball et al. 1998; Katznelson et al. 2001). Hyperacute rejection, however, has not been reported as long as the pretransplant cytotoxic cross-match is negative (Helderman and Goral 2001).

Acute rejection

Historically, approximately 30–50 per cent of renal allograft recipients have an episode of acute rejection within the first 6 months after transplantation. With the introduction of mycophenolate mofetil and anti-IL-2 receptor antibody (anti-IL2R) daclizumab and basiliximab into clinical practice, acute rejection rates of 15–30 per cent or less have now been routinely achieved by most transplant programmes (Pichlmayr 1995; Sollinger 1995; Keown 1996; Nashan 1997; Vincenti et al. 1998; Johnson et al. 2000). In the era of cyclosporin and of potent immunosuppressive agents in general, the classic constitutional symptoms of acute rejection including fever, chills, myalgias, arthralgias, graft swelling, and/or tenderness are often absent. Patients are usually non-oliguric and a rise in serum creatinine may be the only sign of acute rejection. Elevated blood pressure or worsening hypertension may be variably present. Non-invasive imaging studies such as renal Doppler ultrasound or renal radioisotope flow scan is neither sufficiently sensitive nor specific in the diagnosis of acute rejection (Zimmerman et al. 2001). Although invasive, allograft biopsy remains the most accurate means of differentiating acute rejection from other causes of acute deterioration of allograft function.

On the basis of the underlying immunopathogenic mechanisms, acute rejection can be divided into cell-mediated and humoural immunity. Approximately 90 per cent of the episodes of acute rejection are predominantly cell mediated while 20–30 per cent of all acute rejection episodes have a humoural component (Watschinger and Pascual 2002). The histopathological diagnostic criteria and treatment are different for these two types of rejection and are discussed separately. It should be noted, however, that the histopathological findings of acute cellular rejection can be seen in allograft biopsies with acute humoural rejection or vice versa.

Acute cellular rejection

Acute cellular rejection generally occurs after the first post-transplant week and most commonly occurs within the first 3 months after transplantation. It has been suggested that CD4+ T-cells play an important role in the initiation of rejection while CD8+ T-cells are critical at the later stages. Accumulating evidence indicates that the effector pathway of cytotoxic T-lymphocytes killing (CTL) leading to acute renal allograft rejection involves the perforin/granzyme degranulation pathway (Olive et al. 1999). It has recently been shown that perforin mRNA and granzyme B in urinary cells are elevated in acute allograft rejection. Perforin is a molecule that polymerizes to form ring-like transmembrane channels or pores in the target-cell membrane, facilitating the entry of granzyme B into the target cells. Granzyme B in turn induces cell apoptosis through activation of caspase. Perforin is stored in and secreted by the granules of cytotoxic effector cells whereas granzyme B is expressed primarily by activated cytotoxic cells. It has been suggested that measurement of urine perforin mRNA and granzyme B messenger RNA may offer a non-invasive means of diagnosing acute renal allograft rejection with a sensitivity of 79–83 per cent and a specificity of 77–83 per cent (Li et al. 2001). Nevertheless, whether measurement of these cytotoxic proteins may be beneficial in monitoring or in the diagnosis of acute cellular rejection awaits further studies. Table 5 represents the Banff 1997 classification of acute cellular rejection (Racusen et al. 1999). A revised Banff schema that incorporates the criteria for acute humoural rejection is currently underway.

Table 5 Main features of the Banff 1997 classification for acute cellular rejection

Grade	Criteria
IA	Interstitial inflammation (>25% of parenchyma); tubulitis (>4 lymphocytes per tubular cross-section)
IB	Interstitial inflammation (>25% of parenchyma); tubulitis (>10 lymphocytes per tubular cross-section)
IIA	Mild to moderate intimal arteritis
IIB	Moderate to severe intimal arteritis involving >25% of uminal area
III	Transmural arteritis and/or arterial fibrinoid necrosis

Acute humoural rejection

Acute humoural rejection generally occurs within the first 1–3 weeks after transplantation (Mauiyyedi and Colvin 2002). The incidence of acute humoural rejection has been difficult to determine in part due to the lack of well-defined diagnostic criteria. More recently, the immunohistochemical detection of the complement degradation product C4d deposition in peritubular capillaries (PTC) of renal allograft biopsies has been suggested to offer a new tool to aid in the diagnosis of acute humoral rejection. In a series of 232 consecutive kidney transplants performed at a single institution, widespread C4d staining in PTC was found to be present in 30 per cent of all acute rejection episodes occurring within the first 3 months after transplantation. In addition, the detection of C4d has frequently been found to be associated with elevated donor-specific antibodies [90 per cent of C4d(+) versus 2 per cent of C4d(−) acute rejection cases]. The presence of non-HLA, antiendothelial antibodies or subthreshold levels of DSA has been suggested to account for the C4d(+) DSA(−) cases. Literature review reveals that approximately 30–50 per cent of all biopsy-confirmed acute renal allograft rejection episodes have a component of acute humoural rejection (AHR) as defined by PTC staining for C4d. However, Mauiyyedi et al. suggested that a definitive diagnosis of AHR requires demonstration of donor-specific antibodies (DSAs) as PTC C4d staining (atleast focally) has also been found to be present in ischaemic injury (Mauiyyedi and Colvin 2002; Mauiyyedi et al. 2002). The currently proposed pathological criteria for acute humoural rejection are shown in Table 6.

Treatment of acute cellular rejection

Pulse corticosteroid

Pulse corticosteroid is appropriate for the initial treatment of biopsy-proven first episode of acute cellular rejection with mild to moderate allograft dysfunction and without evidence of vascular involvement. There is no standardized 'pulse steroid protocol' and it has been suggested that an oral pulse with prednisone or prednisolone at a dose of 125–250 mg a day may not necessarily be less effective than higher-dose intravenous methylprednisolone pulse (Danovitch 2001).

Table 6 Pathological criteria for acute humoural rejection[a]

1. C4d deposition in peritubular capillaries[b]

2. At least one of the following:[c]
   Neutrophils in peritubular capillaries
   Arterial fibrinoid necrosis, acute tubular injury

3. Circulating donor-specific antibodies

[a] Cases that also meet the criteria of type 1 or 2 acute cellular rejection (Banff) are considered to have both processes.

[b] Bright and diffusely positive staining for C4d in peritubular capillaries (PTCs).

[c] Neutrophils in PTCs, on average, two or more neutrophils per high power field, in PTC, in 10 consecutive 40× (500 μm diameter) fields; fibrinoid necrosis in an artery larger than an arteriole; acute tubular injury, loss of brush borders, flattened epithelium, apoptosis. If only two of the three numbered criteria are present, the term 'suspicious for acute humoural rejection' is recommended (e.g. when donor-specific antibodies are not tested). Adapted from Lehtonen et al. (1997).

Nonetheless, most centres favour an intravenous methylprednisolone pulse which can be given at a dose of 5 mg per kg of body weight or at a fixed dose of 500–1000 mg daily for 3–5 days. After completion of pulse steroid therapy, prednisone can be gradually tapered over a 1–2 week period to its previous level (steroid recycle) or it can be resumed at its previous dose. Rejection reversal is achieved in approximately 70–80 per cent of first acute rejection episodes treated with pulse corticosteroid. Steroid resistant, defined as a failure of the serum creatinine to decrease or a continuing increase in serum creatinine after 3 days of therapy, usually necessitates antibody salvage treatment. Repeat biopsy may be helpful but should be individualized and biopsy is mandatory for those without a prior biopsy particularly if antibody treatment is given.

Antilymphocyte antibody therapy

Currently available monoclonal and polyclonal antibody preparations include OKT3, basiliximab, daclizumab, ATGAM, and thymoglobulin. Basiliximab and daclizumab are humanized monoclonal antibodies that target against the α chain of the IL-2 receptor expressed on alloantigen-reactive T-lymphocytes. They were designed and approved for use as prophylactic therapy against acute rejection episodes, but not for the treatment of acute rejection episodes (Nashan 1997; Vincenti et al. 1998).

The monoclonal antibody OKT3 and the polyclonal antibodies ATGAM and thymoglobulin are highly effective antirejection therapy. Their use as induction therapy is discussed elsewhere. Although the choice and duration of antilymphocyte antibody treatment may differ among centres, the common indications for antibody treatment include steroid-resistant first acute rejection, biopsy confirmed vascular rejection (Banff grade II or III), second episodes of rejection, severe allograft dysfunction at presentation, or rapid deterioration of allograft function despite pulse steroid therapy. During antibody treatment, cyclosporin or tacrolimus should be withheld or dose reduced to avoid over-immunosuppression while oral prednisone is replaced by intravenous methylprednisolone. OKT3 reverses approximately 90 per cent of steroid resistant first acute rejection. The standard dose is 5 mg given intravenously through a peripheral catheter. The first two to three doses must be given in the hospital settings and premedication protocol should be strictly adhered due to the potential life-threatening adverse reactions caused by the cytokine release syndrome. The duration of treatment is not well defined but most centres advocate a 10–14-day course of therapy. The newer antilymphocyte antibody thymoglobulin has been shown to be as effective as OKT3 in reversal of first acute rejection episodes (Danovitch 2001). It is given at a dose of 1.5 mg/kg of body weight infused over 4–8 h through a central venous catheter or into the venous limb of an arteriovenous fistula. Administration of thymoglobulin through a peripheral vein may cause vein thrombosis or thrombophlebitis and should be avoided. ATGAM is given at a dose of 10–15 mg/kg of body weight infused over 4 h, and similar to thymoglobulin, should be given through a central venous catheter or an arteriovenous fistula. Premedication with intravenous methylprednisolone, diphenhydramine hydrochloride, and acetaminophen should be given prior to commencement of antilymphocyte antibody therapy. Results of a double-blind, randomized, multicentre, phase III clinical trial comparing thymoglobulin versus ATGAM in the treatment of acute renal allograft rejection have shown a greater beneficial effect of thymoglobulin compared to that of ATGAM in the rate of

rejection reversal (thymoglobulin versus ATGAM: 88 versus 76 per cent respectively, $P = 0.027$). One-year patient and graft survival were comparable between the two treatment groups as were drug-related adverse events (Gaber et al. 1998).

Treatment of acute humoural rejection

Acute humoural rejection frequently presents with severe allograft dysfunction refractory to conventional antirejection therapy including antilymphocyte antibody and is associated with a high risk of graft loss (1-year graft loss rate of up to 30–50 per cent) (Trpkov et al. 1996; Lederer et al. 2001; Herzenberg et al. 2002; Mauiyyedi et al. 2002). There is currently no well-defined protocol for the treatment of acute humoural rejection and therapy has been largely based on anecdotal reports in small series of patients. In a series of 10 patients who developed severe allograft rejection, four of whom with associated high levels of donor-specific anti-HLA alloantibodies, Jordan et al. (1998) have shown that IVIG treatment resulted in reduction in donor-specific anti-HLA alloantibody level and in rapid improvement in acute rejection episodes and reversal of rejection in all patients within 2–5 days. It is speculated that the effectiveness of IVIG is in part due to the presence of anti-idiotypic antibodies that are potent inhibitors of HLA-specific alloantibodies. IVIG is commonly given at a dose of 2 g/kg of body weight as a single dose infused over 4 h or in divided dose given on two consecutive days. Premedication with acetaminophen, diphenhydramine, and methylprednisolone is recommended. Common side-effects include chills, nausea, headache, fatigue myalgia, arthralgia, back pain, and hypertension, all of which can usually be minimized by reducing the infusion rate. Similar to IVIG, the role of extracorporeal therapies in the removal of immunoglobulins and hence in treating humoural rejection has not been well established. Nonetheless, plasmapheresis and immunoadsorption with protein A have been suggested to be beneficial in acute humoural rejection through removal of DSA alloantibodies (Montgomery et al. 2000; Bohmig et al. 2001). The combination of plasma exchange and tacrolimus–mycophenolate rescue therapy has also been explored as a viable option in controlling alloantibody production (Pascual et al. 1998).

Transplant renal artery stenosis

Transplant renal artery stenosis has been reported to occur in 1–23 per cent of patients and can be an important cause of allograft dysfunction. The wide variation in the incidence reported may in part be due to the difference in the criteria used to define functionally significant stenoses and/or differences in the screening tests performed. Clinically, patients may present with new onset or accelerated hypertension, acute deterioration of graft function, severe hypotension associated with the use of ACEIs, recurrent pulmonary oedema or refractory oedema in the absence of heavy proteinuria, and/or erythrocytosis. The latter, when associated with hypertension and impaired graft function should raise the suspicion of renal artery stenosis (i.e. triad: erythrocytosis, hypertension, elevated serum creatinine). The presence of a bruit over the allograft is neither sensitive nor specific for the diagnosis of graft renovascular disease. However, a change in the intensity of the bruit or the detection of new bruits warrants an evaluation. Although non-invasive, radionuclide scan with and without captopril is neither sufficiently sensitive nor specific for detecting transplant renal artery stenosis (sensitivity and specificity: 75 and 67 per cent, respectively) (Shamlou *et al.* 1994). Colour Doppler ultrasound is highly sensitive and serves well as an initial non-invasive assessment of the transplant vessels. It should be noted, however, that colour Doppler ultrasound is limited by its relatively low specificity. CO_2 angiography avoids nephrotoxic contrast agents but its use is not without limitations. Overestimation of the degree of stenosis, bowel gas artefact, and/or patients' intolerance have been associated with the use of CO_2 angiogram (Hawkins and Maynar 1997). More recently, gadolinium-enhanced magnetic resource angiography has been suggested to be an alternative non-nephrotoxic method in identifying arterial stenosis involving the transplant kidney with high sensitivity and specificity for detecting haemodynamically significant stenoses in iliac arteries, renal allograft arteries and their first branches (sensitivity and specificity: 100 and 93–97 per cent, respectively). However, slight overestimation of the degree of the stenosis still remains and experiences with this technique is currently limited (Huber *et al.* 2001). Although invasive, renal angiography remains the gold standard procedure for establishing the diagnosis of renal artery sterosis. Potential causes of renal artery sterosis and its treatment are discussed under surgical complications.

Common laboratory abnormalities

Haematologic abnormalities

Anaemia

Severe anaemia is uncommon in the era of erythropoietin therapy. Nonetheless, iron deficiency is not infrequently encountered in the dialysis population receiving erythropoietin. After transplantation erythropoietin therapy is generally discontinued and mild anaemia is common in the early post-transplant period and generally improves over several weeks to months. Assessment of baseline iron stores at the time of transplantation may be invaluable. Profound iron deficiency should be treated with intravenous iron as tolerated. Refractory or severe anaemia mandates aggressive evaluation to exclude the possibility of surgical postoperative bleeding, particularly in patients with rapidly falling haemoglobin and haematocrit. Other possibilities may include gastrointestinal bleed, tertiary hyperparathyroidism, underlying inflammatory conditions, or parvovirus infection. Sirolimus and other commonly used drugs including ACEIs and angiotensin receptor blockers (ARBs) may cause or exacerbate anaemia and should not be overlooked. Anaemia secondary to sirolimus may respond to a short course of subcutaneous erythropoietin. Erythropoietin therapy may also be effective in patients who have impaired allograft function and adequate iron stores.

Leucopenia and thrombocytopenia

Leucopenia and thrombocytopenia are not uncommon in transplant recipients and are most commonly related to adverse drug effects including azathioprine (which has been replaced by mycophenolate mofetil by most centres), mycophenolate mofetil, antilymphocyte antibody treatment, sirolimus (Groth *et al.* 1999; Kreis *et al.* 2000), trimethoprim–sulfamethoxazole, among others. Withholding the offending agent or dose reduction generally corrects the haematological abnormalities. Severe leucopenia may be safely treated with granulocyte-stimulating factor (Neupogen). Potential medical complications such as TMA or CMV infection should be excluded. Parvovirus infection may present

with refractory anaemia, pancytopenia, and TMA (Luisa *et al.* 2000; Murer *et al.* 2000).

Erythrocytosis

Renal artery stenosis, polycystic kidney disease, renal cell carcinoma, cerebellar haemangioblastoma, or chronic hypoxia in heavy tobacco users are potential causes of secondary erythrocytosis and should be excluded as clinically indicated.

Post-transplant erythrocytosis (PTE) of varying degrees has been reported to occur in 20–25 per cent of transplant recipients within the first 2 years. Suggested pathogenic mechanism(s) include defective feedback regulation of erythropoietin metabolism, direct stimulation of erythroid precursors by angiotensin II, and/or abnormalities in circulating insulin-like growth factor-1 levels (IGF-1) (Brox *et al.* 1998; Gupta *et al.* 2000; Lezaic *et al.* 2001). Plasma erythropoietin has been shown to be inconsistently elevated. Treatment is generally recommended for haemoglobin greater than or equal to 10.55–11.17 mmol/l or haematocrit greater than or equal to 0.52–0.55 due to the associated risk of thromboembolic complications, hypertension, and headaches. Both ACEIs and ARBs have been shown to be effective although phlebotomy may occasionally be necessary (Julian *et al.* 1998). In a recent study, Wang *et al.* showed that IGF-1 and haemoglobin were elevated in patients with PTE but not in those without PTE, whereas, erythropoietin were similar in both groups. Interestingly, treatment with enalapril 5 mg resulted in a greater reduction in Hb compared to therapy with losartan 50 mg. The reduction in haemoglobin in enalapril-treated patients was associated with a significant reduction in circulating IGF-1, but not in erythropoietin, whereas the reduction in haemoglobin in losartan-treated patients was not associated with any significant reduction in either IGF-1 or erythropoietin (Wang *et al.* 2002). Various pathogenic mechanisms may play a role in the development of PTE and further studies are needed.

Hyperkalaemia

Mild hyperkalaemia is commonly encountered in renal transplant recipients particularly in the early post-transplant period when relatively high-dose CNI is given. It is often associated with mild hyperchloraemic acidosis and an intact capacity to excrete acid urine, a clinical presentation reminiscent of type IV RTA. Suggested mechanism(s) of CNI induced hyperkalaemia include hyporeninism hypoaldosteronism, aldosterone resistance, end-organ defect in potassium excretion, or inhibition of cortical collecting duct potassium secretory channels (Heiring *et al.* 1996). Cyclosporin has been shown to decrease Na^+,K^+-ATPase activity in K^+ secretory cells in the cortical and outer medullary collecting tubules, thereby decreasing intracellular K^+ accumulation required for urinary secretion. In patients receiving cyclosporin or tacrolimus immunosuppression, potassium in the low to mid-five's (5.2–5.5 mmol/l) is typically seen and generally does not require treatment. However, dietary potassium restriction is recommended (2 g per day). Higher potassium levels, especially in the presence of concomitant use of drugs that may exacerbate hyperkalaemia such ACEIs, ARBs, or β-blockers may require treatment at the clinicians' discretion. Caution should be made when potassium-containing phosphorus supplement is prescribed. Although trimethoprim can cause hyperkalaemia through an amiloride-like effect, the routine use of low-dose trimethoprim–sulfamethoxazole (Bactrim) for PCP and urinary tract infections prophylaxis is rarely the cause of severe or refractory hyperkalaemia in recipients of renal allograft transplant.

Depending on the severity and/or acuteness of hyperkalaemia and associated ECG changes, treatment may include diuretics and potassium exchange resin (sodium polystyrene or kayexalate) for mild to moderate hyperkalaemia and the addition of insulin with glucose and calcium gluconate for more severe hyperkalaemia. Diuretics are usually effective in mild to moderate hyperkalaemia and are appropriate therapy for those patients who are also volume overloaded. In life-threatening hyperkalaemia, inhaled β-agonist may be added in patients with low cardiovascular risks and urgent haemodialysis may be required especially for those with poor allograft function.

Hypokalaemia

Unlike cyclosporin or tacrolimus, sirolimus has been suggested to be associated with hypokalaemia. In an early European phase II trial in which sirolimus was compared directly to cyclosporin in renal transplantation (in a triple therapy regimen consisting of either cyclosporin or sirolimus, azathioprine, and steroid), serum potassium was found to be significantly lower in sirolimus-treated compared to cyclosporin-treated patients at weeks 4, 12, 24, and 52 ($P < 0.01$). Moreover, hypokalaemia occurred in 34 per cent, and potassium supplementation was required in 27 per cent of patients among the sirolimus-treated group (Groth et al. 1999). Similar results were obtained in the European phase II trial where sirolimus was compared to cyclosporin in a triple therapy regimen where azathioprine was replaced by mycophenolate mofetil. Serum potassium was significantly lower in sirolimus-treated compared to cyclosporin-treated group at weeks 4, 12, and 52. There was a higher incidence of hypokalaemia in sirolimus-treated compared to cyclosporin-treated group although this did not reach statistical significance (sirolimus versus cyclosporin: 20 versus 16 per cent, respectively) (Kreis et al. 2000).

Hypophosphataemia

Hypophosphataemia is frequently encountered after a successful renal transplantation. The concomitant presence of hypercalcaemia suggests that hypophosphataemia may result from the introduction of a well functioning kidney allograft into a persistently hyperparathyroid milieu whereas the absence of hypercalcaemia or hyperparathyroidism suggests renal phosphate wasting syndrome or even malnutrition (Ward 1997). Mild hypophosphataemia (>0.65 mmol/l) can be managed with high phosphorus dietary intake while oral phosphate replacement is often necessary for more pronounced hypophosphataemia.

Hypercalcaemia

Hypercalcaemia is common after transplantation and is generally due to persistent secondary hyperparathyroidism. The concomitant presence of severe hypophosphataemia particularly in patients with excellent graft function may exacerbate hypercalcaemia through stimulation of renal proximal tubular 1α-hydroxylase. Phosphate supplement is recommended and may be effective in mild post-transplant hypercalcaemia. Adjunctive therapy with 1,25-vitamin D (Rocaltrol) has been suggested to be beneficial. Whether 1α-hydroxyvitamin D_2 (Hectoral), a vitamin D analogue, may be advantageous in post-transplant residual secondary hyperparathyroidism and hypercalcaemia is currently not known and awaits studies. In most cases, hypercalcaemia resolves spontaneously within 6–12 months. Severe hypercalcaemia or persistent hypercalcaemia (≥ 12 months) requires further evaluation and/or intervention. Initial assessment should include an intact parathyroid hormone level. Imaging studies including neck ultrasound or parathyroid technetium 99mTc-sestamibi scan should be done at clinicians' discretion to exclude parathyroid adenoma or parathyroid gland hyperplasia, and/or hyperplastic nodular formation of the parathyroid glands. Parathyroidectomy is warranted in patients with tertiary hyperparathyroidism or persistent severe hypercalcaemia (≥ 3.12 mmol/l for more than 6–12 months), symptomatic or progressive hypercalcaemia, nephrolithiasis, persistent metabolic bone disease, calcium-related renal allograft dysfunction, or progressive vascular calcification and calciphylaxis (Pham and Pham 2002).

Hypomagnesaemia

Hypomagnesaemia was first recognized to occur in renal allograft recipients receiving cyclosporin immunosuppression while it was rarely seen in the precyclosporin era. The association between cyclosporin (or tacrolimus) and hypomagnesaemia is now well established and has been shown to be due to urinary magnesium wasting (Barton 1987). Other factors that may contribute to hypomagnesaemia in the post-transplant settings include loop diuretic therapy, polyuric phase of recovering ATN or following relief of obstructive uropathy, and/or renal tubular acidosis. The propensity towards hypomagnesaemia has also been shown to be more pronounced among patients with diabetes mellitus (Vannini et al. 1999). In the first 3 months after transplantation, a magnesium less than 0.62 mmol/l is commonly seen. Dietary magnesium intake is usually insufficient and oral magnesium supplement is recommended although it may be ineffective due to ongoing magnesuria. Intravenous magnesium should be considered in severe hypomagnesaemia (<0.41 mmol/l) particularly in patients with a prior history of coronary artery disease or cardiac arrythmias and in those taking digitalis. Aggressive treatment of hypomagnesaemia has also been suggested to be beneficial in improving lipid profile ($\downarrow$ total cholesterol, $\downarrow$ low density lipoprotein, and $\downarrow$ total cholesterol/high density lipoprotein ratio) (Gupta et al. 1999), cyclosporin-induced neurotoxicity, and hypertension in hypomagnesaemic renal transplant recipients.

Transaminitis

Elevation of the hepatic enzymes is common in the early post-transplant period and is generally due to drug-related toxicity. Potential culprits include acyclovir, ganciclovir, trimethoprim–sulfamethoxazole, cyclosporin, tacrolimus, HMGCoA reductase inhibitors, and/or proton pump inhibitors. Cyclosporin and less commonly, tacrolimus, may cause transient, self-limited mild hyperbilirubinaemia secondary to defective bile secretion. Drug-related transaminitis generally improve or resolve following drug discontinuation or dose reduction.

Persistent or profound elevation in hepatic liver enzymes should prompt further evaluation to exclude infectious causes of hepatitis including CMV, hepatitis B virus (HBV), and HCV. In high-risk candidates for primary CMV infections (recipient seronegative, donor seropositive), it may occasionally be necessary to initiate CMV therapy while awaiting laboratory results particularly when there is a high index of clinical suspicion (fever, fatigue, malaise, gastroenteritis, leucopenia, and/or thrombocytopenia). Evidence of post-transplant HBV reactivation should be treated with lamivudine (elevated ALT, histological hepatitis, and serum DNA $> 10^5$ copies/ml). Some programmes routinely commence lamivudine prophylaxis in all HbsAg+ candidates at the time of transplantation. Pretransplant lamivudine prophylactic therapy is recommended in renal transplant candidates who have HBV DNA greater than 10^5 copies/ml and active liver disease defined as ALT greater than $2 \times$ ULN or fibrosis greater than stage 2 despite haemodialysis (Gane and Pilmore 2002). There is currently no effective treatment for chronic hepatitis C in renal transplant recipients. Although treatment with IFN-α may result in clearance of HCV RNA in 25–50 per cent of cases, rapid relapse following drug withdrawal is nearly universal (Fabrizio and Martin 2001; Gane and Pilmore 2002). More importantly, IFN-α treatment has been shown to precipitate acute allograft rejection and graft loss and is currently not recommended for renal transplant recipients with HCV infection (Fabrizio and Martin 2001; Gane and Pilmore 2002). Management of HCV infection in this patient population should probably rely on manipulation of immunosuppressive therapy. Experiences gained from liver transplantation indicate that corticosteroid therapy and antilymphocyte antibody treatment are associated with enhanced viral replication and more rapid progression to cirrhosis. On the basis of these observations, it has been suggested that antilymphocyte antibody induction therapy should be avoided in transplant recipients with chronic HCV infection. In addition, steroid should probably be kept at a safe minimum. Interestingly, mycophenolate mofetil, an inosine monophosphate dehydrogenase inhibitor with intrinsic antiviral activities, has recently been shown to reduce HCV replication and delay the recurrence of hepatitis C in Hep C liver transplant recipient (Fasola et al. 2000). Whether mycophenolate mofetil offers similar beneficial effects in renal transplant recipients is currently not known.

Post-transplant infectious complications

The time to occurrence of different infections in any type of solid organ transplantation follows a 'time table' pattern (Fishman and Rubin 1998). Infections within the first month after transplantation are most frequently caused by bacterial microorganisms. In renal transplant recipients, the urinary tract is most commonly involved. Urinalysis should be an integral part of routine laboratory assessment at each clinic visit, at least in the first 1–2 months after transplant. Urine culture should be done in the presence of pyuria as asymptomatic bacteriuria is not uncommon in this patient population. Commonly isolated bacterial pathogens include *Escherichia coli*, *Enterococcus*, *Pseudomonas aeruginosa*, and enterobacteriaceae. However, the prevalence of a particular pathogen may also be centre specific. Open wound, devitalized tissue, indwelling catheters or stents, and/or perinephric fluid collection are other potential sources of infection in renal transplant recipients. With the use of lower steroid dose, strict aseptic surgical technique and routine perioperative antibiotic prophylaxis, wound infection has now been reported to occur in less than 1 per cent of cases. Nonetheless, obese patients are at greater risk for wound complications, and pulmonary infection.

After the first post-transplant month, infections with immuno-modulating viruses including CMV, other human herpes virus, Epstein–Barr virus (EBV), HBV, and HCV may occur due to the overall state of immunosuppression, exogenous infection, or reactivation of latent disease. Repeated courses of antibiotics increase the risk of fungal infections whereas infections with immunomodulating viruses may render patients more susceptible to opportunistic infections due to *Pneumocystis carinii*, aspergillus, and *Listeria monocytogenes*. Beyond 6 months following transplantation, the risk of infection in patients with good allograft function is similar to that of the general population and is discussed under long-term management and complications.

Suggested prophylactic therapy for the commonly encountered infections in the first 6 months is shown in Table 7 (adapted from Pham et al. 2002a,b).

Cytomegalovirus infection

CMV infection occurs primarily after the first month post-transplant and continues to be a significant cause of morbidity in the first 6 months. CMV infection may occur in the setting of primary infection in a seronegative recipient, reactivation of endogenous latent virus, or superinfection with a new virus in a seropositive recipient. Primary CMV infection often results in more severe disease than reactivation or superinfection. The clinical manifestations of CMV infection span the spectrum of asymptomatic seroconversion, mononucleosis-like syndrome, or flu-like illnesses with fever and leucopenia and/or thrombocytopenia to widespread tissue invasive disease. The latter may result in clinical hepatitis, oesophagitis, gastroenteritis, colitis, retinitis, and pneumonitis among others. The transplanted organ appears to be more susceptible to the direct effects of CMV infection than native organs (Ginns et al. 2001). In recipients of renal allograft transplant, CMV may present with an elevated serum creatinine with or without the presence of constitutional symptoms and may mimic allograft rejection or pyelonephritis. Accurate diagnosis rests on biopsy of the transplant kidney. Donor and recipient seropositive status, and the use of blood products from CMV seropositive donor are well-established risk factors for CMV infection. Other factors associated with an increased risk of infection include the use of anti-lymphocyte antibodies, prolonged or repeated courses of antilymphocyte preparations, and episode of allograft rejections. Although the cause/effect of allograft rejection and CMV infection remain largely conjectural, several studies have suggested a bidirectional relationship mediated via inflammatory cytokines. In a recent single-centre retrospective study, CMV sero-mismatched recipients were found to be at higher risk for acute allograft rejection compared to their non-seromismatched counterparts, suggesting that CMV infection or disease is a risk factor for acute rejection (acute rejection rates in sero-mismatched versus non-sero-mismatched recipients: 72.6 versus 54.2 per cent, respectively, $P = 0.05$) (McLaughlin et al. 2002).

Table 7 Suggested prophylactic therapy for recipients of kidney transplants

	Comments
Trimethoprim–sulfamethoxazole (TMP/SMX) (80/400 mg) one tablet q.d. $\times$ 3 months	Its routine use reduces or eliminates incidence of PCP, *L. monocytogenes*, *N. asteroids*, and *T. gondii* in renal transplant recipients, TMP/SMX reduces the incidences of UTI from 30–80% to less than 5–10%
Bimonthly intravenous or aerosolized, pentamidine, dapsone, or atovaquone[a]	Replaces TMP/SMX for patients with sulfa allergies
Nystatin 1,00,000 U/ml, 4 ml q.p.c. and q.h.s.	For fungal prophylaxis
Aciclovir/ganciclovir/ valganciclovir	For CMV prophylaxis

[a] In order of efficacy.

PCP, *Pneumocystis carinii*. Modified from St Peter et al. (2002).

Management of CMV infection consists of preventive (prophylactic and/or pre-emptive therapy) and therapeutic measures. Over the last several years, various prophylactic and pre-emptive protocols have been developed to reduce the rate of CMV infections. Observations drawn from various studies reveal that oral acyclovir provides effective CMV prophylaxis solely in recipients of seronegative donor organ(s) (Pham *et al.* 2002a,b). Oral/intravenous ganciclovir provides superior prophylactic/pre-emptive therapy against CMV reactivation. In a more recent multicentre valacyclovir study (International Valacyclovir Cytomegalovirus Prophylaxis Transplantation Study Group), valacyclovir 2 g orally four times daily for 90 days has been shown to reduce the incidence or delayed the onset of CMV disease in both CMV seronegative and CMV seropositive recipients of CMV positive donor kidneys (Lowance *et al.* 1999). Valganciclovir (valacyclovir) is the valyl ester of ganciclovir with increased bioavailability. When administered orally, valganciclovir has been shown to achieve levels comparable to intravenous ganciclovir. Suggested CMV prophylaxis protocol is shown in Table 8 (modified from Pham *et al.* 2002a,b). The routine use of CMV hyperimmune globulin and intravenous immune globulin result in no added benefit compared to a regimen consisting of antiviral agents alone. Its use should probably be limited to high-risk candidates such as during antilymphocyte therapy in recipients with primary CMV exposure.

Clinical CMV disease should be treated with intravenous ganciclovir and continued until clearance of viraemia as assessed by pp65 antigenaemia or quantitative polymerase chain reaction. The usual course consists of 3 weeks (range 2–4 weeks) of intravenous therapy. In patients with tissue invasive disease, Fishman and Rubin advocate the use of intravenous ganciclovir followed by 2-month course of oral ganciclovir in seropositive individuals and for 3–4 months in those with primary infection (Fishman and Rubin 1998). Relapse may develop as a result of premature discontinuation of intravenous therapy. The use of oral ganciclovir in the presence of high viral load may confer ganciclovir resistance due to low bioavailability achieved by oral ganciclovir therapy (Fishman and Rubin 1998; Ginns *et al.* 2001). Whether oral valganciclovir may be used in such cases awaits further studies.

Management of cardiovascular disease risk factors

Management of cardiovascular disease (CVD) risk factors should begin in the early post-transplant period and should remain as an integral part of long-term care of renal transplant recipients. Although the determinants of CVD risk in renal transplant recipients have not been well defined, both conventional and unconventional risk factors have been suggested to contribute to the increased risk of CVD morbidity and mortality in the transplant population. The former include diabetes mellitus, hypertension, dyslipidaemia, obesity, smoking, and family history. The latter include pre-existing left ventricular hypertrophy, coronary artery vascular calcification, impaired allograft function, and acute rejection episodes (Goodman *et al.* 2000; Kasiske and Chakkera 2000).

Post-transplant dyslipidaemia

Dyslipidaemia is a common occurrence following transplantation. The hyperlipaemic effect of immunosuppressive agents including corticosteroids, cyclosporin, tacrolimus, and sirolimus has been well documented. Tacrolimus-based therapy has been suggested to be associated with better lipid profiles than cyclosporin-based therapy whereas sirolimus has been shown to be associated with a significantly greater incidence and severity of dyslipidaemia than cyclosporin-based therapy, including a higher total cholesterol and more severe hypertriglyceridaemia (Fellstrom and Uppsala 2000). Other potential aetiological factors for post-transplant dyslipidaemia include age, diet, rapid weight gain, pre-existing hypercholesterolaemia, allograft dysfunction, proteinuria, the use of β-blockers and diuretics, and probably hypomagnesaemia. Suggested guidelines for pharmacological treatments of post-transplant dyslipidaemia are shown in Fig. 1.

Post-transplant hypertension

Post-transplant hypertension is common particularly in the early post-transplant period, with a reported prevalence of 67–90 per cent (Midvedt *et al.* 2000). Measurement of blood pressure outside the office is invaluable in assessing the need for instituting antihypertensive

Table 8 CMV prophylaxis protocol

CMV (−) recipients of a CMV (−) organ
A cyclovir 400 mg q.d. or Valcyte 450 mg q.d. for 3 months

CMV (−) recipients of a CMV (+) organ
During antibody treatment DHPG 2.6 mg/kg IV q.d., then following antibody treatment Cytovene 1000 mg tid or Valcyte 900 mg q.d. for 3 months adjusted to renal function. If no antibody treatment: Cytovene 1000 mg tid or Valcyte 900 mg q.d. for 3 months

CMV (+) recipients of a CMV (−) organ
During antibody treatment DHPG 2.5 mg/kg IV q.d., then following antibody treatment: Cytovene 1000 mg tid or Valcyte 900 mg q.d. for 3 months adjusted to renal function. If no antibody treatment: acyclovir 400 mg q.d. or Valcyte 450 mg q.d., CMV DNA q 2 weeks × 3

CMV (+) recipients of a CMV (+) organ
During antibody treatment: DHPG 2.5 mg/kg IV q.d., then following antibody treatment: Cyovene 1000 mg tid or Valcyte 9000 mg q.d. for 3 months adjusted to renal function. If no antibody treatment: acyclovir 400 mg q.d. or Valcyte 450 mg q.d., CMV DNA q 2 weeks × 3

DHPG = 9-(1,3-dihydroxy-2-propoxymethyl)quanine.

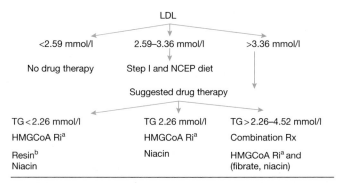

Goals: LDL < 2.59 mmol/l, TG < 2.26 mmol/l, HDL > 0.51 mmol/l. HDL < 0.40 mmol/l: weight management in conjunction with regular exercise programme.

[a] HMGCoA RI (HMGCoA reductase inhibitor) are the most effective drugs and should be the agents of choice. Start at low doses in patients in CSA and FK506. Monitor for myositis and hepatic enzyme elevations, particularly in patients receiving combination therapy.

[b] Bile acid sequestrants should probably not be taken at the same time as CsA.

Fig. 1 Guidelines for pharmacological treatments of post-transplant dyslipidaemia.

therapy and in assessing response to treatment, as well as in detecting 'white coat hypertension'. Hence, patients should be instructed to keep a record of their blood pressure readings particularly in the first month after transplantation. Pre-existing hypertension, cyclosporin, and tacrolimus immunosuppression, high-dose corticosteroid therapy, acute allograft dysfunction due to rejection or ischaemia, renal artery stenosis, and less commonly retained native kidneys have all been implicated in post-transplant hypertension.

Management of post-transplant hypertension should be tailored to each individual patient's need. Controlled clinical trials to determine the superiority of one class of antihypertensive agent over the other in the transplant settings are lacking. All classes of antihypertensive agents including calcium channel blockers, diuretics, β-blockers, ACEIs, ARBs, central and peripheral sympatholytics have been used in various combination therapies with variable results. Non-dihydropyridine calcium channel blockers and diuretics are frequently used in the early post-transplant period, the former due to their salutary effect on renal haemodynamics and the latter due to their beneficial effect in volume expansion state. In a recent single centre retrospective study to identify ischaemic heart disease (IHD) risk after renal transplantation, Kasiske et al. (2000) unexpectedly found an association between the use of dihydropyridine calcium channel antagonists and an increased IHD risk. Although further recommendations await results of large, ongoing, randomized, controlled trials in the general population, dihydropyridine calcium channel antagonists should be used with caution.

The use of ACEIs and/or ARBs has gained popularity due to its safety, efficacy and well-established renoprotective/antiproteinuric and cardioprotective effects. However, an increasing serum creatinine associated with its use should alert clinicians to the possibility of transplant renal artery stenosis. Caution should be excercised when used with diuretics due to exacerbation of nephrotoxicity in the face of volume contraction. In patients with slow or DGF, ACEIs and/or ARBs should probably not be given until recovery of allograft function. Yet, baseline mild to moderate renal allograft dysfunction are not contraindications to its use; however, close monitoring of serum potassium is mandatory particularly given a high incidence of hyperkalaemia associated with cyclosporin and tacrolimus immunosuppression. β-Blockers should be considered in patients with known coronary artery disease or other atherosclerotic vascular disease whereas α-2 blockers may be beneficial in patients with benign prostatic hypertrophy and neurogenic bladder. Although aggressive blood pressure control is vital in reducing cardiovascular morbidities and mortalities as well as improving graft survival, this is not recommended in the early perioperative period due to the risk of precipitating ATN and/or graft thrombosis.

Post-transplant diabetes mellitus

Approximately 30 per cent of renal transplant recipients in North America have a primary diagnosis of endstage renal disease secondary to type I or type II diabetes mellitus (USRDS 2002 Annual Data Report) while new onset post-transplant diabetes mellitus (PTDM) occurs in an additional 3–20 per cent of transplant recipients. Corticosteroid, cyclosporin, and tacrolimus immunosuppression are well-established risk factors for PTDM while the newer immunosuppressive agents mycophenolate mofetil and sirolimus have been shown to be devoid of diabetogenic effects (Jindal and Hjelmesaeth 2000; First et al. 2002). Although clinical trials comparing the incidence of PTDM in cyclosporin- versus tacrolimus-treated patients have yielded mixed

results, a meta-analysis of randomized trials comparing cyclosporin and tacrolimus in renal transplant recipients suggest that tacrolimus has a greater propensity to cause PTDM compared to cyclosporin therapy (Knoll 1999). Other suggested risk factors for PTDM include advanced age, race (African American, Hispanic), family history of diabetes mellitus, pretransplant impaired glucose tolerance, obesity, CMV infection, hepatitis C positivity, rejection episodes, and the use of β-blockers. Although oral hypoglycaemic agents may be effective in many patients with corticosteroid and/or cyclosporin- or tacrolimus-induced PTDM as this is generally associated with relative insulin deficiency and/or peripheral insulin resistance, insulin therapy may be necessary in up to 40 per cent of patients (First et al. 2002). Alternative or adjunctive management has included corticosteroid and/or tacrolimus dose reduction, tacrolimus to cyclosporin conversion therapy, calcineurin withdrawal in a regimen that consists of sirolimus and/or MMF. Nevertheless, it should be emphasized that manipulation of immunosuppressive therapy to alleviate adverse effects must be balanced against the risk of allograft rejection and graft lost. Clinicians must be familiar with the patient's immune status such as prior history of acute rejection, highly sensitized recipients, or recipients of re-allograft transplant prior to manipulating their immunosuppressive regimen.

Although there has been no consensus on the optimal approach to the management of CVD risk in renal transplant recipients, identifying the high-risk patient and implementing primary prevention is probably the best treatment strategy. All transplant recipients should be regarded as coronary heart disease risk equivalent and unless contraindicated, early treatment with statins, ACEIs, +/− β-blockers and antiplatelets should be considered. Target low-density lipoprotein (LDL) concentrations should be maintained less than 100 mg/dl. Interestingly, recent results from the Heart Protection Study showed that in patients with known coronary artery disease, cerebrovascular disease, peripheral vascular disease, diabetes mellitus, or hypertension, statin therapy was beneficial in reducing major vascular events independent of baseline LDL (Collins et al. 2002). Moreover, the beneficial effect of statins was greatest in the lowest LDL subgroups (LDL < 60s). Whether this effect can be extrapolated to renal transplant recipients awaits further studies. In addition to pharmacological treatment, emphasis should be placed on lifestyle modifications including moderation of dietary sodium and saturated fat intake, regular aerobic exercise, weight reduction, and tobacco avoidance.

References

Asaka, M. et al. (2000). Hemolytic uraemic syndrome associated with influenza A virus infection in an adult renal allograft recipient: case report and review of the literature. Nephron 84, 258–266.

Baid, S. et al. (1999). Renal thrombotic microangiopathy associated with anti-cardiolipin antibodies in hepatitis C-positive renal allograft recipients. Journal of the American Society of Nephrology 10, 146–153.

Barrientos, A. et al. (1994). Glomerular hyperfiltration as a nonimmunologic mechanism of progression of chronic renal rejection. Transplantation 57, 753–756.

Barton, C. H. (1987). Hypomagnesemia and renal magnesium wasting in renal transplant recipients receiving cyclosporine. American Journal of Medicine 83, 693–699.

Bohmig, G. A. et al. (2001). C4d-Positive acute humoral renal allograft rejection: effective treatment with immunoadsorption. Journal of the American Society of Nephrology 12, 2482–2489.

Brox, A. G. *et al.* (1998). Erythrocytosis after renal transplantation represents an abnormality of insulin-like growth factor-I and its binding protein. *Transplantation* 66, 1053–1058.

Bryan, C. F. (2001). Cold ischemia time: an independent predictor of increased HLA class I antibody production after rejection of a primary cadaveric renal allograft. *Transplantation* 71, 875–879.

Bryan, C. F. *et al.* (1998). Long-term graft survival is improved in cadaveric renal retransplantation by flow cytometric crossmatching. *Transplantation* 66, 1827–1832.

Cecka, J. M. The Unos Scientific Renal Transplant Registry. In *Clinical Transplants* (ed. J. M. Cecka and P. I. Terasaki), pp. 1–16. Los Angeles, CA: UCLA Tissue Typing Laboratory, 1998.

Collins, R. *et al.* (2002). MRC/BHF Heart Protection Study of cholesterol lowering with simvastatin in 20,536 high-risk individuals: a randomized placebo-controlled trial. Heart Protection Collaborative Group. *Lancet* 360, 7–22.

Danovitch, G. M., ed. Immunosuppressive medications and protocols for kidney transplantation. In *Handbook of Kidney Transplantation*, pp. 61–110. Philadelphia, PA: Lippincott Williams and Wilkins, 2001.

Dawidson, I. *et al.* (1991). Verapamil improves the outcome after cadaver renal transplant. *Journal of the American Society of Nephrology* 2, 983–990.

Dawidson, I. *et al.* (1994). Perioperative albumin and verapamil improve early outcome after cadaver renal transplantation. *Transplantation Proceedings* 26, 3100–3101.

Fabrizio, F. and Martin, P. Hepatitis in kidney transplantation. In *Handbook of Kidney Transplantation* (ed. G. M. Danovitch), pp. 263–271. Philadelphia, PA: Lippincott Williams and Wilkins, 2001.

Fasola, C. *et al.* (2000). Initial clinical evidence that Mycophenolate Mofetil (MMF) antiviral effects may delay the recurrence of hepatitis C in Hep C liver transplant recipients. *Hepatology* 32, 517.

Fellstrom, B. (2000). Impact and management of hyperlipidemia posttransplantation. *Transplantation* 70 (Suppl. 11), SS51–SS57.

First, R. M. *et al.* (2002). Posttransplant diabetes mellitus in kidney allograft recipients: incidence, risk factors, and management. *Transplantation* 73, 379–386.

Fishman, J. A. and Rubin, R. H. (1998). Infection in organ transplant recipients. *New England Journal of Medicine* 338, 1741–1751.

Fotiadis, C. N., Govani, M. V., and Helderman, J. H. Renal allograft dysfunction. In *Textbook of Nephrology* (ed. S. G. Massary and R. J. Glassock), pp. 1617–1635. Philadelphia, PA: Lippincott Williams and Wilkins, 2001.

Gaber, A. O. *et al.* (1998). Results of the double-blind, randomized, phase III clinical trial of thymoglobulin versus Atgam in the treatment of acute allograft rejection episodes after renal transplantation. *Transplantation* 66, 29–37.

Gane, E. and Pilmore, H. (2002). Management of chronic viral hepatitis before and after renal transplantation. *Transplantation* 74, 427–437.

Ginns, L. C., Cosimi, A. B., and Morris, P. J. Infection in the organ transplant recipient. In *Transplantation* (ed. L. C. Ginns, A. B. Cosimi, and P. J. Morris), pp. 749–769. Malden, MA: Blackwell Science, 2001.

Goodman, W. G. *et al.* (2000). Coronary artery calcification in young adults with end stage renal disease who are undergoing dialysis. *New England Journal of Medicine* 342, 1478–1482.

Gritsch, H. A. and Rosenthal, J. M. The transplant operation and its surgical complications. In *Handbook of Kidney Transplantation* (ed. G. M. Danovitch), pp. 146–162. Philadelphia, PA: Lippincott Williams and Wilkins, 2001.

Groth, C. G. *et al.* (1999). Sirolimus (Rapamycin)-based therapy in human renal transplantation. Similar efficacy and different toxicity compared with cyclosporine. *Transplantation* 67, 1036–1042.

Gupta, B. K. and Glicklich, T. V. A. (1999). Magnesium repletion therapy improves lipid metabolism in hypomagnesemic renal transplant recipients. *Transplantation* 67, 1485–1487.

Gupta, M. *et al.* (2000). Expression of angiotensin II type 1 receptor on erythroid progenitors of patients after posttransplant erythrocytosis. *Transplantation* 70, 1188–1194.

Hawkins, I. F. and Maynar, M. Carbon dioxide digital subtraction angiography. In *Interventional Radiology* 3rd edn. (ed. W. R. Castadena-Zuniga), pp. 429–443. Baltimore, MD: Williams and Wilkins, 1997.

Hayes, J. D. and Strange, R. C. (2000). Glutathione S-transferase polymorphisms and their biological consequences. *Pharmacology* 61, 154–166.

Heering, P., Degenhardt, S., and Grabensee, B. (1996). Tubular dysfunction following kidney transplantation. *Nephron* 74, 501–511.

Heering, P. *et al.* (2000). Hemolytic uremic syndrome after renal transplantation: immunosuppressive therapy with rapamycin. *Nephron* 91, 177.

Helderman, J. H. and Goral, S. Transplantation immunobiology. In *Handbook of Kidney Transplantation* (ed. G. M. Danovitch), pp. 17–38. Philadelphia, PA: Lippincott Williams and Wilkins, 2001.

Herzenberg, A. M. *et al.* (2002). C4d deposition in acute rejection: an independent long-term prognostic factor. *Journal of the American Society of Nephrology* 13, 234–241.

Hetzel, G. R. *et al.* (2002). Risk factors for delayed graft function after renal transplantation and their significance for long-term clinical outcome. *Transplantation International* 15, 10–16.

Huber, A. *et al.* (2001). Contrast-enhanced MR angiography in patients after kidney transplantation. *European Radiology* 11, 2488–2495.

Jindal, R. M. and Hjelmesaeth, J. (2000). Impact and management of posttransplant diabetes mellitus. *Transplantation* 70 (Suppl. 11), SS58–SS63.

Johnson, C. *et al.* (2000). Randomized trial of tacrolimus (Prograf) in combination with azathioprine or mycophenolate mofetil versus cyclosporine (Neoral) with mycophenolate mofetil after cadaveric renal transplantation. *Transplantation* 69, 834–841.

Jordan, S. C. *et al.* (1998). Posttransplant therapy using high-dose human immunoglobulin (intravenous gammaglobulin) to control acute humoral rejection in renal and cardiac allograft recipients and potential mechanisms of action. *Transplantation* 66, 800–805.

Julian, B. A. *et al.* (1998). Losartan, an angiotensin II type 1 receptor antagonist, lowers hematocrit in posttransplant erythrocytosis. *Journal of the American Society of Nephrology* 9, 1104–1108.

Kasiske, B. L. and Chakkera, H. A. (2000). Explained and unexplained ischemic heart disease risk after renal transplantation. *Journal of the American Society of Nephrology* 11, 1735–1743.

Katznelson, S., Takemoto, S. K., and Cecka, J. M. Histocompatibility testing, crossmatching, and allocation of cadaveric kidney transplants. In *Handbook of Kidney Transplantation* (ed. G. M. Danovitch), pp. 39–63. Philadelphia, PA: Lippincott Williams and Wilkins, 2001.

Keown, P. A. (1996). A blinded, randomized clinical trial of Mycophenolate Mofetil for the prevention of acute rejection in cadaveric renal transplantation. The Tricontinental Mycophenolate Mofetil Renal Transplant study Group. *Transplantation* 61, 1029–1037.

Kimball, P. *et al.* (1998). Flow crossmatching identifies patients at risk for postoperative elaboration of cytotoxic antibodies. *Transplantation* 65, 444–446.

Knoll, G. A. (1999). Tacrolimus versus cyclosporine for immunosuppression in renal transplantation: meta-analysis of randomized trials. *British Journal of Medicine* 318, 1104–1107.

Kreis, H. *et al.* (2000). Sirolimus in association with mycophenolate mofetil induction for the prevention of acute graft rejection in renal allograft recipients. *Transplantation* 69, 1252–1260.

Lazda, V. A., Pollak, R., Mozes, M. F., and Jonasson, O. (1988). The relationship between flow cytometer crossmatch results and subsequent rejection episodes in cadaver renal allograft recipients. *Transplantation* 45, 562–565.

Lecornu-Heuze, L. *et al.* (1998). Mycophenolate mofetil in cyclosporine-associated thrombotic microangiopathy. *Nephrology, Dialysis, Transplantation* 13, 3212–3213.

Lederer, S. R. *et al.* (2001). Impact of humoral alloreactivity early after transplantation on the long-term survival of renal allografts. *Kidney International* 59, 334–341.

Lehtonen, S. R. K. *et al.* (1997). Long-term graft outcome is not necessarily affected by delayed onset of graft function and early acute rejection. *Transplantation* 64, 103–107.

Lezaic, V. *et al.* (2001). Erythropoiesis after kidney transplantation: the role of erythropoietin, burst promoting activity and early erythroid progenitor cells. *European Medical Research* **6**, 27–32.

Li, B. *et al.* (2001). Noninvasive diagnosis of renal allograft rejection by measurement of messenger RNA for perforin and granzyme B in urine. *New England Journal of Medicine* **344**, 947–954.

Lowance, D. *et al.* (1999). Valacyclovir for the prevention of cytomegalovirus disease after renal transplantation. International Valacyclovir Prophylaxis Transplantation Study Group. *New England Journal of Medicine* **340**, 1462–1470.

Luisa, M. *et al.* (2000). Thrombotic microangiopathy associated with parvovirus B19 infection after renal transplantation. *Journal of the American Society of Nephrology* **11**, 1132–1137.

Marcen, R. *et al.* (1998). Delayed graft function does not reduce the survival of renal transplant allografts. *Transplantation* **66**, 461–466.

Mauiyyedi, S. and Colvin, R. B. (2002). Humoral rejection in kidney transplantation: new concepts in diagnosis and treatment. *Current Opinions of Nephrology and Hypertension* **11**, 609–618.

Mauiyyedi, S. *et al.* (2002). Acute humoral rejection in kidney transplantation. II. Morphology, immunopathology, and pathologic classification. *Journal of the American Society of Nephrology* **13**, 779–787.

McCauley, J. *et al.* (1989). Treatment of cyclosporine-induced haemolytic uremic syndrome with FK506. *Lancet* **30**, 1516.

McLaughlin, K. *et al.* (2002). Cytomegalovirus seromismatching increase the risk of acute allograft rejection. *Transplantation* **74**, 813–816.

Midvedt, K. and Neumayer, H. H. (2000). Management strategies for post-transplant hypertension. *Transplantation* **70** (Suppl. 11), SS64–SS69.

Montgomery R. A. *et al.* (2000). Plasmapheresis and intravenous immune globulin provides effective rescue therapy for refractory humoral rejection and allows kidneys to be successfully transplanted in cross-match positive recipients. *Transplantation* **70**, 887–895.

Murer, L. *et al.* (2000). Thrombotic microangiopathy associated with parvovirus B19 infection after renal transplantation. *Journal of the American Society of Nephrology* **11**, 1132–1137.

Nashan, B. (1997). Randomized trial of basiliximab versus placebo for control of acute cellular rejection in renal allograft recipients. *Lancet* **350**, 1193–1198.

Nast, C. C. and Cohen, A. H. Pathology of kidney transplantation. In *Handbook of Kidney Transplantation* (ed. G. M. Danovitch), pp. 290–312. Philadelphia, PA: Lippincott Williams and Wilkins, 2001.

Ojo, A. O. *et al.* (1997). Delayed graft function: risk factors and implication for renal allograft survival. *Transplantation* **63**, 968–974.

Olive, C., Cheung, C., and Falk, M. C. (1999). Apoptosis and expression of cytotoxic T lymphocyte effector molecules in renal allografts. *Transplant Immunology* **7**, 27–36.

Paff, W. W. *et al.* (1998). Delayed graft function after renal transplantation. *Transplantation* **65**, 219–223.

Pascual, M. *et al.* (1998). Plasma exchange and tacrolimus-mycophenolate rescue for acute humoral rejection in kidney transplantation. *Transplantation* **66**, 1460–1464.

Pham, P. C. and Pham, P. T. Parathyroidectomy. In *Dialysis Therapy* (ed. A. R. Nissenson and R. N. Fine), pp. 410–415. Philadelphia, PA: Hanley and Belfus Inc., 2002.

Pham, P. T., Pham, P. C., and Wilkinson, A. H. Medical and urological complications of pancreas and kidney/pancreas transplantation. In *Pancreas and Islet Transplantation* (ed. N. Hakim, R. Stratta, and D. Gray), pp. 167–189. New York: Oxford University Press, 2002b.

Pham, P. T. *et al.* (2000). Cyclosporine and tacrolimus-associated thrombotic microangiopathy. *American Journal of Kidney Diseases* **36**, 844–850.

Pham, P. T. *et al.* (2003). Inhibitors of ADAMTS13: a potential factor in the etiology of thrombotic microangiopathy in a renal allograft recipient. *Transplantation* **74**, 1077–1080.

Pichlmayr, R. (1995). Placebo-controlled study of mycophenolate mofetil combined with cyclosporin and corticosteroids for prevention of acute rejection. European Mycophenolate Cooperative Study Group. *Lancet* **345**, 1321–1325.

Racusen, L. C. *et al.* (1999). The Banff 97 working classification of renal allograft pathology. *Kidney International* **55**, 713–723.

Ruggenenti, P. (2002). Post-transplant hemolytic uremic syndrome. *Kidney International* **62**, 1093–1104.

Shamlou, K. K. *et al.* (1994). Captopril renogram and the hypertensive renal transplantion patients: a predictive test of therapeutic outcome. *Radiology* **190**, 153–159.

Shokes, D. A. and Cecka, J. M. Effect of delayed graft function on short- and long-term kidney graft survival. In *Clinical Transplants* (ed. J. M. Cecka and P. I. Terasaki), pp. 297–303. Los Angeles, CA: UCLA Tissue Typing Laboratory, 1997.

Shokes, D. A. and Cecka, J. M. (1998). Deleterious effects of delayed graft function in cadaveric renal transplant recipients independent of acute rejection. *Transplantation* **66**, 1697–1701.

Shokes, D. A., Parfrey, N. A., and Halloran, P. F. (1990). Increased major histocompatibility complex antigen expression in unilateral ischemic acute tubular necrosis in the mouse. *Transplantation* **49**, 201–207.

Sollinger, H. W. (1995). Mycophenolate Mofetil for the prevention of acute rejection in primary cadaveric renal allograft recipients. *Transplantation* **60**, 225–232.

St Peter, S. D. *et al.* (2002). Genetic determinants of delayed graft function after kidney transplantation. *Transplantation* **74**, 809–813.

Stone, J. H., Amend, W. J., and Criswell, L. A. (1999). Antiphospholipid antibody syndrome in renal transplantation: occurrence of clinical events in 96 consecutive patients with systemic lupus erythematosus. *American Journal of Kidney Diseases* **34**, 1040–1047.

Takada, M. *et al.* (1998). Effects of explosive brain death on cytokine activation of peripheral organs in the rat. *Transplantation* **65**, 1533–1542.

Troppmann, C. *et al.* (1996). Delayed graft function in the absence of rejection has no long-term impact. *Transplantation* **61**, 1331–1337.

Trpkov, K. *et al.* (1996). Pathologic features of acute renal allograft rejection associated with donor-specific antibody. Analysis using the Banff grading schema. *Transplantation* **61**, 1586–1592.

Vannini, S. D. P. *et al.* (1999). Permanently reduced plasma ionized magnesium among renal transplant recipients on cyclosporine. *Transplantation International* **12**, 244–249.

Vincenti, F. *et al.* (1998). Interleukin-2-receptor blockade with daclizumab to prevent acute rejection in renal transplantation. *New England Journal of Medicine* **338**, 161–165.

Wang, A. Y. H. *et al.* (2002). Effects of losartan or enalapril on hemoglobin, circulating erythropoietin, and insulin-like growth factor-1 in patients with and without posttransplant erythrocytosis. *American Journal of Kidney Diseases* **39**, 600–608.

Ward, H. N. (1997). The renal handling of phosphate by renal transplant recipients: correlation with serum parathyroid hormone, cyclic 3'5'-adenosine monophosphate urinary excretion and allograft function. *Advances in Experimental and Medicinal Biology* **81**, 173–181.

Watschinger, B. and Pascual, M. (2002). Capillary C4d deposition as a marker of humoral immunity in renal allograft rejection. *Journal of the American Society of Nephrology* **13**, 2420–2423.

Zarifian, A. *et al.* (1998). Cyclosporine-associated thrombotic microangiopathy in renal allografts. *Kidney International* **55**, 2457–2466.

Zimmerman, P. *et al.* Diagnostic imaging in kidney transplantation. In *Handbook of Kidney Transplantation* (ed. G. M. Danovitch), pp. 272–289. Philadelphia, PA: Lippincott Williams and Wilkins, 2001.

13.3.3 Long-term medical complications

J. Douglas Briggs

Introduction

There have been two major changes over time in the pattern of medical complications following renal transplantation. First, there has been an overall decrease in fatal complications with a resultant improvement in patient survival. This improvement has continued to the present time despite a trend in recent years towards acceptance for transplantation of more patients in the older age groups and/or with more comorbid disease. Second, there have been relative changes in the types of fatal complications. In the very early days of transplantation as many as 40 per cent of renal allograft recipients died as a consequence of infection. Subsequently, infective deaths have declined dramatically so that now not more than 1–2 per cent of patients die of infection. This decrease in infective deaths is due to the fact that there are now rapid and reliable tests and effective treatment for almost all infections. Nonetheless, many infections are, in the early stages, devoid of obvious clinical features, they may progress rapidly and they may be fatal if treatment is delayed. Thus, a high index of suspicion at the time of presentation combined with efficient investigation is important to avoid unnecessary deaths.

As infective deaths have decreased, cardiovascular disease has become relatively more common as a cause of death and now forms the largest category even in countries with fewer than average cardiovascular deaths in their general population. However, it is encouraging that, as in the general population, cardiovascular deaths in renal allograft recipients are declining in absolute numbers, probably due to more attention being paid to such risk factors as hypertension, hypercholesterolaemia, and smoking. One of the most important but less talked about factors which is harmful to the cardiovascular system is the length of time on dialysis prior to the transplant. During this period, hyperphosphataemia will predispose to vascular calcification and fluid overload and anaemia to left ventricular hypertrophy (LVH) and dysfunction and to remodelling of blood vessel walls. The adverse effect of the dialysis phase on the cardiovascular system is evident from the fact that cardiovascular deaths are several times more common in dialysis patients than in renal allograft recipients even when age is taken into account. Thus, avoidance of dialysis by means of pre-emptive transplantation or even reducing the time spent in the dialysis phase has an important beneficial effect on cardiovascular mortality.

The third major cause of post-transplant mortality is neoplasia. Although in most analyses this accounts for far fewer deaths than cardiovascular disease, most of the deaths occur beyond 10 years. Thus, as the number of allograft recipients with long-term graft function increases, so too will the mortality from neoplasia. Death from neoplasia is a matter of considerable concern because of the increasing incidence in the long term, post-transplant patient and also because, unlike infective and cardiovascular deaths, we are unable at present to take any effective steps to reduce the incidence of neoplasia.

One final point to mention in this introduction is the potentially adverse effect of immunosuppressive therapy on post-transplant medical complications. The heightened risk of infection is well known, as is the adverse effect of calcineurin inhibitors and steroids on such cardiovascular risk factors as serum lipids and blood pressure. With the exception of post-transplant lymphoproliferative disorder, a relationship between the potency of the immunosuppressive regimen and the incidence of neoplasia is as yet unproven but may, nonetheless, exist. At a practical level there are two important points. First, we should try to avoid excessive doses of immunosuppressive drugs. Second, we now have a sufficient variety of drugs that we can devise long term regimens, which can reduce the adverse effect on cardiovascular disease for example by late withdrawal of steroids or calcineurin inhibitors.

Cardiovascular disease

Introduction

Cardiovascular disease is the leading cause of death following renal transplantation, and overall its prevalence is five to 10 times greater than in the general population. This is illustrated in Fig. 1. However, the relative risk of cardiovascular death is as high as 30 times greater in chronic renal failure patients younger than 35 years but much less at around six times greater over the age of 55 years (Brown *et al.* 1994). While renal transplantation may result in additional aetiological factors, the mechanisms contributing to cardiovascular disease begin to operate at an early stage of chronic progressive renal disease, often years before the transplant operation has taken place.

There are two main pathological processes which are responsible for the transplant recipient's cardiovascular disease namely atheroma and the combination of LVH and dysfunction. However, other mechanisms also contribute to the vascular damage, in particular stiffening and calcification of the arterial wall. In turn a number of factors contribute to each of these pathological processes, some of which are preventable or at least in part reversible. There is, therefore, considerable potential for amelioration of cardiovascular disease in the renal transplant recipient. So far this potential has not been fully exploited.

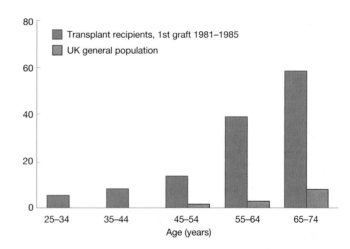

Fig. 1 Age-specific death rates per thousand patient years from myocardial ischaemia and infarction in men in the United Kingdom receiving a first cadaveric graft between 1981 and 1985, compared with that of the male general population in the United Kingdom. Data from the EDTA Registry (reproduced with permission from Raine, A. E. G. (1994). *Kidney Transplantation: Principles and Practice* pp. 339–355).

Ischaemic heart disease

Mechanisms

Those mechanisms which are thought to be most important are listed in Table 1 and the length of the list indicates the potential scope for amelioration.

Hyperlipidaemia

There is a tendency for serum lipid abnormalities to develop following renal transplantation and any pre-existing abnormalities tend to worsen, with a rise in total and LDL cholesterol and in triglycerides. HDL cholesterol is usually not significantly below normal. Although lipid levels tend not to be elevated in dialysis patients, one of the most significant associations of post-transplant hyperlipidaemia is with the pretransplant blood levels. The other important contributory factors to post-transplant hyperlipidaemia are immunosuppressive therapy and the relaxation of dietary restriction and sedentary lifestyle which the patient often adopts. The immunosuppressive drugs which have the most adverse effect are steroids, cyclosporin, and rapamycin while tacrolimus has less effect and mycophenolate mofetil and azathioprine have no effect at all.

Hyperhomocysteinaemia

The association of elevated serum homocysteine and vascular disease in the general population is well established as is the beneficial effect of folic acid in lowering both serum homocysteine and prevalence of coronary artery disease. In renal transplant recipients a similar association exists and this association is independent of other risk factors (Ducloux et al. 2000). There is an inverse correlation between serum homocysteine and glomerular filtration rate but the spontaneous reduction in serum homocysteine following transplantation is less than one would expect in relation to the degree of recovery of renal function. The serum homocysteine concentration in renal transplant recipients falls more readily than in haemodialysis patients in response to folic acid therapy but it remains to be demonstrated that the reduction in serum homocysteine induced by folic acid results in a lowering of cardiovascular mortality.

Smoking

The adverse effect of smoking on cardiovascular mortality, which has been apparent for some time in the general population, has not surprisingly also been confirmed in renal transplant recipients. The relative risk of major cardiovascular events is more than doubled by heavy smoking and this risk is as great as that resulting from the presence of diabetes mellitus (Cosio et al. 1999).

Table 1 Mechanisms of ischaemic heart disease

Potentially remediable	Not remediable
Hyperlipidaemia	Older age
Hyperhomocysteinaemia	Genetic
Smoking	
Hyperglycaemia	
Inflammation	
Oxidative stress	
Immunosuppressive therapy	
Sedentary lifestyle	
Arterial stiffening/vascular calcification	

Hyperglycaemia

This is common even in non-diabetic renal transplant patients, the causes including renal dysfunction, steroids, and calcineurin inhibitors especially tacrolimus. Although the blood glucose can be lowered effectively, mild elevations while still constituting a risk factor, are frequently ignored. Also, hyperglycaemia is often linked with obesity. The latter by itself may also be a cardiovascular risk factor, but this has not yet been proven. Diabetes mellitus, usually as the cause of the patient's renal failure, but less often as an additional co-morbid feature, is an important cardiovascular risk factor. Also the frequency of Type 2 diabetes in renal transplant recipients is slowly increasing in part due to the increasing incidence in the general population but also because the percentage of transplant recipients in the older age groups is increasing.

Inflammation

Epidemiological studies have shown an association between C-reactive protein and cardiovascular disease in the general population and such studies have now been extended to patients with chronic renal failure. The uraemic state is characterized by an altered immune response which is associated with an elevation of acute phase response proteins such as C-reactive protein. This mediator of the inflammatory response is probably linked to atherogenesis through its lipoprotein binding and complement activation functions. Other linked factors are malnutrition, which is common in the renal failure population, and oxidative stress (Stenvinkel et al. 1999).

Oxidative stress

Increased oxidative stress is increasingly seen as having a role in atherogenesis through the generation of lipid peroxidation products. These include oxidized lipoproteins which are consistently found in atheromatous plaques. Oxidative stress represents the balance between the excessive production of free radicals and the depletion of antioxidants which include vitamins C and E. Recent studies have shown a correlation between increased oxidative stress and a raised cardiovascular mortality in dialysis patients and also a reduction in mortality with vitamin E therapy (Boaz et al. 2000). Thus, there is the potential for benefit in the management of cardiovascular disease arising from a further understanding of the role of oxidative stress in the pathogenesis of atheroma.

Immunosuppressive therapy

The increasing number of effective drugs now allows us more choice and we are, therefore, able to use regimens that take into account the adverse effect of some of these drugs on the cardiovascular system. Table 2 shows that steroids and the calcineurin inhibitors have the most adverse effects, while the only disadvantage of rapamycin is its effect on lipid metabolism and both mycophenolate mofetil and azathioprine are free of cardiovascular side-effects. As it is particularly in the long term that one would wish to avoid the cardiovascular side-effects of these drugs, one should consider regimens in which cyclosporin or tacrolimus is withdrawn after the high-risk period for acute rejection is past. With regard to steroids one can reduce their adverse effect on the cardiovascular system by using either a steroid withdrawal regimen or one which is steroid free from the beginning.

Arterial stiffening/vascular calcification

While these two abnormalities often combine in contributing to cardiovascular mortality, they arise through different mechanisms.

Table 2 Adverse influence of immunosuppressive therapy on cardiovascular disease

	Prednisolone	Azathioprine	Cyclosporin	Tacrolimus	Mycophenolate	Rapamycin
Serum cholesterol	+		++	+		++
Blood pressure	+		++	++		
Blood glucose	++		+	++		
Renal function			++	++		
Body weight	++					
Serum uric acid			+	+		

Arterial stiffening represents a remodelling process which is similar to the changes resulting from ageing. The two components are an increase in the volume of the lumen and hypertrophy of the vessel wall. The most obvious consequence is an increase in systolic blood pressure and pulse pressure and this will be further discussed in the subsequent section which deals with hypertension. In addition there is an adverse effect on myocardial perfusion which will contribute to ischaemic heart disease. Vascular calcification has been demonstrated in the majority of dialysis patients even in the 20–30-year-old age group (Goodman *et al.* 2000). The main contributory factors are thought to be hyperphosphataemia and secondary hyperparathyroidism and, therefore, effective serum phosphorus control during the dialysis phase together with early transplantation are the most important measures which can be applied to minimize the presence of vascular calcification.

Management

As an advanced degree of ischaemic heart disease may well exist prior to transplantation, it is important to start by considering management in the pretransplant phase.

Pretransplant management (see also Chapter 13.1)
This falls into two main categories namely assessment of suitability for transplantation and medical and surgical preventive and therapeutic measures.

Assessment of suitability for transplantation is important in order to avoid early post-transplant cardiovascular deaths. The initial screening should include both an electrocardiogram (ECG) and echocardiogram. More detailed investigation is required either if the screening suggests the presence of ischaemic heart disease or routinely in the case of the high-risk patient. Those over 55 years or with diabetes mellitus irrespective of age are the main categories of high risk. Further investigation may consist of an exercise ECG or in the setting of poor exercise tolerance, a dobutamine stress echocardiogram or thallium scan, depending on the preference of the cardiologist. Coronary angiography will be required in the setting of an abnormality of one of these screening tests. If this assessment demonstrates significant coronary artery disease, the insertion of a stent or coronary artery bypass surgery may well be required prior to transplantation. A much higher post-transplant cardiac mortality has been reported following medical as opposed to interventional management of ischaemic heart disease pretransplant (Manske *et al.* 1992). The choice between a stent and surgery depends on the distribution and extent of the coronary artery lesions.

Medical management prior to transplantation follows conventional lines for the patient with ischaemic heart disease but bearing in mind the fact that there are often multiple predisposing factors. The benefit of cessation of smoking and treatment of hyperlipidaemia are beyond dispute. Regular exercise within the patient's tolerance is probably also helpful. It is likely but not so far proven that measures aimed at some of the other factors such as reduction of high homocysteine levels with folic acid and the use of antioxidants such as vitamin E are of some value (Boaz *et al.* 2000). With regard to the high homocysteine levels, it has been found that these are much more resistant to lowering by folic acid than in the setting of normal renal function. High doses are not significantly more effective than moderate doses and one can expect a reduction of around 30 per cent with a dose of 15 mg per day (Sunder-Plassmann *et al.* 2000).

Post-transplant management
The use of antianginal drugs, and revascularization procedures follow conventional lines. A number of studies have confirmed the safety of the statin group of drugs and their ability to lower serum cholesterol (Lepre *et al.* 1999). While it is highly likely that, as in the general population, they will reduce cardiovascular mortality, trials with the aim of proving this are still in progress. Until they have reported, it would be appropriate to restrict the use of statins to patients with a moderate or severe degree of hypercholesterolaemia irrespective of whether there is overt ischaemic heart disease. In addition to their cholesterol lowering effect, statins have been shown to have a beneficial effect on endolethial function, thrombotic mechanisms, and inflammatory markers, all of which have been linked to coronary heart disease (Massy and Guijarro 2001). There may, therefore, be benefit from the use of statins beyond their cholesterol lowering effects. Folic acid has been shown to effectively lower elevated serum homocysteine in transplant recipients. Although such reduction has been shown to reduce cardiovascular deaths in non-renal patients, proof of similar benefit in the post-transplant patient is still awaited. However, in view of the safety of folic acid administration, there is a good argument for its use in the setting of post-transplant hyperhomocysteinaemia. Mention was made earlier of the varying effect of the different immunosuppressive drugs on ischaemic heart disease risk factors (Table 2). The choice of immunosuppressive regimen in relation to its influence on these risk factors is an important component of post-transplant management. The last but certainly not the least important aspect of patient care consists of lifestyle changes. There are four important components some of which are linked namely smoking, diet, lack of exercise, and obesity. The importance of smoking cessation cannot be overemphasized. An excessive calorie intake, associated with lack of exercise and leading to obesity is all too common and leads to much morbidity especially affecting the cardiovascular system. Calorie restriction and an exercise training programme can be highly effective

but are often difficult to achieve because of lack of motivation on the part of the patient.

Cerebrovascular disease

As with coronary artery disease, ischaemic stroke has a much increased frequency in renal transplant recipients in comparison with the general population. Mahoney *et al.* (1982) found that stroke accounted for 12 per cent of deaths over 10 years of post-transplant follow-up and also that in renal transplant patients surviving at 10 years there was a history of stroke or transient ischaemic attack in 8.5 per cent. The mechanisms are similar to those which apply to ischaemic heart disease with the high prevalence of hypertension playing an important role. The management of the transplant patient with cerebrovascular disease follows conventional lines including the importance of looking for carotid artery lesions using ultrasound.

Peripheral vascular disease

For the same reasons as with cerebrovascular disease and ischaemic heart disease, there is a much increased prevalence of this complication in the transplant recipient. Also, there are aspects of management which differ from the standard approach. For example, in the presence of gangrene there is less tendency for transplant patients to auto-amputate and there is an increased risk of superimposed infection. The risk of wound infection is also greater following surgery and prophylactic antibiotic therapy is often indicated. One also needs to bear in mind that proximal vascular disease may impair perfusion of the allograft should there be iliac artery stenosis on the same side as the donor kidney. This may of course mean that a revascularization procedure could benefit perfusion of the kidney as well as the leg. Particular care is needed should angiography be required to avoid interfering with perfusion of the allograft.

Hypertension

Introduction

In a study in my own centre, 42 per cent of transplant patients had hypertension which was well controlled while in 32 per cent it was not well controlled. Thus, only 26 per cent of patients were normotensive (Stewart *et al.* 1999). Other studies of transplant recipients have shown a wide range of blood pressure, but in most analyses, the majority of patients have been hypertensive. Thus, hypertension is clearly a common problem. An association has been demonstrated between hypertension and allograft dysfunction suggesting that hypertension has an adverse effect on graft survival (Schindler *et al.* 2000). One would expect an association as well with cardiovascular mortality. Although this has been found in patients with advanced renal failure (Lazarus *et al.* 1997), no study of renal allograft recipients has as yet addressed this issue.

Mechanisms of hypertension in the renal allograft recipient

There are five clearly defined causes of hypertension in the renal allograft recipient.

Allograft dysfunction

Hypertension is found in almost all patients with chronic allograft dysfunction and there is documentation of its development in previously normotensive patients as allograft dysfunction develops (Olmer *et al.* 1988). Thus, there is good evidence that such dysfunction is one of the causes of post-transplant hypertension. The dysfunction is usually due to chronic allograft nephropathy—previously called chronic rejection—but there are other causes such as recurrent disease. Also, it has been reported that chronic dysfunction more frequently develops in recipients who are hypertensive prior to the transplant compared with previously normotensive recipients (Frei *et al.* 1995). Thus, hypertension can be either a consequence or a cause of chronic allograft dysfunction.

Native kidneys

A number of cross-sectional studies have reported hypertension to be more frequent in patients whose native kidneys were left *in situ*. However, the cause of the native kidney disease is an important factor in that some disease groups such as glomerulonephritis are more frequently associated with hypertension than others such as interstitial nephritis. Also a recent study of 158 live-donor transplants showed no difference in blood pressure between the groups who had and had not been nephrectomized (Midtvedt *et al.* 1996). In any case the question of whether native kidney nephrectomy benefits hypertension is becoming less important as the range of antihypertensive drugs now available has in most patients removed the need to consider the alternative of a major surgical procedure.

Immunosuppressive therapy

As Table 2 shows, steroids, cyclosporin, and tacrolimus can all contribute to post-transplant hypertension. The adverse effect of steroids on blood pressure, while discernible, is small. Some studies which have compared the hypertensive effect of cyclosporin and tacrolimus have shown no significant difference (Meyer *et al.* 1997) while others have shown an advantage in favour of tacrolimus (Margreiter 2002). Thus, overall, the hypertensive effect of tacrolimus may be slightly less than that of cyclosporin. The degree of hypertensive effect of cyclosporin is certainly sufficient to be of clinical importance. In a Glasgow study of cyclosporin withdrawal at 1 year, only 41 per cent of patients in the withdrawal group were receiving antihypertensive therapy 9 years later compared with 85 per cent in those remaining on cyclosporin (MacPhee *et al.* 1998). Cyclosporin or tacrolimus withdrawal should be seriously considered beyond the first year when good blood pressure control is proving difficult to achieve.

Donor kidney

There is evidence both from animal and human studies that a hypertensive tendency can be transmitted by means of the donor kidney. Also one study has shown that the use of kidneys from donors with a family history of hypertension increased the risk of post-transplant hypertension but only in recipients who lacked a family history of hypertension (Guidi 1996). Although transmission of a tendency to hypertension by means of the donor kidney is a proven phenomenon, it has no particular implications with regard to patient management.

Renal artery stenosis

Now that most cadaver transplant operations involve the use of an aortic patch removed with the donor kidney, few centres experience this complication in more than 5 per cent of patients and the reported figure is often lower. Suspicion of renal artery stenosis (RAS) should be aroused by rapid onset of hypertension with or without deterioration in renal function. However, the onset may be insidious and a search for RAS should be considered in any patient with unexplained hypertension and/or renal dysfunction. Colour Doppler ultrasound can be a very useful screening test but needs an experienced operator. Magnetic resonance angiography gives good anatomical information but cannot provide information concerning the gradient across the stenosis. Angiography with injection of contrast is usually only required at the time of an interventional procedure. Stent insertion under angiographic control is the procedure of choice in view of a high recurrence rate with angioplasty on its own. Nowadays, surgical correction of RAS is rarely required.

Management

Post-transplant hypertension is often difficult to control. One of the reasons for this is that the arterial remodelling referred to earlier leads to a disproportionate increase in systolic and pulse pressure (London et al. 1996) and predominantly systolic hypertension is often more difficult to control than diastolic hypertension. Nonetheless, good control is very important in view of the adverse effect of poor control both on graft function and cardiovascular mortality. As an indication of the frequently resistant nature of the hypertension, in a recent analysis from Glasgow it was found that 47 per cent of patients with unsatisfactory blood pressure control were, nonetheless, receiving at least two antihypertensives and 32 per cent were receiving at least three. Also, the target blood pressure now being recommended in chronic renal failure is lower than in the past and the suggested figures which have been put forward by the National Kidney Foundation are 130/85 in the absence of proteinuria and 125/75 in its presence (Levey et al. 1998). It would seem appropriate also to recommend these targets for transplant patients. With regard to the choice of antihypertensive drugs, the angiotensin-converting enzyme (ACE) inhibitors and angiotensin-receptor blockers have a number of advantages. They are usually well tolerated and have an antiproteinuric effect and may have a role in decreasing LVH and improving diastolic dysfunction in transplant recipients. There are also an increasing number of reports that ACE inhibitors have a cardioprotective effect in non-transplant patients. Calcium-channel blockers are also useful but have a number of drawbacks. They may worsen cyclosporin induced gingival hypertrophy, and the non-dihydropyridine types such as diltiazem and verapamil increase cyclosporin blood concentrations through their effect on the cytochrome P450 system. Also, there have been reports of the dihydropyridine types giving rise to an increased incidence of cardiovascular events in high-risk patients (Furberg et al. 1995). Other classes of antihypertensives, in particular the β-blockers, continue to have a useful role. Finally, lifestyle changes have considerable potential to improve blood pressure control, but this potential is usually not fully realized. These lifestyle changes include dietary restriction of calories and salt, regular exercise, and cessation of smoking.

Left ventricular hypertrophy and dysfunction

One of two pathological processes may predominate in the renal failure patient, namely concentric LVH or LV dilatation, and these may lead to diastolic or systolic dysfunction, which in turn predisposes to congestive heart failure. These structural abnormalities begin at an early stage of the patient's chronic renal failure and may have progressed to a considerable degree by the time transplantation takes place. While successful transplantation may result in some regression of these abnormalities, the degree of LVH and LV dysfunction at the time of

the transplant has an important influence on subsequent cardiovascular mortality.

Assessment

Echocardiography is the standard method of assessing LV mass, volume, and function. The measurements derived are, however, influenced in the dialysis patient by the state of hydration, and it is therefore essential that the various indices are measured while the patients are at their dry weights. There are four main measurements. Systolic dysfunction is defined as an ejection fraction of less than 40 per cent and LV dilatation is a cavity volume of greater than 90 ml/m^2. LV mass index represents the degree of muscular hypertrophy and, finally, diastolic dysfunction, which is a consequence of LVH, can be assessed by pulsed Doppler analysis of flow across the mitral valve during diastole.

Left ventricular hypertrophy/dysfunction pretransplant

LVH begins to develop at an early stage of chronic renal failure—initially due to hypertension and later due to anaemia. Once the patient has become dialysis dependent, fluid overload also becomes a factor in the pathogenesis of LVH.

All patients being assessed for renal transplantation should have echocardiography to look for LVH and LV dysfunction in view of the prognostic influence of these two factors. We have found in Glasgow that the post-transplant mortality was higher in patients whose pretransplant echocardiograms showed LVH, increased end-diastolic and end-systolic diameters, and impaired systolic function. The last two of these had the most predictive value for survival (McGregor et al. 1998). The management implications are that during the dialysis phase, every effort should be made to achieve good blood pressure control, avoid fluid overload, and maintain a reasonable haemoglobin (>10 g/dl) if necessary with the help of iron and/or erythropoietin. Also the dialysis phase should be kept as short as possible in view of the almost inevitable deterioration in LV function during this time and pre-emptive transplantation should be the aim as often as possible in order to eliminate the harmful dialysis phase.

Left ventricular hypertrophy and dysfunction following transplantation

Serial echocardiographic studies following renal transplantation have shown benefits in a number of respects. By the end of the first year in the study by Rigatto et al. (2000) the proportion of patients with normal echocardiograms had doubled from 17 to 36 per cent and LV mass and volume had regressed by 17 and 19 per cent, respectively. Systolic function also improved and returned to normal in patients with lesser degrees of damage at the time of the transplant. Further improvement occurred over the second year with maintenance of a stable state thereafter. As one would expect, LVH tended to regress less in older patients and those with poor blood pressure control.

Although LV mass will often to some extent regress spontaneously after renal transplantation, other measures which have the aim of improving LV function may also be worthwhile. Of these, the most important is good blood pressure control as discussed earlier. Fluid overload and anaemia will usually have ceased to exist as significant factors following a successful transplant but the latter may sometimes still be present and require treatment. Finally, those patients who have suffered a severe degree of cardiac damage in the period leading up to the transplant or subsequently may require treatment along the usual lines for cardiac failure.

Neoplasia

The main category of tumour is that which develops *de novo* following the renal transplant. However, two other types which require brief mention are pre-existing cancers in potential transplant recipients and tumours transmitted by the donor organ.

Pre-existing cancer

The recommended interval between treatment of a tumour and a subsequent renal transplant will vary with the tumour type and detailed recommendations have been made by Penn (1993). He suggests that no interval is required in the case of incidentally discovered renal carcinomas, *in situ* carcinomas where there is a small, single focus of tumour such as prostate and uterus, low-grade bladder cancers, and basal cell skin cancers. With most other cancers a 2-year interval is regarded as reasonably safe. However, in the case of those with a high recurrence rate, the interval should be at least 3–5 years. Tumours in this category include symptomatic renal tumours, malignant melanoma, and colorectal, breast, and prostate cancers.

Transmitted tumours

This is an unusual complication but nonetheless every effort should be made to exclude malignancy in the donor. Exceptions are low-grade skin tumours, *in situ* carcinoma of the uterine cervix and most primary intracerebral tumours in which cases it is considered safe to use the donor kidneys. However, in the case of highly malignant primary brain tumours or when craniotomy has taken place, donation should not proceed. Finally, where there is suspicion of a tumour in the donor, it may be possible to resolve the doubt by a postmortem examination while the organs are machine perfused or stored in ice.

De novo cancer

Incidence

The numerous single-centre retrospective analyses in which most of the patients have follow-up of less than 10 years greatly underestimate the longer term risk of cancer. In the Glasgow Transplant Unit, cancer, currently, is second only to cardiovascular disease as a cause of death, accounting for 16 per cent of deaths, and this figure will rise with increasing lengths of follow-up. One of the more frequently quoted assessments of the long-term risks has been from Australia by Sheil (2001) and this is illustrated in Fig. 2. However, in populations with less sun exposure than in Australia the risk of skin cancer will be somewhat less than that shown by Sheil (2001). A high risk of cancer is confined to a small number of tumour types which are listed in Table 3 while, by contrast, the majority of tumours commonly observed in the general population occur with a similar frequency in transplant recipients.

Aetiology

Several factors may predispose the transplant recipient to cancer. Impaired immune surveillance is one such factor and there is support for this from a number of experimental and clinical observations. Immunosuppressive therapy is clearly the main mechanism of the impaired immune response. Another possible cause is that immunosuppressive drugs have a direct oncogenic effect but there is less evidence for this than for the theory that the drugs act through their effect on immune surveillance. There is concern that the introduction of more

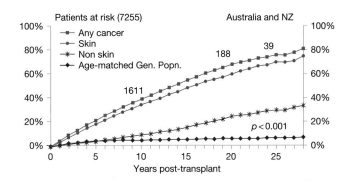

Fig. 2 The risk of the development of skin and non-skin cancer and any cancer following renal transplantation in Australia and New Zealand (reproduced with permission from Sheil, A. G. R. (1997). Cancer report 1997. In the Twentieth Annual Report: Australia and New Zealand Dialysis and Transplant Registry, p. 138).

Table 3 Tumours with a high incidence in renal allograft recipients

Cancer of skin and lips
Post-transplant lymphoproliferative disorder (PTLD)
Kaposi's sarcoma (KS)
Renal carcinoma
Uterine cervical carcinoma
Vulvar carcinoma
Perineal carcinoma
Hepatobiliary carcinoma
Sarcoma (excluding KS)

potent drugs will lead to an increase in the frequency of cancer but there is as yet no direct evidence of this with the exception of post-transplant lymphoproliferative disease (PTLD). A third mechanism is the effect of oncogenic viruses and these are related to PTLD (Epstein–Barr virus or EBV), cancers of the vulva, vagina, and uterine cervix (papilloma virus and herpes simplex), hepatoma (hepatitis B and C), and Kaposi's sarcoma (KS) human herpes virus-8 (HHV-8). The final mechanism that needs to be mentioned is chronic antigen stimulation with respect to lymphoid tumours. There is indirect evidence that malignant lymphoid tumours can develop as a consequence of chronic stimulation of the lymphoreticular system by foreign antigen originating in allografts (Schwartz and Beldotti 1965).

Types of cancer

Skin and lips

A number of aetiological factors in addition to immunosuppression may contribute to these cancers such as ultraviolet (UV) light exposure, virus infection (papilloma virus and herpes viruses), and genetic influences. In contrast to the general population, the squamous cell type is more common than basal cell cancer with a ratio of around 4 : 1. Skin cancer often follows precancerous lesions such as actinic keratoses and viral warts. Also the squamous cell cancers seen in transplant recipients are more often multiple and aggressive with a reported rate of metastasis of 8 per cent compared with 0.6 per cent in the general population in Australia (Sheil 2001).

The importance of exposure to the sun is demonstrated by the preponderance of skin cancers on exposed areas (80 per cent) and the higher incidence in sunny climates. They are also much more common in fair skinned patients. In view of the high incidence and aggressive nature of skin cancer in these patients, transplant follow-up clinics should have a combined counselling and skin surveillance programme (Ramsey et al. 2000) with close links to dermatology and plastic surgery services. Malignant melanoma is also more common in transplant recipients but to a very much lesser degree than is the case with squamous cell cancer.

Post-transplant lymphoproliferative disease

The incidence in renal transplant recipients is around 1 per cent, a risk of lymphoma about 20 times greater than in the general population. The two main aetiological mechanisms are EBV infection and immunosuppression. EBV infection can be detected in about 90 per cent of patients and is almost always a primary infection. Thus, seronegative recipients are those predominantly at risk and this explains why children are commonly affected in contrast to lymphoma in the general population. The EBV attaches to the C3d complement component receptor which is carried by B lymphocytes and the virus transforms these cells into immortalized lymphoblastoid cell lines. Most evidence points to the total amount of immunosuppression rather than any particular drug or drugs as a predisposing factor. Two points which support this argument are the higher frequency of PTLD in heart and heart/lung recipients than in renal patients and the higher frequency in the United States of America where more potent immunosuppressive regimens tend to be used than in Europe. In contrast to most other post-transplant cancers, PTLD commonly occurs during the first year and again this points to the importance of the immunosuppressive dose.

PTLD usually presents as one of four clinical syndromes. An onset similar to acute infectious mononucleosis with constitutional upset and tonsilar and cervical lymph node enlargement is the most common mode of presentation during the first year. Second a fulminating picture with widespread infiltration and ominous prognosis can present within weeks of the transplant. Later, a more indolent presentation may be seen with isolated or multiple tumours often involving the gastrointestinal tract, the lungs, or the allograft. Finally, one may see an EBV-negative type of PTLD which is of late onset and clinically resembles non-Hodgkin's lymphoma. In those patients with localized organ involvement, the brain is frequently involved, much more often than in lymphoma in the general population.

Prevention of PTLD is clearly a more attractive option than treatment of established disease. The most reliable preventive measure is to avoid transplanting donor kidneys from EBV-positive donors into EBV-negative recipients. Although simple in theory this policy is difficult in practice in view of all the other competing priorities in the process of allocating donor kidneys. None of the currently available antiviral drugs are active enough against the EBV to provide effective prophylaxis.

The treatment of established PTLD is often unsatisfactory. The first and universally agreed step should be to eliminate most of the immunosuppression in a stepwise manner but usually with continuation of low-dose steroids. This step alone will sometimes induce remission. It may be possible to successfully treat patients with localized

lymphoma deposits by surgical excision. Also radiotherapy can be of value particularly in the case of PTLD confined to the central nervous system (CNS). Antiviral therapy is often given, the available drugs being acyclovir, gancyclovir, foscarnet, and interferon-α. The consensus view from the observations that have been made is that this approach is of very limited value. γ-Globulin has been used but with not much evidence of benefit. Finally, monoclonal antibody preparations directed against B cells have been used but there is not yet good evidence of benefit. Thus there is not yet a therapeutic regimen of proven value. However, short-term success has been reported in seven consecutive patients from a five-pronged approach consisting of reduction of immunosuppression, acyclovir or gancyclovir, interferon-α, γ-globulins, and an anti-CD19 monoclonal antibody (Schaar et al. 2001). One would expect that it will not be long before further reports appear describing successful treatment regimens.

Kaposi's sarcoma

This tumour is mainly confined to patients whose ethnic origins were Arabic, African, Italian, Jewish, or Greek but it is not confined to their countries of origin. The presence of antibodies to HHV-8 are found in 90 per cent of the cases and their presence confers a 28-fold increase in the likelihood of this disease developing (Farge et al. 1999). Thus, HHV-8 is undoubtedly the main trigger for KS. The use of antibody induction as part of the immunosuppressive regimen has also been reported to predispose. Around half of the cases of KS have presented by the end of the first year. The male to female ratio is around 3 : 1 and the usual clinical presentation is of purple macules or plaques on the skin and oropharyngeal mucosa while in 40 per cent of patients there is also visceral disease involving mainly the gastrointestinal tract, lungs, and lymph nodes. In 27 per cent of patients with visceral disease, skin lesions are absent and as a consequence in these patients the diagnosis is more difficult to make (Penn 1997). Reduction or cessation of immunosuppressive therapy has been reported to result in remission in 53 per cent of patients without visceral involvement and 27 per cent of those with such involvement (Penn 1997). The price is often loss of the allograft and recurrence may follow resumption of immunosuppression or a regraft. There is as yet no other therapeutic measure of proven value.

Genitourinary tumours

There are three groups of tumours under this heading. First, there is a high frequency of anogenital carcinomas involving the vulva, perineum, scrotum, penis, perianal skin, and anus. The sex ratio is reversed compared with most other cancers, women outnumbering men by 2.6 : 1 and these patients are often younger than their counterparts in the general population (Penn 1998). The incidence of these tumours is increased 100-fold compared with the general population, and human papilloma virus (HPV) and herpes simplex virus have an aetiological role in some of these patients. In keeping with the role of viral infection, many of these tumours are preceded by the occurrence of viral warts. The second tumour type which needs mention is carcinoma of the cervix. The reported increase in incidence is around 15-fold and 70 per cent of cases are *in situ*. Clearly, there is a need for regular surveillance in transplant recipients with cervical smears in order to detect these tumours at an early stage. The same viral mechanism applies as with the anogenital cancers. The third group of genitourinary tumours which have a high incidence in transplant recipients are those of the bladder, ureter, and kidney. Risk ratios of around 7 for bladder and kidney and 300 for ureter have been reported (Sheil 2001). Analgesic abuse is known to predispose to urinary tract tumours and may, therefore, have a role in some of these tumours. The other recognized factor in the case of the renal cancers is acquired cystic kidney disease (ACKD). This condition is common in chronic renal failure and has been detected in 31 per cent of patients being screened by ultrasound prior to transplantation (Gulanikar *et al.* 1998). In this study, eight of 206 patients (3.8 per cent) were found to have renal cell carcinoma, seven of whom also had ACKD. This and other similar reports indicate that renal cancer is common and that it usually follows ACKD. Routine native kidney ultrasound is, therefore, a worthwhile procedure in this at risk population. The final point relates to the degree of malignancy of these renal cancers. They are often small and discovered as a result of routine ultrasound examination. However, less commonly they possess a higher degree of malignancy and they have been reported to have metastasized at the time of diagnosis in 9 per cent of cases (Penn 1995).

Hepatobiliary tumours

Epidemiological studies have shown a relative risk of between 20 and 38 compared with the general population. The most common variety of tumour is hepatoma and in a substantial number of these patients there was a past history of hepatitis B. Now that hepatitis C testing is routine, increasing numbers of hepatoma patients are being found to be hepatitis C positive.

Sarcomas

This is the final type of tumour which has a much higher incidence in renal transplant patients than in the general population. These are unrelated to KS and involve mainly visceral organs or soft tissues. A variety of types are found including fibrous histiocytoma, leiomyosarcoma, fibrosarcoma, rhabdomyosarcoma, haemangiosarcoma, and mesothelioma.

Miscellaneous tumours

There is a wide variation in the number of cancers reported from different transplant centres. Some of these differences reflect inaccuracies introduced by small patient numbers. The larger transplant registries of which the best known is the Cincinnati Transplant Tumour Registry have reported that the remaining tumour types which are not included in Table 3 do not occur with any significant increase in frequency in the renal transplant population.

Effect of post-transplant cancer on survival

As a general rule the virus related tumours present early post-transplant and in the case of PTLD and KS often within the first year. By contrast many of the solid organ tumours, other than the virus related ones, often present more than 10 years after the transplant but also late in the course of the disease and/or with metastases at the time of diagnosis and carry a life expectancy of only a few months.

Patient management

Prevention and early diagnosis are clearly worth pursuing. The main preventive measures relate to such carcinogens as smoking and sunlight, surveillance to detect patients at risk of the various relevant viral infections, and avoidance of unnecessarily heavy immunosuppression. Early diagnosis can be assisted by various screening procedures. There are potentially a large number of these including relevant viral studies, cervical smears, mammography, ultrasound of native kidneys, and skin surveillance with especially close observation of patients with warts such as vulvar warts.

In the setting of established cancer, cure may be a realistic aim especially in the case of some of the virus related varieties described above. In other less favourable circumstances it is common practice to considerably reduce or even eliminate immunosuppression although there is no good evidence that this will slow down or prevent further tumour growth. It has been observed in a number of studies that patients destined to develop late onset tumours often have less than average early rejection, presumably due to a degree of immune hyporesponsiveness. Thus, radically reducing immunosuppression is less likely to induce late-onset rejection in these patients than in those without tumours.

Infection

The incidence of infection and the resulting mortality have declined considerably over the past 40 years. In the 1960s, there were reports of 40 per cent of all renal allograft recipients dying of infection. By the late 1970s a typical mortality from infection was 5–10 per cent, and by the 1990s the equivalent figure in our centre had fallen to 0.5 per cent. However, this very low mortality does not mean that infection has ceased to be a major problem. The reduction in mortality has resulted from greater appreciation of the types of infection and modes of presentation, together with more sophisticated methods of diagnosis and treatment (Fishman and Rubin 1998). In addition, there is a better awareness of when to accept failure of a graft and stop drugs such as the high-dose steroids which are used in the treatment of acute rejection. There has, however, been a trend over the past decade towards the use of more powerful immunosuppressive drugs such as tacrolimus, mycophenolate mofetil, and rapamycin and we will have to be on guard in case this is followed by an increased incidence of infection.

There are three main factors predisposing to post-transplant infection: immunodepression caused by the uraemia of the previous renal failure, immunosuppressive therapy, and major surgery involving vascular and urological procedures (Cohen *et al.* 2001). In addition, there are now more older patients receiving transplants as well as other high-risk groups such as those with diabetes mellitus or poor graft function.

Prevention

A number of useful measures can be taken and these can be divided into those applicable before and at the time of the transplant procedure.

Before transplantation

Screening should be carried out for active or occult infection, both bacterial and viral. The main sites of bacterial infection are the chest and urinary tract. Chronic respiratory infection, especially bronchiectasis, is not a contraindication to transplantation but gives rise to increased risk. Pulmonary tuberculosis, if active, should of course be treated before proceeding to transplantation. Asymptomatic bacteriuria is not necessarily an indication for antibiotic therapy. However, if there is established infection in one or both kidneys, or persistent bacteriuria associated with gross ureteric reflux, removal of the affected kidney(s) prior to transplantation should be considered. Screening for viral infection should include hepatitis B and C, human immunodeficiency virus (HIV), and cytomegalovirus (CMV). In addition, EBV and varicella serology can be very useful although not yet considered essential. All patients with negative hepatitis B serology should have active immunization.

During the transplant operation

First, one has to consider the possible transmission of pathogens with the allograft. Bacterial contamination of the kidney at the time of removal is always a possibility but is very uncommon. More important is the carriage of bacteria in the kidney due to bacteraemia in the donor. This is very unlikely to result in transmission of infection provided there has been careful donor selection and antibiotic therapy has been given if indicated to the donor for at least 24 h. Testing of the donor for HIV and hepatitis B virus must always be carried out: a positive result would rule out kidney and other organ and tissue donation as there is every likelihood of virus transmission, with the development of disease in the recipient. Also donation from high-risk individuals, such as drug addicts, should not be considered even if these virus tests are negative. Testing for hepatitis C is also essential, although some centres would consider using a kidney from a positive donor but only for a positive recipient. CMV and EBV testing is useful, as will be discussed below, but a positive test does not contraindicate donation.

Presentation of infection

Sophisticated tests and effective drugs allow accurate diagnosis, followed by cure, for most of the infections encountered following transplantation. However, diagnosis can be difficult, partly due to the paucity of clinical features in the immunosuppressed patient. In many cases a fever is the only sign until a late stage, and one has to have a high level of awareness of the most likely infections in a patient at any

time. In this regard the 'timetable' of infection developed by Rubin *et al.* (1981) is useful. Rubin's later modification of this timetable is reproduced in Fig. 3.

During the first month, bacterial infections in the lungs, wound, urinary tract, and arising from intravenous lines constitute the most important group. From the second to the sixth month post-transplant the main additional pathogens are CMV and other herpes viruses. Infection with these predisposes to the classic opportunistic pathogens, namely *Pneumocystis carinii*, *Listeria monocytogenes*, fungi (mainly Candida and Aspergillus), and *Mycobacterium tuberculosis*. Beyond 6 months these viral and opportunistic pathogens listed still occur and one also sees the typical infections encountered in the general community. A final but important point to note is that infection tends to develop not at the time of peak dose of antirejection therapy but a few weeks later.

Pulmonary infection

Table 4 lists the pathogens which most often cause pulmonary infection. Bacteria account for the majority of cases but the patient who presents several weeks or months after transplantation with a fever and radiological shadowing is more difficult to diagnose. In such cases the rate of progression of the illness and its radiological pattern are useful pointers. Most of the infections progress rapidly unless treated quickly, apart from tuberculosis and, to a lesser degree, aspergillosis. On radiological investigation both CMV and Pneumocystis cause diffuse or segmental infiltrates, while the distribution is more lobar in most other types of infection.

In view of the often rapid progression of infection, investigation should be carried out with urgency. If the routine tests such as sputum

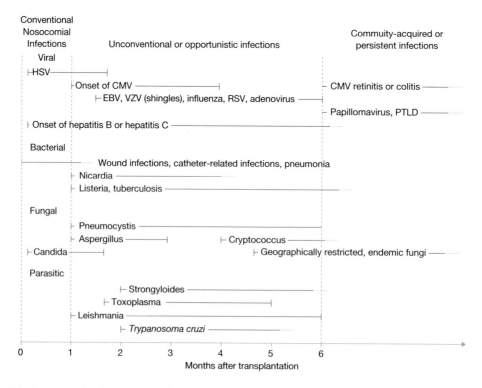

Fig. 3 The timetable of infections occurring after renal transplantation which has been drawn up by Rubin *et al.* (1981) [reproduced with permission from Fishman, J. A. and Rubin, R. H. (1998). *New England Journal of Medicine* **338**, 1741–1751].

Table 4 Main causes of pulmonary infection

Bacteria	Viruses
Pneumococcus	Cytomegalovirus
Haemophilus influenzae	
Staphylococcus aureus	**Fungi**
Legionella spp.	Pneumocystis carinii
Mycobacterium spp.	Aspergillus spp.
Nocardia spp.	Candida spp.

culture for bacterial pathogens fail to establish the diagnosis, sputum obtained spontaneously or assisted by hypertonic saline aerosols can be examined by a variety of techniques. These include histochemistry and immunofluorescence techniques, solid phase immunoassays for microbial antigens, and DNA amplification by polymerase chain reaction (PCR). In the absence of a diagnosis, bronchoscopy should be performed to obtain aspirate or a biopsy. Computed tomography (CT) guidance of the needle can be useful, particularly in the case of nodular lesions.

Pneumocystis carinii

This pathogen often, but by no means always, follows CMV infection. A fever and dry cough are often followed by dyspnoea and hypoxia which develop prior to any radiological changes. When radiological changes do develop, they may be diffuse, segmental, or nodular and by this time the patient will be seriously ill. The diagnostic tests have been summarized in the preceding paragraph and once the diagnosis has been established, the first line of treatment consists of cotrimoxazole, orally or intravenously. Inhaled pentamidine can be useful as a follow-up to the cotrimoxazole while intravenous pentamidine is an option in the case of a poor response to cotrimoxazole.

Other types of pulmonary infections

Aspergillosis usually differs from *P. carinii* infection in that its rate of progression is less rapid and the radiograph shows a discrete area of consolidation, sometimes with cavitation. The liposomal form of amphotericin-B usually provides effective therapy.

Legionella may also complicate renal transplantation, its typical features being sparse sputum, a variable distribution of consolidation and sometimes CNS and gastroenterological features and renal impairment. Erythromycin is usually the drug of choice but the addition of rifampicin may be helpful.

Nocardia is a Gram-positive organism which produces pneumonia with a tendency to cavitation. Cotrimoxazole is the drug of choice.

Septicaemia

Staphylococcus aureus is usually cultured when the septicaemia arises from central venous lines or wound infections. By contrast Gram-negative bacteraemia usually follows infection in the biliary or urinary tract. Septicaemia is one of the most common infections encountered following transplantation and is always potentially serious in view of the patient's immunosuppressed state. The risk is heightened if the organism is of an antibiotic resistant strain such as MRSA.

Urinary infections

These are common particularly during the first 3 months post-transplant, when an incidence of 50 per cent has been reported (Prát

et al. 1985), although the incidence later declines. Such infections are important as a common cause of bacteraemia and also because of the possibility of spread from the bladder, producing pyelonephritis in the allograft. The bacteriuria is usually asymptomatic. Transplant recipients who have a neurogenic bladder are particularly predisposed to bacteriuria, irrespective of whether they have a urinary diversion or their own bladders are being used. Other predisposing factors include the presence of a stent, instrumentation of the urinary tract, and urinary tract abnormalities such as obstructive uropathy, ureteric reflux, and infection in the native kidneys. Pretransplant removal of one or both native kidneys with or without ureterectomy is sometimes indicated in the presence of persistent kidney infection but is not often required.

Acute pyelonephritis in the allograft is relatively uncommon, with a reported incidence of around 2 per cent (Thomalla *et al.* 1988). Its presence is suggested by the occurrence of fever, graft tenderness, and bacteriuria, often with bacteraemia and deterioration in renal function. A search for a predisposing factor is important in view of the potential for progressive allograft dysfunction.

There are no clear guidelines for antibiotic administration in those patients whose urinary infection is usually or consistently asymptomatic. In these circumstances, it would seem reasonable to adopt a more active policy than in healthy individuals, in whom asymptomatic bacteriuria can often be ignored. Antibacterial therapy should be given for 5–7 days to patients with symptomatic or persistent asymptomatic bacteriuria if this occurs within the few months following the transplant. In the longer term, asymptomatic bacteriuria does not routinely require antibiotic therapy, particularly if there is no pyuria. Long-term antibacterial therapy is indicated for patients who have had more than one episode of acute pyelonephritis or those with frequent recurrence of bacteriuria following antibiotic therapy. With regard to the choice of drug for long-term therapy, nitrofurantoin or trimethoprim are worth considering as an option rather than a broad-spectrum antibiotic.

Central nervous system infections

Although an unusual site of infection, it is an important one to remember because of the high mortality—overall around 50 per cent—and the paucity of physical signs. In the immunosuppressed patient with an unexplained fever, one should consider a CT or magnetic resonance imaging (MRI) scan and lumbar puncture even in the absence of clear-cut clinical signs. A typical presentation may include some of the following: headaches, fever, confusion, impaired consciousness, focal signs, and seizures. Three main syndromes of CNS infection may be seen. Meningitis is usually due to conventional bacteria, Listeria, or Cryptococcus. Focal brain abscess may result from Aspergillus or Nocardia, and less frequently from Candida. Finally, encephalitis may occur with Aspergillus, Toxoplasma, or the herpes simplex or varicella viruses.

Gastrointestinal infection

Stomatitis is most often due to *Candida albicans* and is potentially serious as it may spread to the oesophagus. Candida infection presents with the typical creamy white patches on the mucosa and routine prophylaxis for the first few post-transplant weeks with amphotericin lozenges is worthwhile in view of the safety and simplicity of this precaution. If oesophageal or gastric candidiasis does develop, nystatin is usually curative but can be supplemented if necessary by fluconazole.

The transplant patient can develop a variety of enteric infections, of which one of the more common is that due to *Clostridium difficile*. This usually follows antibiotic therapy and presents with diarrhoea, sometimes accompanied by abdominal pain and tenderness. The diagnosis is made by finding the clostridial toxin in the faeces and a course of oral vancomycin and/or metronidazole will usually eradicate the infection. There is a tendency for this infection to occur in outbreaks and also to relapse in 15–50 per cent of patients.

Viral infections

Cytomegalovirus

Cytomegalovirus is the most important of the viruses which infect transplant recipients. Although there is doubt whether it exhibits true latency, it certainly can persist in the healthy carrier for many years without producing symptoms. In Western Europe and North America, around 30 per cent of young adults are seropositive with the figure increasing to 50–60 per cent beyond the age of 50 years. The virus is known to reside in a number of cell types, including the kidney, and it is through the donor kidney that most transplant recipients become infected.

CMV infection usually occurs during the second to fourth month after transplantation and may either be asymptomatic or cause illness of varying severity, with a 2 per cent overall mortality from disseminated disease. The main factor determining the occurrence of infection is the viral status of both the donor and recipient. Infection will occur in about 70–80 per cent of seronegative patients who receive a kidney from a positive donor, and symptomatic illness will develop in 90 per cent of those infected. If both donor and recipient are positive for the virus, the recipient will experience infection with approximately the same frequency. These are usually re-infections caused by the transmitted donor strain of virus. Virological studies show reactivation of latent infection in a much smaller number of these patients (Grundy *et al.* 1988). Reactivation will occur in around 20 per cent of seropositive patients who receive a seronegative kidney, and is almost always asymptomatic, while, of course, if both donor and recipient are negative for the virus the incidence of infection is negligible. Another factor influencing the incidence and severity of overt illness is the immunosuppressive therapy. The more powerful the immunosuppressive regimen being used, the more symptomatic infection will occur.

Clinical features and other sequelae

The most common features are fever with malaise, leucopenia, and elevated hepatic enzymes. Other less common manifestations include arthralgia and splenomegaly while in the more seriously ill patients, thrombocytopenia, pneumonitis, gastrointestinal bleeding, and encephalitis may occur. The pneumonitis is characterized by hypoxia and usually by bilateral infiltrates predominantly in the lower lobes; gastrointestinal bleeding can occasionally occur due to ulceration in the caecum or ascending colon.

There are three other proven or suspected effects of CMV infection. First, it further depresses the immune response, with a resultant predisposition to other opportunistic infections, especially that due to *P. carinii*. Second, it has been shown to increase the expression of HLA antigens and adhesion molecules on cell surfaces. While one would expect this to predispose to rejection, there is no clear evidence of an increased rejection rate. Third, a link has been described between CMV and a glomerulopathy (Richardson *et al.* 1981), but it is not certain whether this glomerulopathy is of importance clinically.

Diagnosis

Although serological tests such as detection of CMV-specific IgM are still in use, one can obtain earlier warning of infection by means of one of the tests which detect the CMV antigen. Qualitative PCR testing has been available for some time but the more recently introduced quantitative tests hold the promise of being more useful in making an early diagnosis. Other techniques for antigen detection include DNA hybrid capture and the pp65 antigen test. The ideal diagnostic outcome would be to detect prior to the onset of illness those at-risk patients who are going to become symptomatic. This would enable treatment to be given only to those patients rather than giving all at-risk patients prophylaxis for several months. However, it has not yet been demonstrated that the currently available techniques for antigen detection enable one to achieve this aim. In patients with suspected invasive CMV disease, a number of rapid diagnostic techniques are now available to detect virus in sputum or bronchial aspirate including the use of fluorescence and monoclonal antibodies.

Prophylaxis and treatment

A number of approaches to prophylaxis are possible. First, CMV-negative recipients could be given kidneys from CMV-negative donors. However, this is associated with major logistic problems and also it is not applicable to the problem of reinfection in CMV-positive recipients. Active immunization may prove useful in the future but an effective vaccine is not yet routinely available. High titre CMV immunoglobulin has been shown to reduce the rate of disease to 10 per cent when used in conjunction with oral acyclovir (Nicol *et al.* 1993) but it is cumbersome to use and expensive. At present, therefore, the most practical approach to prophylaxis is either oral acyclovir or gancyclovir. Valacyclovir, the prodrug, has superior bioavailability, and 2 g four times daily has been shown to be effective and has also been reported to halve the acute rejection rate (Lowance *et al.* 1999). However, this effect on acute rejection has yet to be confirmed by others. Gancyclovir has greater anti-CMV activity than acyclovir and its prodrug, which is now becoming available, may well turn out to be the prophylactic drug of choice. In the meantime, the choice lies between valacyclovir and oral gancyclovir. Although the latter has bioavailability of less than 10 per cent, it has been found to reduce the rate of CMV disease to less than 5 per cent (Smith *et al.* 2001). With regard to who should be given prophylactic antiviral drugs, an appropriate policy is that when the donor is CMV-positive, CMV-negative recipients together with those CMV-positive patients who are being heavily immunosuppressed should receive prophylaxis. An evidence based set of practice guidelines for CMV prophylaxis has been published fairly recently (Jassal *et al.* 1998).

The drug of choice for the treatment of established CMV disease is gancyclovir given intravenously for 6 weeks, and followed by oral therapy in view of a high relapse rate. In the uncommon event of gancyclovir resistance, foscarnet may be of value.

Herpes simplex

Reactivation of latent virus will result in ulcers or vesicles in 15–45 per cent of seropositive transplant recipients (Smith *et al.* 2001). Most cases are relatively mild with oral or anogenital lesions but occasionally serious systemic infection occurs for example encephalitis, hepatitis, or pneumonitis. Confirmation of the diagnosis can be obtained by examination of scrapings or fluid from the vesicles using PCR or fluorescence techniques. Acyclovir is usually effective and can be used topically for localized lesions, orally in the case of more widespread lesions or intravenously in the case of the more seriously ill patient or in the presence of systemic virus infection.

Varicella zoster

This viral infection is about 10 times more common in renal allograft recipients than in healthy individuals. While serious illness is unusual it tends to be slow to resolve and is often followed by postherpetic neuralgia. Treatment should be initiated promptly with either oral or intravenous acyclovir. Much more serious, though uncommon, is the occurrence of chickenpox in those who do not possess immunity to the virus. Ideally, testing for immunity to varicella zoster virus should be carried out prior to transplantation and immunization considered for susceptible patients (Cohen *et al.* 2001). Should a non-immune allograft recipient be exposed to chickenpox or zoster, prophylactic immunoglobulin should be given as soon as possible. Exposure to chickenpox can result in a disseminated infection whose features include a haemorrhagic rash, encephalitis, pneumonia, hepatic failure, and pancreatitis. Treatment consists of intravenous acyclovir and immunoglobulin, but despite this therapy the mortality is high. In a report which described four deaths in five patients, the importance of early acyclovir therapy at an adequate dose was stressed (Bradley *et al.* 1987).

Hepatitis

Hepatitis B

This virus usually exists in a carrier state in dialysis patients. Within Europe the carrier rate varies from negligible in some countries to more than 20 per cent in others. The most common sources of infection are blood and blood products and intravenous drug use, but the virus can also be transmitted by organ donation. Preventive measures should focus on screening of all blood and organ donors, segregation of hepatitis positive dialysis patients, and immunization of those at risk. In dialysis units where hepatitis B carriers are being treated, it is especially important that all patients and staff are offered immunization. However, seroconversion rates among dialysis patients are suboptimal, usually in the region of 65 per cent (Szmuness *et al.* 1981). Patient survival rates following transplantation are significantly worse in hepatitis B positive patients in comparison with those who are seronegative, for example Hiesse *et al.* (1992) reported a 10-year survival of 80 and 64 per cent in seronegative and seropositive patients, respectively. Also, seropositive transplant patients progress more often to chronic hepatitis than do those being treated by haemodialysis (Parfrey *et al.* 1985). Renal transplantation is not contraindicated in all hepatitis B positive patients but there is a good argument for liver biopsy in all potential recipients and certainly in all with abnormal hepatic enzymes. Transplantation should not be advised if there is more than mild histological abnormality.

Hepatitis C

In most countries the carrier rate of this virus is greater than that of hepatitis B. The EDTA registry has given a mean figure of 21 per cent for all centre haemodialysis patients but with a range from a few per cent in some countries to more than 60 per cent in others (Geerlings *et al.* 1994). More recent figures are not available but it is likely that the prevalence is declining with more effective preventive measures such as screening of donated blood. Hepatitis C differs in a number of respects from hepatitis B. It is less readily transmitted, but nonetheless, more than 90 per cent of patients receiving an organ from a hepatitis C positive donor will subsequently test positive for hepatitis C RNA (Pereira *et al.* 1995). In view of the organ shortage it has been suggested that hepatitis C positive recipients could receive kidneys from serologically positive donors. In the short term, this has not increased morbidity (Morales *et al.* 1995), but the long-term effects are still unknown. A second point of difference between the B and C viruses is that the liver disease of the latter appears to pursue a more indolent course. However, the long-term outcome remains uncertain and in the study of Chan *et al.* (1994), potentially life-threatening liver disease developed in half of hepatitis C positive transplant recipients. The same recipient selection policy should probably apply as for hepatitis B. Finally, although interferon-α has a therapeutic role in hepatitis C affecting non-transplant patients, it is not at present advised in transplant recipients in view of its side-effects, in particular that of renal dysfunction (Thervet *et al.* 1994).

Human immunodeficiency virus

Transmission of this virus by organ allografts is well documented but can be avoided by testing of potential donors and avoidance of the use of organs from high-risk groups such as intravenous drug users. With regard to transplantation in asymptomatic HIV carriers, the experience prior to the introduction of antiviral therapy was of a high mortality and accelerated course to acquired immunodeficiency syndrome (AIDS) (Rubin *et al.* 1987). While the prognosis will improve as antiviral therapy becomes increasingly effective, the consensus view at present is that HIV-positive patients are better managed by dialysis than by transplantation (Rubin *et al.* 1987).

Epstein–Barr virus

Primary infection is uncommon in transplant recipients as most patients have been infected previously, but as a consequence when it does occur it is more often in children than adults. The allograft is the usual although not invariable source of the virus. The infection may be asymptomatic, run a typical glandular fever course, or rarely pursue a fulminant course. The main risk of infection is PTLD and this is three to four times more common with primary than secondary infection. Overall PTLD occurs in around 1 per cent of renal transplant recipients but the amount of immunosuppression used is crucial in determining the risk. PTLD is discussed in more detail in the section on 'Neoplasia'.

Other viral infections

Influenza and parainfluenza may affect transplant recipients and while there are few reported studies, serious sequelae would appear to be rare. Nonetheless, transplant patients should be immunized annually.

There is increasing documentation of adenovirus infection in allograft recipients. Serious infection may occur, usually involving the respiratory or urinary tract and sometimes the transplanted kidney and the reported mortality is as high as 17 per cent (Hierholzer 1992).

Polyomavirus infection in transplant recipients mainly involves the BK subtype which is trophic for the urinary tract and can cause haemorrhagic cystitis, ureteric stricture, and interstitial nephritis (Smith *et al.* 2001).

The main relevance of papilloma virus is its aetiological role in squamous cell skin cancer and cervical cancer and these conditions are discussed in the section on cancer. Finally HHV-8 is of importance mainly because of its link with KS and again this is discussed under the heading of cancer.

Tuberculosis

This infection will occur in a few per cent of transplant recipients. In most patients the infection is pulmonary, presenting with a cough and fever, but a review of the literature showed disseminated infection to occur in just under 40 per cent (Quinibi *et al.* 1990). The diagnosis can usually be confirmed by culture of sputum or bronchoalveolar aspirate; however, chemotherapy should be given in the setting of a suggestive clinical presentation but negative cultures. A high frequency of atypical mycobacteria has been a common finding. A good response to antituberculous therapy can be expected in most patients, and the main hazard found in one study was allograft rejection due to a reduction in immunosuppressive therapy (Higgins *et al.* 1991). Reducing the dose of the immunosuppressive drugs is probably only necessary in the setting of disseminated infection. The drugs commonly used for initial treatment are isoniazid 300 mg daily, rifampicin 600 mg daily and pyrazinamide 2 g daily with or without ethambutol, 15 mg/kg daily. Initial treatment should be continued for 2 months and followed by isoniazid and rifampicin on their own for a further 4 months. It is common practice in renal transplant recipients to continue with these two drugs for a full year because of their immunosuppressed status but there is no evidence that treatment beyond 6 months is necessary. The dose of ethambutol should be reduced if renal function is impaired and one should remember that the blood levels of the calcineurin inhibitors will fall in the presence of rifampicin therapy. Prophylactic antituberculous therapy in the post-transplant period is indicated for those at risk and the most commonly used regimen is isoniazid, 300 mg/day for 6 months. The main risk groups are those with a history of tuberculosis, even if treated and those from communities with a high incidence. Mantoux testing is not of diagnostic value as the immunosuppressive therapy may lead to false-negative results.

Liver disease

The reported incidence of liver disease in renal allograft recipients has varied widely. A representative figure from the early 1990s is that of Rao and Anderson (1992). Among 785 patients, they found acute liver disease in 23 per cent and chronic disease in 14 per cent. However, the incidence is falling and the current figures will be less.

Acute liver disease

Acute liver dysfunction is usually seen in the early post-transplant period and is most often due to viral infection or drug toxicity. CMV is the most common viral cause with EBV or one of the herpes viruses being the cause less often.

A wide range of drugs can be hepatotoxic and one has to be aware of the higher risk drugs in the renal transplant recipient as in any other patient. The group of drugs to specifically mention are the immunosuppressive agents. Hepatotoxicity used to be highlighted as one of the important side-effects of cyclosporin but with the currently used dosages it is uncommon. Hepatotoxicity is even less common with tacrolimus and is rare with mycophenolate mofetil and rapamycin.

Acute hepatotoxicity is not a problem with azathioprine and chronic azathioprine hepatotoxicity will be discussed in the next section.

Chronic liver disease

By far the most widely documented cause of chronic liver disease is viral hepatitis, mainly B and C. With the introduction of hepatitis B immunization, screening of blood and organ donors, careful selection of recipients, and other preventative measures, there has been a sharp decline in the frequency of viral hepatitis and thus of the consequent chronic hepatic damage. Much of the data in the literature is, therefore, only of historical interest.

There are two important general points about chronic liver disease. First, as effective therapy in established disease is very limited in its efficacy, it is important to carefully assess patients before transplantation and counsel those whose liver disease is thought likely to considerably worsen as the result of a transplant to remain on dialysis. The second point which is related is that liver histology is much more useful prognostically than clinical or biochemical assessment.

Among renal failure patients who acquire the hepatitis B virus, 80 per cent will remain chronically infected (Fornairon *et al.* 1996). Overall such patients have a 30-fold increased risk of developing chronic hepatitis post-transplant when compared with hepatitis B-negative patients. However, in those with normal liver histology or minimal abnormality the risk of progression is low and transplantation is justified. In contrast, patients with histological hepatitis or cirrhosis should be advised against transplantation. Even where pretransplant liver biopsy shows a less aggressive type of hepatitis such as the chronic persistent type, the 5 year mortality from liver failure alone is 26 per cent (Rao and Anderson 1992). There is less long-term information available regarding hepatitis C. The chronic liver disease resulting from this virus pursues a less aggressive course than that following hepatitis B infection in the short-term with a four-fold increase in liver disease over the first 4 years when compared with hepatitis C-negative patients (Pereira *et al.* 1995). Thus, one can recommend transplantation to hepatitis C-positive patients with histologically mild liver disease but not to those with advanced disease. With regard to therapy, interferon-α has some activity against hepatitis C but may precipitate graft rejection and is, therefore, not recommended in transplanted patients.

In the setting of progressive liver dysfunction of viral origin, immunosuppression should be reduced with the aim of diminishing virus replication. This can often be accomplished without graft rejection as the immune response of these patients is lowered. Apart from the above specific recommendations, the treatment of chronic hepatic dysfunction is along standard lines.

Other than viral infections, there are no other common causes of chronic liver disease in transplant recipients. Occasionally azathioprine can be hepatotoxic with a variety of histological appearances including veno-occlusive disease and nodular regenerative hyperplasia. Finally, haemosiderosis is being seen much less frequently now that erythropoietin has been in routine use for a number of years.

Gastrointestinal complications

Stomach and duodenum

Troublesome dyspepsia has declined in frequency in renal transplant patients with the lowering of steroid doses and the widespread use of proton pump inhibitors and H_2-receptor antagonists. In 1993, Teenan *et al.* found that 61 per cent of an unselected group of transplant patients had dyspeptic symptoms and that 65 per cent of these symptomatic patients had gastric colonization with *Helicobacter pylori*, compared to 23 per cent of an asymptomatic group (Teenan *et al.* 1993). In conclusion, although post-transplant dyspepsia has declined considerably as a problem, it still exists and should be managed by endoscopy, a search for *H. pylori*, and thereafter the appropriate therapy. Management should include consideration as to whether steroids could be withdrawn or reduced to as low a dose as possible.

Pancreatitis

Acute pancreatitis is an uncommon but serious complication. Chapman *et al.* (1991) reported an incidence of 1.4 per cent with the complication of pseudocyst in 10 of 16 patients and a 50 per cent mortality among the patients with pseudocysts. Badalamenti *et al.* (1994) noted a high prevalence of silent gallstone disease in a group of dialysis patients and cholelithiasis and/or steroid therapy are probably both causative factors for post-transplant pancreatitis.

Colonic complications

Antibiotic related (or pseudomembranous) colitis should be considered in the patient with profuse diarrhoea, particularly in the setting of recent antibiotic therapy. Diagnosis and therapy follow the usual lines, namely a search for *C. difficile* toxin in the faeces and the use of oral vancomycin or metronidazole.

Bowel haemorrhage, usually from the caecum or ascending colon, may complicate severe CMV infection.

Finally, diverticulitis may occur particularly in the older patient and be complicated by colonic perforation and faecal peritonitis.

The danger of acute abdominal complications is increased by the masking of physical signs resulting from immunosuppressive therapy and, in particular, steroids. Thus, a high index of suspicion should exist when assessing abdominal symptoms in the renal allograft recipient.

Post-transplant diabetes mellitus

In addition to a genetic predisposition and an excessive calorie intake another important factor which may give rise to post-transplant diabetes mellitus (PTDM) is the immunosuppressive regimen. The three relevant drugs are steroids, cyclosporin, and tacrolimus. The effect of all three is dose dependent and this applies especially to steroids. This adverse effect of steroids provides another argument in favour of steroid avoidance or withdrawal if possible, but failing this, the use of a low maintenance dose. Most studies suggest that the frequency of PTDM is greater with tacrolimus than with cyclosporin, typical figures being an occurrence of 20 and 4 per cent respectively (Pirsch *et al.* 1997). In the long-term patient with a reduction in drug dosage, the prevalence of PTDM will also fall. However, if PTDM persists, consideration should be given to withdrawal of the calcineurin inhibitor. With the availability of rapamycin and mycophenolate mofetil, such withdrawal may well be possible without jeopardizing the graft. If the patient is obese, a low calorie diet and exercise are also worthwhile.

There tends to be a latent interval from the time of onset of diabetes mellitus before the majority of its complications become manifest and this also applies to PTDM. As a consequence, morbidity and mortality may be no higher in the first few post-transplant years in these patients than in non-diabetics. An analysis in Glasgow has, however,

shown poorer patient survival in the longer term with a figure of 49 per cent at 10 years in a group of 48 PTDM patients compared with 75 per cent in the non-diabetic group (Revanur *et al.* 2001).

Bone disease

Three important types of bone disease can become apparent after renal transplantation, these being osteopenia, tertiary hyperparathyroidism, and bone necrosis.

Osteopenia

Bone mineral density tends to be low at the time of transplantation as a consequence of uraemia. It will usually fall further over the subsequent 2 years then remain fairly stable thereafter. Little difference has been found between men and women and no major influence of parathormone levels but the loss of bone mineral density occurs at a faster rate in the early post-transplant period when steroid doses are at their highest than in subsequent months (Grotz *et al.* 1995). The main adverse effect of osteopenia is bone fractures and they have been recorded in 17 per cent of transplant patients overall with a higher frequency in women (23 per cent) than in men (12 per cent) and in patients with diabetes mellitus (40 per cent) compared with non-diabetics (11 per cent) (Nisbeth *et al.* 1999). There are a number of possible approaches to the prevention of progressive osteopenia. First, the steroid dose can be kept low. Second, biphosphonates are of value—for example, pamidronate given intravenously at the time of transplantation and again 1 month later has been shown to prevent early bone loss in men (Fan *et al.* 2000). Other biphosphonates include etidronate and alendronate, the latter having the advantages of greater potency and the ease of daily oral administration. Next, hormone replacement therapy will almost certainly limit bone loss in postmenopausal women although there have been few reports of studies in transplant patients. This approach has the additional potential benefit of reducing cardiovascular morbidity. Finally, calcitonin by subcutaneous injection or nasal spray may prove useful but has not yet undergone detailed evaluation. Moe (1997) has reviewed the treatment of post-transplant osteopenia.

Tertiary hyperparathyroidism

Following renal transplantation, the secondary hyperparathyroidism associated with renal failure often, but not always, lessens or fully resolves. Should hypercalcaemia develop, even if the serum parathormone level is not markedly elevated, tertiary hyperparathyroidism has to be considered. If the hypercalcaemia persists or progressively worsens, parathyroidectomy may be required. It is unwise to allow hypercalcaemia to persist too long in view of the potential for vascular calcification or nephrotoxicity.

Bone necrosis

This complication is almost always due to steroid therapy and it has, therefore, become much less common since low-dose steroid regimens were adopted. It affects mainly the weight-bearing joints and presents with joint pain. The initial radiological feature is structural failure of the articular surface. When there is persistent troublesome pain and/or extensive joint damage, the insertion of a prosthetic joint has to be considered.

2116 13 THE TRANSPLANT PATIENT

Haematological complications

Bone marrow depression

In transplant recipients this is usually manifested by neutropenia only but less often there is also thrombocytopenia and/or anaemia. Both azathioprine and mycophenolate mofetil may depress the bone marrow. With an azathioprine dose of around 1 mg/kg body weight, fewer than 5 per cent of patients become leucopenic and with higher doses the figure may rise to just over 10 per cent (Bergan et al. 1998). The combination of allopurinol and azathioprine will often result in profound leucopenia and if allopurinol is prescribed, azathioprine should be discontinued and another immunosuppressive drug substituted if required. A typical frequency of leucopenia with mycophenolate mofetil is 14 per cent at a dose of 2 g/day with anaemia in 7 per cent and thrombocytopenia in 6 per cent (European Mycophenolate Mofetil Cooperative Study Group 1999). A number of viral infections, especially CMV, may cause neutropenia with or without thrombocytopenia and the effects of the infection and the immunosuppressive drugs may be additive. Rarely, a thrombotic microangiopathy may complicate an unresponsive acute rejection episode and sometimes in such circumstances immediate transplant nephrectomy is indicated following which the low white blood and platelet counts will usually rapidly return to normal.

Erythrocytosis

This phenomenon has been reported to occur following transplantation in 10–15 per cent of patients according to the review by Gaston et al. (1994) although in one subsequent report the incidence was as high as 22 per cent (Kessler et al. 1996). It usually presents during the first year, is commoner in men than women and tends to occur predominantly in patients with good renal function. It has also been reported to be commoner in patients not treated with erythropoietin while on dialysis (Kessler et al. 1996). The type of immunosuppression used would not seem to be an aetiological factor. The mechanism of the erythrocytosis is thought to be inappropriately high erythropoietin production possibly, but not certainly, by the native kidneys (Gaston et al. 1994). Assessment of the risk of thromboembolic events varies but the majority view is that the risk is small. Nonetheless, it is wise to lower the haematocrit, particularly as treatment is simple and effective. ACE inhibitors and angiotensin-II receptor antagonists are equally effective and are usually required on a long-term basis. Their mechanism of action is not yet fully understood.

Dermatological complications

A wide variety of conditions affecting the skin occur in transplant recipients, and the main ones can be grouped under the headings of immunosuppressive drug side-effects, infections including viral, bacterial, and fungal, and skin cancer. The last of these has already been discussed in the section 'Neoplasia'.

Immunosuppressive drug side-effects

Steroids may have considerable adverse effects on the skin including striae, purpura, telangiectasia, atrophic changes, impaired wound healing, acne, and sometimes more deep-seated infections. A reduction in steroid dose and treatment of infection are the main aspects of management. Cyclosporin has two main mucocutaneous side-effects, gum hypertrophy and hypertrichosis. A typical figure for the frequency of each of these is 9 per cent (Pirsch et al. 1997). Calcium-channel blocking antihypertensives may aggravate the gum hypertrophy. In view of the range of immunosuppressive drugs now available, the development of gum hypertrophy or severe hypertrichosis should often be an indication to change to another drug such as tacrolimus, which is free of these two side-effects. The two main effects of tacrolimus on the skin are pruritus and alopecia. They have been recorded in 15 and 11 per cent of patients, respectively (Pirsch et al. 1997).

Infections

A wide range of bacterial infections may be encountered ranging from acne to folliculitis, abscesses, cellulitis, and erysipelas. The most common organisms are *S. aureus* and group A streptococci. There is also a wide range of viral infections which may involve the skin and the more important of these have been discussed in the section 'Infection'.

Obesity

Although obesity is not usually classified as a pathological entity, it can have such an adverse influence on morbidity and patient survival that it justifies separate comment. Studies which have examined the relationship between body mass index (BMI) at the time of transplantation and outcome have usually found an adverse effect of obesity. One such recent study has used the USRDS database (Meier-Kriesche et al. 2002). This study showed an adverse effect of obesity on death with a functioning graft, on cardiovascular and infectious death, and on graft loss. Incidentally, a BMI less than the ideal range was also associated in this study with these same adverse outcomes although the association with graft loss was weaker. The BMI with lowest risk was in the range 22–32 kg/m^2. Another analysis has looked at nine published studies in which obesity has been related to transplant outcome. Here again, obesity was associated with poorer patient and graft survival but not with immunological graft loss (Pischon and Sharma 2001). Thus, there is a strong body of evidence indicating an adverse effect of obesity on both patient and graft survival. The implications of these studies are, first that patients who are considerably obese, that is, with a BMI of more than 35 kg/m^2 should be advised to lose weight before acceptance on to the transplant waiting list. Those with lesser degrees of obesity (i.e. BMI of 30–35 kg/m^2) can usually be advised to have their names placed on the waiting list but they should also be advised to lose weight while awaiting their transplant. Following transplantation, all patients should be counselled regarding diet and regular exercise in an effort to avoid excessive weight gain.

References

Badalamenti, S. *et al.* (1994). High prevalence of silent gallstone disease in dialysis patients. *Nephron* **66**, 225–227.

Bergan, S. *et al.* (1998). Monitored high-dose azathioprine treatment reduces acute rejection episodes after renal transplantation. *Transplantation* **66**, 334–339.

Boaz, M. *et al.* (2000). Secondary prevention with antioxidants of cardiovascular disease in endstage renal disease (SPACE): randomised placebo-controlled trial. *Lancet* **356**, 1213–1218.

Bradley, J. R., Wreghitt, T. G., and Evans, D. B. (1987). Chickenpox in adult renal transplant recipients. *Clinical Transplantation* **1**, 242–245.

Brown, J. H. *et al.* (1994). Comparative mortality from cardiovascular disease in patients with chronic renal failure. *Nephrology, Dialysis, Transplantation* **9**, 1136–1142.

Chan, T.-M. *et al.* (1994). Clinicopathological features of hepatitis C virus infection in renal allograft recipients. *Transplantation* **58**, 996–1000.

Chapman, W. C. *et al.* (1991). Pancreatic pseudocyst formation following renal transplantation: a lethal development. *Clinical Transplantation* **5**, 86–89.

Cohen, J., Hopkin, J., and Kurtz, J. Infectious complications after renal transplantation. In *Kidney Transplantation: Principles and Practice* 5th edn. (ed. P. J. Morris), pp. 468–494. Philadelphia, PA: W.B. Saunders, 2001.

Cosio, F. G. *et al.* (1999). Patient survival after renal transplantation: II. The impact of smoking. *Clinical Transplantation* **13**, 336–341.

Ducloux, D. *et al.* (2000). Serum total homocysteine and cardiovascular disease occurrence in chronic, stable renal transplant recipients: a prospective study. *Journal of the American Society of Nephrology* **11**, 134–137.

European Mycophenolate Mofetil Cooperative Study Group (1999). Mycophenolate mofetil in renal transplantation: 3-year results from the placebo-controlled trial. *Transplantation* **68**, 391–396.

Fan, S. L.-S. *et al.* (2000). Pamidronate therapy as prevention of bone loss following renal transplantation. *Kidney International* **57**, 684–690.

Farge, D. *et al.* (1999). Human herpes virus-8 and other risk factors for Kaposi's sarcoma in kidney transplant recipients. *Transplantation* **67**, 1236–1242.

Fishman, J. A. and Rubin, R. H. (1998). Infection in organ-transplant recipients. *New England Journal of Medicine* **338**, 1741–1751.

Fornairon, S. *et al.* (1996). The long-term virologic and pathologic impact of renal transplantation on chronic hepatitis B virus infection. *Transplantation* **62**, 297–299.

Frei, U. *et al.* (1995). Pre-transplant hypertension: a major risk factor for chronic progressive renal allograft dysfunction? *Nephrology, Dialysis, Transplantation* **10**, 1206–1211.

Furberg, C. D., Psaty, B. M., and Meyer, J. V. (1995). Nifedipine: dose related increase in mortality in patients with coronary heart disease. *Circulation* **92**, 1326–1331.

Gaston, R. S., Julian, B. A., and Curtis, J. J. (1994). Posttransplant erythrocytosis: an enigma revisited. *American Journal of Kidney Diseases* **24**, 1–11.

Geerlings, W. *et al.* (1994). Report on management of renal failure in Europe, XXIII. *Nephrology, Dialysis, Transplantation* **9** (Suppl. 1), 6–25.

Goodman, W. G. *et al.* (2000). Coronary-artery calcification in young adults with end-stage renal disease who are undergoing dialysis. *New England Journal of Medicine* **342**, 1478–1483.

Grotz, W. H. *et al.* (1995). Bone mineral density after kidney transplantation. *Transplantation* **59**, 982–986.

Grundy, J. E. *et al.* (1988). Symptomatic cytomegalovirus infection in seropositive kidney recipients: reinfection with donor virus rather than reactivation of recipient virus. *Lancet* **ii**, 132–135.

Guidi, E. (1996). Hypertension may be transplanted with the kidney in humans: a long-term historical prospective follow-up of recipients grafted with kidneys coming from donors with or without hypertension in their families. *Journal of the American Society of Nephrology* **7**, 1131–1138.

Gulanikar, A. C. *et al.* (1998). Prospective pretransplant ultrasound screening in 206 patients for acquired renal cysts and renal cell carcinoma. *Transplantation* **66**, 1669–1672.

Hierholzer, J. C. (1992). Adenoviruses in the immunocompromised host. *Clinical Microbiology Reviews* **5**, 262–274.

Hiesse, C. *et al.* (1992). Impact of HB$_s$ antigenemia on long-term patient survival and causes of death after renal transplantation. *Clinical Transplantation* **6**, 461–467.

Higgins, R. M. *et al.* (1991). Mycobacterial infections after renal transplantation. *Quarterly Journal of Medicine* **78**, 145–153.

Jassal, S. V. *et al.* (1998). Clinical practice guidelines: prevention of cytomegalovirus disease after renal transplantation. *Journal of the American Society of Nephrology* **9**, 1697–1708.

Kessler, M. *et al.* (1996). Factors predisposing to post-renal transplant erythrocytosis. A prospective matched-pair control study. *Clinical Nephrology* **45**, 83–89.

Lazarus, J. M. *et al.* (1997). Achievement and safety of a low blood pressure goal in chronic renal disease. The modification of diet in renal disease study group. *Hypertension* **29**, 641–650.

Lepre, F. *et al.* (1999). A double-blind placebo controlled trial of simvastatin for the treatment of dyslipidaemia in renal allograft recipients. *Clinical Transplantation* **13**, 520–525.

Levey, A. S. *et al.* (1998). Controlling the epidemic of cardiovascular disease in chronic renal disease: what do we know? What do we need to learn? Where do we go from here? National Kidney Foundation Task Force on Cardiovascular Disease. *American Journal of Kidney Diseases* **32**, 853–906.

London, G. M. *et al.* (1996). Cardiac and arterial interactions in end-stage renal disease. *Kidney International* **50**, 600–608.

Lowance, D. *et al.* (1999). Valacyclovir for the prevention of cytomegalovirus disease after renal transplantation. *New England Journal of Medicine* **340**, 1462–1470.

MacPhee, I. A. M. *et al.* (1998). Long-term outcome of a prospective randomized trial of conversion from cyclosporine to azathioprine treatment one year after renal transplantation. *Transplantation* **66**, 186–192.

Mahoney, J. F. *et al.* (1982). Delayed complications of renal transplantation and their prevention. *Medical Journal of Australia* **2**, 426–429.

Manske, C. L. *et al.* (1992). Coronary revascularisation in insulin-dependent diabetic patients with chronic renal failure. *Lancet* **340**, 998–1002.

Margreiter, R. (2002). Efficacy and safety of tacrolimus compared with cyclosporin microemulsion in renal transplantation: a randomised multicentre study. *Lancet* **359**, 741–746.

Massy, Z. A. and Guijarro, C. (2001). Statins: effects beyond cholesterol lowering. *Nephrology, Dialysis, Transplantation* **16**, 1738–1741.

McGregor, E. *et al.* (1998). Pre-operative echocardiographic abnormalities and adverse outcome following renal transplantation. *Nephrology, Dialysis, Transplantation* **13**, 1499–1505.

Meier-Kriesche, H.-U., Arndorfer, J. A., and Kaplan, B. (2002). The impact of body mass index on renal transplant outcomes: a significant independent risk factor for graft failure and patient death. *Transplantation* **73**, 70–74.

Meyer, A. D. *et al.* (1997). Multicenter randomized trial comparing tacrolimus (FK506) and cyclosporine in the prevention of renal allograft rejection. *Transplantation* **64**, 436–443.

Midtvedt, K. *et al.* (1996). Bilateral nephrectomy simultaneously with renal allografting does not alleviate hypertension 3 months following living-donor transplantation. *Nephrology, Dialysis, Transplantation* **11**, 2045–2049.

Moe, S. M. (1997). The treatment of steroid-induced bone loss in transplantation. *Current Opinions in Nephrology and Hypertension* **6**, 544–549.

Morales, J. M. *et al.* (1995). Transplantation of kidneys from donors with hepatitis C antibody into recipients with pre-transplantation anti-HCV. *Kidney International* **47**, 236–240.

Nicol, D. L. *et al.* (1993). Reduction by combination prophylactic therapy with CMV hyperimmune globulin and acyclovir of the risk of primary CMV disease in renal transplant recipients. *Transplantation* **55**, 841–846.

Nisbeth, U. *et al.* (1999). Increased fracture rate in diabetes mellitus and females after renal transplantation. *Transplantation* **67**, 1218–1222.

Olmer, M. *et al.* (1988). Hypertension in renal transplantation. *Kidney International* **34** (Suppl. 25), S129–S132.

Parfrey, P. S. *et al.* (1985). Chronic hepatitis in end-stage renal disease: comparison of HB$_s$Ag-negative and HB$_s$Ag-positive patients. *Kidney International* **28**, 959–967.

Penn, I. (1993). The effect of immunosuppression on pre-existing cancers. *Transplantation* **55**, 742–747.

Penn, I. (1995). Primary kidney tumours before and after renal transplantation. *Transplantation* **59**, 480–485.

Penn, I. (1997). Kaposi's sarcoma in transplant recipients. *Transplantation* **64**, 669–673.

Penn, I. (1998). *De novo* cancers in organ allograft recipients. *Current Opinion in Organ Transplantation* 3, 188–196.

Pereira, B. J. G. *et al.* (1995). A controlled study of hepatitis C transmission by organ transplantation. *Lancet* 345, 484–487.

Pirsch, J. D. *et al.* (1997). A comparison of tacrolimus (FK506) and cyclosporine for immunosuppression after cadaveric renal transplantation. *Transplantation* 63, 977–983.

Pischon, T. and Sharma, A. M. (2001). Obesity as a risk factor in renal transplant patients. *Nephrology, Dialysis, Transplantation* 16, 14–17.

Prát, V. *et al.* (1985). Urinary tract infection in renal transplant patients. *Infection* 13, 207–210.

Quinibi, W. Y. *et al.* (1990). Mycobacterial infection after renal transplantation—report of 14 cases and review of the literature. *Quarterly Journal of Medicine* 77, 1039–1060.

Ramsey, H. M. *et al.* (2000). Clinical risk factors associated with nonmelanoma skin cancer in renal transplant recipients. *American Journal of Kidney Diseases* 36, 167–176.

Rao, K. V. and Anderson, W. R. (1992). Liver disease after renal transplantation. *American Journal of Kidney Diseases* 19, 496–501.

Revanur, V. K. *et al.* (2001). Influence of diabetes mellitus on patient and graft survival in recipients of kidney transplantation. *Clinical Transplantation* 15, 89–94.

Richardson, W. P. *et al.* (1981). Glomerulopathy associated with cytomegalovirus viraemia in renal allografts. *New England Journal of Medicine* 305, 57–63.

Rigatto, C. *et al.* (2000). Long-term changes in left ventricular hypertrophy after renal transplantation. *Transplantation* 70, 570–575.

Rubin, R. H. *et al.* (1981). Infection in the renal transplant recipient. *American Journal of Medicine* 70, 405–411.

Rubin, R. H. *et al.* (1987). The acquired immunodeficiency syndrome and transplantation. *Transplantation* 44, 1–4.

Schaar, C. G. *et al.* (2001). Successful outcome with a 'quintuple approach' of posttransplant lymphoproliferative disorder. *Transplantation* 71, 47–52.

Schindler, R., Tanriver, Y., and Frei, U. (2000). Hypertension and allograft nephropathy—cause, consequence, or both? *Nephrology, Dialysis, Transplantation* 15, 8–10.

Schwartz, R. S. and Beldotti, L. (1965). Malignant lymphomas following allogenic disease: transition from an immunological to a neoplastic disorder. *Science* 149, 1511–1514.

Sheil, A. G. R. Cancer in dialysis and transplant patients. In *Kidney Transplantation: Principles and Practice* 5th edn. (ed. P. J. Morris), pp. 558–570. Philadelphia, PA: W.B. Saunders, 2001.

Smith, S. R., Butterly, D. W., Alexander, B. D., and Greenberg, A. (2001). Viral infections after renal transplantation. *American Journal of Kidney Diseases* 37, 659–676.

Stenvinkel, P. *et al.* (1999). Strong association between malnutrition, inflammation and atherosclerosis in chronic renal failure. *Kidney International* 55, 1899–1911.

Stewart, G. A. *et al.* Graft and patient survival following renal transplantation: new targets for blood pressure control. In *Cardionephrology* Vol. 5 (ed. M. Timio, V. Wizeman, and S. Venanzi), pp. 357–361. Cosenza: Editoriale Bios, 1999.

Sunder-Plassmann, G. *et al.* (2000). Effects of high dose folic acid therapy on hyperhomocysteinaemia in haemodialysis patients: results of the Vienna multicenter study. *Journal of the American Society of Nephrology* 11, 1106–1116.

Szmuness, W. *et al.* (1981). The immune response of healthy adults to a reduced dose of hepatitis B vaccine. *Journal of Medical Virology* 8, 123–129.

Teenan, R. P. *et al.* (1993). *Helicobacter pylori* in renal transplant recipients. *Transplantation* 56, 100–102.

Thervet, E. *et al.* (1994). Low-dose recombinant leucocyte interferon α treatment of hepatitis C viral infection in renal transplant recipients. *Transplantation* 58, 625–628.

Thomalla, J. V. *et al.* (1988). Renal transplant pyelonephritis. *Clinical Transplantation* 2, 299–302.

13.3.4 Recurrent disease and *de novo* disease

Chas G. Newstead

Introduction

The disease that causes the failure of a patient's native kidneys may result in failure of a subsequent transplant. Establishing the true frequency of recurrent disease and its impact on outcome is difficult for a number of reasons. The aetiology of endstage renal failure is often not established. The renal transplant biopsy specimen may not undergo full immunofluorescence and electron microscopic examination. The possibility of *de novo* glomerulonephritis as well as the inevitability that some donors may have suffered from undiagnosed glomerulonephritis or other renal parenchymal disease makes precise estimation of the risk of recurrent disease impossible. For these reasons, data on the incidence of recurrent disease in transplant recipients must be an underestimate.

If recurrent disease can be reliably identified there often remains doubt about the contribution it makes to progressive transplant dysfunction. The relative contribution of recurrent disease, drug nephrotoxicity, hypertension, and rejection to allograft failure is often impossible to accurately apportion. Recurrent disease of all types, including diabetes mellitus, metabolic disorders, and glomerulonephritis, was established in only 6.3 per cent of a large single centre report of 1557 renal transplants performed between 1984 and 1999. This emphasizes that recurrent disease in a single centre will be a rare diagnosis (Hariharan *et al.* 1998).

At present, recurrent glomerulonephritis is thought to be a minor contributor to graft failure, being responsible for only 3 per cent of all grafts lost in Australia and New Zealand between 1979 and 1998 (unpublished, quoted in Chadban 2001), similar to reports from the United Kingdom (Kotanko *et al.* 1997) and United States (Hariharan *et al.* 1999). Recurrent disease usually develops after a period of years and, as graft survival has improved over the past two decades, the proportion of patients experiencing graft loss due to recurrent disease has increased, as is illustrated by data derived from the Australia and New Zealand registry (Fig. 1) (Chadban 2001).

There are certain subgroups for whom recurrent disease may be a particularly important problem. Paediatric registries report high rates of graft loss due to recurrent disease at 6 per cent in first and 12 per cent of subsequent graft losses (Baqi and Tejani 1997). Patients who have graft failure due to recurrent glomerulonephritis in a first graft have a risk of recurrent disease in a subsequent graft of the order of 48 per cent (Briggs and Jones 1999a).

Clinical features of recurrent disease

In general, recurrence of disease affecting the renal transplant mimics the features of the original disease. The possibility of *de novo* glomerulonephritis or recurrent systemic disease will require careful characterization of the native renal disorder. Extrarenal features such as cutaneous vasculitis or haemolysis and thrombocytopenia in haemolytic–uraemic syndrome (HUS) may be diagnostic. Similarly serological examination for antibodies, hepatitis viruses, and complement may be necessary. The

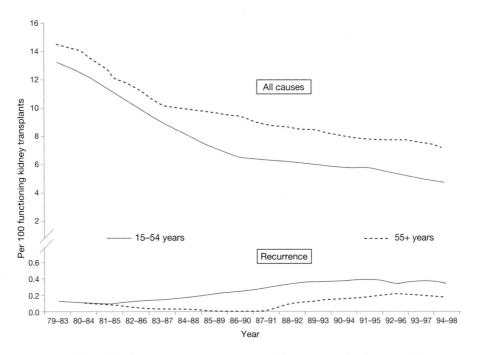

Fig. 1 Incidence of graft loss: Australia 1979–1998, all causes versus recurrent disease. The incidence of graft loss has fallen progressively over the past 20 years, largely as a result of reductions in loss from acute and chronic rejection. In contrast, graft loss caused by recurrent disease has increased over the same period ($P < 0.05$), particularly in the 14–55-year recipient age group (Briganti and Chadban, unpublished data presented in Chadban 2001).

discrimination of allograft dysfunction due to recurrent disease from that due to acute or chronic rejection, drug nephrotoxicity or pyelonephritis usually involves standard investigations such as urine culture, urine protein estimation, measurement of drug concentrations and ultrasound examination. A renal transplant biopsy is required to most accurately define the problem. If recurrent renal disease is a likely diagnosis, then full electron microscopy and immunohistological processing will be necessary to reach a diagnosis.

Minimal-change glomerulonephritis (see also Chapter 3.5)

A small number of cases of renal transplant recipients developing nephrotic syndrome with minimal glomerular abnormalities have been reported, but not all include venography or other imaging to exclude renal vein thrombosis and drug associated effects are impossible to exclude. The detail of the histological diagnosis has not always been reported. The prognosis is variable and often follow-up in published cases is very short, but in some reports there is progression to renal failure which is, of course, unlike the syndrome of minimal-change disease in the native kidney (Hoyer *et al.* 1972; Gephardt *et al.* 1988).

It is notable that rebiopsy in two patients showed focal–segmental glomerulosclerosis (FSGS) (Hoyer *et al.* 1972). This diagnosis as well as transplant glomerulopathy could easily be confused with minimal-change disease unless an adequate number of glomeruli were available and comprehensive histological examination performed. This means that it is very difficult to be confident that this syndrome has truly been identified in renal transplant recipients.

Focal–segmental glomerulosclerosis (see also Chapter 3.5)

Focal–segmental glomerulosclerosis is an especially important problem in paediatric practice. The prognosis is poor with about one-third of patients progressing to endstage renal failure within 5 years. The absolute recurrence rate post-transplantation in children varies with different series; a large North American experience reported 27 of 132 patients (20.5 per cent) (Tejani and Stablein 1992), and in Europe a rate of 20 per cent was reported by the Paediatric European and Transplant Association (Broyer *et al.* 1992). Recurrence of proteinuria is associated with a poor outcome compared with those individuals who do not experience clinical signs of recurrent disease (Dall'Amico *et al.* 1999). In the latter group, normal renal function 'after a mean follow-up of 44 months' was reported. In contrast, some individuals will have proteinuria but adequate renal function for a number of years. Even biopsy-proven recurrent disease is not invariably associated with a dire prognosis. Five of eight patients aged less than 25 years who lost first grafts to recurrent FSGS had prolonged function of between 4 and 10 years (Stephanian *et al.* 1992).

Although one review article has recommended bilateral native nephrectomy as a prophylactic measure prior to transplantation the only reference is to a paper, which points out the manoeuvre will make diagnosis of recurrent FSGS post-transplantation easier (Srivasta *et al.* 1994; Cochat *et al.* 1996). More recently published data, albeit a retrospective non-randomized series, compared 20 patients who had undergone nephrectomy with 93 who had not undergone nephrectomy prior to transplantation (Odorico *et al.* 1996). The frequency of recurrence FSGS was higher at 40 per cent in those who had undergone nephrectomy compared with 16 per cent in those who had not undergone a nephrectomy, although of course it is possible that patients who proceeded to bilateral nephrectomy were a subgroup with more aggressive disease.

Certain general factors, particularly age less than 15 years (Ingulli and Tejani 1991), aggressive clinical course of the original disease with the interval from diagnosis to endstage renal failure less than approximately 3 years (Cheong et al. 2000), and diffuse mesangial proliferation on native biopsy (Dantal et al. 1991) are considered predictive of relapse. The influence of native glomerular histology was carefully explored in a publication that reported 24 children who received 37 transplants. Their native renal histology was divided into three groups, pure FSGS, FSGS with focal mesangial proliferation, and FSGS with diffuse mesangial proliferation. The rate of graft loss from recurrence increased from 12–50 to 70 per cent in these small subgroups divided by histology (Striegel et al. 1986). Although age less than 15 years is considered to have a poor prognosis, there is evidence that within the paediatric group those aged over 6 years do somewhat better (Rizzoni et al. 1991). In a North Italian experience, the mean interval between diagnosis and endstage renal failure was significantly shorter at 3.5 years compared with 6 years in the group with recurrence post-transplantation (Dall'Amico et al. 1999).

Given the high frequency of recurrent disease it is important to carefully advise patients and families about the relative merits of living verses cadaveric transplant donor source. Data from the North American Paediatric Renal Transplant Cooperative Study, which registers and follows all children who undergo renal transplant in the United States and Canada, show that patients with FSGS have the highest overall graft failure rate. Patients whose primary disease was FSGS were on average 90 per cent more likely to lose a graft from a live donor and 50 per cent more likely to lose a graft from a cadaveric donor compared with patients with 'structural disorders'. Overall, however, recipients of a living donor kidney had a better graft survival at 74 per cent compared with 59 per cent for recipients of cadaveric renal transplants at 50 months (Kashtan et al. 1995). My practice would be to avoid a living donor organ source as a primary transplant if the clinical course of the original disease was less than 3 years or if the patient was aged less than 15 years, and/or the FSGS was accompanied with diffuse mesangial proliferation. If the primary transplant is lost to recurrent disease a living related transplant should be avoided for the subsequent grafting as the recurrence rate is in the order of 80 per cent (Striegel et al. 1986). If the first graft was lost from rejection or another complication with no evidence of recurrence, authorities have stated that there is little risk of recurrence in a subsequent graft (Stephanian et al. 1992). It would follow that a live donor would be a good choice in this situation. It should be appreciated, however, that this is based on the experience of six cases, one of which lost the graft from rejection within one month of transplantation, so there is clearly no absolute guarantee the recurrence will not occur. Other anecdotes that urge for caution when utilizing living donors are three cases where FSGS and endstage renal failure developed in donors who had a normal work up with no urinary abnormalities and who then donated a kidney to a sib with FSGS (Ismail-Allouch et al. 1993; Winn et al. 1999).

It would be a significant clinical advance to be able to predict those patients who were at particular high risk of recurrent disease. It has been demonstrated that a circulating protein with a molecular weight between 30 and 50 kDa removed by therapeutic apheresis from patients with recurrent FSGS can cause an immediate and profound increase in the albumin permeability of isolated rat glomeruli (Savin et al. 1996). A North Italian group examined pretransplant serum samples found FSGS reoccurred in 11 of 13 children whom tested positive for the permeability factor and four of 12 patients with a negative test (Dall'Amico et al. 1999). However, using a different measure of glomerular permeability other authors have failed to find any predictive value of pretransplant measurements on the risk of recurrence (Godfrin et al. 1997). Given the relative rarity of this disease it will clearly require a collaborative effort to assess the potential of this type of investigation.

Treatment of recurrent FSGS is clearly an important area. Immunoabsorption by protein A column followed by intravenous immunoglobulin has been used, but only one patient of eight treated showed a sustained response (Dantal et al. 1994a). Treatment with angiotensin-converting enzyme (ACE) inhibitors will reduce proteinuria to approximately one-third. However, there is no difference in mean allograft survival for treated compared with untreated patients (Artero et al. 1992). Some authors have reported control of proteinuria in paediatric transplant patients with presumed relapse of FSGS with high dose cyclosporin. However, only two patients have been reported (Ingulli and Tejani 1991), the dose of cyclosporin was large at 15–35 mg/kg/day, and the published follow-up short at 16–24 months. One review has recommended intravenous cyclosporin early in the post-transplant course to maintain levels of 200–300 ng/ml both as prophylaxis and for treatment (Cochat et al. 1996). However, the only published experience known to me is limited to four children, all of whom showed complete remission soon after the intravenous cyclosporin and two were free of proteinuria with follow-up of 9–15 months. One individual, however, relapsed at 9 months and this relapse did not respond to another course of intravenous cyclosporin and a fourth patient lost the graft at 3.5 months from rejection (Ranchin et al. 1996). This unfortunately is not compelling evidence for the efficacy of this strategy. Where cyclosporin use was delayed until after induction antibody therapy cyclosporin had no effect on proteinuria that was already present (Dantal et al. 1994b). The fact that the frequency of relapse of FSGS has not altered since the introduction of cyclosporin in the early 1980s again suggests that cyclosporin at least at conventional oral dose is unlikely to be helpful (Dantal et al. 1994b). Conversion of cyclosporin to tacrolimus after early recurrence of nephrotic syndrome unfortunately was unsuccessful in 10 cases (MacCauley et al. 1993). A single case report of a 30-year-old man with FSGS who developed nephrotic syndrome 5 years after renal transplantation due to recurrent disease that coincided with being switched from cyclosporin to tacrolimus suggests at least in adults that cyclosporin in this setting may be more protective than tacrolimus (Kessler et al. 1999).

Plasmapheresis is the technique most widely used in the treatment of recurrent nephrotic syndrome post-transplantation. Usually this is in combination with other treatments, such as cyclophosphamide, occasionally high dose cyclosporin, ACE inhibitors, or Indomethacin. It is an important question whether treatment with plasma exchange needs to be augmented with cyclophosphamide. Plasma exchange alone in children with recurrent disease leads to remission in approximately two-thirds of cases. However, the duration of follow-up is only available in a minority of reports (Lanfer et al. 1988; Artero et al. 1992; Mowry et al. 1993; Artero et al. 1994; Kawaguchi et al. 1994; Dall'Amico et al. 1999). In a series of 11 patients treated with plasmapheresis and cyclophosphamide 2 mg/kg for 2 months, in seven of 11 children remission was obtained with 'normal renal function' after a mean of 32 months follow-up. The other four children lost their graft after an average of 15 months (Dall'Amico *et al.* 1999). These results are relatively good and similar to that seen by others (Savin *et al.* 1996) and I would interpret as encouraging the early institution of both plasma exchange and cyclophosphamide. One group of authors used an approach that is a mixture of both prophylaxis and treatment in children who received live donor transplants, eight had three sessions of plasma exchange prior to transplantation and six did not. Recurrence was seen in three of the eight who received prior plasma exchange and four of the six who did not. Subsequently five of the patients had plasma exchange as treatment which was 'effective in four'. The duration of follow-up is unclear. Clearly this prior treatment is a logical approach, but only practical in recipients of live donor kidneys. It is still associated with a high early relapse rate (Kawaguchi *et al.* 1994).

Familial FSGS, although rare, is important to recognize it is a different syndrome to idiopathic FSGS of childhood. Patients generally present in their third or fourth decade and post-transplantation recurrent disease is extremely rare with an overall 10-year graft survival of 62 per cent. Key to making the diagnosis, of course, is careful family history.

Adults with 'secondary' FSGS, for example due to renal artery stenosis or some other long standing conditions that lead to renal insufficiency, would not be expected to be at risk of recurrent disease following renal transplantation.

De novo FSGS in renal transplants

This histological appearance is most commonly reported associated with other pathology, particularly chronic allograft nephropathy, or transplant glomerulopathy and occasionally cyclosporin toxicity or IgA disease. In a recent review of a database of 1706 transplant kidney biopsies, 293 patients had a biopsy diagnosis of chronic allograft nephropathy of which 30 per cent also had *de novo* FSGS. The diagnosis was made relatively late at a mean of 57 months post-transplantation. There were no differences between those with FSGS and chronic allograft nephropathy and those with chronic allograft nephropathy alone with respect to donor age, gender, race, cold ischaemia time, or recipient characteristics such as age, gender, race, weight, presence of diabetes, panel reactive antibody peak, or HLA mismatch (Cosio *et al.* 1999). Again in contrast to FSGS affecting native kidneys only 24 per cent of those with biopsy-proven glomerular disease had nephrotic syndrome and the mean 24 h protein excretion was relatively modest at 2.4 g. There was an important impact on graft survival of the diagnosis of *de novo* FSGS with these patients having a 40 per cent graft survival at 5 years postdiagnosis compared with 60 per cent in those with chronic allograft nephropathy alone. The pathogenesis and whether this is truly separate from a chronic rejection process is unclear.

IgA mesangial glomerulonephritis (see also Chapter 3.6)

IgA glomerulonephritis is almost certainly the most common glomerular disease leading to chronic renal failure in the world (D'Amico 1987). Berger and colleagues were among the first to report that IgA nephropathy can reoccur in renal transplants (Berger *et al.* 1975). The absolute risk of recurrence of IgA glomerulonephritis in transplanted kidneys has been estimated at ranging between approximately 13 per cent and more than 60 per cent (Omacht *et al.* 1997; Freese *et al.* 1999). These variable results are of course greatly influenced by the different indications for renal transplant biopsy and the relatively small number of patients investigated and variable length of follow-up. The risk of recurrence is difficult to predict but must be common. In the only series in which all patients were biopsied recurrence was found in 58 per cent (Odum *et al.* 1994). In a series of 104 primary renal transplant recipients with biopsy-proven IgA disease there were 11 cases with unequivocal IgA disease on transplant biopsy. The duration of the original disease until endstage renal failure was significantly shorter in patients with recurrence at a median of 5 years compared with those without recurrence at median of 10 years (Freese *et al.* 1999). However, this information does not give good data to advise individual patients about the risk of recurrent disease.

A large retrospective study of 106 adults transplanted because of biopsy proven IgA disease and 212 patients who were transplanted immediately before and after the patients with IgA disease were matched 1 : 2 according to the source of the donor, cadaveric, or living. Immunosuppressive therapies were different over the long period of the study between 1973 and 1999, but was similar in the two groups. Clearly critical is the interpretation of the transplant histology. The authors attempted to separate recurrent disease by requiring diffuse mesangial proliferation in the glomeruli along with segmental necrosis of the tuft and extracapillary proliferation in order to define IgA disease. In contrast, chronic rejection required diffuse interstitial fibrosis and transplant arteriopathy. Neither interstitial fibrosis nor tubular atrophy alone was considered supportive of the diagnosis of either recurrent glomerulonephritis or chronic rejection. Graft failures in the first 6 months were excluded, as the authors were interested in the long-term impact of recurrent disease. IgA disease was demonstrated in 35 per cent of patients at a median of 49 months post-transplantation. Importantly, 10-year survival probability of the two groups was the same (Ponticelli *et al.* 2001). Previous authors have reported either little impact or worst outcome in patients with recurrent IgA disease, but in none of these series (Lim and Terasaki 1992; Almartine *et al.* 1994; Floege *et al.* 1998) have the same care given to defining the control group as that reported most recently.

The use of living related donors for recipients with IgA disease has been avoided by some authors. Ponticelli and colleagues (2001), in conjunction with most of the more up to date reports, failed to find a significant difference in long-term graft survival between living transplants in patients with IgA nephropathy and controls (Kessler *et al.* 1996; Freese *et al.* 1999).

In summary, at least 35 per cent of patients with IgA nephropathy are expected to show histological recurrence of the disease in the transplanted kidney and the proportion may be as high as 60 per cent. This generally becomes clinically evident within 6 years. Younger patients are at greater risk of recurrence as are those with a shorter duration of disease in the native kidneys. Graft survival at 10 years is similar to an appropriate control group of patients and living donor transplants give similar results to that seen in patients who do not have IgA disease.

Henoch–Schönlein purpura (see also Chapter 4.5.2)

Because of the very small numbers of patients documented, it is very difficult to accurately describe the clinical syndrome of recurrence of this condition. In a report from Belgium, 10 patients were reported and the clinical course of 64 other transplants that had been reported in the literature were summarized (Meulders *et al.* 1994). Overall the actuarial risk for renal recurrence and graft loss due to recurrence was 35 and 11 per cent at 5 years after transplantation. Importantly, recurrence occurred despite a more than 12-month delay between disappearance of purpura and transplantation in five of eight cases. This means that the common advice to delay for a year between disappearance of purpura and transplantation seems to be inappropriate. For the majority of patients who experience recurrence the interval between last onset of purpura and transplantation was generally around 36 months. This, I would suggest, argues for an interval of 3 years postdisappearance of the purpura before embarking on live donor transplantation. As in this situation the consequences of early recurrence may be considered especially unfortunate.

Once recurrence has been demonstrated, the graft survival is poor at only 57 per cent at 2 years (Briggs and Jones 1999b). Although some authors have reported a greater risk of recurrence in living related donor grafts than cadaver kidney recipients (Nast *et al.* 1987), this is not confirmed by the most comprehensive review at present available (Meulders *et al.* 1994).

Mesangial IgG glomerulonephritis

Glomerular deposition of IgG can be seen in a number of primary and secondary glomerulonephritides. Approximately 30 cases of primary IgG glomerulonephritis have been reported to date. The condition has been most often recognized in young people, 10 in the literature were reported from a paediatric service (Yoshikawa *et al.* 1994), and the mean age at diagnosis in the largest series of 14 cases was 19 years (Fakhouri *et al.* 2002). In this series of 14 cases, seven patients developed chronic renal failure after a mean follow-up of 11 years and four progressed to endstage renal failure. In one patient recurrence of the disorder was diagnosed in a renal transplant 4 years after grafting.

Membranous nephropathy (see also Chapter 3.7)

As is usual for the diseases discussed in this section, data on recurrent membranous glomerulonephritis is difficult to assess because of the small number of published cases. For this condition there is the added complication of the relative frequency of *de novo* membranous glomerulonephritis. The frequency that recurrent disease is diagnosed will depend greatly on the duration of follow-up. In adults the rate of recurrence is approximately 30 per cent (Odorico *et al.* 1996; Cosyns *et al.* 1998). In the latter report, which is an amalgamation from two centres giving a total of 30 patients, no risk factor for recurrence was identified including the duration of membranous glomerulonephritis in the native kidneys, the need for pretransplant haemodialysis, presence of HLA DR3, use of cyclosporin, nor whether the transplant was of cadaveric or live donor origin. The maximum risk of recurrence peaked at 3 years and plateaus for the next 7 years of follow-up. The outcome for graft survival was poor as graft loss was 38 and 52 per cent at 5 and 10 years, respectively. The clinical syndrome seems to be similar to the disease in native kidneys with progressively more severe nephrotic syndrome. The management is usually based on extrapolation of data from management of native kidney disease and similar to

that situation spontaneous remission, failures of immunosuppressive treatment as well as clinical response coincident with change of treatment have all been reported (Marcen *et al.* 1996). There are three cases reported of membranous glomerulonephritis recurring within the first few months following living related transplantation (Berger *et al.* 1983). Caution in using a live donor in the rare instance of membranous glomerulonephritis affecting children or in adults where there is a fulminant native presentation or where a primary graft has been lost through recurrent disease is warranted. However, in other circumstances live donor transplantation appears to be an appropriate treatment choice.

De novo membranous glomerulonephritis

De novo membranous glomerulonephritis is second only to rejection-associated transplant glomerulopathy as a cause of nephrotic syndrome after renal transplantation. In a single centre study of just over 1000 renal transplants *de novo* membranous glomerulonephritis was seen in 30 biopsy specimens in 21 patients giving an incidence of approximately 2 per cent. There was no important effect of the introduction of cyclosporin in the historical series on the incidence of disease and strikingly hepatitis B antigenaemia, hepatitis C antibody, or human immunodeficiency virus was found in eight of the 21 patients. The mean time of diagnosis was late at approximately 63 months post-transplantation and, as expected the incidence increased significantly with time. Proteinuria was on average 3 g/day and noted at approximately 50 months post-transplantation. The addition of pulsed steroid therapy to the baseline immunosuppression in heavily nephrotic patients made no obvious impact on outcome. Interestingly, patients with *de novo* membranous glomerulonephritis did not differ from the much larger group without membranous glomerulonephritis with regard to graft survival. These authors regarded *de novo* membranous glomerulonephritis as a late, often asymptomatic complication (Schwarz *et al.* 1994).

The data regarding the association of infection with hepatitis B or C in patients with *de novo* membranous glomerulonephritis is contradictory. One report in 1983 found 12 of 19 patients with *de novo* membranous glomerulonephritis were seropositive for either hepatitis B or C virus, although the frequency in the control population was not reported (Levy and Charpentier 1983). A more recent study found the incidence of hepatitis C infection no different in patients with *de novo* membranous glomerulonephritis compared to the total transplant population (Hammond *et al.* 1996). In contrast, membranous glomerulonephritis was found to be more prevalent among hepatitis C positive patients at 3.6 per cent compared with hepatitis C negative patients at 0.36 per cent (Morales *et al.* 1997b). In this series of 15 cases of presumed hepatitis C virus associated membranous glomerulonephritis, nephrotic syndrome was present in the absence of complement activation, cryoglobulinaemia or circulating immune complexes. The outcome was poor with eight of 15 patients returning to dialysis an average time of 2 years after diagnosis.

Mesangiocapillary glomerulonephritis (see also Chapter 3.8)

There are marked histological similarities between chronic allograft nephropathy and chronic rejection associated transplant glomerulopathy and mesangiocapillary glomerulonephritis (MCGN). For this reason to achieve an accurate diagnosis full assessment of transplant biopsies as well as a clear diagnosis of the native kidney disease is critical. Immunofluorescence in recurrent type I MCGN shows a greater intensity of C3 staining in contrast to IgM, which is more prominent in transplant glomerulopathy. Electron microscopy can be very useful as in type I MCGN there are subendothelial electron dense deposits in contrast to transplant glomerulopathy where an electrolucent zone in the subendothelial space is seen (Andresdottir *et al.* 1998).

Mesangiocapillary glomerulonephritis type I

In the situation where MCGN type I is thought to be mediated by glomerular deposition of immune complexes generated after exposure, for example, to native DNA in systemic lupus erythematosus (SLE) or hepatitis antigens, the antigens are not removed by transplantation so recurrence of disease in this situation would be predicted. The clinical syndrome is that usually of haematuria, proteinuria, hypertension, and progressive renal impairment. A relatively large European series of 32 patients with type I MCGN who had received first transplants between 1977 and 1994 have been reported. Recurrence was detected in Nine of 27 recipients of the first graft (33 per cent) and cumulative incidence increased to 48 per cent at 4 years post-transplantation. The proteinuria was first observed at a median of 20 months postgrafting and mean duration of graft survival after the diagnosis of recurrence was only 40 months. There were no clear clinical predictors from the progression of native disease that were useful to anticipate subsequent transplant course. Four individuals received a HLA identical graft from a living related donor with recurrence occurring in three patients. Five of the patients with recurrence in the first graft received a second transplant and recurrence was observed in no less than four of these patients (Andresdottir *et al.* 1997). The European and North American experience implies type I MCGN will recur after renal transplantation in half the patients and that this frequency may be even greater in recipients of identical living related donor grafts. Furthermore, recurrence in a second transplant after recurrence in the first graft is extremely common and once diagnosed this disease has an important detrimental impact on graft survival. Interestingly, the risk of recurrence may be considerably less in Japanese patients with a rate of only 3 per cent in one published series (Shimizu *et al.* 1998). It is not possible to give any evidence-based advice with regard to treatment. Lamivudine would be logical in persistent hepatitis B antigenaemia. Single case reports of cyclophosphamide treatment in conjunction with standard immunosuppression with satisfactory 3-year follow-up and an anecdote of plasmapheresis in conjunction with cytotoxic therapy with a functioning renal graft 2 years post-transplantation have been reported.

Mesangiocapillary glomerulonephritis type II

The clinical presentation of this condition is similar to that seen in MCGN type I. The intramembranous electron dense deposits and C3 on immunofluorescence in the basal lamina surrounding these deposits and the mesangium is similar to that seen in the original disease. The condition is rare and 13 patients at a single European centre receiving a first allograft between 1983 and 1994 represents the largest series (Andresdottir *et al.* 1999). Importantly, light microscopy was relatively unremarkable, but glomerular deposits compatible with recurrence of MCGN type II were found in all 11 patients that were biopsied. Eight of these patients progressed to endstage renal failure 14 months post-transplantation with recurrence as the sole cause of

graft loss in three patients who had particularly aggressive histology with glomerular crescents. Clearly, the histological recurrence rate of MCGN type II is extremely high and one-fourth of the patients with recurrent disease lost their grafts because of this. In contrast it would appear that patients with C3 deposition confined to the mesangium have a better prognosis. No treatments are known to be effective, although individual examples of plasma exchange and immunosuppression have been described as case reports.

Mesangiocapillary glomerulonephritis type III

A single case of recurrence of type III MCGN has been reported in a renal transplant received after 3 years of dialysis therapy. Proteinuria appeared after 13 months and 7 years postgrafting the patient returned to haemodialysis (Morales *et al.* 1997a).

Haemolytic–uraemic syndrome (see also Chapter 10.6.3)

It is important in this syndrome to discriminate between 'classical' diarrhoea-associated HUS, familial HUS, and *de novo* HUS. It seems likely that recurrence in 'atypical' or familial HUS is much the most common problem. This is well illustrated by single centre data from a Children's Department in the southern United States. Eighteen patients with atypical HUS received 28 transplants and 12 of those grafts experienced recurrent disease (Miller *et al.* 1997). In contrast in the three patients with diarrhoea-associated HUS recurrent disease occurred on one occasion. There were no significant differences between recurrence and non-recurrence patients in the interval between the onset of HUS and the first renal transplant. Neither was there any clear relationship between immunosuppressive therapy and HUS recurrence.

A meta analysis including 10 studies comprising 159 grafts in 127 patients was published in 1998 (Ducloux *et al.* 1998). Overall 1-year graft survival was 76.6 per cent in patients without recurrence and 33.3 per cent in patients with recurrence. As the meta analysis does not discriminate between atypical and diarrhoea-associated HUS this data should be taken as a guide only. Recurrence of HUS is usually an early phenomenon most often within 2 months of transplantation, though occasionally it can be delayed by several years. The use of a living related donor in atypical HUS needs to be approached with great caution. There is a single case report of a sibling donor developing HUS within a week of donation and clearly now most practitioners would avail themselves of the available immunogenetic studies and explore complement factor H before progressing that option.

The clinical presentation may be gradual or relatively abrupt with marked thrombocytopenia, and haemolysis associated with progressive renal dysfunction. In the early transplant period this needs to be distinguished from graft versus host disease. Hypertension is also associated and the differential diagnosis between HUS, whether recurrent or *de novo*, and microangiopathy associated with malignant hypertension can cause confusion. Therapeutic options are limited with little evidence that altering calcineurin inhibitors changes prognosis. In severe thrombocytopenia most practitioners would adopt treatment strategies similar to that used in classic HUS with plasma fraction infusions and plasma exchange. In the event of life-threatening thrombocytopenia or haemolysis, particularly in the presence of severe allograft dysfunction, stability may be restored by transplant nephrectomy.

De novo haemolytic–uraemic syndrome

De novo HUS has been attributed to OKT3, tacrolimus, vascular rejection, as well as cyclosporin postrenal transplantation. In addition, HUS complicating cyclosporin therapy has been recognized in bone marrow, liver, heart, as well as renal transplant recipients. This syndrome occurs most frequently within a month of transplantation and is associated with graft loss in around 60 per cent and patient death in 20 per cent of cases. Cyclosporin dose reduction is usually adopted and there has been single case of tacrolimus substitution coincident with clinical resolution (Richardson *et al.* 1996), although others have described HUS occurring in patients treated with tacrolimus. A treatment strategy similar to that used in diarrhoea-associated HUS is usually adopted.

Antiglomerular basement membrane disease (see also Chapter 3.11)

The histological hallmark of this disease with linear deposits of IgG on glomerular capillary walls occurs in approximately 50 per cent of patients who receive transplants while circulating antiglomerular basement membrane (anti-GBM) antibodies are present (Glassock 1997). The histological changes are seen in approximately 10 per cent of patients who received transplants 6 months or more after the disappearance of anti-GBM antibodies (Cameron 1982). Clinical disease is significantly less common than histological recurrence and rarely leads to graft loss. The standard practice is to measure circulating anti-GBM antibodies periodically and most would advise a waiting a 12-month interval from when antibodies were negative before offering transplantation, whether from a cadaveric or a live donor source.

De novo anti-GBM nephritis

Approximately 15 per cent of patients with Alport's syndrome develop anti-GBM antibodies in response to what is for them the neoantigen of α chain of type IV collagen. Most commonly the IgG deposition along the GBM does not have any effect on allograft function. However, a small fraction, possibly as many as 5 per cent of Alport patients, develop immunization leading to a severe crescentic glomerulonephritis. Treatment is usually with intensive plasma exchange, but despite this the outlook is poor. However, the largest series known to me is from a European centre and had 30 patients with 1- and 5-year graft survival that was better than a control group. Thirty-four biopsies were available from 21 kidneys in 15 patients. Anti-GBM nephritis was not detected in any of these biopsies and no grafts were lost due to this disease. These authors felt that allograft anti-GBM nephritis was a rare complication or Alport's syndrome and the data could be used to argue for prompt transplantation, whether from a live donor or a cadaveric source (Gobel *et al.* 1992).

Antineutrophil cytoplasmic antibody associated vasculitis

A pooled analysis of several series of recurrent antineutrophil cytoplasmic antibody (ANCA) associated vasculitis including 127 patients and excluding single case reports has been published (Nachman *et al.* 1999). The authors justified a pooled approach in part because of the marked difference in reported recurrence rates ranging from 11 to 50 per cent in series of small numbers of patients. Overall relapse was seen in 22 representing 17.3 per cent. There was no statistically significant difference in the relapse rate between patients treated and not treated with cyclosporin. The rate in the more recent series treated with cyclosporin was 20 per cent. Data regarding ANCA titres at the time of transplantation is available in 59 patients. However, because identifying patients with relapsing disease was incomplete the important analysis of the relapse rate among patients with circulating ANCA at the time of transplantation could only be explored in 39 patients. Recurrent vasculitis affected extrarenal organs in approximately half the occasions that relapse occurred and affected the renal transplant in the other half. There appeared to be no important difference, albeit on very small numbers, on the duration of pretransplant dialysis prior to transplantation and any influence that could have on relapse. In the 39 patients known to have circulating ANCA at the time of transplantation recurrent disease occurred in 10 individuals, giving a relapse rate of 25.6 per cent, which is not statistically significantly different to the rate seen in patients without circulating ANCA at the time of transplantation. The average time from transplantation to relapse was 31 months after transplantation and the presentation varied depending on the organ system involved. The number of patients for whom details on treatment were given is small at 16. The majority, 12, received cyclophosphamide, three azathioprine, and one high-dose methylprednisolone alone. Treatment of recurrent disease resulted in long-term remission in 11 patients. Two relapses were associated with graft loss. Another patient had remission of extrarenal vasculitis, but continued to experience deterioration in renal function and one patient died as a consequence of relapse. The disease subtype, whether Wegener's granulomatosis, microscopic polyarteritis, or idiopathic necrotizing crescentic glomerulonephritis, had no detectable impact on the recurrence rate, although the numbers in each subgroup are inevitably small.

The need to wait for clinical remission before embarking on transplantation has not been prospectively examined and in almost all reports patients did not receive a transplant until they were in clinical remission. It appears that the rate of relapse of ANCA-associated vasculitis is approximately half that seen compared with the untransplanted ANCA-associated vasculitis population.

There is clearly a high potential for relapse and it is difficult to select any characteristics that may provide a useful prognosis. Despite this, transplantation appears to be a good mode of treatment for patients with renal failure associated with ANCA vasculitis. The potential for late relapse should be borne in mind and clearly haematuria and renal impairment as well as symptoms due to extrarenal vasculitis need monitoring. The presence of positive ANCA at the time of transplantation does not preclude transplantation and subsequent serological monitoring would seem to be relatively unhelpful for predicting outcome.

Cyclophosphamide and corticosteroids are the most well established treatment (Ramos *et al.* 1994). Overall the survival rate in graft function, at least in patients with Wegener's granulomatosis, appears to be similar to other kidney transplant recipients (Briggs and Jones 1999b).

Systemic lupus erythematosus (see also Chapter 4.7.2)

The rate of recurrent lupus nephritis is low. The biggest series is of 97 consecutive SLE patients who underwent 106 renal transplants between January 1984 and 1996 (Stone *et al.* 1998). The mean transplant follow-up was 63 months. Nine patients had pathological evidence of recurrent lupus nephritis. This occurred on average of 3.5 years post-transplantation. For all 97 patients lupus was clinically and serologically quiescent at the time of transplantation. Three of the individuals with recurrence on histology had serological evidence of active lupus, only one had symptoms, in this case arthritis. Three of the nine individuals lost their graft because of recurrent lupus and underwent a second renal transplant with follow-up of approximately 20 months with no relapse to date. This recurrence rate is somewhat more common on histological grounds than previously reported in the literature, but the histological recurrence of lupus was not always associated with allograft loss and was frequently present in the absence of clinical or serological evidence of active SLE. In a review by the same authors that encompassed 20 original reports of the outcome of renal transplantation following lupus, allograft survival rates were superior in comparison to the control groups in six and approximately equivalent in three. In the largest series 1-year allograft survival rate in lupus patients for cadaveric renal transplants was a disappointing 67 per cent. This was significantly lower than the rate for the other 14 disease subgroups examined. In this review, recurrence of lupus nephritis was rare at approximately 2 per cent and as before did not invariably result in allograft failure. Importantly pretransplantation serological parameters were unreliable predictors of the likelihood of recurrence and also may not accurately reflect disease activity in the post-transplantation interval. Important to note is that nine of 20 studies reported an increased risk of early graft loss among lupus transplant recipients. This may be because of an increased frequency of acute rejection and/or thrombotic events associated with antiphospholipid antibodies (Stone *et al.* 1998).

As would be expected from the small case experience, there are no formal studies of the management of recurrent lupus nephritis. Most clinicians would opt for management that mirrored that of native disease based on steroids, cyclophosphamide, plasma exchange, and mycophenolate mofetil. Anticoagulation during the early perioperative and early post-transplantation phase should be considered for patients with a history of thrombosis or those with the presence of lupus anticoagulant. It does appear that recurrent lupus nephritis is somewhat more frequent than early reports indicated and the outcome seem to be somewhat worse, particularly as the majority of the lupus population transplanted are young. However, given the low probability of recurrence in the published series where the disease was quiescent by the time of surgery, transplantation whether from a living donor or cadaveric source, remains a good treatment option.

Systemic sclerosis (see also Chapter 4.8)

A retrospective review of data collected from the United Network for Organ Sharing in North America over a 10-year period from 1987 to 1997 identified 86 patients with systemic sclerosis who had a renal transplant (Chang and Spiera 1999). The 1- and 5-year graft survival rates were 62 and 47 per cent, respectively. Of 14 cases where the cause of graft failure was known, three had recurrence of scleroderma. This rate of recurrence is similar to that reported in an earlier and equally small series (Kotanko *et al.* 1997). Clearly, the evidence base for making recommendations here is extremely slight. Most clinicians would manage patients with systemic sclerosis in a similar way to patients

with systemic lupus and recommend renal transplantation as a treatment option. Most would use ACE inhibitors for antihypertensive control and from the outset in patients who had renal failure secondary to scleroderma renal crisis. Although given the mortality rate of this subgroup on dialysis treatment, it is likely few individuals who present in this way come to transplantation.

Hepatitis B associated glomerulonephritis

Concomitant hepatitis B infection has an important impact on survival of renal transplant patients. The issue of glomerulonephritis secondary to hepatitis B postrenal transplantation has very rarely been an important clinical problem. The number of cases described is too small to allow informed advice. Membranous glomerulonephritis is the most common form of glomerular disease associated with hepatitis B this has a far from benign prognosis (Lai *et al.* 1991), a similar prognosis would be expected in renal transplant recipients who develop nephrotic syndrome.

Hepatitis C associated glomerulonephritis (see also Chapters 3.8 and 4.6)

Cryoglobulinaemic nephritis with MCGN has been described after transplantation in patients infected with hepatitis C virus. In a report of six patients all had nephrotic range proteinuria, microhaematuria, and activation of serum complement by the classical pathway with very low levels of cryoglobulins (<4 per cent) (D'Amico and Fornasieri 1995). The very low level of cryoglobulins presumably explains the lack of systemic signs and the authors ascribed this phenomenon to the immunosuppressive therapy. It is possible, of course, that MCGN is being confused with transplant glomerulopathy as electron microscopy would be necessary to separate the diagnoses. Other authors of five cases reported *de novo* MCGN in hepatitis C infected renal transplant recipients, but on this occasion failed to find evidence of cryoglobulinaemia and circulating immune complexes (Morales *et al.* 1997b). Overall the prognosis is poor as hepatitis C virus associated type I MCGN frequently progressed to graft failure (Roth *et al.* 1995; Hammoud *et al.* 1996).

Treatments with interferon-α have a poor reputation in renal transplant medicine, as it is known to have the capability to induce acute rejection and renal dysfunction. Treatment with low-dose ribavirin seems to be more promising and has been reported to be an effective treatment for hepatitis C associated nephrotic syndrome in liver transplant recipients (Pham *et al.* 1998).

Mixed cryoglobulinaemic nephritis (see also Chapter 4.6)

This very rare disease is characterized by systemic vasculitis and glomerular changes, most typically MCGN. Although usually associated with chronic hepatitis C virus, there a number of well-characterized cases where it has not been possible to conclusively demonstrate such an infection. A publication from Italy reported two patients who received a renal transplant with histological recurrence at five and 10 months post-transplantation. One graft was lost because of chronic rejection at 13 months and the other has a functioning kidney at 4 years. From the natural history of the condition in native kidneys it may be predicted that recurrent disease in renal allografts may have a modest impact on subsequent graft function (Tarantino et al. 1994).

Lipoprotein glomerulopathy

In this condition, a qualitative change in plasma apolipoprotein E is associated with intracapillary lipoprotein deposits associated with proteinuria and renal failure. Only 27 cases have been described. However, recurrence has been reported both in living kidney and cadaveric kidney recipients. In one case although there was histological disease and nephrotic syndrome at 4-year follow-up, the patient had satisfactory graft function (Mourad et al. 1998).

Fibrillary glomerulonephritis and immunotactoid glomerulonephritis (see also Chapter 4.2.2)

In this rare condition there is extracellular deposition of non-branching microfibrils or microtubules within the mesangium and capillary walls of the renal glomerulus. Electron microscopy is required to reach a diagnosis. Patients present with proteinuria and often the nephrotic syndrome, haematuria, hypertension, and chronic progressive renal failure. After careful assessment for monoclonal gammopathy and cryoglobulins a few have progressed to renal transplantation. In a series treated at a single centre in North America, four patients received five renal transplants with follow-up varying between 4 and 11 years. The recurrence rate was high as it was documented in three allografts. The authors point out that the rate of deterioration in glomerular filtration rate (GFR) was slower in allografts than in native kidneys and argued that immunosuppression may be a treatment option. However, the difference in rate of decline of renal function is very modest (Pronovost et al. 1996). Although renal transplantation seems a reasonable treatment option a single case report of very early graft failure due to recurrent disease (Palanichamy et al. 1998), may imply that the rate of native renal failure should be taken into account when assessing how appropriate it is to offer renal transplantation.

Amyloidosis (see also Chapter 4.2.1)

The published experience is of about 100 patients with both primary and secondary amyloidosis. The rate of recurrent disease varies between 10 and 40 per cent (Heering et al. 1989; Hartmann et al. 1992). Graft survival appears to be about 74 per cent at 1 year and 62 per cent at 5 years in a series with a 50 per cent rate of living donation. It would be logical to expect the rate of recurrence in secondary amyloid to be determined by how well the underlying disease is controlled. Importantly the patient survival rates are poor at 79 per cent at 1 year and 65 per cent at 5 years with patient death with a functioning graft causing 16 out of 25 graft losses.

Amyloidosis secondary to familial Mediterranean fever was examined in a publication from Israel, which included 21 patients. Proteinuria, which the authors interpreted as due to renal transplant amyloid, developed in 11 patients at a median of 3 years post-transplantation. However, in another 10 patients there was no proteinuria at a median of 5 years post-transplantation. The group retrospectively analysed the colchicine dose that patients had received and observed that a dose of 1.5 mg/day provided complete protection from proteinuria, which did not occur at a dose of 0.5 mg/day or less. In the patients who received 1 mg/day some developed proteinuria and some did not. This important finding implies that colchicine can offer very good protection against amyloidosis in this setting (Livneh et al. 1992).

Light chain deposition disease

In this condition, κ- or λ-immunoglobulin light chains are deposited in the kidneys as well as other organs. At the time of renal diagnosis, one-third of the patients have no known systemic disease whereas in two-thirds there was associated multiple myeloma or a lymphoplasmacytic disorder. Given that remission of the underlying haematological malignancy is often difficult to guarantee and the prognosis of patients with combined renal failure and myeloma is poor, the case experience of patients who have undergone transplantation is small. There are approximately nine reported cases in the literature where remission of the gammopathy had been demonstrated following chemotherapy and steroids for several years after which cadaveric renal transplant was performed with no premature failure of the graft from recurrent disease (Gerlag et al. 1986).

Diabetic nephropathy (see also Chapter 4.1)

Histological recurrence of diabetic renal disease with arteriolar lesions, mesangial expansion and glomerular basement thickening are seen in 100 per cent of patients within 4 years of transplantation (Najarian et al. 1979). Although the histological recurrence rate is very high the frequency with which diabetic nephropathy is ascribed as a cause of graft loss is small and was only 1.8 per cent in the largest series (Basadonna et al. 1992). A diagnosis of diabetic glomerulosclerosis, however, was made in one series of 14 patients at an average 97 months after transplantation. There were marked arteriolar lesions, and the diagnosis was associated with a high rate of allograft failure with seven of 14 patients experiencing graft failure due to the recurrent diabetes (Hariharan et al. 1996).

In isolated renal transplantation, the majority would argue for strict glycaemic control with the early use of ACE inhibitors in an attempt to slow any progression of renal disease.

De novo diabetic nephropathy

Renal transplant recipients are at risk of new onset diabetes, particularly because of treatment with corticosteroids, tacrolimus, and cyclosporin. In a series of 40 patients who developed post-transplantation diabetes 12-year graft survival was only 50 per cent compared with 70 per cent in a control group. Only two individuals, however, had the loss of their renal transplants ascribed to diabetic nephropathy. Given the long interval between onset of diabetes and renal failure from diabetic nephropathy it is not surprising that renal transplantation loss due to *de novo* diabetic nephropathy is rare. It is of course the case, however, that renal transplant recipients have markedly reduced renal mass and often hypertension and nephrotoxic drug therapy. It is therefore sensible to argue for good glycaemic control and the liberal use of ACE inhibitors as renal protection irrespective of the favourable impact this management would be expected to have on cardiovascular disease (Miles *et al.* 1998).

Sarcoidosis (see also Chapter 4.4)

Although as many as 20 per cent of patients with sarcoidosis show a granulomatous interstitial nephritis, endstage renal failure is uncommon. Postrenal transplantation relapse of sarcoid resulting in renal impairment that was improved by increasing steroid treatment has been reported with reasonable evidence on rare occasions (Shen *et al.* 1986; Brown *et al.* 1992). These few cases would suggest to me that an individual with endstage renal failure due to sarcoidosis who receives a renal transplant should be treated with steroid therapy long-term.

References

Almartine, E. *et al.* (1994). Actuarial survival rate of kidney transplant patients in patients with IgA glomerulonephritis: a one-center study. *Transplantation Proceedings* 26, 272.

Andresdottir, M. B., Assmann, K. J., Hoitsma, A. J., and Koene, R. A. (1997). Recurrence of type 1 membranoproliferative glomerulonephritis after renal transplantation: analysis of the incidence, risk factors, and impact on graft survival. *Transplantation* 63, 1628–1633.

Andresdottir, M. B., Assmann, K. J., Koene, R. A., and Wetzels, J. F. (1998). Immunohistological and ultrastructural differences between recurrent type I membranoproliferative glomerulonephritis and chronic transplant glomerulopathy. *American Journal of Kidney Diseases* 32, 582–588.

Andresdottir, M. B., Assmann, K. J., and Hoitsma, A. J. (1999). Renal transplantation in patients with dense deposit disease: morphological characteristics of recurrent disease and clinical outcome. *Nephrology, Dialysis, Transplantation* 14, 1723–1731.

Artero, M., Biava, C., Amend, W., Tomlanovich, S., and Vincenti, F. (1992). Recurrent focal glomerulosclerosis: natural history and response to therapy. *American Journal of Medicine* 92, 375–383.

Artero, M. L., Sharma, R., Savin, V. J., and Vincenti, F. (1994). Plasmapheresis reduces proteinuria and serum capacity to injure glomeruli in patients with recurrent focal glomerulosclerosis. *American Journal of Kidney Diseases* 23, 574–581.

Baqi, N. and Tejani, A. (1997). Recurrence of the original disease in pediatric renal transplantation. *Journal of Nephrology* 10, 85–92.

Basadonna, G. *et al.* (1992). Transplantation in diabetic patients: the University of Minnesota experience. *Kidney International* 42, S193–S198.

Berger, B. E. *et al.* (1983). *De novo* and recurrent membranous glomerulopathy following kidney transplantation. *Transplantation* 35, 315–319.

Berger, J., Janeva, H., Nabarra, B., and Barbanel, C. (1975). Recurrence of mesangial deposition of IgA after renal transplantation. *Kidney International* 7, 232–241.

Briggs, J. D. and Jones, E. on behalf of the Scientific Advisory Board of the ERA-EDTA Registry (1999a). Recurrence of glomerulonephritis following renal transplantation. *Nephrology, Dialysis, Transplantation* 14, 564–565.

Briggs, J. D. and Jones, E. (1999b). Renal transplantation for uncommon diseases. *Nephrology, Dialysis, Transplantation* 14, 570–575.

Brown, J. H., Jos, V., Newstead, C. G., and Lawler, W. (1992). Sarcoid like granulomata in a renal transplant. *Nephrology, Dialysis, Transplantation* 7, 173.

Broyer, M., Selwood, N., and Brunner, F. (1992). Recurrence of primary renal disease on kidney graft: a European pediatric experience. *Journal of the American Society of Nephrology* 2 (Suppl. 12), S255–S257.

Cameron, J. S. (1982). Glomerulonephritis in renal transplants. *Transplantation* 34, 237.

Chadban, S. J. (2001). Glomerulonephritis recurrence in the renal graft. *Journal of the American Society of Nephrology* 12, 394–402.

Chang, Y. J. and Spiera, H. (1999). Renal transplantation in scleroderma. *Medicine* 78, 382–385.

Cheong, H., II *et al.* (2000). Early recurrent nephrotic syndrome after renal transplantation in children with focal segmental glomerulosclerosis. *Nephrology, Dialysis, Transplantation* 15 (1), 78–81.

Cochat, P. *et al.* (1996). Management of recurrent nephrotic syndrome after kidney transplantation in children. *Clinical Nephrology* 46 (1), 17–20.

Cosio, F. G. *et al.* (1999). Focal segmental glomerulosclerosis in renal allografts with chronic nephropathy: implications for graft survival. *American Journal of Kidney Diseases* 34 (4), 731–738.

Cosyns, J. P., Couchoud, C., Pouteil-Noble, C., and Squifflet, J. P. (1998). Recurrence of membranous nephropathy after renal transplantation: probability, outcome and risk factors. *Clinical Nephrology* 50, 144–153.

Dall'Amico, R. *et al.* (1999). Prediction and treatment of recurrent focal segmental glomerulosclerosis after renal transplantation in children. *American Journal of Kidney Diseases* 34 (6), 1048–1055.

D'Amico, G. (1987). The commonest glomerulonephritis in the world: IgA nephropathy. *Quarterly Journal of Medicine* 64, 707–727.

D'Amico, G. and Fornasieri, A. (1995). Cryoglobulinemic glomerulonephritis: a membranoproliferative glomerulonephritis induced by hepatitis C virus. *American Journal of Kidney Diseases* 25, 361–369.

Dantal, J. *et al.* (1991). Recurrent nephrotic syndrome following renal transplantation in patients with focal glomerulosclerosis. *Transplantation* 52, 827–831.

Dantal, J. *et al.* (1994a). Effect of plasma protein adsorption on protein excretion in kidney-transplant recipients with recurrent nephrotic syndrome. *New England Journal of Medicine* 330, 7–14.

Dantal, J. *et al.* (1994b). Recurrent focal glomerulosclerosis: natural history and response to therapy. *American Journal of Medicine* 92, 375–383.

Ducloux, D. *et al.* (1998). Recurrence of hemolytic–uremic syndrome in renal transplant recipients. *Transplantation* 65 (10), 1405–1407.

Fakhouri, F. *et al.* (2002). Mesangial IgG glomerulonephritis: a distinct type of primary glomerulonephritis. *Journal of the American Society of Nephrology* 13, 379–387.

Floege, J., Burg, M., and Kliem, V. (1998). Recurrent IgA nephropathy after kidney transplantation: not a benign condition. *Nephrology, Dialysis, Transplantation* 13, 1933–1935.

Freese, P., Svalander, C., Nordén, G., and Nyberg, G. (1999). Clinical risk for recurrence of IgA nephropathy. *Clinical Transplantation* 13, 313–317.

Gephardt, G. N. *et al.* (1988). Nephrotic range proteinuria with 'minimal change glomerulopathy' in human renal allografts: report of four cases. *American Journal of Kidney Diseases* 12, 51–61.

Gerlag, P. G. G., Koene, R. A. P., and Berden, J. H. M. (1986). Renal transplantation in light chain nephropathy: case report and review of the literature. *Clinical Nephrology* 25, 101–104.

Glassock, R. J. Crescentic glomerulonephritis. In *Treatment of Primary Glomerulonephritis* (ed. C. Poticelli and R. J. Glassock), pp. 234–254. Oxford: Oxford University Press, 1997.

Gobel, J. *et al.* (1992). Kidney transplantation in Alport's syndrome: long-term outcome and allograft anti-GBM nephritis. *Clinical Nephrology* 38 (6), 299–304.

Godfrin, Y. *et al.* (1997). Study of the *in vitro* effect on glomerular albumin permselectivity of serum before and after renal transplantation in focal segmental glomerulosclerosis. *Transplantation* 64, 1711–1715.

Hammoud, H. et al. (1996). Glomerular disease during HCV infection in renal transplantation. Nephrology, Dialysis, Transplantation 11 (Suppl. 4), 54–55.

Hariharan, S., Adams, M. B., Brennan, D. C., and Davis, C. L. (1999). Recurrent and de novo glomerular disease after renal transplantation: a report from Renal Allograft Disease Registry (RADR). Transplantation 68, 635–641.

Hariharan, S. et al. (1996). Diabetic nephropathy after renal transplantation. Transplantation 62, 632–635.

Hariharan, S. et al. (1998). Recurrent and de novo renal diseases after renal transplantation: a report from the renal allograft disease registry. American Journal of Kidney Diseases 31 (6), 928–931.

Hartmann, A. et al. (1992). Fifteen years' experience with renal transplantation in systemic amyloidosis. Transplant International 5 (1), 15–18.

Heering, P. et al. (1989). Renal transplantation in amyloid nephropathy. International Urology and Nephrology 21 (3), 339–347.

Hoyer, J. R. et al. (1972). Recurrence of idiopathic nephrotic syndrome after renal transplantation Lancet II, 344–448.

Ingulli, E. and Tejani, A. (1991). Incidence, treatment, and outcome of recurrent focal segmental glomerulosclerosis post-transplantation in 42 allografts in children—a single-center experience. Transplantation 51, 401–405.

Ismail-Allouch, M. et al. (1993). Rapidly progressive focal segmental glomeruloclerosis occurring in a living related kidney transplant donor. Case report and review of 21 cases of kidney transplants for primary FSGS. Transplantation Proceedings 25, 2176–2177.

Kashtan, C. E. et al. (1995). Renal allograft survival according to primary diagnosis: a report of the North American Pediatric Renal Transplant Cooperative Study. Pediatric Nephrology 9, 679–684.

Kawaguchi, H. et al. (1994). Recurrence of focal glomerulosclerosis of allografts in children: the efficacy of intensive plasma exchange therapy before and after renal transplantation. Transplantation Proceedings 26, 7–8.

Kessler, M. et al. (1996). Recurrence of immunoglobulin A nephropathy after renal transplantation in the cyclosporine era. American Journal of Kidney Diseases 28, 99–104.

Kessler, M. et al. (1999). A renal allograft recipient with late recurrence of focal and segmental glomerulosclerosis after switching from cyclosporin to tacrolimus. Transplantation 76, 641–643.

Kotanko, P., Pusey, C. D., and Levy, J. B. (1997). Recurrent glomerulonephritis following renal transplantation. Transplantation 63, 1045–1052.

Lai, K. N. et al. (1991). Membranous nephropathy related to hepatitis B virus. New England Journal of Medicine 324, 1457–1463.

Lanfer, J. et al. (1988). Plasma exchange for recurrent nephrotic syndrome following renal transplantation. Transplantation 46, 540–542.

Levy, M. and Charpentier, B. (1983). De novo membranous glomerulonephritis in renal allografts: report of 19 cases in 1550 transplant recipients. Transplantation Proceedings 15, 1099–1101.

Lim, E. and Terasaki, P. I. (1992). High survival rate of kidney transplants in IgA nephropathy patients. Clinical Transplantation 6, 100–105.

Livneh, A. et al. (1992). Colchicine prevents kidney transplant amyloidosis in familial Mediterranean fever. Nephron 60, 418–422.

MacCauley, J. et al. (1993). FK506 in the management of nephrotic syndrome after renal transplantation. Transplantation Proceedings 25, 1351–1354.

Marcen, R. et al. (1996). Membranous nephropathy: recurrence after kidney transplantation. Nephrology, Dialysis, Transplantation 11, 1129–1133.

Meulders, Q. et al. (1994). Course of Henoch–Schönlein nephritis after renal transplantation. Report on ten patients and review of the literature. Transplantation 58 (11), 1179–1186.

Miles, A. M. V. et al. (1998). Diabetes mellitus after renal transplantation. Transplantation 65, 380–384.

Miller, R. B. et al. (1997). Recurrence of haemolytic uraemic syndrome in renal transplants: a single-centre report. Nephrology, Dialysis, Transplantation 12, 1425–1430.

Morales, J. M., Martinez, M. A., and Munoz de Bustillo, E. (1997a). Recurrent type III membranoproliferative glomerulonephritis after kidney transplantation. Transplantation 63, 1186–1188.

Morales, J. M. et al. (1997b). Membranous glomerulonephritis associated with hepatitis C virus infection in renal transplant recipients. Transplantation 63, 1634–1639.

Mourad, G., Djamali, A., Turc-Baron, C., and Cristol, J. P. (1998). Lipoprotein glomerulopathy: a new cause of nephrotic syndrome after renal transplantation. Nephrology, Dialysis, Transplantation 13, 1292–1294.

Mowry, J. et al. (1993). Treatment of recurrent focal segmental glomerulosclerosis with high dose cyclosporine A and plasmapheresis. Transplantation Proceedings 25, 1345–1346.

Nachman, P. H., Segelmark, M., Westman, K., and Hogan, S. L. (1999). Recurrent ANCA-associated small vessel vasculitis after transplantation: a pooled analysis. Kidney International 56, 1544–1550.

Najarian, J. S. et al. (1979). Ten year experience with renal transplantation in juvenile onset diabetes. Annals of Surgery 197, 487–500.

Nast, C. C., Ward, H. J., Koyle, M. A., and Cohen, A. H. (1987). Recurrent Henoch–Schönlein purpura following renal transplantation. American Journal of Kidney Diseases 9, 39–43.

Odorico, J. S. et al. (1996). The influence of native nephrectomy on the incidence of recurrent disease following renal transplantation for primary glomerulonephritis. Transplantation 61 (2), 228–234.

Odum, J. et al. (1994). Recurrent mesangial IgA nephritis following renal transplantation. Nephrology, Dialysis, Transplantation 9, 309–312.

Omacht, C. et al. (1997). Recurrent immunoglobulin A nephropathy after renal transplantation. Transplantation 64, 1493–1496.

Palanichamy, V., Saffarian, N., Jones, B., and Nakhleh, R. E. (1998). Fibrillary glomerulonephritis in a renal allograft. American Journal of Kidney Diseases 32, E4.

Pham, H. P. et al. (1998). Effects of ribavirin on hepatitis C-associated nephrotic syndrome in four liver transplant recipients. Kidney International 54, 1311–1319.

Ponticelli, C. et al. (2001). Kidney transplantation in patients with IgA mesangial glomerulonephritis. Kidney International 60, 1948–1954.

Pronovost, P. H., Brady, H. R., Gunning, M. E., and Espinoza, O. (1996). Clinical features, predictors of disease progression and results of renal transplantation in fibrillary/immunotactoid glomerulopathy. Nephrology, Dialysis, Transplantation 11, 837–842.

Ramos, E. and Tisher, C. C. (1994). Recurrent disease in kidney transplant. American Journal of Kidney Diseases 24, 142–154.

Ranchin, B. et al. (1996). Value of cyclosporine in the treatment of the recurrence of nephrosis after renal transplantation. Nephrologie 17 (8), 441–445.

Richardson, D. et al. (1996). The successful conversion to tacrolimus (FK506) of a renal transplant recipient with. Cyclosporin induced haemolytic uraemic syndrome. Nephrology, Dialysis, Transplantation 11, 2498–2500.

Rizzoni, G. et al. (1991). Combined report on regular dialysis and transplantation of children in Europe, 1990. Nephrology, Dialysis, Transplantation 6, 31–42.

Roth, D. et al. (1995). De novo membranoproliferative glomerulonephritis in hepatitis C virus-infected renal allograft recipients. Transplantation 59, 1676–1682.

Savin, V. et al. (1996). Circulating factor associated with increased glomerular permeability to albumin in recurrent focal segmental glomerulosclerosis. New England Journal of Medicine 334, 878–883.

Schwarz, A., Krause, P. H., Offermann, G., and Keller, F. (1994). Impact of de novo membranous glomerulonephritis on the clinical course after kidney transplantation. Transplantation 58, 650–654.

Shen, S. Y., Hall-Craggs, M., Posner, J. N., and Shabazz, B. (1986). Recurrent sarcoid granulomatous nephritis and reactive tuberculin skin test in a renal transplant recipient. American Journal of Medicine 80, 699–702.

Shimizu, T. et al. (1998). Recurrence of membranoproliferative glomerulonephritis in renal allografts. Transplantation Proceedings 30, 3910–3913.

Stephanian, E. et al. (1992). Recurrence of disease in patients retransplanted for focal segmental glomerulosclerosis. Transplantation 53, 755–757.

Stone, J. H., Amend, W. J., and Criswell, L. A. (1997). Outcome of renal transplantation in systemic lupus erythematosus. Seminars in Arthritis and Rheumatism 27, 17–26.

Stone, J. H., Millward, C. L., Olson, J. L., and Amend, W. J. (1998). Frequency of recurrent lupus nephritis among ninety-seven renal transplant patients during the cyclosporine era. *Arthritis and Rheumatism* **41**, 678–686.

Striegel, J. E. *et al.* (1986). Recurrence of focal segmental sclerosis in children following renal transplantation. *Kidney International* **19**, S44–S50.

Srivasta, R. N. *et al.* (1994). Prompt remission of post-renal transplant nephrotic syndrome with high-dose cyclosporine. *Pediatric Nephrology* **8**, 94–95.

Tarantino, A. *et al.* (1994). Renal replacement therapy in cryoglobulinaemic nephritis. *Nephrology, Dialysis, Transplantation* **9**, 1426–1430.

Tejani, A. and Stablein, D. H. (1992). Recurrence of focal segmental glomeruosclerosis posttransplantation: a special report of the North American Pediatric Renal Transplant Cooperative Study. *Journal of the American Society of Nephrology* **2** (Suppl. 2), S258–S263.

Winn, M. P. *et al.* (1999). Focal segmental glomerulosclerosis: a need for caution in live-related renal transplantation. *American Journal of Kidney Diseases* **33**, 970–974.

Yoshikawa, N. *et al.* (1994). IgG-associated primary glomerulonephritis in children. *Clinical Nephrology* **42**, 281–287.

13.3.5 Outcome of renal transplantation*

Brian Junor

Introduction

Patient and graft survival in renal transplantation have improved considerably over the last 20 years. In recent years, however, the rate of improvement has inevitably diminished and analysis of factors, which may change the outcome, has become more difficult. With a 1 year graft survival of 87 per cent, a study, for example, of a new immunosuppressive agent, would require patient numbers of more than 1000 to be able to demonstrate a statistically significant improvement to 90 per cent. This size of study is now beyond the organizational and resource capabilities of most companies, let alone individual units and would also require standardization of the other features of management. As success rates have improved, studies have had to rely more on secondary markers such as the number of acute rejection episodes.

The problem is compounded further when looking at factors affecting the outcome at 5 years, 10 years, and beyond. Such studies now depend on the large Transplant Registries, as single centre studies are not powerful enough to prove the significance of a small difference in survival rate.

Live donor transplantation

HLA matching

Since the first successful renal transplant performed between identical twins by Merrill and his colleagues in 1954 (Murray *et al.* 1958), the

---

* In this chapter graft loss includes death with a functioning graft unless otherwise specified.

use of kidneys from genetically related live donors has become firmly established. The closer the genetic relationship, the more successful is the subsequent outcome. Of 41 transplants between monozygotic twins reported to the European Dialysis and Transplant Registry in 1981 (Kramer *et al.* 1982), none had been lost due to rejection and 21 of the recipients were not receiving immunosuppression.

All studies of the results of living related donor transplantation have confirmed the specially privileged position of the graft from an HLA identical sibling. One-year patient and graft survival rates were over 90 per cent using azathioprine and steroids but Opelz (1989) reported an improved graft survival at 95 per cent at 3 years with the introduction of cyclosporin. The most striking advantage of the HLA identical sibling graft appears to be in the longer term with a 5 year graft survival of 87 per cent (Cecka 1998) and a half life (calculated from those surviving to the end of the first year) ranging from 19.1 to 26.5 years for patients transplanted between 1971 and 1986, compared to parental donor grafts in the same time period of 9.3–11.8 years (Cho and Terasaki 1998). However, the half-life for HLA identical sibling grafts carried out between 1991 and 1997 is essentially unchanged at an estimated 24.8 years (Cecka 1998).

With one haplotype sibling or parental donors, the graft success rate is less with a 5 year survival rate of 75 per cent and a half-life of 13.9 years (Cecka 1998). The results for siblings with no shared haplotype were indistinguishable from those with one shared haplotype in this UNOS Registry Report. It was also noted in this report that the graft survival rates and half-lives of these HLA mismatched family members were superior to zero mismatched cadaver grafts, but this may have been influenced by the selection process and the age of the recipients. With more distant relatives who have a much lower chance of sharing antigens, the 5 year success rate was 75 per cent with an estimated half-life of 14.8 years. The figures were essentially identical for unrelated live donor transplants, mostly from spouses, which were carried out in the same time period (Cecka 1998).

Numbers of live donor transplants

The results from recent live donor transplants of all types in the United States in 1997 and 1998 remain highly encouraging with a 94.5 per cent 1 year graft survival and a 97.6 per cent patient survival (UNOS Report 2000). For live donor transplants in the United Kingdom in 1996–1997, the 2 year graft survival rate was 92 per cent (UKT 2001). These success rates of live donor transplantation, with the lack of evidence of significant harm to donors and falling cadaver donor rates in many countries, have led to an increase in the numbers of live donor grafts performed. In the United States in 1990, 22 per cent of recipients received live donor grafts compared to 36 per cent in 1999 and in Australia, the rise was from 9.1 per cent in 1985 to 36.9 per cent in 1999 and in the United Kingdom from 5 per cent in 1990 to 21 per cent in 2001. The figures are all approaching the 38.3 per cent achieved in Norway of an overall transplant rate of 45.9 per million of the population in 1998, similar to the United States (48.4 pmp in 1998) but much higher than either Australia (28 pmp in 2000) or the United Kingdom (30.5 pmp in 2001).

Delayed graft function and rejection

Delayed graft function is uncommon in live donor transplants but the incidence has fallen from 10.2 per cent (1980–1984) to 3 per cent (1995–1999) for first grafts and from 18.2 to 7 per cent for re-grafts

(ANZ Registry 2000). The ANZ Registry Report of 2001 records a statistically greater chance of rejection in the first 3 months in first living donor transplants, compared to first cadaver transplants despite the better short- and long-term survival of living donor transplants.

Pre-emptive live donor transplantation

Live donor transplantation before dialysis avoids the need for access surgery and the possible adverse effects of dialysis. In 1999, 19 per cent of live donor transplants were pre-emptive in Australia (ANZ Report 2001) while it had been previously reported that the figure for the United States was approximately 25 per cent (Mange *et al.* 1998). The graft survival of pre-emptive live donor transplantation has been reported in two large series from the Collaborative Transplant Study and the USRDS (Donnelly *et al.* 1996; Mange *et al.* 2001) to be superior to live donor transplantation after the initiation of dialysis. A previous study in cadaver grafts had suggested a lower incidence of delayed graft function and acute rejection in patients transplanted within 6 months of starting dialysis compared to those transplanted after longer periods of dialysis. In the USRDS study (Mange *et al.* 2001), there was a significant increase in the risk of rejection within the first 6 months with increasing duration of dialysis compared to the pre-emptive transplant group. There was a 52 per cent reduction in the risk of allograft failure in the first year of transplantation in the pre-emptive group but this increased to 82 per cent in the second year and 86 per cent in the third year. The increasing difference over the first 3 years post-transplant was also seen in the earlier collaborative transplant study (Donnelly *et al.* 1996) without any obvious explanation. Wherever possible, it appears appropriate to recommend pre-emptive live donor transplantation, principally for patient benefit in terms of the excellent results, but also for the reduced pressure on dialysis facilities.

Cadaver donor transplantation

First cadaver grafts

There has been a striking improvement in both patient and graft survival since the early days of cadaver renal transplantation. Results from the ERA–EDTA Registry demonstrate a progressive improvement of both patient and graft survival in 5 year cohorts of first cadaver grafts between 1980 and 1999 (van Dijk *et al.* 2001). A similar improvement has been seen since 1984 in graft survival in the United Kingdom (Fig. 1) but the difference has essentially occurred in the first year after transplantation. Inevitably, the annual improvements in 1 year survival rates have diminished with 1 year survival for grafts in 1996–1997 being 85 per cent and patient survival 96 per cent. Corresponding figures for the UNOS Registry for the same time period for graft survival were 89.4 per cent and for grafts carried out in Australia in 1999 the patient survival was 95 per cent and graft survival 90 per cent. The greatest improvement in graft survival has been in the first 3 months post-transplant as is evident in Fig. 2, which shows the percentage of grafts failing at different time periods in the first year since 1981. The major change occurred in the mid-1980s with the more widespread use of cyclosporin in the United Kingdom.

Graft survival beyond 1 year has only shown a modest improvement in the last two decades (Fig. 3). In Australia, the annual graft loss in relation to grafts at risk was constant between 1996 and 2000 at

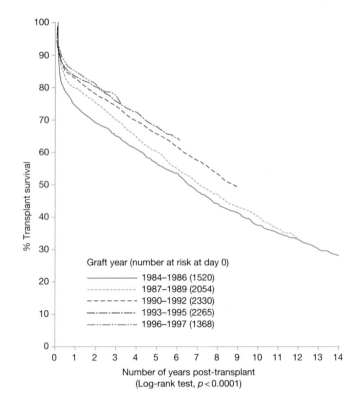

Fig. 1 Long-term transplant survival after first adult cadaveric kidney only transplant, 1 January 1984–31 December 1997, by graft year. Reproduced by permission of UK Transplant.

5.5 per cent, with an equal loss in 2000 from graft failure and from death of a function graft (ANZ Registry 2001).

The graft survival rate beyond 5 years for both first cadaver and living donor transplants has not changed in Australia between 1970 and 1994 (Fig. 4). The longer term pattern of graft survival for this combined group shows an expediential decay out to 25 years (Fig. 5). In the ANZ Registry Report of 2001, there has been a small improvement in the annual death rate beyond 5 years from 3.7 per cent per year (1970–1974) to 3.3 per cent per year in the cohort since 1985.

Second and subsequent grafts

Second and subsequent renal allografts pose particular problems including the risk of sensitization from the first graft. This may require closer matching and more than 25 per cent of multiple re-grafted patients in the UNOS Database had no HLA antigens mismatched (Cecka 1998). This normally means a longer wait for a suitable kidney. The success rate of second grafts has improved even more dramatically than those of primary grafts with 5 year survival curves identical for first and second grafts in the United Kingdom between 1990 and 1997 (Fig. 6). The half-life of second grafts in the UNOS Database was 9.3 years compared to 9.5 years for first grafts (Cecka 1998).

Success rates for third and subsequent grafts are poorer but the difference appears to be established within the first year after transplantation (Fig. 6). Due to the increased risk of rejection occurring despite better tissue matching, most transplant units adopt a more intensive immunosuppressive protocol for second and subsequent grafts.

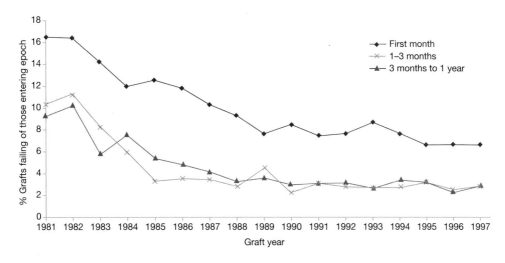

Fig. 2 Graft failures occurring in each epoch as a percentage of the grafts entering the epoch for each year, 1 January 1981–31 December 1997. Reproduced by permission of UK Transplant.

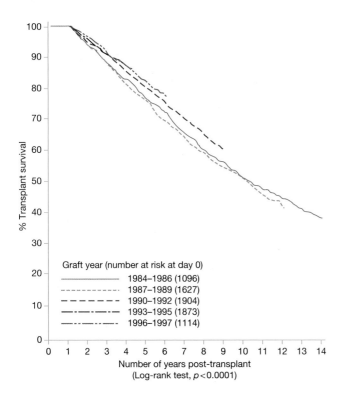

Fig. 3 Long-term transplant survival for those adult recipients having survived the first year after their first cadaveric kidney only transplant, by graft year. Reproduced by permission of UK Transplant.

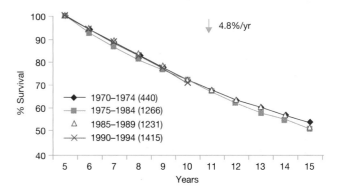

Fig. 4 Australia primary cadaver and living donor graft survival beyond five years; the decline is the same in each selected time period. Reproduced by permission of ANZDATA Registry.

Factors affecting outcome of transplantation

Factors affecting outcome can be divided into those related to the donor, those related to the recipient and those influenced by features involving both donor and recipient. Many of these factors such as age, sex, and cause of death of donors cannot be influenced while others such as matching for age, tissue typing, and immunosuppression can be altered.

Donor factors

Age

The age of the donor has a clear effect on the 5 year graft survival in the United Kingdom as shown in Fig. 7 with the best results coming from donors in the 18–34 age group and a progressive decline in survival with increasing donor age. Paediatric donors under the age of 11 show a different pattern from the other age groups suggesting that once the technical problems of using small kidneys are overcome, these grafts are very successful in the long term. A similar pattern was seen in the UNOS Registry Report with a half-life of cadaver grafts progressively shortening from 11.2 years for donors aged 19–30 years to 5.3 years for those over the age of 60 years (Cecka 1998).

The age of donors has increased in all Registries. The median age in Australia increased from 38.5 years in 1996 to 44.1 years in 2000 (ANZ Registry 2001). The percentage of donors over the age of 50 years increased from 16.2 per cent in 1990 to 30.1 per cent in 1999 in the United States (UNOS Report 2000) and from 29 to 33 per cent from 1990 to 1998 in the United Kingdom (UKT 2001). Cecka (1998)

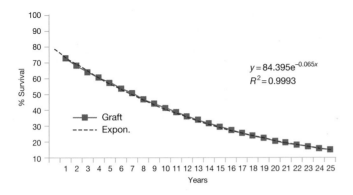

Fig. 5 Primary cadaver and living donor graft survival; Australia 1970–1994 ($n = 7623$); the decay is exponential. Reproduced by permission of ANZDATA Registry.

In the figure: $y = 84.395e^{-0.065x}$, $R^2 = 0.9993$

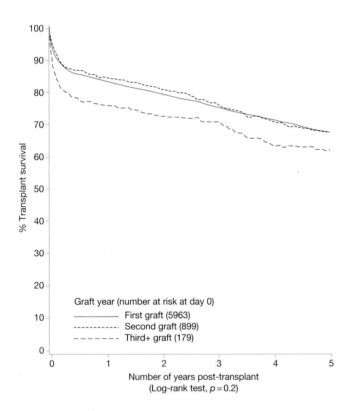

Fig. 6 Five year transplant survival after adult cadaveric kidney only transplant, 1 January 1990–31 December 1997, by graft number. Reproduced by permission of UK Transplant.

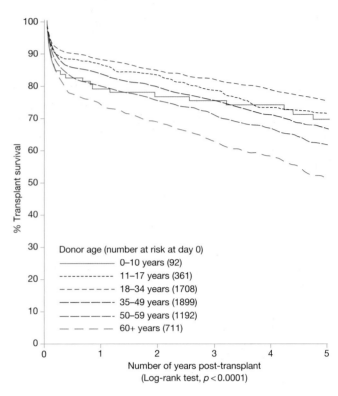

Fig. 7 Five year transplant survival after first adult cadaveric kidney only transplant, 1 January 1990–31 December 1997, by donor age. Reproduced by permission of UK Transplant.

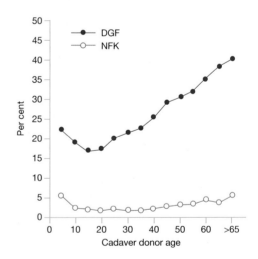

Fig. 8 Incidence of delayed graft function (DGF) and primary non-function (NFK) with age. Reproduced by permission of J.M. Cecka for the UNOS Registry.

reported an increase in the incidence of both delayed graft function and primary non-function with increasing age of the donor as shown in Fig. 8.

Sex

A number of reports have suggested a poorer graft survival rate in male recipients of kidneys from female donors. It has been thought that this might be due to a functionally inadequate supply of nephrons

but under these circumstances, graft failures might be expected to occur late rather than early in the post-transplant period. In a single centre study in New York, Neugarten *et al.* (1996) found no difference in precyclosporin results between recipients of male and female donor kidneys but a difference was present in cyclosporin-treated patients. The difference occurred within the first 24 months and the rate of graft loss thereafter was the same. The authors suggested the pattern might be related to susceptibility to the effect of cyclosporin.

Cause of death

In Australia in 2000, a cerebral vascular accident was the cause of death in 78 per cent of the donors aged more than or equal to 55 years, whereas trauma accounted for 64 per cent of all deaths in the 15–34 age group. When age was taken into account, there was no statistically significant difference in graft survival between traumatic and non-traumatic death in transplants performed in the United Kingdom between 1990 and 1997. This suggests that it is the age rather than the cause of death that has produced the differences noted in the past.

Heart beating and non-heart-beating donors

To try to compensate for the reduction in donors whose death has been confirmed by brain stem testing several transplanting units in the United Kingdom and Europe have introduced a non-heart-beating donor programme. Although comparable results have been reported by individual units (Wijnen et al. 1995; Balapuri et al. 2001; Metcalfe et al. 2001), the composite results from the United Kingdom from 1990 to 1997 show a 1 year graft survival of 72 per cent in asystolic donors compared to 84 per cent for donors whose death had been confirmed by brain stem tests. The subsequent failure rate was very similar for the two groups.

Cold ischaemia

Longer cold ischaemic times lead to an increasing incidence of delayed graft function from 17 per cent for kidneys grafted within 12 h to 35 per cent when the ischaemia time extends to 49–72 h. The effect is accentuated in older donors with delayed graft function occurring in 34 per cent of kidneys from donors over the age of 60 years even when transplanted within 12 h (Cecka 1998).

The movement of kidneys from one centre to another to achieve a better degree of tissue matching inevitably contributes to longer cold ischaemic times. Analysis of UK data showed a significant detrimental effect (relative risk 1.45) of exchanging kidneys but only in the first 3 months following transplantation (UKT 2001). Thereafter, the rate of graft loss appeared identical. As the difference in early graft survival between well and poorly tissue matched kidneys is now relatively small, this has lead to discussion about the value of moving kidneys to better-matched recipients. As the current analysis includes locally transplanted well-matched kidneys, further analysis is required to compare the longer term survival of well-matched exchanged kidneys against poorly matched transplants carried out locally.

Recipient factors

Age

Although UK Transplant Data shows recipients of first cadaver grafts aged more than 60 years to have a significantly poorer graft survival than recipients in the age group of 18–34 years, this effect is solely due to the deaths of recipients with functioning grafts (UKT 2001). In the United States, the half-life for grafts in recipients over the age of 60 years was 7.7 years compared to 10.2 years in the 31–45 age group,

while the patient survival half lives are 29.4 years for recipients aged 31–45 compared to 9.7 years for those aged over 60.

When deaths were censored, there was a highly significantly reduced risk of graft loss for recipients over the age of 50 years in the ANZ Registry Report 2001 consistent with a hypothesis of a less competent immune system in older transplant recipients. A similar finding has been reported for UK Transplant recipients with a decreasing risk of 1 year graft failure up to the age of 60 years when censored for technical failure and death with a functioning graft (Bradley 2000).

Diagnosis

In the UNOS Annual Report for 2000, there was only a 4 per cent variation in the 1 year graft survival for patients with different primary renal diseases ranging from 88.2 per cent for diabetes to 92.2 for those with polycystic disease of the kidneys. By 5 years, the differences have widened with the survival being less than 60 per cent for those with diabetes, hypertensive nephrosclerosis and renovascular disease compared to 74.8 for those with polycystic disease. Patients with glomerular disease, tubular and interstitial disease, and congenital, familial, and metabolic disease were also found to have better 5 year graft survival with figures between 65 and 70 per cent. UK Transplant Data (2001) show less than 10 per cent 1 year graft survival difference between diabetics and non-diabetics but the difference increases over the next 4 years.

Dialysis

An analysis was carried out in the ANZ Registry Report of 2000 of the incidence of delayed graft function according to the mode of dialysis prior to transplantation in more than 2500 recipients. There was a 23 per cent incidence of delayed graft function in patients receiving haemodialysis compared to 12 per cent in those on peritoneal dialysis. Although the effect could be due to a better intravascular volume status, there may be confounding factors such as age and degree of sensitization.

Body mass index

Obesity increases the risk of both mortality and morbidity in most surgical procedures (Pasulka et al. 1986) and this has been confirmed in renal transplantation (Holley et al. 1990). Modlin et al. (1997) recommended that all potential transplant recipients with a body mass index (BMI) of greater than 30 should lose weight before transplantation but those with a cardiac history should not be transplanted until this BMI was achieved. A multi-centre review confirmed the increased risks of obesity but also demonstrated an increased risk of both graft loss and death with a functioning graft for those with a low BMI (Meier-Kiresche et al. 2002). Howard et al. (2002) found no increased risk with a BMI of greater than or equal to 30, compared to groups with BMIs of greater than or equal to 25 to less than 30 and less than 25 and suggested that even if obese patients did have a poorer outcome, they should not be considered differently from other high-risk patients such as diabetics, multiple graft recipients, those with high panel reactive antibodies (PRA) and the elderly.

Antibody status

The presence of PRA tends to increase the delay in finding a graft with a negative cross match and also increases the risk of rejection and graft loss. The 1 year graft survival for cadaver transplants in 1997–1998 reported by UNOS was 89.8 per cent for PRA levels of 0–19 per cent, 85.4 per cent for 20–79 per cent, and 84.2 per cent for more than 80 per cent (UNOS Report 2000). Beyond the first year, Cecka (1998) reported the UNOS Database to show half lives of 9.7 years for 0–10 per cent PRA, 8.7 years for 11–50 per cent and 8.8 years for greater than 50 per cent showing a slightly accelerated rate for later graft loss for broadly sensitized patients.

Blood transfusion

The literature on the magnitude and mechanism of the effect of blood transfusion on renal transplantation remains confusing. During the 1960s, attempts were made to limit blood transfusion in patients on transplant waiting lists to reduce the risk of HLA sensitization. Opelz *et al.* (1973) showed that pretransplant blood transfusion produced a marked improvement in graft survival. This work was confirmed by other studies and led to transplant centres adopting a policy of deliberate blood transfusion, usually up to 5 units. Following the introduction of cyclosporin, Albrechtsen *et al.* (1988) suspended routine blood transfusion and found no significant difference in 1 year graft survival between transfused and non-transfused patients. Larger studies still showed a beneficial effect of transfusion in cyclosporin-treated patients but to a much smaller degree. Opelz (1989) found only a 5 per cent difference in cyclosporin-treated patients compared to a previous difference of 20 per cent but he also reported that the difference in azathioprine-treated patients had fallen to 5 per cent.

Many different mechanisms have been suggested for the effect of blood transfusion on renal allograft survival but none has been unequivocally established. One theory, discounted by Opelz *et al.* in 1981, was the negative selection of patients who developed cytotoxic antibodies in response to blood transfusion. This could virtually exclude 'reactive' patients from transplantation and necessitate better-matched grafts for others. Opelz *et al.* (1981) felt that this could not explain the magnitude of the effect seen at that time but as the difference is now small this could be an explanation. Donor-specific transfusion was reported by Salvatierra *et al.* (1980) to be beneficial in improving 1 year graft survival rates in live donor transplantation but they found that 30 per cent of patients developed cytotoxic antibodies to the potential donor and were unable to be transplanted.

In practice, most units have now abandoned elective blood transfusion protocols with either third party or donor-specific blood and have returned to the policy of the 1960s. There is now the added factor that transfusion for symptoms of anaemia are less frequently required with the availability of erythropoietin.

Factors involving both donor and recipient

Delayed graft function

Both delayed graft function and the level of function obtained have been consistently shown to affect graft survival. Cecka (1998) reported from the UNOS Registry a half-life of 8.9 years for recipients of grafts from 19 to 30-year-olds when function was delayed compared to 11.9 years for those with immediate function. This effect was also evident in a 10 per cent difference in graft survival at 9 years in patients

transplanted in Australia between 1990 and 1999 (ANZ Registry 2001). However, when the delayed graft function group was divided into those requiring dialysis for more or less than 7 days, there was no adverse effect on outcome in the latter patients.

The incidence of delayed graft function in Australia in 1999 and in the patients reported to UNOS in the first 6 months of 2000 was 24 per cent with an incidence of 42 per cent for re-grafts in the ANZ Database. Delayed graft function is more common in re-grafts, recipients with high levels of PRA, with increasing ischaemic time, older donors, and those with impaired renal function at the time of organ retrieval. It may also be more common in haemodialysis than peritoneal dialysis patients. Delayed graft function has a significant adverse effect on 12 month serum creatinine, whether the delayed function is short or prolonged, with mean creatinine values of immediately functioning grafts being 141 μmol/l compared to 158 μmol/l when function was delayed less than 7 days and 188 μmol/l for longer than 7 days (ANZ Registry 2000).

Level of function

The serum creatinine on discharge from hospital is a strong predictor for graft survival. With impaired function (creatinine 2.6–4.5 mg/dl), the 5 year graft survival was around 60 per cent whether the kidney was from a cadaver or living donor. For creatinine values of less than 1.5 mg/dl, the half-life for cadaver donor kidneys was 11.5 years and for living donor grafts, 17.2 years (Cecka 1998).

HLA matching

Following the recognition of antigens on the leucocyte and their subsequent classification, attempts were made to correlate the results of related donor transplants with the degree of matching for HLA-A and B loci. The first large series showed a 6-month graft survival of 96 per cent for HLA identical sibling grafts compared to 68 per cent survival for mismatched grafts suggesting that although matching for these antigens improved results it was not mandatory for graft survival (Singal *et al.* 1969). When similar attempts were made to assess the outcome of cadaveric grafts in relation to HLA-A and B matching, the results were less clear. An initial large-scale study failed to show any significant improvement in graft survival with matching (Opelz and Terasaki 1982), but later studies revealed a small but significant beneficial effect of 10 per cent when comparing 0 antigen mismatched with 4 antigen mismatched grafts (Bashir and d'Apice 1982).

With the introduction of HLA-DR typing, closer matching between donor and recipient became possible. However, with the availability of more powerful immunosuppressants, the differences in the early graft survival related to matching have diminished and there is no universal agreement on the benefits of HLA matching on 1 and 2 year graft survival. In the UK Transplant Audit (2001), the results of non-favourably matched (>2 HLA-A or B mismatches) were significantly worse than either 000 mismatched or favourably matched grafts at 3 months but, in later epochs, there was no significant difference.

In the larger UNOS Database, the 5 year graft survival rates decreased in a stepwise fashion from 69 per cent for HLA matched grafts to 57 per cent for completely mismatched grafts but only a few percentage points separated the individual mismatched levels. The graft half-lives also declined with each additional HLA antigen mismatch from 12.7 years for 0 mismatched grafts to 8.0 years for completely mismatched grafts.

Immunosuppression

Considerable differences of opinion exist on the importance of HLA matching but there is even greater variation in views on the best form of immunosuppression both in the short and long term. Immunosuppressive agents are discussed in Chapter 13 but it is remarkable that despite the differences in the usage of monoclonal antibodies, other induction agents, cyclosporin or tacrolimus, azathioprine or mycophenolate and rapamycin and steroids, the 1 year graft success rates for different transplant units in Australia, Europe, and North America are very similar.

The long-term results of different immunosuppressive protocols are more difficult to establish but may in time reflect a reduction in acute rejection seen with more recent drugs. However, this has to be balanced against the likely increased risks of death from infection and malignancy with increased immunosuppression.

Concern about long-term nephrotoxicity demonstrated by graft loss beyond 5 years at 5.3 per cent per year for patients on cyclosporin compared to 3.8 per cent per year for those not on cyclosporin (ANZ Registry Report 2001) has led to studies of conversion from cyclosporin to azathioprine during the first year after transplant. Serum creatinine and urate levels tended to fall in those successfully converted and blood pressure control improved but there were variable results in relation to graft survival (Pedersen *et al.* 1993; Ponticelli *et al.* 1996, 1997; McPhee *et al.* 1998).

The desire to avoid steroid toxicity has led to attempts to withdraw steroids at intervals from 3 months to many years after transplantation. Although steroid withdrawal is successful in the majority of patients, some require re-introduction of steroids due to a loss in graft function with the concern that late rejection leads to progressive deterioration (Almond *et al.* 1993). In a retrospective uncontrolled study of more than 12,000 renal graft recipients initially treated with cyclosporin, Azathioprine, and steroids, Opelz (1995) found a significantly increased graft and patient survival in patients changed to a steroid-free regime. Caution must be observed, however, in interpretation of these results due to the nature of the study and the bias introduced by 'successful' as opposed to 'unsuccessful' withdrawal of steroids. With the increasing number and combinations of immunosuppressive drugs and the inevitable long-term nature and size of studies of chronic allograft loss, it will be extremely difficult to determine the optimum long-term immunosuppression for individual patients. The goal must be the minimum immunosuppression consistent with avoidance of rejection. Both the 'immunological status' and 'immunological challenge' are different for each individual and their graft. An older patient receiving a HLA identical graft is less likely to reject the transplant than a young patient with a completely mismatched graft and, therefore, different levels of immunosuppression are appropriate but are not catered for in many protocols. The ultimate aim must be to tailor the immunosuppressive regime to match the risk of rejection but, at present, there is no suitable test to establish the correct management.

Rejection

With the advances in immunosuppression, early acute rejection has occurred less frequently and is a less common cause of early graft failure. Early graft rejection, before hospital discharge, occurred in 16 per cent of more than 40,000 cadaver transplants in the UNOS Database leading to a 10 per cent reduction in the 5 year graft survival rate. A similar reduction in 5 year graft survival was seen in 13 per cent of live donor transplants experiencing early rejection (Cecka 1998). The number of acute rejections has a marked effect on long-term graft survival. Massey *et al.* (1995) reported a 10 year survival free from chronic rejection of 54 per cent in patients with more than one rejection episode compared to 88 per cent for one acute rejection episode and 96 per cent if there was no episode of acute rejection. Other studies have suggested that a single early acute rejection does not affect graft survival, but there is agreement that late rejection carries a poor prognosis for graft function. Acute rejection can occur even beyond 10 years after transplantation (Rao *et al.* 1989; Shoker *et al.* 1994) and long-term graft survival is not synonymous with a graft tolerance.

Late graft failure often referred to as chronic rejection, increased 24 per cent in the ANZ Registry (2001) from a failure rate of 2.69 grafts per 100 graft years in 1970–1984 to a rate of 3.35 in 1985–1994. As many late graft failures do not appear to be immunologically based as there is little response to immunosuppressive manipulation, and because the aetiology of these graft failures is uncertain, it is best referred to as chronic allograft dysfunction.

An important, but often neglected, element of graft loss is patient compliance. Lack of compliance was observed by Didlake *et al.* (1988) in all patients who lost their grafts more than 3 years after transplantation.

Viral infections

The effect of cytomegalovirus (CMV) infection on graft and patient survival remains unclear. A small but significantly better graft survival was previously noted in UK Transplant Data when the donor was CMV negative with the difference being established by 100 days after transplant. However, in a later audit, donor or recipient status did not influence the 5 year survival although the data were incomplete (UKT 2001). CMV infection has been noted coincident with acute rejection (Rubin 1989). Humar *et al.* (1999) found the impact of CMV infection on long-term graft survival to be only associated with acute rejection. Trials of antiviral prophylaxis in the prevention of long-term graft loss remain inconclusive.

More recently, polyoma virus infection has been associated with chronic graft dysfunction (Mylonakis *et al.* 2001). Further studies are required to evaluate the contribution of viral infections to this syndrome, as treatment usually requires a reduction in immunosuppression.

Death with a functioning graft

For patients to die with a functioning graft is the aim of all transplant units but the challenge is to prevent that death being premature. Both pre- and post-transplant management must be addressed to attempt to achieve this aim. Satisfactory control of hypertension and the calcium/phosphate product are required before as well as during dialysis treatment to prevent irreversible damage. The contribution of lipid control remains uncertain partly due to the poor survival of patients who are undernourished and have low cholesterol levels.

In the first 4 weeks, cardiac-related causes were responsible for 39 per cent of deaths in the United Kingdom but infection became the most common cause at 39 per cent of deaths between 4 weeks and 1 year. Thereafter, malignancy accounted for 13 per cent and cardiac causes 21 per cent of the deaths (UKT 2001). In the ANZ Registry (2001), only 1 per cent of the causes of death were not reported compared to 34 per cent in the United Kingdom. In 2000, 29 per cent of deaths in patients with a functioning graft were due to cardiac causes, 16 from infection, and 27 from malignancy.

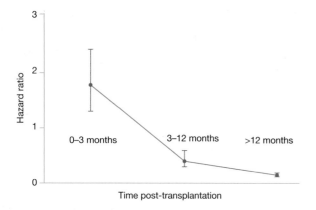

Fig. 9 Hazard ratios for transplant recipients (relative to dialysis = 1.0). Reproduced by permission of ANZDATA Registry.

Comparison of transplantation with dialysis

Quality of life

The popular concept is of a vast improvement in the quality of life following renal transplantation but this is not always confirmed by subjective measurement with patients with a failed transplant doing particularly badly. In a study comparing the quality of life of recipients of organs from non-heart-beating donors with those from conventional cadaver donors, live donors, and patients remaining on the waiting list, Metcalfe *et al.* (2001) found no difference between the transplant recipients and all were better than those on the waiting list.

Studies of sexual function in transplant recipients have all suggested an improvement following transplantation. The clearest indication is the ability to have successful pregnancies compared to dialysis (Geerlings *et al.* 1991).

Survival

Comparisons of survival between transplant recipients and patients remaining on the waiting list are subject to problems including bias but where tissue typing is used to allocate kidneys the process is similar to randomization. Wolfe *et al.* (1999) found a long-term relative risk of dying of 0.32 beyond 12 months for transplant recipients compared to those on the waiting list but in the post-operative period the relative risk increased to 2.8. The change in the hazard ratio with time in the ANZ Database (2001) is shown in Fig. 9. An early increased risk of death from infection is replaced by an improved long-term survival compared to patients remaining on dialysis.

References

Albrechtsen, D. *et al.* Impact of blood transfusion and HLA matching on national kidney transplant programs; the Swedish–Norwegian study of cyclosporine. In *Cyclosporine: Therapeutics in Transplantation* (ed. B. D. Kahan), pp. 257–260. Orlando: Grune and Stratton, 1988.

Almond, P. S. *et al.* (1993). Risk factors for chronic rejection in renal allograft recipients. *Transplantation* **55**, 752–756.

ANZDATA Registry Report (2000). Australia and New Zealand Dialysis and Transplant Registry. Adelaide, South Australia.

ANZDATA Registry Report (2001). Australia and New Zealand Dialysis and Transplant Registry. Adelaide, South Australia.

Balapuri, S. *et al.* (2001). Machine perfusion and viability assessment of non-heart beating donor kidneys—a single-centre result. *Transplantation Proceedings* **33**, 1119–1120.

Bashir, H. V. and d'Apice, A. (1982). Cadaver renal transplantation and HLA matching in Australia from 1971 to 1980. *Transplantation* **34**, 183–189.

Bradley, B. A. (2000). Does the risk of acute rejection really decrease with increasing recipient age? *Transplantation International* **13** (Suppl. 1), S42–S44.

Cecka, J. M. The UNOS Scientific Renal Transplant Registry. In *Clinical Transplants 1998* (ed. J. M. Cecka and P. M. Terasaki), pp. 1–16. Los Angeles: UCLA Tissue Typing Laboratory, 1998.

Cho, Y. W. and Terasaki, P. I. Long term survival. In *Clinical Transplants 1988* (ed. P. M. Terasaki), pp. 277–282. Los Angeles: UCLA Tissue Typing Laboratory, 1998.

Didlake, R. H. *et al.* (1988). Patient non-compliance: a major cause of late graft failure in cyclosporine-treated renal transplants. *Transplantation Proceedings* **20** (Suppl. 3), S63–S69.

Donnelly, P. *et al.* (1996). Living donor kidney transplantation in predialysis patients; experience of marginal donors in Europe and the United States. *Transplantation Proceedings* **28**, 3566–3570.

Geerlings, W. *et al.* (1991). Combined report on regular dialysis and transplantation in Europe, XXI, 1990. *Nephrology, Dialysis, Transplantation* **6** (Suppl. 4), S5–S29.

Holley, J. L. *et al.* (1990). Obesity as a risk factor following cadaveric renal transplantation. *Transplantation* **49**, 387–389.

Howard, R. J. *et al.* (2002). Obesity does not portend a bad outcome for kidney transplant recipients. *Transplantation* **73**, 53–55.

Humar, A. *et al.* (1999). Association between cytomegalovirus disease and chronic rejection in kidney transplant recipients. *Transplantation* **68**, 1879–1883.

Kramer, P. *et al.* (1982). Combined report on regular dialysis and transplantation in Europe, XII, 1981. Proceedings of the European Dialysis and Transplant Association—European Renal Association, pp. 4–59.

Mange, K. C., Joffe, M., and Feldman, H. I. (1998). Pre-emptive living donor kidney transplantation in the United States. *Journal of the American Society of Nephrology* **9** (Suppl.), 686A.

Mange, K. C., Marshall, M. J., and Feldman, H. I. (2001). Effect of the use or nonuse of long-term dialysis on the subsequent survival of renal transplants from living donors. *New England Journal of Medicine* **344**, 726–731.

Massey, Z. A., Guijarro, C., and Kasiske, B. L. (1995). Clinical predictors of chronic renal allograft rejection. *Kidney International* **48** (Suppl. 52), S85–S88.

McPhee, I. A. M. *et al.* (1998). Long-term outcome of a prospective randomised controlled trial of conversion from cyclosporine to azathioprine treatment one year after renal transplantation. *Transplantation* **66**, 1186–1192.

Meier-Kriesche, H., Arndorfer, J. A., and Kaplan, B. (2002). The impact of body mass index on renal transplant outcomes: a significant independent risk factor for graft failure and patient death. *Transplantation* **73**, 70–74.

Metcalfe, M. S. *et al.* (2001). A case–control comparison of the results of renal transplantation from heart-beating and non-heart-beating donors. *Transplantation* **71**, 1556–1559.

Modlin, C. S. *et al.* (1997). Should obese patients lose weight before receiving a kidney transplant? *Transplantation* **64**, 599–604.

Murray, J. E., Merrill, J. P., and Harrison, J. H. (1958). Kidney transplantation between seven pairs of identical twins. *Annals of Surgery* **148**, 343–359.

Mylonakis, E. *et al.* (2001). BK virus in solid organ transplant recipients: an emerging syndrome. *Transplantation* **72**, 1587–1592.

Neugarten, J. *et al.* (1996). The effect of donor gender on renal allograft survival. *Journal of the American Society of Nephrology* **7** (2), 318–324.

Opelz, G. (1989). The role of HLA matching and blood transfusion in the cyclosporin era. *Transplantation Proceedings* **21**, 609–612.

Opelz, G. (1995). For the Collaborative Transplant Study. Effect of maintenance immunosuppressive drug regimen on kidney transplant outcome. *Transplantation* **58**, 443–446.

Opelz, G. and Terasaki, P. L. (1982). International study of histocompatibility in renal transplantation. *Transplantation* **33**, 87–95.

Opelz, G., Graver, O., and Terasaki, P. I. (1981). Induction of high kidney graft survival rate by multiple transfusions. *Lancet* **1**, 1223–1225.

Opelz, G. et al. (1973). Effect of blood transfusion on subsequent kidney transplants. *Transplantation Proceedings* **5**, 252–259.

Pasulka, P. S. et al. (1986). The risks of surgery in obese patients. *Annals of Internal Medicine* **104**, 540–546.

Pedersen, E. B. et al. (1993). Long-term survival after conversion from cyclosporin to azathioprine 1 year after renal transplantation: a prospective randomised study from 1 to 6 years after transplantation. *Nephrology, Dialysis, Transplantation* **8**, 250–254.

Ponticelli, C. et al. (1996). Randomized study with cyclosporine in kidney transplantation: 10 year follow-up. *Journal of the American Society of Nephrology* **7**, 792–797.

Ponticelli, C. et al. (1997). A randomised study comparing three cyclosporine-based regimens in renal transplantation. *Journal of the American Society of Nephrology* **8**, 638–646.

Rao, K. V., Kasiske, B. L., and Bloom, P. M. (1989). Acute graft rejection in the late survivors of renal transplantation. *Transplantation* **47**, 290–292.

Rubin, R. H. (1989). The indirect effect of cytomegalovirus infection on the outcome of renal transplantation. *Journal of the American Medical Association* **261**, 3607–3609.

Salvatierra, O. et al. (1980). Deliberate donor specific blood transfusion prior to living related renal transplantation. A new approach. *Annals of Surgery* **192**, 543–552.

Shoker, A. S. et al. (1994). Can acute cellular rejection occur 27 years after a successful renal transplant? *Transplantation* **58**, 1131–1133.

Singal, D. P., Mickey, M. R., and Terasaki, P. I. (1969). Serotyping for homo-transplantaion, XXIII. Analysis of kidney transplants from parental versus sibling donors. *Transplantation* **7**, 246–258.

U.K. Transplant. Renal Transplant Audit 1990–1998 (2001). UK Transplant, Bristol.

UNOS Annual Report (2000) (http://www.unos.org/Data/anrpt00/ar00).

Van Dijk, P. C. W. et al. (2001). Renal replacement therapy in Europe: the results of a collaborative effort by the ERA–EDTA registry and six national or regional registries. *Nephrology, Dialysis, Transplantation* **16**, 1120–1129.

Wijnen, R. M. et al. (1995). Outcome of transplantation of non-heart-beating donors. *Lancet* **345**, 1067–1070.

Wolfe, R. A. et al. (1999). Comparison of mortality in all patients on dialysis, patients on dialysis awaiting transplantation, and recipients of a first cadaveric transplant. *New England Journal of Medicine* **341**, 1725–1730.

14

Specific problems in chronic renal insufficiency

14.1 Chronic renal failure in children

Uwe Querfeld

Introduction

This chapter reviews the clinical aspects of chronic renal failure (CRF), dialysis, and transplantation that are of special relevance to children and adolescents, that is, the age group of 0–18 years. The period of life from birth to the completion of puberty is characterized by growth and development; if these fundamental processes are disturbed by chronic illness, it becomes evident that children are not 'small adults', but instead, have specific clinical problems which vary with the age of the patient. Medical and psychosocial care for children and adolescents with endstage renal disease (ESRD) is demanding and requires considerable investments of human and financial resources.

Biochemical abnormalities, diminished linear growth, and hormonal disturbances may become noticeable in children with a glomerular filtration rate (GFR) less than 60 ml/min/1.73 m^2. However, in slowly progressive diseases (e.g. juvenile nephronophthisis, oligomeganephronia, and others) patients may remain asymptomatic until more severe stages of renal impairment have been reached. The terms 'mild renal insufficiency' and 'moderate renal insufficiency' have been used for a GFR in the range of 25–50 and 10–25 per cent of normal, respectively. A more uniform classification of chronic kidney disease (CKD), including five clinical stages based on GFR, has been introduced in the United States for adult patients. Since this classification has not been officially adopted by paediatric nephrology guidelines, the traditional term CRF is used throughout this chapter. Usually ESRD is reached at GFR of less than 5 per cent (<3–5 ml/min/1.73 m^2); at this stage of renal function, life becomes dependent on renal replacement therapy (RRT) in the form of dialysis or transplantation.

Incidence

The true incidence of CRF in children is unknown and can only be indirectly estimated by calculating the incidence rates for ESRD. However, not all children may reach ESRD—because of intermittent complications and/or insufficient treatment—and dialysis and transplantation may not be offered to all children with CRF, due to various ethical, cultural, or economic circumstances.

Data regarding the incidence of ESRD in children have been collected by national and international registries. In Germany, the prevalence of ESRD in 1996 was 11 (children under the age of 18 treated with any form of RRT) per million population (p.m.p.) (Frei and Schober-Halstenberg 1999). The annual incidence of ESRD (defined as start of RRT) in the same year was 1.7 p.m.p., which was only a fraction of that seen in adults (156 p.m.p.). The prevalence of

RRT in children was similarly only a very small portion of the adult population (713 p.m.p.). To make national data more comparable, international registries have expressed incidence rates in per million *child* population (p.m.c.p.). In Europe, the annual incidence in children under the age of 15 in 1990 was 2.8 p.m.c.p. (Ehrich *et al.* 1992) and in 1995, 5.4 p.m.c.p. (Vanrenterghem and Jones 1996). Reported *averaged* incidence rates should be regarded with caution; they may be very different from national incidence rates and may not truly reflect morbidity from ESRD because of differences in medical care and access to RRT. In addition, these data are biased by gross underreporting (Mehls *et al.* 1996). In the United States, annual incidence rates adjusted for age, race, and sex, average 10–12 p.m.c.p. in patients aged 0–19 years (USRDS 1993) and have remained stable over many years (Wassner and Baum 2002).

The European Dialysis and Transplant Association (EDTA) registry, which has started data collection on paediatric ESRD patients in 1970, reported a steady increase in paediatric patients admitted to RRT over more than 25 years. The relative proportion of very young patients (<2 years) has increased almost 80-fold and that of children aged 2–5 years 15-fold, whereas the proportion of patients aged 10–14 years decreased from 75 to 51 per cent (Loirat *et al.* 1994). It is, therefore, not surprising that the spectrum of underlying renal diseases has changed over the years, with the most frequent diseases now being obstructive uropathy/renal hypoplasia/dysplasia (36 per cent), followed by glomerulopathies (26 per cent) and hereditary nephropathies (16.3 per cent) (Loirat *et al.* 1994). If congenital and hereditary diseases are grouped together, these entities account for 41.5 per cent of ESRD cases in the North American Pediatric Renal Transplant Cooperative Study (NAPRTCS) database and 19.1 per cent and 22.2 per cent in the United States and Canadian national registries, respectively (Wassner and Baum 2002). In the United States and Canadian registries, congenital and hereditary diseases were exceeded by glomerular diseases, which accounted for 37.6 and 23.5 per cent of the total. Nevertheless, these two groups of diseases make up the bulk of the total of underlying diagnoses, and this is in contrast to the adult population, where diabetic nephropathy and chronic glomerulonephritis are by far the most frequent causes of ESRD.

Approach to the child with chronic renal failure

Today, most children with CRF in countries with 'high-tech' medical care are referred by other medical services. In infants, cystic kidneys, obstructed kidneys or other malformations are frequently detected *in utero*. Older children are usually seen on a routine basis by paediatricians in private practice and these should work in close collaboration with paediatric facilities for RRT to avoid delayed referral. Nevertheless, CRF is still occasionally discovered by accident in children and adolescents admitted for reasons other than renal disease. If it is not immediately apparent whether a child has renal failure of longer or shorter duration or is in acute renal failure, the following findings point to the presence of CRF: sonographic renal abnormalities (e.g. hypoplasia/dysplasia, but not hyperechogenicity, which may be present in acute renal failure), anaemia, renal osteodystrophy [increased parathyroid hormone (PTH), radiological bone disease], growth failure, pubertal delay, and secondary effects of hypertension, for example, left ventricular hypertrophy, arterial changes on fundoscopy.

Where possible, a *renal biopsy* should be performed to establish the histological diagnosis and to allow for a better prognostic estimate of disease progression.

An approach to the paediatric patient with CRF is essentially an approach to a family with a lifetime problem. It takes skill and experience to deal with this situation especially when CRF is first discovered and the consequences of renal failure are explained to the child and/or the parents. These discussions which will eventually transform the lives of a whole family need to be conducted by an experienced clinician. One should be prepared for very specific questions regarding practical details of dialysis and the overall prognosis of the child. If the facility is not equipped with dialysis and transplantation modalities for children, a neighbouring paediatric centre for the treatment for ESRD should be consulted. It is common experience that a family will consult other doctors for treatment alternatives and it is very important that trust and confidence are maintained from the beginning. It is imperative to document the *'family background'*, including details of parental care and responsibilities, school attendance, as well as legal, financial, and ethical considerations.

History

In a child with CRF, the following questions are relevant. Is there a family history of renal disease (any form), are there family members treated with dialysis or transplantation? Has the child experienced changes in appetite, behaviour, activity, weight gain, growth? What is the normal frequency of voiding, and have there been changes? How much does the child drink during the day and night (families count in terms of bottles and cans, not in metric units)? Is incontinence, bedwetting (primary, secondary enuresis) or nocturia present? Additional questions concerning sexual development (menarche, sexually transmitted disease) and use of 'recreational drugs' should be asked if the patient is an adolescent. Medications taken must be documented.

Physical examination

The physical examination should document any malformations and other disturbances (e.g. visual or auditory), movement disorders and muscular tone, skeletal abnormalities, signs of anaemia, and cardiac insufficiency. It should state the level of cooperation in very young children (if difficult to examine) and in handicapped patients. It must always include the systolic and diastolic blood pressure (measured on both arms). A 24 h ambulatory blood pressure measurement (ABPM) should always be performed as a baseline assessment of blood pressure, and it may surprisingly show nocturnal hypertension in seemingly normotensive patients and normotensive 24 h profiles in children with 'white coat hypertension'.

Measurements of *height* will yield drastically false results if no attention is paid to detail. In view of the importance of an early diagnosis of growth retardation in CRF, it is inexcusable to use data reported by parents or to have the child measured with a yardstick or tape by inexperienced staff. The height of a child is properly measured with the patient in standing position (except in infants) with the help of a stadiometer. The headboard of the stadiometer is lowered and gentle upward pressure under the mastoids is applied to minimize diurnal varations in height which can amount to as much as 2 cm. In patients unable to stand, height is measured with the help of an assistant on a supine-length table and in infants with a neonatometer. Measurements should always be plotted on a percentile chart for follow-up and future comparison.

Weight should be measured with the patient nude or with a minimum of clothing (underwear, no shoes, and socks) on a scale with 0.1 kg precision, preferably an electronic scale. Younger children need attendance and older children and adolescents need observation. Self-reported weights should not be trusted. In infants, baby scales have to be used. The time of measurement (preferably in the morning) and relation to dialysis (before/after) should be recorded.

Head circumference is measured with a flexible metric tape as the maximum head circumference, which shows good reproducibility if the mean of three measurements is taken.

Skinfold measurements performed with skinfold calipers measure subcutaneous fat and can be used to estimate total body fat. Skinfolds yielding good reproducibility of measurements are found in the subscapular and triceps area (midpoint between acromion and olecranon). Measured at the same location, the upper arm circumference provides an estimate of muscle mass.

The *pubertal stage* should be assessed in adolescents according to Tanner (1962); in girls by stages of breast and pubic hair development and in boys by genital and pubic hair development. Most paediatric text books contain graphic illustrations of typical developmental stages for comparison. Testicular size should be estimated by palpation of each testis and comparison with the size of wooden or plastic beads of known volume (orchidometer). The volume before puberty is usually less than 3 ml; this increases to 12–25 ml during adolescents. Standard charts are available (Zachmann *et al.* 1974). The time of menarche if present should be recorded and girls should be asked about irregularities of the menstrual cycle.

Bone age is evaluated (in 12 months intervals in growing children) by X-ray of the hand and wrist. Especially infants and preschool children should be assessed for neurological and developmental milestones.

Special clinical and therapeutic aspects of chronic renal failure in children
Failure to thrive and malnutrition

CRF resembles a state of malnutrition. Previous work by Holliday and Chantler has shown that dramatic decreases in weight, height, head circumference, midarm muscle circumference, body fat mass, and other anthropometric parameters are frequently observed in children with CRF compared to healthy controls (Holliday 1973; Chantler *et al.* 1974). Children with CRF have a low spontaneous calorie intake, perhaps favoured by altered taste sensation (Shapera *et al.* 1986). Abdominal distension by ascites or peritoneal dialysis fluid, gastric reflux, dysphagia, and behavioural problems are other known contributing factors. It is important to note that longitudinal growth is slowed if the energy intake is less than 80 per cent of the recommended dietary allowance (RDA; Arnold *et al.* 1983). Increasing energy intake from this level results in a temporary increase in growth velocity; however, increasing energy intake to levels greater than 100 per cent of the RDA is not associated with additional benefit (Wassner *et al.* 1986).

It is one of the most challenging tasks to assure adequate nutritional intake in children with CRF. There are several issues involved here: (1) the prescription of an adequate diet by the physician, (2) the monitoring of nutrition by parents and caretakers, and (3) the feeding of the child.

1. In healthy children the RDA in an infant is about 100 kcal/kg and in a 5-year old it is 70 kcal/kg; it further decreases to about 40 kcal/kg in adolescents. Prescribing 100 per cent of the RDA, which is derived from the mean intake of healthy children of the same age, may seriously underestimate the needed caloric intake, especially if the child is in fact malnourished. Therefore, the dietary intake of children with CRF should be approximately 100 per cent of the RDA *for height age* and may be further increased if malnutrition is present (Nelson and Stover 2002; Wassner and Baum 2002). The term height age refers to the mean age corresponding to the patient's measured height, as derived from growth charts for the particular population. Infants with CRF should receive at least 100 kcal/kg and may require additional calories (up to 140 kcal/kg) during periods of recovery. Infants are usually fed with formulas containing fixed amounts of total energy, protein, carbohydrates, and fats as well as essential amino acid supplements. In addition, energy supplements are frequently necessary and can be added in the form of glucose polymers ('Polycose', 'Maltodextrin'), medium chain triglyceride oil (MCT oil), or unsaturated vegetable oil.

Older children eat solid foods varying in nutritional content and develop individual eating patterns, sometimes dominated by 'junk food'. These patients and their families need to be educated and trained to establish healthier lifestyles.

It is essential to provide enough *protein* for the growing child and dietary prescriptions are focused on protein requirements which have to be adjusted to the degree of renal dysfunction and to protein losses, for example, in patients treated with peritoneal dialysis. In infants, protein requirements are highest and usually met by breast feeding and later by cow-milk-based formulas. Healthy infants need about 2.2 g/kg during the first 6 months and 1.6 g/kg later on (Wassner and Baum 2002) and this amount should be given to infants with mild to moderate CRF. Protein intake can be slightly less in the predialysis stage (1.2–1.6 g/kg) to prevent azotaemia if the child continues to thrive and total energy intake is sufficient. However, if the infant is placed on peritoneal dialysis, protein requirements will increase dramatically and 3–4 g/kg is recommended, sometimes necessitating the use of protein supplements ('Promix', 'Protifar') (Nelson and Stover 2002). Protein supplements are also required in infants and young children (but usually not in older children) with the nephrotic syndrome. In infants with congenital or infantile nephrotic syndrome, protein losses are enormous and cannot be sufficiently replaced; these

children require unilateral or bilateral nephrectomy to assure growth and development (Holmberg *et al.* 1996; Licht *et al.* 2000). In older children, protein requirements correspond to the RDA for height age, but again, are increased in the situation of peritoneal dialysis (1.5–3 g/kg).

Cow-milk-based formulas are usually sufficient to supply protein as well as *sodium* in adequate amounts. However, children with salt-wasting and infants on peritoneal dialysis require sodium supplements that may be as high as 10 mEq/kg/day (and more). In the predialytic and dialytic stage, the *phosphorus* content of cow-milk-based formula is too high; low phosphate formulas ('PM 60/40', 'SMA', 'Renamil') should be used. However, hyperphosphataemia usually cannot be avoided at this stage of renal insufficiency, necessitating treatment with phosphate binders. *Potassium* intake also has to be limited in pre-terminal renal failure and on dialysis, since more than 1–2 mmol/kg daily can result in hyperkalaemia. Potassium intake may be dangerously high in infants fed formula and in older children eating fruits and 'junk food', necessitating routine application of potassium exchange resins ('Sorbisterit', 'Kayexalate'). In addition, *calcium supplements* are frequently needed to correct overt osteopenia and hypocalcaemia. Substitution of water-soluble *vitamins*, usually given as multivitamin preparations once daily, has been recommended (Nelson and Stover 2002). Unfortunately, few data are available documenting the efficacy of these medications in children. While vitamin contents of most food items seem sufficient not to warrant vitamin substitution in CRF, this may well be indicated on dialysis. At any rate, vitamin A-containing preparations should be avoided to prevent vitamin A toxicity; levels are usually high in children with CRF (Warady *et al.* 1994). In view of the frequent presence of hyperhomocysteinaemia, treatment with *folic acid* and *B-vitamins* seems indicated, but therapeutic guidelines have not been established in children. Metabolic acidosis, which can contribute to growth failure, should be corrected by *bicarbonate* supplements, which can be given in soluble form (1 mEq/ml) to children fed formula.

2. In addition, prescribed caloric intake has to be *monitored*. This is best achieved by 3-day *dietary protocols* recorded by the caretaker of the child during average weekdays. In practice, instructions of the caretaker and evaluation of these protocols should be performed by a dietitian experienced in translating brand names and quantities of foods recorded into caloric equivalents. The dietary intake of energy, protein, carbohydrate, and fat as well as the calcium and phosphate contents of this regime are calculated, usually at monthly intervals in patients with CRF and on dialysis. Besides weight and height, specialized centres now record sets of *anthropometric parameters* which may better reflect nutritional state, including measurements of longitudinal and transversal diameters, skin folds, body fat content, and muscular strength (Zivicnjak *et al.* 2000). The most important parameter for monitoring preschool children and especially infants is the *head circumference*. Head growth in infants is a sensitive parameter corresponding to brain size and intellectual development. Microcephaly is seen with malnutrition, but may also develop independently in syndromal conditions and after ischaemic brain injury, for example asphyxia at birth. Since intellectual development is essential for rehabilitation and quality of life the overall prognosis of such infants is problematic even if renal function is not much impaired. If microcephaly develops in a dialysed infant with adequate nutrition (e.g. after renal failure at birth associated with asphyxia), it usually indicates a dismal prognosis.

3. Many infants with CRF do not have a sufficient spontaneous oral intake to meet dietary requirements. Parents and caretakers often report difficulties with feeding and frequent vomiting. For the physician, it is all-important to carefully observe that the child will continue to grow. Infants with CRF need to be seen at least once a month, and weight, height, and head circumference should be plotted on a percentile chart. If deviations from the percentile curve occur and/or dietary and feeding difficulties seem to persist, feeding by *nasogastric, nasojejunal* or *gastrostomy tube* should be considered (Behrens *et al.* 1997). Other authors have reported favourable experiences with a gastrostomy button device (Watson *et al.* 1992). Although parents may initially be opposed to the idea, tube feeding often results in much relief of the anxiety surrounding the futile feeding attempts, which may appear in the form of a battle between mother and child that may consume most of the day. Results of tube feeding are often dramatic, and even catch-up growth has been reported (Claris-Appiani *et al.* 1995). We prefer feeding by nasogastric or gastrostomy tube at night with continuation of oral feeding during the day to continue oral stimulation. Nevertheless, many children further decrease their oral intake and have to be fed completely by tube. Some children later regain normal eating patterns whereas others need the help of feeding clinics (DelloStrologo *et al.* 1997). Gastrostomies may spontaneously close after renal transplantation but sometimes have to be closed by surgery. If conservative therapy and tube feeding does not result in adequate weight gain, therapy with growth hormone (GH), which at this age may mainly be effective as an anabolic hormone, may be considered (Maxwell and Rees 1996).

Remarkably, Proesmans's group has reported a contrasting experience, observing acceptable growth rates in children with CRF and on dialysis with the use of behavioural feeding therapy with strict conservative treatment (without tube feeding or GH) over a period of 3 years (Van Dyck *et al.* 1999).

Neurological and developmental problems

About 50 per cent of postnatal brain growth occurs in the first year of life, making this period especially vulnerable for irreversible brain damage. Adequate nutrition is, therefore, critical and even short-term malnutrition can be catastrophic. Head circumference is closely associated with brain development. Early reports of children with CRF with onset in infancy have described a high prevalence of microcephaly, brain atrophy, seizures, and mental retardation (Rotundo *et al.* 1982; McGraw and Haka-Ikse 1985). Onset of CRF in the first year of life carries the greatest risk for neurological impairment and deterioration of cognitive function has been documented in this age group (Bock *et al.* 1989).

Although malnutrition may be the most important specific factor in infants with CRF, the following conditions (alone or in combination) may at any age contribute to the impairment of neurological function: hypertensive encephalopathy, drug-induced encephalopathy, electrolyte imbalances (water intoxication, hypocalcaemia, acidaemia), aluminium encephalopathy, central nervous system (CNS) infections, and pre-existing neuropsychiatric disorders such as seizure disorders, CNS vasculitis, and behavioural problems (Polinsky 1996).

Newborns

In 1987, a review of published reports on a total of 85 patients with severe CRF from infancy showed that microcephaly and developmental delay were present in 65 and 63 per cent, respectively, and that motor and language developmental delay was most pronounced. Surprisingly, neither prevalence nor severity of developmental delay was correlated with age and severity of CRF at the time of diagnosis (Polinsky *et al.* 1987). However, these results, reflecting a 'learning experience' with treatment of CRF in infancy, may have been influenced by various factors, specifically varying degrees of aggressiveness in the treatment of malnutrition, anaemia, and hyperparathyroidism. Furthermore, the use of aluminium-containing phosphate binders was prevalent, which is now banned in children. It should be noted that recent reports have shown a much more encouraging picture (Elzouki *et al.* 1994). In 1999, Warady and colleagues published a review of 34 infants with ESRD treated with a combination of aggressive nutrition, dialysis and transplantation, and strict avoidance of aluminium-containing phosphate binders. At 1 year of age, 28 patients had a mean head circumference standard deviation score (SDS) of -0.96 ± 1.2. The mental developmental score of 22 (79 per cent) patients fell in the average range, while only 1 (4 per cent) child was significantly delayed. Of 19 children retested at not less than 4 years of age, 15 (79 per cent) performed in the average range. Of 16 patients, not less than 5 years of age, 15 (94 per cent) attended school full time and in age-appropriate classrooms (Warady *et al.* 1999). Neurological development in infants and young children with CRF should be monitored at least every 6 months by a paediatric neurologist; examinations include head ultrasound, developmental milestones, and reflex patterns.

Aluminium

Importantly, the dismal results of treatment outcomes in infants with ESRD reported in early observations included many infants treated with aluminium-containing phosphate binders (Rotundo *et al.* 1982). Several reports have clearly linked the use of these preparations to the occurrence of a progressive encephalopathy; elevated aluminium concentrations were found in serum, bone, and brain.

If urinary excretion is absent, progressive accumulation of aluminium occurs mainly in the cortical grey matter. By interfering with brain energy metabolism and neurotransmitter synthesis, aluminium leads to a characteristic encephalopathy with seizures, abnormal motor function, and microcephaly, and with progression, to deterioration of intellectual and motor development and ultimately to a chronic vegetative state with brain atrophy (Polinsky 1996). If suspected, aluminium overload may best be diagnosed by bone biopsy (Norris *et al.* 1986). High serum levels and the presence of microcytic anaemia may be further indicators, but are much less reliable. Mobilization of stored aluminium by intravenous (IV) desferrioxamine test dose (suspected high aluminium burden) may result in redistribution and neurological deterioration (Van Landeghem *et al.* 1997), and chelation therapy with IV desferrioxamine is fraught with the risk of allergic reactions, ocular and auditory toxicity, as well as exotic infections. Alternatively, desferrioxamine can be given intraperitoneally in peritoneal dialysis (PD) patients (Andreoli and Cohen 1989).

In view of these serious iatrogenic effects, avoidance of all aluminium-containing medications in children with CRF is essential. Traces of aluminium may also be present in infant formulas (especially if soybean-based), parenteral nutrition, and dialysis solutions and these preparations should likewise not be used. Intestinal aluminium resorption is facilitated by ingestion of citrate, iron deficiency, 1,25 vitamin D3 and hyperparathyroidism (Polinsky 1996).

Older children and adolescents

In older children with CRF and ESRD, *cognitive function adjusted to age, gender, and parental education* was shown to be within normal limits, but vigilance and memory were impaired, suggesting an attention deficit (Polinsky 1996). Newer methods can discriminate subtle changes in cognitive and motor abilities, but the picture is not uniform (Zivicnjak *et al.* 2001).

The clinical experience indicates that in contrast to adults, *uraemic peripheral neuropathy* is apparently rare in children. Although studies have shown delayed nerve conduction in children with CRF, undergoing dialysis, and after transplantation (de Beaufort *et al.* 1989), these findings do not seem to correspond to clinical symptoms. Most centres, therefore, have abandoned nerve conduction velocity testing in children since this procedure is painful. Other neurological problems include nocturnal muscle cramps, restless legs, and paraesthesias which are frequently seen in haemodialysis (HD) patients and often correspond to periods of electrolyte imbalances.

Muscle weakness is probably underdiagnosed in children with CRF. It should be noted that it often coexists with vitamin D deficiency; overt myopathy with immobilization may be observed if vitamin D is not presribed or not given by the caretakers in children with ESRD. However, myopathy (as part of the affected 'bone muscle unit') may be present in a less dramatic form as decreased muscle strength (Tenbrock *et al.* 2000). A specific distal *vacuolar myopathy* has been described in children with nephropathic cystinosis (Charnas *et al.* 1994; Vester *et al.* 2000). Children experience their environment by crawling, running, climbing, jumping, etc.—muscle strength is, therefore, a factor contributing to normal motor and psychosocial development. Sports and gymnastics should by all means be encouraged in children with CRF to facilitate this development (exceptions include boxing and other 'heavy contact' sports as well as swimming in public pools for PD patients).

Seizures may occur at any stage of CRF. They may indicate a coexisting neurological disorder (involvement of the CNS by syndromal conditions), CNS infection, a hypertensive crisis, biochemical imbalances (hypocalcaemia, hyponatraemia, hypomagnesaemia, aluminium intoxication), uraemic encephalopathy, and pseudotumour cerebri (incidence increased in CRF). Seizures are also part of the dialysis disequilibrium syndrome.

Developmental delay is often serious in children with syndromal conditions involving the brain or the cranial nerves. For instance, CRF may be associated with blindness, deafness, microcephaly, or other neurological problems. In a single centre study of medical and psychosocial rehabilitation of adults with childhood-onset ESRD, we found disabilities in 37 per cent of patients, in all but two consisting of some degree of visual and auditory impairment (Querfeld *et al.* 1997). A cross-sectional analysis in 151 children with CRF found hearing loss in 47 per cent (Bergstrom and Thompson 1983). Sensoneural hearing loss is often under-reported and hearing aids are often not used because of the fear of stigmatization by other children. Being 'handicapped' adds additional insults to the fragile self-esteem, especially of adolescents.

Growth

Normal growth

In assessing growth it is important to document all properly taken measurements of height by plotting measurements on a growth chart referring to the normal population of children with the same genetic background. Normal variation of growth in this population is depicted on these charts as percentiles, with the 50th percentile indicating mean height and the 3rd and 97th percentile indicating approximately 2SD of the mean and, therefore, the statistically defined normal limits of height. Similar percentile charts can be used for other relevant measurements, for example, head circumference, weight, and growth velocity, etc.; the latter is defined as centimetres of height gain per year. Usually, height measurements are plotted in monthly intervals in infants and 3-monthly intervals in older children as dots on these charts, and the line connecting these measurements allows graphical description of growth progression, which is much more informative than single measurements.

The final height of the child is strongly determined by inheritance. A calculation of the *approximate final height* can be performed by the following formula if the heights of both parents are known: (mid-parental height) +10 cm for boys and −2.6 cm for girls (Molinari *et al.* 1985). However, height prediction in children with CRF has a tendency for overprediction (Schaefer *et al.* 1989); predictions may obviously become inaccurate during the course of CRF, for example, due to complications of renal osteodystrophy or steroid therapy after transplantation.

With impaired growth, height and growth velocity eventually fall below normal in periods of chronic illness; the reversal of this process is termed catch-up growth. Full or complete catch-up occurs if acceleration of growth restores height to normal; unfortunately, final height is more often compromised due to incomplete catch-up growth. It is for this reason that early recognition and treatment of growth failure is so important in CRF.

Growth retardation in CRF can be diagnosed if the measured height and/or growth velocity (during the previous year) is below the 3rd percentile of the normal reference population. For comparison, height is best expressed as the SDS of height, defined as

$$\text{Height SDS} = \frac{\text{Height} - \text{mean height for age}}{\text{Standard deviation of height for age}}$$

In a normal population, the SDS by definition ranges between −2 and +2 with a mean of zero and an SD of ±1. This also allows us to express growth by assessing the difference in height SDS between measurements—if growth is accelerated, the difference will be positive. Another problem arises if in a clinical study, for example assessing the effect of GH, children of various ages are recruited. Simply calculating a mean change in height SDS will not sufficiently evaluate the effects of treatment, since growth velocity is different at various ages. Therefore, changes in growth rate are compared by calculating the *SDS for height velocity* in a similar manner as height SDS.

Growth in chronic renal failure

Growth is essential for quality of life and rehabilitation in adulthoood, and growth retardation is, therefore, one of the most important complications of CRF in children, occuring with a prevalence of approximately 40 per cent (Mehls and Scharer 2002). Figure 1 shows the typical picture of untreated growth retardation observed in children with congenital CRF. Relative loss of height occurs dramatically in the first year of life with a decrease to less than the 3rd percentile. Growth then continues approximately parallel to and underneath the 3rd percentile, only to fall off further from this line during puberty resulting in a severely diminished final adult height ('stunting').

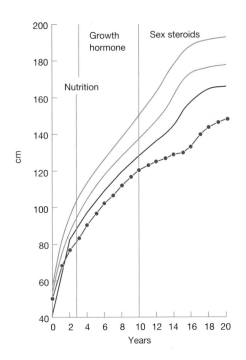

Fig. 1 Typical growth failure in congenital CRF (dotted line) shows distinct abnormalities if not treated with rhGH. Normal growth is represented by the 3rd, 50th, and 97th percentile of height. From Mehls, O., Chantler, C., and Fine, R. N. Chronic renal failure in children. In *Oxford Textbook of Clinical Nephrology* 2nd edn. (ed. A. M. Davison, J. S. Cameron, J.-P. Grünfeld, D. N. S. Kerr, E. Ritz, and C. G. Winearls), pp. 2219–2244. Oxford: Oxford University Press, 1998.

Before the introduction of therapy with recombinant human growth hormone (rhGH), stunting was frequently seen in children with CRF. The EDTA registry has documented a diminished final height in 50 per cent of patients. Boys were more severely affected than girls, and mean final height was lower in patients with congenital renal disorders (Chantler *et al.* 1981). Besides age at onset, the type of underlying renal disease has an effect on growth. Proteinuria is severe in congenital and infantile nephrotic syndrome, and causes protein–energy malnutrition if not adequately replaced; infections and hormonal imbalances due to losses of binding proteins in the urine may further contribute to growth failure. In hereditary tubular disorders (Fanconi syndrome, Bartter's syndrome, cystinosis, etc.), growth impairment may be especially severe (Haffner *et al.* 1999). Other factors contributing to growth retardation are metabolic acidosis, sodium chloride deficiency, disturbed glucose metabolism, anaemia, renal osteodystrophy, and hormonal disturbances.

The work of the Heidelberg group has largely elucidated the pathophysiology of *disturbances of the GH axis* in CRF. GH, is secreted from the anterior pituitary in a pulsatile fashion. In children with CRF, normal or even elevated GH are measured in serum. This is a result of a reduced metabolic clearance of GH by the kidney resulting in a similarly increased half-life in serum (Haffner *et al.* 1994), whereas the secretion of GH is actually low-normal or reduced. Moreover, in puberty, GH secretion normally increases three-fold due to an increase in circulating sex steroid levels. Such an increase is absent in patients with CRF (Schaefer and Mehls 1999). The lack of response to normal or even high circulating GH indicates insensitivity to the actions of GH in peripheral tissues. This hypothesis is further supported by the finding of reduced hepatic GH receptor expression in an animal model of CRF (Tonshoff *et al.* 1994) and decreased GH-binding protein (serum protein derived from the extracellular part of the GH receptor) in children (Tonshoff *et al.* 1997). In addition, a postreceptor defect (impaired signal transduction) has been found in uraemic animals (Schaefer *et al.* 2001).

Not only is the interaction of GH with receptors impaired, but also its metabolic actions. These are mediated by a family of peptides named insulin-like growth factors (IGF); the most important is IGF-I, which is generated in the liver following the GH signal; IGF-I production is low in CRF (Blum *et al.* 1991). It could be demonstrated that CRF causes an imbalance between IGF 1, 2, and 3 and their respective binding proteins (IGFBPs) in serum, which are elevated in CRF due to diminished renal clearance (Tonshoff *et al.* 1995). The net result is diminished bioactivity of IGFs despite normal plasma concentration. Taken together, uraemia produces disturbances in the GH–IGF axis on several distinct levels, resulting in a state of GH resistance.

Disturbances in the gonadal hormone axis may also contribute to growth retardation in CRF. Thus, pubertal patients with CRF derive little benefit from the normal pubertal growth spurt, which is preserved in these patients, but diminished in magnitude and duration, resulting in relatively fast closure of epiphyses. On average, the pubertal growth spurt is delayed by about 2–2.5 years and shortened by about 1.5 years in children with CRF (Schaefer *et al.* 1990). This phenomenon seems to be preserved inspite of treatment with rhGH; regardless of rhGH treatment, pubertal height gain in children with CRF was only 65 per cent of that observed in healthy children (Haffner *et al.* 2000).

Children do not grow well on dialysis. In fact, the majority of children on HD experience further decrease in growth velocity (Fennell *et al.* 1984). There seems to be little, if any, influence of caloric intake or dialysis efficacy on growth on maintenance HD. Theoretically, PD might improve growth, due to better nutrition (little restriction of oral intake, glucose absorption from the dialysate), and some single-centre studies (Stefanidis *et al.* 1983; Fennell *et al.* 1984) indeed found better growth of patients on PD compared to patients on HD. Better growth was found in children switched from HD to PD (Stefanidis *et al.* 1983) and a larger uncontrolled multicentre study could demonstrate stable growth rates in children on PD for at least 6 months (Southwest Pediatric Nephrology Study Group 1985). Unfortunately, however, studies following patients on continuous ambulatory peritoneal dialysis (CAPD)/continuous cyclic peritoneal dialysis (CCPD) for longer periods (Fine and Salusky 1986; Potter *et al.* 1986) found a loss of height SDS, and this was also shown in infants given adequate nutrition (Warady *et al.* 1988).

A contrasting experience has been reported from Finland, where an improvement in height SDS and even catch-up growth could be demonstrated (over 6 and 9 months, respectively) especially in younger children (<5 years) on PD; however, most of these patients had congenital nephrotic syndrome and, therefore, better growth could reflect normalization of protein balance after bilateral nephrectomy (Holtta *et al.* 2000).

Treatment

The first principle of treatment of growth failure in CRF is to assure adequate caloric intake. This is most crucial in the first 2 years of life. Catch-up growth can often be observed if there was pre-existent malnutrition. Unfortunately, catch-up growth is rarely ever seen in later life inspite of adequate nutrition. Other factors contributing to growth retardation (metabolic acidosis, renal osteodystrophy, renal anaemia, protein, and electrolyte losses) should of course be adequately treated.

Second, one should not attempt to delay dialysis by admininistration of low-calorie diets (to avoid high urea concentrations). Concerns about quality of life with dialysis treatment are unwarranted from a medical standpoint, because 'buying time' with low-calorie diets may result in (further) delay of growth and development and eventually in diminished adult height. Instead, it is in the best interest of the patient to start rhGH treatment early (see below), assure good nutrition, and start dialysis whenever necessary; fears that rhGH treatment could result in further loss of renal function have not been substantiated (Tonshoff et al. 1992).

Therapy with rhGH is now the treatment of choice in CRF and on dialysis, regardless of the mode of treatment (PD, HD). In pioneering studies, Mehls et al. showed that long-term administration of porcine and human GH was able to normalize length and weight of uraemic rats, thus proving that uraemic GH resistance can be overcome by supraphysiological GH concentrations (Mehls and Ritz 1983; Mehls et al. 1988). These observations spurred many clinical trials when rhGH became available for use. Controlled and uncontrolled studies in children with CRF uniformly demonstrated the efficacy of this therapy, resulting in catch-up growth and an average height improvement of +2SDS. During the first year of treatment, growth is often dramatic, but the effect seems to be significantly diminished in the following years. This underscores the importance of long-term observations and raises the question of an improvement in final adult height compared to untreated controls. Meanwhile, several studies have reported adult height data (Haffner and Schaefer 2001). The average benefit in final height seems to be 1–1.5 SDS although the range of height gained in these studies only corresponds to between 2 and 10 cm. Untreated children with CRF experience a loss in relative height, which should be added to absolute height gain to fully appreciate the efficacy of rhGH treatment. In a prospective multicentre trial in Germany, mean adult height was 165.2 cm in boys and 156.2 cm in girls in rhGH treated patients and significantly greater than in untreated controls; two-thirds of treated children reached an adult height above the 3rd percentile, but mean adult height was still more than 10 cm below the genetic target height (Haffner et al. 2000).

The success of rhGH treatment is markedly influenced by several important factors such as the degree of renal insufficiency, age, height SDS at the start of treatment, pretreatment height velocity (negative predictors), and the duration of rhGH therapy (positive predictor). A daily subcutaneous dose of 4 IU/m^2 had been recommended and was found to be more efficient than 2 IU/m^2 and equally effective as 8 IU/m^2 (Hokken-Koelega et al. 1994). Unfortunately, rhGH is much less effective in dialysed children, in whom only about 50 per cent of the height gain attained in patients with CRF could be observed during 2 years of treatment (Wuhl et al. 1996). There is still controversy regarding the efficacy of rhGH in pubertal patients and in infants.

Growth failure is especially severe in *nephropathic cystinosis*. In cross-sectional surveys in Europe, mean adult height was 136.5 cm in boys and 124 cm in girls (Broyer et al. 1987) and only few patients reached 150 cm final height (Ehrich et al. 1991). Cystine-depleting agents (cysteamine), if administered from the onset of the disease may prevent growth retardation, but do not achieve catch-up growth. In these patients, long-term rhGH treatment has proven safe and effective and should be started early in the course of the disease if adequate nutrition and cysteamine treatment fail to prevent growth retardation (Wuhl et al. 2001).

Side-effects

Apart from promoting growth, rhGH is an anabolic hormone affecting carbohydrate, lipid, and protein metabolism. Treatment increases insulin secretion, but impaired glucose tolerance in CRF is unchanged during treatment and no cases of irreversible diabetes mellitus have been observed in children with CRF treated with rhGH (Schaefer and Mehls 1999). GH can modulate the metabolism of lipoproteins by affecting both their secretion and uptake by the liver and their catabolism by lipolytic enzymes in plasma. Clinical studies in adults indicate that patients with GH deficiency have atherogenic lipoprotein profiles which are ameliorated by GH administration. However, in children with CRF only modest changes in total plasma lipids and lipoprotein profiles have been observed (Querfeld 1996). In contrast, GH administration results in a significant increase in Lp(a) that does not seem to be mediated by IGF-I but rather by the direct effect of GH on hepatic secretion. In patients with CRF, Lipoprotein(a) [Lp(a)] is frequently elevated and GH administration may lead to a further increase in plasma levels. This highly atherogenic particle should be monitored during rhGH treatment (Querfeld et al. 1996).

The most important side-effect of rhGH treatment is intracranial hypertension (pseudotumour cerebri), which may occur soon after start of treatment, but also after many years of therapy. An incidence of 1–2 : 15,000 has been recorded in all patients treated with rhGH, but the incidence may be higher in patients with CRF (Malozowski et al. 1993). The so-called 'benign' intracranial hypertension is by no means always a benign condition and, although usually reversible with discontinuation of rhGH, lasting neurological damage and blindness have been reported. Regular fundoscopic examinations have been recommended, but heightened awareness is perhaps the most important part of prevention. Visual disturbances, headaches, and vomiting are suggestive symptoms and have to be taken seriously in patients treated with rhGH. Other infrequent side-effects are slipped epiphysis and necrosis of the femoral head.

Delayed puberty

The onset of puberty can be delayed for years in children with CRF. Early data from the EDTA registry showed lack of pubertal development at age 14 in about 25 per cent of boys and delayed menarche in more than 50 per cent of girls with CRF (Scharer et al. 1976). Testosterone levels are generally normal in pubertal male patients and estradiol levels low-normal in females; it is not yet known how adult fertility is affected by childhood-onset CRF (Schaefer and Mehls 1999). Delayed puberty in phenotypically female patients with CRF should be an indication for chromosomal studies to rule out syndromal conditions affecting sexual maturation, for example, Turner's syndrome or Frasier syndrome.

Metabolic disturbances

Anaemia (see also Chapter 11.3.8)

Anaemia, defined as a decrease of haemoglobin to less than 12 g/dl, is regularly observed in children if the GFR decreases to less than

35 ml/min/1.73 m^2. The pathogenesis is multifactorial, but decreased erythropoietin (EPO) production by the diseased kidneys plays a decisive role. Other contributing factors are hypoplasia of the bone marrow, decreased red blood cell survival, deficiency of iron, folate, and B-vitamins, aluminium, PTH-excess, and blood loss. The latter is often due to frequent blood sampling and repeated small blood losses during HD procedures; this should be minimized especially in young patients by using micromethods for biochemical laboratory tests and a complete reinfusion of blood at the end of each session. Another source of blood loss which should not be unterestimated is gastro-intestinal bleeding. A prospective study using upper gastrointestinal endoscopy found bleeding lesions in 4.9 per cent, peptic ulcers without bleeding in 12 per cent, and mild esophagitis, gastritis, or duodenitis in 44 per cent, thus demonstrating a high prevalence of mucosal lesions (Gupta *et al.* 1987). Haemodynamically significant bleeding has also been described associated with gastrostomy tube feeding in young children (Ramage *et al.* 1999).

Treatment with recombinant human EPO has been of greater benefit for the quality of life of children with CRF and on dialysis than any other medication. Before EPO was available, red blood cell transfusions were often needed to counterbalance the effects of anaemia: fatigue, lack of appetite, hypotensive episodes, decreased school performance, and physical capability. Transfusions were usually given if the haemoglobin levels decreased to values less than 5 g/dl. Transfusions carried the risk of hepatitis C transmission, which became endemic in dialysis units, transmission of other viruses [cytomegalovirus (CMV), Epstein–Barr virus (EBV)], iron overload, and sensitization to HLA antigens. The EDTA registry documented that the frequency of transfusions was higher in children than in adults. It was, therefore, not unusual to see children with hepatospenomegaly and excessive serum ferritin levels (Querfeld *et al.* 1988a) who required treatment with chelation agents on dialysis with all the inherent risks of this form of therapy (Müller-Wiefel *et al.* 1985).

Clinical studies in children and adolescents have shown that correction of anaemia by EPO resulted in improved exercise performance (Baraldi *et al.* 1990), reduction of left ventricular hypertrophy, and improved intellectual performance. A beneficial effect of EPO on growth in children with CRF has been observed in some patients but a consistent dose-dependent effect has not been confirmed.

Care should be taken to provide enough iron for the increased demand of a stimulated erythropoiesis. Uraemic patients, even with low iron storage pools, resorb much less iron than healthy persons, and oral iron supplements are frequently not effective. In addition, constipation and nausea are frequent with these medications and liquid iron preparations used in small children lead to unsightly tooth discolorations. Intravenous iron supplementations are, therefore, needed frequently, especially in dialysed patients, and in our experience, appear to be safe in children at a starting dose of 1 mg/kg/week in the form of ferrogluconate administered after HD sessions (Tenbrock *et al.* 1999). Others have used IV iron dextran (4 mg/kg) in consecutive haemodialysis sessions without apparent side-effects (Greenbaum *et al.* 2000). Patients on PD can also be treated on a weekly basis if needed, but IV iron is usually not required in patients with CRF.

In routine clinical practice, a haematocrit in the range of 28–33 per cent is usually maintained with EPO. Whether normalization of the haematocrit (>36 per cent) in children might offer additional benefits for growth is unknown. The usual maintenance dose in children with CRF and on dialysis is 150 U/kg/week, but some children, especially with a weight less than 20 kg may require higher doses. This is given by once weekly subcutaneous injection in outpatients (CRF, PD) and for practical purposes in 2 or 3 divided doses IV in HD patients. Intraperitoneal administration is also feasible, but carries the risk of peritonitis (Kausz *et al.* 1999) and much higher doses are required; it may be considered, however, in children who simply do not tolerate subcutaneous injections.

The most frequent side-effects of treatment with EPO are hypertension, clotting of the vascular access, and hyperkalaemia. Similar to adult patients, hypertension has been observed in roughly a third of paediatric patients treated with EPO (Brandt *et al.* 1999) and blood pressure should, therefore, be carefully monitored after initiation of therapy. Clotting of vascular access in children (Bianchetti *et al.* 1991) has been linked to an increase in procoagulant activity; however, clotting could not be conclusively linked to EPO therapy in prospective studies in adults. Nevertheless, some authors recommend withholding EPO therapy during times of vascular surgery, which seems to be appropriate in view of the sometimes tiny calibres of arteriovenous (AV) fistulas in children. Hyperkalaemia is frequent in dialysis patients, and in EPO-treated patients with rising haematocrit values it may reflect underdialysis and/or increased potassium ingestion with better appetite. In practice, some children require concomitant treatment with potassium-binding resins ('Kayexalate'). It is better to give resins than to reduce caloric intake.

If the response to EPO is inaedquate, several clinical problems should be ruled out or corrected. The most frequent cause, iron deficiency, should be avoided by giving iron supplements (see above); according to current recommendations, the serum ferritin should exceed 100 ng/ml, the transferrin saturation 20 per cent, and the hypochromic red cell count should be less than 10 per cent (Fishbane and Maesaka 1997). Aluminium overload, the presence of infections or malignancies, or vitamin deficiency must be ruled out. Severe (tertiary) hyperparathyroidism is increasingly recognized in children and as a factor suppressing erythropoiesis (by promoting bone marrow fibrosis); especially in small children, parathyroid imaging may be negative and even bone biopsies can be misleading (Muller-Berghaus *et al.* 1997); nevertheless, the consequences may be devastating and one should not hesitate to perform subtotal parathyroidectomy.

Renal osteodystrophy (see also Chapter 11.3.9)

Children and adolescents with CRF have specific problems of bone metabolism which can be described in a simplified manner as the situation of a growing skeleton without adequate supply of active vitamin D facing an excess of PTH; in addition, the physiological demands for mineralization and bone growth are often not supplied sufficiently because of lack of energy intake (diminished nutrition) and functional GH deficiency. Therefore, severe osteodystrophy may be accompanied by stunting of growth and even 'renal dwarfism'. Inadequate therapy may result in severe consequences with growth failure, skeletal deformities, and as a long-term result, disability.

The skeleton of the child has a physiological demand for vitamin D, which has to be supplemented in infancy (normally 500 U vitamin D3 per day, combined with fluoride in many countries). Calcium and phosphorus are adequately supplied by breast milk or formula in infants, and infants and children have physiologically greater calcium and phosphorus concentrations, which later decline to values seen in adolescents and adults (Table 1). In Western countries the normal intake of regular foods and milk products is sufficient for older children to supply sufficient vitamin D, calcium, and phosphorus.

CRF is characterized by diminished synthesis of $1,25(OH)_2D_3$, causing increased PTH and a deficit of active vitamin D. Therefore, vitamin D metabolites must be prescribed to all children and adolescents with CRF. If active vitamin D is not prescribed or not given, clinical symptoms will develop. In infants and small children one can see the full-blown picture of rickets with craniotabes, Harrison's groove and rachitic rosary as well as thickening of wrists and ankles (Figs 2–4). With progressive disease, bone deformities become apparent and the combination of bone pain and myopathy may lead to immobilization and neurodevelopmental delay (Figs 5 and 6). Older children may present with bowing of the diaphysis of long bones, knock knees, ulnar deviation of the hands, and a waddling gait. Fractures occur easily in these poorly mineralized bones and can also lead to immobilization; vertebral fractures can be disabling.

Further symptoms of renal osteodystrophy in children include pruritus and red-eye syndrome (PTH-excess, hyperphosphataemia), dental abnormalities (enamel hypoplasia), brown tumours, and epiphyseal slipping. With long-term elevations of the calcium–phosphate

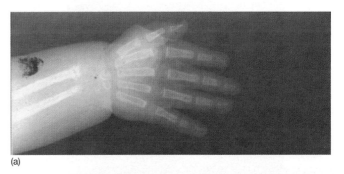
(a)

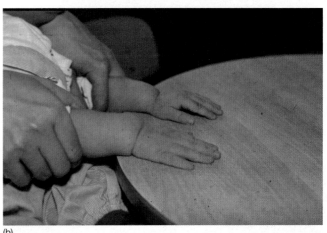
(b)

Fig. 3 (a) Same patient, severe defective mineralization of all bones, cupping and fraying of distal ends of radius and ulna. The epiphyses are actually enlarged (b) but invisible because of defective calcification. Little spontaneous activity due to bone pain. (b) Same patient, note swelling and bajonette-like shape of wrists.

Table 1 Age-dependent upper normal levels of calcium, phosphate, and calcium–phosphate product

Age (years)	Calcium		Phosphorus		Ca × P[a]	
	mmol/l	mg/dl	mmol/l	mg/dl	mmol²/l²	mg²/dl²
<1	2.8	10.9	2.25	6.8	6.3	74
1–3	2.7	10.8	2.1	6.5	5.6	70
4–11	2.7	10.8	1.8	5.6	4.9	60
12–15	2.7	10.8	1.75	5.4	4.7	58
>16	2.6	10.4	1.6	4.8	4.2	50

[a] Calculated from published normal values in children (Nelson Textbook of Pediatrics).

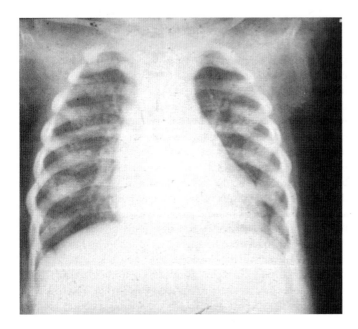

Fig. 2 Chest X-ray of a 2-year-old boy with CRF due to obstructive uropathy: florid rickets with 'rachitic rosary' (enlargement of costochondral junctions).

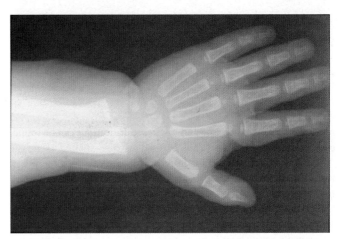

Fig. 4 Same patient, healing rickets with high-dose calcitriol therapy: mineralization much improved, but apparent ulnar deviation and bowing of bones; increased physical activity.

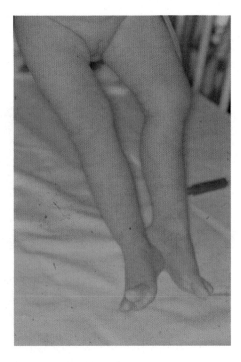

Fig. 5 Immobilized child with bone pain, severe renal osteodystrophy, and displacement of hip joints.

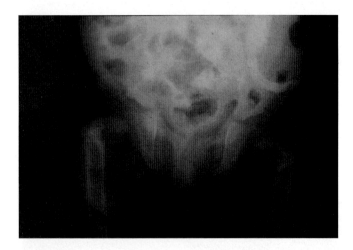

Fig. 6 Pelvic X-ray of the same child as in Fig. 5.

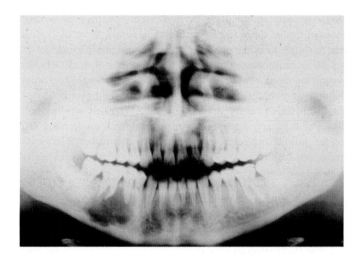

Fig. 7 Brown tumour of the mandibula in a 16-year-old uncompliant adolescent with tertiary hyperparathyroidism. She complained of occasional pain with chewing.

product in serum, soft tissue and vascular calcifications can be found even in childhood (Milliner et al. 1990).

While florid rickets can be diagnosed on clinical grounds, radiological studies are indispensable to detect more subtle changes. Continuous monitoring of bone disease is advised in all patients with CRF (Mehls and Salusky 1987). In general, X-rays of the hands and wrists serve as surrogate markers for the severity of renal osteodystrophy, but occasionally, severe bone lesions can be diagnosed only by an extensive X-ray survey of bones and joints, and even the cranial bones may be affected by osteodystrophy (Fig. 7). Radiological changes may not go in parallel with biochemical abnormalities (alkaline phosphatase, PTH, calcium, phosphate), which are generally of limited value in the assessment of the severity and response to treatment of renal osteodystrophy (Mehls and Salusky 1987). In addition, an X-ray of the hand and wrist serves to determine the bone age of the patient, since the degree of skeletal maturation corresponds to the ossification state of the hand and wrist bones. Bone age may be very different from chronological age because of delayed skeletal maturation in CRF. Specific scoring systems (Tanner et al. 1975) should be preferentially used in children with CRF. Knowledge of the bone age allows an estimation of the remaining growth potential, and an approximation of adult final height to be calculated.

Treatment

Treatment of renal osteodystrophy is mainly empirical. Phosphate retention as a direct result of diminished GFR is observed even in early stages of CRF. It is difficult if not impossible to provide a low phosphorus diet in children, especially infants, who need milk-based formulas with high phosphorus content. As a rule, all patients with CRF, therefore, need phosphate-binding drugs to reduce intestinal phosphate absorption, and these should be given in the form of calcium carbonate or calcium acetate together with meals. The usual dose is 0.5–2 g given three times a day and is adjusted to the serum phosphorus. One should remember that calcium-containing phosphate binders further increase the calcium load in patients with ESRD; in dialysis patients the calcium balance is highly positive, contributing to an elevated calcium–phosphate product which may result in ectopic calcifications. Preliminary experience suggests that sevelamer, a calcium-free phosphate binder can be safely given to children, but results of controlled studies have to be awaited.

Vitamin D3, calcitriol, alpha-calcidol, and dihydrotachysterol (DHT) are commonly used as vitamin D preparations. While in early CRF a daily dose of 1000 U of vitamin D3 (cholecalciferol) is sufficient to prevent vitamin D deficiency, approximately 5000 U of vitamin D3 per square metre body surface area are required with more advanced renal failure. With further decrease of renal $1,25(OH)_2D_3$ production, this may not be sufficient to suppress PTH, and calcitriol or alpha-calcidol should be given; the usual calcitriol dose is 0.25 μg per day. We try to dose vitamin D or its active metabolites according to radiological changes as well as plasma PTH and bone alkaline phosphatase. The PTH concentration should not be lower than 150 pg/ml (reduce calcitriol dose) or even 100 (discontinue calcitriol). Lower PTH concentrations are often associated with adynamic bone disease which can only be diagnosed reliably by bone biopsy. Frequent complications are hypercalcaemia and vascular calcifications. Since PTH is necessary for bone growth, both oversuppression and adynamic bone disease should be avoided to prevent any impairment of longitudinal growth of the child.

It has become clear that vitamin D should be given on a daily basis, because intermittent application was found to be associated with diminished longitudinal growth (Kuizon *et al.* 1998). If slipped epiphysis or bone deformities have developed, surgical correction should only be performed after stabilization of bone lesions (documented radiologically); attempts at surgical interventions in situations of florid osteodystrophy have been disastrous.

Side-effects of osteodystrophy treatment

The landmark report by Milliner *et al.* (1990), based on autopsy data of children with ESRD treated during 1960–1983, revealed soft tissue calcifications in 72 out of 120 patients (60 per cent) and systemic calcinosis in 43 patients (36 per cent). Twelve patients had coronary artery calcifications, 30 had non-myocardial vascular calcifications, and 19 had myocardial calcifications, with extensive involvement of the conductance system in one patient. It is of note that in this study, of all variables considered, the use of active vitamin D preparations and especially calcitriol had the strongest correlation with calcinosis (Milliner *et al.* 1990). In a small series of 12 adolescents aged 11–17 years receiving haemodialysis, intimal thickening, microcalcifications, and atheromatous plaques were described in iliac artery specimens (obtained at the time of transplantation) in six patients; these patients had higher serum phosphorus and a higher serum calcium–phosphate product than patients without arterial changes (Nayir *et al.* 2001).

Vitamin D or its derivatives may be a unique risk for children and adolescents with ESRD. Large doses of vitamin D are known to produce media calcifications as shown experimentally (Tshibangu *et al.* 1975; Price *et al.* 2000). Recent studies in children and young adults have demonstrated severe calcifications in the coronary arteries by electron beam computed tomography (EBCT) and spiral CT, respectively (Eifinger *et al.* 2000; Goodman *et al.* 2000; Oh *et al.* 2002). In two studies, the amount of calcification was correlated to the serum calcium–phosphate product and the cumulative amount of prescribed calcium-containing phosphate binders.

The therapy of renal osteodystrophy in paediatric patients remains a challenge. On the one hand, vitamin D underdosing will aggravate secondary hyperparathyroidism and may lead to rickets, myopathy, and even immobilization. On the other hand, overdosing of vitamin D preparations can result in adynamic bone disease, hypercalcaemia, diminished longitudinal growth, and ectopic calcifications.

Cardiovascular disease and risk factors (see also Chapter 11.3.5)

Children and adolescents with ESRD usually have no clinical symptoms suggestive of heart disease, but young adults with ESRD die primarily of cardiac causes. The relative mortality risk from cardiac causes is excessively elevated in young patients compared to the background population and approximately equal to the risk in 75–80-year-old subjects without ESRD (Meyer and Levey 1998). Similarly, cardiac death is the single most important contributor to mortality in young patients after renal transplantation. In transplanted US children aged 0–19 years (USRDS report 1997) death from cardiac causes combined was approximately 35 per cent more frequent than death from other causes (infection 24 per cent, malignancy 7 per cent). Only 4 per cent of the total mortality, however, was due to myocardial infarction, and another 6 per cent due to cardiovascular disease (CVD).

Uraemia poses a high risk for vascular disease because of the unique accumulation of risk factors for atherosclerosis. Prospective studies establishing a link of these risk factors with morbidity and mortality from CVD in the ESRD population have been performed in adults. In the paediatric ESRD population information is emerging that these risk factors are similarly present in younger patients.

Risk factors

Hypertension is frequent in children and adolescents with renal disease. The prevalence has been estimated between 38 and 78 per cent based on measurements of casual blood pressure (Drukker 1991). However, diagnostic sensitivity has increased considerably with the advent of 24-h ABPM, for which normal ranges for children of different age, race, and gender have now been established (Harshfield *et al.* 1994; Soergel *et al.* 1997). The experience with ABPM shows a high prevalence of 'white coat hypertension' in paediatric patients (Nishibata *et al.* 1995; Sorof 2000), the need for reclassification of blood pressure status (normotensive/hypertensive) in about a third of children on dialysis (Lingens *et al.* 1995), and a high prevalence of nocturnal hypertension, particularly after renal transplantation (Lingens *et al.* 1996). Moreover, hypertension is often insufficiently controlled; the EDTA survey of 1992 found that 55 per cent of children on maintenance dialysis in Europe received antihypertensive drugs, and that despite this treatment one-third of all patients had blood pressure levels above the 95th percentile (Scharer *et al.* 1999). Hypertension frequently persists after transplantation, although to a different degree. The prevalence is influenced by age group, race, rejection episodes, nephrectomy of the native kidneys, and time after transplantation (Sorof *et al.* 1999).

Pharmacological treatment of hypertension is basically similar in children and adolescents, but dose recommendations have to be followed closely.

Hyperlipidaemia is common in patients with CRF. A typical lipoprotein pattern of abnormal lipoprotein composition (dyslipidaemia) is found, which is characterized by hypertriglyceridaemia and low high-density lipoprotein (HDL)-cholesterol levels. In addition, serum total cholesterol, very low-density lipoprotein (VLDL)-cholesterol, LDL-cholesterol, and apolipoprotein B are frequently elevated in children. The underlying mechanisms are complex and mainly involve a diminished catabolism of triglyceride-rich lipoproteins (Querfeld 1993). Recent *in vitro* data demonstrating antagonistic effects of calcitriol and PTH on adipose tissue synthesis of lipoprotein lipase suggest that hyperlipidaemia may be linked to abnormal calcium–phosphate metabolism (Querfeld *et al.* 1999).

The prevalence of hyperlipidaemia varies widely, depending on the presence of proteinuria, the degree of renal failure, and the use of drugs with direct or indirect effects on lipoprotein concentrations. Although lipoprotein profiles are different on PD, HD, and after transplantation, as a rule, the composition of lipoproteins is always atherogenic.

Treatment with PD deserves some special consideration since protein losses and glucose absorption may further aggravate dyslipidaemia. At the start of PD, elevated triglyceride and cholesterol levels were present in 90 and 69 per cent of the patients, respectively (Querfeld et al. 1988b). Serial measurements of serum lipid levels in 68 children treated by PD showed that although fasting mean triglyceride and cholesterol at the start of PD were elevated above the 95th percentile by 102 and 19 per cent, respectively, no significant change in mean lipid levels was observed during a follow-up period of 2 years. Since protein loss into the peritoneal dialysate is relatively high in children, this might also adversely affect lipoproteins, especially loss of the protective HDL. A detailed analysis of lipoprotein fractions, however, confirmed atherogenic lipoprotein profiles, cholesterol ratios, and apolipoprotein ratios, but cholesterol in the high-density fraction and apo A-I were normal despite considerable apo A-I loss into the dialysate (Querfeld et al. 1991).

In the general population total mortality and morbidity from CVD show a continuous and graded relationship with serum cholesterol (Stamler et al. 2000). Vice versa, therapeutic lowering of cholesterol with statins has resulted in a consistent decrease in morbidity and mortality (Gotto 1997). In adult patients with CRF, plasma lipids were correlated with cardiovascular complications in a prospective study (Jungers et al. 1999). In contrast, in the dialysis population no significant correlation with CVD has been found in most prospective studies.

Treatment with lipid-lowering drugs, especially with statins, causes significant reduction in mortality and morbidity from CVD in the general population. In patients with ESRD and after renal transplantation the risk modification by treatment has not been proven, although several trials are currently under way. It should be noted that the use of statins is not recommended in prepubertal children because of uncertainties regarding long-term safety of blocking endogenous cholesterol synthesis in a growing organism with a high demand of cholesterol for hormonal and cell membrane synthesis. In animal experiments, when high doses of statins were administered to young rats, stunted growth and severe myopathy were observed (Reijneveld et al. 1996). Preliminary data from small paediatric cohorts suggest that statins are effective and do not have many immediate side-effects; however, long-term studies will be needed to determine the long-term benefit (Kronn et al. 2000). For the time being, patients in the adolescent age group with unremitting steroid-resistant nephrotic syndrome and progressive renal failure as well as transplanted patients are obvious candidates for lipid-lowering therapy.

Lp(a) is an inherited independent risk factor for atherosclerosis. Its role in childhood thromboembolism is established (Nowak-Gottl et al. 1997). Lp(a) is an LDL-like particle with an additional unique protein component, apolipoprotein(a) [apo(a)]. Apo(a) occurs in multiple isoforms which can be identified by electrophoretic separation. Lp(a) is under genetic control by the apo(a) gene: isoforms of low molecular weight (LMW) are associated on average with high Lp(a) blood concentrations whereas isoforms of high molecular weight (HMW) present usually with low Lp(a) (Scanu 1992).

Lp(a) is elevated in CRF, on dialysis, and after transplantation (Querfeld et al. 1993) and the individual plasma level is highly dependent on the apo(a) phenotype (Kronenberg et al. 2000). Lp(a) is an atherogenic and thrombogenic lipoprotein with unknown physiological properties and a unique metabolism different from other lipoproteins; it is, therefore, resistant to treatment with lipid-lowering drugs.

In HD patients, Lp(a) correlates with survival in some, but not all prospective studies. LMW apo(a) phenotypes are also a sensitive predictor of carotid artery atherosclerosis (Kronenberg et al. 1994). In addition, Lp(a) may be a significant risk factor for chronic rejection; LMW apo(a) isoforms are an inherited risk factor for long-term renal transplant survival in young renal transplant recipients, especially below the age of 35 years, possibly by promoting vascular changes that drive chronic rejection (Wahn et al. 2001).

Hyperhomocysteinaemia is also prevalent in children with CRF and on dialysis. In a cross-sectional analysis of 29 children with various degrees of renal failure, total serum homocysteine (tHcy) was significantly greater than in controls and hyperhomocysteinaemia was seen in 62.0 per cent of patients and 5.2 per cent of controls (Merouani et al. 2001). Children with renal failure treated with HD or PD also have elevated tHcy concentrations, but this could be significantly reduced after administration of 2.5 mg folic acid daily for 4 weeks (Schroder et al. 1999). Clearly, more long-term studies are necessary to establish the optimal dose and prove a beneficial effect of this therapy. It should be mentioned that like most other risk factors, hyperhomocysteinaemia is also present after transplantation, even in young patients (Krmar et al. 2001).

Treatment of risk factors in children with chronic renal failure

Even in the absence of published studies in adolescents, it is obvious that the classical risk factors are targets for treatment. An elevated blood pressure should be lowered to values within the normal range, probably even into the low-normal range. Hyperlipidaemia should be treated in adolescent (postpubertal) nephrotic patients and transplanted patients, preferably with statins. Physical activity should be encouraged and there should be a 'zero tolerance approach' to smoking. The tHcy concentration can be somewhat lowered by supplementation with folic acid and vitamin B6 and B12, although usually not normalized; this treatment is essentially without side-effects (Sunder-Plassmann et al. 2000). Both DOQI and European Best Practice guidelines now recommend that anaemia should be treated to achieve a target haematocrit of 33–36 per cent. In addition, the calcium–phosphate product should be kept in the low-normal range, but this may be in practice the most difficult recommendation to follow.

Progression of chronic renal failure to endstage renal disease

In most patients CRF is characterized by relentless progression to ESRD. In a graphic plot of the rate of loss of renal function, an extrapolation of the slope of 1/serum creatinine can be used to predict progression if the progress is linear (Arbus and Bacheyie 1981). The serum creatinine reflects muscle mass which may be highly variable in children and, although routinely used in clinical practice, is therefore not a good marker for estimating the degree of renal dysfunction. Serum cystatin C may be a more sensitive indicator and reference values for infants and children have been published (Harmoinen et al. 2000); however, this method has not found wide acceptance in clinical practice. Measurements of creatinine clearance by 24-h urine collection are notoriously inaccurate but this method remains in use for the routine clinical evaluation. The calculation of creatinine clearance from serum creatinine according to the formula described by Schwartz has found widespread acceptance [$k \times$ height (cm) : serum creatinine (mg/dl); with the constant k being 0.30 in preterm infants, 0.45 in full-term infants, 0.55 in children and adolescent girls, and 0.70 in adolescent boys] (Schwartz *et al.* 1987). A more accurate estimation is possible with clearance studies using injections of inulin or chromium-EDTA and *p*-aminohippuric acid for the determination of GFR and renal plasma flow, respectively. In children, these methods are mainly confined to clinical studies because they are cumbersome and involve the application of radioactive substances.

Much work has been devoted to the question of whether a *low-protein diet* can retard the progression of CRF. In the modification of diet in renal disease (MDRD) study of more than 1500 adult patients with CRF, a low-protein diet had no significant effect on the decline of renal function when the data were examined by intent to treat (Klahr *et al.* 1994). Secondary analysis of these data as well as meta-analyses of other studies, however, suggest some benefit of dietary intervention (Pedrini *et al.* 1996; Levey *et al.* 1999). In children, the issue is even more critical since low protein diets carry the risk of inadequate nutrition and diminished linear growth. A European multicentre study on the effect of low-protein diet on the progression of renal failure (Wingen *et al.* 1997) recruited 191 patients aged 2–18 years. After a run-in period of at least 6 months, patients were stratified into either progressors or non-progressors based on the change in creatinine clearance. The patients were also stratified into renal-disease categories and randomly assigned to a control or a diet group receiving the lowest recommended (i.e. 'safe') dietary protein content of 0.8–1.1 g/kg daily. All patients were advised to have a caloric intake of at least 70 per cent of the WHO recommendations. Compliance to the dietary prescriptions was checked by dietary protocols and by urinary nitrogen excretion. The results of this study showed that the low-protein diet did not affect growth and that there was no effect of diet on the mean decline in creatinine clearance over 2 years. In contrast, the degree of proteinuria and the systolic blood pressure were independent predictors of the change in GFR (Wingen *et al.* 1997). In view of these data and the often encountered difficulties of providing a sufficient daily caloric intake, it seems inappropriate to generally recommend dietary protein restriction in children with CRF. Temporary dietary protein restriction can be helpful in older children and adolescents with sufficient caloric intake to lower high urea levels in the terminal stage of CRF. However, in a small child with feeding difficulties and failure to thrive, every effort should be made to increase caloric intake (even at the expense of high urea nitrogen levels) and dialysis should not be postponed.

Dialysis

History

It was the adaptation of HD techniques to paediatric needs in the early 1970s that allowed survival of children and adolescents with ESRD. Initial fears that RRT would be unethical especially in young children because of the physical and psychological burden imposed by ESRD

were superceded by the technical advancements in dialysis and renal transplantation. Although not all questions raised early on have been definitely answered, there is now general acceptance of ESRD treatment in children. In fact, today it would be considered unethical by many physicians to withhold therapy for ESRD even in very young children; a multinational survey of paediatric nephrologists found that replacement therapy was offered by 41 per cent to all infants less than 1 month of age and by 53 per cent to all infants between 1 and 12 months without significant differences between countries (Geary 1998). Nevertheless, in selected patients, for example, with multiorgan failure, severe brain damage, or untreatable genetic disease, RRT should be withheld, preferably after reaching consensus in an ethical committee.

Choosing a dialysis modality (see also Chapters 12.1 and 12.3)

The modality of dialysis should be discussed with the family well before terminal renal failure is reached and the advantages and disadvantages of PD and HD should be explained in detail. Infants and small children usually fare much better with PD. Nevertheless, HD can be performed even in small infants if necessary. Reasons for choosing HD at this age are the presence of congenital abdominal disease (omphalocele, diaphragmatic hernia, gastroschisis) making PD impossible. A surgically placed stoma (e.g. gastrostomy, vesicostomy) is not a contraindication to PD. Technical or anatomical limitations in the surgical creation of a sufficient AV fistula can be overcome by placement of a permanent double lumen catheter for HD. However, HD is still demanding at this age and constant supervision during the procedures is mandatory. Apart from these exceptions, PD clearly is the method of choice for this age group and even premature babies have now been successfully dialysed for prolonged periods of time.

Since the considerations for choosing an appropriate mode of dialysis are slightly different in children from adults, these are outlined in Table 2. To facilitate this choice and to better prepare the family especially for PD, many paediatric centres perform visits to the family

Table 2 Priority considerations for choosing dialysis modalities in paediatric patients

	Haemodialysis	Peritoneal dialysis
PRO[a]	Medical supervision	Little limitations of fluid intake
	No daily dialysis	No pain with punctures
	Body image preserved	No dysequilibrium
	Sports allowed	No systemic anticoagulation
	Less infections	Home-based
		Better school attendance
		Freedom during day
Contra	Dysequilibrium	Infectious complications
	Dietary problems (potassium)	Daily dialysis
	Limited fluid intake	Body image not preserved
	Pain (fistula punctures)	Swimming problematic
	Systemic anticoagulation	
	More rapid loss of renal function	
	Hospital-based	

[a] Some of these considerations do not apply if venous catheters are implanted for HD.

home to assure realistic planning for the dialysis procedure. This simple manoeuvre contributes valuable insights into practical details related to dialysis, such as storage of PD fluids (bags), hygienic precautions, and not the least, living conditions, which have to be considered in planning for home dialysis.

Haemodialysis

Although transplantation is the treatment of choice for children with ESRD, maintenance HD can provide satisfactory life expectancy for patients with no possibility of transplantation or highly sensitized patients. The 5 year patient survival rate for children receiving chronic HD was 95 per cent, being comparable with the results of living-related donor transplantation (92 per cent) (Avner et al. 1981). Long-term results of chronic HD in infants are worse; in one single-centre report (including 20 infants with 11 receiving transplants) the overall 14 year survival was 60 per cent and significantly better in children weighing greater than 5 kg (73 per cent) than those weighing less (20 per cent) at initiation of HD (Knight et al. 1993).

While an AV fistula is the most common *dialysis access* in adult patients, the surgical creation of a fistula with sufficient blood flow is often impossible in children. In fact, the most common type of vascular access in children on HD is now the dual lumen venous catheter. The NAPRTCS registry 1996 report showed that among 682 patients, 76 per cent were maintained with an external percutaneous catheter, mostly placed into the subclavian vein. Only 11.4 per cent of patients were maintained with internal AV fistulas, and 12.3 per cent with internal AV grafts. Shunts, fistulas, and grafts were located in the lower arm in 56 per cent, the upper arm 31 per cent, and the thigh in 13 per cent (Lerner et al. 1999). The external percutaneous catheters were preferably double lumen cuffed catheters, which seem to have superior outcome in children. However, the size and length of catheters have to be adapted to the individual need of the patient. These data reflect the difficulty of establishing a trouble-free AV fistula in children, although this remains the safest access for patients. In specialized surgical centres, 75–85 per cent of radial AV fistulas are functioning after 1 year (Brittinger et al. 1997). Thus, pain due to needle punctures can be minimized by applying anaesthetic cream locally.

The major complications of external percutaneous catheters are *venous stenosis*, which seems to be less frequent with internal jugular placement and *infection*, which may be difficult to prevent in spite of rigorous infection control techniques. The median survival of percutaneous catheters is disturbingly short: in the NAPRTCS study, the median survival was 204 days (Lerner et al. 1999), although this may partially reflect removal of catheters at the time of renal transplantaton.

Regarding *dialysis technique*, the extracorporeal circuit ('tubing') must be adapted to the size of the patient. The entire circuit volume should not exceed 10–15 per cent of the total blood volume of the child. In small children and infants, dialyser and tubing should be 'primed' with blood to prevent circulatory collapse.

Dialysis machines can be standard HD machines used for adults, but must allow small flow rates, which may be as low as 20 ml/min in infants, and single needle monitoring (also with continuous dialysis techniques). Ultrafiltration control devices are necessary for accurate balancing of fluid status. We have frequently used the BM 11/BM 14 (manufacturer: Baxter Dialysetechnik, Germany), which allows excellent monitoring of fluid balance even in infants and can also be used for continuous dialysis

techniques. Dialysers for paediatric patients have areas ranging from 0.2 to 1.5 m^2 with a filling volume of less than 100 ml. Dysequilibrium is a complication occurring mainly during the first dialysis sessions with high osmolar shifts due to high blood urea levels; it can be prevented by decreasing the efficiency of dialysis or by infusion of mannitol (0.5 g/kg given as a 20–25 per cent solution) during the first hour of dialysis.

Most paediatric centres now use polysulfone capillary dialysers, which reportedly have better biocompatibility, less need for anticoagulation and improved outcome in adult patients. In the past, dialysis prescriptions were based on predialysis urea concentrations, and later on urea kinetic modelling. The recently developed evidence-based guidelines (DOQI) for dialysis adequacy and minimum delivered dose for adult patients should be applied to children. The recommended target Kt/V is at least 1.2 per session (Harmon and Jabs 1999). These recommendations need to be prospectively evaluated in children.

Heparin is used to prevent clotting in the extracorporeal circuit. The usual loading dose at initiation of HD is 2000 U/m^2, the maintenance dose 400 U/m^2/h; monitoring is usually performed by measuring activated clotting times (ACT). In patients with high risk of bleeding or heparin-induced thrombopenia, regional citrate anticoagulation should be used.

The continuous dialysis modalities for example, continuous veno-venous haemofiltration (CVVH) are mainly used in patients with acute renal failure, and have a place in treatment in children with severe fluid overload, circulatory disturbances, and multiorgan failure (Klee et al. 1996).

Peritoneal dialysis (see also Chapter 12.4)

Although in the 1960s PD had been used in the treatment of acute renal failure, it was the development of the permanent peritoneal catheter and later of CAPD that brought PD to widespread use in the treatment of childhood ESRD. Either in the form of CAPD, CCPD or intermittant PD (IPD), it is now the preferred treatment for dialysis in children, especially infants and young children. Between 1988 and 1992, 66 per cent of paediatric patients were treated with CAPD/CCPD and 10 per cent with IPD according to the EDTA registry (Mehls et al. 1996). In a German survey, 59 per cent of children less than 15 years and 28 per cent of adolescents between 15 and 18 years, were treated with some form of PD (Frei and Schober-Halstenberg 1999). While in the early 1980s CAPD was usually performed, the development of automated 'cycler' devices has gained increased acceptance and today, more than 80 per cent of paediatric PD patients are performing CCPD, mostly in the form of nocturnal IPD (Schaefer et al. 1999b).

It is important to realize that PD is dependent on a functioning catheter. Regardless of the details of catheter placement, the dedication of a specialized surgical team using standardized procedures is essential for satisfactory results of this often underestimated procedure. The length and type of catheter may vary with the age of the patient and catheters and the location of the exit site are, therefore, selected by the paediatrician after assessing the patient. Close communication with the operating team is essential. Many centres have the paediatrician present in the operating theatre during the procedure and this practice is more than justified in view of the importance of this lifeline for the patient.

Most centres now use curled catheters ('pigtail'), which seem to cause less displacement and omental wrapping. Placement of the exit site is usually performed far away from a vesicostomy, ureterostomy, colostomy, or gastrostomy, if present. In some centres, omentectomy is routinely performed at the time of catheter placement. Many centres use straight tunnels with a single cuff, but according to the NAPRTCS database, significantly lower peritonitis rates are observed with double-cuff catheters (one infection per 15.1 patient-months versus 12.6 patient-months with one cuff) (Warady et al. 1997). Swan-neck catheters with a downward-pointing opening have significantly less exit site infections (Lerner et al. 1999). There is also some preliminary experience with peritoneoscopic catheter placement in children, but this is limited to a few centres; this relatively new method has not yet found widespread acceptance.

Following catheter placement, PD is started with a low exchange volume (300 ml/m^2 or 10 ml/kg). We add small amounts of heparin (200 IE/l) to prevent catheter obstruction by fibrin clots. The exchange volume is slowly increased over several days and the exit site is repeatedly checked for leakage of dialysis fluid. The exchange volumes are increased to 1000–1500 ml/m^2, the final volume, during the second week. Some centres have gained experience with intra-abdominal pressure measurements, which may be helpful in adjusting the dialysis dose to the individual need of the patient (Fischbach et al. 1997).

Regarding the *dialysis prescription*, the paediatric experience has shown that a CAPD regimen consisting of 4–5 exchanges per day with an exchange volume of about 1000 ml/m^2 (35–45 ml/kg) of 2.5 per cent dextrose is associated with sufficient ultrafiltration and biochemical control. The same was found for a CCPD regimen consisting of 8–10 exchanges of the same volume per night. These empirical doses have given way recently to more precisely calculated dialysis prescriptions reflecting the published experience on dialysis adequacy. Studies in adult PD patients have clearly shown that survival on PD is dependent on the prescribed dialysis dose (measured in *Kt/V*) in a dose-dependent manner [Canada-USA (CANUSA) Peritoneal Dialysis Study Group 1996]. Similar or even increased target clearances are probably needed for children, although this is not possible to prove with survival data in children. While paediatric outcome variables need yet to be defined and tested in prospective studies, it seems justified to recommend that the DOQI guidelines for adults should also be applied to children: the total creatinine clearance should be at least 60 l/week/1.73 m^2 and the *Kt/V* at least 2.0. Dialysis adequacy is also dependent on peritoneal transport characteristics. The peritoneal equilibration test (PET) for a standard 2 l exchange has been adapted for use in children. The use of this standardized test by the Mid-European Peritoneal Dialysis (MEPPS) group showed that the peritoneal transport properties affected growth and nutritional status in children on PD; the rapid transporter state was associated with decreased growth (Schaefer et al. 1999a). The PET test should, therefore, be performed shortly after the initiation of PD treatment for baseline evaluation of transport kinetics and it is also useful to repeat this test routinely especially after repeated peritonitis episodes.

Complications

Obstruction of the catheter by omental wrapping is the most frequent complication leading to failure and replacement. Catheter obstruction may be caused by fibrin clots which sometimes can be removed by intra-luminal administration of fibrinolytic agents (urokinase, 5000 U/ml). Umbilical, inguinal, and scrotal hernias can occur as a consequence of increased intra-abdominal pressure, and this is seen more frequently in the first months after initiation of PD and in younger patients.

Other mechanical complications are disconnection of the external catheter tubing, sometimes provoked by pulling or playing. We find it safe to tape the catheter firmly to the abdominal wall with surgical dressing fixed with adhesive tape. Unfortunately, routine surgical material may cause severe skin irritations, especially in infants. Hypoallergenic surgical wound dressing should, therefore, be used.

Peritonitis is the main complication of PD. The incidence of peritonitis is higher in children than in adults and especially in children less than 6 years of age (Schaefer et al. 1999c). Data of the NAPRTCS show an annual peritonitis rate of 0.9 per patient per year (Warady et al. 1996). Gram-positive infections, especially with *Staphylococcus aureus*, were the most frequent (up to 80 per cent of all cases) (Schaefer et al. 1999c). Gram-negative bacteria are found in about 20 per cent of cases, but in many instances, dialysis cultures remain sterile. After prolonged antibiotic treatment, fungal peritonitis can be found with an incidence of about 1–2 per cent (Warady et al. 1996).

Peritonitis can usually be diagnosed on clinical grounds. The patient feels ill and may be in acute distress, has abdominal pain sometimes with fever; the effluent dialysate is cloudy. Physical examination of a patient with suspected peritonitis should include inspection of the exit site and careful palpation of the catheter tunnel, which may be red and oedematous. Especially with CCPD, however, children may be relatively asymptomatic. The diagnosis can be made if greater than 100 WBC per millilitre dialysate are found with greater than 50 per cent polymorphonuclear cells. The so-called lymphocytic or eosinophilic peritonitis (with negative cultures and mainly lymphocytes or eosinophils in a differential WBC) is usually accompanied by minor clinical symptoms and does not justify treatment. The current *recommendations for treatment* of peritonitis vary between centres but usually include a cephalosporin, often combined with a glycopeptide (Fig. 8). Consensus guidelines for drugs of choice and dosing regimens in children have been published (Warady et al. 2000).

Exit site infections are usually caused by *S. aureus*. There are large variations in the rate of exit site infections between centres. This may be caused by staphylococcal nasal carriage of caretakers and by different practices regarding wound dressing and exit site care. It is our experience that iodine or alcohol-containing solutions are destructive to skin integrity and of no value in eradicating these infections. Instead, daily non-occlusive sterile dressing changes with mild disinfectants (e.g. octenidine) should be used. In the case of tunnel infections, the application of dressings with a 2 per cent NaCl solution is helpful. Prospective studies in adults have established an association between exit site infections, tunnel infections, and peritonitis with nasal carriage of *S. aureus*. In children, *S. aureus* nasal carriage rates in patients and caretakers are high and can be significantly reduced by intranasal mupirocin treatment (Kingwatanakul and Warady 1997). The preferred mode of administration of mupirocin (timing, local ointment treatment of exit site) has yet to be defined by prospective studies in children.

Exit site infection may lead the way to propagation of bacteria into the catheter tunnel leading to tunnel infections, which again may cause peritonitis. *Tunnel infections* can be diagnosed by clinical inspection or tunnel ultrasound, which shows oedema around the catheter. Tunnel infections can be cured by oral doses of antibiotics with staphylococcal coverage; however, the catheter has to be replaced if this is not successful or peritonitis is present; ultrasound follow-up examinations may help with making this decision. Replacement of the catheter necessitates intermittent HD usually for 2 weeks with systemic antibiotic treatment.

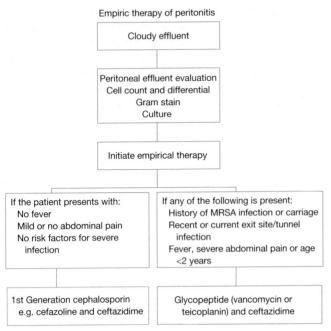

MRSA, methicillin-resistant *Staphylococcus aureus*.

Fig. 8 Current recommendations for empiric therapy of peritonitis. From Warady *et al.* (2000). Consensus guidelines for the treatment of peritonitis in paediatric patients receiving peritoneal dialysis. *Peritoneal Dialysis International* **20**, 600–624.

Some children and adolescents remain on PD for longer times due to various reasons. A decrease in ultrafiltration may be noticed after 2–3 years (Schaefer *et al.* 1999a). In addition, *sclerosing peritonitis* associated with a high mortality has been infrequently observed in paediatric patients (Afthentopoulos *et al.* 1998). The reasons for the loss of ultrafiltration and sclerosing peritonitis are not clear, but long-term bioincompatibility of dialysis solutions may be a major contributing factor. Usually patient survival is satisfactory with this method of treatment. The average patient mortality after 4 years was 10 per cent (Warady *et al.* 1997). Many children learn to adjust well to life with PD. In the NAPRTCS study, 77 per cent were attending full-time school and 15 per cent part-time or at home (Warady *et al.* 1997).

Transplantation in children (see also Section 13)

Transplantation is the treatment of choice for all children and adolescents with ESRD. A functioning transplant terminates the burden of dialysis, leads to better rehabilitation, better school performance, and overall, a much improved quality of life (Morel *et al.* 1991). Contraindications to transplantation include human immunodeficiency virus (HIV) infection, malignancy, and incurable disease (genetic disorders). Worldwide, most kidneys are transplanted from cadaveric donors; however, the relative percentage of living-related donation (LRD) has steadily increased in many countries. In North America, LRD increased from 43 per cent in 1987 to 53 per cent in 1996, the great majority of kidneys coming from parent donors and only occasionally from siblings or unrelated donors (Benfield *et al.* 1999).

Pre-emptive transplantation (before dialysis becomes necessary) has gained increasing acceptance. According to the NAPRTCS registry 26 per cent of children were tranplanted pre-emptively in 1987–1992

and 70 per cent of these received LRD kidneys. There were initially fears that pre-emptive transplantation would result in increased non-compliance rates because the patients have not experienced life with dialysis, but such concerns have proved to be unwarranted (Fine *et al.* 1994). The rate of pre-emptive transplantation has remained constant in the United States in the 1990s, but has steadily increased in Europe; during 1990–1992, pre-emptive LRD transplantation was performed in 42 per cent and pre-emptive cadaveric kidney transplantation in 20 per cent of patients less than 15 years of age (Mehls *et al.* 1996).

Historically, it was believed that cadaveric kidneys from *child donors* would be ideally suited for child recipients. However, the experience of most centres has been dismal with kidneys from donors less than 2 years of age and this is also reflected by data from the NAPRTCS registry (Harmon *et al.* 1992; Tejani *et al.* 1998). Regardless of recipient age, an age-dependent donor effect resulting in a significantly decreased transplant survival could be demonstrated for kidneys from young donors, mostly due to vascular thrombosis, primary non-function, or other technical causes. Many centres have, therefore, adopted an age restriction to donors and do not accept kidneys from donors under the age of 5 years (Benfield *et al.* 1999). In the United States, about 90 per cent of cadaveric transplants in children are now from donors older than 10 years. However, more favourable transplant survival using young donors has been reported from single centres, which use specialized operative techniques (Filler *et al.* 1997).

For the *recipient*, a minimum weight of 10 kg has long been accepted as the lower limit for a successful transplant outcome although satisfactory results have been reported with even smaller children. Besides surgical difficulties, problems in young recipients include increased rates of infection, differences in pharmacokinetis of immunosuppressants, and most importantly, thrombosis of the graft. Regardless of age, preoperative evaluation of the recipient must include Doppler studies of blood flow in iliacal vessels (to be used for arterial and venous anastomoses) and subclavian/cervical veins (to be used for central venous lines) to assure normal patency; blood flow may be diminished due to previous catheterizations, anatomical malformation, or thrombotic events. Histocompatibility issues in children are similar to adults: matching for ABO and HLA compatibility as well as a negative cross-match of donor and recipient are preconditions for successful transplantation. Data are now emerging that inherited or acquired thrombophilia is frequently involved in primary non-function, vascular thrombosis, and even diminshed long-term outcome of transplantation (Wahn *et al.* 2001; Hocher *et al.* 2002). One should, therefore, check for the most common prothrombotic factors in the recipient: Factor V Leiden anomaly, low levels of protein C or protein S, prothrombin gene mutations, and antiphospholipid antibodies. The role of Lp(a) is not clear (Querfeld and Wahn 2002), but it is of note that thrombotic events in childhood are associated with high Lp(a) levels and especially frequent if more than one prothrombotic risk factor is present (Nowak-Gottl *et al.* 1997). In high-risk patients, we use perioperative prophylaxis with low-molecular-weight heparin.

The urological evaluation of the recipient deserves special consideration. Children with ESRD frequently suffer from congenital anomalies of the urinary tract, such as vesicoureteral reflux, posterior urethral valves, or neuropathic bladder. Therefore, as a rule, children considered for renal transplantation have to be carefully evaluated by voiding cystourethrography (VCUG), cystoscopy, and often urodynamic studies. The planned operative procedures should be outlined in detail after reviewing all relevant diagnostic studies with the surgical team. If the patient's bladder cannot be used (e.g. due to scarring after surgical interventions or malformations), urinary diversion has to be constructed, preferably with a continent stoma. Some centres have reported excellent results with continent stomal urinary reservoirs such as the Mainz pouch, which uses the umbilicus as a self-closing stoma which can be catheterized (Gerharz *et al.* 1998). Small capacity bladders due to prolonged anuria, which have not been operated on previously, will usually distend once urinary flow is established and can be used for transplantation. However, this may require catheter drainage for a limited time. Intermittent catheterization is the method of choice for patients with a neurological bladder.

Small children weighing less than 15 kg are best transplanted intraperitoneally, whereas routine extraperitoneal placement of the graft can be performed in older children. Most kidneys today function intraoperatively or during the first 24 h after the operation. However, *acute tubular necrosis* is still seen occasionally, favoured by longer cold ischaemia times and associated with significantly impaired graft function, especially in very young recipients (Sarwal *et al.* 2000). *Graft thrombosis* remains a special risk in renal tranplantation with an overall incidence of 2–4 per cent and is the third most common cause of graft failure. Established predisposing conditions are young donor age (<5 years), young recipient age (incidence almost 10 per cent in recipients <2 years) and a cold ischaemia time greater than 24 h (Singh *et al.* 1997).

For *immunosuppression*, most paediatric centres use a triple therapy consisting of prednisone or methylprednisolone, a calcineurin inhibitor [cyclosporin A (CsA) or tacrolimus (TAC)] and azathioprine or mycophenolate mofetil (MMF). In a recent report of the NAPRTCS registry of 1351 transplants since 1996, 95 per cent of children received prednisone, 82 per cent CsA, 53 per cent azathioprine, 11 per cent TAC, and 35 per cent MMF (Seikaly *et al.* 2001). CsA is given in an induction dose of 400–500 mg/m^2 in two divided doses followed by gradual dose reduction to a maintenance dose of approximately 5–8 mg/kg or 120–220 mg/m^2. Children need higher doses per kilogram body weight than adults because of more rapid metabolism of the drug. Even with the more stable kinetics of the Neoral preparation, some children, especially the very young, require thrice daily dosing. Because of the high pharmacokinetic variability, CsA levels must be monitored; 12 h trough levels in the range of 180–230 ng/ml [enzyme multiplied immunoassay technique (EMIT) assay] in the first 3 months after transplantation and of 100–150 ng/ml thereafter are considered appropriate. In addition, the use of 'C2' and 'C3' levels (2 or 3 h after dose ingestion) have gained some acceptance lately, because they correlate better with the area under the curve (AUC) of the blood concentration and therefore with drug exposure. However, clinical superiority of such 'abbreviated AUC' estimations over conventional trough levels has not been proven by prospective studies. Besides nephrotoxicity, the most common side-effects are hypertension, dyslipidaemia, tubular dysfunction including magnesium wasting, neurotoxicity, hypertrichosis, and gingival hyperplasia. Some patients have to be switched to TAC because of these side-effects; hypertrichosis can be a disturbing feature especially in adolescent patients. In many centres, the main reason for converting patients to TAC is 'rescue therapy' (for acute steroid-resistant rejection), which is frequently so successful that the much more aggressive antirejection therapies with OKT-3 and ATG have been virtually abandoned (Shapiro *et al.* 1995). TAC is usually given in a dose of 10 mg/m^2/day in two divided doses with trough levels [by enzyme-linked immunosorbent assay (ELISA)]

in the range of 10–15 ng/l in the first 4 weeks after transplantation and maintenance trough levels of 3–8 ng/l. TAC has also been increasingly used as the primary calcineurin inhibitor in recent years (22 per cent of transplants in North America in 1998), and is associated with a significantly reduced incidence of acute rejections (Trompeter *et al.* 2002). Other advantages of TAC-based immunosuppression seem to be the potential of steroid-free immunosuppression, resulting in better growth, and a decreased incidence of post-transplant hypertension. Side-effects include nephrotoxicity, diabetes mellitus, and the development of post-transplant lymphoproliferative disease.

MMF has gained increasing acceptance in paediatric immunosuppressive protocols and was used in 70 per cent of patients transplanted in 1998 in North America; similar to results in adult patients it is associated with a significantly decreased rate of acute rejections (compared to azathioprine) in children (Staskewitz *et al.* 2001). The usual dose is 1200 mg/m^2 divided into two daily doses. The most important side-effects are opportunistic infections and gastrointestinal complaints. Azathioprine is still used by many centres and should be used if MMF is not tolerated. It is given in a once daily dose of 1–2 mg/kg.

Steroids (IV methylprednisolone) are given in high doses at the time of transplantation (300 mg/m^2) with a daily tapering schedule thereafter to about 4 mg/m^2/day after 6–8 weeks. Almost all paediatric centres still use maintenance therapy with steroids although they interfere with growth. Unfortunately, attempts to discontinue steroids with CsA-based immunosuppressive protocols have resulted in high rates of rejection (and thus, more steroid exposure with antirejection treatment) (Ingulli *et al.* 1993). Steroid-free immunosuppression is feasible with TAC, however, and current studies are evaluating if steroids can be safely discontinued in paediatric patients maintained on CsA and MMF. Steroids remain the mainstay of treatment of acute rejection, usually given in doses of 10 mg/kg (or 200–400 mg/m^2) for 3–4 days.

In general, graft and patient survival are excellent in paediatric patients. In the period 1987–1998, 1-, 3-, and 5-year graft survival were 91, 85, and 80 per cent for LRD grafts and 83, 73, and 65 per cent for cadaveric grafts in the NAPRTCS database; patient survival was in the range of 92–94 per cent over 5 years for all patients, but significantly lower in children under 3 years of age (Seikaly *et al.* 2001). In Europe, 3 year graft survival was 75 per cent for LRD grafts transplanted during 1980–1985 and between 77 and 84 per cent (depending on age) in patients transplanted in 1986–1991. Three-year graft survival of cadaveric kidneys was 53 per cent in 1980–1985 and 65 per cent during 1986–1991. The 3 year patient survival was 92–95 per cent for LRD grafts and 94 per cent for cadaveric grafts during 1986–1991 (Loirat *et al.* 1994).

The main complications of transplantation are infections and the development of malignancy. CMV is the single most frequent infectious complication after transplantation and carries a high risk if it occurs as a primary infection in seronegative children. It can appear in the form of a systemic infection with fever often with leucopenia, pneumonia, enteritis/colitis, or retinitis. In addition, CMV can trigger transplant rejection and is sometimes found as the only cause of increasing serum creatinine in an asymptomatic patient necessitating renal biopsy. CMV prophylaxis with immunoglobulin and ganciclovir is routinely performed in seronegative recipients. Oral preparations of ganciclovir are available; the dose has to be adjusted to renal function (Filler *et al.* 1998). CMV monitoring [antigenaemia, polymerase chain reaction (PCR), shell vial assay] should be performed regularly (Kunzle *et al.* 2000).

Varicella infection is frequent in the paediatric age group. Patients should be vaccinated before transplantation. Exposure to varicella in seronegative patients is treated with IV hyperimmunglobulin and symptomatic infection is treated with IV acyclovir. Prophylaxis for pneumocystis carinii pneumonia is common in the United States but less widely practiced in other countries. Pneumocystis produces diffuse pneumonia accompanied by hypoxaemia and usually rapid dissemination which may be fatal. Treatment should not be delayed and high-dose TMP/SMZ is the drug of choice.

Post-transplant lymphoproliferative disease (PTLD) has emerged as a major complication of immunosuppressive treatment and is usually associated with EBV infection. About 50 per cent of paediatric graft recipients are seronegative for EBV and it is estimated that 10–15 per cent acquire PTLD after transplantation, usually occurring with a delay of 6–12 months (Shapiro *et al.* 1999). However, PTLD can also develop with EBV reactivation in seropositive recipients. Importantly, PTLD in children may be localized in extranodal lymphatic tissues in the lung, the liver, or intestinum as well as in 'unusual' sites such as adenoids, tonsils, or larynx. PTLD in children is characterized by a higher incidence (10.1 per cent in a large series, compared to 1.2 per cent in adults), a more benign clinical course (high percentage of graft survival), and a high potential for reversibility following reduction of immunosuppression (almost 100 per cent patient survival) (Ellis *et al.* 1999).

Non-compliance is an important issue in paediatric patients and especially in adolescents, in whom non-compliance rates as high as 70 per cent have been reported (Wolff *et al.* 1998). Non-compliance seems particularly frequent in the transition period when patients move from paediatric to adult centres. Besides age, other factors such as poor socioeconomic status and communication problems have been identified in these patients. Emotional and educational support should be provided but may be of limited success; it seems that many issues involved are beyond the control of the physician.

References

Afthentopoulos, I. E., Passadakis, P., Oreopoulos, D. G., and Bargman, J. (1998). Sclerosing peritonitis in continuous ambulatory peritoneal dialysis patients: one center's experience and review of the literature. *Advances in Renal Replacement Therapy* 5, 157–167.

Andreoli, S. P. and Cohen, M. (1989). Intraperitoneal deferoxamine therapy for iron overload in children undergoing CAPD. *Kidney International* 35, 1330–1335.

Arbus, G. S. and Bacheyie, G. S. (1981). Method for predicting when children with progressive renal disease may reach high serum creatinine levels. *Pediatrics* 67, 871–873.

Arnold, W. C., Danford, D., and Holliday, M. A. (1983). Effects of caloric supplementation on growth in children with uremia. *Kidney International* 24, 205–209.

Avner, E. D., Harmon, W. E., Grupe, W. E., Ingelfinger, J. R., Eraklis, A. J., and Levey, R. H. (1981). Mortality of chronic hemodialysis and renal transplantation in pediatric end-stage renal disease. *Pediatrics* 67, 412–416.

Baraldi, E., Montini, G., Zanconato, S., Zacchello, G., and Zacchello, F. (1990). Exercise tolerance after anaemia correction with recombinant human erythropoietin in end-stage renal disease. *Pediatric Nephrology* 4, 623–626.

Behrens, R., Lang, T., Muschweck, H., Richter, T., and Hofbeck, M. (1997). Percutaneous endoscopic gastrostomy in children and adolescents. *Journal of Pediatric Gastroenterology and Nutrition* 25, 487–491.

Benfield, M. R., McDonald, R., Sullivan, E. K., Stablein, D. M., and Tejani, A. (1999). The 1997 Annual Renal Transplantation in Children Report of the North American Pediatric Renal Transplant Cooperative Study (NAPRTCS). *Pediatric Transplantation* 3, 152–167.

Bergstrom, L. and Thompson, P. (1983). Hearing loss in pediatric renal patients. *International Journal of Pediatric Otorhinolaryngology* 5, 227–234.

Bianchetti, M. G., Hammerli, I., Roduit, C., Neuhaus, T. J., Leumann, E. P., and Oetliker, O. H. (1991). Epoetin alfa in anaemic children or adolescents on regular dialysis. *European Journal of Pediatrics* 150, 509–512.

Blum, W. F., Ranke, M. B., Kietzmann, K., Tonshoff, B., and Mehls, O. (1991). Growth hormone resistance and inhibition of somatomedin activity by excess of insulin-like growth factor binding protein in uraemia. *Pediatric Nephrology* 5, 539–544.

Bock, G. H., Conners, C. K., Ruley, J., Samango-Sprouse, C. A., Conry, J. A., Weiss, I., Eng, G., Johnson, E. L., and David, C. T. (1989). Disturbances of brain maturation and neurodevelopment during chronic renal failure in infancy. *Journal of Pediatrics* 114, 231–238.

Brandt, J. R., Avner, E. D., Hickman, R. O., and Watkins, S. L. (1999). Safety and efficacy of erythropoietin in children with chronic renal failure. *Pediatric Nephrology* 13, 143–147.

Brittinger, W. D., Walker, G., Twittenhoff, W. D., and Konrad, N. (1997). Vascular access for hemodialysis in children. *Pediatric Nephrology* 11, 87–95.

Broyer, M., Tete, M. J., and Gubler, M. C. (1987). Late symptoms in infantile cystinosis. *Pediatric Nephrology* 1, 519–524.

Canada-USA (CANUSA) Peritoneal Dialysis Study Group (1996). Adequacy of dialysis and nutrition in continuous peritoneal dialysis: association with clinical outcomes. Canada-USA (CANUSA) Peritoneal Dialysis Study Group. *Journal of the American Society of Nephrology* 7, 198–207.

Chantler, C., Broyer, M., Donckerwolcke, R. A., Brynger, H., Brunner, F. P., Jacobs, C., Kramer, P., Selwood, N. H., and Wing, A. J. (1981). Growth and rehabilitation of long-term survivors of treatment for end-stage renal failure in childhood. *Proceedings of the European Dialysis and Transplantation Association* 18, 329–342.

Chantler, C., Lieberman, E., and Holliday, M. A. (1974). A rat model for the study of growth failure in uremia. *Pediatric Research* 8, 109–113.

Charnas, L. R., Luciano, C. A., Dalakas, M., Gilliatt, R. W., Bernardini, I., Ishak, K., Cwik, V. A., Fraker, D., Brushart, T. A., and Gahl, W. A. (1994). Distal vacuolar myopathy in nephropathic cystinosis. *Annals of Neurology* 35, 181–188.

Claris-Appiani, A., Ardissino, G. L., Dacco, V., Funari, C., and Terzi, F. (1995). Catch-up growth in children with chronic renal failure treated with long-term enteral nutrition. *Journal of Parenteral and Enteral Nutrition* 19, 175–178.

de Beaufort, C. E., Andre, J. L., Heimans, J. J., van der Eerden, H. A., van Diemen, N. G., Duc, M. L., and Pierson, M. (1989). Peripheral nerve function in children with end-stage renal failure. *Pediatric Nephrology* 3, 175–178.

DelloStrologo, L., Principato, F., Sinibaldi, D., Appiani, A. C., Terzi, F., Dartois, A. M., and Rizzoni, G. (1997). Feeding dysfunction in infants with severe chronic renal failure after long-term nasogastric tube feeding. *Pediatric Nephrology* 11, 84–86.

Drukker, A. (1991). Hypertension in children and adolescents with chronic renal failure and end-stage renal disease. *Child Nephrology and Urology* 11, 152–158.

Ehrich, J. H., Loirat, C., Brunner, F. P., Geerlings, W., Landais, P., Mallick, N. P., Margreiter, R., Raine, A. E., Selwood, N. H., and Tufveson, G. (1992). Report on management of renal failure in children in Europe, XXII, 1991. *Nephrology, Dialysis, Transplantation* 7 (Suppl. 2), 36–48.

Ehrich, J. H., Rizzoni, G., Brunner, F. P., Brynger, H., Geerlings, W., Fassbinder, W., Raine, A. E., Selwood, N. H., and Tufveson, G. (1991). Combined report on regular dialysis and transplantation of children in Europe, 1989. *Nephrology, Dialysis, Transplantation* 6 (Suppl. 1), 37–47.

Eifinger, F., Wahn, F., Querfeld, U., Pollok, M., Gevargez, A., Kriener, P., and Gronemeyer, D. (2000). Coronary artery calcifications in children and young adults treated with renal replacement therapy. *Nephrology, Dialysis, Transplantation* 15 (11), 1892–1894.

Ellis, D., Jaffe, R., Green, M., Janosky, J. J., Lombardozzi-Lane, S., Shapiro, R., Scantlebury, V., Vivas, C., and Jordan, M. L. (1999). Epstein–Barr virus-related disorders in children undergoing renal transplantation with tacrolimus-based immunosuppression. *Transplantation* 68, 997–1003.

Elzouki, A., Carroll, J., Butinar, D., and Moosa, A. (1994). Improved neurological outcome in children with chronic renal disease from infancy. *Pediatric Nephrology* 8, 205–210.

Fennell, R. S., III, Orak, J. K., Hudson, T., Garin, E. H., Iravani, A., Van Deusen, W. J., Howard, R., Pfaff, W. W., Walker, R. D., III, and Richard, G. A. (1984). Growth in children with various therapies for end-stage renal disease. *American Journal of Diseases of Children* 138, 28–31.

Filler, G., Lampe, D., von Bredow, M. A., Lappenberg-Pelzer, M., Rocher, S., Strehlau, J., and Ehrich, J. H. (1998). Prophylactic oral ganciclovir after renal transplantation-dosing and pharmacokinetics. *Pediatric Nephrology* 12, 6–9.

Filler, G., Lindeke, A., Bohme, K., Devaux, S., Schonberger, B., and Ehrich, J. H. (1997). Renal transplantation from donors aged <6 years into children yields equal graft survival when compared to older donors. *Pediatric Transplantation* 1, 119–123.

Fine, R. N. and Salusky, I. B. (1986). CAPD/CCPD in children: four years' experience. *Kidney International* 19 (Suppl.), S7–S10.

Fine, R. N., Tejani, A., and Sullivan, E. K. (1994). Pre-emptive renal transplantation in children: report of the North American Pediatric Renal Transplant Cooperative Study (NAPRTCS). *Clinical Transplantation* 8, 474–478.

Fischbach, M., Terzic, J., Dangelser, C., Schneider, P., Roger, M. L., and Geisert, J. (1997). Improved dialysis dose by optimizing intraperitoneal volume prescription thanks to intraperitoneal pressure measurements in children. *Advances in Peritoneal Dialysis* 13, 271–273.

Fishbane, S. and Maesaka, J. K. (1997). Iron management in end-stage renal disease. *American Journal of Kidney Diseases* 29, 319–333.

Frei, U. and Schober-Halstenberg, H. J. (1999). Annual Report of the German Renal Registry 1998. QuaSi-Niere Task Group for Quality Assurance in Renal Replacement Therapy. *Nephrology, Dialysis, Transplantation* 14, 1085–1090.

Geary, D. F. (1998). Attitudes of pediatric nephrologists to management of end-stage renal disease in infants. *Journal of Pediatrics* 133, 154–156.

Gerharz, E. W., Kohl, U. N., Weingartner, K., Kleinhans, B. J., Melekos, M. D., and Riedmiller, H. (1998). Experience with the Mainz modification of ureterosigmoidostomy. *British Journal of Surgery* 85, 1512–1516.

Goodman, W. G., Goldin, J, Kuizon, B. D., Yoon, C., Gales, B., Sider, D., Wang, Y., Chung, J., Americk, A., Greaser, L., Elashoff, R. M., and Salusky, I. B. (2000). Coronary artery calcification in young adults with end-stage renal disease who are undergoing dialysis. *New England Journal of Medicine* 342, 1478–1483.

Gotto, A. M. J. (1997). Results of recent large cholesterol-lowering trials and implications for clinical management. *The American Journal of Cardiology* 79, 1663–1666.

Greenbaum, L. A., Pan, C. G., Caley, C., Nelson, T., and Sheth, K. J. (2000). Intravenous iron dextran and erythropoietin use in pediatric hemodialysis patients. *Pediatric Nephrology* 14 (10–11), 908–911.

Gupta, S., Walker, D. L., Keshavarzian, A., and Hodgson, H. J. (1987). Upper endoscopy for occult bleeding in renal failure. *Journal of Clinical Gastroenterology* 9, 43–45.

Haffner, D. and Schaefer, F. (2001). Does recombinant growth hormone improve adult height in children with chronic renal failure? *Seminars in Nephrology* 21, 490–497.

Haffner, D., Schaefer, F., Girard, J., Ritz, E., and Mehls, O. (1994). Metabolic clearance of recombinant human growth hormone in health and chronic renal failure. *Journal of Clinical Investment* 93, 1163–1171.

Haffner, D., Schaefer, F., Nissel, R., Wuhl, E., Tonshoff, B., and Mehls, O. (2000). Effect of growth hormone treatment on the adult height of children with chronic renal failure. German Study Group for Growth

Hormone Treatment in Chronic Renal Failure. *New England Journal of Medicine* 343 (13), 923–930.

Haffner, D., Weinfurth, A., Manz, F., Schmidt, H., Bremer, H. J., Mehls, O., and Scharer, K. (1999). Long-term outcome of paediatric patients with hereditary tubular disorders. *Nephron* 83, 250–260.

Harmoinen, A., Ylinen, E., Ala-Houhala, M., Janas, M., Kaila, M., and Kouri, T. (2000). Reference intervals for cystatin C in pre- and full-term infants and children. *Pediatric Nephrology* 15, 105–108.

Harmon, W. E. and Jabs, K. Hemodialysis. In *Pediatric Nephrology* 4th edn. (ed. T. M. Barratt, E. D. Avner, and W. E. Harmon), pp. 1267–1287. Philadelphia, PA: Lippincott Williams and Wilkins, 1999.

Harmon, W. E., Alexander, S. R., Tejani, A., and Stablein, D. (1992). The effect of donor age on graft survival in pediatric cadaver renal transplant recipients—a report of the North American Pediatric Renal Transplant Cooperative Study. *Transplantation* 54, 232–237.

Harshfield, G. A., Alpert, B. S., Pulliam, D. A., Somes, G. W., and Wilson, D. K. (1994). Ambulatory blood pressure recordings in children and adolescents. *Pediatrics* 94, 180–184.

Hocher, B., Slowinski, T., Hauser, I., Vetter, B., Fritschel, L., Bachert, D., Kulozik, A., and Neumayer, H. H. (2002). Association of Factor V Leiden mutation with delayed graft function, acute rejection episodes and long-term graft dysfunction in kidney transplant recipients. *Thrombosis and Haemostasis* 87 (2), 194–198.

Hokken-Koelega, A. C., Stijnen, T., de Jong, M. C., Donckerwolcke, R. A., de Muinck Keizer-Schrama, S. M., Blum, W. F., and Drop, S. L. (1994). Double blind trial comparing the effects of two doses of growth hormone in prepubertal patients with chronic renal insufficiency. *Journal of Clinical Endocrinology and Metabolism* 79, 1185–1190.

Holliday, M. A. (1973). Growth in children with renal disease with particular reference to the effects of calorie malnutrition: a review. *Clinical Nephrology* 1, 230–242.

Holmberg, C., Laine, J., Ronnholm, K., Ala-Houhala, M., and Jalanko, H. (1996). Congenital nephrotic syndrome. *Kidney International* 53 (Suppl.), S51–S56.

Holtta, T., Ronnholm, K., Jalanko, H., and Holmberg, C. (2000). Clinical outcome of pediatric patients on peritoneal dialysis under adequacy control. *Pediatric Nephrology* 14 (10–11), 889–897.

Ingulli, E., Sharma, V., Singh, A., Suthanthiran, M., and Tejani, A. (1993). Steroid withdrawal, rejection and the mixed lymphocyte reaction in children after renal transplantation. *Kidney International* 43 (Suppl.), S36–S39.

Jungers, P., Khoa, T. N., Massy, Z. A., Zingraff, J., Labrunie, M., Descamps-Latscha, B., and Man, N. K. (1999). Incidence of atherosclerotic arterial occlusive accidents in predialysis and dialysis patients: a multicentric study in the Ile de France district. *Nephrology, Dialysis, Transplantation* 14, 898–902.

Kausz, A. T., Watkins, S. L., Hansen, C., Godwin, D. A., Palmer, R. B., and Brandt, J. R. (1999). Intraperitoneal erythropoietin in children on peritoneal dialysis: a study of pharmacokinetics and efficacy. *American Journal of Kidney Diseases* 34, 651–656.

Kingwatanakul, P. and Warady, B. A. (1997). *Staphylococcus aureus* nasal carriage in children receiving long-term peritoneal dialysis. *Advances in Peritoneal Dialysis* 13, 281–284.

Klahr, S., Levey, A. S., Beck, G. J., Caggiula, A. W., Hunsicker, L., Kusek, J. W., and Striker, G. (1994). The effects of dietary protein restriction and blood-pressure control on the progression of chronic renal disease. Modification of Diet in Renal Disease Study Group. *New England Journal of Medicine* 330, 877–884.

Klee, K. M., Greenleaf, K., Fouser, L., and Watkins, S. L. (1996). Continuous venovenous hemofiltration with and without dialysis in pediatric patients. *ANNA Journal* 23, 35–39.

Knight, F., Gorynski, L., Bentson, M., and Harmon, W. E. (1993). Hemodialysis of the infant or small child with chronic renal failure. *ANNA Journal* 20, 315–323.

Krmar, R. T., Ferraris, J. R., Ramirez, J. A., Galarza, C. R., Waisman, G., Janson, J. J., Llapur, C. J., Sorroche, P., Legal, S., and Camera, M. I. (2001). Hyperhomocysteinemia in stable pediatric, adolescents, and young adult renal transplant recipients. *Transplantation* 71 (12), 1748–1751.

Kronenberg, F., Kathrein, H., Konig, P., Neyer, U., Sturm, W., Lhotta, K., Grochenig, E., Utermann, G., and Dieplinger, H. (1994). Apolipoprotein(a) phenotypes predict the risk for carotid atherosclerosis in patients with end-stage renal disease. *Arteriosclerosis Thrombosis* 14, 1405–1411.

Kronenberg, F., Kuen, E., Ritz, E., Junker, R., Konig, P., Kraatz, G., Lhotta, K., Mann, J. F., Muller, G. A., Neyer, U., Riegel, W., Reigler, P., Schwenger, V., and Von Eckardstein, A. (2000). Lipoprotein(a) serum concentrations and apolipoprotein(a) phenotypes in mild and moderate renal failure. *Journal of the American Society of Nephrology* 11 (1), 105–115.

Kronn, D. F., Sapru, A., and Satou, G. M. (2000). Management of hypercholesterolemia in childhood and adolescence. *Heart Disease* 2 (5), 348–353.

Kuizon, B. D., Goodman, W. G., Juppner, H., Boechat, I., Nelson, P., Gales, B., and Salusky, I. B. (1998). Diminished linear growth during intermittent calcitriol therapy in children undergoing CCPD. *Kidney International* 53, 205–211.

Kunzle, N., Petignat, C., Francioli, P., Vogel, G., Seydoux, C., Corpataux, J. M., Sahli, R., and Meylan, P. R. (2000). Preemptive treatment approach to cytomegalovirus (CMV) infection in solid organ transplant patients: relationship between compliance with the guidelines and prevention of CMV morbidity. *Transplant Infectious Disease* 2 (3), 118–126.

Lerner, G. R., Warady, B. A., Sullivan, E. K., and Alexander, S. R. (1999). Chronic dialysis in children and adolescents. The 1996 annual report of the North American Pediatric Renal Transplant Cooperative Study. *Pediatric Nephrology* 13, 404–417.

Levey, A. S., Greene, T., Beck, G. J., Caggiula, A. W., Kusek, J. W., Hunsicker, L. G., and Klahr, S. (1999). Dietary protein restriction and the progression of chronic renal disease: what have all of the results of the MDRD study shown? Modification of Diet in Renal Disease Study group. *Journal of the American Society of Nephrology* 10, 2426–2439.

Licht, C., Eifinger, F., Gharib, M., Offner, G., Michalk, D. V., and Querfeld, U. (2000). A stepwise approach to the treatment of early onset nephrotic syndrome. *Pediatric Nephrology* 14 (12), 1077–1082.

Lingens, N., Dobos, E., Lemmer, B., and Scharer, K. (1996). Nocturnal blood pressure elevation in transplanted pediatric patients. *Kidney International* 55 (Suppl.), S175–S176.

Lingens, N., Soergel, M., Loirat, C., Busch, C., Lemmer, B., and Scharer, K. (1995). Ambulatory blood pressure monitoring in paediatric patients treated by regular haemodialysis and peritoneal dialysis. *Pediatric Nephrology* 9, 167–172.

Loirat, C., Ehrich, J. H., Geerlings, W., Jones, E. H., Landais, P., Mallick, N. P., Margreiter, R., Raine, A. E., Salmela, K., and Selwood, N. H. (1994). Report on management of renal failure in children in Europe, XXIII, 1992. *Nephrology, Dialysis, Transplantation* 9 (Suppl. 1), 26–40.

Malozowski, S., Tanner, L. A., Wysowski, D., and Fleming, G. A. (1993). Growth hormone, insulin-like growth factor I, and benign intracranial hypertension. *New England Journal Medicine* 329, 665–666.

Maxwell, H. and Rees, L. (1996). Recombinant human growth hormone treatment in infants with chronic renal failure. *Archives of Disease in Childhood* 74, 40–43.

McGraw, M. E. and Haka-Ikse, K. (1985). Neurologic-developmental sequelae of chronic renal failure in infancy. *Journal of Pediatrics* 106, 579–583.

Mehls, O. and Ritz, E. (1983). Skeletal growth in experimental uremia. *Kidney International* 15 (Suppl.), S53–S62.

Mehls, O. and Salusky, I. B. (1987). Recent advances and controversies in childhood renal osteodystrophy. *Pediatric Nephrology* 1, 212–223.

Mehls, O. and Scharer, K. Chronische Niereninsuffizienz. In *Pädiatrische Nephrologie* 1st edn. (ed. K. Scharer and O. Mehls), pp. 373–390. Berlin: Springer, 2002.

Mehls, O., Rigden, S., Ehrich, J. H., Berthoux, F., Jones, E. H., and Valderrabano, F. (1996). Report on management of renal failure in Europe, XXV, 1994. The child–adult interface. The EDTA–ERA Registry.

European Dialysis and Transplant Association–European Renal Association. *Nephrology, Dialysis, Transplantation* 11 (Suppl. 1), 22–36.

Mehls, O., Ritz, E., Hunziker, E. B., Eggli, P., Heinrich, U., and Zapf, J. (1988). Improvement of growth and food utilization by human recombinant growth hormone in uremia. *Kidney International* 33, 45–52.

Merouani, A., Lambert, M., Delvin, E. E., Genest, J. J., Robitaille, P., and Rozen, R. (2001). Plasma homocysteine concentration in children with chronic renal failure. *Pediatric Nephrology* 16 (10), 805–811.

Meyer, K. B. and Levey, A. S. (1998). Controlling the epidemic of cardiovascular disease in chronic renal disease: report from the National Kidney Foundation Task Force on cardiovascular disease. *Journal of the American Society of Nephrology* 9, S31–S42.

Milliner, D. S., Zinsmeister, A. R., Lieberman, E., and Landing, B. (1990). Soft tissue calcification in pediatric patients with end-stage renal disease. *Kidney International* 38, 931–936.

Molinari, L., Largo, R. H., and Prader, A. Target height and secular trend in the Swiss population. In *First Zurich Longitudinal Study of Growth and Development* (ed. J. Borms), pp. 193–200. New York, NY: Plenum Press, 1985.

Morel, P., Almond, P. S., Matas, A. J., Gillingham, K. J., Chau, C., Brown, A., Kashtan, C. E., Mauer, S. M., Chavers, B., and Nevins, T. E. (1991). Long-term quality of life after kidney transplantation in childhood. *Transplantation* 52, 47–53.

Muller-Berghaus, J., Hoppe, B., Schmidt, R., Wagner, M., and Querfeld, U. (1997). A transplanted child with severe hypercalcaemic hyperparathyroidism despite only modest bone lesions. *Nephrology, Dialysis, Transplantation* 12, 2445–2446.

Müller-Wiefel, D. E., Vorderbrugge, U., and Scharer, K. (1985). Iron removal by desferrioxamine during haemodialysis: *in vitro* studies. *Proceedings of the European Dialysis and Transplant Association European Renal Association* 21, 377–381.

National Kidney Foundation (2002). K/DOQI clinical practice guidelines for chronic kidney disease: evaluation, classification, and stratification. Kidney Disease Outcome Quality Initiative. *American Journal of Kidney Diseases* 39 (Suppl. 2), S1–S246.

Nayir, A., Bilge, I., Kilicaslan, I., Ander, H., Emre, S., and Sirin, A. (2001). Arterial changes in paediatric haemodialysis patients undergoing renal transplantation. *Nephrology, Dialysis, Transplantation* 16 (10), 2041–2047.

Nelson, P. and Stover, J. Nutritional assessment and management of the child with ESRD. In *End Stage Renal Disease in Children* 1st edn. (ed. R. N. Fine and A. B. Gruskin), pp. 209–226. Philadelphia, PA: W.B. Saunders, 2002.

Nishibata, K., Nagashima, M., Tsuji, A., Hasegawa, S., Nagai, N., Goto, M., and Hayashi, H. (1995). Comparison of casual blood pressure and twenty-four-hour ambulatory blood pressure in high school students. *Journal of Pediatrics* 127, 34–39.

Norris, K. C., Goodman, W. G., Howard, N., Nugent, M. E., and Coburn, J. W. (1986). Iliac crest bone biopsy for diagnosis of aluminum toxicity and a guide to the use of deferoxamine. *Seminars in Nephrology* 6, 27–34.

Nowak-Gottl, U., Debus, O., Findeisen, M., Kassenbohmer, R., Koch, H. G., Pollmann, H., Postler, C., Weber, P., and Vielhaber, H. (1997). Lipoprotein(a): its role in childhood thromboembolism. *Pediatrics* 99, E11.

Oh, J., Wunsch, R., Turzer, M., Bahner, M., Raggi, P., Querfeld, U., Mehls, O., and Schaefer, F. (2002). Advanced coronary and carotid arteriopathy in young adults with childhood-onset chronic renal failure. *Circulation* 106 (1), 100–105.

Pedrini, M. T., Levey, A. S., Lau, J., Chalmers, T. C., and Wang, P. H. (1996). The effect of dietary protein restriction on the progression of diabetic and nondiabetic renal diseases: a meta-analysis. *Annals of Internal Medicine* 124, 627–632.

Polinsky, M. S. Neurologic manifestations of renal disease. In *Principles of Child Neurology* 1st edn. (ed. B. O. Berg), pp. 1327–1342. New York: McGraw-Hill, 1996.

Polinsky, M. S., Kaiser, B. A., Stover, J. B., Frankenfield, M., and Baluarte, H. J. (1987). Neurologic development of children with severe chronic renal failure from infancy. *Pediatric Nephrology* 1, 157–165.

Potter, D. E., San Luis, E., Wipfler, J. E., and Portale, A. A. (1986). Comparison of continuous ambulatory peritoneal dialysis and hemodialysis in children. *Kidney International* **19** (Suppl.), S11–S14.

Price, P. A., Faus, S. A., and Williamson, M. K. (2000). Warfarin-induced artery calcification is accelerated by growth and vitamin D. *Arteriosclerosis, Thrombosis, and Vascular Biology* **20** (2), 317–327.

Querfeld, U. (1993). Disturbances of lipid metabolism in children with chronic renal failure. *Pediatric Nephrology* **7**, 749–757.

Querfeld, U. (1996). Is the impact of recombinant human growth hormone (rhGH) on the plasma lipid profile beneficial or harmful? *British Journal of Clinical Practice* **85** (Suppl.), 54–55.

Querfeld, U. and Wahn, F. (2002). Should lipoprotein(a) be measured in pediatric renal transplant recipients? *Pediatric Transplantation* **6** (2), 87–90.

Querfeld, U., Dietrich, R., Taira, R. K., Kangarloo, H., Salusky, I. B., and Fine, R. N. (1988a). Magnetic resonance imaging of iron overload in children treated with peritoneal dialysis. *Nephron* **50**, 220–224.

Querfeld, U., Haffner, D., Wuhl, E., Wingen, A. M., Wolter, K., Friedrich, B., Michalk, D. V., and Mehls, O. (1996). Treatment with growth hormone increases lipoprotein(a) serum levels in children with chronic renal insufficiency. *European Journal of Pediatrics* **155**, 913.

Querfeld, U., Hoffmann, M. M., Klaus, G., Eifinger, F., Ackerschott, M., Michalk, D., and Kern, P. A. (1999). Antagonistic effects of vitamin D and parathyroid hormone on lipoprotein lipase in cultured adipocytes. *Journal of the American Society of Nephrology* **10**, 2158–2164.

Querfeld, U., Korten, B., Naumann, G., and Michalk, D. V. (1997). Medical and psychosocial rehabilitation of young adults receiving renal replacement therapy since childhood: a single-centre experience. *Nephrology, Dialysis, Transplantation* **12**, 33–37.

Querfeld, U., Lang, M., Friedrich, J. B., Kohl, B., Fiehn, W., and Scharer, K. (1993). Lipoprotein(a) serum levels and apolipoprotein(a) phenotypes in children with chronic renal disease. *Pediatric Research* **34**, 772–776.

Querfeld, U., LeBoeuf, R. C., Salusky, I. B., Nelson, P., Laidlaw, S., and Fine, R. N. (1991). Lipoproteins in children treated with continuous peritoneal dialysis. *Pediatric Research* **29**, 155–159.

Querfeld, U., Salusky, I. B., Nelson, P., Foley, J., and Fine, R. N. (1988b). Hyperlipidemia in pediatric patients undergoing peritoneal dialysis. *Pediatric Nephrology* **2**, 447–452.

Ramage, I. J., Harvey, E., Geary, D. F., Hebert, D., Balfe, J. A., and Balfe, J. W. (1999). Complications of gastrostomy feeding in children receiving peritoneal dialysis. *Pediatric Nephrology* **13**, 249–252.

Reijneveld, J. C., Koot, R. W., Bredman, J. J., Joles, J. A., and Bar, P. R. (1996). Differential effects of 3-hydroxy-3-methylglutaryl-coenzyme A reductase inhibitors on the development of myopathy in young rats. *Pediatric Research* **39**, 1028–1035.

Rotundo, A., Nevins, T. E., Lipton, M., Lockman, L. A., Mauer, S. M., and Michael, A. F. (1982). Progressive encephalopathy in children with chronic renal insufficiency in infancy. *Kidney International* **21**, 486–491.

Sarwal, M. M., Cecka, J. M., Millan, M. T., and Salvatierra, O. J. (2000). Adult-size kidneys without acute tubular necrosis provide exceedingly superior long-term graft outcomes for infants and small children: a single center and UNOS analysis. United Network for Organ Sharing. *Transplantation* **70** (12), 1728–1736.

Scanu, A. M. (1992). Lipoprotein(a). A genetic risk factor for premature coronary heart disease. *Journal of the American Medical Association* **267**, 3326–3329.

Schaefer, F. and Mehls, O. Endocrine and growth disturbances. In *Pediatric Nephrology* 4th edn. (ed. T. M. Barratt, E. D. Avner, and W. E. Harmon), pp. 1197–1230. Philadelphia, PA: Lippincott Williams & Wilkins, 1999.

Schaefer, F., Chen, Y., Tsao, T., Nouri, P., and Rabkin, R. (2001). Impaired JAK-STAT signal transduction contributes to growth hormone resistance in chronic uremia. *Journal of Clinical Investigation* **108** (3), 467–475.

Schaefer, F., Gilli, G., and Scharer, K. Pubertal growth and final height in chronic renal failure. In *Growth and Endocrine Changes in Children and Adolescents with Chronic Renal Failure* (ed. K. Scharer), pp. 59–69. Basel: Karger, 1989.

Schaefer, F., Klaus, G., and Mehls, O. (1999a). Peritoneal transport properties and dialysis dose affect growth and nutritional status in children on chronic peritoneal dialysis. Mid-European Pediatric Peritoneal Dialysis Study Group. *Journal of the American Society of Nephrology* **10**, 1786–1792.

Schaefer, F., Klaus, G., Muller-Wiefel, D. E., and Mehls, O. (1999b). Current practice of peritoneal dialysis in children: results of a longitudinal survey. Mid-European Pediatric Peritoneal Dialysis Study Group (MEPPS). *Peritoneal Dialysis International* **19** (Suppl. 2), S445–S449.

Schaefer, F., Klaus, G., Muller-Wiefel, D. E., and Mehls, O. (1999c). Intermittent versus continuous intraperitoneal glycopeptide/ceftazidime treatment in children with peritoneal dialysis-associated peritonitis. The Mid-European Pediatric Peritoneal Dialysis Study Group (MEPPS). *Journal of the American Society of Nephrology* **10**, 136–145.

Schaefer, F., Seidel, C., Binding, A., Gasser, T., Largo, R. H., Prader, A., and Scharer, K. (1990). Pubertal growth in chronic renal failure. *Pediatric Research* **28**, 5–10.

Scharer, K., Chantler, C., Brunner, F. P., Gurland, H. J., Jacobs, C., Parsons, F. M., Seyfart, G., and Wing, A. J. (1976). Combined report on regular dialysis and transplantation of children in Europe, 1974. *Proceedings of the European Dialysis and Transplant Association* **12**, 65–108.

Scharer, K., Schmidt, K. G., and Soergel, M. (1999). Cardiac function and structure in patients with chronic renal failure. *Pediatric Nephrology* **13**, 951–965.

Schroder, C. H., de Boer, A. W., Giesen, A. M., Monnens, L. A., and Blom, H. (1999). Treatment of hyperhomocysteinemia in children on dialysis by folic acid. *Pediatric Nephrology* **13**, 583–585.

Schwartz, G. J., Brion, L. P., and Spitzer, A. (1987). The use of plasma creatinine concentration for estimating glomerular filtration rate in infants, children, and adolescents. *Pediatric Clinics of North America* **34**, 571–590.

Seikaly, M., Ho, P. L., Emmett, L., and Tejani, A. (2001). The 12th Annual Report of the North American Pediatric Renal Transplant Cooperative Study: renal transplantation from 1987 through 1998. *Pediatric Transplantation* **5** (3), 215–231.

Shapera, M. R., Moel, D. I., Kamath, S. K., Olson, R., and Beauchamp, G. K. (1986). Taste perception of children with chronic renal failure. *Journal of the American Dietetic Association* **86**, 1359–1362, 1365.

Shapiro, R., Nalesnik, M., McCauley, J., Fedorek, S., Jordan, M. L., Scantlebury, V. P., Jain, A., Vivas, C., Ellis, D., Lombardozzi-Lane, S., Randhawa, P., Johnston, J., Hakala, T. R., Simmons, R. L., Fung, J. J., and Starzl, T. E. (1999). Posttransplant lymphoproliferative disorders in adult and pediatric renal transplant patients receiving tacrolimus-based immunosuppression. *Transplantation* **68**, 1851–1854.

Shapiro, R., Scantlebury, V. P., Jordan, M. L., Vivas, C., Tzakis, A. G., Ellis, D., Gilboa, N., Hopp, L., McCauley, J., and Irish, W. (1995). FK506 in pediatric kidney transplantation—primary and rescue experience. *Pediatric Nephrology* **9** (Suppl.), S43–S48.

Singh, A., Stablein, D., and Tejani, A. (1997). Risk factors for vascular thrombosis in pediatric renal transplantation: a special report of the North American Pediatric Renal Transplant Cooperative Study. *Transplantation* **63**, 1263–1267.

Soergel, M., Kirschstein, M., Busch, C., Danne, T., Gellermann, J., Holl, R., Krull, F., Reichert, H., Reusz, G. S., and Rascher, W. (1997). Oscillometric twenty-four-hour ambulatory blood pressure values in healthy children and adolescents: a multicenter trial including 1141 subjects. *Journal of Pediatrics* **130**, 178–184.

Sorof, J. M. (2000). White coat hypertension in children. *Blood Pressure Monitoring* **5** (4), 197–202.

Sorof, J. M., Sullivan, E. K., Tejani, A., and Portman, R. J. (1999). Antihypertensive medication and renal allograft failure: a North American Pediatric Renal Transplant Cooperative Study report. *Journal of the American Society of Nephrology* **10**, 1324–1330.

Southwest Pediatric Nephrology Study Group (1985). Continuous ambulatory and continuous cycling peritoneal dialysis in children. A report of the Southwest Pediatric Nephrology Study Group. *Kidney International* 27, 558–564.

Stamler, J., Daviglus, M. L., Garside, D. B., Dyer, A. R., Greenland, P., and Neaton, J. D. (2000). Relationship of baseline serum cholesterol levels in 3 large cohorts of younger men to long-term coronary, cardiovascular, and all-cause mortality and to longevity. *Journal of the American Medical Association* 284, 311–318.

Staskewitz, A., Kirste, G., Tonshoff, B., Weber, L. T., Boswald, M., Burghard, R., Helmchen, U., Brandis, M., and Zimmerhackl, L. B. (2001). Mycophenolate mofetil in pediatric renal transplantation without induction therapy: results after 12 months of treatment. German Pediatric Renal Transplantation Study Group. *Transplantation* 71 (5), 638–644.

Stefanidis, C. J., Hewitt, I. K., and Balfe, J. W. (1983). Growth in children receiving continuous ambulatory peritoneal dialysis. *Journal of Pediatrics* 102, 681–685.

Sunder-Plassmann, G., Fodinger, M., Buchmayer, H., Papagiannopoulos, M., Wojcik, J., Kletzmayr, J., Enzenberger, B., Janata, O., Winkelmayer, W. C., Paul, G., Auinger, M., Barnas, U., and Horl, W. H. (2000). Effect of high dose folic acid therapy on hyperhomocysteinemia in hemodialysis patients: results of the Vienna multicenter study. *Journal of the American Society of Nephrology* 11 (6), 1106–1116.

Tanner, J. M. *Growth at Adolescence.* Oxford: Blackwell, 1962.

Tanner, J. M., Whitehouse, R. H., Marshall, W. A., Healey, M. J. R., and Goldstein, H. *Assessment of Skeletal Maturity and Prediction of Adult Height.* London: Academic Press, 1975.

Tejani, A. H., Stablein, D. M., Sullivan, E. K., Alexander, S. R., Fine, R. N., Harmon, W. E., and Kohaut, E. C. (1998). The impact of donor source, recipient age, pre-operative immunotherapy and induction therapy on early and late acute rejections in children: a report of the North American Pediatric Renal Transplant Cooperative Study (NAPRTCS). *Pediatric Transplantation* 2, 318–324.

Tenbrock, K., Kruppa, S., Mokov, E., Querfeld, U., Michalk, D., and Schoenau, E. (2000). Analysis of muscle strength and bone structure in children with renal disease. *Pediatric Nephrology* 14 (7), 669–672.

Tenbrock, K., Muller-Berghaus, J., Michalk, D., and Querfeld, U. (1999). Intravenous iron treatment of renal anemia in children on hemodialysis. *Pediatric Nephrology* 13, 580–582.

Tonshoff, B., Blum, W. F., Wingen, A. M., and Mehls, O. (1995). Serum insulin-like growth factors (IGFs) and IGF binding proteins 1, 2, and 3 in children with chronic renal failure: relationship to height and glomerular filtration rate. The European Study Group for Nutritional Treatment of Chronic Renal Failure in Childhood. *Journal of Clinical Endocrinology and Metabolism* 80, 2684–2691.

Tonshoff, B., Cronin, M. J., Reichert, M., Haffner, D., Wingen, A. M., Blum, W. F., and Mehls, O. (1997). Reduced concentration of serum growth hormone (GH)-binding protein in children with chronic renal failure: correlation with GH insensitivity. The European Study Group for Nutritional Treatment of Chronic Renal Failure in Childhood. The German Study Group for Growth Hormone Treatment in Chronic Renal Failure. *Journal of Clinical Endocrinology and Metabolism* 82, 1007–1013.

Tonshoff, B., Eden, S., Weiser, E., Carlsson, B., Robinson, I. C., Blum, W. F., and Mehls, O. (1994). Reduced hepatic growth hormone (GH) receptor gene expression and increased plasma GH binding protein in experimental uremia. *Kidney International* 45, 1085–1092.

Tonshoff, B., Tonshoff, C., Mehls, O., Pinkowski, J., Blum, W. F., Heinrich, U., Stover, B., and Gretz, N. (1992). Growth hormone treatment in children with preterminal chronic renal failure: no adverse effect on glomerular filtration rate. *European Journal of the Pediatrics* 151, 601–607.

Trompeter, R., Filler, G., Webb, N. J., Watson, A. R., Milford, D. V., Tyden, G., Grenda, R., Janda, J., Hughes, D., Ehrich, J. H., Klare, B., Zacchello, G., Bjorn, B. I., McGraw, M., Perner, F., Ghio, L., Balzar, E., Friman, S.,

Gusmano, R., and Stolpe, J. (2002). Randomized trial of tacrolimus versus cyclosporin microemulsion in renal transplantation. *Pediatric Nephrology* 173, 141–149.

Tshibangu, K., Oosterwijck, K., and Doumont-Meyvis, M. (1975). Effects of massive doses of ergocalciferol plus cholesterol on pregnant rats and their offspring. *Journal of Nutrition* 105, 741–758.

USRDS report (1997). Excerpts from United States Renal Data System 1997 Annual Data Report. *American Journal of Kidney Diseases* 30, S1–213.

Van Dyck, M., Bilem, N., and Proesmans, W. (1999). Conservative treatment for chronic renal failure from birth: a 3-year follow-up study. *Pediatric Nephrology* 13, 865–869.

Van Landeghem, G. F., D'Haese, P. C., Lamberts, L. V., Barata, J. D., and De Broe, M. E. (1997). Aluminium speciation in cerebrospinal fluid of acutely aluminium-intoxicated dialysis patients before and after desferrioxamine treatment; a step in the understanding of the element's neurotoxicity. *Nephrology, Dialysis, Transplantation* 12, 1692–1698.

Vanrenterghem, Y. and Jones, E. H. (1996). Report on management of renal failure in Europe, XXVI, 1995. Report based on the Centre Questionnaire, 1995. The ERA-EDTA Registry. *Nephrology, Dialysis, Transplantation* 11 (Suppl. 7), 28–32.

Vester, U., Schubert, M., Offner, G., and Brodehl, J. (2000). Distal myopathy in nephropathic cystinosis. *Pediatric Nephrology* 14 (1), 36–38.

Wahn, F., Daniel, V., Kronenberg, F., Opelz, G., Michalk, D. V., and Querfeld, U. (2001). Impact of apolipoprotein(a) phenotypes on long-term renal transplant survival. *Journal of the American Society of Nephrology* 12 (5), 1052–1058.

Warady, B. A., Belden, B., and Kohaut, E. (1999). Neurodevelopmental outcome of children initiating peritoneal dialysis in early infancy. *Pediatric Nephrology* 13, 759–765.

Warady, B. A., Hebert, D., Sullivan, E. K., Alexander, S. R., and Tejani, A. (1997). Renal transplantation, chronic dialysis, and chronic renal insufficiency in children and adolescents. The 1995 Annual Report of the North American Pediatric Renal Transplant Cooperative Study. *Pediatric Nephrology* 11, 49–64.

Warady, B. A., Kriley, M., Lovell, H., Farrell, S. E., and Hellerstein, S. (1988). Growth and development of infants with end-stage renal disease receiving long-term peritoneal dialysis. *Journal of Pediatrics* 112, 714–719.

Warady, B. A., Kriley, M., Alon, U., and Hellerstein, S. (1994). Vitamin status of infants receiving long-term peritoneal dialysis. *Pediatric Nephrology* 8, 354–356.

Warady, B. A., Schaefer, F., Holloway, M., Alexander, S., Kandert, M., Piraino, B., Salusky, I., Tranaeus, A., Divino, J., Honda, M., Mujais, S., and Verrina, E. (2000). Consensus guidelines for the treatment of peritonitis in pediatric patients receiving peritoneal dialysis. *Peritoneal Dialysis International* 20 (6), 610–624.

Warady, B. A., Sullivan, E. K., and Alexander, S. R. (1996). Lessons from the peritoneal dialysis patient database: a report of the North American Pediatric Renal Transplant Cooperative Study. *Kidney International* 53 (Suppl.), S68–S71.

Wassner, S. J. and Baum, M. Physiology and management. In *Pediatric Nephrology* 4th edn. (ed. T. M. Barratt, E. D. Avner, and W. E. Harmon), pp. 1155–1182. Philadelphia, PA: Lippincott Williams & Williams, 2002.

Wassner, S. J., Abitbol, C., Alexander, S., Conley, S., Grupe, W. E., Holliday, M. A., Rigden, S., and Salusky, I. B. (1986). Nutritional requirements for infants with renal failure. *American Journal of Kidney Diseases* 7, 300–305.

Watson, A. R., Coleman, J. E., and Taylor, E. A. (1992). Gastrostomy buttons for feeding children on continuous cycling peritoneal dialysis. *Advances in Peritoneal Dialysis* 8, 391–395.

Wingen, A. M., Fabian-Bach, C., Schaefer, F., and Mehls, O. (1997). Randomised multicentre study of a low-protein diet on the progression of chronic renal failure in children. European Study Group of Nutritional Treatment of Chronic Renal Failure in Childhood. *Lancet* 349, 1117–1123.

Wolff, G., Strecker, K., Vester, U., Latta, K., and Ehrich, J. H. (1998). Non-compliance following renal transplantation in children and adolescents. *Pediatric Nephrology* 12, 703–708.

Wuhl, E., Haffner, D., Nissel, R., Schaefer, F., and Mehls, O. (1996). Short dialyzed children respond less to growth hormone than patients prior to dialysis. German Study Group for Growth Hormone Treatment in Chronic Renal Failure. *Pediatric Nephrology* 10, 294–298.

Wuhl, E., Haffner, D., Offner, G., Broyer, M., van't Hoff, W., and Mehls, O. (2001). Long-term treatment with growth hormone in short children with nephropathic cystinosis. *Journal of Pediatrics* 138 (6), 880–887.

Zachmann, M., Prader, A., Kind, H. P., Hafliger, H., and Budliger, H. (1974). Testicular volume during adolescence. Cross-sectional and longitudinal studies. *Helvetica Paediatrica Acta* 29, 61–72.

Zivicnjak, M., Franke, D., Ehrich, J. H., and Filler, G. (2000). Does growth hormone therapy harmonize distorted morphology and body composition in chronic renal failure? *Pediatric Nephrology* 15 (3–4), 229–235.

Zivicnjak, M., Zebec, M., Franke, D., Filler, G., Szirovica, L., Haffner, D., Querfeld, U., Ehrich, J. H., and Rudan, P. (2001). Analysis of cognitive and motor functioning during pubertal development: a new approach. *Journal of Physiological Anthropology and Applied Human Science* 20 (2), 111–118.

14.2 Chronic renal failure in the elderly

J. Stewart Cameron and Juan F. Macías-Núñez

Do not go gentle into that good night,
Old age should burn and rave at close of day;
Rage, rage against the dying of the light.

Dylan Thomas (1914–1953)

Introduction

The growth of the elderly population

In developed countries, endstage renal disease (ESRD) is predominantly a condition of the elderly: but who are they? In this chapter, we will consider 'the elderly' to be any patient aged more than 65 years, although geriatricians would regard this as late middle age, or the beginning of the 'young elderly' (65–75 years). However, the age of 65 years has the advantage that in many countries it is also the age at which retirement from employment occurs and pensions begin. However, increasing attention is turning to the treatment (almost always by some form of dialysis), of the 'elderly elderly'—octogenarians and older when they enter ESRD.

In all developed countries, the elderly are the fastest-growing group, and renal failure is much more common in the elderly than in the young. In 2000, 15–20 per cent of the population were aged over 65 years in most developed countries and 4–7 (mean 5.9) per cent were over 75. This increase will continue for another 20 years at least, by which time 8.3 per cent (58 million) of the European and 6.7 per cent (24 million) of the North American populations will be aged more than 75 years. In Asia, there will be 134 million people aged over 75 in 2020 (UN World Population Prospects 1999). Numbers of males and females are approximately equal up to the age of 65, but thereafter the mortality of males is greater, with the ratio reaching eight females to each male at 100 years of age. This is counterbalanced somewhat by the fact that many causes of chronic renal failure are more common in males than females, but nevertheless, there is a predominance of women amongst elderly patients in ESRD.

The appropriate comparison for mortality at all ages is a similar cohort of healthy individuals matched for age (Table 1). At 75 years of age, dialysis increases the risk of death less than threefold, whereas at 45 years of age, it is *20 times greater* than expected (Mignon *et al.* 1993) and the number of 'lost years' of life correspondingly greater. In most developed countries today, a 65-year-old has a life expectancy of 12–15 years (Table 1).

Endstage renal disease in the elderly

Despite these data, in past decades elderly patients were rarely referred for ESRD treatment, largely because of the extreme shortage of dialysis places in the 1960s and even the 1970s, and the feeling that the elderly simply would not tolerate dialysis well. This reluctance has now largely been overcome in almost all developed countries but some patients with ESRD are still not considered for treatment in many countries, particularly for transplantation.

The incidence of new adult patients devloping chronic renal failure increases steadily with age (Feest *et al.* 1990; USRDS 2001), to 10 times more at 75 than 15–45 (Table 2), and the mean age of incident patients is now 60–65 years in almost all developed countries (see below). Apart from widening of criteria of acceptance, there are multiple

Table 1 Expected remaining lifetime in the normal elderly American Caucasian individuals (US 1996), compared with expected survival of dialysed patients of similar age (1999 data)

At age	Males			Females		
	Life expectancy (RDT)	Estimated age at death	'Lost' years	Life expectancy (RDT)	Estimated age at death	'Lost' years
65	15.7 (3.1)	80.7 (68.1)	12.6	19.1 (3.1)	84.1 (68.1)	14.0
70	12.5 (2.7)	82.5 (72.7)	9.8	15.4 (2.7)	85.4 (72.7)	12.7
75	9.7 (2.3)	84.7 (77.3)	7.4	12.0 (2.3)	87.0 (77.3)	9.7
80	7.2 (1.9)	87.2 (81.9)	5.3	8.9 (2.0)	88.9 (82.0)	7.9
85	5.2 (1.6)	90.2 (86.6)	3.6	6.3 (1.6)	91.3 (86.6)	4.7

Data from the United States statistical reports 1996 (all figures in years). Data for different countries in Europe is similar, but with slightly longer survival, as are Japanese data. Estimated survival of dialysis patients from USRDS report (2001). Estimated survival of African-Americans on dialysis is 0.8–0.2 years longer with increasing age.

Table 2 Age-related incidence of:

(a) Chronic renal failure, and treatment rate in the United Kingdom[a]

Age (years)	Population rate/million/year (95% confidence intervals) 1989	Age (years)	Accepted for ESRD treatment 1991–1993 rate/million total population/year
		16–24	26
0–19	6 (2–14)	25–34	47
20–49	58 (38–78)	35–44	61
50–59	160 (96–224)	45–54	113
60–69	282 (197–271)	55–64	175
70–79	503 (370–636)	65–74	272
80–	588 (422–754)	75–84	314
		85–	56

(b) Patients entering ESRD in the United States, 1999[b]

Age (years)	n/year	n/million population (p.m.p.)/year
0–19	1,292	15
20–44	13,006	119
45–64	31,014	603
65–74	22,171	1317
>75	20,608	1434
Total	88,091	Mean 315 p.m.p./year

[a] From Feest *et al.* 1990.

[b] US intake rates are approximately twice those of UK population rates at all ages (USRDS Report 2001).

Notes: The UK Registrar-General's death certificate data suggests that just before the introduction of treatment for ESRD in the United Kingdom (1961), the death rate from all forms of renal failure was 137/million total population/year (~7000 deaths/year).

Subsequent studies have revealed the expected higher incidence of renal failure in immigrant populations of Afro-Caribbean and Asian origin, who now form about 5% of the total population, but with a very local distribution. These groups have an average incidence of ESRD three to five times that of the long-term Caucasian population at all ages.

Since 1991–1993, the overall intake rate on to ESRD in the United Kingdom has risen from 67 p.m.p./year to just over 100 p.m.p./year in 1999.

For comparison, the certificated overall incidence of death from renal failure in the United States (US Census data 1960) was almost twice the figure for the United Kingdom: 268/million total population/year (60,000 deaths/year). These data and contemporary intake rates suggest a real rise in the incidence of ESRD in the population since 1960—or undercertification in 1960.

additional factors which have fuelled the 'greying' of the dialysis population in the 1980s and 1990s which has been termed an 'epidemic' by some (Piccoli *et al.* 1996): treatment facilities have increased in number, and technical improvements have allowed better tolerance of dialysis and less intradialytic morbidity. Most importantly, family and general physicians now regard renal insufficiency in the elderly as a treatable condition (Mignon *et al.* 1993).

In the United States, the Federal Age Discrimination Act was followed by a sharp increase in the number of elderly patients with ESRD receiving renal replacement therapy. By 1985, 36 per cent of

ESRD patients in the United States were older than 65 years and the treatment rate overall was 124 per million population (Port 1992); by the end of the century, more than half (51 per cent) of those entering ESRD treatment in the United States (44,779 of 88,091, 315 p.m.p.) were over 65, and more than one in five (23.4 per cent) were over 75 years of age. Of prevalent ESRD patients (340,261) 35 per cent were over 65 and one in seven (14.3 per cent) over 75 years in 1999. Focusing on dialysed patients only, 45.6 per cent were over 65 and one in five (19.8 per cent) over 75 (USRDS report 2001). Although the maximum increases were during the 1980s (Port 1992; Latos 1996), the elderly still represent the fastest growing population of those entering ESRD in the United States and in Europe (Salamone *et al.* 1995): during 1995–1999 the incidence of American patients aged 65–75 years still increased by 8.2 per cent, and those over 75 years by 12.5 per cent compared with 5 per cent for younger incident patients. Even these figures are exceeded in Germany however, where already 58 per cent of prevalent ESRD patients are over 65 years (Fig. 1); most developed countries have proportions above 40 per cent and even in the United Kingdom, in contrast to the past (Challah *et al.* 1984) the mean age at entry is over 60, and Williams and Antao (1989) reported from Wales that 17 per cent of their incident patients were more than 75 years of age. In 1995, the last year for which overall (but incomplete) data are available for Europe, 52 per cent of incident patients were aged more than 60 years (Brunner *et al.* 1995).

The median and mode age of patients entering or under treatment for ESRD seems at last to be stabilizing somewhat with the largest cohort of incident patients aged between 65 and 70 years of age and prevalent patients, 60–65 years. In Japan, whose population is older than any European population and dialysis is readily available, the numbers of incident patients aged 65–70 years only just exceeded those for 70–75 years in 1999, and the mode age for prevalent patients was already 65–70 years (Nakai *et al.* 2001). Where will all this stop? Given the multiplying effect of an ageing population and the increase in incidence of ESRD with age, the US Renal Data System (1989) and Nissenson (1993) both calculated that by 2000 at least 60 per cent of new patients treated for ESRD in the United States would be over 65 years; the figure in 1999 however was 'only' 51 per cent, and the rate of increase is slowing from 1997 to 1999, showing the fragility of calculations of future demand, but a plateau in numbers seems unlikely until 2010, or even 2015. Xue *et al.* (2001) predict that by 2010, there will be 700,000 patients under ESRD treatment in the United States, with 129,000 incident patients annually. Again this may be an over-gloomy outlook because after their database closed in 1998 there have been some signs of a slowing in the rate.

Who can and should be treated?

Elderly patients have an increasing burden of comorbidity which may be overwhelming in some instances. Added to physical problems is the spectre of dementia, which affects an increasing proportion of people with age, especially those over 80 years. This burden of ill-health is unequally borne by the elderly population, with some individuals in their 80s or even 90s apparently both mentally and physically unimpaired, whilst others suffer a heavy load of complicated medical illnesses, sensory impairment or dementia, from robust good health to almost total decrepitude. This marked heterogeneity amongst the elderly contrasts with relative homogeneity of young populations. Social factors are important also, with an increasing

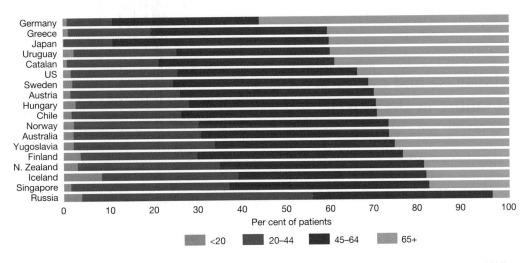

Fig. 1 Proportion of prevalent patients under treatment for ESRD at different ages in different countries in 1999 (USRDS Report 2001).

number of elderly indivduals in Western urban societies leading isolated lives, with no surviving family or distant from relatives and few social contacts.

In addition, the elderly adjust to dialysis regimens more slowly, take longer to learn techniques, are more fragile in their responses to fluid changes, spend more time in hospital, have an increased mortality principally from infection and cardiovascular disease, and inevitably survive for shorter periods than younger patients. Treatment costs consequently are higher per patient than younger controls (Grün *et al.* 2003). As individuals of greater frailty are considered for ESRD treatment, inevitably questions arise as to whether *all* elderly patients in ESRD can benefit from or should be submitted to dialysis. Almost all nephrologists accept that *some* elderly patients are unsuitable for treatment. The ethical and medical background to these questions has much in common with withdrawal from dialysis, and indeed the two problems are often intertwined by the policy of 'trial of dialysis' in 'marginal' patients: the patient and her or his family enter into a contract with the dialysis unit to attempt treatment, and judge the outcome after some few weeks or months—with the stated implication that treatment may well cease (see below on withdrawal).

Treatment of the elderly with ESRD has clearly improved today compared with the recent past (see Berlyne 1982 versus Oreopoulos 1994). Chronological age alone is certainly not a reason to exclude patients from dialysis—or transplantation (Pollini and Teissier 1990; Salamone *et al.* 1995). Nevertheless, the elderly are in practice often excluded from many life-saving treatments, of which dialysis is only one (Hamel *et al.* 1999), as part of a widepread cultural phenomenon. Since exclusion by chronological age *per se* is not possible, the concept of 'biological age' (how young or old in relation to chronological age the individual patient seems to be) is sometimes used. Whilst psychometry and some physical factors (as an example, cardiac ejection fraction) can be measured, this type of judgement tends to be subjective at best and arbitrary at worst. As well as age, for inevitable actuarial reasons, some indicators such as race, gender, severe vascular disease, and diabetes mellitus are associated with poor prognosis in the elderly. At the time of first evaluation, the possibility of survival and rehabilitation is strongly influenced by these other comorbid states, particularly diabetes and cardiovascular disease (Khan *et al.* 1993;

Blagg and Fitts 1994; Foley *et al.* 1994; Kutner *et al.* 1994). Diabetes is a common associate of death during or withdrawal from dialysis (Nelson *et al.* 1994). Older Black patients with ESRD treated by haemodialysis had a lower risk of death than White patients (Ismail *et al.* 1993), just the opposite to younger ages, and Oriental patients fare better than either (USRDS Report 2001). Other non-physical factors such as social and psychological support (Kutner *et al.* 1994) may be more crucial than even 'biological' age in determining survival.

As yet, no firm advice can be given for de-selecting any but the most obvious cases of 'untreatable' renal failure in the elderly, although general guidelines are needed badly (Mulkerrin *et al.* 2000; Renal Physicians Association 2000); in many countries such as the United Kingdom, nephrologists are often protected from this seemingly impossible task by their colleagues in family practice and internal medicine, who simply do not refer many of the more frail patients in the age group between 70 and 90 years for treatment (Challah *et al.* 1984; Woodhouse *et al.* 1987; Feest *et al.* 1990). However, it is clear that overt or covert rationing of treatment in the elderly remains prevalent today in almost all countries within the developed world (Kjellstrand 1988; Singer 1992; Kjellstrand and Moody 1994; McKenzie *et al.* 1998; Chadna *et al.* 1999). Few detailed studies of the numbers and characteristics of excluded patients have been done (Hirsch *et al.* 1994; Main 2000; Joly *et al.* 2003) and usually go unrecorded. Even in the United States whose unique permissive legislation has been mentioned above, age selection has been shown to be present (Singer 1992; Friedman 1994; Hamel *et al.* 1999) and some appropriate or inappropriate exclusion of the elderly from treatment *is* practised. In that country more than in others, the opposite problem has been raised, of whether patients who should not be dialysed by most criteria are sometimes submitted to treatment, for reasons of emotional involvement or even of profit; but this for obvious reasons is even less well documented.

Finally, the question has been raised in recent years whether by renoprotective strategies the elderly might avoid dialysis altogether, given the rather poor survival even when compared with their peers of similar age (Table 1 and below). However, a glance at Tables 1 and 4 shows that such conservative treatment would have to offer even an 80–85-year-old a mean extra survival of at least 3–4 years to compete with dialysis, and of more than 5 years to allow full expected survival. The younger elderly would require even longer.

Chronic renal disease and causes of chronic renal failure in the elderly

The pattern and causes of ESRD in the elderly differ substantially from those in younger populations (Martinez-Maldonado *et al.* 1996; Lusvarghi *et al.* 1997; Maisonneuve *et al.* 2000). The patterns of glomerular disease (Vendemia *et al.* 2001) and underlying causes of the nephrotic syndrome (Cameron 1998) again differ. The most common disorders leading to renal failure at this age are vascular diseases, including that assciated with hypertension (nephrosclerosis), diabetes mellitus, and obstructive uropathy, although in as many as one-third of patients in many series reported it proved impossible to identify any specific cause (Table 3). Many of these latter patients have small coarsely granular kidneys without major scars and show trivial proteinuria with or without hypertension. These kidneys may be the end result of vascular nephrosclerosis. Correspondingly, patients diagnosed as having 'glomerulonephritis' form a smaller proportion of elderly ESRD patients. The limitations of the analysis by Maissonneuve *et al.* (2000) must be remembered: these data are from a past era (1980–1994) during which selection and criteria for and rates of acceptance changed rapidly: many of the detailed differences in Table 3 represent patterns of behaviour and not biology, and several groups are vague (e.g. 'glomerulonephritis not confirmed by biopsy'), but

Table 3 Distribution of causes of renal failure in the elderly from three major ESRD registries

Patients aged over 65	USRDS 236,639 (42%)	EDTA-ERA 84,353 (27%)	Australasian 2448 (18% of total[a])
Arteriopathic diseases	89,407 (38%)	13,987 (17%)	416 (17%)
Diabetes	65,018 (28%)	11,621 (14%)	246 (10%)
Uncertain/unknown	30,035 (13%)	24,761 (29%)	296 (12%)
Glomerulonephritis	25,174 (10%)	5,090 (6%)	685 (28%)
Infective and obstructive uropathies	12,464 (5%)	14,612 (17%)	33 (1%)
Neoplastic disease	5,118 (2.5%)	3,330 (4%)	57 (2%)
Hereditary diseases	4,411 (2%)	4,487 (5%)	148 (6%)
Miscellaneous	2,980 (1%)	1,741 (2%)	33 (1%)
Toxic nephropathies	1,802 (1%)	3,797 (5%)	433 (18%)
Congenital diseases	1,145 (0.5%)	134 (0.2%)	1–

[a] Of those who entered ESRD 1980–1994.

Note: Toxic nephropathies mainly analgesic nephropathy and (in Europe) gouty nephropathy. Neoplastic disease includes all amyloid and light chain disease. Glomerulonephritis includes both primary glomerulonephritis and that secondary to systemic disease, e.g. lupus vasculitis, etc. (Calculated from the data of Maissonneuve *et al.* 2000.)

other differences are almost certainly significant—for example the greater incidence of toxic nephropathies (including analgesic nephropathy) in Europe and especially Australasia when compared with the United States.

Vascular disease of the main renal arteries (see Chapters 1.6.2 and 10.6.5) (Safian and Textor 2001) is present in 15–20 per cent of many series of patients with ESRD, especially those older than 60 (Mailloux *et al.* 1994). In the registry data of Table 3, however, this was recorded only in about 1 per cent of cases. Generalized atheroma is common in the elderly, and renal arterial disease should be suspected as a cause of or a factor contributing to renal failure in any patient with kidneys of unequal size. However, in the presence of aortic atheroma, the renal disease may be bilateral and the diagnosis is not obvious. Bruits over any major vessel, particularly the femoral arteries or the renal arteries themselves, are a valuable clue. Equally, any patient with either claudication and peripheral vascular disease, or known myocardial disease on whatever evidence, has a one in three chance of having renal artery stenosis.

Thus, it is worth searching for treatable renal artery stenosis in almost all elderly patients whose cause of chronic renal failure is obscure (see Chapter 10.6.5). A lesion susceptible to angioplasty with or without stenting, or occasionally surgery, may be found on one or both sides. Obviously the risks and benefits for each individual must be balanced, since there is a risk of atheroembolism, damaging the vessel, or of thrombosis, with precipitation of ESRD or at least worsening of the uraemia. However, the potential of current medical therapy are not well studied.

Even more important in elderly males is *prostatic obstruction*. This should never be allowed to lead to ESRD, but remains a common finding in all renal replacement programmes. It is often not recognized, either by the patient or by his family physician, until it is too late (Sacks *et al.* 1989), largely because the patient becomes polyuric rather than oliguric. However, catheterization followed by transurethral resection when renal function ceases to improve can be most rewarding even in patients with severe uraemia, including those requiring dialysis; although recovery of renal function may be incomplete and postponement, rather than prevention, of renal failure is all that can be achieved.

A further problem worth noting in the elderly is that of *amyloidosis* (see Chapter 4.2.1). Like its fellow myelopathies, primary amyloidosis becomes increasingly common with age; one of the three most common causes of the nephrotic syndrome in the elderly is primary amyloid (Cameron 1998). Apart from age, clinical clues to the presence of amyloid are increased atrial pressures and subcutaneous haemorrhages, often around the eyes (see Fig. 10, Chapter 4.2.1). Many of these patients have monoclonal 'spikes' in their plasma or a urine protein electrophoresis pattern which should suggest this diagnosis, but many do not. Since amyloid infiltration affects all vessels, including the heart, severe cardiac problems may also affect this group of patients, and death from cardiac failure before endstage renal failure supervenes is common; they may also suffer adrenal failure and bleeding from affected blood vessels.

A final group of elderly patients is worth noting—those who present in acute renal failure (see Chapter 10.7.4) but fail to recover function—sometimes called 'acute irreversible renal failure'. This outcome is almost unknown under the age of 50, but becomes more common with older age.

General problems present in elderly patients with endstage renal disease

Cardiovascular disease

Cardiovascular disease is the single greatest problem in patients in ESRD (Luke 1998; Baigent *et al.* 2000; Loscalzo and London 2000) and it becomes even more common with age. As Table 3 shows, the actual cause of ESRD in 58 per cent of American, 44 per cent of European and 39 per cent of Australasian patients aged over 65 was classified as 'arteriopathic' (Maisonneuve *et al.* 2000). Table 4 gives the comorbidity already afflicting patients *of all ages* starting dialysis in the United States in 1999; many more elderly individuals can be expected to develop these complications after starting long-term dialysis (Bonal *et al.* 1997), and for a considerable proportion will be the cause of death (see below). The USRDS data show that the prevalence of vascular disease is greater in those aged 60 or 65 years than in younger subjects, as in previous data. Previous hypertension is undoubtedly one of the most important age-related risk factors. It is known also that systolic hypertension correlates very well with left ventricular hypertrophy, and that in turn left ventricular hypertrophy is associated with sudden death, arrhythmias, and myocardial infarction (Silverberg *et al.* 1989; Foley *et al.* 1992). Anaemia is important in determining left ventricular hypertrophy, and treatment with epoetin to a haemoglobin of at least 10–12 g/dl is mandatory (see Chapter 11.3.8). Whether further increases in haemoglobin confer benefit remains contentious, especially in the presence of vascular disease (European Guidelines for the Management of the Anaemia of Renal Failure 1999).

Clearly, good control of hypertension in the elderly has a high priority: modest salt restriction to a maximum of 5 g/24 h can be used, but salt depletion occurs easily in these patients before starting dialysis and they often do not adhere to restriction. Antihypertensive agents such as calcium-channel blockers are preferable; low doses of angiotensin-converting enzyme inhibitors should be tried, but the high incidence of renal artery stenosis in the elderly uraemic must not be forgotten—although this becomes less relevant after starting dialysis. β-Blockers are not the first choice in elderly patients with hypertension; bradycardia, bronchospasm, and coldness of feet and hands frequently occur as a result of peripheral artery disease.

A common and major problem in elderly patients with ESRD is dialysis intolerance because of unstable circulation, which is itself the result of poor cardiac output associated with a dilated ischaemic cardiomyopathy (Parfrey *et al.* 1988). Non-invasive techniques such as a thallium scintiscan and echocardiography can be used to investigate abnormal ventricular wall motion and perfusion. As good correlation is found between ventricular wall hypomotility and coronary disease, patients with ventricular wall dysfunction may be selected for angiography and later percutaneous transluminal angioplasty, or even open bypass coronary artery surgery if survival or quality of life are threatened and the general condition of the patient suggests that it will be useful (Opsahl *et al.* 1988).

Peripheral vascular problems are common in the elderly population with ESRD, and associated renal vessel disease is the major cause of the ESRD in some patients. These patients are vulnerable to major ischaemia of the toes and feet, particularly if they are also diabetic. It is always worth investigating such patients by Doppler techniques and angiography, because it may be possible to use bypass surgery or angioplasty to alleviate or palliate focal blockage. However, amputation is frequently necessary and, if it is necessary to remove more than a toe, it is almost always below the knee or sometimes even above.

Malnutrition

Atrophy of the intestinal villi and atrophy of the intestinal mucosa which interferes with the normal processes of reabsorption is present in normal elderly subjects. In addition, there is a tendency for the diet of the elderly to shift towards an increased carbohydrate intake (potatoes, pasta, cakes). Apart from personal preferences, proteins such as meat and fish are more expensive and may not be affordable on a retirement income. In addition, elderly patients who become confused, for whatever reason (see below), or depressed may not eat or drink appropriately, sometimes for long periods.

The presence of all or many of these factors means that, in some series of elderly patients, more than half have been judged to be malnourished (Chaveau *et al.* 2001) and up to one-third of deaths among patients on haemodialysis have been attributed to 'cachexia' (Hakim and Levin 1993; Piccoli *et al.* 1993). This 'death in cachexia' is a nonspecific clinical term defining death as a consequence of a progressive impairment of clinical condition without a single identifiable cause (Verdery 1990). This diagnosis has been used more frequently in older patients suffering from neoplasia or diffuse vasculopathy or on dialysis. This increase is probably due to the increasing age and vulnerability of new patients on dialysis and more open acceptance of vulnerable patients for ESRD treatment (Collins *et al.* 1990; Disney 1990; Posen *et al.* 1990a).

Severe hypertension, diffuse vascular disease, severe cardiopathy, active tuberculosis, severe urinary tract infection, liver cirrhosis, collagen diseases, amyloidosis, diabetes mellitus, psychosis, epilepsy, chronic lung disease, and HIV positivity have all been considered as risk factors for cachexia. An age of over 70 is generally believed to be a risk *per se* in the absence of pathology, but in the analysis of Piccoli *et al.* (1993) age was *not* a comorbid risk factor, nor did it emerge strongly in the Netherlands Cooperative Study (Merkus *et al.* 2000) with a relative risk in those aged over 65 years of only 1.8 compared with younger patients, and age was not included in their mutivariate prediction model. Age *per se* also is not a determinant of malnutrition (Kopple *et al.* 1986).

Early markers of malnutrition are not always easy to identify, but non-fluid weight loss in the absence of intercurrent illnesses is the best

Table 4 Cardiovascular comorbidity in the cohort of incident patients starting dialysis in 1999 in the United States

	Over 65 years % with specified comorbidity		
	Starting haemodialysis		Starting peritoneal dialysis
Hypertension	74		
Congestive cardiac failure	33		23
Ischaemic heart disease	24	m 37, f 14	19
Previous myocardial infarct	8	m 14, f 10	7
Cerebrovascular disease	8		6
Peripheral vascular disease	14		12

USRDS report 2001.

clinical predictor of insidious malnutrition. Clinial guidelines for the assessment and management of nutrition have been published (DOQI 2000). Of routine laboratory tests, a reduction in serum albumin is the most powerful independent factor indicating risk of mortality (Lowrie and Lew 1990; Merkus *et al.* 2000) but is method-dependent, and local normal ranges must be established. Even when serum albumin has only declined to between 35 and 40 g/l the relative risk of death is doubled, and between 30 and 35 g/l it is increased fivefold. Other rapid-turnover proteins such as transferrin and prealbumin can be measured, but there is no evidence they are better predictors than albumin. A low plasma creatinine is also a pointer to low muscle mass and poor outlook.

In general, a dietary protein intake of 1 g/kg/day with at least 6.3 g of essential amino acids should prevent malnutrition in elderly haemodialysis. A maintenance standard diet for old persons undergoing dialysis should provide at least 35 kcal/kg/24 h and a protein intake of 1 g/kg/24 h, of which 70–75 per cent should be of high biological value. In addition, piridoxine (10 mg/24 h), folic acid (1 mg/24 h), and $1,25(OH)_2$-vitamin D_3 (0.25–0.75 μg/24 h) are required together with a sufficient quantity of fluid to preclude more than 5 per cent inter-dialytic weight gain. If malnutrition appears despite this type of diet, it can be treated by intravenous feeding (fats, amino acids, and carbohydrates) during haemodialysis, although the evidence that this is effective is contentious (see Chapters 12.3 and 12.6). One formulation for intravenous feeding consists of 500 ml of 50 per cent dextrose, 500 ml of 8.5 per cent amino acids, and 200 ml of 20 per cent lipids infused over a period of 3–4 h during the dialysis (Ismail *et al.* 1993).

Neuropsychiatric disorders and psychosocial problems

The cerebral ageing process is characterized by parenchymal cerebral atrophy, diminished cerebral blood flow and the frequent finding of cerebral amyloidosis at autopsy. Neurological problems frequently develop in older haemodialysed patients. In addition, atherosclerosis of the carotid or cerebral circulation may predispose to transient ischaemic attacks during intradialytic episodes of hypotension. Malnourishment contributes to the increased incidence of Wernicke's syndrome (ataxia, mental confusion, loss of recent memory, and alterations in ocular motility) in the elderly. Binswanger's encephalopathy may also appear as a result of hypertension and atherosclerosis.

Dementia becomes progressively more common with age, and affects one woman in two and one man in three of the population aged over 85 years. Thus development of dementia in a proportion of patients undergoing dialysis is inevitable. An increased incidence of the development of Alzheimer's disease in uraemic or dialysed subjects has not been reported so far (although the problem has been surprisingly little studied) surprising also since cerebral atrophy is common even in younger dialysed patients (Savazzi *et al.* 1985). Screening of the dialysis population using the mini mental status (MMS) test is useful; if abnormal, more formal studies and exclusion or treatable intracerebral lesions and general conditions can be done. The management of such patients is outlined in Chapter 11.3.14, and withdrawal from dialysis under these circumstances is discussed later in this chapter.

In the absence of any of these factors, the patient with intellectual deterioration should be investigated for a silent subdural haematoma, perhaps precipitated or worsened by the regular heparin administration of haemodialysis. Episodes of overt cerebral vascular accidents (thrombosis, embolism, or haemorrhage) or intracerebral bleeding are major causes of death among elderly subjects on haemodialysis. If these events are not terminal and the patient recovers, a low-dose heparin regimen should be given in order to maintain a Lee and White clotting time of 12 min or less during haemodialysis, or transfer to continuous ambulatory peritoneal dialysis (CAPD) considered if this is feasable. As dialyser clotting may occur under these circumstances, it is useful to clamp the arterial line every hour and perform a saline washout of the dialyser. Newer heparin preparations (e.g. fragmin) or other methods of anticoagulation may be useful in these patients.

Another far from minor problem problem faced by many elderly subjects is *poor eyesight* in which subjects lack the skills acquired by the truly blind, but are have such poor vision that they cannot function normally because of this handicap. In some cases, this is simply the result of inappropriate prescriptions for spectacles, as the long sight which begins in middle age worsens and fine close work becomes impossible. In others, cataracts may be present which can be dealt with by surgical removal and plastic lens emplacement even in the immuno-suppressed elderly transplant patient, despite the obvious risks of haemorrhage and infection. Of course, elderly diabetics present special problems in this respect.

Depression, which is common in the otherwise healthy aged, is even more common and pronounced in those with ESRD, particularly those on long-term haemodialysis. It forms a potent associate and probable cause of death in elderly patients on dialysis (Kimmel *et al.* 2000) and suicide is markedly more common in the elderly on dialysis than in younger subjects. The situation may be triggered or aggravated by loss of social role, decreased mobility outside the home, poverty, or anxiety, or it may be a reaction to treatment (machine dependence) (Rife *et al.* 1979). All the above problems increase if complications, particularly with vascular access, are allowed to develop. However, elderly ESRD patients may feel that their need to go to the hospital for haemodialysis keeps them 'employed' and gives them a new role in life. Many also feel 'safer' under the care of the nephrological team and use the unit as a sort of social club. Measures such as flexibility in the arrangement of dialysis sessions, periodic psychological support during the dialysis period, moderate physical exercise, and meetings which involve relatives, social workers, nurses, and doctors may help to reduce depression and anxiety (Jennekens and Jennekens-Schinkel 1983).

Social support may also be a problem; even the fit isolated old person may have problems, particularly in inner-city environments, and these may become overwhelming when renal failure is added. Other patients may be able to cope with their own problems, but may have an aged spouse who has sickness, mobility, or mental difficulties. Occasionally a dialysis patient in his or her seventies may be caring for an even more dependent parent in his or her 90s.

Bone disease

Ageing itself is accompanied by alterations in calcium, phosphate, and bone metabolism (see Chapter 1.5). Poor calcium absorption leads to reduction in plasma calcium which together with increased plasma phosphate stimulates release of parathyroid hormone. Osteopenia and reduction of bone trabecular volume also occur in the elderly, particularly in postmenopausal women and men aged over 65. In addition, an unbalanced diet, reduced physical activity, and lack of exposure to sunlight worsen the condition. Prophylaxis and management of bone disease in the elderly does not differ from younger patients, and is reviewed in Chapter 11.3.9. A protein intake of no less than 1 g/kg/24 h, moderate exercise such as walking and passive musculoskeletal rehabilitation in patients who are not physically active are also of importance in the management of osteodystrophy.

Rheumatological problems

Age is a strong risk factor for dialysis β-2 microglobulin amyloidosis (see Chapter 11.3.10), as well as time on dialysis (van Ypersele *et al.* 1991) and (possibly) the type of haemodialysis membrane used. Generally, this manifests itself in periarticular structures. Although data on prevalence rates in elderly populations are not available, the blunt fact is that most elderly patients do not survive the 5–7 years or more on haemodialysis required for the development amyloidosis (see below). There is now hope that adsorption techniques will permit really effective control of β-2 microglobulin plasma concentrations (see Chapter 11.3.10).

Arthritis and osteoporosis are both common in non-uraemic elderly patients, and up to one-third of the elderly population take non-steroidal anti-inflammatory drugs. Hypertension, gastrointestinal bleeding, and other well-known complications of these drugs are discussed elsewere in this book (Chapter 6.3); the reversible decline in glomerular filtration rate and the interstitial nephritis which may occur are important also. It is always worth obtaining a careful history of the use of these drugs in any older patient at presentation, particularly as they are widely available without prescription.

The main impact of rheumatological conditions on dialysis is on mobility with its secondary effects on bone as noted above, and on dexterity. Many elderly patients have difficulty with fine movements, such as those required in performing CAPD because of arthritis in their hands; this problem is often compounded by poor eyesight. 'Frozen shoulder' may be seen in the elderly after shunt or fistula emplacement, and active steps should be taken to keep the limb mobile.

Rehabilitation

Dialysis that can only be done for a short period without improving the quality of life (Westlie *et al.* 1984) may be worse than death. Active rehabilitation is provided routinely to persons suffering from events such as stroke or amputation to prevent complications and maximize functional status. In contrast, rehabilitation is infrequently provided for elderly ESRD patients, perhaps because these disabilities are less obvious than motor deficits (Blagg and Fitts 1994).

Improvement in the rehabilitation of ESRD patients requires monitoring using standarized measures and periodic intervention, ideally beginning at the diagnosis of chronic renal insufficiency. Measures may include a history of recent falls, assessment using the Karnofsky scale, and functional assessements such as grip strength, range of motion, and the 2-min walk test (Stewart *et al.* 1990; Kutner *et al.* 1992). Timely intervention should identify and treat anaemia, bone disease, depression, and any other intercurrent illness interfering with physical activity, and should promote exercise and active lifestyle. Vocational counselling and therapeutic recreation may motivate patients towards physical activity. An example of such intervention is that the level of exercise does not reduce suddenly but gradually deteriorates during the course of chronic renal failure. This should be prevented by identifying and maintaining a normal level of physical activity for age, and treating anaemia. Prevention of 'fraility' (Woodhouse *et al.* 1987) will improve quality of life, reduce hospital confinement, help independence, and reduce costs associated with loss of employment in the younger elderly.

Dialysis in the elderly (Latos 1996)

Because of inability to perform self-dialysis at home either from frailty or lack of support, most elderly patients find themselves on in-centre haemodialysis and most remain on that treatment (see Chapter 12.1). Thus, in the United States in 1999, 88 per cent of patients aged 65–74 were on dialysis, 80 per cent on haemodialysis and 8 per cent using CAPD. Over the age of 75 years, 98.4 per cent were on dialysis, all but 4.7 per cent using haemodialysis (USRDS 2001) and less than 1 per cent were using haemodialysis at home. The overall pattern is similar in Europe (Valderrábano *et al.* 1995) although there are international contrasts. Questions surrounding the selection of elderly patients for transplantation are dealt with later in this chapter.

Haemodialysis in the elderly: technical problems

Many clinicians find that a majority of patients older than 65 years undergoing hospital haemodialysis have a high incidence of adverse symptoms (Ponticelli *et al.* 1987): acute hypotension, hypoxaemia, and arrhythmias, and chronic malnutrition, inadequate dialysis, amyloidosis, increased incidence of infections, gastrointestinal bleeding, depression, and subdural haematomas are the most common (Stacy and Sica 1985; Roy *et al.* 1990; Niu *et al.* 1992).

Vascular access (see also Chapter 12.2)

In the elderly peripheral arterial disease may be severe, the veins fragile, and fistula formation difficult, resulting in immediate thrombosis or chronic poor flow. Nevertheless, many observers find that patency and complications of vascular access for haemodialysis in the elderly not a major problem (Didlake *et al.* 1991; Bernardelli and Vegeto 1997) with modifications to technique such as an increased used of fistulas at the elbow rather than the wrist, and results can be comparable with those in younger populations (Pourchez *et al.* 1990; Didlake *et al.* 1991). However, others have had much less satisfactory results (Porush and Faubert 1991) and Hinsdale *et al.* (1985) found that a Cimino–Brescia fistula was possible in only 25–30 per cent of their 119 patients with a mean age of 63.5 years, and that all fistulas in patients older than 65 years lasted for a maximum of 1 year.

If the fistula should thrombose immediately after creation, we have found it useless to perform recanalization by the Fogarty technique; it is generally necessary to create a new vascular access. If all local access fails, transposition of a saphenous vein graft to the radial or cubital artery in a loop may allow haemodialysis, and seems to give better results than other artificial grafts. Gore-Tex® arteriovenous grafts have a short life in the elderly, and they usually clot; when implanted as an arterio-arterial loop such grafts last longer. Studies with prosthetic fistulae have shown a survival of 60–80 per cent at 1 year and 50–70 per cent at 2 years in patients aged 50–55 years using PTFE (Munda *et al.* 1983; Palder *et al.* 1985), poorer results than younger patients. When all of these vessels have been used, a Thomas' shunt in the femoral artery and vein may be required. Because of all these findings, greater use is now made of long-term tunnelled subclavian lines, which can function for a year or more successfully (Canaud *et al.* 1997); there was no difference in useful survival of this type of access with age of the subject.

Intradialytic complications

Arrhythmias are very frequent in the elderly during dialysis (Morrison *et al.* 1980; Jacobs *et al.* 1985) because metastatic calcification, amyloid infiltration, coronary heart disease, cardiac hypertrophy, and hypertension are more frequent than in younger patients. Hypokalaemia, acidosis, and hypoxaemia which may develop early during dialysis using bio-incompatible cellulosic membranes (de Broe 1994) contribute to this. In some countries, digitalis is commonly used to control cardiac dysfunction; arrythmias are even more frequent in elderly patients treated with this drug (Blumberg et al. 1983) and it should be avoided.

Cardiovascular instability occurs during 20–30 per cent of dialyses in the elderly and is multifactorial in origin (Daugirdas 1991; Sherman 1992; Maggiore et al. 2000). Transient cerebral ischaemic episodes and angina are not unusual in this situation. Atherosclerosis and a rigid vascular tree, more frequent with age, interfere with the vascular adaptation to volume depletion and make cardiovascular instability more common. Autonomic dysfunction and poor cardiac reserve also contribute. In many patients, hypotension occurs after meals even when they are off dialysis.

Such episodes can be alleviated by maintenance of a haemoglobin greater than 10–11 g/dl and an albumin of more than 40 g/l, careful titration of 'dry' weight, slow gentle ultrafiltration, avoidance of vasodilator drugs in the predialysis period, and no food just before or during dialysis. Sequential ultrafiltration–dialysis and the use of bicarbonate dialysis fluid may help; some patients improve if high-sodium (>140 mmol/l) dialysis fluid is used. If hypotension appears despite these measures, rapid infusion of small quantities of saline (i.e. 200 ml) will restore blood pressure. Profiled haemodialysis, if available, is valuable in avoiding this complication (Coli et al. 1998).

Angina: aged patients with coronary insufficiency are more prone to episodes of angina during haemodialysis, and this may be aggravated by anaemia, left ventricular hypertrophy, and perhaps the greater free radical production of the elderly treated by haemodialysis. Many such episodes can be prevented by maintaining the haemoglobin concentration using epoietin at whatever level is required to alleviate symptoms although the increase in haematocrit during the haemo-concentration immediately following haemodialysis may be dangerous (Mignon et al. 1993). Slow-release cutaneous glyceryl trinitrate patches may help and in general have no side-effects.

Gastrointestinal bleeding: elderly patients are more prone to gastrointestinal bleeding during dialysis because of the high incidence of diverticulosis and carcinoma, the angiodysplasia of old age, and perhaps occult increased consumption of non-steroidal anti-inflammatory drugs. If needed for rheumatological complaints, Cox-2 inhibitors are preferable. More serious blood loss may occur in patients with angiodysplasia (Porush and Faubert 1991). If this is acute, administration of deamino-D-arginine vasopressin (DDAVP) and transfusion may be necessary. In some cases, the angiodysplastic area can be identified at endoscopy and treated with laser cauterization, but on occasion even coeliac axis angiography fails to identify the lesion and resection may be needed.

Interdialytic problems

Interdialytic problems have been discussed above under the heading of 'general problems of the elderly with ESRD'. Excessive fluid weight gain is the major problem.

Peritoneal dialysis and its problems in the elderly

Peritoneal dialysis (see Chapter 12.4) in one of its several current forms has been strongly advocated as the ideal method of treatment for ESRD in older patients (Nissenson 1990; Issad et al. 1995; Brown 1999; Winchester 1999), but even today only about 15 per cent of elderly European, and a smaller proportion (8 per cent of 65–74 year olds and only 4 per cent of those over 75 years) amongst American patients have been being treated by this method during the 1990s (Ponticelli et al. 1987; Gokal 1990). Nevertheless, today CAPD is the first choice for treatment of ESRD in the elderly in many renal units, including our own (Gokal 1990; Nolph et al. 1990; Segoloni et al. 1990; Nissenson 1991).

Among the *advantages* of CAPD are a reduction of cardiovascular instability and arrhythmias, rather better (but still inadequate) removal of β-2-microglobulin (particularly if cellulose membranes are used for haemodialysis), better control of disequilibrium syndromes, no need for permanent vascular access, longer and better maintenance of residual kidney function, and better removal of middle molecules and parathyroid hormone (Issad et al. 1995; Brown 1999; Winchester 1999). In diabetics, intraperitoneal insulin is more effective and easier to control. Moreover, a better quality of life, less associated illness, and treatment-related stress, and more stable behaviour have been reported in comparison with patients on haemodialysis (see below).

The *disadvantages* are that arthritic, poorly sighted, haemiplegic, mildly demented, or depressed individuals or patients with poor social support find it difficult to perform self-care CAPD adequately. Machine-assisted APD in one of its several forms (see Chapter 12.4) may render the technique more widely available, but many patients are not able to carry out any form of CAPD on their own, and assistance from a relative or a non-relative helper is unavoidable.

In general, the contraindications to beginning CAPD are the same in the elderly as in younger patients (see Chapter 12.4) (Michel et al. 1990; Nolph 1991). Hernias and some degree of uterine prolapse, which are both common in the elderly, are only relative contraindications provided that they can be dealt with surgically before dialysis begins.

Complications related to the performance of peritoneal dialysis in the elderly

These complicate peritoneal dialysis at any age (Chapter 12.4). *Peritonitis* has the same incidence as in the young (1.09/year versus 0.9/year, range 0.46–1.28; Ismail et al. 1993). In some reports, its incidence was actually less in older patients (Bennett-Jones et al. 1987; Nolph et al. 1990; Posen et al. 1990b; Nissenson 1991). For treatment netilmicin, which has a lower ototoxicity than other aminoglycosides, together with vancomycin is preferable in the elderly. Rates for catheter removal are also identical in older and younger patients on CAPD, at 0.25 removals per patient per year (Nolph et al. 1990), or 1.47 and 1.48 removals per patient per year (Maiorca et al. 1990). *Exit site and tunnel infections* are again no more frequent in old than in younger patients (0.43/year versus 0.55/year) (Nolph et al. 1990), and catheter survival is also similar (Nissenson et al. 1986). The number of days in hospital did not differ significantly between young and elderly dialysis populations in either this study or that of Mion et al. (1981).

Dialysate leakage: laxity of the abdominal wall and small muscle bulk in elderly patients makes leakage more frequent than in young patients, however (Ponce et al. 1982). To overcome this, the catheter can be inserted 1 or 2 weeks before it is required or a neck line can be used for immediate haemodialysis, with the catheter being used only after it has healed in (Ponticelli et al. 1987); this technique is used in our unit in London. In Salamanca, we start a continuous exchange regimen with gradually increasing volumes and frequency from the time of catheter placement. *Hernia formation* is favoured by diminished muscular tone in elderly patients. Kyphosis produces a widening of the diaphragm, leading to hiatus hernias, which are also more common in this age group (Oreopoulos *et al.* 1982).

The insidious development of *underdialysis* is a major danger to all patients on CAPD, and has many causes reviewed in Chapter 12.4. *Diverticulosis and constipation* are common, and both are almost universal in the elderly on dialysis in developed countries eating a Western diet, and may predispose to diverticulitis, intestinal perforation, and faecal peritonitis. Perforation of colonic diverticula may give an obscure clinical picture with only insidious abdominal pain with fever as the initial symptom (Lipschutz and Easterling 1973). This complication is very serious, and laparotomy should be indicated by the suspicion of colonic perforation before the picture of acute peritonitis becomes evident.

Some elderly patients present with intolerable *shoulder and back pain* during CAPD; these complications are also seen in young patients. Pre-existing lumbar disc disease may worsen during CAPD, making discal hernia a relative contraindication to this treatment. Shoulder pain may be due to phrenic nerve irritation. *Dialysate draining pain* occurs in the elderly with the same frequency as in younger patients. Its management is discussed in Chapter 12.4.

Many elderly patients show a very narrow 'window' of body weight (and hence body water), above which they are *breathless* or in frank pulmonary oedema, and below which they are *hypotensive* when upright. This is the result of poor cardiac output and a rigid vascular tree. Meticulous attention to weight gain and loss can cope with this problem but renders the patient's life intolerable in some cases. Restriction of inappropriate salt intake may be a help, and preservation of residual renal function excretion by diuretics may help to broaden the 'window'. CAPD may aggravate *inferior limb ischaemia* in patients with atherosclerosis involving femoroiliac vessels. The reason for this is obscure, but pressure exerted by the dialysis fluid upon vessels may hamper the blood supply to limbs which are already ischaemic. Hypotension exacerbates the problem.

Nutritional problems have been discussed in general above, but peritoneal dialysis imposes an additional nutritional stress in that 8–15 g of first-class protein, mainly albumin, are lost each day in dialysate, and this amount increases during and following episodes of peritonitis (see Chapter 12.4). In contrast, approximately 1500 kcal of energy are supplied each day through the metabolism of glucose absorbed from the peritoneum. Serum albumin concentrations in elderly patients on CAPD are usually less than 40 g/l and, distressingly, often less than 30 g/l. It is essential to ensure a good intake of first-class protein, and this will often involve the prescription of protein supplements. Malnutrition makes all the other complications of CAPD more likely. Oral iron is usually sufficient in CAPD patients as an adjunct to epoetin therapy, but some advocate intermittent intravenous dosing (European Best Practice Guidelines 1999). Hyperlipidaemia is found in both elderly and younger patients during CAPD. Little work has been done on this in older patients, and its significance and correlates are not known.

Infections are more frequent in the elderly, perhaps owing to immunosenescence (see below) and malnutrition, the most common being lung infection and septicaemia. The most frequent life-threatening infections are infections of vascular access followed by Gram-negative organisms coming from the bowel or genitourinary tract. Opportunistic infections are an unusual but serious problem. In a setting of iron overload and treatment with deferrioxamine, *Yersinia enterocolitica* infections should be excluded (Boelaert *et al.* 1988).

Another cause of hospital admission is sepsis from *Escherichia coli*, which may run a fulminant course in haemodialysis patients (Goldman and Vanherweghen 1990).

Depression is common in the elderly on dialysis including CAPD, especially as there is little or no hope for many of escape through transplantation. Many other factors impinge, however, including loss of autonomy, effects of comorbidity, social isolation, and poor economic circumstances. Compared with patients being seen thrice a week on centre haemodialysis, CAPD patients receive relatively little on-going contact with, and support from, unit staff. Failure of CAPD and transfer to haemodialysis in the elderly is at least as commonly the result of pyschological as physical problems (Issad *et al.* 1995). Nevertheless in a major meta-analysis, a comparison of mental state and quality of life in patients doing CAPD appeared to show superior status to those receiving haemodialysis (Cameron *et al.* 2000).

Iatrogenic problems: the low and variable clearance of many drugs through CAPD is often forgotten by physicans caring for peritoneal dialysis patients, and this should always be considered in any sick patient, or in those failing to thrive.

Outcomes of dialysis in the elderly

Survival

Quantity of survival, which is relatively easy to measure, and the quality of survival, which is not, are both crucial (Gokal 1994). There may also be purely technical considerations which can affect the apparent results of treatment quite profoundly and make comparisons difficult. The best known of these is the exclusion by the US Renal Data System of any patient who enters dialysis but dies during the first 90 days of treatment; in addition, some of the fittest patients leave dialysis through transplantation, although as we shall see this proportion is quite small in those aged over 65 years. The relative non-availablity of transplantation in Japan is bound to have a positive effect on the survival of their dialysis population. In many countries, frail patients are excluded from treatment who might be accepted elsewhere.

Overall survival of elderly patients on dialysis improved considerably during the 1980s, and (although attenuated) this trend has continued during the 1990s. Many individual authors (some cited in the tables) and a number of large national and international registries (United States, Europe, Japan, Australia, and Canada) have reported results in the treatment by dialysis of elderly patients with ESRD in terms of survival (Tables 5 and 6). Of course, these tables give the outcomes of only those patients who were taken on for treatment. The exclusion processes operating in the various countries before the patients were admitted were discussed in the introduction, and can only be guessed at, but are known to be considerable (Kjellstrand and Logan 1987; Feest *et al.* 1990).

Recently attention has turned to the increasing number of patients being accepted for dialysis treatment (the number transplanted at the moment is negligible) aged 75–80 years of age or even more (Issad *et al.* 1995; Sturm *et al.* 1998; Schaefer and Röhrich 1999; Lamping *et al.* 2000; Dimkovic *et al.* 2001; Joly *et al.* 2003). Such octagenarian patients (Table 1) should have a life expectancy of 5–9 years, but no series published so far has achieved anything like this survival (Tables 1 and 7). European and Japanese data from the 1980s are somewhat better than even recent American results (Table 7); unfortunately, few data are avilable for Europe as a whole during the 1990s.

The actuarial survival of patients treated by either haemodialysis or CAPD, of course, shows an increased mortality with increasing age

Table 5 Survival of elderly patients in ESRD treated by haemodialysis: national/international registries

	Age (years)	'Young' elderly actuarial survival at				Age (years)	'Elderly' elderly actuarial survival at			
		1 year	2 years	3 years	5 years		1 year	2 years	3 years	5 years
Europe	65–74	76	62	51	30	75–84	75	55	20	—
USA	65–	72	46	36	15	75–79	65	41	12	—
	70–74	68	47	17	—	80–84	60	34	9	—
						85–	54	28	4	—
Japan	60–74	73	63	38	—	75–89	54	40	18	—
						90–	45	35	24	—
Australasia	65–74	83	66	51	29	75–84	68	55	<10	—
Canada	65–	68	50	20	—					
European countries										
Belgium	65–74	—	64	—	32	75–84	—	44	—	
Germany	65–74	—	65	—	34	75–84	—	58	—	22
France	65–74	—	68	—	37	75–84	—	55	—	19
Italy	65–74	—	65	—	30	75–84	—	50	—	14
Netherlands	65–74	—	65	—	33	75–84	—	45	—	—
Spain	65–74	—	71	—	40	75–84	—	50	—	—
Catalan	65–70	91	—	74	67					
UK	65–74	—	56	—	27	75–84	—	44	—	—
Large individual series of 'elderly elderly'										
Piccoli (1996)	Italy					>75	76	33	—	10[a]
Röhrich (1996)	Germany					>80	71	51	—	19[b]
Chadna (1999)	UK					>75	66	48	—	19
Lampling (2000)	UK					>75–79	69	—	—	—
						>80	53	—	—	—
Chaveau (2001)	France					>75	80	65	—	—
Munshi (2001)	UK					>75	54	37	12	2

[a] 1981–1985 cohort; other data for 1991–1993.

[b] Röhrich reports much better survivals post-1990 than before (1 year 80%, 2 years 61%, 5 years but numbers are small (46 versus 36 pre-1990).

All series 80–250 patients except Munshi et al. (n = 58).

All figures in percentages; Europe: 1981–1987, Brunner et al. 1995; USA: 1993, 1993–1998, USRDS 1995, 2000; Japan: 1980–1988, Odaka (1990); Canada: 1981–1987, Posen 1990; Australia: 1987–1996, Disney 1998; Catalan: Bonal et al. (1997).

Table 6 Survival of elderly patients in ESRD treated by CAPD

		n	1 year	3 years	5 years
Registry reports					
Europe		65–69	72	44	—
Canada		60–	73	35	15
Australasia		65–74	81	49	17
Individual series with >100 patients included					
Gokal		60–		60[a]	
Segoloni		60–		40	16
Nissenson		60–		49	32
Maiorca		60–	89	73	46
Gentile		60–	89	64	
Lupo		60–			45
Older patients					
De Vecchi	63	70–	85	44	21
Dimkovic	31	80–	72	39	0

[a] = 2y survival.

Table 7 Observed and expected percentage survival of elderly US patients under treatment for ESRD, 1987–1991

Age (years)	Expected (US population) and observed (ESRD Rx) % survival					
	1 year		2 years		5 years	
	ESRD	US	ESRD	US	ESRD	US
65	71.0	98.2	54.3	96.4	21.7	93.3
70	65.3	97.3	47.3	94.7	15.4	76.1
75	60.2	96.0	35.3	92.1	10.5	66.3
80	54.9	94.0	27.4	88.3	6.6	53.7

All treatments included: ~5% transplanted and ~8% on CAPD, remainder (~86%) on haemodialysis.

Modified from Latos (1996) and derived from 1993 national US statistics and USRDS data for the relevant years.

See also Table 1 for life expectancy data.

(Ponticelli *et al.* 1987) (Tables 1 and 4, Fig. 2). Part of this relates to inevitable actuarial facts, but the greater mortality also relates to technical difficulties and other factors, including poverty and race, discussed by Kjellstrand and Logan (1987), and Kimmel *et al.* (2000). There is a tendency to give less dialysis to elderly patients, perhaps because of the misinterpretation that their lower plasma creatinine suggests the need for less dialysis. This underdialysis may contribute to

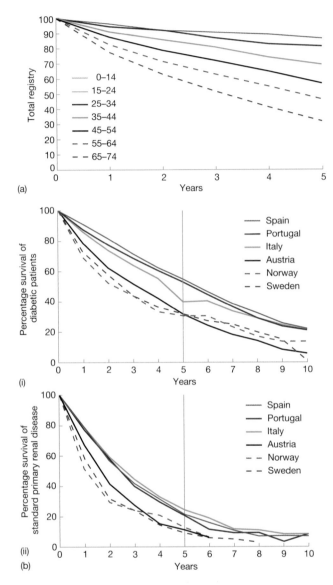

Fig. 2 Survival of elderly ESRD patients in Europe 1986–1991 (all treatments). As expected, the absolute survival decreases with increasing age at entry to treatment. Curves for peritoneal dialysis and haemodialysis are not significantly different, and the contribution of transplantation to these overall survival curves is small in the elderly groups because of the small numbers transplanted in most European countries (see text). (b) Survival of patients over the age of 60 years in various European countries (1983–1992) with (i) standard primary renal diseases and (ii) diabetes mellitus, almost exclusively type II. As in all data sets, the survival of diabetics is markedly poorer than that of patients with standard primary renal disease. Interestingly, survival in both groups is better in Mediterranean countries than in Northern European countries (data with permission from the European Renal Association Registry).

the shortfall in survival of the elderly (Tables 5 and 6) compared with control populations of a similar age (Table 2). However, it must be emphasized again that the number of life-years of life lost at any point following dialysis in the elderly is much less than in younger patients (Maiorca *et al.* 1991, 1993), and at least some populations of elderly patients can achieve the same mortality as a control elderly population when treated by regular haemodialysis (Rotellar *et al.* 1985) or transplantation (Becker *et al.* 2000).

Causes of death in elderly patients on dialysis

Causes of death in the elderly on dialysis (Fig. 3) do not differ markedly from younger patients, with cardiovascular disease and infections forming the two major groups. However, these and similar data from North America conceal the fact that 5–15 per cent or more of deaths in those over the age of 65 are preceded by withdrawal from dialysis, which although not technically the 'cause of death', clearly has role in precipitating it (see below). As well as a major problem at the onset of ESRD treatment, the proportion of those elderly with cardiovascular disease increases (Bonal *et al.* 1997) (Fig. 4) especially in the elderly. However, the increase in *relative* risk of dying of cardiovascular disease in the elderly is slight compared with the huge increase in younger patients. Fatal infections are probably more common in the elderly because of their altered immune status (see below) although there is little direct evidence for this. Malignancy is, perhaps surprisingly, not a major hazard in those without it when beginning dialysis. Although there have been suggestions that neoplasia are more common in patients on dialysis (Mainsonneuve *et al.* 1999), this increase is small (RR 1.2 in those over 65 years) and (again surprisingly) mainly concentrated on younger (RR 2.5) rather than older patients.

Hospital admission rates

Habach *et al.* (1995) examined data from all the 221,301 patients in the US Renal Data System in 1993, of whom 87 per cent were receiving

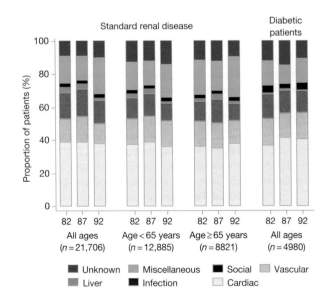

Fig. 3 Causes of death in the European ESRD population over 65 years of age in Europe compared with younger patients (EDTA-European Renal Association data) [with permission from: Mallick, N. P. and Gokal, R. (1999). Haemodialysis. *Lancet* **353**, 737–742].

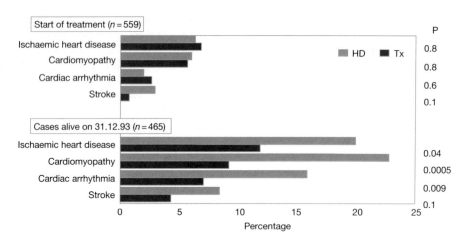

Fig. 4 Proportion of elderly patients on long-term dialysis or with a transplant showing vascular disease at start of treatment, and up to 10 years later. Data from the Catalan Registry (Bonal et al. 1997).

haemodialysis and 37.6 per cent were over the age of 65. They confirmed previous reports (Westlie et al. 1984; Gokal 1987; Ismail et al. 1993) that the elderly on dialysis come into hospital a little more frequently than their younger counterparts (2.2 versus 1.9 times/year), but stay a little longer on each admission (21.9 versus 17.3 days, CAPD figures being greater than for those on haemodialysis). There are few data for admissions in the very elderly: Lamping et al. (2000) noted 2.2 admissions per patient in the first year and 1.8 in subsequent years in 174 patients aged more than 70 years in North London, the mean hospital stay being 9.5 days. These very elderly patients had no longer or more frequent admissions than those aged 'only' 65–70.

Quality of life

Quality of life is difficult to compare because of the great variety of rather imprecise instruments used to assess it (Stewart and Ware 1992; Gokal 1994; McGee and Bradley 1994; Carvar and Rockwood 1995). As with absolute survival, the effect of selection for treatment in the elderly is unknown. Westlie et al. (1984) found that 73 per cent of their 157 patients aged 70–87 had a Karnovsky index of greater than 80, and 93 per cent were at home, having good social contact (90 per cent), spending time outdoors (86 per cent), and 'enjoying life' (71 per cent). This landmark retrospective study was followed by a prospective study (Husebye and Kjellstrand 1987). Fifty-four per cent of the original patients had died by this time, and the predictors of survival were all psychosocial: compliance (as judged by weight gain), Karnofsky score, ability to dialyse at home, and less frequent request for a transplant. Similar overall results have been obtained by others (Kutner et al. 1994) in the dialysis population as a whole (data reviewed by Gokal 1994), with some observers finding that the elderly adjust even better than younger patients (Auer et al. 1990). In the North Thames study (Lamping et al. 2000), using the SF-36 questionnaire, it was found that in those over 70 on dialysis the mental component summary (MCS) was no different from local controls of the same age, although as expected the physical (PCS) scores were lower (34 versus 41); the haemoglobin concentrations and use of epoetin were, unfortunately, not given. Rebollo et al. (1998) found that SF-36 scores were better in older (>65 years) dialysis patients than younger.

However, other reports have not been so hopeful. Kutner et al. (1991) found that 40 per cent of their dialysis patients in Georgia aged

over 60 spent all day in a bed or a chair at home, and almost half (twice the proportion of non-dialysed elderly controls) reported symptoms of depression. Even so, life was reported as 'very satisfying' or 'satisfying' by 55 per cent of respondents. McKevitt et al. (1986) assessed only 32 per cent of their 60 patients aged 60–78 as having a Karnofsky score of 70 or more; 33 per cent had 'mild to severe' intellectual impairment (Pfeiffer questionnaire) and 62 per cent were judged to be depressed. Ifudu et al. (1994) studied 104 patients aged 65–90 years living in Brooklyn and undergoing in-centre haemodialysis, of whom one-third were diabetic and 60 per cent were Black; 87 were receiving erythropoietin. They described their results as 'dismal'. The mean Karnofsky score for the whole group was 66 ± 12, with 14 requiring a wheelchair. The authors concluded that 'few elderly diabetic haemodialysis patients conduct any substantive portion of their lives outside their homes'. Munshi et al. (2000) reported from the United Kingdom that 20 per cent of the survival time of 58 elderly patients (>65 years) had been spent in hospital.

These studies emphasize yet again that support and environment, as well as selection for treatment, may be crucial factors in determining the degree of rehabilitation observed. It should also be noted that all of these data except those of Ifudu et al. (1994) and Munshi et al. (2000), were obtained in the period before the introduction of erythropoietin, which has universally been found to improve quality of life in dialysed patients when used appropriately (Canadian Erythropoietin Study Group 1990). Surprisingly, the only data of the impact of this on QOL in the elderly is in a prospective study by Moreno et al. (1996), who found improved Karnofsky scores and a decrease in sickness impact profile in patients whose haemoglobin was raised only from 7 to 9.6 g/dl. No data are available on whether further increments in haemoglobin to 11–12 g/dl as recommended, or even higher concentrations, might confer benefit or disadvantage in the elderly and such studies are needed.

Choice of dialysis modality for the elderly endstage renal disease patient

Obviously, independent CAPD or even automated peritoneal dialysis at home requires skills which passive in-centre dialysis does not, and some patients will exclude themselves immediately from home self-dialysis of any form. Holley and Foulks (1991) showed that the failure of home CAPD in elderly patients could be predicted with some accuracy by a simple inventory of visual acuity, personal hygiene, manual dexterity, family support, adaptability to change, learning ability, motivation, compliance, and wish for dialysis in a home setting. In many elderly patients, however, there are no strong pointers either way. All units should strive to provide an integrated and balanced programme for all their patients, including the elderly, which allows choice of treatment and change of treatment should this become necessary or desirable. This is far from the case in many countries and many centres, even where fiscal restraints do not operate.

There are many pitfalls in attempting any comparison between CAPD and haemodialysis, including in the elderly (Biesen et al. 2000), but almost all carefully adjusted registry and single-centre comparisons (e.g. Burton and Walls 1987; Bloembergen et al. 1995; Fenton et al. 1997) show that the survival of elderly uraemic patients is similar whether haemodialysis or CAPD is used (Tables 4, 5, and Fig. 4). However, the Canadian registry analysis (Fenton et al. 1997) found a lower relative risk of death on CAPD in those aged over 65 (0.76, CI 0.68–0.84) in non-diabetics compared to that in those on haemodialysis; in diabetics, the RR was 0.88 (CI 0.73–1.06); the benefit was all during the first 2 years of treatment. In two other important studies, survival was also better during peritoneal dialysis in a 6-year follow-up in patients aged more than 65 years after adjustment of comorbid factors (US Renal Data System 1992; Vonesh and Maiorca 1993); this was reversed in younger patients. Other studies, however, have shown worse outcomes for the elderly on CAPD than on haemodialysis (Gentile et al. 1990; Gokal et al. 1990). True prospective randomized trials comparing peritoneal dialysis of either type and haemodialysis for ESRD patients are lacking, and likely to remain so since true randomization is almost impossible to achieve.

What about quality of life? One careful attempt to compare by meta-analysis the quality of life in 49 published comparisons (Cameron et al. 2000) showed that patients on CAPD in their own home had better psychological well being and less mental distress than comparable patients underging haemodialysis in dialysis centres, but was unable to eliminate effects of differences in case-mix as a major factor in this difference.

Peritoneal dialysis is clearly better for patients with major cardiovascular instability (Vlachoyannis et al. 1988). However, the disadvantages of this method mean that those with lower-limb ischaemic disease, extensive abdominal surgery, diverticulitis, intractable hernias, or poor social support are best treated by in-centre haemodialysis (Ross and Rutsky 1990). Haemodialysis is obviously better for those only marginally competent to manage the technique of CAPD for reasons of physical or mental illness. Technique survival favours haemodialysis, but shows different time dependency in haemodialysis and CAPD (see Maiorca et al. 1994 for a detailed review). In data censored for death, fallout from peritoneal dialysis is considerable and linear with time, whereas fallout from haemodialysis generally occurs during the first year and is relatively stable thereafter. In the US Renal Data System data, 12.5 per cent of patients transferred from CAPD to haemodialysis whilst only 1.7 per cent transferred the other way (Port 1992).

The final choice of treatment modality may depend as much on local facilities as on individual patient characteristics. As noted above, the high proportion of elderly British uraemics treated by CAPD during the 1980s (Gokal 1990) reflected at least in part a severe shortage of in-centre dialysis places, but also reflected a positive choice of British

nephrologists and the patients themselves for self-care. Interestingly, the opposite trend is seen in the United States, where the proportion of patients over 65 years of age treated by peritoneal dialysis (6–8 per cent) has always been lower than that of younger patients (Gentile et al. 1990; USRDS 2001). This may be related, at least in part, to local funding systems and physician reimbursement. Although obviously patient preference should be paramount, this does not always achieve the attention it deserves, the individual in ESRD receiving most commonly what is 'on offer' as preferred treatment in their local unit.

Withdrawal of or from dialysis in elderly patients

The problem of withdrawal from ESRD treatment first surfaced in North America during the early 1980s (Rodin et al. 1981; Kaye and Lella 1986; Neu and Kjellstrand 1986) and must be increasingly faced as more and more very fragile elderly patients begin dialysis. Also those who are capable and competent may later become incapable, often from dementia and, if conscious of their state, unhappy to the point of suicide (Kjellstrand 1988; Chazan 1990; Mailloux et al. 1993). It is difficult to get reliable statistics on just how large the problem of actual *suicide* may be, because deliberate underdialysis in the case of those doing self-care may precipitate death from other causes, and because in many units similar deaths are not recorded as such. Deliberate suicide has always been more common in the dialysis population than the general population but accounts for less than 1 per cent of dialysis deaths (Haemel et al. 1983).

Discontinuation of dialysis is much more common, and even given the reservations above, is the second most common 'cause' of death in the elderly on dialysis after cardiovascular disease in the United States, Canada, and Australasia (Oreopoulos 1995). In 1995 (USRDS 1996), the US Renal Data System gave an overall rate of 82.3 withdrawals/1000 patient-years in over 65-year-old Whites, compared with only 35.8 in African-Americans, with a total death rate of about 317/1000 patient-years for all those aged 65–74 years, and 472 in over 75-year-olds, withdrawal preceding death in 17.6 per cent of cases. Since 1990, the US Renal Data System has recognized the fact that withdrawal of dialysis is not of itself an actual *cause* of death, which occurs later from uraemia, usually complicated by systemic illness. This was present in 35 per cent of withdrawals in 1995, whilst the largest group (42 per cent) were put down as 'failure to thrive'. Some earlier individual accounts gave similar high figures (18 per cent, Kjellstrand 1988; Mailloux et al. 1993) but in contrast, other reports considered it rare (Porush and Faubert 1991), and in Europe as a whole only 3.1 per cent of dialysis deaths were preceded by withdrawal (Kjellstrand 1992). However, in the single study from the United Kingdom, Catalano et al. (1996) gave a figure of 17 per cent of deaths at all ages, similar to higher American estimates. In all Western societies, discontinuation is much more common in the elderly, but interestingly this trend is reversed in Japan where a lower level of withdrawal throughout of only 1.4 per cent is found (Kjellstrand 1992). Risk factors apart from increasing age are female sex, White race rather than African-American or Asian, and the presence of chronic fatal disease (malignancy or dementia) (Leggat et al. 1997). Clearly, the number of such terminations of dialysis will increase if the policy of 'trial of dialysis' is adopted more widely at onset in marginal, vulnerable uraemic patients (see above).

The management of this situation is full of difficulties. The subject has been much discussed (Sessa 1995; Singer et al. 1995; Cohen et al. 1996;

Tobe and Senn 1996; Brody *et al.* 1997; Auer 1998; Moss 2000) and the American Renal Physicians' Association has published guidelines recently (Renal Physicians Association 2000) which are useful, but almost every patient presents some unique combination of circumstances. Clearly, any action must start from discussions involving the patient him- or herself together with their family if available (Muñoz Silva and Kjellstrand 1988; Holley *et al.* 1989).

Two broad groups of patients can be distinguished: the first is the patient who is conscious and competent in the legal sense; here the request to withdraw usually will come from him or herself. More commonly, however, patients will signal in an indirect fashion that dialysis has become intolerable; they may covertly or even actively try to kill themselves, but may later be grateful for having been prevented from this (Kaye *et al.* 1987). It is always necessary to allow time for reflection; intercurrent but treatable illnesses (particularly those likely to precipitate temporary dementia or depression), social problems, or lack of psychological or family support may induce patients to feel temporarily that they wish to withdraw from treatment, and active steps to treat these are needed (Campbell 1991). Shared decision making, informed consent (including likely prognosis) and resolution of any conflicts between patient, relatives/carers and staff are central to good management.

The second, even more difficult situation arises when the patient is judged not to be competent in either a legal or a social sense, usually because of advancing dementia. This is often fluctuant to begin with, and ascertaining the patients' own inner feelings difficult in the extreme and finally impossible. Advance directives ('living wills') are a great help in this situation and all patients, especially those indetifiable as at risk of withdrawal should be encouraged to make one. In this situation, the request to stop treatment will usually arise from the family or carer, or from the unit medical and nursing staff. In the latter case, the family may oppose what seems reasonable to the doctors and nurses, to the point of threatening litigation if treatment is stopped, but the opposite situation may arise also, with relatives requesting discontinuation when staff are unwilling. In many such patients, intercurrent illness may solve the problem within a short while, and it may be easier to wait for this resolution rather than trying to force the issue. Some units also practise 'gradual' withdrawal of dialysis, that is, progressive underdialysis, in an attempt to blunt the hurt of apparent withdrawal of care for all concerned, both family and staff (Kjellstrand 1988) but this approach is inconsistent and difficult to defend.

In either case, with or without the patient's participation, if a decision to withdraw dialysis is made this should be followed by a carefully planned, *active* regimen of alternative management (Cohen *et al.* 2000a), including involvement of the palliative care team if one is available. Patients usually take from 8 to about 12 days to die following cessation of dialysis (Neu and Kjellstrand 1986) and today many renal physicians have forgotten—or never knew—how to manage the often distressing symptoms of terminal uraemia. Certainly, we are not yet as good as we should be at achieving the goal of a 'good' death; even in a unit with much experience of, and a major interest in this subject, Cohen *et al.* (2000b) suggested from a survey of 131 patients that only 38 per cent had 'good' deaths and 15 per cent 'bad' deaths, whilst 42 per cent experienced some pain, severe in 5 per cent. There is no doubt that the questions of the grounds on which treatment may be withheld in the first place, and whether and when to stop treatment and on what grounds, will quite rightly continue to excite interest not only among those directly involved in dialysis, but also among lawyers, ethicists, and the general public (Rothenberg 1993).

Transplantation in the elderly recipient

Renal transplantation in the elderly remains even today somewhat controversial (Taube *et al.* 1987; Becker *et al.* 1996; Ponticelli 2000; Jacobs and Mignon 2002). This is despite it being recognized as the most successful and cost-effective treatment for patients with ESRD in general, and even today, the elderly are rarely treated by what is generally accepted as the best method available. The proportion of patients receiving a transplant falls from more than half in childhood and adolescence (Table 8), to less than 1 per cent in those over 70 years of age. Why is this?

In our view, the optimum mode of therapy for the otherwise fit elderly up to the age of 70 or even 75 years should be transplantation (Taube *et al.* 1987). The relative neglect of the elderly uraemic seems to be a continuation of behaviour built into the history of the management of elderly patients from the beginning of ESRD programmes (Taube *et al.* 1987) but it is worth noting here that until the early 1980s patients as young as 45 years of age were considered to be a 'high-risk' group; indeed allograft survival in this age group was only 20 per cent at 1 year in 1970.

Nevertheless, an increasing proportion of transplanted patients are now over 65 years of age, and an increasing number of grafts are allocated each year to older patients. In Europe, the proportion of recipients of grafts aged over 60 increased from 2.9 per cent in 1983 to 10.2 per cent in 1992. The United States has shown a striking increase also: in 1984, only 1.6 per cent of those aged 65–74 years and 0.1 per cent of those aged 75 bore a successful transplant. By 1988, this was 4 per cent and 0.3 per cent, and a decade later in 1999, 13.0 and 2.2 per cent (Table 9). In that year of 8.4 per cent of 8019 cadaver and 5.4 per cent of 3513 living donors grafts were placed in those aged 65–74 years, and also 42 (0.5 per cent) cadaver grafts—but less than 10 living donor grafts—to those over 75 years. However, the proportion of grafts placed into and borne by older recipients varies considerably from country to country: in 1999 of those aged greater than 60 years, only 2.2 per cent in Australia, 2.5 per cent in Italy, 2.1 per cent in France, and 5.8 per cent in Canada, compared with 30.4 per cent in Norway and 19.5 per cent in Switzerland bore grafts (Valderrábano *et al.* 1995). In our unit in London, England, the proportion of those over 60 amongst those transplanted is now 21 per cent (Cameron *et al.* 1994; Cameron 2000) and is still increasing.

Some of the continued reluctance to transplant the elderly arises from memories of gloomy results before 1980 (Roodnat *et al.* 1999). The report of the US Renal Data System noted in 1991 that the *actual*

Table 8 Transplanted ESRD patients in the United States 1999

	Total ESRD	**Per cent with transplant**
All patients on ESRD treatment at 12.99	340,261	29.6
0–19 years	6,154	70.5
20–44 years	80,854	50.0
45–64 years	135,960	33.9
65–74 years	68,349	13.0
>75 years	48,944	2.2

From USRDS Report 2001 [*American Journal of Kidney Diseases* **38** (Suppl. 3), s18].

Table 9 Results of cadaver transplantation in recipients over the age of 60 years. I: recent registry data

	n	Age	1 year	5 years	10 years
Patient survival					
Collaborative transplant study (Opeltz 1998)	4254	60–65	86	66	41
USRDS 1999	?	>65	86	68	
UNOS 1994	1353	>65	85	74 (3 years)	
Canadian registry (Schaubel et al. 1995)	284	>60	87	68	
Catatan registry (Bonal et al. 1997)	222	55–70	88	87	
Combined series (from Table 10)	1948	>60	88	71	
Overall			87	70	
Living donors USRDS 1999		>65	82		
Graft survival					
Collaborative transplant study (Opelz 1998)	4254	60–65	77	58	33
USRDS 1998		>65	71	56	
UNOS 1994	1353	>65	77	64 (3 years)	
UK Transplant SSA (Belger 1998)	630	>60	73	52	
Combined series (from Table 10)	1948	>60	79	62	
Overall			75	57	
Living donors USRDS 1999		>65	72		

Note: The CTS data as given in Jassal et al. (1997) differ in detail from those in Opeltz (1998). The ages of patients included in these data differ: some are only 60–64 years, others >60 year of age, the UNOS data >65 years of age. Obviously, the UNOS and USRDS data must overlap to a considerable extent and with the CIS data to an unknown extent.

Updated from Cameron 2000.

10-year survival for transplant recipients (i.e. those transplanted during the 1980s) aged 50–59 years was only 22 per cent, 10.5 per cent for those aged 60–64, and 8 per cent for those aged 65–69 (Ismail *et al.* 1993; USRDS 1993); fortunately, this is no longer the case (Roodnat *et al.* 1999 and see below). However, the major factor today has to be the seemingly intractable shortage of cadaver kidneys: when young, fit patients with decades of potential survival are waiting on dialysis for a graft, is it fair or reasonable to use a graft for a 70-year-old with a life expectancy of only 10 years or so. Recipient survival is inevitably less with increasing age and although transplant outcomes today are much better than in the past (see Tables 10–12) they are still substantially worse than for control populations of similar age: as noted in Table 1, the average life expectancy for a 65-year-old is 13–15 years in developed countries. Maximization of *the number of successful transplant-years* would require that patients aged more than 70 be not transplanted at all. However, this does not apply so forcefully to those aged 60–70 years, particularly remembering that the usual half-life for a cadaver transplant remains less than 10 years (Opelz *et al.* 1992; Opelz 1998).

Selection of older patients for transplantation

The heterogeneity of elderly populations of similar chronological age contrasted with the homgeneity of younger populations has been emphasized above and in Chapter 1.5. Since, as we shall see, the principal cause of lost grafts in the elderly is patients bearing a functioning graft lost through death, clearly selection of potential recipients who are physically more robust has a considerable role to play in improving the use of scarce cadaver kidneys, as well as reducing individual morbidity and overall mortality. Although it is true that when considered globally, the aged have a greater rate of complications than the younger, and survive much less well (Taube *et al.* 1987; Takemoto and Terasaki 1988; Velez *et al.* 1991; Raine *et al.* 1992; USRDS 2001), when patients are stratified by risk, with 'low risk' defined as absence of diabetes or cardiovascular disease, 1-year survival rates of 91 per cent for the patient and 84 per cent for the graft have been recorded (Schulak and Hricik 1991; Tesi *et al.* 1994) (see below).

Selection consists mainly in screening for *cardiovascular disease*, both cardiac and peripheral (Cameron *et al.* 1994; Helderman *et al.* 1995; Cameron 2000; Stewart *et al.* 2000), since this is the principal cause of death following transplantation in the elderly (see below). Cardiac assessment consists at a minimum of a careful history and examination, and a resting ECG. Smoking should cease (Doyle *et al.* 2000) but is not always possible to achieve. Blood lipids may need correction. In addition, even elderly patients without any signs of vascular disease on clinical evaluation should have non-invasive investigation of their heart such as a thallium stress test using dipyridamole, and an echocardiogram including assessment of the left ventricular ejection fraction and hypertrophy, both of which were found by Basu *et al.* (2000) to be useful discriminants. Coronary angiography is only necessary if any of these, or the clinical examination, are abnormal. Most clinicians regard severe cerebrovascular disease as a contraindication. Severe peripheral arterial disease is also a controversial issue and a Doppler ultrasound evaluation of femoro-iliac vessels is necessary also. Disease affecting the iliac arteries is a complication for the surgeon (Geis *et al.* 1976), but can be treated by prior endarterectomy or even by grafting onto aortoiliac Dacron bypass protheses, a technique which we have used in several patients. An obvious risk in these patients is a 'steal' of blood from an already ischaemic limb, but in our experience this is a rare complication (Taube *et al.* 1987). Clearly, to optimize results, any elderly patient with any sign of vascular disease should be excluded from transplantation; in practice, this is not possible, and we have found ourselves transplanting patients with previous coronary angioplasty or aortoiliac bypass grafts. Nevertheless, most clinicians would consider patients with severe coronary artery disease in whom revascularization or angioplasty is not possible unsuitable for kidney transplant (Schulak and Hricik 1991), and also those with a left ventricular ejection fraction less than 35 per cent (Basu *et al.* 2000).

In many units, patients aged over 60 or 65 years with a diagnosis of *diabetes mellitus* are unlikely to receive a transplant. For example, in our local data from 1986 to 1989, only three such patients (1.8 per cent) were transplanted from a pool of 169 patients over 60 years of age (Cameron *et al.* 1994), although in large American series (Tesi *et al.* 1994; Doyle *et al.* 2000) 18–25 per cent of elderly recipients had diabetes, and more patients with type II diabetes are being considered for transplantation today (Mieghem *et al.* 2001) (see Table 11). In many units, routine coronary angiography is performed in all diabetic

Table 10 Results of cadaver transplantation in recipients over the age of 60 years. II: Single-centre data using immunosuppression including cyclosporin

Year	Author	Age	% Diabetes	n	Survival (%)					
					Patient			Graft		
					1 year	5 years	10 years	1 year	5 years	10 years
1989	Pirsch	>60	6	36	91	—		72	—	—
1989	Fauchald[a]	>60	?	122	87	—		67	—	—
1990	Schulak	>60	24	26	79	—		79	—	
1991	Morris	>60	7	45	73	59		71	59	
1992	Andreu	>60	7	33	88	—		88	—	
1994	Cameron	>60	2	169	80	60		71	42	
1994	Tesi[a]	>60	25	133	85	68		80	60	
1994	Cantarovich	>60	2	121	92	80		86	80	
1994	Benedetti	>60	19	76	91	77 (3 years)	—	83	68 (3 years)	
1995	Nyberg	>60	6	70	89	—		75	—	
1995	Albrechtsen	55–69	3 CD	340	81	59		72	51	
	Albrechtsen	*(for comparison LD*		159	92	70		86	62)	
1999	Meier–Kriesche[b]	>60	18	93	89	84 (3 years)	—	87	80	—
2000	Basu	>60	?	69	96	87	41	68	42	—
2000	Johnson	>60	5	67	98	90	—	—	—	—
2000	Doyle	>60	25	206	90	68	—	86	60	—
2001	Saudan	>60	4	49	92	78	44	84	64	32
2001	Kappes	>60		63	92	80	—	88	82	—
Tacrolimus instead of cyclosporin:										
1999	Basar	>60	22	230	90	76	—	84	64	—
Weighted mean				1948	88	71		79	62	
Recipients over 65 years										
1989	Roza	>65	0	17[c]	65	—	—	59	—	—
1989	Fehrman	>65	?	38[c]	71	—	—	63	—	—
1992	Vivas	>65	5	22	89	—	—	71	—	—
1994	Cameron	>65	0	77	74	—	—	60	—	—
1996	Barry	>65	8	24	91	86	—	77	77	—
1998	Bendtdal	>65		244	—		—	78	54	—
2000	Lufft	>65	?	91	94	73	50	87	65	42
Weighted mean				513	77			64	—	—
Recipients over 70 years										
1995	Albrechtsen	>70	3	CD 106	81	54	—	78	52	—
				(LD 20	80	74	—	80	73	—)

[a] These series contain a significant number of living related grafts whose data cannot be extracted: Fauchald, 26/122; Tesi 24/133; Nyberg 13/70. Others series contained only occasional living related grafts. There is overlap between the series of Fauchald, Albrechtsen, and Bentdal (Norwegian national data). CD, cadaver transplant donor; LD, living transplant donor.

[b] Half the recipients received mycophenolate instead of azathioprine with no difference in survivals.

[c] Four patients (Roza) and 17 patients (Fehrman) did not receive cyclosporin (updated from Cameron 2000).

potential recipients irrespective of symptoms or age, and lesions requiring correction are dealt with prophylactically.

In males, *prostatic obstruction* must be looked for. *Diverticulitis* is very common amongst the elderly in Western societies and colonic perforation is a serious, although no longer invariably fatal, complication in the elderly immunosuppressed recipient (Church *et al.* 1986). A problem arises when patients have had *neoplasia*, but appear to have been cured in that they have survived a year or several years without recurrence. In general, the evidence is that common epithelial tumours such as lung, breast, and gut (with the exception of skin) are not affected by immunosuppression (Brunner *et al.* 1995). Those with *dementia* from Alzheimer's disease or multiple cerebral infarcts, *physical incapacity* due to severe musculoskeletal pathology, those with *hemiplegia*, and those

unable to eat, walk, and care for themselves would not normally be selected for transplant therapy.

The immunological system and immunosuppression in the older recipient

The immune system in the aged

In elderly subjects, complex changes of the immune system appear with increasing age, so called 'immunosenescence' (Ginaldi *et al.* 1999a–c) or rather remodelling of the immune system, exemplified by the atrophy of the thymus from puberty. Problems arise, however, in both the description and the interpretation of observed alterations in immune reponses, since many elderly suffer from disease states which may

Table 11 Causes of death in elderly transplant recipients: the Collaborative Transplant Study data

	First year	2–5 years	5–10 years
Patients under 50 years of age			
	n = 404	n = 515	n = 418
Infection	40.1	14.6	11.5
Cardiac disease	24.3	30.7	29.4
Cardiovascular disease	7.4	8.5	9.8
Malignancy	~.0	20.0	23.7
Others	23.2	26.2	25.6
Patients over 50 years of age			
	n = 412	n = 501	n = 622
Infection	36.4	17.8	13.4
Cardiac disease	21.4	24.2	31.2
Cardiovascular disease	6.1	9.0	11.7
Malignancy	4.6	13.8	12.5
Others	31.5	35.2	31.2

All figures percentages of number of deaths during period indicated (data of Jassal et al. 1997).

Table 12 Death rates (/1000 patient years) in patients dying with a functioning graft in the USRDS data

Age	20–44 years	45–64 years	>65 years
All causes	17	45.3	94.5
Acute myocardial infarction	1.1	3.2	5.0[a]
Other cardiac causes	0.7	3.2	5.0[a]
Cardiac arrest	1.3	3.4	5.9[a]
Septicaemia	1.1	2.8	5.1[b]
Pulmonary infection	0.4	1.0	2.0[b]
Cerebrovascular accident	0.6	1.6	2.7[a]
Malignant disease	0.7	2.7	6.6

[a] All cardiovascular disease 37.3.

[b] All infections 16.7 in those over 65 years of age (Meier-Kriesche et al. 2001).

From Jacobs and Mignon (2002) derived from USRDS data (2000 report).

contribute to the alterations (Francheschi *et al.* 1996; Castle 2000). What role if any the 'immunosenescence' of the healthy elderly may play in clinical states such as the increased incidence of malignant disease and increased susceptibility to infections has been much debated, some (Voets *et al.* 1997) suggesting they play a negligible role, others (Burns and Goodwin 1997; Khanna and Markham 1999) that significant clinical effects follow. It is clear that even healthy elderly patients have different immune reponses from younger subjects, however. The changes in the elderly immune response can be summarized as first, alterations in the humoral B lymphocyte system, with a decrease in the numbers of peripheral B cells, alterations in the balance of antibody subclasses, and of the antibody response to antigens (Ginaldi *et al.* 1999a). However, cell-mediated immunity shows abnormalities also, with a decrease in numbers of circulating T cells, alterations in T cell phenotype with a decrease in naive T cells and an increase in 'memory' cells, which is

associated with poor responses to new antigens. Macrophage function is subnormal compared with younger subjects, and there is a complex dysregulation of the cytokine network, with increase in secretion of some cytokines and decreases in others (Ginaldi *et al.* 1999b). Finally, most granulocyte functions are depressed but NK cell activity is probably upregulated (Ginaldi *et al.* 1999c). Indeed, it is difficult to find any aspect of the immune reponse that does not alter with age.

In addition, uraemic patients suffer a complex immunosuppressive state (see Chapter 11.3.11) involving almost all aspects of the immune reponse. On this, in the case of patients maintained by haemodialysis, are superimposed effects of repeated exposure of cells and mediator systems to the dialysis membrane. These effects will be present also in the early phases following transplantation.

Two posssible consequences of this immune dysregulation in the elderly are immediately obvious. First, it is well known that the elderly tend to have fewer and milder early episodes of acute rejection (Takemoto and Terasaki 1988; Raine *et al.* 1992; Tesi *et al.* 1994) (see Fig. 8) only 10–20 per cent showing rejection episodes with using cyclosporin as immunosuppression, compared with 30–40 per cent in younger recipients. In our London series (Cameron 2000), in recipients aged 18–30 years a mean of 1.7 rejection episodes were noted in the first year, compared with only 0.9 in those aged 61–75 years. This is associated with a decreased graft loss from rejection (Fig. 5, and see below). However Lufft *et al.* (2000) found no difference in late or in chronic rejection between older (>65 years) and younger recipients in a careful case–control study, or in the number of grafts lost to rejection. Second, older patients are more prone to infections of almost all types, from bacteria, intracellular bacteria and viruses whilst under immunosuppression (Vivas *et al.* 1992; Meier-Krieschke *et al.* 2001), which results in a much higher death rate from infection (see below).

Immunosuppressive regimes in elderly transplant recipients

Obviously, these changes have major implications when one comes to consider immunosuppressive therapy to be used in older recipients (Morales *et al.* 2000). Given the increased risk of infection and the reduced rate of graft loss from rejection, most clinicians have felt it prudent to avoid side-effects in this vulnerable group by the use of lower doses of drugs. In particular, avoidance of long-term high-dose prednisolone seems essential since this drug as well as immunosuppressive effects has a particularly rapid and severe deleterious effect on elderly skin, bone, and other tissues (Fig. 5).

The P450 microsomal system, which is responsible for the removal of both prednisolone and cyclosporin (P450 IIIA), is less active in the elderly (Cohen 1986). Thus, although a triple therapy regimen of prednisolone, azathioprine, and cyclosporin (all in relatively low doses) as used in many transplant units can be used also in the elderly without much modification (see Chapter 13.2.2 for details), it is prudent to reduce the dose of both cyclosporin and prednisolone to avoid toxicity. Some transplant units favour using corticosteroids for an induction period only (Morales *et al.* 1994), or using cyclosporin monotherapy from the time of transplantation onwards (Morris *et al.* 1991; Andreu *et al.* 1992). However, a controlled trial of cyclosporin monotherapy in older patients showed higher rejection rates than when corticosteroids were used in addition (Spanish Monotherapy Study Group 1994), so no clear guidance has emerged as yet. It is unclear also whether antilymphocyte globulin (Pirsch *et al.* 1989) or monoclonal antibodies such as muromonab CD3 (OKT3) or newer agents such as infliximab

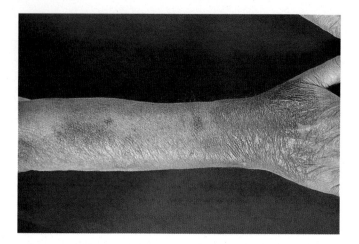

Fig. 5 The arm of a patient aged 72 years taking only 10 mg prednisolone per day following transplantation. The skin is thin and friable, and large persistent eccymoses cover much of the outer aspect of the forearm.

or basiliximab (see Chapter 13.2.2) should be used in the elderly, but in view of the very powerful effects exerted by muromonab CD3, we feel it should only be used with great caution, if at all. Pirsch *et al.* (1989) used antilymphoblast globulin together with a triple regime of cyclosporin, a rather generous dose of prednisolone (10–30 mg daily) and azathioprine. Their patient and allograft survivals at 3 years were excellent, 91 and 74 per cent, respectively. Rejection was less common than in younger recipients, but surgical complications were more likely to lead to graft loss.

There is little experience with newer forms of immunosuppression in elderly recipients as yet. Basar and colleagues (1999) reported experience of 230 patients over 60 years of age who were transplanted using tacrolimus and corticosteroids: results were comparable with cyclosporin-treated recipients, with 9 per cent death rate from cardiovascular causes and 7 per cent from infection and comparable graft survival. In this study, only 25 per cent of patients experienced rejection episodes compared with 73 per cent in the Spanish monotherapy group, and 41 per cent in their prednisolone–cyclosporin patients. Meier-Krieschke *et al.* (1999) give a worrying report on use of 2G of mycophenolate mofetil in recipients over 60 years of age in a consecutive but well-matched cohort compared to azathioprine, both in a triple regime with predinsolone and cyclosporin. Twenty-seven episodes of serious infection occurred in 45 patients using mycophenolate, 85 per cent of whom had at least one infection, compared with only 10 in 46 receiving azathioprine only 32 per cent of whom suffered any infection (RR 3.2); infection included bacterial and fungal causes, and cytomegalovirus. There was, perhaps surprisingly, no benefit in terms of the already low number of patients with rejection epsiodes—only 5/41 (12 per cent) in the azathioprine group and 7/38 (18 per cent) in the mycophenolate group, and neither graft nor patient survival differed. Thus, this agent should be used with caution if at all in the elderly—or perhaps at even lower dosage.

Outcomes of transplantation in elderly patients

Survival of the elderly recipient

Information from large registry data bases is available on the survival of older recipients (Table 9). These data show 5-year patient survivals

of about 70 per cent for those aged 60–64 years. Surprisingly, figures for smaller numbers of 65–69-year-olds are similar. The CTS data extend to 10 years for significant numbers of older patients (>65 years) and show as expected that longer term results are poorer in terms of survival in these oldest recipients: at 10 years, recipient survival was only 34 ± 6 per cent compared with 81 ± 1 per cent in those aged 16–40. However, even though survival of the elderly transplant recipient is necessarily shorter than that of younger recipients in absolute terms, the relevant comparison is with the expected survival: in the case of 60-year-olds, 13–15 years (Table 1). In the careful long-term analysis of Becker *et al.* (2000), 57 per cent of 146 recipients (124 CD and 24 LD) aged over 60 years achieved their expected life span, derived from locally based population statistics, a result comparable to 21–60-year-olds. This is in agreement with the limited 10-year data from other series (Tables 10 and 11) showing approximately 50 per cent survival at 10 years, compared with the 34 per cent of the CTS data.

Additional data for patients over the age of 60 years from recent *single centre series* are summarized in Table 10. These data are undoubtedly affected by publication bias towards successful outcomes. Results obtained in the elderly improved sharply with the introduction of cyclosporin, as they did for younger recipients (Taube *et al.* 1987; Eggers *et al.* 1988; Lundgren *et al.* 1989) and previous data (Taube *et al.* 1987) are now of historical interest only. The weighted means of patient survival in nearly 2000 patients aged over 60 in collected series are 88 per cent at 1 year, and 71 per cent at 5 years. The rather scanty results yet available for 513 recipients aged 65–82 years are also shown: 1-year survival was 77 per cent. It is clear that outcomes for the graft are similar at all patients up to about the age of 70 years, a point emphasized in the introduction, and in a recent careful proportional hazard study by Roodnat *et al.* (1999).

Only one study addresses the outcome of patients over 70 years of age in any detail (Albrechtsen 1995) (although over 1000 such grafts have been performed in the United States). Five-year survivals of patient and graft were 54 and 52 per cent, respectively. Twenty patients received living donor grafts (see below) and in these long-term graft and patient survival was better (74 per cent). Figure 6 shows a comparison of 5-year patient and graft survival of recipients at various ages in Norway, a country unique in the world because 41 per cent of its transplantation is done from living donors and almost every candidate for transplantation receives a graft (Bentdal *et al.* 1998). This shows that the advantage of living donor grafts well-known in younger recipients is present also in the older recipient (Albrechtesen *et al.* 1995; Opeltz 1998).

Graft survival in the elderly recipient

Tables 9 and 10 give also data on 1- and 5-year survival of *grafts* together with limited data for 10 years' follow-up. In those recipients aged over 60, four of every five of grafts survive after 1 year and almost two-thirds after 5 years. These figures are worse than for younger recipients (85 and 70 per cent) especially in the early period, largely the result of deaths in recipients with functioning grafts.

The striking feature of graft survival data in the elderly is, however, that in almost every data set (Takemoto and Terasaki 1988; Schulak and Hricik 1991; Helderman *et al.* 1995; ERA data 1996; Jassal *et al.* 1997; Becker *et al.* 1998; Cameron 2000; Lufft *et al.* 2000) if the graft survival data is censored for *death with a functioning graft*, then the rate of graft loss in the elderly becomes equal to—or even better than—that found in younger recipients (Fig. 7). In the longer term, however the excess death rate of the elderly tips the balance against actual long-term graft survival and (e.g.) 20-year graft survival in a 60–65-year-old recipient is unlikely; the limited data on Tables 9 and 10 suggest 10-year patient survival is 45–50 per cent and graft survival 40 per cent in recipients aged over 60–65 years. These different ways of calculating graft survival, with and without censorship, have great bearing on the debate over the use of scarce donor kidneys in the elderly recipient (see below).

Causes of patient and graft loss in the elderly

The causes of graft loss in the elderly differ from those in younger recipients in a dramatic way: in the younger the predominant cause of graft loss (68 per cent) is *rejection*; in the elderly, as already noted, it is the *death of the recipient with a functioning graft* (Fig. 8), which occurs in about 50 per cent of cases (Takemoto and Terasaki 1988; Vivas *et al.* 1992; Cameron *et al.* 1994), with rejection the cause in only 13–28 per cent of cases (Vivas *et al.* 1992; Cameron *et al.* 1994). In the Norwegian data from 1989 to 1997 (Bentdal *et al.* 1998) 75 per cent graft loss in older recipients aged greater than 65 years was from death of the recipient compared with 45 per cent in younger recipients. These deaths have been attributed in terms of frequency first to cardiovascular disease (Cardella *et al.* 1986), followed by infections in the majority of series. This is true of our series (Cameron 2000): in those aged over 60 at transplant, vascular disease accounted for 29 of 51 deaths (25/39 with a functioning graft). In Albrechtsen *et al.*'s (1995) series of recipients aged over 70 years, 83 per cent of graft losses were from death of the recipient, again the majority from cardiovascular disease. However, in a number of older studies infections were the predominant cause (Taube *et al.* 1987) including some more recent data (Velez *et al.* 1991; Bonal *et al.* 1997).

Some of the differences between these data probably arise from different lengths of follow-up. One of the most detailed studies of causes of death in older recipients is that of the Collaborative Transplant Study (Jassal *et al.* 1997) (Table 11). Although infection was the most common early cause of death, by 5 years, this had been replaced by vascular disease. Meier-Kriesche *et al.* (2001) compared death rates following transplantation in patients in the USRDS data with similar data from wait-listed patients; mortality from all causes at all ages was greater in the wait-listed patients, and the increase in deaths from infection was exponential with age, rather than linear as were all other causes of death studied. Jacobs and Mignon (2002) give an analysis of the URDS data (2000) for death rates in recipients of different ages (Table 12): almost all causes of death are about five times more frequent in the elderly (>65 years) recipients than those aged 20–44 years, but particularly malignancy (10 times greater) is even more common. The possible causes of susceptibility to infection and malignancy have

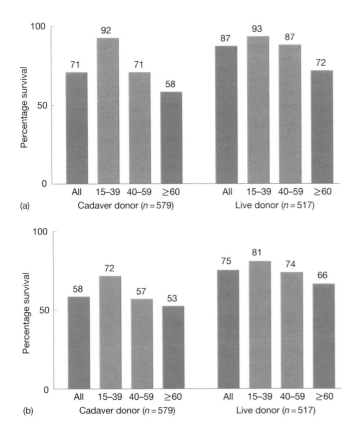

(a) Cadaver donor (n = 579) Live donor (n = 517)

(b) Cadaver donor (n = 579) Live donor (n = 517)

Fig. 6 Five-year graft and patient survival according to age in Norway: a comparison of cadaver (left) and living donor transplants (right). Patient survival is shown in the upper panels, uncensored graft survival in the lower panel. The figures over each column give the 5-year actuarial survival in per cent. Data from the European Renal Association registry, presented at the 32nd Congress of the ERA, Athens 1995, with permission. See also Fauchald *et al.* (1991), Albrechtsen *et al.* (1995), and Bentdal *et al.* (1998).

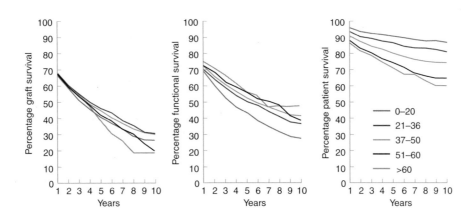

Fig. 7 Long-term survival of recipients of cadaver allografts at different ages. The left-hand panel shows overall *graft* survival from 1 to 10 years. The centre panel *shows graft survival censored for the death of recipients with a functioning graft;* those over 60 years of age do as well as or better than younger recipients. The right-hand panel shows *recipient* survival; as expected, there is a marked effect of recipient age on survival. Reproduced with permission from Takemoto and Terasaki (1988).

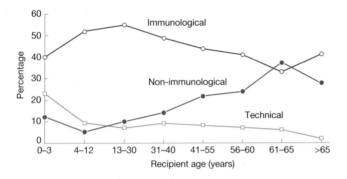

Fig. 8 Recipient age and causes of graft failure. The proportion of graft losses from immunological reasons declines with increasing recipient age (reproduced from Takemoto and Terasaki 1988 with permission).

been discussed above. This large difference in malignant disease, however, is not reflected in the CTS data for 5–10-year deaths (Jassal *et al.* 1997) nor in the analysis of Roodnat *et al.* (1999), in both of which studies the ratio was only about 2 : 1. However, these different studies were on populations analysed using different age discriminants and different statistical analyses. In our London series (Cameron 2000), cumulative tumour incidence (42/563, 7.4 per cent up to December 1995) was increased approximately fourfold in all age groups of transplant recipients, when compared to age-matched controls from the general population. In addition, there was a clear trend for the tumour incidence to increase with increasing age, both in the general and in the transplant populations ($p < 0.01$ for all data points). Skin cancers were the most common malignancy (59 per cent of total) resulting in two fatalities. Of the remaining 13 tumour-related deaths, the commonest cause was from lymphoma (five), which was the most common non-skin malignancy, with a 183-fold risk of development compared to the general population.

Comparison with elderly patients on dialysis: survival, hospitalization, quality of life

Clearly such comparisons are rendered difficult by the fact that fitter elderly patients with less comorbidity tend to be transplanted. However, the first of several recent attempts to assess this point using patients wait-listed for a graft but who did not receive one as controls is that of Fauchald *et al.* (1991): outcomes were identical. The Catalan registry showed better survival in those transplanted compared with transplant patients still on the waiting list on dialysis (Bonal *et al.* 1997). Ismail *et al.* (1994) examined the outcomes of those who had been transplanted but whose transplants then failed with return to dialysis, as well as those listed but never transplanted, all from the US Renal Data System database for 1992. Standardized mortality rates were 9 per cent less for those previously transplanted than those never transplanted, suggesting a small but significant extra morbidity in those denied access to grafting, which overcame any risks of immunosuppression. Those with a functioning graft had only 30 per cent of the mortality of those on dialysis. However, perhaps the best data in this area are those from the Canadian registry (Schaubel *et al.* 1995) and recent analyses of the URSRDS data (Wolff *et al.* 1999; Meier-Kriesche *et al.* 2001). In the Canadian data, a multivariate comorbidity-corrected and controlled comparison showed a reduced hazard for death (risk ratio 0.47, CI 0.33–0.97) for those transplanted

compared with those who continued dialysis. In the USRDS study, patients aged 60–74 years given a cadaver transplant had a 4-year increment in survival and a 61 per cent decrease in risk of death compared with waiting list patients still on dialysis. Meier-Kriesche *et al.* (2001) analysed causes of death in detail, and found all causes to be more common in waiting list patients with the exception of malignancy, which was 25 per cent greater in transplanted patients. Similar conclusions were reached from studies in Catalonia (Bonal *et al.* 1997) and Australia (Johnson *et al.* 2000). The Catalan data (Bonal *et al.* 1997) include important data that there was a smaller increase in the prevalence of cardiovascular disease in elderly patients following transplantation, compared with those who remained on dialysis (Fig. 4), and in the study of Johnson *et al.* (2000) the transplanted group had a 5-year survival of 90 per cent compared to only 17 per cent in the waiting group. Thus there seems no doubt that transplantation does benefit the elderly in terms of survival more than a comparable cohort remaining on dialysis.

There are few data on *hospitalization* following transplantation in the elderly, but in our London series (Cameron 2000), patients transplanted aged greater than 60 required a significantly longer period in hospital in the first year post-transplantation than younger patients (43 days versus 25 days); no data from dialysed patients were available for comparison. However, the data of Benedetti and colleagues (1994) showed no effect of recipient age on hospitalization; this arose because although the initial stay in hospital was longer, there were fewer subsequent admissions in the elderly. *Quality of life* has been compared in elderly patients in at least three studies: that of Benedetti *et al.* (1994) used a general questionnaire on satisfaction, and also the SF-36 questionnaire. Scores in the latter were less than control non-transplanted individuals of the same age but were in general good; data were not compared with those on dialysis. Bonal *et al.* (1997) used the Karnofsky index of functional autonomy, and found that this was significantly better in transplanted patients than dialysed patients. Rebollo *et al.* (1998) performed a formal QOL assessment using the HF-36 and SIP questionnaires. The HRQOL was better in transplanted patients than in haemodialysis patients, which partly depended upon comorbidity. Finally Nyberg *et al.* (1995a,b) assessed muscular strength after transplantation in elderly patients, but rather surprisingly found no improvement after 1 year of transplantation, whilst younger recipients did show an improvement. Perhaps the extra myotoxicity of corticosteroids in the elderly played a role in these data.

Kidneys for the elderly; 'age-matching' of cadaver kidneys, and living donor transplantation in the elderly

The use of 'marginal'/older kidneys in the elderly—'age matching'

Given the continuing shortage of cadaver kidneys for transplantation, it has been argued that the elderly should receive kidneys which might be considered marginal for younger recipients: in particular those from older donors, that is, *matching the recipient and donor age* (Donnelly *et al.* 1990; Newstead *et al.* 1992). In our London series, although no formal policy was in place, two thirds of kidneys placed in those over the age of 60 years were judged to be 'marginal', whilst only 40 per cent were so designated in 18–30-year-old recipients. There is no doubt that the use of kidneys from 'marginal' donors results in poorer graft outcomes than when younger donor kidneys are used (Thorogood *et al.* 1990; Jassal *et al.* 1997; Belger 1998; Opeltz 1998; Basar *et al.* 1999; Doyle *et al.* 2000; Schratzberger and Mayer 2003) both in terms of delayed function, graft survival and plasma creatinine concentrations, at all recipient ages including the elderly (Fig. 9); however, patient survival is not compromised (Basar *et al.* 1999). In the UKTSSA data (Belger 1998) 5-year graft survival was twice as good in recipients over 60 if donors aged less than 40 years were used, compared with donors over 60 (56 per cent versus 29 per cent) similar to data in younger recipients, and simlar figures emerge from Eurotransplant (Fig. 9). In our series in London, graft survivals in those over 60 receiving (almost always young) multi-organ donor kidneys were 86, 78, and 75 per cent at 1, 3, and 5 years; comparable figures for those receiving 'marginal' kidneys were 75, 55, and 44 per cent. One series is at variance with these data, that of Waiser *et al.* (2000) who found older (> 50 years) donor/recipient matches did as well as young, with old kidneys in young recipients doing worst.

Thus, there seems little doubt that if the *total number of life-years with a functioning graft* is taken as the goal of a transplant programme, age matching can be justified even if the *individual* elderly patient is given a less than optimum chance. The dilemma of organ allocation to individual elderly recipients (who naturally want the best chance obtainable for themselves) is enhanced in the continuing presence of an organ shortage, not resolved. Moreover, the dilemma becomes worse because expanding the donor pool can best—perhaps solely—be achieved today by using donors over the age of 60 years, as in the success achieved by the Spanish ONT during the past decade, where the increased donation rate almost entirely depended upon use of such organs (Matesanz, personal communication 2000). However, it is worth remembering that *any* transplant, even one from a 'marginal' donor, is superior in terms of survival than comparable patients remaining on dialysis, at least in the US Renal Data System data (Ojo *et al.* 2001). Thus, there are at present insufficient data upon which a strategy for optimum use of the current donor pool can be constructed, and any decision must to a large extent be arbitrary and based on local circumstances, particularly the overall availablity of donors, policy with regard to 'marginal' kidneys and the number of transplants done. The vexed question of assessing the quality of 'marginal' kidneys is discussed in Chapter 13.3.1.

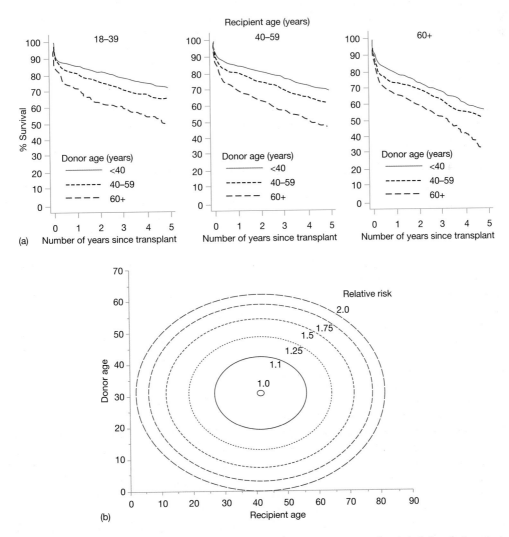

Fig. 9 (a) Graft outcome in transplantation using donors of different ages into recipients of different ages. Survival of all grafts in patients over 60 is poorer if aged donors are used, as for younger age groups (data of the UKTSSA from Belger 1998). (b) Zones of equal risk for graft loss with donors and recipients of various ages. Again, result in the elderly are best if younger donors are used (from Thorogood *et al.* 1990 with permission).

A new approach has been the suggested use of double kidney transplants from elderly donors (Remuzzi *et al.* 1999; Andres *et al.* 2000; Gridelli and Remuzzi 2000; Lu *et al.* 2000) to compensate for the lower number of nephrons and decreased function of the elderly organ. Few such transplants have yet been done into elderly recipients, but this approach deserves attention.

Living donor transplantation in the elderly

Given the reluctance to use cadaver kidneys in the middle-aged or elderly, what about living donors? In the past numbers were small, and patient and allograft survivals were not significantly different compared to the results of cadaver transplantation in the elderly (Taube *et al.* 1987). In the United States in 1985, for example, only 66 of 1654 living donor grafts involved recipients aged more than 55 years, and only 3 (0.02 per cent) were performed in the 65–74 years age group; in 1998 however, 4.4 per cent of living donor grafts (160) were placed into those over 65.

Only in Norway has transplantation of elderly recipients from living donors—many of them also elderly—been pursued actively, in line with the high overall use of living donor grafts in that country. Albrechtsen *et al.* (1995) and Fauchald *et al.* (1988) have reported the Norwegian experience (Fig. 8): of 368 patients over 60 years of age who were studied between 1981 and 1985, 127 were transplanted, 26 from living donors. In 12 of these living donor transplants, both the recipient and the donor were over 60 years, and graft survival at 2 years was 73 per cent. One-third of all living donors in Norway between 1985 and 1987 were aged over 60 years. In 1995, Albrechtsen *et al.* reported also on their experience of tranplantation in 70-year-olds: 20 had received a living donor graft from four siblings, 11 adult offspring and five unrelated individuals (spouses): 74 per cent of patients were alive with functioning grafts after 5 years (Bentdal 1998). The deleterious effect of age on survival of living donor transplants has not been studied so intensively as it has for cadaver grafts, but older living donors' kidneys appear to survive less well irrespective of the age of the recipient (Ivanovski *et al.* 2001; Toma *et al.* 2001).

Choice of treatment for the elderly patient in endstage renal disease (Mignon *et al.* 1995)

Choice of treatment modality for endstage renal disease in the elderly

The balance of treatment modalities used in the elderly with ESRD vary from country to country depending not on realities of treatment but on economic resources, distribution of renal units, number of specialists, and patterns of reimbursement of both hospitals and physicians (Mattern *et al.* 1989). For example in the United Kingdom, there were only 0.8 renal units/p.m.p. compared with 3.9–6.4 in other European countries and the number of nephrologists (2.5 p.m.p.) is also less than a quarter of that found elsewhere. Given this paucity of renal units and nephrologists, self-treatment at home was over-emphasized (Nicholls *et al.* 1984). In practice, this meant that many frail elderly patients barely able to cope with CAPD were pressured into undertaking this form of treatment, when in-centre dialysis would have been more appropriate. Thus, 70 per cent of patients aged more than 65 years were on peritoneal dialysis in the United Kingdom by 1989. During the 1990s,

many such patients returned or transferred to centre haemodialysis, and new patients were treated more frequently by this means. In contrast, in some other countries, CAPD has rarely been undertaken because little or no physician reimbursement follows.

Elderly patients who begin and continue dialysis need assessment for independent dialysis at home using a standard protocol of assesment of medical, psychological, motor, and social factors. Chronological age is much less important than the presence or absence of significant comorbidity. Some will begin such treatment but the remainder—probably the majority—will stay on in-centre dialysis. The need for temporary or permanent back-up in-centre dialysis for those at home is paramount. The choice between home haemodialysis and CAPD is largely one of preference on the part of the local team and the patient. Those with more stable and robust cardiovascular systems will generally be more suitable for haemodialysis. In all patients, haemoglobin should be optimized. Patients with poor cardiac performance and/or angina will require assessment, medical treatment, and, if appropriate, surgical treatment or angioplasty.

Transplantation should be considered in all reasonably fit patients aged less than 70 years, and in selected patients over that age. Screening should consist of a cardiovascular, respiratory, and urological assessment, with a low threshold for coronary angiography. Only the continuing shortage of suitable kidneys limits our ability to treat all those who could benefit from this type of treatment—a situation sadly identical to that which faces their younger counterparts. All older diabetics, even if symptomless, should have a full cardiovascular assessment including coronary angiography; others need only non-invasive assessment. Kidney transplantation offers real benefit in terms of both survival and quality of life for selected recipients up to an age of 70 years and beyond.

Transplantation should be performed with a favourably matched cadaver, or in some cases, an available living donor kidney. Immunosuppression should be light, and there is a strong case for avoiding or minimizing the use of corticosteroids. A low threshold for abandoning grafts and returning to dialysis needs to be maintained in the unlikely event of vigorous repeated rejections. Mycophenolate should be avoided until more data emerge. Antilymphocyte globulin may be considered, but muromonab CD3 (OKT3) should be avoided.

References

Albrechtsen, D. *et al.* (1995). Kidney transplantation in patients older than 70 years of age. *Transplantation Proceedings* **27**, 986–988.

Andres, A. *et al.* (2000). Double versus single renal allografts from aged donors. *Transplantation* **69**, 2060–2066.

Andreu, J. *et al.* (1992). Renal transplantation in elderly recipients. *Transplantation Proceedings* **24**, 120–121.

Auer, J. (1998). Issues surrounding the withdrawal of dialysis treatment. *Nephrology, Dialysis, Transplantation* **13**, 1149–1151.

Auer, J. *et al.* (1990). The Oxford–Manchester study of dialysis patients. *Scandinavian Journal of Urology and Nephrology* **131**, 31–37.

Baigent, C., Burbury, K., and Wheeler, D. (2000). Premature cardiovascular disease in chronic renal failure. *Lancet* **356**, 147–152.

Barry, J. M., Lemmers, M. J., Meyer, M. M., De Mattos, A., Bennett, W. M., and Norman, D. J. (1996). Cadaver kidney transplantation in patients more than 65 years old. *World Journal of Urology* **14**, 243–248.

Basar, H. *et al.* (1999). Renal transplantation in recipients over the age of 60. The impact of donor age. *Transplantation* **67**, 1191–1193.

Basu, A. *et al.* (2000). Renal transplantation in patients above 60 years of age in the modern era: a single center experience with a review of the literature. *International Urology and Nephrology* **32**, 171–176.

Becker, B. N., Ismail, N., Becker, Y. T., MacDonnell, R. C., and Helderman, J. H. (1996). Renal transplantation in the older end stage renal disease patient. *Seminars in Nephrology* **16**, 353–362.

Becker, B. N. *et al.* (2000). Using renal transplantation to evaluate a simple approach for predicting the impact of end-stage renal disease therapies on patient survival: observed/expected life span. *American Journal of Kidney Diseases* **35**, 653–659.

Belger, M. (1998). UK Transplant Services Special Authority newsletter, UKTSSA, Bristol.

Benedetti, E. *et al.* (1994). Renal transplantation for patients 60 years or older: a single institution experience. *Annals of Surgery* **220**, 445–458.

Bennett-Jones, D. *et al.* (1987). A comparison of intraperitoneal and oral/intravenous antibiotics in CAPD peritonitis. *Peritoneal Dialysis Bulletin* **7**, 31–33.

Bentdal, O. H. *et al.* The national kidney transplant program of Norway still results in unchanged waiting lists. In *Clinical Transplants* (ed. P. I. Terasaki), pp. 221–228. Los Angeles: University of California at Los Angeles, 1998.

Berlyne, G. M. (1982). Over 50 and uremic = death. *Nephron* **31**, 189–190.

Bernardelli, L. and Vegeto, A. (1997). Lesssons from 494 permanent accesses in 348 haemodialysis patients older than 65 years of age: 19 years of experience. *Nephrology, Dialysis, Transplantation* **13** (Suppl. 7), 73–77.

Biesen, W., Vanholder, R., Debacker, G., and Lameire, N. (2000). Comparison of survival on CAPD and haemodialysis: statistical pitfalls. *Nephrology, Dialysis, Transplantation* **15**, 307–311.

Blagg, C. R. and Fitts, S. S. (1994). Dialysis, old age, and rehabilitation. *Journal of the American Medical Association* **271**, 67–68.

Bloembergen, W., Port, F. K., Mauger, E. A., and Wolfe, R. A. (1995). A comparison of mortality between patients treated with hemodialysis and peritoneal dialysis. *Journal of the American Society of Nephrology* **6**, 177–183.

Blumberg, A. *et al.* (1983). Cardiac arrhythmias in patients on maintenance haemodialysis. *Nephron* **33**, 91–95.

Boelaert, J. R., Van Roost, G. F., Vergauwe, P. L., Verbanck, J. J., De Vroey, C., and Segaert, M. F. (1988). The role of desferrioxamine in dialysis-associated mucormycosis: report of three cases and review of literature. *Clinical Nephrology* **29**, 261–266.

Bonal, J., Clèries, M., Velea, E., and the Renal Registry Committee (1997). Transplantation versus haemodialysis in elderly patients. *Nephrology, Dialysis, Transplantation* **12**, 261–264.

Brody, H., Campbell, M. L., Faber-Langendoen, K., and Ogle, K. S. (1997). Withdrawing intensive life-sustaining treatment—recommendations for compassionate clinical management. *New England Journal of Medicine* **336**, 652–657.

Brown, E. A. (1999). Peritoneal dialysis versus haemodialysis in the elderly. *Perintoneal Dialysis International* **19**, 311–312.

Brunner, F. P., Landais, P., and Selwood, N. H. (1995). Malignancies after renal transplantation: the EDTA-ERA Registry experience. *Nephrology, Dialysis, Transplantation* **10** (Suppl. 1), 74–80.

Burns, E. A. and Goodwin, J. S. (1997). Immunodeficiency of aging. *Drugs and Aging* **11**, 394–397.

Burton, P. R. and Walls, J. (1987). A selection-adjusted comparison of life expectancy of patients on continuous ambulatory peritoneal dialysis, haemodialysis and renal transplantation. *Lancet* **i**, 1115–1119.

Cameron, J. S. (1998). Nephrotic syndrome in the elderly. *Seminars in Nephrology* **16**, 319–329.

Cameron, J. S. (2000). Renal transplantation in the elderly. *International Urology and Nephrology* **32**, 193–201.

Cameron, J. I., Whiteside, C., Katz, J., and Devins, G. M. (2000). Differences in quality of life across renal replacement therapies: a meta-analytic comparison. *American Journal of Kidney Diseases* **35**, 629–637.

Cameron, J. S., Compton, F., Koffman, G., and Bewick, M. (1994). Transplantation in elderly recipients. *Geriatric Nephrology and Urology* **4**, 93–99.

Campbell, M. L. (1991). Terminal care of ESRD patients forgoing dialysis. *Dialysis and Transplantation* **18**, 202–204.

Canadian Erythropoietin Study Group (1990). Association between recombinant erythropoietin and quality of life and exercise capacity of patients receiving haemodialysis. *British Medical Journal* **300**, 573–578. Canadian Organ Replacement Register 1989.

Canaud, B., Leray-Moragues, V., Garrigues, V., and Mion, C. (1997). Permanent twin catheter: a vascular access option of choice for haemodialysis in elderly patients. *Nephrology, Dialysis, Transplantation* **13** (Suppl. 7), 82–88.

Cantarovich, D. *et al.* (1994). Cadaveric renal transplantation after 60 years of age. A single center experience. *Transplantation Proceedings* **7**, 33–38.

Cardella, C. J., Oreopoulos, D. G., Honey, J., and Deveber, G. A. (1986). Renal transplantation in patients 60 years or older. *Transplantation Proceedings* **18**, 151–152.

Carvar, D. J. and Rockwood, K. R. (1995). Evaluation of methods for measuring quality of life in the elderly with end stage renal disease. *Geriatric Nephrology and Urology* **4**, 165–171.

Castle, S. C. (2000). Clinical relevance of age-related immune dysfunction. *Clinical Infectious Diseases* **31**, 578–585.

Catalano, C. *et al.* (1996). Withdrawal of renal replacement therapy in Newcastle upon Tyne: 1964–1993. *Nephrology, Dialysis, Transplantation* **11**, 133–139.

Challah, S., Wing, A. J., Bauer, R., Morris, R. W., and Schroeder, S. A. (1984). Negative selection of patients for dialysis in the United Kingdom. *British Medical Journal* **288**, 1119–1122.

Chandna, S. M., Schulz, J., Lawrence, C., Greenwood, R. N., and Farrington, K. (1999). Is there a rationale for rationing chronic dialysis? A hospital-based cohort study of factors affecting survival and morbidity. *British Medical Journal* **318**, 217–223.

Chaveau, P. *et al.* for the French study group for nutrition in dialysis (2001). Factors influencing survival in hemodialysis patients aged older than 75 years: 2.5 year outcome study. *American Journal of Kidney Diseases* **37**, 997–1003.

Chazan, J. A. (1990). Elective withdrawal from dialysis: an important cause of death among patients with renal failure. *Dialysis and Transplantation* **19**, 530–553 (discontinuous pages).

Church, J. M. *et al.* (1986). Perforation of the colon in renal homograft recipients. *Annals of Surgery* **203**, 69–76.

Cohen, J. L. (1986). Pharmacokinetic changes in ageing. *American Journal of Medicine* **80** (Suppl. A), 31–38.

Cohen, L. M., McCul, J. D., German, M., and Kjellstrand, C. M. (1995). Dialysis discontinutation: a good death? *Archives of Internal Medicine* **155**, 42–47.

Cohen, L. M. *et al.* (2000a). Dialysis discontinuation and palliative care. *American Journal of Kidney Diseases* **36**, 140–144.

Cohen, L. M. *et al.* (2000b). Dying well after discontinuing the life-support treatment of dialysis. *Archives of Internal Medicine* **160**, 2513–2518.

Coli, L. *et al.* (1998). Evidence of profiled hemodialysis efficiency in the treatment of intra-dialytic hypotension. *International Journal of Artifical Organs* **21**, 389–402.

Collins, A. J., Hanson, G., Umen, A., Kjellstrand, C., and Keshaviah, P. (1990). Changing risk factor demographics in end-stage renal disease patients entering haemodialysis and the impact on long-term mortality. *American Journal of Kidney Diseases* **15**, 422–432.

Daugirdas, J. T. (1991). Dialysis hypotension. *Kidney International* **39**, 233–246.

De Broe, M. E. (1994). Haemodialysis-induced hypoxaemia. *Nephrology, Dialysis, Transplantation* **9** (Suppl. 2), 173–175.

Dessner, G. H. (1986). Stopping long-term dialysis. *New England Journal of Medicine* **314**, 1449–1450.

Didlake, R., Raju, S., Rhodes, R. S., and Bower, J. Dialysis access in patients older than 65 years. In *Vascular Access for Haemodialysis—II* (ed. B. G. Sommer and M. L. Henry), pp. 166–172. Boston, MA: Precept Press, 1991.

Dimkovic, N. B. *et al.* (2001). Chronic peritoneal dialysis in octogenarians. *Nephrology, Dialysis, Transplantation* **16**, 2034–2040.

Disney, A. P. (1998). Some trends in chronic renal replacement therapy in Australia and New Zealand, 1997. *Nephrology, Dialysis, Transplantation* **13**, 854–859.

Disney, A. P. S. (1990). Dialysis treatment in Australia 1982 to 1988. *American Journal of Kidney Diseases* **25**, 402–409.

Donnelly, P. K. *et al.* (1990). Age-matching improves the results of renal transplantation with older donors. *Nephrology, Dialysis, Transplantation* **5**, 808–811.

DOQI™ (2000a). Clinical practice guidelines for nutrition in renal failure: evaluation of protein-energy nutritional status. *American Journal of Kidney Diseases* **16** (Suppl. 1), s17–s36.

DOQI™ (2000b). Management of protein and energy intake in maintenance hemodialysis and peritoneal dialysis patients. *American Journal of Kidney Diseases* **16** (Suppl. 1), s40–s46.

Doyle, S. E., Matas, A. J., Gillingham, K., and Rosenberg, M. E. (2000). Predicting clinical outcome in the elderly renal transplant recipient. *Kidney International* **57**, 2144–2150.

Eggers, P. W. *et al.* (1988). Effect of transplantation on the Medicare end stage renal disease program. *New England Journal of Medicine* **318**, 223–229.

European Best Practice Guidelines for the Management of Anaemia in Patients with Chronic Renal Failure (1999). *Nephrology, Dialysis, Transplantation* **14** (Suppl. 5), 1–50.

European Renal Association Registry (1996). Report on management of renal failure in Europe XXV, 1994. *Nephrology, Dialysis, Transplantation* **11** (Suppl. 1), 1–47.

Evans, R. W. *et al.* (1985). The quality of life of patients with end-stage renal disease. *New England Journal of Medicine* **312**, 553–559.

Fauchald, P., Sodal, G., Albrechtsen, D., Leivestad, T., Berg, K. J., and Flatmark, A. (1991). The use of elderly living donors in renal transplantation. *Transplant International* **4**, 51–53.

Fauchald, P. *et al.* (1988). Renal replacement therapy in patients over 60. *Transplantation Proceedings* **20**, 432–433.

Feest, T. G., Mistry, C. D., Grimes, D. S., and Mallick, N. P. (1990). Incidence of advanced chronic renal failure and the need for end-stage renal replacement treatment. *British Medical Journal* **301**, 897–903.

Fehrman, I., Brattstgrom, C., Duraj, F., and Groth, C. G. (1989). Kidney transplantation in patients between 65 and 75 years of age. *Transplantation Proceedings* **21**, 2018–2019.

Fenton, S. S. *et al.* (1997). Hemodialysis versus peritoneal dialysis: a comparison of adjusted mortality rates. *American Journal of Kidney Diseases* **30**, 334–342.

Fisher, S. H., Curry, E., and Batuman, V. (1986). *New England Journal of Medicine* **314**, 1449–1450.

Foley, R. N., Parfrey, P. S., and Harnett, J. D. (1992). Left ventricular hypertrophy in dialysis patients. *Seminars in Dialysis* **5**, 34–41.

Foley, R. N. *et al.* (1994). Advance prediction of early death in patients starting maintenance haemodialysis. *American Journal of Kidney Diseases* **23**, 836–842.

Francheshi, C. *et al.* (1996). Successful immunosenescence and the remodelling of immune reponses with ageing. *Nephrology, Dialysis, Transplantation* **11** (Suppl. 9), 18–25.

Friedman, E. A. (1992). Rationing of uremia therapy. *Artificial Organs* **16**, 90–97.

Friedman, E. A. (1994). The best and worst times for dialysis are now. *ASAIO Journal* **40**, 107–108.

Geis, P. W. *et al.* (1976). Technical considerations in elderly renal allograft recipient. *American Journal of Surgery* **132**, 332–335.

Gentile, D. E. and the Geriatric Advisory Committee (1990). Peritoneal dialysis in geriatric patients. A survey of clinical practice. *Advances in Peritoneal Dialysis* **6** (Suppl. 6), 29–32.

Ginaldi, L. *et al.* (1999a). The immune system in the elderly: I specific humoral immunity. *Immunological Research* **20**, 101–108.

Ginaldi, L. *et al.* (1999b). The immune system in the elderly: II specific cellular immunity. *Immunological Research* **20**, 109–115.

Ginaldi, L. *et al.* (1999c). The immune system in the elderly: III natural immunity. *Immunological Research* **20**, 117–126.

Gokal, R. (1990). CAPD in the elderly—European and UK experience. *Advances in Peritoneal Dialysis* **6** (Suppl.), 38–41.

Gokal, R. Quality of life. In *The Textbook of Peritoneal Dialysis* (ed. R. Gokal and K. D. Nolph), pp. 678–698. Dordrecht: Kluwer, 1994.

Gokal, R. *et al.* (1987). Multicentre study on outcome of treatment in patients on continuous ambulatory peritoneal dialysis and haemodialysis. *Nephrology, Dialysis, Transplantation* **2**, 172–178.

Goldman, M. and Vanherweghen, J. L. (1990). Bacterial infections in chronic haemodialysis: epidemiologic and pathophysiologic aspects. *Advances in Nephrology* **19**, 315–332.

Gridelli, B. and Remuzzi, G. (2000). Strategies for making more organs available for transplantation. *New England Journal of Medicine* **343**, 404–410.

Grün, R. P. *et al.* (2003). Costs of dialysis for elderly people in the UK. *Nephrology, Dialysis, Transplantation* **18**, 2122–2127.

Habach, G., Bloembergen, W. E., Mauger, E. A., Wolfe, R. A., and Port, F. K. (1995). Hospitalization among United States dialysis patients: haemodialysis versus peritoneal dialysis. *Journal of the American Society of Nephrology* **5**, 1940–1948.

Haemel, T., Brunner, F., and Battegay, R. (1983). Renal dialysis and suicide: occurrence in Switzerland and Europe. *Comprehensive Psychiatry* **21**, 140.

Hakim, R. M. and Levin, N. L. (1993). Malnutritrion in haemodialysis patients. *American Journal of Kidney Diseases* **21**, 125–137.

Hamel, M. B. *et al.* for the SUPPORT Investigators (1999). Patient age and decisions to withold life-sustaining treatments from seriously ill hospitalized adults. *Annals of Internal Medicine* **130**, 116–125.

Helderman, J. H. (1995). Transplantation in the elderly. *Nephrology, Dialysis, Transplantation* **10**, 773–774.

Hinsdale, J. G., Lipcouritz, G. S., and Hoover, E. L. (1985). Vascular access in the elderly. Results and perspectives in a geriatric population. *Dialysis and Transplantation* **14**, 560–562.

Hirsch, D. J., West, M. L., Cohen, A. D., and Jindal, K. K. (1994). Experience with not offering dialysis to patients with a poor prognosis. *American Journal of Kidney Diseases* **23**, 463–466.

Holley, J. L. and Foulks, C. J. (1991). The utility of structured evaluation of elderly patients for continuous peritoneal dialysis. *Peritoneal Dialysis International* **11**, 162–165.

Holley, J. L., Finucane, T. E., and Moss, A. H. (1989). Dialysis patients' attitudes about cardiopulmonary resuscitation and stopping dialysis. *American Journal of Nephrology* **9**, 245–250.

Husebye, D. G. and Kjellstrand, C. M. (1987). Old patients and uraemia: rates of acceptance to and withdrawal from dialysis. *International Journal of Artificial Organs* **10**, 160–172.

Ifudu, O., Mayers, J., Matthew, J., Tan, C. C., Cambridge, A., and Friedman, E. A. (1994). Dismal rehabilitation in geriatric inner-city haemodialysis patients. *Journal of the American Medical Association* **271**, 29–33.

Ismail, N., Hakim, R. M., Oreopoulos, D. G., and Patrikaerea, A. (1993). Renal replacement therapies on the elderly. Part I. Haemodialysis and chronic peritoneal dialysis. *American Journal of Kidney Diseases* **22**, 759–782.

Ismail, N., Hakim, R. M., and Helderman, J. H. (1994). Renal replacement therapies in the elderly: part II: transplantation. *American Journal of Kidney Diseases* **23**, 1–15.

Issad, B. *et al.* (1995). 213 elderly uremic patients over the age of 75 years of age treated with long-term peritoneal dialysis: a French multicenter study. *Peritoneal Dialysis International* **16** (Suppl. 1), s414–s418.

Ivanovski, N. *et al.* (2001). Living related renal transplantation—the use of advanced age donors. *Clinical Nephrology* **55**, 309–312.

Jacobs, C. and Mignon, F. Optimal renal replacement therapy in elderly patients. Oxford: Oxford University Press, pp. 147–174, 2002.

Jacobs, C., Diallo, A., Balas, E. A., Nectoux, M., and Etienne, S. (1985). Maintenance haemodialysis treatment in patients aged over 60 years. Demographic profile, clinical aspects and outcome. *Proceedings of the European Dialysis and Transplant Association* **22**, 447–489.

Jassal, J. V., Opeltz, G., and Cole, E. (1997). Transplantation in the elderly: a review. *Geriatric Nephrology and Urology* **7**, 157–165.

Jennekens, F. G. I. and Jennekens-Schinkel, A. Neurological aspects of dialysis patients. In *The Replacement of Renal Function by Dialysis* (ed. A. Drukker, F. M. Parsons, and J. F. Maher), pp. 724–741. The Hague: Nijhoff, 1983.

Johnson, D. W. *et al.* (2000). A comparison of the effects of dialysis and renal transplantation on the survival of older uremic patients. *Transplantation* **60**, 794–799.

Joly, D. *et al.* (2003). Octagenarians reaching end-stage renal disease: cohort study of decision-making and clinical outcomes. *Journal of the American Society of Nephrology* **14**, 1012–1021.

Kappes, U., Schanz, G., Gerhardt, U., Matzkies, F., Suwelak, B., and Hohage, H. (2001). Influence of age on the prognosis of renal transplant recipients. *American Journal of Nephrology* **21**, 259–263.

Kaye, N. and Lella, J. W. (1986). Discontinuation of dialysis therapy in the demented patient. *American Journal of Nephrology* **6**, 75–79.

Kaye, M., Bourgouin, P., and Low, G. (1987). Physician's noncompliance with patients' refusal of life-sustaining treatment. *American Journal of Nephrology* **7**, 304–312.

Khan, I. H. *et al.* (1993). Influence of co-existing disease on survival on renal replacement therapy. *Lancet* **341**, 415–418.

Khanna, K. V. and Markham, R. B. (1999). A perspective on cellular immunity in the elderly. *Cinical Infectious Diseases* **4**, 710–713.

Kimmel, P. L. *et al.* (2000). Multiple measurement of depression predict mortality in a longitudinal study of chronic hemodialysis patients. *Kidney International* **57**, 1093–1098.

Kjellstrand, C. M. (1988). Giving life—giving death. Ethical problems of high-technology medicine. *Acta Medica Scandinavica* **725** (Suppl.), 5–88.

Kjellstrand, C. M. Practical aspects of stopping dialysis and cultural differences. In *Ethical Problems in Dialysis and Transplantation* (ed. C. M. Kjellstrand and J. B. Dossetor), pp. 103–116. Dordrecht: Kluwer Academic, 1992.

Kjellstrand, C. M. and Logan, G. M. (1987). Racial, sexual and age inequalities in chronic dialysis. *Nephron* **45**, 257–263.

Kjellstrand, C. M. and Moody, H. (1994). Hemodialysis in Canada: a first-class medical crisis. *Canadian Medical Association Journal* **150**, 1067–1071.

Kopple, J. D., Grosvenor, M. B., and Roberts, C. E. Nutritional needs of the elderly haemodialysis patient. In *Geriatric Nephrology* (ed. D. G. Oreopoulos), pp. 127–134. Boston, MA: Nijhoff, 1986.

Kutner, N. G., Brogan, D., Fielding, B., and Hall, W. D. (1991). Older renal dialysis patients and quality of life. *Dialysis and Transplantation* **20**, 171–175.

Kutner, N. G., Cardenas, D. D., and Bower, J. D. (1992). Rehabilitation, ageing, and chronic renal disease. *American Journal of Physical Medical Rehabilitation* **71**, 97–101.

Kutner, N. G., Lin, J. S., Fielding, B., Brogman, D., and Hall, W. D. (1994). Continued survival of older haemodialysis. Investigation of psychosocial predictors. *American Journal of Kidney Diseases* **24**, 42–49.

Lamping, D. L. *et al.* (2000). Clinical outcomes, quality of life, and costs of the North Thames dialysis study of elderly people on dialysis: a prospective cohort study. *Lancet* **356**, 1543–1550.

Latos, D. L. (1996). Chronic dialysis in patients over age 65. *Journal of the American Society of Nephrology* **7**, 637–646.

Leggat, J. E., Jr., Bloembergen, W. E., Levine, G., Hulbert-Shearon, T. E., and Port, F. K. (1997). An analysis of risk factors for withdrawal from dialysis before death. *Journal of the American Society of Nephrology* **8**, 1755–1763.

Liptschutz, D. E. and Easterling, R. E. (1973). Spontaneous perforation of the colon in chronic renal failure. *Archives of Internal Medicine* **132**, 758–759.

Loscalzo, J. and London, G., ed. *Cardiovascular Disease in End-Stage Renal Failure*. Oxford: Oxford University Press, 2000.

Lowrie, E. G. and Lew, H. L. (1990). Death risk in haemodialysis patients: the predictive value of commonly measured variables and an evaluation of death rate differences between facilities. *American Journal of Kidney Diseases* **15**, 458–482.

Lu, A. D. *et al.* (2000). Outcome in recipients of dual transplants. *Transplantation* **69**, 281–285.

Lufft, V., Kleim, V., Tusch, G., Dannenberg, B., and Brunkhorst, R. (2000). Renal transplantation in older adults. Is graft survival affected by age? A case control study. *Transplantation* **69**, 790–794.

Luke, R. G. (1998). Chronic renal failure—a vasculopathic state. *New England Journal of Medicine* **339**, 841–843.

Lundgren, G. *et al.* (1989). Recipient age—an important factor for the outcome of cadaver renal transplants in patients treated with cyclosporin. *Transplantation Proceedings* **21**, 1653–1654.

Lupo, A. *et al.* (1992). Comparison of survival in CAPD and haemodialysis: a multicenter study. *Advances in Peritoneal Dialysis* **8**, 136–140.

Lusvarghi, E., Cappelli, G., and Davison, A. M., ed. (1998). Renal disease and ageing. Second international congress. *Nephrology, Dialysis, Transplantation* **13** (Suppl. 7), 1–101.

McGee, H. and Bradley, C. *Quality of Life Following Renal Failure*. Chur, Switzerland: Harwood Academic Publishers, 1994.

McKenzie, J. K., Moss, A. H., Feest, T. G., Stocking, C. B., and Siegler, M. (1998). Dialysis decision making in Canada, the United States and the United Kingdom. *American Journal of Kidney Diseases* **31**, 12–18.

Maggiore, Q., Pizzarelli, F., Dattolo, P., Maggiore, U., and Cerrai, T. (2000). Cardiovascular stability during haemodialysis, haemofiltration and haemodiafiltration. *Nephrology, Dialysis, Transplantation* **15** (Suppl. 1), 68–73.

Mailloux, L. U., Bellucci, A. G., Napolitano, B., Massey, R. T., Wilkes, B. M., and Bluestone, P. A. (1993). Death by withdrawal from dialysis: a twenty year clinical experience. *Journal of the American Society of Nephrology* **3**, 1631–1637.

Mailloux, L. U. *et al.* (1994). Survival estimates for 683 patients starting dialysis from 1970 through 1989: identification of risk factors for survival. *Clinical Nephrology* **42**, 127–135.

Main, J. (2000). Deciding not to start dialysis—a one year prospective study in Teesside. *Journal of Nephrology* **13**, 137–141.

Maiorca, R., Cancarini, G. C., Camerini, C., Manili, C., and Brunori, G. (1990). Modality selection for the elderly: medical factors. *Advances in Peritoneal Dialysis* **61** (Suppl. 6), 18–25.

Maiorca, R. *et al.* (1991). A multicenter, selection adjusted comparison of patients and techniques survival on CAPD and haemodialysis. *Peritoneal Dialysis International* **11**, 118–127.

Maiorca, R. *et al.* (1993). Continuous ambulatory peritoneal dialysis in the elderly. *Peritoneal Dialysis International* **13** (Suppl. 2), 165–171.

Maiorca, R. *et al.* (1994). Rational choice of haemodialysis treatment in the elderly. *Contributions to Nephrology* **109**, 25–32.

Maisonneuve, P. *et al.* (1999). Cancer in patients on dialysis for end-stage renal disease: an international collaborative study. *Lancet* **354**, 93–99.

Maisonneuve, P. *et al.* (2000). Distribution of primary renal diseases leading to end-stage renal failure in the United States, Europe and Australia/New Zealand: results from an international comparative study. *American Journal of Kidney Diseases* **35**, 157–165.

Martinez-Maldonado, M. *et al.*, ed. (1996). Renal disease in the elderly. *Seminars in Nephrology* **16**, 263–362.

Mattern, W. D. *et al.* (1989). Selection of end-stage renal disease treatment: an international study. *American Journal of Kidney Diseases* **13**, 457–464.

McKevitt, D. M., Jones, J. J. F., and Marion, R. R. (1986). The elderly on dialysis: physical and psychosocial functioning. *Dialysis Transplantation* **15**, 130–137.

Meier-Kriesche, H.-U., Friedman, G., Jacobs, M., Mulgaonkar, S., Vaghela, M., and Kaplan, B. (1999). Infectious complications in geriatric renal transplant patients: comparison of two immunosuppressive protocols. *Transplantation* **68**, 1496–1502.

Meier-Kriesche, H.-U., Akinlolu, O. O., Hanson, J. A., and Kaplan, B. (2001). Exponentially increased risk of infectious death in older renal transplant recipients. *Kidney International* **59**, 1539–1543.

Merkus, M. P., Jager, K. J., Dekker, F. W., de Haan, R. J., Boetshoten, E. W., and Krediet, R. T. for the NECOSAD study group (2000). Predictors of poor outcome in chronic dialysis patients: the Netherlands cooperative study on the adequacy of dialysis. *American Journal of Kidney Diseases* **35**, 69–78.

Michel, C., Bindi, P., and Viron, B. (1990). CAPD with private home nurses: an alternative treatment for elderly and disabled patients. *Advances in Peritoneal Dialysis* **6** (Suppl.), 92–94.

Mieghem, A. V. *et al.* (2001). Outcome of cadaver kidney transplantation in 23 patients with type 2 diabetes mellitus. *Nephrology, Dialysis, Transplantation* **16**, 1686–1691.

Mignon, F., Michel, C., Mentre, F., and Viron, B. (1993). Worldwide demographics and future trends of the management of renal failure in the elderly. *Kidney International* **43** (Suppl. 41), S18–S26.

Mignon, F., Siohan, P., Legallicier, R., Khayat, B., Viron, B., and Michel, C. (1995). The management of uraemia in the elderly: treatment and choices. *Nephrology, Dialysis, Transplantation* **10** (Suppl. 6), 55–59.

Mion, C., Slingeneyer, A., Canaud, B., and Elie, M. (1981). A review of seven years' home peritoneal dialysis. *Proceedings of the European Dialysis and Transplant Association* **17**, 91–107.

Morales, J. M., Campistol, J. M., Andres, A., and Herrero, J. C. (2000). Immunosuppression in older renal transplant patients. *Drugs and Aging* **16**, 279–287.

Morales, J. M. *et al.* (1994). Renal transplantation in older patients with double therapy with optional change to cyclosporin monotherapy. *Transplantation Proceedings* **26**, 2511–2512.

Moreno, F., Aracil, J., Perez, R., and Valderrábano, F. (1996). Controlled study on the improvement of quality of life in elderly haemodialysis patients after correcting endstage disease-related anemia with erythropoietin. *American Journal of Kidney Diseases* **27**, 548–556.

Morris, G. E., Jamieson, N. V., Small, J., Evans, D. B., and Calne, R. (1991). Cadaveric renal transplantation in elderly recipients: is it worthwhile? *Nephrology, Dialysis, Transplantation* **6**, 887–892.

Morrison, G., Michelson, E. L., Brown, S., and Morgan Roth, J. J. (1980). Mechanism and prevention of cardiac arrhythmias in chronic haemodialysis patients. *Kidney International* **17**, 811–819.

Moss, A. H. (2000). Shared decision-making in dialysis: the new RPA/ASN guideline on appropriate initiation and withdrawal of treatment. *American Journal of Kidney Diseases* **37**, 1081–1091.

Mulkerrin, E. C. (2000). Rationing renal replacement therapy to older patients—agreed guidelines are needed. *Quarterly Journal of Medicine* **93**, 253–255.

Munda, R., First, M. R., Alexander, J. W., Linnemann, C. C., Jr., Fidler, J. P., and Kuttur, D. (1983). Polytetrafluoro-ethylene graft survival in haemodialysis. *Journal of the American Medical Association* **249**, 219–222.

Muñoz-Silva, E. J. and Kjellstrand, C. M. (1988). Withdrawing life support. Do families and physicians decide as patients do? *Nephron* **48**, 201–205.

Munshi, S. K., Visayakumar, N., Taub, N. A., Bhullar, H., Nelson Lo, T. C., and Warwick, G. (2000). Outcome of renal replacement therapy in the very elderly. *Nephrology, Dialysis, Transplantation* **16**, 128–133.

Nakai, S. *et al.* (2001). An overview of dialysis treatment in Japan as of 31st December 1999. *Journal of the Japanese Society for Dialysis Therapy* **34**, 1121–1147.

Nelson, C. B., Port, F. K., Wolfe, R. A., and Guire, K. E. (1994). The association of diabetic status, age and race to withdrawal from dialysis. *Journal of the American Society of Nephrology* **4**, 1608–1614.

Neu, S. and Kjellstrand, C. M. (1986). Stopping long-term dialysis: an empirical study of stopping life-supporting treatment. *New England Journal of Medicine* **314**, 14–20.

Newstead, C. G. and Dyer, P. (1992). The influence of increased age and age matching on graft survival after first cadaver renal transplantation. *Transplantation* **54**, 441–443.

Nicholls, A. L. *et al.* (1984). Impact of continuous ambulatory peritoneal dialysis treatment of renal failure in patients over 60. *British Medical Journal* **288**, 18–19.

Nissenson, A. R., ed. (1990). Peritoneal dialysis in the geriatric patient. *Advances in Peritoneal Dialysis* **6** (Suppl.), 1–95.

Nissenson, A. R. (1991). Chronic peritoneal dialysis in the elderly. *Geriatric Nephrology and Urology* **1**, 3–12.

Nissenson, A. R. (1993). Dialysis therapy in the elderly patient. *Kidney International* **43** (Suppl. 40), s51–s57.

Nissenson, A. R., Gentile, D. E., Soderblom, R., and Brax, C. CAPD in the elderly—regional Axperience. In *Frontiers in peritoneal Dialysis* (ed. J. F. Maher and J. F. Winchester), pp. 312–317. New York: Field Rich, 1986.

Niu, P. C., Roberts, M., Tabibian, B., Brautbar, N., and Lee, D. B. N. (1992). How can the care of elderly dialysis patients be improved? *Seminars in Dialysis* **5**, 31–33.

Nolph, K. D. Peritoneal dialysis. In *The Kidney* Vol. I (ed. B. N. Brenner and F. C. Rector), pp. 2299–2335. Philadelphia, PA: W. B. Saunders, 1991.

Nolph, K. D., Lindblad, A. S., Novak, J. W., and Steinberg, S. M. (1990). Experiences with the elderly in the National CAPD registry. *Advances in Peritoneal Dialysis* **6** (Suppl.), 33–38.

Nyberg, G., Hallste, G., Nordén, G., Hadimeri, H., and Wrammer, L. (1995a). Physical performance does not improve in elderly patients following transplantation. *Nephrology, Dialysis, Transplantation* **10**, 86–90.

Nyberg, G., Nilsson, B., Nordén, G., and Karlberg, I. (1995b). Outcome of renal transplantation in patients over the age of 60: a case–control study. *Nephrology, Dialysis, Transplantation* **10**, 91–94.

Ojo, A. O. *et al.* (2001). Survival in recipients of marginal cadvaeric donor kidneys compared with other recipients and wait-listed patients. *Journal of the American Society of Nephrology* **12**, 589–597.

Okada, M. (1990). Mortality in chronic dialysis patients in Japan. *American Journal of Kidney Diseases* **15**, 410–413.

Opeltz, G. (1998). The influence of recipient age on kidney transplant outcome. *Nephrology* **2** (Suppl. 1), s211–s214.

Opelz, G. and the Collaborative Transplant Group (1992). Collaborative transplant study—10 year report. *Transplantation Proceedings* **24**, 2342–2355.

Opsahl, J. N., Husebye, D. G., Helseth, H. K., and Collins, A. J. (1988). Coronary artery bypass surgery in patients on maintenance haemodialysis: long term survival. *American Journal of Kidney Diseases* **12**, 271–274.

Oreopoulos, D. G. (1994). Should the elderly be denied dialysis? *Peritoneal Dialysis International* **14**, 105–107.

Oreopoulos, D. G. (1995). Withdrawing from dialysis: when letting die is better than helping to live. *Lancet* **346**, 3–4.

Oreopoulos, D. G., Khanna, R., Williams, P., and Vas, S. I. (1982). Continuous ambulatory peritoneal dialysis—1981. *Nephron* **20**, 298–303.

Palder, S. B., Kirkman, R. L., Whittemore, A. D., Hakim, R. M., Lazarus, J. M., and Tilney, N. L. (1985). Vascular access for haemodialysis: patency rates and results of revision. *Annals of Surgery* **202**, 235–239.

Parfrey, P. S., Harnett, J. D., Griffiths, S. M., Gault, M. H., and Barre, P. E. (1988). Congestive heart failure in dialysis patients. *Archives of Internal Medicine* **148**, 1519–1525.

Piccoli, G. *et al.* (1990). Dialysis in the elderly: comparison of different dialytic modalities. *Advances in Peritoneal Dialysis* **6** (Suppl.), 72–81.

Piccoli, G. *et al.* (1993). Death in conditions of cachexia: the price for the dialysis treatment of the elderly? *Kidney International* **43** (Suppl. 41), S282–S286.

Piccoli, G. *et al.* (1996). Elderly patients on dialysis: epidemiology of an epidemic. *Nephrology, Dialysis, Transplantation* **11** (Suppl. 9), s26–s30.

Pirsch, J. D. *et al.* (1989). Cadaveric renal transplantation with cyclosporine in patients more than 60 years of age. *Transplantation* **47**, 259–261.

Pollini, J. and Teissier, M. (1990). Un dileme difficile à résoudre: les malades âgés réfusés pour la dialyse chronique. Problèmes éthiques ou choix médical? *Néphrologie* (Suppl.), 341–347.

Ponce, S. P. *et al.* (1982). Comparison of the survival of three permanent peritoneal dialysis catheters. *Peritoneal Dialysis Bulletin* **2**, 82–86.

Ponticelli, C. (2000). Should renal transplantation be offered to older patients? *Nephrology, Dialysis, Transplantation* **15**, 315–317.

Ponticelli, C., Graziani, G., Cantaluppi, A., and Moore, R. Dialysis treatment of end-stage renal disease. In *Renal Function and Disease in the Elderly* (ed. J. F. Macías and J. S. Cameron), pp. 509–528. London: Butterworth, 1987.

Port, F. K. (1992). The end-stage renal disease program: trends over the past 18 years. *American Journal of Kidney Diseases* **20**, 3–7.

Porush, J. G. and Faubert, P. F. Chronic renal failure. In *Renal Disease in the Aged* (ed. J. G. Porush and P. F. Faubert), pp. 285–313. Boston, MA: Little Brown, 1991.

Posen, G. A., Fenton, S. S. A., Arbus, G. S., Churchill, D. N., and Jeffery, J. R. (1990a). The Canadian experience with peritoneal dialysis in the elderly. *Advances in Peritoneal Dialysis* **6** (Suppl.), 47–50.

Posen, G. A., Jeffery, J. R., Fenton, S. S. A., and Arbus, G. S. (1990b). Results from the Canadian Renal Failure Registry. *American Journal of Kidney Diseases* **15**, 397–401.

Pourchez, T., Moriniere, P., and St. Priest, A. (1990). Outcome of vascular access for haemodialysis in the elderly (<75 years). *Proceedings of the European Dialysis Transplant Association* **27**, 160 (abstract).

Raine, A. E. G. et al. (1992). Report on management of renal failure in Europe XXII, 1991. *Nephrology, Dialysis, Transplantation* **7**, 7–35.

Rebollo, P. et al. (1998). Health-related quality of life (HRQOL) in end stage renal disease (ESRD) patients over 65 years. *Geriatric Nephrology and Urology* **8**, 85–94.

Remuzzi, G. et al. (1999). Early experience with dual kidney transplantation in adults using expanded donor criteria. *Journal of the American Society of Nephrology* **10**, 2591–2598.

Renal Physicians Association and the American Society of Nephrology (2000). *Shared Decision-Making in the Appropriate Initiation and Withdrawal from Dialysis.* Clinical practice guideline no. 2. Renal Physicians Association, Rockville, MD.

Rife, M. et al. (1979). The dependent elderly on dialysis. *Dialysis and Transplantation* **8**, 867–878.

Rodin, G. M., Charma, J., Ennis, J., Fenton, S., Lockin, N., and Steinhouse, K. (1981). Stopping life-sustaining medical treatment: psychiatric considerations in the termination of renal dialysis. *Canadian Journal of Psychiatry* **26**, 540–544.

Roodnat, J. I. et al. (1999). The vanishing importance of age in renal transplantation. *Transplantation* **67**, 576–580.

Ross, C. J. and Rutsky, E. A. (1990). Dialysis modality selection in the elderly patient with end stage renal disease: advantages and disadvantages of peritoneal dialysis. *Advances in Peritoneal Dialysis* **6** (Suppl.), 11–17.

Rotellar, E., Lubelza, R. A., Rotellar, C., Martinez-Camps, E., and Valls, R. (1985). Must patients over 65 be haemodialysed? *Nephron* **41**, 152–156.

Rothenberg, L. S. (1993). Withholding and withdrawing dialysis from elderly endstage renal disease patients: part 2—ethical and policy issues. *Geriatric Nephrology and Urology* **3**, 23–41.

Roy, A. T., Johnson, L. E., Lee, D. B. N., Brautbar, N., and Morley, J. E. (1990). Renal failure in older people. *Journal of the American Geriatric Society* **39**, 239–253.

Roza, A. M., Gallagher-Lepak, S., Johnson, C. P., and Adams, M. B. (1989). Renal transplantation in patients more than 65 years old. *Transplantation* **48**, 689–690.

Sacks, S. H., Aparicio, S. A. J. R., Bevan, A., Oliver, D. O., Will, E. J., and Davison, A. M. (1989). Late renal failure due to prostatic out flow obstruction: a preventable disease. *British Medical Journal* **298**, 180–189.

Safian, R. D. and Textor, S. C. (2001). Renal-artery stenosis. *New England Journal of Medicine* **344**, 431–442.

Salamone, M. et al. (1995). Dialysis in the elderly: improvement of survival results in the eighties. *Nephrology, Dialysis, Transplantation* **10** (Suppl. 6), 60–64.

Saudan, P., Berney, T., Leski, M., Orel, P., Bollee, J.-F., and Martin, P.-Y. (2001). Renal transplantation in the elderly: a long-term, single-centre experience. *Nephrology, Dialysis, Transplantation* **16**, 824–828.

Savazzi, G. M., Gusmano, G., and Degasperi, T. (1985). Cerebral atrophy in patients on long-term regular haemodialysis treatment. *Clinical Nephrology* **23**, 89–95.

Schaefer, K. and Röhrich, B. (1999). The dilemma of renal replacement therapy in patients over 80 years of age: dialysis should not be withheld. *Nephrology, Dialysis, Transplantation* **14**, 35–36.

Schaubel, D., Desmeules, M., Mao, Y., Jeffrey, J., and Fenton, S. (1995). Survival experience among elderly end-stage renal disease patients. *Transplantation* **60**, 1389–1394.

Schratzberger, G. and Mayer, G. (2003). Age and renal transplantation: an interim analysis. *Nephrology, Dialysis, Transplantation* **18**, 471–476.

Schulak, J. A. and Hricik, D. E. (1991). Kidney transplantation in the elderly. *Geriatric Nephrology and Urology* **1**, 105–112.

Schulak, J. A., Mayes, J. T., Johnston, K. H., and Hrickik, D. E. (1990). Kidney transplantation in patients aged sixty years and older. *Surgery* **108**, 726–733.

Segoloni, G. P., Salomone, M., and Piccoli, G. B. (1990). CAPD in the elderly: Italian multicenter study experience. *Advances in Peritoneal Dialysis* **6** (Suppl.), 41–46.

Sessa, A. (1995). When dialysis becomes worse than death. *Nephrology, Dialysis, Transplantation* **10**, 1128–1130.

Sherman, R. A. (1992). The pathophysiologic basis for haemodialysis-related hypotension. *Seminars in Dialysis* **1**, 136–142.

Silverberg, J. S., Barre, P. E., Prichard, S. S., and Sniderman, A. D. (1989). Impact of left ventricular hypertrophy on survival in end-stage renal disease. *Kidney International* **36**, 286–290.

Singer, P. A. (1992). Nephrologists' experience with and attitudes towards decisions to forego dialysis. *Journal of the American Society of Nephrology* **2**, 1235–1240.

Singer, J. et al. (1995). Life-sustaining treatment preferences of hemodialysis patients: implications for advance directives. *Journal of the American Society of Nephrology* **6**, 1410–1417.

Spanish Monotherapy Study Group (1994). Cyclosporine monotherapy versus OKT3 and cyclosporine versus prednisone and cyclosporine as induction therapy in older renal transplant patients: a multicenter randomized study. *Transplantation Proceedings* **26**, 2522–2524.

Stacy, W. and Sica, D. Dialysis of the elderly patient. In *Geriatric Nephrology and Urology* (ed. E. T. Zawada and D. A. Sica), pp. 229–251. Littleton, MA: PSG Publishing, 1985.

Stewart, A. L. and Ware, J. E. *Measuring Functioning and Well-Being.* Durham, NC: Duke University Press, 1992.

Stewart, D. A., Burns, J. M. A., Dunn, S. G., and Roberts, M. A. (1990). The 2-minute walking test: a sensitive index of mobility in the rehabilitation of elderly patients. *Clinical Rehabilitation* **4**, 273–276.

Stewart, G., Jardine, A. G., and Briggs, J. D. (2000). Ischaemic heart disease following renal transplantation. *Nephrology, Dialysis, Transplantation* **15**, 269–277.

Sturm, J. M., Maurizi-Balsan, J., Foret, M., and Cordonnier, D. (1998). Dialysis in octogenarians: search for mortality risk factors. Consecutive series of 30 patients. *Presse Médicale* **16**, 748–752.

Takemoto, S. and Terasaki, P. I. Donor and recipient age. In *Clinical Transplants* (ed. P. I. Terasaki), pp. 345–356. Los Angeles, CA: UCLA Tissue Typing Laboratory, 1988.

Taube, D., Cameron, J. S., and Challah, S. Renal transplantation in older patients. In *Renal Function and Diseases in the Elderly* (ed. J. F. Macías and J. S. Cameron), pp. 509–528. London: Butterworth, 1987.

Tesi, R. J., Elkhmammas, E. A., Davies, E. A., Henry, M. L., and Ferguson, R. M. (1994). Renal transplantation in older people. *Lancet* **343**, 461–464.

Tobe, S. W. and Senn, J. S. for the end-stage renal disease group (1996). Foregoing renal dialysis: case study and review of ethical issues. *American Journal of Kidney Diseases* **28**, 147–153.

Toma, H., Tanabe, K., Tokumoto, T., Shimizu, T., and Shimamura, H. (2001). Time-dependent factors influencing the long term outcome in living renal allografts: donor age is a crucial risk factor for long-term graft survival more than 5 years after transplantation. *Transplantation* **72**, 940–947.

Thorogood, J., Persijn, C. G., Zantvoort, F. A., van Houwelingen, M., and van Rood, J. J. (1990). Matching for age in renal transplantation. *New England Journal of Medicine* 322, 852–853.

United States Network for Organ Sharing and Division of Organ Transplantation 1994 report (1988–1993) (1994). Bethesda, MD: Bureau of Health Services Development, US Dept of Health and Human Services.

US Renal Data System (1989). *Annual Data Report*, pp. 17–20. Bethesda, MD: National Institutes of Health NIDDK.

US Renal Data System (1992). Annual data report. Comorbid conditions and correlation with mortality risk among 3399 incident hemodialysis patients. *American Journal of Kidney Diseases* 20 (Suppl. 2), 32–39.

US Renal Data System (1993). *Annual Report*. Bethesda, MD: National Institutes of Health, National Institute of Diabetes and Digestive and Kidney Diseases.

US Renal Data System Report (2001). *American Journal of Kidney Diseases* 38 (Suppl. 3), 32–39.

Valderrábano, F., Jones, E. H. P., and Mallick, N. P. (1995). Report on management of renal failure in Europe XXIV 1993. *Nephrology, Dialysis, Transplantation* 10 (Suppl. 5), 1–25.

Van Ypersele de Strihou, C., Jadoul, C. M., Malghem, J., Maldague, B., and Jamart, J. (1991). Effects of dialysis membranes and patients' age on signs of dialysis-related amyloidosis. The working party on dialysis amyloidosis. *Kidney International* 39, 1012–1019.

Velez, R. L. *et al.* (1991). Renal transplantation with cyclosporine in the elderly population. *Transplantation Proceedings* 23, 1749–1752.

Vendemia, F., Gesualdo, L., Schena, F. P., and D'Amico, G. on behalf of the Renal Immunopathology Study Group of the Italian Society of Nephrology (2001). *Journal of Nephrology* 14, 34–52.

Verdery, R. B. (1990). Wasting away of the old: can—and should—it be treated? *Geriatrics* 45, 26–31.

Vivas, C. A. *et al.* (1992). Renal transplantation in patients 65 years old or older. *Journal of Urology* 147, 990–993.

Vlachoyannis, J., Kurtz, P., and Hoppe, D. (1988). CAPD in elderly patients with cardiovascular risk. *Clinical Nephrology* 30, 513–517.

Voets, A. J., Tulner, L. R., and Ligthart, G. J. (1997). Immunosenescence revisited. Does it have any clinical significance? *Drugs and Aging* 11, 394–397.

Vonesh, E. F. and Maiorca, R. (1993). A multicenter, selection-adjusted comparison of patient and technique survival on CAPD and haemodialysis. *Peritoneal Dialysis International* 13, 71–72.

Waiser, J. *et al.* (2000). Age-matching in renal transplantation. *Nephrology, Dialysis, Transplantation* 15, 696–700.

Westlie, L., Umen, A., Nestrud, S., and Kjellstrand, C. M. (1984). Mortality, morbidity, and life satisfaction in the elderly dialysis patient. *ASAIO Transactions* 30, 21–30.

Wetzels, J. F. M., Hoitsma, A. J., and Koene, R. A. P. (1986). Influence of cadaver donor age on renal graft survival. *Clinical Nephrology* 25, 256–259.

Williams, A. J. and Antao, A. J. O. (1989). Referral of elderly patients with end-stage renal failure for renal replacement therapy. *Quarterly Journal of Medicine* 72, 749–756.

Winchester, J. F. (1999). Peritoneal dialysis in older individuals. *Geriatric Urology and Nephrology* 9, 147–152.

Wolff, R. A. *et al.* (1999). Comparison of mortality in patients on dialysis, patients on dialysis awaiting tranplantation and recipients of a first cadaveric transplant. *New England Journal of Medicine* 341, 1725–1730.

Woodhouse, K. W., Wynne, H., Baillie, S., James, O. F. W., and Rawlins, M. (1987). Who are the frail elderly? *Quarterly Journal of Medicine* 68, 505–506.

Xue, J. L., Ma, J. Z., Louis, T. A., and Collins, A. J. (2001). Forecast of the numbers of patients with end-stage renal disease in the United States to the year 2010. *Journal of the American Society of Nephrology* 12, 2753–2758.

14.3 The diabetic patient with impaired renal function

Ralf Dikow and Eberhard Ritz

Terminal renal failure used to be a death sentence for the diabetic patient. Maintenance haemodialysis (HD) was used in diabetic patients as early as 1966 (Avram 1966), but results were poor. In one famous paper entitled 'The sad truth about hemodialysis in diabetic nephropathy' (Ghavamian *et al.* 1972) the authors arrived at the conclusion that 'dialysis for such patients . . . carries little likelihood of long-term survival or improvement in quality of life'. Mean patient survival was 11 months. Survival of even less than 7 months was reported for elderly diabetics (Blagg *et al.* 1971). Although survival of uraemic diabetic patients has improved dramatically in recent years, such historical experience underlines the particular susceptibility of the diabetic patient to cardiovascular (CV) complications and infectious episodes. In the pioneer report on kidney transplantation combined with pancreatic–duodenal allotransplantation only two of 10 patients with juvenile onset diabetes were alive 7 months postoperatively (Lillehei *et al.* 1970). Meanwhile, the outcome of combined pancreas–kidney transplantation has improved dramatically and this alternative has become the procedure providing best survival and quality of life (Becker *et al.* 2000) in the patient with type 1 diabetes mellitus.

Chronic ambulatory peritoneal dialysis (CAPD) is a complementary modality, which may in certain situations be superior to HD (Van Biesen *et al.* 2000). Today a majority of patients who are accepted for renal replacement therapy have diabetes and most suffer from diabetic nephropathy. It is therefore essential that the nephrologist is familiar with the principles of treating diabetes and its major complications, particularly retinopathy, the diabetic foot, and cardiac problems. The latter are the major cause of morbidity and mortality.

Magnitude of the problem

There has been a secular trend of decreasing prevalence of nephropathy in type 1 diabetic patients (Bojestig *et al.* 1994), presumably because of progressively better management of glycaemia and hypertension. Although aggressive early intervention definitely reduces the frequency of CV and renal endpoints in type 2 diabetic patients (Gaede *et al.* 2003), there is no evidence of a decreasing incidence of advanced nephropathy in such patients. On the contrary, endstage renal failure with diabetes as a comorbid condition has become the single most frequent diagnosis for patients entering renal replacement programmes in the Western world (Ritz *et al.* 1999; Dikow and Ritz 2003a,b; Schwenger *et al.* 2003). Follow-up of the United Kingdom Prospective Diabetes Study (Adler *et al.* 2003) showed that approximately 2 per cent of patients per year progress from normo- to microalbuminuria, from

micro- to macroalbuminuria and from macroalbuminuria to impaired renal function or terminal renal failure, respectively. It is notable that the risk of the type 2 diabetic patient to succumb to CV disease is greater than the risk to go into endstage renal failure.

In the past decades, a continuous and consistent increase in the incidence of patients with diabetes as a comorbid condition entering renal replacement programmes has been observed (Lippert *et al.* 1995; Ritz and Orth 1999; Ritz *et al.* 1999). This is the result of an absolute increase of the prevalence of type 2 diabetes in the general population, the ageing of the population (because diabetes becomes more frequent with increasing age), but most importantly is the result of better survival of diabetic patients with nephropathy.

According to the United States Renal Data System (USRDS) (2001), diabetic nephropathy was the primary diagnosis in 42.8 per cent of incident patients (i.e. 38.160 out of 89.252). This was an increase by 238 per cent compared to the year 1990. In the year 2000, the actual proportion of diabetic patients amongst those admitted for renal replacement therapy varied considerably between different countries as illustrated in Table 1. Registry figures, for example, those from

Table 1 Incidence of patients admitted to renal replacement programmes with diabetes as a comorbid condition according to national registries [data are given as patients per million population (pmp) or per cent]

Country	Year	New patients total (pmp)	Diabetes (% of total)	Diabetes (pmp)
Australia	2000	93.7	22	20.3
Catalunya	2000	146	19.8	28.9
Denmark	2000	67.5	15.8	28.8[b]
Germany	2001	73.3	36	26.4
Heidelberg[a]	2001	183	48.9	101[c]
New Zealand	2000	91.8	35	32.0
Poland	2000	67.5	15.8	10.6
Turkey	2001	89.7	25.3	22.7
United States	2001	317	42.8	136

[a] According to Schwenger *et al.* (2001).

[b] Type 1 diabetes, 14.8 pmp; type 2 diabetes, 14.0 pmp.

[c] Type 1 diabetes, 6 pmp; type 2 diabetes, 92 pmp.

Germany tend to underestimate the renal burden of diabetes: we found that diabetes was present in no less than 48.9 per cent of patients admitted for renal replacement therapy in Heidelberg (Schwenger *et al.* 2001). Clinical features of classical Kimmelstiel Wilson's disease were found only in 60 per cent, however. Atypical presentation consistent with ischaemic nephropathy accounted for 13 per cent and known primary renal disease (e.g. polycystic kidney disease, analgesic nephropathy, glomerulonephritis) with superimposed diabetes for 27 per cent of the cases. Survival of the diabetic patient on HD is similar (Koch *et al.* 1993), however, whether or not diabetic or primary non-diabetic renal disease accounts for endstage renal failure. In the Heidelberg series, diabetes had not been diagnosed at the time of admission in 11 per cent of the diabetic patients with renal failure, presumably because the patient had lost weight secondary to anorexia, thus self-correcting hyperglycaemia. A great majority, that is, 94 per cent suffered from type 2 diabetes (Schwenger *et al.* 2001) and in all countries it is primarily patients with type 2 diabetes whose number is consistently on the increase (Ritz *et al.* 1999). The annual per cent increase of type 2 diabetic patients entering renal replacement programmes in the European sample reported by the European Renal Association and European Dialysis and Transplant Association (ERA–EDTA) registry (Stengel *et al.* 2003) was on average +13.6 per cent per year ranging from +10 per cent in Austria to +20.9 per cent in Francophone Belgium. Such rapid recent increase explains why our recent local evaluation (Schwenger *et al.* 2001) yielded substantially higher values compared to the data of an earlier analysis of the ERA–EDTA registry, where the incidence of type 2 diabetic patients in the period 1990–1999 ranged from 9.4 pmp in Denmark to 32.8 pmp in Austria, compared to 98 pmp in Heidelberg as of 1999.

There is a substantial discrepancy between the incidence and prevalence of diabetic patients on dialysis. This is explained by the fact that survival of diabetic patients is considerably worse than in non-diabetic patients as illustrated by Fig. 1 giving the results of a prospective study on incident dialysis patients in Germany (Koch *et al.* 1993). The 5-year survival of 5 per cent in type 2 diabetic patients corresponds to the survival in patients with metastasising gastrointestinal carcinoma. Survival rates in dialysed diabetic patients are much better in countries such as Japan (Iseki *et al.* 2002), presumably related to the generally lower rate of CV death in Japan.

It is known that between 5 and 10 per cent of patients (Ritz and Stefanski 1996) develop diabetes *de novo* on dialysis, presumably because they had been prediabetic to begin with. They had presumably a temporary reversal of hyperglycaemia following weight loss from anorexia in the predialytic stage and recurrence after weight gain on dialysis. Recently, it has been found (Gilbertson *et al.* 2002) that in the United States by the end of the first year of renal replacement therapy, close to two-thirds of patients have the diagnosis of recognized diabetes, particularly patients in whom when the primary diagnosis had been hypertensive nephropathy. It is of importance that an increasing proportion of patients present as acute irreversible renal failure, mostly acute on chronic renal failure, usually after cardiac or septic complications with or without administration of radiocontrast or non-steroidals. This was seen in 27 per cent of the diabetic patients in the Heidelberg series (Schwenger *et al.* 2001). Patients admitted as emergencies with acute renal failure have a particularly poor prognosis (Chantrel *et al.* 1999; Schwenger *et al.* 2001). Late referral continues to be a problem (Jungers 2002; Schwenger *et al.* 2003). In Heidelberg, the median interval between referral and start of dialysis was 17 weeks. One-year mortality was 37 per cent in diabetic and 30.6 per cent, in non-diabetic patients for those referred less than 17 weeks and only 7.3 per cent and 4.1 per cent, respectively, for those referred greater than 17 weeks (Fig. 2). Patients referred late have particularly insufficient control of risk factors (see Table 2) and have more frequently no vascular access. The latter is the main factor causing increased morbidity and mortality.

The causes of death in haemodialysed diabetic patients are given in Table 3.

Evaluation of the diabetic patient with preterminal renal failure

Evaluation of the diabetic patient with preterminal renal failure has the following aims:

(1) to assess the cause of renal failure;

(2) to assess the rate of progression and the magnitude of proteinuria;

(3) to recognize the presence of acute renal failure or acute on chronic renal failure;

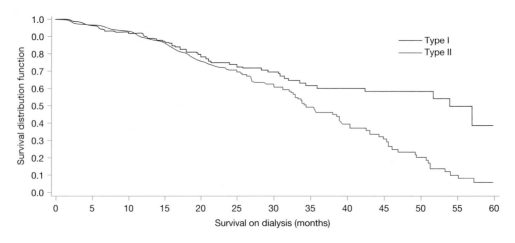

Fig. 1 Survival distribution function of 412 diabetic patients (181 type 1 and 231 type 2) with end-stage renal disease (after Koch *et al.* 1997).

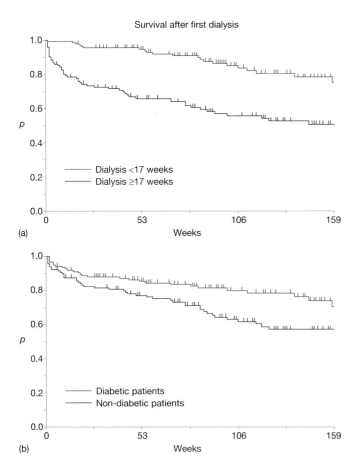

Fig. 2 Actuarial survival on dialysis as a function of the interval between referral and start of dialysis—comparison of overall cohort (a) with diabetic patients (b) (after Schwenger et al. 2003).

Table 2 Characteristics of diabetic patients at the time of admission to the renal unit (after Keller et al. 2000)

Known duration of diabetes (years)	
Type 1 ($n = 16$)	19 (10–26)
Type 2 ($n = 157$)	11 (0–44)
Body mass index (kg/m²)	
Type 1	23.1 (21.4–28.7)
Type 2	28.7 (18.4–44.4)
HbA1c (%)	7.9 (4.9–15.7)
Insulin treatment (%)	49
LDL-cholesterol (mg/dl)	170 (67–307)
ACE inhibitors (%)	52
No antihypertensive treatment (%)	18
Systolic BP (mmHg)	170 (120–260)

(4) to recognize renal problems other than diabetic nephropathy, for example, ischaemic nephropathy, diabetic cystopathy, urinary tract infection;

(5) to monitor the patient for clinical evidence of extrarenal microvascular and macrovascular complications (Table 4).

Table 3 Most frequent causes of death in diabetic haemodialysed patients (rates per 1000 patient-years at risk in the years 1996–1998) (after Dikow et al. 2002a,b)

Cardiac arrest	59.4
Septicaemia	30.5
Myocardial infarction	26.7
Cardiac arrythmia	16.0
Stroke	16.8
Other	46.5

Table 4 Major microvascular and macrovascular complications in patients with diabetic nephropathy

Microvascular complications
Retinopathy
Polyneuropathy including autonomic neuropathy (gastroparesis, diarrhoea/obstipation, detrusor paresis, painless myocardial ischaemia, erectile impotence; supine hypertension/orthostatic hypotension)

Macrovascular complications
Coronary heart disease, left ventricular hypertrophy, congestive heart failure
Cerebrovascular complications (stroke)
Peripheral artery occlusive disease

Mixed complications
Diabetic foot (neuropathic, vascular)

Diabetic nephropathy versus other causes of renal failure

The overwhelming majority of diabetic patients reaching endstage renal failure suffer from diabetic nephropathy. This is the ultimate consequence of microvascular damage to the kidney. A minority of patients, however, suffer from specific renal problems with or without superimposed diabetic glomerulosclerosis. Renal ischaemia or atherosclerotic renal artery stenosis is much more common in diabetic patients than was previously assumed (Table 5). In our experience, more than one-third of patients presenting for percutaneous transluminal dilatation of renal arteries suffer from diabetes.

In the past, urinary tract infection frequently led to renal parenchymatous infection with purulent papillary necrosis and intrarenal abscess formation. This has now become rare, presumably due to the frequent use of antibiotics and better management of urinary tract infection. We have observed this complication only once in the past two decades, but it is still important to consider this possibility in the acutely ill febrile uraemic diabetic patient. Urinary tract infection may be more frequent in the diabetic patient, particularly when residual urine is present in the bladder as a consequence of autonomous polyneuropathy, but the issue whether the frequency is truely increased is still moot. There is no doubt, however, that symptomatic urinary tract infections are more severe in the diabetic compared to the non-diabetic patient.

Glomerulonephritis, particularly membranous glomerulonephritis, was thought to be more common in diabetic patients than in

Table 5 Common renal problems in diabetics

Diabetic nephropathy (Kimmelstiel–Wilson)

Renovascular (ischaemic) disease (renal artery stenosis, cholesterol embolism)

Urinary tract infection ($\pm$ papillary necrosis)

Glomerulonephritis (membranous glomerulonephritis)?

Acute renal failure after administration of contrast media

Table 6 Frequent therapeutic challenges in the diabetic patient with renal failure

---

Hypertension (blood pressure amplitude, circadian rhythm)

Hypervolaemia

Glycaemic control (insulin half-life, cumulation of oral hypoglycaemic agents)

Malnutrition

Bacterial infections (diabetic foot)

Timely creation of vascular access

---

the general population (Amoah *et al.* 1988; Parving *et al.* 1992), but this has not been our experience (Waldherr *et al.* 1992) and no excess frequency was reported in a meta-analysis by Olsen and Mogensen (1996). The clinician should suspect the presence of non-diabetic renal disease if a nephritic urinary sediment is found, and if urinary abnormalities and/or renal dysfunction occur early (in the patient with type 1 diabetes). Retinopathy is present in virtually all patients with type 1 diabetes and diabetic nephropathy. In type 2 diabetic patients, absence of diabetic retinopathy does not argue against the presence of diabetic nephropathy, however, since retinopathy is found only in 60–70 per cent of patients with terminal renal failure.

Diabetic patients with nephropathy are particularly prone to develop acute renal failure after administration of radiocontrast media (Parfrey *et al.* 1989). The risk is similar for ionic and non-ionic radiocontrast media (Schwab *et al.* 1989), but it has recently been described that the renal risk is less for dimeric radiocontrast media (Aspelin *et al.* 2003). The risk can be reduced considerably by attention to preventive measures including administration of fluid, as well as temporary omission of diuretics and possibly angiotensin-converting enzyme (ACE) inhibitors. Radiographic techniques should be chosen which reduce the required dose of radiocontrast media. In the future radiocontrast administration will presumably be superseded by CO_2 angiography or magnetic resonance angiography. To reduce the risk of radiocontrast adjusting the dose in proportion to renal function has been proposed (Cigarroa *et al.* 1989).

The search for extrarenal complications caused by micro- and macroangiopathy

The diabetic patient with advanced renal failure has usually a much higher burden of micro- and macrovascular complications (Table 4) than the diabetic patient without or with early stages of diabetic nephropathy. The morbidity of these diabetic patients with advanced renal failure is usually more severe than that of the average patient seen in a diabetes outpatient clinic. The major clinical problem is accelerated and premature atherosclerosis, frequently causing coronary heart disease: This may take the form of myocardial infarction (often silent), angina pectoris or ischaemic cardiomyopathy. There is also an excess frequency of cerebrovascular disease and (particularly in smokers) peripheral artery disease. The diabetic patient with advanced renal impairment, even if he or she is asymptomatic, must therefore be monitored at regular intervals for timely detection of the above complications (ophthalmological examination at half-yearly intervals;

cardiac and angiological status including imaging of the carotid artery yearly; foot inspection preferable at each visit).

The physician in charge of the diabetic patient with impaired renal function has to face a spectrum of therapeutic challenges which are listed in Table 6.

Diabetic retinopathy

In the 1970s a large proportion of diabetic patients on HD was blind (Leonard *et al.* 1973). This has become very rare. In the 1300 German diabetic patients currently examined in the 4D trial, blindness was reported only in 5 per cent of patients (Wanner *et al.* 1999). This decrease is presumably to a major extent the result of better blood pressure control and also of better ophthalmological care. While visual problems in the type 1 diabetic patients are usually due to proliferative retinopathy as a late complication, in elderly type 2 diabetic patients in whom the diagnosis of diabetes is made late in the course of the disease, retinopathy may be present even at the time of diagnosis (Walsh *et al.* 1975). The effect of optimal glycaemic control and lowering of blood pressure, particularly with ACE inhibitors, is of proven benefit. In contrast, the effect of many popular medications is unproven including piracetam, carbacobrom, ruticide, and calcium-dobesilate. The elderly diabetic patient may also have visual problems because of cataract (which is more frequent in diabetic patients), macular degeneration, and glaucoma.

Diabetic neuropathy

Disturbance of both the sensor and motor and autonomous nervous systems is a major complication in the diabetic patient with advanced nephropathy. Diabetic neuropathy may be aggravated by superimposed neuropathy of renal failure. Patients with diabetic polyneuropathy first lose sensation of pain and temperature (conducted by small fibres) and later lose the sensation of light touch or vibration (conducted by large fibres): sensory loss delops in a characteristic 'glove and stocking' pattern. When motor fibres are affected, wasting and weakness of intrinsic foot muscles cause flexor/extensor imbalance, while wasting gives rise to foot deformities including claw toes. Muscular dysfunction contributes to the development of the diabetic foot. Loss of pain and perception of temperature carries the risk of trauma and thermal injury, which further contribute to the genesis of diabetic foot problems or gangrene. The salient features of diabetic neuropathy are summarized in Table 7. Pain of the leg is usually present at night-time, in contrast to the patin from arterio-occlusive disease. It can severely impair the quality of life. Recently, some short-term benefit has been shown from administration of the antioxidant α-lipoic acid (Ziegler *et al.* 1995; Ametov *et al.* 2003). Tricyclic antidepressants or carbamazepine may be helpful, and, as an ultima ratio, mexiletine has been tried. This necessitates tight electrocardiogram (ECG) monitoring (Luft 1999). The neuropathic Charcot joint is usually the result of minor injury, for example, tripping, and gives rise to a hot and swollen, but often painless foot. The extremity should be rested until swelling has resolved. Sequential radiographs usually show fragmentation of bones and reactive new bone formation resulting in a more or less advanced disorganization of the joint (Fig. 3). Neuropathic ulcers (mal perforant) are common in diabetic patients with renal failure (Fig. 4). They are usually found under the metatarsal head and the tips of the toes and in the region of the heels. They are the result of haematomata and tissue necrosis underneath a callus. Predisposing factors are repetitive painless injury, for instance by wearing ill fitting shoes. Infection and gangrene are major complications. The management is discussed in the next paragraph.

Mononeuritis multiplex, wasting and paresis of skeletal muscles are relatively rare complications. Sudden sensory and motor loss may occur in a distribution corresponding to single peripheral nerves, presumably as a result of vascular damage. In patients with high fistula flow, usually PTFE grafts, ischaemia resulting from a steal phenomenon may cause monomeric neuropathy (Miles 1999).

Diabetic amyotrophy is also relatively rare: this is thought to be a primary myopathic disturbance, symmetrically affecting muscles, most commonly of the shoulder girdle. Autonomic neuropathy poses the most difficult and most serious clinical problems in the diabetic patient with endstage renal failure. In the initial stages it can be recognized by the lack of heart rate variation in response to respiration or upright posture (beat-to-beat-variation). This can be documented by ECG. Common clinical problems resulting from autonomic denervation are:

(1) neurogenic bladder with residual urine formation;

(2) gastroparesis with reduced gastric motility and vomiting;

(3) episodes of prolonged constipation interrupted by explosive nocturnal diarrhoea; and

(4) erectile impotence (the relative contributions of vascular and neurogenic factors in the genesis of impotence vary from patient to patient).

To exclude residual urine in a neurogenic bladder, postvoiding bladder ultrasonography should be performed in every diabetic patient with renal failure. In the elderly male with prostatic adenoma, the distinction between neurogenic bladder, subvesical obstruction, and the combination of both is difficult and requires urodynamic investigation. Unless infection is present, even considerable volumes of the residual urine are remarkably well tolerated and are best left alone. Delayed and irregular gastric emptying may make metabolic control difficult because of the temporal dissociation between food ingestion and food absorption.

Table 7 Clinical consequences of diabetic neuropathy

Sensorimotor neuropathy
Loss of pain and thermal sensation
Lancinating (nocturnal) pain
Sensory loss (stocking-glove pattern)
Muscular wasting and paresis (lower limb)
(Mononeuritis multiplex)
(Diabetic amyotrophy)

Autonomous neuropathy
Loss of beat-to-beat variation
Orthostatic hypotension (with supine hypertension)
Gastroparesis
Constipation (nocturnal diarrhoea)
Neurogenic bladder
Impotence
Increased peripheral blood flow ('hot' extremities)
Reduced sweating
Neuropathic oedema
Neuropathic foot ulcer
Neuropathic (Charcot) joint

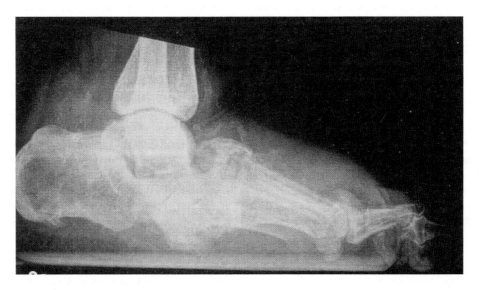

Fig. 3 Destruction of foot skeleton in a diabetic patient with a 'Charcot joint'.

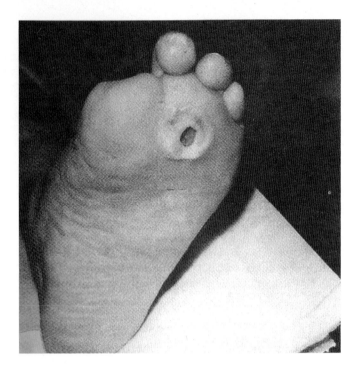

Fig. 4 Mal perforant of a 46-year-old female diabetic. Type 2 diabetes known for 11 years. Pulses were palpable. Ulceration developed following subepidermal haematoma.

Gastroparesis is also a common cause of nausea and vomiting in the diabetic patient with renal failure. It may respond to the administration of the dopamine antagonist metoclopramide or treatment with erythromycin which stimulates intestinal motility. Gastroparesis may render glycaemic control difficult because of the temporal dissociation between absorption of food from the gastrointestinal tract and resorption of postprandially administered subcutaneous insulin. It may also make antihypertensive treatment problematic because of delayed transport of antihypertensive medication out of the stomach into the intestine where the medication is absorbed. In diabetic patients with relatively modest elevation of blood urea nitrogen, vomiting as a result of documented gastroparesis which had failed to respond to drug treatment may promptly disappear after starting dialysis treatment. Among the consequences of autonomic polyneuropathy some problems may seriously interfere with patient comfort and social function, for example, constipation, diarrhoea, and incontinence. Diarrhoea is often nocturnal, may be explosive and result from disturbed intestinal motility with or without bacterial overgrowth. Bacterial overgrowth may respond to intermittent doses of doxycycline or metronidazole. Constipation may respond to cascara and psyllium seeds. Diarrhoea may respond to loperamide.

The consequences of sympathetic denervation of the limb are increased blood flow and reduced swetting typically producing a hot pink dry foot with thick plaques of hyperkeratotic material that predisposes to fissure formation, ulceration, and infection (see next paragraph).

The most dire complications of autonomic polyneuropathy are the result of cardiac denervation (Margolis *et al.* 1973) which is associated with silent ischaemia (Murray *et al.* 1990) and silent myocardial infarction (Acharya *et al.* 1991). It is commonly thought that autonomic neuropathy increases the risk of cardiac death in diabetic (Chen *et al.* 2001) and in non-diabetic patients (La Rovere *et al.* 1998), although the underlying mechanisms are still controversial (Airaksinen 2001). The clinical hallmarks are low variability of the heart rate and abnormal cardiocirculatory reflexes, which carry an adverse prognosis (Maser *et al.* 1990), particularly when this is combined with postural hypotension (Luukinen *et al.* 1999). Diabetics with severe autonomic polyneuropathy are prone to incidents during general anaesthesia with respiratory arrest (Knüttgen *et al.* 1990). When such patients are on HD they tolerate volume removal poorly and develop intradialytic hypotension. Finally, autonomic polyneuropathy is thought to contribute to hypoglycaemia and hypoglycaemia unawareness, although this issue is currently moot.

The foot in diabetes (Figs 3–5)

Foot lesions are the single most commonly mismanaged problem of the diabetic patient with renal insufficiency. They account to a large extent for more frequent and prolonged hospitalization in these patients. Even today, many unnecessary amputations are performed (Schömig *et al.* 2000). Most foot problems result from neuropathy, a smaller proportion result from ischaemia secondary to peripheral arterial disease and many are due to a combination of both. The latter carry a particularly adverse prognosis. Table 8 summarizes the main distinguishing features. The rate of amputations in diabetic patients with uraemia is 10 times higher than in the diabetic population at large. In an ongoing German study in patients with type 2 diabetes on dialysis (4D study), 16 per cent of incident patients had a history of amputation and 44 per cent had clinical evidence of peripheral arterial disease (Wanner *et al.* 1999). The proportion of patients requiring amputation on dialysis is approximately 4 per cent per year (Eggers *et al.* 1999).

Amputation is much feared tragedy in the life of a diabetic patient. Above ankle amputation carries a postoperative mortality of 30 per cent, presumably because 40 per cent of patients with diabetic foot lesions have coronary heart disease (Schömig *et al.* 2000). More than one-third of the patients remain unable to care for themselves. The potential for rehabilitation after amputation is much poorer in diabetic compared to non-diabetic amputees. Patients may lose self-management to a degree that necessitates institutional care (Schömig *et al.* 2000). The best evidence that appropriate management prevents an excess of amputations comes from Sweden (Larsson *et al.* 1995), where so-called 'foot clinics' providing appropriate interdisciplinary care for patients with diabetic foot lesions reduced amputations, particularly above ankle amputations (mostly resulting from peripheral arterial disease) by up to 80 per cent, but also below ankle amputations (mostly resulting from neuropathic foot lesions) by up to 50 per cent.

The distinction between neuropathic and ischaemic foot lesions is important, because the interventional strategies are different.

Neuropathy disrupts the equilibrium of muscle forces as a result of atrophy of the anterior muscles of the lower leg and of the lumbrical and intraosseous muscles, thus destabilizing the metatarsophalangeal joint. The forefoot is also exposed to unphysiologically high pressures because of the aductor varus position of the toes. Mechanical trauma is further aggravated by reduced viscoelasticity resulting from stiffening of connective tissue, loss of fat tissue, and oedema formation as a result of capillary hypertension. Because of lower limb muscle dysfunction and disturbed innervation, the foot hits the ground in an

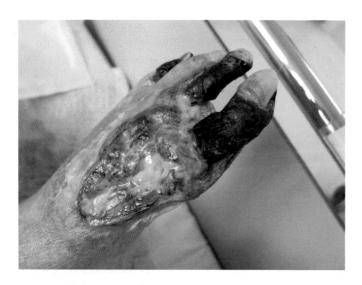

Fig. 5 Acral necrosis (ischaemic foot) in a 64-year-old female diabetic patient with end-stage renal failure.

Table 8 Foot lesions in diabetic patients

Neuropathic	Ischaemic
Painless	Painful (intermittent claudication)
Foot warm, pink	Foot cold, livid
Foot pulses + + (unless severe oedema)	Foot pulses − (+)
Sensation impaired	Sensation unimpaired
Painless metatarsal ulcer, necrosis below callus	Acral necrosis of tip of toe and of heel

Table 9 Characteristics of peripheral arterial disease of the lower extremity in diabetes mellitus

Accelerated course
Frequency similar in men and women
Lower limb vessels affected in 70%
Frequent involvement of deep femoral artery
Frequent calcification of media of arteries
Intermittent claudication often absent

uncoordinated manner. Further factors predisposing to ulcers are anhidrosis causing dry skin with formation of cracks and fissures as well as capillary hypertension with formation of oedema.

Characteristic for the diabetic with ischaemic foot lesions is the preferential involvement of the lower leg and the frequent involvement of the deep femoral artery (Table 9). Frequently multiple arterial segments are stenosed. Patients frequently fail to report claudication because of denervation by polyneuropathy. Calcification of the media is a risk predictor for severe atherosclerotic lesions of the intima. It is also important because it makes measurements of arterial pressure unreliable.

In both the neuropathic and ischaemic variety the catastrophe is often triggered by trivial events, for example, tight shoes, minor trauma, inadequate foot care (e.g. inadvertent cuts during nail trimming) etc. The initial lesion in the neuropathic foot is usually a metatarsal hyperkeratotic plaque with necrosis underneath, whereas the ischaemic lesion usually starts as a superficial blister or ulcer of toes or heel. The major aggravating factor is infection. Ports of entry are often ingrowing nails, paronychia, fissures, and interdigital mycosis. The most feared complication is spread of infection to ligaments, tendons, and bones. The diagnosis of osteomyelitis by X-ray is difficult. The distinction from Charcot's foot (see preceding paragraph) is often

difficult. The major antibiotics currently used for systemic treatment include chinolones, betalactan antibiotics with or without clavulanic acid, cephalosporines, clindamycin, and metronidazole. Recently, an increasing prevalence of MRSA has been noted. The most feared complication is spread of infection to ligaments, tendons, and bones. Patients with diabetic gangrene should be hospitalized and managed according to recently standardized guidelines (Pinzur *et al.* 1999) with the aim to control infection, to assess the potential need for revascularization or amputation and to provide long-term adequate foot care and foot wear to prevent recurrence (Schömig *et al.* 2000).

If correctable ischaemia is present this intervention has priority. Otherwise surgical debridement, removal of necrotic tissue, and antiseptic measures are indicated. One has to remove callus and luxuriant growth and has to relieve pressure from massive tissue infiltration by broad incisions. If tendons and bones are affected, minimal surgery should be considered, for example, resection of metatarsal heads or toes. To increase fibroblast proliferation moist wound dressings should subsequently be applied. To promote epithelialization tulle gras dressings should be used. In contrast, ischaemic gangrenous toes must be kept dry and the surrounding skin must be cleaned. If at all possible one should wait for spontaneous demarcation.

Prophylaxis of the diabetic foot syndrome requires adequate education and motivation of the patient. The salient features are summarized in Table 10.

Cardiac problems in the diabetic patient

Even prior to dialysis (Stack and Bloembergen 2001) heart disease is more frequent in diabetic (46.4 per cent) than non-diabetic patients (32.2 per cent). This includes myocardial infarction, angina pectoris, necessity for coronary artery bypass grafting (CABG), or percutaneous transluminal coronary angioplasty (PTCA), or a pathological coronary angiogram, and congestive heart failure. In preterminal diabetic patients compared to non-diabetic patients, the odds ratio for a new CV event is 5.3 (Levin *et al.* 2001) and progression, that is, either new events or worsening of existing pathology is seen in 20 per cent of the patients over a 23-month follow-up period. The odds ratio for a new event in diabetic compared to non-diabetic patients is 5.3 and this difference was highly significant. In 433 Canadian patients, 116 of whom were diabetics, the latter had more frequently left ventricular hypertrophy (LVH), ischaemic heart disease, and congestive heart failure (Table 11). No difference between diabetic and non-diabetic patients was found with respect to *de novo* appearance or progression of LVH and congestive heart failure. In contrast, the relative risks to develop ischaemic heart disease *de novo* and to die from CV causes were

Table 10 Prevention of diabetic foot problems in the diabetic patient

Avoid walking barefoot to prevent trauma
Avoid tight footwear
Use orthopedic shoes to relieve pressure on deformed foot
Use correct technique (filing) to trim toenails
Have corns treated by physician or chiropodist only
Treat fungal infections
Use foot powder for sweaty feet
Use lanolin ointment for dry skin
Inspect feet regularly
Exercise daily to improve collateral blood flow

Table 11 Cardiac findings in diabetic patients on dialysis (after Foley et al. 1997)

Baseline	Diabetic patients ($n = 116$) (%)	Non-diabetic patients ($n = 317$) (%)	p
Concentric left ventricular hypertrophy	50	38	0.04
Ischaemic heart disease	32	18	0.003
Cardiac failure	48	24	0.00001

Follow-up	Adjusted relative risk (diabetic/non-diabetic)	p
Ischaemic heart disease	3.2	0.0002
Overall mortality	2.3	0.0001
Cardiovascular mortality	2.6	0.0001

significantly greater in dialysed diabetic compared to non-diabetic patients suggesting accelerated atherogenesis. It is of note that although transplantation reduces the risk of CV death it does not completely abrogate it. It was recently found that the hazard ratio to develop an acute coronary syndrome after transplantation was still 0.38 and the rate of new events was 0.79 per patient-year compared to 1.67 prior to transplantation (Hypolite et al. 2002).

If the diabetic patient on dialysis develops an acute coronary syndrome, his or her chances of survival are very poor (Herzog et al. 1998). Cardiac mortality at 1 year is 42 and at 5 years 75 per cent. Unfortunately, up to date interventions including lysis, PTCA, or CABG are not widely used in the high risk population of renal patients irrespective of the presence or absence of diabetes (Shlipak et al. 2002). The DIGAMI study documented the benefit of intensified insulin and glucose treatment (Malmberg et al. 1999), but this strategy has not been widely adopted in diabetic patients with renal failure although insulin resistance is present, even in non-diabetic uraemic patients (Dikow et al. 2002a). The risk of an adverse cardiac outcome in the diabetic patient with ischemic heart disease is amplified because of the coexistance of more severe LVH (Foley et al. 1997), congestive heart failure (Foley et al. 1998), disturbed sympathetic innervation (Standl and Schnell 2000), and microvessel disease (Amann and Ritz 2000).

Table 12 Comparison of cardiac intervention in diabetic and non-diabetic dialysis patients (after Herzog et al. 2002)

	Relative risk of all-cause death compared to PTCA without stent	
	PTCA + stent	Coronary artery bypass surgery
Non-diabetic	0.9 (0.86–0.97)	0.79 (0.7–0.85)
Diabetic	0.99[a] (0.91–1.08)	0.81[b] (0.75–0.86)

[a] $p = $ N.S.

[b] $p = 0.0001$.

A particular dilemma concerns the diagnosis of coronary heart disease. Because of autonomic polyneuropathy, coronary disease is often silent with episodes of silent myocardial ischaemia and silent myocardial infarction. Coronary heart disease is not well predicted by baseline or exercise ECG (the latter is difficult to perform in polyneuropathic patients with muscular atrophy or arterial occlusive disease). Conventional screening tests such as treadmill or exercise ECG are therefore unreliable. Dipyridamol thallium scans predict myocardial ischaemia, but are not well correlated to the findings on coronarography, that is, do not predict the presence of lesions necessitating intervention well. It has been recommended as a screening test, however. Unfortunately, the best approach is still to study the patient directly with coronary angiography if there is a suspicion of coronary heart disease, for example, LV dilatation on echocardiography, regional contraction abnormalities on echocardiography, sudden deterioration of cardiac function with pulmonary oedema, arrhythmia or an increase in troponin T concentration. Troponin T is excreted via the kidney and it has long been controversial whether it is a faithful predictor of myocardial ischaemia in the presence of renal failure, but this issue has recently been settled (Aviles et al. 2002). Troponin T concentrations are predictive of cardiac death (Mallamaci et al. 2002) even in the absence of overt coronary heart disease, presumably reflecting diffuse myocardial microvascular ischaemia. Nevertheless an acute major increase is a reliable indicator of myocardial infarction in the uraemic diabetic patient as well.

Much new information on interventions has become available. There is no doubt that interventional management is superior to conservative management with β-blockers (Manske et al. 1992). It had remained controversial, however, whether PTCA ($\pm$ stent) or coronary bypass is the preferred modality of treatment. Although prospective data are not available, very compelling observational informations in a large patient sample indicate that CABG has the disadvantage of higher in-hospital death rates (12.5 versus 5.4 per cent in PTCA), but the advantage of better long-term survival (56.9 versus 52.9 per cent) (Herzog et al. 1999). The most powerful predictors of cardiac death are old age and diabetes, the relative risk being 1.37 in diabetic compared to non-diabetic patients. Table 12 compares the results of cardiac intervention in diabetic and non-diabetic dialysis patients (Herzog et al. 2002). Compared to PTCA without stent, PTCA plus stent was superior in non-diabetic, but not in diabetic patients. Similar to the result of the BARI study in non-renal patients [The Bypass Angioplasty Revascularization Investigation (BARI) Investigators 1996] CABG was superior in both non-diabetic and diabetic patients. It is important that such benefit was seen only when internal mammary grafts were used and not saphenous bypass grafts. There is some discussion concerning the use of β-blockers and statines. Norepinephrine is predictive of cardiac death in dialysis patients (Zoccali *et al.* 2002). In dialysis patients with congestive heart failure, a prospective trial documented functional improvement by administration of carvedilol compared to placebo (Cice *et al.* 2001). We had strongly advocated more liberal use of β-blockers in patients with diabetes (Zuanetti *et al.* 1997), based on the observation that only 3 per cent of dialysed type 2 diabetic patients who died from cardiac causes had been on β-blockers, but no less than 30 per cent of those who survived (Koch *et al.* 1993). Survival benefit from administration of β-blockers has meanwhile also been suggested by an observational study indicating that the mortality was substantially lower in β-blocker treated dialysed patients, including diabetic patients (Bragg *et al.* 2002).

Concerning the prevention of cardiac disease current recommendation suggest that low-density lipoprotein (LDL)-cholesterol should be lowered to values less than 100 mg/dl in diabetic patients. An ongoing prospective trial examines whether tatines are also indicated in diabetic patients with advanced renal disease (Wanner *et al.* 1999). Table 13 summarizes the recommended measures to prevent coronary heart disease in the diabetic patient. Several predictors of cardiac death had been identified in diabetic patients, that is, a history of vascular disease, specifically myocardial infarction or angina pectoris (Koch *et al.* 1997), proliferative retinopathy and polyneuropathy (presumably inducing unbalanced autonomic cardiac innervation; Koch *et al.* 1993) and serum lipid levels (Tschöpe *et al.* 1992). The latter observation is remarkable because in non-diabetic patients on HD, an inverse relation exists between cholesterol and survival, presumably because low cholesterol is an index of malnutrition (Chertow *et al.* 2000). In prospective studies, strong predictors of CV death were smoking (Foley *et al.* 2003) as well as poor glycaemic control prior to dialysis (Wu *et al.* 1997) or on HD (Morioka *et al.* 2001).

Hypertension

At any given level of (glomerular filtration rate, GFR), blood pressure tends to be higher in diabetic compared to non-diabetic patients with renal failure.

Because of their beneficial effect on CV complications (The Heart Outcomes Prevention Evaluation Study Investigators 2000) and progression (Lewis *et al.* 1993, 2001; Brenner *et al.* 2001). ACE inhibitors or angiotensin receptor blockers are obligatory unless there are contraindications, for example, an acute increase in serum creatinine (renal artery stenosis, hypovolaemia, congestive heart failure) or hyperkalaemia

Table 13 Suggested preventive manoeuvres in diabetic patients with renal failure and risk of cardiovascular disease

Start intervention in early stage of renal disease
ACE inhibitors or angiotensin receptor blockers
Low target blood pressure values
Aspirin
Control of hypervolaemia (low salt intake, diuretics)
Statins (LDL-cholesterin < 100 mg/dl)
Treat anaemia

resistant to corrective manoeuvres such as administration of loop diuretics, dietary potassium restriction or correction of metabolic acidosis. Because pharmacological blockade of the RAS will lower glomerular capillary pressure and by implication GFR, an increase in serum creatinine is expected and should not deter from the administration of ACE inhibitors or angiotensin receptor blockers unless the serum creatinine concentration increases by more than approximately 50 per cent. In patients with initially very high serum creatinine concentrations, approximately 6 mg/dl if muscle mass is normal, administration of ACE inhibitors may lower GFR to such an extent that acute dialysis becomes necessary. At this stage of renal dysfunction these drugs are therefore, no longer the antihypertensive medication of first choice. In the IDNT trial (Lewis *et al.* 2001), administration of angiotensin receptor blockers extended the time until patients required dialysis. Therefore, the widely practised habit to withdraw ACE inhibitors or angiotensin receptor blockers in advanced renal failure in the hope of decreasing the serum creatinine concentration does not make sense, unless there has been an abrupt recent increase in serum creatinine. Because of their marked propensity to retain salt, patients with diabetic nephropathy are prone to develop hypervolaemia and oedema. Therefore dietary salt restriction and administration of loop diuretics are usually indicated. At least in monotherapy, thiazides are no longer sufficient once GFR is less than 30–50 ml/min. When the serum creatinine concentration is elevated, usually multidrug therapy on average with 3–5 antihypertensive agents is necessary to normalize blood pressure.

Glucose control

On the one hand, renal failure causes insulin resistance, amongst others by cumulation of a (hypothetical) circulating factor interfering with the action of insulin. As a result, patients tend to develop impaired glucose tolerance and hyperglycaemia. Since the hypothetical low circulating insulin inhibitor is apparently dialysable, insulin resistance is improved after the start of dialysis.

On the other hand, the half-life of insulin is prolonged, predisposing the patient to develop hypoglycaemic episodes. This risk is further compounded by anorexia and by cumulation of most sulfonylurea compounds (with the exception of gliquidone or glimerpiride). Glinides and glitazones do not cumulate, but long-term safety data in renal failure are not available.

It follows from the above that the net result of these opposing influences is difficult to predict, so that close monitoring of glycaemia is advisable. In the treatment of these patients there is an increasing tendency to use short acting insulins with or without a basis of long acting insulin more liberally to prevent catabolism and malnutrition. Insulin administration is obligatory during intercurrent illness, infection, surgery, or myocardial infarction (Malmberg 1999).

Malnutrition

Diabetic patients with renal failure are often severely catabolic and tend to develop malnutrition. This risk is particularly high during periods of intercurrent illness and fasting, but may also be the result of ill-advised recommendations to restrict protein intake, particularly when these anorectic patients concomitantly reduce energy intake. Malnutrition is a potent independent predictor of mortality (Flanigan *et al.* 2001) and its presence justifies an early start of renal replacement treatment. Anorectic obese patients with type 2 diabetes and advanced renal failure often undergo massive weight loss, leading to normalization of fasting flucose and even of glycaemia after a glucose load. The diagnosis of Kimmelstiel–Wilson's glomerulosclerosis then requires documentation of retinopathy or renal biopsy. Low muscle mass because of wasting is an important cause why physicians misjudge the severity of renal failure, since at any given level of GFR the serum creatinine concentration will then be spuriously low. Misjudgement of the extent of renal impairment may contribute to dosing errors of drugs which cumulate in renal failure and may also delay the start of renal replacement therapy. In cases of doubt, it is advised to measure or estimate (Cockroft–Gault formula) the creatinine clearance.

Anaemia

Patients with diabetic nephropathy tend to have more severe anaemia than non-diabetic patients. In a small series of type 1 diabetic patients (Bosman *et al.* 2001) nearly 50 per cent of the patients were anaemic, compared to matched control patients with glomerulonephritis. More severe anaemia in type 2 diabetic patients with more advanced renal disease compared to matched non-diabetic controls was also found by Ishimura *et al.* (1998) and by ourselves (Schwenger *et al.* 2001). A multivariate analysis in a retrospective cohort found that diabetes increased the odds of anaemia in renal disease (Kazmi *et al.* 2001). Interestingly diabetic patients have a similar increase in plasma erythropoietin (EPO) in response to hypoxia compared to healthy individuals (Bosman *et al.* 2002), but inadequately low EPO concentrations in relation to the degree of anaemia (Dikow *et al.* 2002b). Interestingly, a low EPO concentration is a predictor of more rapid loss of renal function (Inomata *et al.* 1997). There is some evidence that anaemia is associated with more severe diabetic retinopathy (Shorb 1985) and that reversal of anaemia causes regression of macula oedema (Friedman *et al.* 1995). The role of anaemia and its reversal by EPO in patients with peripheral artery disease is unclear. One retrospective study claimed an adverse effect (Wakeen and Zimmermann 1998), but the relative roles of improving oxygen supply versus increasing viscosity and potential adverse effects on microrheology have not been worked out. Anaemia has also been claimed to either improve (Spaia *et al.* 2000) or aggravate (Rigalleau *et al.* 1998) insulin resistance, but confounding effects of EPO treatment on appetite and food intake have not been excluded. There are some intriguing suggestions that reversal of anaemia even ameliorates the rate of progression of renal disease (Kuriyama *et al.* 1997; Jungers *et al.* 2001), but controlled evidence with sufficient biostatistical power is not available.

Current guidelines suggest work-up for anemia when Hb is less than 12 g/dl in adult males and postmenopausal females and less than 11 g/dl in premenopausal females (European Best Practice Guidelines 1999). Two major studies currently investigate whether prevention of anaemia by administration of EPO ameliorates CV surrogate markers and improves outcome. Currently expert groups recommend a target Hb of 12 g/dl.

Management of terminal renal failure

Vascular access

Timely creation of a vascular access is of over-riding importance. This should be considered when the GFR is approximately 20–25 ml/min.

Although venous run-off problems are not unusual because of hypoplastic veins, particularly in elderly female diabetics or venous occlusion from infections or infusions, inadequate arterial inflow is increasingly recognized as a major cause of fistula malfunction (Konner *et al.* 2003). If radial arteries are severely sclerotic, anastomosis at a more proximal level may be necessary. Use of native vessels is clearly the first choice (Konner 2000) and results of PTFE grafts are definitely inferior. It is often necessary to create an upper arm av fistula (Konner 2000; Revanur *et al.* 2000; Dixon *et al.* 2002) or use sophisticated surgical approaches (Gefen *et al.* 2002). The underlying cause is the inability of a sclerotic radial artery to undergo vasodilatation and remodelling to permit an increase in blood flow from 10–20 ml/min to 1000 ml/min (Konner *et al.* 2003). Arteriosclerosis of arm arteries not only jeopardizes fistula flow, but also predisposes to a 'steal phenomenon' with finger gangrene (Yeager *et al.* 2002).

Initiation of renal replacement therapy

Most nephrologists agree that in diabetic compared to non-diabetic patients renal replacement therapy should be started earlier at a GFR of approximately 15 ml/min. An even earlier start may be justified when hypervolaemia and blood pressure become uncontrollable, when the patient is severely anorectic or cachectic and when the patient vomits as the combined result of uraemia and gastroparesis. Clinical findings are more important than laboratory values.

Haemodialysis

In recent years, survival of diabetic patients on HD has tended to improve. Several years ago, the 5-year survival in type 2 diabetic patients on HD did not exceed 10 per cent, but was 40 per cent in the younger type 1 diabetic patients (Koch *et al.* 1997). Recently, however, it has risen to approximately 30 per cent and astonishingly good survival rates, that is, 50 per cent in 5 years in dialysed diabetic patients have been reported from East Asia. To a large extent these differences between countries reflect the frequency of CV death in the background population.

Inter- and intradialytic blood pressure

Dialysed diabetic patients tend to be more hypertensive than dialysed non-diabetic patients. In diabetic patients blood pressure is exquisitely volume-dependent. The problem is compounded by the fact that patients are predisposed to intradialytic hypotension, so that it is very difficult to reach the target 'dry weight' by ultrafiltration. Nevertheless, reduced dietary salt intake and ultrafiltration often permit to control hypertension without medication, but most patients need antihypertensive drugs. The main causes of intradialytic hypotension are disturbed counterregulation (autonomic polyneuropathy) on the one hand and disturbed left ventricular compliance with an abrupt decrease of cardiac output when left ventricular filling pressure diminishes during ultrafiltration on the other hand (Daugirdas 2001). One or more of the following approaches are useful to avoid intradialytic hypotension: omission of antihypertensive agents immediately before dialysis sessions, long dialysis sessions, lowering of dialysate temperature, controlled ultrafiltration, correction of anemia by EPO therapy. If nothing works, however, alternative treatment modalities such as haemofiltration and CAPD should be considered. Intradialytic hypotension increases the risk of cardiac death by a factor of 3 (Koch *et al.* 1993). It also predisposes to myocardial ischaemia, arrhythmia, deterioration of maculopathy and, particularly in the elderly, non-thrombotic mesenteric infarction. Sudden death on dialysis is preceded by a hypotensive episode in up to 30 per cent of patients (Karnik *et al.* 2001). Pulse pressure and impaired elasticity of central arteries are major predictors of CV events and of death in non-uraemic patients and in non-diabetic dialysed patients, but for uncertain reasons not so in diabetic patients on dialysis (Tozawa *et al.* 2002).

Metabolic control on haemodialysis

Dialysis treatment partially reverses insulin resistance, so that insulin requirements are often less than before dialysis. Even patients with type 1 diabetes may occasionally lose their need for insulin, at least transiently, upon institution of HD. In other patients, however, insulin requirements increase, presumably because anorexia is reversed so that appetite and food consumption increase. It is most convenient to use a dialysate which contains glucose usually about 200 mg/dl. This allows insulin to be administered at the usual times of the day, reduces the risk of hyper- or hypoglycaemic episodes and also causes less hypotensive episodes (Simic-Ogrizovic *et al.* 2001).

Adequate control of glycaemia is important because hyperglycaemia causes thirst, high fluid intake and hypervolaemia as well as an osmotic shift of water and K^+ from the intracellular to the extracellular space. The consequences are circulatory congestion and hyperkalaemia. Diabetics with poor glucose control are also more susceptible to infection. Finally, in dialysed diabetic patients poor glycaemic control definitely increases the risk of death, mainly from CV causes (Morioka *et al.* 2001).

Asssessment of glycaemic control using HbA1c is confounded by carbamylation of Hb and by altered red blood cell survival (Joy *et al.* 2002). Hba1c values above 7.5 per cent cause modest overestimation of hyperglycaemia in diabetic patients with (end-stage renal disease) ESRD. Diminished insulin-mediated glucose uptake as evidence of insulin resistance has been noted in the hearts of uraemic animals (Ritz and Koch 1993) and this has been related to reduced ischaemia tolerance of the heart (Amann and Ritz 2000). Insulin should presumably be administered more generously and this might also be beneficial to control malnutrition and anaemia management (Pinero-Pilona *et al.* 2002).

In view of the dramatic results of insulin and glucose administration after myocardial infarction (Malmberg 1997) and of the impressive benefit from intensive insulin therapy in critically ill patients, particularly in those with acute renal failure (Van den Berghe *et al.* 2001), administration of insulin is advisable in diabetic patients with ischaemic heart disease.

Malnutrition on haemodialysis

Because of anorexia and prolonged habituation to dietary restriction, the dietary intake of diabetic patients on HD often falls short of the required intake of energy (30–35 kcal/kg/d) and protein (1.3 g/kg/d). By X-ray absorptiometry, Okuno *et al.* (2001) documented a decrease in body fat mass in diabetic compared to non-diabetic patients on HD. This finding is particularly problematic because malnutrition is a potent predictor of mortality. It is also of concern that malnutrition and/or microinflammation tend to be more common in diabetic patients (Suliman *et al.* 2002). Indicators of malnutrition predict survival of diabetic patients on HD (Cano *et al.* 2002).

Peritoneal dialysis

According to the United States Renal Data System (USRDS) (2001) 7.1 per cent of all patients with diabetes receiving renal replacement therapy are treated with peritoneal dialysis (PD), whilst 75.4 per cent receive maintenance HD and 17.5 per cent undergo transplantation. The proportion of diabetic patients treated by PD varies widely between countries, illustrating that selection of treatment modalities is also strongly influenced by logistics and reimbursement policies. There are often good a priori reasons to offer initially CAPD treatment to diabetic patients. In diabetic patients with ESRD, forearm vessels are often sclerosed, so that it is not easy to create a fistula. The alternative of HD via intravenous catheters (instead of using av fistulas or grafts) is not sufficient in the long run, because blood flow is low and the risk of infections high. Long-term dialysis via catheters was identified as one major predictor of poor survival on HD (Sehgal *et al.* 2002).

There are further reasons to offer PD as the initial mode of renal replacement therapy to the diabetic patient. According to Heaf *et al.* (2002), during the first 2 years survival is better for patients treated with PD compared to HD and this was also true for diabetic patients except in the very elderly (Winkelmayer *et al.* 2002). The survival advantage was no longer demonstrable beyond the second year (presumably because by then residual renal function has decayed). Moreover, PD provides low and sustained ultrafiltration without rapid fluctuations of fluid volume and electrolyte concentrations (features which are advantageous for blood pressure control and prevention of heart failure).

An interesting concept has been proposed by Van Biesen *et al.* (2000). When patients started PD and were then transferred to HD after residual renal function had decayed, they had better long-term survival compared to patients who started on HD and remained on HD throughout. As a potential explanation it has been proposed that early start on CAPD prevents cumulative organ damage in the late stages of uraemia. Survival of patients who had remained on CAPD for more than 48 months, however, was inferior when compared to patients on HD, presumably because CAPD is no longer sufficiently effective once residual renal function has gone, at least in heavy patients. These optimistic views have recently been challenged by the result of a national survey in the United States, which showed that even in the initial years of treatment survival on CAPD was worse, particularly in diabetic patients with coronary heart disease (Winkelmayer *et al.* 2002). It is relevant that CAPD treatment is not a contraindication to renal transplantation.

In the past it was felt to be an attractive concept to administer insulin by injection into the CAPD fluid with the goal of providing insulin via the more physiological portal route. Unfortunately there are many practical problems: uncertainties of dosage, since insulin binds to the surface of dialysis bags and tubing (Twardowski *et al.* 1983) and is degraded by insulinases in the peritoneum (Khanna and Oreopoulos 1986). Moreover, absorption from the peritoneal cavity shows large interindividual variations. There is no firm evidence that the procedure permits better control of glycaemia or dyslipidaemia (Nevalainen *et al.* 1996). As a result, most nephrologists do no longer use this approach.

Although protein is lost across the peritoneal membrane, the main nutritional problem is gain of glucose and calories, because high glucose concentrations in the dialysate are necessary for the osmotic removal of excess body fluid. This leads to weight gain and obesity. Daily glucose absorption is 100–150 g and a CAPD patient is exposed to 3–7 tons of fluid containing 50–175 kg glucose per year. The use of glucose-containing fluid has another interesting disadvantage. Heat sterilization of glucose under acid conditions creates highly reactive glucose degradation products (GDPs) such as methylglyoxal, glyoxal-formaldehyde, deoxyglucosone and 3,4-dideoxyglucosone-3-ene (Linden et al. 2002). GDPs are cytotoxic and lead also to the formation of advanced glycation end products (AGE). Even in non-diabetic patients on CAPD, deposits of AGE are found in the peritoneal membrane and this is accompanied by fibrogenesis and neoangiogenesis with deterioration of peritoneal membrane properties. These observations led to the snappy, but misleading, term 'local diabetes mellitus'. Heat sterilization using two compartment bags circumvents the generation of toxic GDP. In prospective studies, CAPD fluid thus sterilized was much less toxic than conventional CAPD fluids despite the high glucose concentration (Rippe et al. 2001).

Transplantation in the diabetic patient (kidney alone and pancreas plus kidney)

Outcome of kidney transplantation

There is consensus that medical rehabilitation of the diabetic patient with uraemia is best after transplantation (Wolfe et al. 1999). Although survival of the diabetic patient with a kidney graft is worse compared with a grafted non-diabetic patient the gain in life expectancy of the diabetic patient with a graft, compared with the dialysed diabetic patient on the waiting list, is proportionally much greater than in the non-diabetic patients. This is so because survival of the diabetic patient is so poor on dialysis. The higher mortality of the diabetic compared to the non-diabetic patient with a kidney graft is mainly explained as the consequence of pre-existing vascular disease (Hypolite et al. 2002), LVH and post-transplant hypertension. Wolfe et al. (1999) calculated the adjusted relative risk of death of transplant recipients as compared with patients on the waiting list. It was 0.27 for diabetic patients compared to 0.39 in non-diabetic patients with glomerulonephritis. Obviously, the perioperative risk is greater in diabetic than in non-diabetic patients, but nevertheless in diabetic patients the predicted survival on the waiting list was only 8 years and after transplantation no less than 19 years. The majority of diabetic patients receiving a transplant are currently C-peptide negative type 1, although in carefully selected type 2 diabetic patients without vascular disease who had received kidney grafts, graft and patients survival are impressive (Mieghem et al. 2001). Diabetic patients must be subjected to rigorous pretransplantation evaluation which includes in most centres routine coronary angiography (Zeier and Ritz 2002). As an alternative Manske et al. (1993) have devised an algorithm to identify the diabetic patient who should receive coronarography. Patients should also be examined by Doppler sonography of pelvic arteries and if necessary angiography to avoid placement of a renal allograft into an iliac artery with compromised arterial flow risking ischaemia of the extremity and amputation.

Kidney plus pancreas transplantation

Despite great excitement about the seminal double transplantation by Kelly et al. (1967) in Minneapolis the results of simultaneous pancreas

and kidney transplantation (SPK) had remained disappointing for a long time. The breakthrough came with the introduction of calcineurin inhibitors and low steroids protocols. In an impressivly large single-centre experience comprising 335 patients Becker et al. (2000) recently showed that survival of patients with SPK approached that of patients transplanted for non-diabetic renal disease and was clearly superior to diabetic recipients of living donor kidney grafts and particularly of cadaver kidney grafts (Fig. 6). The Kaplan–Meier estimate of patient survival in 215 SPK versus 111 live donor kidney graft recipients after 10 years was 82 versus 71 per cent. The annual mortality rate was 1.5 per cent for SPK recipients, 3.65 per cent for living donor kidney grafts recipients and 6.27 per cent for cadaver donor kidney grafts recipients. Reversibility of established microvascular complications after SPK is minor at best, with the important exception of autonomic polyneuropathy (Tyden et al. 1999), particularly improved cardiorespiratory reflexes potentially contributing to increased survival (Nvarro et al. 1996) and some improvement in nerve conduction velocity (Solders et al. 1995). Further benefits include improved gastric and bladder function (Hathaway et al. 1994), as well as superior quality of life, better metabolic control (Kahl et al. 2001a,b), improved survival (Becker et al. 2000). Consequently, today SPK should be the preferred treatment modality for the type 1 diabetic who meets the selection criteria. As of 2002, 17,000 pancreas transplants have been performed, the majority in the United States. There is an increasing tendency for early or even pre-emptive SPK. Because graft outcome is progressively more adverse with increasing time spent on HD (Mange et al. 2001) this strategy is sensible. In the United States, diabetics less than 55 years of age are usually considered for SPK at a GFR less than 40 ml/min, while criteria in Europe are more conservative with a GFR less than 20 ml/min (Kahl et al. 2001a,b). Exclusion criterias are amongst others active smoking, morbid obesity, (uncorrected) CV disease etc. The indications for pancreas transplantation in non-uraemic patients have not been established.

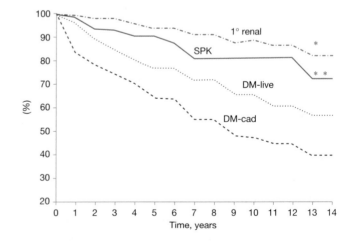

Fig. 6 Kaplan–Meier patient survival estimates in diabetic patients after simultaneous pancreas–kidney (SPK), cadaveric (DM-cad), or live-donor kidney transplantation (DM-live), compared to patients with non-diabetic primary renal disease undergoing cadaveric kidney transplantation (1° renal) (after Becker et al. 2000). * p = 0.0029 1° versus all others; ** p = 0.004 SPK versus DM-Cad, DM-Live.

Pancreas after kidney transplantation

An alternative strategy must be considered in the diabetic patient who has a life kidney donor: to first transplant the living donor kidney, and subsequently, once stable renal function is achieved (GFR > 50 ml/min), to transplant a cadaver donor pancreas. The outcomes are quite satisfactory (Hariharan *et al.* 2002).

Transplantation of pancreas segments obtained from living donors is still an experimental procedure (Gruessner *et al.* 2001).

Procedure and management

Today the preferred SPK technique is enteric drainage. Bladder drainage has been increasingly abandoned because of irritation of mucosa, development of strictures, bicarbonate wasting with metabolic acidosis, recurrent urinary tract infections and reflux pancreatitis.

Oral glucose tolerance normalizes unless the graft is damaged by ischaemia or subclinical rejection related to HLA-DR mismatch (Pfeffer *et al.* 1996). Most investigators find either normalization of insulin sensitivity (Cottrell 1996) or some impairment of insulin stimulated non-oxidated glucose metabolism (Christiansen *et al.* 1996) with hepatic insulin resistance (Rooney and Robertson 1996) possibly related to insulin delivery into the systemic circulation (as opposed to the physiological delivery into the portal circulation) (Barrou *et al.* 1994). Impressive normalization of lipoprotein lipase activity and of the lipid spectrum pointing to reduced atherogenic risk (Hughes *et al.* 1995; Foger *et al.* 1996) have also been reported. Finally, insulin mediated protein turnover is normalized (Luzi *et al.* 1994). An interesting issue is whether rejection affects kidney and pancreatic grafts in parallel. Although this is mostly so (permitting to use the renal function as a surrogate marker of rejection of the pancreas) it is by no means obligatory, but episodes of isolated rejection of the pancreas are rare so that monitoring the kidney graft is the usual procedure. The pancreatic graft can be monitored by duplex sonography, if necessary, or pancreas graft biopsy. Pancreas grafts are usually lost because of alloimmunity reactions, but in rare cases graft loss resulting from destruction by autoimmune mechanisms (with GAD-antibodies and IA2-antibodies) has been observed (Tyden *et al.* 1996). Recurrence of autoimmune inflammation with selective loss of insulin producing β-cells (while sparing glucagon, somatostatin, and pancreatic polypeptide secreting cells) and lymphocytic infiltration have been noted in the pioneer era when segmental pancreatic grafts were performed in monozygotic twins and when insulitis often recurred in the recipient (Sutherland *et al.* 1997). Today this has become rare, presumably because immunosuppression keeps autoimmunity under control. Rejection of the pancreas responds poorly to steroid treatment. Its treatment should always include T-cell antibodies. Poorly understood late problems after SPK include carpal tunnel syndrome (Mueller-Felber *et al.* 1993) and fracturing bone disease (Smets *et al.* 1998).

At present, an immunosuppression protocol based on tacrolimus and mycophenolate mofetil (MMF) is used as the standard in most centers around the world (International Pancreas Transplantation Registry Newsletter 2000). In 72 per cent of patients treated with a combination of tacrolimus/MMF it is possible to withdraw steroids within the first year after SPK (Kahl *et al.* 2001a,b). One-year rejection rates of 20 per cent are reported for SPK patients remaining on tacrolimus/MMF immunosuppression (Kaufmann *et al.* 1999). The role of sirolimus is currently under investigation.

Islet cell transplantation

Although more advanced procedures such as transplantation of stem cells or precursor cells, transplantation of encapsulated islet cells, islet xenotransplants, or insulin gene therapy are still beyond the horizon, islet cell transplantation has so far yielded some interesting, but not yet definitive results. As of 2002 worldwide 439 cases received islet cell transplants, mainly in eight centres. Patient survival was 79 per cent and 14 per cent of patient were off insulin, but measureable C-peptide greater than 0.5 ng/ml as evidence of residual islet function was noted in 45 per cent. Minor intraportal insulin secretion may be relevant because it may normalize hepatic glucose production (Luzi *et al.* 2001). This area got a major boost by the observation of Shapiro *et al.* (2000) who reported on successful islet transplantation achieving insulin independence in seven consecutive patients using a steroid-free immunosuppression regimen consisting of sirolimus, tacrolimus, and taclizumab. The generalizability of the results is currently evaluated by a multicentre study.

Diabetes in non-diabetic kidney graft recipients

A new aspect is the recent recognition that de novo appearance of type 2 diabetes is a frequent occurrence after renal transplantation of non-diabetic patients which is seen in up to 20 per cent of patients (Cosio *et al.* 2002). This is presumably the combined result of the diabetogenic action of calcineurin inhibitors, particularly tacrolimus, and unmasking of diabetes in individuals genetically predisposed to diabetes mellitus. It is interesting that *de novo* type 2 diabetes was particularly associated with hepatitis C infection in several series (Baid *et al.* 2002).

It is also of note that recently—contrasting with past teaching—transplantation of the kidneys of diabetic cadaver donors has been proposed as a measure to expand the donor pool (Becker *et al.* 2002).

References

Acharya, D. U., Shekhar, C., Aggarwal, A., and Annand, I. S. (1991). Lack of pain during myocardial infarction in diabetics—is autonomic dysfunction responsible? *American Journal of Cardiology* **68**, 793–796.

Adler, A. I., Stevens, R. J., Manley, S. E., Bilous, R. W., Cull, C. A., and Holman, R. R. (2003). Development and progression of nephropathy in type 2 diabetes: the United Kingdom Prospective Diabetes Study (UKPDS 64). *Kidney International* **63**, 225–232.

Airaksinen, K. E. J. (2001). Silent coronary artery disease in diabetes—a feature of autonomic neuropathy or accelerated atherosclerosis? *Diabetologia* **44**, 259–266.

Amann, K. and Ritz, E. (2000). Microvascular disease—the Cinderella of uraemic heart disease. *Nephrology, Dialysis, Transplantation* **15**, 1493–1503.

Ametov, A. S., Barinov, A., Dyck, P. J., Hermann, R., Kozlova, N., Litchy, W. J., Low, P. A., Nehrdich, D., Novosadova, M., O'Brien, P. C., Reljanovic, M., Samigullin, R., Schuette, K., Strokov, I., Tritschler, H. J., Wessel, K., Yakhno, N., and Ziegler, D. (2003). SYDNEY Trial Study Group: the sensory symptoms of diabetic polyneuropathy are improved with alpha-lipoic acid: the SYDNEY trial. *Diabetes Care* **26**, 770–776.

Amoah, E., Glickman, J. L., Maclchoff, C. D., Sturgill, B. C., Kaiser D. L., and Bolton, W. K. (1988). Clinical identification of nondiabetic renal disease in diabetic patients with type I and type II disease presenting with renal dysfunction. *American Journal of Nephrology* **8**, 204–211.

Aspelin, P., Aubry, P., Fransson, S. G., Strasser, R., Willenbrock, R., and Berg, K. J. (2003). Nephrotoxic effects in high-risk patients undergoing angiography. *New England Journal of Medicine* **348**, 491–499.

Aviles, R. J., Askari, A. T., Lindahl, B., Wallentin, L., Jia, G., Ohman, E. M., Mahaffey, K. W., Newby, L. K., Califf, R. M., Simoons, M. L., Topol, E. J., Berger, P., and Lauer, M. S. (2002). Troponin T levels in patients with acute coronary syndromes, with or without renal dysfunction. *New England Journal of Medicine* 346, 2047–2052.

Avram, M. M. *Proceedings of the Conference on Dialysis as a Practical Workshop.* National Union Catalogue, 1966.

Baid, S., Tolkoff-Rubin, N., Farrell, M., Delmonico, F., Williams, W., Hayden, D., Ko, D., Cosimi, A., and Pascual, M. (2002). Tacrolimus-associated post-transplant diabetes mellitus in renal transplant recipients: role of hepatitis C infection. *Transplantation Proceedings* 34, 1771.

Barrou, Z., Seaquist, E. R., and Robertson, R. P. (1994). Pancreas transplantation in diabetic humans normalizes hepatic glucose production during hypoglycemia. *Diabetes* 43, 661–666.

Becker, B. N., Brazy, P. C., Becker, Y. T., Odorico, J. S., Pintar, T. J., Collins, B. H., Pirsch, J. D., Leversen, G. E., Heisey, D. M., and Sollinger, H. W. (2000). Simultaneous pancreas–kidney transplantation reduces excess mortality in type 1 diabetes patients with end-stage renal disease. *Kidney International* 57, 2129–2135.

Becker, Y. T., Leverson, G. E., D'Alessandro, A. M., Sollinger, H. W., and Becker, B. N. (2002). Diabetic kidneys can safely expand the donor pool. *Transplantation* 74, 141–145.

Blagg, C. R., Eschbach, J. W., Sawyer, T. K., and Casaretto, A. A. (1971). Dialysis for end-stage diabetic nephropathy. *Proceedings of the Dialysis and the Transplantation Forum* 1, 133–135.

Bojestig, M., Arnquist, H. J., Hermansson, G., Karlberg, B. E., and Ludvigsson, J. (1994). Declining incidence of nephropathy in insulin-dependent diabetes mellitus. *New England Journal of Medicine* 330, 15–18.

Bosman, D. R., Winkler, A. S., Marsden, J. T., MacDougall, I. C., and Watkins, P. J. (2001). Anemia with erythropoietin deficiency occurs early in diabetic nephropathy. *Diabetes Care* 24, 495–499.

Bosman, D. R. *et al.* (2002). Erythropoietin response to hypoxia in patients with diabetic autonomic neuropathy and non-diabetic chronic renal failure. *Diabetic Medicine* 19, 65–69.

Bragg, J. L., Mason, N. A., Maroni, B. J., Held, P. J., and Young, E. W. (2002). Beta-adrenergic antagonist utilization among hemodialysis patients. Data from the DOPPS study. Lecture from the Annual Meeting of the American Society of Nephrology, Philadelphia.

Brenner, B. M., Cooper, M. E., De Zeeuw, D., Keane, W. F., Mitch, W. E., Parving, H. H., Remuzzi, G., Snapinn, S. M., Zhang, Z., and Shahinfar, S. (2001). Effects of losartan on renal and cardiovascular outcomes in patients with type 2 diabetes and nephropathy. *New England Journal of Medicine* 345, 861–869.

Cano, N. J., Roth, H., Aparicio, M., Azar, R., Canaud, B., Chauveau, P., Combe, C., Foque, D., Laville, M., and Leverve, X. M. (2002). Malnutrition in hemodialysis diabetic patients: evaluation and prognostic influence. *Kidney International* 62, 593–601.

Chantrel, F., Enache, I., Bouiller, M., Kolb, I., Kunz, K., Petitjean, P., Moulin, B., and Hannedouche, T. (1999). Abysmal prognosis of patients with type 2 diabetes entering dialysis. *Nephrology, Dialysis, Transplantation* 14, 129–136.

Chen, H. S., Hwu, C. M., Kuo, B. I., Chiang, S. C., Kwok, C. F., Lee, S. H., Lee Y. S., Weih, M. J., Hsiao, L. C., Lin, S. H., and Ho, L. T. (2001). Abnormal cardiovascular reflex tests are predictors of mortality in type 2 diabetes mellitus. *Diabetic Medicine* 18, 268–273.

Chertow, G. M., Johansen, K. L., Lew, N., Lazarus, J. M., and Lowrie, E. G. (2000). Vintage, nutritional status, and survival in hemodialysis patients. *Kidney International* 57, 1176–1181.

Christiansen, E. *et al.* (1996). Impaired insulin-stimulated nonoxidative glucose metabolism in pancreas–kidney transplant recipients: dose–response effects of insulin on glucose turnover. *Diabetes* 45, 1267–1275.

Cice, G., Ferrara, L., Di Benedetto, A., Russo, P. E., Marinelli, G., Pavese, F., and Iacono, A. (2001). Dilated cardiomyopathy in dialysis patients—beneficial effects of carvedilol: a double-blind, placebo-controlled trial. *Journal of the American College of Cardiology* 37, 407–411.

Cigarroa, R., Lange, R., Williams, R., and Willis, D. (1989). Dosing of contrast media to prevent contrast nephropathy in patients with renal disease. *American Journal of Medicine* 86, 649–652.

Cosio, F. G., Pesavento, T. E., Kim, S., Osei, K., Henry, M., and Ferguson, R. M. (2002). Patient survival after renal transplantation. IV. Impact of post-transplant diabetes. *Kidney International* 62, 1440–1446.

Cottrell, D. A. (1996). Normalization of insulin sensitivity and glucose homeostasis in type 1 diabetic pancreas transplant recipients: a 48-month cross-sectional study. A clinical research study. *Journal of Clinical Endocrinology and Metabolism* 81, 3513–3519.

Daugirdas, J. T. (2001). Pathophysiology of dialysis hypotension: an update. *American Journal of Kidney Diseases* 38, S11–S17.

Dikow, R. and Ritz, E. (2003a). Cardiovascular complications in the diabetic patient with renal disease—an update in 2003. *Nephrology, Dialysis, Transplantation* 18, 1993–1998.

Dikow, R. and Ritz, E. Hemodialysis and CAPD in type 1 and type 2 diabetic patients with endstage renal disease. In *The Kidney and Hypertension Diabetes Mellitus* 6th edn. (ed. C. E. Mogensen), 2003b.

Dikow, R., Adamczak, M., Henriquez, D. E., and Ritz, E. (2002a). Strategies to decrease cardiovascular mortality in patients with end-stage renal disease. *Kidney International* 80, 5–10.

Dikow, R., Schwenger, V., Schömig, M., and Ritz, E. (2002b). How should we manage anaemia in patients with diabetes? *Nephrology, Dialysis, Transplantation* 17 S67–S72.

Dixon, B. S., Novak, L., and Fangman, J. (2002). Hemodialysis vascular access survival: upper-arm native arteriovenous fistula. *American Journal of Kidney Diseases* 39, 92–101.

EBPG (1999). European Best Practice Guidelines for the management of anemia in patients with chronic renal failure. *Nephrology, Dialysis, Transplantation* 14 (Suppl. 5), 1–5.

Eggers, P. W., Gohdes, D., and Pugh, J. (1999). Nontraumatic lower extremity amputations in the Medicare end-stage renal disease population. *Kidney International* 56, 1524–1533.

Flanigan, M. J., Frankenfield, D. L., Prowant, B. F., Bailie, G. R., Frederick, P., and Rocco, M. V. (2001). Nutritional markers during peritoneal dialysis: data from the 1998 Peritoneal Dialysis Core Indicators Study. *Peritoneal Dialysis International* 21, 345–354.

Foger, B. *et al.* (1996). Effects of pancreas transplantation on distribution and composition of plasma lipoproteins. *Metabolism* 45, 856–861.

Foley, R. N., Culleton, B. F., Parfrey, P. S., Harnett, J. D., Kent, G. M., Murray, D. C., and Barre, P. E. (1997). Cardiac disease in diabetic end-stage renal disease. *Diabetologia* 40, 1307–1312.

Foley, R. N., Parfrey, P. S., and Sarnak, M. J. (1998). Epidemiology of cardiovascular disease in chronic renal disease. *Journal of the American Society of Nephrology* 9, S16–S23.

Foley, R. N., Herzog, C. A., and Collins, A. J. (2003). Smoking and cardiovascular outcomes in dialysis patients: the United States Renal Data System Wave 2 Study. *Kidney International* 63, 1462–1467.

Friedman, E. A., Brown, C. D., and Berman, D. H. (1995). Erythropoietin in diabetic macular edema and renal insufficiency. *American Journal of Kidney Diseases* 26, 202–208.

Gaede, P., Vedel, P., Larsen, N., Jensen, G. V., Parving, H. H., and Pedersen, O. (2003). Multifactorial intervention and cardiovascular disease in patients with type 2 diabetes. *New England Journal of Medicine* 348, 383–393.

Gefen, J. Y., Fox, D., Giangola, G., Ewing, D. R., and Meisels, I. S. (2002). The transposed forearm loop arteriovenous fistula: a valuable option for primary hemodialysis access in diabetic patients. *Annals of Vascular Surgery* 16, 89–94.

Ghavamian, M., Gutch, C. G., Kopp, K. F., and Kolff, W. J. (1972). The sad truth about hemodialysis in diabetic nephropathy. *Journal of the American Medical Association* 222, 1386–1389.

Gilbertson, D. T., Xue, J. L., and Collins, A. J. (2002). The increasing burden of diabetes in United States ESRD patients. *Journal of the American Society of Nephrology* 13, 646A.

Gruessner, R. W., Sutherland, D. E., Drangstveit, M. B., Bland, B. J., and Gruessner, A. C. (2001). Pancreas transplants from living donors: short- and long-term outcome. *Transplantation Proceedings* **33**, 819–820.

Hariharan, S., Pirsch, J. D., Lu, C. Y., Chan, L., Pesavento, T. E., Alexander, S., Bumgardner, G. L., Baasadona, G., Hricik, D. E., Pescovitz, M. D., Rubin, N. T., and Stratta, R. J. (2002). Pancreas after kidney transplantation. *Journal of the American Society of Nephrology* **13**, 1109–1118.

Hathaway, D. K. *et al.* (1994). Improvement in autonomic and gastric function following pancreas–kidney versus kidney-alone transplantation and the correlation with quality of life. *Transplantation* **57**, 816–822.

Heaf, J. G., Lokkegaard, H., and Madsen, M. (2002). Initial survival advantage of peritoneal dialysis relative to haemodialysis. *Nephrology, Dialysis, Transplantation* **17**, 112–117.

Herzog, C. A., Ma, J. Z., and Collins, A. J. (1998). Poor long-term survival after acute myocardial infarction among patients on long-term dialysis. *New England Journal of Medicine* **339**, 799–805.

Herzog, C. A., Ma, J. Z., and Collins, A. J. (1999). Long-term outcome of dialysis patients in the United States with coronary revascularization procedures. *Kidney International* **56**, 324–332.

Herzog, C. A., Ma, J. Z., and Collins, A. J. (2002). Comparative survival of dialysis patients in the United States after coronary angioplasty, coronary artery stenting, and coronary artery bypass surgery and impact of diabetes. *Circulation* **106**, 2207–2211.

Hughes, T. A. *et al.* (1995). Kidney–pancreas transplantation: the effect of portal versus systemic venous drainage of the pancreas on the lipoprotein composition. *Transplantation* **60**, 1406–1412.

Hypolite, I. O., Bucci, J., Hshieh, P., Cruess, D., Agodoa, L. Y., Yuan, C. M., Taylor, A. J., and Abbott, K. C. (2002). Acute coronary syndromes after renal transplantation in patients with end-stage renal disease resulting from diabetes. *American Journal of Transplantation* **2**, 274–281.

Inomata, S., Itoh, H., and Imai, H. (1997). Serum levels of erythropoietin as a novel marker reflecting the severity of diabetic nephropathy. *Nephron* **75**, 426–430.

International Pancreas Transplantation Registry (2000). *Newsletter* **12**, 4–23.

Iseki, K., Tozawa, M., Iseki, C., Takishita, S., and Ogawa, Y. (2002). Demographic trends in the Okinawa Dialysis Study (OKIDS) registry (1971–2000). *Kidney International* **61**, 668–675.

Ishimura, E. *et al.* (1998). Diabetes mellitus increases the severity of anemia in non-dialyzed patients with renal failure. *Journal of Nephrology* **11**, 83–86.

Joy, M. S., Cefalu, W. T., Hogan, S. L., and Nachman, P. H. (2002). Long-term glycemic control measurements in diabetic patients receiving hemodialyis. *American Journal of Kidney Diseases* **39**, 297–307.

Jungers, P. (2002). Late referral: loss of chance for the patient, loss of money for society. *Nephrology, Dialysis, Transplantation* **17**, 371–375.

Jungers, P. *et al.* (2001). Beneficial influence of recombinant human erythropoietin therapy on the rate of progression of chronic renal failure in predialysis patients. *Nephrology, Dialysis, Transplantation* **16**, 307–312.

Kahl, A., Bechstein, W. O., and Frei, U. (2001a). Trends and perspectives in pancreas and simultaneous pancreas and kidney transplantation. *Current Opinion in Urology* **11**, 165–174.

Kahl, A. *et al.* (2001b). Long term prednisolons withdrawal after pancreas and kidney transplantation in patients treated with ATG, tacrolimus and mycophenolate mofetil. *Transplantation Proceedings* **33**, 1694–1695.

Karnik, J. A., Young, B. S., Lew, N. L., Herget, M., Dubinsky, C., Lazarus, J. M., and Chertow, G. M. (2001). Cardiac arrest and sudden death in dialysis units. *Kidney International* **60**, 350–357.

Kaufman, D. B. *et al.* (1999). Mycophenolate mofetil and tacrolimus as primary maintenance immunosuppression in simultaneous pancreas–kidney transplantation: initial experience in 50 consecutive cases. *Transplantation* **67**, 586–593.

Kazmi, W. H. *et al.* (2001). Anemia: an early complication of chronic renal insufficiency. *American Journal of Kidney Diseases* **38**, 803–812.

Keller, C., Ritz, E., Pommer, W., Stein, G., Frank, J., and Schwarzbeck, A. (2000). Quality of treatment of diabetics with renal failure in Germany. *Deutsche Medizinische Wochenschrift* **125**, 240–244.

Kelly, W. D. *et al.* (1967). Allotransplantation of the pancreas and duodenum along with the kidney in diabetic nephropathy. *Surgery* **61**, 827–837.

Khanna, R. and Oreopoulos, D. G. CAPD in patients with diabetes mellitus. In *Continuous Ambulatory Peritoneal Dialysis* Vol. 12 (ed. R. Gokal), pp. 291–306. London: Churchill Livingstone, 1986.

Knüttgen, D., Weidmann, D., and Doehn, M. (1990). Diabetic autonomic neuropathy: abnormal cardiovascular reactions under general anesthesia. *Klinische Wochenschrift* **68**, 1168–1172.

Koch, M., Kutkuhn, B., Grabensee, B., and Ritz, E. (1997). Apolipoprotein A, fibrinogen, age, and history of stroke are predictors of death in dialysed diabetic patients: a prospective study in 412 subjects. *Nephrology, Dialysis, Transplantation* **12**, 2603–2611.

Koch, M., Thomas, B., Tschope, W., and Ritz, E. (1993). Survival and predictors of death in dialysed diabetic patients. *Diabetologia* **36**, 1113–1117.

Konner, K. (2000). Primary vascular access in diabetic patients: an audit. *Nephrology, Dialysis, Transplantation* **15**, 1317–1325.

Konner, K., Nonnast-Daniel, B., and Ritz, E. (2003). The arteriovenous fistula. *Journal of the American Society of Nephrology* **14**, 1669–1680.

Kuriyama, S. *et al.* (1997). Reversal of anemia by erythropoietin therapy retards the progression of chronic renal failure, especially in non-diabetic renal patients. *Nephron* **77**, 176–185.

La Rovere, M. T., Bigger, J. T., Jr., Marcus, F. I., Mortara, A., and Schwartz, P. J. (1998). Baroreflex sensitivity and heart-rate variability in prediction of total cardiac mortality after myocardial infarction. ATRAMI (Autonomic Tone and Reflexes After Myocardial Infarction) Investigators. *Lancet* **351**, 478–484.

Larsson, J., Apelquist, J., Agardh, C. D., and Stenström, A. (1995). Decreasing incidence of major amputation in diabetic patients: a consequence of a multidisciplinary foot care team approach. *Diabetic Medicine* **12**, 770–776.

Leonard, A., Comty, C. M., Raji, L., Rattazzi, T., Wathen, R., and Shapiro, F. (1973). The natural history of regularly dialyzed diabetics. *Transactions of the American Society for Artificial Internal organs* **19**, 282–286.

Levin, A., Djurdjev, O., Barrett, B., Burgess, E., Carlisle, E., Ethier, J., Jinda, K., Mendelssohn, D., Tobe, S., Singer, J., and Thompson, C. (2001). Cardiovascular disease in patients with chronic kidney disease: getting to the heart of the matter. *American Journal of Kidney Diseases* **38**, 1398–1407.

Lewis, E. J., Hunsicker, L. G., Bain, R. P., and Rohde, R. D. (1993). The effect of angiotensin-converting-enzyme inhibition on diabetic nephropathy. *New England Journal of Medicine* **329**, 1456–1462.

Lewis, E. J., Hunsicker, L. G., Clarke, W. R., Berl, T., Pohl, M. A., Lewis, J. B., Ritz, E., Atkins, R. C., Rohde, R., and Raz, I. (2001). Renoprotective effect of the angiotensin-receptor antagonist irbesartan in patients with nephropathy due to type 2 diabetes. *New England Journal of Medicine* **345**, 851–860.

Lillehei, R. C., Simmons, R. L., and Najarian, J. S. (1970). Pancreaticduodenal allotransplantation: experimental and clinical experience. *Annals of Surgery* **172**, 405–436.

Linden, T., Cohen, A., Deppisch, R., Kjellstrand, P., and Wieslander, A. (2002). 3,4-Dideoxyglucosone-3-ene (3,4-DGE): a cytotoxic glucose degradation product in fluids for peritoneal dialysis. *Kidney International* **62**, 697.

Lippert, J., Ritz, E., Schwarzbeck, A., and Schneider, P. (1995). The rising tide of endstage renal failure from diabetic nephropathy type II—an epidemiological analysis. *Nephrology, Dialaysis, Transplantation* **10**, 462–467.

Luft, D. (1999). Neuropathic pain in diabetic nephropathy—update on analgesic strategies. *Nephrology, Dialysis, Transplantation* **14**, 2285–2288.

Luukinen, H., Koski, K., Laippala, P., and Kivela, S. L. (1999). Prognosis of diastolic and systolic orthostatic hypotension in older persons. *Archives of Internal Medicine* **159**, 273–280.

Luzi, L., Perseghin, G., Brendel, M. D., Terruzzi, I., Batteizzati, A., Eckhard, M., Brandhorst, D., Brandhorst, H., Friemann, S., Socci, C., Di Carlo, V., Piceni Sereni, L., Benedini, S., Secchi, A., Pozza, G., and Bretzel, R. G.

(2001). Metabolic effects of restoring partial beta-cell function after islet allotransplantation in type 1 diabetic patients. *Diabetes* **50**, 277–282.

Luzi, L. *et al.* (1994). Combined pancreas and kidney transplantation normalizes protein metabolism in insulin-dependent diabetic-uremic patients. *Journal of Clinical Investigation* **93**, 1948–1958.

Mallamaci, F., Zoccali, C., Parlongo, S., Tripepi, G., Benedetto, F. A., Cutrupi, S., Bonanno, G., Fatuzzo, P., Rapisarda, F., Seminara, G., Stancanelli, B., Bellanuova, I., Cataliotti, A., and Malatino, L. S. (2002). Troponin is related to left ventricular mass and predicts all-cause and cardiovascular mortality in hemodialysis patients. *American Journal of Kidney Diseases* **40**, 68–75.

Malmberg, K. (1997). Prospective randomised study of intensive insulin treatment on long term survival after acute myocardial infarction in patients with diabetes mellitus. DIGAMI (Diabetes Mellitus, Insulin Glucose Infusion in Acute Myocardial Infarction) Study Group. *British Medical Journal* **314**, 1512–1515.

Malmberg, K., Norhammer, A., Wedel, H., and Ryden, L. (1999). Glycometabolic state at admission: important risk marker of mortality in conventionally treated patients with diabetes mellitus and acute myocardial infarction. *Circulation* **99**, 2626–2632.

Mange, K. C., Joffe, M. M., and Feldman, H. I. (2001). Effect of the use or nonuse of long-term dialysis on the subsequent survival of renal transplants from living donors. *New England Journal of Medicine* **344**, 726–731.

Manske, C. L. *et al.* (1992). Coronary revascularization in insulin-dependent diabetic patients with chronic renal failure. *Lancet* **340**, 998–1002.

Manske, C. L. *et al.* (1993). Screening diabetic transplant candidates for coronary artery disease: identification of a low risk subgroup. *Kidney International* **44**, 617–621.

Margolis, J. R., Kannel, W. B., Feinleib, M., Dawber, T. R., and McNamara, P. M. (1973). Clinical features of unrecognized myocardial infarction—silent and symptomatic. *American Journal of Cardiology* **32**, 1–7.

Maser, R. E., Pfeifer, M. A., Dorman, J. S., Kuller, L. H., Becker, D. J., and Orchard, T. J. (1990). Diabetic autonomic neuropathy and cardiovascular risk. Pittsburgh epidemiology of diabetes complications study III. *Archives of Internal Medicine* **150**, 1218–1223.

Mieghem, A. V., Fonck, C., Coosemans, W., Vandeleene, B., Venrenterghem, Y., Squifflet, J. P., and Pirson, Y. (2001). Outcome of cadaver kidney transplantation in 23 patients with type 2 diabetes mellitus. *Nephrology, Dialysis, Transplantation* **16**, 1686–1691.

Miles, A. M. (1999). Vacular steal syndrome and ischaemic monomelic neuropathy: two variants of upper limb ischaemia after haemodialysis vascular access surgery. *Nephrology, Dialysis, Transplantation* **14**, 297–300.

Morioka, T., Emoto, M., Tabata, T., Shoji, T., Tahara, H., Kishimoto, H., Ishimura, E., and Nishizawa, Y. (2001). Glycemic control is a predictor of survival for diabetic patients on hemodialysis. *Diabetes Care* **24**, 909–913.

Mueller-Felber, W. *et al.* (1993). High incidence of carpal tunnel syndrome in diabetic patients after combined pancreas and kidney transplantation. *Acta Diabetologica* **30**, 17–20.

Murray, D., O'Brien, T., Mulrooney, R., and O'Sullivan, D. (1990). Autonomic dysfunction and silent myocardial ischemia on exercise testing in diabetes mellitus. *Diabetic Medicine* **7**, 580–584.

Navarro, X. *et al.* (1996). Neuropathy and mortality in diabetes: influence of pancreas transplantation. *Muscle and Nerve* **19**, 1009–1016.

Nevalainen, P. I., Lahtela, J. T., Mustonen, J., and Pasternak, A. (1996). Subcutaneous and intraperitoneal insulin therapy in diabetic patients on CAPD. *Peritoneal Dialysis International* **16**, S288–S291.

Okuno, S., Ishimura, E., Kim, M., Izumotani, T., Otoshi, T., Maekawa, K., Yamakawa, T., Morii, H., Inaba, M., and Nishizawa, Y. (2001). Changes in body fat mass in male hemodialysis patients: a comparison between diabetics and nondiabetics. *American Journal of Kidney Diseases* **38**, S208–S211.

Olsen, S. and Mogensen, C. E. (1996). How often is NIDDM complicated with non-diabetic renal disease? An analysis of renal biopsies and the literature. *Diabetologia* **39**, 1638–1645.

Parfrey, P. *et al.* (1989). Contrast material induced renal failure in patients with diabetes mellitus, renal insufficiency or both. *New England Journal of Medicine* **320**, 143–149.

Parving, H. H. *et al.* (1992). Prevalence and causes of albuminuria in non-insulin-dependent diabetic patients. *Kidney International* **41**, 758–762.

Pfeffer, F. *et al.* (1996). Determinants of a normal (versus impaired) oral glucose tolerance after combined pancreas–kidney transplantation in IDDM patients. *Diabetologia* **39**, 462–468.

Pinero-Pilona, A., Litonjua, P., Deveraj, S., Aviles-Santa, L., and Raskin, P. (2002). Anemia associated with new-onset diabetes: improvement with blood glucose control. *Endocrine Practice* **8**, 276–281.

Pinzur, M. S., Slovenkai, M. P., and Trepman, E. (1999). Guidelines for diabetic foot care. The Diabetes Committee of the American Orthopaedic Foot Ankle Society. *Foot & Ankle International* **20**, 695–702.

Revanur, V. K., Jardine, A. G., Hamilton, D. H., and Jindal, R. M. (2000). Outcome for arterio-venous fistula at the elbow for haemodialysis. *Clinical Transplantation* **14**, 318–322.

Rigalleau, V. *et al.* (1998). Erythropoietin can deteriorate glucose control in uremic non-insulin dependent diabetic patients. *Diabetic Medicine* **24**, 62–65.

Rippe, B., Simonsen, O., Heimburger, O., Christensson, A., Haraldsson, B., Stelin, G., Weiss, L., Nielsen, F. D., Bro, S., Friedberg, M., and Wieslander, A. (2001). Long-term clinical effetcs of a peritoneal dialysis fluid with less glucose degradation products. *Kidney International* **59**, 348–357.

Ritz, E. and Koch, M. (1993). Morbidity and mortality due to hypertension in patients with renal failure. *American Journal of Kidney Diseases* **21**, 113–118.

Ritz, E. and Orth, S. M. (1999). Nephropathy in patients with type 2 diabetes mellitus. *New England Journal of Medicine* **341**, 1127–1133.

Ritz, E. and Stefanski, A. (1996). Diabetic nephropathy in type II diabetes. *American Journal of Kidney Diseases* **27**, 167–194.

Ritz, E., Rychlik, I., Locatelli, F., and Halimi, S. (1999). End-stage renal failure in type 2 diabetes: a medical catastrophe of worldwide dimensions. *American Journal of Kidney Diseases* **34**, 795–808.

Rooney, D. P. and Robertson, R. P. (1996). Hepatic insulin resistance after pancreas transplantation in type 1 diabetes. *Diabetes* **45**, 134–138.

Schömig, M., Ritz, E., Standl, E., and Allenberg, J. (2000). The diabetic foot in the dialyzed patient. *Journal of the American Society of Nephrology* **11**, 1153–1159.

Schwab, S. T. *et al.* (1989). Contrast nephrotoxicity: a randomized controlled trial of non-ionic and ionic radiographic contrast agent. *New England Journal of Medicine* **320**, 149–153.

Schwenger, V., Mussig, C., Hergesell, O., Zeier, M., and Ritz, E. (2001). Incidence and clinical characteristics of renal insufficiency in diabetic patients. *Deutsche Medizinische Wochenschrift* **126**, 1322–1326.

Schwenger, V., Hofmann, A., Khalifeh, N., Meyer, T., Zeier, M., Hörl, W. H., and Ritz, E. (2003). Uremic patients: late referral—early death. *Deutsche Medizinische Wochenschrift* **128**, 1216–1220.

Sehgal, A. R., Leon, J. B., Siminoff, L. A., Singer, M. E., Bunosky, L. M., and Cebul, R. D. (2002). Improving the quality of hemodialysis treatment: a community-based randomized controlled trial to overcome patient-specific barriers. *Journal of the American Medical Association* **287**, 1961–1967.

Shapiro, A. M., Lakey, J. R., Ryan, E. A., Korbutt, G. S., Toth, E., Warnock, G. L., Kneteman, N. M., and Rajotte, R. V. (2000). Islet transplantation in seven patients with type 1 diabetes mellitus using a glucocorticoid-free immunosuppressive regimen. *New England Journal of Medicine* **343**, 230–238.

Shlipak, M. G., Heidenreich, P. A., Noguchi, H., Chertow, G. M., Browner, W. S., and McClellan, M. B. (2002). Association of renal insufficiency with treatment and outcomes after myocardial infarction in elderly patients. *Annals of Internal Medicine* **137**, 555–562.

Shorb, S. R. (1985). Anemia and diabetic retinopathy. *American Journal of Ophthalmology* **100**, 434–436.

Simic-Ogrizovic, S., Backus, G., Mayer, A., Vienken, J., Djukanovic, L., and Kleophas, W. (2001). The Influence of different glucose concentrations in haemodialysis solutions on metabolism and blood pressure stability in diabetic patients. *International Journal of Artificial Organs* 24, 863–869.

Smets, Y. F. C. *et al.* (1998). Low bone mass and high incidence of fractures after successful simultaneous pancreas–kidney transplantation. *Nephrology, Dialysis, Transplantation* 13, 1250–1255.

Solders, G. *et al.* (1995). Improvement in nerve conduction 8 years after combined pancreatic and renal transplantation. *Transplantation Proceedings* 27, 3091.

Spaia, S. *et al.* (2000). Effect of short-term rhu-EPO treatment on insulin resistance in hemodialysis patients. *Nephron* 84, 320–325.

Stack, A. G. and Bloembergen, W. E. (2001). A cross-sectional study of the prevalence and clinical correlates of congestive heart failure among incident US dialysis patients. *American Journal of Kidney Diseases* 38, 992–1000.

Standl, E. and Schnell, O. (2000). A new look at the heart in diabetes mellitus: from ailing to failing. *Diabetologia* 43, 1455–1469.

Stengel, B., Billon, S., Van Dijk, P. C., Jager, K. J., Dekker, F. W., Simpson, K., and Briggs, J. D. (2003). Trends in the incidence of renal replacement therapy for end-stage renal disease in Europe, 1990–1999. *Nephrology, Dialysis, Transplantation* 18, 1824–1833.

Suliman, M. E., Stenvinkel, P., Heimburger, O., Barany, P., Lindholm, B., and Bergstrom, J. (2002). Plasma sulfur amino acids in relation to cardiovascular disease, nutritional status, and diabetes mellitus in patients with chronic renal failure at start of dialysis treatment. *American Journal of Kidney Diseases* 40, 480–488.

Sutherland, D. E. R. *et al.* Pancreas transplantation. In *Ellenberg and Rifkin's Diabetes Mellitus* 5th edn. (ed. D. Porte and R. S. Scherwin), pp. 1255–1279. Stanford: Appleton & Lange, 1997.

The Bypass Angioplasty Revascularization Investigation (BARI) Investigators (1996). Comparison of coronary bypass surgery with angioplasty in patients with multivessel disease. *New England Journal of Medicine* 335, 217–225.

The Heart Outcomes Prevention Evaluation Study Investigators (2000). Effects of ramipril on cardiovascular and microvascular outcomes in people with diabetes mellitus: results of the HOPE and MICRO-HOPE substudy. *Lancet* 355, 253–259.

Tozawa, M., Iseki, K., Iseki, C., and Takishita, S. (2002). Pulse pressure and risk of total mortality and cardiovascular events in patients on chronic hemodialysis. *Kidney International* 61, 717–726.

Tschöpe, W., Koch, M., Thomas, B., and Ritz, E. (1992). Serum lipids predict cardiac death in diabetic patients on maintenance hemodialysis. *Nephron* 64, 354–358.

Twardowski, Z. J., Nolph, K. D., McGary, T. J., Moore, H. L., Collin, P., Ausman, R. K., and Slimack, W. S. (1983). Insulin binding to plastic bags: a methodologic study. *American Journal of Hospital Pharmacy* 40, 575–579.

Tyden, G. *et al.* (1996). Recurrence of autoimmune diabetes mellitus in recipients of cadaveric pancreas grafts. *New England Journal of Medicine* 335, 860–863.

Tyden, G. *et al.* (1999). Improved survival in patients with insulin-dependent diabetes mellitus and end-stage diabetic nephropathy 10 years after combined pancreas and kidney transplantation. *Transplantation* 67, 645–648.

United States Renal Data System (USRDS). *Annual Data Report.* Bethesda: The National Institute of Health, National Institute of Diabetes and Digestive and Kidney Diseases, 2001.

Van Biesen, W., Vanholder, R. C., Veys, N., Dhondt, A., and Lameire, N. (2000). An evaluation of an integrative care approach for end-stage renal disease patients. *Journal of the American Society of Nephrology* 11, 116–125.

Van den Berghe, G., Wouters, P., Weekers, F., Verwaest, C., Bruyninckx, F., Schetz, M., Vlasselaers, D., Ferdinande, P., Lauwers, P., and Bouillon, R. (2001). Intensive insulin therapy in the critically ill patients. *New England Journal of Medicine* 345, 1359–1367.

Wakeen, M. and Zimmermann, S. W. (1998). Association between human recombinant EPO and peripheral vascular disease in diabetic patients receiving peritoneal dialysis. *American Journal of Kidney Diseases* 32, 488–493.

Waldherr, R., Ilkenhans, C., and Ritz, E. (1992). How frequent is glomerulonephritis in diabetes mellitus type II? *Clinical Nephrology* 37, 271–273.

Walsh, C. H., Fitzgerald, M. G., Soler, N. G., and Malins, J. M. (1975). Association of foot lesions with retinopathy in patients with newly diagnosed diabetes. *Lancet* ii, 878.

Wanner, C., Krane, V., Ruf, G., März, W., and Ritz, E. (1999). Rationale and design of a trial improving outcome of type 2 diabetics on hemodialysis. *Kidney International* 56, S222–S226.

Winkelmayer, W. C., Glynn, R. J., Mittleman, M. A., Levin, R., Pliskin, J. S., and Avorn, J. (2002). Comparing mortality of elderly patients on hemodialysis versus peritoneal dialysis: a prospective score approach. *Journal of the American Society of Nephrology* 13, 2353–2362.

Wolfe, R. A., Ashby, V. B., Milford, E. L., Ojo, A. O., Ettenger, R. E., Agodoa, L. Y. C., Held, P. J., and Port, F. K. (1999). Comparison of mortality in all patients on dialysis, patients on dialysis awaiting transplantation, and recipients of a first cadaveric transplant. *New England Journal of Medicine* 341, 1725–1730.

Wu, M. S., Yu, C. C., Yang, C. W., Wu, C. H., Haung, J. Y., Hong, J. J., Fan Chiang, C. Y., Huang, C. C., and Leu, M. L. (1997). Poor pre-dialysis glycaemic control is a predictor of mortality in type II diabetic patients on maintenance haemodialysis. *Nephrology, Dialysis, Transplantation* 12, 2105–2110.

Yeager, R. A., Moneta, G. L., Edwards, J. M., Landry, G. J., Taylor, L. M., Jr., McConnell, D. B., and Porter, J. M. (2002). Relationship of hemodialysis access to finger gangrene in patients with end-stage renal disease. *Journal of Vascular Surgery* 36, 245–249.

Zeier, M. and Ritz, E. (2002). Preparation of the dialysis patient for transplantation. *Nephrology, Dialysis, Transplantation* 17, 552–556.

Ziegler, D. *et al.* (1995). Treatment of symptomatic diabetic peripheral neuropathy with the anti-oxidant α-lipoic acid. *Diabetologia* 38, 1425–1433.

Zoccali, C., Mallamaci, F., Parlongo, S., Cutrupi, S., Benedetto, F. A., Tripepi, G., Bonanno, G., Rapisarda, F., Fatuzzo, P., Seminara, G., Cataliotti, A., Stancanelli, B., Malatino, L. S., and Cateliotti, A. (2002). Plasma norepinephrine predicts survival and incident cardiovascular events in patients with end-stage renal disease. *Circulation* 105, 1354–1359.

Zuanetti, G., Maggioni, A. P., Keane, W., and Ritz, E. (1997). Nephrologists neglect administration of betablockers to dialysed diabetic patients. *Nephrology, Dialysis, Transplantation* 12, 2497–2500.

15

The pregnant patient

15.1 The normal renal physiological changes which occur during pregnancy

Chris Baylis and John M. Davison

Introduction

The striking anatomical and physiological changes that occur in the urinary tract during normal pregnancy lead to marked deviations from non-pregnant 'physiological' norms. An understanding why and how these alterations occur is essential in order to recognize and manage both normal and compromised pregnancies (Lindheimer *et al.* 2001). Information on these changes has been obtained from clinical practice and animal studies, providing insights into the mechanisms controlling the altered renal function of normal pregnancy as well as the long-term renal consequences of pregnancy in health and disease.

Structural changes in the urinary tract

The kidneys of normal pregnant women enlarge because both vascular volume and interstitial space increase (Brown 1990) with the microscopic structure unchanged. Evidence from intravenous urography (IVU) performed immediately after delivery reveals that renal size is consistently greater than that predicted by standard height–weight nomography and that by 6 months postpartum, renal length has decreased by approximately 1 cm. Ultrasound studies demonstrate an increase in renal parenchymal volumes during pregnancy, by 70 per cent at the beginning of the third trimester with a slight reduction during the first weeks postpartum.

Dilatation of the calyces, renal pelvis, and ureter (Fig. 1), invariably more prominent on the right side, can sometimes be seen in the first trimester, and by the third trimester are present in 90 per cent of women (Cietak and Newton 1985). The cause of the dilatation is disputed; some advocate hormonal effects and others, obstruction (Croce *et al.* 1994). There is no doubt that, as pregnancy progresses, the supine or upright posture may cause partial ureteric obstruction as the enlarged uterus compresses the ureter at the pelvic brim, where dilatation terminates as the ureter crosses the iliac artery, and at this point a filling defect termed the 'iliac sign' can be demonstrated (Fig. 1). Interestingly, there is increased tone in the upper ureter, hypertrophy of the ureteric smooth muscle, and hyperplasia of its connective tissue, no decrease in pacemaker activity for ureteral peristalsis, and no decrease in the frequency and amplitude of the ureteric contraction complex, so that it is erroneous to think of toneless, floppy ureters. These structural changes have the following important clinical implications:

1. Dilatation of the urinary tract may lead to collection errors in tests based on timed urine volume; for example 24-h creatinine

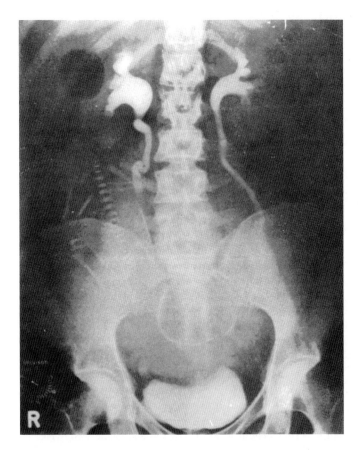

Fig. 1 Intravenous excretory urogram showing ureteral dilatation of pregnancy. The right ureter is abruptly cut off at the pelvic brim where it crosses the iliac artery (the so-called 'iliac sign').

clearance and/or protein excretion. Such errors are minimized if the pregnant woman is sufficiently hydrated to give a high urine flow and/or if she lies down on her side for an hour before and at the end of the collection.

2. Acceptable norms of kidney size should be increased by 1 cm if radiography is undertaken during pregnancy or immediately after delivery. Dilatation of the ureters may persist until the 16th postpartum week, and elective IVU during this period should be deferred (Rasmussen and Nielsen 1988). Ureteric dilation is permanent in up to 11 per cent of parous women with no history of urinary tract infection (Fried *et al.* 1982).

3. Very occasionally, there can be massive dilation of the ureters and renal pelvis (as well as slight reduction in cortical width), but this is without ill-effect (Brown 1990). Rarely, the changes may be extreme and precipitate the 'overdistension syndrome' (see Chapter 15.2) and/or hypertension (Khauna and Nguyn 2001).

4. Urinary stasis within the ureters may contribute to the propensity of pregnant women with asymptomatic bacteriuria to develop frank pyelonephritis.

Renal haemodynamic changes in normal human pregnancy

Time course and magnitude of renal haemodynamic changes

In the normal pregnant woman, effective renal plasma flow increases by 70–80 per cent between conception and midpregnancy, decreasing close to term, but remaining above the non-pregnant value (Dunlop 1976). The decrease in renal blood flow during the third trimester is not solely a postural artefact because pregnant women in lateral recumbency have a significant reduction in renal plasma flow too (Ezimokhai et al. 1981).

It is generally accepted that inulin clearance increases by about 50 per cent during pregnancy (Fig. 2), reaching a maximum at the end of the first trimester and being maintained at this level until at least the 36th gestational week.

Since glomerular filtration rate (GFR) increases less than renal plasma flow during early pregnancy, the filtration fraction must decline. Late pregnancy is associated with an increase in filtration fraction to values similar to those of the non-pregnant normal woman (Roberts et al. 1996; Milne et al. 2002). The probable mechanism of this alteration will be discussed in more detail later.

Changes in creatinine clearance

Endogenous 24-h creatinine clearance is a convenient, non-invasive method to assess changes in GFR when infusion studies are impracticable (see Chapter 1.3 for a critique). Increase in 24-h creatinine clearance by 25 per cent occurs 4 weeks after the last menstrual period and by 45 per cent at 9 weeks (Davison and Noble 1981) (Fig. 3).

During the third trimester, a decrease towards non-pregnant values precedes delivery (Davison et al. 1980), with a small increase during the first few days of the puerperium (Davison and Dunlop 1984).

Values for GFR estimated from 24-h creatinine clearances are consistently less than those obtained from inulin clearances, despite the fact that creatinine is secreted into the tubule and therefore tends to overestimate GFR by about 10 per cent (Davison and Hytten 1974). Although 24-h creatinine clearance may not give an exact measure of GFR, it is a valuable gauge in serial assessment.

Renal haemodynamic changes in pregnant animals

Pregnancy-induced increases in GFR have been reported in a number of animal species, including the rat, dog, rabbit, and sheep (Conrad 1987), and the rat is a particularly good animal model for both renal and systemic haemodynamic studies in pregnancy.

Time course and magnitude of renal haemodynamic changes

Gestation in the rat lasts 22 days. As shown in Fig. 4(a), GFR increases early in the conscious rat and has reached a maximum increase of 30–40 per cent by midterm, close to term a return towards the non-pregnant value occurs (Conrad 1984). A similar pattern of increase in GFR has been detected in the pregnant, anaesthetized, volume-maintained rat prepared for micropuncture [Fig. 4(b)], a preparation which allows measurement of the intrarenal mechanisms responsible for the renal haemodynamic changes in pregnancy.

Determinants of glomerular filtration (see also Chapter 1.3)

There is no change in glomerular number in pregnancy; thus, the increased GFR is due to increases in single nephron GFR. The net filtration pressure is a major determinant of single nephron GFR and, as

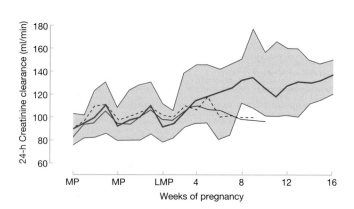

Fig. 3 Changes in 24-h creatinine clearance measured weekly before conception and through to uncomplicated spontaneous abortion in two women. The solid line represents the mean and the stippled area the range for nine women with successful obstetric outcome. MP, menstrual period; LMP, last menstrual period (reproduced from Davison and Noble 1981, with permission).

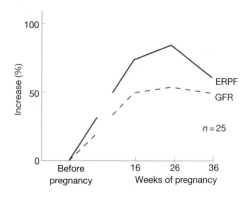

Fig. 2 Relative changes in renal haemodynamics during normal human pregnancy (calculated from the data of Davison and Hytten 1975; Dunlop 1976; Ezimokhai et al. 1981; Davison 1985).

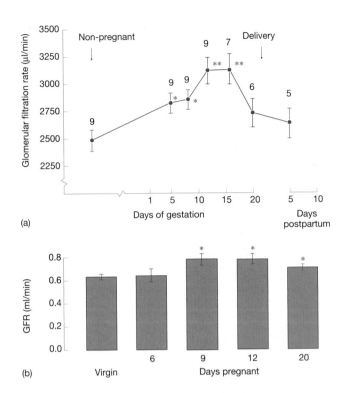

(a)

(b)

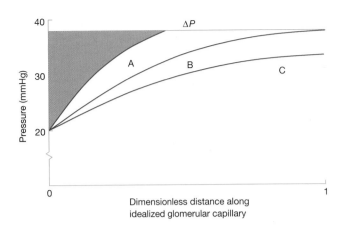

Fig. 4 (a) Magnitude and time course of the gestational change in GFR measured in the conscious, chronically catheterized Long–Evans rat by Conrad (1984); reproduced with permission. (b) GFR (left kidney) measured in the anaesthetized, euvolaemic Munich–Wistar rat before and during pregnancy by Baylis (1984); reproduced with permission. In both (a) and (b) data are shown as mean ± SE. A significant difference from the virgin value is denoted by * ($p < 0.05$) and ** ($p < 0.001$). This composite is reproduced from Baylis (1994), with permission.

Fig. 5 Several possible profiles (curves A–C) of the intraglomerular oncotic pressure (II) for a given transcapillary hydrostatic pressure difference (ΔP) along an idealized glomerular capillary. Curves A and B are obtained under conditions of filtration pressure equilibrium; curve C is obtained at filtration pressure disequilibrium. The shaded area between ΔP and oncotic pressure curve A denotes the net ultrafiltration pressure obtained under these hypothetical conditions.

shown by the shaded area in Fig. 5, this is the difference between the glomerular hydrostatic pressure gradient (favouring filtration) and the glomerular oncotic pressure gradient (opposing filtration). The other determinants are the filtration surface area and the water permeability of the glomerular capillary wall, which together can be calculated (from micropuncture measurements) as the glomerular capillary ultrafiltration coefficient, K_f (Baylis 1986).

In normal non-pregnant rats, the net filtration pressure and the glomerular wall water permeability are high and filtration proceeds rapidly. Not all the available filtration surface area is utilized, that is, the glomerular oncotic pressure (which increases along the length of the capillary as protein free filtrate is removed) has increased to a value which equals (and opposes) the hydrostatic pressure gradient, somewhere before the end of the glomerulus (Fig. 5, curve A). This state is known as filtration pressure equilibrium.

In animals, at filtration pressure equilibrium, the single nephron GFR is highly dependent on glomerular plasma flow, and an increase in plasma flow will elicit a proportional increase in filtration rate with no change in filtration fraction. This is achieved by increasing net filtration pressure with a shift in the glomerular oncotic pressure profile, for example, from curve A to curve B (for a full explanation see Baylis 1986). In addition to plasma flow, the hydrostatic pressure gradient and systemic oncotic pressure also control the single nephron GFR by changing the net glomerular filtration pressure. Alterations in the glomerular

capillary ultrafiltration coefficient (K_f) will not influence the single nephron GFR provided that filtration pressure equilibrium is maintained (Fig. 5, curve A). At filtration pressure disequilibrium, where a positive net ultrafiltration pressure persists over the entire length of the glomerular capillary (Fig. 5, curve C), the single nephron GFR is influenced by changes in K_f (for a full discussion see Baylis 1986).

Glomerular haemodynamics in pregnancy in the rat

Micropuncture studies performed in the euvolaemic pregnant Munich–Wistar rat demonstrated increases of 30–40 per cent in superficial cortical single nephron GFR by midterm (day 9 and 12). As shown in Fig. 6, the increase in single nephron GFR (solid symbols, upper panel) is the result exclusively of an increase in glomerular plasma flow rate (open symbols, upper panel). As shown in the middle panel of Fig. 6, the oncotic pressure of systemic blood (at the beginning of the glomerulus, π_A) and the glomerular hydrostatic pressure gradient are unchanged by pregnancy. Pregnant rats remain at filtration pressure equilibrium, and the glomerular capillary ultrafiltration coefficient, K_f, does not change markedly with pregnancy.

Systemic oncotic pressure is constant throughout the first part of pregnancy in the rat, although reductions in plasma albumin concentration have been reported beyond about day 12 (Beaton *et al.* 1961). This contrasts with pregnant women, where plasma albumin concentration decreases early and remains low through to term (Milne *et al.* 2002). Although a decline in systemic oncotic pressure (due to reduced plasma albumin) is predicted to increase GFR by lowering glomerular oncotic pressure, this effect is offset in practice since reductions in plasma protein concentration also lower K_f (Baylis *et al.* 1977). Thus, a reduction in plasma protein concentration results in two offsetting changes in the determinants of glomerular ultrafiltration with little net change in filtration rate.

In euvolemic Munich–Wistar rats (Baylis 1979/1980, 1980, 1982, 1994; Deng *et al.* 1996), there is no sustained increase in glomerular

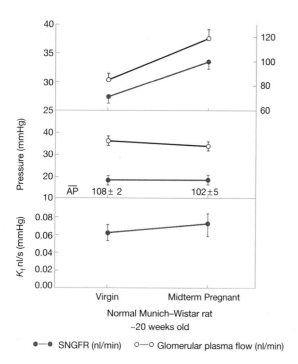

Fig. 6 Determinants of glomerular filtration in the virgin and midterm pregnant Munich–Wistar rat studied under anaesthetized, euvolaemic conditions. In the upper panel, single nephron GFR is given by the solid circles and glomerular plasma flow by open circles. The middle panel summarizes the ultrafiltration pressures; the transglomerular hydrostatic pressure difference (ΔP) and the preglomerular (systemic) oncotic pressure (π_A). Mean arterial blood pressure (AP) is also given. The lower panel shows the glomerular capillary ultrafiltration coefficient, K_f, and data throughout are given as mean $\pm$ SE (reproduced from Baylis and Reckelhoff 1991, with permission).

capillary blood pressure at any time during the gestation period, despite the renal vasodilation of pregnancy, due to proportional reductions in tone in the pre- and postglomerular resistance vessels. This means that increased plasma flow is the sole determinant of the increased GFR. In humans, neutral dextran sieving curves and mathematical modelling combined with measured GFR, effective renal plasma flow, and plasma oncotic pressure, give indirect estimates of glomerular haemodynamics and membrane porosity can be obtained. Glomerular hydrostatic pressure give gradient and K_f remain unchanged endorsing the predominant role for increased plasma flow in mediating the gestational increase in GFR (Roberts *et al.* 1996).

In some situations prolonged periods of renal vasodilation may damage the glomerulus. The primary damaging stimulus is the prolonged increase in glomerular blood pressure secondary to preferential vasodilation of the preglomerular arteriole, as seen in a variety of progressive glomerulopathies (Brenner *et al.* 1982; Meyer *et al.* 1987). Pregnancy is a state in which the kidneys are chronically vasodilated, although pregnancy is a physiological condition which proceeds without loss of nephron number or underlying disease and is reversible. Also, there is no sustained increase in glomerular blood pressure during a single gestation period because of the parallel falls in pre- and postglomerular arteriolar resistances (Baylis 1994). Studies in the rat have demonstrated that five successive, closely spaced pregnancies, which represents continual renal vasodilation for approximately half of the rats life, had no adverse effects on glomerular or renal haemodynamics. So, effectively, there was no elevation in glomerular blood

pressure, proteinuria, or morphological damage despite the prolonged renal vasodilation (Baylis and Rennke 1985). Thus, pregnancy *per se* does not lead to any acceleration in the non-specific age-dependent deterioration seen in renal function in animals whose kidneys were previously normal. In humans, the evidence also argues against glomerular injury resulting from normal pregnancy. The gestational rise in GFR is similar in later compared with first pregnancies, and there are no long-term inputs of pregnancy in normal women on GFR and protein excretion (Davison 1989). Indeed, it is well known that women do not show any tendency for GFR to decline during the reproductive years and overall show far less of an age-dependent decline than men.

In summary, therefore, the gestational increase in GFR in the rat is entirely due to renal vasodilation with consequent increases in renal plasma flow. The increase in GFR in the pregnant woman is the result of a selective rise in renal plasma flow (Roberts *et al.* 1996) and a decrease in oncotic pressure, especially in late pregnancy (Milne *et al.* 2002). The available evidence indicates that the chronic renal vasodilation of pregnancy has no long-term damaging effects on the maternal kidney.

Functional characteristics of the renal vasculature in pregnant animals

Despite substantial plasma volume expansion and increases in cardiac output, arterial blood pressure declines by midterm, due to marked reductions in total peripheral vascular resistance (Chesley 1978). Serial studies before and during pregnancy have indicated that the maximal reductions in both renal and systemic vascular resistances have occurred by 6 weeks after conception (Chapman *et al.* 1998). A progressive and massive increase in plasma volume also occurs in the gravid rat, with an early decline in total peripheral resistance (Baylis 1994).

Renal autoregulation during pregnancy

The normal kidney maintains blood flow and GFR over a range of systemic blood pressure (i.e. autoregulates) and variation in preglomerular arteriolar tone is the main mechanism of this autoregulatory maintenance of renal plasma flow and glomerular blood pressure (Robertson *et al.* 1972; Navar 1978). Despite the haemodynamic changes of normal pregnancy, renal autoregulatory ability is intact in pregnant rats (Reckelhoff *et al.* 1992) and rabbits (Woods *et al.* 1987). Thus, the gestational renal vasodilation does not alter intrinsic renal autoregulation ability. In late-pregnant rats, when the gestational reduction in blood pressure has occurred, there is some indication of a downward resetting in the 'threshold' for renal autoregulation of blood flow. This may represent a protective mechanism whereby late-pregnant animals are protected from periods of renal hypoperfusion (Reckelhoff *et al.* 1992). It has been reported that renal autoregulation of blood flow in the ovine kidney is impaired during pregnancy (Cha *et al.* 1993). There has been no direct assessment in pregnant women but the routinely elevated GFR of normal pregnancy makes it likely that autoregulation is well maintained.

Renal autoregulation involves a tubuloglomerular feedback component as well as a myogenic component (Navar 1978). The tubuloglomerular feedback system provides a mechanism whereby the rate of delivery of fluid (or some constituent of tubular fluid) controls the rate of filtration (single nephron GFR) at the glomerulus of the same nephron (Blantz and Pelayo 1984). When fluid delivery in the early distal nephron increases (e.g. in response to an abrupt increase in blood pressure) this is sensed by the macula densa; a signal is sent to the parent glomerulus, which results in a vasoconstriction with a consequent reduction in single nephron GFR and restoration of early distal fluid delivery. In midterm-pregnant rats, tubuloglomerular feedback activity is normal, not suppressed, having reset to recognize the elevated single nephron GFR as normal (Baylis and Blantz 1985), thus this component of the autoregulatory response is intact.

Responsivity of the renal vasculature in pregnancy; renal vasodilatory capacity

In normal non-pregnant humans and experimental animals, a high protein meal or amino acid infusion elicit substantial increases in GFR due to a selective renal vasodilation and increased renal plasma flow (Meyer et al. 1983; Hostetter 1984). The normal midterm-pregnant rat, which exhibits the maximal gestational renal vasodilation, responds to an acute amino acid infusion with further substantial increases in both GFR and single nephron GFR, due solely to further increases in plasma flow (Baylis 1988), indicating significant reserve vasodilatory capacity despite the chronic renal vasodilation of pregnancy. To date, studies in normal women have been conflicting, since one group observed a substantial increase in endogenous creatinine clearance following a meat meal in the third trimester (Brendolan et al. 1985), whereas others have suggested that inulin and p-aminohippurate clearances increase marginally, if at all (Barron and Lindheimer 1995). Differences in intake of dietary protein influence the renal response to acute protein feeding in pregnant women, which may explain the differences in the literature (Woods and Gaboury 1995). In response to intravenous amino acids, however, normal pregnant women show a marked renal vasodilatory response (Sturgiss et al. 1996; Milne et al. 2002).

It is interesting that in women with single kidneys, where compensatory renal hypertrophy has already occurred, pregnancy still causes a significant augmentation of renal haemodynamics, unmasking renal reserve. Surprisingly, GFR increases in renal allograft recipients during pregnancy, where in addition to hypertrophy the kidney is ectopic, at best partially innervated, possibly from an old and/or male donor, potentially damaged by previous ischaemia, and immunologically different from both mother and fetus (Davison 1985).

Overall, the kidney in pregnancy exhibits significant renal vasodilatory reserve capacity, showing further acute renal vasodilatory responses to amino acids or a fall in blood pressure. Also, despite chronic compensatory renal vasodilation secondary to nephron loss, pregnancy remains an effective renal vasodilatory stimulus.

Mechanism(s) initiating the gestational increase in GFR

The first question, whether the renal vasodilatory stimulus in pregnancy arises from the mother or from fetoplacental sources, has been easy to study in the rat. In pseudopregnancy, a state characterized by

cessation of the oestrous cycle, rats exhibit identical changes in whole kidney and outer cortical single nephron function to those seen in pregnant rats (Baylis 1982). Also, peripheral vasodilation and the plasma volume expansion which attends normal pregnancy is evident in pseudopregnant rats (Baylis 1982; Slangen et al. 1997). In women, marked renal and peripheral vasodilation is evident early in pregnancy prior to complete placentation (Chapman et al. 1998). Similar changes occur in nonpregnant women in the luteal phase of the menstrual cycle (Davison and Noble 1981; Chapman et al. 1997). These studies suggest that the fetoplacental unit is not necessary for the increase in GFR (or the volume expansion) of pregnancy and indicate that some maternal stimulus must initiate these gestational changes.

Although the placenta is not involved in the initiation of the gestational increase in GFR, there may be some role for placental factors in maintenance of the elevated GFR later in pregnancy, since removal of the placenta from midterm-pregnant rats leads to reduction in GFR and renal plasma flow (Matthews and Taylor 1960).

Possible hormonal mediators

Renin–angiotensin system and other vasoconstrictors

The renin–angiotensin II system is substantially modified during pregnancy and although increases occur in plasma renin activity and plasma angiotensin II, a decreased responsivity to the vasopressor action of administered angiotensin II is also seen (Gant et al. 1987; Broughton-Pipkin 1988; Brown and Venuto 1988). Whether this loss of sensitivity to the vasoconstrictor actions of angiotensin II extends to the renal resistance vessels and the glomerulus is not clear. In vitro studies in pregnant rabbits and rats suggest downregulation of glomerular angiotensin II receptors (Brown and Venuto 1986; Barbour et al. 1990) but no difference in angiotensin II receptors in rabbit renal preglomerular vessels from pregnant and virgin animals (Brown and Venuto 1988). Some studies report a blunting of the renal vasoconstrictor response to administered angiotensin II in pregnant rabbits (Brown and Venuto 1991) and rats (Conrad and Colpoys 1986; Novak et al. 1997), although others show normal renal vascular responsiveness to administered angiotensin II in pregnant rats, despite loss of pressor responsivity (Sicinska et al. 1971; Masilamani and Baylis 1992). Also indirect, functional studies suggest that the glomeruli of midterm-pregnant rats do not develop a reduced responsivity to angiotensin II, since the glomerulotoxic effects of gentamicin (mediated by angiotensin II) are not blunted by pregnancy (Baylis 1989). Furthermore, since renal haemodynamics are not dependent on angiotensin II in the normal, unstressed animal (Baylis and Collins 1986; Baylis et al. 1993), loss of renal responsivity to endogenous angiotensin II cannot be the mechanism of the renal vasodilation of pregnancy. Also, studies in rats have indicated that angiotensin II-mediated renal vasoconstriction is unlikely to cause the close-to-term reduction in GFR and renal plasma flow (Baylis and Collins 1986; Conrad et al. 1989).

Vascular sensitivity to other vasoconstrictors is also influenced during pregnancy, and some workers report reduced peripheral responsivity to administered noradrenaline and arginine vasopressin (AVP) (Conrad and Colpoys 1986). Not everyone agrees that vascular responsiveness to α-adrenergic agonists is depressed in pregnancy (McLaughlin et al. 1989; Pan et al. 1990), but it does seem that baroreflex-mediated bradycardia is enhanced (Magness and Rosenfeld 1988; Crandall and Heesch 1990; Conrad and Russ 1992; Brooks *et al.* 1995). These systems have not been extensively studied with regard to control of renal haemodynamics in pregnancy; however, acute α_1-adrenoceptor blockade has similar depressor and renal vasoconstrictor effects on virgin, midterm, and late-pregnant, conscious rats (Baylis 1995), and acute blockade of the vascular AVP (V_1) receptor is without blood pressure or renal haemodynamic effect in conscious virgin, mid- and late-pregnant rats (Baylis 1993). In contrast to other vasoconstrictors, pressor responses to administered thromboxane A2 are potentiated in pregnant rabbits and rats while the renal vasoconstriction is also slightly enhanced (Kriston *et al.* 1999). Overall, alterations in the various vasoconstrictor systems are *unlikely* to contribute to the gestational renal vasodilation.

Prostaglandins

It is well documented that urinary prostaglandins increase in normal pregnant women, rats, and rabbits, and in pseudopregnant rats (Conrad and Colpoys 1986; Paller *et al.* 1989), and this has been generally assumed to reflect increased renal synthesis. One group has reported increased glomerular prostaglandin production in late-pregnant rats (Gregoire *et al.* 1987), and another that prostaglandin production by isolated glomeruli, and by cortical and papillary slices, was not elevated in pregnancy (Conrad and Dunn 1987), despite an increase in urine prostaglandin excretion in pregnant rats. Studies with acute cyclo-oxygenase inhibition in the pregnant rat suggest that the prostaglandins are not the renal vasodilators of pregnancy, since cyclo-oxygenase inhibition does not obliterate the gestational increase in GFR in either anaesthetized rats or in the conscious, chronically catheterized preparation (Conrad and Colpoys 1986; Baylis 1987). Chronic administration of cyclo-oxygenase inhibitors to pregnant rabbits (for 3 days) does not blunt the gestational increase in GFR (Venuto and Donker 1982). The *in vitro* data on prostaglandin production in pregnancy does not support a role for an increase in prostaglandins as primary mediators of the gestational increase in GFR. It has been suggested that prostaglandins can be 'recruited' as gestational renal vasodilators when the nitric oxide (NO) system is chronically inhibited (see below) (Danielson and Conrad 1996), although our observations indicate that cyclo-oxygenase products cannot compensate for the complete lack of NO in the pregnant rat (Baylis 2002).

Other vasodilator systems

Dopamine produces a selective renal vasodilation, and it has been suggested as the gestational renal vasodilatory agent since elevated urinary dopamine excretion has been reported during pregnancy (Perkins *et al.* 1981; Gregoire *et al.* 1990). At present, there is no evidence for a causal relationship between dopamine and the gestational renal vasodilation.

In the rat, plasma atrial natriuretic peptides (ANPs) and vascular and renal haemodynamic responsiveness to ANP are unchanged during gestation (Kristensen *et al.* 1986; Nadel *et al.* 1988; Masilamani and Baylis 1994), whereas normal women show moderate increases in plasma ANP during the second and third trimesters, although there is substantial variability in the data (Gregoire *et al.* 1990; Steegers *et al.* 1991). The glomerular haemodynamic mechanisms by which ANP increases GFR (Dunn *et al.* 1986) are different to that of normal pregnancy and administered ANP causes renal vasoconstriction in normal pregnant women (Irons *et al.* 1996), therefore ANP is unlikely to be involved in the renal haemodynamic alterations of pregnancy.

Nitric oxide

A number of studies have investigated whether enhanced production and/or sensitivity to NO occurs in normal pregnancy. In women, 24-h urinary excretions of cyclic guanosine monophosphate (cGMP) and plasma cGMP increase in normal pregnancy (Kopp *et al.* 1977; Begum *et al.* 1996; Boccardo *et al.* 1996; López-Jaramillo *et al.* 1996) although the persistence of this increased cGMP excretion long after delivery (Kopp *et al.* 1977) may reflect the prolonged postpartum rise in plasma ANP (Gregoire *et al.* 1990), rather than stimulation by NO. In fact, cGMP in the plasma and urine may have little prognostic value regarding activity of NO; for example, tissue but not plasma cGMP correlate inversely with blood pressure during graded doses of NO synthesis inhibitors in the non-pregnant rat (Arnal *et al.* 1992).

NO is unstable *in vivo* and is rapidly oxidized to NO_2 and NO_3 (NO_X) and the NO_X content of body fluids can be analysed, providing an index of NO production, after correction for dietary NO_X intake. Plasma and urinary NO_X excretions have been reported as unchanged and increased in normal pregnant women (Baylis *et al.* 1998). Of note, only one study has been conducted on a controlled low NO_X intake, a requirement for interpretation of NO_X values in the context of NO activity (Baylis and Vallance 1998), and here no difference was seen in plasma or 24-h urinary NO_X excretion in late pregnancy versus the non-pregnant state (Conrad *et al.* 1999). It is important to recognize that an increased NO_X production does not necessarily demonstrate an increased 'haemodynamically active' NO, and conversely, failure to demonstrate increased NO_X does not rule out local increases in regional vascular NO production (Baylis and Vallance 1998; Baylis *et al.* 1998). There have been a number of *in vitro* studies to assess abundance and/or activity of vascular nitric oxide synthase (NOS) in pregnancy, with variable results and these have been reviewed in detail elsewhere (Baylis *et al.* 1988; Poston *et al.* 1995; Sladek *et al.* 1997).

The *in vivo* response to acute systemic NOS inhibition in pregnant rats is also variable (Baylis *et al.* 1998) although an exaggerated local vasoconstriction is seen with intra-arterial NOS inhibition in the hand circulation of normal pregnant women, suggesting increased tonic NO release in the skin vasculature in pregnancy (Williams *et al.* 1997). Acute NOS inhibition in rats suggests that increased NO is responsible for the pregnancy-associated refractoriness to administered vasoconstrictors (Molnar and Hertelendy 1992). There is general agreement that chronic systemic NOS inhibition in the pregnant rat causes hypertension (Baylis et al. 1998) and this is noteworthy since in other models of genetic and experimentally induced hypertension in the rat, pregnancy is invariably associated with profound reduction in blood pressure (Takeda 1964).

Normal pregnant rats exhibit signs of relative arginine deficiency since orotic acid excretion increases progressively during pregnancy (Milner and Visek 1978) and plasma arginine is approximately 40 per cent reduced in the basal state (Raij 1994). There is also evidence that arginine deficiency develops in normal pregnant women since maternal plasma arginine concentrations decline although levels in cord blood are maintained (Ghadimi and Pecora 1964; Domenech *et al.* 1986) and orotic acid excretion increases markedly (Wood and O'Sullivan 1973). The possible impact on NO synthesis of this reduction in arginine availability is offset by a parallel decline in the circulating endogenous NOS inhibitor, asymmetric dimethyl arginine (Fickling *et al.* 1993).

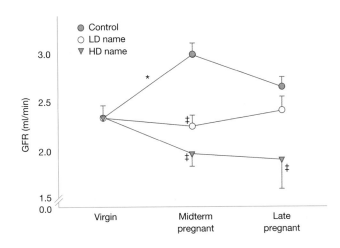

Fig. 7 Glomerular filtration rate (GFR) in conscious, chronically catheterized rats studied in the virgin state, midterm, and late pregnancy. Data are given for normal controls (solid circles), rats given chronic low-dose NOS inhibitor (oral L-NAME, 50 mg/l drinking water; open circles) and rats given chronic high-dose NOS inhibitor (oral L-NAME, 100 mg/l drinking water; closed triangles) (reproduced from Baylis and Engels 1992, with permission).

Although a role for increased NO production has not been established in the generalized peripheral vasodilation of normal pregnancy, animal studies suggest that increased NO production does play a role in the renal vasodilation of pregnancy. NO is a physiologically important, renal vasodilator (Raij and Baylis 1995) and acute NOS inhibition in pregnant rats selectively abolishes the midterm renal vasodilation, suggesting a specific role for NO (Danielson and Conrad 1995). We have found increased midterm renal NOS activity, *in vitro*, which has characteristics of both the inducible and neuronal NOS (Santmyire and Baylis 1998, 1999). *In vivo* and *in vitro* studies by others have implicated NO derived from both inducible NOS and neuronal NOS (Alexander *et al.* 1999, 2002; Abram *et al.* 2001) and it seems likely that a novel cytosolic NOS may be upregulated in the kidney during pregnancy, as suggested by Singh *et al.* (1997). Irrespective of the isoform responsible, nonselective chronic NOS inhibition during pregnancy leads to suppression of the renal vasodilation, with failure of the GFR to increase (Fig. 7), proteinuria, and increased maternal and fetal morbidity and mortality (Baylis and Engels 1992; Deng *et al.* 1996; Baylis 2002) in a pattern that closely resembles the symptoms of pre-eclampsia. Thus, studies in the rat suggest that increased NO production is responsible for the renal vasodilation in the normal pregnant rat, but at present there are no clinical studies which address this issue. Furthermore, an elegant recent study has suggested a key role for the ovarian hormone relaxin, which may signal increased NO in rat pregnancy (Danielson *et al.* 1999) although this remains to be confirmed.

Influence of the plasma volume expansion on the gestational increase in GFR

Plasma volume expansion will cause renal vasodilation with resultant increases in renal plasma flow and GFR in non-pregnant rats, provided

the volume expansion is of sufficient magnitude. A cumulative volume expansion occurs during pregnancy in both women and rats, such that, close to term, plasma volume is enormously expanded (Lindheimer and Katz 1985b; Baylis 1994). There is, however, a dissociation between the plasma volume increase and the elevation in renal plasma flow and GFR in pregnancy well before the maximum increase in plasma volume. It therefore seems that the plasma volume expansion of pregnancy is not the primary determinant of the gestational increase in GFR.

Renal tubular function in human and animal pregnancy

The physiological plasma volume expansion of pregnancy leads to small decrements in plasma concentration of many plasma constituents, despite which their filtered load increases due to the large rise in GFR. Modest increments in excretion are seen for some substances but increases in tubular reabsorption often occur, preventing depletion. Intake also frequently increases, with net retention leading to positive balance for many of the key constituents. The renal handling of a number of solutes is altered in normal pregnancy, as discussed below.

Renal handling of sodium

Renal sodium handling is the prime determinant of volume homeostasis and will be discussed in detail later.

Renal handling of uric acid (see Chapter 6.4)

Plasma uric acid concentration decreases by 25 per cent during early pregnancy, so that normal values range from 149 to 298 μmol/l with 298–327 μmol/l being an acceptable upper limit of normal. It has been suggested that this reflects alterations in the fractional excretion of uric acid (uric acid clearance/GFR) due to a decrease in net tubular reabsorption (Dunlop and Davison 1977). The changes are greatest in early gestation because as pregnancy advances, the kidney appears to excrete a smaller proportion of the filtered uric acid load, and this increase in net reabsorption is associated with an increasing plasma uric acid concentration which returns towards the non-pregnant value.

There may be racial variations for the normal range as well as diurnal variations during pregnancy, with the highest values noted in the morning and lowest in the evening (Barry *et al.* 1992). Also, plasma concentrations tend to be higher in the presence of multiple fetuses (Fischer *et al.* 1995).

Renal handling of glucose

Excretion of glucose increases soon after conception and may exceed non-pregnant rates by a factor of 10 (Sturgiss *et al.* 1994). The glycosuria varies markedly, both from day to day and within 24h, but the intermittency is unrelated to either blood glucose concentrations or duration of gestation. Normal non-pregnant values are re-established within a week of delivery.

Renal handling of glucose is complex. There is normally extensive proximal reabsorption of filtered glucose until the maximal reabsorptive capacity (T_mG) is reached. In non-pregnant women, the T_mG averages 1.6–1.9 mmol/min (300–350 mg/min), which, at normal blood glucose values, sufficiently exceeds filtered load to result in excretion of an almost glucose-free urine. The original concept of a fixed T_mG is now known to be incorrect (Davison and Cheyne 1972) because trace quantities of glucose are always present in normal urine and T_mG varies with changes in extracellular fluid volume and GFR (see below).

The glycosuria of pregnancy could be due to the inability of the renal tubules to cope with the increased filtered glucose load, a change in tubular reabsorption *per se*, or both. Serial studies of the renal handling of glucose under infusion conditions in women with varying degrees of glycosuria have shown that glucose reabsorption is less complete during pregnancy than when non-pregnant (Davison and Hytten 1975). Reabsorption was always less complete in pregnant women with obvious glycosuria, and these women, although no longer clinically glycosuric following pregnancy, still had less complete reabsorption under infusion conditions when they were not pregnant, that is, all women demonstrated decrements in the fractional reabsorption of glucose (T/F glucose) in pregnancy; that is, the T_mG declined (Fig. 8).

Renal handling of other sugars

The excretion of lactose, fructose, xylose, and fucose are increased in pregnancy, but not that of arabinose (Davison 1975). Some oligosaccharides, which (similar to lactose) are presumably of mammary gland origin, appear in the urine of pregnant women.

Lactosuria is a benign condition of pregnancy of no clinical importance except as a possible source of confusion with glycosuria. It is easy to distinguish between glucose and lactose, since lactose does not react with glucose oxidase paper test strips.

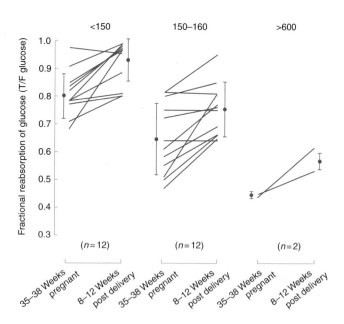

Fig. 8 Twenty-four-hour glucose excretion during pregnancy. Fractional reabsorption of glucose under infusion conditions (individual values and means ± SD) in 26 women studied during late pregnancy and after the puerperium. Women were divided into three groups according to their 24-h glucose excretion (mg) during pregnancy. The within-groups significance (paired student's *t*-test) for less than 150 mg/24 h was $p < 0.005$; and for 150–600 mg/24 h was $p < 0.005$. The between-groups significance (student's *t*-test) was $p < 0.001$ (data were calculated from Davison and Hytten 1975).

Renal handling of water-soluble vitamins

Nicotinic acid, ascorbic acid, and folic acid are all excreted in increased amounts during pregnancy (Davison 1975). In the case of folic acid, this is due to less efficient tubular reabsorption because plasma folate declines in pregnancy and, despite the increase in GFR, the filtered load is unlikely to be increased. These increases in renal excretion of vitamins emphasizes the need for adequate vitamin supplementation in pregnancy.

Renal handling of amino acids

Urinary excretion of most, but not all, amino acids increases in pregnancy. There are several patterns of amino acid excretion (Hytten and Cheyne 1972). Excretion of glycine, histidine, threonine, serine, and alanine increases in early pregnancy and remains elevated through to term. The excretion of lysine, cystine, taurine, phenylalanine, valine, leucine, and tyrosine also increases markedly in early pregnancy but thereafter tends to decline. Glutamic acid, methionine, and ornithine are excreted in slightly greater amounts than before pregnancy, isoleucine excretion is unchanged, and that of arginine tends to decrease. The reduction in arginine excretion is consistent with reduced arginine availability, discussed earlier in the context of increased NO production (see above). The increased excretion of most amino acids, together with reduced blood concentrations and the elevated GFR of pregnancy, point to the possibility of diminished tubular reabsorption. Overall, urinary total amino acid excretion during pregnancy may reach 2 g/day.

Renal regulation of acid–base (see Chapter 2.6)

In pregnancy, the daily amount of acid generated is increased due both to an increased basal metabolism and greater food intake. Despite this increased acid load, the blood concentrations of hydrogen ions *decrease* by 2–4 mmol/l early in pregnancy, a decrement which is sustained until term. Thus, arterial pH averages 7.44 in pregnant women, compared to 7.40 in non-pregnant women. This mild alkalaemia is respiratory in origin, since pregnant women normally hyperventilate and their arterial P_{CO_2} decreases from approximately 39 mmHg when non-pregnant to approximately 31 mmHg in pregnancy. A secondary, compensatory fall in plasma bicarbonate concentration occurs so that values between 18 and 22 mmol/l are normal (Lucius *et al.* 1970).

The renal capacity to reabsorb bicarbonate and excrete H^+ is unchanged by pregnancy (Lim *et al.* 1976), but since steady-state plasma bicarbonate and P_{CO_2} are less than in non-pregnant women, the pregnant woman is at a disadvantage when threatened by sudden metabolic acidosis, such as lactic acidosis in pre-eclampsia, diabetic ketoacidosis, or acute renal failure.

Renal handling of protein

Both total protein excretion (TPE) and urinary albumin excretion (UAE) are significantly elevated after 20 weeks in normal pregnancy, with pregnancy means (and upper limits) for 24-h TPE and UAE as 200 mg (300 mg) and 12 mg (29 mg), respectively (Higby *et al.* 1994; Taylor and Davison 1997). These gestational increases may be due to the increment in GFR, alteration in glomerular barrier permeability/change and/or altered tubular handling of filtered proteins (Roberts *et al.* 1996; Milne *et al.* 2002).

Potassium excretion

Despite the high aldosterone values and relatively alkaline urine of pregnancy, potassium excretion is decreased during gestation, which together with the increased potassium intake leads to significant net potassium retention of approximately 350 mmol of potassium, most of which enters the enlarging tissues of mother and fetus. Furthermore, pregnant women are resistant to the kaliuretic effects of a combination of exogenous mineralocorticoids and a high sodium intake (Lindheimer *et al.* 1987). The gestational tendency to conserve potassium despite increased concentrations of potent mineralocorticoids has been ascribed to the antimineralocorticoid effect of the increased progesterone of pregnancy (Brown *et al.* 1986).

The tubular handling of potassium is complex and the final urinary potassium excretion is independent of the filtered load of potassium and is determined largely by the magnitude of potassium secretion in the distal nephron (Giebisch *et al.* 1986). Probably, inhibition of potassium secretion in the collecting duct, and/or enhanced potassium recycling, provides the final mechanism of urinary potassium conservation by the gravida.

The resistance of pregnant women to the potassium-losing effects of steriods may benefit those with certain potassium-losing diseases. There are reports that hypokalaemia is ameliorated during pregnancy in women with Conn's syndrome (primary aldosteronism) and Bartter's syndrome (Klaus *et al.* 1971). On the other hand, renal resistance to kaliuretic stimuli in women with underlying disorders impairing potassium excretion could jeopardize pregnancy, as with sickle-cell anaemia (Lindheimer *et al.* 1987).

Calcium excretion

An increase in the filtered load of calcium accompanies the increased GFR of pregnancy and despite an increase in tubular reabsorption, urinary calcium excretion increases two- to threefold during pregnancy (Howarth *et al.* 1977). The hypercalciuria may be secondary to increased plasma 1,25-dihydroxy vitamin D_3 (calcitriol), a hormone which increases intestinal reabsorption of calcium and is known to cause hypercalciuria (Maikranz *et al.* 1994). Calcitriol can suppress serum parathyroid hormone (directly and by increased serum calcium) such that renal calcium reabsorption is reduced in the thick ascending limb of the loop of Henle.

As well as increased calcium excretion in pregnancy, urinary supersaturation is increased, predisposing to the formation of calcium stones. However, magnesium and citrate, known inhibitors of calcium kidney stones, also increase and afford some protection against nephrolithiasis (Maikranz *et al.* 1994). In addition, during pregnancy there is increased excretion of acidic glycoproteins, including Tamm–Horsfall protein (Nakagawa *et al.* 1989) and nephrocalcin (Davison *et al.* 1993), which inhibit calcium oxalate stone formation.

Osmoregulation in pregnancy

Very early in pregnant women, plasma osmolality decreases by about 10 mOsm/kg below the non-pregnant norm (Davison *et al.* 1981) due to a reduction in plasma sodium and associated anions (Fig. 9). This hypo-osmolality would inhibit antidiuretic hormone (AVP) release in non-pregnant individuals, leading to a state of continuous diuresis.

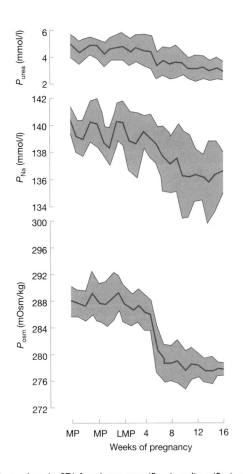

Fig. 9 Mean values (± SD) for plasma urea (P_{urea}), sodium (P_{Na}), and osmolality (P_{osm}) measured at weekly intervals from before conception through the first trimester in nine women with successful obstetric outcome. MP, menstrual period; LMP, last menstrual period (reproduced from Davison *et al.* 1981, with permission).

However, this does not happen in pregnancy because the osmotic thresholds for AVP release and thirst also decrease during the initial weeks of pregnancy (Davison *et al.* 1988) (Fig. 10). The decrement in thirst threshold may precede that for hormone release, resulting in mild transient polyuria early in pregnancy. The rat exhibits similar reductions in plasma osmolality and the osmotic threshold for AVP release during pregnancy, while basal plasma AVP and urinary concentrating and diluting capacity remain unchanged (Durr *et al.* 1981; Barron *et al.* 1985).

Human chorionic gonadotrophin (hCG) may influence osmoregulation in pregnancy, since small increments in circulating hCG decrease the osmotic thresholds for thirst and AVP secretion in non-pregnant women (Davison *et al.* 1988).

Osmoregulation may also be affected by changes in AVP metabolism which are apparent by midpregnancy. The metabolic clearance rate of AVP is similar to non-pregnant values in early pregnancy, but increases fourfold during the second and third trimesters (Davison *et al.* 1989b). The blood of pregnant women contains a cystine aminopeptidase enzyme (vasopressinase) of placental origin, capable of inactivating large quantities of AVP *in vitro*. Increments in the metabolic clearance rate of AVP correlate with the appearance and increase in plasma vasopressinase after midpregnancy (Davison *et al.* 1989b), suggesting that

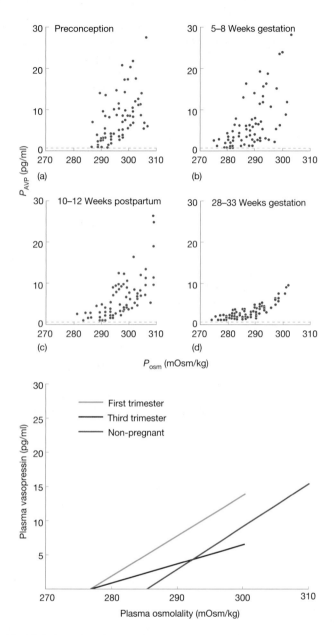

Fig. 10 Relationship of P_{AVP} to P_{osmol} during several 5% saline infusions of eight women before pregnancy and during pregnancy. Each part, (a)–(d), represents an individual plasma measurement. Highly significant mean regression lines from first and third trimesters and non-pregnant tests show the marked decrease in osmotic threshold for AVP release (abscissal intercept) during pregnancy. Volumes for the osmotic threshold for thirst (not shown) were always 2–5 mOsm/kg above AVP release and were also 10 mOsm/kg lower in pregnancy (from data given in Davison *et al.* 1981, 1988).

the placental vasopressinase is also active *in vivo*. Furthermore, the metabolic clearance rate of 1-desamino-(8-D-arginine) vasopressin, an AVP analogue resistant to *in vitro* degradation by vasopressinase, does not increase during human gestation (Davison *et al.* 1993). In addition, the placenta can degrade AVP *in situ*, and studies with *in vitro* perfusion of term placentas suggest that this organ may be responsible for at least one-third of the increased hormonal disposal rates during pregnancy (Landon *et al.* 1988).

Volume status is a separate, non-osmotic determinant of AVP release (Lindheimer and Davison 1995). Hypovolaemia stimulates AVP secretion, and although this is much less sensitive than the osmotic control, when activated (by greater than about 10 per cent haemorrhage), volume depletion provides a powerful stimulus to AVP release. Absolute blood volume increases significantly in pregnancy, but how 'effective volume' is sensed is controversial (see below), and it has been postulated that the osmoregulatory changes are due to 'underfilling' of the dilated intravascular compartment (Schrier 1988). Hypovolaemia can diminish osmotic thresholds for AVP release and thirst, however, central volume expansion (by water immersion) in pregnancy has no effect on the reduced plasma osmolality or the lowered osmotic thresholds (Davison *et al.* 1989a). In the late-pregnant rat, where blood volume is almost twice normal, the relation between AVP secretion and percentage volume depletion, by graded haemorrhage, is similar to that in the virgin (Barron *et al.* 1984), indicating resetting of the non-osmotic release of AVP during pregnancy to sense the expanded volume as normal.

Volume homeostasis and tubular function in human and animal pregnancy

In normal pregnant women, the average weight gain is 12.5 kg, much of which is fluid, since total body water increases by 6–8 l, of which 4–6 l are extracellular. There are increases in plasma volume (maximum during the second trimester and approaching 50 per cent above non-pregnant values) and in fluid accumulations within the fetal and maternal interstitial spaces, which are greatest in late pregnancy (Gallery and Brown 1987). During normal pregnancy, there is a gradual cumulative retention of about 900 mmol of sodium, distributed between the products of conception and maternal extracellular space.

Renal handling of sodium

In pregnant women, the filtered sodium load increases from about 20,000 to about 30,000 mmol/day, due to increases in GFR and despite a slight reduction in plasma sodium concentration. The adaptive increment in renal tubular reabsorption not only equals the increase in filtered load, but an additional 2–6 mmol of sodium are reabsorbed daily for fetal and maternal stores (Gallery and Brown 1987). Nevertheless, it is usual for sodium excretion to increase during pregnancy, reflecting an increase in intake. The pregnant woman handles ingested salt as she would when she is not pregnant.

It has not been possible to determine how sodium is handled at individual nephron segments during pregnancy. Using lithium clearance (with simultaneous measurement of GFR and urinary volume) as an index of proximal tubular sodium reabsorption, studies in normal women indicate enhanced sodium reabsorption in the proximal tubule and distal nephron segments in late pregnancy (Atherton *et al.* 1988). However, caution should be employed in interpretation of lithium clearance studies, since animal studies have shown that lithium may be reabsorbed in the ascending limb of the loop of Henle as well as in the proximal tubule (Kirchner 1987).

The reason for the net renal sodium retention in pregnancy is not known and, in fact, sodium homeostasis in pregnancy remains an enigma. As shown in Table 1, there are many factors operating to both increase and to decrease sodium excretion, and exactly how the normal balance of net retention is achieved remains a mystery.

Factors influencing sodium excretion

Hormones

Antinatriuretic hormones

Several hormones that enhance sodium reabsorption (i.e. antinatriuretic hormones) are increased in pregnancy (August and Lindheimer 1995).

Angiotensin There are marked increased in plasma angiotensin II levels in normal pregnancy. In addition to stimulating aldosterone release (see below), physiological concentrations of angiotensin II act directly on the proximal tubule to increase sodium reabsorption. However, a refractoriness develops to the vascular and possibly tubular actions of angiotensin II in normal pregnancy which may nullify any net sodium retention by this mechanism (August and Lindheimer 1995).

Aldosterone Values are elevated and often exceed those measured in patients with primary aldosteronism (Lindheimer and Katz 1985a), but without causing potassium depletion, oedema, or hypertension. Despite these high values, aldosterone still serves a homeostatic function in pregnancy, as it does in non-pregnant subjects, since sodium depletion results in further increases of aldosterone, while expansion of body fluid volume decreases the concentration of aldosterone appropriately.

Desoxycorticosterone Concentrations increase continuously throughout normal pregnancy, but most markedly in the third trimester (MacDonald *et al.* 1982; August and Lindheimer 1995). This pattern of change is similar to that for aldosterone, progesterone, and oestradiol, and correlations are often emphasized in discussion of renal salt balance. Whereas aldosterone is loosely bound to plasma proteins so that increasing plasma concentrations with advancing pregnancy result in comparable increments in the biologically active free steroid, each of the other hormones is bound to carrier protein

(globulins). Since concentrations of these globulins also increase during pregnancy, the biologically free moiety may not increase above non-pregnant values. The situation is more complex in the case of desoxycorticosterone, which is bound to cortisol-binding globulin with an avidity similar to that of cortisol and probably greater than that of progesterone, and alteration in the concentrations of these two hormones may influence the values of plasma-free desoxycorticosterone. In this respect, both urinary free desoxycorticosterone and the free desoxycorticosterone in plasma are substantially increased during gestation.

Some of the increased desoxycorticosterone during pregnancy may be from a fetal source, but the current view is that most arises by extra-adrenal 21-hydroxylation of circulating progesterone. Oestrogen enhances the activity of the enzyme responsible for 21-hydroxylation of progesterone to desoxycorticosterone (MacDonald *et al.* 1982). Also, steroid 21-hydroxylase activity, present in human kidneys, is increased in the kidney in pregnancy (Winkel *et al.* 1980); consequently, much of the increased desoxycorticosterone during pregnancy may be produced in the vicinity of its renal receptor. Furthermore, these extra-adrenal factors may also be the reason why the increased plasma desoxycorticosterone of pregnancy is not suppressible by sodium loading and ACTH or dexamethasone administration (Nolten *et al.* 1980).

The role in pregnancy of several other hormones with potentially antinatriuretic activity remains to be elucidated. Oestrogens, known to induce sodium retention in the rat, increase markedly during human pregnancy (Lindheimer and Katz 1985a). Increased oestrogen may also enhance the extra-adrenal 21-hydroxylase activity and, thus, increase the conversion of natriuretic progesterone to salt-retaining desoxycorticosterone (MacDonald *et al.* 1982). Prolactin is a sodium-retaining and osmoregulatory hormone in lower animals (Ensor 1978) but its role in mammals is less clear. In addition to prolactin, human placental lactogen, growth hormone, ACTH, and cortisol may also cause renal sodium retention, but their roles in gestational sodium retention are not clear.

Natriuretic hormones

The concentration of several potentially natriuretic hormones increases in pregnancy. Progesterone increases by 10- to 100-fold and these concentrations are potently natriuretic, and cause a natriuresis in non-pregnant subjects by an antimineralocorticoid effect as well as a direct inhibitory effect on proximal tubular reabsorption. The significance of increased neurophysins, melanocyte-stimulating hormone, AVP, oxytocin, and the vasodilatory prostaglandins is uncertain, but all can be natriuretic under certain circumstances (August and Lindheimer 1995).

ANP and its metabolic clearance increase in human pregnancy, although plasma ANP increments are small relative to the marked intravascular volume expansion (Castro *et al.* 1994). Furthermore, the pregnant rat develops resistance to the natriuretic effects of ANP (Masilamani and Baylis 1994), although this is not reported in normal women (Irons *et al.* 1996). ND is also a potent natriuretic agent, both by virtue of its renal vasodilatory action and by direct inhibition of sodium reabsorption in the collecting duct (Stoos *et al.* 1995), and NO increases in normal rat and possibly human pregnancy (see above). Both ANP and NO signal through cGMP and it is possible that there may be a generalized adaptation of the tubular epithelium which opposes natriuretic stimuli that act via cGMP. We have preliminary observations in normal late pregnant rats which demonstrate an

Table 1 Factors that influence sodium excretion in pregnancy

Increase	Decrease
Marked increase in GFR	Elevated plasma aldosterone
Increased progesterone production	concentration
Natriuretic hormone(s)	Increased concentration of
Possible increments in neurophysins, prostaglandins, and melanocyte-stimulating hormone	other potential salt-retaining hormones (oestrogen, cortisol, placental lactogen, prolactin)
Physical factors	Physical factors
Decreased plasma albumin (possible postglomerular oncotic pressure decreased)	Possible filtration fraction increase (possible postglomerular oncotic pressure increase)
Decreased vasular resistance	Placenta may simulate arteriovenous shunt
Possible increased renin activity	Exaggerated influence of upright and supine posture
	Increased ureteral pressure
	Possible increased renin activity

increased activity of the cGMP-degrading enzyme, phosphodiesterase 5, in the inner medulla, and this will inhibit all cGMP-mediated natriuretic signals (Ni *et al.* 2001a). Of note, this same alteration is associated with the pathological renal sodium retention and volume expansion that are characteristic of liver cirrhosis and nephrotic syndrome (Valentin *et al.* 1992; Ni *et al.*, 2001b). It has even been suggested that a globalantinatriuretic event occurs in late pregnancy involving a ubiquitous increase in Na^+,K^+-ATPase activity. There is evidence of enhanced activity of Na^+,K^+-ATPase and Na–Li countertransport in red cells from pregnant women (Gallery 1984) and increased renal Na^+,K^+-ATPase activity has been observed in late pregnant rats (Lindheimer and Katz 1971). However, a more recent, extensive study by us revealed no increase in either Na^+,K^+-ATPase subunit abundance or enzyme activity in the kidney of the late pregnant rat; in fact, some declines were observed (Mahaney *et al.* 1998). Furthermore, the plasma levels of oubain-like inhibitors of Na^+,K^+-ATPase are also increased in normal pregnant women (Phelps *et al.* 1988); thus, the net effect of pregnancy on renal tubular Na^+,K^+-ATPase is not known.

Physical factors

Antinatriuretic

Physical factors which have antinatriuretic potential in women are the elevated intraureteral pressure (in the upright or supine positions) and the presence of the newly formed uterine vasculature (August and Lindheimer 1995), which has been likened to an arteriovenous shunt. Maternal posture is another physical factor influencing sodium handling during pregnancy. Supine and upright positions are strongly antinatriuretic and standing may decrease sodium excretion more in a pregnant than in a non-pregnant woman. Finally, the decrease in mean arterial blood pressure that also occurs in normal pregnancy is antinatriuretic.

Natriuretic

Increased GFR leads to increased filtration of sodium which will increase sodium excretion. Decreases in plasma albumin concentration and the increment in effective renal plasma flow during pregnancy will also enhance sodium excretion by inhibiting tubular sodium reabsorption (Baylis 1984). The slightly decreased filtration fraction and consequent reduction in postglomerular and thus renal interstitial colloid osmotic (oncotic) pressure in pregnant women will reduce proximal tubular sodium reabsorption via a direct action on the tubule (Wilcox *et al.* 1992).

It is evident that there are many conflicting stimuli to sodium excretion in pregnancy but net sodium retention and marked plasma volume expansion is the norm. In fact, there is a strong positive correlation between the maternal plasma volume expansion and a successful obstetrical outcome (Brown and Gallery 1994). In the normal non-pregnant steady state, plasma volume expansion and renal sodium retention cannot coexist, but pregnancy is not a steady state, and the volume sensing and regulatory systems are dramatically readjusted throughout pregnancy to accommodate and maintain the volume expansion (see below).

Volume sensing systems in pregnancy

Volume sensing and control in pregnancy is different from that in non-gravid states. Despite the progressive extracellular fluid volume expansion of normal pregnancy, the volume receptors sense these large gains as normal and when diuretics or salt restriction limit volume expansion, the maternal response is similar to that observed in salt-depleted non-pregnant women (Lindheimer and Katz 1985a). Below, we consider how various volume sensing and regulatory systems respond in pregnancy.

Plasma renin activity, concentration (mainly in the form of 'big' or inactive renin), and substrate, as well as plasma angiotensin II, increase markedly in pregnancy, and pregnant women and rats are resistant to the pressor and renal effects of infused angiotensin II (Broughton-Pipkin 1988; Baylis 1994). In non-pregnant animals and humans, increased plasma renin, angiotensin II, and aldosterone is associated with volume depletion (Ballerman *et al.* 1986), whereas in pregnancy, elevated renin, angiotensin II, and aldosterone coexist with a plasma volume which, in absolute terms, is expanded.

It is unclear exactly how the changes in the renin–angiotensin system during pregnancy are associated with the alterations in volume homeostasis. For example, baseline renin activity, already elevated despite increased effective renal plasma flow and absolute blood volume, is increased further by sodium restriction (Hsueh *et al.* 1984) or assumption of the supine or upright posture (Lindheimer and Katz 1985a) and is decreased by volume expansion, data consistent with a new 'set point' in the system. On the other hand, it has been suggested that the enhanced renin secretion in pregnancy is secondary to increments in vasodilatory prostaglandins (Friedman 1988), which originate from both the uterus and vascular endothelium. The prostaglandins could contribute to the decreased blood pressure and dilated vascular compartment of normal pregnancy, and both the vasodilation and the direct action of increased prostacyclin concentration could lead to compensatory stimulation of the renin–angiotensin system (Broughton-Pipkin 1988). This might explain why angiotensin and aldosterone values are increased despite the absolute hypervolaemia of pregnancy. Indeed, increased renin/angiotensin in pregnancy has been cited as evidence that pregnancy is actually a state of 'underfill', that is, suboptimal blood volume despite the marked increase in blood volume that occurs in absolute terms (Schrier and Durr 1987; Schrier 1988). This view is supported by the observation that in early pregnancy an infusion of angiotensin-converting enzyme inhibitors leads to exaggerated decrements in blood pressure (Taufield *et al.* 1988), while graded infusions of angiotensin II lead to greater increments in aldosterone than similar doses evoke in non-pregnant individuals.

In contrast, and as discussed in detail above, both osmotic and non-osmotic control of antidiuretic hormone release are dramatically altered in normal pregnancy in a manner indicating that the expanded volume of pregnancy is sensed as normal.

The ANP system is activated in response to increased extracellular fluid volume (Ballerman and Brenner 1986). In the late pregnant rat, the cardiac content of ANP and plasma ANP are similar to those in the virgin, despite an absolute increase in plasma volume of 70–80 per cent (Kristensen *et al.* 1986; Nadel *et al.* 1988). Plasma ANP increases slightly in late-pregnant women, but this is unlikely to reflect a physiological response to volume expansion because:

1. atrial size does not change during normal pregnancy (Steegers *et al.* 1991);

2. plasma ANP remains elevated long after delivery (Gregoire *et al.* 1990), when plasma volume has returned to normal; and

3. even greater increases in ANP are seen in pre-eclamptic pregnancies, which also exhibit volume contraction (Irons *et al.* 1997).

Thus, the ANP system appears to recognize the expanded volume in pregnancy as 'normal'.

The tubuloglomerular feedback system also functions as an intra-renal volume sensing and regulatory system, in which the delivery of tubular fluid is sensed by the macula densa (a specialized region in the early distal nephron). When fluid delivery increases, a signal is sent to the parent glomerulus, resulting in vasoconstriction with a consequent reduction in single nephron GFR and, thus, restoration of early distal fluid delivery. In some states of chronic volume expansion in the non-gravid animal, tubuloglomerular feedback activity is suppressed (Blantz and Pelayo 1984), an adaptation which allows the volume-expanded organism to excrete the excess volume load efficiently. However, in pregnancy, the tubuloglomerular feedback system is not suppressed but is reset to recognize the expanded volume and increased GFR as normal (Baylis and Blantz 1985).

Taken in concert, the various volume sensing and control systems are dramatically altered in normal pregnancy. Despite clear evidence of an absolute expansion in the plasma volume, the majority of body-volume sensor systems are perceiving the maternal plasma volume as normal or contracted. This raises the concept of 'effective' rather than absolute vascular volume (Schrier and Durr 1987; Schrier 1988). In normal, physiological pregnancy, the peripheral vasculature is markedly vasodilated; this is the only mechanism by which the elevated cardiac output of pregnancy could be accommodated without increasing arterial blood pressure. This vasodilation produces pooling of blood in the venous side of the circulation, which means arterial volume receptors sense the 'effective' blood volume as less expanded. Also, in non-gravid animals, the presence of an arteriovenous fistula causes renal sodium retention, suggesting that the 'effective' blood volume may be sensed as reduced. As indicated in a recent rat study, the responses of the ANP system in late pregnancy are consistent with the presence of an arteriovenous fistula (the uteroplacental perfusion circuit) while the abrupt increase in atrial peptide immediately following parturition is consistent with closure of the same 'arterio-venous fistula' (Nadel et al. 1988).

Clinical relevance of renal alterations

The altered milieu of pregnancy means that haemodynamic and biochemical markers of normal functions are substantially altered. Table 2 summarizes how a number of these common normal values are altered by pregnancy.

Assessment of renal function

Plasma creatinine decreases from a non-pregnant value of 73 μmol/l to 65, 51, and 47 μmol/l, respectively, in successive trimesters; plasma urea declines from non-pregnancy values of 4.3 mmol/l to pregnancy values of 3.5, 3.3, and 3.1 mmol/l, respectively. Familiarity with the changes is vital, because values considered normal in non-pregnant women may signify decreased renal function in pregnancy. As a rough guide, values of plasma creatinine and urea greater than 75 μmol/l and of 4.5 mmol/l, respectively, should alert the clinician to assess renal function further. It should be remembered, however, that caution is necessary when assessing renal function serially on the basis of plasma creatinine alone, especially in the presence of renal disease. Even when up to 50 per cent of renal function has been lost, it is still possible to have a plasma creatinine of less than 130 μmol/l.

Table 2 Changes (means) in some common indices during pregnancy

	Non-pregnant	Pregnancy
Hct (vol/dl)	41	33
$P_{protein}$ (g/dl)	7.0	6.0
P_{osm} (mOsm/kg)	285	275
P_{Na} (mEq/l)	140	135
P_{cr} mmol/l (mg/dl)	73 (0.8)	45 (0.5)
P_{urea} mmol/l (mg/dl)	4.5 (27)	3.3 (20)
pH units	7.40	7.44
P_{CO_2} (kPa)	40	30
P_{HCO_3} (mEq/l)	25	20
$P_{uric\ acid}$ μmol/l (mg/dl)	250 (0.40)	190 (0.32) early 259 (0.43) late
Systolic BP (mmHg)	115	105
Diastolic BP (mmHg)	70	60

Creatinine clearance in clinical practice (see also Chapter 1.3)

Although plasma (or serum) creatinine, its reciprocal, or its logarithm is often used to estimate GFR (in relation to age, height, and weight) (Trolifors et al. 1987), this approach has been questioned for pregnancy (Sturgiss et al. 1994), where in any case it is not ideal, because body weight or size do not reflect kidney size. Ideally, evaluation of renal function in pregnancy should be based on the clearance rather than the plasma concentration of creatinine. To overcome such problems as 'washout' from changes in urine flow, and to avoid difficulties caused by diurnal variations, 24-h urine samples should be used for clearances. Many methods of determining creatinine concentration in plasma also measure non-creatinine chromogens, leading to overestimates that must be taken into account when calculating creatinine clearances. In addition, recent intake of cooked meat can increase plasma creatinine by up to 16 μmol/l (because prolonged cooking converts preformed creatine into creatinine) and awareness of this governs the timing of blood sampling during a clearance period.

Changes in plasma uric acid

From the clinical viewpoint it is of interest that plasma uric acid concentration and renal absorption are significantly greater in pregnancies complicated by pre-eclampsia or intrauterine growth retardation. At a critical blood value of greater than 350 μmol/l there is significant perinatal mortality in hypertensive patients and serial measurements can be used to monitor progress in pre-eclampsia (Redman et al. 1976). It must be remembered that there is diurnal variation in plasma concentrations, that variability is such that some healthy women have hyperuricaemia without problems, that single random measurements are of no use clinically, and that concentrations tend to be greater with multiple pregnancy (see above).

Changes in glucose excretion

Glycosuria of pregnancy reflects alteration in renal function rather than alteration in carbohydrate metabolism (Sturgiss et al. 1994). The testing of random urine samples during pregnancy is unhelpful in the diagnosis or control of diabetes mellitus and unrepresentative as to the degree of glycosuria present.

Proteinuria

Urine flow normally varies over a wide range from moment to moment so that the protein concentration of a random specimen can give only a semiquantitative appraisal. Proteinuria on dipstick testing is notoriously unreliable (Halligan et al. 1999) and '1+' will not represent significant proteinuria in 50 per cent. In normal pregnancy proteinuria may well be up to 500 mg in 24 h (twice the upper limit in non-pregnancy), but for the purposes of definition 300 mg in 24 h is considered abnormal (Brown et al. 2001). Some now advocate 'near-bedside' urinalysis devices to quantify spot urine protein/creatinine ratios, with greater than 30 mg protein/mmol creatinine being the optimal discriminant value for true proteinuria, with sensitivity 93 per cent, specificity 92 per cent, positive predictive value 95 per cent, and negative predictive value 90 per cent (Sandan et al. 1997).

Currently, there is debate about the independent effect of normal pregnancy on long-term renal function, using microalbuminuria to detect any damage (Davison 1987; Baylis 1994; Sturgiss et al. 1994). As discussed in detail elsewhere in this chapter, the consensus is that pregnancy does not damage the kidney, and in any case, better markers are needed than albumin excretion alone.

The proteinuria of pre-eclampsia is non-selective, and from a variety of research approaches the data endorse the concept of an attenuated K_f in association with reduced renal blood flow, a significant non-discriminatory shunt (ω_o), some loss of glomerular charge but no increase in intraglomerular pressure (ΔP) (Naiker et al. 1997; Lafayette et al. 1998; Moran et al. 2003).

Renal function tests in pregnancy

Serial data on renal function are often needed to supplement routine antenatal observations. Tests available for use in routine clinical practice include the estimation of plasma urea and electrolytes, creatinine clearance determination, and urinary concentration and dilution assessment. Serial surveillance of 24-h creatinine clearance and protein excretion (24-h collections and protein–creatinine ratios) should be performed and, where possible, compared with non-pregnant values.

If renal function deteriorates at any stage of pregnancy, reversible causes such as urinary tract infection or obstruction, subtle dehydration, or electrolyte imbalance (perhaps secondary to inadvertent diuretic therapy) should be sought. Near term, a decrease in function of 15 per cent (which affects plasma creatinine minimally) is probably normal. If hypertension accompanies any observed decrease in renal function, the outlook is usually more serious. Immediate decisions and action may be required and the patient should be admitted to hospital.

Volume homeostasis and diuretics

Optimal maternal extracellular fluid volume in pregnancy is associated with successful perinatal outcome, implying that this adaptation is associated with optimal uteroplacental perfusion. In pre-eclampsia, intravascular volume is decreased (Gallery and Brown 1987; Irons et al. 1997) with compromised placental perfusion and function, diuretics could reduce placental function further. Proplylactic diuretics do not reduce the incidence of pre-eclampsia. Many diuretics affect the renal handling of uric acid and, with few exceptions, cause hyperuricaemia,

which can obviously be confusing (Kahn 1988). Furthermore, diuretics are not without risk, and can cause maternal pancreatitis, severe hypokalaemia, neonatal electrolyte imbalance, cardiac arrhythmias, and thrombocytopenia.

Disorders of water metabolism in pregnancy

Diabetes insipidus in pregnancy

The causes of diabetes insipidus antedating pregnancy are discussed in Chapter 5.6. Patients are rarely treated with synthetic forms of AVP, but, if they are, the increase in hormone disposal rates will obviously require an increase in the AVP dosage. Currently, however, virtually all women with known central diabetes insipidus are managed with desmopressin, the metabolic clearance rate of which, as mentioned, is not altered during pregnancy (Davison et al. 1989c). However, there have been reports of increased desmopressin requirements in pregnancy where symptoms associated with the threshold for thirst seem to have been misinterpreted as desmopressin 'escape'. When such cases were appropriately studied, however, the preconception replacement dose has proved sufficient throughout gestation (Lindheimer and Barron 1994).

Nephrogenic diabetes insipidus in pregnancy

This is quite rare, although carriers of the X-linked variety may become polyuric in pregnancy. Diuretics, the mainstay of therapy in this disorder, work by depleting intravascular volume which results in increased proximal reabsorption of sodium and the delivery of less filtrate to the diluting site. The maintenance of hypovolaemia may not be optimal for pregnancy, when the polyuria is massive such agents may have to be used.

Transient diabetes insipidus of pregnancy

On occasion, polyuria and polydipsia may develop late in pregnancy, disappearing postpartum. It seems likely that in these women the disorder might reflect massive in vivo destruction of AVP by extremely elevated concentrations and/or exaggerated effects of vasopressinase (Lindheimer and Davison 1995). However, the use of desmopressin produces a concentrated urine.

There is a second form of transient diabetes insipidus of pregnancy in which some women with partial central diabetes insipidus, asymptomatic when non-pregnant, manifest polyuria after mid-pregnancy coincident with the normal fourfold increase in the metabolic clearance rate of AVP. This disorder also remits postpartum. Some patients with transient diabetes insipidus postpartum can be resistant to both AVP and desmopressin, where both plasma AVP and urinary prostaglandin E_2 are markedly elevated.

References

Abram, S. R., Alexander, B. T., Bennett, W. A., and Granger, J. P. (2001). Role of neuronal nitric oxide synthase in mediating renal hemodynamic changes during pregnancy. *American Journal of Physiology* **281**, R1390–R1393.

Alexander, B. T., Cockrell, K., Cline, F. D., and Granger, J. P. (2002). Inducible nitric oxide synthase inhibition attenuates renal hemodynamics during pregnancy. *Hypertension* **36**, 586–590.

Alexander, B. T., Miller, M. T., Kassab, S., Novak, J., Reckelhoff, J. F., Kruckeberg, W. C., and Granger, J. P. (1999). Differential expression of renal nitric oxide synthase isoforms during pregnancy in rats. *Hypertension* **33**, 435–439.

Arnal, J.-F., Warin, L., and Michel, J.-B. (1992). Determinants of aortic cyclic guanosine monophosphate in hypertension induced by chronic inhibition of NO synthase. *Journal of Clinical Investigation* **90**, 647–652.

Atherton, J. C., Bielinska, A., Davison, J. M., Haddon, I., Kay, C., and Samuels, R. (1988). Sodium and water reabsorption in the proximal and distal nephron in conscious pregnant rats and third trimester women. *Journal of Physiology* **396**, 457–470.

August, P. and Lindheimer, M. D. Pathophysiology of preeclampsia. In *Hypertension: Pathophysiology, Diagnosis and Management* 2nd edn. (ed. J. H. Laragh and B. M. Brenner), pp. 2407–2426. New York: Raven Press, 1995.

Ballerman, B. J., Levenson, D. J., and Brenner, B. M. Renin, angiotensin, kinins, prostaglandins and leukotrienes. In *The Kidney* (ed. B. M. Brenner and F. C. Rector, Jr.), pp. 281–340. Philadelphia: W. B. Saunders, 1986.

Barbour, C. J., Stonier, C., and Aber, G. M. (1990). Pregnancy-induced changes in glomerular angiotensin II receptors in normotensive and spontaneously hypertensive rats. *Clinical and Experimental Hypertension* **B9**, 43–56.

Barron, W. M. and Lindheimer, M. D. (1995). Effect of oral protein loading on renal hemodynamics in human pregnancy. *American Journal of Physiology* **269**, R888–R895.

Barron, W. M., Durr, J. A., Stamoutsos, B. A., and Lindheimer, M. D. (1985). Osmoregulation during pregnancy in homozygous and heterozygous Brattleboro rats. *American Journal of Physiology* **248**, R229–R237.

Barron, W. M., Stamoutsos, B. A., and Lindheimer, M. D. (1984). Role of volume in the regulation of vasopressin secretion during pregnancy in the rat. *Journal of Clinical Investigation* **73**, 923–932.

Barry, C. I., Royle, G. A., and Lake, Y. (1992). Racial variation in serum uric acid concentration in pregnancy. A comparison between European, New Zealand Maori and Polynesian women. *Australian and New Zealand Journal of Obstetrics and Gynaecology* **32**, 17–19.

Baylis, C. (1979/1980). Effect of early pregnancy on glomerular filtration rate and plasma volume in the rat. *Renal Physiology* **2**, 333–339.

Baylis, C. (1980). The mechanism of the increase in glomerular filtration rate in the 12 day pregnant rat. *Journal of Physiology* **305**, 405–414.

Baylis, C. (1982). Glomerular ultrafiltration in the pseudopregnant rat. *American Journal of Physiology* **243**, F300–F305.

Baylis, C. (1984). Renal hemodynamics and volume control during pregnancy in the rat. *Seminars in Nephrology* **4**, 208–220.

Baylis, C. Glomerular filtration dynamics. In *Advances in Renal Physiology* (ed. C. J. Lote), pp. 33–83. London: Croom Helm, 1986.

Baylis, C. (1987). Renal effects of cyclooxygenase inhibition in the pregnant rat. *American Journal of Physiology* **253**, F158–F163.

Baylis, C. (1988). Effect of amino acid infusion as an index of renal vasodilatory capacity in pregnant rats. *American Journal of Physiology* **254**, F650–F656.

Baylis, C. (1989). Gentamicin-induced glomerulotoxicity in the pregnant rat. *American Journal of Kidney Diseases* **13**, 108–113.

Baylis, C. (1993). Blood pressure and renal hemodynamic effects of acute blockade of vascular actions of AVP in normal pregnancy in the rat. *Hypertension in Pregnancy* **12**, 93–102.

Baylis, C. Glomerular filtration and volume regulation in gravid animal models. In *Baillière's Clinical Obstetrics and Gynaecology* 2nd edn. Chapter 2, Vol. 8 (ed. M. D. Lindheimer and J. M. Davison), pp. 235–264. London: Baillière Tindall, 1994.

Baylis, C. (1995). Acute blockade of α-1-adrenoceptors has similar effects in pregnant and nonpregnant rats. *Hypertension in Pregnancy* **14**, 17–25.

Baylis, C. (2002). Cyclooxygenase products do not contribute to the gestational renal vasodilation in the NO synthase inhibited pregnant rat. *Hypertension in Pregnancy* **21**, 109–114.

Baylis, C. and Blantz, R. C. (1985). Tubuloglomerular feedback activity in virgin and pregnant rats. *American Journal of Physiology* **249**, F169–F173.

Baylis, C. and Collins, R. C. (1986). Angiotensin II inhibition on blood pressure and renal hemodynamics in pregnant rats. *American Journal of Physiology* **250**, F308–F314.

Baylis, C. and Rennke, H. G. (1985). Renal hemodynamics and glomerular morphology in repetitively pregnant, aging rats. *Kidney International* **28**, 140–145.

Baylis, C. and Engels, K. (1992). Adverse interactions between pregnancy and a new model of systemic hypertension produced by chronic blockade of EDRF in the rat. *Clinical Experimental Hypertension* **B11**, 117–129.

Baylis, C. and Reckelhoff, J. F. (1991). Renal hemodynamics in normal and hypertensive pregnancy; lessons from micropuncture. *American Journal of Kidney Diseases* **17**, 98–104.

Baylis, C. and Vallance, P. (1998). Editorial review: measurement of nitrite and nitrate (NO_x) levels in plasma and urine; what does this measure tell us about the activity of the endogenous NO. *Current Opinion in Nephrology and Hypertension* **7**, 1–4.

Baylis, C. and Wilson, C. B. (1989). Sex and the single kidney. *American Journal of Kidney Diseases* **13**, 290–298.

Baylis, C., Beinder, E., Suto, T., and August, P. (1998). Recent insights into the roles of NO and renin-angiotensin in the pathophysiology of pre-eclampsia pregnancy. *Seminars in Nephrology* **18**, 208–230.

Baylis, C., Engels, K., Harton, P., and Samsell, L. (1993). The acute effects of endothelial derived relaxing factor (EDRF) blockade in the normal conscious rat are not due to angiotensin II. *American Journal of Physiology* **264**, F74–F78.

Baylis, C., Ichikawa, I., Willis, W. T., Wilson, C. B., and Brenner, B. M. (1977). Dynamics of glomerular ultrafiltration. IX. Effects of plasma protein concentration. *American Journal of Physiology* **232**, F58–F71.

Beaton, G. H., Selby, A. E., and Vene, M. J. (1961). Starch gel electrophoresis of serum proteins: II. Slow α2-globulins and other serum proteins in pregnant, tumor bearing and young rats. *Journal of Biological Chemistry* **236**, 2005–2008.

Begum, S., Yamasaki, M., and Mochizuki, M. (1996). The role of NO metabolites during pregnancy. *Kobe Journal of Medical Science* **42**, 131–141.

Blantz, R. C. and Pelayo, J. C. (1984). A functional role for the tubuloglomerular feedback mechanism. *Kidney International* **25**, 739–746.

Boccardo, P. *et al.* (1996). Systemic and fetal-maternal NO synthesis in normal pregnancy and pre-eclampsia. *British Journal of Obstetrics and Gynaecology* **103**, 879–886.

Brendolan, A. *et al.* (1985). Renal functional reserve in pregnancy. *Kidney International* **28**, 232A.

Brenner, B. M., Meyer, T. W., and Hostetter, T. H. (1982). Dietary protein intake and the progressive nature of kidney disease: the role of hemodynamically mediated glomerular injury in the pathogenesis of progressive glomerular sclerosis in ageing, renal ablation and intrinsic renal disease. *New England Journal of Medicine* **307**, 652–659.

Brooks, V. L., Quesnell, R. R., Cumbee, S. R., and Bishop, V. S. (1995). Pregnancy attenuates activity of the baroreceptor reflex. *Clinical Experimental Pharmacology and Physiology* **22**, 152–156.

Broughton-Pipkin, R. The renin–angiotensin system in normal and hypertensive pregnancies. In *Handbook of Hypertension* Vol. 10 (ed. P. C. Rubin), pp. 117–151. Amsterdam: Elsevier, 1988.

Brown, M. A. (1990). Urinary tract dilatations in pregnancy. *American Journal of Obstetrics and Gynecology* **164**, 641–643.

Brown, M. A. and Gallery, E. D. M. (1994). Volume homeostasis in normal pregnancy and pre-eclampsia: physiology and clinical implications. *Clinical Obstetrics and Gynecology (Baillière)* **8**, 287–310.

Brown, G. P. and Venuto, R. C. (1986). Angiotensin II receptor alterations during pregnancy in rabbits. *American Journal of Physiology* **251**, E58–E64.

Brown, G. P. and Venuto, R. C. (1988). Angiotensin II receptors in rabbit renal preglomerular vessels. *American Journal of Physiology* **255**, E16–E22.

Brown, G. P. and Venuto, R. C. (1991). Renal blood flow response to angiotensin II infusions in conscious pregnant rabbits. *American Journal of Physiology* **261**, F51–F59.

Brown, M. A., Lindheimer, M. D., de Swiet, M., van Assche, F. A., and Moutquin, J.-M. (2001). The classification and diagnosis of the hypertensive disorders of pregnancy: statement from the International Society for the Study of Hypertension in Pregnancy (ISSHP). *Hypertension in Pregnancy* **20**, ix–xiv.

Brown, M. A., Sinosich, M. J., Saunders, D. M., and Gallery, E. D. M. (1986). Potassium regulation and progesterone–aldosterone interrelationships in human pregnancy. *American Journal of Obstetrics and Gynecology* **155**, 349–353.

Castro, L. C., Hobel, C. J., and Gornbein, J. (1994). Plasma levels of atrial natriuretic peptide in normal and hypertensive pregnancies: a meta-analysis. *American Journal of Obstetrics and Gynecology* **171**, 1642–1651.

Cha, S. C., Aberdeen, G. W., Mukaddam-Daher, S., Quillen, E. W., Jr., and Nuwayhid, B. S. (1993). Autoregulation of renal blood flow during ovine pregnancy. *Hypertension in Pregnancy* **12**, 71–83.

Chapman, A. B., Zamudio, S., Woodmansee, W., Merouani, A., Osorio, F., Johnson, A., Moore, L. G., Dahms, T., Coffin, C., Abraham, W. T., and Schrier, R. W. (1997). Systemic and renal hemodynamic changes in the luteal phase of the menstrual cycle mimic early pregnancy. *American Journal of Physiology* **273**, F777–F782.

Chapman, A. B., Abraham, W. T., Zamudio, S., Coffin, C., Merouani, A., Young, D., Johnson, A., Osorio, F., Goldberg, C., Moore, L. G., Dahms, T., and Schrier, R. W. (1998). Temporal relationships between hormonal and hemodynamic changes in early human pregnancy. *Kidney International* **54**, 2056–2063.

Chesley, L. C. Blood pressure and circulation. In *Hypertensive Disorders in Pregnancy* (ed. L. C. Chesley), pp. 119–154. New York: AppletonCentury-Crofts, 1978.

Cietak, K. A. and Newton, J. R. (1985). Serial qualitative nephronosonography in pregnancy. *British Journal of Radiology* **58**, 399–404.

Conrad, K. (1984). Renal hemodynamics during pregnancy in chronically catheterized conscious rats. *Kidney International* **26**, 24–29.

Conrad, K. (1987). Possible mechanisms for changes in renal hemodynamics during pregnancy: studies from animal models. *American Journal of Kidney Diseases* **9**, 253–259.

Conrad, K. P. and Colpoys, M. C. (1986). Evidence against the hypothesis that prostaglandins are the vasodepressor agents of pregnancy. *Journal of Clinical Investigation* **77**, 236–245.

Conrad, K. P. and Dunn, M. J. (1987). Renal synthesis and urinary excretion of eicosinoids during pregnancy in the rat. *American Journal of Physiology, Renal Physiology* **253**, F1197–F2001.

Conrad, K. P. and Russ, R. D. (1992). Augmentation of baroreflex-mediated bradycardia in conscious pregnant rats. *American Journal of Physiology* **262**, R472–R477.

Conrad, K. P., Kerchner L. J., and Mosher, M. D. (1999). Plasma and 24-h NO_x and cGMP during normal pregnancy and preeclampsia in women on a reduced NO_x diet. *American Journal of Physiology, Renal Physiology* **277**, F48–F57.

Conrad, K. P., Morganelli, P. M., Brinck-Johnsen, T., and Colpoys, M. C. (1989). The renin–angiotensin system during pregnancy in chronically instrumented, conscious rats. *American Journal of Obstetrics and Gynecology* **161**, 1065–1072.

Crandall, M. E. and Heesch, C. M. (1990). Baroreflex control of sympathetic outflow in pregnant rats: effects of captopril. *American Journal of Physiology* **258**, R1417–R1423.

Croce, J. F., Signorelli, P., and Chapparini, I. (1994). Hydronephrosis in pregnancy. Ultrasonographic study (Ital). *Minerva Ginicologica* **46**, 147–153.

Danielson, L. A. and Conrad, K. P. (1995). Nitric oxide mediates renal vasodilation and hyperfiltration during pregnancy in chronically instrumented, conscious rats. *Journal of Clinical Investigation* **96**, 482–490.

Danielson, L. A., and Conrad, K. P. (1996). Prostaglandins maintain renal vasodilation and hyperfiltration during chronic NO synthase.blockade in conscious pregnant rats. *Circulation Research* **79**, 1161–1166.

Danielson, L. A., Sherwood, O. D., and Conrad, K. P. (1999). Relaxin in a potent renal vasodilator in conscious rats. *Journal of Clinical Investigation* **103**, 525–533.

Davison, J. M. (1975). Renal nutrient excretion with emphasis on glucose. *Clinics in Obstetrics and Gynaecology* **2**, 365–380.

Davison, J. M. (1985). The effect of pregnancy on kidney function in renal allograft recipients. *Kidney International* **27**, 74–79.

Davison, J. M. (1987). Kidney function in pregnant women. *American Journal of Kidney Diseases* **9**, 248–252.

Davison, J. M. (1989). The effect of pregnancy on long term function in women with chronic renal disease and single kidneys. *Clinical and Experimental Hypertension* **B8**, 226.

Davison, J. M. and Cheyne, G. A. (1972). Renal reabsorption of glucose. *Lancet* **i**, 787–788.

Davison, J. M. and Hytten, F. E. (1974). Glomerular filtration during and after pregnancy. *Journal of Obstetrics and Gynaecology of the British Commonwealth* **81**, 588–595.

Davison, J. M. and Hytten, F. E. (1975). The effect of pregnancy on the renal handling of glucose. *Journal of Obstetrics and Gynaecology of the British Commonwealth* **82**, 374–381.

Davison, J. M. and Noble, M. C. B. (1981). Serial changes in 24-hour creatinine clearance during normal menstrual cycles and the first trimester of pregnancy. *British Journal of Obstetrics and Gynecology* **88**, 10–17.

Davison, J. M. and Dunlop, W. (1984). Changes in renal haemodynamics and tubular function induced by normal human pregnancy. *Seminars in Nephrology* **4**, 198–207.

Davison, J. M., Dunlop, W., and Ezimokhai, M. (1980). Twenty-four hour creatinine clearance during the third trimester of normal pregnancy. *British Journal of Obstetrics and Gynaecology* **87**, 106–109.

Davison, J. M., Shiells, E. A., Barron, W. M., Robinson, A. G., and Lindheimer, M. D. (1989b). Changes in the metabolic clearance of vasopressin and in plasma vasopressinase throughout human pregnancy. *Journal of Clinical Investigation* **83**, 1313–1318.

Davison, J. M., Shiells, E. A., and Lindheimer, M. D. (1989a). The influence of humoral and volume factors on the altered osmoregulation of normal human pregnancy. *American Journal of Physiology* **258**, F900–F908.

Davison, J. M., Shiells, E. A., Philips, P. R., and Lindheimer, M. D. (1988). Serial evaluation of vasopressin release and thirst in human pregnancy: the role of chorionic gonadotropin in the osmoregulatory changes of gestation. *Journal of Clinical Investigation* **81**, 798–806.

Davison, J. M., Shiells, E. A., Philips, P. R., and Lindheimer, M. D. (1993). Metabolic clearance rate of vasopressin and an analogue resistant to vasopressin in human pregnancy. *American Journal of Physiology* **264**, F348–F353.

Davison, J. M., Vallotton, M. B., and Lindheimer, M. D. (1981). Plasma osmolatity and urinary concentrating and dilution during and after pregnancy: evidence that lateral recumbency inhibits maximal urinary concentrating ability. *British Journal of Obstetrics and Gynaecology* **88**, 472–479.

Deng, A., Engels, K., and Baylis, C. (1996). Increased NO production plays a critical role in the maternal blood pressure and glomerular hemodynamic adaptations to pregnancy in the rat. *Kidney International* **50**, 1132–1138.

Domenech, M., Gruppuso, P. A., Nishino, V. T., Susa, J. B., and Schwartz, R. (1986). Preserved fetal plasma aminoacid concentrations in the presence of maternal hypoaminoacidemia. *Pediatric Research* **20**, 1071–1076.

Dunlop, W. (1976). Investigations into the influence of posture on renal plasma flow and glomerular filtration rate during late pregnancy. *British Journal of Obstetrics and Gynaecology* **83**, 17–23.

Dunlop, W. and Davison, J. M. (1977). The effect of normal pregnancy upon the renal handling of uric acid. *British Journal of Obstetrics and Gynaecology* **84**, 13–21.

Dunn, B. R., Ichikawa, I., Pfeffer, J. M., Troy, J. L., and Brenner, B. M. (1986). Renal and systemic hemodynamic effects of synthetic atrial natriuretic peptide in the anesthetized rat. *Circulation Research* **59**, 237–246.

Durr, J. A., Stamoutsos, B., and Lindheimer, M. D. (1981). Osmoregulation during pregnancy in the rat: evidence for resetting of the threshold for vasopressin secretion during gestation. *Journal of Clinical Investigation* **68**, 337–346.

Ensor, D. M. *Comparative Endocrinology of Prolactin*. London: Chapman & Hall, 1978.

Ezimokhai, M., Davison, J. M., Philips, P. R., and Dunlop, W. (1981). Non-postural serial changes in renal function during the third trimester of normal pregnancy. *British Journal of Obstetrics and Gynaecology* **88**, 465–471.

Fickling, S. A., Williams, D., Vallance, P., Nussey, S. S., and Whitley, G. St. J. (1993). Plasma concentrations of endogenous inhibitor of NO synthesis in normal pregnancy and pre-eclampsia. *Lancet* **342**, 242–243.

Fischer, R. L. *et al.* (1995). Maternal serum uric acid levels in twin gestations. *Obstetrics and Gynecology* **85**, 60–64.

Fried, A. M., Woodring, J. H., and Thompson, D. S. (1982). Hydronephrosis in pregnancy. A prospective sequential study of course of dilatation. *Journal of Ultrasound and Medicine* **2**, 255–259.

Friedman, S. A. (1988). Pre-eclampsia: a review of the role of prostaglandins. *Obstetrics and Gynecology* **71**, 122–137.

Gallery, E. D. M. (1984). Volume homeostasis in normal and hypertensive human pregnancy. *Seminars in Nephrology* **4**, 221–231.

Gallery, E. D. M. and Brown, M. (1987). Volume homeostatis in normal and hypertensive human pregnancy. *Clinical Obstetrics and Gynaecology* **1**, 835–851.

Gant, N. F., Whalley, P. J., Everett, R. B., Worley, R. J., and MacDonald, P. C. (1987). Control of vascular reactivity in pregnancy. *American Journal of Kidney Diseases* **9**, 303–307.

Ghadimi, H. and Pecora, P. (1964). Free aminoacids of cord plasma as compared with maternal plasma during pregnancy. *Pediatrics* **33**, 500–506.

Giebisch, G., Malnic, G., and Berliner, R. W. Renal transport and control of potassium excretion. In *The Kidney* 3rd edn (ed. B. M. Brenner and F. C. Rector Jr.), pp. 177–205, Pennsylvania: W. B. Saunders, 1986.

Gregoire, I., Dupouy, J. P., Fievet, P., Sraer, J. D., and Fournier, A. (1987). Prostanoid synthesis by isolated rat glomeruli: effect of oestrous cycle and pregnancy. *Clinical Science* **73**, 641–644.

Gregoire, I. *et al.* (1990). Plasma atrial natriuretic factor and urinary excretion of a ouabain displacing factor and dopamine in normotensive pregnant women before and after delivery. *American Journal of Obstetrics and Gynecology* **162**, 71–76.

Halligan, A. W. F., Bell, S. C., and Taylor, D. J. (1999). Dipstick proteinuria: caveal emptor. *British Journal of Obstetrics and Gynaecology* **106**, 1113–1115.

Higby, K. *et al.* (1994). Normal values of urinary albumin and total protein excretion during pregnancy. *American Journal of Obstetrics and Gynecology* **171**, 984–989.

Hostetter, T. H. (1984). Human renal response to a meat meal. *American Journal of Physiology* **250**, F613–F618.

Howarth, A. T., Morgan, D. B., and Payne, R. B. (1977). Urinary excretion of calcium in late pregnancy and its relation to creatinine clearance. *American Journal of Obstetrics and Gynecology* **239**, 499–503.

Hsueh, W. A., Leutcher, J. A., Carlson, E. J., Frifles, G., Fraze, E., and McHargue, A. (1984). Changes in active and inactive renin in pregnancy. *Journal of Clinical Endocrinology and Metabolism* **54**, 1010–1015.

Hytten, F. E. and Cheyne, G. A. (1972). The aminoaciduria of pregnancy. *Journal of Obstetrics and Gynaecology of the British Commonwealth* **79**, 424–432.

Irons, D. W., Baylis, P. H., and Davison, J. M. (1996). Effect of atrial natriuretic peptide on renal hemodynamics and sodium excretion during human pregnancy. *American Journal of Physiology* **271**, F239–F242.

Irons, D. W., Baylis, P. H., and Davison, J. M. (1997). Atrial natriuretic peptide in preeclampsia: metabolic clearance, sodium excretion and renal hemodynamics. *American Journal of Physiology* **273**, F483–F487.

Kahn, A. M. (1988). Effect of diuretics on the renal handling of urate. *Seminars in Nephrology* **8**, 305–314.

Khauna, N. and Nguyn, H. (2001). Reversible acute renal failure in association with bilateral ureteral obstruction and hydronephrosis in pregnancy. *American Journal of Obstetrics and Gynecology* **184**, 239–240.

Kirchner, K. A. (1987). Lithium as a marker for proximal tubular marker for proximal tubular delivery during low salt intake and diuretic infusion. *American Journal of Physiology* **253**, F188–F196.

Klaus, D., Klumpp, F., and Rossier, R. (1971). Effects of pregnancy on Bartter's syndrome. *Klinische Wochenschrift* **49**, 1280–1282.

Kopp, L., Paradiz, G., and Tucci, J. R. (1977). Urinary excretion of cyclic 3′,5′-adenosine monophosphate and cyclic 3′,5′-quanosine monophosphate during and after pregnancy. *Journal of Clinical Endocrinology and Metabolism* **44**, 590–594.

Kristensen, C. G., Nakagawa, Y., Coe, F. L., and Lindheimer, M. D. (1986). Effect of atrial natriuretic factor in rat pregnancy. *American Journal of Physiology* **250**, R589–R594.

Kriston, T. Venuto, R. C., Baylis, C., and Losonczy, G. (1999). Hemodynamic and renal effects of U-46619, a TXA2/PGH2 analog, in late-pregnant rats. *American Journal of Physiology* **276**, R831–R837.

Lafayette, R. A. *et al.* (1998). Nature of glomerular dysfunction in pre-eclampsia. *Kidney International* **54**, 1240–1249.

Landon, M. J., Copas, D. K., Shiells, E. A., and Davison, J. M. (1988). Degradation of radiolabelled arginine vasopressin (I-AVP) by the human placenta perfused *in vitro*. *British Journal of Obstetrics and Gynaecology* **95**, 488–492.

Lim, V. S., Katz, A. I., and Lindheimer, M. D. (1976). Acid–base metabolism in pregnancy. *American Journal of Physiology* **231**, 1764–1769.

Lindheimer, M. D. and Katz, A. I. (1971). Kidney function in the pregnant rat. *Journal of Laboratory Clinical Medicine* **78**, 633–641.

Lindheimer, M. D. and Katz, A. I. Normal and abnormal pregnancy. In *Fluid, Electrolyte and Acid–Base Disorders* (ed. A. I. Arieff and R. DeFronzo), pp. 1041–1080. New York: Churchill Livingstone, Inc., 1985a.

Lindheimer, M. D. and Katz, A. I. Renal physiology in pregnancy. In *The Kidney: Physiology and Pathophysiology* Vol. 2 (ed. D. W. Seldin and G. Geibisch), pp. 2017–2042. New York: Raven Press, 1985b.

Lindheimer, M. D. and Barron, W. M. (1994). Water metabolism and vasopressin secretion during pregnancy. *Clinical Obstetrics and Gynaecology (Baillière)* **8**, 311–331.

Lindheimer, M. D. and Davison, J. M. (1995). Osmoregulation, the secretion of arginine vasopressin and its metabolism during pregnancy (minireview). *European Journal of Endocrinology* **132**, 133–143.

Lindheimer, M. D., Davison, J. M., and Katz, A. I. (2001). The kidney and hypertension in pregnancy: twenty exciting years. *Seminars in Nephrology* **21**, 173–189.

Lindheimer, M. D., Richardson, D. A., Ehrlich, E. N., and Katz, A. I. (1987). Potassium homeostasis in pregnancy. *Journal of Reproductive Medicine* **32**, 517–520.

López-Jaramillo, P. *et al.* (1996). Cyclic guanosine 3′,5′ monophosphate concentrations in pre-eclampsia: effects of hydralazine. *British Journal of Obstetrics and Gynaecology* **103**, 33–38.

Lucius, H., Gahlenbeck, H., Kleine, H. O., Fabel, H., and Bartels, H. (1970). Respiratory functions, buffer system and electrolyte concentrations of blood during human pregnancy. *Respiration Physiology* **9**, 311.

MacDonald, P. C., Cutter, S., MacDonald, S. C., Casey, M. L., and Parker, O. R., Jr. (1982). Regulation of extra-adrenal steroid 21hydroxylase activity: increased conversion of plasma progesterone during estrogen treatment of women pregnant with a dead fetus. *Journal of Clinical Investigation* **69**, 469–474.

McLaughlin, M. K., Keve, T. M., and Cooke, R. (1989). Vascular catecholamine sensitivity during pregnancy in the ewe. *American Journal of Obstetrics and Gynecology* **160**, 47–53.

Magness, R. R. and Rosenfeld, C. R. (1988). Mechanisms for attenuated pressor responses to alpha-agonists in ovine pregnancy. *American Journal of Obstetrics and Gynecology* **159**, 252–261.

Mahaney, J., Felton, C., Taylor, D., Fleming, W., Kong, J. Q. and Baylis, C. (1998). Renal Na-K ATPase activity and abundance is decreased in normal mid and late pregnant rats. *American Journal of Physiology* **275**, F812–F817.

Maikranz, P., Lindheimer, M., and Coe, F. Nephrolithiasis in pregnancy. In *Baillière's Clinical Obstetrics and Gynaecology* 2nd edn., Chapter 8, Vol. 8 (ed. M. D. Lindheimer and J. M. Davison), pp. 375–386. London: Baillière Tindall, 1994.

Masilamani, S. and Baylis, C. (1992). The renal vasculature does not participate in the peripheral refractoriness to administered angiotensin II in the late pregnancy rat. *Journal of the American Society of Nephrology* **3**, 566A.

Masilamani, S. and Baylis, C. (1994). Pregnant rats are refractory to the natriuretic action of atrial natriuretic peptide. *American Journal of Physiology* **267**, R1611–R1616.

Matthews, B. M. and Taylor, D. W. (1960). Effects of pregnancy on inulin and para-aminohippurate clearances in the anesthetized rat. *Journal of Physiology* **151**, 385–389.

Meyer, T. W., Anderson, S., Rennke, H. G., and Brenner, B. M. (1987). Reversing glomerular hypertension stabilizes glomerular injury. *Kidney International* **31**, 752–759.

Meyer, T. M., Ichikawa, I., Zatz, R., and Brenner, B. M. (1983). The renal hemodynamic response to amino acid infusion in the rat. *Transactions of the Association of American Physicians* **96**, 76–83.

Milne, J. E., Lindheimer, M. D., and Davison, J. D. (2002). Glomerular heteroporous membrane modeling in third trimester and postpartum before and during amino acid infusion. *American Journal of Physiology. Renal Physiology* **282**, F170–F175.

Milner, J. A. and Visek, W. J. (1978). Orotic aciduria in the female rat and its relation to dietary arginine. *Journal of Nutrition* **108**, 1281–1288.

Molnar, M. and Hertelendy, F. (1992). Nw-nitro-L-arginine, an inhibitor of NO synthesis, increases blood pressure in rats and reverses the pregnancy-induced refractoriness to vasopressor agents. *American Journal of Obstetrics and Gynecology* **166**, 1560–1567.

Moran, P., Baylis, P. H., Lindheimer, M. D., and Davison, J. M. (2003). Glomerular ultrafiltration in normal and preeclamptic pregnancy. *Journal of the American Society of Nephrology* **14**, 648–652.

Mujais, S. K., Nora, N. A., and Chen, Y. (1993). Regulation of the renal Na : K pump—role of progesterone. *Journal of the American Society of Nephrology* **3**, 1488–1495.

Nadel, A. S., Ballerman, B. J., Anderson, S., and Brenner, B. M. (1988). Interrelationships among atrial peptides, renin and blood volume in pregnant rats. *American Journal of Physiology* **254**, R793–R800.

Naiker, T. *et al.* (1997). Correlation between histological changes and loss of anionic change of the glomerular basement membrane in early onset preeclampsia. *Nephron* **75**, 201–207.

Nakagawa, Y., Sirivongs, D., Maikranz, P., Linheimer, M. D., and Coe, F. L. (1989). Excretion of Tamm–Horsfall glycoprotein (THP) during pregnancy: a defense against nephrolithiasis. *Kidney International* **33**, 203A.

Navar, L. G. (1978). Renal autoregulation: perspectives from whole kidney and single nephron studies. *American Journal of Physiology* **234**, F357–F370.

Ni, X.-P., Rishi, R., Safai, M., Baylis, C., and Humphreys, M. H. (2001a). Increased activity of cGMP-specific phosphodiesterase (PDE5) contributes to renal resistance to atrial natriuretic peptide (ANP) in the pregnant rat. *Journal of the American Society of Nephrology* **12**, 574A.

Ni, X.-P., Safai, M., Gardner, D. G., and Humphreys, M. H. (2001b). Increased cGMP phosphodeisterase activity mediates renal resistance to ANP in rats with bile duct ligation. *Kidney International* **59**, 1284–1273.

Nolten, W. E., Holt, L. H., and Ruerckert, P. (1980). Desoxycorticosterone in normal pregnancy. III. Evidence of a fetal source of desoxycorticosterone. *American Journal of Obstetrics and Gynecology* **139**, 477–481.

Novak, J., Reckelhoff, J., Bumgarner, L., Cockrell, K., Kassab, S., and Granger, J. P. (1997). Reduced sensitivity of the renal circulation to angiotensin II in pregnant rats. *Hypertension* **30**, 580–584.

Paller, M. S., Gregorini, G., and Ferris, T. F. (1989). Pressor responsiveness in pseudopregnant and pregnant rats: role of maternal factors. *American Journal of Physiology* **257**, R866–R871.

Pan, Z.-R., Lindheimer, M. D., Bailin, J., and Barron, W. M. (1990). Regulation of blood pressure in pregnancy: pressor system blockade and stimulation. *American Journal of Physiology* **258**, H1559–H1572.

Perkins, C. M., Hancock, K. W., Cope, C. F., and Lee, M. R. (1981). Urine free dopamine in normal primigrand pregnancy and women taking oral contraceptives. *Clinical Science* **61**, 423–427.

Phelps, S. J., Cochran, E. B., Gonzales-Ruiz, A., Tolley, E. A., Hammond, K. D., and Sibai, B. H. (1988). The influence of gestational age and preeclampsia on the presence and magnitude of digoxin-like immunoreactive substances. *American Journal of Obstetrics and Gynecology* **158**, 34–38.

Poston, L., McCarthy, L., and Ritter, J. M. (1995). Control of vascular resistance in the maternal and feto-placental arterial beds. *Pharmacology and Therapeutics* **65**, 215–239.

Raij, L. (1994). Glomerular thrombosis in pregnancy: role of the L-arginine-NO pathway. *Kidney International* **45**, 775–781.

Raij, L. and Baylis, C. (1995). Nitric oxide and the glomerulus. Editorial review. *Kidney International* **48**, 20–32.

Rasmussen, P. E. and Nielsen, F. R. (1988). Hydronephrosis during pregnancy: a literature survey. *European Journal of Obstetrics, Gynaecology, and Reproductive Biology* **27**, 249–259.

Reckelhoff, J. F., Yokota, S., and Baylis, C. (1992). Renal autoregulation in midterm and late pregnant rats. *American Journal of Obstetrics and Gynecology* **166**, 1546–1550.

Redman, C. W. G., Beilin, L. J., Bonnar, J., and Wilkinson, R. H. (1976). Plasma-urate measurements in predicting fetal death in hypertensive pregnancy. *Lancet* i, 1370–1373.

Roberts, M., Lindheimer, M. D., and Davison, J. M. (1996). Alterations in glomerular hemodynamics and barrier function in normal pregnancy: assessment using neutral dextrans and heteroporous membrane modelling. *American Journal of Physiology* **270**, F338–F343.

Robertson, C. R., Deen, W. M., Troy, J. L., and Brenner, B. M. (1972). Dynamics of glomerular ultrafiltration in the rat. III. Hemodynamics and autoregulation. *American Journal of Physiology* **223**, 1191–1200.

Santmyire, B. R. and Baylis, C. (1998). Isoform specific changes in kidney NOS activity during rat pregnancy. *Journal of the American Society of Nephrology* **9**, 346.

Santmyire, B. R. and Baylis, C. (1999). The inducible nitric oxide synthase inhibitor aminoguanidine inhibits the pregnancy induced renal vasodilation and increase in kidney NOS activity in the rat. *Journal of the American Society of Nephrology* **10**, 386A.

Sandan, P. J., Brown, M. A., Farrell, T., and Shaw, L. (1997). Improved methods of assessing proteinuria in hypertensive pregnancy. *British Journal of Obstetrics and Gynaecology* **104**, 1159–1164.

Satin, S. A., Seikin, G. L., and Cunningham, F. G. (1993). Reversible hypertension in pregnancy caused by obstructive uropathy. *Obstetrics and Gynecology* **81**, 823–825.

Schrier, R. W. (1988). Pathogenesis of sodium and water retention in high-output and low-output cardiac failure, nephrotic syndrome, cirrhosis and pregnancy. Part 11. *New England Journal of Medicine* **319**, 1127–1134.

Schrier, R. W. and Durr, J. A. (1987). Pregnancy: an overfill or underfill state. *American Journal of Kidney Diseases* **4**, 284–289.

Sicinska, J., Bailie, M. D., and Rector, F. C. (1971). Effects of angiotensin on blood pressure and renal function in pregnant and non pregnant rats. *Nephron* **8**, 375–381.

Singh, R., Pervin, S., Rogers, N. E., Ignarro, L. J., and Chaudhurri, G. (1997). Evidence for the presence of an unusual nitric oxide- and citrulline-producing enzyme in rat kidney. *Biochemical and Biophysical Research Communications* **232**, 672–677.

Sladek, S. M., Magness, R. R., and Conrad, K. P. (1997). Nitric oxide and pregnancy. *American Journal of Physiology* **272**, R441–R463.

Slangen, B. F. M., Out, I. C. M., Verkeste, C. M., Smits, J. F. M., and Peeters, L. L. H. (1997). Hemodynamic changes in pseudopregnancy in chronically instrumented conscious rats. *American Journal of Physiology* **272**, H695–H700.

Steegers, E. A. P. *et al.* (1991). Atrial natriuretic peptide and atrial size during normal pregnancy. *British Journal of Obstetrics and Gynaecology* **98**, 202–206.

Stoos, B. A., Garcia, N. H., and Garvin, J. L. (1995). Nitric oxide inhibits sodium reabsorption in the isolated perfused cortical colecting duct. *Journal of the American Society of Nephrology* **6**, 89–94.

Sturgiss, S. N., Dunlop, W., and Davison, J. M. (1994). Renal haemodynamics and tubular function in human pregnancy. *Clinical Obstetrics and Gynaecology (Ballière)* **8**, 209–234.

Sturgiss, S. N., Wilkinson, R., and Davison, J. M. (1996). Renal hemodynamic reserve in pregnancy in health and disease. *American Journal of Physiology* **271**, F16–F20.

Takeda, T. (1964). Experimental study on the blood pressure of pregnant hypertensive rats. *Japanese Circulation Journal* **28**, 49–54.

Taufield, P. A., Mueller, F. B., Edersheim, T. G., Druzen, M. L., Laragh, J. H., and Sealy, J. E. (1988). Blood pressure regulation in normal pregnancy: unmasking the role of the renin–angiotension system with captopril. *Clinical Research* **36**, 433A.

Taylor, A. A. and Davison, J. M. (1997). Albumin excretion in normal pregnancy. *American Journal of Obstetrics and Gynecology* **177**, 1559–1560.

Trolifors, B., Alestig, K., and Jagenburg, R. (1987). Prediction of glomerular filtration rate from serum creatinine, age, sex and body weight. *Acta Medica Scandinavica* **221**, 495–498.

Valentin, J.-P., Qiu, C., Muldowney, W. P., Ying, W.-Z., Gardner, D. G., and Humphreys, M. H. (1992). Cellular basis for blunted volume expansion natriuresis in experimental nephrotic syndrome. *Journal of Clinical Investigation* **90**, 1302–1312.

Venuto, R. C. and Donker, A. J. M. (1982). Prostaglandin E2, plasma renin activity and renal function throughout rabbit pregnancy. *Journal of Laboratory and Clinical Medicine* **99**, 239–246.

Williams, D. J. *et al.* (1997). Nitric oxide-mediated vasodilation in human pregnancy. *American Journal of Physiology* **272**, H748–H752.

Wilcox, C. S., Baylis, C., and Wingo, C. S. Glomerular tubular balance and proximal regulation. In *The kidney. Physiology and Pathophysiology* 2nd edn., Chapter 50 (ed. D. W. Seldin and G. Giebisch), pp. 1807–1841. New York: Raven Press, 1992.

Winkel, C. A., Simpson, E. R., Milewich, L., and MacDonald, P. C. (1980). Deoxycorticosterone (DOC) biosynthesis in human kidney: potential for the formation of potent mineralocorticoid in its site of action. *Proceedings of the National Academy of Sciences of the USA* **77**, 7069–7073.

Wood, M. H. and O'Sullivan, W. J. (1973) The orotic aciduria of pregnancy. *American Journal of Obstetrics and Gynecology* **116**, 57–61.

Woods, L. L. and Gaboury, C. L. (1995). Importance of baseline diet in modulating renal reserve in pregnant women. *Journal of the American Society of Nephrology* **6**, 688.

Woods, L. L., Mizelle, H. L., and Hall, J. E. (1987). Autoregulation of renal blood flow and glomerular filtration rate in the pregnant rabbit. *American Journal of Physiology* **252**, R69–R72.

15.2 Renal complications that may occur in pregnancy

John M. Davison

The anatomical and physiological changes in the urinary tract that occur during pregnancy and the various diagnostic pitfalls for the unwary clinician are discussed in Chapter 15.1. This chapter focuses on some renal complications that can arise *de novo* in the antenatal period or in the puerperium. Urinary tract infection, mechanical problems, and acute renal failure will be dealt with in detail, discussing the effects on obstetric management decisions, perinatal outcome and the long-term implications.

Infection of the urinary tract (see also Section 7)

The analysis of urine specimens during pregnancy is especially likely to be hampered by contamination at the time of collection with bacteria from urethra, vagina, or perineum. This problem can be overcome by suprapubic aspiration of bladder urine, but this rather inconvenient procedure is unacceptable to many patients and clinicians. It is best to obtain a fresh midstream urine specimen (MSU) collected by a clean-catch technique. Traditionally, true bacteriuria is still defined as the presence of more than 100,000 bacteria of the same species per millilitre of urine in two consecutive MSUs (or in a single suprapubic aspiration) even though there is a view that lower colony counts may represent active infection (Stamm *et al.* 1991). There are several presumptive tests based on changes in chemical indicators, but these are not reliable enough for clinical practice.

Asymptomatic or covert bacteriuria designates true bacteriuria in the absence of symptoms or signs of acute urinary tract infection. Symptomatic infection is divided into lower urinary tract infection or cystitis, and upper tract infection or acute pyelonephritis. It must be remembered, however, that pregnant women often complain of, or will admit to, frequency of micturition, dysuria, urgency, or nocturia, singly or in combination, and such symptoms are not in themselves diagnostic of urinary tract infection.

It is probable that bacteria originate from the large bowel and colonize the urinary tract transperineally. By far the most common infecting organism is *Escherichia coli*, which is responsible for 75–90 per cent of bacteriuria seen during pregnancy. The pathogenic virulence of this bacterium, which is not the predominant organism in faeces, appears to derive from a number of factors, including resistance to vaginal acidity, rapid division in urine, the presence of Dr operons coding for Dr adhesins (Goluszko *et al.* 2001) which allow adherence to uroepithelial cells, and production of chemicals which decrease ureteric peristalsis and inhibit phagocytosis (Cunningham and Lucas 1994; Gilstrap and Ramin 2001; Shelton *et al.* 2001). Other organisms frequently responsible for urinary tract infection include *Klebsiella*, *Proteus*, coagulase-negative staphylococci, and *Pseudomonas*.

The stasis associated with ureteropelvic dilatation and/or partial ureteric obstruction increases the nutrient content of the urine, and although potential pathogens are present in most women, only a small minority develop bacteriuria. Susceptible women may differ immunologically from those who resist infection: they are less likely to express antibody to the O antigen of *E. coli* on the bladder epithelium and may display less effective leucocyte activity against the organism.

Asymptomatic bacteriuria

Site of infection

Asymptomatic or covert bacteriuria is a heterogeneous entity. Methods that have been used to try to differentiate between upper and lower urinary tract bacteriuria include renal biopsy, ureteral catheterization, bladder washout tests, urinary concentration tests, and serum antibody tests. The first two methods are too invasive for clinical practice and the remainder are too imprecise to localize infection confidently. The usefulness of another predictor of the presence and site of infection, the determination of antibody-coated bacteria in the urine, also remains controversial.

Importance of diagnosis

About 5 per cent of young women have covert bacteriuria acquired during childhood, but only 1.2 per cent are infected at any one time (Gilstrap and Ramin 2001). The incidence increases after puberty and is approximately equal in both the pregnant and non-pregnant populations (2–10 per cent), but is two to three times more common in pregnant diabetic patients or transplant recipients. During pregnancy, 40 per cent of the infected group, if left untreated, develop acute symptomatic infections. Thus, treating pregnant women with covert bacteriuria should prevent approximately 70 per cent of all potential cases of symptomatic urinary tract infection in pregnancy (Pedler and Orr 2000). However, about 1.5 per cent of those with initially negative cultures develop acute infections, and these account for the remaining 30–40 per cent of acute urinary tract infections in pregnancy. One antenatal study (Stenquist *et al.* 1989), in which 99 per cent of women participated in at least one screening, suggested that bacteriuria was greatest between the 9th and 17th week of pregnancy, calculated on the number of bacteria-free gestational weeks gained by treatment.

Asymptomatic bacteriuria has been alleged to be associated with several complications of pregnancy, notably low birth weight, fetal loss, pre-eclampsia, and maternal anaemia. Several of these apparent correlations may have resulted from inaccuracies in matching cases and controls. There is also a view that underlying chronic pyelonephritis may be present in some cases and may be responsible for the reported increased incidences of pre-eclampsia, prematurity, and fetal loss (Graham *et al.* 2001).

Not all untreated bacteriuric women will develop symptoms of acute infection during pregnancy, and those who have sterile urine when screened at antenatal booking will contribute substantially to the pool of symptomatic women. It has therefore been argued that screening programmes are not cost-effective (literature cited in Pedler and Orr 2000). Interestingly, it has been suggested that women with a history of previous urinary tract infection, as well as those with current bacteriuria, were 10 times more likely to develop symptoms during pregnancy than women without either feature. Women with renal scarring and persistent reflux constitute another group where acute pyelonephritis is more likely to develop.

Management in pregnancy

Choice of drug and duration of therapy

Most clinicians treat asymptomatic bacteriuria despite the screening controversy and the choice of drug should be determined by the sensitivity of the isolated organism. A 2-week course is usually adequate and short-acting sulfonamides or nitrofurantoin derivatives are satisfactory (Cunningham and Lucas 1994; Pedler and Orr 2000). Other antibiotics are reserved for treatment of failures and for symptomatic infection. Ampicillin and the cephalosporins produce few known adverse reactions in the fetus and can be used safely throughout pregnancy. Tetracyclines are contraindicated; they can cause staining of the teeth of infants by binding with orthophosphates, as well as the rare maternal complication of acute fatty liver or pregnancy. If sulfonamides are still being prescribed in late pregnancy, they should be withheld during the last 2–3 weeks since they compete with bilirubin for albumin binding sites, increasing the risk of fetal hyperbilirubinaemia and kernicterus. Nitrofurantoin used during the last few weeks may precipitate haemolysis due to erythrocyte phosphate dehydrogenase deficiency in the newborn. There is still controversy about very short (especially single high dose) courses in pregnancy (Wing *et al.* 1999).

Many of the new antibiotics that have been introduced during the past decade have been administered to pregnant women: the clinician should limit administration to those with a proven record during pregnancy (Pfau and Sacks 1992; Pedler and Orr 2000). Follow-up urine cultures should be obtained 1 week after therapy is discontinued and then at regular intervals throughout the pregnancy (every 4 weeks).

Relapses and reinfection

Relapse is the recurrence of bacteriuria caused by the same organism, usually within 6 weeks of the initial infection. Reinfection is the recurrence of bacteriuria involving a different strain of bacteria, after successful eradication of the initial infection. Most reinfections are limited to the bladder, and they usually occur at least 6 weeks after therapy.

Approximately 30 per cent of patients will have a recurrence during pregnancy and a second course of treatment should be given, based on a repeat culture with sensitivity testing. After a second course of treatment, about 15 per cent continue to have positive urinary cultures. Since *E. coli* causes the majority of initial infections as well as

recurrences, it is sometimes desirable to employ an *E. coli* serotyping system to distinguish different strains precisely.

Long-term management

Need for follow-up

As the interval between treatment of bacteriuria in pregnancy and postpartum follow-up becomes longer, the influence of the bacteriuria becomes less noticeable. Ten or more years after an initial episode of bacteriuria of pregnancy, the prevalence of bacteriuria is virtually the same in untreated (25 per cent) and treated (29 per cent) women. Women who never had bacteriuria during pregnancy have rates of bacteriuria of around 5 per cent. Thus, a single course of treatment during the index pregnancy does not appear to protect against persistent or recurrent bacteriuria years later (Dempsey *et al.* 1992). Few prospective studies are available, but there is no evidence that persistent asymptomatic bacteriuria in a woman with a normal urinary tract causes long-term renal damage, or that treatment reduces the incidence of chronic renal disease (Gilstrap and Ramin 2001).

Postpartum evaluation

There is no consensus regarding the need for postpartum evaluation, including intravenous urography. Twenty per cent of all patients with asymptomatic bacteriuria have radiological abnormalities and the proportion is increased among patients with acute infections and/or infections difficult to eradicate during pregnancy (Dempsey *et al.* 1992). The significance of this is not so certain; it may indicate a predisposition to infection, it may result from infection, or it may be unrelated to infection. Most abnormalities are minor and neither result from nor cause the renal infection, and so the exact relationship is unclear.

An intravenous urogram and renal ultrasound should be performed on one occasion, no earlier than 4 months after delivery, to document a non-obstructed urinary tract in women who have had asymptomatic bacteriuria during pregnancy and who fulfil the following additional criteria:

(1) difficulty in eradicating the bacteriuria;

(2) episode(s) of acute symptomatic urinary tract infection;

(3) history of acute symptomatic urinary tract infections prior to pregnancy; and

(4) persistent and/or recurrent asymptomatic bacteriuria or acute infection postpartum.

In this way, about 90 per cent of women with major urinary tract abnormalities will be detected.

Symptomatic infection

Acute cystitis

This occurs in about 1 per cent of pregnant women, 60 per cent of whom have a negative initial urine screening. The symptoms are often difficult to distinguish from those due to pregnancy itself. Features indicating a true infection include haematuria, dysuria, and suprapubic discomfort, as well as a positive urine culture. The bacteriology is the same as in women with asymptomatic bacteriuria (Pedler and Orr 2000). Similar treatment is recommended, with the aims of abolishing symptoms and preventing occurrence of acute pyelonephritis. It is too early to gauge the success of single-dose therapy for pregnant women with cystitis, and a standard 2-week course of treatment is still the recommendation.

Acute pyelonephritis (see also Chapter 7.1)

Importance of diagnosis

The differential diagnosis includes other urinary tract pathology, other causes of pyrexia, such as respiratory tract infection, viraemia, or toxoplasmosis (appropriate serological screening should be performed), and other causes of acute abdominal pain, such as acute appendicitis, biliary colic, gastroenteritis, uterine fibroid degeneration, or abruptio placentae. Acute appendicitis can be a difficult diagnosis to make, especially in the third trimester. At the onset of the appendicitis, the pain is usually referred to the centre of the abdomen, vomiting is not a marked feature, the pyrexia is not as high as in acute pyelonephritis, and rigors rarely occur.

Pneumonia on the affected side should present no difficulties if attention is paid to the type of respiration, the respiratory rate, and the physical signs in the chest. It should be noted, however, that so-called adult respiratory distress syndrome, with accompanying liver and haematopoietic dysfunction, can be a significant complication of pyelonephritis (Cunningham et al. 1987; Pruett and Faro 1987) (Table 1) in 10–20 per cent of cases. In addition, pelvic cellulitis and abscess, as well as septicaemic shock, can be life-threatening (Cunningham and Lucas 1994). In all such cases, prompt recognition and appropriate respiratory support may be necessary to prevent severe hypoxaemia that may cause fetal death (Weinberger 1993).

Table 1 Comparison of clinical factors associated with acute pyelonephritis in pregnancy with and without respiratory distress

	With respiratory distress (n=15)	Without respiratory distress (n=30)
Duration of symptoms[a] (days)	2.6	2.5
Maximum temperature (°C)	39.7	39.1
Duration of pyrexia[a] (days)	3.2	1.9
Tachypnoea (>28/min) (%)	100	16
Blood creatinine > 90 μmol/l (%)	57	20
Haematocrit (%)[a]		
Initial	30.1	32.3
Decrement	4.9	4.7
Platelets[a] (×10^9/l)		
Initial	215,000	277,000
Lowest	153,000	242,000
<100,000	40	0
Highest leucocytes (×10^9/l)[a]	18,100	14,000
Positive blood culture (%)	43	22
Preterm labour (%)	21	4

[a] Mean values.

Modified from Cunningham et al. (1987).

Management in pregnancy

An MSU should be sent immediately for culture and sensitivities. Treatment should be aggressive, undertaken in a hospital setting, and backed up with good nursing care. Causative organisms are similar to those in the general population, with P-fimbriated E. coli representing approximately 75 per cent. A patient dehydrated due to vomiting and sweating will require intravenous fluid therapy and regular assessment of renal function (Twickler et al. 1994). Infection episodes during pregnancy can cause marked but transient decrements in creatinine clearance.

Choice of drug

Dogmatic statements cannot be made regarding the type of antimicrobial therapy for acute urinary tract infection and the appropriate duration of treatment is also debatable (Pedler and Orr 2000). Treatment should aim at administering the most effective drug to eradicate a particular infection without exposing the fetus to an unnecessarily harmful agent.

Antibiotics producing high blood concentrations and resulting in high renal parenchymal concentrations are favoured: two antibiotics that give appropriate blood concentrations are ampicillin and cephalosporins. E. coli is usually sensitive to these antibiotics. Until the patient is afebrile, it is preferable to give intravenous antibiotics, to be continued orally thereafter.

Duration of therapy

There is some evidence to suggest that intravenous therapy once a day as opposed to multiple daily doses is satisfactory (Sanchez-Ramos et al. 1995), but most would still advocate that the duration of treatment should be 2 weeks for lower-tract symptomatic infection and a minimum of 3 weeks for acute pyelonephritis. Antibiotic sensitivity should be reviewed within 48 h. In patients showing no improvement within 48 h, clinical deterioration, or whose urine cultures reveal bacterial resistance to the selected antibiotic, a repeat urine culture is necessary and alternative antibiotic therapy should be considered (Hart et al. 2001). In severely ill patients, blood cultures should be taken. After the completion of treatment, urine culture should be performed at every antenatal visit for the remainder of the pregnancy. Continuous antimicrobial suppression with close follow-up until term may be used in a potentially non-compliant patient or when an underlying urinary tract abnormality is present or suspected, if further assessment of this can safely be postponed until the puerperium.

Gram-negative sepsis

This can occur in severely ill patients with acute pyelonephritis, but is more commonly associated with instrumentation of an infected urinary tract. An aminoglycoside antibiotic is best because it is effective against nearly all of the Gram-negative urinary bacteria. Enterococci less commonly cause bacteraemia but, because of their resistance to aminoglycosides, ampicillin should be used in combination with the aminoglycoside until culture results are available.

Perinatal implications

Controversy still abounds about the link to adverse outcomes in the offspring. The difficulty of performing controlled studies in humans has promoted the use of animal models: in the murine model there was invariably evidence of metritis, which is important in terms of uterine activity because until now preterm labour and delivery were thought to be associated with systemically mediated 'toxic' mechanisms (Mussalli *et al.* 2000).

Urinary infections in pregnancy may influence cognitive development in the offspring. In a recent cohort study (McDermott *et al.* 2000), 41,090 Medicaid-linked maternal and infant records were analysed along with collected and non-collected prescriptions, with 23 per cent of pregnant women without antibiotics revealing a significant association between maternal urinary infection and mental retardation in childhood. Furthermore, the fetal death rate was 5.2 per cent compared to no deaths in the group whose antibiotics were taken.

Haematuria during pregnancy (see also Chapter 1.6.2.i)

Spontaneous gross or microscopic haematuria can be due to a variety of causes. If associated with congenital anomalies, the urinary tract infection can be difficult to eradicate and may predispose to haematuria. Rupture of small veins in the dilated renal pelvis may also cause bleeding and, indeed, the haematuria may recur in subsequent pregnancies. Very rarely, haematuria may be secondary to glomerulonephritis, primary or metastatic neoplasm, haemangiomas, calculi, or fungal diseases. Endometriosis, inflammatory bowel lesions, leucoplakia, amyloidosis, and granulomas may involve the urinary tract and produce haematuria. A bleeding ureteral stump after a nephrectomy (for either benign or malignant disease), should not be forgotten.

Investigation of haematuria includes ultrasound, radiology, magnetic resonance imaging, and endoscopic assessment; this may, however, be deferred until after delivery. The clinician should assess all the circumstances to decide, whether or not it takes absolute priority. In the absence of any demonstrable cause, haematuria can be classified as idiopathic, and recurrences are unlikely in the current or subsequent pregnancy. It has been suggested, however, that haematuria is associated with an increased likelihood of adverse maternal outcomes including preterm labour and pre-eclampsia (Stehman-Breen *et al.* 2000) because a retrospective case controlled study showed an eight-fold increased risk of pre-eclampsia with mean duration from dipstick detection to diagnosis of around 11 weeks.

Acute hydroureter and hydronephrosis

Very occasionally, the anatomical changes associated with normal pregnancy (see Chapter 15.1) can be exaggerated, with massive ureteral and renal pelvis distension (as well as slight reduction in cortical width), but this is invariably without ill-effect (Brown 1990). Rarely, the changes may be extreme and precipitate the so-called 'overdistension syndrome', hypertension and/or reversible acute renal failure (Khauna and Nguyn 2001). In fact, there is a broad spectrum of this syndrome (Satin *et al.* 1993) with obstruction occurring at varying levels at or above the pelvic brim (Tables 2 and 3). Women who have had surgery for vesicoureteric reflux in childhood (especially bilateral) can develop distal ureteric obstruction even in early pregnancy, which can masquerade as pre-eclampsia and/or severe renal insufficiency (Thorpe *et al.* 1999).

Some women only have transient mild loin pain whereas others have recurrent episodes of severe loin pain or lower abdominal pain

Table 2 Clinical entities associated with urinary tract dilatation during pregnancy

Clinical entity	Clinical features
Overdistension syndrome	Flank pain, renal colic
Pyelonephritis	Flank pain, fever, bacteriuria
Urinary tract rupture	
Retroperitoneal	
Parenchymal	Flank pain
	Mass: abscess, haematoma
	Anaemia/hypotension due to blood loss
	Haematuria
Collecting system	Flank pain
	Mass: perinephric or subcapsular urinoma
	Haematuria (microscopic)
Intraperitoneal	
Parenchymal	Peritonitis
Collecting system	Flank pain
	Anaemia/hypotension due to blood loss
	Haematuria

Table 3 Rupture of the urinary tract

Traumatic
Non-traumatic
Parenchymal
Tumour, especially haematoma
Abscess
Vasculitides: polyarteritis nodosa
Cystic disease
Congenital: tuberous sclerosis
Non-parenchymal
Obstruction due to urolithiasis,
infection, reflux, or stricture
Pregnancy related

radiating to the groin. Urinalysis shows few or no red cells, and repeat midstream urine specimens are sterile (Fig. 1).

Variation in symptoms with changes in posture and position are hallmarks of this condition. Diagnosis can be confirmed using limited excretory urography or ultrasound sonar scanning (Delakas *et al.* 2000). Positioning of the patient in lateral recumbency or the knee–chest position often gives relief, but if this fails, ureteral catheterization or nephrostomy may be necessary. Corrective surgery is best delayed until the postpartum period.

Non-traumatic rupture of the urinary tract

The intrusion of unremitting pain and haematuria upon the course of pyelonephritis or the 'overdistension syndrome' suggests rupture of the urinary tract (Tables 2 and 3). This complication can masquerade as other obstetric and surgical abdominal catastrophies, including appendicitis, pelvic abscess, cholecystitis, urolithiasis (see Chapter 15.3), or abruptio placentae. Prompt recognition may prevent extrusion or expansion or both of a small tear and urine leak, treatable by postural or tube drainage (Nielson and Rasmussen 1998). Rupture of the renal

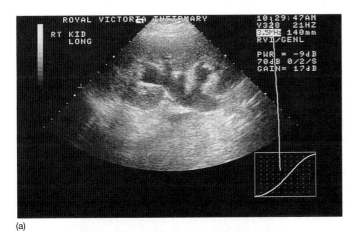

(a)

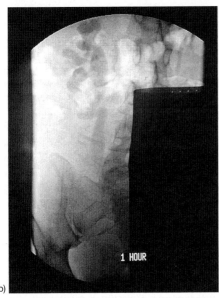

(b)

Fig. 1 Over 3 days this 26-week pregnant patient was diagnosed as having acute right-sided pyelonephritis, with gradually increasing loin pain radiating into her groin. Repeated midstream urine specimens were, however, negative. Renal ultrasonography (a) and an intravenous urogram (b) were undertaken. The former reveals a grossly dilated pelvicalyceal system and the latter acute kinking of the dilated right ureter above the level of the pelvic brim. Cystoscopy and ureteric stenting immediately resolved the situation. The stent was removed 1 month postpartum. There were no residual problems.

parenchyma, with haemorrhagic shock, formation of a flank mass, or dissection of urinary tract contents intraperitoneally compels prompt surgical intervention, usually with nephrectomy.

Obstetric acute renal failure

Perspective (Table 4) (see Chapter 10.7.2)

For the most part, acute renal failure occurs in women with previously healthy kidneys, but it may also complicate the course of women with pre-existing renal disease (Krane and Cucuzzella 1995; Nzerue *et al.* 1998). Before anuria or oliguria is ascribed to acute renal failure, obstruction of the urinary tract must be excluded, usually by ultrasound examination or infusion urography. This is particularly pertinent in

Table 4 Some causes of obstetric acute renal failure

Volume contraction/hypotension
Antepartum haemorrhage due to placenta praevia
Postpartum haemorrhage: from uterus or extensive soft tissue trauma
Abortion
Hyperemesis gravidarum
Adrenocortical failure; usually failure to augment steroids to cover delivery

Volume contraction/hypotension and coagulopathy
Antepartum haemorrhage due to abruptio placentae
Pre-eclampsia/eclampsia
Amniotic fluid embolism
Incompatible blood transfusion
Drug reaction(s)
Acute fatty liver
Haemolytic–uraemic syndrome

Volume contraction/hypotension, coagulopathy, and infection
Septic abortion
Chorioamnionitis
Pyelonephritis
Purpural sepsis

Urinary tract obstruction
Damage to ureters: during caesarean section or repair of cervical/vaginal lacerations
Pelvic and/or broad ligament haematomas

obstetric practice, since it is all too easy to damage the urinary tract unwittingly when performing emergency surgery for obstetric disasters, such as postpartum haemorrhage, which are themselves causes of acute renal failure.

In recent years, there has been a marked decline in cases of acute renal failure related to obstetric causes, and currently cases severe enough to require dialysis occur in fewer than 1 in 20,000 pregnancies, although complications with transient mild to moderate glomerular filtration rate (GFR) decrements occur in about 1 in 8000 deliveries (Pertuiset and Grünfeld 1994). This decrease has been attributed chiefly to a decline in the number of septic abortions and improvements in perinatal care, with clinicians ready to intervene quickly and aggressively in situations that could potentially lead to renal failure. Such situations include placental abruption, acute pyelonephritis, pre-eclampsia, postpartum haemorrhage, and any disease that may lead to systemic infection, dehydration, and/or hypotension (Chugh *et al.* 1994; Pertuiset and Grünfeld 1994). The reasons for this disposition remain unknown. Two entities associated with pregnancy—acute fatty liver and idiopathic postpartum renal failure [haemolytic–uraemic syndrome (HUS)]—are, fortunately, rare.

The pathology, diagnosis, and management are detailed elsewhere (Chapter 10.7.2) and while the principles are similar in non-pregnant and pregnant women, certain precautions warrant emphasis.

Diagnostic pitfalls

A carefully taken history and physical examination may reveal a background of abortion, severe hyperemesis gravidarum, haemorrhage, sensitization to drugs, incompatible blood transfusion, and/or pre-eclampsia–eclampsia. Once the diagnosis of acute renal failure has been considered a possibility, then a full initial assessment is essential, remembering that antepartum a decision will also be needed regarding the timing and route of delivery. Abnormal laboratory values should be interpreted in terms of 'pregnancy norms'. For example, normal values for arterial pH, and serum sodium and bicarbonate are 7.44, 135 mmol/l, and 20 mmol/l, respectively, whereas P_{CO_2} is only 37–40 kPa (see Chapter 15.1, Table 2).

It is difficult, and often impossible, to decide on the aetiology of the renal failure. Total anuria or alternating periods of anuria and polyuria are strongly suggestive of obstruction, but normal urine volumes do not exclude obstruction. Complete anuria and/or evidence of disseminated intravascular coagulation are suggestive of acute cortical necrosis, but this diagnosis can only be firmly established by renal biopsy.

Acute renal failure and septic shock (see Section 10)

Septicaemia associated with pregnancy is usually due to septic abortion, whereas chorioamnionitis, pyelonephritis, and puerperal sepsis occur less frequently.

Septic abortion, especially when due to clostridia, may result in a striking life-threatening syndrome (Pertuiset and Grünfeld 1994). Onset may be sudden, from hours to 2 days after the abortion, and is characterized by an abrupt increase in temperature (40°C or above), myalgia, vomiting, and bloody diarrhoea. Muscular pains are most intense in the arms, thorax, and abdomen. The clinical picture may be confused with intra-abdominal inflammatory disease, especially when a history of provoked abortion is denied or not sought for. Vaginal bleeding may be absent, and clostridia difficult to culture or to detect in the smear; the situation is further confounded by the normal presence of clostridium in the female genital tract. The patient is often jaundiced, and may have a peculiar bronze colour due to the association of jaundice with cutaneous vasodilation, cyanosis, and pallor. Once signs and symptoms develop, hypotension, dyspnoea, and progression to shock occur rapidly.

Characteristic laboratory findings include severe anaemia with markedly elevated bilirubin (due to haemolysis), evidence of disseminated intravascular coagulation, and a striking leucocytosis ($\geq$50,000 mm³). Hypocalcaemia sufficiently severe to provoke tetany has been described, and abdominal radiography may demonstrate air in the uterus or abdomen due to gas-forming organisms and/or perforation.

Death occurs in hours in a small percentage of patients; most respond to antibiotic treatment and volume replacement, and they then require treatment for acute renal failure. The clinical cause of the latter is usually that of tubular necrosis in general, but on occasion the more ominous cortical necrosis may occur. The oliguric phase in women with tubular necrosis due to septic abortion may last 3 weeks or more, and anuria may occur in this period. In fact, the diuretic phase often begins just when there are fears that the patient has underlying cortical rather than tubular necrosis.

The initial phase of the therapy requires vigorous supportive therapy and antibiotics. Use of antitoxin, hyperbaric oxygen, and exchange transfusion in the treatment of clostridial infections remains controversial, and there are major disagreements on the role of surgical intervention. As the uterus is a huge culture medium for bacterial growth and toxin formation, resistant to treatment, hysterectomy may need to be considered if the mother is to survive. Usually, however, modern-day antibiotic therapy suffices, and surgery in these critically ill women could be too risky and counterproductive.

Acute renal failure and pyelonephritis (see Section 10)

Acute pyelonephritis is the most common renal complication of pregnancy. In the absence of complicating features such as obstruction, calculi, papillary necrosis, and analgesic nephropathy, acute pyelonephritis is an extremely rare cause of acute renal failure in non-pregnant subjects, but appears more commonly in pregnant women, although the reason is obscure. It is known that in pregnant women acute pyelonephritis is accompanied by marked decrements in GFR and significant increments in plasma creatinine, in contrast to the situation in non-pregnant patients. It has been suggested that the vasculature in pregnancy may be more sensitive to the vasoactive effect of bacterial endotoxins and/or cytokines (Petersson et al. 1994).

Acute renal failure and pre-existing renal disease

The literature suggests that in some women with underlying renal disease but well-preserved GFR, acute tubular necrosis can develop when pregnancy is complicated by severe superimposed pre-eclampsia with its intense vasoconstriction, hypovolaemia, and generalized endothelial dysfunction (Sibai and Ramadan 1993; Friedman et al. 1995). Certainly, in women with moderate–severe renal disease [serum creatinine > 180 μmol/l (2 mg/dl)] gestational loss of renal function occurs in almost 50 per cent of pregnancies with 10 per cent of women progressing to endstage renal failure within a year of delivery (Jones and Hayslett 1996). In some of the more severe cases dialysis has to be introduced during pregnancy to 'buy' time for the fetus (Jungers et al. 1996).

Acute tubular necrosis

Volume depletion is the precipitating cause of acute tubular necrosis complicating hyperemesis gravidarum or when severe vomiting occurs with pyelonephritis (Pertuiset and Grünfeld 1994); in pregnancy the increased sensitivity of the vasculature to antitoxin also plays a role. Uterine haemorrhage is another major cause of renal failure in late pregnancy and the immediate puerperium. Antepartum bleeding may be difficult to diagnose or be underestimated when most of the blood loss remains behind the placenta ('concealed haemorrhage'), and suspicion requires rapid ultrasonic assessments. Uterine haemorrhage most often leads to acute tubular necrosis, and cortical necrosis may ensue, especially when associated with abruption (see below). Pre-eclampsia, characterized by generalized vasoconstriction, when neglected and accompanied by a marked coagulopathy, could progress to tubular and even cortical necrosis (Gaber and Lindheimer 1999).

Acute cortical necrosis

Fortunately, cortical necrosis, characterized by tissue death throughout the cortex with sparing of the medullary portions of the kidney, is a rare cause of acute renal failure, but it is more common in pregnancy. It is most common late in pregnancy, most frequently after placental abruption, and less commonly following prolonged intrauterine death or with pre-eclampsia. Abruption should always be borne in mind when renal failure develops suddenly, between the 26th and 30th gestational weeks.

Although acute cortical necrosis may involve the entire renal cortex with resultant irreversible renal failure, the incomplete or 'patchy' variety occurs more often in pregnancy, characterized by an initial episode of severe oliguria and even anuria, lasting longer than uncomplicated tubular necrosis. This is followed by a variable return of function and a stable period of moderate renal insufficiency, which in some cases progresses years later to endstage disease (Pertuiset and Grünfeld 1994).

It is not known why pregnant women are more susceptible to develop cortical necrosis than non-pregnant patients. Many of the women are older multiparas (>30 years) who have pre-existing nephrosclerosis, suggesting that their kidneys are more 'vulnerable' to the inciting factor(s) such as ischaemia or disseminated intravascular coagulation. It is interesting that the Sanarelli–Shwartzman reaction can be more easily produced in pregnant animals than in non-pregnant controls (Conger et al. 1981).

Acute renal failure particular to pregnancy

Acute fatty liver of pregnancy

This disease of the third trimester or puerperium is characterized by jaundice and severe hepatic dysfunction (Usta et al. 1994) occurring in 1 in 13,000 deliveries. The earliest manifestations are nausea and vomiting, important clues that are frequently overlooked and considered 'functional' because the woman is pregnant. Laboratory investigation often reveals evidence of disseminated intravascular coagulation, including decrements in antithrombin III. Serum urate concentrations may be elevated out of proportion to the degree of renal dysfunction, and hyperuricaemia may precede the clinical onset of the disease. Ultrasonography and computed tomography may also aid in the diagnosis. Since this disease is uncommon, it may be misdiagnosed as septicaemia or as pre-eclampsia complicated by liver involvement— some authors suggest that acute fatty liver and pre-eclampsia frequently coexist (see later and Chapter 10.7.2).

The aetiology of acute fatty liver of pregnancy is unknown, although in the past tetracycline toxicity was implicated in several instances. Reversible urea cycle enzyme abnormalities resembling those seen in Reye's syndrome have also been described, and it has been suggested that this condition may be an adult form of Reye's syndrome provoked by the metabolic stress of pregnancy (Rolfes and Ishak 1985). Against this, however, is that surviving women may have subsequent uneventful pregnancies (Pertuiset and Grünfeld 1994). More recently, there have been reports noting that patients with acute fatty liver of pregnancy harbour a long-chain 3-hydroxyacyl-co-enzyme A dehydrogenase deficiency or carry mutations of the enzyme's gene resulting in deficiencies in the fetus (Ibdah et al. 1999).

The hepatic lesion is characterized by deposition of fat microdroplets within the hepatocytes. Inflammation and necrosis are usually absent, although there are exceptions, and some cases may be misdiagnosed as hepatitis. Such errors can be avoided by studying freshly frozen tissue, using special fat stains.

The incidence of acute renal failure in women with acute fatty liver of pregnancy, once as high as 60 per cent, is now considerably less, possibly due to earlier recognition of the disease followed by rapid intervention to end the pregnancy. The renal lesion is mild: kidney structure may be within normal limits or abnormalities may be limited to fatty vacuolization and other non-specific changes of the tubule cells. The cause of the renal failure is obscure and may be due to haemodynamic factors, as in the 'hepatorenal syndrome', or perhaps a consequence of the disseminated intravascular coagulation. The mortality rate for mother and fetus, once quoted as exceeding 70–75 per cent, probably reflected an older literature selective of patients with the poorest outcome. Currently, the prognosis is improving, with survival exceeding 80–90 per cent, possibly because milder forms of the disease are being recognized. Irreversible forms still occur, however, and in such circumstances orthoptic liver transplantation may be lifesaving (Ockner et al. 1990).

Haemolytic–uraemic syndrome (see Chapter 10.6.4)

Various other names have been used for this condition, including idiopathic postpartum renal failure, irreversible postpartum renal failure, and postpartum malignant sclerosis.

HUS may occur between 1 day and several weeks after delivery. A typical patient presents with oliguria, or sometimes anuria, rapidly progressive azotaemia, and often evidence of microangiopathic haemolytic anaemia or a consumption coagulopathy. Blood pressure on admission varies from normal or only minimally elevated to severe hypertension. Some patients exhibit extrarenal manifestations involving the cardiovascular system (cardiac dilatation and congestive heart failure) and central nervous system (lethargy, convulsion) which appear disproportionate to the degree of uraemia, hypertension, or volume overload present.

The aetiology of HUS is unknown, but suggestions include a viral illness prior to the onset of the disease, retained placental fragments, or drugs such as ergotamine compounds, oxytocic agents, and/or oral contraceptives prescribed shortly after delivery (Pertuiset and Grünfeld 1994). Several women have manifested hypocomplementaemia, suggesting a possible immunological cause, and deficiencies in prostaglandin production and antithrombin III akin to those described in non-pregnant patients have been ascribed to the postpartum renal variant.

The pathophysiology of HUS has been compared to that of thrombotic thrombocytopenic purpura, other disease characterized by disseminated intravascular coagulation and the generalized Sanarelli–Shwartzman reaction, which, as noted above, develops more readily in pregnant animals (Conger et al. 1981). The renal pathology, detailed elsewhere (Pertuiset and Grünfeld 1994), differs substantially in various reports but falls into two general categories: changes in the glomerular capillaries resembling those seen in HUS in the nonpregnant patient (Fig. 2), and arteriolar lesions reminiscent of malignant nephrosclerosis or scleroderma. Some believe that glomerular lesions suggesting *thrombotic microangiopathy* are more apt to be noted in specimens obtained soon after the disease begins, while those resembling *accelerated nephrosclerosis* are seen in biopsy material taken later in the course. An increased incidence of postbiopsy bleeding has also been reported.

The prognosis of this disease is guarded. Most women have either succumbed, required chronic dialysis, or have survived with severely reduced renal function, and only a few have recovered. Of interest is

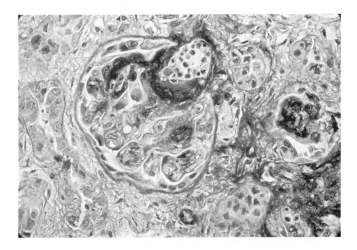

Fig. 2 The patient had an influenza-like illness on the third day after delivery. Blood pressure, initially normal, rose rapidly. She developed a severe microangiopathic anaemia (with anisocytosis, numerous schistocytes, high reticulocyte count, and a low serum haptoglobin level) and thrombocytopenia. There was rapidly progressive oliguria proceeding to anuric renal failure. The renal biopsy (after which she bled) revealed glomerular endothelial swelling and depositions of fibrin with capillary obstruction, thrombi, and fibrinoid necrosis.

a woman reported to have had a mild form of 'postpartum haemolytic syndrome', whose disease occurred in two successive pregnancies (Gomperts *et al.* 1978).

Treatment is primarily reduction of the high blood pressure, when present, with the general supportive measures used for all patients with acute renal failure. In the past, bilateral nephrectomy was used as a life-saving measure in a few women with accelerated hypertension unresponsive to treatment. This should be unnecessary today when potent vasodilators, converting enzyme inhibitors, and calcium-channel-blocking agents are available. The early use of anticoagulants, such as heparin and fibrinolytic agents, may reverse the renal failure, but data thus far have not been convincing, and such drugs are not harmless. In view of the possible contributing role of retained placental fragments, dilatation and curettage should be considered for women in whom the syndrome occurs close to delivery. Other regimens, including antiplatelet therapy (which may be of use in a possible variant of postpartum renal failure linked to circulating lupus anticoagulants), infusion of blood products, including antithrombin III concentrates, or exchange transfusions, have been advocated on the basis of their alleged success in patients with thrombotic thrombocytopenic purpura.

Acute renal failure and pre-eclampsia/eclampsia

Pre-eclampsia is accompanied by a characteristic renal lesion in which the glomeruli enlarge and become ischaemic because of swelling of the intracapillary cells—glomerular endotheliosis and mesangiosis. Most pre-eclamptic patients experience moderate decreases in GFR (Moran *et al.* 2003), but occasionally this decrease is accompanied by acute renal failure. The kidney failure is usually due to acute tubular necrosis, but acute cortical necrosis may also occur. It is possible that acute tubular necrosis is the obligatory outcome of glomerular cell

swelling and loss of anionic change along with complete obliteration of the capillary lumen (Friedman *et al.* 1995; Naicker *et al.* 1997) (see Chapter 15.3). This might be aggravated by inappropriate drug therapy, abruption placentae, or haemorrhage in the antenatal and peripartum periods (Brown *et al.* 1990). If the renal failure is related solely to pre-eclampsia without chronic hypertension, renal disease, or both before pregnancy, long-term normal renal function is evident in about 80 per cent of cases (Suzuki *et al.* 1997). Underlying chronic problems reduce this to 20 per cent, with the rest needing long-term dialysis (Sibai *et al.* 1990) and perinatal mortality is increased to 40 per cent (Drakeley *et al.* 2002).

Treatment should follow the standard approach (Lieberthal 1997) (see later), with intensive haemodynamic intervention; recently, more specific therapies for this group of patients have been tested, such as prostacyclin infusion. Interestingly, in the recent series of Drakeley *et al.* (2002), only 10 per cent required temporary dialysis and there were no cases of endstage renal failure needing permanent dialysis or renal transplant, contrasting with higher figures quoted by others, for example, 80 and 7 per cent, respectively (Selcuk *et al.* 2000).

HELLP syndrome (haemolysis, elevated liver enzymes and low platelets) was originally thought to be a rare complication of severe pre-eclampsia, but as more attention is paid to liver and haematological functions, it is now diagnosed more often (Gaber and Lindheimer 1999). The incidence of acute renal failure with the HELLP syndrome seems to be considerably higher for that with pre-eclampsia in general, but this may reflect the experience of tertiary care centres that receive the most complicated cases in transfer. In one recent series of 72 women with a median maximum serum creatinine of 340 μmol/l (3.85 mg/dl) 50 per cent had HELLP syndrome (Drakeley *et al.* 2002), and in another of 39 women with renal failure [median serum creatinine of 496 μmol/l (5.6 mg/dl)] 36 per cent had HELLP (Selcuk *et al.* 2000). It is not clear, however, whether acute renal failure is a specific component of the HELLP syndrome itself or a complication of a particularly severe multisystem condition. Certainly, it may occur without haemolysis (referred to by some as ELLP syndrome) (Sibai and Ramadan 1993; Sibai *et al.* 1994).

Miscellaneous causes

Acute renal failure has occurred after intra-amniotic saline administration, after amniotic fluid embolism, and following illnesses or accidents unrelated to the pregnancy, such as drug ingestion, bacterial endocarditis, and incompatible blood transfusions. Sudden acute renal failure during pregnancy has also complicated sarcoidosis (Warren *et al.* 1988), various nephritides, or collagen disorders, and can also be due to obstructive uropathy related to the enlarged uterus with or without polyhydramnios (Brandes and Fritsche 1991). Most of the latter problems have been in women with solitary kidneys, but there have also been instances of bilateral obstruction, which can be managed conservatively by placement of intraureteral stents under local anaesthesia (Delekas *et al.* 2000).

Principles of management (see Chapters 10.3 and 10.4)

Treatment of sudden renal failure resembles that in non-pregnant populations and aims at retarding the appearance of uraemic symptomatology, acid–base and electrolyte disturbances, and volume problems (i.e. overhydration when the patient is oliguric and dehydration during the polyuric phase) (Lieberthal *et al.* 1997; Drakeley *et al.* 2002). One must also be aware of the propensity of patients with acute renal failure to acquire infection, a complication that can be serious in pregnant women. Most of the aforementioned problems respond to judicious conservative management, but if such an approach is unsuccessful, dialysis will be necessary.

Dialysis in patients with acute renal failure is prescribed 'prophylactically' (i.e. prior to the appearance of electrolyte, acidaemic, or uraemic symptoms). Such prophylactic dialysis appears even more necessary in prepartum patients with an immature fetus and in whom temporization is desired (Jungers and Chauveau 1997; Hou and Firanek 1998). Problems during dialysis peculiar to pregnancy were discussed in detail earlier.

Peritoneal dialysis is effective and safe as long as the catheter is inserted high in the abdomen under direct vision through a small incision. In fact, as discussed earlier, chronic ambulatory peritoneal dialysis may become the preferred dialysis approach in the prepartum woman because it minimizes rapid metabolic perturbations. Volume shifts during haemodialysis should be minimized to avoid impairment of uteroplacental blood flow.

Controlled anticoagulation with heparin (preferably including monitoring to verify that activated clotting time is maintained between 150 and 180 s) is desirable during haemodialysis. Observation for vaginal bleeding is also important.

As discussed previously, premature contractions or the onset of labor frequently occurs during or immediately after dialysis. Therefore, when possible, early delivery (as dictated by fetal maturity) should be undertaken. Blood losses should be replaced quickly to the point of overtransfusing slightly, because in the pregnant patient uterine bleeding may be concealed and, thus, underestimated.

When delivery is imminent, nursery personnel should be advised that the neonate could be subject to rapid dehydration, due to increased fetal levels of urea and other solutes that precipitate an osmotic diuresis shortly after birth.

References

Brandes, J. C. and Fritsche, C. (1991). Obstructive acute renal failure by a gravid uterus: a case report and review. *American Journal of Kidney Diseases* **18**, 398–401.

Brown, M. A. (1990). Urinary tract dilatation in pregnancy. *American Journal of Obstetrics and Gynecology* **164**, 641–643.

Chugh, K. S., Singhal, P. C., and Kher, V. K. (1994). Acute renal cortical necrosis. A study of 113 patients. *Renal Failure* **16**, 37–47.

Conger, J. D., Falk, S. A., and Guggenheim, S. J. (1981). Glomerular dynamics and morphologic changes in the generalized Schwartzman reaction in postpartum rats. *Journal of Clinical Investigation* **67**, 1334–1336.

Cunningham, F. G. and Lucas, M. J. (1994). Urinary tract infections complicating pregnancy. *Clinics in Obstetrics and Gynaecology* **8**, 353–373.

Cunningham, F. G., Lucas, M. J., and Hankins, G. D. V. (1987). Pulmonary injury complicating antepartum pyelonephritis. *American Journal of Obstetrics and Gynecology* **156**, 797–807.

Delekas, D., Karyotis, I., and Loumbakis, P. (2000). Ureteral drainage by double-J-catheters during pregnancy. *Clinical and Experimental Obstetrics and Gynaecology* **27**, 200–202.

Dempsey, C., Harrison, R. F., and Maloney, A. (1992). Characteristics of bacteriuria in a homogeneous maternity hospital population. *European Journal of Obstetrics, Gynaecology and Reproductive Biology* **44**, 189–194.

Drakeley, A. J. *et al.* (2002). Acute renal failure complicating severe preeclampsia requiring admission to an obstetric intensive care unit. *American Journal of Obstetrics and Gynecology* **186**, 253–259.

Friedman, S. A., Schiff, E., Emeis, J. J., Dekker, G. A., and Sibai, B. M. (1995). Biochemical corroboration of endothelial involvement in severe preeclampsia. *American Journal of Obstetrics and Gynecology* **172**, 202–203.

Gaber, L. W. and Lindheimer, M. D. Pathology of the kidney, liver and brain. In *Chesley's Hypertensive Disorders in Pregnancy* 2nd edn. (ed. M. D. Lindheimer, J. M. Roberts, and F. G. Cunningham), pp. 231–252. Stamford, Connecticut: Appleton and Lange, 1999.

Gilstrap, L. S. and Ramin, S. M. (2001). Urinary tract infections during pregnancy. *Obstetric and Gynecological Clinics* **28**, 581–591.

Goluszko, P. *et al.* (2001). Dr operon-associated invasiveness of *Escherichia coli* from pregnant patients with pyelonephritis. *Infection and Immunity* **69**, 4678–4680.

Gomperts, D., Sessel, L., DuPlessis, V., and Hersch, C. (1978). Recurrent postpartum haemolytic uraemic syndrome. *Lancet* **i**, 48.

Graham, J. C. *et al.* (2001). Analysis of *Escherichia coli* strains causing bacteriuria during pregnancy: selection for strains that do not express Type 1 fimbriae. *Infection and Immunity* **69**, 794–799.

Hart, A. *et al.* (2001). Ampicillin-resistant *Escherichia coli* in gestational pyelonephritis: increased occurrence and association with the colonization faction Dr adhesin. *Journal of Infectious Diseases* **183**, 1526–1529.

Hou, S. and Firanek, C. (1998). Management of the pregnant dialysis patient. *Advances in Renal Replacement Therapy* **5**, 24–30.

Ibdah, J. A., Bennett, M. J., Rinaldo, P., Zhoo, Y., Sims, H., Gibson, B., and Strauss, A. W. (1999). A fetal fatty acid oxidation disorder as a cause of liver disease in pregnant women. *New England Journal of Medicine* **346**, 1723–1731.

Jones, D. C. and Hayslett, J. P. (1996). Outcome of pregnancy in women with moderate or severe renal insufficiency. *New England Journal of Medicine* **335**, 226–230.

Jungers, P. and Chauveau, D. (1997). Pregnancy in renal disease. *Kidney International* **52**, 871–882.

Jungers, P. *et al.* (1996). Pregnancy in women with reflux nephropathy. *Kidney International* **50**, 593–598.

Khauna, N. and Nguyen, H. (2001). Reversible acute renal failure in association with bilateral ureteral obstruction and hydronephrosis in pregnancy. *American Journal of Obstetrics and Gynecology* **184**, 239–240.

Krane, K. and Cucuzzella, A. (1995). Acute renal insufficiency in pregnancy: a review of 30 cases. *Journal of Maternal-Fetal Medicine* **4**, 12–18.

Lieberthal, W. (1997). Biology of acute renal failure: therapeutic implications. *Kidney International* **52**, 1102–1107.

McDermott, S. *et al.* (2000). Urinary tract infections during pregnancy and mental retardation and developmental delay. *Obstetrics and Gynecology* **96**, 113–119.

Moran, P., Baylis, P. H., Lindheimer, M. D., and Davison, J. M. (2003). Glomerular ultrafiltration in normal and preeclamptic pregnancy. *Journal of the American Society of Nephrology* **14**, 648–652.

Mussalli, G. M. *et al.* (2000). Preterm delivery in mice with renal abscess. *Obstetrics and Gynecology* **95**, 453–456.

Naicker, T. *et al.* (1997). Correlation between histological changes and loss of anionic change of the glomerular basement membrane in early onset preeclampsia. *Nephron* **75**, 201–206.

Neilson, R. F. and Rasmussen, P. E. (1998). Hydronephrosis during pregnancy: 4 cases of hydronephrosis causing symptoms during pregnancy. *European Journal of Obstetrics, Gynecology and Reproductive Biology* **3**, 245–249.

Nzerue, C. M., Hewan-Lowe, K., and Nwawka, C. (1998). Acute renal failure in pregnancy: a review of clinical outcomes at an inner city hospital from 1986–1996. *Journal of the National Medical Association* **90**, 486–491.

Ockner, S. A., Brunt, E. M., and Cohen, S. M. (1990). Fulminant hepatic failure caused by acute fatty liver of pregnancy treated by orthotopic liver transplantation. *Hepatology* **11**, 59–64.

Pedler, S. J. and Orr, K. E. Bacterial, fungal and parasitic infections. In *Medical Disorders During Pregnancy* 3rd edn. (ed. W. M. Barron and M. D. Lindheimer), pp. 411–495. Mosby-Year Book: St Louis, 2000.

Pertuiset, N. and Grünfeld, J. P. (1994). Acute renal failure in pregnancy. *Clinics in Obstetrics and Gynaecology* 8, 333–351.

Petersson, C., Hedges, S., and Stenquist, K. (1994). Suppressed antibody and interleukin-6 response to acute pyelonephritis in pregnancy. *Kidney International* 45, 571–577.

Pfau, A. and Sacks, T. G. (1992). Effective prophylaxis for recurrent urinary tract infections during pregnancy. *Clinics in Infectious Diseases* 14, 810–814.

Pruett, K. and Faro, S. (1987). Pyelonephritis associated with respiratory distress. *Obstetrics and Gynecology* 69, 444–446.

Rolfes, D. B. and Ishak, K. G. (1985). Acute fatty liver of pregnancy: a clinico-pathologic study of 35 cases. *Hepatology* 5, 1149–1158.

Sanchez-Ramos, L., McAlpine, K. J., Adair, D., Kaunitz, A. M., Delke, I., and Briones, D. K. (1995). Pyelonephritis in pregnancy: once-a-day ceftriax-one versus multiple doses of cefazolin. *American Journal of Obstetrics and Gynecology* 172, 129–133.

Satin, S. A., Seikin, G. L., and Cunningham, F. G. (1993). Reversible hypertension in pregnancy caused by obstructive uropathy. *Obstetrics and Gynecology* 81, 823–825.

Selcuk *et al.* (2000). Outcome of pregnancies with HELLP syndrome complicated by acute renal failure (1989–1999). *Renal Failure* 22, 319–327.

Shelton, S. D. *et al.* (2001). Urinary interleukin-8 with asymptomatic bacteriuria in pregnancy. *Obstetrics and Gynecology* 97, 583–586.

Sibai, B. M. and Ramadan, M. (1993). Acute renal failure in pregnancies complicated by hemolysis, elevated liver enzymes and low platelets. *American Journal of Obstetrics and Gynecology* 168, 1682–1690.

Sibai, B. M., Kustermann, L., and Velasco, J. (1994). Current understanding of severe pre-eclampsia, pregnancy-associated hemolytic uremic syndrome, thrombotic thrombocytopenic purpura, hemolysis, elevated liver enzymes and low platelet syndrome and postpartum acute renal failure: different clinical syndromes or just different names? *Current Opinion in Nephrology and Hypertension* 3, 436–445.

Stamm, W. E., McKevitt, M., Roberts, P. L., and White, N. J. (1991). Natural history of recurrent urinary tract infections in women. *Review of Infectious Disease* 13, 77.

Stehman-Breen, C. *et al.* (2000). Preeclampsia and premature labour among pregnant women with haematuria. *Paediatric Perinatal Epidemiology* 14, 136–139.

Stenquist, K., Dahlin-Nilsson, I., and Lidin-Janson, G. (1989). Bacteriuria in pregnancy. Frequency and risk of acquisition. *American Journal of Epidemiology* 129, 372–379.

Suzuki, S. *et al.* (1997). Post-partum renal lesions in women with pre-eclampsia. *Nephrology, Dialysis, Transplantation* 12, 2488–2491.

Thorp, J. A., Davis, B. E., and Klingele, C. (1999). Severe early onset pre-eclampsia secondary to bilateral ureteral obstruction reversed by stenting. *Obstetrics and Gynecology* 94, 806–807.

Twickler, D. M., Lucas, M. J., Bowe, L., McIntire, D. D., Barron, J., and Cunningham, F. G. (1994). Ultrasonic evaluation of central and end-organ hemodynamics in antepartum peylonephritis. *American Journal of Obstetrics and Gynecology* 179, 814–818.

Usta, I. M., Barton, J. R., Amon, E. A., Gonzalez, A., and Sibai, B. M. (1994). Acute fatty liver of pregnancy: an experience in the diagnosis and management of fourteen cases. *American Journal of Obstetrics and Gynecology* 171, 1342–1347.

Warren, G. V., Sprague, S. M., and Corwin, H. C. (1988). Sarcoidosis presenting as acute renal failure in pregnancy. *American Journal of Kidney Diseases* 12, 161–167.

Weinberger, S. E. (1993). Recent advances in pulmonary medicine. *New England Journal of Medicine* 328, 1462–1470.

Wing, D. A. *et al.* (1999). Outpatient treatment of acute pyelonephritis in pregnancy after 24 weeks. *Obstetrics and Gynecology* 94, 683–688.

15.3 Pregnancy in patients with underlying renal disease

John M. Davison and Chris Baylis

Women with underlying renal disease contemplating pregnancy and those already pregnant ask straightforward questions.

1. Is pregnancy advisable?

2. Will the pregnancy be complicated?

3. Will I have a live and healthy baby?

4. Will I come to any harm in the long term?

The answers should be equally straightforward and should be based on fact, not on anecdote. The clinician must, therefore, have an up-to-date knowledge of renal physiology in pregnancy, as described in Chapter 15.1, as well as an awareness of recent advances in nephrological, obstetric, and neonatal practice. This chapter highlights new information and the prevailing controversies and attempts to provide the answers for women with chronic renal disease, dialysis patients, and renal transplant recipients. The key to success is close scrutiny during antenatal care, with cooperation between nephrologist, obstetrician and, eventually, paediatrician in a centre with all the necessary facilities for dealing with 'high-risk' patients.

Chronic renal disease

The majority view (Lindheimer *et al.* 2001), is now that, provided non-pregnant renal function is only mildly compromised, proteinuria is not in the nephrotic range, and hypertension is absent or minimal, then obstetric outcome is usually successful with little or no adverse effect on long-term renal prognosis, except in a few specific disease entities (see below).

Clinical implications of renal dysfunction in pregnancy

An individual may lose approximately 50 per cent of renal function and still maintain a plasma creatinine less than 130 μmol/l (1.5 mg/dl) (Fig. 1). However, if renal function is more severely compromised, small further decreases in glomerular filtration rate (GFR) will cause plasma creatinine to increase markedly. Nevertheless, a patient who has lost 75 per cent of her nephrons may have lost only 50 per cent of renal function and may have a deceptively normal plasma creatinine due to hyperfiltration by the remaining nephrons. Evaluation of renal function should therefore be based on the clearance of creatinine rather than on its plasma concentration, or better still on measurement of GFR itself (see Chapter 1.3).

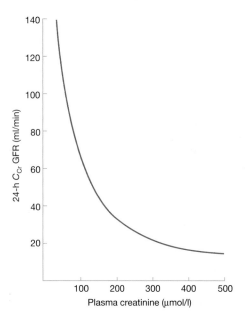

Fig. 1 Relationship between GFR (ml/min), deterimined by clearance of creatinine (24-h C_{Cr}), and plasma creatinine concentration (μmol/l) assuming a constant 24-h creatinine excretion of about 11.5 mmol (J.M. Davison, unpublished observations).

In patients with renal disease, pathological conditions may be both biochemically and clinically silent. Most individuals remain symptom free until their GFR declines to less than 25 per cent of normal, and many plasma constituents are frequently normal until a late stage of disease (Parmar 2002). As renal function declines, the ability to conceive and to sustain a viable pregnancy decreases (Cunningham *et al.* 1990). Degrees of functional impairment that do not cause symptoms or appear to disrupt homoeostasis in non-pregnant individuals can jeopardize pregnancy.

Normal pregnancy is rare when renal function declines, such that the non-pregnant plasma creatinine and urea exceed 275 and 10 μmol/l, respectively. Although only moderately increased over non-pregnant concentrations, these values represent considerable loss of renal function. The basic question for a woman with renal disease must be: is pregnancy advisable? If it is, then the sooner she starts to have her family the better, since in many cases renal function will decline with time. Women with suspected or known renal disease are not always counselled prior to pregnancy and may therefore present already pregnant, as a *fait accompli*; then the question must be: 'does pregnancy continue?'

Renal impairment and the impact of pregnancy

Obstetric and long-term renal prognoses differ in women with different degrees of renal insufficiency, and the impact of pregnancy is best considered by categories of functional renal status prior to pregnancy (Tables 1 and 2).

Preserved/mildly impaired renal function

Women with normal or only mildly decreased renal function at conception [serum creatinine < 125 μmol/l (1.4 mg/dl)] usually have a successful obstetric outcome, and pregnancy does not appear to adversely affect the course of their disease (Davison 1989; Jungers and Chauveau 1997; Lindheimer and Katz 1999a; Baylis 2003). Although this holds true for most patients, there are exceptions. Most authors strongly advise against pregnancy in women with scleroderma and periarteritis nodosa. Others express reservations when the underlying renal disorder is lupus nephropathy, membranoproliferative glomerulonephritis, and perhaps IgA and reflux nephropathies.

Most women whose prepregnancy creatinine is less than or equal to 1.4 mg/dl (≤125 μmol/l) manifest increments in GFR, but less than those of normal pregnant women (Fig. 2). Increased proteinuria is common, occurring in 50 per cent of pregnancies (although this is unusual in women with chronic pyelonephritis), and exceeding the nephrotic range (3 g in 24 h) in 50 per cent of gravidas. Perinatal outcome is said to be jeopardized by the presence of uncontrolled hypertension and for some when nephrotic range proteinuria is already present in early pregnancy (Jungers and Chauveau 1997; Rashid and Rashid 2003). In one study where creatinine clearances were available, a value less than 70 ml/min prior to conception was associated with poorer outcomes, even when serum concentrations were in the 'minimal dysfunction' range (Abe 1996). Finally, gestation does not appear to influence the natural history of the renal disease when preconception renal function is only minimally impaired.

Moderate and severe renal insufficiency

Outlooks are more guarded when renal function is moderately impaired [serum creatinine 125–250 μmol/l (1.4–2.5 mg/dl)] before

pregnancy and is very definitely affected with severe renal dysfunction [serum creatinine > 250 μmol/l (2.8 mg/dl)] (Hou 1999). These women do, however, become pregnant. Prior to 1996, there were few reports, all of limited size, but of particular interest is a study that assessed maternal and fetal outcomes of 82 pregnancies in 62 women (Jones and Hayslett 1996), all of whom had serum creatinine exceeding 125 μmol/l (1.4 mg/dl). The incidence of hypertension increased from 28 per cent at the baseline to 48 per cent by the third trimester, and the presence of significant proteinuria (urinary protein excretion > 3 g in 24 h) increased from 23 to 41 per cent. Of these pregnancies, 43 per cent were associated with a deterioration in renal function, at times rapid and substantial, and in 10 per cent of these instances the deterioration did not reverse postpartum. Although the infant survival rate was high (93 per cent), rates of premature delivery (59 per cent), and fetal growth restriction (37 per cent) underscored the very high potential for obstetric complications in these women (see Table 3).

The results reported by Jones and Hayslett (1996) actually confirm the previous reports of limited size in which one-third to one-half of women with moderate to severe renal insufficiency experienced functional loss more rapidly than would have been expected from the natural course of their renal disease (Cunningham et al. 1990). A surprising observation from Jones and Hayslett (1996) was that good blood pressure control did not guarantee the preservation of maternal renal function, data that require confirmation.

Another recent study (Jungers et al. 1997) remains optimistic. Awareness of progress in obstetric and neonatal care means that more women with impaired renal function will contemplate pregnancy and anticipate a good obstetric outcome. It is suggested that this view holds as long as the serum creatinine is less than 200 μmol/l (<2.3 mg/dl). Once creatinine exceeds 250 μmol/l (2.8 mg/dl), however, there is a substantial risk of both an unsuccessful fetal outcome and accelerated loss of maternal renal function (Table 4). Also, we lack reliable and convincing data allowing prediction of which women will experience a rapid loss of renal function, and when function starts to decrease, terminating the pregnancy does not necessarily reverse the decline.

Table 1 Prepregnancy assessment: categories of renal functional status

Classification	Plasma creatinine (μmol/l)
Preserved/mildly impaired renal function	≤125
Moderately renal insufficiency	≥125
Severe renal insufficiency	≥250

Table 2 Pregnancy prospects for women with chronic renal disease (%)

Problems in pregnancy	Successful obstetric outcome	Problems in long term	Endstage renal failure within 1 year
90 (81–97)	84 (65–93)	50 (30–57)	15 (10–23)

Mean (range): data are from 107 women in 125 pregnancies (Jones and Hayslett 1996; Jungers et al. 1997).

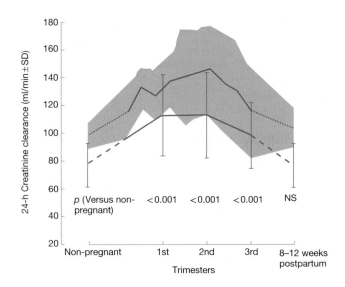

Fig. 2 Serial 24-h creatinine clearances (mean ± 1 SD) before, during, and after pregnancy in 26 women with chronic renal disease where renal function was preserved or mildly impaired (solid line). Data from 10 healthy pregnant women (mean ± 1 SD) shown by hatched area (taken from Katz et al. 1980, with permission).

Table 3 Effect of blood pressure on pregnancy complications (%)

	Intrauterine growth retardation	Preterm delivery	Renal deterioration
Normotension	4	12	3
Hypertension	16	20	15

Derived from Cunningham et al. (1990), Abe (1996), Jones and Hayslett (1996), Jungers et al. (1996, 1997), and Jungers and Chauveau (1997).

Table 4 Effect of blood pressure and/or renal deterioration on fetal mortality (%)

	Hypertension	Renal deterioration	Both
Absent throughout pregnancy	6	7	7
Present at some time during pregnancy	12	12	19
Present and managed from first trimester	10	—	13
Present from first trimester and not managed or management inadequate	50	40	55
Present only during third trimester	8	9	10

Derived from Cunningham et al. (1990), Abe (1996), Jones and Hayslett (1996), Jungers et al. (1996, 1997), and Jungers and Chauveau (1997).

The worries about moderate and severe dysfunction continue to be reiterated. A recent single centre experience (Bar et al. 2000) documents short- and long-term outcomes in 38 patients in 46 pregnancies. Successful outcome was defined as a live healthy infant without handicap by 2 years of age. This was the case in 96 per cent of pregnancies from women with diabetic nephropathy and 89 per cent from those with transplants. Again, poorly controlled pre-existing hypertension was the harbinger of poor outcome, but the influences of serum creatinine and of proteinuria were more variable. In general, a worse outcome and poorer renal prognosis occurred in those with the moderate and severe renal dysfunction (Baylis 2003).

Dialysis has also been instituted prophylactically during pregnancy to increase the chances of successful outcome (Bagon et al. 1998; Chan et al. 1998; Okundaye et al. 1998). Obviously, 'buying time' for fetal maturation in this way is independent of the inexorable further declines in renal function ultimately to endstage failure. Nevertheless, extreme prematurity and/or disturbing, life-threatening maternal problems are still commonplace and such additional health risks are difficult to justify. The aim should be to preserve what little renal function remains and to achieve renal rehabilitation via dialysis and transplantation, after which the question of pregnancy can be considered if appropriate. Some women, however, will be prepared to take a chance and even seek assisted conception in the face of their infertility. This obsessional pursuit of pregnancy and the issues surrounding the clinician's obligation to accede to (or refute) care that poses a risk to the woman's health have been discussed elsewhere (Stotland and Stotland 1997; Kimmel and Patel 2003; Palmer 2003).

Finally, and of utmost importance to this discussion, the literature that forms the basis of our views is primarily *retrospective*. Most patients described had only mild dysfunction, women with severe disease being limited in number. Confirmation of guidelines, therefore, requires further adequate prospective trials.

Antenatal strategy and decision-making

Patients should be seen at 2-week intervals until 32 weeks' gestation, after which assessment should be weekly. Routine serial antenatal observations should be supplemented with:

(1) assessment of renal function by 24-h creatinine clearance and protein excretion (see Chapter 15.1);

(2) careful monitoring of blood pressure for early detection of hypertension and then assessment of its severity;

(3) early detection of pre-eclampsia;

(4) biophysical/ultrasound assessment of fetal size, development, and well being; and

(5) early detection of covert bacteriuria or confirmation of urinary tract infection.

The crux of management is the balance between maternal prognosis and fetal prognosis—the effect of pregnancy on a particular disease and the effect of that disease on pregnancy. The various problems specifically associated with particular kidney diseases are summarized in Table 5; the following guidelines apply to all clinical situations.

Renal function

If renal function deteriorates significantly at any stage of pregnancy, then reversible causes, such as urinary tract infection, subtle dehydration, or electrolyte imbalance (occasionally precipitated by inadvertent diuretic therapy) should be sought. Near term, as in normal pregnancy, a decrease in function of 15–20 per cent, which affects blood creatinine minimally, is permissible. Failure to detect a reversible cause of a significant decrement is grounds to end the pregnancy by elective delivery. When proteinuria occurs and persists, but blood pressure is normal and renal function preserved, pregnancy can be allowed to continue.

Blood pressure

Blood pressure should be measured in the sitting position with a cuff which is large enough for a particular patient's arm. Phases I and V of the Korotkoff sounds are used. Hypertension is not a disease but one end of a continuous distribution of all individuals' blood pressures. The conventional dividing line for obstetric hypertension is 140/90.

Most of the specific risks of hypertension in pregnancy appear to be related to superimposed pre-eclampsia (see Chapter 15.4). There is confusion about the true incidence of superimposed pre-eclampsia in women with pre-existing renal disease. This is because the diagnosis cannot be made with certainty on clinical grounds alone; hypertension and proteinuria may be manifestations of the underlying renal disease. Treatment of mild hypertension (diastolic blood pressure <95 mmHg in the second trimester or <100 mmHg in the third) is not necessary during normal pregnancy, but many would treat women

Table 5 Specific kidney diseases and pregnancy

Renal disease	Effects and outcomes
Chronic glomerulonephritis	Usually no adverse effect in the absence of hypertension. One view is that glomerulonephritis is adversely affected by the coagulation changes of pregnancy. Urinary tract infections may occur more frequently
IgA nephropathy	Risks of uncontrolled and/or sudden escalating hypertension and worsening of renal function
Pyelonephritis	Bacteriuria in pregnancy can lead to exacerbation. Multiple organ system derangements may ensue, including adult respiratory distress syndrome
Reflux nephropathy	Risks of sudden escalating hypertension and worsening of renal function
Urolithiasis	Infections can be more frequent, but ureteral dilatation and stasis do not seem to affect natural history. Limited data on lithotripsy, thus best avoided
Polycystic disease	Functional impairment and hypertension usually minimal in childbearing years
Diabetic nephropathy	Usually no adverse effect on the renal lesion, but there is increased frequency of infection, oedema, and/or pre-eclampsia
Systemic lupus erythematosus	Controversial; prognosis most favourable if disease in remission > 6 months prior to conception. Steroid dosage should be increased postpartum
Periarteritis nodosa	Fetal prognosis is dismal and maternal death often occurs
Scleroderma	If onset during pregnancy then there can be a rapid overall deterioration. Reactivation of quiescent scleroderma may occur postpartum
Previous urinary tract surgery	Might be associated with other malformations of the urogenital tract. Urinary tract infection common during pregnancy. Renal function may undergo reversible decrease. No significant obstructive problem but Caesarean section often needed for abnormal presentation and/or to avoid disruption of the continence mechanism if an artificial sphincter is present
After nephrectomy, solitary kidney, and pelvic kidney	Might be associated with other malformations of the urogenital tract. Pregnancy well tolerated. Dystocia rarely occurs with pelvic kidney
Wegener's granulomatosis	Limited information. Proteinuria ($\pm$ hypertension) is common from early in pregnancy. Immunosuppressives are safe but cytotoxic drugs are best avoided
Renal artery stenosis	May present as chronic hypertension or as recurrent isolated pre-eclampsia. If diagnosed then transluminal angioplasty can be undertaken in pregnancy if appropriate

with underlying renal disease more aggressively, believing that this preserves kidney function. Most patients can be taught to take their own blood pressure, but there are still debates about the accuracy of automated devices and the role of ambulatory blood pressure measurements (Shennan *et al.* 1996; Gupta *et al.* 1997; Brown *et al.* 1998).

Fetal surveillance and timing of delivery

Serial assessment of fetal well being is essential since renal disease can be associated with fetal growth restriction and, when complications do arise, the judicious moment for intervention can be assessed by fetal status. Current technology should minimize the incidence of intrauterine fetal death as well as neonatal morbidity and mortality. Regardless of gestational age, most babies weighing 1500 g or more survive better in a special care nursery than in a hostile intrauterine environment. Planned preterm delivery may be necessary if (a) there are signs of impending intrauterine fetal death, (b) renal function deteriorates substantially, (c) uncontrollable hypertension supervenes, or (d) eclampsia occurs.

Clinicians are still searching for antenatal tests that identify the fetus at risk of intrauterine hypoxia and death. Ideally, such a test should not only be reliable but performed easily and repeatedly. It is now recognized that biochemical tests, such as estimations of oestriol and human placental lactogen are poor predictors of fetal outcome.

Antenatal fetal heart rate monitoring is the most widely accepted diagnostic test for assessing fetal well being. Non-stress antenatal cardiotocography (CTG) (the non-stress test) is the most commonly used and needs to be done frequently to identify the changing fetal heart rate pattern associated with hypoxia. A normal test predicts a normal outcome in 80–90 per cent of cases, whereas an abnormal test, especially one where there is repeated loss of variability with decelerative patterns, is associated with fetal compromise in nearly all cases. The exogenous oxytocin challenge test is problematical and is not used and nipple stimulation tests are currently being investigated.

Dynamic ultrasound imaging has now advanced from merely assessing gestational age (fetal biometry) to examination of placental architecture and fetal biophysical profile scoring. Doppler ultrasound also allows cardiovascular assessments, especially in the umbilical vessels, the fetal cerebral circulation and aorta, as well as the uterine and arcuate arteries.

Role of renal biopsy in pregnancy

Experience with renal biopsy in pregnancy is sparse, mainly because clinical circumstances rarely justify the risks. Reports of excessive bleeding and other complications in pregnant women have led some to consider pregnancy as a relative contraindication to renal biopsy (Kuller *et al.* 2001), although others have not observed any increased morbidity

(Chen *et al.* 2001). New debates prevail about ethical issues surrounding renal biopsy in pregnant women, let alone the clinical justification (de Swiet and Lightstone 2004; Gallery 2004; Lindheimer and Mahowald 2004; Stevens *et al.* 2004). When renal biopsy is undertaken immediately after delivery in women with well-controlled blood pressure and normal coagulation indices, the morbidity is certainly similar to that reported in non-pregnant patients (Lindheimer and Davison 1987).

The classical report of Packham and Fairley (1987) described 111 preterm biopsies in pregnant women and showed that the risks of the procedure resemble those in the non-pregnant population. In fact, the incidence of transient gross haematuria (all patients undergoing biopsy have microscopic haematuria unless the kidney has been missed), was 0.9 per cent, considerably less than in non-pregnant patients, where it is 3–5 per cent. Such excellent statistics no doubt reflect the experience and technical skills of the unit and careful prebiopsy evaluation of the patient; they should not be used to encourage inexperienced physicians to undertake biopsy in pregnant patients.

Nevertheless, it is still important to have specific indications for renal biopsy in pregnancy. Packham and Fairley (1987) suggest that closed (percutaneous) needle biopsy should be undertaken more often, because they believe that certain glomerular disorders are adversely influenced by pregnancy and that specific therapy, such as antiplatelet agents, might be beneficial. The consensus, however, goes against such broad indications and reiterates that renal biopsy should be performed infrequently during pregnancy (Lindheimer and Davison 1987). Indeed, even in the non-pregnant individual the reasons for renal biopsy are not clearly defined and experts categorize indications as 'most useful', 'possibly useful', and/or 'of little or no use' (see Chapter 1.7).

The few widely agreed indications for antepartum biopsy are as follows:

1. Sudden deterioration of renal function before 30–32 weeks' gestation with no obvious cause. Certain forms of rapidly progressive glomerulonephritis may respond to aggressive treatment with steroid 'pulses', chemotherapy, and perhaps plasma exchange, when diagnosed early.

2. Symptomatic nephrotic syndrome before 30–32 weeks' gestation. While some might consider a therapeutic trial of steroids in such cases, it is best to determine beforehand whether the lesion is likely to respond to steroids, because pregnancy is itself a hypercoagulable state prone to deterioration by such treatment. On the other hand, proteinuria alone, in a non-eclamptic pregnant woman with well preserved renal function and without gross oedema and/or hypoalbuminaemia, suggests the need for close monitoring; biopsy can be deferred until the puerperium.

3. Presentation with active urinary sediment, proteinuria, and borderline renal function in a woman who has not been evaluated in the past. This is a controversial area and it could be argued that diagnosis of a collagen disorder such as scleroderma or periarteritis would be grounds for terminating the pregnancy, or that classifying the type of lesion in a woman with lupus would determine the type and intensity of therapy.

Differentiating between renal diseases, essential hypertension, and/or pre-eclampsia

There are diagnostic dilemmas for the clinician when a patient presents with hypertension and proteinuria in the third trimester (Lindheimer *et al.* 2001). In most cases it represents either a disease specific to pregnancy—pre-eclampsia—or essential hypertension, which may only become permanently manifest decades later. In other cases it is an exacerbation of an underlying renal disease, alone or with superimposed pre-eclampsia. Very rarely it is due to secondary causes such as acute glomerulonephritis, primary aldosteronism, phaeochromocytoma (the diagnosis of which relies on careful history-taking as well as a full medical and laboratory assessment), or renal artery stenosis (Heybourne *et al.* 1991). With the exception of these last examples, treatment is usually similar but knowledge of the exact cause is, nevertheless, useful, given the varying impact of different disease states on the outcome of future pregnancies as well as the remote renal and cardiovascular prognoses for the woman herself (Lindheimer *et al.* 1999b).

It must be remembered that dipstick testing for proteinuria can give false-positive results (see Chapter 15.1); nevertheless, any positive result (1+ or more) should be further evaluated in a midstream sample of urine. If urinary infection is excluded, then the amount of proteinuria should be measured—ideally over 24 h, but nowadays as a 'spot' protein/creatinine ratio. Obviously, the time course of concomitant hypertension and any escalation must also be considered.

If the cause is pre-eclampsia then there will usually be other features. At present there is controversy about whether significant proteinuria is preceded by a phase of microalbuminuria, undetected by the crude techniques of clinical screening, or not (see Chapter 15.4). Early involvement of the renal system does, however, lead to reduced uric acid clearance despite a normal GFR. Plasma uric acid will increase and hyperuricaemic hypertension in the second half of pregnancy is therefore more likely to be pre-eclamptic than not. As a rough guide, values greater than 0.30, 0.35, 0.40, and 0.45 mmol/l at 28, 32, 36, and 40 weeks' gestation, respectively, are likely to reflect abnormality, but occasionally the situation can be muddled by constitutional hyperuricaemia. As plasma uric acid increases, the plasma concentrations of creatinine and urea initially remain steady, tending to increase slowly after proteinuria has become established. The significance and usefulness of changes in serum Cystatin-C levels remain to be established. Overall therefore, pre-eclampsia is characteristically variable in its presentation, certainly more than is commonly recognized, and eclampsia has been documented without proteinuria, that is, neurological complications can be severe without apparent renal involvement.

An increased blood pressure in the first half of pregnancy tends to reflect a permanent state—chronic hypertension. In the second half, it identifies in addition those who have an acquired pregnancy-induced hypertension, including cases with pre-eclampsia. This group comprises women with essential hypertension, renal hypertension, and hypertension caused by the miscellaneous, but rare conditions previously mentioned. Women with essential hypertension tend to be older, parous, and heavier, with a family history of hypertension. A woman with chronic hypertension may appear normotensive when she starts antenatal care and then may show an increase in blood pressure in the third trimester of a degree resembling pre-eclampsia. This has led to considerable diagnostic confusion, but explains why third trimester hypertension segregates into two groups: non-recurrent, affecting primigravidae (with an increased perinatal mortality) and recurrent, affecting multiparae (with a good perinatal outcome).

The only sure way to detect chronic hypertension in pregnancy is to refer to readings taken before pregnancy, or if, as is usual, these are not available, to reassess the blood pressure at a remote time after delivery. If blood pressures are consistently at or greater than 140/90 mmHg in the first half of pregnancy, then chronic hypertension can be inferred.

However, it may not be possible to distinguish chronic hypertension from pre-eclampsia with absolute certainty and, furthermore, women with chronic hypertension and/or renal disease are three to seven times more likely to develop high blood pressure and proteinuria (superimposed pre-eclampsia) than normotensive women (Lindheimer *et al.* 1999b; Sibai 2002). Thus two conditions, which in their pure forms are easily separable, may commonly occur together. Further increases in the blood pressure, progressive hyperuricaemia, or abnormal activation of the clotting system are suggestive of superimposed pre-eclampsia with the appearance of proteinuria sooner or later.

In women with pre-existing hypertension, renal disease, or both, there may be genuine acute exacerbations of the hypertension and proteinuria in the second half of pregnancy. Sometimes these episodes are labelled superimposed pre-eclampsia and sometimes they are perceived only as an underlying medical problem coinciding with pregnancy. Often the disorders affect second and later pregnancies and, on this basis alone, a pre-eclamptic process is discounted. Without a specific diagnostic test for pre-eclampsia it is sometimes difficult or impossible to disentangle those elements of proteinuric hypertension caused by a chronic medical problem from those arising from superimposed pre-eclampsia. If a woman is permanently proteinuric, there are no accepted criteria for diagnosing proteinuric pre-eclampsia. For the present, if the episode is transient, confined to the second half of pregnancy, and associated with evidence of placental disease such as intrauterine growth retardation, it may be reasonably called pre-eclampsia superimposed on whatever chronic disorder has been identified.

Renal biopsy is never indicated to resolve the differential diagnosis of pre-eclampsia, although as mentioned earlier new arguments have emerged outside in research studies. It is rarely needed anyway in pregnancy and is usually reserved for those who continue to have significant proteinuria and renal impairment at a remote time after delivery. It has been claimed and denied that the glomerular lesions are pathognomic (see Lindheimer *et al.* 1999a,b; Stevens et al. 2003a,b; Lindheimer and Mahowald 2004). The glomerular pathology apparently correlates with the degree of hyperuricaemia. Normal renal histology has been found in some cases of eclampsia. Since it may not exclude the diagnosis, renal biopsy does not provide a completely specific or sensitive diagnosis for pre-eclampsia. Interestingly, where pre-eclampsia has been diagnosed on clinical grounds, such a diagnosis was incorrect in 25 per cent of primigravidae and in over 50 per cent of multiparae from the renal biopsy evidence, which revealed that a surprisingly large number had unsuspected renal disease (Fisher *et al.* 1981). In fact, it has been suggested that the majority of pregnant women classified as pre-eclamptic prior to the thirty-seventh gestational week must have glomerular disease (see Jungers and Chauveau 1997). The message behind all of this is simply that all women developing hypertension and proteinuria for the first time during pregnancy require close postpartum scrutiny. Some may eventually need evaluation for underlying renal disease, including a renal biopsy.

Specific renal diseases and pregnancy

Table 5 lists specific diseases associated with pregnancy, the information having been derived from publications over the past 10 years. To recap, the crucial balance between obstetric outcome and long-term renal prognosis depends on prepregnancy renal functional status, the absence or presence of hypertension (and its management) and the kidney pathology itself, as well as better fetal surveillance, more timely delivery and ever improving neonatal care.

Acute and chronic glomerulonephritis

Acute poststreptococcal glomerulonephritis is a very rare complication of pregnancy, and if it occurs late in pregnancy can be mistaken for pre-eclampsia. With chronic glomerulonephritis, one view warns of aggravation because of the hypercoagulable state accompanying pregnancy, with patients more prone to superimposed pre-eclampsia, or hypertensive crises earlier in pregnancy. The consensus, however, is that if renal function is stable and hypertension is absent, most pregnancies are successful.

Complications do develop more frequently in women who already have some dysfunction or hypertension in early pregnancy. In 25 per cent there is *de novo* hypertension or worsening of pre-existing hypertension usually reverting after delivery, suggesting superimposed pre-eclampsia, a diagnosis that is not easy to confirm in this group of patients. In 10 per cent, however, hypertension persists after delivery, especially in focal and segmental glomerulosclerosis, membranoproliferative glomerulonephritis, and IgA nephropathy. The increased rate of fetal loss observed in these gravidas can be accounted for by the greater prevalence of severe hypertension and renal insufficiency.

The recent literature endorses these messages. For example: (a) pregnancy is well tolerated without effect on the course of the disease, if blood pressure is normal and GFR is greater than 70 ml/min before conception and (b) with hypertension the rate of live births is lower if it exists before pregnancy, or if it is not well controlled during gestation (Abe 1996; Jungers and Chanveau 1997).

Hereditary nephritis (see Chapters 16.4.1 and 16.4.2), an uncommon disorder, may first become manifested or exacerbated during pregnancy, but most gestations succeed. Of interest is a variant of hereditary nephritis, involving disordered platelet morphology and function. In these cases, pregnancy has been successful but at times complicated by bleeding problems, especially at delivery.

Pyelonephritis (tubulointerstitial disease)

Acute pyelonephritis has been dealt with in Chapter 15.2. The chronic condition in pregnancy may be either infectious or non-infectious and the prognosis is similar to that for patients with glomerular disease, in that outcome is best in women with adequate renal function and normal blood pressure. Compared with non-pregnant women, pregnant women have a higher frequency of symptomatic infections, but these patients may have a more benign antenatal course than do women with glomerular disease. Of interest, is a report suggesting that women who develop frank pyelonephritis manifest greater degrees of pelvicalyceal dilatation in pregnancy, that may not regress after delivery, underscoring the need for postpartum investigation of this population (Twickler *et al.* 1994).

Reflux nephropathy

Reflux nephropathy is used to describe the renal structural and functional changes that relate to past (and usually present) vesicoureteric reflux, often complicated by recurrent infection. Opinions were once controversial, but with preserved renal function and no hypertension, both fetal and maternal outcomes appear to be excellent (Jungers *et al.* 1996). Vigilance is still necessary to detect and treat infection in these patients. Unfortunately, reflux nephropathy is often associated with hypertension and moderate or severe renal dysfunction by the time these patients reach childbearing age; as discussed earlier, such a scenerio adversely affects pregnancy outcome. Specific obstetric concerns in affected patients include severe fetal growth restriction and the risk of sudden rapid worsening of hypertension and renal function with accelerated progression to renal failure.

Urolithiasis

In pregnancy the prevalence of urolithiasis is 0.03–0.35 per cent (Butler et al. 2000). Renal and ureteric calculi are common causes of non-uterine abdominal pain severe enough to necessitate hospital admission during pregnancy. Most calculi are the more benign calcium types (oxalate and brushite), but occasionally the more malicious struvite stones (e.g. infected and staghorn) are seen. Uric acid and cystine are much more infrequent.

All stone patients should be evaluated frequently for asymptomatic urinary tract infections and rapidly treated when such complications are diagnosed. Management of stone symptoms should be conservative initially, with adequate hydration, appropriate antibiotic therapy, and pain relief with systemic analgesics (Evans and Wollin 2001). The use of continuous segmental (T11 to L2) epidural block has been advocated, as in non-pregnant patients with ureteric colic, and may even favourably influence spontaneous passage of the stones, especially as the ureter is dilated during gestation. With good pain relief, patients micturate without difficulty, move without assistance, and are less at risk from thromboembolic problems than if they are drowsy, nauseated, and bedridden with pain.

Pregnancy should not be a deterrent to intravenous urography (IVU), especially when there are complications that might require surgical intervention. The absence of ureteric jets may be significant if urolithiasis is suspected (Asrat et al. 1998). Specific clinical criteria suggested before a limited IVU is done are: microscopic haematuria, recurrent urinary tract symptoms, sterile urine culture when pyelonephritis is suspected and the presence of two of these criteria indicates a diagnosis of calculi in a substantial percentage of women (Bucholz et al. 1998). Ultrasonography may be useful, but it is less efficient in detecting very small calculi (<5 mm diameter) and/or in defining the degree or site of obstruction (Shokeir et al. 2000).

Obstruction of the ureters by calculi can be treated by the cystoscopic placement of an internal ureteral tube, or stent, between the bladder and kidney under local anesthesia, a procedure that has been successfully used in pregnant women for decades with little or no reports of excess morbidity. The stent retains its position because it has a pigtail or J-like curve at each end (double-J) and can be changed every 8 weeks to prevent encrustation (Delekas et al. 2000). Early empirical use for presumed stone obstruction in pregnant women with flank pain is recommended, by some (Butler et al. 2000) especially when hydration, analgesia, and antibiotics do not resolve pain or fever, and when the pregnancy is over, the usual X-ray evaluation is obtained and standard management is resumed.

Sonographically guided percutaneous nephrostomy is another effective method of treating gravidas with ureteric colic or symptomatic obstructive hydronephrosis (Van Sonnenberg et al. 1992). The procedure is rapid, requires minimal anaesthesia, and is perhaps a preferable alternative to retrograde stenting or more invasive surgery. Information on lithotripsy during pregnancy is limited and until more is known the procedure is best avoided.

As noted, the relatively benign history of stone disease relates to patients with uncomplicated calcium stones, while anecdotally those with struvite (infected) stones do worse, in part because of functional loss and severe infections. Unfortunately, the pregnancy literature on struvite stones is sparse, such women requiring close management with stone specialists. Finally, in patients with cystinuria, assiduous maintenance of high fluid intake is the mainstay of management. Although D-penicillamine appears relatively safe, it should be used only for severe cases, when urinary cystine excretion is known to be very high.

Autosomal dominant polycystic kidney disease (see Chapter 16.2.2)

Autosomal dominant polycystic kidney disease (ADPKD) is the most frequent genetic renal disorder, affecting one of 400–1000 persons, but may remain undetected during pregnancy (Gabow 1993). Careful questioning for a history of familial problems and the use of ultrasonography may lead to earlier detection. Patients do well when functional impairment is minimal and hypertension is absent, as is often the case in childbearing years (Morgan and Grunfeld 1998); they do, however, have an increased incidence of hypertension late in pregnancy and a higher perinatal mortality compared with that in pregnancies of sisters unaffected by this autosomal dominant disease (Chapman et al. 1994).

If one or the other prospective parent has evidence of polycystic renal disease, the couple may seek genetic counselling. There is a 50 per cent chance of transmitting the disease to the offspring. Deoxyribonucleic acid (DNA) probe techniques (Calvet and Grantham 2001) are now being developed, so that antenatal diagnosis is possible by chorionic villus biopsy (CVB) allowing women to consider selective termination of pregnancy.

Diabetic nephropathy (see also Chapter 4.1)

Many women have had diabetes since childhood, so probably already have microscopic changes in the kidneys (Hayslett and Reece 1994). During pregnancy, diabetic women have an increased prevalence of asymptomatic bacteriuria (and may be more susceptible to symptomatic urinary tract infection), peripheral oedema, and pre-eclampsia (Jungers and Chauveau 1997).

The consensus is that most women with diabetic nephropathy demonstrate normal GFR increments (and perhaps significant proteinuria), and pregnancy does not accelerate renal deterioration. There is, however, a report of diabetic women with moderate renal dysfunction [serum creatinine above 125 μmol/l ($\geq$1.4 mg/dl)] whose renal function permanently deteriorated in pregnancy in comparison to the changes before and afterward (Purdy et al. 1996). Such changes occurred despite good metabolic control and might have been related to hypertension, which often accelerates in the third trimester but one uncontrolled report suggested that the best predictor of renal and pregnancy outcome is proteinuria, less than 1 g/24 h having better outcomes (Gordon et al. 1996; Ekban et al. 2001).

Diet and insulin therapy

Based on the estimated excess 'caloric cost' of pregnancy, a diet (45 per cent carbohydrates, 15–20 per cent protein) is advised that provides 30–32 kcal/kg ideal body weight during the first trimester and 38 kcal/kg body weight thereafter. Calories are distributed between three evenly spaced meals and a bedtime snack, which is included to reduce the overnight fast to less than 12 h. With regard to insulin therapy the usual aim is fasting and premeal plasma glucose of 4–5 mmol/l and postprandial levels that are generally less than 8 mmol/l during the latter part of pregnancy. These glycaemic limits cannot be achieved in all women and are not relentlessly pursued at the expense of recurrent or severe hypoglycaemia. No single pattern of insulin administration can be advised for all diabetic patients: regimens range from twice-daily injections of intermediate and regular insulin to continuous subcutaneous infusions, depending on prepregnancy management.

Monitoring diabetic control

Self-measurement of capillary whole blood glucose using reagent-impregnated strips (self-glucose monitoring) is a standard approach to metabolic monitoring, which allows rapid assessment of glycaemia at any time, permits outpatient adjustment of insulin doses, and reduces the need for frequent hospital admission. Patient accuracy needs to be reviewed frequently, constant encouragement to be meticulous is essential, and premeal testing is probably best. Glycosylated haemoglobin measurements can be used to assess overall metabolic control, reflecting average glycaemia during the preceding 6–8 weeks. This may back up increased efforts at better control, but is not of any day-to-day utility.

Blood pressure control

Aggressive treatment of high blood pressure is extremely important in diabetic care and pregnancy is no exception where even mild hypertension should be treated (Leguizaman and Reece 2000). Diabetic women prepregnancy will frequently have been prescribed angiotensin-converting enzyme (ACE) inhibitors or angiotensin receptor blockers, which should be discontinued prior to conception and at the latest in early pregnancy (Hod *et al.* 1995). They cause fetopathies and neonatal anuria with renal failure, but their association with malformations is less certain.

Systemic lupus erythematosus

This has a predilection for women of childbearing age. Its coincidence with pregnancy poses complex clinical problems because of the profound disturbance of the immunological system, multiple-organ involvement, and complicated immunology of pregnancy itself (Nicklin 1991; Jungers and Chauveau 1997). Transient improvements, no change, and a tendency to relapse have all been reported (see Chapter 4.7.2).

Decisions regarding the importance of having a baby to the patient and her partner and the status of the disease should be made on an individual basis. Most pregnancies succeed, especially when the maternal disease has been in complete clinical remission for 6 months prior to conception, even if there were marked pathological changes in the original renal biopsy and heavy proteinuria in the early stages of the disease (Hayslett 1992). Continued signs of disease activity or increasing renal dysfunction reduces the likelihood of an uncomplicated pregnancy and the clinical course thereafter. Obviously, prepregnancy counselling must take account of the actual form of lupus nephritis (mild versus aggressive) as well as the medications being used, either separately or in combination, for example, glucocorticoids, cyclophosphamide, azathioprine, and nowadays, mycophenolate mofetil (MMF; CellCept) (Falk 2000; Armenti *et al.* 2002).

The effects of gestation on systemic lupus erythematosus (SLE) activity and on the course of lupus nephritis have long been debated. Taking into account both extrarenal manifestations and renal changes,

at least 50 per cent of women show some change in clinical status, often called 'lupus flare' (Petri 1994). Admittedly, increments in proteinuria or blood pressure could be due to pre-eclampsia. From recent reviews, however (Lockshin and Sammaritane 2000; Thi Huong *et al.* 2001), it appears that as many as 20 per cent (progressive in 8 per cent) and 40 per cent experience decrements in GFR and hypertension, respectively. The figures become worse if renal insufficiency [serum creatinine >125 μmol/l (>1.4 mg/dl)] antedates the pregnancy.

Lupus nephropathy may sometimes become manifest during pregnancy and, when accompanied by hypertension and renal dysfunction, may be mistaken for pre-eclampsia. Some patients tend to experience relapse, occasionally severely in the puerperium; therefore, some clinicians prescribe or increase steroids at this time (Le Thi Huong *et al.* 2001). Rarely, a particularly severe postpartum syndrome may develop, consisting of pleural effusion, pulmonary infiltration, fever, electrocardiogram (ECG) abnormalities, and even cardiomyopathy, with extensive IgG, IgM, IgA, and C3 deposition in the myocardium. Of note, the disturbing complications above, especially that of a 'stormy puerperium', are disputed. In fact, many now observe postpartum patients and do not institute or increase steroid therapy unless signs of increased disease activity are noted.

SLE sera may contain a bewildering array of autoantibodies (lupus serum factor) against nucleic acids, nucleoproteins, cell-surface antigens, and phospholipids. Antiphospholipid antibodies (APLA) exert a complicated effect on the coagulation system (Cowchock *et al.* 1992). This led to the rather enigmatic definition of a lupus anticoagulant, found in 5–10 per cent of patients with SLE (see Chapters 4.7.1 and 4.7.2). Because treatment with low molecular weight heparin and aspirin may lead to successful pregnancies, it is important to screen for lupus anticoagulant in women with SLE and perhaps in those with a history of recurrent intrauterine death or thrombotic episodes in order to identify this particular cohort. A decision to use prophylactic aspirin, however, must be weighed against the knowledge that this drug may cause decreases in GFR in lupus patients.

An increased incidence of congenital cardiac anomalies occurring in the offspring of women with SLE, and particularly in patients with antiRo (SS-A) antibodies, is discussed in Chapter 4.7.2.

The course of pregnancy in women with renal involvement due to periarteritis nodosa is very guarded, largely because of the associated hypertension, frequently malignant. The literature, however, is anecdotal comprising selective case reports, but many of them involved maternal demise. Nevertheless, a few successful pregnancies have been reported. Still, in the absence of new data early therapeutic termination may be a strong recommendation because of maternal risk.

Systemic sclerosis

Scleroderma is a term that includes a heterogeneous group of limited and systemic conditions causing hardening of the skin. Systemic sclerosis implies involvement of both skin and other sites, particularly certain internal organs. Renal involvement is thought to occur in about 60 per cent of these patients, usually within 3–4 years of diagnosis. The presentation may take one of three forms: sudden onset of malignant hypertension, rapidly progressive renal failure, or slowly increasing azotaemia (Steen 1999).

The combination of systemic sclerosis and pregnancy is infrequent because the disease occurs most often in the fourth and fifth decades and affected patients are usually infertile. When disease onset is during pregnancy, there appears to be a greater tendency for deterioration. Here, too, data are from selective case reports, some where patients with scleroderma and no evidence of renal involvement prior to conception have developed severe kidney disease in gestation. There are also instances in which pregnancy has been uneventful and successful, but marked reactivation occurred unexpectedly in the puerperium. Most maternal deaths involve rapidly progressive scleroderma with severe pulmonary complications, infections, hypertension, and renal failure (Steen 1999).

The extent of systemic involvement is probably more important than the duration of the disease, and limited mild disease carries a better prognosis. Sclerosis usually spares the abdominal wall skin, but theoretically thickened skin and decreased abdominal wall compliance could be troublesome.

Wegener's granulomatosis

Information on the outcome of pregnancy in women with granulomatosis is scarce. Proteinuria (with or without hypertension) is common from early in pregnancy (Auzary *et al.* 2000), and reports to date have described both complicated and uneventful pregnancies. Experience with cyclophosphamide (cytoxan) in pregnancy is limited, and the risks to the embryo and fetus must be weighed in relation to the course of the disease if such therapy were to be withheld from the mother (Harber *et al.* 1999).

Previous urinary tract surgery

Permanent urinary diversion is still used in the management of patients with congenital lower urinary tract defects, but its use for neurogenic bladder has declined since the introduction of self-catheterization. The most common complication of pregnancy is urinary infection. Premature labour occurs in 20 per cent; the use of prophylactic antibiotics throughout pregnancy may reduce its incidence. Decline in renal function may occur, invariably related to infection or intermittent obstruction or both. With an ileal conduit or augmentation cystoplasty, elevation and compression by the expanding uterus can cause outflow obstruction, whereas with a ureterosigmoid anastomosis, actual ureteral obstruction may occur (Hill *et al.* 1990). The changes usually reverse after delivery.

The mode of delivery is dictated by obstetric factors. Abnormal presentation accounts for a cesarean section rate of 25 per cent. Vaginal delivery is safe, but because the continence of a ureterosigmoid anastomosis depends on an intact anal sphincter, this area must be protected with a mediolateral episiotomy.

During the past decade, urinary tract reconstruction by means of augmentation cystoplasty, with or without artificial genitourinary sphincter, has become more commonplace. Deterioration of renal function as well as urinary tract obstruction or infection can occur at any time in pregnancy. Delivery by cesarean section is recommended for these gravidas because of the potential for disruption of the continence mechanism.

Solitary kidney

Some patients have either a congenital absence of one kidney or marked unilateral renal hypoplasia. Most, however, have had a previous nephrectomy because of pyelonephritis (with abscess or hydronephrosis), unilateral tuberculosis, congenital abnormalities, a tumour or nowadays,

kidney donation (Wrenshall *et al.* 1996). It is important to know the indication for and the time elapsed since nephrectomy. In patients with an infectious or a structural renal problem, sequential prepregnancy investigation is needed to detect any persistent infection.

It makes no difference whether the right or left kidney remains, as long as it is located in the normal anatomic position. If function is normal and stable, women with this problem seem to tolerate pregnancy well despite the superimposition of GFR increments on already hyperfiltering nephrons. The rare occurrence of acute renal failure in pregnancy due to obstruction is most often associated with the presence of a single kidney.

Ectopic kidneys (usually pelvic) are more vulnerable to infection and are associated with decreased fetal salvage, probably because of associated malformations of the urogenital tract. If infection occurs in a solitary kidney during pregnancy and does not quickly respond to antibiotics, termination may have to be considered for preservation of renal function.

Human immunodeficiency virus-associated nephropathy (see also Chapter 3.12)

The worldwide pandemic of human immunodeficiency disease appears to be involving greater numbers of pregnant women. This disease has a renal component including nephrotic syndrome and severe renal impairment (Rao 2001). Human immunodeficiency virus-associated nephropathy (HIVAN) may be seen in patients who are HIV-seropositive patients, patients with acquired immunodeficiency syndrome (AIDS), or patients with AIDS-related complex. HIVAN is characterized by severe proteinuria and rapid progression to endstage renal disease, possibly slowed down by the use of an ACE inhibitor (a drug that cannot be used in pregnancy) and steroids (Szczech *et al.* 2002). The distinctive features seen on histological evaluation of renal biopsy are glomerulosclerosis, visceral epithelial cell hypertrophy, and variable tubulointerstitial nephritis. Currently there appears to be no HIVAN literature in pregnancy, but given the ravages of this epidemic note that the disease should be considered when nephritic proteinuria appears suddenly, especially in patients who have not been screened for the virus.

Nephrotic syndrome in pregnancy (see Chapter 3.5)

Pre-eclampsia is the most common cause of nephrotic syndrome in late pregnancy, and fetal prognosis declines with increasing proteinuria. Other causes of nephrotic syndrome include proliferative or mesangiocapillary glomerulonephritis, minimal-change nephrosis, lupus nephropathy, hereditary nephritis, diabetic nephropathy, renal vein thrombosis, and amyloidosis. Some of these do not respond to steroid therapy and may even be seriously aggravated by their use, emphasizing the importance of making a diagnosis on the basis of histology before initiating steroid therapy.

If renal function is adequate and hypertension is absent, there should be few complications during pregnancy. Several of the physiological changes occurring during pregnancy may, however, simulate aggravation or exacerbation of the disease. For example, increments in renal haemodynamics and increases in renal vein pressure may enhance protein excretion. Serum albumin usually decreases by 5–10 g/l during normal pregnancy, and further reductions due to nephrotic syndrome may enhance the tendency toward fluid retention. Because of decreased intravascular volume, diuretic therapy could compromise uteroplacental perfusion or aggravate the increased tendency to thrombotic episodes. Low birth weight correlates with decrements in maternal serum albumin.

Long-term effects of pregnancy in women with renal disease

Pregnancy does not cause any deterioration or otherwise affect the rate of progression of the disease beyond what might be expected in the non-pregnant state, provided that kidney dysfunction was minimal and/or very well-controlled before pregnancy and hypertension is absent during pregnancy (Jungers and Chauveau 1997). An important factor in long-term prognosis could be the sclerotic effect that prolonged renal vasodilation might have in the residual (intact) glomeruli of the kidneys of these women (Baylis 1994). The situation may be worse in a single diseased kidney, where more sclerosis has usually occurred within the fewer (intact) glomeruli. Although the evidence in healthy women and those with mild renal disease argues against hyperfiltration-induced damage in pregnancy, there is little doubt that in some women with moderate dysfunction there can be unpredicted, accelerated, and irreversible renal decline in pregnancy or immediately afterwards.

Dialysis patients

Clinical implications of haemodialysis in pregnancy

Despite reduced libido and relative infertility, women receiving haemodialysis can conceive and must therefore use contraception if they wish to avoid pregnancy (Schmidt and Holley 1998). Although conception is not common (an incidence of one in 200 patients has been quoted), its true frequency is unknown because most pregnancies in dialysis patients probably end in early spontaneous abortion. The high therapeutic abortion rate in this group of patients, although decreased from 40 per cent in 1989 to under 20 per cent today, still suggests that those who become pregnant do so inadvertently, probably because they are unaware that pregnancy is possible.

Many authorities do not advise conception or continuation of pregnancy, if present, when the women has severe renal insufficiency. Clinicians are reluctant to publish unsuccessful cases as well as those that end in disaster, but the literature has expanded in recent years (Okundaye et al. 1998; Ramão et al. 1998; Hou 1999). Pregnancy poses big risks for the mother who is prone to volume overload and severe exacerbation of her hypertension and/or superimposed pre-eclampsia, with only a 40–50 per cent chance of producing a healthy infant.

Antenatal strategy and decision-making

Women on dialysis, if they become pregnant, may present for care in advanced pregnancy because it was not suspected by either the patient or her doctors. Irregular menstruation is common in dialysis patients and missed periods are usually ignored. Urine pregnancy tests are unreliable (even if there is any urine available). Ultrasonic evaluation is needed to confirm and to date the pregnancy. For a successful

outcome, scrupulous attention must be paid to increased dialysis, fluid balance, blood pressure control, and provision of good nutrition (Hou and Firanek 1998; Hussey and Pombar 1998).

Dialysis policy

Some patients show increments in GFR despite the fact that the actual degree of renal function is insufficient to sustain life without haemodialysis. The planning of dialysis strategy has several aims:

1. Maintain plasma urea less than 20 mmol/l (60 mg/dl). Some would argue less than 15 mmol/l (45 mg/dl), as intrauterine death is more likely if values are much in excess of 20 mmol/l. [Success has occasionally been achieved despite levels of 28 mmol/l (84 mg/dl) for many weeks.]

2. Avoid hypotension during dialysis, which could be damaging to the fetus. In late pregnancy, the gravid uterus and the supine posture may aggravate this by decreasing venous return.

3. Ensure rigid control of blood pressure.

4. Avoid rapid fluctuations in intravascular volume, by limiting interdialysis weight gain to about 1 kg until late pregnancy.

5. Scrutinize carefully for preterm labour, as dialysis and uterine contractions are associated.

6. Watch plasma calcium closely to avoid hypercalcaemia. Pregnant women with endstage renal disease usually require a 50 per cent increase in hours and frequency of dialysis, a policy which renders dietary management and control of weight gain much easier.

Anaemia

Dialysis patients are usually anaemic; this is invariably aggravated further in pregnancy. Blood transfusion may be needed, especially before delivery. Caution is necessary because transfusion may exacerbate hypertension and impair the ability to control circulatory overload, even with extra dialysis. Fluctuations in blood volume can be minimized if packed red cells are transfused during dialysis.

Treatment of anaemia with low-dose rHuEpo has been used in pregnancy without ill-effect (Braga et al. 1996). The theoretical risks of hypertension and thrombotic complications have so far not been encountered and no adverse neonatal effects have been reported (Vora and Grushin 1998). Unnecessary blood sampling should be avoided in the face of anaemia and lack of venepuncture sites. The protocol for tests usually performed in one's own unit should be followed strictly, with no more blood removed per venepuncture than is absolutely necessary.

Hypertension

A normotensive prepregnancy state is reassuring. Some patients have abnormal lipid profiles and possibly accelerated atherogenesis, so it is difficult to predict whether the patient possesses the cardiovascular capacity required to tolerate pregnancy. Patients with diabetic nephropathy who become pregnant are those in whom cardiovascular problems are most evident. As a generalization, blood pressure tends to be labile and hypertension is common, although control may be possible by careful dialysis.

Nutrition

Despite more frequent dialysis, an uncontrolled dietary intake should be discouraged. A daily oral intake of 70 g protein, 1500 mg calcium,

50 mmol potassium, and 80 mmol sodium is advised, with supplements of dialysable vitamins. Vitamin D supplements can be difficult to judge in patients who have had parathyroidectomy (Brookhyser and Wiggins 1998). All this poses risks for fetal nutrition: in addition, the exact impact of the uraemic environment is difficult to assess.

Fetal surveillance and timing of delivery

What has been said regarding chronic renal disease applies here. Preterm labour is generally the rule and this may commence during haemodialysis. Caesarean section should be necessary only for purely obstetric reasons. It could be argued, however, that elective caesarean section in all cases would minimize potential problems during labour.

Continuous ambulatory peritoneal dialysis

Young women can be managed with this approach and a few successful pregnancies have now been reported (Okundaye *et al.* 1998; Castillo *et al.* 1999). Although anticoagulation and some of the fluid balance and volume problems of haemodialysis are avoided in these gravidas, they nevertheless face the same problems of hypertension, anaemia, placental abruption, premature labour, and sudden intrauterine death. There are no differences in outcome dependent on mode of dialysis (haemodialysis versus peritoneal dialysis) but there may be greater infertility in women receiving continuous ambulatory peritoneal dialysis (CAPD) (Okundaye *et al.* 1998).

It should be remembered that peritonitis can be a severe complication of chronic ambulatory peritoneal dialysis, accounting for the majority of therapy failures. This superimposed on a pregnancy can present a confusing diagnostic picture as well as a whole series of management dilemmas.

Renal transplantation

Clinical implications of renal transplantation and pregnancy

Renal, endocrine, and sexual functions return rapidly after transplantation and assisted conception techniques are also available (Lockwood *et al.* 1995). About one in 50 women of childbearing age with a functioning transplant become pregnant during their remaining childbearing era. Of the conceptions, about 35 per cent do not go beyond the initial trimester because of spontaneous or therapeutic abortion; however, 95 per cent of pregnancies that do continue past early pregnancy end successfully (Table 6).

Transplants have even been performed with the surgeons unaware that the recipient was in early pregnancy (Pergola *et al.* 2001). Obstetric success in such cases does not negate the importance of contraception counselling for all renal failure patients and the exclusion of pregnancy prior to transplantation.

Preconception counselling

A woman should be counselled from the time the various treatments for renal failure and the potential for optimal rehabilitation are discussed (Armenti *et al.* 1998; Kimmel and Patel 2003). Couples who want a child should be encouraged to discuss all of the implications, including the harsh realities of maternal survival prospects (Table 7). Individual centres have their own guidelines. In most, a wait of 18 months to 2 years post-transplant is advised. By then, the patient will have recovered from the surgery and any sequelae, graft function will have stabilized, and immunosuppression will be at maintenance levels (Jungers and Chauveau 1997; Hou 2003). Also, if function is well maintained at 2 years, there is a high probability of allograft survival at 5 years.

A suitable set of guidelines is given here, but the criteria are only relative: (a) good general health for about 2 years post-transplant; (b) stature compatible with good obstetric outcome; (c) no, or minimal, proteinuria; (d) no or minimal (well controlled) hypertension; (e) no evidence of graft rejection; (f) no pelvicalyceal distension on a recent intravenous urogram; (g) stable renal function with plasma creatinine of 180 µmol/l (2 mg/dl) or less, preferably less than 125 µmol/l (1.4 mg/dl); and (h) immunosuppressive drug therapy reduced to maintenance levels: prednisone, 15 mg/day or less, azathioprine 2 mg/kg/day or less and cyclosporin A 2–4 mg/kg/day. Experience is limited for the more recently introduced immunosuppressants.

Ectopic pregnancy

This occurs in about 0.3 per cent of all conceptions. The diagnosis can be difficult because of irregular bleeding and amenorrhoea accompanying deteriorating renal function or even an intrauterine pregnancy. These patients may be at greater risk of ectopic pregnancy because of pelvic adhesions due to previous urological surgery, peritoneal dialysis, pelvic inflammatory disease, or the overzealous use of intrauterine contraceptive devices. The main clinical problem is that symptoms secondary to genuine pelvic pathology are erroneously attributed to the transplant.

Antenatal strategy and decision-making

Management requires serial assessment of renal function, early diagnosis and treatment of rejection, blood pressure control, early diagnosis

Table 6 Pregnancy prospects for renal allograft recipients[a]

Problems in pregnancy	Successful obstetric outcome	Problems in the long-term
49%	95% (75%)[b]	12% (25%)

[a] Estimates are based on data from 5670 women in 7510 pregnancies that attained at least 28 weeks' gestation (1961–2001).

[b] Numbers in parentheses refer to implications when complications developed prior to 28 weeks' gestation.

Table 7 Antenatal guidelines in pregnant renal transplant patients

Serial surveillance of renal function

Hypertension/pre-eclampsia

Graft rejection

Maternal infection

Fetal surveillance/intrauterine growth retardation

Premature rupture of membranes

Preterm labour

Decisions on timing and method of delivery

Effects of drugs on fetus and neonate

or prevention of anaemia, treatment of any infection, and meticulous assessment of fetal well being (Table 8). As well as regular renal assessments, liver function tests, plasma protein, and calcium and phosphate should be checked at 6-weekly intervals. Cytomegalovirus and herpes hominis virus status should be checked during each trimester and HIV should be determined at the first attendance. Haematinics are needed if the various haematological indices show deficiency.

Transplant function

Serial renal function data are needed to supplement routine antenatal assessments, and several points should be borne in mind (Davison 1994):

1. The sustained increase in GFR characteristic of early pregnancy in normal women is evident in renal transplant recipients, even though the transplant is ectopic, denervated, often derived from a male donor, potentially damaged by previous ischaemia, and immunologically different from both the recipient and her fetus.

2. Immediate graft function after transplantation and the better the prepregnancy GFR, the greater the increment in pregnancy. In one series, the stable problem-free group had a mean prepregnancy serum creatinine of 80 μmol/l (0.9 mg/dl) in contrast to 212 μmol/l (2.4 mg/dl) in the group with gestational problems (Nojima et al. 1996). Furthermore, in two single-centre analysis of 33 and 48 pregnancies in 29 and 24 women, respectively, those with serum greater than 200 μmol/l (>2.25 mg/dl) had progression of renal impairment and required dialysis within 2–3 years of delivery (Crowe et al. 1999; Thompson et al. 2003).

3. Transient reductions in GFR can occur during the third trimester and do not usually represent a deteriorating situation with permanent impairment.

4. Significant renal functional impairment develops in 15 per cent of patients during pregnancy, and this may persist following delivery. However, as a gradual decline in function is common in non-pregnant patients it is difficult to delineate the specific role of pregnancy. Subclinical chronic rejection with declining renal function may occur as a late result of acute rejection or when immunosuppression has not been adequate.

Table 8 Neonatal problems in offspring or renal transplant patients

Preterm delivery/small for gestational age

Respiratory distress syndrome

Depressed haematopoiesis

Lymphoid/thymic hypoplasia

Adrenocortical insufficiency

Septicaemia

CMV infection

Hepatitis B surface antigen carrier state

Congenital abnormalities

Immunological problems
 Reduced lymphocyte—PHA reactivity
 Reduced T lymphocytes
 Reduced immunoglobulin levels
 Chromosome aberrations in leucocytes

PHA, phytohaemogglutinin.

5. Proteinuria occurs near term in 40 per cent of patients but disappears postpartum and, in the absence of hypertension, is not significant.

6. Whether or not cyclosporin is more nephrotoxic in the pregnant compared to the non-pregnant patient is not known. Advice to switch to standard immunosupressive regimens in gravidas is based purely on clinical anecdote, and evaluations are urgently needed in pregnancy.

Transplant rejection

Serious rejection episodes occur in 9 per cent of pregnant women. While this incidence is no greater than that seen in non-pregnant individuals during a similar period, it is unexpected because it has been assumed that the privileged immunological status of pregnancy might benefit the allograft. Rejection often occurs in the puerperium and may be due to a return to a normal immune state (despite immunosuppression) or possibly a rebound effect from the altered gestational immunoresponsiveness.

Chronic rejection with a progressive subclinical course may be a problem in all recipients. Whether pregnancy influences the course of subclinical rejection is unknown: no factors consistently predict which patients will develop rejection during pregnancy. There may also be a non-immune contribution to chronic graft failure due to the damaging effect of hyperfiltration through remnant nephrons, perhaps even exacerbated during pregnancy. From the clinical viewpoint the following points are important:

(1) rejection is difficult to diagnose;

(2) if any of the clinical hallmarks are present—fever, oliguria, deteriorating renal function, renal enlargement, and tenderness—then the diagnosis should be considered;

(3) although ultrasound may be helpful, without renal biopsy rejection cannot be distinguished from acute pyelonephritis, recurrent glomerulopathy, possibly severe pre-eclampsia, and even cyclosporin nephrotoxicity;

(4) renal biopsy is indicated before embarking upon antirejection therapy.

Immunosuppressive therapy

Immunosuppressive therapy is usually maintained at pre-pregnancy levels, but adjustments may be needed if the maternal leucocyte or platelet count decreases. When white blood cell counts are maintained within physiological limits for pregnancy, the neonate usually is born with a normal blood count (Davison 1994). Azathioprine liver toxicity has been noted occasionally during pregnancy and responds to dose reduction.

There are many encouraging reports of (non-complicated) pregnancies in patients taking cyclosporin (Armenti et al. 2000; Lessan-Pezeshki 2002). Currently, the National Transplantation Pregnancy Registry (NTPR), maintained by Vincent T. Armenti, MD at Thomas Jefferson University, Philadelphia, is accruing data (Gaughan et al. 1996; Armenti et al. 1998, 2000, 2002). A United Kingdom Registry has also been established as part of an international effort to coordinate data collection (Davison and Redman 1997) and efforts are under way in Japan to audit pregnancies (Toma et al. 1998).

Numerous adverse effects are attributed to cyclosporin in non-pregnant transplant recipients, including renal toxicity, hepatic dysfunction, chronic hypertension, tremor, convulsions, diabetogenic effects, haemolytic–uraemic syndrome, and neoplasia (Gaughan *et al.* 1996). In pregnancy, some of the maternal adaptations that normally occur may theoretically be blunted or abolished by cyclosporin, especially plasma volume expansion and renal haemodynamic augmentation. It will be interesting to monitor the impact of the new cyclosporin preparation Neoral, which is claimed to improve drug bioavailability and have more stable pharmacokinetics. Its use in nonpregnant renal transplant patients appears to permit easier maintenance of trough blood drug concentrations in the therapeutic range. Data from the US National Transplantation Pregnancy Registry suggest that patients treated with cyclosporin may have more hypertension and smaller babies, but it is still too premature for definitive conclusions (Armenti *et al.* 2002).

Finally, newer agents such as tacrolimus (FK506 or Prograf), mycophenolate (MMF/CellCept), antithymocytic globulin, ATG (Atgam), and orthodione, OKTS are being prescribed more frequently for transplant recipients (Newstead 1997; Kainz *et al.* 2000), but there is minimal information about these agents in pregnancy (Ghandour *et al.* 1998). Some of these newer agents were originally considered to have a 'rescue role' only in kidney and kidney–pancreas transplants but nowadays they can be used as primary immunosuppressive agents (Shapiro 2000).

Hypertension and pre-eclampsia

Hypertension, particularly before 28 weeks' gestation, is associated with adverse perinatal outcome (Sturgiss and Davison 1991). This may be due to covert cardiovascular changes that accompany and/or are aggravated by chronic hypertension. The appearance of hypertension in the third trimester, its relationship to deteriorating renal function, and the possibility of chronic underlying pathology and pre-eclampsia is a diagnostic problem (Hou 2003). Pre-eclampsia is actually diagnosed clinically in about 30 per cent of pregnancies.

Infections

Throughout pregnancy patients should be monitored carefully for bacterial and viral infection. Prophylactic antibiotics must be given before any surgical procedure, however trivial.

Diabetes mellitus

As the results of renal transplantation have improved in those women whose renal failure was caused by juvenile onset diabetes mellitus, pregnancies are now being reported in these women. Pregnancy complications occur with at least twice the frequency seen in the non-diabetic patient, and this may be due to the presence of generalized cardiovascular pathology, which is part of the 'metabolic risk factor syndrome' (Dimeny and Fellström 1997). Successful pregnancies have been reported after confirmed pancreas–kidney allograft (Wilson *et al.* 2001).

Fetal surveillance and timing of delivery

The points discussed under chronic renal disease are equally applicable to renal transplant recipients. Preterm delivery is common (45–60 per cent) because of intervention for obstetric reasons and the common occurrence of premature labour or premature rupture of membranes. Premature labour is commonly associated with poor renal function, but in some it has been postulated that long-term steroid therapy may weaken connective tissues and contribute to the increased incidence of premature rupture of the membranes.

Delivery

Vaginal delivery should be the aim; usually there are no obstructive problems and/or mechanical injury to the transplant. Unless there are specific obstetric problems then spontaneous onset of labour can be awaited.

Management during labour

Careful monitoring of fluid balance, cardiovascular status, and temperature is mandatory. Aseptic technique is essential for every procedure. Surgical induction of labour (by amniotomy) and episiotomy warrant antibiotic cover. Pain relief can be conducted as for healthy women. Augmentation of steroids should not be overlooked.

Role of caesarean section

This is necessary for obstetric reasons only. The following points may be important in connection with this delivery route.

1. Transplant patients may have pelvic osteodystrophy related to their previous renal failure (and dialysis) or prolonged steroid therapy, particularly before puberty. Patients with pelvic problems must be recognized antenatally and delivered by caesarean section.

2. If there is a question of kidney disproportion or compression, then simultaneous intravenous urogram and radiographic pelvimetry may be performed at 36 weeks' gestation (Fig. 3).

3. When a caesarean section is performed, a lower segment approach is usually feasible but previous urological surgery may make this difficult. The high section rate (25–35 per cent) in most series probably represents iatrogenous worries more than obstetric necessity.

Paediatric management

Over 50 per cent of live borns have no neonatal problems. Preterm delivery is common (45–60 per cent), small for gestational age infants are delivered in at least 20–30 per cent of pregnancies, and occasionally the two problems coexist (Little *et al.* 2000) (Table 8). Lower birth

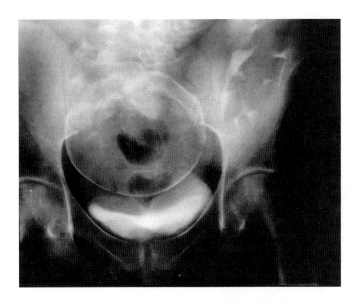

Fig. 3 Single injection intravenous excretory urogram at thirty-seventh week of pregnancy in a renal transplant recipient. The left-sided transplant, in the false pelvis, neither interfered with, nor was damaged by vaginal delivery.

weights are seen in infants born to recipients of less than 2 years post-transplant (Cunningham *et al.* 1983) and the use of cyclosporin in some series is associated with birth weight depression (Armenti *et al.* 2000). Management of the offspring is the same as in neonates of other mothers but there are additional specific worries.

Breast feeding

There are substantial benefits to breast feeding. It could be argued that because the baby has been exposed to azathioprine and its metabolites in pregnancy, breast feeding should not be allowed, however, little is known about the quantities of azathioprine and its metabolites in breast milk and whether the levels are biologically trivial or substantial. Even less is known about cyclosporin in breast milk except that levels are usually greater than those in a simultaneously taken blood sample. Until the many uncertainties are resolved, breast feeding should not be encouraged (Nyberg *et al.* 1998).

Long-term assessment

Azathioprine can cause abnormalities in the chromosomes of leucocytes, which may take almost 2 years to disappear spontaneously. In tissues not yet studied, however, these anomalies may not be as temporary. The sequelae could be eventual development of malignant tumours in affected offspring, autoimmune complications, and/or abnormalities in the reproductive performance in the next generation (Scott *et al.* 2002). This latter effect must be initiated in the offspring when *in utero*. It is unlikely that such damage would be eliminated or repaired, as seems to happen in somatic cells, because synthesis of DNA stops when the germ cells are arrested in the prophase of the first meiotic division *in utero* and no new DNA is synthesized until after fertilization.

Any child exposed to immunosuppressants *in utero* must have evaluation of the immune system and paediatric follow-up. To date, information about general progress in early childhood has been good (Willis *et al.* 2000). A recent study has evaluated 175 children from 133 gravidas on cyclosporin at 4 months–12 years (mean 4.4 years) (Stanley *et al.* 1999), who at birth had a mean gestational age of 36 weeks and mean birth weight of 2.49 Kg. Twenty-nine children (16 per cent) had 'delays' or needed educational support, with a much higher incidence of preterm delivery in this group too. Amongst US children, 11 per cent in state schools had special educational needs.

Maternal follow-up after pregnancy

The ultimate measure of transplant success is the long-term survival of the patient and the graft. As it is only 30 years since this procedure became widely employed in the management of endstage renal failure, few long-term data from sufficiently large series exist from which to draw conclusions. Furthermore, the long-term results for renal transplants relate to a period when many aspects of management would be unacceptable by present-day standards. Average survival figures of large numbers of patients worldwide indicate that about 87 per cent of recipients of kidneys from related living donors are alive 5 years after transplantation (Andrews 2002). With cadaver kidneys, the figure is approximately 50 per cent. If renal function was normal 2 years after transplant, survival increased to about 80 per cent. This is why women are counseled to wait about 2 years before considering a pregnancy.

A major concern is that the mother may not survive or remain well enough to rear the child she bears. Pregnancy occasionally and sometimes unpredictably causes irreversible declines in renal function.

However, the consensus is that pregnancy has no effect on graft function or survival (First *et al.* 1995; Sturgiss and Davison 1995; Nojima *et al.* 1996). Also, repeated pregnancies do not adversely affect graft function or fetal development, provided that renal function is well preserved at the time of conception (Ehrich *et al.* 1996; Owda *et al.* 1998).

Despite continuing improvement there is still substantial early mortality as well as debilitating morbidity in transplant populations (Kok *et al.* 2002). Nevertheless, many women will choose parenthood in an effort to re-establish a normal life and possibly in defiance of the sometimes negative attitudes of the medical establishment. Psychiatrists are now asking the questions why women in such circumstances get pregnant and why there is such overwhelming maternalism? As mentioned in relation to chronic renal disease, the so-called 'burning building syndrome' defines this maternal obsession and tries to differentiate between healthy and pathological levels of assumed risk (Stotland and Stotland 1997; Kimmel and Patel 2003).

Contraception

It is unwise to offer the option of sterilization at the time of transplantation. Oral contraception can cause or aggravate hypertension or thromboembolism and can also produce subtle dangers to the immune system, but this does not necessarily contraindicate its use. Careful surveillance is essential.

An intrauterine contraceptive device may aggravate menstrual problems, which in turn may obscure symptoms and signs of early pregnancy abnormalities, such as threatened miscarriage or ectopic pregnancy. The increased risk of chronic pelvic infection in an immunosuppressed patient with an intrauterine device is a substantial problem. Indeed, as the insertion or replacement of a coil is associated with bacteraemia of vaginal origin in at least 13 per cent of cases, antibiotic cover is essential at this time (Murray *et al.* 1987). Lastly, the efficacy of the intrauterine device is reduced in women taking immunosuppressive and anti-inflammatory agents. Nevertheless, many request this method.

Gynaecological problems

There is a danger that symptoms secondary to genuine pelvic pathology may be erroneously attributed to the transplant, due to its location near the pelvis. Transplant recipients receiving immunosuppressive therapy have a malignancy rate estimated to be 100 times greater than normal and the female genital tract is not an exceptional site (Newstead 1998). This association is probably related to factors such as loss of immune surveillance, chronic immunosuppression allowing tumour proliferation, and/or prolonged antigenic stimulation of the reticuloendothelial system. Regular gynaecological assessment is therefore essential. Management should be on conventional lines, with the outcome unlikely to be influenced by stopping or reducing immunosuppression.

Concluding remarks

At the beginning of the Chapter the questions usually asked by women with underlying problems contemplating pregnancy or those already pregnant were listed:

1.   Is pregnancy advisable?

2.   Will the pregnancy be complicated?

3. Will I have a live healthy baby?

4. Will I come to any harm in the long term?

The answers to those questions, provided during the course of the chapter, can be summarized as follows.

Chronic renal disease

Provided kidney dysfunction is minimal and hypertension is absent prepregnancy, then pregnancy is not contraindicated and a successful and healthy obstetric outcome is usually the rule. Pregnancy does not adversely affect the course of the renal disease. This statement must be tempered somewhat, as certain nephropathies, such as lupus nephropathy and perhaps mesangiocapillary glomerulonephritis, appear more sensitive to intercurrent pregnancy, and it does not apply to women who have scleroderma and periarteritis nodosa, in whom pregnancy should be discouraged. Furthermore, there is some disagreement as to whether or not pregnancy adversely influences the natural history of IgA nephropathy, focal–segmental glomerulosclerosis, and reflux nephropathy.

It must be emphasized that the degree of renal dysfunction and/or hypertension prior to pregnancy influences the incidence of both maternal and fetal complications. Poorer prognosis is associated with poorer renal function (see Tables 1 and 2). The main dangers are that women with moderate, and certainly those with severe, dysfunction will experience serious deterioration in renal function and/or accelerated progression of the underlying disease postdelivery.

Dialysis

These patients are usually infertile, but contraception should not be neglected. On balance, pregnancy is probably contraindicated, since it is invariably complicated and poses excessive risk to the mother, with an uncertain and low chance of success. Even when therapeutic terminations are excluded, the live birth outcome, at best, is 40–50 per cent. Realistically, these women should not take any health risks, and might be persuaded to pursue rehabilitation into a transplant programme, with the question of pregnancy being reconsidered thereafter.

Renal transplantation

Taking into account the criteria used in chronic renal disease—prepregnancy renal status and/or hypertension—certain generalizations can be made. If, according to a suitable set of guidelines, prepregnancy assessment is satisfactory, then pregnancy can be advised. Despite an overall complication rate of 46 per cent, the chances of success are 95 per cent (Table 6). If complications (usually hypertension, renal deterioration, and/or rejection) occur before 28 weeks then successful obstetric outcome is reduced by 20 per cent. More information is needed about the intrauterine effects and neonatal aftermath of immunosuppression which, at maintenance levels, is apparently harmless. From data available it seems that pregnancy does not compromise long-term graft prognosis.

References

Abe, S. (1996). Pregnancy in glomerulonephritic patients with decreased renal function. *Hypertension in Pregnancy* **15**, 305–313.

Andrews, P. A. (2002). Renal transplantation. *British Medical Journal* **324**, 530–534.

Armenti, V. T., Moritz, M. J., and Davison, J. M. (1998). Medical management of the pregnant transplant recipient. *Advances in Renal Replacement Therapy* **5**, 14–21.

Armenti, V. T. et al. (2000). Pregnancy and transplantation. *Graft* **3**, 59–64.

Armenti, V. T., Moritz, M. J., Cardonick, E. H., and Davison, J. M. (2002). Immunosuppression in pregnancy: choices for infant and maternal health. *Drugs* **62**, 2361–2375.

Asrat, T., Roossin, M. C., and Miller, E. I. (1998). Ultrasonographic detection of ureteral jets in normal pregnancy. *American Journal of Obstetrics and Gynecology* **178**, 1194–1196.

Auzary, C. et al. (2000). Pregnancy in patients with Wegener's granulomatosis: report of 5 cases in 3 women. *Annals of the Rheumatic Diseases* **59**, 800–805.

Bagon, J. A. et al. (1998). Pregnancy and dialysis. *American Journal of Kidney Diseases* **31**, 756–760.

Bar, J. et al. (2000). Prediction of pregnancy outcome in subgroups of women with renal disease. *Clinical Nephrology* **53**, 437–441.

Baylis, C. (1994). Glomerular filtration and volume regulation in gravid animal models. *Clinical Obstetrics and Gynaecology* **8**, 235–264.

Baylis, C. (2003). Impact of pregnancy on underlying renal disease. *Advances in Renal Replacement Therapy* **10**, 31–39.

Braga, J. et al. (1996). Maternal and perinatal implications of the use of recombinant erythropoietin. *Acta Obstetrica Gynecologica Scandinavica* **75**, 449–454.

Brookhyser, J. and Wiggins, K. (1998). Medical nutrition in pregnancy and kidney disease. *Advances in Renal Replacement Therapy* **5**, 53–58.

Brown, M. A. et al. (1998). Ambulatory blood pressure monitoring in pregnancy: what is normal? *American Journal of Obstetrics and Gynecology* **178**, 836–842.

Bucholz, N.-P. et al. (1998). Urolithiasis in pregnancy—a clinical challenge. *European Journal of Obstetrics, Gynecology and Reproductive Biology* **80**, 25–29.

Butler, E. L. et al. (2000). Symptomatic nephrolithiasis complicating pregnancy. *Obstetrics and Gynecology* **96**, 753–758.

Calvet, J. P. and Grantham, J. J. (2001). The genetics and physiology of polycystic kidney disease. *Seminars in Nephrology* **21**, 107–113.

Castillio, A. A., Lew, S. Q., and Smith, A. M. (1999). Women's issues in female patients receiving peritoneal dialysis. *Advances in Renal Replacement Therapy* **6**, 327–332.

Chan, W. S., Okun, N., and Kjellstrand, C. M. (1998). Pregnancy in chronic dialysis: a review of the literature. *International Journal Artificial Organs* **21**, 259–264.

Chen, H.-H., Lin, H.-C., Yeh, J.-C., and Che, C.-P. (2001). Renal biopsies in pregnancies complicated by undetermined renal disease. *Acta Obstetrica Gynaecologica Scandinavica* **80**, 888–893.

Chapman, A. B., Johnson, A. M., and Gabow, P. A. (1994). Pregnancy outcome and its relationship to progression of renal failure in autosomal dominant polycystic kidney disease. *Journal of the American Society of Nephrology* **5**, 1178–1185.

Cowchock, F. S. et al. (1992). Repeated fetal losses associated with antiphospholipid antibodies: a collaborative randomised trial comparing prednisone with low dose heparin treatment. *American Journal of Obstetrics and Gynecology* **166**, 1318–1324.

Crowe, A. V. et al. (1999). Pregnancy does not adversely affect renal transplant function. *Quarterly Journal of Medicine* **92**, 631–636.

Cunningham, F. G., Buszta, C., Brann, W. E., Steinmuller, D., Novick, A. C., and Popowniak, K. (1983). Pregnancy in renal allograft recipients and long-term follow-up of their offspring. *Transplantation* **15**, 1067–1070.

Cunningham, F. G., Cox, S. M., and Harstad, T. W. (1990). Chronic renal disease and pregnancy outcome. *American Journal of Obstetrics and Gynecology* **163**, 453–459.

Davison, J. M. (1989). The effect of pregnancy on longterm renal function in women with chronic renal disease and single kidneys. *Clinical and Experimental Hypertension* **B8**, 226.

Davison, J. M. (1994). Pregnancy in renal allograft recipients: problems, prognosis and practicalities. *Baillière's Clinical Obstetrics and Gynaecology* **8**, 501–525.

Davison, J. M. and Redman, C. W. G. (1997). Pregnancy post-transplant: the establishment of a UK Registry. *British Journal of Obstetrics and Gynaecology* **104**, 1106–1107.

Delekas, D., Karyotis, I., and Loumbakis, P. (2000). Ureteral drainage by double-J-catheters during pregnancy. *Clinical and Experimental Obstetrics and Gynaecology* **27**, 200–202.

de Swiet, M. and Lightstone, L. (2004). Glomerular endotheliosis in normal pregnancy and pre-eclampsia. *British Journal of Obstetrics and Gynaecelogy* **111**, 191–192.

Dimeny, E. and Fellström, B. (1997). Metabolic abnormalities in renal transplant recipients: risk factors and prediction of graft dysfunction? *Nephrology, Dialysis, Transplantation* **12**, 21–26.

Ehrich, J. H. H. *et al.* (1996). Repeated successful pregnancies after kidney transplantation in 102 women. *Nephrology, Dialysis, Transplantation* **11**, 1312–1316.

Ekban, P. *et al.* (2001). Pregnancy outcome in type 1 diabetic women with microalbuminuria. *Diabetes Care* **24**, 1739–1745.

Evans, H. and Wollin, T. A. (2001). The management of urinary calculi in pregnancy. *Current Opinion in Urology* **11**, 379–385.

Falk, R. J. (2000). Treatment of lupus nephritis. *New England Journal of Medicine* **343**, 1182–1183.

First, M. R., Combs, C. A., Weiskittel, P., and Miodovinik, M. (1995). Lack of effect of pregnancy on renal allograft survival or function. *Transplantation* **59**, 472–477.

Fisher, K. A., Luger, A., Spargo, B. H., and Lindheimer, M. D. (1981). Hypertension in pregnancy: clinical–pathological correlation and late prognosis. *Medicine* **60**, 267–276.

Gabow, P. A. (1993). Autosomal dominant polycystic kidney disease. *New England Journal of Medicine* **329**, 332–342.

Gallery, E. D. M. (2004). Glomerular endotheliosis in normal pregnancy and pre-eclampsia. *British Journal of Obstetrics and Gynaecology* **111**, 193.

Gaughan, W. J., Moritz, M. J., Radomski, J. S., Burke, J. F., and Armenti, V. T. (1996). National Transplantation Pregnancy Registry: report on outcomes in cyclosporine-treated female kidney recipients with an interval from transplant to pregnancy of greater than 5 years. *American Journal of Kidney Diseases* **28**, 266–269.

Ghandour, F. Z., Knauss, T. C., and Hricik, D. E. (1998). Immunosuppressive drugs in pregnancy. *Advances in Renal Replacement Therapy* **5**, 31–37.

Gordon, M. *et al.* (1996). Perinatal outcome and long term follow up associated with modern management of diabetic nephropathy. *Obstetrics and Gynecology* **87**, 401–407.

Gupta, M., Shennan, A. H., Halligan, A., Taylor, D. J., and de Swiet, M. (1997). Accuracy of oscillometric blood pressure monitoring in pregnancy and pre-eclampsia. *British Journal of Obstetrics and Gynaecology* **104**, 350–355.

Harber, M. A. *et al.* (1999). Wegener's granulomatosis in pregnancy—the therapeutic dilemma. *Nephrology, Dialysis, Transplantation* **14**, 1789–1790.

Hayslett, J. P. (1992). The effect of systemic lupus erythematosus on pregnancy and pregnancy outcome. *American Journal of Reproductive Immunology* **28**, 199–204.

Hayslett, J. P. and Reece, E. A. (1994). Managing diabetic patients with nephropathy and other vascular complications. *Baillière's Clinical Obstetrics and Gynaecology* **8**, 405–424.

Heybourne, K. D. *et al.* (1991). Renal artery stenosis during pregnancy: a review. *Obstetrical and Gynecological Survey* **46**, 509–512.

Hill, D. E., Chantigan, P. M., and Kramer, S. A. (1990). Pregnancy after augmentation cystoplasty. **170**, 485–487.

Hod, M. *et al.* (1995). Diabetic nephropathy and pregnancy: the effect of ACE inhibitors prior to pregnancy on fetomaternal outcome. *Nephrology, Dialysis, Transplantation* **10**, 2328–2330.

Hon, S. (2003). Pregnancy in renal transplant recipients. *Advances in Renal Replacement Therapy* **10**, 40–47.

Hou, S. (1999). Pregnancy in chronic renal insufficiency and end stage renal disease. *American Journal of Kidney Diseases* **32**, 235–240.

Hou, S. and Firanek, C. (1998). Management of the pregnant dialysis patient. *Advances in Renal Replacement Therapy* **5**, 24–29.

Hussey, M. J. and Pombar, X. (1998). Obstetric care for renal allograft recipients or for women treated with hemodialysis or peritoneal dialysis during pregnancy. *Advances in Renal Replacement Therapy* **5**, 3–8.

Jones, D. C. and Hayslett, J. P. (1996). Outcome of pregnancy in women with moderate or severe renal insufficiency. *New England Journal of Medicine* **335**, 226–231.

Jungers, P. and Chauveau, D. (1997). Pregnancy in renal disease. *Kidney International* **52**, 871–880.

Jungers, P. *et al.* (1996). Pregnancy in women with reflux nephropathy. *Kidney International* **50**, 593–596.

Jungers, P., Chauveau, D., Fouget, D., Houllier, P., and Grünfeld, J.-P. (1997). Pregnancy in women with impaired renal function. *Clinical Nephrology* **47**, 281–288.

Kainz, A. *et al.* (2000). Analysis of 100 pregnancy outcomes in women treated systemically with tacrolimus. *Transplant International* **13**, S299–S303.

Katz, A. I., Davison, J. M., Hayslett, J. P., Singson, E., and Lindheimer, M. D. (1980). Pregnancy in women with kidney disease. *Kidney International* **18**, 192–206.

Kimmel, P. L. and Patel, S. S. (2003). Psychosocial issues in women with renal disease. *Advances in Renal Replacement Therapy* **10**, 61–70.

Kok, T. P. *et al.* (2002). Effect of pregnancy on renal graft function and material survival in renal transplant recipients. *Transplantation Proceedings* **34**, 1161–1163.

Kuller, J. A., D'Andrea, N., and McMahon, M. J. (2001). Renal biopsy and pregnancy. *American Journal of Obstetrics and Gynecology* **184**, 1093–1096.

Leguizaman, G. and Reece, E. A. (2000). Effect of medical therapy on progressive nephropathy: influence of pregnancy, diabetes and hypertension. *Journal of Maternal–Fetal Medicine* **9**, 70–76.

Lessan-Pezeshki, M. (2002). Pregnancy after renal transplantation: points to consider. *Nephrology, Dialysis, Transplantation* **17**, 703–705.

Lindheimer, M. D. and Davison, J. M. (1987). Renal biopsy during pregnancy: 'To b … or not to b'. *British Journal of Obstetrics and Gynaecology* **94**, 932–934.

Lindheimer, M. D. and Katz, A. I. Renal physiology and disease in pregnancy. In *The Kidney: Pathology and Pathophysiology* 3rd edn. (ed. D. W. Seldin and G. Giebisch), Philadelphia, PA: Lippincott Williams & Wilkins, 1999a.

Lindheimer, M. D. and Mahowald, M. B. (2004). Glomerular endotheliosis in normal pregnancy and pre-eclampsia. *British Journal of Obstetrics and Gynaecology* **111**, 191.

Lindheimer, M. D., Roberts, J. M., and Cunningham, F. G. In *Chesley's Hypertensive Disorders in Pregnancy* 2nd edn. (ed. M. D. Lindheimer, J. M. Roberts, and F. G. Cunningham), Stamford, CT: Appleton & Lange, 1999b.

Lindheimer, M. D., Davison, J. M., and Katz, A. I. (2001). The kidney and hypertension in pregnancy: twenty exciting years. *Seminars in Nephrology* **21**, 173–180.

Little, M. A. *et al.* (2000). Pregnancy in Irish renal transplant recipients in the cyclosporine era. *Irish Journal of Medical Science* **169**, 19–23.

Lockshin, M. D. and Sammaratino, L. R. Rheumatic disease. In *Medical Disorders During Pregnancy* 2nd edn. (ed. W. M. Barron and M. D. Lindheimer), pp. 335–391. St Louis: Mosby-Year Book, 2000.

Lockwood, G. M., Ledger, W. L., and Barlow, D. H. (1995). Successful pregnancy outcome in a renal transplant patient following *in vitro* fertilization. *Human Reproduction* **10**, 1528–1531.

Morgan, S. H. and Grünfeld, J. P., ed. *Inherited Disorders of the Kidney*. Oxford: Oxford University Press, 1998.

Murray, S., Hickey, J., and Houange, E. (1987). Significant bacteriuria associated with replacement of intrauterine contraceptive device. *American Journal of Obstetrics and Gynecology* **156**, 698–699.

Newstead, C. G. (1997). Tacrolimus in renal transplantation. *Nephrology, Dialysis, Transplantation* **12**, 1342–1343.

Newstead, C. G. (1998). Assessment of risk of cancer after renal transplantation. *Lancet* **351**, 610–611.

Nicklin, J. L. (1991). Systemic lupus erythematosus and pregnancy at the Royal Women's Hospital, Brisbane 1979–1989. *Australian and New Zealand Journal of Obstetrics and Gynaecology* **31**, 128–133.

Nojima, M. *et al.* (1996). Influence of pregnancy on graft function after renal transplantation. *Transplantation Proceedings* **28**, 1582–1585.

Nyberg, G. *et al.* (1998). Breast feeding during treatment with cyclosporin. *Transplantation* **65**, 253–254.

Okundaye, I. B., Abrinko, P., and Hou, S. H. (1998). Registry of pregnancy in dialysis patients. *American Journal of Kidney Diseases* **31**, 766–774.

Owda, A. K. *et al.* (1998). No evidence of functional deterioration of renal graft after repeated pregnancies—a report on 3 women with 17 pregnancies. *Nephrology, Dialysis, Transplantation* **13**, 1281–1283.

Packham, D. and Fairley, K. F. (1987). Renal biopsy: indications and complications in pregnancy. *British Journal of Obstetrics and Gynaecology* **94**, 935–939.

Palmer, B. F. (2003). Sexual dysfunction in men and women with chronic kidney disease and end-stage kidney disease. *Advances in Renal Replacement Therapy* **10**, 48–60.

Parmar, M. S. (2002). Chronic renal disease. *British Medical Journal* **325**, 85–89.

Pergola, P. E., Kancharla, A., and Riley, D. J. (2001). Kidney transplantation during the first trimester of pregnancy: immunosuppression with mycophenolate mofetil, tacrolimus and prednisone. *Transplantation* **71**, 994–997.

Petri, M. (1994). Systemic lupus erythematosus and pregnancy. *Rheumatic Diseases Clinics of North America* **20**, 87.

Purdy, L. P. *et al.* (1996). Effect of pregnancy on renal function in patients with moderate-to-severe diabetic renal insufficiency. *Diabetes Care* **19**, 1067–1072.

Rao, T. K. (2001). Human immunodeficiency virus infection and renal failure. *Infectious Disease Clinics of North America* **15**, 833–842.

Rashid, M. and Rashid, H. M. (2003). Chronic renal insufficiency in pregnancy. *Saudi Medical Journal* **24**, 709–714.

Romão, J. E. *et al.* (1998). Pregnancy in women on chronic dialysis. *Nephron* **78**, 416–419.

Schmidt, R. J. and Holley, J. L. (1998). Fertility and contraception in end-stage renal disease. *Advances in Renal Replacement Therapy* **5**, 38–45.

Scott, J. R., Branch, D. W., and Holman, J. (2002). Autoimmune and pregnancy complications in the daughter of a kidney transplant patient. *Transplantation* **73**, 815–816.

Shapiro, R. (2000). Tacrolimus in renal transplantation—a review. *Graft* **3**, 64–69.

Shennan, A., Gupta, M., Halligan, A., Taylor, D. J., and de Swiet, M. (1996). Lack of reproducibility in pregnancy of Korotkoff phase IV as measured by mercury sphygmomanometry. *Lancet* **347**, 139–142.

Shokeir, A. A., Makran, M. R., and Abdulmaaboud, M. (2000). Renal colic in pregnancy women: role of renal resistive index. *Urology* **55**, 344–346.

Sibai, B. M. (2002). Chronic hypertension in pregnancy. *Obstetrics and Gynecology* **100**, 369–377.

Stanley, C. W. *et al.* (1999). Developmental well-being in offspring of women receiving cyclosporine post-renal transplant. *Transplantation Proceedings* **31**, 241–243.

Steen, V. D. (1999). Pregnancy in women with systemic sclerosis. *Obstetrics and Gynecology* **94**, 15–19.

Stevens, H. *et al.* (2003a). Serum Cystatin-C reflects endotheliosis in normal hypertensive and pre-eclamptic pregnancy. *British Journal Obstetrics and Gynaecology* **110**, 825–830.

Stevens, H. *et al.* (2003b). Glomerular endotheliosis in normal pregnancy and pre-eclampsia. *British Journal of Obstetrics and Gynaecology* **110**, 831–836.

Stevens, H., Wide-Swensson, D., Ingemarsson, I., and Grubb, A. (2004). Glomerular endotheliosis in normal pregnancy and pre-eclampsia. *British Journal of Obstetrics and Gynaecology* **111**, 193–195.

Stotland, N. L. and Stotland, N. E. (1997). The mother and the burning building. *Obstetrical and Gynecological Survey* **53**, 1–3.

Sturgiss, S. N. and Davison, J. M. (1991). Perinatal outcome in renal allograft recipients: prognostic significance of hypertension and renal function before and during pregnancy. *Obstetrics and Gynecology* **78**, 573–577.

Sturgiss, S. N. and Davison, J. M. (1995). Effect of pregnancy on the long-term function of renal allografts: an update. *American Journal of Kidney Diseases* **26**, 54–56.

Szczech, L. A. *et al.* (2002). Predictors of proteinuria and renal failure among women with HIV infection. *Kidney International* **61**, 195–198.

Thi Huong, D. *et al.* (2001). Pregnancy in past or present lupus nephritis: a study of 32 pregnancies from a single center. *Annals of the Rheumatic Diseases* **60**, 599, 2001–2006.

Thompson, B. C. *et al.* (2003). Pregnancy in renal transplant recipients: the Royal Free Hospital experience. *Quarterly Journal of Medicine* **96**, 837–844.

Toma, H. *et al.* (1998). A nationwide survey on pregnancies in women on renal replacement therapy in Japan. *Nephrology, Dialysis, Transplantation* **13**, A163.

Twickler, D. *et al.* (1994). Renal pelvicalyceal dilatation in antepartum pyelonephritis: ultrasonographic findings. *American Journal of Obstetrics and Gynecology* **165**, 1115–1117.

Van Sonnenberg, E. *et al.* (1992). Symptomatic renal obstruction or urosepsis during pregnancy: treatment by sonographically guided percutaneous nephrostomy. *American Journal of Roentgenology* **158**, 91–94.

Vora, M. and Grushin, A. (1998). Erythropoietin in obstetrics. *Obstetrical and Gynecological Survey* **53**, 500–506.

Willis, F. R. *et al.* (2000). Children of renal transplant recipient mothers. *Journal Paediatrics and Child Health* **36**, 230–234.

Wilson, G. A. *et al.* (2001). National Transplantation Pregnancy Registry: post-pregnancy graft loss among female pancreas–kidney recipients. *Transplantation Proceedings* **33**, 1667–1670.

Wrenshall, L. E. *et al.* (1996). Pregnancy after donor nephrectomy. *Transplantation* **62**, 1934–1938.

15.4 Pregnancy-induced hypertension

Ian A. Greer

Introduction

Pregnancy-induced hypertension remains a major cause of maternal death in the United Kingdom today (The National Institute for Clinical Excellence 2001, http://www.cemd.org.uk/); it is also a major contributor to maternal and perinatal morbidity and perinatal mortality. The aetiology of this condition remains obscure despite increasing knowledge of its pathophysiological processes. What must be appreciated, however, is that pregnancy-induced hypertension is not simply an hypertensive problem, but is a disease that can affect virtually every system and organ in the body, hypertension representing just one facet of the disease process. The common pathological feature of the disease, whether in the placental bed or in the renal microcirculation, is vascular endothelial damage and dysfunction. Failure to appreciate the multisystem nature of this disease and its alternative presentations, which make it one of the great imitators, is a major source of potential morbidity and mortality for women with this problem.

Definitions, classification, and diagnosis

The classification of hypertension in pregnancy is confusing. A variety of conditions make up the hypertensive disorders of pregnancy and there is not only a lack of knowledge of their aetiology, but a lack of agreement on their nomenclature and classification. To compound this confusion, the true diagnosis, and therefore the classification, may only be evident retrospectively several months after the pregnancy is completed. The clinician faced with the problem during pregnancy must, therefore, make a provisional diagnosis. Here, some form of classification is essential to make diagnoses consistent, to help quantify the risk to mother and fetus, and to guide decisions on the patient's management. The lack of an agreed classification and nomenclature has also hampered research in this area by preventing comparisons between centres and between countries.

There are three possible types of hypertension that can occur in pregnancy. First, there are women who have hypertensive problems antedating the pregnancy. This will usually be essential hypertension, although some women with chronic hypertension will have an underlying problem such as renal disease. Second, and rarely, hypertension in pregnancy may represent the coincidental development of a new medical cause of hypertension occurring in pregnancy, such as phaeochromocytoma. Third, there are women who are normotensive before pregnancy and in early pregnancy, but who develop hypertension during pregnancy that remits within a few months of delivery; these women have pregnancy-induced hypertension. The simplest classification of these disorders is on the basis of two clinical features—hypertension and proteinuria. The classification of the International Society for the Study of Hypertension in Pregnancy (ISSHP) (Davey and MacGillivray 1988) is a useful and widely used system (Table 1). This chapter will concentrate on pregnancy-induced hypertensive problems. Even within this group of patients, the terminology is somewhat confusing. Pre-eclampsia, a term that is often loosely applied to these patients regardless of the severity of their hypertension or degree of proteinuria, appears to mean different things to different people, leading to further confusion. Traditionally, pre-eclampsia is associated with three classical clinical features: hypertension, proteinuria, and oedema. However proteinuria is really an indicator of severe disease as it reflects target organ damage. Pre-eclampsia should, therefore, be reserved for proteinuric (severe) pregnancy-induced hypertension. Gestational hypertension without proteinuria should be termed pregnancy-induced hypertension and such hypertension may be mild/moderate (140–165/90–105 mmHg) or severe (170/110 mmHg). The absence of proteinuria does not imply that the problem is not severe. For example, eclampsia, the most severe form of the disorder, and severe hypertension sufficient to precipitate a cerebrovascular accident, can occur without proteinuria.

Table 1 Summary of the ISSHP classification (Davey and MacGillivray 1988)

Hypertension
Diastolic BP of ≥110 mmHg on any one occasion
or
Diastolic BP of ≥90 mmHg on any two or more
    consecutive occasions ≥4 h apart

Severe hypertension
Diastolic BP ≥120 mmHg on any one occasion
or
Diastolic BP ≥110 mmHg on two or more
    consecutive occasions ≥4 h apart

Proteinuria
One 24-h urine collection with a total protein excretion
    of ≥300 mg/24 h
or
Two midstream or catheter specimens of urine (collected
    ≥4 h apart) with ≥ '++' protein on reagent strip testing
or
3 '+' protein (if urine SG < 1.030 *and* pH ≤ 8)

Diagnostic criteria

Cardiovascular changes in pregnancy, pregnancy-induced hypertension, and diagnosis of hypertension

During normal pregnancy, blood pressure starts to decline in the first trimester reaching a nadir in mid-pregnancy, before increasing during the third trimester to values compatible with those in the non-pregnant state. Cardiac output increases by around 40 per cent in the first trimester and is maintained through pregnancy, although a reduction can be seen in the third trimester when measured in the supine position, due to diminished venous return arising from obstruction by the gravid uterus. The fall in blood pressure must, therefore, reflect a reduction in peripheral resistance in excess of the increased cardiac output. Hypertension results from an increase in systemic vascular resistance in the face of an unchanged cardiac output. Thus, blood pressure is really a 'second-hand' measure of one of the pathological features of pregnancy-induced hypertension, namely vasoconstriction, although it remains one of the mainstays of diagnosis.

In pregnancy, just as in the non-pregnant population, blood pressure is continuously distributed and the dividing line between normotension and hypertension is arbitrary and artificial. A diastolic blood pressure of 90 mmHg after 20 weeks of pregnancy is usually considered the threshold for diagnosis. There is merit in this as the perinatal mortality rate increases when maternal diastolic blood pressure exceeds this level. In addition, it falls in line with statistical descriptions of the distribution of blood pressure in the population. A diastolic pressure of 90 mmHg is 3 SD greater than the mean for mid-pregnancy, 2 SD above the mean for 34 weeks' gestation but only 1.5 SD above the mean at term, reflecting the physiological increase in blood pressure towards term (MacGillivray et al. 1969). In late pregnancy, this can lead to overdiagnosis of the problem and may precipitate unnecessary intervention, indeed over 20 per cent of pregnant women will have a blood pressure of 140/90 mmHg at least once in pregnancy (Redman 1995). While in the late second trimester a 90 mmHg threshold may lead to under-diagnosis. This threshold excludes women who have a substantial increase in blood pressure (over the preconception or early pregnancy measurement), but where the diastolic pressure does not exceed 90 mmHg, and will include some women with mild chronic hypertension who have a minimal increase in blood pressure (Redman and Jeffries 1988). It has been proposed that a threshold of 90 mmHg together with an increase of 25 mmHg should be used, as this will improve the diagnosis when compared with either measurement alone (Redman and Jeffries 1988). Repeated measures of blood pressure should be made to obtain an accurate diagnosis. The ISSHP definitions require that a value of greater than 90 mmHg be recorded on two measurements at least 4 h apart or a single value greater than 110 mmHg. It was customary to use Korotkoff phase IV (K4) as the measure of diastolic pressure since Korotkoff phase V (K5) was not thought to occur always in pregnancy. However, it is now accepted that K5 is a more accurate, reproducible, and reliable measure of diastolic pressure, which corresponds more closely to the true mean arterial pressure and, furthermore, does not have any adverse impact on the association between diastolic pressure and maternal or fetal outcome (Brown and De Swiet 1999). The use of K5 has recently been endorsed by the ISSHP. It is also important to use the correct technique and appropriate cuff size [arm circumference over 33 cm requires a large adult (15 cm) cuff] (Table 2). The systolic blood pressure is considered abnormal if it exceeds 140 mmHg, but has not been widely used in classifications as it is considered more variable. However, it does correlate with perinatal mortality and inversely with birthweight (Tervila et al. 1973). Although not used for classification of the disorder, this does not mean that the systolic pressure is unimportant clinically, as pressures in excess of 160 mmHg will place the woman at risk of vascular complications. Thus, in terms of clinical management the systolic pressure is important, and should precipitate treatment to lower blood pressure if values of 165 mmHg are obtained. An increase in systolic and diastolic blood pressures of 30 and 15 mmHg, respectively, or readings over the thresholds of 140 mmHg systolic and 90 mmHg diastolic, on at least two occasions 6 h or more apart, has been employed as an alternative diagnostic criterion for hypertension by the American College of Obstetricians and Gynecologists. This increment in diastolic pressure is probably too modest as the average increase in diastolic pressure in normal pregnancy is around 10–12 mmHg (MacGillivray et al. 1969). Diurnal variation also exists, with the greatest pressures being recorded in the afternoon and early evening, and the lowest pressures being obtained between midnight and 4 a.m. (Redman et al. 1976a). This nocturnal reduction can be lost or even reversed in patients with pregnancy-induced hypertension (Redman et al. 1976c). Because of the diurnal variation and short-term variability of blood pressure, multiple measures of blood pressure are required to obtain a true assessment of the situation.

Measurement of blood pressure is fraught with sampling errors of various forms such as inter- and intraobserver variation, digit preference, threshold avoidance, and poor technique. Automated and ambulatory blood pressure measurement may be of value in pregnancy overcoming sampling errors and factors such as 'white coat hypertension' (Bellomo et al. 1999) and also taking account of the diurnal rhythm of blood pressure in pregnancy, so avoiding many of the problems associated with conventional blood pressure measurement. It is important that such devices are appropriately validated in pregnancy such as has

Table 2 Measurement of blood pressure in pregnancy

Use a bell stethoscope as it better amplifies the Korotkoff sounds

Use a well-maintained sphygmomanometer

A range of sphygmomanometer cuff sizes must be available. Too small a cuff will overestimate blood pressure, too large a cuff will underestimate (ideally, bladder length should encompass 80% of the arm circumference and bladder width should be 40% of the arm circumference)

Measurements should be taken with the woman sitting after a period of rest with the arm supported at heart level. Measurements are not significantly altered if the woman is lying with lateral tilt provided that the arm is at heart level

When the cuff is first inflated an approximation of systolic pressure should be taken by palpation of the radial pulse

During auscultation, the cuff should initially be inflated to a pressure 20 mmHg higher than the estimated systolic pressure determined by palpation

Systolic pressure is recorded as the level where repetitive sounds are first heard (Korotkoff I) (rounded, upwards, to the nearest 2 mmHg)

The diastolic pressure is recorded at the point of disappearance of these sounds (Korotkoff V) rounded to the nearest 2 mmHg been carried out with the Spacelabs device (Greer 1993; Halligan *et al.* 1995). In particular, it should be noted that some automated systems will significantly underestimate blood pressure in pre-eclampsia, particularly, at extremes of blood pressure (Natarajan *et al.* 1999). Thus, when managing women with severe hypertension, it is useful to check automated readings with traditional manual techniques.

Central haemodynamic studies in pregnancy-induced hypertension (Clark and Cotton 1988) show that cardiac output and heart rate remain normal while the systemic vascular resistance and arterial pressure are increased. The left ventricle is usually hyperdynamic and the pulmonary capillary-wedge pressures are normal to low. The central venous pressure (CVP) is also usually normal or low but does not always correlate with the wedge pressure. The wedge pressures are sometimes high due to an excessive afterload, producing depressed left ventricular function, or due to fluid overload. Pulmonary oedema can occur because of depressed left-ventricular function, capillary leakage, and reduced colloid osmotic pressure due to hypoalbuminaemia. These multiple possible mechanisms mean that pulmonary oedema can occur without any significant elevation in CVP.

Proteinuria

Proteinuria is easier to quantify than hypertension and is indicative of severe disease as it reflects damage to the kidney. The degree of proteinuria has been shown in the past to correlate with perinatal mortality (Naeye and Friedman 1979) and incidence of growth restriction (Tervila *et al.* 1973). The proteinuria can be severe enough to result in nephrotic syndrome. However, a recent South African Study (Hall *et al.* 2002) found that neither the rate of increase, nor the amount of proteinuria, in women with heavy or moderate proteinuria, affected maternal or perinatal outcomes in women with pre-eclampsia managed conservatively. The accepted threshold for significant proteinuria in pregnancy is 0.3 g/24 h (Davey and MacGillivray 1988). Formal quantification of proteinuria was traditionally obtained by a 24-h collection. However, the delay in collecting the sample and obtaining the result often means that management decisions need to be based on dipstick testing or by measuring the urine protein–creatinine ratio. A value of more than 30 mg protein/mmol creatinine reflects quantitative proteinuria of greater than 0.3 g/24 h (Saudan *et al.* 1997). The protein–creatinine ratio has greater clinical utility than the 24-h assessment and has been shown to correlate strongly with 24-h urine protein excretion (Robert *et al.* 1997). Random urine samples assessed by 'dipstick' may produce false-positive results due to contamination of the urine by vaginal discharge, chlorhexidine preparations, or if the urine is highly alkaline or very concentrated (specific gravity > 1.030). False-negative results may occur if the urine is very dilute (specific gravity < 1.010). However, as noted above, in the clinical situation, most management decisions are made on 'dipstick' testing of urine as the evolution of the disease, particularly the severe proteinuric form, may occur at a speed at which formal laboratory quantification of proteinuria by 24-h assessments may be unable to keep pace. On the semi-quantitative dipstick testing a 'trace' corresponds to around 0.1 g/l, 1+ to 0.3 g/l, 2+ to 1.0 g/l, 3+ to 3 g/l, and 4+ to 10 g/l of protein and clinicians need to be aware of the limitations of dipstick testing noted above.

While proteinuria is indicative of severe disease, the absence of proteinuria does not preclude a severe form of pregnancy-induced hypertension. Eclampsia and severe hypertension can occur without proteinuria (Sibai *et al.* 1981). Further, proteinuria in the absence of significant hypertension can still be a manifestation of pre-eclampsia and can be associated with severe growth restriction. In addition, microalbuminuria is present in a many women with milder forms of the disease (Thong *et al.* 1991) suggesting that there is a spectrum of renal damage and dysfunction ranging from an absence of proteinuria through microalbuminuria to gross proteinuria.

Additional diagnostic features

Oedema is part of the classical definition of pre-eclampsia and has been used as a diagnostic feature. Such use should be abandoned. While pathological oedema, associated with a rapid increase in weight, occurs commonly in pre-eclampsia, severe pre-eclampsia and eclampsia can occur without oedema. Perinatal mortality has been shown to be greater in pre-eclampsia without oedema compared to pre-eclampsia with oedema. Furthermore, significant oedema occurs in around 70 per cent of normal pregnancies and in a prospective study, the incidence of hypertension was no different between those with and without oedema (Robertson 1971). Although rapid weight gain has been employed to identify women developing pre-eclampsia, this can occur without pre-eclampsia. In one series, only 10 per cent of patients with eclampsia had a rapid weight gain (Chesley 1978). Thus, oedema is of little value as an objective diagnostic sign.

Hyperuricaemia is a useful diagnostic feature as it precedes proteinuria and is of value in distinguishing women with pregnancy-induced hypertension from those with chronic hypertension. Elevated plasma urate together with hypertension is associated with a substantial increase in perinatal mortality compared to pregnancies with the same degree of hypertension, but with normal plasma urate values (Redman *et al.* 1976a). Elevated plasma urate is not specific to pregnancy-induced hypertension, and values normally increase with gestation: Redman (1989) showed that plasma urate concentrations 2 SD above the mean at 16, 28, 32, and 36 weeks were 0.28, 0.29, 0.34, and 0.39 mmol/l, respectively. Urea increases in parallel with uric acid, but both urea and creatinine generally stay within the normal non-pregnant range in mild/moderate disease while with severe disease associated with renal compromise urea can be expected to be more than 7 mM/l and creatinine more than 100 mM/l.

Platelet consumption occurs in pregnancy-induced hypertension. It is often an early feature, present in the second trimester. Since there is a wide range of platelet counts in normal pregnancy and also because platelet count falls in normal pregnancy, the absolute count is not usually of diagnostic value unless combined with other features. Serial counts are more helpful. Thrombocytopenia is also an inconsistent feature of the disease.

The clinical diagnosis

Hypertensive disorders in pregnancy are difficult to diagnose and classify, reflecting the problem of using two signs of the disorder to define the problem. Despite this, the clinician must make management decisions based on the prognostic implications of the suspected problem. The diagnosis made during pregnancy is always provisional and may be modified on longer-term follow-up. Clinical practice is, however, essentially concerned with only a few diagnostic groups.

Chronic hypertension

Chronic hypertension is found in around 1.5 per cent of pregnancies and is associated with a persistently elevated blood pressure (>90 mmHg diastolic) occurring in the first or early second trimester where rare causes of pre-eclampsia such as hydatidiform mole are excluded. It may be present preconceptually, but diagnosed for the first time in pregnancy. Over 95 per cent of women with chronic hypertension have essential hypertension. In women with chronic hypertension, blood pressure shows the same physiological changes as in normal pregnancy. This may not be apparent if the woman is not seen until later in pregnancy. This can confuse the diagnosis when her blood pressure exhibits the normal physiological increase in the third trimester. Plasma urate is useful in helping to distinguish chronic from pregnancy-induced hypertension. An assessment of underlying medical conditions should be made including the exclusion of renal and connective tissue disease. It must be remembered that such woman have around a 10-fold increased risk of developing superimposed pregnancy-induced hypertension or pre-eclampsia (15–25 per cent of these women will develop superimposed pre-eclampsia), where proteinuria and/or increased plasma uric acid will usually be present. When pre-eclampsia does occur in women with chronic hypertension, it is more commonly severe and early onset in nature and is likely to be recurrent in future pregnancies. Intrauterine growth restriction (IUGR) is also more frequent and occurs in around 10 per cent of cases of chronic hypertension even in the absence of pre-eclampsia. Most of the excess maternal and fetal morbidity associated with chronic hypertension relates to the development of superimposed pre-eclampsia. However, where the hypertension is secondary to a problem such as chronic renal disease, a deterioration in the condition may occur in the absence of superimposed pre-eclampsia. Women with chronic hypertension at highest risk of developing superimposed pre-eclampsia are those with severe hypertension, a diastolic pressure of greater than 100 mmHg before 20 weeks gestation, and those with evidence of target organ damage such as left ventricular hypertrophy or renal compromise. In such situations, the risk of pre-eclampsia may be over 40 per cent. Thus, where chronic hypertension has been present for several years, an assessment of target organ damage should be made.

With chronic hypertension, it is often possible to discontinue antihypertensive therapy in the first half of pregnancy in these women, although it may require to be reintroduced in the third trimester as blood pressure rises from its physiological nadir in mid-pregnancy. Such treatment should be instituted if diastolic pressure is 100 mmHg or 90 mmHg if there is underlying renal disease or evidence of target organ damage. Ideally, these women should be seen prepregnancy in order to review the level of risk, assess end-organ damage, and review antihypertensive therapy as some agents such as angiotensin-converting enzyme (ACE) inhibitors and angiotensin II (AII) receptor antagonists are best avoided in pregnancy.

Pregnancy-induced hypertension and pre-eclampsia

Pregnancy-induced hypertension is the diagnosis applied to women who are normotensive in the first 20 weeks of pregnancy, but who develop hypertension in the second half of pregnancy. In association with significant proteinuria, it is termed pre-eclampsia. Proteinuria is not a constant feature of severe disease and a persistent diastolic blood pressure of greater than 110 mmHg should also be considered severe pregnancy-induced hypertension (Davey and MacGillivray 1988). It is associated with variable systemic upset including disturbance of coagulation, renal, and hepatic functions.

Eclampsia

Eclampsia can be regarded as the inevitable consequence of disease progression in pregnancy-induced hypertension. However, it can be the first clinical manifestation of the condition. It is characterized by grand mal seizures, which cannot be attributed to epilepsy or any other problem. It arises without any obvious symptoms in 15–20 per cent of cases (Villar and Sibai 1988). A UK survey reported that almost 40 per cent of cases occurred before hypertension or proteinuria was documented (Douglas and Redman 1994). In the UK survey, 38 per cent of cases occurred antepartum, 44 per cent of cases occurred postpartum, and the rest intrapartum (Douglas and Redman 1994). This is similar to North American reports where approximately 50 per cent of cases occur before labour, 25 per cent during labour, and 25 per cent postpartum (Villar and Sibai 1988). Postpartum eclampsia usually occurs, within the first 48 h but may occur up to 2–3 weeks later (Villar and Sibai 1988). Eclampsia is usually accompanied by hypertension, although not always severe, and proteinuria is absent in 20–40 per cent of cases (Villar and Sibai 1988). Where prodromal symptoms occur, those most commonly encountered are headache, epigastric pain, and visual disturbance. Hyperuricaemia, deranged liver function tests, thrombocytopenia, and coagulation disturbances can also be seen. An awareness of the diverse presentations is important. Women with headache, epigastric pain, and vomiting in pregnancy should be considered to have fulminating pre-eclampsia until proven otherwise. Hypertension and proteinuria in pregnancy must be treated seriously. Routine laboratory testing including plasma urate and liver function tests, a platelet count, and blood film should help resolve the diagnosis and allow suitable therapeutic measures to be taken. It is noteworthy that most cases in the United Kingdom occur despite the patient having antenatal care with 75 per cent occurring in hospital. The majority did not have liver function assessed before the seizure and only two-thirds after the seizure (Douglas and Redman 1994) suggesting that investigation of such patients is often inadequate. This is in keeping with the findings of the Confidential Enquiries into Maternal Deaths in the United Kingdom.

Epidemiology

Incidence and risk factors

The incidence of pregnancy-induced hypertension and pre-eclampsia has been difficult to establish due to various definitions and classification systems, but using ISSHP definitions is considered to be around 5 and 2 per cent, respectively, in the United Kingdom. Pregnancy-induced hypertension is traditionally regarded as a disorder of the primigravida; previous pregnancies offer some protection, although it has become clear that primipaternity is a more accurate description with the length of sexual cohabitation being inversely related to the risk (Robillard and Hulsey 1996). A first trimester abortion (either spontaneous or induced) does not protect against pre-eclampsia in a second pregnancy. A late miscarriage reduces the risk of pre-eclampsia in a subsequent pregnancy by around 75 per cent. If the first pregnancy reaches term without any hypertensive complication, the risk of pre-eclampsia in the subsequent pregnancy is reduced by almost 90 per cent. However, if the first pregnancy is complicated by pre-eclampsia, then the incidence in the second pregnancy is similar to the first and the risk is increased if the first pregnancy is also complicated by a low birth-weight baby (<2.5 kg) (Campbell and MacGillivray 1985). Thus, while the incidence of pre-eclampsia is reduced overall in a second pregnancy, the protective effect is modified by the presence of hypertensive complications, gestation at delivery, and birthweight of the first pregnancy. Woman with chronic hypertension have around a 10-fold increased risk of developing superimposed pregnancy-induced hypertension or pre-eclampsia, which is more commonly severe and early onset in nature and is likely to be recurrent in future pregnancies (Table 3).

Pre-eclampsia is associated with maternal age under 20 years and over 35 years; the former may be associated with primiparity and the latter to an increased prevalence of underlying chronic hypertensive problems, which increase the risk of, or may be misdiagnosed as pregnancy-induced hypertension. There does not appear to be an association with social class *per se*, but geographical and racial differences exist that may reflect an interaction between genes and environment such as dietary factors leading to insulin resistance and obesity. Obese women are more likely to have both pre-eclampsia and chronic hypertension. Women with pre-existing insulin dependent and gestational diabetes (Sermer *et al.* 1998; Sibai 2000) are at increased risk of pre-eclampsia although the risk is variable as such patients are predisposed to chronic hypertension and diabetic nephropathy. With gestational diabetes, the risk is about 10 per cent. For women with diabetes of short duration without nephropathy or retinopathy, the risk is about 8 per cent, but for those with target organ damage (nephropathy, hypertension, or retinopathy) the risk increases to 16 per cent. (Landon and Gabbe 1996). A history of migraine is also a maternal risk factor. In addition, a family history of pre-eclampsia on the maternal side is important due to the genetic component of the process (see below). Fetal factors are also important: twin pregnancies (Thornton and Macdonald 1999), fetal hydrops, hydatidiform moles, and triploidy and trisomy 13 are all associated with an increased risk of pregnancy-induced hypertension. Smoking has been consistently shown to be protective with regard to pre-eclampsia even after adjusting for body mass index, social class, and race. The relative risk of developing pre-eclampsia and gestational hypertension has been estimated at 0.5 (95% CI 0.4–0.7) and 0.6 (95% CI 0.4–0.9), respectively, in women smoking 10 cigarettes a day compared to women who have never smoked (Zhang *et al.* 1999). The risk reduction correlates with the duration of smoking and the amount of cigarettes smoked. Furthermore, it persists after cessation of smoking. As smokers are more at risk of complications such as IUGR, it would appear that smoking alters the maternal response to placental problems that might otherwise lead to pre-eclampsia. The mechanism underlying the protective effect of smoking is not established.

Eclampsia is uncommon in the United Kingdom occurring in 4.9/10,000 (95% CI 4.5–5.4) maternities (Douglas and Redman 1994). This is similar to the incidence in North America. The risk of eclampsia is threefold higher in women under 19 years of age, but in contrast to pregnancy-induced hypertension there is no increase in risk in women aged 35 and over (Douglas and Redman 1994). Multiple pregnancy enhances the risk sixfold (Douglas and Redman 1994). Around 25 per cent of women with eclampsia are parous and only about 25 per cent have a past history of pre-eclampsia. Thus, it is important to appropriately assess parous women with any symptoms or signs which might be related to pre-eclampsia. Around 2 per cent of cases will be associated with maternal death, and over one-third will have serious complications such as disseminated intravascular coagulation (DIC), adult respiratory distress syndrome (ARDS), and renal failure. In addition, there is a high level of perinatal morbidity and mortality related independently to both the pre-eclampsia–eclampsia disease process and preterm delivery. Following eclampsia, the risk of problems in future pregnancies has been estimated at around 20 per cent for pre-eclampsia, and around 2 per cent each for recurrent eclampsia, abruption, and perinatal death.

Maternal outcome

We have accurate data on the incidence and nature of deaths from pre-eclampsia and eclampsia in the United Kingdom due to the Reports on Confidential Enquiries into Maternal Deaths in England and Wales. Although there has been a dramatic improvement in deaths from pre-eclampsia/eclampsia since the 1950s, this remains one of the major causes of maternal mortality, second only to pulmonary thrombo-embolism in the United Kingdom (National Institute of Clinical Effectiveness 2001). The most frequent mode of death is currently intracranial haemorrhage reflecting a failure of adequate antihypertensive therapy. However, over the last few reports, pulmonary oedema and the development of ARDS have also been important. ARDS is rare in pre-eclampsia unless other complications are present, such as disseminated intravascular coagulation, pulmonary oedema, fluid overload, or over transfusion (Mabie *et al.* 1992; Catanzarite and Wilms 1997). Pulmonary oedema can easily arise due to fluid overload especially as vascular permeability is increased due to the endothelial damage. Clearly aside form fatal events, these complications are associated with increased morbidity for the mother. Other major causes of mortality and morbidity are cerebral oedema, cerebral infarction, disseminated intravascular coagulation, renal failure, liver damage including hepatic necrosis and liver rupture.

The early work by Chesley and others (Chesley *et al.* 1976; Fisher *et al.* 1981) suggested that women with pregnancies complicated by pregnancy-induced hypertension and eclampsia did not develop

Table 3 Risk factors for pre-eclampsia

Positive risk factors	Negative risk factors
First pregnancy	Previous pregnancy reaching the
Previous pre-eclampsia	second trimester and not
Central obesity	complicated by pre-eclampsia
Migraine	Long period of sexual cohabitation
Age <20 and >35 years	Smoking
Maternal family history of	
pre-eclampsia	
Diabetes	
Congenital and acquired	
thrombophilia	
Renal and connective tissue disease	
Essential hypertension	
Multiple pregnancy	
Hydrops and molar pregnancy	
Fetal trisomy	

chronic hypertension later, but others (Sibai *et al.* 1986a) have found an increase in risk of hypertension especially where the hypertensive problem arises before 30 weeks gestation. There does appear to be agreement, however, that mothers who experience uncomplicated pregnancies have a lower incidence of subsequent hypertension compared with the general population of similar age and race. Recent studies demonstrate that women with a history of pre-eclampsia have higher circulating levels of fasting insulin, lipid, and coagulation factors postpartum relative to body mass index matched controls (Laivouri *et al.* 1996; He *et al.* 1999). They also appear to exhibit a specific defect in endothelial-dependent vascular function relative to women with a history of a healthy pregnancy, independent of maternal obesity, blood pressure, and metabolic disturbances associated with insulin resistance or dyslipidaemia (Chambers *et al.* 2001). This pattern of metabolic and vascular changes in women with a history of pre-eclampsia is near identical to the abnormalities seen in this condition at diagnosis, namely exaggerated lipid and insulin levels, disturbed haemostatic parameters, and endothelial dysfunction (Sattar *et al.* 1996). It is not surprising, therefore, that the specific vascular lesion of pre-eclampsia, acute atherosis with lipid laden foam cells, seen in the placental bed (see below) is similar to that observed in atherosclerosis (Sattar and Greer 2002). Thus, the genotypes and phenotypes underlying vascular disease may also underlie pre-eclampsia. The above changes in surrogate risk markers in women with a history of pre-eclampsia would predict an increased coronary heart disease (CHD) risk. Jonsdottir *et al.* (1995) examined causes of death in 374 women with a history of hypertensive complications and noted that their death rate from CHD complications was significantly higher [1.47 (95% CI 1.05–2.02)] than expected from analysis of population data from public health and census reports during corresponding periods. Moreover, they noted that the relative risk (RR) of dying from CHD was significantly higher among eclamptic women (RR = 2.61; 95% CI 1.11–6.12) and those with pre-eclampsia (RR = 1.90; 95% CI 1.02–3.52) than those with hypertension alone (Jondottir *et al.* 1995). A prospective cohort study using the Royal College of General Practitioners Oral Contraceptive Study Data reported that a history of pre-eclampsia increased the risk of cardiovascular conditions in later life. For ischaemic heart disease, the RR was 1.7 (1.3–2.2). Furthermore, they found that the increased risk could not be explained by underlying chronic hypertension alone (Hannaford *et al.* 1997). A retrospective cohort study from Scotland using hospital discharge data (Smith *et al.* 2001) has also recently reported an association between pre-eclampsia and subsequent ischaemic heart disease in the mother (hazard ratio 2.0 95% CI 1.5–2.5). Prospective evaluation of women in pregnancy with long-term follow-up is now required to elaborate the mechanisms underlying this association. It is also important to determine whether this finding represents a new source of identifying risk that might not have been evident otherwise or whether these women would have been identified as 'at risk' from the use of established risk factors such as hypertension and obesity (Sattar and Greer 2002). Only then will we know if this finding represents an opportunity for primary prevention.

Fetal outcome

Pre-eclampsia and eclampsia are associated with IUGR, intrauterine asphyxia, and iatrogenic prematurity. The British Births Survey of 1970 (Chamberlain *et al.* 1978) showed a perinatal mortality rate in severe pregnancy-induced hypertension (and eclampsia) of 33.7/1000 compared to the rate of 19.2/1000 in normotensive pregnancies. The perinatal mortality rate was not increased in mild/moderate disease and was 15.6/1000 in chronic hypertension. When chronic hypertension was complicated by superimposed pre-eclampsia, the perinatal mortality rate rose to 30.7/1000. Thus, the severity of hypertension is important. Modern maternal and neonatal care has substantially improved these figures, and perinatal mortality is no a longer useful measure of the fetal effects of pre-eclampsia. A more recent Australian report reflecting practice in the 1990s found a small rate for gestational age infants of 24 per cent in pre-eclampsia and a perinatal mortality rate of 38/1000, this fell to 17 per cent for SGA infants and 6/1000 perinatal mortality rate for gestational hypertension using the ISSHP criteria (Brown and Buddle 1997). With regard to eclampsia, the British Eclampsia Survey (Douglas and Redman 1994) found a stillbirth rate of 22.2/1000 and a neonatal death rate of 34.1/1000. The presence of IUGR is important as it is associated with a reduced risk of survival independently of other variables such as gestation and severity of maternal disease (Witlin *et al.* 2000). There is an association between severe disease and neurodevelopmental disability in childhood. There is now plentiful evidence linking low birthweight, due to IUGR, to increased risk of vascular disease and type 2 diabetes in later adult life. This is considered to be due in part to fetal programming through fetal nutrition (Godfrey *et al.* 2000). Such programming, interacting with the genotype relating to insulin resistance and birthweight, may provoke selective changes in body composition, metabolism, and hormonal axes (Lawlor *et al.* 2002). For example, birthweight of offspring is inversely related to maternal insulin resistance in later life (Lawlor *et al.* 2002). These data support the hypothesis that pregnancy outcome in terms of birthweight is linked to the infant's subsequent health; thus, emphasizing the importance of intrauterine well being to adult health.

Pathology and pathophysiology

The three stages of the pathophysiological process in pre-eclampsia

Although pre-eclampsia is a very variable disorder in both its presenting features, reflecting the multisystem nature of the disorder, and in the rate of progression, it is valuable to consider the pathological process in three stages (Redman 1995). The first stage or primary pathology is placental in origin. This reflects that pre-eclampsia is a disorder specific to pregnancy requiring the presence of the placenta, it resolves following delivery and can occur in conditions such as hydatidiform mole where there is no fetus. It is associated with both an abnormal, inadequately implanted placenta such as is seen with growth restriction where placental ischaemia and infarction can occur and also with large placentas such as in twin pregnancy or in hydrops fetalis. These associations suggest that the placental trigger may arise from either placental mass or dysfunction with ischaemia. Stage two or the secondary pathology is the maternal response to the placental trigger, the syndrome that we call pregnancy-induced hypertension or pre-eclampsia. This is manifest as hypertension and multisystem disturbance including renal dysfunction with proteinuria, and metabolic disturbances such as hyperlipidaemia. These changes might be regarded as an attempt at a maternal compensatory response to provide greater placental blood flow and nutrient delivery to meet the need of the developing baby. This response, however, can harm the mother. The third stage or tertiary pathology occurs when the organs and systems affected by the pathological processes can no longer cope and serious complications arise such as eclampsia, cerebral haemorrhage, hepatic haematoma or rupture, renal failure, DIC, and pulmonary problems such as pulmonary oedema and ARDS. Thus, symptoms such as epigastric pain and visual disturbance indicate that the tertiary pathology is imminent or present.

While these stages are sequential, a problem may not be apparent clinically until stage three is reached. This does not mean that stages one and two were absent, only that they were subclinical or not recognized or that progress through the stages was so rapid as to avoid clinical detection. However, from a clinical perspective, the object should be to avoid, mainly by control of blood pressure, prevention of seizures and timely delivery, progress to stage three of the disorder.

The placental pathology

In normal pregnancy, the spiral arteries of the placental bed undergo a series of physiological changes. They are invaded by the cytotrophoblast (Robertson and Khong 1987), which breaks down the endothelium, internal elastic lamina, and muscular coat of the vessel which are largely replaced by fibrinoid. Virtually every spiral artery in the decidua basalis would have undergone these physiological changes by the end of the first trimester (Brosens and Dixon 1966). Early in the second trimester, a second wave of cytotrophoblast invasion occurs and transforms the myometrial segments of the spiral arteries, and occasionally the distal segments of the radial arteries. These physiological changes convert the vessels supplying the placenta from muscular end arteries to wide-mouthed sinusoids. The vascular supply is thus transformed from a high-pressure–low-flow system to a low-pressure–high-flow system to meet the needs of the fetus and placenta. Loss of the endothelial and muscular layers render these vessels unable to respond to vasomotor stimuli.

In pre-eclampsia, only about one-half to two-thirds of the decidual spiral arteries undergo these physiological changes (Khong et al. 1986), and the conversion of myometrial components of the spiral arteries fails to occur, even in vessels where the decidual segments have undergone physiological change (Sheppard and Bonnar 1981). Thus, the primary invasion of trophoblast is partially impaired, and the second wave fails to occur or is limited. This qualitative and quantitive restriction of normal physiological changes results in restricted placental blood flow, which becomes more critical with advancing gestation as the demands of the conceptus increases. In addition, the vessels maintain their muscular coats, and so remain sensitive to vasomotor stimuli (Figs 1–4). These changes are not specific to pre-eclampsia and also occur in IUGR without pre-eclampsia.

The typical, though non-specific, vascular lesion found in the placental bed in pregnancy-induced hypertension has been termed 'acute atherosis' because of the presence of foam cells in the damaged vessel wall (Labarrere 1988). This can be seen in the intramyometrial segments of the spiral arteries in the placental bed, the basal arteries, and the decidua parietalis, but is not seen in the intradecidual vessels of the placental bed, which have undergone physiological change. Acute atherosis is a necrotizing arteriopathy characterized by fibrinoid necrosis, accumulation of lipid laden macrophages and damaged cells, fibroblast proliferation, and a mononuclear cell perivascular infiltrate.

Again, it is not specific to pre-eclampsia being present in IUGR also. In the early stages, this lesion is characterized by endothelial damage. Evidence of endothelial damage can be seen ultrastructurally in the decidua at sites outside the placental bed throughout the maternal fetal boundary (Shanklin and Sibai 1989) and this correlates with the degree of maternal hypertension. Plasma urate, a marker of disease severity correlates with these vascular changes in the placental bed (McFadyen et al. 1986). Ischaemia of the fetal placenta will occur because of the restricted blood flow and lead to infarcts, patchy necrosis, and intracellular damage of the syncitiotrophoblast, an increase in villous cytotrophoblastic cells, and an obliterative endarteritis of the fetal stem arteries (Fox 1988). More recently, it has been suggested that there is incomplete development of the fetal placental microvasculature in

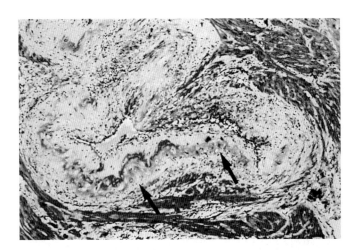

Fig. 1 Intramyometrial segment of a spiral artery in the placental bed during the third trimester. The uteroplacental artery is artefactually collapsed but shows the normal marked dilatation. The vessel wall contains a large amount of fibrinoid material with incorporated fibroblasts (arrows) and fibrous tissue, with the musculoelastic tissue of the vessel having been largely destroyed (reproduced from Robertson et al. 1975, with permission). H and E, 130×.

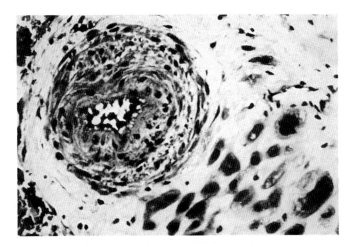

Fig. 2 Intramyometrial segment of a spiral artery in the placental bed in a patient suffering from pre-eclampsia. The vessel has not undergone the physiological changes noted in Fig. 1, with no invasion of the vessel at this site by endovascular trophoblast (reproduced from Robertson et al. 1967, with permission). H and E, 360×.

pre-eclampsia associated with IUGR, which could account for reduced perfusion of the fetal placenta seen in this condition (Macara *et al.* 1995).

The kidney

The glomeruli enlarge and sometimes bulge and protrude into the proximal tubule due to swelling and lipid vacuolation of the cytoplasm of the glomerular endothelial cells in the capillary loops (Fig. 5). This swelling narrows the lumen. These glomerular changes are termed 'glomerular endotheliosis'. The epithelial cells of the glomerulus and their foot processes appear normal except for a few intracytoplasmic hyaline droplets. The mesangium, however, widens and shows an increase in mesangial matrix, with expansion of the mesangial cell cytoplasmic foot processes which can grow round the capillary between the endothelium and the basement membrane (Tribe *et al.* 1979). This interposition is associated with deposition of mesangial matrix in the

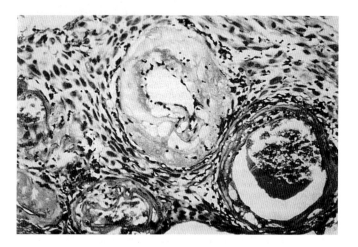

Fig. 3 Acute atherosis in a spiral artery in the decidua in a patient with pre-eclampsia. Fibrinoid necrosis around the vessel and intramural lipophages and a mild perivascular lymphocytic infiltrate are seen (reproduced from Robertson **1976**, with permission). H and E, 250×.

area between the basement membrane and the endothelium, which may be mistaken for apparent thickening of the basement membrane (Fox 1987). Deposits of IgM and fibrin may also be found, but there is no evidence of deposition of any other immunoglobulin or of complement (Fox 1987). Again, these changes are characteristic, but not specific to pre-eclampsia, as similar changes can be seen in abruption; they may be related to low-grade disseminated intravascular coagulation and fibrin deposition which can occur in both conditions. There is no major tubular damage in pregnancy-induced hypertension, although dilatation and epithelial thinning of the proximal tubules, hyaline deposition related to protein reabsorption, and tubular necrosis have been noted. The renal damage can be severe enough to produce acute renal failure, either through tubular or cortical necrosis (Lindheimer and Katz 1986). Although uncommon, this is more likely when there is further circulatory compromise such as when abruption complicates pre-eclampsia.

This damage results in a reduced glomerular filtration rate. Although creatinine clearance is reduced, the serum creatinine does not usually increase noticeably, because of the geometric relationship between clearance and serum creatinine. Plasma urea increases, again usually modestly. The most obvious evidence of glomerular dysfunction is proteinuria which reflects disease severity. It may be severe enough to lead to nephrotic syndrome. The mechanism underlying proteinuria is unclear, but it may be related to loss of the strong negative charge which normally repels proteins from the glomerular basement membrane. In addition, hypocalciuria is seen (Thong *et al.* 1991). While glomerular dysfunction is manifest as proteinuria, tubular dysfunction is associated with hyperuricaemia (Chesley and Williams 1945) due to increased resorption of uric acid, which is coupled to tubular sodium reabsorption. It has been proposed that the hyperuricaemia is of benefit as it acts as an antioxidant (Moran and Davison 1999). This reduction in uric acid clearance precedes the proteinuria and the decline in glomerular filtration rate indicative of glomerular damage (Moran and Davison 1999). Tubular, red cell, hyaline, and granular casts are also seen within the urine consistant with both tubular and glomerular damage (Leduc *et al.* 1991).

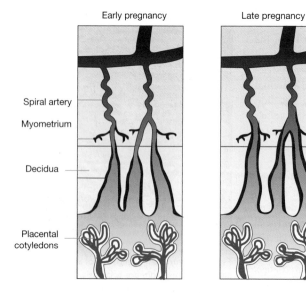
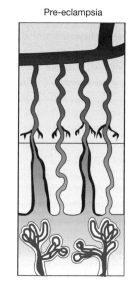

Fig. 4 Schematic representation of trophoblast invasion into the placental bed in normal early pregnancy, normal late pregnancy, and pre-eclampsia and IUGR (reproduced from Greer, I.A., Cameron, I.T., Kitchener, H.C., and Prentice, A. *Mosby's Color Atlas and Text of Obstetrics and Gynaecology*, with permission from the publisher).

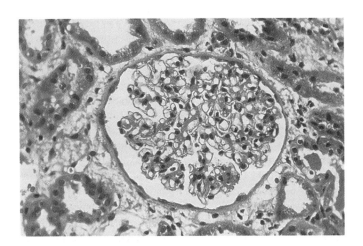

Fig. 5 Typical glomerular appearances in a patient with pre-eclampsia (H and E, 40×) (kindly provided by Dr George Smart, Edinburgh Royal Infirmary, UK).

The liver

The hepatic lesions seen in pre-eclampsia include lake haemorrhages, periportal fibrin deposition, and areas of infarction and necrosis (Sheehan and Lynch 1973). Thrombosis of the capillaries of the portal tract and small branches of the hepatic arteries is seen. These haemorrhages are thought to arise in the arteries of the portal tract, which show evidence of vascular damage similar to that seen in other sites. The hepatic lesions are likely to be secondary to activation of the coagulation system, endothelial damage, and vasoconstriction. The lesions are not specific to pre-eclampsia, as similar changes can be seen in obstetric haemorrhage.

Liver enzymes (transaminases and γ-glutamyl transferase) and plasma bilirubin are elevated. Clinical jaundice occasionally occurs, and may progress to hepatic failure. Subcapsular haematoma or hepatic rupture can also occur. Clinically, these changes may produce vomiting and epigastric pain and tenderness and are usually indicative of a fulminating disease process; however, they may be absent, and screening for hepatic dysfunction should, therefore, be performed. The epigastric pain and tenderness is thought to be caused by stretching of Glisson's capsule. Shoulder tip pain can occur with hepatic rupture and internal bleeding. Deranged liver function tests occur in around 20 per cent of cases, and are associated with severe disease and an increased risk of premature delivery IUGR (Romero *et al.* 1988). As associated neonatal morbidity is independent of the severity of hypertension and the presence of proteinuria, hepatic dysfunction may be an independent risk factor for both the mother and the fetus (Romero *et al.* 1988).

The brain

Eclampsia is an extreme clinical manifestation of pre-eclampsia. It is associated with cerebral vasospasm. A significant increase in cerebrovascular resistance occurs, but subsequent loss of cerebral autoregulation is associated with a fall in resistance and over-perfusion similar to hypertensive encephalopathy (Williams and Wilson 1999). This can persist for several days following the seizure. This alteration in perfusion contrasts with pre-eclampsia where there is increased perfusion pressure and increased cerebral resistance with no change in blood flow. The pathological features include cerebral oedema, cerebral haemorrhage, petechial haemorrhages, perivascular microinfracts, thrombotic lesions, and fibrinoid necrosis, secondary to endothelial dysfunction and

vascular damage. Cerebral oedema is not a constant feature, but may be seen on computerized tomography scanning of the brain in eclamptic patients. This correlates with the duration of intermittent seizures, suggesting that oedema is not the primary cause of the symptoms and signs of eclampsia or the cause of the seizures, but it is a secondary feature occurring after seizures. Magnetic resonance imaging also shows areas consistent with patchy cerebral oedema. Abnormalities are most commonly seen in the parietal and occipital lobes, in the watershed areas between the middle and posterior cerebral artery territories. It is not clear whether this oedema is intracellular, reflecting focal ischaemia or extracellular reflecting capillary leakage. Cortical blindness can occur, which may be due to oedema and/or petechial haemorrhages again resulting from vasospasm in the posterior cerebral circulation.

Vasomotor function

In contrast to the normal pregnant situation, a contracted plasma volume occurs in pre-eclampsia. This is associated with an increase in systemic vascular resistance, a normal or reduced cardiac output, and reduced cardiac preload (Clarke and Cotton 1988; Wallenburg 1988). This reflects increased peripheral resistance due to vasoconstriction.

Despite increases in plasma renin concentration, renin substrate, and AII in normal pregnancy, blood pressure falls. This is due to acquired vascular insensitivity to AII which is maximal in the second trimester, after which it slowly returns towards the non-pregnant situation (Gant *et al.* 1974) and is associated with downregulation of AII receptors (Baker *et al.* 1991). In pre-eclampsia, there is a loss of the acquired insensitivity to AII, which antedates clinical disease, and an increase in AII receptors (Gant *et al.* 1974; Baker *et al.* 1991). The insensitivity is not specific to AII and is found with other agonists such as noradrenaline. *Ex vivo* studies suggest that endothelium-dependant vascular relaxation is reduced, so implicating the endothelium in the increased vasomotor activity of pre-eclampsia (Ashworth *et al.* 1997). Furthermore, circulating plasma factor(s) may be involved in altering the endothelial response (Ashworth *et al.* 1997). The mechanism may be due to disturbance of or damage to key processes relating to vasomotor control.

Reduced production of endothelial-derived vasodilator prostaglandins, particularly prostacyclin, has been proposed, although the evidence is conflicting. Deficiency of the vasodilator nitric oxide, which is produced by the endothelium, has been evaluated, but results are again inconsistent. Similar inconsistent results have been obtained when the highly potent vasoconstrictor peptide endothelin has been measured in pre-eclampsia. Accurate measurement of these substances or their metabolites to reflect accurately the *in vivo* situation is difficult and the conflicting evidence may represent methodological difficulties. However, taken together, these results, assessing a variety of vasomotor agonists, are consistent with endothelial damage and/or dysfunction in pre-eclampsia, which is responsible for vasoconstriction and the increased peripheral resistance.

Coagulation, fibrinolysis, and platelets

The endothelium is intimately associated with the regulation of haemostasis and thrombosis; thus, its dysfunction will trigger activation of the haemostatic system as well as disturbance of the vasomotor system (see above). Platelet consumption in pre-eclampsia was pivotal in identifying that endothelial dysfunction, the key underlying pathophysiological mechanism in the disorder, was present. The coagulation disturbance ranges from subclinical disturbance to disseminated intravascular coagulation.

In normal pregnancy, there are significant changes to the coagulation system (Clark *et al.* 1998a). Coagulation factors such as fibrinogen, FVIII, and von Willebrand factor (vWF) increase. Fibrinolysis is reduced as there is an increase in inhibitors of fibrinolysis, particularly plasminogen activator inhibitor type 2 (PAI-2), which is produced by the placenta. There is a reduction in the activity of the endogenous anticoagulant system as resistance to protein C is acquired and proteins S levels fall (Clark *et al.* 1998a). Despite increased procoagulant potential, there is only a minor degree of activation of the coagulation and fibrinolytic systems with generation of fibrin and subsequent fibrinolysis resulting in increased fibrin-degradation products (FDPs) and there is no evidence of endothelial damage.

In pre-eclampsia, the widespread deposition of fibrin associated with vascular damage, such as acute atherosis, has long been known to be a pathological feature indicating that the coagulation system is activated, and the activation of which is more marked in the uteroplacental circulation (Higgins *et al.* 1998). There are also increases in coagulation factors such as FVIII and vWF, which exceed the changes seen in normal pregnancy. Platelet activation and consumption occur and progresses as the disorder advances, markers of platelet activation correlate with disease severity. Coagulation activation is unlikely to be a primary phenomenon in the disorder, and probably represents a secondary event consequent upon endothelial activation or damage. Nonetheless, it will still contribute to this damage, promoting positive feedback through further endothelial damage. Increased levels of thrombomodulin and fibrinectin reflect endothelial damage and correlate with disease severity. The possibility has been raised that fibrinectin and thrombomodulin levels in early pregnancy may be a predictive marker for the development of pre-eclampsia (Halligan *et al.* 1994; Boffa *et al.* 1998). Antithrombin, which binds to and inactivates thrombin, is reduced, in keeping with the thrombin generation and correlates with maternal and perinatal outcome. In particular, there is evidence that antithrombin levels correlate inversely with both the level of proteinuria and fibrinectin linking the consumption of antithrombin to endothelial damage and subsequent renal dysfunction (Clark *et al.* 1998a). The key trigger to coagulation disturbance may be tissue factor expression on endothelial cells. Tissue factor, which is now recognized as the major activation step of coagulation, is increased in pre-eclampsia (Bellart *et al.* 1999).

Interestingly, tissue factor expression is stimulated by cytokines such as tumour necrosis factor. This links coagulation activation to increase cytokine production and a proinflammatory state, which are now recognized to be present in pre-eclampsia. Concentrations of specific markers of fibrinolysis such as D-dimer are increased indicating that the fibrinolytic system is activated. There is an increase in the endothelial derived tissue plasminogen activator (tPA) in plasma reflecting endothelial activation. This increase in tPA is accompanied by an increase in PAI-1, again, reflecting endothelial activation, and a reduction in PAI-2, reflecting impaired placental function and/or mass (Halligan *et al.* 1994; Clark *et al.* 1998a). Routine coagulation tests are essentially normal, unless pre-eclampsia is complicated by disseminated intravascular coagulation. The normal prothrombin time and activated partial thromboplastin time and slightly prolonged thrombin time do not imply that significant coagulation activation is not occurring, as these tests are relatively insensitive.

Thrombophilia and pre-eclampsia

The widespread vascular damage of pre-eclampsia associated with endothelial dysfunction, enhanced coagulation, and fibrin deposition (Fig. 6) plays a role in the vascular insult leading to end organ damage such as in the kidney, brain, and placenta (Greer 1999a). IVGR is associated with thrombosis and placental infarction on the maternal side. Thus, thrombophilias could predispose a woman to these pregnancy complications. It is already appreciated that acquired thrombophilia, in the form of antiphospholipid antibody syndrome (APS), is associated with pre-eclampsia. Recent studies have shown that such an association occurs with several of the congenital thrombophilias, namely Factor V Leiden, the prothrombin gene variant, and hyperhomocysteinaemia found in MTHFR C677T homozygotes (Greer 1999b) with a concomitant dietary deficiency in B vitamins. These conditions are prevalent in around 2–7, 2, and 10 per cent respectively, of Western populations. For example, case–control studies have reported a two- to fivefold increased carrier rate for FVL (or abnormal APC resistance) in subjects with a history of pre-eclampsia and IUGR (Kupferminc *et al.* 1999; Greer 1999b; Martinelli *et al.* 2001). However, a recent large population-based study, published in conjunction with a meta-analysis,

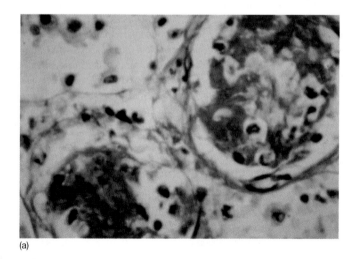

(a)

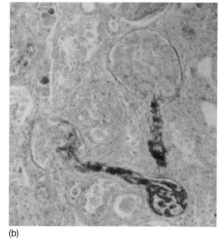

(b)

Fig. 6 (a) Fibrin in capillaries of the glomerular tuft in pre-eclampsia (Picro-Mallory 325×). (b) Fibrin thrombi in intralobular artery and afferent arteriole of the glomerulus in pre-eclampsia (John Bonnar, MD Thesis, University of Glasgow, 1970, with kind permission from the author).

did not find an association between pre-eclampsia and Factor V Leiden, prothrombin G20210A, MTHFR C677T, or platelet collagen receptor, $\alpha 2\beta 1$C807T, in a population of 404 women with a history of pre-eclampsia compared to 303 with gestational hypertension and 164 controls (Morrison *et al.* 2002). The meta-analysis of studies of pre-eclampsia and thrombophilia with appropriate inclusion criteria (Morrison *et al.* 2002) reported that there was no overall association between pre-eclampsia and Factor V Leiden, prothrombin G20210A, and MTHFR C677T homozygotes. However, when analysis was restricted to severe pre-eclampsia, there was a significant association with Factor V Leiden and with MTHFR C677T homozygotes with pooled odds ratio of 2.84 (95% CI 1.95–4.14) and 1.5 (95% CI 1.02–2.23), respectively. No association was found between severe pre-eclampsia and prothrombin G20210A (Table 4).

Another recent large case–control study has also cast doubt on the association between IUGR and thrombophilia (Infante-Rivard *et al.* 2002). This study of 493 newborns with IUGR and 472 controls found no increase in risk of IUGR (defined as birthweight below the 10th centile for gestation) among mothers carrying MTHFR C677T, Factor V Leiden, or prothrombin G20210A with odd ratios (ORs) of 1.55 (95% CI 0.83–2.90), 1.18 (95% CI 0.54–2.35), and 0.92 (95% CI 0.36–2.35), respectively. Even when the birthweight centile was reduced to the 5th centile and the analysis repeated, there was no relationship, suggesting that unlike pre-eclampsia there is no relation to disease severity. However, there was an association between MTHFR C677T homozygotes and IUGR in the subgroup of mothers not taking vitamin supplements (OR 12.3, 95% CI 1.2–126.2). Thus, the lack of association between IUGR and MTHFR C677T homozygotes may reflect the widespread use of multivitamins in pregnancy and emphasizes the need for consideration of plasma homocysteine rather than the genotype alone. In addition, there was no association with fetal thrombophilic genotype; indeed, homozygosity in the fetus for MTHFR C677T was associated with a reduced risk of growth restriction (OR 0.52, 95% CI 0.29–0.94). The difference between this study and previous reports are, firstly the size, and, secondly, the possibility of selection bias for subjects as the prevalence of various polymorphism was similar in the control populations in previous studies.

The reason underlying differences in results with regard to the association between thrombophilia and pregnancy complications are unclear. It may reflect different diagnostic criteria, small sample size, and reported bias as many studies had relatively low levels of heterozygosity for Factor V Leiden in the control groups studied. Nonetheless, these data suggest that prothrombotic genotypes may not be causative factors for pre-eclampsia, but may be linked to the severity of disease expression once the condition arises.

Acquired thrombophilic problems other than APS may also be relevant. Acquired resistance to APC occurs in around 40 per cent of pregnancies (Clark *et al.* 1998a) in Factor V Leiden negative subjects, and has been associated with around a threefold risk of pre-eclampsia (Clark *et al.* 2001). The underlying mechanism may be thrombin generation as acquired APC resistance correlates with levels of thrombin–antithrombin complexes, which correlate inversely with birthweight (Clark *et al.* 1999).

With regard to screening for thrombophilic abnormalities, there may be a place in *severe* pre-eclampsia to consider evaluating the woman for heritable thrombophilia and hyperhomocysteinaemia including their B vitamin status (folic acid, vitamin B_6, and B_{12}). However, if we do establish that a patient with a history of pre-eclampsia has an underlying thrombophilia, management is uncertain, except in hyperhomocysteinaemia, where B vitamin supplements, particularly folic acid, can correct the hyperhomocysteinaemia. Some extrapolation can be made from the benefits of the combination of aspirin and heparin in women with APS and recurrent miscarriage, but we have no evidence that such intervention, although logical, is effective in patients at risk of pre-eclampsia. Thus, if heritable screening is to be employed, it is important that we develop appropriate trials to determine the effectiveness of the intervention. Only when such evidence becomes available, can we weigh the advantages, disadvantages, and cost-effectiveness of screening and intervention for thrombophilia in pre-eclampsia.

Metabolic factors

High body mass index is an established risk factor for pre-eclampsia, in particular central obesity, which is in turn associated with insulin resistance. Pre-eclampsia is associated with insulin resistance and a dramatic increase in free fatty acids (antedating clinical expression of the disorder), and plasma triglycerides, well above that seen in normal pregnancy (Lorentzen *et al.* 1995). These changes are compatible with those seen in patients with coronary artery disease in terms of the pattern of lipoprotein subfractions (Kaaja *et al.* 1995; Sattar *et al.* 1997). The dramatic increase in triglycerides results in an increase in very low density lipoprotein (VLDL), small dense low density lipoprotein (LDL III), and decreased high density lipoprotein. Such hyperlipidaemia can directly induce vascular damage and dysfunction, and indirectly through enhanced oxidative stress, and also by potentiating insulin resistance (Hayman *et al.* 1999; Sattar and Greer 1999). For example, VLDL1 can stimulate endothelial expression of proinflammatory adhesion molecules such as VCAM-1, which in turn is involved with monocyte activation and transformation into macrophages. These macrophages may then take up lipid and so lead to the characteristic vascular lesion acute atherosis. The disturbance in lipoproteins is likely to be triggered or contributed to by a placentally derived factor such as increased cytokine expression, for example, the proinflammatory cytokine interleukin-6, which is elevated in pre-eclampsia (Greer *et al.* 1995; Clark *et al.* 1998b) and which enhances lipolysis. Alternatively or additionally, there may be reduced hepatic β-oxidation as there is a link between defects in maternal β-oxidation and HELLP syndrome, and pre-eclampsia (Sattar *et al.* 1996).

Thus, pre-eclampsia may be the pregnancy-associated maternal expression of an underlying metabolic syndrome. This response is revealed in pregnancy by a change in insulin resistance with subsequent enhanced free fatty acid flux, hypertriglyceridaemia, and

Table 4 Odds ratios for risk of pre-eclampsia on meta-analysis (Morrison *et al.* 2002)

Thrombophilia	Pre-eclampsia		Severe pre-eclampsia	
	Pooled odds ratio	95% CI	Pooled odds ratio	95% CI
Factor V Leiden	1.38	0.97–1.99	2.84	1.95–4.14
Prothrombin 20210A	1.15	0.62–2.15	1.76	0.79–3.91
MTHFR C677T homozygotes	1.03	0.83–1.28	1.5	1.02–2.23

subsequent endothelial dysfunction. Acute atherosis seen in the placental bed, similar to that seen in atherosclerosis in the non-pregnant, and the lipid accumulation in the glomerular endothelial cells noted above, would be in keeping with such a metabolic disturbance. The recent association between pre-eclampsia and cardiovascular disease in later life (Hannaford *et al.* 1997) might be due to similar pathological features or predispositions such as genetic polymorphism for key steps in the lipid metabolism pathway or cytokine function.

Inflammatory changes and oxidative stress

There is substantial evidence of inflammatory changes in pre-eclampsia. Neutrophil activation, confined to the maternal circulation, occurs (Greer *et al.* 1989a, 1991b; Barden *et al.* 1997; Redman *et al.* 1999) and may be an early part of the disease process. Neutrophils have also been localized to the placental bed in women with pre-eclampsia and this correlates with disease severity (Butterworth *et al.* 1991). Neutrophil activation results in release of a variety of substances capable of mediating vascular damage, including proteases, oxygen radicals, and leukotrienes. Neutrophil activation markers correlate with vWF levels (Greer *et al.* 1991a) so linking neutrophil activation to vascular damage. Monocyte activation is also present (Oian *et al.* 1985; Sacks *et al.* 1998). These inflammatory changes are over and above those associated with normal pregnancy (Sacks *et al.* 1998).

The leucocyte activation may be related to increased expression of cell adhesion molecules, which control leucocyte capture and activation, on the endothelium as increased E-selectin and VCAM-1 have been found in pre-eclampsia (Clark *et al.* 1998b). VCAM-1 is important in monocyte activation. As monocytes transform into macrophages which in turn can take up lipid, particularly where hypertriglyceridaemia is present, and become the lipid-laden macrophages characteristic of acute atherosis this may be a critical process in the vascular lesion of pre-eclampsia. There is an increase in proinflammatory cytokines in pre-eclampsia (Greer *et al.* 1995; Vince *et al.* 1995), which can stimulate adhesion molecule expression and leucocyte activation. As discussed previously, these cytokines may also influence the metabolic changes of pre-eclampsia. The associated increase in oxidative stress in pre-eclampsia is accompanied by a reduced antioxidant potential, so allowing the antioxidants to potentially provoke a greater degree of damage to the vessel wall, which is relevent to endothelial dysfunction.

The endothelium

The endothelium, as evident from the above discussion, is the victim of activation of many of the disease mechanisms in pre-eclampsia; increased free fatty acids, deranged lipoproteins, increased oxidative stress, increased cytokine production, coagulation activation, and leucocyte activation. It is not an innocent bystander, however, as such damage will trigger expression of adhesion molecules and promote coagulation activity so amplifying the response. The endothelium is consequently responsible for the wide diversity of presentations of this condition as endothelial damage accounts for all aspects of the pathophysiology (Roberts *et al.* 1989). Evidence of endothelial activation and damage include increased endothelin production, elevated levels of fibrinectin, increased concentrations of von Willebrand's factor, and PAIs.

Genetics of pregnancy-induced hypertension

Susceptibility to pre-eclampsia has an inherited maternal component, although its precise nature is unclear. Indeed, there is likely to be

a variety of genetic predispositions which can influence the maternal response to pregnancy of defective trophoblast invasion and lead to the clinical expression of pre-eclampsia. An association between eclampsia and miscarriage has been found (Cooper *et al.* 1988), suggesting that there may be a genetic basis for disturbance of the normal feto-maternal interaction in the placental bed that may predispose not only to pre-eclampsia but other pregnancy complications also. Segregation analysis had suggested that a single autosomal recessive gene model was consistant with pre-eclampsia (Chesley and Cooper 1986; Arngrimsson *et al.* 1990); however, it is now clear that it is likely to be a polygenic disorder with genetic heterogeneity (Broughton-Pipkin 1999). Genome-wide linkage studies or candidate gene association studies, such as the angiotensin gene variant M235T, have also been utilized. For example, possible linkage has been established for a region on chromosome 4q in Australian families (Harrison *et al.* 1987) but was not found in Icelandic families (Arngrimsson *et al.* 1999). The latter study identified a region on chromosome 2p13, which was confirmed in Australian and New Zealand families (Moses *et al.* 2000).

Thus, there are a wide variety of possible genetic associations. This reflects the multifactorial nature of pre-eclampsia. Pre-eclampsia is likely to represent a range of maternal response to abnormal placentation rather than a single disease entity. The various genetic components will contribute to a maternal phenotype which when challenged with the appropriate placental trigger will result in the clinical expression of the pre-eclampsia syndrome. The nature of this trigger is unknown at present, but could involve the paternal or fetal genotype possibly influencing the immunological response to placentation.

The pathophysiological process

Pre-eclampsia has a complex pathophysiology. However, what we see clinically as pre-eclampsia are simple facets to an abnormal or possibly exaggerated maternal response to pregnancy. The primary pathology in the placenta is not unique to pre-eclampsia. Nonetheless, there is clearly a placental trigger as the disorder is dependant on the presence of trophoblast. The trigger may be a signal which is important for the normal physiological response to pregnancy, but which is overexpressed in situations of placental damage or abnormality. Such is seen in 'classic' cases of pre-eclampsia where a small, infarcted placenta, which has not adequately invaded the maternal circulation is present. The signal may also be overexpressed in situations of increased placental mass such as twins or molar pregnancy which are associated with pre-eclampsia. Candidate triggers include placental cytokine production.

It is not simply the placental trigger which is important as IUGR which shares the same placental pathology often occurs without accompanying pre-eclampsia. Thus, the mother's response to the trigger is critical. Her response may depend on her genotype and/or phenotype. For example, women with central obesity and insulin resistance may be more at risk with an exaggerated metabolic response, women with congenital thrombophilia will have an exaggerated coagulation reponse or women with an underlying inflammatory condition such as systemic lupus erythematosus (SLE) will have an exaggerated inflammatory response. On first impressions, these mechanisms seem too diverse to explain pre-eclampsia. However, as discussed above, all these mechanisms are inter-related. An exaggerated metabolic response in terms of increased small dense LDL can trigger endothelial dysfunction with expression of adhesion molecules, coagulation activation, and leucocyte activation leading to further vascular damage. An enhanced procoagulant response to the placental trigger can similarly lead to endothelial damage with proinflammatory changes which may trigger metabolic change. An enhanced inflammatory response to pregnancy will result in similar endothelial responses. As all these mechanisms are inter-related and provide positive feedback loops leading to further vascular damage, a vicious circle is established. The vicious circle can be triggered from any point as the interrelations will ensure that the other processes are activated with the extent of each component dependant on the particular maternal genotype or phenotype. Those women who do not have a susceptible phenotype for pre-eclampsia might develop IUGR alone. This model, dependant on both a trophoblast trigger which could be of varying magnitude and maternal genetic and phenotypic susceptibility, can provide the wide spectrum of pathology seen from pre-eclampsia with gross multiorgan dysfunction, through to IUGR without secondary maternal pathology. One might ask why such responses occur. It is possible that pre-eclampsia is an attempt by the mother to compensate for poor placentation by increasing blood pressure to improve perfusion (this would be in line with the association between chronic antihypertensive therapy and low birthweight), and increasing lipids in an attempt to provide the fetus with a better supply of nutrients. These changes are at the mother's expense as they lead to vascular damage. Other women may develop pre-eclampsia not because of an abnormal placenta but rather a greater placental mass and/or maternal sensitivity, in this situation there may be no disturbance of fetal growth. In contrast, in IUGR alone the mother fails to compensate for abnormal placentation and shows no increase in blood pressure and fails to show even the normal lipid response seen in pregnancy (Sattar *et al.* 1999). Thus, her genotype or phenotype allows her to 'neglect' the growth-restricted fetus.

Management

Prediction and prevention

Although we know many risk factors for pre-eclampsia such as obesity, family history, and high blood pressure in early pregnancy, we have, at least at present, no specific or sensitive enough test to determine pregnancies at high risk. Hypertension is a risk factor for pre-eclampsia, but the clinical utility of a blood pressure measurement in early pregnancy has not been useful in practice, at least in part because of measurement errors such as digit preference and rapid cuff deflation. Ambulatory blood pressure monitoring has not improved upon this situation (Higgins *et al.* 1997). Biochemical tests that may have some benefit in prediction of pre-eclampsia when used very early in pregnancy include, inhibin, P-selectin, circulating interleukin-2 receptor, PAI-1 and PAI-2, leptin, and uric acid. The so-called 'roll-over' test assessing change in blood pressure on rolling the women on to her side was one of the earliest predictive tests (Gant *et al.* 1974). However, subsequent studies have shown that it is of little predictive value (Dekker *et al.* 1990). Increased pressor sensitivity to AII was considered to be one of the better predictors of pre-eclampsia (Gant *et al.* 1973) and was used to select patients in trails of prophylaxis (Wallenburg *et al.* 1986; Kyle *et al.* 1995). However, the test is impractical as a screening test for the general obstetric population, and Kyle *et al.* (1995) have reported a low positive predictive value (19 per cent). Isometric exercise, using a hand-grip exercise, provokes an increase in systemic arterial pressure in healthy adults. In pregnancy, an increase in diastolic pressure greater than 20 mmHg at 28–32 weeks gestation was associated with an increased incidence of pre-eclampsia (Degani *et al.* 1985) with a sensitivity of 81 per cent and specificity of 96 per cent. However, it is

time-consuming limiting its clinical value in practical terms. Thrombophilia screening (discussed above) may be relevant in women with a past history of severe disease but further information is required to establish the strength of the relationship and whether screening would be of value. High body mass index is an established risk factor for pre-eclampsia, in particular central obesity, which is, in turn, associated with insulin resistance. As pre-eclampsia is associated with insulin resistance and a dramatic increase in free fatty acids, antedating clinical expression of the disorder this may offer an opportunity for screening. Waist circumference in early pregnancy, a measure of central obesity and insulin resistance, is directly associated with risk of pre-eclampsia, emphasizing the contribution of metabolic factors to this disorder (Sattar *et al.* 2001). Women with pre-existing and gestational diabetes (Sermer *et al.* 1998; Sibai 2000) are at increased risk of pre-eclampsia. For gestational diabetes, the risk is about 10 per cent. For women with diabetes of short duration without renal or retinal complications, the risk is about 8 per cent, but for those with target organ damage such as nephropathy, hypertension, or retinopathy the risk increases to 16 per cent (Landon and Gabbe 1996). Women with pre-existing hypertension have an increased risk of superimposed pre-eclampsia compared to controls (21.2 versus 2.3 per cent) (Rey and Couturier 1994). However, the degree of risk varies with the severity of hypertension, for example, with a diastolic pressure of 110 mmHg before 20 weeks gestation the risk of pre-eclampsia is over 40 per cent (McCowen *et al.* 1996). SLE is associated with an increased risk of pre-eclampsia, which is mostly attributable to the presence of antiphospholipid antibodies, renal involvement, and disease activity at conception. APS with or without underlying SLE is associated with an increased risk of pre-eclampsia, which is more likely to be of early onset, ranging from 11 to 51 per cent depending on the underlying clinical manifestation (Moodley *et al.* 1995; Backos *et al.* 1999). Renal impairment regardless of its aetiology is associated with an increased risk of early onset pre-eclampsia with IUGR (Epstein 1996; Jones and Hayslett 1996; Jungers and Chauveau 1997).

Although epidemiological studies have shown a three- to fivefold increase in the incidence of pre-eclampsia in first-degree relatives of index cases (Mogren *et al.* 1999), this relationship is not consistent with a single gene disorder (see above) but rather a polygenic disorder with genetic heterogeneity (Broughton-Pipkin 1999). At present, the prediction by genotyping is not viable but a larger-scale genetic study of pre-eclampsia is underway at present.

The disturbance in placentation with a resultant increase in uteroplacental vascular resistance can be assessed by Doppler arterial waveform analysis from the maternal uterine arteries in the second trimester. Such studies have shown an association between high-resistance waveform patterns, particularly the so-called diastolic notch pattern, and pre-eclampsia (Bower *et al.* 1993), where the presence of persistent bilateral notching has been demonstrated to be associated with more severe complications (Bower *et al.* 1993; Harrington *et al.* 1996). Women with persistent bilateral notching, for example, have a 30-fold increased risk of requiring delivery before 34 weeks gestation for severe pre-eclampsia. In addition, 57 per cent of women with bilateral notching at 18–20 weeks, and 72 per cent of women with bilateral notching at 22–24 weeks had an adverse pregnancy outcome such as pre-eclampsia, or IUGR (Mires *et al.* 1998). Most of the studies in this area have been in women at increased risk as determined by known risk factors and recent studies have suggested that uterine arterial Doppler flow velocimetry has limited accuracy in predicting pre-eclampsia in low risk women (Chien *et al.* 2000).

Combinations of risk factors have also been used for prediction of pre-eclampsia. Stamilio *et al.* (2000) assigned a score based on the presence or absence of predictive factors clinical and biochemical risk factors but obtained limited sensitivity for prediction. In a recent study, Chappell *et al.* (2002) evaluated the predictive power of a combination of markers to predict pre-eclampsia in women already known to be at risk on the basis of their uterine artery waveform analysis. This study strongly suggested that a combination of a haemodynamic variable such as uterine artery Doppler waveform analysis and biochemical markers such as leptin or PAI-1/PAI-2 ratio may be useful in the prediction of pre-eclampsia.

Numerous clinical trials have been undertaken in the last 20 years with the aim of preventing pre-eclampsia, but have been hindered by the lack of a definitive predictive test. Primary prevention would involve identification and modification of the pre-pregnancy risk factors and some, such as obesity, may be more amenable to intervention than others. Secondary prevention by way of identifying mothers at risk and treating them accordingly is also disappointing.

The use of low-dose aspirin (60–75 mg per day) to prevent pre-eclampsia was based upon the rationale that pre-eclampsia is associated with alterations in the production of prostacyclin and thromboxane, secondary to activation of the clotting system and changes in platelet function. A recent meta-analysis (Duley *et al.* 2001), reported on 42 randomized trials involving over 32,000 women comparing antiplatelet agents to placebo or no treatment. Trials were subgrouped by maternal risk. Taking the cohort as a whole there was a 15 per cent reduction (RR 0.85, 95% CI 0.78–0.92) in the risk of pre-eclampsia associated with the use of antiplatelet agents. It was concluded that there are small to moderate benefits with antiplatelet agents in the prevention of pre-eclampsia, but further information was required to identify which women were most likely to benefit, when treatment should be started and what dose should be used. In practical terms, aspirin should be considered in the management of women with a history of severe or early onset pre-eclampsia or specific underlying medical conditions that place them at increase risk such as chronic hypertension, connective tissue, or renal disease—it seems likely that these women should begin prophylactic treatment early in the second trimester or sooner if they have a problem such as APS. It is clear from the randomized controlled trials that low-dose aspirin is not associated with adverse maternal or fetal outcome and in particular is not associated with an increased risk of abruption.

Low calcium intake has been linked to mechanisms that could provoke vasoconstriction and hypertension and pre-eclampsia appears less common in populations with high calcium intake. Calcium supplementation has, therefore, been considered in the prevention of pre-eclampsia. A meta-analysis of 10 trials of calcium supplementation in 6864 women, subdividing into low and high risk (Atallah *et al.* 2001), found a moderate reduction in the risk of pre-eclampsia (RR 0.70, 95% CI 0.58–0.83), but this was not significant for women with adequate calcium intake (RR 0.86, 95% CI 0.71–1.05) and less pronounced in women at low risk (RR 0.79, 95% CI 0.65–0.94). There is likely, therefore, to be no role for calcium supplementation for pre-eclampsia prevention in developed countries with normal calcium intake.

Observational studies showing lower rates of pre-eclampsia in populations with a high fish intake led to interest in using fish oil supplements (containing $n - 3$ fatty acids), to modify prostanoid production, and prevent pre-eclampsia. However, several trials have shown no reduction in the incidence of pre-eclampsia in the fish-oil-treated groups.

Most interest at present is focussed on antioxidant vitamin supplements, which may be of value because of the oxidative stress and reduced antioxidant capacity associated with pre-eclampsia. A recent randomized controlled trial investigated the early administration of antioxidants to over 300 women at risk of pre-eclampsia, identified using uterine artery Doppler ultrasound in mid-pregnancy or previous pre-eclampsia. The women were randomized to 1000 mg vitamin C and 400 IU vitamin E daily or placebos until delivery. The primary outcome of the study was a reduction in a biochemical index of the disease process, the PAI-1–PAI-2 ratio (reflecting endothelial and placental function), and the secondary outcome was pre-eclampsia. Vitamin supplementation was associated with a significant reduction in the PAI-1–PAI-2 ratio and an adjusted odds ratio of 0.24 for pre-eclampsia (Chappell *et al.* 1999). Although encouraging, this work urgently requires to be repeated on a larger scale. In women with established severe, early onset pre-eclampsia use of 1000 mg vitamin C, 800 IU vitamin E, and 200 mg allopurinol per day was not found to be of benefit (Gulmezoglu *et al.* 1997).

Assessment

There is no clear pattern to the timing of antenatal visits in relation to the development of pre-eclampsia. Many cases develop rapidly and can progress to a severe form within days of an adequate antenatal assessment. In view of the rapid development of some cases, even with regular antenatal assessment, it is important to ensure that antenatal education makes women aware of the types of symptoms associated with pre-eclampsia, its importance, and the need to obtain formal assessment. There is also a need for continued education of medical and midwifery staff, particularly, in the community, with regard to the implications of pre-eclampsia and the need for accurate diagnosis, assessment, and prompt referral, especially when proteinuria or severe hypertension is present.

It is clearly important to make a correct diagnosis (Fig. 7), being constantly aware of the multiplicity of possible presentations of this

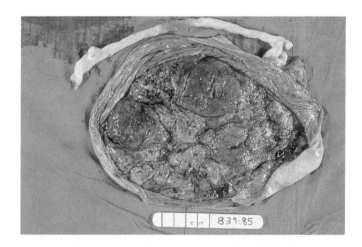

Fig. 7 An infarcted placenta: most of the cotyledons have been replaced by calcified and fibrous tissue and only two or three healthy cotyledons exist to sustain the fetus *in utero*. This patient had severe pre-eclampsia and intrauterine growth retardation and went on to have an iatrogenic preterm delivery because of fetal compromise.

disorder. The severity of the disease and rate of progression must also be assessed, necessitating not only a blood pressure profile and assessment and quantification of proteinuria, but also a full blood and platelet count along with biochemical assessment of urea and electrolytes, plasma urate, and liver function. Patients with fulminating disease will also require a coagulation screen.

The fetus should also be assessed, using methods appropriate for gestational age and the clinical problem. Ultrasound assessment of growth will be required in pregnancies where growth restriction is suspected. Regular assessment of fetal well being by cardiotocography or biophysical profile is also required. Doppler ultrasound assessment of the umbilical artery flow velocity waveform is helpful in identifying fetuses at high risk and has been shown to improve perinatal outcome (Figs 8 and 9).

The initial assessment can often be carried out in a day assessment unit especially in patients whose mild/moderate hypertension is picked up at a routine antenatal visit. Those who are symptomatic or severely hypertensive clearly require immediate admission and treatment, as do those with significant proteinuria or evidence of gross systemic disturbances. Patients with mild/moderate (non-proteinuric)

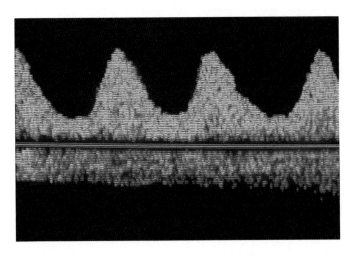

Fig. 8 Normal Doppler ultrasound flow velocity waveform from the umbilical artery in the third trimester.

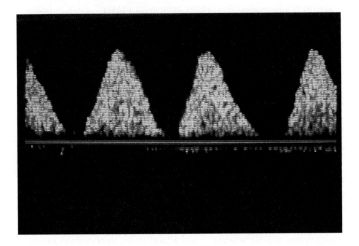

Fig. 9 Abnormal Doppler ultrasound flow velocity waveform in pre-eclampsia with loss of diastolic flow due to high resistance in the fetal placenta.

hypertension can usually be monitored as outpatients. The frequency and type of monitoring tests requires to be tailored to the patients' needs, determined by the severity of the disease and presence of fetal growth retardation. These investigations will provide information about the rate of progression of the disease. This will allow the obstetrician to make informed management decisions, including when to admit outpatients to hospital, how frequently maternal and fetal monitoring is required, whether antihypertensive therapy is required, the need for antenatal steroids to reduce the risk of respiratory distress syndrome, and when and by what route the baby should be delivered.

The aims of treatment are to protect the mother and fetus from the consequences of hypertension and to prolong the pregnancy, where required, to avoid the problems of prematurity. There is no doubt that substantial prolongation of pregnancy even in severe cases remote from term can be obtained by conservative management, with antihypertensive therapy and careful monitoring, in a significant number of cases. This will require a constant evaluation of the risks to mother and fetus of continuing the pregnancy against those of delivery, to optimize the situation for both patients. There is little place for conservative mangement of women with proteinuric disease at 34 weeks gestation. In women with eclampsia, symptomatic disease (e.g. visual disturbance or epigastric pain), pulmonary oedema, gross hepatic dysfunction, coagulopathy, and renal compromise are usually indications for immediate delivery.

Antihypertensive therapy

Pregnancy-induced hypertension and pre-eclampsia are curable: delivery will remove the disease. The philosophy of treatment is to protect the mother from the effects of severe hypertension, such as cerebrovascular haemorrhage and eclampsia, and to attempt to reduce the disease progression and prolong the pregnancy, where this is desirable, reducing the risks of iatrogenic prematurity. The earlier in pregnancy the patient presents, the greater the justification in attempting conservative management, even in those with severe hypertension.

Antihypertensive treatment is essential in severe hypertension. It is important to treat both systolic and diastolic hypertensions. Sometimes systolic hypertension is ignored inadvertently as the focus on the disease classification is on diastolic pressure. A systolic blood pressure of 170 mmHg or a diastolic pressure of 110 mmHg requires antihypertensive treatment to protect the mother from cerebral haemorrhage, cardiac failure, and placental abruption. Treatment should aim to reduce the blood pressure to less than 160/110 mmHg or mean arterial pressure less than 125 mmHg.

The value of antihypertensives in mild/moderate disease (blood pressure < 160/110 mmHg) is unclear. There may be a reduction in the development of proteinuria, severe hypertension, and IRDS, but there is no benefit in terms of gestation at delivery or obstetric intervention (Duley 1994; Magee *et al.* 1999). There is also no compelling evidence to suggest that any one drug is better than another (Magee *et al.* 1999). Recently, a meta-analysis has shown that reduction in blood pressure is associated with an increased risk of IUGR (von Dadelszen *et al.* 2000). Thus, the risk–benefit profile in mild/moderate disease requires to be re-examined.

A stepwise approach to the use of antihypertensive therapy is required with first-line, second-line, and third-line agents. First-line therapy is either methyldopa or an adrenoceptor antagonist such as labetalol, atenolol, or oxprenolol. Second-line therapy is usually a vasodilator such as nifedipine. Third-line therapy will be either an adrenoceptor antagonist or methyldopa, depending on which of these agents was employed as first-line therapy. A suitable regime is labetalol 200 mg thrice daily increasing to 300 mg four times daily as required. If blood pressure is not controlled, then nifedipine is added, using long-acting preparations such as Nifedipine LA 30–60 mg once daily. Such therapy is usually sufficient; if blood pressure is not adequately controlled on this combination, the disease is usually sufficiently advanced to warrant delivery. However, occasionally a third-line agent is required and in this situation methyldopa is added, at a dose of 0.25 g two to three times daily increasing up to 1.0 g three times per day. Where an adrenoceptor antagonist is contraindicated, methyldopa is used as first-line therapy. ACE inhibitors and AII receptor antagonists should not be used antenatally.

Methyldopa

Methyldopa is the most extensively studied drug in the treatment of hypertension in pregnancy. Although now little used in the non-pregnant, its safety profile and efficacy allow it to maintain its position in pregnancy. It is the preferred agent for chronic therapy in pregnancy as β-blockers were considered to be associated with reduced fetal growth. However, this phenomenon appears on the basis of a meta-analysis to be related more to reduction in blood pressure rather than an effect of any one class of drug (von Dadelszen et al. 2000). This might be due to reduced placental perfusion and would fit with the hypothesis that increased blood pressure is an attempt by the mother to enhance placental perfusion and compensate for the failure in adequate implantation.

Although effective in blood pressure control, one drawback to the use of methyldopa is the frequency of side-effects reported in around 15 per cent of patients in one study (Redman et al. 1976b, 1977), including tiredness, loss of energy, dizziness, depression, flushes, headache, vomiting, and palpitations. However, only the incidence of loss of energy and dizziness were significantly different between the treatment and control groups. Long-term follow-up on the children from this study (Cockburn et al. 1982) has confirmed that there is no long-term adverse effect.

Adrenoceptor antagonists

There is a wide range of adrenoceptor antagonists, with varying receptor specificity and varying degrees of intrinsic sympathomimetic activity. Only atenolol, labetalol, and oxprenolol have been studied to any great extent in pregnancy (Rubin et al. 1983; Gallery et al. 1985; Pickles et al. 1989). These agents are often preferred by clinicians, due to the low incidence of side-effects associated with their use compared to methyldopa. They are highly effective as first-line antihypertensives and do not appear to adversely affect fetal monitoring tests, in particular cardiotocography (Rubin et al. 1984). Long-term use of adrenoceptor antagonists has been subject to several reports of an association with growth restriction, particularly atenolol (Butters et al. 1990), although labetalol has also been implicated (Sibai et al. 1987). As discussed above, this is likely to be related to reduction of blood pressure rather than an effect confined to a single class of drugs.

Infants exposed to atenolol *in utero* (Rubin et al. 1983) have been followed up after 1 year, and no harmful effects of treatment found (Reynolds et al. 1984). Thus, at least in the short term these agents appear to be safe for the fetus, although they have not yet been subject to the same extent of long-term paediatric assessment as methyldopa.

Both methyldopa and adrenoceptor antagonists are, therefore, suitable agents for the treatment of hypertension in pregnancy. The adrenoceptor antagonists cause fewer side-effects than methyldopa, and within the adrenoceptor antagonist group, labetalol has several theoretical advantages, such as an α-adrenoceptor antagonist function, over atenolol, although these are unproven value in the clinical setting. Atenolol does, however, have a slower onset of action and a flatter dose–response curve than labetalol. It is probably best for the clinician to use the agent he/she is most familiar with to obtain good control of hypertension.

Hydralazine

Hydralazine is used for severe and acute hypertension, and may be given by intramuscular injection, intravenous boluses, and continuous intravenous infusions; it is also administered orally in the chronic situation as a second-line antihypertensive agent. It acts by inhibiting contraction of vascular smooth muscle, although the precise mechanism of this is not clear. It has a delay in onset of action of 20–30 min, even when given intravenously, and is associated with tachycardia brought about by two mechanisms—a baroreceptor-mediated reflex tachycardia and prolonged stimulation of noradrenaline release. The stimulation of noradrenaline release may account for symptoms such as the anxiety and restlessness, as well as tachycardia seen following administration. Headache is a significant side-effect and may be due to dilatation of the cerebral venous circulation. These side-effects are unwelcome in the management of severe pre-eclampsia: the headache and noradrenaline-related effects may mimic the prodromal symptoms of eclampsia, confusing the situation. These side-effects can be reduced if hydralazine is used in conjunction with methyldopa or an adrenoceptor antagonist, which will inhibit the sympathetic effects and reflex tachycardia.

Hydralazine, although effective in reducing blood pressure, is far from ideal as a parenteral first-line antihypertensive, and labetalol and nifedipine are superior in terms of episodes of maternal hypertension, incidence of abruption, and caesarean section (Magee et al. 1999) and side-effects.

Calcium-channel blocking agents

Calcium-channel blocking agents such as nifedipine are established as first- and second-line agents in hypertension in the non-pregnant and pregnant (Constantine et al. 1987; Allen et al. 1989; Greer et al. 1989b). These drugs are potent vasodilators with a rapid onset of action when given orally (or sublingually). They act by blocking calcium influx into smooth muscle cells, so interfering with excitation–contraction coupling. A useful attribute of these agents is that the degree of reduction in blood pressure which they produce appears to be directly proportional to the pretreatment pressure. They have been shown to reduce vascular sensitivity to AII infusions in pregnant sheep (Lawrence and Broughton-Pipkin 1986) and also produce cerebral vasodilatation which may reduce cerebral ischaemia in eclampsia or severe disease.

They have no major maternal or fetal adverse effects. Despite the vasodilator effect of these agents, there appears to be little problem with tachycardia. Transient facial flushing, headache, and warm, sweaty extremities appear to be the most common side-effects. The action of nifedipine is potentiated by magnesium sulfate, producing profound hypotension, muscle weakness, and fetal distress, thus caution must be exercised in their concomitant use although the risk of serious interaction appears small.

Mild/moderate hypertension

Mild/moderate hypertension is usually picked up as a blood pressure between 90 and 110 mmHg diastolic with no proteinuria at antenatal check. These women should have a repeat BP measurement 4 h later. If hypertension is confirmed, basic surveillance of twice weekly monitoring of blood pressure/urine and clinical assessment of maternal and fetal well being is required. Full blood count, urea, and electrolytes and urate should be obtained. Enhanced surveillance is required if (i) the diastolic blood pressure is greater than 100 mmHg at gestations less than 37 weeks; (ii) the blood pressure increment is greater than 25 mmHg; (iii) there is clinical suspicion of IUGR; (iv) concern over maternal or fetal well being; or (v) abnormal biochemistry. This can take the form of thrice weekly assessment of blood pressure, urine and full blood count, urea and electrolytes and urate, and liver function tests. An assessment of the fetus should also be made including fetal growth, CTG, or biophysical profile (SOGAP 1997). There is no indication for admission or bed rest for these women unless further abnormalities are found such as evidence of fetal compromise or abnormal biochemistry, for example, deranged liver function tests or HELLP syndrome. Thus, care can be managed, effectively both clinically and in terms of cost, through a day care unit and/or in the community (Twaddle and Harper 1992; Duley 1993). The value of antihypertensive therapy is these women is uncertain. Meta-analyses suggest that it leads to a reduction in the development of proteinuric disease, severe hypertension, and IRDS, but there is no benefit in terms of gestation at delivery or obstetric intervention (Duley 1994; Magee et al. 1999). Thus, perhaps antihypertensive therapy should be reserved for early onset disease (<32 weeks) or diastolic blood pressure greater than 100 mmHg, although the reduction in proteinuria and severe hypertension may be of value in reducing the perceived need for intervention. The usual first-line antihypertensive agents are methyldopa or labetalol. As these women are at increased risk of chronic hypertension in later life, persistent hypertension 6 weeks after delivery will require investigation.

Severe hypertension and the fulminating pre-eclamptic patient

Severe disease usually requires admission to hospital for careful assessment. The mother's blood pressure should be recorded at least 4 hourly, proteinuria should be quantitated, and a regular enquiry made for symptoms. Investigations should include: urea, urate, and electrolytes, liver function, and full blood count. Coagulation screen should be performed if there is clinical concern or there is significantly abnormal or deteriorating laboratory parameters. The chest should be auscultated if there is suspicion of pulmonary oedema and a chest X-ray performed. Fetal growth and well being should be assessed.

Antihypertensive treatment is required and a target blood pressure should be set. Stepwise therapy is recommended with methyldopa, labetalol, or atenolol as first line followed by nifedipine which is best given as a long-acting form. As severe disease is often of early onset, the key objective is to prolong pregnancy without risk to the mother. An average prolongation of 2 weeks can be achieved with associated reduction in neonatal morbidity (Magee et al. 1999), but careful maternal surveillance is required with delivery if there is significant maternal compromise.

The use of anticonvulsants for primary prevention of eclampsia in women with severe disease has until recently been controversial and obstetricians varied in the anticonvulsant regime they employed (Duley et al. 1998; Gülmezoglu and Duley 1998). However, the international MAGPIE trial studying the primary prevention of eclampsia with magnesium sulfate has recently been published (The Magpie Trial Collaborative Group 2002). In this trial, 10,141 women with blood pressure greater than or equal to 90 mmHg diastolic or greater than or equal to 140 mmHg systolic, proteinuria greater than or equal to 1+, and with clinical uncertainty about whether magnesium sulfate would be beneficial were randomly allocated to receive either magnesium sulfate or placebo, given as a loading dose plus 24 h maintenance therapy. Maintenance therapy was either intravenous or intramuscular. Women in the magnesium sulfate group had a 58 per cent lower risk of eclampsia (95% CI, 40–71 per cent reduction) than those allocated placebo. This translates to 11 fewer women with eclampsia per 1000 women. Twenty-four per cent allocated magnesium sulfate reported side-effects (mostly flushing) compared to 5 per cent allocated placebo. There were no differences between the groups in any measure of maternal morbidity or perinatal mortality except for a 30 per cent lower RR of placental abruption. Thus, magnesium sulfate significantly reduces the risk of eclampsia for women with pre-eclampsia.

In view of the risks to the mother, conservative management is rarely if ever indicated in severe disease beyond 34 weeks' gestation.

These patients are also at risk of venous thromboembolism and prophylaxis with TED stockings and low molecular weight heparin should be considered both ante- and postpartum.

Fulminating pre-eclampsia, where the woman is symptomatic, with epigastric pain, headache, and visual disturbance, or where blood pressure is uncontrolled, or where haematological and biochemical investigations are rapidly deteriorating requires urgent, usually operative, delivery. The woman will be in high dependency care in a labour ward equipped and staffed for such patients. Management is best carried out by an experienced obstetrician and an anaesthetist. The patient must be rapidly assessed, treated, and monitored: monitoring, in addition to emergency biochemistry and coagulation status, will require automated blood pressure measurement, CVP monitoring, and hourly urine output. Although venous access is essential, minimal fluids (maximum 500 ml over 6 h) should be given to maintain access as these patients are overloaded with extracellular fluid, although they have a contracted intravascular volume. Excessive administration of fluids, such as dilute drug solutions, can easily result in fluid overload which is a serious complication of treatment as it can be followed by pulmonary oedema and/or ARDS which may be fatal. It is important to appreciate that oliguria is a common feature postpartum in severe pre-eclampsia. Fluid management can be extremely difficult in these cases and requires input from experienced senior staff and optimal assessment of fluid balance, circulatory status, and in particular, assessment for possible pulmonary oedema. Fluid management requires to be coordinated as a wide variety of infusions may be given such as blood products for coagulation failure and dilute drug solutions to control blood pressure and prevent seizures. One member of staff should, therefore, take responsibility for the overall fluid management. If a coagulopathy complicates the situation, this is best corrected by delivery combined with supportive administration of blood products such as platelet concentrate and fresh-frozen plasma as required.

Central haemodynamic monitoring in pre-eclampsia shows that cardiac output and heart rate remain normal while the systemic vascular resistance and arterial pressure are increased. The left ventricle is usually hyperdynamic and the pulmonary capillary wedge pressures are normal to low. The CVP is also usually normal or low but does not always correlate with the wedge pressure. The wedge pressures are sometimes high due to an excessive afterload, producing depressed left ventricular function or due to fluid overload. Pulmonary oedema can occur due to depressed left ventricular function, capillary leakage, and reduced colloid osmotic pressure due to hypoalbuminaemia. These possible multiple mechanisms mean that pulmonary oedema can occur without any significant elevation in CVP.

Prophylactic anticonvulsant therapy (magnesium sulfate) should be administered, and clearly blood pressure should be controlled. Hydralazine has been the main therapy employed in the past, but intravenous labetalol is highly effective and has several advantages, including a more rapid onset and fewer side-effects. The dose should be titrated to control the patient's blood pressure. A suitable regime is a loading dose of 50 mg labetalol intravenous, then continuing the infusion at 60 mg/h doubling the dose every 15–30 min (maximum 480 mg/h) until control is achieved. When good control is not obtained by labetalol or hydralazine, sodium nitroprusside infusions are highly effective but potentially toxic to the fetus: this is best used following delivery or immediately prepartum. Calcium-channel blockers can also be given in this situation. These can be used in addition to or as an alternative to labetalol or hydralazine.

Volume expansion and oliguria

As pre-eclampsia is associated with a contracted intravascular volume, volume expansion has been explored in severe disease in an attempt to lower blood pressure and increase renal and placental blood flow. The mechanism underlying the hypotensive effect of volume expansion with plasma protein solutions is not clear and appears not to be related to plasma volume expansion *per se* (Gallery *et al.* 1984). Although volume expansion has been reported as being of value, there are insufficient data to provide any reliable estimate of its effectiveness (Duley 1992; Magee *et al.* 1999). It is potentially dangerous, as it may provoke circulatory overload and pulmonary oedema. If it is to be employed, then central monitoring with at least a CVP line is mandatory to guide therapy. Volume expansion is usually combined with vasodilator therapy to facilitate the administration of volume expansion to an already contracted vascular compartment under high pressure.

As discussed above, the usual haemodynamic status of women with severe pre-eclampsia is an increased systemic vascular resistance, a hyperdynamic left ventricle, and normal pulmonary vascular resistance (Clark and Cotton 1988): this will usually be improved by volume expansion coupled with a vasodilator. If, however, the left ventricular function is impaired, due to the increased systemic vascular resistance, and pulmonary artery pressures are increased, as occurring sometimes, then volume expansion can potentially worsen the situation. Similarly, if there is increased pulmonary capillary permeability (diagnosed by pulmonary oedema on chest radiographs, with normal left ventricular function and pulmonary artery pressure), then again volume expansion with plasma protein solutions will worsen the pulmonary oedema by increasing the extravascular colloid osmotic pressure. Hence, the need for central monitoring.

Oliguria is common in severe disease due to reduced intravascular volume, vasospasm, and sometimes the effect of antihypertensive therapy. Prerenal failure can occur especially if there is a sudden reduction in blood volume such as with major obstetric haemorrhage. This may tip the patient into renal failure and acute tubular necrosis particularly if DIC occurs with haemoglobinuria. In the woman with pre-eclampsia

where urinary output is less than 25 ml/h for 4 h, the situation should initially be managed expectantly, if persistent over a further 4 h, then a fluid challenge should be considered. Recurrent fluid challenges require CVP monitoring. If the CVP is less than 4 mmHg and oliguria persists, then a further fluid challenge can be given. If the CVP is greater than 8 mmHg, then a careful assessment for pulmonary oedema (basal crepitations and oxygen saturation <92 per cent plus signs on chest X-ray) should be made. If pulmonary oedema is present, treat with frusemide 20 mg intravenous and if no response, give a further dose of 40 mg frusemide. With a CVP greater than 4 mmHg and no pulmonary oedema, the initial managment is expectant but a further fluid challenge should be considered. A dopamine infusion (1 μg/kg/min increasing up to 5 μg/kg/min) to enhance renal blood flow should be used in persistent oliguria unresponsive to volume expansion. Clearly, the urea and creatinine must be monitored in all cases and where there is any suspicion of renal failure developing, a renal physician should be involved.

Delivery

Delivery must be expedited by the most suitable route, decided upon by the obstetrician, who must assess the relative risks of abdominal and vaginal delivery, taking into account both the maternal and fetal state and length of gestation. In the absence of a coagulopathy, epidural analgesia is ideal for both abdominal and vaginal delivery. It will aid blood pressure control by reducing catecholamine release in response to pain, but should not be considered a primary treatment for hypertension. General anaesthesia can be hazardous in these patients: not only will they often have laryngeal oedema, making intubation difficult, but laryngoscopy may provoke extreme hypertension, with the risk of cerebral complications. This response can be ameliorated effectively by pretreatment with intravenous labetalol. Ergometrine containing preparations must be avoided in the management of the third stage of labour as this will substantially worsen the hypertension.

Pulmonary oedema and ARDS

Pulmonary oedema may complicate up to 3 per cent of severe cases with a mortality less than 10 per cent, around 70 per cent of cases occur postpartum. It is uncommon in well-managed cases. The preeclamptic mother is at risk of pulmonary oedema because of increased capillary permeability and reduced oncotic pressure. When hypertension is severe, the high afterload may also precipitate pulmonary oedema. It can occur with a normal CVP. It is unusual without other complications such as excess fluid or colloid administration, massive transfusion, sepsis, anaemia, or DIC. Dyspnoea and difficulty maintaining adequate oxygen saturation on pulse oximetry will usually raise suspicion, although other complications such as pulmonary embolism must be considered. It will require oxygen and diuretic therapy along with vasodilator and antihypertensive therapy for hypertension and associated high afterload. ARDS can complicate pre-eclampsia and is more common postpartum. Again it is very unusual without the presence of additional complications such as fluid overload, HELLP syndrome, aspiration, eclampsia, or underlying medical problem. Management is supportive therapy in an ITU with ventilation, maintainence of cardiac and renal function treatment of DIC and any infection. Mortality is around 50 per cent usually due to multiorgan failure.

HELLP syndrome

Haemolysis, abnormalities of liver function, and thrombobocytopenia have long been recognized as complications of pre-eclampsia, although they may exist without severe hypertension or gross coagulation disturbance. In 1982, Weinstein described 29 cases of severe pre-eclampsia or eclampsia complicated by microangiopathic haemolytic anaemia, elevated liver enzymes, and low platelet count. He derived the acronym HELLP; haemolysis (characteristic red cell morphology and lactate dehydrogenase >600 U/l), elevated liver enzymes (aspartate aminotransferase >70 U/l,), and low platelets (<100 × 10^9/l). The liver will show periportal haemorrhage and necrosis, fibrin deposition, and, in some cases, steatosis, emphasizing the overlap with acute fatty liver of pregnancy. This is not a distinct entity, but rather a constellation of well-recognized pathological features associated with pre-eclampsia. Nonetheless, the recognition of this syndrome is of value since it draws the clinician's attention to the wider ramifications of the disease process, which may be present even when blood pressure is not grossly elevated. These patients, regardless of blood pressure, must be regarded as having severe disease. They have a high incidence of further complications including DIC [although there will be underlying activation of the coagulation system which is not apparent on basic coagulation screening (Greer et al. 1985)], pulmonary oedema, ARDS, abruption, acute renal failure, eclampsia, and maternal death. There is also a high risk of neonatal morbidity and mortality, although this may not be higher than for women with pre-eclampsia when gestation at delivery is taken into account (Abramovici et al. 1999).

The most common symptoms are malaise in the days leading up to presentation and diagnosis, epigastric or right hypochondrial pain, nausea and vomiting, and visual disturbance. All pregnant women presenting with such symptoms should have this syndrome excluded, regardless of blood pressure, as up to 50 per cent may be normotensive by conventional criteria. This syndrome can present for the first time postpartum. Full blood count and a blood film are essential for diagnosis: a platelet count must be obtained and red cell fragmentation looked for. Biochemical tests are required: increased urate and elevated transaminases, and bilirubin are present. Various diagnostic criteria for thrombocytopenia (<100 × 10^9/l or <150 × 10^9/l) and AST (>30 to >70 U/l) levels have been used, but the author favours that of Sibai et al. (1986b) (platelet count < 100, LDH > 600 U/l, and AST 70 U/l) while recognizing that these criteria should not be slavishley followed in view of the very variable presentation of the disorder. A coagulation screen should be performed, as disseminated intravascular coagulation can occur. In clinical practice, this condition is frequently misdiagnosed. Conditions that may be confused with HELLP syndrome include viral hepatitis, cholestasis of pregnancy, cholecystitis, hyperemesis, ITP, thrombotic thrombocytopenic purpura, haemolytic uraemic syndrome, SLE, or acute fatty liver of pregnancy. Interestingly, a rare complication of HELLP syndrome that can obscure the diagnosis is mephrogenic diabetes insipidus due to resistance to AVP brought about by high levels of vasopressinase, which may, in turn, be the result of impaired hepatic breakdown of the enzyme.

These patients are best managed at tertiary referral centres in view of the complex nature of their condition and need for access to various medical disciplines. Management of such patients usually requires urgent delivery in the maternal interest, although conservative management especially remote from term has been utilized and is associated with an improved neonatal outcome. Conservative management must be balanced against the high risk of serious maternal morbidity, thus, delivery is the safest option for the mother. Blood pressure control, seizure prophylaxis, and careful maternal and fetal monitoring is required, and supportive therapy for coagulation disorders may be

needed. Abdominal ultrasound is useful if there is any suspicion of liver haematoma. High-dose steroid (10 mg dexamethasone 12-hourly) therapy may improve the haematological and biochemical parameters antenatally and may hasten the resolution of HELLP postpartum and reduce morbidity and need for additional interventions (Martin et al. 1997). There have also been reports of plasma exchange being beneficial in patients with severe problems and delayed resolution of the condition although the overall value of this therapy is unclear.

In the longer term, these women are at increased risk of pre-eclampsia (19 per cent) and IUGR (12 per cent) in future pregnancies, but risk of recurrent HELLP syndrome is low (3 per cent) (Sibai et al. 1995). There is no evidence, at least as yet, to suggest that these women are at increased risk of chronic hypertension and no evidence to contraindicate the subsequent use of oral contraceptives. However, if the woman has underlying chronic hypertension with superimposed HELLP syndrome, then the risk of recurrence is 75 per cent for pre-eclampsia and 5 per cent for HELLP as well as the increased risk of other complications, such as IUGR and abruption associated with chronic hypertension (Sibai et al. 1995).

Management of eclampsia

Eclampsia may be asymptomatic or may be preceded by the classical prodrome of headache, visual disturbance, and epigastric pain. Hypertension and proteinuria may not previously have been noted. It is important to be aware of the possible presentations to allow prompt and adequate treatment to be provided, especially in view of the limited experience that obstetricians now have of this uncommon condition. Our inadequacies in diagnosis of patients at risk are highlighted by the finding that most women have their first seizure while in hospital and have inadequate investigation prior to the siezure and also in many cases afterwards also (Douglas and Redman 1994). The need for support from regional teams with special knowledge of the problem has been highlighted in the past. The differential diagnosis will include epilepsy, coincidental cerebrovascular accident, a space-occupying lesion, infection, or metabolic disturbance, and such conditions may need to be considered and excluded, especially in patients with atypical or late onset presentation.

Guidelines for the management of eclampsia have been produced (Royal College of Obstetricians and Gynaecologists 1996). The objectives are to control convulsions and blood pressure, stabilize the situation, and effect delivery. The patient should be placed in the left lateral position, the airway secured, and oxygen given. Senior medical and midwifery staff should be alerted immediately. Intravenous access should be secured and intravenous magnesium sulfate given to treat the seizures (Table 5). An alternative to halt seizures is Diazemuls 10–20 mg intravenous bolus followed by magnesium sulfate to prevent further seizures. Secondary prophylaxis should be continued for at least 24 h after the last seizure.

Hypertension should be controlled with intravenous labetalol or hydralazine. A urinary catheter should be inserted and strict recording and control of fluid balance maintained. Pulse oximetry should be employed. A chest X-ray and arterial blood gases should be performed if pulmonary oedema is suspected. Frequent monitoring of full blood count to pick up red cell fragmentation indicative of microangiopathic haemolytic anaemia which can occur, coagulation screen, liver function tests, and urea and creatinine should be performed. Once seizures and hypertension are controlled, fetal well being can be assessed and

Table 5 Magnesium sulfate for treatment and prophylaxis of eclamptic seizures

Regimen for the intravenous administration of magnesium sulfate
Loading dose of 4 g given slowly over 5–10 min
Maintenance of intravenous infusion of 1 g/h
Recurrent seizures should be treated with a further intravenous bolus of 2 g
Serum magnesium levels can be monitored (therapeutic range 2–4 mmol/l)

Features of magnesium toxicity
Double vision
Slurred speech
Loss of deep tendon reflexes
Respiratory depression and respiratory arrest (treat with 10 ml of 10% calcium gluconate)

arrangements made for delivery. Caesarean section is usually required especially in primigravid women remote from term with an unfavourable cervix. Cerebral imaging is required to exclude haemorrhage in women with focal neurological signs or prolonged coma. After delivery, high dependency care should be given for at least 24 h.

In the past, other agents such as phenytoin and diazepam were preferred to control seizures. However, following the Eclampsia Trial Collaborative Group (1995) report demonstrating the superiority of magnesium sulfate over diazepam and phenytoin for the secondary prevention of eclampsia, magnesium sulfate has become the first and preferred choice for treatment and prevention of seizures. This study found that the incidence of recurrent seizure was reduced by 52 and 67 per cent when magnesium sulfate was compared with diazepam and phenytoin, respectively. There were no problems with magnesium toxicity despite no monitoring of magnesium levels being performed.

Magnesium sulfate does not cause maternal or neonatal sedation. Although its precise mechanism of action is unclear, it appears to have a peripheral site of action at the neuromuscular junction and does not cross the intact blood/brain barrier. It may, however, relax the constricted cerebral circulation in eclampsia.

Care following delivery

Following delivery, pre-eclampsia will resolve although the hypertension and proteinuria may take several weeks to do so. In the immediate postpartum period, pre-eclampsia may initially worsen; indeed, many cases of eclampsia occur at this time, before resolving and intensive monitoring should continue for at least 24–48 h. Thus, hypertension often worsens in the first week postpartum often reaching a peak 3–4 days following delivery. The antihypertensive regime used antenatally can be continued and dose adjusted and second- and third-line agents introduced as required to control blood pressure. Where there is a poor response, agents such as ACE inhibitors can be employed alone or in combination. As blood pressure settles, therapy can be withdrawn under supervision and monitoring, usually as an outpatient at the Day Care Unit. Methyldopa is best avoided where possible in the postnatal period as a side-effect is depression. Antihypertensive medication, including the ACE inhibitors are not contraindicated in breastfeeding. Women with a history of essential hypertension can recommence their prepregnancy antihypertensive therapy postnatally. Oliguria can be managed as discussed above.

Where the blood pressure remains elevated or severe disease has occurred, the patient should be investigated to exclude an underlying medical condition such as connective tissue disease, thrombophilia, or renal disease. This is usually organized around 6 weeks after delivery and counselling about future pregnancies and contraception will be required at this time also.

Pre-eclampsia increases the risk of venous thrombosis and these women should be assessed with regard to their thromboembolic risk and treated with low molecular weight heparin and/or graduated elastic compression stocking as required.

Conclusions

Pre-eclampsia is a multisystem disorder that represents an abnormal or exaggerated maternal response to pregnancy. Clinically, it is usually manifest as hypertension, proteinuria, and placental insufficiency, although its protean nature allows a wide variety of presentations. Pathophysiologically, the clinical features result from vascular endothelial damage and dysfunction. The trigger for the condition originates from the placenta, and is associated with defective trophoblast invasion and placental ischaemia or excessive placental mass. The trigger initiates metabolic, inflammatory, and coagulation disturbances, but the nature of these responses and their severity appear to relate to the maternal genotype and phenotype. Thus, problems such as congenital thrombophilia or central obesity may influence the way in which the disorder is expressed. It is essential to appreciate the widespread nature of the potential clinical problem to accurately diagnose it and determine the depth of the problem. Management at present focuses on controlling blood pressure and monitoring mother and fetus to optimize the timing and mode of delivery. However, antihypertensive therapy is not aimed primarily at the disease process, but rather at one of its manifestations. There is no established prophylactic therapy, although several areas, including antioxidant vitamin supplementation are under investigation. The development and application of primary preventive therapy is hampered by our lack of a reliable means of identifying women at risk. Much research is required to further unravel the enigma of pre-eclampsia, research which will require wide collaboration to address the problem in a coordinated and systematic way.

References

Abramovici, D., Friedman, S., Mercer, B. M., Audibert, F., Kao, L., and Sibai, B. (1999). Neonatal outcome in severe preeclampsia at 24–36 weeks gestation: does the HELLP syndrome matter? *American Journal of Obstetrics and Gynecology* **180**, 221–225.

Allen, J. *et al.* (1989). Acute effects of nitrendipine in pregnancy-induced hypertension. *British Journal of Obstetrics and Gynaecology* **94**, 222–226.

Arngrimsson, R., Bjornsson, S., Geirsson, R. T., Bjornsson, H., Walker, J. J., and Snaedel, G. (1990). Familial and genetic predisposition to eclampsia and preeclampsia in a defined island population. *British Journal of Obstetrics and Gynaecology* **97**, 762–770.

Arngrimsson, R. *et al.* (1999). A genome-wide scan reveals a maternal susceptibility locus for pre-eclampsia on chromsome 2p13. *Human Molecular Genetics* **8**, 1799–1805.

Ashworth, J., Warren, A. Y., Baker, P. N., and Johnson, I. R. (1997). Loss of endothelium dependent relaxation in myomertial resistance arteries in preeclampsia. *British Journal of Obstetrics and Gynaecology* **104**, 1152–1159.

Atallah, A. N., Hofmeyr, G. J., and Duley, L. (2001). Calcium supplementation during pregnancy for preventing hypertensive disorders and related problems (Cochrane Review). In *The Cochrane Library* Issue 2. Oxford: Update Software.

Backos, M., Rai, R., Baxter, N., Chilcott, I. T., Cohen, H., and Regan, L. (1999). Pregnancy complications in women with recurrent miscarriage associated with antiphospholipid antibodies treated with low dose aspirin and heparin. *British Journal of Obstetrics and Gynaecology* 106, 102–107.

Baker, P. N., Broughton Pipkin, F., and Symonds, E. M. (1991). Platelet angiotensin II binding sites in normotensive and hypertensive pregnancy. *British Journal of Obstetrics and Gynaecology* 98, 436–440.

Barden, A. *et al.* (1997). Neutrophil CD11b expression and neutrophil activation in preeclampsia. *Clinical Science* 92, 37–44.

Bellart, J. *et al.* (1999). Tissue factor levels and high ratio of fibrinopeptide A: D-dimer as a measure of endothelial procoagulant disorder in preeclampsia. *British Journal of Obstetrics and Gynaecology* 106, 594–597.

Bellomo, G. *et al.* (1999). Prognostic value of 24 hour blood pressure in pregnancy. *Journal of the American Medical Association* 282, 1447–1452.

Boffa, M. C. *et al.* (1998). Predictive value of plasma thrombomodulin in pre-eclampsia and gestational hypertension. *Haemostasis and Thrombosis* 79, 1092–1095.

Bower, S., Bewley, S., and Campbell, S. (1993). Improved prediction of preeclampsia by two stage screening of the uterine arteries using the early diastolic notch as colour Doppler imaging. *British Journal of Obstetrics and Gynaecology* 82, 78–83.

Brosens, I. and Dixon, H. G. (1966). The anatomy of the maternal side of the placenta. *Journal of Obstetrics and Gynaecology of the British Commonwealth* 73, 357–363.

Broughton-Pipkin, F. (1999). Genetics of preeclampsia: ideas at the turn of the millennium. *Current Obstetrics and Gynaecology* 9, 178–182.

Brown, M. A. and Buddle, M. L. (1997). What's in a name? Problems with the classification of hypertension in pregnancy. *Journal of Hypertension* 15, 1049–1054.

Brown, M. A. and De Swiet, M. (1999). Classification of hypertension in pregnancy. *Baillieres Clinical Obstetrics and Gynaecology* 13, 27–39.

Butters, L., Kennedy, S., and Rubin, P. C. (1990). Atenolol in essential hypertension in pregnancy. *British Medical Journal* 301, 587–589.

Butterworth, B., Greer, I. A., Liston, W. A., Haddad, N. G., and Johnston, T. A. (1991). Immunolocalisation of neutrophil elastase in term decidua and myometrium in pregnancy-induced hypertension. *British Journal of Obstetrics and Gynaecology* 98, 929–933.

Campbell, D. M. and MacGillivray, I. (1985). Pre-eclampsia in second pregnancy. *British Journal of Obstetrics and Gynaecology* 92, 131–140.

Catanzarite, V. A. and Willms, D. (1997). Adult respiratory distress syndrome in pregnancy: report of three cases and review of the literature. *Obstetrical and Gynecological Survey* 52, 381–392.

Chamberlain, G., Phillipp, E., Howlett, B., and Masters, K. *British Births 1970*, Volume 2: *Obstetric Care* 7, pp. 80–100. London: William Heinemann Medical Books Limited, 1978.

Chambers, J. C., Fusi, L., Malik, I. S., Haskard, D. O., De Swiet, M., and Kooner, J. S. (2001). Association of maternal endothelial dysfunction with preeclampsia. *Journal of the American Medical Association* 285, 1607–1612.

Chappell, C. *et al.* (1999). Effect of antioxidants of preeclampsia in women at increased risk: a randomized trial. *Lancet* 354, 810–816.

Chappell, L. C., Seed, P. T., Briley, A., Kelly, F. J., Hunt, B. J., Charnock-Jones, D. S., Mallet, A. I., and Poston, L. (2002). A longitudinal study of biochemical variables in women at risk of preeclampsia. *American Journal of Obstetrics and Gynaecology* 187 (1), 127–136.

Chesley, L. C. *Hypertensive Disorders in Pregnancy*. New York: Appleton-Century-Crofts, 1978.

Chesley, L. C. and Cooper, D. W. (1986). Genetics of hypertension in pregnancy: possible single gene control of pre-eclampsia and eclampsia in the descendents of eclamptic women. *British Journal of Obstetrics and Gynaecology* 93, 898–908.

Chesley, L. C. and Williams, L. O. (1945). Renal glomerular and tubular functions in relation to the hyperuricemia of preeclampsia and eclampsia. *American Journal of Obstetrics and Gynecology* 50, 367–375.

Chesley, L. C., Annitto, J. E., and Cosgrove, R. A. (1976). The remote prognosis of eclamptic women: sixth periodic report. *American Journal of Obstetrics and Gynecology* 124, 446–459.

Chien, P. F. W. *et al.* (2000). How useful is uterine arterial Doppler flow velocimetry in the prediction of pre-eclampsia, intrauterine growth retardation and perinatal death? An overview. *British Journal of Obstetrics and Gynaecology* 107, 196–208.

Clark, P., Brennand, J., Conkie, J. A., McCall, F., Greer, I. A., and Walker, I. D. (1998a). Activated protein C sensitivity, protein C, protein S and coagulation in normal pregnancy. *Thrombosis and Haemostasis* 79, 1166–1170.

Clark, P., Boswell, F., and Greer, I. A. The neutrophil and pre-eclampsia. In *The Endocrinology of Pre-eclampsia. Seminars in Reproductive Endocrinology* Vol. 16 (ed. S. Walsh), pp. 57–64. New York: Thieme Medical Publishing Inc., 1998b.

Clark, P., Sattar, N., Walker, I. D., and Greer, I. A. (2001). The Glasgow Outcome, APCR and Lipid (GOAL) pregnancy study: significance of pregnancy associated activated protein C resistance. *Haemostasis and Thrombosis* 85, 30–35.

Clark, P., Walker, I. D., and Greer, I. A. (1999). The acquired activated protein C resistance of pregnancy is associated with an increase in thrombin generation and is inversely associated with fetal weight. *Lancet* 353, 292–293.

Clarke, S. L. and Cotton, D. B. (1988). Clinical indications for pulmonary artery catheterisation in the patient with severe preeclampsia. *American Journal of Obstetrics and Gynecology* 158, 453–458.

Cockburn, J., Moar, V. A., Ounsted, M., and Redman, C. W. G. (1982). Final report of study on hypertension during pregnancy: the effects of specific treatment on the growth and development of the children. *Lancet* I, 647–649.

Constantine, G., Beevers, D. G., Reynolds, A. L., and Luesley, D. M. (1987). Nifedipine as a second line antihypertensive drug in pregnancy. *British Journal of Obstetrics and Gynaecology* 94, 1136–1142.

Cooper, D. W., Hill, J. A., Chesley, L. C., and Iverson Bryans, C. (1988). Genetic control of susceptibility to eclampsia and miscarriage. *British Journal of Obstetrics and Gynaecology* 95, 644–653.

Davey, D. A. and MacGillivray, I. (1988). The classification and definition of the hypertensive disorders of pregnancy. *American Journal of Obstetrics and Gynecology* 158, 892–898.

Degani, S. *et al.* (1985). Isometric exercise test for predicting gestational hypertension. *Journal of Obstetrics and Gynecology* 65, 652–654.

Dekker, G. A., Makovitz, J. W., and Wallenburg, H. C. S. (1990). Prediction of pregnancy-induced hypertensive disorders by angiotensin II sensitivity and supine pressor test. *British Journal of Obstetrics and Gynaecology* 97, 817–821.

Duley, L. (1992). Plasma volume expansion in pregnancy-induce hypertension. In *Pregnancy and Childbirth Module Cochrane Database of Systematic Reviews*. (ed. M. W. Enkin, M. J. N. C. Keirse, and J. P. Neilson). Review No. 05734, Cochrane Updates on Disc. Oxford: UpdateSoftware, Disc Issue 1.

Duley, L. Hospitalisation for non-proteinuric pregnancy hypertension. In *The Pregnancy and Childbirth Module*. The Cochrane Collaboration Issue 2. Oxford: Update Software, 1993.

Duley, L. Any hypertensive therapy for pregnancy hypertension. In *The Pregnancy and Childbirth Module*. The Cochrane Collaboration Issue 2. Oxford: Update Software, 1994.

Douglas, K. and Redman, C. W. G. (1994). Eclampsia in the United Kingdom. *British Medical Journal* 309, 1395–1400.

Duley, L., Gulmezoglu, A. M., and Henderson-Smart, D. Anticonvulsants for women with preeclampsia (Cochrane review). In *The Cochrane Library*. Issue 1. Oxford: Update Software, 1998.

Duley, L., Henderson-Smart, D., Knight, M., and King, J. (2001). Antiplatelet drugs for prevention of pre-eclampsia and its consequences: systematic review. *British Medical Journal* 322, 329–333.

Eclampsia Trial Collaborative Group (1995). Which anticonvulsant for women with eclampsia? Evidence from the collaborative eclampsia trial. *Lancet* 345, 1455–1463.

Epstein, F. H. (1996). Pregnancy and renal disease. *New England Journal of Medicine* **335**, 277–278.

Fisher, K. A., Luger, A., Spargo, B. H., and Lindheimer, M. D. (1981). Hypertension in pregnancy, clinical-pathological correlations and remote prognosis. *Medicine* **60**, 267–276.

Fox, H. Histopathology of pre-eclampsia and eclampsia. In *Hypertension in Pregnancy* (ed. F. Sharp and E. M. Symonds), pp. 119–130. Ithaca, NY: Perinatology Press, 1987.

Fox, H. The placenta in pregnancy hypertension. In *Handbook of Hypertension, Hypertension in Pregnancy* Vol. 10 (ed. P. C. Rubin), pp. 16–37. Amsterdam: Elsevier Science, 1988.

Gallery, E. D. M., Mitchell, M. D. M., and Redman, C. W. G. (1984). Fall in blood pressure in response to volume expansion in pregnancy associated hypertension (preeclampsia): why does it occur? *Journal of Hypertension* **2**, 117–182.

Gallery, E. D. M., Ross, M. R., and Gyory, A. Z. (1985). Anti-hypertensive treatment in pregnancy: analysis of different responses to oxprenolol and methyldopa. *British Medical Journal* **291**, 563–566.

Gant, N. F. *et al.* (1973). A study of angiotensin II pressor response throughout primigravid pregnancy. *Journal of Clinical Investigation* **52**, 2682–2689.

Gant, N. F. *et al.* (1974). A clinical test useful for predicting the development of acute hypertension in pregnancy. *American Journal of Obstetrics and Gynecology* **120**, 1–7.

Godfrey, K. M. and Barker, D. J. (2000). Fetal nutrition and adult disease. *American Journal of Clinical Nutrition* **71**, 1344S–1352S.

Grandone, E., Margagilione, M., Colazzo, D., Cappucci, G., Paladini, D., Martinelli, P., Montanaro, S., Pavone, G., and Di Minno, G. (1997). Factor V Leiden. C>TMTHFR polymorphism and genetic susceptibility to pre-eclampsia. *Thrombosis and Haemostasis* **77**, 1052–1054.

Greer, I. A. (1993). Ambulatory blood pressure in pregnancy: measurements and machines. *British Journal of Obstetrics Gynaecology* **100**, 887–889.

Greer, I. A. (1999a). Thrombosis in pregnancy: maternal and fetal issues. *Lancet* **353**, 1258–1265.

Greer, I. A. Platelets and coagulation abnormalities in pre-eclampsia. In *Handbook of Hypertension: Hypertension in Pregnancy* (ed. P. Rubin), pp. 163–181. Amsterdam: Elsevier Science, 1999b.

Greer, I. A., Cameron, A. D., and Walker, J. J. (1985). HELLP syndrome: pathologic entity or technical inadequacy? *American Journal of Obstetrics and Gynecology* **152**, 113–114.

Greer, I. A., Haddad, N. G., Dawes, J., Johnstone, F. D., and Calder, A. A. (1989a). Neutrophil activation in pregnancy induced hypertension. *British Journal of Obstetrics and Gynaecology* **96**, 978–982.

Greer, I. A., Walker, J. J., Bjornsson, S., and Calder, A. A. (1989b). Second line therapy with nifedipine in severe pregnancy induced hypertension. *Clinical and Experimental Hypertension* **B8**, 277–292.

Greer, I. A., Leask, R., Hodson, B. A., Dawes, J., Kirkpatrick, D., and Liston, W. A. (1991a). Endothelin elastase and endothelial dysfunction in pregnancy induced hypertension. *Lancet* **337**, 558.

Greer, I. A., Dawes, J., Johnston, T. A., and Calder, A. A. (1991b). Neutrophil activation is confined to the maternal circulation in pregnancy induced hypertension. *Obstetrics and Gynecology* **78**, 28–32.

Greer, I. A., Lyall, F., Perera, T., Boswell, F., and Macara, L. M. (1995). Increased concentrations of cytokines IL-6 and IL-1ra in plasma of women with preeclampsia: a mechanism for endothelial dysfunction. *Obstetrics and Gynecology* **84**, 937–940.

Gülmezoglu, A. M. and Duley, L. (1998). Use of anticonvulsants in eclampsia and preeclampsia: survey of obstetricians in the United Kingdom and Republic of Ireland. *British Medical Journal* **316**, 975–976.

Gülmezoglu, A. M., Hofmeyr, G. J., and Oostuizen, M. M. (1997). Antioxidants in the treatment of severe pre-eclampsia: an explanatory randomized controlled trial. *British Journal of Obstetrics and Gynaecology* **104**, 689–696.

Hall, D. R. *et al.* (2002). Urinary protein excretion and expectant management of early onset, severe pre-eclampsia. *International Journal of Gynaecology and Obstetrics* **77** (1), 1–6.

Halligan, A., Bonnar, J., Sheppard, B., Darling, M., and Walshe, J. (1994). Haemostatic, fibrinolytic and endothelial variables in normal pregnancies and preeclampsia. *British Journal of Obstetrics and Gynaecology* **101**, 488–492.

Halligan, A., Shennan, A., Thurston, H., de Swiet, M., and Taylor, D. (1995). Ambulatory blood pressure measurement in pregnancy: the current state of the art. *Hypertension in Pregnancy* **14**, 1–16.

Hannaford, P., Ferry, S., and Hirsch, S. (1997). Cardiovascular sequelae of toxaemia of pregnancy. *Heart* **77** (2), 154–158.

Harlan, J. D. (1987). Neutrophil-mediated vascular injury. *Acta Medica Scandinavica* **715** (Suppl.), 123–129.

Harrington, K., Cooper, D., Lees, K., Hecher, K., and Campbell, S. (1996). Doppler ultrasound of the uterine arteries: the importance of bilateral notching in the prediction of preeclampsia, placental abruption or delivery of a small for gestational age baby. *Ultrasound Obstetrics and Gynecology* **7**, 182–188.

Harrison, G. A. *et al.* (1997). A genomewide linkage study of pre-eclampsia/eclampsia reveals evidence for a candidate region on 4q. *American Journal of Human Genetics* **60** (5), 1158–1167.

Hayman, R. G., Sattar, N., Warren, A. Y., Greer, I. A., Johnson, I. R., and Baker, P. N. (1999). Relationship between myometrial resistance artery behaviour and circulating lipid composition. *American Journal of Obstetrics and Gynecology* **180**, 381–386.

He, S., Silveira, A., Hamsten, A., Blomback, M., and Bremme, K. (1999). Haemostatic, endothelial and lipoprotein parameters and blood pressure levels in women with a history of pre-eclampsia. *Thrombosis and Haemostasis* **81**, 538–542.

Higgins, J. R., Walshe, J. J., Halligan, A., O'Brien, E., Conroy, R., and Darling, M. R. (1997). Can 24-hour ambulatory blood pressure measurement predict the development of hypertension in primigravidae? *British Journal of Obstetrics and Gynaecology* **104**, 356–362.

Higgins, J. R., Walshe, J. J., Darling, M. R. N., Norris, L., and Bonnar, J. (1998). Hemostasis in the uteroplacental and peripheral circulations in normotensive and preeclamptic pregnancies. *American Journal of Obstetrics and Gynecology* **179** (2), 520–526.

Infante-Rivard, C. *et al.* (2002). Absence of association of thrombophilic polymorphism with intrauterine growth restriction. *New England Journal of Medicine* **347**, 19–25.

Jones, D. C. and Hayslett, J. P. (1996). Outcome of pregnancy in women with moderate or severe renal insufficiency. *New England Journal of Medicine* **335**, 226–232.

Jonsdottir, L. S., Arngrimsson, R., Geirsson, R. T., Sigvaldason, H., and Sigfusson, N. (1995). Death rates from ischaemic heart disease in women with a history of hypertension in pregnancy. *Acta Obstetrica Gynaecologica Scandinavica* **74**, 772–776.

Jungers, P. and Chauveau, D. (1997). Pregnancy in renal disease. *Kidney International* **52**, 871–885.

Kaaja, R., Tikkanen, M. J., Viinikka, L., and Ylikorkala, O. (1995). Serum lipoproteins, insulin and urinary prostanoid metabolites in normal and hypertensive pregnant women. *Obstetrics and Gynecology* **85** (3), 353–356.

Khong, T. Y., de Wolf, F., Robertson, W. B., and Brosens, I. (1986). Inadequate maternal vascular response to placentation in pregnancies complicated by preeclampsia and by small-for-gestational-age infants. *British Journal of Obstetrics and Gynecology* **93**, 1049–1059.

Kupferminc, M. J. *et al.* (1999). Increased frequency of genetic thrombophilia in women with complications of pregnancy. *New England Journal of Medicine* **340**, 9–13.

Kyle, P. M., Buckley, D., Kissane, J., de Swiet, M., and Redman, C. W. (1995). The angiotensin sensitivity test and low-dose aspirin are ineffective methods to predict and prevent hypertensive disorders in pregnancy. *American Journal of Obstetrics and Gynecology* **173**, 865–872.

Labarrere, C. A. (1988). Acute atherosis. A histopathological hallmark of immune aggression. *Placenta* **9**, 95–108.

Laivuori, H., Tikkanen, M. J., and Ylikorkala, O. (1996). Hyperinsulinaemia 17 years after pre-eclamptic first pregnancy. *Journal of Clinical Endocrinology and Metabolism* **81**, 2908–2911.

Landon, M. B. and Gabbe, S. G. Diabetes mellitus. In *High Risk Pregnancy: Management Options* (ed. D. K. James, P. J. Steer, C. P. Weiner, and B. Gonik). Philadelphia: W.B. Saunders Company Ltd., 1996.

Lawlor, D. A., Davey Smith, G., and Ebrahim, S. (2002). Birth weight of offspring and insulin resistance in late adulthood: a cross sectional survey. *British Medical Journal* **325**, 359–362.

Lawrence, M. R. and Broughton-Pipkin, F. (1986). Effects of nitrendipine on cardiovascular parameters in conscious pregnant sheep. *Abstracts of the 5th International Congress of the International Society for the Study of Hypertension in Pregnancy*, Nottingham.

Leduc, L., Lederer, E., Lee, W., and Cotton, D. B. (1991). Urinary sediment changes in severe preeclampsia. *Obstetrics and Gynecology* **77**, 186–189.

Lindheimer, M. D. and Katz, A. I. The kidney in pregnancy. In *The Kidney* (ed. B. M. Brenner and F. C. Rector), pp. 1253–1295. Philadelphia: W.B. Saunders, 1986.

Lorentzen, B., Drevon, C. A., Endresen, M. J., and Henriksen, T. (1995). Fatty acid pattern of esterified and free fatty acids in sera of women with normal and pre-eclamptic pregnancy. *British Journal of Obstetrics and Gynaecology* **102**, 530–537.

Magee, L. A., Ornstein, M. P., and van Dadelszen, P. (1999). Management of hypertension in pregnancy. *British Medical Journal* **318**, 1322–1336.

Mabie, W. C., Barton, J. R., and Sibai, B. M. (1992). Adult respiratory distress syndrome in pregnancy. *American Journal of Obstetrics and Gynecology* **167**, 950–957.

Macara, L., Kingdom, J. C. P., Kohnen, G., Bowman, A. W., Greer, I. A., and Kaufman, P. (1995). Elaboration of stem villous vessels in growth restricted pregnancies with abnormal umbilical artery doppler waveforms. *British Journal of Obstetrics and Gynaecology* **102**, 807–812.

McFadyen, I. R., Greenhouse, P., Price, A. B., and Geirsson, R. T. (1986). The relation between plasma urate and placental bed vascular adaptation to pregnancy. *British Journal of Obstetrics and Gynaecology* **93**, 482–487.

McCowan, L. E. *et al.* (1996). Perinatal morbidity in chronic hypertension. *British Journal of Obstetrics and Gynaecology* **103**, 123–129.

MacGillivray, I., Rose, G. A., and Rowe, D. (1969). Blood pressure survey in pregnancy. *Clinical Science* **37**, 395–407.

Moran, P. and Davison, J. M. (1999). The kidney and the pathogenesis of preeclampsia. *Current Obstetrics and Gynaecology* **9**, 196–202.

Martin, J. N. *et al.* (1997). Better maternal outcomes are achieved with dexamethasone therapy for postpartum HELLP syndrome. *American Journal of Obstetrics and Gynecology* **177**, 1011–1017.

Martinelli, P. *et al.* (2001). Familial thrombophilias and the occurrence of fetal growth restriction. *Haematologica* **86**, 428–431.

Mogren, I., Hogberg, U., Winkvist, A., and Stenlund, H. (1999). Familiar occurrence of preeclampsia. *Epidemiology* **10**, 18–22.

Morrison, E. R. *et al.* (2002). Prothrombotic genotypes are not associated with preeclampsia and gestational hypertension: results from a large population-based study and systematic review. *Thrombosis and Haemostasis* **87**, 779–785.

Moses, E. K. *et al.* (2000). A genome scan in Australian and New Zealand families confirms the presence of a maternal susceptibility locus for pre-eclampsia on chromosome 2. *American Journal of Human Genetics* **67**, 1581–1585.

Moodley, J. *et al.* (1995). The association of APA with severe early-onset pre-eclampsia. *South African Medical Journal* **85**, 105–107.

Mires, G. J., Williams, F. L. R., Leslie, J., and Howie, P. W. (1998). Uterine notching as a screening test for adverse pregnancy outcome. *American Journal of Obstetrics and Gynecology* **179**, 1317–1323.

Naeye, R. L. and Friedman, E. A. (1979). Causes of perinatal death associated with gestational hypertension and proteinuria. *American Journal of Obstetrics and Gynecology* **133**, 8–10.

Natarajan, P., Shennan, A. H., Penny, J., Halligan, A. W., de Swiet, M., and Anthony, J. (1999). Comparison of auscultatory and oscillometric automated blood pressure monitors in the setting of preeclampsia. *American Journal of Obstetrics and Gynecology* **181** (5), 1203–1210.

National Institute of Clinical Excellence, Welsh Office, Scottish Home and Health Department and Department of Health and Social Services Northern Ireland. *Confidential Enquiries into Maternal Deaths in the United Kingdom 1997–1999*. London: RCOG, 2001.

Oian, P., Omsjo, I., Maltau, J. M., and Osterud, B. (1985). Increased sensitivity to thromboplastin synthesis in blood monocytes from preeclamptic patients. *British Journal of Obstetrics and Gynaecology* **92**, 511–517.

Pickles, C. J., Symonds, E. M., and Broughton Pipkin, F. (1989). The fetal outcome in a randomised double blind controlled trial of labetalol versus placebo in pregnancy-induced hypertension. *British Journal of Obstetrics and Gynaecology* **96**, 38–43.

Redman, C. W. G. Hypertension in pregnancy. In *Medical Disorders in Obstetric Practice* (ed. M. de Swiet), pp. 249–305. Oxford: Blackwell Scientific Publications, 1989.

Redman, C. W. G. Hypertension in pregnancy. In *Turnbull's Obstetrics* (ed. G. Chamberlain), pp. 441–469. Edinburgh: Churchill Livingstone, 1995.

Redman, C. W. G. and Jeffries, M. (1988). Revised definition of pre-eclampsia. *Lancet* I, 809–812.

Redman, C. W. G., Beilin, L. J., Bonnar, J., and Ounsted, M. K. (1976a). Plasma urate measurements in predicting fetal death in hypertensive pregnancy. *Lancet* I, 1370–1373.

Redman, C. W. G., Beilin, L. J., Bonnar, J., and Ounsted, M. K. (1976b). Fetal outcome in trial of antihypertensive treatment in pregnancy. *Lancet* II, 753–756.

Redman, C. W. G., Beilin, L. J., and Bonnar, J. Variability of blood pressure in normal and abnormal pregnancy. In *Hypertension in Pregnancy* (ed. M. D. Lindheimer, A. I. Katz, and F. P. Zuspan), pp. 53–60. New York: Wiley, 1976c.

Redman, C. W. G., Beilin, L. J., and Bonnar, J. (1977). Treatment of hypertension in pregnancy with methyldopa: blood pressure control and side effects. *British Journal of Obstetrics and Gynaecology* **84**, 419–426.

Redman, C. W. G., Sacks, G. P., and Sargent, I. L. (1999). Preeclampsia: an excessive maternal inflammatory response to pregnancy. *American Journal of Obstetrics and Gynecology* **180** (2), 499–506.

Rey, E. and Couturier, A. (1994). The prognosis of pregnancy in women with chronic hypertension. *American Journal of Obstetrics and Gynecology* **171**, 410–416.

Reynolds, B., Butters, L., Evans, J., Adams, T., and Rubin, P. C. (1984). First year of life after the use of atenolol in pregnancy associated hypertension. *Archives of Diseases of Children* **59**, 1061–1063.

Robert, M., Sepandi, F., Liston, R. M., and Dooley, K. C. (1997). Random protein–creatinine ratio for the quantification of proteinuria in pregnancy. *American Journal of Obstetrics and Gynecology* **90**, 893–895.

Roberts, J. M., Taylor, R. N., Musci, T. J., Rodgers, G. M., Hubel, C. A., and McLaughlin, M. K. (1989). Preeclampsia: an endothelial cell disorder. *American Journal of Obstetrics and Gynecology* **161**, 1200–1204.

Robertson, E. G. (1971). The natural history of oedema during pregnancy. *Journal of Obstetrics and Gynaecology of the British Commonwealth* **78**, 520–529.

Robertson, W. B. and Khong, T. Y. Pathology of the uteroplacental bed. In *Hypertension in Pregnancy* (ed. F. Sharp and E. M. Symonds), pp. 101–113. Ithaca, NY: Perinatology Press, 1987.

Robillard, P. Y. and Hulsey, T. C. (1996). Association of pregnancy-induced hypertension, preeclampsia and eclampsia with duration of sexual cohabitation before conception. *Lancet* **374**, 619.

Romero, R. *et al.* (1988). Clinical significance of liver dysfunction in pregnancy-induced hypertension. *American Journal of Perinatology* **5**, 146–151.

Royal College of Obstetricians and Gynaecologists. *Management of Eclampsia*. RCOG Guideline Number 10. RCOG Press: London, 1996.

Rubin, P. C. *et al.* (1983). Placebo controlled trial of atenolol in treatment of pregnancy associated hypertension. *Lancet* I, 431–434.

Rubin, P. C. *et al.* (1984). Obstetric aspects of the use in pregnancy-associated hypertension of the β-adrenoceptor antagonist atenolol. *American Journal of Obstetrics and Gynecology* **150**, 389–392.

Sacks, G. P., Studena, K., Sargent, I. L., and Redman, C. W. (1998). Normal pregnancy and preeclampsia both produce inflammatory changes in peripheral blood leukocytes akin to those of sepsis. *American Journal of Obstetrics and Gynecology* **179**, 80–86.

Sattar, N. and Greer, I. A. (1999). Lipids and the pathogenesis of pre-eclampsia. *Current Obstetrics and Gynecology* **9**, 190–195.

Sattar, N. and Greer, I. A. (2002). Pregnancy complications and maternal cardiovascular risk: opportunities for intervention and screening? *British Medical Journal* **325**, 157–160.

Sattar, N., Clark, P., Lean, M., Holmes, A., Walker, I., and Greer, I. A. (2001). Antenatal waist circumference and hypertension risk. *Obstetrics and Gynaecology* **97** (2), 268–271.

Sattar, N., Gaw, A., Packard, C. J., and Greer, I. A. (1996). Potential pathogenic roles of aberrant lipoprotein and fatty acid metabolism in pre-eclampsia. *British Journal of Obstetrics and Gynaecology* **103**, 614–620.

Sattar, N., Greer, I. A., Packard, C. J., Kelly, T., and Mathers, A. M. (1999). A failure of LDL-cholesterol rise in pregnancies complicated by intrauterine growth restriction. *Journal of Clinical Endocrinology and Metabolism* **84**, 128–130.

Sattar, N. *et al.* (1997). Lipoprotein subfraction concentrations in pre-eclampsia: pathogenic parallels to atherosclerosis. *Obstetrics and Gynecology* **89**, 403–408.

Saudan, P. J., Brown, M. A., Farrel, T., and Shaw, L. (1997). Improved methods of assessing proteinuria in hypertensive pregnancy. *British Journal of Obstetrics and Gynaecology* **104**, 159–164.

Sermer, M. *et al.* (1998). The Toronto Tri-Hospital Gestational Project. *Diabetes Care* **21** (Suppl. 2), B33–B42.

Shanklin, D. R. and Sibai, B. M. (1989). Ultrastructural aspects of pre-eclampsia. *American Journal of Obstetrics and Gynecology* **161**, 735–741.

Sheehan, H. L. and Lynch, J. B. *Pathology of Toxaemia of Pregnancy*. London: Churchill Livingstone, 1973.

Sheppard, B. L. and Bonnar, J. (1981). An ultrastructural study of uteroplacental spiral arteries in hypertensive and normotensive pregnancy and fetal growth retardation. *British Journal of Obstetrics and Gynaecology* **88**, 695–705.

Sibai, B. A. (2000). Risk factors, pregnancy complications, and prevalence of hypertensive disorders in women with pregravid diabetes mellitus. *The Journal of Maternal–Fetal and Neonatal Medicine* **9**, 62–65.

Sibai, B. M., El-Nazer, A., and Gonzalez-Ruiz, A. (1986a). Severe pre-eclampsia–eclampsia in young primigravid women: subsequent pregnancy outcome and remote prognosis. *American Journal of Obstetrics and Gynecology* **155**, 1011–1016.

Sibai, B. M., Taslimi, M. M., El-Nazar, A., Amen, E., Mabie, B. C., and Ryan, G. M. (1986b). Maternal–perinatal outcome associated with the syndrome of hemolysis, elevated liver enzymes and low platelets in severe pre-eclampsia eclampsia. *American Journal of Obstetrics and Gynecology* **155**, 501–509.

Sibai, B. M., Gonzalez, A. R., Mabie, W. C., and Moretti, M. (1987). A comparison of labetalol plus hospitalisation alone in the management of pre-eclampsia remote from term. *Obstetrics and Gynecology* **70**, 323–327.

Sibai, B. M., McCubbin, J. H., Anderson, G. D., Lipschitz, J., and Dilts, P. V. (1981). Eclampsia: observations from 67 recent cases. *Obstetrics and Gynecology* **58**, 609–613.

Sibai, B. M., Ramadan, M. K., Chari, R. S., and Friedman, S. A. (1995). Pregancies complicated by HELLP syndrome: subsequent pregnancy outcome and long term prognosis. *American Journal of Obstetrics and Gynecology* **172**, 125–129.

Smith, G. C. S., Pell, J. P., and Walsh, D. (2001). Pregnancy complications and maternal risk of ischaemic heart disease: a retrospective cohort study of 129,290 births. *Lancet* **357**, 2002–2006.

SOGAP (1997). The Management of mild, non-proteinuric hypertension in pregnancy. A clinical practice guideline for professionals involved in maternity care in Scotland. Scottish Obstetric Guidelines and Audit Project. Scottish Programme for Clinical Effectiveness in Reproductive Health.

Stamilio, D. M., Sehdev, H. M., Morgan, M., Propert, K., and Macones, G. (2000). Can antenatal clinical and biochemical markers predict the development of severe preeclampsia. *American Journal of Obstetrics and Gynecology* **182**, 589–594.

Tervila, L., Groecke, C., and Timonen, S. (1973). Estimation of gestosis of pregnancy (EPH-gestosis). *Acta Obstetricia et Gynecologica Scandinavica* **52**, 235–243.

The Magpie Trial Collaborative Group (2002). Do women with pre-eclampsia, and their babies, benefit from magnesium sulphate? The Magpie Trial: a randomised placebo controlled trial. *Lancet* **359**, 1877–1890.

Thong, J., Howie, F., Smith, A. F., Greer, I. A., and Johnstone, F. D. (1991). Microalbuminuria in random daytime specimens in pregnancy induced hypertension. *Journal of Obstetrics and Gynecology* **11**, 324–327.

Thornton, J. G. and Macdonald, A. M. (1999). Twin mothers, pregnancy hypertension and preeclampsia. *British Journal of Obstetrics and Gynaecology* **106**, 570–575.

Tribe, C. R., Smart, G. E., Davies, D. R., and Mackenzie, J. C. (1979). A renal biopsy study in toxaemia of pregnancy using light microscopy linked with immunofluorescence and immuno-electron microscopy. *Journal of Clinical Pathology* **32**, 681–692.

Twaddle, S. and Harper, V. (1992). Day care and pregnancy hypertension. *Lancet* **339**, 813–814.

Villar, M. A. and Sibai, B. M. (1988). Eclampsia. *Obstetrics and Gynecology Clinics of North America* **15**, 355–377.

Vince, G. S., Starkey, P. M., Austgulen, R., Kwiatkowski, D., and Redman, C. W. G. (1995). Interleukin-6, tumour necrosis factor and soluble tumour necrosis factor receptors in women with pre-eclampsia. *British Journal of Obstetrics and Gynaecology* **102**, 20–25.

Von Dadelszen, P., Ornstein, M. P., Bull, S. B., Logan, A. G., Koren, G., and Magee, L. A. (2000). Fall in mean arterial pressure and fetal growth restriction in pregnancy hypertension: a meta-analysis. *Lancet* **355**, 87–92.

Wallenburg, H. C. S. Hemodynamics in hypertensive pregnancy. In *Hypertension in Pregnancy* (ed. R. Rubin), pp. 66–101. New York: Elsevier, 1988.

Wallenburg, H. C. S., Dekker, G. A., Makovitz, J. W., and Rotmans, P. (1986). Low dose aspirin prevents pregnancy-induced hypertension and pre-eclampsia in angiotensin sensitive primigravidae. *Lancet* **I**, 1–3.

Weinstein, L. (1982). Syndrome of hemolysis, elevated liver enzymes and low platelet count: of severe consequences of hypertension in pregnancy. *American Journal of Obstetrics and Gynecology* **142**, 159–167.

Williams, K. P. and Wilson, S. (1999). Persistence of cerebral hemodynamic changes in patients with eclampsia: a report of three cases. *American Journal of Obstetrics and Gynecology* **181** (5), 1162–1165.

Witlin, A. G., Saade, G. R., Mattar, F., and Sibai, B. M. (2000). Predictors of neonatal outcome in women with severe preeclampsia or eclampsia between 24 and 33 weeks' gestation. *American Journal of Obstetrics and Gynecology* **182** (3), 607–611.

Zhang, J., Klebanoff, M., Levines, R. J., Puri, M., and Moyer, P. (1999). The puzzling association between smoking and hypertension during pregnancy. *American Journal of Obstetrics and Gynecology* **181**, 1407–1413.

16

The patient with inherited disease

16.1 Strategies for the investigation of inherited renal disease

Friedhelm Hildebrandt and Edgar Otto

Gene–protein–phenotype

The flow of genetic information

In every cell in the human body, the nucleus contains about 35,000 structural genes that represent the entirety of genetic information (with the exception of the very small mitochondrial genome) (Boheler and Stern 2003). Tissue specificity, external stimuli, developmental stage, and the current functional state of a cell determine which of these genes are actively expressed, that is, transcribed into messenger RNA (mRNA) and translated into protein (Fig. 1a). Thus, in each cell there is a, virtually deterministic, flow of genetic information from the gene to the phenotype as formulated in the central dogma of molecular biology (Crick 1958), where a gene is transcribed into a mRNA, which is translated into a protein, which through its function, determines a phenotype of a cell, a tissue, or an organism.

Monogenic diseases

Several hundred renal diseases represent so-called 'monogenic diseases'. Monogenic diseases are defined by the fact that in a given patient the disease is caused by mutations in a single gene only. In other words, in this patient a mutation in one nucleotide (nt) of the 3,000,000,000 nt that the human genome contains is sufficient to cause the disease in this patient. In *recessive diseases* a mutation needs to be present on both parental chromosomes, while in *dominant disorders*, a defect on one parental chromosome is sufficient to cause the disease. The term 'monogenic' does not exclude, however, that in different patients different genes can cause a similar disease, such as in polycystic kidney disease types 1 and 2. Monogenic diseases are usually rare disorders in the range of 1 : 1000–1 : 10,000 individuals.

In a monogenic disease (Fig. 1b), a gene defect leads to a mutated mRNA, and an altered protein causing a process, which we commonly refer to as 'pathogenesis', which in turn determines a disease phenotype. A very important characteristic of monogenic diseases is the fact that the mutation itself represents the aetiology (i.e. the primary cause) of the disease. From this ensue the following opportunities if a gene for a monogenic disorder has been identified. Since in a monogenic disease, the gene defect represents the aetiology, gene identification allows for:

(1) unequivocal molecular genetic diagnostics,

(2) new insights into pathogenesis and physiology of this gene,

(3) studies on genotype/phenotype correlation, and

(4) might provide inroads into new ways of therapy.

Polygenic diseases

In contrast to *monogenic* diseases, in *polygenic* diseases, for a given patient, only the actions of different genes *together* lead to the disease phenotype through interaction of the proteins encoded (Fig. 2). A prominent example of polygenic inheritance in nephrology is represented by essential hypertension. It has been proposed that some of the genes that alter blood pressure regulation in monogenic diseases might be the same ones in which certain alleles in concert with other genes give rise to polygenic hypertension (Lifton 1996). Polygenic disorders are usually frequent diseases occurring in the range of up to 1 : 5 (essential hypertension) to 1 : 1000 individuals.

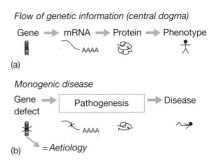

Fig. 1 *Central dogma of molecular biology and its relation to monogenic disease mechanisms.* (a) In each cell there is a flow of genetic information from the gene to the phenotype as formulated in the central dogma of molecular biology, where a gene is transcribed into a mRNA, which is translated into a protein which, through its function, determines a phenotype. (b) In a monogenic disease, a gene defect leads to a mutated mRNA, and an altered protein, causing a process commonly described as 'pathogenesis', which in turn determines a disease phenotype. In a monogenic disease, the genetic defect represents the aetiology.

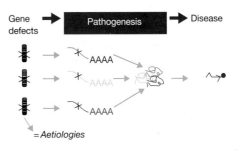

Fig. 2 *The flow of genetic information in polygenic diseases.* In a given patient, only the action of different genes *together* leads to the disease phenotype, through interaction of the proteins encoded. See also legend to Fig. 1.

Very recently, a fascinating new concept of a potential continuum between monogenic and polygenic disease mechanisms has been described for the Bardet–Biedl syndrome (BBS), the association of renal anomalies with obesity, retinitis pigmentosa, polydactyly, hypogenitalism, and mental retardation (OMIM 3209900; http://www.ncbi.nlm.nih.gov/entrez/query.fcgi?db=OMIM). Six gene loci have been mapped for the BBS, and the genes for BBS 2, 4, 6, and 8 have been identified. It was discovered that in this recessive disease, where mutations should be present in both alleles of the same gene of an affected individual, in a few patients a third mutation in another BBS gene was necessary for expression of the disease (Burghes *et al.* 2001; Katsanis *et al.* 2001). In this seeming violation of Mendelian inheritance, one may regard the second gene carrying a mutation as a modifier gene; one may refer to this phenomenon as 'triallelic inheritance', or one may view it as the first indication for a blurred border between monogenic and polygenic inheritance. Direct identification of genes for polygenic diseases is a very complex task involving statistics, and for 15 years many groups have tried to positionally clone such genes with only very recent success (Glazier *et al.* 2002; Korstanje and Paigen 2002). Therefore, it is well worth hunting for further monogenic disease genes as candidate genes for polygenic diseases.

Genes

In the description of strategies for the investigation of inherited renal diseases we will follow the flow of genetic information, describing first genes, then proteins, before moving on to phenotypic studies of proteins, cells, and the entire organism in describing the disease phenotype of a patient.

Positional cloning of disease genes

Family studies and haplotype analysis

In the paradigm of *positional cloning* of disease genes, one is working backwards against the flow of genetic information, starting from its end point, that is, the phenotype, and jumping to the disease-causing gene by studying the segregation of chromosomal segments in families affected with the disease. The approach used, termed *linkage analysis*, applies the prior knowledge that the set of 46 human chromosomes consists of two sex chromosomes and a double set of 22 autosomes, one of which is inherited from the individual's father and one from the mother. In addition, it is based on the fact that cross-overs between parental homologous chromosomes can occur in meioses of the gametes that lead to a newborn child. In family studies, these cross-overs can be observed by examination of genomic DNA extracted from blood samples of family members of families affected by the disease. This method is called *haplotype analysis*. In a 'total genome search for linkage' haplotype analysis is applied to the entire human genome, which is scanned with about 400 polymorphic DNA markers, which are evenly spaced along all chromosomes (Hildebrandt 1999) (Fig. 3).

After a disease gene has been mapped by haplotype analysis to a certain chromosomal region, this critical region is narrowed down by demonstration of more crossing-overs in additional families, until only a few genes can be accommodated in this region. The exons of those genes will have to be examined by direct sequencing of DNA for loss-of-function mutations in individuals affected with the disease in question. Identification of such mutations in a specific gene will then identify this gene as responsible for the disease. Even in the ages of availability of the almost complete genomic sequence of the human genome (http://www.ensembl.org), this process might still require

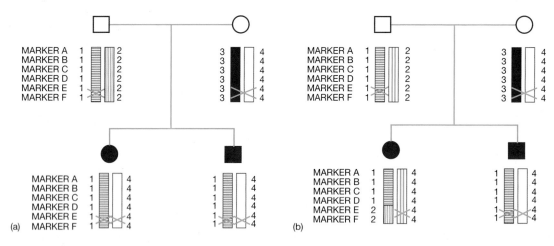

Fig. 3 *The principle of haplotype analysis.* Examination of DNA extracted from blood samples of members of families, in which a monogenic disease segregates, is examined by polymerase chain reaction (PCR) for about 400 polymorphic DNA markers, which are evenly spaced along all chromosomes, as shown here for the example of six markers on one chromosome. PCR products for markers are detected as different size bands on size resolution, and are here represented by numbers. They represent the two different alleles of each marker from the two parental chromosomes. Thus, markers allow discerning in each child the paternal chromosomes, as symbolized here by differently hatched bars. This process is termed 'haplotype analysis'. (a) In this example of a family with two children affected by a recessive disease (filled symbols), marker alleles indicate that the recessively affected children inherited the same chromosomes from the parents. This is compatible with the hypothesis that the gene in question would, for instance, be localized at the position indicated, and the children would be carrying a mutation in this gene on both parental chromosomes, as symbolized by an 'X'. (In fact, in this example, the gene could be positioned anywhere on this chromosome.) (b) If, however, a crossing-over had occurred in the meiosis leading to one of these children (the girl on the left), the disease-causing gene cannot be positioned in the region indicated, because only the mutation ('X') from the mother can have segregated to this child, which is not sufficient to cause a recessive disease. In this way one can exclude the gene in question from large regions of the whole genome, and, by examining more families, can localize the disease gene to the only region in the human genome that has not been excluded in this way.

years of research. The key to disease gene identification by positional cloning is still the availability of clinically very accurately characterized families in which the respective disease segregates. Since many of the approximately 35,000 genes in the human genome have only been identified by structure and not by function, there is still an immense opportunity to identify novel genes of renal diseases using the strategy of positional cloning. One of the strengths of positional cloning, although it is a very tedious process, is its ability to identify genes which are completely novel, and therefore may provide new insights into kidney function. Such disease genes will not have been found by approaches other than positional cloning, since there is no prior knowledge about their function.

Known monogenic causes of renal disease

The past few years have been very successful in identifying the causes of many monogenic renal disorders through positional cloning. An incomplete list of renal disease genes that were identified by positional cloning or by candidate gene approaches is shown in Table 1. There are *renal cystic diseases*, such as autosomal dominant polycystic kidney disease (ADPKD) and autosomal recessive polycystic kidney disease (ARPKD), and nephronophthisis. There are *glomerular diseases*, with the podocin gene responsible for steroid-resistant nephrotic syndrome, and genes for *renal tumours*, renal *tubular disorders*, and causes of *nephrolithiasis*, for which genes have been identified. Disease gene identification by positional cloning in many instances has led to novel insights into the pathophysiology of renal diseases as well as to some understanding of novel physiological mechanisms.

Molecular genetic diagnostics

Monogenic disorders are unique, in that the disease is caused by a defect in a *single* gene. Since in a monogenic disease, the gene defect represents the primary cause or 'aetiology' of this disorder, gene identification allows for unequivocal molecular genetic diagnosis. It is due to the quasi-deterministic nature of the monogenic defects (Fig. 1) that molecular genetic diagnosis in most cases is definite.

Table 1 Renal disease genes identified by positional cloning

Glomerular	Tubular
Congenital nephrotic syndrome, Finnish type	Bartter syndrome 1, 2, 3
	Bartter syndrome with deafness
Steroid-resistant nephrotic syndrome	Gitelman syndrome
	PHA1, Gordon, Liddle syndrome
Alport syndrome	Familial hypomagnesaemic hypercalciuric nephrocalcinosis
Nail patella syndrome	
Familial Mediterranean fever	Nephrogenic diabetes insipidus
Cystic	Cystinosis
ADPKD 1, 2, ARPKD	*Nephrolithiasis*
Nephronophthisis 1–4	Dent's disease
Glomerulocystic kidney disease	Cystinuria 1, 2
Bardet–Biedl type 2, 4, 6, 8	Hyperoxaluria types 1, 2
Renal tumours	APRTase-deficiency
Wilms tumour	Xanthinuria
Von-Hippel–Lindau disease Tuberous sclerosis 1, 2	Osteopetrosis with proximal renal tubular acidosis 1 (RTA)
	Distal renal tubular acidosis +/− deafness

In molecular genetic diagnostics two approaches are discernable:

(1) *direct genetic testing*, which can be applied if the disease-causing gene is known; and

(2) *indirect genetic testing*, which is employed if the causative gene is unknown but has been localized to a specific chromosomal region by linkage analysis.

There are a number of limitations to both approaches, which are outlined in Table 2.

Direct genetic testing

Direct sequencing

In diseases where the responsible gene is known, relevant mutations may be detected directly in affected individuals following amplification of exons by PCR and consecutive direct sequencing using the chain termination method (Deichmann 1999). An example of a sequence readout from direct sequencing of an exon sequence amplified from genomic DNA is given in Fig. 4.

Conditions that need to be met to allow for *direct molecular genetic diagnosis* are as follows:

1. The disease gene must have been identified.

2. The functional relevance of mutations detected must be proven by absence from 100 healthy controls, or by a functional test.

3. The mutation may have been shown to be relevant for the disease phenotype from its occurrence in an affected sibling or from the literature.

4. If there are multiple affected individuals, the mutation must segregate within the pedigree.

For molecular genetic testing prior genetic counselling is mandatory, and ethical guidelines should be observed (http://www.faseb.org/genetics/ashg/policy/pol-00.htm). A main advantage of molecular genetics diagnostics is that, due to the deterministic nature of the monogenic defects, diagnosis in most cases is definite. A major problem, however, is the fact that there is still a wide gap between identification of disease genes and availability of molecular genetic diagnostics. The GeneTests database provides help in finding laboratories all over the world that offer molecular genetic diagnostics for inherited renal diseases (www.GeneTests.org). In many instances, there has been a considerable time lag in many diseases between the discovery of the causative gene and the availability of molecular genetic diagnostics. In ADPKD, the most frequent life-threatening disease of autosomal dominant inheritance, the large number of exons and the presence of

Table 2 Comparison of direct and indirect molecular genetic diagnostics

	Direct	**Indirect**
Requirement	Single individual	(Large) pedigree
Method	Mutational analysis	Haplotype analysis
Disadvantage	Screening of many exons	Affecteds to be known, needs statistics to evaluate
Advantage	Safe, if positive	Safe exclusion is possible, if there is no more than one gene locus known for the disease

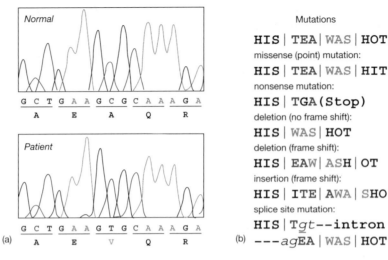

Fig. 4 *The principle of mutational analysis by direct sequencing.* (a) Sequence chromatogram readout from cDNA sequence of the *NPHS2* (podocin) gene in a patient with focal–segmental glomerulosclerosis (FSGS) (lower panel) in comparison with a normal control (upper panel). In the nucleotide sequence of the podocin gene, the patient carries a homozygous point mutation, replacing a cytosine (___) for a thymine (___). The altered triplet codon (GTG for GCG) is translated into a different amino acid (valine for alanine). This will disrupt the function of the podocin protein, which is essential for proper glomerular function, thus leading to FSGS in this patient. (b) Types of mutations detected by direct sequencing of the exon sequence. Within exons genomic DNA encodes translation products (proteins) as triplet codons for amino acids. Mutations will disrupt the function of the translation product by altering 'sense' during translation, as symbolized here by using meaningful words of three letters instead of three-letter codons. Mutations change codons in different ways: In a *missense mutation* an amino acid (aa) is exchanged. In a *nonsense mutation*, one of three possible STOP codons (TAA, TAG, or TGA) is introduced into the reading frame. In a *frame-shift mutation* the amino acid sequence following the mutation is garbled, either by loss of a nucleotide(s) (*deletion*) or by *insertion*. In a *splice site mutation* the obligatory consensus sequence is altered at the splice donor or splice acceptor sites, where introns are excised and exons are joined before translation. This leads to an altered translation product.

four very similar pseudogenes have made the development of molecular genetic diagnostics very difficult. Recently, an approach to its molecular genetic diagnostics has become available (Phakdeekitcharoen *et al.* 2001).

New genotyping techniques

Heteroduplex chromatography using denaturing high pressure liquid chromatography (dHPLC) is being employed in mutational analysis as an alternative to direct sequencing. However, the need to develop very specific amplification conditions to detect heteroduplexes resulting from mutations still limits the efficacy of dHPLC as an inexpensive screening technique.

Indirect genetic testing

If the causative gene for a monogenic disorder is unknown, but a gene locus has been localized to a chromosomal region by positional cloning, indirect genetic testing can be performed for diagnosis, employing haplotype analysis at this gene locus in affected families (Fig. 3).

Conditions that need to be met to allow for *indirect molecular genetic diagnosis* are as follows:

1. If there is more than one gene locus known to cause similar diseases ('genetic locus heterogeneity'), a sufficient number of affected relatives must exist (i.e. seven or more affected relatives in autosomal dominant or recessive diseases, and four or more affected siblings of consanguineous parents in recessive diseases).

2. If there exists only one gene locus for an inherited disease, exclusion by haplotype analysis may be possible even in small pedigrees.

3. DNA from unaffected individuals may also be needed in order to correctly infer segregation of haplotypes.

Animal models of genetic renal disease

Transgenic mouse models have proved to be extremely helpful in the study of human genetic disorders, and are greatly facilitated by sequencing of most of the human and mouse genomes (http://www. ensembl.org). Mouse models are particularly useful for the study of human genetic disease, since a comparison of mouse chromosome Mmu16 with the human genome demonstrated that about only 2 per cent of all mouse genes had no counterpart in the human genome. Mouse models of renal disease have become available through identification of disease phenotypes that are based on spontaneously arisen mutations as exemplified by renal cystic diseases (Guay-Woodford *et al.* 2000). Alternatively, mouse models of human renal genetic disease have been generated by targeted disruption of specific disease-causing genes. Databases of genes that have been targeted to create mouse models of human disease are available (TBASE at http://tbase.jax.org; LexiconGenetics™ at http:// www.lexgen.com; GeneTrap project at http://tikus.gsf.de).

Zebrafish

As a lower vertebrate the zebrafish (*Danio rerio*) has proved to be a very useful model for the study of kidney organogenesis and human renal cystic diseases (Drummond *et al.* 1998).

Caenorhabditis elegans

Many genes which, if mutated, give rise to renal cystic disease show conservation of sequence homology and of function in the nematode *C. elegans*, the genome of which has been fully sequenced (http://www. wormbase.org). This includes the genes causing PKD types 1 and 2

Table 3 Electronic databases of genes, proteins, and phenotypes of human and animal model diseases (URLs are given in parentheses)

Genes
Genomic sequence of human, mouse, and other model organisms
  (www.ensembl.org)
Genomic DNA exon prediction
  GeneScan (www.genome.dkfz-heidelberg.de)
  BCM search launcher (www.hgsc.bcm.tmc.edu)
Expression databases
  Serial analysis of gene expression (www.sagenet.org)
Diagnostics
  Gene tests (www.GeneTests.org)
Mutations
  HUGO mutation (ariel.ucs.unimelb.edu.au:80)
  Human gene mutation database (HGMD) (archive.uwcm.ac.uk)

Proteins
Protein databases
  Expasy (www.expasy.org)
Proteomics (http://base-peak.wiley.com)

Animal models and genomes
Comparative transcript maps
  Human–mouse homology (www.ncbi.nlm.nih.gov/Homology)
Mouse
  TBASE (tbase.jax.org)
  Lexicon Genetics (www.lexgen.com)
  Gene trap project (tikus.gsf.de)
Zebrafish (www.ensembl.org/Danio_rerio)
C. elegans (www.wormbase.org/) (www.sanger.ac.uk/Projects/C_elegans/)

Disease phenotypes
Genetic diseases
  OMIM (www3.ncbi.nlm.nih.gov/OMIM)

(*PKD1* and *PKD2*) (Barr *et al.* 2001; Yoder *et al.* 2002) and juvenile nephronophthisis (*NPHP1*) (Otto *et al.* 2000). Since the cell lineage of every cell in the development of *C. elegans* can be followed under a microscope using Nomarski optics from the zygote to the adult organisms, *C. elegans* will prove to be a very useful model for the study of physiological and pathophysiological mechanisms.

Electronic databases

Electronic databases on the Internet are very valuable resources for genomic, proteomic, and disease-related information. Two very useful starting points are (www.ncbi.nlm.nih.gov) and (www.ncbi.nlm.nih.gov/LocusLink) (Table 3).

Proteins

Generation and use of antibodies as molecular probes

Western blotting

In Western blotting, proteins or peptides are first size separated by SDS-polyacrylamide gel electrophoresis (PAGE), then electroblotted onto a suitable membrane (nitrocellulose or Immobilon) to yield a spatial representation of the result from size separation. This representation can then be visualized by staining with amido black or Ponceau S. The membrane is overlaid with a so-called 'primary' antibody directed against the protein of interest. Unbound antibody is then washed away, and secondary antibodies recognizing the Fc fragments of the primary antibody is added. The secondary antibody has been coupled to a colour detection tool, for example, by using horse radish peroxidase or enhanced luminescence, which allows us to document detection of the secondary antibody in its bound state to the primary antibody, and thereby of the band representing the protein of interest. If a suitable antibody is available, Western blotting allows detection of a protein of interest out of a complex protein mixture, such as total cell lysates from cell culture. Since the size of the protein of interest is known, it can be detected as a band in comparison to bands of size markers (Reilly 1999). As an example, Western blotting can be employed for detection of proteins from coimmunoprecipitation experiments (see below) (Fig. 5). In very complex protein mixtures, size separation by SDS-PAGE alone may not yield sufficient resolution. Under these circumstances, two-dimensional gel electrophoresis may be used. In this method, proteins are first separated by their characteristic isoelectric point through isoelectric focusing in a tube gel. Thereafter, the linear tube gel is loaded onto an SDS-PAGE gel and proteins are size separated in a direction at 90° to the direction for isoeletric focusing. Thereby, two-dimensional size separation is achieved according to two independent characteristics: isoelectric point and molecular weight.

Protein–protein interaction

Coimmunoprecipitation (*in vivo* assays)

Aspects of protein–protein interaction are of considerable interest when studying novel physiological and pathophysiological mechanisms of genetic renal disease, as exemplified by the identification of protein interaction partners of nephrocystin 1, the product of the *NPHP1* gene, mutations in which cause juvenile nephronophthisis (Benzing *et al.* 2001; Mollet *et al.* 2002). Protein–protein interaction can be demonstrated by coimmunoprecipitation experiments. Usually, both proteins or fragments thereof are co-expressed in a suitable cell line through transfection of this cell line with expression-plasmids containing inserts encoding these proteins. If no cognate antibody is available for these proteins, they can be expressed as fusion proteins containing a peptide tag for which antibodies are available, such as myc-tags or FLAG-tags. After transfection and cell lysis, the lysates are incubated with the antibody directed against (the tag of) one protein. Antibodies with bound protein are precipitated and the precipitate isolated. The precipitate is then size separated by SDS-PAGE, and protein–protein interaction partners that are expected to coprecipitate are detected by Western blot analysis of the precipitate (Fig. 5a). The results usually have to be corroborated in the reciprocal form (Fig. 5), that is, if protein 'A' precipitated with protein 'B', protein 'B' should also coprecipitate with protein 'A' (Fig. 5a and b).

Coimmunoprecipitation data are more reliable if antibodies are directed against the protein rather than against a tag marker. Data are even more meaningful if coprecipitation of *endogenous* protein can be detected, by directing an antibody against a protein expressed from transfection and showing coprecipitation of the endogenously expressed protein. In an ideal situation, the antibody should be directed against one endogenously expressed protein and Western blot detection should also be directed against an endogenous protein. Due to low endogenous

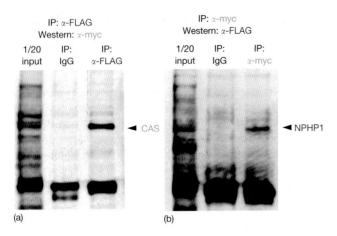

(a)   (b)

Fig. 5 *Coimmunoprecipitation of nephrocystin and p130CAS.*
(a) Myc-tagged murine p130CAS and FLAG-tagged human nephrocystin
were co-expressed in baby hamster kidney cells. When nephrocystin was
precipitated (IP) with the anti α-FLAG-antibody, p130CAS was shown in a
Western blot to coprecipitate with anti-myc-ab (right lane; CAS). Also
shown is 1/20 of the cell lysate input as positive control (left lane), and IP
with an irrelevant antibody (middle lane). Strong bands at 60 kDa are
immunoglobulin heavy chains. (b) Vice versa, if p130CAS was precipitated,
nephrocystin (NPHP1) was coprecipitated, as detected by Western blot
using an anti-FLAG-tag antibody.

expression levels of most proteins in suitable cell cultures, the latter result
often can only be achieved if the coprecipitating protein is detected after
radioactive metabolic labelling of proteins and detection by autoradio-
graphy rather than Western blotting.

Pull-down assays (*in vitro* assays)

In so-called 'pull-down assays' *in vitro* protein interaction is examined
by adsorption of one protein binding partner as fusion protein to a
solid phase, for example, in a column of this solid phase material. The
column is then equilibrated with a lysate that contains the binding
partner under high salt conditions allowing the binding partner to
interact. Other non-binding proteins from the lysate are washed out.
Finally, the binding partner is eluted under low salt conditions and
detected, for example, by Western blot analysis. In this way, interaction
of the proteins polycystin 1 and 2, the gene of which cause ADPKD
types 1 and 2, respectively, has been demonstrated (Qian *et al.* 1997).

Mapping of protein–protein interaction domains

In vitro protein–protein interaction assays from *in vitro* interaction
assays or from coimmunoprecipitation can be used to map protein–
protein interaction domains. For this purpose, specific constructs
containing full-length of the protein and others that contain only
fragments of the protein are tested for interaction. Depending on
the result, regions necessary and sufficient for interaction can be
delineated.

Identification of new protein–protein interaction partners

In order to identify novel binding partners to a protein or peptide, the
yeast-2-hybrid system can be employed (Fig. 6). In this way, the
protein p130CAS has been identified as a binding partner to nephrocystin, the product of the *NPHP1* gene, which, if defective, gives rise to

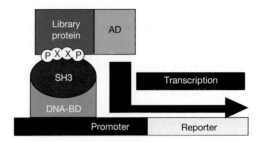

Fig. 6 *Identification of protein–protein interaction partners with the yeast-2-hybrid
system.* The protein domain for which a binding partner is sought (the 'bait'), in
this case a 'src-homology 3 (SH3) domain', is cloned into an expression vector
as a fusion protein with a *GAL4* DNA binding domain (DNA-BD). SH3 domains
are known to recognize cognate peptides on other proteins with the minimal
binding consensus P–x–x–P (proline–any amino acid–any amino acid–proline).
This expression construct is cotransfected into yeast cells, where each yeast
cell contains a single copy of specific cDNA fragment (the 'prey'), for example,
from a human kidney cDNA library. These cDNA fragments are expressed as
fusion proteins with an activation domain of transcription (AD). In the yeast
cell, the DNA-BD of the 'bait' will bind to a promoter of the reporter gene
β-galactosidase. If then, in some of the yeast cell clones, an interaction partner
('prey') will bind to the 'bait' (in this case, the SH3 domain), this binding
partner will bring the fused AD into close proximity to the reporter gene,
thereby activating transcription of the β-galactosidase reporter gene, and the
respective yeast colonies will turn blue. By this colour detection, yeast cells
expressing binding partners can be identified, the respective clones shuttled
into *E. coli* hosts, their inserts sequenced, and the binding partner recognized
by sequence comparison to pertinent databases.

juvenile nephronophthisis type 1 (Hildebrandt *et al.* 1997; Donaldson
et al. 2000; Hildebrandt and Otto 2000; Otto *et al.* 2003).

Proteomics

In analogy to the term 'genomics' that refers to work on the entirety of
an organism's genome, its structure, expression, and regulation, the term
'proteomics' has been coined to represent the science of studying the
entirety of all proteins translated within a certain cell type or organism.
The proteome of an organism is more complex than the genome, since
each gene may be transcribed into alternative splice forms, leading to distinct translation products. Furthermore, post-translational modification, such as cleavage of a signal peptide, gylcosylation, etc., lead to
additional protein products derived from the same gene. Modern techniques of protein biochemistry, such as high-resolution two-dimensional
electrophoresis allow rapid access to comparison of very complex protein expression patterns from whole cell extracts in a two-dimensional
pattern of protein 'spots'. The high sensitivity of mass spectrometry
enables sequence-based identification of these spots. This, together with
sequence comparisons to genetic and protein databases, provides a very
powerful approach to studying differential protein expression (Jackson
et al. 2000; Pasa-Tolic *et al.* 2002). As an example, the total protein
expression pattern of primary cilia from human trachea has been
resolved by mass spectrometry (Ostrowski *et al.* 2002). This data set will
be very valuable for the study of renal cystic disease, since virtually all
proteins, which if defective cause renal cystic disease in humans and
mice, are expressed in the primary cilia of renal distal tubular cells
(Igarashi and Somlo 2002; Nauli *et al.* 2003). High-throughput protein
analysis can also be performed with the help of microarray technique
(MacBeath and Schreiber 2000).

Phenotyping

Cell biological phenotyping

Immunofluorescence studies

Studies on subcellular localization of proteins encoded by genes which, if defective, cause genetic renal diseases can be very helpful in answering questions regarding the physiological and pathophysiological role of newly discovered proteins. This is exemplified by subcellular localization studies of barttin, the product of the BSND gene, responsible for Bartter syndrome with sensorineural deafness (SND) (Birkenhager *et al.* 2001; Estevez *et al.* 2001).

Clinical phenotyping

Correct definition of the clinical disease phenotype is of paramount importance for studies of positional cloning of disease genes. This is the case, since data on cosegregation of the affected status, on one hand, and hundreds of polymorphic markers distributed over the entire genome, on the other hand, can only be correctly interpreted, if there is an *a priori* definition of which member of a pedigree is affected and which one is not. All attempts to evaluate haplotype data following *a posteriori* redefinition of clinical 'subgroups' are bound to lead to false positive results. With renal disease genes being sought for more and more subtle phenotypes, good collaboration between molecular geneticists and clinician scientists becomes increasingly important and promising.

Genotype–phenotype correlation

Some genotype–phenotype correlations are emerging in monogenic renal diseases. They can be based on:

(1) genetic locus heterogeneity, that is, different genes cause a similar but not identical phenotype (as in PKD types 1 and 2, the latter of which has a slightly later median onset of terminal renal failure);

(2) allelic differences of the same gene, that is, different mutations decide on phenotypic differences (as in Alport syndrome) (Jais *et al.* 2000); and

(3) the effect of modifier genes (as in *pcy* mice with renal cystic disease) (Woo *et al.* 1997).

In about 28 per cent of all children with steroid-resistant nephrotic syndrome due to focal–segmental glomerulosclerosis (FSGS), the disease is caused by mutations in the *NPHS2* (podocin) gene (Boute *et al.* 2000; Karle *et al.* 2002; Winn 2002). There may be an emerging genotype–phenotype correlation in this disorder in the sense that patients with mutations in the *NPHS2* gene show primary steroid resistance and do not show recurrence in the renal transplant (Boute *et al.* 2000; Ruf *et al.* 2004). If these data hold up to testing of larger patient cohorts, this might have far reaching consequences for patients carrying podocin-mutations, since it might be warranted to avoid steroids and cytotoxic drugs in their treatment in the first place. In addition, one might be able to plan living related donor transplantation without having to fear the 1 : 3 recurrence rate that commonly complicates renal transplantation in FSGS.

From positional cloning to novel (patho)physiology

One of the advantages of positional cloning, although it is a very tedious process, is its ability to identify genes that are completely novel, and may thus provide new information about kidney function. An example is given below for Bartter syndrome with SND.

Bartter syndrome with deafness

Since positional cloning of a disease genes directly leads to the cause of a disease, one knows from the outset that one will end up identifying the aetiology of the disease. One will then be able to study and line up along this causal axis from gene to the disease, the related pathogenesis. Novel physiological principals have been identified by this approach for many kidney diseases as exemplified by the Bartter syndrome: Antenatal Bartter syndrome is an autosomal recessive salt-losing nephropathy, which by fetal polyuria leads to polyhydramnios and premature birth. Postnatally, massive polyuria, renal salt loss, and dehydration occur. Biochemical hallmarks are hypokalaemic metabolic alkalosis and hyperreninaemic hyperaldosteronism with hypercalciuria and nephrocalcinosis.

By positional cloning, mutations in three genes, the proteins of which are all expressed in the medullary thick ascending tubule (mTAL) of Henle's loop, have been shown to cause BS types 1–3, respectively. This has led to new insights into the pathophysiology of Na/Cl reabsorption (Fig. 7), where Cl reabsorption is driven by the primary action of the Na,K-ATPase. Na, K, and Cl follow on the luminal side via the secondary active Na/K/2Cl cotransporter (which is the protein through which furosemide exerts its action), which is defective

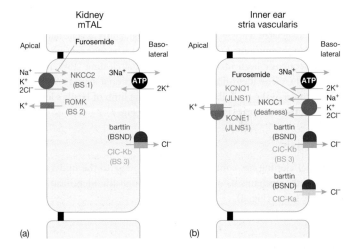

Fig. 7 *Pathomechanisms in kidney and inner ear of Bartter syndrome with deafness.* (a) In the medullary thick ascending limb, mutations in the apical NKCC2 cotransporter cause Bartter syndrome (BS) type 1. Its inhibition by furosemide mimics Bartter syndrome. For recycling of potassium, NKCC2 requires ROMK, which is responsible for BS type 2. Cl^- exits basolaterally through the ClC–Kb chloride channel. Mutations in ClC–Kb cause BS type 3. Since barttin acts as a β-subunit to this channel, mutations in the barttin gene *BSND* also cause BS. (b) In stria vascularis cells of the inner ear, basolateral NKCC1 raises the intracellular K^+ concentration, requiring KCNQ1 and its β-subunit KCNE1 to produce the high potassium concentration of cochlear endolymph. Mutations in both genes cause JLNS. Mutations in NKCC1 cause deafness in mice, which explains the deafness occurring in overdoses of furosemide. In contrast to the kidney, stria vascularis cells in the ear express chloride channels, ClC–Kb and ClC–Ka. Barttin acts as a β-subunit for both of them. Hence, if there is a mutation in ClC–Kb, BS will result, but no deafness, since in the inner ear there is additional expression of ClC–Ka, which can substitute for ClC–Kb. However, if there is a mutation in barttin, in addition to BS, deafness will result, since barttin is necessary for the function of both chloride channels.

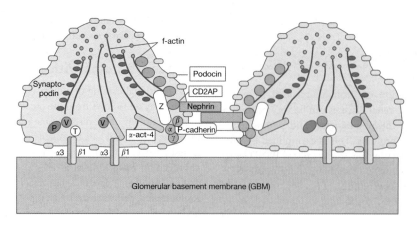

Fig. 8 *Pathomechanisms of nephrotic syndrome (NS).* This cartoon shows two podocyte foot processes, which are anchored to the glomerular basement membrane (blue) by integrin molecules, and between them form the glomerular slit membrane, which represents the critical filter of the glomerulus. Proteins of the slit membrane and proteins anchoring them to the cytoskeleton are shown in colour. The components shown here in boxes have been identified as functionally critical by disease gene identification through positional cloning, such as nephrin (NS Finnish type) (Kestila *et al.* 1998), podocin (Boute *et al.* 2000), α-actinin-4 (SRNS) (Kaplan *et al.* 2000), and CD2 associated protein from a mouse model (Shih *et al.* 1999). In this way, essential structural features of glomerular function may be constructed from the knowledge of disease genes (reproduced with permission and modified from Somlo and Mundel 2000).

in BS type 1. The driving force for this cotransporter is strongly dependent on K recycling back to the lumen. Genetic defects in the K channel ROMK are responsible for BS type 2. In this way, BS types 1 and 2 are the genetic equivalent of fursemide action. Cl exits from the cell on the basolateral side via the Cl channel, ClC–Kb. Genetic defects in its gene are responsible for BS type 3. For a fourth variant of aBS, which is associated with SND and chronic renal failure, a gene had been localized to chromosome 1 (Brennan *et al.* 1998). The gene causing BSND has subsequently been identified by positional cloning (Birkenhager *et al.* 2001). Gene identification revealed functional aspects on NaCl reabsorption in the medullary thick ascending limb of Henle's loop as well as in the inner ear (Estevez *et al.* 2001) (Fig. 7).

Nephrosis

Positional cloning has contributed most strongly to the understanding of pathomechanisms of nephrosis, through the identification of causative genes (Fig. 8).

New developments

From the Human Genome Projects, some new developments are already emerging, such as the use of single nucleotide polymorphisms (SNPs) for the definition of genetic variability, highly parallel approaches to the study of gene expression, and three-dimensional resolution of protein structure. In the near future, molecular genetics might help to differentiate more clearly different variants of a disease, which might result in more specific treatment.

Single nucleotide polymorphisms

A very powerful development within the Human Genome Projects is the identification of SNPs. There are about 3–5 million nt positions in the human genome at which individuals may differ from each other (~0.1 per cent of the genome). New research demonstrates that stretches of about 200,000 base pairs have been inherited 'en bloc' over

thousands of generations with no crossing over. Therefore, by testing only the alleles of two informative SNPs, one may infer the whole block of 200 kb (Patil *et al.* 2001; Stoll *et al.* 2001; Gabriel *et al.* 2002). This approach has already been very helpful for studies in polygenic diseases (Glazier *et al.* 2002; Korstanje and Paigen 2002). These SNPs can be detected by DNA microarray analysis.

Highly parallel expression studies

Developments within the Human Genome Projects have greatly facilitated the simultaneous detection of expression of tens of thousands of genes at the mRNA level. This is achieved by a technique called simultaneous analysis of gene expression (SAGE) (Boheler and Stern 2003), but also by using microarrays of expressed gene tags in automated systems, where the 'transcriptome' of the ten thousands of genes expressed by a cell line can be detected through simultaneous hybridization to a glass microchip. In this way, differential mRNA expression under two different (patho)physiological conditions can be hybridized using two different colour detections. The genes that are up- or down-regulated can then be identified in a cluster analysis of the hybridization results and new hypotheses on their functional roles can be generated. *In situ* hybridization data of gene expression can be rendered in a three-dimensional fashion, so that the spatial distribution can be appreciated well from the animated picture. Studies like this now help us to understand complicated spatial/temporal relationships of gene expression. This is exemplified in a three-dimensional rendition of a ninth day mouse embryo for expression of the *MSX2* gene at URL: http://genex.hgu.mrc.ac.uk/Documentation/SamplePics/#Movies.

Three-dimensional resolution of protein structure

Knowledge of the coding sequences for many functional domains of human proteins has been gained from the Human Genome Projects. These data provide a very powerful basis for the determination of three-dimensional structure by X-ray crystallography. An example is given for the SH3 domain (src-homology 3 domain) of murine c-src, which mediates protein–protein interactions with proline rich peptides in signal proteins at URL: http://www.ncbi.nlm.nih.gov/Structure/cdd/cddsrv.cgi?uid=pfam00018. In the long run, it may be possible to design new drugs that very specifically interact with structures that have been resolved at the three-dimensional level.

Genetic component in renal diseases

Positional cloning of disease genes will remain a very strong paradigm for many years to come. The gene identification process is far from being over. The rate at which renal genes are being identified by positional cloning is still in its exponential phase as shown in Fig. 9.

Most childhood renal diseases are probably due to monogenic causes as indicated by the following aspects:

1. Virtually all disorders of renal *tubular* transport are caused by monogenic defects (for an example see Bartter syndrome).

2. Twenty-eight per cent of all childhood steroid-resistant nephrotic syndromes are caused by podocin mutations, and there are many more genes known or to be identified as causes for renal *glomerular* diseases.

3. Multiple monogenic causes have been identified for *nephrolithiasis*.

4. All renal *cystic* diseases represent monogenic diseases.

5. Diseases genes have been identified for renal tumours (see Table 1).

Many genes involved in rare cases of monogenic renal disorders might play a role in frequent polygenic disorders such as hypertension (Lifton 1996).

There are many more genes to be found for renal diseases, and even at a time when the human genome is fully sequenced, the rate-limiting step for disease identification is the availability of clinically well characterized familial cases. Therefore, the three most important courses of actions for nephrologists in the process of gene identification of renal diseases are the following:

1. Take a family history and sketch a pedigree.

2. If in doubt, check on the internet, if the gene for the disorder in question is known and molecular genetic diagnostics is available (www3.ncbi.nlm.nih.gov/OMIM; www.Genetests.org; www.renalgenes.org).

3. If the gene has not been identified and if a pedigree is informative (AR: 3+ affecteds of consanguineous parents, AD: 10+ affecteds), contacting a positonal cloning laboratory can initiate the exciting process of gene identification of a novel gene causing renal disease and its subsequent functional evaluation.

References

Barr, M. M. *et al.* (2001). The *Caenorhabditis elegans* autosomal dominant polycystic kidney disease gene homologs lov-1 and pkd-2 act in the same pathway. *Current Biology* **11** (17), 1341–1346.

Benzing, T. *et al.* (2001). Nephrocystin interacts with Pyk2, p130(Cas), and tensin and triggers phosphorylation of Pyk2. *Proceedings of the National Academy of Sciences USA* **98** (17), 9784–9789.

Birkenhager, R. *et al.* (2001). Mutation of BSND causes Bartter syndrome with sensorineural deafness and kidney failure. *Nature Genetics* **29** (3), 310–314.

Boheler, K. R. and Stern, M. D. (2003). The new role of SAGE in gene discovery. *Trends in Biotechnology* **21** (2), 55–57.

Boute, N. *et al.* (2000). NPHS2, encoding the glomerular protein podocin, is mutated in autosomal recessive steroid-resistant nephrotic syndrome. *Nature Genetics* **24** (4), 349–354.

Brennan, T. M. *et al.* (1998). Linkage of infantile Bartter syndrome with sensorineural deafness to chromosome 1p. *American Journal of Human Genetics* **62** (2), 355–361.

Burghes, A. H., Vaessin, H. E., and De La Chapelle, A. (2001). Genetics. The land between Mendelian and multifactorial inheritance. *Science* **293** (5538), 2213–2214.

Crick, F. H. C. (1958). The biological replication of macromolecules. *Symposia of the Society Experimental Biology* **XII**, 138.

Deichmann, K. A. Sequencing. In *Techniques in Molecular Medicine* (ed. F. Hildebrandt and P. Igarashi), pp. 186–206. Berlin: Springer, 1999.

Donaldson, J. C. *et al.* (2000). Crk-associated substrate p130(Cas) interacts with nephrocystin and both proteins localize to cell–cell contacts of polarized epithelial cells. *Experimental Cell Research* **256** (1), 168–178.

Drummond, I. A. *et al.* (1998). Early development of the zebrafish pronephros and analysis of mutations affecting pronephric function. *Development* **125** (23), 4655–4667.

Estevez, R. *et al.* (2001). Barttin is a Cl-channel beta-subunit crucial for renal Cl-reabsorption and inner ear K$^+$ secretion. *Nature* **414** (6863), 558–561.

Gabriel, S. B. *et al.* (2002). The structure of haplotype blocks in the human genome. *Science* **296** (5576), 2225–2229.

Glazier, A. M., Nadeau, J. H., and Aitman, T. J. (2002). Finding genes that underlie complex traits. *Science* **298** (5602), 2345–2349.

Guay-Woodford, L. M. *et al.* (2000). Quantitative trait loci modulate renal cystic disease severity in the mouse bpk model. *Journal of the American Society of Nephrology* **11** (7), 1253–1260.

Hildebrandt, F. Positional cloning and linkage analysis. In *Techniques in Molecular Medicine* (ed. F. Hildebrandt and P. Igarashi), pp. 352–366. Berlin: Springer, 1999.

Hildebrandt, F. and Otto, E. (2000). Molecular genetics of nephronophthisis and medullary cystic kidney disease. *Journal of the American Society of Nephrology* **11** (9), 1753–1761.

Hildebrandt, F. *et al.* (1997). A novel gene encoding an SH3 domain protein is mutated in nephronophthisis type 1. *Nature Genetics* **17**, 149–153.

Igarashi, P. and Somlo, S. (2002). Genetics and pathogenesis of polycystic kidney disease. *Journal of the American Society of Nephrology* **13** (9), 2384–2398.

Jackson, P. E., Scholl, P. F., and Groopman, J. D. (2000). Mass spectrometry for genotyping: an emerging tool for molecular medicine. *Molecular Medicine Today* **6** (7), 271–276.

Jais, J. P. *et al.* (2000). X-linked Alport syndrome: natural history in 195 families and genotype–phenotype correlations in males. *Journal of the American Society of Nephrology* **11** (4), 649–657.

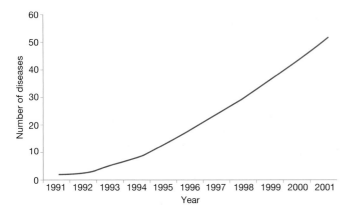

Fig. 9 *Time course on the identification of renal disease causing genes by positional cloning.* The number of genetic renal diseases that have been identified by positional cloning is shown on the vertical axis. Note that the rate at which renal genes are being identified by positional cloning is still in its exponential phase.

Kaplan, J. M. *et al.* (2000). Mutations in ACTN4, encoding alpha-actinin-4, cause familial focal segmental glomerulosclerosis. *Nature Genetics* **24** (3), 251–256.

Karle, S. M. *et al.* (2002). Novel mutations in *NPHS2* detected in both familial and sporadic steroid-resistant nephrotic syndrome. *Journal of the American Society of Nephrology* **13** (2), 388–393.

Katsanis, N. *et al.* (2001). Triallelic inheritance in Bardet–Biedl syndrome, a Mendelian recessive disorder. *Science* **293** (5538), 2256–2259.

Kestila, M. *et al.* (1998). Positionally cloned gene for a novel glomerular protein—nephrin—is mutated in congenital nephrotic syndrome. *Molecular Cell* **1** (4), 575–582.

Korstanje, R. and Paigen, B. (2002). From QTL to gene: the harvest begins. *Nature Genetics* **31** (3), 235–236.

Lifton, R. P. (1996). Molecular genetics of human blood pressure variation. *Science* **272** (5262), 676–680.

Macbeath, G. and Schreiber, S. L. (2000). Printing proteins as microarrays for high-throughput function determination. *Science* **289** (5485), 1760–1763.

Mollet, G. *et al.* (2002). The gene mutated in juvenile nephronophthisis type 4 encodes a novel protein that interacts with nephrocystin. *Nature Genetics* **32** (2), 300–305.

Nauli, S. M. *et al.* (2003). Polycystins 1 and 2 mediate mechanosensation in the primary cilium of kidney cells. *Nature Genetics* **33** (2), 129–137.

Ostrowski, L. E. *et al.* (2002). A proteomic analysis of human cilia: identification of novel components. *Molecular Cell Proteomics* **1** (6), 451–465.

Otto, E. *et al.* (2000). Nephrocystin: gene expression and sequence conservation between human, mouse, and *Caenorhabditis elegans*. *Journal of the American Society of Nephrology* **11** (2), 270–282.

Otto, E. *et al.* (2003). Mutations in INVS encoding inversion cause nephronophthisis type 2, concerning renal optic disease to the function of primary cilia and left–right axis development. *Nature Genetics* **34**, 413–420.

Pasa-Tolic, L. *et al.* (2002). Gene expression profiling using advanced mass spectrometric approaches. *Journal of Mass Spectrometry* **37** (12), 1185–1198.

Patil, N. *et al.* (2001). Blocks of limited haplotype diversity revealed by high-resolution scanning of human chromosome 21. *Science* **294** (5547), 1719–1723.

Phakdeekitcharoen, B., Watnick, T. J., and Germino, G. G. (2001). Mutation analysis of the entire replicated portion of PKD1 using genomic DNA samples. *Journal of the American Society of Nephrology* **12** (5), 955–963.

Qian, F. *et al.* (1997). PKD1 interacts with PKD2 through a probable coiled-coil domain. *Nature Genetics* **16** (2), 179–183.

Reilly, R. F. Protein techniques. In *Techniques in Molecular Medicine* (ed. F. Hildebrandt and P. Igarashi). Berlin: Springer, 1999.

Ruf, R. G. *et al.* (2004). Patients with mutations in podocin do not respond to standard steroid treatment of nephrotic syndrome. *Journal of the American Society of Nephrology* **15**, 722–732.

Shih, N. Y. *et al.* (1999). Congenital nephrotic syndrome in mice lacking CD2-associated protein. *Science* **286** (5438), 312–315.

Somlo, S. and Mundel, P. (2000). Getting a foothold in nephrotic syndrome. *Nature Genetics* **24** (4), 333–335.

Stoll, M. *et al.* (2001). A genomic-systems biology map for cardiovascular function. *Science* **294** (5547), 1723–1726.

Winn, M. P. (2002). Not all in the family: mutations of podocin in sporadic steroid-resistant nephrotic syndrome. *Journal of the American Society of Nephrology* **13** (2), 577–579.

Woo, D. D. *et al.* (1997). Genetic identification of two major modifier loci of polycystic kidney disease progression in pcy mice. *Journal of Clinical Investigation* **100** (8), 1934–1940.

Yoder, B. K., Hou, X., and Guay-Woodford, L. M. (2002). The polycystic kidney disease proteins, polycystin-1, polycystin-2, polaris, and cystin, are co-localized in renal cilia. *Journal of the American Society of Nephrology* **13** (10), 2508–2516.

16.2 Cystic diseases

16.2.1 Polycystic kidney disease in children

Marie-France Gagnadoux

Introduction

Renal cysts occur in a wide variety of renal diseases, of both dysplastic and genetic origin. Genetic counselling requires a clear differentiation to be made between these types of cysts, and the former classification of Osathanondh and Potter, which combined inherited diseases and developmental abnormalities, must be discarded. The term 'polycystic kidney disease' should be reserved for two hereditary cystic diseases: autosomal-recessive and autosomal-dominant polycystic kidney diseases (ARPKD and ADPKD). These are clearly distinguishable by their mode of inheritance and by their pathological characteristics, and, although both of these forms of polycystic disease may occur in children, it is the recessive form that usually manifests in childhood. The recessive condition was commonly called the 'infantile form', while dominant polycystic disease was commonly known as the 'adult form'. However, nowadays, the development of renal imaging techniques, particularly ultrasonography, allows early detection of the dominant form, which is increasingly recognized in childhood and even *in utero*. The expression of these two forms in children will be described, and the problems of differential diagnosis will be discussed.

Autosomal-recessive polycystic kidney disease

Definition

This disease is characterized by an autosomal-recessive mode of inheritance and its constant association with a biliary dysgenesis known as 'congenital hepatic fibrosis'. It is usually recognized in young children, but may also be discovered in late childhood or early adulthood. ARPKD is a rare condition. Its incidence has been estimated as about 1/20,000 individuals (Zerres *et al.* 1998).

Pathology

Renal lesions

Renal involvement is invariably bilateral and generally symmetrical, with a characteristic finding of enlarged and normally shaped kidneys

with many microcysts lying beneath the capsule. The urinary tract is normal. On section, there is no clear limit between the cortex and the medulla, and the kidney has a spongy appearance (Fig. 1).

Histologically, there is a marked ectasia of the collecting ducts, which appear in a radial arrangement from the calyx to the capsule and which are lined by a cuboidal or flat epithelium. Immunochemical or histochemical stainings demonstrate that the cysts originate from collecting ducts. In fetal kidneys studied at an early stage, however, proximal tubular cysts (up to 30 per cent) may be found in addition to collecting duct dilatations until the thirty-fourth week of gestation. Glomerular cysts are never found. The proportion of nephrons affected with cystic dilatations may vary from 20–30 per cent to more than 90 per cent, in correlation with the clinical severity (Blyth and Ockenden 1971).

The morphological picture of striation produced by ectasia of the collecting ducts loses its uniformity with increasing age, as larger cysts develop and compress the calices of the renal pelvis. There are small areas of normal parenchyma in the superficial cortex and no evidence of dysplasia in these kidneys.

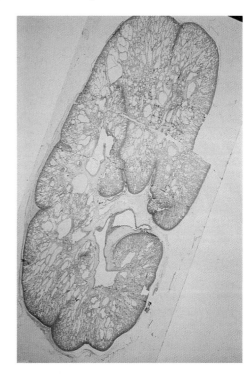

Fig. 1 Macroscopic features of the kidney in recessive polycystic disease.

Hepatic lesions

Liver disease is always present and is often incorrectly called 'congenital hepatic fibrosis'. Biliary dysgenesis or 'biliary fibroadenomatosis' are more precise terms to describe the peculiar characteristics of this fibrosis. The macroscopic appearance of the liver is unique, with white stellar spots over a smooth or finely granular surface. The histological lesions are also characteristic: the portal spaces are enlarged by varying amounts of periportal fibrosis and there is proliferation of biliary ducts, which are dilated and tortuous and frequently contain biliary casts (Fig. 2). The hepatic cells themselves are normal.

Clinical features

The clinical presentation varies with the age of onset and the predominance of renal or hepatic symptoms. Within a sibship, there may be a complete dissimilarity in the age at onset, clinical presentation, and evolution of the disease (Kaplan *et al.* 1988; Deget *et al.* 1995; Fonck *et al.* 2001). The disease cannot therefore be separated into several genetically distinct forms—perinatal, neonatal, and infantile, with renal predominance, and juvenile forms with hepatic predominance—as was proposed by Blyth and Ockenden (1971).

Age and symptoms at discovery

Over the last 20 years, progress in ultrasonography, allowing earlier detection, and development of neonatal intensive care have modified the age at discovery and the short-term outcome of the disease. The former classification into forms of perinatal, infantile, and juvenile onset has therefore become largely obsolete. The only relevant distinction is between immediately lethal cases and patients who survive the neonatal period.

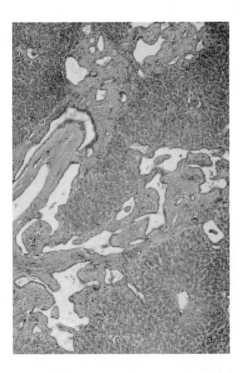

Fig. 2 Histology of the liver in a case of recessive polycystic kidney disease with typical biliary fibroadenomatosis.

Pre- and perinatally lethal disease

The proportion of children with ARPKD who die *in utero* or in the perinatal period has been estimated at about 75 per cent (Kääriäinen 1987). These fetuses, who have extensive and widespread tubular dilatation, present with huge kidneys, oligohydramnios, and pulmonary hypoplasia or atelectasia. If born alive, they usually die within the first few hours or days, from respiratory distress rather than from renal failure. Nowadays, these severe forms are recognized by ultrasonography in the second trimester of pregnancy and usually lead to pregnancy termination in case of anamnios attesting to anuria. In a recent French obstetrical survey of 20 ARPKD fetuses with large hyperechoic kidneys detected prenatally from 1985 to 1996, 10 underwent termination of pregnancy because of severe oligohydramnios, four died neonatally and only six, who presented with normal or moderately decreased amniotic fluid, survive (Tsatsaris *et al.* 2002).

Children who survive the neonatal period

Among the survivors, the disease, if undetected *in utero*, is now most often recognized in the newborn because of some degree of respiratory distress or a distended abdomen, or at a systematic examination, which reveals the enlarged kidneys. In the mildest forms, it may be discovered later, in infants or in older patients, by palpation of enlarged kidneys either during systematic examination or during investigation of symptoms such as hypertension, abdominal pain, proteinuria, haematuria, pyuria, or liver abnormality.

Renal involvement

Clinical renal symptoms

Enlargement of kidneys

The kidneys are always palpable and are occasionally visible in newborn infants, but are often no longer palpable some years later. However, at the endstage of renal failure, the absence of enlarged kidneys, and even their small size, is not inconsistent with the diagnosis.

Hypertension

High blood pressure is a main feature of ARPKD and in two recent surveys, 60–70 per cent of patients required antihypertensive medication during the course of the disease (Zerres *et al.* 1996; Roy *et al.* 1997). In half of the patients of Zerres *et al.*, hypertension appeared early, during the first year of life, with a mean age of 0.5 years at initiation of therapy. At this age, hypertension may be very severe and its cardiovascular complications are the main cause of death in infants with ARPKD (Gagnadoux 1997). In some cases, blood pressure normalizes during childhood, but may reappear at adolescence.

The mechanism of high blood pressure in ARPKD is not yet clearly understood. As plasma renin activity is not increased and many infants present with hyponatraemia during the first months, an intravascular volume expansion has been suggested, at least in infants (Kaplan *et al.* 1989). However, this explanation is not relevant in older children with normal urine dilution, and in clinical practice, the almost constant efficacy of angiotensin-converting enzyme (ACE) inhibitors to normalize blood pressure argues for a hyperreninaemic form of hypertension.

Other symptoms

Recurrent urinary tract infections, not explained by urinary tract malformations, are not uncommon during the first years of life and usually disappear later in childhood. Haematuria is quite uncommon, except following trauma, and proteinuria is rare.

Functional disturbances

The glomerular filtration rate (GFR) is more or less reduced at the onset of disease, depending on the severity of the renal involvement, but most patients exhibit an increase in clearance throughout the first 2 years (Cole *et al.* 1987); it then remains stable, but usually less than the normal range. Progression of renal insufficiency is generally slow and occurs late in most series. With adequate conservative management and antihypertensive therapy, no more than one-third of patients reach endstage renal failure before adulthood (Gagnadoux *et al.* 1989; Roy *et al.* 1997).

The most frequent functional disturbance is a loss of concentrating ability, with maximum urinary osmolality being between 300 and 500 mOsm/l in all the patients studied before the onset of advanced renal failure (Gagnadoux *et al.* 1989). This abnormality does not usually deteriorate with time and rarely gives rise to massive polyuria. Disturbance of H^+ excretion with metabolic acidosis may be observed before the onset of endstage renal failure, and is characterized by a decreased urinary excretion of ammonia with a persistent ability to decrease urinary pH.

Hyponatraemia is frequently observed in the first months of life; it was reported in 15 of 19 infants aged less than 3 months and was related to inappropriately high urine osmolality (Kaplan *et al.* 1989). This disorder may be difficult to manage (mainly with water restriction) in some severe cases but regresses spontaneously and is not observed in older children.

Ultrasonography and radiology

Ultrasonography is now the basic diagnostic tool and is often sufficient on its own, for example, in the familial forms. The kidneys are invariably enlarged (>+2 SD > mean, often >+4 SD). They are uniformly hyperechogenic in newborns, while the renal medulla may appear more echogenic in older children. Disseminated small cysts, generally smaller than 15 mm, are frequently visible and may be present from the neonatal period. In adolescent and young adults, kidneys may appear normal sized, but remain hyperechoic with loss of corticomedullary differentiation and presence of multiple small cysts (Nicolau *et al.* 2000). The development of cysts similar to those seen in ADPKD have been described in some cases.

Excretory urography shows very large kidneys with radial streaks of contrast material, sometimes persisting for as long as 48 h after injection; this streaky appearance is very suggestive of ARPKD. On computed tomography (CT) after contrast injection, which has now replaced urography, tubular dilatations appear as fusiform or 'lace-like' medullary hypodensities radiating from the papilla (Kääriäinen *et al.* 1988) (Fig. 3).

Magnetic resonance (MR) imaging and particularly RARE-MR urography also seem a valuable tool, allowing to disclose the characteristic dilated collecting ducts as a hyperintense linear radial pattern (Kern *et al.* 2000).

Liver involvement

Liver involvement, characterized by biliary dysgenesis, is constantly present in patients with ARPKD. There is, however, a wide spectrum of severity, from completely silent to major and predominant liver

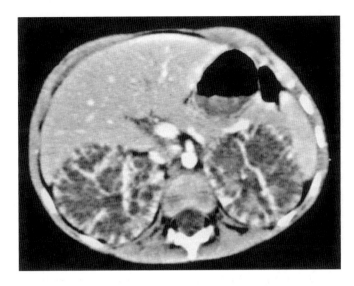

Fig. 3 Computed tomography in a case of polycystic kidney disease, showing the 'lace-like' appearance of medulla (by courtesy of Pr Nivet, University of Tours, France).

disease. Clinical expression of the liver and kidney disease can be different in siblings (Kaplan *et al.* 1988).

Forms with predominant liver involvement

Hepatomegaly with predominant enlargement of the left lobe is usually found in these patients, often with splenomegaly. Portal hypertension is the main consequence of the liver disease, resulting in oesophageal varices and possibly gastrointestinal bleeding. Thrombocytopenia, either isolated or associated with neutropenia due to hypersplenism, is also a common finding in these forms. Biliary-duct abnormalities may be complicated with cholangitis, which may result in lethal septicaemia. Hepatocellular decompensation has never been reported and liver enzymes are normal, or slightly elevated as regards γ-glutamyl transpeptidase (Zerres *et al.* 1996).

Abdominal ultrasonography shows dilatation of the biliary ducts or even true cysts, a heterogeneous looking liver or at least symptoms of portal hypertension (Alvarez *et al.* 1981; Davies *et al.* 1986). CT and MR-cholangiography are currently the best means to reveal dilatation of intrahepatic biliary ducts and characteristic duplication of the intrahepatic branches of the portal vein (Ernst *et al.* 1998) (Fig. 4).

In patients with predominantly liver symptoms, renal involvement may be discovered only after systematic imaging investigation (Alvarez *et al.* 1981). However, there is no 'balance' between renal and hepatic disease and early occurrence of severe renal failure in children with severe portal hypertension has been reported by several authors. It has been recently stressed that portal-systemic shunts may be harmful in anephric dialysis patients, with development of hyperammoniaemia resulting in fatal hepatic encephalopathy (Tsimaratos *et al.* 2000). In case of severe portal hypertension in endstage renal disease (ESRD) patients, early combined liver–kidney transplantation should be considered, although successful renal transplantation in two children with a portal-systemic shunt had been reported (McGonigle *et al.* 1981).

Detection of asymptomatic liver involvement

In patients with apparently isolated ARPKD, liver involvement is usually detected by a specific investigation. Clinical examination seeks

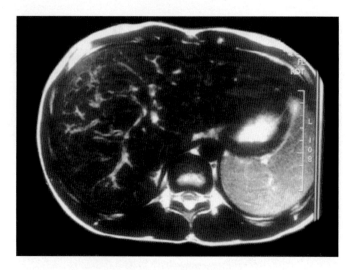

Fig. 4 MR-cholangiography in a child with ADPKD without apparent liver involvement, showing dilatation of intrahepatic bile ducts.

hepatomegaly and splenomegaly. Abdominal ultrasonography must be systematic, with particular attention paid to looking for biliary-duct ectasia. In the Enfants Malades series, systematic ultrasonography of the abdomen demonstrated unequivocal dilatation of the peripheral intrahepatic biliary ducts in 16 of 24 ARPKD children without clinical symptoms of liver involvement (66 per cent), and signs of portal hypertension in a further case.

Abdominal CT or MR-cholangiography may also be performed to affirm the liver involvement, necessary for an unequivocal diagnosis. Liver histology is now rarely used for ascertaining the diagnosis, because portal lesions may be irregularly distributed within liver.

Prognosis and long-term evolution

The prognosis essentially depends on the renal component of the disease and is not as poor as previously considered. In the past, the prognosis of ARPKD detected at birth was considered to be lethal. Now most of children born alive survive. In three recently published series, the actuarial probability of survival with functioning kidneys for children who survived the neonatal period was 86–93 per cent at 2 years of age, 78–83 per cent at 5 years, 75–82 per cent at 10 years, 67–79 per cent at 15 years, and 50–60 per cent at 20 years (Gagnadoux et al. 1989; Kaplan et al. 1989; Roy et al. 1997).

The prevention of early death, particularly by good control of hypertension, explains much of the improvement in the prognosis of this disease. It is important, therefore, not to be too pessimistic about the prognosis when the disease is detected in a newborn or in utero (except in case of oligoamnios).

Long-term survival beyond the second decade and adult-onset forms of the disease have also been reported (Shaikewitz and Chapman 1993; Perez et al. 1998; Fonck et al. 2001). The series reported by Fonck et al. (2001) comprises 16 patients followed beyond 18 years of age (age at latest follow-up: 18–55 years, mean 27 ± 10). Three of them ultimately reached ESRD at 20, 22, and 29 years of age; 11 others, aged 20–55 years, are in chronic renal failure, and two, aged 18–21 years, still have normal GFR. In patients with renal failure, the yearly decline in creatinine clearance was estimated to 2.9 ± 1.6 ml/min.

The prognosis of the liver involvement depends on the risks of portal hypertension and of cholangitis, which can be largely prevented or treated. However, long-term morbidity and mortality due to liver involvement was significant in the two series with follow-up to the adult age: four deaths from gastrointestinal bleeding and one portal-systemic encephalopathy at 46 years in the British series (Roy et al. 1997) and five cases of gastro-oesophageal bleeding with one death at 47 years in the French series (Fonck et al. 2001). No death from hepatocellular insufficiency has been so far reported.

Genetics

Since 1994, genetic linkage studies have mapped the gene for ARPKD (named *PKDH1*) to the 6p21.1–p12 region of chromosome 6 (Zerres et al. 1994; Guay-Woodford et al. 1995). With linkage studies, no genetic heterogeneity had been found whatever the clinical spectrum of the disease, particularly regarding hepatic involvement and severity of initial presentation (Guay-Woodford et al. 1995; Alvarez et al. 2000).

In 2002, two teams, by two different approaches, identified the gene *PKDH1*. Ward et al. (2002) have mapped the gene for a rodent disease similar to human ARPKD, described in the *pck* rat, on rat chromosome 9 and have subsequently cloned and sequenced the human ortholog of this gene on chromosome 6, which is in fact *PKDH1*. By screening the 66 coding exons of this gene, they found mutations in 11 of 14 families with ARPKD. Simultaneously, Onuchic et al. (2002), by positional cloning of the candidate region, identified a gene including at least 86 exons and detected various mutations across this gene in 12 families with ARPKD. In the two series, most patients were compound heterozygotes, and no clear genotype–phenotype correlation could be evidenced.

The main *PKDH1* transcript is expressed in fetal and adult kidney and is predicted to encode a novel transmembrane protein (named fibrocystin or polyductin), belonging to a superfamily of proteins involved in regulation of cellular adhesion and repulsion and of cell proliferation. The mechanism by which the absence or the alteration of this protein results in the tubular and biliary lesions of ARPKD remains to be elucidated.

Prenatal diagnosis

Until recently, only ultrasonography could allow to detect ARPKD before birth, by showing kidney enlargement greater than 2 SD, increased renal echogenicity and, in severe cases, oligoamnios due to fetal oliguria. However, these signs are not manifest before 18 weeks of pregnancy at the best, and they may not be detected before 30 weeks or even be completely missed when amniotic fluid is normal (Gagnadoux 1997; Zerres et al. 1998). Moreover, ultrasound criteria are not pathognomonic and may be observed in other cystic renal diseases, and even without patent renal disease after birth (Slovis et al. 1993; Guay-Woodford et al. 1998).

Therefore, in families with a previously deceased child, the demand is great for a molecular genetic testing in early pregnancy, allowing for early termination of pregnancy in case of affected sibling. Since the mapping of the gene to 6p21.1–p12, indirect haplotype-based genetic testing has been performed in two series reporting, respectively, 65 and 35 prenatal analyses (Zerres et al. 1998; Gagnadoux et al. 2000); both series demonstrate that reliable prenatal diagnosis of further pregnancies is possible in nearly 80 per cent of affected families, provided several conditions are gathered: definitive diagnosis in the index case, availability of index case and parents' DNA, and genetic informativity of the family at the ARPKD locus. It seems premature to hope that the identification of *PKHD1* gene will permit direct genetic diagnosis by mutation finding in the near future, given the very large size of the gene.

Autosomal-dominant polycystic kidney disease (see 16.2.2)

Definition

ADPKD is defined genetically by its dominant inheritance and pathologically by cystic dilatation of all parts of the nephron. In contrast with the recessive disease, liver involvement, usually characterized by macrocysts, is not constant. This disease is much more common than ARPKD in the general population, affecting 1/500 to 1/1000 individuals.

Theoretically, ADPKD is present from the beginning of fetal life, but usually it does not become clinically evident until adulthood. However, it has long been known that the disease could appear in childhood and even in fetal life. In addition, modern imaging techniques or genetic markers may now provide the diagnosis in asymptomatic children or fetuses. ADPKD, therefore, being 40 times more prevalent, is now as commonly diagnosed as the autosomal-recessive disease in children (Zerres *et al.* 1995; Gagnadoux 1997).

Pathology

Macroscopically, the kidneys are almost always bilaterally enlarged, with grossly visible cysts disseminated in the cortex and in the medulla affecting all or part of the parenchyma. In contrast with ARPKD, the cysts may be derived from any segment of the nephrons, including Bowman's space, proximal tubules, loops of Henle, and collecting ducts. Glomerular cysts are particularly abundant in very early-onset ADPKD (Reeders *et al.* 1986; Bernstein 1993; Guay-Woodford *et al.* 1998).

Extrarenal cysts, involving mainly liver and sometimes pancreas, which may develop in older patients, particularly in females, are exceptional in children (Perrone 1997). In the vast majority of cases of ADPKD, there is no biliary dysgenesis similar to that observed in the recessive polycystic disease. However, several cases of ADPKD patients, both adults and children, presenting with some degree of portal fibrosis and bile-duct proliferation have been described (Grünfeld *et al.* 1985; Cobben *et al.* 1990). In addition, MR imaging of liver show that intrahepatic bile ducts dilatations are present in 28 per cent of adult ADPKD patients (Dranssart *et al.* 2002).

Clinical presentation in childhood

The clinical spectrum of childhood dominant polycystic kidney disease is very wide, ranging from asymptomatic children detected by routine ultrasonography to fetuses presenting *in utero* with massive renal enlargement and oligoamnios. Before sonographic detection, two clinical forms could be described: a juvenile form revealed in later childhood, generally paucisymptomatic, and a neonatal form, simulating the recessive form. Nowadays, owing the wide use of ultrasonography, which allows detection of the disease at an infraclinical stage, ADPKD is increasingly recognized in young children and fetuses and asymptomatic forms have become more and more common.

Child form

Sonographic detection in childhood

The ultrasonographic diagnosis is easy when macrocysts are bilaterally distributed in more or less enlarged kidneys and when the family history is suggestive. The diagnosis may be more difficult to ascertain, especially if the disease has not yet been recognized in the family, in case of single or unilateral cysts in normal-sized kidneys, what is not uncommon in children (Fick-Brosnahan *et al.* 1999, 2001). As far as, in the general population, the sonographic detection of 'simple renal cysts' is exceptional before 30 years of age (Ravine *et al.* 1993), the diagnosis of simple cyst in a child should not be accepted before an accurate family inquiry. In doubtful cases, kidney CT may help by showing the presence of other smaller cysts.

Several studies have been devoted to the systematic detection of cysts in high-risk children belonging to families with an affected adult member. In the usual form linked to the gene located on chromosome 16 (*PKD1*), the detection rate has been estimated to be as high as 62 per cent of affected children aged 0–5 years, 82 per cent of children 6–10 years of age, 86 per cent of children 10–15 years of age, 90 per cent at 20 years of age, and 100 per cent at 30 years of age (Bear *et al.* 1992; Gabow *et al.* 1997). In the rare families affected with the form linked to the gene located on chromosome 4 (*PKD2*), the reliability of ultrasonography was found to be only 50 per cent before the age of 15, but 100 per cent at the age of 30 (Demetriou *et al.* 2000).

Most of the affected children detected by systematic examination are completely asymptomatic, and routine ultrasonographic screening is not ethically justified in children at risk, at least in the first decade. Some of these children, however, develop hypertension in later childhood and adolescence, and annual blood pressure measurement is recommended in at-risk children.

Symptomatic forms in children

Clinical onset of the disease in childhood has been reported by several teams (Sedman *et al.* 1987; Kääriäinen *et al.* 1988b; Gagnadoux *et al.* 1989; Fick *et al.* 1994). Some patients were referred because of symptoms such as haematuria, hypertension, flank pain, or urinary infection, mostly after 10 years of age. Some others were detected by a systematic ultrasonographic screening and were found to be actually symptomatic (30 per cent of the Sedman series and 55 per cent of the Fick series).

Hypertension is the most common symptom in children with ADPKD (47 per cent in the series of Fick-Brosnahan *et al.* 2001). It is usually easily controlled by antihypertensive drugs, for example β-blockers or ACE inhibitors. Renal function is not generally modified in these patients, but a reduced GFR was reported in some cases (Sedman *et al.* 1987; Parfrey *et al.* 1990). A defect of concentrating ability may also be found in the absence of a reduction in GFR (Fick *et al.* 1994). Proteinuria was present in 28 per cent of affected children in the series of Fick-Brosnahan, whereas gross haematuria occurred in only 10 per cent of children.

Extrarenal manifestations observed in adult patients (liver cysts, cerebral aneurysms, valvular abnormalities) are exceptional in paediatric patients (Perrone 1997). Only one patient among 62 affected children studied by Fick *et al.* (1994) had a single liver cyst, at the age of 16 years. Rupture of cerebral aneurysms occurs exceptionally during childhood (Proesmans 1982; Perrone 1997). The minimum age from which periodic screening for aneurysms by MR-angiography is indicated, in families with history of intracranial aneurysms, remains a matter of debate.

Prognosis and evolution

The long-term prognosis in children with ADPKD detected during childhood, because of symptoms or through systematic detection, is largely unknown. In most cases, it is impossible, with the present follow-up, to know if these children will ultimately develop renal failure at an earlier age than the patients detected at the adult age. The study of Fick-Brosnahan *et al.* (2001) found, in a large series of ADPKD children, a correlation between structural progression of the disease (marked by increase in cysts number and renal growth) and development of hypertension. 'Risk factors' were defined as early renal enlargement, presence of more than 10 cysts before the age of 12, and blood pressure above the seventy-fifth percentile. However, in that study, no decline in GFR was observed in any child or young adult up to 25 years of age, whatever the increase in renal volume, and the relevance of these 'risk factors' for the prognosis of renal failure remains questionable.

Infantile form

Symptomatic newborns and infants

The early-onset form of ADPKD has been known for a long time; more than 80 such cases had been reported up to 1998 (Mc Dermot *et al.* 1998). In these forms, it is not rare that the family is not aware of the inherited disease and the diagnosis is made after ultrasonography of the parents.

The presentation of these cases, *in utero* or after birth, mimics the recessive form, both clinically (enlarged kidneys, respiratory distress, high blood pressure ± renal failure) and sonographically (large hyperechoic kidneys). The presence of macrocysts, suggestive of the dominant form, is uncommon, and imaging findings are often equivocal (Cole *et al.* 1987; Kääriäinen *et al.* 1988a). On intravenous pyelography, the prolonged excretion and the accumulation of contrast material in multiple, small cystic structures typically give a 'mottled' or 'puddled' appearance to the parenchyma. Presently, CT seems the more useful tool to differentiate the round cysts, affecting both cortex and medulla, of the dominant form from the fusiform tubular dilatations, radiating from the medulla, of the recessive disease (Kääriäinen *et al.* 1988a) (Fig. 5).

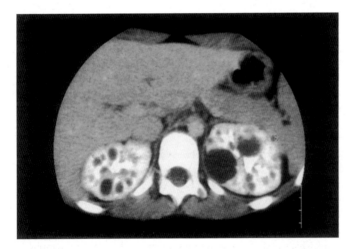

Fig. 5 Computed tomography of kidneys in a child with ADPKD, showing the round cysts disseminated within cortex and medulla.

The rare cases of biliary dysgenesis associated with ADPKD may present as infantile forms, the liver involvement adding to the similarity with the recessive form (Cobben *et al.* 1990; Torra *et al.* 1997).

Some early-onset cases are lethal *in utero* or at birth, or undergo now termination of pregnancy when there are huge kidneys with oligoamnios; it was the case in three of eight fetuses with prenatally detected ADPKD in the obstetrical survey of Tsatsaris *et al.* (2002). However, most of these newborns survive. They present usually with early hypertension and renal failure; however, their outcome does not seem to be as poor as it appeared from previous reports, which found near 50 per cent mortality within the first year (Mc Dermot *et al.* 1998).

Sonographic prenatal detection of mild forms

The routine detection, by the third trimester ultrasonography, of moderately large and hyperechoic kidneys, with normal amniotic fluid, in a fetus whose one parent is affected with ADPKD, is increasingly frequent. This discovery should not lead to an excessive concern. Indeed, most of these children appear completely asymptomatic, at least in their first decade (Gagnadoux 1997; Tstsaris *et al.* 2002). After birth a transient normalization of renal sonography may be observed in some cases, but cysts develop within the first year (Jeffery *et al.* 1998).

Prognosis and evolution

Forms with clinical manifestations in early life were thought to have a poor prognosis, with a more rapid progression to ESRD than in the recessive form (Gagnadoux *et al.* 1989; Fick *et al.* 1993). However, more recent series do not support this pessimistic view. In a series of 16 dominant forms recognized before 1 year of age (eight *in utero*), only one developed endstage renal failure and the survival rate with functioning kidneys was 87 per cent at 5 years of age (Gagnadoux 1997). In another series of 11 children with sonographic prenatal diagnosis, five had renal failure at birth but only three remained with mild renal failure after a mean follow-up of 4 years, the other eight having normal GFR (Pecoraro *et al.* 2001).

As regards infants detected *in utero* with mild forms, their long-term prognosis is not yet known; most of them remain asymptomatic at the present follow-up of 10–15 years. However, they should be followed annually, particularly regarding their blood pressure.

Genetics (see Chapters 16.1 and 16.2.2)

All families with early-onset ADPKD analysed to date have shown linkage to the *PKD1* gene, without difference from the adult-onset form (Michaud *et al.* 1994; Mc Dermot *et al.* 1998). A strong familial recurrence of these neonatal forms has been reported by several investigators (Kääriäinen 1987; Zerres *et al.* 1993), which has important implications for genetic counselling. Furthermore, a predominance of maternal transmission in the early-onset forms has been found in two important series (Fick *et al.* 1993; Zerres *et al.* 1993). These observations favour the role of genetic anticipation and imprinting in the pathogenesis of early manifestation of the disease (Zerres *et al.* 1995).

Prenatal diagnosis

Molecular biological techniques allow the diagnosis to be reached in embryos only a few weeks old in certain informative families (Reeders *et al.* 1986; Michaud *et al.* 1994). However, genetic prenatal screening seems ethically justified only in families with a high risk of recurrence of the early-onset form, and even in those families, a large variation in the clinical presentation within a family may be observed, leading to caution in deciding termination of pregnancy.

Ultrasonography is in fact the best tool of prenatal diagnosis of ADPKD; it allows to differentiate, from about 20 weeks of pregnancy, between the mild forms, with normal amniotic fluid and moderately enlarged kidneys, which will not cause symptoms during childhood, and the severe forms, with very large kidneys and oligoanamnios, which will result in neonatal renal failure or termination of pregnancy. It is still unknown whether only particularly early forms, or almost all affected children, can be detected *in utero* by modern imaging techniques.

Differential diagnosis

ARPKD and ADPKD do not represent the unique cause of renal cysts in children. There are many other clinical circumstances in which renal cysts may be found, namely cystic dysplasias (particularly multicystic kidney), multiple malformations syndromes, and several other inherited diseases (Zerres *et al.* 1984; Bernstein 1987; Woolf *et al.* 2002). Many of these conditions present *in utero* with large hyperechoic kidneys and may be falsely diagnosed as ARPKD (Slovis *et al.* 1993; Guay-Woodford *et al.* 1998; Tsatsaris *et al.* 2002). After birth, associated clinical symptoms and ultrasonographic features (normal or reduced-sized kidneys and presence of large cysts) allow usually to differentiate these conditions from the two forms of polycystic kidney disease. However tuberous sclerosis, in its form linked to the *TSC2* gene, may appear in infants as a cystic renal disorder, clinically and macroscopically similar to neonatal forms of ADPKD, several years before the appearance of neurological and cutaneous signs. In these forms, large deletions involving the two contiguous genes, *PKD1* and *TSC2*, have been reported (Brook-Carter *et al.* 1994; Sperandio *et al.* 2000). An accurate familial anamnesis and a complete clinical investigation are therefore mandatory to establish the diagnosis of ARPKD or ADPKD.

References

Alvarez, F. *et al.* (1981). Congenital hepatic fibrosis in children. *Journal of Pediatrics* 99, 370–375.

Alvarez, V. *et al.* (2000). Analysis of chromosome 6p in Spanish families with recessive polycystic kidney disease. *Pediatric Nephrology* 14, 205–207.

Bear, J. C. *et al.* (1992). Autosomal dominant polycystic kidney disease: new information for genetic counselling. *American Journal of Medical Genetics* 43, 548–553.

Bernstein, J. *et al.* (1987). Renal hepatic pancreatic dysplasia: a syndrome reconsidered. *American Journal of Medical Genetics* 26, 391–403.

Blyth, H. and Ockenden, B. G. (1971). Polycystic disease of kidneys and liver presenting in childhood. *Journal of Medical Genetics* 8, 257–284.

Brook-Carter, P. T. *et al.* (1994). Deletion of the *TSC2* and *PKD1* genes associated with severe infantile polycystic kidney disease—a contiguous gene syndrome. *Nature Genetics* 8, 328–332.

Cobben, J. M. *et al.* (1990). Congenital hepatic fibrosis in autosomal dominant polycystic kidney disease. *Kidney International* 38, 880–885.

Cole, B. R. *et al.* (1987). Polycystic kidney disease in the first year of life. *Journal of Pediatrics* 111, 693–699.

Davies, C. H. *et al.* (1986). Congenital hepatic fibrosis with saccular dilatations of intrahepatic bile ducts and infantile polycystic kidneys. *Pediatric Radiology* 16, 302–305.

Deget, F., Rudnik-Schöneborn, S., and Zerres, K. (1995). Course of autosomal recessive polycystic kidney disease (ARPKD) in siblings: a clinical comparison of 20 sibships. *Clinical Genetics* 47, 248–253.

Demetriou, K. *et al.* (2000). Autosomal dominant polycystic kidney disease—type 2. Ultrasound, genetic and clinical correlations. *Nephrology, Dialysis, Transplantation* 15, 205–211.

Dranssart, M. *et al.* (2002). MR choloangiography in the evaluation of hepatic and biliary abnormalities of autosomal dominant polycystic kidney disease: study of 93 patients. *Journal of Computer Assisted Tomography* 26, 237–242.

Ernst, O. *et al.* (1998). Congenital hepatic fibrosis: findings at MR cholangiopancreatography. *American Journal of Roentgenology* 170, 409–412.

Fick, G. M. *et al.* (1993). Characteristics of very early onset autosomal dominant polycystic kidney disease. *Journal of the American Society of Nephrology* 3, 1863–1870.

Fick, G. M. *et al.* (1994). The spectrum of autosomal dominant polycystic kidney disease in children. *Journal of the American Society of Nephrology* 4, 1654–1660.

Fick-Brosnahan, G. M. *et al.* (1999). Renal assymetry in children with autosomal dominant polycystic kidney disease. *American Journal of Kidney Diseases* 34, 639–645.

Fick-Brosnahan, G. M. *et al.* (2001). Progression of autosomal-dominant polycystic kidney disease in children. *Kidney International* 59, 1654–1662.

Fonck, C. *et al.* (2001). Autosomal recessive polycystic kidney disease in adulthood. *Nephrology, Dialysis, Transplantation* 16, 1648–1652.

Gabow, P. *et al.* (1997). Utility of ultrasonography in the diagnosis of autosomal dominant polycystic kidney disease in children. *Journal of the American Society of Nephrology* 8, 105–110.

Gagnadoux, M. F. (1997). Diagnostic et évolution des polykystoses rénales découvertes dans la première année de vie. *Annales de Pediatrie (Paris)* 44, 660–666.

Gagnadoux, M. F. *et al.* (1989). Cystic renal diseases in children. *Advances in Nephrology* 18, 33–57.

Gagnadoux, M. F. *et al.* (2000). Diagnostic prenatal de la polykystose renale autosomique. *Archives de Pediatrie* 7, 942–947.

Grünfeld, J. P. *et al.* (1985). Liver changes and complications in adult polycystic kidney diseases. *Advances in Nephrology* 14, 1–20.

Guay-Woodford, L. M. *et al.* (1995). The severe perinatal form of autosomal recessive polycystic kidney disease maps to chromosome 6p21.1–p12: implications for genetic counseling. *American Journal of Human Genetics* 56, 1101–1107.

Guay-Woodford, L. M. *et al.* (1998). Diffuse renal cystic disease in children: morphologic and genetic correlations. *Pediatric Nephrology* 12, 173–182.

Jeffery, S. *et al.* (1998). Apparent normalization of fetal renal size in autosomal dominant polycystic kidney disease (PKD1). *Clinical Genetics* 53, 303–307.

Kääriäinen, H. (1987). Polycystic kidney disease in children: a genetic and epidemiological study of 82 Finnish patients. *Journal of Medical Genetics* 24, 474–481.

Kääriäinen, H. *et al.* (1988a). Dominant and recessive polycystic kidney disease in children: classification by intravenous pyelography, ultrasound and computed tomography. *Pediatric Radiology* 18, 45–50.

Kääriäinen, H. *et al.* (1988b). Dominant and recessive polycystic kidney disease in children: evaluation of clinical features and laboratory data. *Pediatric Nephrology* 2, 296–302.

Kaplan, B. S. *et al.* (1988). Variable expression of autosomal recessive polycystic kidney disease and congenital hepatic fibrosis within a family. *American Journal of Medical Genetics* 29, 639–647.

Kaplan, B. S. *et al.* (1989). Autosomal recessive polycystic kidney disease. *Pediatric Nephrology* 3, 43–49.

Kern, S. *et al.* (2000). Appearance of autosomal recessive polycystic kidney disease in magnetic resonance imaging and RARE-MR-urography. *Pediatric Radiology* 30, 156–160.

MacDermot, K. D. *et al.* (1998). Prenatal diagnosis of autosomal dominant polycystic kidney disease (PKD1) presenting *in utero* and prognosis for very early onset disease. *Journal of Medical Genetics* **35**, 13–16.

McGonigle, R. J. S. *et al.* (1981). Congenital hepatic fibrosis and polycystic kidney disease: role of portacaval shunting and transplantation in 3 patients. *Quarterly Journal of Medicine* **199**, 269–278.

Michaud, J. *et al.* (1994). Autosomal dominant polycystic kidney disease in the fetus. *American Journal of Medical Genetics* **51**, 240–246.

Nicolau, C. *et al.* (2000). Sonographic pattern of recessive polycystic kidney disease in young adults. Differences from the dominant form. *Nephrology, Dialysis, Transplantation* **15**, 1373–1378.

Onuchic, L. F. *et al.* (2002). PKDH1, the polycystic kidney and hepatic disease 1 gene, encodes a novel large protein containing multiple immunoglobulin-like plexin-transcription-factor domains and parallel beta-helix 1 repeats. *American Journal of Human Genetics* **70**, 1305–1317.

Parfrey, P. S. *et al.* (1990). The diagnosis and prognosis of autosomal dominant polycystic kidney disease. *New England Journal of Medicine* **323**, 1085–1090.

Pecoraro, C. *et al.* (2001). Prognosis for autosomal dominant polycystic kidney disease (ADPKD) presenting *in utero*. *Pediatric Nephrology* **16**, C50.

Perez, L. *et al.* (1998). Autosomal recessive polycystic kidney disease presenting in adulthood. Molecular diagnosis of the family. *Nephrology, Dialysis, Transplantation* **13**, 1273–1276.

Perrone, R. (1997). Nephrology forum: extrarenal manifestations of ADPKD. *Kidney International* **51**, 2022–2036.

Proesmans, W. *et al.* (1982). Autosomal dominant polycystic kidney disease in the neonatal period; association with a cerebral arteriovenous malformation. *Pediatrics* **70**, 971–975.

Ravine, D. *et al.* (1993). An ultrasound renal cyst prevalence survey; specific data for inherited renal cystic diseases. *American Journal of Kidney Diseases* **22**, 803–807.

Reeders, S. T. *et al.* (1986). Prenatal diagnosis of autosomal dominant polycystic kidney disease with a DNA-probe. *Lancet* **ii**, 6–8.

Roy, S. *et al.* (1997). Autosomal recessive polycystic kidney disease: long-term outcome of neonatal survivors. *Pediatric Nephrology* **11**, 302–306.

Sedman, A. *et al.* (1987). Autosomal dominant polycystic kidney disease in childhood: a longitudinal study. *Kidney International* **31**, 1000–1005.

Shaikewitz, S. T. and Chapman, A. (1993). Autosomal recessive polycystic kidney disease: issues regarding the variability of clinical presentation. *Journal of the American Society of Nephrology* **3**, 1858–1862.

Slovis, T. L., Bernstein, J., and Gruskin, A. (1993). Hyperechoic kidneys in the newborn and young infant. *Pediatric Nephrology* **7**, 294–302.

Sperandio, M. *et al.* (2000). Cutaneous white spots in a child with polycystic kidneys: a clue to TSC2/PKD1 gene mutation. *Nephrology, Dialysis, Transplantation* **15**, 909–912.

Torra, R. *et al.* (1997). Autosomal dominant polycystic kidney disease with anticipation and Caroli's disease associated with a PKD1 mutation. *Kidney International* **52**, 33–38.

Tsatsaris, V. *et al.* (2002). Prenatal diagnosis of bilateral fetal hyperechoic kidneys. Is it possible to predict long-term outcome? *British Journal of Obstetrics and Gynaecology* **109**, 1388–1393.

Tsimaratos, M. *et al.* (2000). Chronic renal failure and portal hypertension—is portosystemic shunt indicated? *Pediatric Nephrology* **14**, 856–858.

Ward, C. *et al.* (2002). The gene mutated in autosomal recessive polycystic kidney disease encodes a large, receptor-like protein. *Nature Genetics* **30**, 259–269.

Woolf, A. S., Feather, S. A., and Bingham, C. (2002). Recent insights into kidney diseases associated with glomerular cysts. *Pediatric Nephrology* **17**, 229–235.

Zerres, K. and Rudnik-Schöneborn, S. (1995). On genetic heterogeneity, anticipation and imprinting in polycystic kidney diseases. *Nephrology, Dialysis, Transplantation* **10**, 7–19.

Zerres, K. *et al.* (1984). Cystic kidneys: genetics, pathologic anatomy, clinical picture, and prenatal diagnosis. *Human Genetics* **68**, 104–135.

Zerres, K. *et al.* (1993). Childhood onset autosomal dominant polycystic kidney disease in sibs: clinical picture and recurrence risk. *Journal of Medical Genetics* **30**, 583–588.

Zerres, K. *et al.* (1994). Mapping of the gene for autosomal recessive polycystic kidney disease (ARPKD) to chromosome 6p21-cen. *Nature Genetics* **7**, 429–432.

Zerres, K. *et al.* (1996). Autosomal recessive polycystic kidney disease in 115 children: clinical presentation, course and influence of gender. *Acta Paediatrica* **85**, 437–445.

Zerres, K. *et al.* (1998). Prenatal diagnosis of autosomal recessive polycystic kidney disease (ARPKD): molecular genetics, clinical experience and fetal morphology. *American Journal of Medical Genetics* **76**, 137–144.

16.2.2 Autosomal-dominant polycystic kidney disease

Yves Pirson, Dominique Chauveau, and Olivier Devuyst

Autosomal-dominant polycystic kidney disease (ADPKD) is an inherited disorder usually manifest in adulthood and essentially characterized by the development of multiple renal cysts typically leading to endstage renal disease (ESRD) in the sixth decade. Renal involvement is variably associated with a number of extrarenal abnormalities (mainly hepatic and cardiovascular).

ADPKD is genetically heterogeneous. The gene responsible in about 85 per cent of families (*PKD1*) is located on chromosome 16p13.3. There is another gene (*PKD2*) located on chromosome 4q22 accounting for virtually the remainder (Wu 2001). The resulting disease phenotypes are very similar, except that renal disease is typically less severe in *PKD2* families. A very small number of families have been reported with ADPKD unlinked to either *PKD1* or *PKD2*, raising the possibility of a third gene. However, the existence of a third locus is currently questioned, because a number of potential confounders could lead to false exclusion of linkage, best exemplified by bilineal disease (transheterozygous mutations involving both *PKD1* and *PKD2*) (Pei *et al.* 2001).

Epidemiology

ADPKD is by far the most frequent inherited kidney disease. In White populations, its prevalence ranges from one in 400 to one in 1000 (Gabow 1993). Though the corresponding figure in Blacks is not yet available, the incidence of ESRD due to ADPKD is similar in American Blacks and Whites (Yium *et al.* 1994). There is a significant level of *de novo* mutations with a reported rate of 3.6 per cent in a series of pedigrees with a *PKD1* mutation (Rossetti *et al.* 2001). At large, ADPKD currently accounts for 3–10 per cent of all patients admitted for maintenance dialysis in the Western countries. The annual incidence rate of patients with ADPKD treated for ESRD in the United States has not changed over the last decade (United States Renal Data System 2001).

Renal pathology

ADPKD is pathologically characterized by innumerable fluid-filled cysts scattered in both cortex and medulla. They develop in less than 1 per cent of the one million nephrons from any segment, including the collecting duct. Individual cyst wall consists of a single layer of epithelial cells surrounded by a basement membrane. Cyst forms up as a focal outgrowth of renal tubule. As cyst grows, it becomes disconnected from the tubule. Its size enlarges at a variable rate. The basement membrane undergoes progressive thickening.

Molecular genetics

The *PKD1* and *PKD2* genes

The *PKD1* gene spans 53 kb of genomic DNA and encodes a transcript of 14 kb composed of 46 exons (European Polycystic Kidney Disease Consortium 1994). A large portion of the 5′ region of the gene (exons 1–33) is replicated at least five times further proximally on chromosome 16 (European Polycystic Kidney Disease Consortium 1994). The biological function of these *PKD1*-like genes remains unknown. The replicated portion of *PKD1*, as well as the large size of the gene, explain why mutation detection in *PKD1* has been particularly difficult. Until recently, the search for mutations was restricted to the non-replicated portion of the gene. The establishment of specific methods, including high-performance liquid chromatography, has allowed to overcome

the difficulty and screen the entire *PKD1* gene with a mutation detection rate of at least 60 per cent (Rossetti *et al.* 2001, 2002a). A wide variety of different mutations was detected throughout *PKD1*, although they were twice more common in the 3′ compared to the 5′ half of the gene. No clear hotspot was found and most mutations are private (Rossetti *et al.* 2001). The majority of mutations are predicted to truncate the protein due to nonsense or frameshifting changes, but a significant number of missense or in-frame mutations have been described (Rossetti *et al.* 2001).

The second gene, *PKD2*, spans 68 kb of genomic DNA and encodes a transcript of 5.4 kb composed of 15 exons (Mochizuki *et al.* 1996). The mutation detection rate in *PKD2* has been higher (70–80 per cent) than *PKD1*, due to its smaller transcript and lack of homologous loci. Like *PKD1*, the mutations are scattered throughout the gene and most are private. Apart from a few missense, most of the mutations are predicted to result in null alleles or truncated proteins caused by nonsense, frameshifting, or aberrant splicing (Wu 2001).

The *PKD1* protein, polycystin-1

The *PKD1* gene encodes for polycystin-1, a large protein of 4302 amino acids (for review, see Wu 2001; Harris 2002; Igarashi and Somlo 2002). Polycystin-1 is predicted to be an integral membrane protein with 11 transmembrane domains, a short cytoplasmic tail, and a large extracellular region (Fig. 1).

The cytoplasmic *C*-terminus contains approximately 200 amino acids and has an α-helical coiled-coil structure (Qian *et al.* 1997) as

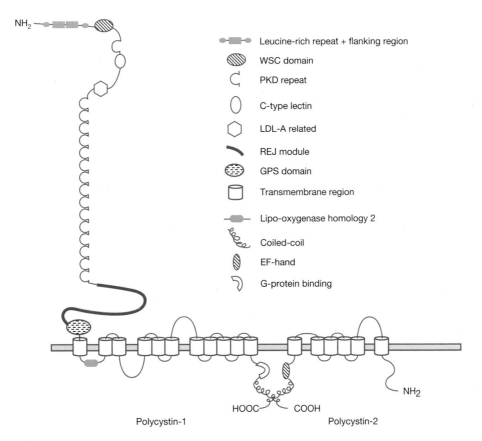

Fig. 1 Predicted topology, conserved domains, and possible interaction between polycystin-1 and polycystin-2. WSC, cell wall integrity and stress response component; LDL-A, low-density lipoprotein A; REJ, receptor for egg jelly; GPS, G-protein coupled receptor proteolytic site (adapted from Peters and Breuning 2001; Harris 2002).

well as consensus sites for phosphorylation that appears essential to mediate interactions between polycystin-1 and intracellular signalling molecules. The long (~3000 amino acids) extracellular *N*-terminus of polycystin-1 contains several domains involved in protein–protein or protein–carbohydrate interactions (Fig. 1) (for review, see Harris 2002). One of them is a large (~1000 amino acids) segment homologous to the sea urchin sperm receptor for egg jelly (REJ) domain. In sea urchins, the binding of the REJ receptor located on the sperm head to the extracellular matrix of the egg triggers the acrosomial reaction, an essential step for fertilization that is associated with ion-channel activation (Moy *et al.* 1996). Thus, the interaction of the REJ domain of polycystin-1 with the extracellular matrix may regulate the ion-channel activity of polycystin-2 (see below).

The cytoplasmic tail of polycystin-1 interacts via its coiled-coil domain with the *C*-terminus of polycystin-2 (Qian *et al.* 1997) and intermediate filament proteins (Xu *et al.* 2001). Several studies have suggested that polycystin-1 regulates G-protein signalling pathways (Kim *et al.* 1999) and modulates Wnt signalling (Igarashi and Somlo 2002). Interestingly, the expression of the *C*-terminus of polycystin-1 triggers branching morphogenesis in inner medullary collecting duct cells (Nickel *et al.* 2002).

The *PKD2* protein, polycystin-2

The *PKD2* gene encodes a 968 amino acids protein, polycystin-2 (Mochizuki *et al.* 1996). Polycystin-2 is predicted to have six transmembrane domains and cytoplasmic *N*- and *C*-termini (Fig. 1). The transmembrane region of polycystin-2 is approximately 50 per cent homologous to polycystin-1 and shows even higher homology to voltage-activated and transient receptor potential (TRP) channel subunits. The region of homology extends to the *C*-terminus and includes an EF-hand domain that has calcium-binding activity (Mochizuki *et al.* 1996). Electrophysiological studies have confirmed that polycystin-2 is a non-selective cation channel that can conduct calcium ions (Igarashi and Somlo 2002). Polycystin-2 appears to be predominantly expressed in the endoplasmic reticulum.

Taken together, these data suggest that both polycystins participate in signalling pathways that regulate normal renal tubule function. Thus, binding of an unknown ligand to the extracellular, *N*-terminus of polycystin-1 may activate, via the cytosolic *C*-terminus, the polycystin-2 cation channel. This activation may result in transient and localized increases in calcium levels that are susceptible to affect many pathways (Harris 2002; Igarashi and Somlo 2002). The nearly identical clinical profile that results from mutations in either *PKD1* or *PKD2* is in line with this hypothesis.

Since the polycystins belong to a family of proteins conserved in vertebrates as well as in non-vertebrates, studies performed in model organisms will undoubtedly provide further insights on the signalling pathways involved (Barr 2001).

Expression of the polycystins

The *PKD1* and *PKD2* transcripts are widely expressed in most tissues (Mochizuki *et al.* 1996; Ward *et al.* 1996). The expression of *PKD1* and *PKD2* transcripts concords with their respective proteins during human embryogenesis and renal development (Chauvet *et al.* 2002). Both *PKD1* and *PKD2* are widely expressed in human 5–6-week-old embryos, mainly in neural tissue, cardiomyocytes, endodermal derivatives, and

mesonephros. This expression pattern is in agreement with the cardiovascular and liver manifestations of the disease.

Polycystin-1 is expressed at a low level in normal tubular epithelial cells and is developmentally regulated, with highest levels during renal development and a decrease after birth, with renal expression limited to collecting ducts and distal tubules (Geng *et al.* 1996; Ward *et al.* 1996; Ong *et al.* 1999a). The expression of polycystin-2 is quite similar to that of polycystin-1, the protein being also detected in the ascending loop of Henle and the distal convoluted tubule, with delayed and low expression in the collecting duct (Ong *et al.* 1999a). Both polycystins were recently found to colocalize in the primary cilia expressed on most renal tubular epithelial cells (Yoder *et al.* 2002). A coordinate expression of polycystins 1 and 2 has been documented in the developing and mature epithelia lining biliary and pancreatic ducts (Ibraghimov-Beskrovnaya *et al.* 1997; Ong *et al.* 1999a), as well as in the heart and the vasculature (Ong *et al.* 1999a; Chauvet *et al.* 2002).

A significant immunoreactivity for polycystin-1 has been detected in PKD1 cystic epithelia (Ward *et al.* 1996; Ong *et al.* 1999b), although negative cysts have also been reported (Geng *et al.* 1996; Ibraghimov-Beskrovnaya *et al.* 1997). Staining for polycystin-2 has also been detected in a majority of kidney and liver cysts from PKD2 patients (Ong *et al.* 1999a). The interpretation of this finding in relation with the two-hit hypothesis is discussed below.

Pathophysiology

Mechanism of cyst formation: the two-hit hypothesis

The fact that renal cysts develop in a limited segment of a small percentage of nephrons (see above) suggested that the germline mutation, which is present in every tubular cell, is not sufficient to produce a cyst and that a second mutation ('second hit') in the remaining wild-type allele of the *PKD* gene may be necessary for cyst formation. The demonstration that epithelial cells isolated from renal cysts are monoclonal, and the detection of loss of heterozygosity for the wild-type allele of *PKD1* in a fraction of renal and liver cysts concur with this theory (Qian *et al.* 1996; Watnick *et al.* 1998). Somatic mutations in *PKD2* have also been described in cystic epithelia from PKD2 patients (Pei *et al.* 1999). In all instances, the somatic mutations were shown to affect the wild-type allele derived from the unaffected parent. Inactivation of both copies of the *PKD* gene by successive germline and somatic mutations within a renal tubular epithelial cell would result in a loss of functional protein below a critical level, a disruption of the tubular maturation pathway, and clonal proliferation into a cyst.

Though the two-hit hypothesis is supported by studies in ADPKD mouse models (see below), it remains controversial for two reasons. First, a somatic mutation has been found in only 30–40 per cent of studied cysts; however, this could be due to the low sensitivity of the techniques. Second, a strong immunoreactivity for polycystins has been found in cyst-lining epithelia. This could be explained either by a lack of specificity of antibodies, or the detection of a mutant protein that is non-functional (e.g. missense mutation) or with prolonged half-life or increased expression (Pei 2001). Alternatively, the recent demonstration that inactivating somatic mutations in *PKD1* (Watnick *et al.* 2000) may occur in cysts with germline mutation in *PKD2* shows that a transheterozygous two-hit model may also be involved.

Mechanisms of cyst growth

The renal failure in ADPKD is attributed at least in part to the progressive enlargement of renal cysts, which extend from a single tubular dilation to a macroscopically visible, fluid-filled cavity bordered by a single-layer epithelium. The process necessitates both cell proliferation and fluid accumulation within the cyst lumen. Several lines of evidence suggest that dysregulation of epithelial cell growth occurs in ADPKD. Cyst-lining cells are hyperproliferative and show a high mitotic rate (Nadasdy et al. 1995). Furthermore, overexpression of polycystin-1 downregulates the proliferation of renal cells in culture (Boletta et al. 2000), and it has been shown that polycystin-1 induces cell-cycle arrest in G0/G1, secondary to the activation of the Janus kinase–signal transducers and activators of transcription (JAK-STAT) pathway (Bhunia et al. 2002). The fact that the majority of renal cysts in ADPKD are isolated from the nephron segment of origin implies that cyst fluid primarily derives from a net secretion across the cystic epithelium (for review, see Sullivan et al. 1998). A cyclic adenosine monophosphate (cAMP)-stimulated fluid secretion, primarily driven by Cl^-, has been demonstrated in isolated cyst walls or cultured ADPKD cells (Sullivan et al. 1998). Cyst fluid secretion in ADPKD cysts appears to be mediated, at least in part, by the cystic fibrosis transmembrane conductance regulator (CFTR) chloride channel operating at the apical pole of the cell. Mechanisms for chloride entry at the basolateral pole of the cells include the bumetanide-sensitive Na^+–K^+–$2Cl^-$ (NKCC1) cotransporter (Lebeau et al. 2002). The secretory phenotype of ADPKD cyst cells may be triggered by the chronic activation of cAMP, which activates CFTR and regulates its expression (Sullivan et al. 1998).

The ADPKD cyst-lining cells retain some characteristics of their nephron segment of origin, including the expression of water channels or ion transporters (Devuyst et al. 1996; Lebeau et al. 2002). Accordingly, a majority of cysts contain Na^+ and H^+ concentrations similar to those of plasma ('non-gradient' cysts), suggesting a proximal tubule origin, whereas others show low Na^+ and high H^+ concentrations ('gradient' cysts), probably related to collecting duct origin (Huseman et al. 1980). ADPKD cysts also present alterations of tubular basement membrane that may alter the compliance and/or participate in the abnormal tubular morphogenesis (Carone et al. 1992). A more generalized defect in basement membranes might also account for the extrarenal changes in ADPKD, but this hypothesis has not been substantiated thus far. The recent finding that polycystins colocalize in primary cilia of renal tubular cells (Yoder et al. 2002) may also prove important since mutations disrupting the structure or function of cilia may result in a renal cystic phenotype (Igarashi and Somlo 2002).

Animal models of autosomal-dominant polycystic kidney disease

Homologous recombination was used to create mutant alleles and provide murine models of ADPKD. The first *Pkd1* knock-out mouse was generated by targeting exon 34 (Lu et al. 1997). Homozygous $Pkd1^{-/-}$ mice died *in utero* or in the perinatal period with massive cystic kidneys, pancreatic ductal cysts, and pulmonary hypoplasia. Renal development progressed normally until embryonic day (E) 14.5 (E14.5), indicating that polycystin-1 is not required during the earliest stages of murine renal development. Renal cysts appeared in proximal tubules at E15.5, rapidly progressing to replace the entire parenchyma. Renal cysts from all nephron segments, as well as liver cysts were observed in aging $Pkd1^{+/-}$ mice (Lu et al. 1999). Interestingly, polycystin-1 expression was found to be absent in some cysts.

Three additional *Pkd1* knock-out mice have been described that are targetted in exon 4 ($Pkd1^{null}$) (Lu et al. 2001); exons 17–21 ($Pkd1^{del17-21bgeo}$) (Boulter et al. 2001); or exon 44 ($Pkd1^L$) (Kim et al. 2000). In addition to kidney and pancreatic cysts, these mice show evidence for vascular fragility including subcutaneous oedema, vascular leaks, and haemorrhage, as well as impairment in skeletal development, indicating a role for polycystin-1 in cardiac development, vascular integrity, and collagen and bone development.

A true null allele of *Pkd2* was generated by disruption of exon 1 (Wu et al. 1998, 2000). Mice heterozygous for this allele ($Pkd2^{+/-}$) developed occasional renal and hepatic cysts and had decreased long-term survival (Wu et al. 2000). The homozygous, $Pkd2^{-/-}$ mice died *in utero* between E13.5 and parturition. These embryos had normal kidney development until E14.5 but showed progressive cyst formation from E15.5. $Pkd2^{-/-}$ embryos were also characterized by pancreatic cysts, as well as oedema and focal haemorrhages related to severe defects in cardiac septation (Wu et al. 2000). The same investigators also generated a second, unstable allele of *Pkd2* (WS25) that is prone to acquire somatic mutations via intragenic homologous recombination (Wu et al. 1998). Heterozygous ($Pkd2^{WS25/+}$) and homozygous ($Pkd2^{WS25/WS25}$) mice developed renal cystic disease. Hepatic cysts arising from the bile duct epithelium were also observed in $Pkd2^{WS25/WS25}$ mice. Of note, immunostaining studies showed that the majority of renal cysts in $Pkd2^{WS25/WS25}$ mice lacked polycystin-2. An intercross of $Pkd2^{+/-}$ mice with mice carrying the unstable allele ($Pkd2^{WS25/+}$ or $Pkd2^{WS25/WS25}$) produced compound *cis*-heterozygous mice ($Pkd2^{WS25/-}$). The $Pkd2^{WS25/-}$ mice survived to birth and by 11 weeks had developed significant, bilateral renal cystic disease as well as hepatic cysts. As predicted by the model, the renal phenotype was most severe in $Pkd2^{WS25/-}$ mice (one null allele + one unstable allele) than in the $Pkd2^{WS25/WS25}$, $Pkd2^{+/-}$, and $Pkd2^{WS25/+}$ mice (Wu et al. 1998). These mouse models recapitulate the human disease and suggest that loss of functional polycystin-1 or -2 below a critical threshold results in a block in the differentiation programme of the kidney. They also support the view that cyst formation occurs through a cellular recessive mechanism (Lu et al. 1997; Wu et al. 1998).

Inherited cystic kidney disease has been described in several species, and renal cyst formation can be triggered by chemicals and drugs. However, genetic and phenotypic differences limit the relevance of these experimental models to ADPKD.

Clinical presentation

The disease may be revealed by a renal or extrarenal complication or discovered at clinical examination or by imaging technique, either incidentally, or during familial investigation. The main clinical manifestations are listed in Table 1.

Renal manifestations

Renal involvement may be totally asymptomatic at the early stage. On random examination, only 25 per cent of people with ADPKD have microscopic haematuria and 18 per cent overt proteinuria (most often <1 g/day) (Chapman et al. 1994a). Just as in other kidney diseases, overt proteinuria is preceded by microalbuminuria.

Table 1 Clinical manifestations of ADPKD

Manifestations	Prevalence (%)
Renal	
Hypertension	60 before renal failure
	90 at ESRD
Pain (acute and chronic)	60
Gross haematuria	50
Urinary tract infection	Men 20; women 70
Calculus	20
Renal failure	≅50 by age 70
Hepatobiliary	
Asymptomatic liver cysts	80 at age 60
Symptomatic polycystic liver disease	Uncommon (male : female ratio 1 : 10)
Congenital hepatic fibrosis	Rare
Caroli disease	Rare
Cardiovascular	
Mitral valve prolapse	25
Intracranial aneurysm	8
Intracranial dolichoectasia	2
Ascending aortic dissection	Rare
Other	
Pancreatic cyst	9
Arachnoid cyst	8
Hernia	
Inguinal	13
Umbilical	7

Renal clinical manifestations include pain, bleeding, infection, calculus, cancer, hypertension, and renal failure.

Flank or abdominal pain

Flank or abdominal pain is the presenting symptom in 20–30 per cent of the patients and occurs at some time in at least 50–60 per cent, its frequency increasing with age and with the size of the cysts (Milutinovic et al. 1984).

Acute pain is suggestive of intracystic haemorrhage, urinary tract obstruction (by clot or stone), or infection (associated with fever) (Table 2). Chronic pain, often described as abdominal discomfort and fullness, is frequently observed.

Common chronic pain is believed to be due to compression of kidney cysts on the surrounding tissues, traction on the pedicle of the kidney, and stretching of the renal capsule (Bajwa et al. 2001). The pain severity generally correlates with the size of the kidneys, but there are some exceptions. Coping with chronic pain may be difficult in some patients. Collaboration with a pain clinic may be helpful. Expectations should not be set too high, rather patients should be allowed to adjust to the chronic pain (Bajwa et al. 2001). Pharmacological therapy includes, in a stepwise sequence, acetaminophen and more potent analgesics such as tramadol, trying to avoid opioids. Non-steroidal anti-inflammatories are not suitable for long-term use (Bajwa et al. 2001).

In a small minority of patients in whom pain is resistant to analgesics, surgical intervention may be considered. Percutaneous aspiration of a single or a few dominant painful cyst(s) can relieve pain, but only temporarily because of reaccumulation of fluid. Instillation of a sclerosing agent has been successfully performed in a few such cases.

Table 2 Specific causes of acute abdominal pain in patients with ADPKD

Cause	Frequency	Fever
Renal		
Cyst bleeding	+++	Mild (<38°C, max 2 days) or none
Stone	++	With pyonephrosis (rare)
Infection	+	High, prolonged with cyst involved
Liver		
Cyst infection	Rare	High, prolonged
Cyst bleeding	Very rare	Mild (<38°C, max 2 days) or none

For patients with large kidneys with many cysts, decortication (deroofing and collapse of cysts) surgery has been performed, either open or more recently laparoscopic (Dunn et al. 2001) with similar results with respect to the number of cysts unroofed (150–200) and the proportion of patients with pain relief (60–70 per cent at 2 years), but also with a similar quite high rate of complications (37–47 per cent) including haemorrhage and urine leakage. These procedures do not appear to significantly alter blood pressure control and renal function. Laparoscopic renal denervation has been recently proposed as an alternative approach (Valente et al. 2001). More experience with all these procedures is needed before recommending their use in clinical practice. In patients having reached endstage renal failure, nephrectomy may be the best option for pain control (see below).

Other causes of flank or back pain should not be missed. Severe pain in the right flank may be related to massive liver cysts (see below). Chronic back pain may be caused by disc disease facilitated by increased lumbar lordosis due to increasing abdominal girth.

Cyst bleeding

Cyst bleeding is a common event in patients with ADPKD. Propensity to cyst bleeding is explained by the rich vascular network of cyst walls, including aneurysmal vessels and neoformation of capillaries (Bello-Reuss et al. 2001). Typical presentation of intracystic haemorrhage is either gross haematuria (with or without pain) or acute renal pain without haematuria according to the existence or non-existence of a communication between the bleeding cyst and the collecting system. Gross haematuria is the presenting symptom in 15–20 per cent and occurs at least once in 30–50 per cent of patients with ADPKD (Milutinovic et al. 1984; Gabow et al. 1992a). It occurs less frequently in PKD2 than in PKD1 patients (Hateboer et al. 1999a). Its incidence increases with the degree of kidney enlargement. It may follow strenuous physical activity or minor trauma but often occurs spontaneously. Depending on the amount of bleeding, intracystic haemorrhage can produce transient moderate fever (Table 2) and leucocytosis in the absence of infection. Bleeding into the perirenal space and the peritoneum has been very rarely reported.

Rest is the best management for cyst bleeding. Gross haematuria rarely lasts for more than 7 days (Gabow et al. 1992a). Blood transfusion is rarely required. Very rarely, bleeding may be severe and persistent, notably in dialysed patients, necessitating uninephrectomy.

Intracystic haemorrhage is responsible for most high-density cysts and wall calcifications demonstrated by computed tomography (CT).

Other causes of gross haematuria include urinary-tract infection and nephrolithiasis (see below). Late-onset and/or prolonged or recurrent haematuria should also raise the possibility of an unrelated problem such as bladder cancer, especially in patients with increased risk factors for this neoplasm.

Infection

Prevalence and organisms

Symptoms consistent with lower urinary tract infection were the initial manifestation in 3 per cent of men and 42 per cent of women, and occurred at least once in 19 per cent of men and 68 per cent of women with ADPKD studied by Milutinovic *et al.* (1984). The exact prevalence of upper urinary tract infection has not been well evaluated. Renal infection may occur whatever the renal function. Causal organisms generally reach the kidneys by the ascending route, as suggested by the following observations: (a) upper urinary tract infection is often preceded by symptoms of lower urinary tract infection, (b) 90 per cent of renal infections occur in women, just as for lower urinary tract infection, and (c) upper urinary tract infections are mostly caused by the organisms (enterobacteriaceae) commonly responsible for lower urinary tract infection. Occasionally, infection is caused by Gram-positive and anaerobic bacteria. Renal infection is potentially severe since it may be complicated by septic shock or perirenal abscess.

Diagnosis

Renal infection is the first diagnosis to consider in a febrile patient with ADPKD (Table 3). It may involve the upper collecting system, renal parenchyma, or cyst. The diagnosis of acute infection of the upper collecting system associated with ureteric obstruction must not be missed: it is suggested by renal colic and, in patients with compromised renal function, by a rapid deterioration of renal function. Initial differentiation between parenchymal and cyst infection is not always easy. The former is evidenced by a positive urine culture and prompt response to antibiotic therapy. The latter is characterized by the development of discrete, new palpable area(s) of renal tenderness, a quite often negative urine culture (as infected cysts may not communicate with the pelvis), a very high proportion of positive blood cultures, and apparent refractoriness to antibiotic therapy (Gibson and Watson 1998). In the bacteraemic patient with a negative urine culture, sources of infection other than renal cysts must be excluded, since clinical presentation may be misleading; pain in the upper right quadrant of the abdomen may reveal an infected liver cyst; pain in the left lower quadrant may be due to diverticulitis of the sigmoid colon (Table 3). In difficult cases, imaging techniques may provide valuable information. Ultrasonography or, more often, CT may show the heterogeneous contents and irregularly thickened walls of infected cysts. However, identification of the infected cyst(s) may be inconclusive, particularly in patients with advanced disease whose cysts have previously been the sites of repeated infection or bleeding. Comparison with previous scans may be extremely helpful, hence the usefulness of a baseline CT performed at diagnosis. Scintigraphy with gallium-67

or leucocytes labelled with indium-111 is positive in only about half of the cases.

Management

The response to antibiotics is not uniform. In some patients, the infection is rapidly controlled, while in others, fever is still present after a 5-day treatment, despite adequate doses and *in vitro* sensitivity of the responsible microorganism. Poor clinical response is indicative of renal cyst infection or ureteric obstruction and requires hospital evaluation. The refractory nature of cyst infection has been shown to be largely due to poor penetration of commonly used antibiotics into cyst fluid (Bennett *et al.* 1985). A major route for antibiotic penetration into the cyst is indeed diffusion across the cyst wall, a property dependent on lipid solubility. Lipophilic antibiotics (such as trimethoprim, fluoroquinolones, chloramphenicol, and metronidazole) rapidly achieve high intracystic concentrations (Bennett *et al.* 1985). The poor liposolubility of other common antibiotics active against common Gram-negative enteric bacteria (i.e. aminoglycosides, ampicillin, and cephalosporins) requires 5–8 days of administration of the drug for adequate intracystic concentrations to be achieved. The choice of antibiotics will also depend on the clinical presentation. In severe renal infection with septicaemia, rapid control of sepsis is the first goal: parenteral administration of a fluoroquinolone or a third-generation cephalosporin is recommended as initial therapy. Antibiotic therapy is subsequently adapted according to the bacteriological findings, and oral administration of antibiotics with good intracyst penetration, such as cotrimoxazole or preferably a fluoroquinolone such as ciprofloxacine, may be substituted. Oral fluoroquinolone can be the primary therapy in patients with a less severe presentation. The optimal duration of antibiotic administration is unclear. There is no evidence that giving antibiotics for more than 3 weeks has significant advantage in common cases of parenchymal infection. We recommend a 6-week course in proven or suspected cyst infection. If the infection recurs after withdrawal of antibiotics, treatment should be reinstituted and continued for 12 weeks.

The management of refractory renal infection is difficult. Drainage is rarely needed and feasible; it should be considered in large infected cysts if transcutaneous access is possible as well as in perinephric abscess. Provided infection is not life-threatening, perseverance with symptomatic management is advisable: we have observed remission of infection after 2–3 weeks. Nephrectomy should be limited to cases with uncontrolled renal infection and/or perirenal infection.

Prophylactic measures against as well as prompt treatment of lower urinary tract infection apply to patients with ADPKD (see Chapter 7.1). Urinary tract instrumentation should particularly be avoided, or done under cover of prophylactic antibiotics (such as a fluoroquinolone) before and for 24 h after the procedure.

Calculi

Nephrolithiasis occurs in approximately 20 per cent of patients with ADPKD. It is as common in women as in men and is asymptomatic in 50 per cent of patients. The composition of stones is most frequently uric acid and/or calcium oxalate (Torres *et al.* 1993). A combination of both anatomic and metabolic abnormalities caused by ADPKD are responsible for stone formation. The role of urinary stasis due to cysts compression is demonstrated by the presence of greater number of cysts in stone-forming kidneys compared with kidneys without stones (Grampsas *et al.* 2000). Furthermore, precalyceal tubular ectasia, a

Table 3 Main causes of fever in patients with ADPKD

Renal infection (including cyst infections)
Upper renal collecting-system infection due to obstructive stone or clot
Liver cyst infection (rare)
Angiocholitis complicating biliary-tract dilatation (rare)
Colonic diverticulitis (essentially after transplantation)

condition clearly associated with calcium nephrolithiasis, was observed in 15 per cent of the patients (Torres *et al.* 1993). While urinary excretion of both calcium and uric acid is in the normal range, a decreased urinary excretion of citrate and magnesium, which are powerful inhibitors of crystal formation is frequently found (Torres *et al.* 1993; Grampsas *et al.* 2000). The frequency and nature of the stones encountered in these patients have some practical implications. Generous water intake must be recommended as a general prophylactic measure for every patient with normal renal function. Nephrolithiasis must always be considered in the patient with flank pain. Excretory urograms and/or CT are mostly needed to locate obstructive radiolucent or faintly opaque stones.

Obstructive or symptomatic stones may be treated by the techniques commonly used in the general population, including percutaneous and extracorporeal lithotripsy. Torres *et al.* (1993) reported on 23 extracorporeal lithotripsies in 16 patients with ADPKD: 82 per cent were successful and no complications (including perirenal, subcapsular, and intracystic haemorrhage) occurred. There were, however, residual fragments in half of the patients.

Calcification in renal stones should be distinguished (usually with CT) from cystic calcifications, a common finding in patients with more advanced cystic disease, probably resulting from previous intracystic haemorrhage (Fig. 2).

Cancer

The incidence of renal-cell carcinoma in ADPKD does not appear to be increased as compared to the general population (Keith *et al.* 1994). However, there are some specific features of renal cancer in ADPKD. As compared to the general population, it is more often concurrently bilateral (12 versus 1–5 per cent), multicentric (28 versus 6 per cent), and sarcomatoid in type (33 versus 1–5 per cent) (Keith *et al.* 1994). Though a bias in favour of reporting uncommon renal cancers in ADPKD cannot be totally excluded, those peculiarities led

Keith *et al.* (1994) to suggest either a malignant potential restricted to a small subset of patients with the disease or an alteration in the biology of renal cancer when it develops in that setting.

The diagnosis of kidney carcinoma in a patient with ADPKD is not easy since clinical presentation (haematuria and flank pain in nearly half of the cases; fever in one-third) mimics banal intracystic haemorrhage or infection. An association with anorexia and weight loss should raise the suspicion of cancer (Keith *et al.* 1994). Diagnostic imaging also remains difficult, even with the improvements in CT and magnetic resonance imaging (MRI). Interpretation in a given patient may be facilitated by comparing this with previous imaging studies. Cyst calcification should not be considered as a sign of neoplasm (see above). Renal cancer may elicit an increased uptake of gallium- or indium-labelled white blood cells (Keith *et al.* 1994).

Occasionally, polycystic kidney disease is the presenting manifestation of von Hippel–Lindau disease (see below), a disorder in which the incidence of renal carcinoma is high. Therefore, the diagnosis of von Hippel–Lindau disease should always be considered in patients with polycystic kidney disease and renal carcinoma, especially when other familial members developed renal carcinoma.

Hypertension

Hypertension is an early and frequent manifestation of ADPKD, being the presenting clinical finding in 13–20 per cent of patients and occurring in approximately 60 per cent of the patients before the renal function has become impaired (Ecder and Schrier 2001). Hypertension is four times more prevalent in PKD1 than in PKD2 patients (Hateboer *et al.* 1999a).

A subtle, albeit detectable elevation of blood pressure precedes manifestation of hypertension and renal failure by several years or decades. As compared with 20 unaffected relatives, 19 individuals with ADPKD aged 16–35 years had a higher blood pressure (123/74 versus 115/71 mmHg on average) despite similar glomerular filtration rates (Harrap *et al.* 1991). Circadian blood pressure was also greater in 12 individuals aged 15–25 years with ADPKD and normal renal function than in matched controls (Zeier *et al.* 1993). Not unexpectedly, there is an increased incidence of new-onset hypertension revealed by pregnancy (16 per cent of pregnant women with the disease versus 6 per cent in their controls) (Chapman *et al.* 1994b). This early raised blood pressure, even within the normal range, probably accounts for the increase in left ventricular mass found in young people with ADPKD (Zeier *et al.* 1993; Valero *et al.* 1999).

The prevailing opinion is that the growth of cysts induces hypertension through intrarenal ischaemia resulting from vascular compression and stretching (for review, see Wang and Strandgaard 1997; Ecder and Schrier 2001). This in turn activates the renin–angiotensin system with an attendant increased arteriolar resistance, sodium retention, and increased sympathetic activity. In agreement with this hypothesis, an inappropriately high level of plasma renin activity as well as an abnormal intrarenal distribution of renin-secreting cells, an early expansion of the extracellular fluid volume, and an increased level of plasma catecholamines have been documented in hypertensive patients with ADPKD well before the onset of renal failure (Wang and Strandgaard 1997; Ecder and Schrier 2001). Endothelial dysfunction might also play a role, through both an activation of the renal endothelin system and an impaired nitric oxide (NO) synthase-dependent relaxation of small resistance vessels (Wang *et al.* 2000). In patients with ADPKD, other coincidental causes of hypertension have been

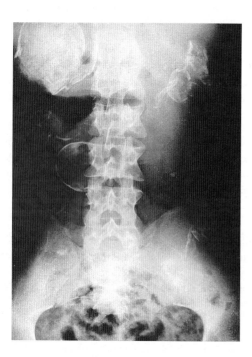

Fig. 2 Calcified cyst walls seen on abdominal plain film in a 33-year-old patient with ADPKD on haemodialysis for 7 years.

reported, including stenosis of the renal artery, primary aldosteronism, and phaeochromocytoma.

The early control of hypertension is mandatory, as cardiovascular complications are a leading cause of death in these patients (Fick *et al.* 1995). In the early stage, a moderate reduction of salt intake is advisable. Owing to the pathogenetic role of the renin–angiotensin system, β-blockers and angiotensin-converting enzyme (ACE) inhibitors or angiotensin II-receptor antagonists appear as the first-choice drugs. There is so far no study showing that ACE inhibitors do better than other antihypertensive agents on the progression of renal failure. ACE inhibitors must be used cautiously in patients with advanced ADPKD and chronic renal insufficiency, as acute deterioration of renal function has occasionally been observed in this setting. As a general rule, this treatment should be started at low dose in patients who are not severely volume-depleted. A target blood pressure of 130/85 mmHg is desirable. A lower goal could even be recommended in patients with left ventricular hypertrophy: in this category, left ventricular hypertrophy was indeed decreased by 35 per cent over a 7-year period in patients assigned to rigourous control (<120/80 mmHg) versus only 21 per cent in those assigned to standard control (135–140/85–90 mmHg) (Schrier *et al.* 2002). With an educational programme developed at the University of Colorado for both ADPKD patients and their primary care physicians, the rate of blood pressure control increased from 38 to 64 per cent over a 10-year period (Ecder and Schrier 2001).

Renal failure

Progressive renal failure is the most serious renal complication of ADPKD. The majority of affected patients reach endstage renal failure during their sixth decade. In our experience, regular dialysis was initiated between 40 and 59 years of age in 68 per cent of the patients, earlier than this in 11 per cent, and later in 21 per cent (Persu *et al.* 2002). There is, however, a wide variation in the pattern of progression, both between families and within affected family members, resulting from both genetic and environmental factors, only a part of which have been identified.

Patterns of progression

In general, glomerular filtration rate remains within the normal range for decades despite the progressive development and growth of kidney cysts. The rate of the early decline in glomerular filtration rate has not been thoroughly examined. Once glomerular filtration rate is lower than 50 ml/min, its rate of decline is about 5 ml/min/year (Choukroun *et al.* 1995; Modification of Diet in Renal Disease Study Group 1995), which is faster than in other primary renal diseases.

Not all individuals affected with ADPKD progress to endstage renal failure. In three studies including 1832 patients from France, Canada, and the United States, the probability of being alive without endstage renal failure was 71–78 per cent by the age of 50 and 23–66 per cent by the age of 70 (Churchill *et al.* 1984; Simon *et al.* 1989; Gabow *et al.* 1992b). A minority of patients die at 80 years or more, in whom ADPKD is only recognized at the time of autopsy. Conversely, very early progression has been reported in a few young children. Possible risk factors for early-onset disease are a parental new mutation and the maternal inheritance of the disease (Fick *et al.* 1993; Zerres *et al.* 1993) as well as the nature of mutation (Watnick *et al.* 1999). The risk of recurrence for sibs reached 43 per cent (Zerres *et al.* 1993).

Determinants of progression

One of the most striking features in ADPKD is the substantial variability in the severity of renal phenotype, primarily assessed by the age

at ESRD. This variability is observed among families, family members, and even dizygotic twins (Peters and Breuning 2001). *Interfamilial* phenotypic variability is first explained by genetic heterogeneity (*PKD1* versus *PKD2*).

In two large series comprising 620 patients with PKD1 disease and 335 with PKD2 disease, the median age at renal death, remarkably concordant, was 53 and 54 years in the former group, versus 68 and 74 years in the latter (Johnson and Gabow 1997; Hateboer *et al.* 1999a). However, age range at renal death substantially overlapped in both groups of families occurring between 35 and 78 years in PKD1 individuals and between 44 and 81 years in PKD2 individuals (Johnson and Gabow 1997; Hateboer *et al.* 1999a).

Since a wide variety of mutations have been reported in both genes, the type of mutation might be a further determinant of progression. This has been suggested by significant differences in renal survival between 10 large PKD1 families which, on the basis of having unique disease-associated haplotypes, were likely to be associated with a heterogeneous range of *PKD1* mutations (Hateboer *et al.* 1999b). In a recent study including 80 families with a characterized *PKD1* mutation, only the location of the mutation, but not the type, was associated with the age at onset of ESRD; however, the effect was modest, with only a 3-year difference in renal survival between patients with a mutation in the 5′ region compared to those with a mutation in the 3′ region (Rossetti *et al.* 2002b). No correlation was found between age at endstage renal failure and type or location of *PKD2* mutation (Deltas 2001).

A large deletion disrupting both *PKD1* and *TSC2* [the second gene for tuberous sclerosis (TSC), see below] has been identified in a few children with TSC and severe polycystic kidney disease (Brook-Carter *et al.* 1994). In other children with early-onset ADPKD but without TSC, a variety of *PKD1* mutations have been found, in both the 5′ and the 3′ area of the gene (Rossetti *et al.* 2002b). The same variety was found in families with mild disease (Rossetti *et al.* 2002b). The substantial intrafamilial heterogeneity in the course of renal disease could thus result from a combination of genetic and environmental factors, which might influence all steps leading to the disease.

The two-hit model implies that the rate of somatic mutation, which itself can be influenced by common environmental factors, is critical for individual cyst formation. Furthermore, modifier loci have been demonstrated in mouse models of polycystic kidney disease (Peters and Breuning 2001). These modifying genes may influence the rate of second hit (detoxification of mutagens, DNA repair); affect the polycystin signal transduction pathway; regulate factors involved in cyst progression and/or fluid accumulation; or influence more general mechanisms involved in renal disease progression such as hypertension or fibrosis (Persu *et al.* 2000; Peters and Breuning 2001).

Given the implication of the renin–angiotensin system in the genesis of hypertension (see above) the role of the insertion/deletion (I/D) polymorphism in the ACE gene has been examined, with conflicting results (Peters and Breuning 2001; Rossetti *et al.* 2002b). More convincingly, male ADPKD patients with the Glu 298 Asp polymorphism of *ENOS*, the gene encoding for endothelial NO synthase (eNOS), were shown to have a 5-year lower mean age at renal death. This deleterious effect could be due to partial cleavage of eNOS and decreased vascular production of NO, worsening the endothelial dysfunction associated with ADPKD (Persu *et al.* 2002). Contrary to previous reports, black race is not associated with a faster progression to endstage renal failure in ADPKD (Freedman *et al.* 2000). Male gender has been associated with an earlier age at endstage renal failure in the whole

ADPKD population (Neugarten *et al.* 2000). However, this gender effect has not been found in several series of PKD1 patients (Hateboer *et al.* 1999a; Persu *et al.* 2002; Rossetti *et al.* 2002b).

Does hypertension accelerate the course of renal failure just as in other renal diseases? Presumably, uncontrolled hypertension can do so, but this has not been rigorously demonstrated in ADPKD. It has been shown that hypertensive patients have significantly worse renal function for a given age than normotensive patients, but the relationship between blood pressure and renal function may not be causal. Moreover, others failed to find a significant correlation between mean arterial pressure and the rate of progression of renal failure (Choukroun *et al.* 1995). In two, randomized prospective trials enrolling, respectively, 200 and 64 patients with ADPKD with a glomerular filtration rate between 13 and 60 ml/min, neither assignment to a low blood pressure (125/75 mmHg) (Modification of Diet in Renal Disease Study Group 1995), nor the administration of an ACE inhibitor (Maschio *et al.* 1996) slowed the rate of decline of glomerular filtration rate over 3 years. A recent prospective study in 75 patients with no or mild renal failure also failed to show any difference in the 7-year course of renal function between those assigned to rigorous (<120/80 mmHg) versus standard (135–140/85–90 mmHg) blood pressure control (Schrier *et al.* 2002). This does not mean that earlier intervention and a longer follow-up would not have been beneficial and does not detract from the need to carefully control blood pressure in this disease.

Other factors that may affect renal progression include diet, smoking, and urinary tract infection. The other aim of the large prospective study cited above (Modification of Diet in Renal Disease Study Group 1995) was to assess the effect of a low (0.6 g/kg/day) or very low (0.3 g/kg/day) protein diet: the rate of progression of renal failure was not affected. In a retrospective multicentre case–control study including patients with ADPKD, cigarette smoking was associated with a faster progression to endstage renal failure in males. The effect was dose-dependent and disappeared in the patients treated with an ACE inhibitor (Orth 2002). The role of urinary tract infection in the progression of renal failure in man remains unclear. A detrimental effect of urinary tract infection on renal function was found by Gabow *et al.* (1992b) in men but not in women. Progression to renal failure is not quicker in affected women in whom upper urinary tract infection is more frequent.

Pregnancy does not seem to alter significantly the course of ADPKD, although a mild negative effect was found in a subgroup of hypertensive women with four or more pregnancies (Chapman *et al.* 1994b). Not unexpectedly, 25 per cent of women developed a hypertensive complication during pregnancy, including new or worsening hypertension, with 11 per cent developing pre-eclampsia (Chapman *et al.* 1994b). As in other renal diseases, renal insufficiency and uncontrolled hypertension are the main determinants of poor fetal prognosis.

Prospects for therapy

No specific treatment currently prevents or slows the progression towards renal failure in ADPKD. With the growing body of knowledge on genetics and pathophysiology (see below), no doubt that novel therapies will be tested within the next decade. The availability of cellular and animal models will allow high-throughput screening of compounds that may slow the progression of the renal cystic phenotype. At the stage of clinical trials, the most convenient surrogate marker in patients with failing kidneys is the slope of glomerular filtration rate.

Earlier in the course of the disease, when renal function is still preserved, predictive markers of progression include blood pressure level, microalbuminuria or proteinuria, and increase in cyst number and volume as assessed by CT or MRI (King *et al.* 2000; Sise *et al.* 2000).

Associated clinical features

The altered architecture of the renal medulla, with an attendant reduction of the corticomedullary concentration gradient, most likely explains both the urinary concentrating defect and the decreased urinary excretion of ammonia found in the early stage of the disease. Microalbuminuria may precede hypertension and frank proteinuria in some individuals with the disease. The rare patients developing nephrotic-range proteinuria have a superimposed glomerular disease.

Contrary to common belief, ADPKD is not associated with an increased tendency to salt wasting. Non-azotaemic patients can indeed appropriately lower their sodium excretion. In contrast, patients with ADPKD and advanced renal failure commonly have slight or mild salt loss, as may occur in many other renal diseases. Severe sodium restriction is not indicated at this stage.

Erythrocytosis is occasionally observed in non-azotaemic patients. This is likely accounted for by an increased production of erythropoietin by interstitial cells adjacent to cyst walls induced by ischaemia.

Extrarenal manifestations

Liver involvement

Liver cysts

Liver cysts represent the most frequent extrarenal manifestation of ADPKD. They result from abnormal remodelling of the ductal plate. They arise from two different structures. Most of them originate from overgrowth of bile ductules called biliary microhamartomas that become disconnected from the bile ducts from which they derive. The epithelial lining retains the distinctive characteristics of biliary epithelia. By contrast-enhanced CT, these cysts exhibit intraparenchymatous location, and their size varies from less than 5 mm to more than 10 cm. Other cysts result from the dilatation of the peribiliary glands surrounding large intrahepatic bile ducts. They are typically tiny and located in the hepatic hilum or around large portal tracts.

Epidemiology and risk factors In the general population, the prevalence of simple liver cysts detected by ultrasonography increases with age, from 0 per cent in individuals less than 20 years old to 4 per cent around 70 years of age, with a maximum of three cysts. In ADPKD, liver cysts develop later than renal cysts. They are very rare before 20 years of age. Their prevalence increases dramatically from the third to the sixth decade of life, reaching a plateau of 80 per cent thereafter. Liver cysts are easily diagnosed by ultrasonography. Enhanced CT or MRI may, however, reveal small cysts undetected by ultrasonography. Occasionally, massive polycystic liver disease contrasts with mild cystic involvement of the kidneys and is the presenting manifestation of either PKD1 or PKD2 disease (unpublished observations). Epidemiological evidence suggests that liver phenotype is strongly influenced by hormonal environment, with a clear female predisposition. Liver cysts are indeed recognized earlier and are more numerous and larger in women than in men. Among 37 patients referred to us for massive polycystic liver disease, 35 were females. In postmenopausal women with ADPKD, a 1-year course of an equine oestrogen was associated with a 7 per cent increase in liver volume resulting from both cystic and parenchymal volumes. Whether use of non-equine oestrogens, as is currently practised in most European countries, carries a similar risk is not known (for review, see Chauveau *et al.* 2000).

Clinical manifestations Liver cysts are asymptomatic in the vast majority of patients. Even some patients with massive polycystic liver have no symptoms. Schematically, acute complications involve a single cyst, while chronic complications occur in massive polycystic liver disease (Chauveau *et al.* 2000).

Acute complications include infection and haemorrhage. They occur much less frequently in the liver than in the kidney. Cyst infection presents with fever and right abdominal pain (Tables 2 and 3). An elevation of liver enzymes is common. Identification of the causative micro-organism relies on blood culture and puncture of the infected cyst. Gram-negative enterobacteriaceae or Haemophilus are most often involved. Localization of the infected cyst may be difficult, even with extensive imaging evaluation. For treatment, a combination of antibiotics is recommended, relying on drugs with good penetration in cysts such as ciprofloxacin and amikacin. Drainage is not a prerequisite to successful treatment. Should antibiotic therapy fail, drainage or hepatic resection would be promptly considered. Optimal duration of treatment is unclear. We recommend a 6-week course. Relapses or recurrence are not uncommon. Their occurrence should raise the suspicion for associated intrahepatic bile duct abnormalities (see below). In these cases, selective hepatic resection can eradicate the infection.

Intracystic haemorrhage may cause severe abdominal pain. It occurs less frequently than infection in our experience. MRI best differentiates haemorrhage from infection. Rarely, rupture of a cyst into the peritoneal cavity leads to haemoperitoneum. Massively enlarged polycystic liver presents with continuous or intermittent pain in the upper abdomen and abdominal heaviness or distension. Mechanical compression of the adjacent organs may be responsible for early satiety, heartburn, dyspnoea, abdominal hernias, and uterine prolapse. A two- to fivefold increase in serum γ-glutamyl transferase or alkaline phosphatase is found in half the patients, whereas serum levels of aminotransferase and bilirubin are elevated in only a minority of patients. As liver parenchyma is preserved, liver cysts never cause liver failure. Therefore, signs or symptoms of liver failure should prompt investigation for another, superimposed liver disease.

Treatment of massive cystic liver disease Severe symptoms may be improved by reducing liver size. Percutaneous cyst fluid aspiration should be considered if up to four medium-sized cysts have to be treated. It is always combined with instillation of a sclerosing agent, alcohol or minocycline, so as to minimize recurrence. Sustained improvement is observed in half of the patients, with a second attempt being effective in half of the primary non-responders. Fenestration of cyst walls may apply to large cysts exposing a great proportion of their wall in anterior, lateral, or even superior location. Laparoscopic fenestration reduces subsequent adhesions (Kabbej *et al.* 1996).

Postoperative ascites is troublesome in nearly half of the patients, especially those with chronic renal failure in whom resorption capacity of the peritoneum is altered. In the long term, symptoms recur in 23–57 per cent of cases. However, since morbidity is low, cyst fenestration may be offered to patients with few symptomatic large superficial cysts, optimally when serum creatinine is less than 200 μmol/l.

Liver resection best applies to massive enlargement by numerous small cysts. On average, three to four segments are removed. Most patients experience sustained improvement. However, the mortality rate is 7.5 per cent and early morbidity includes ascites and bile leaks. Long-lasting ascites is frequent in patients with severe renal failure or on dialysis. Liver resection is thus preferably considered when serum creatinine is below 200 μmol/l (Chauveau *et al.* 2000).

Liver transplantation should be reserved for patients with severely disabling polycystic liver disease with diffuse cystic involvement and for those in whom liver resection has failed or cannot be used. In a review of 51 cases 1-year mortality rate was 18 per cent, mostly predicted by poor nutritional status prior to transplantation (Chauveau *et al.* 2000). Combined liver/kidney transplantation is the best option for patients with concomitant advanced kidney failure.

Uncommon complications Ascites is uncommon in patients with ADPKD. When massively enlarged cystic liver is present, hepatic venous outflow obstruction is the most likely diagnosis. Obstruction is related to compression of hepatic veins or the inferior vena cava, or both by one or multiple posterior cysts, best shown by Doppler ultrasound and CT. Ascitic fluid is exudative and intractable (Torres *et al.* 1994a).

In the rare patients presenting with variceal bleeding and portal hypertension, two diagnoses should be considered. Mechanical compression of portal venous flow by liver cysts may selectively affect the main portal vein, or intrahepatic portal branches. Alternatively, when only a few or no liver cysts are demonstrable, the most likely diagnosis is congenital hepatic fibrosis. A constant feature in the recessive form of polycystic kidney disease, congenital hepatic fibrosis has been recognized in more than 20 patients with ADPKD, most often in early childhood or before 25 years of age. Spleen enlargement and variceal bleeding are prominent features. If present, ascites is transudative. Congenital hepatic fibrosis is not vertically transmitted along with the renal disease, but siblings can be affected. The molecular mechanism is not elucidated. All reported cases are in PKD1 families. Congenital hepatic fibrosis may be associated with focal or diffuse cystic dilatation of the segmental bile ducts (Caroli's syndrome), best detected by cholangio-CT or magnetic resonance cholangiography. Conventional treatment of portal hypertension, including non-selective β-blockers, is indicated (Chauveau *et al.* 2000).

Other rare liver complications include jaundice resulting from bile duct compression, acute hepatic vein thrombosis or Budd–Chiari syndrome following uni- or bilateral nephrectomy and a few cases of cholangiocarcinoma.

Intracerebral aneurysm

Epidemiology and risk factors

An asymptomatic intracerebral aneurysm is found by screening in 8 per cent of patients with ADPKD, that is, a rate four to five times above that found in the general population (Pirson *et al.* 2002a). Just as in the general population, 90 per cent of them are found in the anterior circulation. Of note, most of them are small, in majority less than 6 mm in diameter, a finding to take into account when the usefulness of screening is discussed (see below). The only clinical characteristic clearly associated with the presence of intracerebral aneurysm is a family history of intracerebral aneurysm. The relative risk for harbouring intracerebral aneurysm is indeed 2.6 higher among patients with a definite family history of intracerebral aneurysm or subarachnoid haemorrhage than in those without. This suggests that specific types of mutation may predispose to the development of intracranial aneurysm. Conversely, the absence of intracranial aneurysm in other relatives with ADPKD within such families indicates that other factors, genetic or non-genetic (smoking, arterial hypertension) also play a role in the formation and rupture of intracranial aneurysm.

Aneurysm rupture

The natural history of intracerebral aneurysm in ADPKD remains largely unknown. The risk of rupture seems quite similar to that observed in the general population (Pirson *et al.* 2002a). The profile of the patient with ADPKD admitted for intracerebral aneurysm rupture has been delineated on the basis of three studies that included 191 patients (Pirson *et al.* 2002a).

Age at the time of rupture averages 41 years, with 10 per cent of the patients less than 21 years old (Chauveau *et al.* 1994). Occasionally, intracerebral aneursym rupture is the presenting manifestation of ADPKD. As expected from the mean age at rupture, 54 per cent of the patients still have a normal renal function at that time and 26 per cent had a blood pressure within the normal range before rupture (Chauveau *et al.* 1994).

Intracerebral aneurysm rupture results in subarachnoid haemorrhage. Blood tracks into cerebrospinal fluid and may extend into brain (cerebral haematoma) and ventricles (ventricular haemorrhage). Early recognition of subarachnoid haemorrhage is crucial, since any delay adversely affects patients' outcome.

The cardinal feature of subarachnoid haemorrhage is a sudden intense headache, often described as a blow or an explosion inside the head, the worst ever experienced by the patient. Headache is more often diffuse than local. It subsequently radiates into the occipital or cervical region. Doctors should be alerted by the unusual character of headaches. Between 20 and 50 per cent of patients admitted for subarachnoid haemorrhage have a history of acute and transient headache in the days or weeks before the index episode of bleeding. This 'warning headache' is most likely due to a first, limited leak from the intracerebral aneurysm. It is frequently overlooked both by the patient and the doctor. Nonetheless, the majority of acute neurological events affecting ADPKD patients do not result from intracerebral aneurysm rupture but from hypertensive intracranial haemorrhage or ischaemic stroke (Chapman *et al.* 1993). Other symptoms or signs of subarachnoid haemorrhage include nausea and vomiting, photophobia, focal neurological deficit, seizures, lethargy, and transient loss of consciousness. Physical examination may show neck stiffness, focal neurologic signs, and retinal haemorrhages.

The first diagnostic step to assess the possibility of subarachnoid haemorrhage should be non-contrast cerebral CT with very thin cuts. Haemorrhage appears as areas of increased density, the degree of which depends on the haemoglobin concentration. Blood is rapidly cleared from the subarachnoid space; the sensitivity of CT in detecting haemorrhage thus decreases over time, from 92 per cent on the day of rupture to 86 per cent 1 day, 76 per cent 2 days, and 58 per cent 5 days later (Pirson *et al.* 2002a). If subarachnoid haemorrhage is strongly suspected on clinical grounds but not confirmed by CT, a lumbar puncture should be performed. If both CT scan and cerebrospinal fluid are normal, the diagnosis of subarachnoid haemorrhage is very unlikely.

Once established, subarachnoid haemorrhage should be further investigated under the direction of a neurologist/neurosurgeon team. Conventional angiography is usually performed as soon as possible, in order to localize the ruptured intracerebral aneurysm, delineate its size

and neck, assess the degree of vasospasm, and detect other unruptured intracerebral aneurysms. Multiple intracerebral aneurysms are indeed found in 24–31 per cent of ADPKD patients with intracerebral aneurysm rupture (Schievink *et al.* 1992; Chauveau *et al.* 1994).

For patients with chronic renal failure or on renal replacement therapy, the neurosurgeon and the nephrologist should closely cooperate to prescribe medical therapy and take decisions about intracerebral aneurysm treatment. The classical intervention is surgical clipping of the intracerebral aneurysm neck. Endovascular treatment has been recently developed as an alternative to surgery. The currently favoured technique is the placement of detachable platinum coil into the intracerebral aneurysm dome, inducing thrombosis by electrothermocoagulation. The long-term results of endovascular treatment are awaited.

As in the general population, intracerebral aneurysm rupture in ADPKD patients entails a combined mortality–morbidity rate of 35–55 per cent (Schievink *et al.* 1992; Chauveau *et al.* 1994). In the long term, survivors are threatened by recurrent rupture arising from the remnant neck of a previously treated intracerebral aneurysm, or from another intracerebral aneurysm, either left untreated, or developed *de novo* after the first intracerebral aneurysm rupture (Chauveau *et al.* 1990). Several steps may prevent a second rupture. First, any intact intracerebral aneurysm detected at the time of first rupture should be treated together with (or shortly after the treatment of) the ruptured intracerebral aneurysm, whenever feasible. Second, the result of treatment should be assessed with an angiography 3–6 months later. Third, patients should be screened for a further intracerebral aneurysm, so as to allow prophylactic treatment. The optimal interval for screening is not defined. We suggest a 2–3-year interval.

Screening

Given the grave prognosis of ruptured aneurysm and the possibility of detecting and repairing one before it ruptures, the screening for asymptomatic intracerebral aneurysm followed by prophylactic treatment has to be considered. The risks of this strategy should be weighted against the risks of spontaneous rupture. Several investigators have addressed this issue with a Markov decision model comparing the expected outcomes (gain in life expectancy, or better gain in years of good functional health) of screening versus no screening. It appeared very unlikely that the screening of all asymptomatic patients with ADPKD followed by prophylactic intervention would be cost effective (Pirson *et al.* 2002a).

Because ADPKD patients with a family history of intracerebral aneurysm have a higher prevalence of intracerebral aneurysm and may be at increased risk for rupture, we currently recommend periodic screening (every 3–5 years) only for patients with such a family history and a reasonable estimated life expectancy, recognizing that the natural history of incidental intracerebral aneurysm in this subgroup of patients remains to be defined with accuracy. In practice, the decision of screening should also take into consideration patients' knowledge and feeling about the respective risks of intracerebral aneurysm rupture and prophylactic treatment. Some patients with a distressful family history of intracerebral aneurysm rupture will require screening for either reassurance or treatment. Others will choose not to be screened because they prefer to avoid the immediate risk of treatment, even at the cost of a later risk of bleeding.

Our current approach may be summarized as follows. Patients without family history of intracerebral aneurysm are not screened, except that rare individuals who firmly request it. In patients with a positive family history (documented ruptured intracerebral aneurysm or stroke before the age of 50) we explain the risks of harbouring an unruptured intracerebral aneurysm, as well as the benefits and risks of screening: in case of negative screening, reassurance but also the risk of missing a tiny intracerebral aneurysm and therefore the need for further periodic screening; in case of positive screening, periodic surveillance of a small intracerebral aneurysm, or arteriography followed by appropriate treatment of intracerebral aneurysms more than 10 mm in diameter. Reassurance, re-evaluation at yearly intervals, smoking cessation, and strict control of hypertension and hyperlipidaemia are recommended for intracerebral aneurysms measuring less than 5 mm diameter. Some physicians argue and current data in the general population support that asymptomatic unruptured intracerebral aneurysms 5–9 mm in diameter should also be managed medically. However, considering that more than 50 per cent of ruptured intracerebral aneurysms in ADPKD are less than 10 mm in diameter, we increasingly consider the treatment of aneurysms more than 5 mm in diameter, especially in young individuals with an intracerebral aneurysm, easily treatable by coil embolization.

Other vascular abnormalities

Intracranial arterial dolichoectasia (elongation and dilatation of an arterial segment, most commonly in the posterior circulation) has been found in 2.2 per cent of ADPKD patients (versus 0.06 per cent in the general population). In some cases, it is a sequela of arterial dissection. It may mimic a fusiform or even saccular aneurysm on radiographic studies. Arterial dolichoectasia may be a cause of stroke (Schievink et al. 1997).

Patients with ADPKD could be at increased risk to develop dissection of cervicoencephalic arteries and thoracic aorta. An increased prevalence of coronary aneurysms has reported in a single limited series. These complications are, however, uncommon and their prevalence is unknown (Bobrie et al. 1998).

The previously reported association with abdominal aortic aneurysms was not supported by a large, control-matched study (Torra et al. 1996).

Cardiac valvular abnormalities

Once considered as important extrarenal manifestations of ADPKD, cardiac valvular abnormalities have been reported with a highly variable prevalence in different ADPKD subgroups, ranging from their absence to involvement of almost one-third of patients (reviewed by Perrone 1997). Differences in study design, methodology, or genetic background probably account for this discrepancy. In the single study of patients with a uniform genotype (PKD1), only mitral valve prolapse was clearly associated with ADPKD, with a prevalence rate of 26 per cent; mitral regurgitation was likely to be secondary to elevated blood pressure; the prevalence of aortic and tricuspid abnormalities was not increased (Lumiaho et al. 2001). Prophylaxis for bacterial endocarditis is indicated in the presence of valvular regurgitation but not for valvular prolapse without regurgitation (Perrone 1997). Valvular replacement is rarely needed.

Other abnormalities

Cysts in organs other than kidney and liver have been reported in some patients with ADPKD. However, an increased prevalence has been established only for intracranial arachnoid (8 per cent), pancreatic (9 per cent), and seminal vesicle (60 per cent) cysts (Perrone 1997). Cystic involvement of these organs remains asymptomatic in the vast majority of affected patients.

Whether ADPKD is associated with colonic diverticula is disputed. This is clearly not the case in patients without ESRD in whom prevalence rate, number of diverticula, and size of the largest diverticula do not differ from age-matched controls (Sharp et al. 1999). After renal transplantation, however, an increased incidence of diverticulitis and colon perforation has been reported (Andreoni et al. 1999) (see later).

ADPKD predisposes to abdominal wall hernia: as compared to unaffected family members, patients with the disease have an increased prevalence of inguinal (13 versus 4 per cent) and umbilical (7 versus 2 per cent) hernias (Gabow 1990).

Diagnosis

Diagnosing ADPKD is generally easy in the adult. Ultrasonography reveals bilaterally enlarged kidneys with multiple contiguous cysts of various sizes in the cortex and medulla. This is undoubtedly ADPKD if it is associated with a positive family history and/or cysts in the liver.

Diagnosis may be less easy in two settings: the first is the establishment of presymptomatic diagnosis in a young individual at risk of the disease; the second is the recognition of the disease in an adult patient with renal cysts but without a family history. In this section, we review the value of the two diagnostic tools, that is, imaging techniques and genetic analyses, for presymptomatic diagnosis and the differential diagnosis of the main renal cystic diseases in the adult.

Positive diagnosis

Imaging techniques

Ultrasonography is the primary diagnostic tool in ADPKD since it is rapid, non-invasive, cheap, and provides information on the location of other cysts. CT with contrast and T2-weighted MRI are more sensitive than ultrasonography because of their superior power of resolution (roughly, ultrasound can detect cysts of 1.0 cm, enhanced-CT cysts of 0.5 cm and T2-weighted MRI cysts of 0.3 cm in diameter).

However, no robust studies currently detail the sensitivity and specificity of CT and MRI in screening at-risk individuals for ADPKD. Moreover, enhanced CT implies the injection of contrast material and both CT and resonance imaging techniques are much more expensive than ultrasonography. Currently, CT and resonance imaging are largely reserved for the diagnosis of complications such as haemorrhage or infection (see above).

Ultrasonography thus remains the mainstay for screening. On the basis of both the prevalence of simple renal cysts in the general population (see below) by ultrasonography and the ultrasound results in individuals with a proven PKD1 disease, Ravine et al. (1994) have developed specific age-dependent criteria for diagnosing ADPKD: the diagnosis is made when at least two cysts (unilateral or bilateral) are present in at-risk family members aged 15–29 years, at least two cysts in each kidney in those aged 30–59 years, and at least four cysts in each kidney in those aged 60 years and above. In less than 15 years old at-risk individuals from PKD1 families, any renal cyst is highly suspect for the disease (Gabow et al. 1997). Conversely, in PKD1 families, the absence of cyst rules out the diagnosis in at-risk individuals older than 30 years, but not in those younger than 30 years.

The same diagnostic criteria has been recently tested in proven PKD2 families: as expected, the sensitivity of ultrasonography was lower in this milder form of the disease, with a false-negative rate of 23 per cent in individuals less than 30 years old, versus only 5 per cent in the same age category individuals belonging to PKD1 families (Nicolau *et al.* 1999). Just as in the PKD1 form, there was, however, no false-negative case in subjects aged 30 years or older (Nicolau *et al.* 1999). Of note, only a small number of PKD2 families has been studied so far.

In practice, the question of presymptomatic diagnosis usually arises in subjects older than 18 years (see later). In subjects older than 30 years with a negative ultrasound, the diagnosis of the disease may confidently be ruled out in PKD1 families and is very unlikely in PKD2 families as well in (the many) families in whom the genetic form is unknown. If sonography is negative or equivocal in someone under 30 years of age, especially if PKD2 disease is suspected or proven, the next step could be CT examination or MRI, keeping in mind, however, that the value of these techniques has not been adequately studied as a screening procedure. A preliminary study with *T*2-weighted magnetic resonance suggests that for someone 18–29 years of age, at least five cysts are required to make the diagnosis of ADPKD (Nascimento *et al.* 2001). If imaging findings remain doubtful a follow-up examination is proposed. Alternatively, gene testing may be considered.

Genetic analyses

Identification of mutation in both PKD genes is now achievable, with a detection rate of ≅60 per cent for *PKD1* and 70–80 per cent for *PKD2* (see above). However, mutational screening of the *PKD1* gene remains uniquely difficult, and for both genes, most mutations are private with no clear hotspot identified (see above). Therefore, although direct mutational analysis is increasingly yielding, it is not yet largely available for routine clinical use. In the meantime, genetic analysis is performed through the usual indirect approach, that is, linkage analysis.

Before advising linkage analysis, the clinician must be aware of both the feasibility and the limits of this diagnostic method. First of all, this analysis requires that a sufficient number of other affected and unaffected family members are available for study, in order to identify the genetic markers associated with the *PKD* gene. Thus, it cannot be used in families that have only a single affected member or in which relatives are unavailable for testing or unwilling to be tested. Second, as this approach is limited by potential errors due to recombination events, the use of a sufficient number of markers on both sides of the genes is required. Currently, linkage studies require the availability of at least two affected and one unaffected relative. When these conditions are met, a diagnosis can be made with 99 per cent accuracy. Linkage to *PKD1* is tested first, as it accounts for at least 85 per cent of the cases. As recently evidenced, the possibility of bilineal disease must be considered in the families apparently unliked to *PKD1* and *PKD2* (Pei *et al.* 2001).

Differential diagnosis in adults (for children, see Chapter 16.2.1)

There is a great variety of cystic kidney diseases which are usually classified as genetic or non-genetic disorders (Pirson and Chauveau 1999) (Table 4) keeping in mind that some of the latter could still be found to have a genetic basis.

Table 4 Classification of cystic diseases of the kidney (adapted from Pirson and Chauveau 1999)

Non-genetic

Acquired
Simple renal cysts (solitary or multiple)
Cysts of the renal sinus (or peripelvic lymphangiectasis)
Acquired renal cystic disease (in patients with failing kidneys)
Multilocular cysts
Hypokalaemia-related cysts

Developmental disorders
Medullary sponge kidney
Multicystic dysplastic kidneys (including *HNF-1β* related nephropathy)
Pyelocalyceal cysts

Genetic

Autosomal dominant
Autosomal-dominant polycystic kidney disease
Tuberous sclerosis complex
von Hippel–Lindau disease
Medullary cystic disease
Glomerulocystic kidney disease

Autosomal recessive
Autosomal-recessive polycystic kidney disease
Nephronophthisis
Glomerulocystic kidney disease included in multiple malformation syndrome: Meckel syndrome, Jeune asphyxiating thoracic dystrophy, Zellweger cerebrohepatorenal syndrome, Goldston syndrome, lissencephaly, etc.

X-linked
Orofaciodigital syndrome, type I

Chromosomal disorders
Trisomy 21, trisomy 13, trisomy 18, trisomy C

Non-genetic cystic diseases of the kidney

Acquired disorders

The prevalence of simple cysts increases with age in the general population. By ultrasonography, at least one renal cyst is found in 1.7 per cent of normal people aged 30–49, in 11.5 per cent of those aged 50–70, and in 22.1 per cent of those aged more than 70, and at least one cyst in each kidney in 1, 4, and 9 per cent of these age groups, respectively (Ravine *et al.* 1993). By newer imaging technique, a higher number of cysts is detected: thus, with *T*2-weighted single-shot fast spin–echo MRI, at least one cyst in each kidney is found in 12 per cent of women and 20 per cent of men aged 18–29, in 17 per cent of women and 18 per cent of men aged 30–44, and 27 per cent of women and 50 per cent of men aged 45–59 years (Nascimento *et al.* 2001). The differential diagnosis with ADPKD may arise in a young individual with a few cysts (see above) or in an elderly subject with multiple simple cysts: in the latter case, the kidneys are not enlarged, the cysts are usually large with no adjacent smaller cysts disseminated in either kidney, and liver cysts are absent. It should, however, be recalled that so far no specific morphological pattern has been documented in slowly progressive forms of ADPKD (either PKD1 or PKD2).

Cysts of the renal sinus (also known as peripelvic or parapelvic cysts, or hilar lymphangiectasis) consists of dilated hilar lymph channels. Found in 1 per cent at autopsy in the general population they are usually asymptomatic. In some cases, they may be multiple and bilateral, surrounding the entire collecting system and causing urinary obstruction of the pelvis. Distinction from ADPKD is easily made by ultrasonography (Fig. 3) and CT scan.

The term acquired renal cystic disease refers to the development of cysts in the patients with long-standing chronic renal failure or maintenance dialysis. In the early stage, kidneys are small or even shrunken and cysts are usually smaller than 0.5 cm. With time, cyst number and kidney volume may increase to such an extent that advanced forms may mimic ADPKD. Usually the two conditions are easily distinguished by familial and clinical data.

Multilocular cyst or multilocular cystic nephroma are rare, unilateral, and solitary tumour. They are increasingly detected in adults (as more imaging procedures are performed) as a complex mass characteristically divided by septa into multiple sonolucent locules (Fig. 4). This disease seems to represent one end of a spectrum of neoplasia with Wilms' tumour containing a few cysts at the other end.

Chronic potassium depletion such as in primary aldosteronism may induce the development of kidney cysts, predominantly in the medulla. Renal cysts observed in primary distal tubular acidosis could also be explained by hypokalaemia.

Developmental disorders

Medullary sponge kidney consists of small cystic dilatations involving the medullary collecting ducts (see Chapter 17.5): typical findings on excretory urogram (precalyceal brush-like striations or small cysts) clearly differ from those found in ADPKD, athough an interesting association between the two conditions has been reported (see above).

Multicystic dysplasic kidney or congenital multicystic kidney is the most common form of cystic disease in infants. Bilateral disease is incompatible with life. Unilateral form may incidentally be encountered in adults: diagnosis is generally easy as the multicystic kidney has no excretory function (the ureter is atretic) while the controlateral kidney is not cystic but may be hydronephrotic due to obstruction at the ureteropelvic or ureterovesical junction. The familial occurrence of some cases, together with renal agenesis and/or dysplasia, strongly suggests the existence of a genetic form with variable expression. This is the case, for example, in *HNF-1β* related nephropathy, an autosomal-dominant condition with diabetes (so-called MODY5 or maturity-onset diabetes of the young) and abnormal liver tests and genital tract malformation (Bellané-Chantelot *et al.* 2003).

Very rare cases of sporadic unilateral polycystic disease strikingly resembling ADPKD, radiologically and pathologically, have been reported. The origin of this disorder is unknown.

Genetic cystic diseases of the kidney

Correct identification of the various and rare forms of genetic cystic kidney disease other than ADPKD is clinically important for genetic counselling. These different inherited forms suggest that cyst formation and progression may depend on various molecular defects.

Renal cysts may be found in multiple systemic syndromes with autosomal-dominant inheritance (Table 4). TSC is the most frequent with a prevalence estimate of 1 : 14,500. It is caused by a mutation either on chromosome 9 (*TSC1*) or 16 (*TSC2*), each accounting for about 50 per cent of affected families. About 70 per cent of cases could be new mutations. Renal involvement occurs in 40–80 per cent of patients and consists mainly of angiomyolipomas. Cysts are the second most common renal manifestation of the disease and may predominate or occur in the absence of angiomyolipomas (Torres *et al.* 1994b). Moreover, liver cysts may also be observed in TSC. In a few cases, the aspect is indistinguishable from ADPKD. Interestingly, *TSC2* and *PKD1* are contiguous genes on chromosome 16, and in a rare phenotype of TSC with severe polycystic kidney disease in childhood, large deletions disrupting both *TSC2* and *PKD1* have been described (see above). The diagnosis of TSC should be considered in a patient with presumed ADPKD when the mutation apparently occurs *de novo* and in the presence of radiologically solid masses coexisting with cysts. Assessment should include the search for skin lesions (facial and ungueal fibromas) and central nervous involvement (mainly periventricular calcification on CT). Last, various malignant lesions may rarely involve the kidney in TSC.

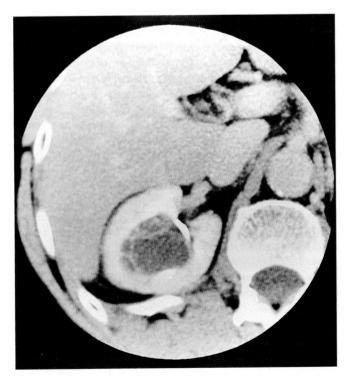

Fig. 4 CT showing a multilocular cyst (with characteristic septa) in the right kidney of a 70-year-old man (by courtesy of Drs P. François and A. Dardenne).

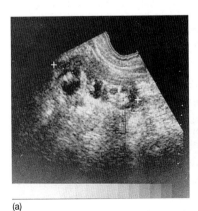 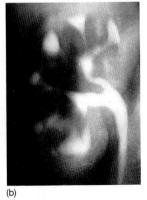

(a)   (b)

Fig. 3 Multiple parapelvic cysts of the right kidney seen on:
(a) ultrasonography and (b) an excretory urogram. Confinement of the cysts to the peripelvic area in a normal-sized kidney clearly differentiates this entity from ADPKD.

von Hippel–Lindau disease is a rare (prevalence estimate 1 : 40,000) hereditary cancer syndrome with autosomal-dominant inheritance. It is caused by germline mutations in *VHL*, a tumour suppressor gene. The disease is characterized by the development of various tumours involving cerebellum, spinal cord and retina (haemangioblastoma), adrenal gland (phaeochromocytoma), pancreas (mostly cysts), endolymphatic sac, and kidney (Richard *et al.* 2000). Renal lesions arise in about 50 per cent of the cases and includes cysts and, importantly, renal cell carcinomas. Bilateral multiple kidney cysts may simulate ADPKD. Liver cysts are very rare. The diagnosis of von Hippel–Lindau disease should always be considered in a patient with presumed ADPKD and renal cell carcinoma.

Medullary cystic disease (described in Chapter 16.3) is a genetically heterogeneous condition characterized by hyperuricaemia, chronic interstitial nephropathy, and late-onset medullary cysts. The kidneys are not enlarged or are even contracted. Endstage renal failure may occur in early adulthood. At least two genes are involved (Scolari *et al.* 1999).

Glomerulocystic kidney disease is an uncommon condition, predominantly described in children, but also reported in adults. The disorder is characterized by prominent cystic dilatation of Bowman's space, forming a glomerular cyst that contains abortive or primitive-appearing glomeruli (Fig. 5). The disease exists as a familial form with an apparently autosomal-dominant transmission. Some of these cases are ascribed to mutations in *HNF-1β* (Kolatsi-Joannou *et al.* 2001). The cysts may or may not be detected by ultrasonography: when they are, they may be distinguished from ADPKD by their smaller size and location in the cortex, as well as the absence of distortion and significant enlargement of the renal contour. The disease may progress to renal failure. It is of note that some glomerular cysts may be found in most renal cystic diseases, including ADPKD with early onset.

Autosomal-recessive polycystic kidney disease (ARPKD), (described in Chapter 16.2.1) is differentiated from ADPKD on the basis of the following characteristics: a recessive pattern of inheritance (absence of renal cysts in the parents is decisive), earlier age at presentation (most frequently during infancy or childhood), and, constantly, congenital hepatic fibrosis on liver biopsy, (leading to portal hypertension with an attendant risk of bleeding from oesophageal varices) sometimes associated with dilatation (sometimes cystic) of intrahepatic biliary ducts (Caroli's disease) with an attendant risk of cholangitis. The gene was recently characterized, with no evidence for heterogeneity (Ward *et al.* 2002). Nephrologists may be faced with the diagnosis of ADPKD in a young adult patient since renal failure may be delayed or become symptomatic only in adulthood (Fonck *et al.* 2001).

Nephronophthisis (NPH), formerly joined to medullary-cystic kidney disease (MCKD) in the NPH–MCKD complex is now recognized as a separate entity with autosomal-recessive inheritance and genetic heterogeneity (see Chapter 16.3). Cysts are a late albeit not constant finding. They are located at the corticomedullary junction.

Orofaciodigital syndrome, type I, is a rare X-linked dominant disorder with prenatal lethality in males. Approximately 75 per cent of cases are sporadic. The condition may include polycystic kidney disease. Central nervous system involvement with mental retardation, agenesis of the corpus callosum with cerebral and cerebellar atrophy, or porencephaly and cerebral cysts has been observed in some patients (Odent *et al.* 1998). In rare case, in some families, both the mother and the daughter had both cystic kidneys and orofaciodigital syndrome. Renal size is not increased, and cysts are less than 1 cm in size (Fig. 6). Most derive from the glomeruli. Endstage renal failure is reached at

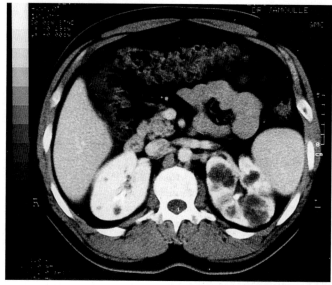

(a)

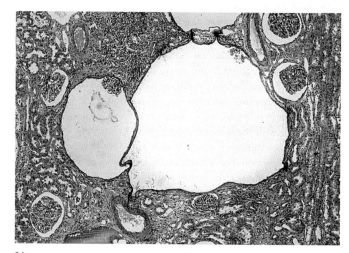

(b)

Fig. 5 (a) Multiple renal cysts found on CT in a 44-year-old man presenting with the nephrotic syndrome. Kidney biopsy showed both membranous nephropathy and glomerulocystic disease: cysts consisted of a dilatation of Bowman's space, as shown by the presence (b) of a primitive-looking glomerulus in the cysts (by courtesy of Drs P. Bernis and J. Hamels).

variable age, from the second decade (Feather *et al.* 1997). The diagnosis rests on extrarenal abnormalities: cleft tongue, cleft lip, cleft palate, hypertrophic lingular and buccal frenulae, hypoplasia of alonasal cartilage, brachydactyly, syndactyly, and alopecia (Fig. 6).

The autosomal recessive malformation syndromes (listed in Table 4) are observed in infants or children, and may be associated with glomerulocystic kidney disease.

Genetic counselling

The inheritance pattern of ADPKD means that the offspring of an affected individual are at a 50 per cent risk of having the disease. Adequate genetic and clinical information should be given to affected

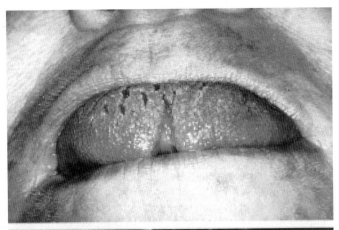

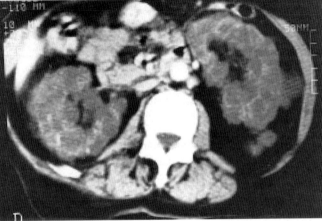

Fig. 6 Orofaciodigital syndrome type 1: (upper) cleft tongue in an affected woman; (lower) kidney CT showing multiple cysts. The kidneys are less enlarged and deformed, and the cysts are more uniform in size, than in ADPKD (reproduced by courtesy of Drs J. P. Méry and F. Daniel).

families. Individuals should be informed about the implications of a positive diagnosis before undergoing screening. A negative testing may provide some degree of survivor guilt or the feeling of ostracism from affected relatives (Marsick *et al.* 1998). For the 50 per cent cases tested positive, early detection of the disease aims at providing optimal health care and genetic counselling. However, it may carry severe burden, including anxiety and depression because no specific treatment is as yet available, concerns for passing the disease to offspring, difficulty in obtaining employment, and disqualification for medical and life insurance. Since there is a wide intrafamilial variability in the severity of the phenotype, it would not be wise to predict the course of the disease on the basis of family history.

Geneticists have developed comprehensive policy on presymptomatic genetic testing. At-risk individual should be given understandable oral and written information from experienced physician, including advantages and drawbacks of testing; he or she may refuse the test, or even refuse knowledge of the results. The offer of testing should be separated in time from the laboratory appointment. Tests results should be given by a physician (geneticist) with ample opportunity to ask questions and to be offered support for the patient and his/her relatives. Since consequences of ultrasound screening share many similarities with genetic testing—or even requires more sophisticated interpretation, as exemplified by the absence of definite

conclusion in the absence of cyst in childhood—we plead for similar information both prior and after the decision of making any imaging procedure for the purpose of presymptomatic screening.

Presymptomatic screening before the age of majority raises a number of ethical and legal issues (Levy 2001). With the exception of direct benefit from the test, we do not recommend to screen before the majority, so as to preserve the patient's own decision to decide for himself. However, we encourage families to inform their general practitioner/paediatrician of the risk of the disease in the offspring of affected individuals. The strategy for presymptomatic imaging screening is detailed above (see section on 'Positive diagnosis').

In concordance with the guidelines provided by the National Kidney Foundation in the United States of America, we consider gene testing (a) in potential living related kidney donors with equivocal MRI, (b) in those in whom early management would be altered by establishment of the diagnosis (e.g. in those with a family history of early intracranial aneurysm), (c) and in at-risk individuals who have reached their majority, request the test and have an appropriate understanding of the potential benefits and drawbacks of a positive diagnosis.

Prenatal diagnosis by genetic analysis (see above) on a sample of chorionic villi has been achieved at approximately the ninth week of pregnancy in a small number of cases, and parents may elect to have the pregnancy terminated. Affected parents should be informed about the feasibility of prenatal genetic diagnosis, but should also be advised that this does not predict the natural history of the disease; it should be remembered that ADPKD usually manifests late in life and that the majority of people affected are alive, without endstage renal failure, at the age of 50 (see above). Actually, the frequency of elective abortion was not greater in women with ADPKD than in a control group in a large American series (Chapman *et al.* 1994b), which is in keeping with a survey demonstrating that only 4 per cent of affected adults would have an abortion if the fetus had the disease (Sujansky *et al.* 1990).

Renal replacement therapy

Survival

Despite the existence of specific renal and extrarenal manifestations, ADPKD has no negative impact on overall survival in renal replacement therapy. Compared to age-matched patients with other primary chronic renal diseases, those with ADPKD were even found to have a 10–20 per cent greater 5-year survival both in the European and North American Registers (Pirson *et al.* 1996; Perrone *et al.* 2001). Most of this survival advantage accrued to the time on dialysis, because no significant difference in mortality rate between ADPKD and control patient was found after transplantation both in large surveys and single-centre studies (Pirson *et al.* 1996; Perrone *et al.* 2001).

Whether some extrarenal manifestations of ADPKD contributed to mortality in renal replacement therapy was examined using data from the United States Renal Data System. The only category in which mortality in ADPKD patients significantly exceeded control patients was polycystic liver disease. For other potentially ADPKD-related causes of death, mortality was actually significantly lower in ADPKD patients (ischaemic heart disease, cardiac valvular disease) or not significantly different (ruptured vascular aneurysm, bowel perforation) (Perrone *et al.* 2001).

Renal complications

Kidney size tends to increase with time on long-term haemodialysis—probably due to superimposed development of acquired cystic disease—whereas it gradually decreases after successful renal transplantation (Pirson *et al.* 2002b).

Every renal manifestation of ADPKD described above may be encountered during renal replacement therapy. Only the prevalence of the most frequent manifestations and some specific aspects of management are emphasized here.

On haemodialysis, renal pain (requiring medical evaluation and/or analgesic use), gross haematuria, and renal infection are observed in 57, 51, and 12 per cent of patients within 5 years following initiation of treatment (Pirson *et al.* 1996). Both gross haematuria and renal infection occur more frequently among patients with such a history before the initiation of haemodialysis than among those without. A close monitoring of heparinization is advised during bleeding episodes. Renal infection can be controlled by appropriate antibiotics such as fluoroquinolones in most patients. A 4-week course is recommended, especially in haemodialysed patients with permanent dialysis catheters or prosthetic grafts (Norby and Torres 2000).

Rarely, intractable pain, recurrent haematuria, or severe infection require nephrectomy. Excluding preparation for kidney transplantation, nephrectomy was needed in only 4 per cent of our patients on haemodialysis (Pirson *et al.* 1996). With a policy of selective removal of problematic kidneys before transplantation (see below), complication due to polycystic kidneys are infrequent after transplantation, leading to post-transplant nephrectomy in only 7 per cent of patients in our experience (Pirson *et al.* 1996). Laparoscopic nephrectomy has been successfully used in patients in renal replacement therapy; however, this challenging procedure requires an experienced surgeon and may not be advisable for infected kidneys (Seshadri *et al.* 2001).

Renal cell carcinoma has been reported in very few ADPKD patients in renal replacement therapy.

Extrarenal complications

Liver cysts are rarely symptomatic. Acute pain or infection occur in less than 5 per cent of patients on renal replacement therapy (Pirson *et al.* 1996). Low cardiac output with recurrent hypotension during the haemodialysis session may result from compression of inferior vena cava by a cyst. In the occasional patient with either incapacitating or complicated massive polycystic liver or symptomatic Caroli's disease, liver transplantation is increasingly considered, especially when a kidney transplantation is concurrently planned (see above). Cardiac valvular disease does not contribute significantly to morbidity in the ADPKD population in renal replacement therapy (Pirson *et al.* 1996).

The prevalence of strokes among ADPKD patients on renal replacement therapy has been found either similar or slightly increased compared to control patients (Pirson *et al.* 1996; Norby and Torres 2000). Whether this is accounted for by rupture of intracranial aneurysm is not established. When intracranial aneurysm rupture occurs in a patient on haemodialysis, heparinization should be closely monitored and hypotension or hypovolaemia should be avoided (see above).

Though an excess of colon complications among ADPKD patients has not been found in most groups (Pirson *et al.* 1996; Norby and Torres 2000), an increased incidence of colonic perforation (4.8 versus 1.4 per cent in control patients) was reported in a large single-centre series of transplanted patients (Andreoni *et al.* 1999).

Selection of renal replacement modality (Fig. 7)

Since kidney transplantation provides both a better quality of life and a higher long-term survival (Perrone *et al.* 2001), this option should be considered in any ADPKD patient with a reasonable life expectancy (at least 5 years in our opinion) and with no contraindication to surgery or immunosuppression.

Pretransplant work-up should include abdominal CT, echocardiography, myocardial stress scintigraphy and, in patients with signs or symptoms of arteriosclerosis, aortoiliac angiography. As regard screening for intracranial aneurysm, our approach does not differ from that applied in the ADPKD population in general (see above). We do not screen our transplant candidates for diverticular disease since post-transplant colonic perforation is not predicted by the presence of pretransplant diverticula (Pirson *et al.* 1996); pretransplant elective colon resection should only be considered in patients with symptomatic, severe diverticular disease.

Since most kidneys left *in situ* do not lead to major complications after transplantation, pretransplant nephrectomy, once routinely performed, is now restricted to patients with a history of recurrent cyst infection, recurrent major bleeding, or complicated lithiasis (Pirson *et al.* 2002b).

Living-related donor transplantation may be considered, provided the existence of ADPKD has been formally excluded on clinical or genetic grounds (see above).

Patients either awaiting kidney transplantation or not eligible for this treatment may opt for haemodialysis or peritoneal dialysis. Short-term survival and complication rates on peritoneal dialysis were found

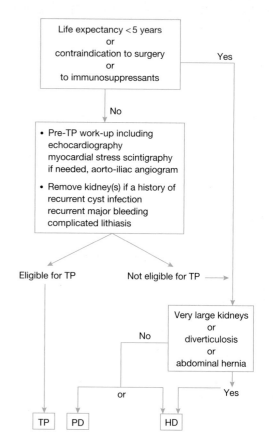

HD, haemodialysis; PD, peritoneal dialysis; TP, kidney transplantation.

Fig. 7 Selection of renal replacement modality in patients with ADPKD.

similar in ADPKD and age-matched controls (Hadimeri et al. 1998). Peritoneal dialysis is, however, less desirable for patients with very large kidneys, since the larger the kidney volume the lesser the available effective peritoneal surface area. Furthermore, tolerance of peritoneal dialysis may be affected by excessive abdominal distension. Haemodialysis should also be preferred in patients with colonic diverticular disease or abdominal hernia. A 15 per cent rate of late peritoneal leakage has been reported in a small series of ADPKD patients treated by peritoneal dialysis (De Vecchi et al. 2002).

In summary, most patients with ADPKD are excellent candidates for any form of renal replacement therapy. Kidney transplantation is the treatment of choice. Renal and extrarenal complications do not significantly impact survival on renal replacement therapy. Mean prolongation of life with such therapy has been estimated at 14 years (Barrett and Parfrey 1991).

References

Andreoni, K. A. et al. (1999). Increased incidence of gastrointestinal surgical complications in renal transplant recipients with polycystic kidney disease. Transplantation 67, 262–266.

Bajwa, Z. H. et al. (2001). Pain management in polycystic kidney disease. Kidney International 60, 1631–1644.

Barr, M. M. et al. (2001). The Caenorhabditis elegans autosomal dominant polycystic kidney disease gene homologs lov-1 and pkd-2 act in the same pathway. Current Biology 11, 1341–1346.

Barrett, B. J. and Parfrey, P. S. (1991). Autosomal dominant polycystic kidney disease and end stage renal disease. Seminars in Dialysis 4, 26–32.

Bellanné-Chantelot, C., Chauveau, D., Gautier, J. F., Dubois-Laforgue, D., Clauin, S., Beaufils, S., Wilhelm, J. M., Boitard, C., Noël, L. H., Velho, G., and Timsit, J. (2004). Multiple organ involvement in patients with HNF-1B related Maturity-Onset Diabetes of the Young (MODY5). Annals of Internal Medicine (in press).

Bello-Reus, E., Holubeck, K., and Rajaraman, S. (2001). Angiogenesis in autosomal-dominant polycystic kidney disease. Kidney International 60, 37–45.

Bennett, W. M. et al. (1985). Cyst fluid antibiotic concentrations in autosomal-dominant polycystic kidney disease. American Journal of Kidney Diseases 6, 400–404.

Bhunia, A. K. et al. (2002). PKD1 induces p21(waf1) and regulation of the cell cycle via direct activation of the JAK-STAT signaling pathway in a process requiring PKD2. Cell 109, 157–168.

Bobrie, G. et al. (1998). Spontaneous artery dissection: is it part of the spectrum of autosomal dominant polycystic kidney disease? Nephrology, Dialysis, Transplantation 13, 2138–2141.

Boletta, A. et al. (2000). Polycystin-1, the gene product of PKD1, induces resistance to apoptosis and spontaneous tubulogenesis in MDCK cells. Molecular Cell 6, 1267–1273.

Boulter, C. et al. (2001). Cardiovascular, skeletal, and renal defects in mice with a targeted disruption of the Pkd1 gene. Proceedings of the National Academy of Sciences of the United States of America 98, 12174–12179.

Brook-Carter, P. T. et al. (1994). Deletion of the TSC2 and PKD1 genes associated with severe infantile polycystic kidney disease a contiguous gene syndrome. Nature Genetics 8, 328–332.

Carone, F. A. et al. (1992). Sequential tubular cell and basement membrane changes in polycystic kidney disease. Journal of the American Society of Nephrology 3, 244–253.

Chapman, A. B., Johnson, A. M., and Gabon, P. A. (1993). Intracranial aneurysms in autosomal dominant polycystic disease. New England Journal of Medicine 327, 916–920.

Chapman, A. B. et al. (1994a). Overt proteinuria and microalbuminuria in autosomal dominant polycystic kidney disease. Journal of the American Society of Nephrology 5, 1349–1354.

Chapman, A. B., Johnson, A. M., and Gabow, P. A. (1994b). Pregnancy outcome and its relationship to progression of renal failure in autosomal dominant polycystic kidney disease. Journal of the American Society of Nephrology 5, 1178–1185.

Chauveau, D., Fakhouri, F., and Grunfeld, J. P. (2000). Liver involvement in autosomal-dominant polycystic kidney disease: therapeutic dilemma. Journal of the American Society of Nephrology 11, 1767–1775.

Chauveau, D. et al. (1990). Recurrent rupture of intracranial aneurysms in autosomal dominant polycystic kidney disease. British Medical Journal 301, 966–967.

Chauveau, D. et al. (1994). Intracranial aneurysms in autosomal dominant polycystic kidney disease. Kidney International 45, 1140–1146.

Chauvet, V. et al. (2002). Expression of PKD1 and PKD2 transcripts and proteins in human embryo and during normal kidney development. American Journal of Pathology 160, 973–983.

Choukroun, G. et al. (1995). Factors influencing progression of renal failure in autosomal dominant polycystic kidney disease. Journal of the American Society of Nephrology 6, 1634–1642.

Churchill, D. N. et al. (1984). Prognosis of adult onset polycystic kidney disease re-evaluated. Kidney International 26, 190–193.

Deltas, C. C. (2001). Mutations of the human polycystic kidney disease 2 (PKD2) gene. Human Mutation 18, 13–24.

De Vecchi, A. F. et al. (2002). Polycystic kidney disease and late peritoneal leakage in CAPD: are they related? Peritoneal Dialysis International 22, 82–86.

Devuyst, O. et al. (1996). Expression of aquaporins-1 and -2 during nephrogenesis and in autosomal dominant polycystic kidney disease. American Journal of Physiology 271, F169–F183.

Dunn, M. D. et al. (2001). Laparoscopic cyst marsupialization in patients with autosomal dominant polycystic kidney disease. Journal of Urology 165, 1888–1892.

Ecder, T. and Schrier, R. W. (2001). Hypertension in autosomal-dominant polycystic kidney disease: early occurrence and unique aspects. Journal of the American Society of Nephrology 12, 194–200.

European Polycystic Kidney Disease Consortium (represented by Ward, C. J. et al.) (1994). The polycystic kidney disease 1 gene encodes a 14 kb transcript and lies within a duplicated region on chromosome 16. Cell 77, 881–894.

Feather, S. A. et al. (1997). The oral–facial–digital syndrome type 1 (OFD1), a cause of polycystic kidney disease and associated malformations, maps to Xp22.2–Xp22.3. Human Molecular Genetics 6, 1163–1167.

Fick, G. M. et al. (1993). Characteristics of very early onset autosomal dominant polycystic kidney disease. Journal of the American Society of Nephrology 3, 1863–1870.

Fick, G. M. et al. (1995). Causes of death in autosomal dominant polycystic kidney disease. Journal of the American Society of Nephrology 5, 2048–2056.

Fonck, C. et al. (2001). Autosomal recessive polycystic kidney disease in adulthood. Nephrology, Dialysis, Transplantation 16, 1648–1652.

Freedman, B. I. et al. (2000). Racial variation in autosomal dominant polycystic kidney disease. American Journal of Kidney Diseases 35, 35–39.

Gabow, P. A. (1990). Autosomal dominant polycystic kidney disease—more than a renal disease. American Journal of Kidney Diseases 16, 403–413.

Gabow, P. A. (1993). Autosomal dominant polycystic kidney disease. New England Journal of Medicine 329, 332–342.

Gabow, P. A., Duley, I., and Johnson, A. M. (1992a). Clinical profiles of gross hematuria in autosomal dominant polycystic kidney disease. American Journal of Kidney Diseases 20, 140–143.

Gabow, P. A. et al. (1992b). Factors affecting the progression of renal disease in autosomal-dominant polycystic kidney disease. Kidney International 41, 1311–1319.

Gabow, P. A. et al. (1997). Utility of ultrasonography in the diagnosis of autosomal dominant polycystic kidney disease in children. Journal of the American Society of Nephrology 8, 105–110.

Geng, L. et al. (1996). Identification and localization of polycystin, the PKD1 gene product. Journal of Clinical Investigation 98, 2674–2682.

Gibson, P. and Watson, M. L. (1998). Cyst infection in polycystic kidney disease: a clinical challenge. *Nephrology, Dialysis, Transplantation* **13**, 2455–2457.

Grampsas, S. A. *et al.* (2000). Anatomic and metabolic risk factors for nephrolithiasis in patients with autosomal dominant polycystic kidney disease. *American Journal of Kidney Diseases* **36**, 53–57.

Hadimeri, H. *et al.* (1998). CAPD in patients with autosomal dominant polycystic kidney disease. *Peritoneal Dialysis International* **18**, 429–432.

Harrap, S. B., Davies, D. L., Macnicol, A. M., Dominiczak, A. F., Fraser, R., Wright, A. F., Watson, M. L., and Briggs, J. D. (1991). Renal, cardiovascular and hormonal characteristics of young adults with autosomal dominant polycystic kidney disease. *Kidney International* **40**, 501–508.

Harris, P. C. (2002). Molecular basis of polycystic kidney disease: PKD1, PKD2 and PKHD1. *Current Opinion in Nephrology and Hypertension* **11**, 309–314.

Hateboer, N. *et al.* (1999a). Comparison of phenotypes of polycystic kidney disease types 1 and 2. European PKD1–PKD2 Study Group. *Lancet* **353**, 103–107.

Hateboer, N. *et al.* (1999b). Familial phenotype differences in PKD1. *Kidney International* **56**, 34–40.

Huseman, R. *et al.* (1980). Macropuncture study of polycystic disease in adult human kidneys. *Kidney International* **18**, 375–385.

Ibraghimov-Beskrovnaya, O. *et al.* (1997). Polycystin: *in vitro* synthesis, *in vivo* tissue expression, and subcellular localization identifies a large membrane-associated protein. *Proceedings of the National Academy of Sciences of the United States of America* **94**, 6397–6402.

Igarashi, P. and Somlo, S. (2002). Genetics and pathogenesis of polycystic kidney disease. *Journal of the American Society of Nephrology* **13**, 2384–2398.

Johnson, A. M. and Gabow, P. A. (1997). Identification of patients with autosomal dominant polycystic kidney disease at highest risk for end-stage renal disease. *Journal of the American Society of Nephrology* **8**, 1560–1567.

Kabbej, M. *et al.* (1996). Laparoscopic fenestration in polycystic liver disease. *British Journal of Surgery* **83**, 1697–1701.

Keith, D. S. *et al.* (1994). Renal cell carcinoma in autosomal dominant polycystic kidney disease. *Journal of the American Society of Nephrology* **4**, 1661–1669.

Kim, E. *et al.* (1999). Interaction between RGS7 and polycystin. *Proceedings of the National Academy of Sciences of the United States of America* **96**, 6371–6376.

Kim, K. *et al.* (2000). Polycystin 1 is required for the structural integrity of blood vessels. *Proceedings of the National Academy of Sciences of the United States of America* **97**, 1731–1736.

King, B. F. *et al.* (2000). Quantification and longitudinal trends of kidney, renal cyst, and renal parenchyma volumes in autosomal dominant polycystic kidney disease. *Journal of the American Society of Nephrology* **11**, 1505–1511.

Kolatsi-Joannou, M. *et al.* (2001). Hepatocyte nuclear factor-1β: a new kindred with renal cysts and diabetes and gene expression in normal human development. *Journal of the American Society of Nephrology* **12**, 2175–2180.

Lebeau, C. *et al.* (2002). Basolateral chloride transporters in autosomal dominant polycystic kidney disease. *Pflügers Archiv* **444**, 722–731.

Levy, M. (2001). How well do we manage and support patients and families with dominantly inherited renal disease? *Nephrology, Dialysis, Transplantation* **16**, 1–4.

Lu, W. *et al.* (1997). Perinatal lethality with kidney and pancreas defects in mice with a targeted *Pkd1* mutation. *Nature Genetics* **17**, 179–181.

Lu, W. *et al.* (1999). Late onset of renal and hepatic cysts in Pkd1-targeted heterozygotes. *Nature Genetics* **21**, 160–161.

Lu, W. *et al.* (2001). Comparison of *Pkd1*-targeted mutants reveals that loss of polycystin-1 causes cystogenesis and bone defects. *Human Molecular Genetics* **10**, 2385–2396.

Lumiaho, A. *et al.* (2001). Mitral valve prolapse and mitral regurgitation are common in patients with polycystic kidney disease type 1. *American Journal of Kidney Diseases* **38**, 1208–1216.

Marsick, R., Limwongse, C., and Kodish, E. (1998). Genetic testing for renal diseases: medical and ethical considerations. *American Journal of Kidney Diseases* **32**, 934–945.

Maschio, G. *et al.* (1996). Effect of the angiotensin-converting-enzyme inhibitor benazepril on the progression of chronic renal insufficiency. The Angiotensin-Converting-Enzyme Inhibition in Progressive Renal Insufficiency Study Group. *New England Journal of Medicine* **334**, 939–945.

Milutinovic, J. *et al.* (1984). Autosomal dominant polycystic kidney disease: symptoms and clinical findings. *Quarterly Journal of Medicine* **53**, 511–522.

Mochizuki, T. *et al.* (1996). *PKD2*, a gene for polycystic kidney disease that encodes an integral membrane protein. *Science* **272**, 1339–1342.

Modification of Diet in Renal Disease Study Group (prepared by Klahr, S. *et al.*) (1995). Dietary protein restriction, blood pressure control, and the progression of polycystic kidney disease. *Journal of the American Society of Nephrology* **5**, 20037–20047.

Moy, G. W. *et al.* (1996). The sea urchin sperm receptor for egg jelly is a modular protein with extensive homology to the human polycystic kidney disease protein, PKD1. *Journal of Cell Biology* **133**, 809–817.

Nadasdy, T. *et al.* (1995). Proliferative activity of cyst epithelium in human renal cystic diseases. *Journal of the American Society of Nephrology* **5**, 1462–1468.

Nascimento, A. B. *et al.* (2001). Rapid MR imaging detection of renal cysts: age-based standards. *Radiology* **221**, 628–632.

Neugarten, J., Acharya, A., and Silbiger, S. R. (2000). Effect of gender on the progression of nondiabetic renal disease: a meta-analysis. *Journal of the American Society of Nephrology* **11**, 319–329.

Nickel, C. *et al.* (2002). The polycystin-1 C-terminal fragment triggers branching morphogenesis and migration of tubular kidney epithelial cells. *Journal of Clinical Investigation* **109**, 481–489.

Nicolau, C. *et al.* (1999). Autosomal dominant polycystic kidney disease types 1 and 2: assessment of US sensitivity for diagnosis. *Radiology* **213**, 273–276.

Norby, S. M. and Torres, V. E. (2000). Complications of autosomal dominant polycystic kidney disease in hemodialysis patients. *Seminars in Dialysis* **13**, 30–35.

Odent, S. *et al.* (1998). Central nervous system malformations and early end-stage renal disease in oro-facio-digital syndrome type I: a review. *American Journal of Medical Genetics* **75**, 389–394.

Ong, A. C. *et al.* (1999a). Coordinate expression of the autosomal dominant polycystic kidney disease proteins, polycystin-2 and polycystin-1, in normal and cystic tissue. *American Journal of Pathology* **154**, 1721–1729.

Ong, A. C. *et al.* (1999b). Characterisation and expression of the PKD-1 protein, polycystin, in renal and extrarenal tissues. *Kidney International* **55**, 2091–2116.

Orth, S. R. (2002). Smoking and the kidney. *Journal of the American Society of Nephrology* **13**, 1663–1672.

Pei, Y. (2001). A 'two-hit' model of cystogenesis in autosomal dominant polycystic kidney disease? *Trends in Molecular Medicine* **7**, 151–156.

Pei, Y. *et al.* (1999). Somatic PKD2 mutations in individual kidney and liver cysts support a 'two-hit' model of cystogenesis in type 2 autosomal dominant polycystic kidney disease. *Journal of the American Society of Nephrology* **10**, 1524–1529.

Pei, Y. *et al.* (2001). Bilineal disease and trans-heterozygotes in autosomal dominant polycystic kidney disease. *American Journal of Human Genetics* **68**, 355–363.

Perrone, R. D. (1997). Extrarenal manifestations of ADPKD. *Kidney International* **51**, 2022–2036.

Perrone, R. D., Ruthazer, R., and Terrin, N. C. (2001). Survival after end-stage renal disease in autosomal dominant polycystic kidney disease: contribution of extrarenal complications to mortality. *American Journal of Kidney Diseases* **38**, 777–784.

Persu, A. *et al.* (2000). CF gene and cystic fibrosis transmembrane conductance regulator expression in autosomal dominant polycystic kidney disease. *Journal of the American Society of Nephrology* **11**, 2285–2296.

Persu, A. *et al.* (2002). Modifier effect of ENOS in autosomal dominant polycystic kidney disease. *Human Molecular Genetics* **11**, 229–241.

Peters, D. J. and Breuning, M. H. (2001). Autosomal dominant polycystic kidney disease: modification of disease progression. *Lancet* **358**, 1439–1444.

Pirson, Y. and Chauveau, D. Cystic diseases of the kidney. In *Atlas of Diseases of the Kidney* Vol. 2 (ed. R. W. Schrier, A. H. Cohen, R. J. Glassock, and J. P. Grünfeld), pp. 9.1–9.24. Philadelphia, PA: Current Medicine, 1999.

Pirson, Y., Chauveau, D., and Torres, V. (2002a). Management of cerebral aneurysms in autosomal dominant polycystic kidney disease. *Journal of the American Society of Nephrology* **13**, 269–276.

Pirson, Y., Christophe, J. L., and Goffin, E. (1996). Outcome of renal replacement therapy in autosomal dominant polycystic kidney disease. *Nephrology, Dialysis, Transplantation* **11** (Suppl. 6), 24–28.

Pirson, Y., Cochat, P., and Goffin, E. Treatment of patients with hereditary and congenital disorders. In *Optimal Treatment Strategies in End-stage Renal Failure* (ed. C. Jacobs), pp. 205–228. Oxford: Oxford University Press, 2002b.

Qian, F. *et al.* (1996). The molecular basis of focal cyst formation in human autosomal dominant polycystic kidney disease type I. *Cell* **87**, 979–987.

Qian, F. *et al.* (1997). PKD1 interacts with PKD2 through a probable coiled-coil domain. *Nature Genetics* **16**, 179–183.

Ravine, D. *et al.* (1993). An ultrasound renal cyst prevalence survey: specificity data for inherited renal cystic diseases. *American Journal of Kidney Diseases* **22**, 803–807.

Ravine, D. *et al.* (1994). Evaluation of ultrasonographic diagnostic criteria for autosomal dominant polycystic kidney disease 1. *Lancet* **343**, 824–827.

Richard, S. *et al.* (2000). Central nervous system hemangioblastomas, endolymphatic sac tumors, and von Hippel–Lindau disease. *Neurosurgery Review* **23**, 1–22.

Rossetti, S. *et al.* (2001). Mutation analysis of the entire *PKD1* gene: genetic and diagnostic implications. *American Journal of Human Genetics* **68**, 46–63.

Rossetti, S. *et al.* (2002a). A complete mutation screen of the *ADPKD* genes by DHPLC. *Kidney International* **61**, 1588–1599.

Rossetti, S. *et al.* (2002b). The position of the polycystic kidney disease 1 (PKD1) gene mutation correlates with the severity of renal disease. *Journal of the American Society of Nephrology* **13**, 1230–1237.

Schievink, W. I. *et al.* (1992). Saccular intracranial aneurysms in autosomal dominant polycystic kidney disease. *Journal of the American Society of Nephrology* **3**, 88–95.

Schievink, W. I. *et al.* (1997). Intracranial arterial dolichoectasia in autosomal dominant polycystic kidney disease. *Journal of the American Society of Nephrology* **8**, 1298–1303.

Schrier, R. *et al.* (2002). Cardiac and renal effects of standard versus rigorous blood pressure control in autosomal-dominant polycystic kidney disease: results of a seven-year prospective randomized study. *Journal of the American Society of Nephrology* **13**, 1733–1739.

Scolari, F. *et al.* (1999). Identification of a new locus for medullary cystic disease on chromosome 16p12. *American Journal of Human Genetics* **64**, 1655–1660.

Seshadri, P. A. *et al.* (2001). Transperitoneal laparoscopic nephrectomy for giant polycystic kidneys: a case control study. *Urology* **58**, 23–27.

Sharp, C. K. *et al.* (1999). Evaluation of colonic diverticular disease in autosomal dominant polycystic kidney disease without end-stage renal disease. *American Journal of Kidney Diseases* **34**, 863–868.

Simon, P. *et al.* (1989). Prognosis of adult polycystic kidney disease re-evaluated: results of an investigation in 1112 patients from 369 kindreds. *Nephrology, Dialysis, Transplantation* **4**, 442.

Sise, C. *et al.* (2000). Volumetric determination of progression in autosomal dominant polycystic kidney disease by computed tomography. *Kidney International* **58**, 2492–2501.

Sujansky, E. *et al.* (1990). Attitudes of at-risk and affected individuals regarding presymptomatic testing for autosomal dominant polycystic kidney disease. *American Journal of Medical Genetics* **35**, 510–515.

Sullivan, L. P., Wallace, D. P., and Grantham, J. J. (1998). Epithelial transport in polycystic kidney disease. *Physiology Review* **78**, 1165–1191.

Torra, R. *et al.* (1996). Abdominal aortic aneurysms and autosomal dominant polycystic kidney disease. *Journal of the American Society of Nephrology* **7**, 2483–2486.

Torres, V. E. *et al.* (1993). Renal stone disease in autosomal dominant polycystic kidney disease. *American Journal of Kidney Diseases* **22**, 513–519.

Torres, V. E. *et al.* (1994a). Hepatic venous outflow obstruction in autosomal dominant polycystic kidney disease. *Journal of the American Society of Nephrology* **5**, 1186–1192.

Torres, V. E. *et al.* (1994b). The kidney in the tuberous sclerosis complex. *Advances in Nephrology* **23**, 43–70.

United States Renal Data System (2001). Excerpts from the USRDR 2001 Annual Data Report. *American Journal of Kidney Diseases* **38** (Suppl. 3), S1–S248.

Valente, J. F. *et al.* (2001). Laparoscopic renal denervation for intractable ADPKD-related pain. *Nephrology, Dialysis, Transplantation* **16**, 160.

Valero, F. A. *et al.* (1999). Ambulatory blood pressure and left ventricular mass in normotensive patients with autosomal dominant polycystic kidney disease. *Journal of the American Society of Nephrology* **10**, 1020–1026.

Wang, D. and Strandgaard, S. (1997). The pathogenesis of hypertension in autosomal dominant polycystic kidney disease. *Journal of Hypertension* **15**, 925–933.

Wang, D., Iversen, J., and Strandgaard, S. (2000). Endothelium-dependent relaxation of small resistance vessels is impaired in patients with autosomal dominant polycystic kidney disease. *Journal of the American Society of Nephrology* **11**, 1371–1376.

Ward, C. J. *et al.* (1996). Polycystin, the polycystic kidney disease 1 protein, is expressed by epithelial cells in fetal, adult, and polycystic kidney. *Proceedings of the National Academy of Sciences of the United States of America* **93**, 1524–1528.

Ward, C. J. *et al.* (2002). The gene mutated in autosomal recessive polycystic kidney disease encodes a large, receptor-like protein. *Nature Genetics* **30**, 259–269.

Watnick, T. *et al.* (1999). Mutation detection of PKD1 identifies a novel mutation common to three families with aneurysms and/or very-early-onset disease. *American Journal of Human Genetics* **65**, 1561–1571.

Watnick, T. *et al.* (2000). Mutations of *PKD1* in ADPKD2 cysts suggest a pathogenic effect of trans-heterozygous mutations. *Nature Genetics* **25**, 143–144.

Watnick, T. J. *et al.* (1998). Somatic mutation in individual liver cysts supports a two-hit model of cystogenesis in autosomal dominant polycystic kidney disease. *Molecular Cell* **2**, 247–251.

Wu, G. (2001). Current advances in molecular genetics of autosomal-dominant polycystic kidney disease. *Current Opinion in Nephrology and Hypertension* **10**, 23–31.

Wu, G. *et al.* (1998). Somatic inactivation of Pkd2 results in polycystic kidney disease. *Cell* **93**, 177–188.

Wu, G. *et al.* (2000). Cardiac defects and renal failure in mice with targeted mutations in Pkd2. *Nature Genetics* **24**, 75–78.

Xu, G. M. *et al.* (2001). Polycystin-1 interacts with intermediate filaments. *Journal of Biological Chemistry* **276**, 46544–46552.

Yium, J. *et al.* (1994). Autosomal dominant polycystic kidney disease in Blacks: clinical course and effects of sickle-cell hemoglobin. *Journal of the American Society of Nephrology* **4**, 1670–1674.

Yoder, B. K., Hou, X., and Guay-Woodford, L. M. (2002). The polycystic kidney disease proteins, polycystin-1, polycystin-2, polaris, and cystin, are co-localized in renal cilia. *Journal of the American Society of Nephrology* **13**, 2508–2516.

Zeier, M. *et al.* (1993). Elevated blood pressure profile and left ventricular mass in children and young adults with autosomal dominant polycystic kidney disease. *Journal of the American Society of Nephrology* **3**, 1451–1457.

Zerres, K., Rudnik-Schoneborn, S., and Deget, F. (1993). Childhood onset autosomal dominant polycystic kidney disease in sibs: clinical picture and recurrence risk. German Working Group on Paediatric Nephrology (Arbeitsgemeinschaft fur Padiatrische Nephrologie). *Journal of Medical Genetics* **30**, 583–588.

16.3 Nephronophthisis

Rémi Salomon, Marie-Claire Gubler, and Corinne Antignac

Nephronophthisis and medullary cystic kidney disease (MCKD) constitute a group of chronic tubulointerstitial nephropathies with cyst formation at the corticomedullary junction of the kidney. This group includes renal diseases with various clinical features, different modes of inheritance, and associations with extrarenal disorders. The recent progress made in molecular genetics have helped in the classification of these disorders and have improved the understanding of their pathophysiology.

In 1951, Fanconi first coined the term nephronophthisis to describe a familial renal disease with progression to renal failure before puberty, with prominent polyuria in the absence of haematuria, heavy proteinuria, and hypertension. At autopsy, the kidneys were shrunken and showed diffuse prominent tubulointerstitial lesions. Medullary cysts were not mentioned but were present on one of the micrographs (Fanconi *et al.* 1951). In parallel, other authors have proposed the term MCKD for the same disease. It is now generally admitted that MCKD designates the disease occurring in adults with an autosomal dominant inheritance, while nephronophthisis points out the autosomal recessive form. A further classification has been delineated for the recessive forms, which takes into consideration the age of onset for end-stage renal disease (ESRD) (Hildebrandt and Otto 2000). Three variants have been defined, the juvenile (NPH1), the infantile (NPH2), and the adolescent (NPH3) forms with median ages for onset of ESRD at 13, 1–3, and 19 years, respectively.

Genetically, extensive genetic heterogeneity has also been shown, with at least four different loci detected for nephronophthisis (*NPHP1*, *NPHP2*, *NPHP3*, and *NPHP4*) and two for MCKD (*MCKD1* and *MCKD2*). To date, only two genes, *NPHP1* encoding nephrocystin and *NPHP4* encoding nephrocystin-4/nephroretinin, have been identified for nephronophthisis, and one, *MCKD2* encoding the Tamm–Horsfall protein, for MCKD (Table 1).

Autosomal recessive nephronophthisis

Juvenile and adolescent forms

The condition is rare with an incidence estimated around 1 : 50,000 live births. It is, however, generally considered to be the first cause of terminal renal failure during childhood and adolescence representing 6–10 per cent of children treated for ESRD (Brunner *et al.* 1988). The disease has been mainly described in Europe and in North America, but cases have been reported from all areas around the word.

Clinical symptoms

The commonest presenting complaints are polydipsia and polyuria frequently associated with enuresis. These symptoms occur usually

Table 1 Disease variants, gene loci, gene products, and extrarenal disorders in nephronophthisis and medullary cystic kidney disease

	Inheritance	Locus	Gene	Gene product	Extrarenal associations
Juvenile (NPH1)	AR	2q12–q13	NPHP1	Nephrocystin	RP, OMA
		1p36	NPHP4	Nephrocystin-4/ nephroretinin	OMA
		?	?	?	Skeletal dysplasia, hepatic fibrosis, Joubert sd, Sensenbrenner sd
Infantile (NPH2)	AR	9q22–q31	NPHP2	?	
Adolescent (NPH3)	AR	3q21–q22	NPHP3	?	
SLS	AR	3q21–q22	?	?	Leber amaurosis
		1p36	NPHP4	Nephrocystin-4/ nephroretinin	Leber amaurosis
		?	?	?	
MCKD1	AD	1q21	MCKD1	?	
MCKD2	AD	16p13	MCKD2	TH	

AR, autosomal recessive; AD, autosomal dominant; RP, retinitis pigmentosa; OMA, ocular motor apraxia; sd, syndrome; TH, Tamm–Horsfall protein.

around 4–6 years of age, and are related to a reduced urinary concentrating ability that is the only renal dysfunction during the first years. Polyuria is more or less severe, but is often paid little attention. When hyposthenuria is important, growth retardation may precede the fall in glomerular filtration rate. The other main clinical symptom is a progressive renal failure which is constant, insidious, and which often remains undetected until an advanced stage, probably because of normal urinanalysis: haematuria is never found; proteinuria is usually absent, except for a mild protein loss never exceeding 1 g/day in the presence of advanced renal failure. Probably because of sodium wasting, blood pressure remains normal until the onset of ESRD, when it may be elevated. Glomerular filtration rate is usually reduced at presentation except for a few patients with dramatic polyuria and for children who are systematically examined after detection of an affected sibling. The other clinical and biological findings, that is, anaemia, acidosis, and osteodystrophy, are directly related to renal failure. There is no evidence of abnormal proximal tubular dysfunction: glucosuria, hypophosphataemia, and excessive aminoaciduria are absent. ESRD usually occurs around 12–13 years of age in juvenile nephronophthisis (median age of 12 years—range 4–20 years—in a cohort of 33 patients from Germany; Hildebrandt *et al.* 1992).

Radiological findings

Ultrasonography can be helpful in the diagnosis, showing medullary cysts and loss of corticomedullary differentiation in kidneys of normal or slightly reduced size (Garel *et al.* 1984). In a child with renal failure, these signs are highly suggestive of nephronophthisis, but they are usually observed in patients with ESRD. They may be lacking even in advanced stages, and are rarely found in earlier stages, when ultrasonographic investigations may be normal, or show only a loss of corticomedullary differentiation (Blowey *et al.* 1996). The most important contribution of radiology is that it allows the exclusion of some other causes of renal failure with hyposthenuria, such as renal hypoplasia and urinary tract malformations.

Pathology

Macroscopically, the prominent feature is a diffuse but slight contraction of both kidneys, which have a finely granular surface. Cut sections typically show grossly visible cysts of variable size irregularly distributed at the corticomedullary junction and in the outer medulla (Fig. 1).

In advanced stages of renal failure, when most of the renal samples are obtained, light microscopy shows diffuse lesions of the renal parenchyma, with shrinking of both the cortex and the medulla. At low magnification, the most striking feature is the severe involvement of the tubules with a radial distribution of changes. Groups of atrophic tubules with thickened basement membrane stain strongly with periodic acid–Schiff and alternate with groups of viable tubules showing dilatation or marked compensatory hypertrophy and with groups of collapsed tubules. Although identification of individual segments of the nephron is often impossible because of the dedifferentiation of the epithelial lining of the tubules, it seems that all segments of the nephron are affected (Fig. 2). Higher magnification shows that the basement membrane thickening in atrophic tubules (and rarely, in normal tubules) is sometimes homogeneous, sometimes layered or laminated (Figs 3 and 4). The inner linear layer is separated from the outer wrinkled layer by a lucent area. Other tubules may show considerable attenuation or even disintegration of the basement membrane. As underlined by Cohen and Hoyer (1986), there may be an abrupt

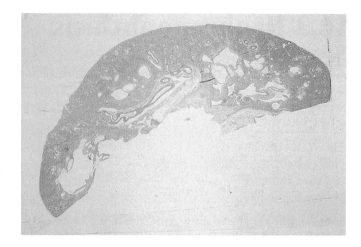

Fig. 1 Macroscopic appearance. Cortex and medulla are both shrunken. Note the presence of irregularly distributed cysts of variable size at the corticomedullary junction and in the outer medulla.

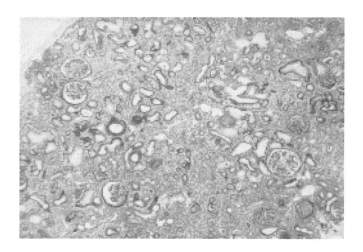

Fig. 2 Cortex. Massive interstitial fibrosis separating groups of atrophic tubules. Most glomeruli are surrounded by periglomerular fibrosis (light microscopy; magnification 60×).

transition from one abnormality to another. These various changes in the tubular basement membrane (TBM) are the hallmark of the disease and, according to Zollinger *et al.* (1980) and Cohen and Hoyer (1986), although non-specific, they occur in nephronophthisis more extensively than in any kidney disorders with abnormal tubules.

Between the atrophic tubules, and surrounding the groups of hypertrophied tubules, there is moderate to massive interstitial fibrosis, without significant cell infiltration. In some cases the interstitium may contain protein casts that stain positively for Tamm–Horsfall protein.

Glomeruli are often normal by light and electron microscopy (Zollinger *et al.* 1980; Waldherr *et al.* 1982; Cohen and Hoyer 1986), although some are completely sclerosed and others show periglomerular fibrosis.

The arteries and arterioles are usually normal, and no abnormality of the juxtaglomerular apparatus is recorded.

In the early stages of the disease, in the rare available renal biopsies, the first abnormality observed is the presence of groups of atrophic

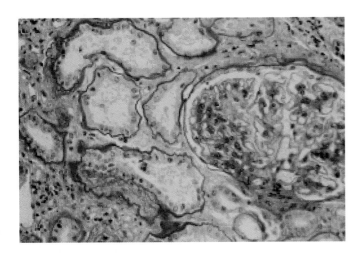

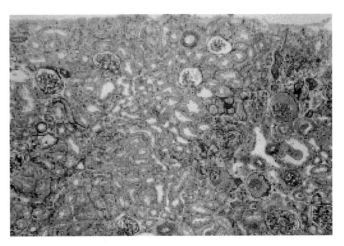

Fig. 3 Cortex. At a higher magnification, various tubular changes are present. Some tubules are collapsed, others are surrounded by thickened TBMs. Note the laminated and wrinkled appearance of some TBM segments as well as the abrupt attenuation of others in the same tubule (light microscopy; magnification 360×).

Fig. 5 Early stage of the disease. Segmental zone of interstitial fibrosis containing atrophic tubules with thickened basement membranes (light microscopy; magnification ×130).

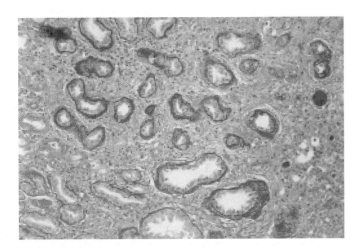

Fig. 4 Cortex. All the TBMs are irregularly thickened and the tubules are separated by a marked interstitial fibrosis (light microscopy; magnification 280×).

tubules with irregularly thickened TBM, which suggests that the disease is primarily tubular (Fig. 5).

By immunofluorescence, various patterns of staining were observed with antibodies to laminin and type IV collagen. Normal and increased staining of the thick TBM (Cohen and Hoyer 1986), alternate with decreased labelling of the central portion of the thick TBM, gave a railroad appearance (Gubler *et al.* 1987). However, both investigators using certain human anti-TBM antibodies observed absence of normal and thick TBM labelling. These findings have suggested that the fundamental defect in nephronophthisis might be the production of an abnormal TBM, similar to the glomerular basement membrane lesions of Alport's syndrome. Furthermore, Rahilly and Fleming (1995), studying abnormalities of cell–matrix interactions using immunohistochemistry, found enhanced expression of $\alpha 2$ integrin, which appears to be a common response to tubular injury, and expression of the

$\alpha 5$ integrin fibronectin receptor in nephronophthisis, but not in other renal diseases. These findings, although not confirmed by others to date, suggested to the authors that cell–substratum adhesion contributes to the pathogenesis of nephronophthisis.

Associated disorders

Tapetoretinal degeneration

The most frequently associated anomalies involve the eyes, and these are often the only associated conditions described. Contreras and Espinoza (1960), Løken *et al.* (1961), and Senior *et al.* (1961) were the first to report patients with coarse nystagmus and blindness in early infancy that developed to uraemia in childhood. Senior *et al.* (1961) identified nephropathy as being a nephronophthisis and showed that the early blindness, resulting from tapetoretinal degeneration, presented clinically as Leber's amaurosis with a flat electroretinogram in all the four siblings investigated. When visual impairment is severe and precocious, this association is called Senior–Løken syndrome (SLS), but some patients present with amblyopia or even with normal visual acuity, the ocular disease only then being characterized by dystrophy of the pigmented epithelium shown by fluoroangiography and by low-voltage waves on electroretinogram (Caridi *et al.* 1998). However, there is no clear-cut definition for SLS, and this term is sometimes used for patients with mild and delayed visual impairment. Tapetoretinal degeneration has been estimated to account for 15–20 per cent of the patients with nephronophthisis. A thorough search for ocular anomalies in all patients with known nephronophthisis is warranted including fundus examination and electroretinogram. Since retinopathy can be progressive, ophthalmological examination should be performed on a regular basis. On the other hand, since the first renal symptoms can occur many years after the retinal disease has been discovered (Georges *et al.* 2000), patients with known tapetoretinal degeneration should be evaluated for symptoms of nephronophthisis.

Other rare diseases combine chronic tubulointerstitial nephritis and tapetoretinal degeneration such as mitochondrial cytopathy, Bardet–Biedl syndrome, Zellweger syndrome, and Jeune's thoracic asphyxiating dystrophy, so that the presence of the eye defect cannot be considered as evidence for the diagnosis of nephronophthisis. Specific anomalies or malformations associated with these disorders usually distinguish them from SLS. Several authors have reported patients with SLS associated with congenital hepatic fibrosis (see below). It is to be noted here that some patients with SLS have mental retardation and when a magnetic resonance imaging is performed, it is not rare to notice cerebellar vermis hypoplasia and the 'molar tooth sign' which is characteristic of the Joubert syndrome (see below).

Oculomotor apraxia (Cogan syndrome)

Recently, cases of nephronophthisis have been reported associated with congenital oculomotor apraxia also called Cogan syndrome, which is characterized by defective or absent horizontal voluntary saccade eye movements whereas vertical eye movements are intact. The term congenital saccade initiation failure has been proposed to design this anomaly (Harris *et al.* 1998). During the first months, jerking head movements compensate for the oculomotor deficiency. The disease is not progressive, and older patients may be able to compensate by an over-shooting thrust of the eyeballs rather than by head jerks. Little is known about the mechanism of this disease, lesions located in the oculogyric center have been reported as well as supratentorial abnormalities, but the most common imaging finding is a hypoplasia of the cerebellar vermis (Sargent *et al.* 1997). Similar symptoms can sometimes occur in children with Gaucher disease, ataxia–telangectasia syndrome, and brain tumours. Signs of cerebellar dysfunction such as ataxia and hypotonia and mild mental retardation are present in most patients.

Joubert syndrome and related disorders

Nepronophthisis has also been reported in a complex syndrome named Joubert syndrome which shares some features with Cogan syndrome although far more severe. Joubert syndrome is characterized by cerebellar vermis hypoplasia, ataxia, hypotonia, developmental delay, abnormal respiratory patterns (hyperapnoea intermixed with apnoea in infancy), and abnormal eye movements (Joubert *et al.* 1969). The oculomotor apraxia in Joubert syndrome differs from congenital idiopathic oculomotor apraxia (Cogan syndrome), in that it does not resolve with time and it is not restricted to the initiation of horizontal saccades. Moreover, visual impairment is frequently associated. Most children have a characteristic facial appearance with a large head, prominent forehead, high rounded eyebrows, epicanthal folds, upturned nose, tongue protrusion. Neuroimaging in the axial plane shows the 'molar tooth sign', that is, deep posterior interpeduncular fossa, thick and elongated superior cerebellar peduncles, and hypoplastic or aplastic superior cerebellar vermis (Quisling *et al.* 1999). A classification of patients has been proposed, dividing them into those with retinal dystrophy and those without (Joubert syndrome type B and A, respectively). In the few patients presenting the association of nephronophthisis and Joubert syndrome, retinal dystrophy is always present (Saraiva and Baraister 1992).

Skeletal involvement

Bone anomalies associated with nephronophthisis, particularly phalangeal cone-shaped epiphyses, were first reported by Mainzer *et al.* (1970) and this association is often called Saldino–Mainzer syndrome or conorenal syndrome. Cone-shaped epiphyses have been reported several times, but in most cases with additional skeletal anomalies and sometimes with tapetoretinal degeneration and liver fibrosis. All these features are classically described in Jeune's asphyxiating thoracic dystrophy and in chondroectodermal dysplasia (Ellis-van Creveld syndrome),

suggesting that these syndromes are part of a disease spectrum with a common aetiology (Donaldson *et al.* 1985; Moudgil *et al.* 1998; Ozcay *et al.* 2001). It should be emphasized that other renal diseases have also been described in association with cone-shaped epiphyses (Mendley *et al.* 1995).

Cranioectodermal dysplasia (Sensenbrenner syndrome) is a very rare disorder defined by the association of dolichocephaly due to craniosynostosis, sparse slow growing hair, epicanthal folds, hypodontia or microdontia, brachydactyly, a narrow thorax, and retinitis pigmentosa. Among the 12 reported cases, six have chronic renal failure secondary to a tubulointerstitial nephropathy that resembles nephronophthisis (Savill *et al.* 1997; Tsimaratos *et al.* 1997). Recently, two patients have been described with nephronophthisis associated with retinitis pigmentosa, upper eyelid ptosis, partial hypopituitarism, and mild skeletal dysplasia such as epiphyseal hypoplasia, hypoplastic iliac bones, and thin tubular bones. The acronym RHYNS has been proposed for this association (Bianchi *et al.* 1989; Di Rocco *et al.* 1997).

Liver involvement

Liver involvement was first reported by Boichis *et al.* (1973) who observed hepatosplenomegaly, with liver portal fibrosis but without bile-duct proliferation, in three uraemic siblings with renal lesions consistent with nephronophthisis. Several investigators have since reported nephronophthisis with 'congenital hepatic fibrosis'. In all the reported cases, bile-duct proliferation was mild, and hence different from classical congenital hepatic fibrosis as found in autosomal recessive polycystic kidney disease. In most instances, the eye, brain, or bone were also involved. Moderate portal fibrosis and cholestasis have been also reported in infants, but the histological pattern of tubulointerstitial nephritis seems different from juvenile nephronophthisis and these cases possibly represent the infantile form (see below) (Harris *et al.* 1986; Gagnadoux *et al.* 1989; Popovic-Rolovic *et al.* 1993).

The infantile nephronophthisis

Gagnadoux *et al.* (1989) described a group of infants who reached ESRD before the age of 2 years with tubulointertitial nephritis that shares some features with nephronophthisis although with significant differences. Indeed, renal ultrasonography showed moderately enlarged kidneys, while no cysts were detected, and renal pathology differs from typical nephronophthisis by the presence of cystic dilatations of the cortical tubules and Bowman's spaces and by the absence of prominent thickening of the TBM on the kidney biopsy. In the endstage kidneys, tubules were uniformly collapsed and there were neither cortical nor medullary cysts. One of them had cholestasis and portal fibrosis. Liver biopsy performed in two others was normal.

Later on, an extended Bedouin family with 10 affected subjects was reported, with onset of the disease before 30 months of age in all, and even antenatally with fetal oliguria and oligohydramnios resulting in postnatal respiratory failure and death in one patient (Haider *et al.* 1998). None of the patients had extrarenal symptoms, and renal histology was very reminiscent to the features reported by Gagnadoux. Fourteen other infants have been described as either infantile tubulointerstitial nephropathy (Proesmans *et al.* 1976; Harris *et al.* 1986) or early nephronophthisis (Witzleben *et al.* 1982; Bodaghi *et al.* 1987). Many had extrarenal disorders: two were blind, four had cholestasis and moderate portal fibrosis with or without duct proliferation, and two siblings had 'hepatic fibrosis' in the absence of biliary dysgenesis characteristic of 'congenital hepatic fibrosis' (Parchoux *et al.* 1982; Gruppuso *et al.* 1983).

Molecular biology

Identification of the *NPHP1* gene

As little was known about the pathogenesis of nephronophthisis, a positional cloning approach (Collins *et al.* 1992) was used to identify the gene(s) involved in this nephropathy. A linkage was found between nephronophthisis and microsatellite markers located on chromosome 2, in 18 kindred with nephronophthisis without extrarenal symptoms (Antignac *et al.* 1993), localizing a gene for nephronophthisis, *NPHP1*, on chromosome 2. Mapping of *NPHP1* to chromosome 2q13 was subsequently showed by Hildebrandt *et al.* (1993) in 10 German families with nephronophthisis without associated disorders.

When testing novel families and using additional markers, Medhioub *et al.* (1994) showed genetic heterogeneity between nephronophthisis and SLS. Their results also produced evidence for additional genetic heterogeneity in the purely renal form of nephronophthisis although there were no clinical or pathological features that could separate the families linked to chromosome 2 and the unlinked families.

It then appeared that, within the *NPHP1* region, several markers mapped to different loci and that parts of the region were duplicated on chromosome 2p12, suggesting that large-scale chromosomal rearrangements could occur involving the *NPHP1* gene. Indeed, large homozygous deletions of ~250 kb were detected in 80 per cent of the patients belonging to inbred or multiplex families and in 65 per cent of the sporadic cases (Konrad *et al.* 1996). The sizes and localization of the deletions seemed to be very similar in most patients. As such homozygous deletions have never been found in any parent or unaffected sibling and in any control individual, these data strongly suggested that the *NPHP1* gene lies, at least in part, in the deleted region. The deletion was subsequently shown to measure precisely 290 kb and to be due to a mechanism of unequal recombination between two 45 kb direct repeats flanking the *NPHP1* gene (Saunier *et al.* 2000).

Using the information provided by the characterization of the deletions, two groups independently cloned the *NPHP1* gene (Hildebrandt *et al.* 1997; Saunier *et al.* 1997a), by the identification of point mutations in patients without the large common deletion or with the deletion in the heterozygous state. *NPHP1* contains 20 exons spanning more than 80 kb, is entirely located in the non-duplicated region within the large common deletion, and has a widespread but relatively weak expression (Otto *et al.* 2000). It encodes a novel intracellular protein of 732 amino acids named nephrocystin. Its structural analysis predicts several protein interaction domains, three coil-coiled domains in the *N*-terminus, composed of alpha helices known to be involved in protein–protein interactions, and a SH3 domain (Src homology 3 domain). This domain, found in a great variety of membrane associated or cytosolic proteins, mediates assembly of specific protein complexes involved in signal transduction via binding to proline-rich regions of other proteins. The presence of such domains in nephrocystin suggests a role for nephrocystin in signalling pathways essential for maintenance of basement membrane integrity.

Since the original report, deletions in the *NPHP1* gene, easily detectable by the lack of amplification by PCR of genomic DNA markers, have been reported in a few series in the literature, with similar results in patients with nephronophthisis without extrarenal symptoms. Hildebrandt *et al.* (2001) studied 204 patients with nephronophthisis without extrarenal symptoms, belonging to 127 families, 61 of them being multiplex families. Altogether, they found 115 homozygous deletions in 74 families, and five heterozygous deletions associated with a point mutation on the other allele. Considering only the families in which linkage to the *NPHP1* locus was not excluded and the sporadic cases, the rate of homozygous deletions was 71 per cent (32/45) and 64 per cent (42/66), respectively. Ala-Mello *et al.* (1999) found homozygous deletions in four out of six familes and seven out of 11 sporadic cases in a Finnish population of patients with juvenile nephronophthisis without extrarenal symptoms. In a population of 68 Italian children with clinical and histopathological features of juvenile nephronophthisis, belonging to 57 families, a large homozygous deletion was found in 30 cases (44 per cent) and a heterozygous deletion associated with a point mutation in the other allele in two cases (Caridi *et al.* 2000). The rate of homozygous deletions rises to 57 per cent (17/30) if only the sporadic cases are taken into account. This lower rate of deletions can be explained by the inclusion of patients with extrarenal disorders (cf. infra) and probably of families not linked to the *NPHP1* locus.

These studies also raise the question of the involvement of the *NPHP1* gene in nephronophthisis associated with extrarenal disorders. Indeed, Caridi *et al.* (2000) detected *NPHP1* deletions in seven out of 12 patients with retinal dystrophy. Of note, all the children bearing *NPHP1* deletions had mild ocular impairment. However, no *NPHP1* deletion has been found in the patients with severe retinal involvement.

NPHP1 deletions have also been found in individuals with Cogan syndrome (with or without vermis hypoplasia) associated with nephronophthisis, arguing for a role of the *NPHP1* gene in the aetiology of oculomotor apraxia (Saunier *et al.* 1997b; Betz *et al.* 2000; Graber *et al.* 2001). On the contrary, *NPHP1* deletions were not found in 11 families with Joubert type B (Hildebrandt *et al.* 1998), five cases with liver fibrosis and nephronophthisis (Caridi *et al.* 2000), and in one case with Sensenbrenner syndrome (Tsimaratos *et al.* 1997). Altogether, although the number of patients and families tested is quite low and the extent of the deletion not precisely characterized to verify that the cases with and without extrarenal symptoms bear the same deletion, it seems, from the linkage analysis and deletion studies, that the *NPHP1* gene can be involved in some extrarenal features associated with nephronophthisis, but generally the milder ones.

Only 12 *NPHP1* single base mutations have been reported in patients with isolated nephronophthisis, most of them being loss-of-function mutations and being associated to a heterozygous deletion on the other allele (Hildebrandt *et al.* 1997, 2001; Saunier *et al.* 1997a, 2000; Caridi *et al.* 2000). Actually, given the high rate of homozygous deletions in *NPHP1* and the genetic heterogeneity in nephronophthisis, the mutation screening is not very productive and should not be undertaken if a heterozygous deletion is not suspected either by pulsed-field gel electrophoresis or by genotyping of polymorphisms present in the deletion (Hildebrandt *et al.* 2001).

Mapping of the *NPHP2* and *NPHP3* genes

In parallel to the identification of the *NPHP1* gene, several attempts have been performed to identify new gene loci in nephronophthisis, using the strategy of homozygosity mapping, which relies on the fact that in consanguineous families, the affected individuals are assumed to have inherited a common haplotype from the same ancestor, which allows to test a very few number of inbred families. Along this line, the *NPHP2* gene involved in infantile nephronophthisis was mapped to a 12.9-cM region of chromosome 9q22–31, in a large highly inbred Bedouin family from Israel, with at least 11 affected children showing most of the clinical and histopathological features reported by Gagnadoux *et al.* (1989), four of which being studied by linkage analysis (Haider *et al.* 1998). Conversely, a new gene, *NPHP3*, was mapped to a genetic interval of 2.4 cM on chromosome 3q22 in a large 340-member inbred Venezualian kindred with adolescent nephronophthisis (Omran *et al.* 2000). In this family, in which the affected members present symptoms typical of nephronophthisis without any extrarenal disorders, ESRD occurred significantly later (median age 19 years) than in juvenile nephronophthisis, although there is clearly an overlap between the age of ESRD in *NPHP1* and *NPHP3* patients. More recently, a locus for SLS was mapped to a 14-cM region on chromosome 3, overlapping the *NPHP3* region, in a kindred of German ancestry with extended consanguinity and typical findings of SLS with congenital Leber amaurosis and nephronophthisis (Omran *et al.* 2002). These findings raised the question of the possibilities of both diseases arising by mutations within the same pleiotropic gene or two adjacent genes. Nevertheless, in the same study, Omran *et al.* (2002) also found evidence for genetic heterogeneity in SLS, emphasizing the genetic complexity of SLS.

Identification of the *NPHP4* gene

More recently, a second locus associated with the juvenile form of the disease, *NPHP4*, was mapped to chromosome 1p36 (Schuermann *et al.* 2002) and the underlying gene was subsequently identified by two independent groups by the detection of single base mutations of one gene lying in the critical genetic interval in patients belonging to families not linked to any of the previous known nephronophthisis loci. This new gene contains 29 coding exons and displays, as *NPHP1*, a rather weak expression in a large number of organs including kidney and brain. This gene encodes a new 1426-aminoacid protein, named nephrocystin-4 (Mollet *et al.* 2002) or nephroretinin (Otto *et al.* 2002), of unknown function containing any conserved motif or domain, except for a proline-rich region at position 456–512. Nephrocystin-4 was shown to interact with endogenous nephrocystin in renal cell lines (Mollet *et al.* 2002), which suggest that these two proteins participate in a common signalling pathway. Twelve *NPHP4* mutations have been described to date, either in the homozygous or in the heterozygous state. Most of them represent very likely loss-of-function mutations (six stop-codon mutations, one frameshift mutation, and three obligatory splice-consensus mutations) and eight out of 12 are localized in exons 15–18. Altogether, *NPHP4* mutations have been found in families with juvenile nephronophthisis alone and in families with extrarenal symptoms, in a family with nephronophthisis and Cogan syndrome (Mollet *et al.* 2002), and in two families with SLS (Otto *et al.* 2002) previously described in the literature (Fillastre *et al.* 1976; Polak *et al.* 1977). However, further analyses are needed to know the phenotypic spectrum associated with *NPHP4* mutations.

In summary, *NPHP1* and *NPHP4* mutations are mainly detected in patients with isolated nephronophthisis, except for few patients in whom nephronophthisis is associated with Cogan syndrome (*NPHP1* and *NPHP4* mutations), with late onset retinitis pigmentosa (*NPHP1* deletions), or with congenital Leber amaurosis (*NPHP4* mutations) (Table 1). Although tremendous advances have been made in the

genetics of nephronophthisis, however, there still remain families with nephronophthisis without or with extrarenal symptoms, mainly with liver fibrosis and bone disease, in which linkage to all the known nephronophthisis loci is excluded, indicating that a number of causative genes still need to be identified. The characterization of these genes will be helpful in the classification of the different syndromes. Moreover, it will enhance the comprehension of the disease in the kidney and in the other affected organs.

Pathophysiology

The identification of nephrocystins sheds new lights on the pathophysiology of nephronophthisis. Both nephrocystin and nephrocystin-4/nephroretinin are novel proteins that share no homologies with known mammalian proteins. Nevertheless, the presence of protein-interacting domains in nephrocystin suggested that nephrocystin could be an adapter protein involved in focal adhesion signalling complexes of cell–matrix contacts, which should be in agreement with the early histological findings (i.e. focal alterations of the TBM) observed in nephronophthisis. Actually, nephrocystin has been shown to interact with proteins localized to focal adhesions, such as the adapter protein p130^{cas}, and tensin, and with the proline-rich tyrosine kinase 2 (Pyk2), known to interact with p130^{cas} (Donaldson *et al.* 2000; Benzing *et al.* 2001). Furthermore, it has also been shown that nephrocystin triggers phosphorylation of Pyk2 and subsequent activation of mitogen-activated protein kinases, suggesting that nephrocystin might help to recruit Pyk2 to cell–matrix adhesions, thereby initiating phosphorylation of Pyk2 and Pyk2-dependent signalling (Benzing *et al.* 2001). In addition, it has been shown that nephrocystin colocalizes with P130^{cas} and E-cadherin in MDCK cells and that nephrocystin also interacts with filamins, actin-binding proteins that have been shown to anchor various transmembrane proteins to the actin cytoskeleton at cell–cell contact sites (Donaldson *et al.* 2000, 2002). Thus, nephrocystin could also function as a docking protein belonging to a protein complex involved in regulation of the actin cytoskeleton at adherens junctions and in establishing or maintaining cell polarity. As it has been shown that nephrocystin-4 interacts with nephrocystin (Mollet *et al.* 2002), these results altogether suggest a main role for nephrocystins in cell–cell and cell–matrix adhesions. Cell proliferation and extracellular matrix turnover processes are tightly regulated by the cell adhesion phenomena. Disruption of these processes has been shown to be involved in the fibrosis process and in cyst formation, which could explain the abnormalities observed in nephronophthisis.

Animal models

Several animal models have been reported which share some clinical and histological features with nephronophthisis. The *pcy* mice exhibit cysts in all the segments of the nephron and chronic renal interstitial inflammatory infiltrates at later stages. Interestingly, a synteny between the *pcy* locus and the human *NPHP3* locus has been demonstrated suggesting that the human and mouse diseases are caused by homologous genes (Omran *et al.* 2001). In the tensin knockout mouse, there is a marked TBM disruption with cysts mainly in the proximal tubule and interstitial cell infiltration (Lo *et al.* 1997). Tensin plays a crucial role in the attachment of the tubular epithelium to the extracellular matrix via the focal adhesions. The phenotype of the knockout mice and the interaction between tensin and nephrocystin (cf. above) suggest a direct intervention of these structures in the pathogenesis of nephronophthisis.

Other animal mutants have been reported with renal failure and histological lesions reminiscent of nephronophthisis, but this must be considered with caution. As an example, the renal disease observed in the Japanese black cattle, which appears in many respects similar to that seen in juvenile nephronophthisis is in fact related to a deletion of the paracellin gene (Ohba *et al.* 2000). Along the same line, the kd/kd mice display a hereditary tubulointerstitial disease with mononuclear cell infiltration and cysts formation which have long been considered as the murine homologue of juvenile nephronophthisis (Lyon and Hulse 1971). However, later studies have clearly demonstrated that the disease is an autoimmune disorder (Neilson *et al.* 1984).

Autosomal dominant medullary cystic disease (see also Chapter 16.2.2)

Besides autosomal recessive forms, cases of nephronophthisis, MCKD, or familial interstitial nephritis with a clear autosomal dominant inheritance, often with an incomplete penetrance, have also been described. As previously mentioned, it is now usual to denominate them 'medullary cystic kidney disease'. As in juvenile nephronophthisis, the diagnosis criteria are decreased urinary concentration ability with polyuria, hyposthenuria without haematuria or proteinuria, normal or small-sized kidneys with occasional small medullary cysts, and histological findings characterized by massive tubulointerstitial fibrosis, tubular atrophy, and thickening of the TBM (Scolari *et al.* 1998). However, MCKD is characterized by an onset and an evolution towards ESRD later than in juvenile nephronophthisis, usually in the third to fifth decade of life, with large variations even in the same family, and by the absence of the extrarenal symptoms that can be associated with juvenile nephronophthisis. In addition, hyperuricaemia and gout have been observed in several members from at least four out of 12 kindreds reported in the literature (Thompson *et al.* 1978; Burke *et al.* 1982; Scolari *et al.* 1998; Stavrou *et al.* 1998). In a recent review of six large Cypriot families, Stavrou *et al.* (2002) found hyperuricaemia in 36 out of 72 affected individuals and gout in five of them. Renal cysts were found on renal ultrasonography in 40 per cent of patients and mean age at ESRD was 53.7 years.

Two gene loci have been identified to date. The first locus, *MCKD1*, was mapped on 1q21 initially in two Cypriot families (Christodolou *et al.* 1998) and subsequently in one British family (Fuchshuber *et al.* 1998) and in five Finnish families (Auranen *et al.* 2001), whereas *MCKD2* was mapped to 16p12–p13 in a large Italian family (Scolari *et al.* 1999). Nevertheless, further genetic heterogeneity has been shown, since no linkage to *MCKD1* or *MCKD2* was found in five families of several geographic origin, with, so far, no evidence of hyperuricaemia and gout, indicating the existence of other gene locus (or loci) for MCKD, in particular in families without hyperuricaemia (Kroiss *et al.* 2000; Fuchshuber *et al.* 1998). Intriguingly, a gene locus for familial juvenile hyperuricaemic nephropathy (FJHN) (see Chapter 16.5.3), which shares several clinical, biological, and histological findings with MCKD, although medullary cysts are rarely reported in FJHN, has been localized to a chromosomal region overlapping with the *MCKD2* locus on chromosome 16, raising the question that the two disorders might be allelic (Kamatani *et al.* 2000; Stiburkova *et al.* 2000; Dahan *et al.* 2001). Indeed, this has been recently proved, since mutations in the *UMOD* gene localized to the critical genetic interval have been found both in three families with FJHN and in one family with MCKD with hyperuricaemia (Hart *et al.* 2002). *UMOD* encodes the Tamm–Horsfall protein, also referred as uromodulin, which is a glycosylphosphatidylinositol anchored glycoprotein, localized to the thick ascending limb of the loop of Henle. All the *UMOD* mutations found to date have been found in exon 4 and most of them involve highly conserved cysteine residues, which are amino acids critical for inter- or intramolecular disulfide bond formation. Nevertheless, the function of the Tamm–Horsfall protein remains unclear until now and additional functional studies should be undertaken to understand why specific alterations of this protein leads to hyperuricaemia and tubulointerstitial chronic renal disease.

The genes responsible for the infantile and adolescent forms have been recently identified and encode for inversin and nephrocystin-3 respectively (Otto *et al.* 2003; Olbrich *et al.* 2003).

References

Ala-Mello, S. *et al.* (1999). Nephronophthisis in Finland: epidemiology and comparison of genetically classified subgroups. *European Journal of Human Genetics* 7, 205–211.

Antignac, C. *et al.* (1993). A gene for familial juvenile nephronophthisis (recessive medullary cystic kidney disease) maps to chromosome 2p. *Nature Genetics* 3, 342–345.

Auranen, M. *et al.* (2001). Further evidence for linkage of autosomal-dominant medullary cystic disease on chromosome 1q21. *Kidney International* 60, 1225–1232.

Benzing, T. *et al.* (2001). Nephrocystin interacts with Pyk2, p130(Cas), and tensin and triggers phosphorylation of Pyk2. *Proceedings of the National Academy of Sciences USA* 98, 9784–9789.

Betz, R. *et al.* (2000). Children with ocular motor apraxia type Cogan carry deletions in the gene (NPHP1) for juvenile nephronophthisis. *Journal of Pediatrics* 136, 828–831.

Bianchi, C. G. *et al.* (1989). Juvenile nephronophthisis associated with new skeletal abnormalities, tapetoretinal degeneration and liver fibrosis. *Helvetica Paediatrica Acta* 43, 449–455.

Blowey, D. L. *et al.* (1996). Ultrasound findings in juvenile nephronophthisis. *Pediatric Nephrology* 10, 22–24.

Bodaghi, E., Honarmand, M. T., and Ahmadi, M. (1987). Infantile nephronophthisis. *International Journal of Pediatric Nephrology* 8, 207–210.

Boichis, H. *et al.* (1973). Congenital hepatic fibrosis and nephronophthisis. *Quarterly Journal of Medicine* 42, 221–233.

Brunner, F. P. *et al.* (1988). Demography of dialysis and transplantation in children in Europe, 1985. Report from the European Dialysis and Transplant Association Registry. *Nephrology, Dialysis, Transplantation* 3, 235–243.

Burke, J. R. *et al.* (1982). Juvenile nephronophthisis and medullary cystic disease: the same disease (report of a large family with medullary cystic disease associated with gout and epilepsy). *Clinical Nephrology* 18, 1–8.

Caridi, G. *et al.* (1998). Renal–retinal syndromes: association of retinal anomalies and recessive nephronophthisis in patients with homozygous deletion of the NPH1 locus. *American Journal of Kidney Diseases* 32, 1059–1062.

Caridi, G. *et al.* (2000). Clinical and molecular heterogeneity of juvenile nephronophthisis in Italy: insights from molecular screening. *American Journal of Kidney Diseases* 35, 44–51.

Christodoulou, K. *et al.* (1998). Chromosome 1 localization of a gene for autosomal dominant medullary cystic kidney disease. *Human Molecular Genetics* 7, 905–911.

Cohen, A. H. and Hoyer, J. R. (1986). Nephronophthisis-A primary tubular basement membrane defect. *Laboratory Investigation* **55**, 564–572.

Collins, F. (1992). Positional cloning: let's not call it reverse anymore. *Nature Genetics* **1**, 3–6.

Contreras, C. B. and Espinoza, J. S. (1960). Discusion clinica y anatomopatologica de enfermos que presentaron un problema diagnostico. *Pediatria* **3**, 271–282.

Dahan, K. *et al.* (2001). Familial juvenile hyperuricemic nephropathy and autosomal dominant medullary cystic kidney disease type 2: two facets of the same disease? *Journal of the American Society of Nephrology* **12**, 2348–2357.

Di Rocco, M. P. *et al.* (1997). Retinitis pigmentosa, hypopituitarism, nephronophthisis, and mild skeletal dysplasia (RHYNS): a new syndrome? *American Journal of Medical Genetics* **73**, 1–4.

Donaldson, J. C. *et al.* (2000). Crk-associated substrate p130(Cas) interacts with nephrocystin and both proteins localize to cell–cell contacts of polarized epithelial cells. *Experimental Cell Research* **256**, 168–178.

Donaldson, J. C. *et al.* (2002). Nephrocystin-conserved domains involved in targeting to epithelial cell–cell junctions, interaction with filamins, and establishing cell polarity. *Journal of Biological Chemistry* **277**, 29028–29035.

Donaldson, M. D. C. *et al.* (1985). Familial juvenile nephronophthisis: Jeune's syndrome and associated disorders. *Archives of Disease in Childhood* **60**, 426–434.

Fanconi, G. *et al.* (1951). Die familiare juvenile nephronophthise. *Helvetica Paediatrica Acta* **6**, 1–49.

Fillastre, J. P. *et al.* (1976). Senior–Løken syndrome (nephronophthisis and tapeto-retinal degeneration): a study of 8 cases from 5 families. *Clinical Nephrology* **5**, 14–19.

Fuchshuber, A. *et al.* (1998). Autosomal dominant medullary cystic kidney disease: evidence of gene locus heterogeneity. *Nephrology, Dialysis, Transplantation* **13**, 1955–1957.

Fuchshuber, A. *et al.* (2001). Refinement of the gene locus for autosomal dominant medullary cystic kidney disease type 1 (MCKD1) and construction of a physical and partial transcriptional map of the region. *Genomics* **72**, 278–284.

Gagnadoux, M. F. *et al.* (1989). Infantile chronic tubulo-interstitial nephritis with cortical cysts: variant of nephronophthisis or new disease entity? *Pediatric Nephrology* **3**, 50–55.

Garel, L. A. *et al.* (1984). Juvenile nephronophthisis: sonographic appearance in children with severe uremia. *Radiology* **151**, 93–95.

Georges, B. *et al.* (2000). Late-onset renal failure in Senior–Løken syndrome. *American Journal of Kidney Diseases* **36**, 1271–1275.

Graber, D. *et al.* (2001). Cerebellar vermis hypoplasia with extracerebral involvement (retina, kidney, liver): difficult to classify syndromes. *Archives de Pediatrie* **8**, 186–190.

Gruppuso, P. A. *et al.* (1983). Juvenile nephronophthisis with blindness in a three-month-old infant. Senior's syndrome associated with relative parathyroid insufficiency. *Clinical Pediatric (Philadelphia)* **22**, 114–118.

Gubler, M. C. *et al.* Ultrastructural and immunohistochemical study of renal basement membranes in familial juvenile nephronophthisis. In *Renal Basement Membranes in Health and Disease* (ed. R. G. Price and B. G. Hudson), pp. 389–398. London: Academic Press, 1987.

Haider, N. B. *et al.* (1998). A Bedouin kindred with infantile nephronophthisis demonstrates linkage to chromosome 9 by homozygosity mapping. *American Journal of Human Genetics* **63**, 1404–1410.

Harris, C. M. *et al.* (1998). Familial congenital saccade initiation failure and isolated cerebellar vermis hypoplasia. *Developmental Medicine and Neurology* **40**, 775–779.

Harris, H. W. *et al.* (1986). Progressive tubulointerstitial renal disease in infancy with associated hepatic abnormalities. *American Journal of Medicine* **81**, 169–176.

Hart, T. C. *et al.* (2002). Mutations of the UMOD gene are responsible for medullary cystic kidney disease 2 and familial juvenile hyperuricaemic nephropathy. *Journal of Medical Genetics* **39**, 882–892.

Hildebrandt, F. and Otto, E. (2000). Molecular genetics of nephronophthisis and medullary cystic kidney disease. *Journal of the American Society of Nephrology* **11**, 1753–1761.

Hildebrandt, F., Waldherr, R., Kutt, R., and Brandis, M. (1992). The nephronophthisis complex: clinical and genetics aspects. *The Clinical Investigator* **70**, 802–808.

Hildebrandt, F. *et al.* (1993). Mapping of a gene for familial juvenile nephronophthisis: confirmation of linkage to chromosome 2 and definition of flanking markers. *American Journal of Human Genetics* **53**, 1256–1261.

Hildebrandt, F. *et al.* (1997). A novel gene encoding an SH3 domain protein is mutated in nephronophthisis type 1. *Nature Genetics* **17**, 149–153.

Hildebrandt, F. *et al.* (1998). Lack of large, homozygous deletions of the nephronophthisis 1 region in Joubert syndrome type B. *Pediatric Nephrology* **12**, 16–19.

Hildebrandt, F. *et al.* (2001). Establishing an algorithm for molecular genetic diagnostics in 127 families with juvenile nephronophthisis. *Kidney International* **59**, 434–445.

Joubert, M. *et al.* (1969). Familial agenesis of the cerebellar vermis: a syndrome of episodic hyperpnea, abnormal eye movements, ataxia, and retardation. *Neurology* **19**, 813–825.

Kamatani, N. *et al.* (2000). Localization of a gene for familial juvenile hyperuricemic nephropathy causing underexcretion-type gout to 16p12 by genome-wide linkage analysis of a large family. *Arthritis and Rheumatism* **43**, 925–929.

Konrad, M. *et al.* (1996). Large homozygous deletions of 2q13 region are a major cause of juvenile nephronophthisis. *Human Molecular Genetics* **5**, 367–371.

Kroiss, S. *et al.* (2000). Evidence of further genetic heterogeneity in autosomal dominant medullary cystic kidney disease. *Nephrology, Dialysis, Transplantation* **15**, 818–821.

Lo, S. H. *et al.* (1997). Progressive kidney degenerescence in mice lacking tensin. *Journal of Cell Biology* **136**, 1349–1361.

Løken, A. C. *et al.* (1961). Hereditary renal dysplasia and blindness. *Acta Paediatrica* **50**, 177–184.

Lyon, M. F. and Hulse, E. V. (1971). An inherited kidney disease of mice resembling human nephronophthisis. *Journal of Medical Genetics* **8**, 41–48.

Mainzer, F. *et al.* (1970). Familial nephropathy associated with retinitis pigmentosa, cerebellar ataxia and skeletal abnormalities. *American Journal of Medicine* **49**, 556–562.

Medhioub, M. *et al.* (1994). Refined mapping of a gene causing familial juvenile nephronophthisis and evidence for genetic heterogeneity. *Genomics* **22**, 296–301.

Mendley, S. R. *et al.* (1995). Hereditary sclerosing glomerulopathy in the conorenal syndrome. *American Journal of Kidney Diseases* **25**, 792–797.

Mollet, G. *et al.* (2002). The gene mutated in juvenile nephronophthisis type 4 encodes a novel protein that interacts with nephrocystin. *Nature Genetics* **32**, 300–305.

Moudgil, A. A. *et al.* (1998). Nephronophthisis associated with Ellis-van Creveld syndrome. *Pediatric Nephrology* **12**, 20–22.

Neilson, E. G. *et al.* (1984). Spontaneous interstitial nephritis in kdkd mice. I. An experimental model of autoimmune renal disease. *Journal of Immunology* **133**, 2560–2565.

Ohba, Y. *et al.* (2000). A deletion of the paracellin-1 gene is responsible for renal tubular dysplasia in cattle. *Genomics* **68**, 229–236.

Olbrich, H. *et al.* (2003). Mutations in a novel gene, NPHP3, cause adolescent nephronophthisis, tapeto-retinal degeneration and hepatic fibrosis. *Nature Genetics* **34**, 455–459.

Omran, H. *et al.* (2000). Identification of a new gene locus for adolescent nephronophthisis, on chromosome 3q22 in a large Venezuelan family. *American Journal of Human Genetics* **16**, 755–758.

Omran, H. *et al.* (2001). Human adolescent nephronophthisis: gene locus synteny with polycystic kidney disease in pcy mice. *Journal of the American Society of Nephrology* **12**, 107–113.

Omran, H. *et al.* (2002). Identification of a gene locus for Senior–Løken syndrome in the region of the nephronophthisis type 3 gene. *Journal of the American Society of Nephrology* **13**, 75–79.

Otto, E. *et al.* (2000). Nephrocystin: gene expression and sequence conservation between human, mouse, and *Caenorhabditis elegans*. *Journal of the American Society of Nephrology* **11**, 270–282.

Otto, E. *et al.* (2002). A gene mutated in nephronophthisis and retinitis pigmentosa encodes a novel protein, nephroretinin, conserved in evolution. *American Journal of Human Genetics* **71**, 1161–1167.

Otto, E. A. *et al.* (2003). Mutations in INVS encoding inversin cause nephronophthisis type 2, linking renal cystic disease to the function of primary cilia and left-right axis determination. *Nature Genetics* **34**, 413–420.

Ozcay, F. M. *et al.* (2001). A family with Jeune syndrome. *Pediatric Nephrology* **16**, 623–626.

Parchoux, B. *et al.* (1982). Cécité et insuffisance renale précoce: à propos d'un cas avec néphropathie tubulo-interstitielle et kystes rénaux. *Pédiatrie* **37**, 211–217.

Polak, B. C. P., Hogewind, B. L., and Van Lith, F. H. M. (1977). Tapeto retinal degeneration associated with recessively inherited medullary cystic disease. *American Journal of Ophthalmology* **84**, 645–651.

Popovic-Rolovic, M. *et al.* (1993). Progressive tubulointerstitial nephritis and chronic cholestatic liver disease. *Pediatric Nephrology* **7**, 396–400.

Proesmans, W. *et al.* (1976). Fatal tubulointerstitial nephropathy with chronic cholestatic liver disease. *Acta Paediatrica Belgica* **29**, 231–238.

Quisling, R. G., Barkovitch, A. J., and Maria, B. L. (1999). Magnetic resonance imaging features and classification of central nervous system malformations in Joubert syndrome. *Journal of Children Neurology* **14**, 628–635.

Rahilly, M. A. and Fleming, S. (1995). Abnormal integrin receptor expression in two cases of familial nephronophthisis. *Histopathology* **26**, 345–349.

Saraiva, J. M. and Baraister, M. (1992). Joubert syndrome: a review. *American Journal of Medical Genetics* **43**, 726–731.

Sargent, M. A., Poskitt, K. J., and Jan, J. E. (1997). Congenital ocular motor apraxia: imaging findings. *American Journal of Neuroradiology* **18**, 1915–1922.

Saunier, S. *et al.* (1997a). A novel gene that encodes a protein with a putative src homology 3 domain is a candidate gene for familial juvenile nephronophthisis. *Human Molecular Genetics* **6**, 2317–2323.

Saunier, S. *et al.* (1997b). Large deletions of the NPH1 region in Cogan syndrome (CS) associated with familial juvenile nephronophthisis (NPH). *American Journal of Human Genetics* **61**, A346.

Saunier, S. *et al.* (2000). Characterization of the *NPHP1* locus: mutational mechanism involved in deletions in familial juvenile nephronophthisis. *American Journal of Human Genetics* **66**, 778–789.

Savill, G. A. *et al.* (1997). Chronic tubulo-interstial nephropathy in children with cranioectodermal dysplasia. *Pediatric Nephrology* **11**, 215–217.

Schuermann, M. J. *et al.* (2002). Mapping of gene loci for nephronophthisis type 4 and Senior–Løken syndrome, to chromosome 1p36. *American Journal of Human Genetics* **70**, 1240–1246.

Scolari, F. *et al.* (1998). Autosomal dominant medullary cystic disease: a disorder with variable clinical pictures and exclusion of linkage with the NPH1 locus. *Nephrology, Dialysis, Transplantation* **13**, 2536–2546.

Scolari, F. *et al.* (1999). Identification of a new locus for medullary cystic disease, on chromosome 16p12. *American Journal of Human Genetics* **64**, 1655–1660.

Senior, B., Friedmann, A. I., and Braupo, J. L. (1961). Juvenile familial nephropathy with tapeto retinal degeneration. A new oculo renal dystrophy. *American Journal of Ophthalmology* **52**, 625–633.

Stavrou, C. *et al.* (1998). Medullary cystic kidney disease with hyperuricemia and gout in a large Cypriot family: no allelism with nephronophthisis type 1. *American Journal of Medical Genetics* **77**, 149–154.

Stavrou, C. *et al.* (2002). Autosomal-dominant medullary cystic kidney disease type 1: clinical and molecular findings in six large Cypriot families. *Kidney International* **62**, 1385–1394.

Stiburkova, B. *et al.* (2000). Familial juvenile hyperuricemic nephropathy: localization of the gene on chromosome 16p11.2-and evidence for genetic heterogeneity. *American Journal of Human Genetics* **66**, 1989–1994.

Tsimaratos, M. *et al.* (1997). Chronic renal failure and cranioectodermal dysplasia: a further step. *Pediatric Nephrology* **11**, 785–786.

Thompson, G. R. *et al.* (1978). Familial occurrence of hyperuricemia, gout, and medullary cystic disease. *Archives of Internal Medicine* **138**, 1614–1617.

Waldherr, R. *et al.* (1982). The nephronophthisis complex. *Virchows Archives A, Pathological Anatomy and Histopathology* **394**, 235–254.

Witzleben, C. L. *et al.* (1982). Nephronophthisis: congenital hepatic fibrosis. An additional hepatorenal disorder. *Human Pathology* **13**, 728–733.

Zollinger, H. U. *et al.* (1980). Nephronophthisis (medullary cystic disease of the kidney). *Helvetica Paediatrica Acta* **35**, 509–530.

16.4 Inherited glomerular diseases

16.4.1 Alport's syndrome

*Bertrand Knebelmann and
Jean-Pierre Grünfeld*

Introduction

Alport's syndrome is an inherited renal disorder characterized by familial occurrence, in successive generations, of progressive haematuric nephritis, with ultrastructural changes of the glomerular basement membrane (GBM) and sensorineural hearing loss. The family reported by Dr A. Cecil Alport (Alport 1927) had been studied since the beginning of the twentieth century. Alport clearly noted that 'males develop nephritis and deafness and do not as a rule survive' whereas 'females have deafness and haematuria, and live to old age'. This statement has subsequently been largely confirmed: X-linked dominant inheritance is the most frequent in this disorder (85–90 per cent of the families).

Alport's syndrome is considered to be the cause of approximately 0.6 per cent of endstage renal failure (ESRF) in Europe, 1.1 per cent in India (Chugh *et al.* 1993), and 0.3 per cent in adults and 2.3 per cent in children in the United States, including African-American families (USRDS 1997). This proportion is probably underestimated since Alport's syndrome is underdiagnosed, in small kindreds or in sporadic cases, particularly if hearing defect is lacking. The gene mutation frequency is estimated to be 1/5000–1/10,000.

In recent years, the genetics and pathogenesis of Alport's syndrome have progressed dramatically. It has been shown successively that the primary lesion involves the GBM, and more specifically type IV collagen (which is a major component of basement membranes), and that the primary biochemical defects involve novel α-chains of type IV collagen (whose genes have been located, cloned, and found mutated in the patients). Thus, in two decades, we have moved from a 'syndrome' to different 'diseases' whose clinical, biochemical, and molecular features have, in part, been identified.

Type IV collagen in basement membranes

The primary defect in classical Alport's syndrome involves the α5 chain of type IV collagen, α5(IV), in the GBM and its corresponding gene, *COL4A5*. Consequently, α3(IV), which contains the Goodpasture antigen, is probably not normally incorporated into the GBM.

The GBM is composed of several proteins. Its major component is type IV collagen, which binds to laminins, entactin (or nidogen), and proteoglycans, and whose adjacent molecules interact to form a characteristic network (Fig. 1).

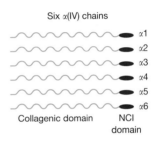

Six α(IV) chains

α1
α2
α3
α4
α5
α6

Collagenic domain   NCl domain

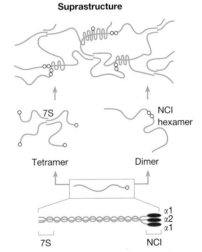

Suprastructure

7S   NCl hexamer

Tetramer   Dimer

α1
α2
α1

7S   NCl

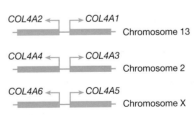

COL4A2 ← → COL4A1
                  Chromosome 13

COL4A4 ← → COL4A3
                  Chromosome 2

COL4A6 ← → COL4A5
                  Chromosome X

Fig. 1 Organization of type IV collagen. The genes encoding the six type IV collagen chains are located pairwise on three different chromosomes (bottom). Each chain has a 7S N-terminal domain, a long collagenous domain (#1400 residues), and a noncollagenous C-terminal domain, NC1 (#230 residues). Three α chains assemble into a triple helix, as exemplified by the $(\alpha 1)_2 \alpha 2$ molecule. Protomers interact head to head and end to end forming a supramolecular network.

The monomer of type IV collagen is a triple helical molecule composed of three α-chains. Each chain contains a long collagenous domain of ~1400 residues containing the repetitive triplet sequence Gly–X–Y, a ~15-residue non-collagenous amino terminus, and a ~230-residue non-collagenous (NC1) globular domain at the carboxyl terminus. Monomers associate at the NC1 domain, forming dimers stabilized by interchain disulfide bonds, and at the amino terminal end, forming tetramers (Fig. 1). Furthermore, a supramolecular assembly forming a supercoiled structure seems to exist resulting in a non-fibrillar network (Hudson *et al.* 1993). Six genetically distinct α-chains contribute to type IV collagen molecules. A large number of different isoforms of type IV collagen molecules can therefore be expected, differing in various basement membranes. Heterotrimers of $(\alpha1)2\ \alpha2$ are probably the most abundant. In the GBM, at least two different networks are found, one of classical $(\alpha1)2\ \alpha2$ type and the other composed of $\alpha3–\alpha5(IV)$ (Kashtan 2000 and references therein).

Six genes encode for the six α-chains (Hudson *et al.* 1993). They have a unique arrangement in that they are located pairwise in a head-to-head fashion on three different chromosomes (Fig. 1). These genes are large, exceeding 200 kb, and contain about 50 exons: *COL4A1* and *A2* on chromosome 13, *COL4A3* and *COLA4* on chromosome 2, and *COL4A5* and *COL4A6* on the Xq chromosome.

While the $\alpha1$ and $\alpha2(IV)$ are ubiquitous, the other chains have a restricted distribution (Table 1). In the kidney, $\alpha1$ and $\alpha2$ chains are formed by mesangial/endothelial cells and are expressed in vascular and tubular basement membranes (TBMs) and, within the glomerulus, in the mesangial matrix and the subendothelial aspect of the GBM. The novel $\alpha(IV)$ chains ($\alpha3–\alpha5$) are supposed to be synthesized by the visceral epithelial cells and are restricted to the GBM and distal TBM (Heidet *et al.* 2000). The $\alpha5(IV)$ is also present in the basement membrane of the collecting duct (Gubler *et al.* 1995). The $\alpha6(IV)$ chain is not found in the GBM but only in Bowman's capsule and in distal TBM. Extrarenal distribution of $\alpha3$, $\alpha4$, and $\alpha5(IV)$ includes the lens capsule, cochlea, and alveolar basement membranes. The $\alpha5$ and

$\alpha6(IV)$ chains are also present in the epidermal basement membrane where $\alpha3/\alpha4(IV)$ are normally absent.

Classical X-linked dominant Alport's syndrome

Renal disease

Alport's syndrome may be detected in infancy or childhood. All affected children have microscopic haematuria, and 50–60 per cent exhibit gross haematuria, often before the age of 5 years (Gubler *et al.* 1981). Recurrence (often following upper respiratory tract infection) is frequent during the first years of life. Gross haematuria does not generally recur after the age of 15.

In early childhood, proteinuria may be absent, intermittent, or permanent and mild; its incidence increases progressively with age. Approximately 40 per cent of patients, mainly boys, develop the nephrotic syndrome, usually mild, after the age of 10 years. The nephrotic syndrome is often accompanied by hypertension and is indicative of poor renal prognosis.

The renal disease found in childhood may progress in adulthood, but it is often first discovered in adults in whom gross haematuria is rarely the presenting symptom. Proteinuria and microhaematuria, with hypertension and/or renal failure, are the presenting abnormalities. The slower the rate of progression, the rarer the nephrotic syndrome.

The rate of progression to renal failure is heterogeneous and depends on sex and genetic factors. All affected males progress to renal failure. ESRF is rarely reached in males before 10 years of age, the median age at ESRF being 20 years. Ninety per cent of male patients develop ESRF before 40 years (Jais *et al.* 2000).

In contrast, most female carriers have intermittent or persistent microhaematuria (90 per cent) with or without proteinuria, and do not progress to renal failure. Proteinuria is found in approximately 75 per cent of affected women. Progression to ESRF occurs in only 12 per cent of females before the age of 40. The youngest age at ESRF reported is 19 years. However, more than 30 per cent develop ESRF after the age of 60 (Jais *et al.* 2003). However, the rate of progression is slower than in males (Gretz *et al.* 1987; Pochet *et al.* 1989). Renal progression is often difficult to predict in women with persistent urinary abnormalities: heavy proteinuria indicates poor prognosis and renal biopsy findings may have a predictive value (Grünfeld *et al.* 1985). Random inactivation of one X chromosome in each cell of the body probably explains some variability of expression of an X-linked disease in females. In a female Alport patient with a severe phenotype, two predisposing genetic factors were found: two missense mutations in the *COL4A5* gene (see below) and, mostly, a preferential inactivation of the normal *COL4A5* allele in the kidney (only mutant COL4A5 mRNA was detected in this tissue) (Guo *et al.* 1995).

Intrafamilial resemblance with regard to age at 'renal death' in males has been emphasized (Grünfeld *et al.* 1973). However, large intrafamilial variability can be observed. In such a family with a proven mutation in the *COL4A5* gene, ESRF in affected males was reached between 30 and 70 years of age (Knebelmann *et al.* 1992). It seems that missense mutations, often involving glycine residues, are more often associated with such a variability than large deletions and nonsense mutations (Jais *et al.* 2000).

The predictive value of extrarenal signs in a given patient is controversial. Correlation between progression of hearing loss and renal

Table 1 Tissue distribution of type IV collagen chains in basement membranes

Type IV collagen disease	Glomerular basement membrane	Bowman's capsule	Collecting duct basement membrane	Epidermal basement membrane
Normal				
$\alpha3/\alpha4(IV)$	+	+	+	−
$\alpha5(IV)$	+	+	+	+
X-linked males				
$\alpha3/\alpha4(IV)$	−	−	−	−
$\alpha5(IV)$	−	−	−	−
X-linked females				
$\alpha3/\alpha4(IV)$	Mosaic			−
$\alpha5(IV)$	Mosaic			Mosaic
Autosomal recessive				
$\alpha3/\alpha4(IV)$	−	−	−	−
$\alpha5(IV)$	−	+	+	+

failure is the rule. Eye defects appear associated with a more rapid progression to renal failure (Perrin *et al.* 1980).

No specific therapy exists for Alport's syndrome. Conflicting results have been presented on the antiproteinuric effect of angiotensin-converting enzyme inhibitors. Surprisingly, cyclosporin was found to be effective in eight children with Alport's syndrome not only to decrease proteinuria, but also to retard renal insufficiency (Callis *et al.* 1999). Confirmatory studies are needed before recommending such a therapy, because of the well-known nephrotoxicity of cyclosporin.

Hearing defect

High-tone sensorineural hearing loss is bilateral and may lead to clinically evident deafness. In its early stage, however, it can only be detected by audiometry, and an audiogram should be performed in any patient with suspected hereditary nephritis because subclinical hearing impairment, involving the non-conversational range (high frequencies), may otherwise be missed. This hearing defect is usually not detected before late childhood in boys with X-linked Alport's syndrome. It may be progressive in children, necessitating the use of a hearing aid.

Of interest, mutations in the *COL4A5* gene have been identified in families with progressive hereditary nephritis but without hearing defect. This shows that these families belong to the spectrum of Alport's syndrome.

Ocular abnormalities

Ocular defects involving the lens and retina occur in 15–40 per cent of patients with Alport's syndrome. Bilateral anterior lenticonus is the most specific eye abnormality; all cases investigated were found to have evidence of nephritis (Govan 1983; Streeten *et al.* 1987). Anterior lenticonus is consistently associated with hearing loss, but is less frequent than hearing defect. Diagnosis is based on biomicroscopy examination, which reveals a lens that looks like an oil droplet in water.

Among lens abnormalities, opacities are rather frequently found but are non-specific. Cataract has been reported in some families. Retinal flecks in the macula and midperiphery have been recognized more recently (Perrin *et al.* 1980; Govan 1983). These flecks are a pale yellow colour, round and symmetrical, and appear to be located in the innermost layer of the retina. Fluorescein angiography of the macular region is normal. Electroretinograms and electro-oculograms are normal (Perrin *et al.* 1980; Govan 1983) and visual acuity is not altered. Retinal changes are more frequent than lens abnormalities and are often associated with lenticonus, but they may also be present when the lens is normal. Their presence is suggestive of Alport's syndrome and should encourage further family investigations.

A group in Thailand described a particular but unspecific lesion of the cornea, called posterior polymorphic dystrophy, in 11 of their 17 Alport patients (Teekhasacnee 1991). Furthermore, recurrent corneal epithelial erosions seem to be abnormally frequent but can be frequently overlooked (Rhys *et al.* 1997).

Pathology, pathogenesis, and molecular genetics

Pathology

Light microscopy shows normal or near-normal renal tissue in young children. With increasing age, increased mesangial matrix, areas of segmental proliferation, thickening of capillary walls, and focal segmental glomerulosclerosis develop. Tubulointerstitial changes appear early. Interstitial foam cells have been considered as suggestive of Alport's syndrome, but these cells are seen in most types of glomerular disease with persistent heavy proteinuria. Conventional immunofluorescence studies are generally negative.

Electron microscopy reveals the most characteristic lesions (Fig. 2). The GBM is irregularly thickened with splitting and splintering of the lamina densa, thus delimiting clear zones containing small granulations. The external aspect of the GBM is irregularly festooned and bordered by hypertrophied podocytes. This ultrastructural lesion, when diffuse and associated with negative immunofluorescence, is highly suggestive of Alport's syndrome (Hinglais *et al.* 1972; Spear and Slusser 1972; Churg and Sherman 1973). The diagnostic value of electron microscopy (as well as of immunohistochemical study; see below) has been repeatedly demonstrated in patients with no positive family history (Hinglais *et al.* 1972; Yoshikawa *et al.* 1987).

GBM thickening is usually diffuse in adults whereas in the child it is segmental, and thinning of GBM with occasional ruptures is associated. Furthermore, diffuse thinning may be the only GBM lesion in patients with progressive nephritis (Gubler *et al.* 1993). Heterozygous females express the GBM defect in a mosaic pattern. Thus, sampling errors may sometimes make it difficult to form a firm histological diagnosis in these women.

The processes leading to the development of progressive renal lesions in Alport's syndrome are poorly understood. In the GBM, there is accumulation of the α1 and α2(IV) chains, along with type V and type VI collagen. Furthermore, abnormal deposition of laminin α2 chain occurs during the progression of the disease (Kashtan 2001). This may represent a compensatory response to the lack of the α3–α5(IV) chains. Interestingly, it has been reported that Alport's syndrome GBM lacking α3–α5(IV) chains is more susceptible to proteolytic degradation (Kalluri *et al.* 1997). Lesions of TBMs may be observed, usually associated with the more severe GBM changes.

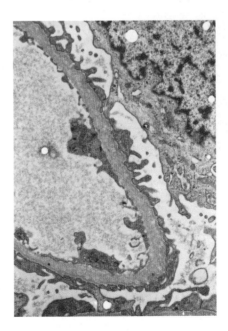

Fig. 2 Renal electron micrography of Alport syndrome ($\times$7000). There is thickening of the GBM with splitting of the lamina densa and irregularities of the epithelial aspect. (By courtesy of Dr L.H. Noël, Hôpital Necker, Paris.)

Basement membranes of retina and cochlea have not been studied by electron microscopy. The histopathological lesions responsible for hearing and ocular defects have not been well delineated.

Immunohistochemical findings

Kidney biopsy

Indirect immunofluorescence or immunoperoxidase analysis of kidney biopsies from patients with Alport's syndrome, using monoclonal antibodies, showed a lack of fixation along the GBM (i.e. a defect in GBM antigenicity) in most, but not all, male patients. In female patients from the same families, binding was either normal or discontinuous, with regions of normal reactivity interspersed with gaps of unreactive basement membrane, suggesting random inactivation of the X chromosome in an X-linked disease (Gubler *et al.* 1995) (Fig. 3).

By using mAb against the $\alpha5$(IV) chain several authors (Kashtan *et al.* 1986; Ding *et al.* 1994a; Yoshioka *et al.* 1994) found that 75 per cent of male patients with Alport's syndrome did not express the $\alpha5$(IV) chain in the GBM and in the epidermal basement membrane. Similarly, a lack of binding of $\alpha3$(IV) monoclonal antibodies was demonstrated in the kidneys of approximately 75 per cent of the patients (Gubler *et al.* 1993). The $\alpha4$(IV) antigenicity was also lacking. These defects were observed predominantly when thick and split rather than thin GBM was the main ultrastructural lesion, and they were correlated with more severe renal disease. Thus, these results suggest that a mutation in the gene encoding for the $\alpha5$(IV) chain leads to a defect of molecular assembly of the $\alpha3$ and $\alpha4$ chains in the basement membranes where these chains are coexpressed. The final consequence is that triple helices involving $\alpha3$(IV) and $\alpha4$(IV) without $\alpha5$(IV) are not formed or are unstable.

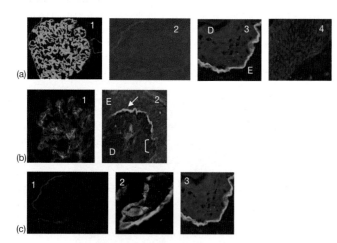

Fig. 3 Immunohistochemistry analysis of Alport syndrome basement membranes. (a) Male patient with X-linked Alport syndrome. (1) In normal kidney, GBM stains strongly for $\alpha3$(IV); similar staining would be seen for $\alpha4$ and $\alpha5$(IV). (2) Staining of the GBM is absent for each of these chains in a male patient. (3) In the normal epidermal basement membrane, staining for $\alpha5$(IV) is present in normal subjects; D, dermis; E, epidermis. (4) No staining for a5(IV) is seen in the EBM of male patients. (b) Female patient with X linked Alport syndrome. (1) A focal distribution is observed for a3–5(IV) in the GBM. (2) Similarly, some areas are negative (bracket) for a5(IV) in the epidermal basement membrane. (c) Patient with autosomal recessive Alport syndrome. (1) There is coabsence of a3–5(IV) in the GBM with persistent staining for a5(IV) in the Bowman's capsule. (2) Staining for a5(IV) persists in the collecting duct. (3) The epidermal basement membrane remains positive for a5(IV). (By courtesy of Dr L.H. Noël, Hôpital Necker, Paris.)

All these immunochemical findings have diagnostic value in X-linked Alport's syndrome. It should be kept in mind, however, that approximately 25 per cent of the male patients have apparently normal basement membrane antigenicity.

Diagnostic value of skin biopsy

As shown in Table 1, $\alpha5$(IV) is normally present in the epidermal basement membrane (EBM) whereas $\alpha3$ and $\alpha4$ are not. In 75 per cent of male patients with X-linked Alport's syndrome, $\alpha5$(IV) is absent in the EBM, as in the GBM. In female heterozygotes, a mosaic pattern of $\alpha5$ expression is found. This pattern can, however, be very heterogeneous, and normal expression cannot rule out a carrier status. It has also been suggested that the extent of defective $\alpha5$ chain in the skin was correlated with progression of renal disease in heterozygous women (Nakanishi *et al.* 1994). In contrast, $\alpha5$ is present in EBM in autosomal recessive Alport's syndrome (Table 1) since $\alpha3$ and $\alpha4$ are not required for its integration. Thus, absence of $\alpha5$ in the skin is diagnostic not only of Alport's syndrome but also of its X-linked mode of inheritance. Normal expression of $\alpha5$ in the skin of a patient suspected of Alport's syndrome has several possible explanations (Kashtan 1999): (a) the patient has a *COL4A5* mutation that allows $\alpha5$ expression in the skin (and the GBM) which is encountered in around 25 per cent of cases; (b) the patient has autosomal recessive Alport's syndrome; (c) the patient has another renal disease. In these cases, kidney biopsy analysis, including by immunofluorescence, would be necessary.

Molecular genetics

The gene responsible for the classical X-linked Alport's syndrome is the *COL4A5* gene located at Xq22 (Table 2). Mutations in *COL4A5* have been found in more than 300 families throughout the world (Lemmink *et al.* 1997). Each family appears to have its own 'private' mutation, making mutation search laborious.

Major rearrangements, mainly deletions, are detected in 5–16 per cent of the kindreds (Antignac *et al.* 1994). Most deletions are associated with early progression to ESRF (Jais *et al.* 2000), before the age of 20, and hearing loss and ocular lesions in more than 50 per cent of the patients.

Small mutations in *COL4A5*, missense, splice site, and small deletions of a few base pairs are the most common lesions. Substitutions for glycine residues in the collagenous domain are a common type of missense mutations (25 per cent) and interfere with the normal folding of the $\alpha5$ chain into triple helices with other α(IV) chains. The severity of the disease associated with such mutations is so far unpredictable.

Table 2 Molecular genetics of Alport's syndrome

Clinical presentation	Defective α(IV) chain	Mutant gene	Chromosomal location
X-linked disease with or without sensorineural hearing loss	$\alpha5$	COL4A5	Xq22
X-linked disease with diffuse leiomyomatosis	$\alpha5$ and $\alpha6$	COL4A5 and COL4A6	Xq22
Autosomal recessive disease	$\alpha3$ $\alpha4$	COL4A3 COL4A4	2q35–q37 2q35–q37
Autosomal dominant disease	$\alpha3$ or $\alpha4$	COL4A3/ COL4A4	2q35–q37

Conversely, frameshift mutations and stop codons are generally associated with early progression to ESRF and hearing defect (Jais *et al.* 2000).

Sporadic cases of Alport's syndrome without positive family history could represent *de novo* mutations. Such mutations have been demonstrated by molecular genetic studies (Knebelmann *et al.* 1996; Lemmink *et al.* 1997). Their incidence has been estimated as up to 12 per cent (Jais *et al.* 2000), but their real incidence is unknown and depends in part on the diagnostic criteria required. Another genetic situation may mimic *de novo* mutation. The mutation may occur in only some gametes of the mother, during mitosis in early germline proliferation, leading to germline mosaicism (Nakazato *et al.* 1994; Plant 2000). In this case, the mother's somatic cells, such as leucocytes, contain two copies of the normal gene and therefore her phenotype is normal. However, she can transmit the disease through her mutated gametes with an unpredictable frequency making genetic counselling uneasy.

X-linked diffuse oesophageal leiomyomatosis and Alport's syndrome

Diffuse leiomyomatosis is a rare tumoural condition characterized by smooth muscle cell proliferation. Sporadic and inherited cases have been described. The association of leiomyomatosis involving the oesophagus, the tracheobronchial tree, and the genital tract (with vulvar and clitoral enlargement), first described by Garcia-Torrès *et al.* (1993), has now been reported in 35 cases with Alport's syndrome, belonging to 19 families. Oesophageal involvement, sometimes limited to the lower third of the oesophagus, is responsible for dysphagia, usually in childhood.

In most cases, surgical treatment is required. Respiratory symptoms may reveal leiomyomatosis. Tracheobronchial leiomyoma should be sought by endoscopy because of the risk of sudden death (Cochat *et al.* 1988). In affected males, the renal disease is of juvenile type. Female patients appear to be as severely affected as males concerning leiomyomatosis, whereas renal involvement is milder than in males. Hearing loss is frequently observed. Another peculiar feature is the high incidence of bilateral congenital cataract, an eye abnormality not commonly found in classical Alport's syndrome.

The transmission of this syndrome is in accordance with an X-linked dominant trait. Molecular studies have shown deletions removing 5′ ends of both the *COL4A5* and *COL4A6* genes, as well as the intergenic region thought to bear the regulatory sequences (Zhou *et al.* 1993; Heidet *et al.* 1995). The absence of either $\alpha 6$(IV) alone or both $\alpha 5$ and $\alpha 6$(IV) should be responsible for smooth muscle cell proliferation. However, some patients with Alport's syndrome but without leiomyomatosis, and bearing deletions in *COL4A5* and *COL4A6*, have been reported (Heidet *et al.* 1995). This observation remains unexplained.

Autosomal recessive Alport's syndrome

Although Alport's syndrome has an X-linked dominant transmission in 85–90 per cent of the families, some features highly suggestive of autosomal recessive inheritance in 10–15 per cent of the families have been reported (Feingold *et al.* 1985). These features are mainly: (a) appearance of the disease in the family after a consanguineous marriage;

(b) equally severe disease in males and females, or more specifically, severe renal diseases in females leading to ESRF before 20 years of age.

Molecular studies have clearly established autosomal recessive inheritance. Linkage analysis using a polymorphism inside the *COL4A5* gene may be useful to exclude a mutation at the X-located Alport locus. More decisively, mutations have been identified in *COL4A3* or *COL4A4* gene in several families (Heidet 2001; Longo 2002). They can be nonsense, frameshift, splicing or missense mutations, the latter frequently affecting glycine residues, as in the $\alpha 5$(IV) chain. Affected patients are true homozygotes or compound heterozygotes, having two different mutations on the two alleles of *COL4A3* or *COL4A4*.

Extrarenal features in these kindreds are similar to those found in X-linked classical Alport's syndrome, that is, hearing defect and eye abnormalities. The GBM ultrastructural lesions are not distinguishable from those of the X-linked form. Immunohistochemical analysis using monoclonal antibodies shows heterogeneity as in the X-linked form; the GBM of most patients with autosomal recessive Alport's syndrome lacks expression of the $\alpha 3$ and $\alpha 4$ chains, but others express these chains normally. In the former cases, $\alpha 3$, $\alpha 4$, and $\alpha 5$ chains are coabsent in the GBM, whereas $\alpha 5$ chain is normally present in a series of basement membranes, including Bowman's capsule, collecting duct, and EBM (Gubler *et al.* 1995). Thus, immunohistochemical analysis of kidney biopsy, alone or coupled with skin biopsy, can be of great value to establish not only the diagnostic of Alport's syndrome, but also its mode of inheritance.

Heterozygous carriers of a *COL4A3* or *COL4A4* mutation usually present with no symptoms or intermittent microscopic haematuria. However, depending on the type of mutation and may be also on environmental factors, they sometimes display more severe symptoms including proteinuria and renal failure (Heidet 2001; Longo *et al.* 2002).

Autosomal dominant Alport's syndrome

Autosomal dominant forms of Alport's syndrome have been reported, characterized by male-to-male transmission. They probably represent less than 5 per cent of all cases. In one such family, a splice site mutation resulting in an in-frame deletion in *COL4A3* has been identified (van der Loop *et al.* 2000). One of the affected individuals reached ESRF at 35 years and had hearing loss. Based on the few families described in the literature, it seems that the renal disease is less severe than in the autosomal recessive form. Thus, autosomal dominant Alport's syndrome is caused by heterozygote mutations affecting only one allele of *COL4A3* or *COL4A4*, the nature of the mutation, may be by a dominant negative effect, being responsible for an intermediary phenotype, between no symptoms or isolated microscopic haematuria in heterozygote carriers of a recessive mutation, and a full blown phenotype in patients having both alleles mutated.

Animal models

Several animal models of Alport's syndrome have been described in dogs, both X-linked and autosomal recessive, which mimic most of the clinical and immunohistological features of Alport's syndrome in humans (see review in Kashtan 2002). Along with knock out mouse models, they could prove valuable to test new therapeutic approaches.

Kidney transplantation

Kidney transplantation in patients with Alport's syndrome

Most Alport patients who have undergone kidney transplantation have achieved satisfactory long-term results (Peten *et al.* 1990; Byrne *et al.* 2002). Approximately 15 per cent of the patients develop transient IgG linear deposition along transplant GBM, in the absence of detectable circulating anti-GBM antibodies, whereas such fixation is found in only 1–2 per cent of other renal transplant patients (Quérin *et al.* 1986; Byrne *et al.* 2002). A small number, about 2.5 per cent, of Alport patients develop immunization against graft GBM (Kashtan 2000; Jais *et al.* 2002). The onset of anti-GBM nephritis occurred mainly in the first year following transplantation. It led to severe crescentic glomerulonephritis and subsequent graft loss in three-fourths of the cases. In the remaining cases, the course is more indolent. Anti-GBM glomerulonephritis recurred in most retransplanted patients. Rapid diagnosis is based on serology and renal biopsy data. Adequate treatment should be promptly initiated, including intensive plasma exchange therapy.

Most cases occurred in X-linked families and thus, obviously, in males (Ding *et al.* 1994b). A similar complication has been described in two female patients with autosomal recessive Alport's syndrome who were transplanted at 10 and 20 years of age, respectively (Ding *et al.* 1995; Kalluri *et al.* 1995).

It is reasonable to think that the alloimmunization of Alport's patients has been triggered by the introduction of the graft GBM antigenic epitopes that were lacking in the native kidney. Most of them are anti-$\alpha5$(IV) antibodies but antibodies against $\alpha3$(IV) have also been described (Kashtan 2000). Of note, the $\alpha3$(IV) chain contains the Goodpasture antigen (Saus *et al.* 1988).

Why is this alloimmunization such a rare event, and can it be predicted in X-linked forms? In the European study (Jais *et al.* 2000), only three of 118 transplanted male patients with identified *COL4A5* mutation developed post-transplant anti-GBM glomerulonephritis. All three had a large deletion. The risk for these patients of developing this complication is 15 per cent, which represents a sixfold increase compared to the total Alport's syndrome population. However, 16 other patients with a large *COL4A5* rearrangement and 32 with mutations expected to produce a truncated protein did not develop anti-GBM glomerulonephritis in the graft, showing that other factors must contribute to alloimmunization.

Kidney donation from female subjects in Alport families

This practical issue is often raised. Clinical detection of heterozygous females in X-linked disease can be difficult, as indicated above. More definite clues can be provided by molecular genetics. Furthermore, the question has been extended to whether non-proteinuric carrier females, with normal GFR, should be excluded from kidney donation. Few data are available on the long-term effect of uninephrectomy in such women. In one carrier female donor, renal function remained stable 2 years after uninephrectomy (Sessa *et al.* 1995). In any case, kidney donation from carrier females should be viewed with caution until additional information is collected, and decision should be made on an individual basis. In contrast, non-proteinuric heterozygous subjects in autosomal recessive Alport's syndrome can be accepted as kidney donors.

Diagnosis

The two most characteristic elements of Alport's syndrome are inherited progressive haematuric nephritis and sensorineural hearing loss. However, genetic deafness (including genetic nerve deafness) is not rare in the general population and sensorineural hearing defect may be associated with various types of renal disease, in addition to Alport's syndrome (Table 3).

Positive diagnosis of Alport's syndrome (covering different genetic diseases) is based on the following criteria: a positive family history of progressive haematuric nephritis (i.e. leading to renal failure), sensorineural hearing loss, specific eye defects, characteristic ultrastructural changes of the GBM, and a defect in GBM antigenicity. Identification of a type IV collagen gene mutation, cosegregating with the disease in the kindred, will become the strongest diagnostic criteria (Table 2). Of note, among 193 families with a proven *COL4A5* mutation in an European study, 14 (7.5 per cent) had only one and 58 (30 per cent) only two diagnostic criteria (Jais *et al.* 2000). Sensorineural hearing loss should only be considered as a feature suggestive, but not pathognomonic, of Alport's syndrome (Pirson 1999). As mentioned above, skin biopsy with study of $\alpha5$(IV) expression has become a very useful tool to diagnose X-linked Alport's syndrome.

Differential diagnosis of haematuria in children

The incidence of asymptomatic haematuria in the paediatric population ranges from 0.5 to 2.0 per cent (Trachtman *et al.* 1984), and the diagnosis of Alport's syndrome should be considered in all of these children; urine testing of first-degree relatives is an essential early part of the investigation. The diagnosis is suggested by the findings of hearing

Table 3 Various inherited conditions in which sensorineural hearing loss has been reported in association with renal disease

Alport's syndrome and variants
Muckle–Wells syndrome (Chapter 4.2)
Refsum disease (Chapter 16.4.2)
Cockayne syndrome (Chapter 16.7)
Renal tubular acidosis
Bartter syndrome (Chapter 5.5)
Ichthyosis, hyperprolinuria
Charcot–Marie–Tooth syndrome
Alström syndrome
Ataxia, hyperuricaemia
Photomyoclonus, diabetes mellitus
Familial spastic paraplegia intellectual retardation (Fitzsimmons *et al.* 1988)
Various syndromes, including renal, genital, and/or digital abnormalities
Various malformative syndromes involving urinary tract and ear, such as branchio-oto-renal dysplasia (or BOR syndrome) and the multiple lentigines syndrome (Chapter 16.7)
Mitochondrial cytopathies (Chapter 16.7)
HDR syndrome (Chapter 16.7)
von Hippel–Lindau disease with endolymphatic sac tumour (Chapter 16.6)

defect, eye abnormalities, and/or positive family history of progressive nephritis, although these findings may be lacking. Alport boys almost invariably have persistent haematuria, whereas intermittent haematuria is a pointer to IgA nephropathy. Thus, renal biopsy with immunofluorescence and electron microscopy examination is of clinical value in these children, as shown in the study by Trachtman *et al.* (1984). In this study, histopathological renal lesions were identified in only 40 per cent of children and young adults with isolated microhaematuria; ultrastructural changes of the GBM (mainly thinning) predominated. Renal biopsy was more often abnormal in children with microscopic and gross haematuria; ultrastructural lesions (mainly thickening) and IgA nephropathy were found with similar frequencies.

In a series of 322 children with persistent haematuria for longer than 6 months, biopsies were classified as IgA nephropathy in 78 patients (24 per cent), Alport's syndrome in 86 (26 per cent), and thin basement membrane in 50 (15 per cent). The biopsies in 48 (15 per cent) patients showed normal glomeruli (Piqueras *et al.* 1998).

Benign familial haematuria

Benign familial haematuria is defined by the familial occurrence of persistent microscopic haematuria, without hearing defect and progression to renal failure in the proband and in his/her kindred. To predict the benign course of the disease, additional criteria are necessary, including absence of gross haematuria, absence of proteinuria, and presence of adult male patients with isolated microhaematuria in the kindred. In rare instances, extensive family investigations have been performed and inheritance has been said to be compatible with autosomal dominant transmission. Renal biopsy shows thinning of the GBM in approximately half of the cases, and various non-specific and minor glomerular changes in the other half (Rogers *et al.* 1973; Blumenthal *et al.* 1988).

The prevalence of microhaematuria in adults is estimated to be between 4 and 13 per cent; in patients with persistent microhaematuria, familial investigation using simple tests may be rewarding (Blumenthal *et al.* 1988). In adults, as well as in children, benign haematuria may be familial or non-familial (Piel *et al.* 1982).

Great caution should be exercised in establishing the diagnosis of benign familial haematuria. This is most difficult in young children; thinning of the GBM may be the prominent, or even isolated, histopathological finding in patients with true Alport's syndrome, and thickening and lamination, if present, may be limited to rare segments of the capillary wall (Gubler *et al.* 1981; Habib *et al.* 1982). The possibility of benign familial haematuria should be excluded when thickening of the GBM and splitting of the lamina densa are found on electron microscopy. The clinical diagnosis may also be difficult in kindreds where only adult women are affected in a kindred. It should be kept in mind that in families with X-linked Alport's syndrome, carrier females may present only with microhaematuria.

Patients with benign familial haematuria are heterozygous for a mutation in *COL4A3/A4* (Badenas *et al.* 2002). However, cases unlinked to this locus have been reported (Piccini *et al.* 1999). Moreover, mutations in *COL4A3/A4* are associated with autosomal recessive Alport's syndrome: heterozygotes may present benign microhaematuria and the mutation appears to have a dominant mode of transmission; in contrast, compound heterozygotes or true homozygotes develop full blown Alport's syndrome (Lemmink *et al.* 1996; Boye *et al.* 1998). The term 'thin basement membrane nephropathy'

has been coined to describe diffuse thinning of the GBM whose definition is controversial. GBM thickness may vary with age and sex. Morita *et al.* (1998) reported that GBM thickness varies from 190 to 440 nm in children aged over 9 years. A GBM of 200 nm or less is generally accepted as 'thin' and between 200 and 250 is considered borderline. The term thin basement membrane nephropathy is misleading: it describes an histopathological lesion, it does not correspond to a clinical entity and is not the guarantee of a benign disease. Indeed, this so-called thin basement membrane disease has been observed in patients with microhaematuria, either in isolation or associated with gross haematuria or substantial proteinuria, in patients with familial or non-familial disease, and in patients who did or did not progress to renal failure (Tiebosch *et al.* 1989). It is well documented that patients with typical Alport's syndrome may present with thin GBM on electron microscopy.

Nephritis, deafness, and macrothrombocytopenia

This assocation was first described by Epstein *et al.* (1972) and has subsequently been observed in several other families. The haematological abnormalities include thrombocytopenia and giant platelets. Different types of granulocyte inclusions may be associated with macrothrombocytopenia. Progression to ESRF occurs usually in early adulthood. Hearing defect is present in most kindreds. This association has been described initially as autosomal dominant Alport's syndrome with macrothombocytopenia. In some families, male carriers may present with thrombocytopenia and/or deafness in the absence of clinical renal involvement, a pattern which is not observed in Alport's syndrome. Molecular genetics has clarified the situation. This syndrome, along with the May Hegglin purely haematological disorder, is associated with mutation in *MYH9*, a gene encoding a non-muscle myosin heavy chain, and does not belong to the spectrum of type IV collagen diseases (Seri *et al.* 2000; Knebelmann *et al.* 2001; Arrondel 2002).

Genetic counselling

The prerequisite for genetic counselling is to identify the inherited nature of the kidney disease. Genetic diagnosis is first based on the family history. Careful establishment of the family pedigree is therefore a crucial step. The clinical difficulties have been illustrated above (see identification of carrier females, diagnostic criteria, and *de novo* mutations).

The second step is to identify the mode of inheritance. In X-linked Alport's syndrome, affected (hemizygous) males transmit the mutant gene to all daughters but not to sons. Affected (heterozygous) females carry a 50 per cent risk to transmit the disease to their offspring, whatever the sex. In the autosomal recessive form, both parents are heterozygous, and the risk of transmission is 25 per cent, whatever the sex. Molecular genetics can be very helpful in counselling: by direct identification of the mutation or by linkage analysis using highly polymorphic repetitive sequences within or close to the gene.

Genetic counselling should be considered a partnership between an at-risk individual and a counsellor. It should be shared by a clinical geneticist and a nephrologist. Indeed, both are able to offer information on the natural history of the disease, options for presymptomatic testing and support, and the at-risk subject or patient makes the decision. Presymptomatic testing using molecular techniques should focus on females who desire it, before they become pregnant. It should be kept in mind that it may have serious drawbacks if the results are misused by third parties, namely other family members, employers, or insurance companies.

Prenatal diagnosis can be considered in the X-linked and autosomal recessive forms. The question may arise whether it is an acceptable option given the partially treatable nature of the condition. This issue has to be discussed between the carrier female and the geneticist. Surveys are necessary to evaluate the attitudes of the families towards prenatal diagnosis.

References

Alport, A. C. (1927). Hereditary familial congenital haemorrhagic nephritis. *British Medical Journal* 1, 504–506.

Antignac, C. *et al.* (1994). Deletions in the COL4A5 collagen gene in X-linked Alport syndrome: characterization of the pathological transcripts in non-renal cells and correlation with disease expression. *Journal of Clinical Investigation* 93, 1195–1207.

Arrondel, C., Vodovar, N., Knebelmann, B., Grunfeld, J. P., Gubler, M. C., Antignac, C., and Heidet, L. (2002). Expression of the nonmuscle myosin heavy chain IIA in the human kidney and screening for MYH9 mutations in Epstein and Fechtner syndromes. *Journal of the American Society of Nephrology* 13, 65–74.

Badenas, C. *et al.* (2002). Mutations in the COL4A4 and COL4A3 genes cause familial benign hematuria. *Journal of the American Society of Nephrology* 13, 1248–1254.

Blumenthal, S. S., Fritsche, C., and Lemann, J., Jr., (1988). Establishing the diagnosis of benign familial hematuria. *Journal of the American Medical Association* 259, 2263–2266.

Boye, E. *et al.* (1998). Determination of the genomic structure of the COL4A4 gene and of novel mutations causing autosomal recessive Alport syndrome. *American Journal of Human Genetics* 63 (5), 1329–1340.

Byrne, M. C., Budisavljevic, M. N., Fan, Z., Self, S. E., and Ploth, D. W. (2002). Renal transplant in patients with Alport's syndrome. *American Journal of Kidney Diseases* 39 (4), 769–775.

Callis, L., Vila, A., Carrera, M., and Nieto, J. (1999). Long-term effects of cyclosporine A in Alport's syndrome. *Kidney International* 55, 1051–1056.

Chugh, K. S., Sakhuja, V., Agarwal, A., Jha, V., Joshi, K., Datta, B. N., Gupta, A., and Gupta, K. L. (1993). Hereditary nephritis (Alport's syndrome), clinical profile and inheritance in 28 kindreds. *Nephrology, Dialysis, Transplantation* 8, 690–695.

Churg, J. and Sherman, R. L. (1973). Pathologic characteristics of hereditary nephritis. *Archives of Pathology* 95, 374–379.

Cochat, P., Guibaud, P., Garcia Torres, R., Roussel, B., Guarner, V., and Larbre, F. (1988). Diffuse leiomyomatosis in Alport syndrome. *Journal of Pediatrics* 113, 339–343.

Ding, J., Kashtan, C. E., Fan, W. W., Kleppel, M. M., Sun, M. J., Kalluri, R., Neilson, E. G., and Michael, A. F. (1994a). A monoclonal antibody marker for Alport syndrome identifies the Alport antigen as the $\alpha5$ chain of type IV collagen. *Kidney International* 46, 1504–1506.

Ding, J., Stitzel, J., Berry, P., Hawkins, E., and Kashtan, C. E. (1995). Autosomal recessive Alport syndrome: mutation in the COL4A3 gene in a woman with Alport syndrome and posttransplant antiglomerular basement membrane nephritis. *Journal of the American Society of Nephrology* 5, 1714–1717.

Ding, J., Zhou, J., Tryggvason, K., and Kashtan, E. (1994b). COL4A5 deletions in three patients with Alport syndrome and posttransplant antiglomerular basement membrane nephritis. *Journal of the American Society of Nephrology* 5, 161–168.

Epstein, C. J. *et al.* (1972). Hereditary macrothrombocytopathia, nephritis and deafness. *American Journal of Medicine* 52, 299–310.

Excerpts from United States Renal Data System (1997). *American Journal of Kidney Diseases* 30, S40–S53.

Feingold, J., Bois, E., Chompret, A., Broyer, M., Gubler, M. C., and Grünfeld, J. P. (1985). Genetic heterogeneity of Alport syndrome. *Kidney International* 27, 672–677.

Fitzsimmons, J. S., Watson, A. R., Mellor, D., and Guilbert, P. R. (1988). Familial spastic paraplegia, bilateral sensorineural deafness, and intellectual retardation associated with a progressive nephropathy. *Journal of Medical Genetics* 25, 168–172.

Garcia-Torres, R. and Orozco, L. (1993). Alport-leiomyomatosis syndrome: an update. *American Journal of Kidney Diseases* 22, 641–648.

Gauthier, B., Trachtman, H., Frank, R., and Valderrama, E. (1989). Familial thin basement membrane nephropathy in children with asymptomatic microhematuria. *Nephron* 51, 502–508.

Govan, J. A. A. (1983). Ocular manifestations of Alport's syndrome: a hereditary disorder of basement membranes? *British Journal of Ophthalmology* 67, 493–503.

Gretz, N. *et al.* (1987). Alport's syndrome as a cause of renal failure in Europe. *Pediatric Nephrology* 1, 411–415.

Grünfeld, J. P. (1985). The clinical spectrum of hereditary nephritis. *Kidney International* 27, 83–92.

Grünfeld, J. P., Bois, E. P., and Hinglais, N. (1973). Progressive and non-progressive hereditary chronic nephritis. *Kidney International* 4, 216–228.

Grünfeld, J. P., Noël, L. H., Hafez, S., and Droz, D. (1985). Renal prognosis in women with hereditary nephritis. *Clinical Nephrology* 23, 267–271.

Gubler, M. C., Antignac, C., Deschênes, G., Knebelmann, B., Hors-Cayla, M. C., Grünfeld, J. P., Broyer, M., and Habib, R. (1993). Genetic, clinical and morphologic heterogeneity in Alport syndrome. *Advances in Nephrology* 22, 15–35.

Gubler, M. C., Knebelmann, B., Beziau, A., Broyer, M., Pirson, Y., Haddoum, F., Kleppel, M. M., and Antignac, C. (1995). Autosomal recessive Alport syndrome: immunohistochemical study of type IV collagen chain distribution. *Kidney International* 47, 1142–1147.

Gubler, M. *et al.* (1981). Alport's syndrome. A report of 58 cases and a review of the literature. *American Journal of Medicine* 70, 493–505.

Guo, C., van Damme, B., Vanrenterghem, Y., Devriendt, K., Cassiman, J. J., and Marynen, P. (1995). Severe Alport phenotype in a woman with two missense mutations in the same COL4A5 gene and preponderant inactivation of the X chromosome carrying the normal allele. *Journal of Clinical Investigation* 95, 1832–1837.

Habib, R. *et al.* (1982). Alport's syndrome: experience at Hôpital Necker. *Kidney International* 21 (Suppl. 11), S-20–S-28.

Heidet, L., Arrondel, C., Forestier, L., Cohen-Solal, L., Mollet, G., Gutierrez, B., Stavrou, C., Gubler, M. C., and Antignac, C. (2001). Structure of the human type IV collagen gene COL4A3 and mutations in autosomal Alport syndrome. *Journal of the American Society of Nephrology* 12, 97–106.

Heidet, L., Cai, Y., Guicharnaud, L., Antignac, C., and Gubler, M. C. (2000). Glomerular expression of type IV collagen chains in normal and X-linked Alport syndrome kidneys. *American Journal of Pathology* 156, 1901–1910.

Heidet, L., Dahan, K., Zhou, J., Xu, Z., Cochat, P., Gould, J. D. M., Leppig, K. A., Proesmans, W., Guyot, C., Guillot, M., Roussel, B., Tryggvason, K., Grünfeld, J. P., Gubler, M. C., and Antignac, C. (1995). Deletions of both $\alpha5(IV)$ and $\alpha6(IV)$ collagen genes in Alport syndrome and in Alport syndrome associated with smooth muscle tumours. *Human Molecular Genetics* 4, 99–108.

Hinglais, N., Grünfeld, J. P., and Bois, E. (1972). Characteristic ultrastructural lesion of the glomerular basement membrane in progressive hereditary nephritis (Alport's syndrome). *Laboratory Investigation* 27, 473–487.

Hudson, B. G., Reeders, S. T., and Tryggvason, K. (1993). Type IV collagen: structure, gene organization, and role in human diseases. *Journal of Biological Chemistry* 268, 26033–26036.

Jais, J. P., Knebelmann, B., Giatras, I., De Marchi, M., Rizzoni, G., Renieri, A., Weber, M., Gross, O., Netzer, K. O., Flinter, F., Pirson, Y., Dahan, K., Wieslander, J., Persson, U., Tryggvason, K., Martin, P., Hertz, J. M., Schroder, C., Sanak, M., Carvalho, M. F., Saus, J., Antignac, C., Smeets, H., and Gubler, M. C. (2003). X-linked Alport syndrome: natural history and genotype–phenotype correlations in girls and women belonging to 195 families: a 'European Community Alport Syndrome Concerted Action' study. *Journal of the American Society of Nephrology* **14** (10), 2603–2610.

Jais, J. P. *et al.* (2000). X-linked Alport syndrome: natural history in 195 families and genotype–phenotype correlations in males. *Journal of the American Society of Nephrology* **11**, 649–657.

Kalluri, R., Shield, C. F., Todd, P., Hudson, B. G., and Neilson, E. G. (1997). Isoform switching of type IV collagen is developmentally arrested in X-linked Alport syndrome leading to increased susceptibility of renal basement membranes to endoproteolysis. *Journal of Clinical Investigation* **99**, 2470–2478.

Kalluri, R., van den Heuvel, L. P., Smeets, H. J. M., Schroder, C. H., Lemmink, H. H., Boutaud, A., Neilson, E. G., and Hudson, B. G. (1995). A COL4A3 gene mutation and post-transplant anti-α3(IV) collagen alloantibodies in Alport syndrome. *Kidney International* **47**, 1199–1204.

Kalluri, R., Weber, M., Netzer, K. O., Sun, M. J., Neilson, E. G., and Hudson, B. G. (1994). COL4A5 gene deletion and production of post-transplant anti-α3(IV) collagen alloantibodies in Alport syndrome. *Kidney International* **45**, 721–726.

Kashtan, C. E. (1999). Alport syndrome: is diagnosis only skin-deep? *Kidney International* **55**, 1575–1576.

Kashtan, C. E. (2000). Alport syndrome: phenotypic heterogeneity of progressive hereditary nephritis. *Pediatric Nephrology* **14**, 502–512.

Kashtan, C. E. (2002). Animal models of Alport syndrome. *Nephrology, Dialysis, Transplantation* **17**, 1359–1362.

Kashtan, C. E., Fish, A. J., Kleppel, M., Yoshioka, K., and Michael, A. F. (1986). Nephritogenic antigen determinants in epidermal and renal basement membranes of kindreds with Alport-type familial nephritis. *Journal of Clinical Investigation* **78**, 1035–1044.

Kashtan, C. E., Kim, Y., Lees, G. E., Thorner, P. S., Virtanen, I., and Miner, J. H. (2001). Abnormal glomerular basement membrane laminins in murine, canine, and human Alport syndrome: aberrant laminin alpha2 deposition is species independent. *Journal of the American Society of Nephrology* **12**, 252–260.

Knebelmann, B., Deschenes, G., Gros, F., Hors, M. C., Grünfeld, J. P., Tryggvason, K., Gubler, M. C., and Antignac, C. (1992). Substitution of arginine for glycine 325 in the collagen α5(IV) chain associated with X-linked Alport syndrome: characterization of the mutation by direct sequencing of PCR-amplified lymphoblast cDNA fragments. *American Journal of Human Genetics* **51**, 135–142.

Knebelmann, B., Fakhouri, F., and Grunfeld, J. P. (2001). Hereditary nephritis with macrothrombocytopenia: no longer an Alport syndrome variant. *Nephrology, Dialysis, Transplantation* **16**, 1101–1103.

Knebelmann, B. *et al.* (1996). Spectrum of mutations in the COL4A5 collagen gene in X-linked Alport syndrome. *American Journal of Human Genetics* **59**, 1221–1232.

Lemmink, H. H., Mochizuki, T., van den Heuvel, L. P. W. J., Schröder, C. H., Barrientos, A., Monnens, L. A. H., van Oost, B. A., Brunner, H. G., Reeders, S. T., and Smeets, H. J. M. (1994). Mutations in the type IV collagen α3 (COL4A3) gene in autosomal recessive Alport syndrome. *Human Molecular Genetics* **3**, 1269–1273.

Lemmink, H. H., Schroder, C. H., Monnens, L. A., and Smeets, H. J. (1997). The clinical spectrum of type IV collagen mutations. *Human Mutation* **9**, 477–499.

Longo, I. *et al.* (2002). COL4A3/COL4A4 mutations: from familial hematuria to autosomal-dominant or recessive Alport syndrome. *Kidney International* **61** (6), 1947–1956.

Mochizuki, T., Lemmink, H. H., Mariyama, M. Antignac, C., Gubler, M. C., Pirson, Y., Verellen-Dumoulin, C., Chan, B., Schröder, C. H., Smeets, H. J., and Reeders, S. T. (1994). Identification of mutations in the α3(IV) and α4(IV) collagen genes in autosomal recessive Alport syndrome. *Nature Genetics* **8**, 77–81.

Morita, M., White, R. H., Raafat, F., Barnes, J. M., and Standring, D. M. (1988). Glomerular basement membrane thickness in children. A morphometric study. *Pediatric Nephrology* **2** (2), 190–195.

Nakanishi, K., Yoshikawa, N., Iijima, K., Kitagawa, K., Nakamura, H., Ito, H., Yoshioka, K., Kagawa, M., and Sado, Y. (1994). Immunohistochemical study of alpha 1–5 chains of type IV collagen in hereditary nephritis. *Kidney International* **46**, 1413–1421.

Nakazato, H., Hattori, S., Ushijima, T., Matsuura, T., Koitabashi, Y., Takada, T., Yoshioka, K., Edo, F., and Matsuda, I. (1994). Mutations in the COL4A5 gene in Alport syndrome: a possible mutation in primordial germ cells. *Kidney International* **46**, 1307–1314.

Perrin, D., Jungers, P., Grünfeld, J. P., Delons, S., Noël, L. H., and Zenatti, C. (1980). Perimacular changes in Alport's syndrome. *Clinical Nephrology* **13**, 163–167.

Peten, E. *et al.* (1991). Outcome of 30 patients with Alport's syndrome after renal transplantation. *Transplantation* **52**, 823–826.

Piel, C. F., Biava, C. G., and Goodman, J. R. (1982). Glomerular basement membrane attenuation in familial nephritis and 'benign' hematuria. *Journal of Pediatrics* **101**, 358–365.

Piqueras, A. I., White, R. H., Raafat, F., Moghal, N., and Milford, D. V. (1998). Renal biopsy diagnosis in children presenting with haematuria. *Pediatric Nephrology* **12**, 386–391.

Pirson, Y. (1999). Making the diagnosis of Alport's syndrome. *Kidney International* **56**, 760–775.

Plant, K. E., Boye, E., Green, P. M., Vetrie, D., and Flinter, F. A. (2000). Somatic mosaicism associated with a mild Alport syndrome phenotype. *Journal of Medical Genetics* **37**, 238–239.

Pochet, J. M., Bobrie, G., Landais, P., Goldfarb, B., and Grünfeld, J. P. (1989). Renal prognosis in Alport's and related syndromes: influence of the mode of inheritance. *Nephrology, Dialysis, Transplantation* **4**, 1016–1021.

Quérin, S. *et al.* (1986). Linear glomerular IgG fixation in renal allografts: incidence and significance in Alport's syndrome. *Clinical Nephrology* **25**, 134–140.

Rhys, C., Snyers, B., and Pirson, Y. (1997). Recurrent corneal erosion associated with Alport's syndrome. Rapid communication. *Kidney International* **52**, 208–211.

Rogers, P. W., Kurtzman, N. A., Bunn, S. M., Jr., and White, M. G. (1973). Familial benign essential hematuria. *Archives of Internal Medicine* **131**, 257–262.

Saus, J., Wieslander, J., Langeveld, J. P. M., Quinones, S., and Hudson, B. G. (1988). Identification of the Goodpasture antigen as the alpha 3(IV) chain of collagen IV. *Journal of Biological Chemistry* **263**, 11374–11380.

Seri, M. *et al.* (2000). Mutations in MYH9 result in the May-Hegglin anomaly, and Fechtner and Sebastian syndromes. The May-Hegglin/Fechtner Syndrome Consortium. *Nature Genetics* **26**, 103–105.

Sessa, A., Pietrucci, A., Carozzi, S., Torri Tarelli, L., Tazzari, S., Meroni, M., Battini, G., Valente, U., Renieri, A., and De Marchi, A. (1995). Renal transplantation from living donor parents in two brothers with Alport syndrome. Can asymptomatic female carriers of the Alport gene be accepted as kidney donors? *Nephron* **70**, 106–109.

Spear, G. S. and Slusser, R. J. (1972). Alport's syndrome: emphasizing electron microscopic studies of the glomerulus. *American Journal of Pathology* **69**, 213–220.

Streeten, B. W., Robinson, M. R., Wallace, R., and Jones, D. B. (1987). Lens capsule abnormalities in Alport's syndrome. *Archives of Ophthalmology* **105**, 1693–1697.

Teekhasaenee, C., Nimmanit, S., Wutthiphan, S., Vareesangthip, K., Laohapand, T., Malasitr, P., and Ritch, R. (1991). Posterior polymorphous dystrophy and Alport syndrome. *Ophthalmology* **98**, 1207–1215.

Tiebosch, A. T. M. G. *et al.* (1989). Thin-basement-membrane nephropathy in adults with persistent hematuria. *New England Journal of Medicine* **320**, 14–18.

Trachtman, H., Weiss, R. A., Bennett, B., and Greifer, I. (1984). Isolated hematuria in children: indication for a renal biopsy. *Kidney International* **25**, 94–99.

van der Loop, F. T. *et al.* (2000). Autosomal dominant Alport syndrome caused by a COL4A3 splice site mutation. *Kidney International* **58**, 1870–1875.

Yoshikawa, N., Matsuyama, S., Ito, H., Hajikano, H., and Matsuo, T. (1987). Nonfamilial hematuria associated with glomerular basement membrane alterations characteristic of hereditary nephritis: comparison with hereditary nephritis. *Journal of Pediatrics* **111**, 519–524.

Yoshioka, K., Hino, S., Takemura, T., Maki, S., Wieslander, J., Takekoshi, Y., Makino, H., Kagawa, M., Sado, Y., and Kashtan, C. E. (1994). Type IV collagen α5 chain. Normal distribution and abnormalities in X-linked Alport syndrome revealed by monoclonal antibody. *American Journal of Pathology* **144**, 986–996.

Zhou, J., Mochizuki, T., Smeets, H., Antignac, C., Laurila, P., De Paepe, A., Tryggvason, K., and Reeders, S. (1993). Deletion of the paired α5(IV) and α6(IV) collagen genes in an inherited smooth muscle cell tumour. *Science* **261**, 1167–1169.

16.4.2 Fabry disease

A. α-Galactosidase A deficiency

Robert J. Desnick

Fabry disease (also known as Anderson–Fabry disease) is an X-linked recessive inborn error of glycosphingolipid catabolism caused by the deficient activity of the lysosomal enzyme, α-galactosidase A (α-Gal A) (Desnick *et al.* 2001; EC 3.2.1.22) (Fig. 1). The enzymatic defect in this lysosomal storage disease results in the progressive systemic accumulation of neutral glycosphingolipids with terminal α-linked galactosyl moieties, predominately globotriaosylceramide (GL-3). In classically affected males who have little, if any, α-Gal A activity, the glycosphingolipid deposition occurs primarily in the lysosomes of vascular endothelial cells (Fig. 2) and in the plasma, as well as in the lysosomes of epithelial, perithelial, and smooth muscle cells throughout the body. The major early clinical manifestations of the disease in classically affected males include angiokeratoma, acroparesthesias, hypohidrosis, and corneal and lenticular changes (Desnick *et al.* 2001). With advancing age, progressive GL-3 accumulation in the microvasculature results in renal, cardiovascular, and cerebrovascular disease in the third to fifth decades of life, leading to premature demise.

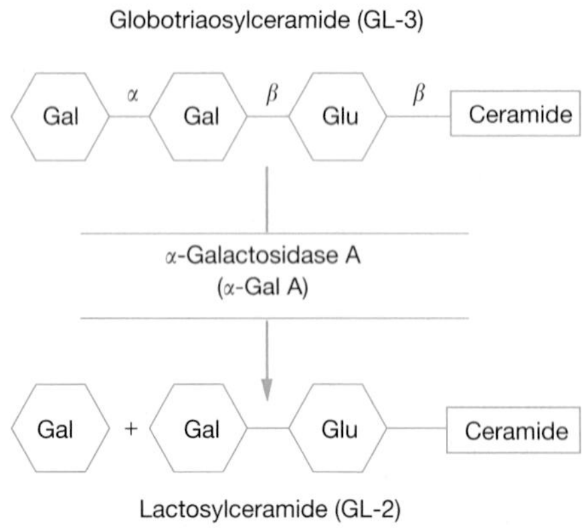

The spectrum of the disease phenotype has been expanded with the recent recognition of 'cardiac' and 'renal' variants who have residual α-Gal A activity, usually due to missense mutations (von Scheidt *et al.* 1991; Nakao *et al.* 1995, 2003; Desnick *et al.* 2001). Males with the 'cardiac' variant phenotype do not manifest the classical disease signs and symptoms (i.e. acroparesthesias, angiokeratoma, hypohidrosis, or corneal/lenticular lesions), and present in the fifth to eighth decades of life with left ventricular hypertrophy, mitral insufficiency and/or cardiomyopathy, and mild to moderate proteinuria with normal renal function for age. They have very low, but sufficient, residual α-Gal A activity to preclude the vascular endothelial glycosphingolipid deposits that are the pathological hallmark of the classical disease phenotype (von Scheidt *et al.* 1991; Desnick *et al.* 2001). 'Renal variants', who were previously diagnosed as having glomerulonephritis or unclassified endstage renal disease, have been identified recently in dialysis clinics (Nakao *et al.* 2003). These variants develop endstage renal failure, but lack the corneal/lenticular lesions angiokeratoma and/or acroparesthesias that usually signal the diagnosis of Fabry disease.

Until recently, the treatment of Fabry disease has been non-specific and directed to the palliative management of disease complications. Now, after extensive preclinical (Ioannou *et al.* 2001) and clinical studies

Globotriaosylceramide (GL-3)

α-Galactosidase A
(α-Gal A)

Lactosylceramide (GL-2)

Fig. 1 The metabolic defect in Fabry disease. The deficient α-galactosidase A activity leads to the accumulation of glycosphingolipids with terminal α-linked galactosyl moieties, including globotriaosylceramide (GL-3), galabiosylceramide, and blood group B substances.

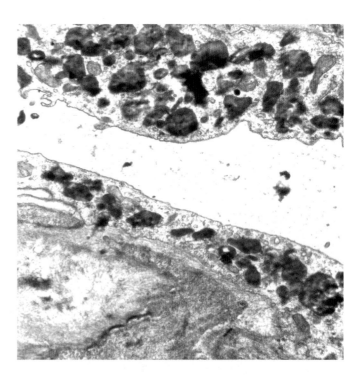

Fig. 2 Electron micrograph of a section of an arteriole from a classically affected male, showing the marked accumulation of concentric lamellar inclusions in the lysosomes of the vascular endothelium. The progressive lysosomal deposition of the glycosphingolipid substrate leads to the narrowing and eventual occlusion of the vascular lumen.

(Schiffmann *et al.* 2000, 2001; Eng *et al.* 2001a,b), the safety and efficacy of recombinant human α-Gal A replacement therapy has been demonstrated. In this review, the clinical, pathological, biochemical and molecular findings in classically affected and variant patients are described, with special emphasis on the renal involvement. In addition, the effectiveness of renal replacement and recombinant enzyme replacement therapy are presented.

The classical disease phenotype

Clinical manifestations in affected males

In classically affected males, who have essentially no α-Gal A activity, the onset of clinical manifestations usually occurs in childhood or adolescence with chronic pain in the extremities (acroparesthesias) periodic crises of severe pain which may last days to weeks the appearance of vascular cutaneous lesions (angiokeratomas), hypohidrosis, and the characteristic corneal and lenticular opacities (Table 1). Progressive glycosphingolipid deposition in the kidney interferes with renal function, resulting in the early onset of proteinuria and the development of azotaemia and renal insufficiency, typically occurring in the third to fifth decades of life. With maturity, most classically affected males experience cardiovascular and/or cerebrovascular disease including myocardial ischaemia and infarctions, transient ischaemic attacks, and/or strokes in middle age. The progressive vascular involvement is a major cause of morbidity and mortality, particularly after treatment of the renal insufficiency by chronic dialysis or transplantation. Each of the major manifestations is discussed briefly below.

Pain (acroparesthesias)

Episodic crises of agonizing, burning pain in the distal extremities most often begin in childhood or early adolescence and signal clinical onset of the disease. These crises typically last from minutes to several days and usually are triggered by exercise, fatigue, emotional stress, or rapid changes in temperature and humidity. Often, the pain will radiate to the proximal extremities and other parts of the body. Attacks of abdominal or flank pain may simulate appendicitis or renal colic. With increasing age, the crises usually decrease in frequency and severity; however, in some patients, they may occur more often, and the pain can be so excruciating and incapacitating that the patient may contemplate suicide. Because the pain usually is associated with a low-grade fever and an elevated erythrocyte sedimentation rate, these symptoms frequently have led to the misdiagnosis of rheumatic fever, neurosis, or erythromelalgia. The acroparesthesias presumably result from glycosphingolipid deposition in the microvasculature that supplies blood to the peripheral nerve cells. The endothelial glycosphingolipid accumulation narrows the vascular lumen and vessel spasms or frank infarction cause the excruciating pain.

Angiokeratoma and hypohidrosis

Angiokeratomas appear as clusters of individual punctate, dark red to blue-black angiectases in the superficial layers of the skin, and are often one of the earliest manifestations of Fabry disease (Fig. 3). The number and size of these cutaneous vascular lesions progressively increase with age. The lesions may be flat or slightly raised and do not blanch with pressure. There is a slight hyperkeratosis notable in larger lesions. The clusters of lesions are most dense between the umbilicus and the knees, most commonly involve the hips, back, thighs, buttocks, penis, and scrotum, and have a tendency toward bilateral symmetry. However, there may be a wide variation in the distribution pattern and density of the lesions. The oral mucosa, conjunctiva, and other mucosal areas are commonly involved. Classically affected patients without any or with only a few isolated skin lesions have been reported. Although the angiectases may not be readily apparent in some patients, careful examination of the skin, especially the scrotum and umbilicus, may reveal the presence of isolated lesions. In addition to these vascular

Table 1 Fabry disease: major manifestations in classical and variant patients

Manifestation	Classical type	'Renal variant'	'Cardiac variant'
Age at onset	4–8 years	>25 years	>40 years
Average age of death	41 years	??	>60 years
Angiokeratoma	++	−/+	−
Acroparesthesias	++	−/+	−
Hypohidrosis/ anhidrosis	++	−/+	−
Corneal/lenticular opacity	+	−/+	−
Heart	LVH/ischaemia/MI	LVH	LVH/myopathy
Brain	TIA/strokes	?	−
Kidney	Proteinuria Renal failure	Proteinuria Renal failure	Mild proteinuria
Residual α-Gal A activity	<1%	>1%	>1%

LVH, left ventricular hypertrophy; MI, myocardial infarction; TIA, transient ischaemic attack; +, present; −, absent.

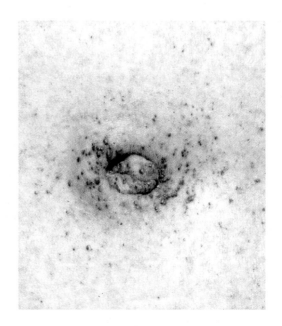

Fig. 3 Clusters of dark-red to blue angiokeratomas (telangiectases) in the umbilical area of a hemizygote with Fabry disease.

lesions, anhidrosis, or more commonly hypohidrosis, is an early and almost constant finding.

Renal involvement (Fig. 4)

The progressive glycosphingolipid accumulation in the kidney interferes with renal function, resulting in azotaemia and renal insufficiency. During childhood and adolescence, protein, casts, red cells, and birefringent lipid globules with characteristic 'Maltese crosses' can be observed in the urinary sediment. Proteinuria, isosthenuria, and a gradual deterioration of tubular reabsorption, secretion, and excretion (Tsakiris *et al.* 1996) occur with advancing age. Polyuria and a syndrome similar to vasopressin-resistant diabetes insipidus occasionally develop. Gradual deterioration of renal function and the development of azotaemia usually occur in the third to fifth decades of life (Branton *et al.* 2002), although renal failure has been reported in the second decade. Death most often results from uraemia, unless chronic haemodialysis or renal transplantation is undertaken. The mean age at death of affected males who were not treated for uraemia was 41 years in one series (Colombi *et al.* 1967), but occasionally a classically affected male has survived into his sixties. With haemodialysis and transplantation, the average age of death was extended about a decade (MacDermot *et al.* 2001a).

Cardiac and cerebrovascular manifestations

Most classically affected males develop cardiovascular and/or cerebrovascular disease in middle age. The progressive vascular involvement is a major cause of morbidity and mortality, particularly after treatment of the renal insufficiency by chronic dialysis or transplantation. Left ventricular enlargement, valvular involvement, and conduction abnormalities are early findings. Mitral insufficiency may be present in childhood or adolescence. Dysrhythmias such as ST segment changes, T-wave inversion, intermittent supraventricular tachycardias, and a short PR interval may be due to infiltration of the conduction system. Myocardial deposition may cause left ventricular hypertrophy. Echocardiographic studies demonstrate an increased incidence of mitral valve prolapse and an increased thickness of the interventricular

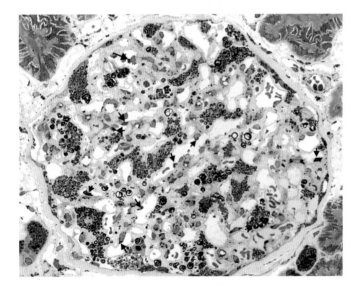

Fig. 4 Photomicrograph of a section of kidney from an affected man with Fabry disease, showing concentric lamellar inclusions within lysosomes.

septum and the left ventricular posterior wall (Desnick *et al.* 2001). In addition, hypertrophic obstructive cardiomyopathy secondary to glycosphingolipid infiltration in the interventricular septum has been reported. Hypertension, angina pectoris, myocardial ischaemia and infarction, congestive heart failure, and severe mitral regurgitation are late signs. Cerebrovascular manifestations result primarily from multifocal small vessel involvement and may include thromboses, transient ischaemic attacks, basilar artery ischaemia and aneurysm, seizures, haemiplegia, haemianaesthesia, aphasia, labyrinthine disorders, or frank cerebral haemorrhage.

Ocular features

The cornea, lens, conjunctiva, and retina all may be involved. A characteristic corneal opacity, observed only by slit-lamp microscopy, is found in classically affected males and most female carriers, and is typically absent in cardiac and renal variants. The earliest corneal lesion is a diffuse haziness in the subepithelial layer. With time, the opacities appear as whorled streaks extending from a central vortex to the periphery of the cornea. Typically, the whorl-like opacities are inferior and cream-coloured; however, they range from white to golden-brown and may be very faint. Lenticular changes include a granular anterior capsular or subcapsular deposit seen in about 30 per cent of affected males, and a unique, possibly pathognomonic, lenticular opacity (the 'Fabry cataract'). The cataracts, which are best observed by retroillumination, are whitish, spoke-like deposits of fine granular material on or near the posterior lens capsule. These lines usually radiate from the central part of the posterior cortex. These lesions do not interfere with visual acuity. Aneurysmal dilatation and tortuosity of conjuctival and retinal vessels also occur.

Other clinical features

In addition to the major clinical features described above, classically affected males may have gastrointestinal, auditory, pulmonary, and other manifestations. Glycosphingolipid deposition in intestinal small vessels and in the autonomic ganglia of the bowel may cause episodic diarrhoea, nausea, vomiting, flank pain, and/or intestinal malabsorption. Achalasia and jejunal diverticulosis, which may lead to perforation of the small bowel, have been described. Radiographic studies may reveal thickened, oedematous colonic folds, mild dilatation of the small bowel, a granular-appearing ileum, and the loss of haustral markings throughout the colon. Hearing difficulties and vestibular abnormalities have been described. In addition, several patients have had pulmonary involvement, which manifested clinically as chronic bronchitis, wheezing, or dyspnoea. Pulmonary function studies may show a mild obstructive component, and primary pulmonary involvement has been reported in the absence of cardiac or renal disease. Pitting oedema of the lower extremities may be present in adulthood in the absence of hypoproteinaemia, varices, or other clinically significant vascular disease. It is thought to be caused by the progressive glycosphingolipid deposition in the lymphatic vessels and lymph nodes. Varicosities, haemorrhoids, and priapism also have been reported.

Clinical manifestations in classic phenotype carrier females

Due to random X-inactivation, markedly variable expression is expected in females heterozygous for X-linked diseases (Desnick *et al.* 2001; MacDermot *et al.* 2001b). Most carriers experience little difficulty in adult life at ages when affected males have severe renal, cardiac, and/or cerebrovascular involvement. However, carriers can manifest symptoms of the disease in an attenuated or milder form. About 70–80 per cent of carriers have the whorl-like corneal dystrophy, many have a few, isolated angiokeratomas, and at least 30 per cent have acroparesthesias, particularly during childhood or adolescence. Most female carriers live a normal lifespan and do not develop azotaemia or renal failure. In late maturity, some carriers develop cardiac involvement.

In contrast, rare female carriers of Fabry disease (<1 per cent of carriers) have been described with clinical manifestations as severe as those of classically affected hemizygous males, including the development of renal failure. However, obligate carriers (i.e. daughters of affected hemizygous males) without any clinical manifestations and with normal levels of leucocyte α-Gal A and urinary sediment glycosphingolipids also have been reported (Desnick et al. 2001).

The cardiac variant phenotype

Clinical manifestations

Affected males with residual α-Gal A activity have been described who were essentially asymptomatic during most of their lives and did not experience the classical disease manifestations including acroparesthesias, angiokeratomas, hypohidrosis, and corneal and lenticular opacities (e.g. Elleder et al. 1990; von Scheidt et al. 1991; Nakao et al. 1995). These variants had cardiomegaly, typically involving the left ventricular wall and interventricular septum, and electrocardiographic abnormalities consistent with a cardiomyopathy. Others had hypertrophic cardiomyopathy and conduction abnormalities. These patients also had mild to moderate proteinuria as their only renal manifestation (Desnick et al. 2001) (Table 1). The frequency of the cardiac variant has been estimated to be up to 3 per cent of patients presenting with left ventricular hypertrophy (Nakao et al. 1995), and up to 6 per cent of patients 40 years or older who have hypertrophic cardiomyopathy (Sachdev et al. 2002). The clinical manifestations in obligate carriers for the cardiac variant have not been delineated. Of note, histological and ultrastructural examination of the endomyocardium, skin and other non-renal tissues from males with the cardiac variant phenotype has consistently shown the absence of the vascular endothelial glycosphingolipid deposits that are the pathological hallmark of the classical disease phenotype (Elleder et al. 1990; von Scheidt et al. 1991; Nakao et al. 1995).

The recently identified 'renal variant'

Clinical manifestations

Renal variants for Fabry disease were identified recently among Japanese chronic haemodialysis patients whose endstage renal disease had been misdiagnosed as chronic glomerulonephritis (Nakao et al. 2003). These patients had absent or low plasma α-Gal A activity, and subsequent DNA analysis identified specific α-Gal A missense mutations in each patient. Of note, five of the six patients did not have angiokeratoma, acroparesthesias, hypohidrosis, or corneal opacities, but did have moderate to severe left ventricular hypertrophy (Table 1). Only one of the patients had a renal biopsy which was examined under light microscopy. In such endstage kidneys, ultrastructural examination may be required to clearly make a morphological diagnosis of Fabry disease. These observations indicated that the early symptoms of classical Fabry

disease may not occur in these variant patients who develop renal insufficiency, and that this variant form of the disease may be under diagnosed among renal dialysis and transplant patients.

Renal variants can be readily detected by determining the plasma α-Gal A activity of male chronic haemodialysis and transplanted patients, especially those diagnosed with chronic glomerulonephritis, hypertension, or unknown causes of renal failure. This is important since these patients are likely to develop vascular disease of the heart or brain which can be treated by enzyme replacement therapy. In addition, detection of renal variants will permit family studies to identify other affected relatives before they progress to renal failure, and will facilitate early intervention, including enzyme replacement therapy (see below).

Renal pathology

In classically affected Fabry patients, birefringent crystalline glycosphingolipid deposits are found in the lysosomes of endothelial, perithelial, and smooth-muscle cells of blood vessels and, to a lesser degree, in histiocytic and reticular cells of connective tissue. Lipid deposits are also prominent in epithelial cells of the cornea, in glomeruli and tubules of the kidney, in muscle fibres of the heart, and in ganglion cells of the autonomic system.

In the kidney, the earliest lesions are due to the accumulation of glycosphingolipids in endothelial and epithelial cells of the glomerulus and of Bowman's space and in the epithelium of the loops of Henle and of distal tubules. In later stages, and to a lesser extent, proximal tubules, interstitial histiocytes, and fibrocytes may show lipid accumulation. Lipid-laden distal tubular epithelial cells desquamate and may be detected in the urinary sediment (Desnick et al. 1971). These cells have been shown to account for about 75 per cent of the urinary cells shed by a classically affected male.

Concurrently, renal blood vessels are involved progressively, and often, extensively. An early finding is arterial fibrinoid deposits, which may result from the necrosis of severely involved muscular cells (Gubler et al. 1978). Other histological changes in the kidney are the sequelae of nonspecific, endstage renal disease with evidence of severe arteriolar sclerosis, glomerular atrophy and fibrosis, pseudotubular proliferation of residual glomerular epithelium, tubular atrophy, and diffuse interstitial fibrosis. Kidney size increases during the third decade of life, followed by a decrease in the fourth and fifth decades. The renal involvement has been the subject of a recent review (Branton et al. 2002). In males with the cardiac variant phenotype, glycosphingolipid deposition has been documented in the lysosomes of myocytes and podocytes (Meehan et al. 2003). Renal biopsies have revealed little, if any, glycosphingolipid deposition in the vascular endothelium, mesangial cells, or interstitial cells. Vascular endothelial involvement has been notably absent (Elleder et al. 1990; von Scheidt et al. 1991; Meehan et al. 2003).

To date, little information is available on the renal manifestations or pathology of the renal variant. Only one patient, a 51-year-old male, had a renal biopsy for proteinuria and that biopsy was interpreted as chronic glomerulonephritis by light microscopy. When examined retrospectively by electron microscopy, the characteristic lysosomal pathology was evident, even in the endstage kidney. Thus, it is likely that the renal manifestations and pathology of the renal variant are similar, if not essentially the same, as those of the classical phenotype described above (Nakao et al. 2003).

The metabolic and molecular defects

Fabry disease is caused by the deficient activity of the lysosomal enzyme, α-Gal A, which leads to the progressive accumulation of GL-3 and related glycosphingolipids with terminal α-galactosyl moieties including galabiosylceramide and the blood group B glycolipids. Classically affected males have essentially no α-Gal A activity, while cardiac and renal variants have residual activity ($>$1 per cent of mean normal activity in cultured cells), consistent with the attenuation or absence of the characteristic clinical manifestations (Desnick et al. 2001).

The full-length cDNA and entire genomic sequence encoding human α-Gal A have been isolated, sequenced (Bishop et al. 1986; Kornreich et al. 1989), and localized to the chromosomal region, Xq22.1. To date, over 300 α-Gal A mutations causing Fabry disease have been reported (Human Gene Mutation Database, http//archive.uwcmac.uk/uwcm/mg/hgmd0.html). Classically affected males had a variety of mutations, including large and small gene rearrangements, splicing defects, and missense or nonsense mutations (e.g. Ashton-Prolla et al. 2000; Germain et al. 2002; Shabbeer et al. 2002). In contrast, most cardiac and renal variants had missense mutations which expressed residual α-Gal A activity (e.g. von Scheidt et al. 1991; Nakao et al. 1995; Ashton-Prolla et al. 2000; Ishii et al. 2002; Sachdev et al. 2002; Nakao et al. 2003). Of note, the N215S mutation was found in several unrelated cardiac variants.

Most mutations have been private, occurring only in single pedigrees. However, mutations at CpG dinucleotides have been found in unrelated families of different ethnic or geographic backgrounds. Haplotype analysis of mutant alleles that occurred in two or more families revealed that those with rare novel alleles were probably related, whereas those with mutations involving CpG dinucleotide 'hot spots' were not (Ashton-Prolla et al. 2000).

Efforts to establish genotype–phenotype correlations have been limited since most Fabry patients have private mutations, and attempts to predict the phenotype requires more extensive clinical information from unrelated patients with the same genotype. Of interest, three missense mutations (R112H, R301Q, and G328R) have been identified in patients with the classical disease and the cardiac variant phenotypes, suggesting that other modifying factors are involved in disease expression (Ashton-Prolla et al. 2000).

Diagnosis

Fabry disease should be considered in males and females with periodic crises of severe pain in the extremities (acroparesthesias), the appearance of vascular cutaneous lesions (angiokeratomas), hypohidrosis, characteristic corneal and lenticular opacities, strokes, cardiac involvement, or renal insufficiency of unknown aetiology. Affected males can be reliably diagnosed by the demonstration of markedly deficient α-Gal A activity in plasma, isolated leucocytes, and/or cultured cells (Desnick et al. 1973a). Classically affected males have essentially no α-Gal A activity, while cardiac and renal variants have residual activity ($>$1 per cent of mean normal activity). Identification of a mutation in the patient's α-Gal A gene confirms the diagnosis of Fabry disease.

Carrier females for the classic or variant phenotypes have markedly variable α-Gal A activities because of random X-chromosomal inactivation and, therefore, measurement of plasma and/or leucocyte α-Gal A activity may be misleading. For example, some obligate carriers (daughters of classically affected males) may have α-Gal A levels ranging from normal to very low activities similar to those of affected males. Many carrier females (70–80 per cent) have the characteristic corneal dystrophy of Fabry disease (Desnick et al. 2001). Accurate diagnosis of heterozygous females requires demonstration of the specific family mutation in the α-Gal A gene. Such testing is recommended for all at-risk females. Prenatal testing can be performed in chorionic villi or amniocytes using either enzymatic or molecular techniques.

Treatment

Medical management

In young classically affected males, the single most debilitating aspect of the disease is the excruciating pain (Desnick et al. 2001). Numerous drugs have been tried to relieve these agonizing pains. With the exception of centrally acting narcotic analgesics such as morphine, which have been only partially effective, conventional analgesic agents have not been helpful. However, prophylactic administration of low maintenance dosages of diphenylhydantoin has been found to provide relief by reducing the frequency and severity of the periodic crises of excruciating pain and constant discomfort in affected males and carriers. Carbamazepine has similar effects. The combination of these two drugs also may significantly reduce the frequency and severity of the pain. The potential side-effects of gingival hypertrophy with diphenylhydantoin and dose-related autonomic complications with carbamazepine, including urinary retention, nausea, vomiting, and ileus, have been recorded. Recently, gabapentin (neurontin) has been used to prevent pain, but long-term experience will determine its effectiveness (Desnick et al. 2001).

Care of patients with regard to cardiac, pulmonary, and cerebrovascular manifestations remains nonspecific and symptomatic. Obstructive lung disease has been documented in older affected males and carriers, with more severe impairment in smokers; therefore, patients should be discouraged from smoking. Patients with reversible obstructive airway disease may benefit from bronchodilation therapy. Prophylactic oral anticoagulants are recommended for stroke-prone patients.

Dialysis and renal transplantation

Since renal insufficiency is the most frequent and serious late complication in classically affected patients and the renal variants, chronic haemodialysis and/or renal transplantation have become life-extending procedures. In the United States Renal Data System (USRDS), there were 42 patients with Fabry disease on dialysis between 1995 and 1998 (Thadhani et al. 2002), while the European Renal Association–European Dialysis and Transplantation Association (ERA–EDTA) identified 83 Fabry patients who began dialysis between 1987 and 1993 (Tsakiris et al. 1996). The frequencies of patients with Fabry disease in the USRDS and ERA–EDTA were 0.0167 and 0.0188 per cent, respectively. Of note, female carriers who developed renal insufficiency accounted for 12 per cent of the Fabry patients in both the American and European studies. The mean age at which Fabry patients started renal replacement therapy was 42 and 38 years in the USRDS and ERA–EDTA studies, respectively. Similar 3 year survival rates for Fabry patients on dialysis, 63 and 60 per cent, were reported in the USRDS ($n = 95$, 1985–1993) and ERA–EDTA ($n = 83$, 1987–1993) studies. In the US study, the survival rate for Fabry patients (63 per cent) was higher than that for diabetic controls (53 per cent), but lower than that for non-diabetic controls (74 per cent). Cardiovascular complications (48 per cent) and cachexia (17 per cent) were the main causes of death. The 3-year survival data for the 42 USRDS Fabry patients who started dialysis from 1995 to 1998 improved: 70 per cent for Fabry patients, 76 per cent for non-diabetic controls, and 40 per cent for diabetic controls.

The first renal transplant in a patient with Fabry disease was performed in 1967. Recent reviews of the registries of the ERA–EDTA (Tsakiris *et al.* 1996) and the USRDS (Ojo *et al.* 2000) support excellent outcomes for renal transplantation in Fabry disease. For example, during the 10 year period from 1988 to 1998, the 93 transplanted Fabry patients reported to the US registry had an equivalent, if not better, 5-year patient (82 versus 83 per cent) and graft (67 versus 75 per cent) survival than a matched control group with the usual nephropathies (Ojo *et al.* 2000). Also, immune function in Fabry affected males has been shown to be similar to that in other uraemic patients, obviating any immunological contraindication to transplantation in this disease (Donati *et al.* 1984).

Successful transplantation corrects renal function, and the engrafted kidney will remain histologically free of glycosphingolipid deposition (e.g. Bannwart 1982) since the normal α-Gal A activity in the allograft will catabolize endogenous renal glycosphingolipid substrates. Rare, isolated glycosphingolipid deposits have been detected in endothelial cells of transplanted cadaveric kidneys by electron microscopy as small myelin figures (e.g. Faraggiana *et al.* 1981; Friedlaender *et al.* 1987). These cells were derived from the recipient and were α-Gal A deficient (Sinclair 1972). The presence of glycosphingolipid was demonstrated in some cells of the allograft in a patient who expired following acute rejection. This recipient was cross-reacting immunological material (CRIM)-negative for the enzyme protein and developed anti-α-Gal A antibodies, which apparently inhibited the endogenous α-Gal A activity and resulted in GL-3 accumulation (Faraggiana *et al.* 1981).

Importantly, transplantation of kidneys from Fabry carriers should be avoided as they already may contain significant substrate deposition. In one reported case, transplantation of an allograft from a carrier to an affected male relative resulted in decreased renal function 5 years later (serum creatinine, 3.0 mg/dl) (Popli *et al.* 1987). Therefore, all potential related donors must be carefully evaluated so that affected males, and carrier females for the Fabry gene are excluded. Since carriers may have low normal to normal α-Gal A activities due to random X-inactivation, it is necessary to demonstrate the absence of the recipient's α-Gal A gene mutation or haplotype in potential female donors.

In addition to treatment of the renal failure, kidney transplantation has been undertaken to determine if the allograft could provide normal α-Gal A for systemic substrate metabolism (Desnick *et al.* 1972). Hypothetically, the normal kidney might metabolize the accumulated substrate by uptake and catabolism within the allograft and/or by the release of the active enzyme into the circulation for uptake and metabolism in other tissues, such as the vascular endothelium. Although biochemical and/or clinical improvement initially was reported (e.g. Desnick *et al.* 1972, 1973b), no clear biochemical effect could be demonstrated (Clarke *et al.* 1972; Grunfeld *et al.* 1975).

Of note, patients with successful engraftment who survived for 10–15 years have expired from complications of vascular disease, for example (Kramer *et al.* 1985) or other unrelated causes. Thus, renal allografts are not effective in altering the rate of progressive systemic substrate accumulation, and patients with allografts should benefit from enzyme replacement therapy to prevent the late cardiac and cerebrovascular complications of the disease.

Enzyme replacement therapy

Over 100 patients with classic Fabry disease participated in recent clinical trials of enzyme replacement therapy using recombinant human α-Gal A produced by two different companies (Schiffmann *et al.* 2000, 2001; Eng *et al.* 2001a,b). A recent study comparing the structural and kinetic properties as well as the cell uptake and *in vivo* pharmacokinetics and biodistribution of the two preparations agalsidase alfa (Replagal™ Transkaryotic Therapies, Inc.) and agalsidase beta (Fabrazyme®, Genzyme Corp.), found that the proteins were essentially the same with comparable glycosylation, specific activities, and *in vivo* pharmacokinetics and biodistribution in the mouse model (Lee *et al.* 2002). Thus, the trials can be taken together as a body of evidence supporting the efficacy of enzyme replacement therapy in Fabry disease.

Phase 1 and 1/2 clinical trials

A Phase 1 trial involving 10 affected males demonstrated that a single dose (0.007–0.1 mg/kg) of recombinant human α-Gal A (r-hαGalA) could reduce the accumulated GL-3 in the liver and urinary sediment (Schiffmann *et al.* 2000). A Phase 1/2 open-label, dose-escalation trial involving 15 classically affected males evaluated the safety and effectiveness of five doses of r-hαGalA in dose regimens of 0.3, 1.0, or 3.0 mg/kg every 14 days or 1.0 or 3.0 mg/kg every 48 h (Eng *et al.* 2001a). The enzyme was well tolerated, and rapid and marked reductions in plasma and tissue GL-3 were observed biochemically, histologically, and ultrastructurally. Mean GL-3 content decreased 84 per cent in liver ($n = 13$) and was markedly reduced in kidney in four of five patients who had pre- and post-treatment biopsies. GL-3 deposits also were reduced in a dose-dependent manner in the vascular endothelium of the kidney, heart, skin, and liver by light and electron microscopic evaluation. The clearance of plasma GL-3 also was dose-dependent. In addition, patients reported decreased pain, increased ability to perspire, and improved quality of life.

Phase 2 and 3 clinical trials

A single centre, double-blind, placebo-controlled Phase 2 trial of r-hαGalA involved 26 male patients selected for neuropathic pain who received 0.2 mg/kg every 2 weeks for 22 weeks (12 doses) (Schiffmann *et al.* 2001). The primary efficacy endpoint was pain at its worst and pain medication was withdrawn before evaluations. The mean (SE) Brief Pain Inventory neuropathic pain severity score declined from 6.2 (0.46) to 4.3 (0.73) in patients treated with r-hαGalA ($n = 14$) versus no significant change in the placebo group ($n = 12$) ($p = 0.02$). Mean creatinine clearance increased by 2.1 ml/min for patients receiving r-hαGalA versus a decrease of 16.1 ml/min for the patients receiving the placebo ($p = 0.02$). One patient in the placebo group advanced to renal failure. Plasma GL-3 levels decreased approximately 50 per cent in patients treated with r-hαGalA.

A Phase 3 multinational, multicentre, randomized placebo-controlled, double-blind study evaluated the safety and effectiveness of r-hαGalA in of 58 patients who received 1 mg/kg of r-hαGalA or placebo every 2 weeks for 20 weeks (11 doses) (Eng *et al.* 2001b). The primary efficacy endpoint was the percentage of patients whose renal capillary endothelial GL-3 deposits cleared to normal or near normal (Fig. 5). Also evaluated were the histological clearance of microvascular endothelial GL-3 deposits in the heart and skin, changes in pain (Short Form McGill Pain Questionnaire), and in quality of life (Short Form-36 Health Status Survey). In this study, 20 of 29 r-hαGalA-treated patients (69 per cent) cleared the accumulated GL-3 from the renal capillary endothelium versus 0 of 29 placebo-treated patients ($p < 0.001$). Compared to the placebo group, r-hαGalA-treated patients also had markedly decreased microvascular endothelial GL-3 in the skin ($p < 0.001$) and heart ($p < 0.001$). Patients receiving r-hαGalA cleared the accumulated GL-3 in plasma to non-detectable levels. Pain and quality of life assessments improved in both treatment groups in comparison to baseline, indistinguishable from a 'placebo effect'. Note that patients in this study were not selected for pain nor were pain medications discontinued during treatment.

All 58 patients who completed the Phase 3 trial received r-hαGalA in an extension study. After 6 months of the open-label therapy, all 22 former placebo and 20 of 21 r-hαGalA-treated patients (42 of 43; 98 per cent) who had optional biopsies achieved or maintained normal or near normal renal capillary endothelial histology. Similar results were observed for skin capillary endothelium; 96 per cent of both former placebo patients (22 of 23) and of r-hαGalA patients (23 of 24) who had optional biopsies achieved normal or near normal histology. In the capillary endothelium of the heart, histology scores improved with duration of treatment. Among patients who had optional heart biopsies, 14 of 17 (82 per cent) of the r-hαGalA patients (12 months of treatment) attained normal or near normal histology versus 10 of the 15 (67 per cent) former placebo patients (6 months of treatment). Also, the accumulated plasma GL-3 in the former placebo group decreased to non-detectable levels after 6 months of r-hαGalA.

Treatment with r-hαGalA was well tolerated; the adverse event incidence and profiles were similar for both treatment groups in the Phase 3 trial, except for mild to moderate infusion reactions to r-hαGalA, which were managed conservatively. While IgG seroconversion occurred in 51 of 58 r-hαGalA-treated patients, GL-3 clearance was not impaired, and titres decreased with continued treatment.

More recent experience has demonstrated that enzyme replacement stabilized deteriorating renal function (De Schoenmakere *et al.* 2003), and improved cardiac function (Waldek 2003; Weidemann *et al.* 2003), peripheral nerve and sweat function (Schiffmann *et al.* 2003), and quality of life (Guffon and Fouilhoux, in press).

In summary, enzyme replacement with α-Gal A has been shown to safely reverse the pathogenesis of the major clinical manifestations, to decrease pain, and to stabilize renal function in patients with Fabry disease. The European Agency for Evaluation of Medical Products approved the treatment in 2003 (both preparations) and the US Food and Drug Administration approved Fabrazyme in 2003.

Studies are underway to determine the long-term clinical benefit of enzyme replacement therapy. Recently, a group of physicians expert in Fabry disease recommended that all affected males and carriers with substantial manifestations should be treated, with treatment being initiated as early as possible to prevent disease manifestations (Desnick *et al.* 2003). Clearly, replacement therapy should be initiated early, prior to evidence of renal impairment. In patients who have early renal compromise, treatment with adequate doses may prevent, stabilize or retard progression. Patients on renal replacement therapy should receive enzyme to prevent the late cardiac and cerbrovascular complications of Fabry disease. Early experience with enzyme replacement therapy suggests that patients on haemodialysis can be infused with the high molecular enzyme during dialysis.

Future directions

The past two decades have witnessed remarkable advances in the understanding, diagnosis, and treatment of Fabry disease. The cloning of the α-Gal A gene has facilitated accurate diagnosis, especially for carrier females, and the production of recombinant enzyme for replacement therapy. Experience with enzyme replacement will determine its

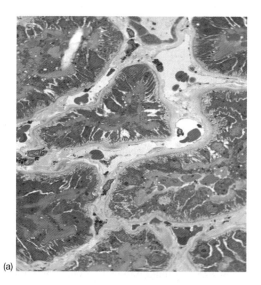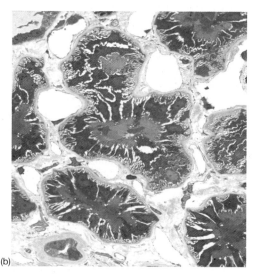

(a)   (b)

Fig. 5 Paired photomicrographs of the renal cortex pretreatment (a) and post-treatment (b) from a patient who received 11 treatments of r-hαGalA in the double-blind study (Eng *et al.* 2001b). Pretreatment the intertubular capillaries demonstrate numerous GL-3 inclusions meeting the criteria for a score = 3. Post-treatment the capillary endothelium has been cleared of GL-3 inclusions resulting in a score = 0.

therapeutic effectiveness for the prevention, reversal or stabilization of the renal disease, which is the major morbid aspect of this X-linked nephropathy. Future efforts are directed at preclinical evaluation of various gene therapy strategies for Fabry disease (Ziegler *et al.* 1999, 2002, 2004; Qin *et al.* 2001; Li *et al.* 2002; Park *et al.* 2003) but these studies remain exploratory. In addition, the use of specific small molecules that act as 'pharmacologic chaperones' and rescue and enhance the activity of mutant α-Gal A enzymes with residual activity may provide effective oral therapy in the future for responsive patients (Fan *et al.* 1999; Frustaci *et al.* 2001; Desnick and Schuchman 2002).

Acknowledgements

Professor Robert Desnick thanks Kenneth H. Astrin for his assistance with this manuscript. This work was supported in part by grants from the National Institutes of Health including a research grant (R37 DK 34045 Merit Award), a grant (5 MO1 RR00071) for the Mount Sinai General Clinical Research Center Program from the National Center of Research Resources, a grant (5 P30 HD28822) for the Mount Sinai Child Health Research Center, and a research grant from the Genzyme Corporation.

B. Other inherited metabolic storage disorders with significant renal involvement

Stephen H. Morgan and
Jean-Pierre Grünfeld

Glucose 6-phosphatase deficiency (Von Gierke's disease—glycogen storage disease type I)

The glycogen storage disorders primarily affect the liver, heart, and muscle. To date, more than 10 distinct metabolic lesions are known to produce this group of diseases (Howell and Williams 1983). Primary renal involvement only occurs in glycogen storage disease type I, although some of the other glycogenoses may indirectly cause renal damage by the development of myoglobinuria (Talente *et al.* 1994). The classification of the glycogenoses are attributed to Cori and Cori (1952), who recognized that the storage disorder described earlier by Von Gierke (1929) was due to a deficiency of the hepatic enzyme glucose 6-phosphatase (EC 3.1.3).

Clinical features of Von Gierke's disease

From early childhood onwards, patients inheriting this autosomal recessive disorder are of short stature, although normally proportioned. There is prominent abdominal enlargement due to massive hepatomegaly and the skeletal musculature is 'flabby' and poorly developed.

Pronounced hypoglycaemia may precipitate convulsions in childhood. Later, cutaneous xanthomas may be found on extensor surfaces, and discrete bilateral symmetrical yellow perimacular lesions may be observed at ophthalmoscopy. Low-grade hypoglycaemia in adolescence and adult life may present a more chronic problem in terms of concentration and cognitive function. Quantitative platelet dysfunction has been described, and this may cause a troublesome bleeding diathesis.

Renal involvement in Von Gierke's disease

Deficient activity of glucose 6-phosphatase in proximal and distal convoluted tubules results in glycogen accumulation within the kidney and progressive renal enlargement (Reitsman-Beirens *et al.* 1992), although this is masked clinically by the gross hepatosplenomegaly. Histologically, tubular cells become vacuolated and biochemically there is a Fanconi-like syndrome with aminoaciduria, glycosuria, and phosphaturia (Garty *et al.* 1974). Renal insufficiency has previously not been considered a major problem in Von Gierke's disease, but progressive renal failure may occur as a result of focal segmental glomerulosclerosis (Chen *et al.* 1988). Recent reviews highlight the heterogeneity of renal disease in this disorder, including amyloidosis which reoccurred in a renal allograft in one patient (Chen and VanHove 1995). Hyperuricaemia, the cause of which is unclear, but which is not necessarily due to uric acid overproduction, may result in the development of a hyperuricaemic nephropathy as well as acute or chronic 'gouty' syndromes (Howell 1965). Uric acid urinary calculi are rare.

Management

The diagnosis of Von Gierke's disease is made by enzyme analysis performed on tissue taken at liver biopsy. There is no specific treatment, but frequent high carbohydrate meals may correct the metabolic abnormalities (Greene *et al.* 1979). Glucose metabolism is not improved by renal transplantation (Emmett and Narins 1978). The use of allopurinol is rational, but theoretically could be complicated by the development of xanthine stones. Hepatic adenomas may develop, and these can be detailed by ultrasonography; malignant change in these lesions should not be overlooked. In the case of proteinuria, angiotensin-converting enzyme (ACE) inhibitors may be used, as in other glomerular diseases. Hepatocyte transplantation has been performed in a patient and may be an alternative to liver transplantation (Muraca *et al.* 2002).

Familial lecithin–cholesterol acyltransferase deficiency

An unusual disease due to deficient activity of the enzyme lecithin–cholesterol acyltransferase (LCAT-phosphatidylcholine: sterol acyltransferase, EC 2.3.1.43) was first described in a Scandinavian family in 1967 (Norum and Gjone 1967). Although many subsequently documented cases are also from Scandinavia, patients with this disease have been identified in Europe and, indeed, within the United Kingdom (Bron *et al.* 1975). In normal individuals, this enzyme plays an important role in lipoprotein metabolism; it is synthesized in the liver and secreted into the plasma compartment, where it catalyzes the transfer of a fatty acid from the 2-position of lecithin to the 3'-hydroxyl group of cholesterol, to form a cholesterol ester (Fig. 1).

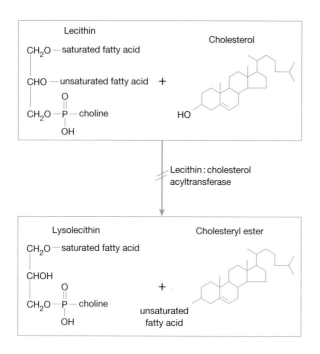

Fig. 1 The metabolic defect in lecithin–cholesterol acyltransferase deficiency.

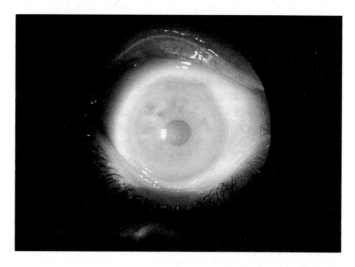

Fig. 2 Corneal changes in lecithin–cholesterol acyltransferase deficiency (by courtesy of E. Gjone).

There is considerable clinical and biochemical heterogeneity within the disease produced by deficiency of LCAT (Norum *et al.* 1989), which causes gross changes in serum lipoprotein structure and in lipid and apolipoprotein composition. In particular, high levels of low density lipoprotein may be generated, causing glomerular capillary endothelial damage.

Clinical features of lecithin–cholesterol acyltransferase deficiency

Corneal opacities (Fig. 2), composed of numerous minute greyish dots throughout the stroma, causing a 'misty' appearance, are detectable from early childhood. The density of these deposits increases towards the limbus, producing a 'pseudo-arcus'. A normochromic normocytic anaemia develops towards the second decade due to low-grade haemolysis as a result of phospholipid abnormalities in the red cell membrane. A reduction in compensatory erythropoiesis contributes to this. The lipid and lipoprotein abnormalities lead to premature diffuse arteriosclerosis, and calcification may be noted in vessel walls before the fourth decade. Neurological abnormalities, organomegaly, and cutaneous lesions, such as xanthomas, have not been described.

Renal involvement in lecithin–cholesterol acyltransferase deficiency

Proteinuria and hyaline casts are found early in life, but renal insufficiency is rarely noted before the fourth decade. Its onset, usually accompanied by hypertension, may be unpredictable and rapid (Gjone 1974). Histologically, foam cells are present in glomerular tufts and there is intimal proliferation and narrowing of the arteriolar lumen. On electron microscopy, capillary lumens may be filled with a meshwork of membranes and particles with an amorphous mottled structure.

There is irregular thickening of basal lamina, often with fusion of endothelial foot processes (Hovig and Gjone 1973).

Genetics of lecithin–cholesterol acyltransferase deficiency

To date, some 30 patients with this disease have been described within 15 families from a variety of geographical locations. Obligate heterozygotes have normal serum lipoprotein levels and no clinical features. They do, however, have half the normal circulating levels of LCAT (Albers *et al.* 1981, 1982). Most studies suggest an autosomal recessive mode of inheritance, and the clustering of cases in Scandinavia may be due to inbreeding. Family linkage studies initially suggest that the enzyme locus is close to the β-haptoglobin gene on the long arm of chromosome 16 (Teisberg and Gjone 1974). A cDNA encoding human LCAT has been cloned, and the structural gene has been mapped to 16q22 (Azoulay 1987). Early linkage studies using a cDNA did not identify any mutations within the structural gene in families with this enzyme deficiency (Humphries *et al.* 1988), but more recently many have been described (Gotada *et al.* 1991; Hill *et al.* 1993; Klein *et al.* 1993).

Management

A low dietary fat intake is recommended to reduce levels of nephrotoxic low-density lipoproteins, although the efficacy of this would be difficult to confirm. The role of blood transfusion and plasma exchange are likewise controversial. Lipid and lipoprotein abnormalities are not reversed by renal transplantation and plasma LCAT activity is not increased. Early reaccumulation of lipid in allografts has been described (Flatmark *et al.* 1977; Myhre *et al.* 1977). Hepatic transplantation has, to the author's knowledge, not been used in the treatment of this disease.

Other inherited storage diseases

Glomerular changes have been observed rarely in other metabolic disorders, such as in Gaucher's disease, where renal involvement is rare and occurs mostly after splenectomy (Smith *et al.* 1978; Chander *et al.* 1979; Faraggiana and Churg 1987). In a patient with Gaucher's disease and nephrotic syndrome, proteinuria virtually disappeared in association with specific enzyme therapy (Santoro *et al.* 2002). In Refsum's disease, where a lack of phytanic acid β-hydroxylase leads to plasma and tissue accumulation of phytanic acid, renal tubular changes usually predominate (Pabico *et al.* 1981; D'Agrosa *et al.* 1988), as is also the case in nephrosialidosis (Maroteaux *et al.* 1978) and in other rare inherited renal lipidoses (reviewed by Faraggiana and Churg 1987). There are also several other storage diseases which appear quite unique (Doitchinov 1988; Newsom *et al.* 1988).

Lipoprotein glomerulopathy is a newly recognized renal disease, first described in Japan in 1989 by Saito (see reference in Saito *et al.* 2002). So far, 32 cases have been reported from different countries, mainly from Japan. The disease is characterized by thrombus-like lipoproteins in the glomerular capillaries and abnormal lipid profiles similar to those of type III hyperlipoproteinaemia. Most patients present with nephrotic syndrome. Half of them progressed to renal failure. The disease recurs in transplanted kidneys. Systemic manifestations of lipidoses (such as corneal arcus or xanthomas) are rarely observed. The disease has been shown to be associated with apoE mutations. A mouse model of the disease has been developed (Saito *et al.* 2002).

References

Albers, J. J., Chen, C. H., and Adolphson, J. (1981). Familial lecithin–cholesterol acyltransferase deficiency. Identification of heterozygotes with half normal enzyme activity. *Human Genetics* **58**, 306–319.

Albers, J. J., Chen, C.-H., Adolphson, J., Sakuma, M., Kodama, T., and Akanuma, Y. (1982). Familial lecithin cholesterol acyltransferase deficiency in a Japanese family: evidence for functionally defective enzyme in homozygotes and obligate heterozygotes. *Human Genetics* **62**, 82–85.

Ashton-Prolla, P., Tong, B., Astrin, K. H., Shabbeer, J., Eng, C. M., and Desnick, R. J. (2000). Twenty-two novel mutations in the α-galactosidase A gene and genotype/phenotype correlations including mild hemizygotes and severely affected heterozygotes. *Journal of Investigative Medicine* **48**, 227–235.

Azoulay, M. (1987). The structural gene for lecithin: cholesterol acyltransferase maps to human chromosome 16q22. *Annals of Human Genetics* **51**, 129–136.

Bannwart, F. (1982). Fabry's disease. Light and electron microscopic cardiac findings 12 years after successful kidney transplantation. *Schweizer Medisinische Wochenschrift* **112**, 1742–1747.

Bishop, D. F., Calhoun, D. H., Bernstein, H. S., Hantzopoulos, P., Quinn, M., and Desnick, R. J. (1986). Human α-galactosidase A: nucleotide sequence of a cDNA clone encoding the mature enzyme. *Proceedings of the National Academy of Sciences USA* **83**, 4859–4863.

Branton, M. H. *et al.* (2002). Natural history of Fabry renal disease: influence of α-galactosidase A activity and genetic mutations on clinical course. *Medicine (Baltimore)* **81**, 122–138.

Bron, A. F., Lloyd, J. K., Fosbrooke, A. S., Winder, A. F., and Tripathy, R. C. (1975). Primary lecithin: cholesterol acyltransferase deficiency disease. *Lancet* **i**, 928–989.

Chander, P. J., Nurse, H. M., and Pirani, C. L. (1979). Renal involvement in adult Gaucher's disease after splenectomy. *Archives of Pathology and Laboratory Medicine* **103**, 440–445.

Chen, Y. T. and VanHove, J. L. K. (1995). Renal involvement in type I glycogen storage disease. *Advances in Nephrology* **24**, 357–365.

Chen, Y. T., Coleman, R. A., Scheiman, J. J., Kolbeck, P. C., and Sidbury, J. B. (1988). Renal disease in type 1 glycogen storage disease. *New England Journal of Medicine* **318**, 7–11.

Clarke, J. T., Guttmann, R. D., Wolfe, L. S., Beaudoin, J. G., and Morehouse, D. D. (1972). Enzyme replacement therapy by renal allotransplantation in Fabry's disease. *New England Journal of Medicine* **287**, 1215–1218.

Colombi, A., Kostyal, A., Bracher, R., Gloor, F., Mazzi, R., and Tholen, H. (1967). Angiokeratoma corporis diffusum—Fabry's disease. *Helvetica Medica Acta* **34**, 67–83.

Cori, G. T. and Cori, C. F. (1952). Glucose-6-phosphatase of the liver in glycogen storage disease. *Journal of Biology and Chemistry* **199**, 661–667.

D'Agrosa, M.-C. *et al.* (1988). Le rein dans la maladie de Refsum. Etude clinique, histologique et ultrastructurale d'une observation. *Nephrologie* **9**, 169–172.

De Schoenmakere, G., Chauveau, D., and Grunfeld, J. P. (2003). Enzyme replacement therapy in Anderson–Fabry's disease: beneficial clinical effect on vital organ function. *Nephrology, Dialysis, Transplantation* **18**, 33–35.

Desnick, R. J. and Schuchman, E. H. (2002). Enzyme replacement and enhancement therapies: lessons from lysosomal disorders. *Nature Reviews. Genetics* **3**, 954–966.

Desnick, R. J., Allen, K. Y., Desnick, S. J., Raman, M. K., Bernlohr, R. W., and Krivit, W. (1973a). Fabry's disease: enzymatic diagnosis of hemizygotes and heterozygotes. α-Galactosidase activities in plasma, serum, urine, and leukocytes. *Journal of Laboratory and Clinical Medicine* **81**, 157–171.

Desnick, R. J. *et al.* (1973b). Fabry disease: correction of the enzymatic deficiency by renal transplantation. *Birth Defects Original Article Series* **9**, 88–96.

Desnick, R. J., Brady, R., Barranger, J., Collins, A. J., Germain, D. P., Goldman, M., Grabowski, G., Packman, S., and Wilcox, W. R. (2003). Fabry disease, an under-recognized multisystemic disorder: expert recommendations for diagnosis, management, and enzyme replacement therapy. *Annals of Internal Medicine* **138**, 338–346.

Desnick, R. J., Dawson, G., Desnick, S. J., Sweeley, C. C., and Krivit, W. (1971). Diagnosis of glycosphingolipidoses by urinary-sediment analysis. *New England Journal of Medicine* **284**, 739–744.

Desnick, R. J., Ioannou, Y. A., and Eng, C. M. α-Galactosidase A deficiency: Fabry disease. In *The Metabolic and Molecular Bases of Inherited Disease* 8th edn. (ed C. R. Scriver, A. L. Beaudet, W. S. Sly, D. Valle, K. E. Kinzler, and B. Vogelstein), pp. 3733–3774. New York: McGraw-Hill, 2001.

Desnick, R. J. *et al.* (1972). Correction of enzymatic deficiencies by renal transplantation: Fabry's disease. *Surgery* **72**, 203–211.

Doitchinov, D. (1988). Lipidose glomérulaire mésangiale avec accumulation de cholestérol. Une nouvelle maladie héréditaire. *Nephrologie* **9**, 273–276.

Donati, D. *et al.* (1984). Immune function and renal transplantation in Fabry's disease. *Proceedings of the European Dialysis and Transplantation Association* **21**, 686.

Elleder, M. *et al.* (1990). Cardiocyte storage and hypertrophy as a sole manifestation of Fabry's disease. Report on a case simulating hypertrophic non-obstructive cardiomyopathy. *Virchows Archiv. A Pathological Anatomy and Histopathology* **417**, 449–455.

Emmett, M. and Narins, R. G. (1978). Renal transplantation in Type I glycogenosis: failure to improve glucose metabolism. *Journal of the American Medical Association* **239**, 1642–1644.

Eng, C. M. *et al.* (2001a). A phase 1/2 clinical trial of enzyme replacement in Fabry disease: pharmacokinetic, substrate clearance, and safety studies. *American Journal of Human Genetics* **68**, 711–722.

Eng, C. M. *et al.* (2001b). Safety and efficacy of recombinant human α-galactosidase A replacement therapy in Fabry's disease. *New England Journal of Medicine* **345**, 9–16.

Fan, J. Q., Ishii, S., Asano, N., and Suzuki, Y. (1999). Accelerated transport and maturation of lysosomal α-galactosidase A in Fabry lymphoblasts by an enzyme inhibitor. *Nature Medicine* **5**, 112–115.

Faraggiana, T. and Churg, J. (1987). Renal lipidoses: a review. *Human Pathology* **18**, 661–679.

Faraggiana, T. *et al.* (1981). Light- and electron-microscopic histochemistry of Fabry's disease. *American Journal of Pathology* **103**, 247–262.

Friedlaender, M. M. *et al.* (1987). Renal biopsy in Fabry's disease eight years after successful renal transplantation. *Clinical Nephrology* **27**, 206–211.

Frustaci, A., Chimenti, C., Ricci, R., Natale, L., Russo, M. A., Pieroni, M., Eng, C. M., and Desnick, R. J. (2001). Improvement in cardiac function in the cardiac variant of Fabry's disease with galactose-infusion therapy. *New England Journal of Medicine* **345**, 25–32.

Flatmark, A. L., Hovig, T., Myhre, E., and Gjone, E. (1977). Renal transplantation in patients with familial lecithin: cholesterol acyltransferase deficiency. *Transplantation Proceedings* **9**, 1665–1671.

Garty, R., Cooper, M., and Tabachnick, E. (1974). The Fanconi syndrome associated with hepatic glycogenosis and abnormal metabolism of galactose. *Journal of Paediatrics* **85**, 821–824.

Germain, D. P., Shabbeer, J., Cotigny, S., and Desnick, R. J. (2002). Fabry disease: twenty novel α-galactosidase A mutations and genotype–phenotype correlations in classical and variant phenotypes. *Molecular Medicine* **8**, 308–315.

Gjone, E. (1974). Familial lecithin: cholesterol acyltransferase deficiency: a clinical survey. *Scandinavian Journal of Clinical and Laboratory Investigation* **33** (Suppl. 137), 73.

Gotada, T. *et al.* (1991). Differential phenotypic expression by three mutant alleles in familial lecithin: cholesterol acyltransferase deficiency. *Lancet* **338**, 778–781.

Greene, H. L., Slonim, A. E., and Burr, I. M. (1979). Type I glycogen storage disease: a metabolic basis for advances in treatment. *Advances in Paediatrics* **26**, 63–92.

Grunfeld, J. P., Le Porrier, M., Droz, D., Bensaude, I., Hinglais, N., and Crosnier, J. (1975). Renal transplantation in patients suffering from Fabry's disease. Kidney transplantation from a heterozygote subject to a subject without Fabry's disease. *Nouvelle Presse Medecine* **4**, 2081–2085.

Gubler, M. C., Lenoir, G., Grunfeld, J. P., Ulmann, A., Droz, D., and Habib, R. (1978). Early renal changes in hemizygous and heterozygous patients with Fabry's disease. *Kidney International* **13**, 223–235.

Guffon, N. and Fouilhoux, A. Clinical benefit in Fabry patients given enzyme replacement therapy—a case series. *Journal of Inherited Metabolic Disease* (in press).

Hill, J. J., Wang, X., and Pritchard, P. H. (1993). Recombinant lecithin–cholesterol acyltransferase containing Thr123 to Ile mutation esterifies cholesterol in low density lipoprotein but not in high density lipoprotein. *Journal of Lipid Research* **34**, 81–88.

Hovig, T. and Gjone, E. (1973). Familial cholesterol: acyltransferase deficiency: ultrastructural aspects of a new syndrome with particular reference to lesions in the kidney and spleen. *Acta Pathologica et Microbiologica Scandinavica* **81**, 681–697.

Howell, R. R. (1965). The interrelationship of glycogen storage disease and gout. *Arthritis and Rheumatism* **8**, 789–795.

Howell, R. R. and Williams, J. C. The glycogen storage diseases. In *The Metabolic Basis of Inherited Disease* (ed. J. B. Stanbury, J. B. Wyngaarden, D. S. Fredrickson, J. L. Goldstein, and M. S. Brown), pp. 141–166. New York: McGraw-Hill, 1983.

Ioannou, Y. A., Zeidner, K. M., Gordon, R. E., and Desnick, R. J. (2001). Fabry disease: preclinical studies demonstrate the effectiveness of α-galactosidase A replacement in enzyme-deficient mice. *American Journal of Human Genetics* **68**, 14–25.

Ishii, S., Nakao, S., Minamikawa-Tachino, R., Desnick, R. J., and Fan, J. Q. (2002). Alternative splicing in the α-galactosidase A gene: increased exon inclusion results in the Fabry cardiac phenotype. *American Journal of Human Genetics* **70**, 994–1002.

Klein, H.-G. *et al.* (1993). Fish eye syndrome: a molecular defect in the lecithin–cholesterol acyltransferase gene associated with normal alpha LCAT specific activity. *Journal of Clinical Investigation* **92**, 479–488.

Kornreich, R., Desnick, R. J., and Bishop, D. F. (1989). Nucleotide sequence of the human α-galactosidase A gene. *Nucleic Acids Research* **17**, 3301–3302.

Kramer, W., Thormann, J., Mueller, K., and Frenzel, H. (1985). Progressive cardiac involvement by Fabry's disease despite successful renal allotransplantation. *International Journal of Cardiology* **7**, 72–75.

Lee, K., Jin, X., Zhang, K., Copertino, L., Andrews, L., Baker-Malcolm, J., Geagan, L., Qiu, H., Seiger, K., Barngrover, D., McPherson, J. M., and Edmunds, T. (2003). A biochemical and pharmacological comparison of enzyme replacement therapies for the glycolipid storage disorder Fabry disease. *Glycobiology* **13**, 305–313.

Li, C. *et al.* (2002). Adenovirus-transduced lung as a portal for delivering α-galactosidase A into systemic circulation for Fabry disease. *Molecular Therapy* **5**, 745–754.

MacDermot, K. D., Holmes, A., and Miners, A. H. (2001a). Anderson–Fabry disease: clinical manifestations and impact of disease in a cohort of 98 hemizygous males. *Journal of Medical Genetics* **38**, 750–760.

MacDermot, K. D., Holmes, A., and Miners, A. H. (2001b). Anderson–Fabry disease: clinical manifestations and impact of disease in a cohort of 60 obligate carrier females. *Journal of Medical Genetics* **38**, 769–775.

Maroteaux, P., Humbel, R., Strecker, G., Michalski, J. C., and Mande, R. (1978). Un nouveau type de sialidose avec atteinte rénale: la néphrosialidose. *Archives Françaises de Pédiatrie* **35**, 819–829.

Meehan, S. M., Junsanto, T., Rydel, J. J., and Desnick, R. J. (2004). Fabry disease: renal involvement limited to podocyte pathology and proteinuria in a septuagenarian cardiac variant. Pathologic and therapeutic implications. *American Journal of Kidney Diseases* **43**, 164–171.

Muraca, M. *et al.* (2002). Hepatocyte transplantation as a treatment for glycogen storage disease type 1a. *Lancet* **359**, 317–318.

Myhre, E., Gjone, E., Flatmark, A., and Hovig, T. (1977). Renal failure in familial lecithin–cholesterol acyltransferase deficiency. *Nephron* **18**, 239–248.

Nakao, S., Kodama, C., Takenaka, T., Tanaka, A., Yasumoto, Y., Yoshida, A., Kanzaki, T., Enriquez, A. L. D., Eng, C. E., Tanaka, H., Tei, C., and Desnick, R. J. (2003). Fabry disease: detection of undiagnosed hemodialysis patients and identification of a 'renal variant' phenotype. *Kidney International* **64**, 801–807.

Nakao, S. *et al.* (1995). An atypical variant of Fabry's disease in men with left ventricular hypertrophy. *New England Journal of Medicine* **333**, 288–293.

Newsom, G. D., Stanbaugh, G. H., Kurtzman, N. A., Brady, R. O., Gal, A. E., and Vorstad, J. (1988). Nephrotic syndrome and renal failure associated with a novel glycolipid disorder. *American Journal of Nephrology* **8**, 316–321.

Norum, K. R. and Gjone, E. (1967). Familial plasma lecithin–cholesterol acyltransferase deficiency. Biochemical study of a new inborn error metabolism. *Scandinavian Journal of Clinical and Laboratory Investigation* **20**, 231–243.

Norum, K. R., Gjone, E., and Glomset, J. A. Familial lecithin–cholesterol acyltransferase deficiency including 'fish eye' disease. In *The Metabolic Basis of Inherited Disease* 6th edn. (ed. C. R. Scriver, A. L. Beaudet, W. S. Sly, and D. Valle), pp. 1181–1194. New York: McGraw-Hill, 1989.

Ojo, A. *et al.* (2000). Excellent outcome of renal transplantation in patients with Fabry's disease. *Transplantation* **69**, 2337–2339.

Pabico, R. C. *et al.* (1981). Renal involvement in Refsum's disease. *American Journal of Medicine* **70**, 1136–1143.

Park, J., Murray, G. J., Limaye, A., Quirk, J. M., Gelderman, M. P., Brady, R. O., and Qasba, P. (2003). Long-term correction of globotriaosylceramide storage in Fabry mice by recombinant adeno-associated virus-mediated gene transfer. *Proceedings of the National Academy of Sciences USA* **100**, 3450–3454.

Popli, S. *et al.* (1987). Involvement of renal allograft by Fabry's disease. *American Journal of Nephrology* **7**, 316–318.

Qin, G. *et al.* (2001). Preselective gene therapy for Fabry disease. *Proceedings of the National Academy of Sciences USA* **98**, 3428–3433.

Reitsman-Beirens, W. C. C., Smit, G. P. A., and Troelstra, J. A. (1992). Renal function and kidney size in glycogen storage disease type I. *Paediatric Nephrology* **6**, 236–238.

Sachdev, B. *et al.* (2002). Prevalence of Anderson–Fabry disease in male patients with late onset hypertrophic cardiomyopathy. *Circulation* **105**, 1407–1411.

Saito, T., Ishigaki, Y., Oikawa, S., and Yamamoto, T. T. (2002). Etiological significance of apolipoprotein E mutations in lipoprotein glomerulopathy. *Trends in Cardiovascular Medicine* **12**, 67–70.

Santoro, D., Rosenbloom, B. E., and Cohen, A. H. (2002). Gaucher disease with nephrotic syndrome: response to enzyme replacement therapy. *American Journal of Kidney Diseases* **40**, E1–E5.

Schiffmann, R., Floeter, M. K., Dambrosia, J. M., Gupta, S., Moore, D. F., Sharabi, Y., Khurana, R. K., and Brady, R. O. (2003). Enzyme replacement therapy improves peripheral nerve and sweat function in Fabry disease. *Muscle Nerve* **28**, 703–710.

Schiffmann, R. *et al.* (2000). Infusion of α-galactosidase A reduces tissue globotriaosylceramide storage in patients with Fabry disease. *Proceedings of the National Academy of Sciences USA* **97**, 365–370.

Schiffmann, R. *et al.* (2001). Enzyme replacement therapy in Fabry disease: a randomized controlled trial. *Journal of the American Medical Association* **285**, 2743–2749.

Shabbeer, J., Yasuda, M., Lucas, M., and Desncik, R. J. (2002). Fabry disease: 45 novel mutations in the α-galactosidase a gene causing the classical phenotype. *Molecular Genetics and Metabolism* **76**, 23–30.

Sinclair, R. (1972). Origin of endothelium in human renal allograft. *British Medical Journal* **11**, 15–16.

Smith, R. R. L., Hutchins, G. M., Sack, G. H., Jr., and Ridolfi, R. L. (1978). Unusual cardiac, renal and pulmonary involvement in Gaucher's disease. Interstitial glucocerebroside pulmonary hypertension and fatal bone marrow embolization. *American Journal of Medicine* **65**, 352–360.

Talente, G. M. *et al.* (1994). Glycogen storage disease in adults. *Annals of Internal Medicine* **120**, 218–226.

Teisberg, P. and Gjone, E. (1974). The lecithin: cholesterol acyltransferase deficiency locus in man: probable linkage to the alpha haptoglobin locus on chromosome 16. *Nature* **249**, 550–551.

Thadhani, R. *et al.* (2002). Patients with Fabry disease on dialysis in the United States. *Kidney International* **61**, 249–255.

Tsakiris, D. *et al.* (1996). Report on management of renal failure in Europe, XXVI, 1995. Rare diseases in renal replacement therapy in the ERA–EDTA Registry. *Nephrology, Dialysis, Transplantation* **11** (Suppl. 7), 4–20.

Von Gierke, E. (1929). Hepato-nephromegalia Glykogenia (Glykogenspeicherkrankheit der Leber und Nieren). *Beiträge zur Pathologischen Anatomie und Allgemeinen Pathologie* **82**, 497–513.

von Scheidt, W. *et al.* (1991). An atypical variant of Fabry's disease with manifestations confined to the myocardium. *New England Journal of Medicine* **324**, 395–399.

Waldek, S. (2003). PR interval and the response to enzyme-replacement therapy for Fabry's disease. *New England Journal of Medicine* **348**, 1186–1187.

Weidemann, F., Breunig, F., Beer, M., Sandstede, J., Turschner, O., Voelker, W., Ertl, G., Knoll, A., Wanner, C., and Strotmann, J. M. (2003). Improvement of cardiac function during enzyme replacement therapy in patients with Fabry disease: a prospective strain rate imaging study. *Circulation* **108**, 1299–1301.

Ziegler, R. J., Li, C., Cherry, M., Zhu, Y., Hempel, D., Van Rooijen, N., Ioannou, Y. A., Desnick, R. J., Goldberg, M. A., Yew, N. S., and Cheng, S. H. (2002). Correction of the nonlinear dose response improves the viability of adenoviral vectors for gene therapy of Fabry disease. *Human Gene Therapy* **13**, 935–945.

Ziegler, R. J., Lonning, S. M., Armentano, D., Li, C., Souza, D. W., Cherry, M., Ford, C., Barbon, C. M., Desnick, R. J., Gao, G., Wilson, J. M., Peluso, R., Godwin, S., Carter, B. J., Gregory, R. J., Wadsworth, S. C., and Cheng, S. H. (2004). AAV2 vector harboring a liver-restricted promoter facilitates sustained expression of therapeutic levels of alpha-galactosidase A and the induction of immune tolerance in Fabry mice. *Molecular Therapy* **9**, 231–240.

Ziegler, R. J. *et al.* (1999). Correction of enzymatic and lysosomal storage defects in Fabry mice by adenovirus-mediated gene transfer. *Human Gene Therapy* **10**, 1667–1682.

16.4.3 Nail-patella syndrome and other rare inherited disorders with glomerular involvement

Guillaume Bobrie and Jean-Pierre Grünfeld

Nail-patella syndrome

The nail-patella syndrome (NPS) (or hereditary osteo-onychodysplasia) is an autosomal dominant condition characterized by nail dysplasia, patellar hypoplasia or aplasia, elbow and iliac abnormalities, and nephropathy. Renal disease is not found in all affected families. When present, nephropathy may represent the most serious complication of this syndrome.

Renal involvement

For unknown reason, renal disease is not always present in patients with NPS. Among some 500 observations of NPS reviewed by Meyrier *et al.* (1990), renal disease occurred in 20 per cent. When the study is limited to families with nephropathy, renal disease occurred in approximately 48 per cent of the subjects with osteo-onychodysplasia (Looij *et al.* 1988). Renal disease is asymptomatic with moderate proteinuria for many years, occasionally with nephrotic syndrome (Bennett *et al.* 1973), or associated with microhaematuria. Progression to endstage renal failure occurred in 15 (Meyrier *et al.* 1990) to 29 per cent of the patients at the age of 33 ± 18 years (mean $\pm$ SD) (Looij *et al.* 1988).

Renal glomerular changes seen on light microscopy are non-specific, with varying degrees of focal and segmental sclerosis, hypercellularity, and thickening of peripheral capillary loops. A characteristic lesion of the glomerular basement membrane has been identified by electron microscopy (Silverman *et al.* 1967; Del Pozo and Lapp 1970; Ben-Bassat *et al.* 1971) and consists of areas of rarefaction, containing bundles of fibrillar type III collagen (Fig. 1). In the review of Meyrier *et al.* (1990), this lesion was constant. The extent of these abnormalities does not correlate with clinical findings, and the tubular basement membrane is not affected. Immunofluorescence has shown discontinuous fixation of anti-IgM antiserum along the glomerular basement membrane (Hoyer *et al.* 1972; Bennett *et al.* 1973) or granular and diffuse fixation (Browning *et al.* 1988). As indicated in Table 1, the ultrastructural lesion has been documented in patients with NPS who had no or slight urinary abnormalities and who belonged to families with or without nephropathy. Surprisingly, this lesion was found in a woman without clinical renal disease, belonging to a family without nephropathy (Silverman *et al.* 1967). Conversely (and as expected), ultrastructure was normal in an unaffected subject from an affected family (Bennett *et al.* 1973). The exact significance of the ultrastructural lesion is therefore not clear.

The pathogenesis of the ultrastructural lesions is probably due to abnormal maturation of collagen or entrapment of collagen precursors within the glomerular basement membrane. Gubler *et al.* (unpublished observations) have detected abnormal distribution of type VI collagen using immunofluorescence techniques, and have suggested that the biochemical composition of the glomerular basement membrane is abnormal. Binding of monoclonal antibodies directed against glomerular basement membrane has been found to be either normal or absent

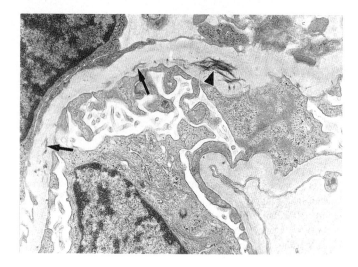

Fig. 1 Hereditary osteo-onychodysplasia (electron microscopy 11,890×). There is irregular thickening of the glomerular basement membrane and isolated (arrowhead) or grouped fibrils (arrows); by courtesy of Drs M.C. Gubler and L.H. Noël; reproduced with permission from Grünfeld, J.-P., ed. *Advances in Nephrology* Vol. 18, pp. 77–94. Chicago: Year Book, 1989.

Table 1 Relationships between the ultrastructural glomerular basement membrane lesion and clinical features in nail-patella syndrome

Families	Patients	Ultrastructural glomerular basement membrane lesion	Series
HOOD+/N+	HOOD+/N+	+	Hoyer et al. (1972) Bennett et al. (1973)
	HOOD+/N−	+	Bennett et al. (1973) (1 case)
	HOOD+/N−	−	Bennett et al. (1973) (1 case)
HOOD+/N−	HOOD+/N−	+	Silverman et al. (1967) (1 case)
HOOD+/N−	HOOD+/N−	+	Taguchi et al. (1998) (1 case)
HOOD−/N+	HOOD+/N+	+	Dombros and Katz (1982) Sabnis et al. (1980)

(as in some Alport patients; Chapter 16.4.1) (Noël *et al.* 1989; Sutcliffe *et al.* 1989). Development of Goodpasture's syndrome in a patient with NPS indicated that, in this case, the corresponding antigen was not altered (Curtis *et al.* 1976). No antiglomerular basement membrane nephritis has so far been reported after kidney transplantation in these patients.

NPS is an autosomal dominant trait, caused by mutations in LMX1B (see infra), encoding an LIM homeodomain transcription factor (Dreyer *et al.* 1998). Lmx1b (−/−) mice show skeletal defects reflecting a disruption of normal dorsoventral patterning of the limb during development, and renal disease, reminiscent of that found in NPS (Chen *et al.* 1998). In these mice, glomerular development in general and the differentiation of podocytes in particular were severely impaired (Miner *et al.* 2002; Rohr *et al.* 2002). Podocytes have reduced number of foot processes and lack typical slit diaphragms. Expression of collagen IV α3 and α4 chains, and podocin was severely reduced whereas expression of nephrin and GBM laminins was preserved (Morello *et al.* 2001; Miner *et al.* 2002; Roh *et al.* 2002). Thus, LMX1B in humans, as lmx1b in mice, is probably involved in the regulation of the expression of multiple genes critical for podocyte differentiation and function.

No osteo-onychodysplasia was found in seven families (Sabnis *et al.* 1980; Dombros and Katz 1982; Gubler *et al.* 1990) and autosomal recessive inheritance was suggested in two of them. Gubler *et al.* (1990) studied eight patients with this form of the disease and showed that it differs from NPS. Collagen fibres were demonstrated by electron microscopy not only within the internal part of the glomerular basement membrane, but also in the mesangial areas. Renal disease developed early in life and was severe, associated with chronic haemolytic anaemia or pulmonary disease in most children. The anomaly in biochemical composition of the glomerular basement membrane may be different from that found in NPS, and may also involve some extrarenal basement membranes (Gubler *et al.* 1990).

Other renal abnormalities described in isolated patients with NPS include membranous nephropathy (Mackay *et al.* 1985), IgA glomerular deposits (Gubler *et al.* 1978), and urinary tract malformations (Silverman *et al.* 1967; Bennett *et al.* 1973; Browning *et al.* 1988).

Osteo-onychodysplasia

The classic tetrad of osteo-onychodysplasia includes ungueal dystrophy, patellar hypoplasia or aplasia, elbow dysplasia, and iliac horns.

Nail dysplasia is the most frequent finding (93–98 per cent of cases) and is present at birth. It predominates on the hands, and is bilateral and symmetrical. Ungueal aplasia may be found, but there is often only moderate hypoplasia, involving the distal and cubital parts of the nail, and particularly affecting the thumb and the index finger.

Patellar dysplasia (approximately 92 per cent of cases) may range from aplasia to hypoplasia, often with fragmentation or a polygonal shape of the patella. Condylar abnormalities may also be found and these may lead to patellar luxation.

Elbow dysplasia (90 per cent of cases) consists of deformities of the radial head and distal humeral extremity, and causes subluxation and limited supination and extension.

Iliac horns are found in 30–70 per cent of cases. They develop from the posterior side of the ileum, may be palpated, and are easily detected on pelvic radiography (Fig. 2). Other osteoarticular abnormalities involving the spine, the shoulders, and the wrist have been reported.

Eye defects including abnormal pigmentation of the iris (40 per cent of cases), aniridia, glaucoma, and microcornea, are present in some patients. Cosegregation of NPS with open angle glaucoma has been documented in some families (Lichter *et al.* 1997).

Genetics

Hereditary osteo-onychodysplasia is transmitted as an autosomal dominant trait. The gene locus is linked to the ABO blood group locus

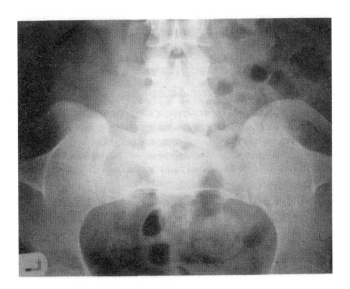

Fig. 2 Pelvic radiograph illustrating iliac horns [courtesy of Drs J.M. Boulton-Jones and C.O.S. Savage; reproduced with permission from *Nephrology, Dialysis, Transplantation* (1989) **4**, 262–265].

focal and segmental glomerulosclerosis in all patients. Electron microscopy of the glomerular basement membrane was normal, in contrast with findings in patients with Alport's syndrome. Half of the patients had sensorineural hearing loss; this is rare in classic Charcot–Marie–Tooth syndrome.

Charcot–Marie–Tooth syndrome is inherited as an autosomal dominant condition, with incomplete penetrance. Only four of the nine patients had a positive family history of nephropathy (Lemieux and Nemeeth 1967; Hanson *et al.* 1970; Gherardi *et al.* 1985). It should be recalled that families with primary glomerular diseases, including focal glomerulosclerosis have been reported (Section 3).

Familial dysautonomia

Familial dysautonomia is a rare, autosomal recessive, neurological disorder due to decreased neuronal numbers in ganglia and diminished axons in peripheral nerves. It predominates in Ashkenazi Jews.

More than 50 per cent of these patients develop renal failure: glomerulosclerosis, associated with glomerular collapse and ischaemic wrinkling of the basement membrane, was the prominent histopathological finding in 10 of the 13 patients studied, all of who were aged less than 33 years. In addition, electron microscopy showed no vessel innervation. Hypotension, impaired rein release, and increased sensitivity to circulating catecholamines could contribute to the renal pathology (Pearson *et al.* 1980).

α1-Antitrypsin deficiency

α1-Antitrypsin deficiency is associated with severe emphysema and liver cirrhosis, and various glomerular changes may also be encountered. Predominantly membranoproliferative glomerulonephritis has been observed in 11 children, while rapidly progressive glomerulonephritis with crescents has been described in three adult patients. This may be associated with disseminated vasculitis, also involving the skin and the colon (Lévy *et al.* 1985; Lewis *et al.* 1985; Lévy 1986). The lack of α1-antitrypsin, a protease involved in the suppression of a number of immunological and inflammatory processes, may facilitate the development of glomerular injury and exaggerate its course (Lewis *et al.* 1985).

Miscellaneous diseases

A familial syndrome characterized by hyalinosis of the small vessel of the kidneys and the digestive tract has been described. Diarrhoea, intestinal bleeding, malabsorption, and protein losing enteropathy are the most prominent features. Retinal ischaemic changes, poikiloderma, early hair greying, cerebral calcification, and subarachnoid haemorrhage due to ruptured cerebral aneurysms are associated abnormalities. Kidney involvement leads to renal failure (Rambaud *et al.* 1986).

Non-specific glomerular changes (including glomerulosclerosis) have been observed in various inherited syndromes, including Bardet–Biedl syndrome, in which renal involvement is a regular finding, and in which glomerular changes with mesangial proliferation and sclerosis are found and may or may not be primary (see Chapter 16.7).

and to the adenylate cyclase locus (Renwick and Lawler 1955; Schleutermann *et al.* 1969), and is assigned to the distal end of the long arm of chromosome 9 (9q34) (McKusik 1988a), between D9S315 and D9S2172 (McIntosh *et al.* 1997). Dreyer *et al.* (1998) demonstrated that NPS is the result of mutations within the LMX1B gene. The great number of loss-of-function mutations suggests that NPS is the result of haploinsufficiency for LMX1B (Clough *et al.* 1999; Hamlington *et al.* 2001). There is a cosegregation of open-angle glaucoma and the NPS (Lichter *et al.* 1997; Vollrath *et al.* 1998).

A large number of families with this syndrome show no renal disease. On the other hand, typical glomerular basement membrane changes have been observed in families with autosomal dominant inheritance without osteo-onychodysplasia (Sabnis *et al.* 1980; Dombros and Katz 1982). The various genetic findings could be explained either by incomplete penetrance of the gene or by the presence of two separate gene defects, one accounting for NPS and the other for nephropathy (McKusik 1988b). The variability of the NPS could be also modulated by the allele contributed by the unaffected parent (Farley *et al.* 1999).

Other rare inherited disorders with glomerular involvement

Charcot–Marie–Tooth syndrome (see Chapters 3.5 and 16.4.4)

This hereditary syndrome is a degenerative neurological disorder, which leads to slowly progressive neuromuscular atrophy. Since 1967, nine patients with this syndrome and renal disease have been reported; renal involvement was revealed by proteinuria and progressed rapidly to endstage renal failure in seven cases. Steroid administration in one patient was ineffective (Hara *et al.* 1984). Two other patients had a more favourable spontaneous course, with partial remission of the nephrotic syndrome in one (Martini *et al.* 1985). Renal biopsy showed

References

Ben-Bassat, M., Cohen, L., and Rosenfeld, J. (1971). The glomerular basement membrane in the nail-patella syndrome. *Archives of Pathology* **92**, 350–355.

Bennett, W. M. *et al.* (1973). The nephropathy of the nail-patella syndrome. *American Journal of Medicine* **54**, 304–319.

Browning, M. C., Weidner, N., and Lorentz, W. B., Jr. (1988). Renal histopathology of the nail-patella syndrome in a two-year-old-boy. *Clinical Nephrology* **29**, 210–213.

Chen, H., Lun, Y., Ovchinnikov, D., Kokubo, H., Oberg, K. C., Pepicelli, C. V., Gan, L., Lee, B., and Johnson, R. L. (1998). Limb and kidney defects in *Lmx1b* mutant mice suggest an involvement of LMX1B in human nail patella syndrome. *Nature Genetics* **19**, 51–55.

Clough, M. V., Hamlington, J. D., and McIntosh, I. (1999). Restricted distribution of loss-of-function mutations within the LMX1B genes of nail-patella syndrome patients. *Human Mutation* **14**, 459–465.

Curtis, J. J., Bhathena, D., Leatch, R. P., Galla, J. H., Lucas, B. A., and Luke, R. G. (1976). Goodpasture's syndrome in a patient with nail-patella syndrome. *American Journal of Medicine* **61**, 401–406.

Del Pozo, E. and Lapp, H. (1970). Ultrastructure of the kidney in the nephropathy of the nail-patella syndrome. *American Journal of Clinical Pathology* **54**, 845–851.

Dombros, N. and Katz, A. (1982). Nail patella-like renal lesions in the absence of skeletal abnormalities. *American Journal of Kidney Diseases* **4**, 237–240.

Dreyer, S. D., Zhou, G., Baldini, A., Winterpacht, A., Zabel, B., Cole, W., Johnson, R. L., and Lee, B. (1998). Mutations in *LMX1B* cause abnormal skeletal patterning and renal dysplasia in nail patella syndrome. *Nature Genetics* **19**, 47–50.

Farley, F. A., Lichter, P. R., Downs, C. A., McIntosh, I., Vollrath, D., and Richards, J. E. (1999). An orthopaedic scoring system for nail-patella syndrome and application to a kindred with variable expressivity and glaucoma. *Journal of Pediatric Orthopaedics* **19**, 624–631.

Gherardi, R., Belghiti-Deprez, D., Hirbec, G., Bouche, P., Weil, B., and Lagrue, G. (1985). Focal glomerulosclerosis associated with Charcot–Marie–Tooth disease. *Nephron* **40**, 357–361.

Gubler, M. C., Levy, M., Loirat, C., and Broyer, M. (1978). Lésions rénales de l'onycho-ostéodystrophie héréditaire. *VII International Congress of Nephrology*, Montreal, Abstract L-11.

Gubler, M. C. *et al.* (1990). Syndrome de 'Nail-Patella' sans atteinte extrarénale. Une nouvelle néphropathie héréditaire glomérulaire. *Annales de Pédiatrie* **2**, 78–82.

Hamlington, J. D., Jones, C., and McIntosh, I. (2001). Twenty-two novel LMX1B mutations identified in nail patella syndrome (NPS) patients. *Human Mutation* **18**, 458.

Hanson, P. A., Farber, R. E., and Armstrong, R. A. (1970). Distal muscle wasting, nephritis and deafness. *Neurology* **20**, 426–434.

Hara, M., Ichida, F., Higuchi, A., Tanizawa, T., and Okada, T. (1984). Nephropathy associated with Charcot–Marie–Tooth disease. *International Journal of Pediatric Nephrology* **5**, 99–102.

Hoyer, J. R., Michael, A. F., and Vernier, R. L. (1972). Renal disease in nail-patella syndrome: clinical and morphologic studies. *Kidney International* **2**, 231–238.

Lemieux, G. and Nemeeh, J. A. (1967). Charcot–Marie–Tooth disease and nephritis. *Canadian Medical Association Journal* **97**, 1193–1198.

Lévy, M. (1986). Severe deficiency of alpha₁-antitrypsin associated with cutaneous vasculitis, rapidly progressive glomerulonephritis, and colitis. *American Journal of Medicine* **81**, 363.

Lévy, M., Gubler, M. C., Hadchouel, M., Niaudet, P., Habib, R., and Odièvre, M. (1985). Déficit en alpha₁-antitrypsine et atteinte rénale. *Néphrologie* **6**, 65–70.

Lewis, M. *et al.* (1985). Severe deficiency of alpha1-antitrypsin associated with cutaneous vasculitis, rapidly progressive glomerulonephritis, and colitis. *American Journal of Medicine* **79**, 489–494.

Lichter, P. R., Richards, J. E., Downs, C. A., Stringham, H. M., Boehnke, M., and Farley, F. A. (1997). Cosegregation of open-angle glaucoma and the nail-patella syndrome. *American Journal of Ophthalmology* **124**, 506–515.

Looij, B. J., Jr., Te Slaa, R. L., Hogewind, B. L., and Van de Kamp, J. J. P. (1988). Genetic counseling in hereditary osteo-onychodysplasia (HOOD, nail-patella syndrome) with nephropathy. *Journal of Medical Genetics* **25**, 682–686.

Mackay, I. G., Doig, A., and Thomson, D. (1985). Membranous nephropathy in patient with nail-patella syndrome nephropathy. *Scottish Medical Journal* **30**, 47–49.

Martini, A., Ravelli, A., and Burgio, G. R. (1985). Focal segmental glomerulo-sclerosis and Charcot–Marie–Tooth disease. *International Journal of Pediatric Nephrology* **6**, 15.

McIntosh, I., Clough, M. V., Schaffer, A. A., Puffenberger, E. G., Horton, V. K., Peters, K., Abbott, M. H., Roig, C. M., Cutone, S., Ozelius, L., Kwiatkowski, D. J., Pyeritz, R. E., Brown, L. J., Pauli, M., McCormick, M. K., and Francomano, C. A. (1997). Fine mapping of the nail-patella syndrome locus at 9q34. *American Journal of Human Genetics* **60**, 133–142.

McKusik, V. A. (1988a). The morbid anatomy of the human genome: a review of gene mapping in the clinical medicine (second of four parts). *Medicine* **66**, 1–63.

McKusik, V. A. *Mendelian Inheritance in Man* 8th edn. Baltimore: The Johns Hopkins University Press, 1988b.

Meyrier, A., Rizzo, R., and Gubler, M. C. (1990). The nail-patella syndrome. A review. *Journal of Nephrology* **2**, 133–140.

Miner, J. H., Morello, R., Andrews, K. L., Li, C., Antignac, C., Shaw, A. S., and Lee, B. (2002). Transcriptional induction of slit diaphragm genes by Lmx1b is required in podocytes differentiation. *Journal of Clinical Investigation* **109**, 1065–1072.

Morello, R., Zhou, G., Dreyer, S. D., Harvey, S. J., Ninomiya, Y., Thorner, P. S., Miner, J. H., Cole, W., Winterpacht, A., Zabel, B., Oberg, K. C., and Lee, B. (2001). Regulation of glomerular basement membrane collagen expression by LMX1B contributes to renal disease in nail patella syndrome. *Nature Genetics* **27**, 205–208.

Noël, L. H., Gubler, M. C., Bobrie, G., Savage, C. O. S., Lockwood, C. M., and Grünfeld, J. P. Inherited defects of renal basement membranes. In *Advances in Nephrology* Vol. 18 (ed. J. P. Grünfeld), pp. 77–94. Chicago: Year Book, 1989.

Pearson, J., Gallo, G., Gluck, M., and Axelrod, F. (1980). Renal disease in familial dysautonomia. *Kidney International* **17**, 102–112.

Rambaud, J. C. *et al.* (1986). Digestive tract and renal small vessel hyalinosis, idiopathic norarteriosclerotic intracerebral calcificatios, retinal ischemic syndrome, and phenotypic abnormalities. *Gastroenterology* **90**, 930–938.

Renwick, J. H. and Lawler, S. D. (1955). Genetical linkage between the ABO and nail-patella loci. *Annals of Human Genetics* **19**, 312–331.

Rohr, C., Prestel, J., Heidet, L., Hosser, H., Kriz, W., Johnson, R. L., Antignac, C., and Witzgall, R. (2002). The LIM-homeodomain transcription factor Lmx1b plays a crucial role in podocytes. *Journal of Clinical Investigation* **109**, 1073–1082.

Sabnis, S. G., Antanovych, T. T., Argy, W. P., Rakowski, T. A., Gandy, D. R., and Salcedo, J. R. (1980). Nail-patella syndrome. *Clinical Nephrology* **14**, 148–153.

Schleutermann, D. A., Bias, W. B., Murdoch, J. L., and McKusick, V. A. (1969). Linkage of the loci for the nail-patella syndrome and adenylate kinase. *American Journal of Human Genetics* **21**, 606–630.

Silverman, M. E., Goodman, R. M., and Cuppage, F. E. (1967). The nail-patella syndrome: clinical findings and ultrastructural observations in the kidney. *Archives of Internal Medicine* **120**, 68–74.

Stuchiffe, N. P., Cashman, S. J., Savage, C. O., Fox, J. G., and Boulton-Jones, J. M. (1989). Variability of the antigenicity of the glomerular basement membrane in nail-patella syndrome. *Nephrology, Dialysis, Transplantation* **4**, 262–265.

Taguchi, T., Takebayashi, S., Nishimura, M., and Tsuru, N. (1988). Nephropathy of nail-patella syndrome. *Ultrastructural Pathology* **12**, 175–183.

Vollrath, D., Jaramillo-Babb, V. L., Clough, M. V., McIntosh, I., Scott, K. M., Lichter, P. R., and Richards, J. E. (1998). Loss-of-function mutations in the LIM-homeodomain gene, LMX1B, in nail-patella syndrome. *Human Molecular Genetics* **7**, 1091–1098.

16.4.4 Congenital nephrotic syndrome

Hannu Jalanko and Christer Holmberg

Introduction

Congenital nephrotic syndrome is defined as proteinuria leading to clinical symptoms and findings soon after birth. An arbitrary age limit of three months has been adopted to separate it from 'infantile nephrotic syndrome' becoming manifest later in the first year of life (Holmberg *et al.* 1999). The best characterized entity in this age group is congenital nephrotic syndrome of the Finnish type (CNF) (Table 1). The next most common variety is diffuse mesangial sclerosis (DMS), which may be isolated or associated with malformation syndromes. In addition, secondary nephroses due to infections as well as minimal-change nephrotic syndrome (MCNS) and focal and segmental glomerulosclerosis (FSGS) may sometimes occur within the first few months of life (Shahin *et al.* 1974; Repetto *et al.* 1982; Rao 1991; Batisky *et al.* 1993; Niaudet 1999; Hamed and Somaf 2001).

During the recent years, our knowledge of the pathophysiology of CNF and the other genetic disorders has greatly increased which helps in understanding the pathogenesis of proteinuria in general (Tryggvason 1999; Wickelgren 1999; Salomon *et al.* 2000; Somlo and Mundel 2000; Jalanko *et al.* 2001). The important role of glomerular podocytes in the kidney filtration has become evident and it seems probable that the molecular mechanisms responsible for proteinuria will gradually be resolved.

Congenital nephrotic syndrome of the Finnish type

CNF originally denoted to a severe form congenital nephrotic syndrome typically seen in the Finnish newborns (Hallman *et al.* 1956; Norio 1966).

Table 1 Nephrotic syndromes appearing in the first months of life

Congenital nephrotic syndrome of the Finnish type
NPHS1 gene mutations
Other glomerular gene defects
Diffuse mesangial sclerosis (DMS)
Isolated
Denys–Drash syndrome
CNS malformations
Focal–segmental glomerulosclerosis (FSGS)
NPHS2 gene mutations
Other gene mutations
Other malformation syndromes
Infections
Congenital syphilis, toxoplasmosis
Rubella, cytomegalovirus
HIV, malaria, hepatitis
Systemic lupus erythematosus

After the gene (named as *NPHS1*) responsible for this disorder was isolated in 1998 it has become evident that not all cases of 'typical' CNF are caused by mutations in *NPHS1* and, on the other hand, mutations in *NPHS1* may sometimes (although rarely) cause milder (atypical) forms of nephrotic syndrome. In this text NPHS1 refers to those cases which are known to be caused by *NPHS1* mutations, and CNF is used for the classical clinically entity.

Epidemiology

NPHS1 is an autosomal recessive disease first described by Hallman *et al.* (1956). The disease is highly enriched in Finland (incidence one in 8200 newborns) (Huttunen 1976), but cases are reported all over the world among various ethnic groups (Bolk *et al.* 1999; Lee *et al.* 1999; Lenkkeri *et al.* 1999; Savage *et al.* 1999; Aya *et al.* 2000; Koziell *et al.* 2002). A very high incidence of NPHS1 was recently reported among the Old Order Mennonites in Lancaster County, Pennsylvania (Bolk *et al.* 1999). In a subgroup of 'Groffdale Conference' Mennonites the incidence was 1/500, which is almost 20 times greater than that observed in Finland.

Clinical features

The clinical features of the classical CNF varies only slightly (Hallman *et al.* 1973; Huttunen 1976; Patrakka *et al.* 2000). Over 80 per cent of these children are born prematurely (<38th week) with a birth weight ranging between 1500–3500 g (Patrakka *et al.* 2000). Amniotic fluid is often meconium stained, but most neonates do not have major pulmonary problems. The index of placental weight/birth weight (ISP) is over 25 per cent in practically all newborns. The patients do not have non-renal malformations. On the other hand, minor functional disorders in central nervous system and cardiac hypertrophy are common during the first months. Most have muscular hypotonia and without nutritional support and albumin substitution, the old classical picture of a CNF child may develop severe oedema, large cranial sutures and fontanelles, abdominal distention, ascites, and hernias.

In CNF proteinuria begins *in utero* and is thus detectable in the first urine sample tested. The urinary protein concentration exceeds 20 g/l when the serum albumin concentration is 15 g/l. Microscopic haematuria and normal serum creatinine values during the first months are observed. Heavy protein losses lead to hypogammaglobulinaemia and increased risk for infections (Ljungberg *et al.* 1997). Low antithrombin III increase the risk for thrombotic complications (Holmberg *et al.* 1999). The plasma thyroxine concentration is low owing to loss of thyroxine-binding globulin (Chadha and Alon 1999). Hyperlipidaemia is often severe (Antikainen *et al.* 1994).

Renal pathology

In typical cases of CNF, the kidneys are large compared to the size of the patient (Huttunen *et al.* 1980). The histological alterations are polymorphic and progressive and no single finding is pathognomonic for CNF. Glomeruli are often normal looking but proliferation of mesangial cells and increase of PAS- and silver-positive matrix are also seen. Dilation of the proximal and sometimes also distal tubules is the most characteristic finding (Huttunen *et al.* 1980; Patrakka *et al.* 2000). The amount of it varies greatly, from an occasional dilation to a universal dispersion throughout the renal cortex. The tubular epithelium is tall in the beginning, but flat and atrophic in advanced cases. In the interstitium, round-cell infiltration and fibrosis increase with age.

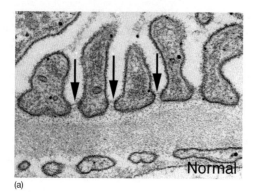

(a)

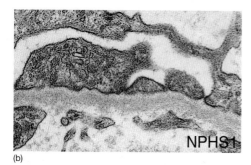

(b)

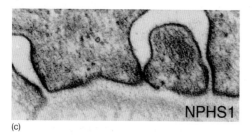

(c)

Fig. 1 Electron microscopic view of the glomerular capillary wall. (a) Normal kidney showing the podocyte foot processes, the glomerular basement mebrane and the fenestrated endothelium. The arrows indicate the filamentous slit diaphragms located at the podocyte pores. (b) NPHS1 kidney shows effacement of the podocyte foot processes, which is a common finding in proteinuric disorders. (c) Higher magnification of podocyte pores in the NPHS1 kidney showing absence of slit diaphragms.

In electron microscopy the principal finding is the effacement of podocyte foot processes in glomeruli (Fig. 1). This is not specific for NPHS1 but seen in many nephrotic kidney diseases. In many NPHS1 patients no slit diaphragms are seen between podocyte foot processes (Fig. 1) (Patrakka *et al.* 2000).

NPHS1 and nephrin

The gene responsible for NPHS1 was first linked by disequilibrium analysis to chromosome 19q13.1 (Kestilä *et al.* 1994). This region was then sequenced and a novel gene—named *NPHS1*—was identified (Kestilä *et al.* 1998). The gene consists of 29 exons and has a size of 26 kb. It codes for a novel protein, nephrin, which is a 1241-residue transmembrane adhesion protein of the immunoglobulin family (Fig. 2). Nephrin is synthesized by glomerular podocytes (Kestilä *et al.* 1998) and localized at the slit diaphragm area between the podocyte foot processes (Ruotsalainen *et al.* 1999) (Fig. 2). A zipper-like model

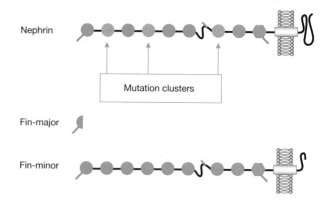

Fig. 2 Nephrin molecule. Nephrin has a size of 1241 amino acid residues. The extracellular part contains eight immunoglobulin like motifs (circles) and one fibronectin type III motif (square). The intracellular part has a unique structure containing eight tyrosine residues taking part in the signal transduction. Over 60 mutations have been found in *NPHS1* coding for nephrin. These mutations span the whole gene. However, mutation clusters are found in exons coding for Ig-motifs 2, 4, and 7. The Finnish patients have two important mutations: the Fin-major mutation is a 2 bp deletion in exon 2 leading to a truncated protein of 90 residues; the Fin-minor mutation is a nonsense mutation in exon 26 leading to a truncated protein of 1109 residue. Neither of the truncated proteins are expressed in the kidney glomerulus.

for nephrin assembly in the slit diaphragm has been proposed (Fig. 3) (Ruotsalainen *et al.* 1999; Tryggvason 1999). These results indicate that the slit diaphragm has an essential role in the normal glomerular filtration barrier.

NPHS1 mutations

Exon sequencing analyses has revealed two important mutations in 94 per cent of the chromosomes of the Finnish NPHS1 patients (Kestilä *et al.* 1998). The first mutation, a 2 bp deletion in exon 2, causes a frameshift resulting in a stop codon within the same exon (Fin-major mutation). The second is a nonsense mutation in exon 26 (Fin-minor). Fin-major leads to a truncated 90-residue protein and Fin-minor leads to a truncated 1109-residue protein (Fig. 2). In addition to Fin-major and Fin-minor, a few missense mutations in the Finnish patients has been found (Lenkkeri *et al.* 1999). The uniform mutation pattern seen in the Finnish population can be explained by the founder effect.

Several reports on *NPHS1* mutations in non-Finnish patients have recently been published (Bolk *et al.* 1999; Lee *et al.* 1999; Lenkkeri *et al.* 1999; Aya *et al.* 2000; Beltcheva *et al.* 2001; Koziell *et al.* 2002). The patients come from Europe, North America, North Africa, Middle East, and Asia. In contrast to the Finnish patients, most non-Finns have 'individual mutations'. These include deletions, insertions, nonsense, missense, and splicing mutations spanning over the whole gene. For the moment, over 60 mutations in *NPHS1* has been identified. To date, missense mutations are all located within the extracellular part and clustering to exons coding for the Ig-like motifs two, four, and seven have been reported (Fig. 2) (Lenkkeri *et al.* 1999; Koziell *et al.* 2002). Interestingly, the Fin-major and Fin-minor mutations are rare outside Finland. Enrichment of other mutations has been reported also in non-Finns. In Mennonites, 1481delC mutation is common and leads to a truncated protein of 547 residues (Bolk *et al.* 1999). On the

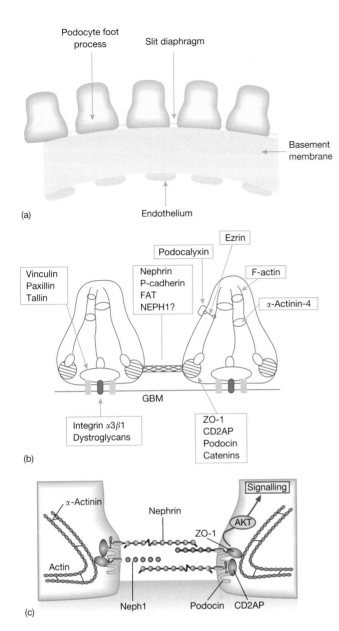

Fig. 3 (a) The structure of glomerular capillary wall. The podocyte foot processes are connected by slit diaphragms that are important in restricting the passage of plasma proteins into urine. (b) A model of the podocyte foot processes showing some of the known components of the slit diaphragm and cytoskeleton. The slit diaphragm and the glomerular basement membrane (GBM) are connected to podocyte cytoskeleton by linker proteins. (c) A hypothetical model for the slit diaphragm. Nephrin and Neph1 proteins from adjacent foot processes probably form the backbone of the slit diaphragm. Adapter proteins podocin, ZO-1 and CD2AP interact with nephrin and Neph1 and take part in the signal transduction from the slit diaphragm into podocyte. The final structure of the slit diaphragm waits to be resolved.

other hand, a homozygous nonsense mutation R1160X in exon 27 has been found in all Maltese cases (Koziell *et al.* 2002).

Genotype/phenotype correlations of *NPHS1* mutations indicate that the majority result in a severe nephrotic syndrome (Koziell *et al.* 2002). The Fin-major and Fin-minor mutations lead to a complete

absence of nephrin and the podocyte slit diaphragm in the kidney glomerulus, which explains the severity of the disorder in the Finnish patients (Fig. 1) (Patrakka *et al.* 2000). Recent work by Liu *et al.* (2001) suggests that also many missense mutations lead to the misfolding of nephrin and a defective intracellular nephrin transport in the podocyte. Thus, even 'mild, non-Finnish mutations' may cause a situation analogous to that seen in the Finns. An interesting exception is the nonsense mutation R1160X found in Maltese patients. About half of these patients (mostly females) have a mild form of NPHS1 (Koziell *et al.* 2002).

Prenatal diagnosis

Proteinuria in classical CNF starts *in utero* and the measurement of α-fetoprotein (AFP) in the amniotic fluid and maternal serum has successfully been used for prenatal screening of CNF and in families with a previous CNF diagnosis (Aula *et al.* 1978). If the AFP concentration in amniotic fluid is very high [>10 multiples of normal medians (MOMs)] and the ultrasound examination does not reveal fetal anencephaly or other malformations, CNF is a very probable diagnosis. However, fetal carriers of *NPHS1* mutations may have elevated values (up to 50 MOMs) and a false positive result in the AFP test (Männikkö *et al.* 1997; Patrakka *et al.* 2002a) This may lead to termination of pregnancy on false grounds. Sequence analysis of the *NPHS1* from placental biopsies is the method of choice for precise prenatal diagnosis of NPHS1. In the Finnish population, analysis of the two major mutations is feasible. Sequencing of the whole *NPHS1* gene is also possible.

Other nephrotic syndromes

CNF not caused by *NPHS1* mutations

Mutations in *NPHS1* are not the only cause of CNF. In the report of Lenkkeri *et al.* (1999), no mutations in *NPHS1* were found in seven of 35 patients (20 per cent) with classical CNF. Similarly, Koziell *et al.* (2002) found no *NPHS1* mutations in eight of 37 CNF cases analysed. In two of these eight patients, mutations were found in *NPHS2* coding for another podocyte protein, podocin (see below). Mutations in genes coding for the other components of the glomerular filtration barrier (Fig. 3) most probably lead to disorders resembling CNF, for example, lack of CD2-associated protein in mice leads to severe nephrotic syndrome at the age of a few weeks (Shih *et al.* 1999). This protein is now known to interact with nephrin and podocin at the podocyte slit diaphragm (Fig. 3) (Shih *et al.* 2001). The slit diaphragm is connected to actin cytoskeleton by several (partly unknown) linker proteins and defects in these may play a role in the appearance of proteinuria, for example, mutations in the gene coding for α-actinin-4 cause nephrotic syndrome in man (Kaplan *et al.* 2000). Understanding of the glomerular filtration barrier and its components increases now rapidly and it is to be expected that new 'nephrosis genes' will be revealed in the near future.

Diffuse mesangial sclerosis

Habib and Bois (1973) originally described infants with nephrotic syndrome and renal histological changes differing distinctly from that seen in CNF. In this entity, DMS, the glomerular capillary tufts are small and contracted and the capillaries are severely occluded. Mesangial sclerosing fibrils are constantly found and epithelial crescents may be present. Tubular atrophy and dilations are common, as is interstitial fibrosis (Habib 1993).

DMS can be a isolated or associated with additional congenital anomalies. In infants with isolated DMS proteinuria can manifest in the first 3 months of life, but it is more often detected later in infancy (Lennert *et al.* 1997; Ito *et al.* 2001). Proteinuria is often moderate, and in contrast to CNF, the patients develop progressive renal insufficiency and endstage renal disease within a few months or years (Habib 1993). Renal transplantation is the only effective treatment. An autosomal recessive inheritance has been suggested in some cases but prenatal diagnosis is not possible (Salomon *et al.* 2000).

Malformations syndromes

During the past decades more than 40 infants having DMS type nephrotic syndrome together with primary microcephaly and mental retardation (Meyers *et al.* 1999) have been reported. Some of the published cases have shown, in addition to microcephaly, other extrarenal disorders such as hiatus hernia (Galloway and Mowat 1968), dysmorphic features (Cooperstone *et al.* 1993), congenital spondylorhizomelic shortness (Opitz *et al.* 1985), and diaphragmatic defects (Shapiro *et al.* 1976). Age at onset of the nephrotic syndrome has varied from the first days of life to the age of some months, or even later childhood. The early manifesting cases are often early lethal while the later manifesting cases show a more variable renal prognosis including totally normal renal function, as reviewed by Meyers *et al.* (1999).

In addition to nephrosis–microcephaly syndomes there are solitary reports on other, unique combinations. They include familial nephrosis, deafness, and hypoparathyroidism (Barakat *et al.* 1977), action myoclonus-renal failure syndrome (Andermann *et al.* 1986; Nishikawa *et al.* 1997), congenital nephrosis with adrenal calcification (Powers *et al.* 1990), nephrosis with infantile sialic acid storage disease (Sperl *et al.* 1990), nephrosis with cardiac manifestations (Grech *et al.* 2000), and neonatal nephrotic syndrome with Dandy–Walker malformation (Mildenberger *et al.* 1998).

Denys–Drash syndrome

DMS is also a feature of Denys–Drash syndrome (DDS) (Schumacher *et al.* 1998). DDS is a nephrotic disorder with a renal histopathological picture of DMS, male pseudohermaphroditism, and Wilms' tumour (Denys *et al.* 1967; Drash *et al.* 1970). Male pseudohermaphroditism in most published cases means karyotype XY, some kind of testes elsewhere than in the scrotum, and ambiguous features of genitalia such as hypospadia and cryptorchidism in children looking like boys, or hypertrophy of the clitoris in patients looking like girls (Eddy and Mauer 1985). Some cases with the karyotype XX with female phenotype have been reported (Coppes *et al.* 1993a,b).

DDS is caused by heterozygous mutations in Wilms' tumour suppressor gene (*WT1*) (Call *et al.* 1990; Gessler *et al.* 1991; Pelletier *et al.* 1991). This gene is located on chromosome 11p13 (Call *et al.* 1990), and it codes for a transcription factor of the zinc finger family. The factor plays a crucial role in the embryonic development of the kidney and genitalia (Pitchard-Jones 1999). In DDS patients, over 60 different *WT1* gene mutations have been reported (Salomon *et al.* 2000). Missense mutations that involve exon 9 corresponding to the third zinc finger of the *WT1* gene are the most common (Jeanpierre *et al.* 1998; Schumacher *et al.* 1998). The correlation of the site and type of the mutation does not unanimously correlate to the clinical picture.

Mutations in *WT1* gene have been described also in patients with isolated DMS (Jeanpierre *et al.* 1998; Schumacher *et al.* 1998) suggesting that DMS and DDS are genetically overlapping. In DMS, *WT1* mutations are seen in less than half of the cases while they are found in most DDS patients. These recent findings suggest that while the clinical entity called DDS seems to be genetically homogeneous, DMS is clearly not. New heterozygous mutations of *WT1* may well be the cause of sporadic cases but, based on old reports of familial cases, autosomal recessive inheritance is also possible.

Familial focal–segmental glomerulosclerosis

During the past few years, familial forms of FSGS (FFSGS) have been repeatedly identified in children and adults. FFSGS has been linked to chromosomes 1, 11, and 19 as well as to mitochondrial genes (Conlon *et al.* 1999; Doleris *et al.* 1999; Win *et al.* 1999a,b). Positional cloning has identified glomerular gene associated with nephrotic disease presenting early in life. This new gene, *NPHS2*, is located on chromosome 1q25–1q32 and encodes for podocin which is a transmembrane protein produced by podocytes (Boute *et al.* 2000). Podocin is able to bind to nephrin and may augment nephrin-induced signal transduction (Huber *et al.* 2001; Schwartz *et al.* 2001). *NPHS2* mutations were originally detected in autosomal recessive FFSGS, which presents between 3 months and 5 years of age. More recently Koziell *et al.* (2002) found *NPHS2* mutations in two infants with severe CNF and no *NPHS1* mutations. They also identified four patients with congenital FSGS who had mutations both in *NPHS1* and *NPHS2* genes. The results clearly indicate that there is a functional link between the two genes (Fig. 3).

Management of congenital nephrotic syndrome

Immunosuppressive therapy with steroids or cyclophosphamide does not bring CNF or the other forms of congenital nephrotic syndrome into remission. Today, the only curative treatment is renal transplantation. A necessary prerequisite for transplantation is aggressive treatment during the first months of life (Table 2). This consists of protein supplementation by daily albumin infusions, hyperalimentation, and thyroxine, calcium, and magnesium supplementation (Mahan *et al.* 1984; Holmberg *et al.* 1999). The avoidance of thrombotic complications by warfarin prophylaxis and aggressive treatment of infections are also essential treatment modalities. In many centres, bilateral nephrectomy is performed and dialysis commenced before transplantation to further improve the nutritional state of the patients (Chadha and Alon 1999; Holmberg *et al.* 1999; Savage *et al.* 1999; van Lieburg and Monnens 2001).

Reduction of protein losses by antiproteinuric drugs, angiotensin-converting enzyme (ACE)-inhibitor and indomethacin, has been reported (Pomeranz *et al.* 1995; Guez *et al.* 1998; Heaton *et al.* 1999; Licht *et al.* 2000). These drugs lower the perfusion pressure in the glomerulus and lead to reduced protein leakage. In our experience, patients who have severe *NPHS1* mutations (e.g. Fin-major and Fin-minor) leading to a total lack of nephrin in glomerular slit diaphragm do not respond to this medication. On the other hand, patients with minor mutations may show a clear reduction in protein excretion and this therapy should be tried in non-Finnish CNF patients.

Table 2 Management of infants with congenital nephrotic syndrome

Nephrotic stage
Parenteral protein supplementation
    20% Albumin infusions daily
    3–4 g/kg of protein
Nutrition
    Hypercaloric diet (130 kcal/kg/day of energy)
    Protein supplementation (4 g/kg/day)
    Rapeseed oil (10–15 ml) and fish oil (2 ml)
    Magnesium (40–60 mg/day) and calcium (500–750 mg/day)
Medication
    Thrombosis prophylaxis
        Oral warfarin (PTT is kept at 20–30%)
        Antithrombin III (50 IU/kg) given before vascular procedures
    Thyroxine supplementation (6.25–30 μg/day)
    Antibiotics
        No prophylaxis
        Aggressive therapy when infection suspected
        Major hospital strains covered

Dialysis
Bilateral nephrectomy when the weight is >7 kg
Peritoneal dialysis (CCPD or Tidal dialysis)

Kidney transplantation
Performed after a few months on dialysis
Patient weight > 9 kg if the graft placed extraperitoneally

Renal transplantation is usually performed when an infant has reached a weight of about 10 kg. The outcome of transplantion is good (Kim *et al.* 1998). The patient and graft survivals in Finnish patients at 5 years are 98 and 82 per cent, respectively (Qvist *et al.* 1999). The growth, neurological development and quality of life of most patients is quite satisfactory (Qvist *et al.* 2002a,b). Recurrence of nephrosis in the kidney graft is a special problem among NPHS1 patients (Laine *et al.* 1993; Barayan *et al.* 2001). In many of these patients circulating autoantibodies against nephrin can be detected (Patrakka *et al.* 2002b). Aggressive treatment of the recurrence with cyclophosphamide and plasma exchange usually resolves the episode.

References

Andermann, E. *et al.* (1986). Action myoclonus-renal failure syndrome: a previously unrecognised neurological disorder unmasked by advances in nephrology. *Advances in Neurology* **43**, 87–103.

Antikainen, M. *et al.* (1994). Pathology of renal arteries of dyslipidemic children with congenital nephrosis. *Acta Pathologica, Microbiologica, et Immunologica Scandinavica* **192**, 129–134.

Aula, P. *et al.* (1978). Prenatal diagnosis of congenital nephrosis in 23 high-risk families. *American Journal of Disease in Childhood* **132**, 984–987.

Aya, K., Tanaka, H., and Seino, Y. (2000). Novel mutation in the nephrin gene of a Japanese patient with congenital nephrotic syndrome of the Finnish type. *Kidney International* **57**, 401–404.

Barakat, A. Y., D'Albora, J. B., Martin, M. M., and Jose, P. A. (1977). Familial nephrosis, nerve deafness, and hypoparathyroidism. *Journal of Pediatrics* **91**, 61–64.

Barayan, S. *et al.* (2001). Immediate post-transplant nephrosis in a patient with congenital nephrotic syndrome. *Pediatric Nephrology* **16**, 547–549.

Batisky, D. L., Roy, S. D., and Gaber. L. W. (1993). Congenital nephrosis and neonatal cytomegalovirus infection: a clinical association. *Pediatric Nephrology* **7**, 741–743.

Beltcheva, O., Martin, P., Lenkkeri, U., and Tryggvason, K. (2001). Mutation spectrum in the nephrin gene (*NPHS1*) in congenital nephrotic syndrome. *Human Mutation* **17**, 368–373.

Bolk, S. *et al.* (1999). Elevated frequency and allelic heterogeneity of congenital nephrotic syndrome, Finnish type, in the old order Mennonites. *American Journal of Human Genetics* **65**, 1785–1790.

Boute, N. *et al.* (2000). *NPHS2*, encoding the glomerular protein podocin, is mutated in autosomal recessive steroid-resistant nephrotic syndrome. *Nature Genetics* **24**, 349–354.

Call, K. *et al.* (1990). Isolation and characterization of a zinc finger polypeptide gene at the human chromosome 11 Wilms' tumor locus. *Cell* **60**, 509–520.

Chadha, V. and Alon, U. (1999). Bilateral nephrectomy reverses hypothyroidism in congenital nephrotic syndrome. *Pediatric Nephrology* **13**, 209–211.

Conlon, P. J. *et al.* (1999). Spectrum of disease in familial focal and segmental glomerulosclerosis. *Kidney International* **56**, 1863–1871.

Cooperstone, B. G., Friedman, A., and Kaplan, B. S. (1993). Galloway-Mowat syndrome of abnormal gyral patterns and glomerulopathy. *American Journal of Medical Genetics* **47**, 250–254.

Coppes, M. J., Campbell, C. E., and Williams, B. R. G. (1993a). The role of WT1 in Wilms tumorigenesis. *FASEB Journal* **7**, 886–895.

Coppes, M. J., Huff, V., and Pelletier, J. (1993b). Denys–Drash syndrome: relating a clinical disorder to genetic alterations in the tumor suppressor gene *WT1*. *Journal of Paediatrics* **123**, 673–678.

Denys, P. *et al.* (1967). De pseudohermaphrodisme masculin, d'une tumeur de Wilms, d'une nephropathie parenchymateuse et d'une mosaicisme XX/XY. *Archives de Pediatrie* **24**, 729–739.

Doleris, L. M. *et al.* (1999). Focal and segmental glomerulosclerosis (FSGS) and mitochondrial cytopathy. *Journal of the American Society of Nephrology* **10**, A2216.

Drash, A., Sherman, F., Hartmann, W. H., and Blizzard, R. M. (1970). A syndrome of pseudohermaphroditism, Wilms' tumor, hypertension, and degenerative renal disease. *Journal of Pediatrics* **76**, 585–593.

Eddy, A. A. and Mauer, S. M. (1985). Pseudohermaphroditism, glomerulopathy, and Wilms' tumor (Drash syndrome): frequency in end-stage renal failure. *Journal of Pediatrics* **106**, 584–587.

Galloway, W. H. and Mowat, A. P. (1968). Congenital microcephaly with hiatus hernia and nephrotic syndrome in two sibs. *Journal of Medical Genetics* **5**, 319–321.

Gessler, M. *et al.* (1990). Homozygous deletion in Wilms tumours of a zinc-finger gene identified by chromosome jumping. *Nature* **343**, 774–778.

Grech, V. *et al.* (2000). Cardiac manifestations associated with the congenital nephrotic syndrome. *Pediatric Nephrology* **14**, 1115–1117.

Guez, S. *et al.* (1998). Adequate clinical control of congenital nephrotic syndrome by enalapril. *Pediatric Nephrology* **12**, 130–132.

Habib, R. (1993). Nephrotic syndrome in the 1st year of life. *Pediatric Nephrology* **7**, 347–353.

Habib, R. and Bois, E. (1973). Hétérogénété des syndromes néphrotiques a debut précoce du nourisson (syndrome néphrotique 'infantilé'), étude anatomoclinique et génétique de 37 observations. *Helvetica Paediatrica Acta* **28**, 91–107.

Hallman, N., Hjelt, L., and Ahvenainen, E. K. (1956). Nephrotic syndrome in newborn and young infants. *Annales Paediatriae Fenniac* **2**, 227–241.

Hallman, N., Norio, R., and Rapola, J. (1973). Congenital nephrotic syndrome. *Nephron* **11**, 101–110.

Hamed, R. and Shomaf, M. (2001). Congenital nephrotic syndrome: a clinico-pathologic study of thirty children. *Journal of Nephrology* **14**, 104–109.

Heaton, P. A., Smales, O., and Wong, W. (1999). Congenital nephrotic syndrome responsive to captopril and indomethacin. *Archives of Disease in Childhood* **81**, 174–175.

Holmberg, C., Jalanko, H., Tryggvason, K., and Rapola, J. Congenital nephrotic syndrome. In *Pediatric Nephrology* 4th edn. Chapter 47 (ed. T. M. Barratt, E. D. Avner, and W. E. Harmon), pp. 765–777. Baltimore: Lippincott Williams & Wilkins, 1999.

Huber, T. *et al.* (2001). Interaction with podocin facilitates nephrin signalling. *Journal of Biological Chemistry* **276**, 41543–41546.

Huttunen, N.-P. (1976). Congenital nephrotic syndrome of Finnish type: study of 75 patients. *Archives of Disease in Childhood* **51**, 344–348.

Huttunen, N.-P., Rapola, J., Vilska, J., and Hallman, N. (1980). Renal pathology in congenital nephrotic syndrome of Finnish type: a quantitative light microscopic study on 50 patients. *International Journal of Pediatric Nephrology* **1**, 10–16.

Ito, S. *et al.* (2001). Isolated diffuse mesangial sclerosis and Wilms' tumor suppressor gene. *Journal of Paediatrics* **138**, 425–427.

Jalanko, H., Patrakka, J., Tryggvason, K., and Holmberg, C. (2001). Genetic kidney diseases disclose the pathogenesis of proteinuria. *Annals of Medicine* **33**, 526–533.

Jeanpierre, C. *et al.* (1998). Identification of constitutional *WT1* mutations in patients with isolated diffuse mesangial sclerosis, and analysis of genotype/phenotype correlations by use of computerized mutation database. *American Journal of Human Genetics* **62**, 824–833.

Kaplan, J. *et al.* (2000). Mutations in *ACTN4*, encoding alpha-actinin-4, cause familial focal segmental glomerulosclerosis. *Nature Genetics* **24**, 251–256.

Kestilä, M. *et al.* (1994). Congenital nephrotic syndrome of the Finnish type maps to the long arm of chromosome 19. *American Journal of Human Genetics* **54**, 757–764.

Kestilä, M. *et al.* (1998). Positionally cloned gene for a novel glomerular protein—nephrin—is mutated in congenital nephrotic syndrome. *Molecular Cell* **1**, 575–582.

Kim, M., Stablein, D., and Harmon, W. (1998). Renal transplantation in children with congenital nephrotic syndrome: a report of the North American Pediatric Renal Transplant Cooperative Study (NAPRTCS). *Pediatric Transplantation* **2**, 305–308.

Koziell, A. *et al.* (2002). Genotype/phenotype correlations of *NPHS1* and *NPHS2* mutations in nephrotic syndrome advocate a functional inter-relationship in glomerular filtration. *Human Molecular Genetics* **11**, 379–388.

Laine, J. *et al.* (1993). Posttransplantation nephrosis in congenital nephrotic syndrome of the Finnish type. *Kidney International* **44**, 867–874.

Lee, H. J., Gribouval, O., and Antignac, C. (1999). *NPHS1* mutations in non-Finnish CNF populations. *Journal of the American Society of Nephrology* **10**, A2206.

Lenkkeri, U. *et al.* (1999). Structure of the gene for congenital nephrotic syndrome of the Finnish type (*NPHS1*) and characterization of mutations. *American Journal of Human Genetics* **64**, 51–61.

Lennert, T. *et al.* (1997). Augenveränderung be diffuser mesangialer Sklerose (DMS). *Monatschrift Kinderheilkunde* **145**, 209–212.

Licht, C. *et al.* (2000). A stepwise approach to the treatment of early onset nephrotic syndrome. *Pediatric Nephrology* **14**, 1077–1082.

Liu, L. *et al.* (2001). Defective nephrin trafficking by missense mutations in the *NPHS1* gene: insight into the mechanisms of congenital nephrotic syndrome. *Human Molecular Genetics* **10**, 2637–2644.

Ljungberg, P., Holmberg, C., and Jalanko, H. (1997). Infections in infants with congenital nephrosis of the Finnish type. *Pediatric Nephrology* **11**, 148–152.

Mahan, J. D., Mauer, S. M., Sibley, R. K., and Vernier, R. L. (1984). Congenital nephrotic syndrome: evolution of medical management and results of renal transplantation. *Journal of Pediatrics* **105**, 549–557.

Männikkö, M. *et al.* (1997). Improved prenatal diagnosis of the congenital nephrotic syndrome of the Finnish type based on DNA analysis. *Kidney International* **51**, 868–872.

Meyers, K. V. C., Kaplan, P., and Kaplan, B. S. (1999). Nephrotic syndrome, microcephaly, and developmental delay: three separate syndromes. *American Journal of Medical Genetics* **82**, 257–260.

Mildenberger, E. *et al.* (1998). Diffuse mesangial sclerosis: associated with unreported congenital anomalies and placental enlargement. *Acta Pediatrica* **87**, 1301–1303.

Niaudet, P. Steroid-resistant idiopathic nephrotic syndrome. In *Pediatric Nephrology* 4th edn. Chapter 46 (ed. T. M. Barratt, E. D. Avner, and W. E. Harmon), pp. 749–763. Baltimore: Lippincott Williams & Wilkins, 1999.

Nishikawa, M. *et al.* (1997). A case of early myoclonic encephalopathy with the congenital nephrotic syndrome. *Brain and Development* **19**, 144–147.

Norio, R. (1966). Heredity in the congenital nephrotic syndrome: a genetic study of 57 Finnish families with a review of reported cases. *Annales Paediatriae Fenniae* **12** (Suppl.), 27–35.

Opitz, J. M. *et al.* (1985). Hutterite Cerebro-osteo-nephrodysplasia: autosomal recessive trait in a Lehlerleut Hutterite family from Montana. *American Journal of Medical Genetics* **22**, 521–529.

Patrakka, J. *et al.* (2000). Congenital nephrotic syndrome (NPHS1): features resulting from different mutations in Finnish patients. *Kidney International* **58**, 972–980.

Patrakka, J. *et al.* (2002a). Proteinuria and prenatal diagnosis of congenital nephrosis in fetal carriers of nephrin gene mutations. *Lancet* **359**, 1575–1577.

Patrakka, J. *et al.* (2002b). Recurrence of nephrotic syndrome in patients with congenital nephrosis (NPHS1): role of nephrin. *Transplantation* **73**, 394–403.

Pelletier, J. *et al.* (1991). Germline mutations in the Wilm's tumor suppressor gene are associated with abnormal urogenital development in Denys–Drash syndrome. *Cell* **67**, 437–447.

Pitchard-Jones, K. (1999). The Wilms tumor gene, WT1, in normal and abnormal nephrogenesis. *Pediatric Nephrology* **13**, 620–625.

Pomeranz, A., Wolach, B., Bernheim, J., and Korzets, Z. (1995). Successful treatment of Finnish congenital nephrotic syndrome with captopril and indomethacin. *Journal of Pediatrics* **126**, 140–142.

Powers, R. J., Cohen, M. L., and Williams, J. (1990). Adrenal calcification and congenital nephrotic syndrome in three American Indians. *Pediatric Nephrology* **4**, 29–31.

Qvist, E. *et al.* (1999). Graft function 5–7 years after renal transplantation in early childhood. *Transplantation* **67**, 1043–1049.

Qvist, E. *et al.* (2002a). Growth after renal transplantation in infancy or rearly childhood. *Pediatric Nephrology* **17**, 438–443.

Qvist, E. *et al.* (2002b). Neurodevelopmental outcome in high-risk patients after renal transplantation in early childhood. *Pediatric Transplantation* **6**, 53–62.

Rao, T. K. (1991). Clinical features of human immunodeficiency virus associated nephropathy. *Kidney International* **40** (Suppl. 35), S13–S18.

Repetto, H. A., Vazquez, L. A., Russ, C., and Costa, J. A. (1982). Late appearance of nephrotic syndrome in congenital syphilis. *Journal of Pediatrics* **100**, 591–592.

Ruotsalainen, V. *et al.* (1999). Nephrin is located in the slit diaphragm of glomerular podocytes. *Proceedings of National Academy of Sciences USA* **96**, 7962–7967.

Salomon, R., Gubler, M., and Niaudet, P. (2000). Genetics of the nephrotic syndrome. *Current Opinion in Pediatrics* **12**, 129–134.

Savage, J. M. *et al.* (1999). Improved prognosis for congenital nephrotic syndrome of the Finnish type in Irish families. *Archives of Disease in Childhood* **80**, 466–469.

Schumacher, V. *et al.* (1998). Spectrum of early onset nephrotic syndrome associated with *WT1* missense mutations. *Kidney International* **53**, 1594–1600.

Schwartz, K. *et al.* (2001). Podocin, a raft-associated component of the glomerular slit diaphragm, interacts with CD2AP and nephrin. *Journal of Clinical Investigation* **11**, 1621–1629.

Shahin, B., Papadopoulou, Z. L., and Jenis, E. H. (1974). Congenital nephrotic syndrome associated with congenital toxoplasmosis. *Journal of Pediatrics* **85**, 366–370.

Shapiro, L. R., Duncan, P. A., Farnsworth, P. B., and Lefkowitz, M. (1976). Congenital microcephaly, hiatus hernia and nephrotic syndrome: an autosomal recessive syndrome. *Birth Defects Original Article Series* **12** (5), 275–278.

Shih, N.-Y. *et al.* (1999). Congenital nephrotic syndrome in mice lacking CD2-associated protein. *Science* **286**, 312–315.

Shih, N.-Y. *et al.* (2001). CD2AP localizes to the slit diaphragm and binds to nephrin via a novel *C*-terminal domain. *American Journal of Pathology* **159**, 2303–2308.

Somlo, S. and Mundel, P. (2000). Getting a foothold in nephrotic syndrome. *Nature Genetics* **24**, 333–335.

Sperl, W. *et al.* (1990). Nephrosis in two siblings with infantile sialic acid storage disease. *European Journal of Pediatrics* **149**, 477–482.

Tryggvason, K. (1999). Unravaling the mechanism of glomerular ultrafiltration: nephrin, a key component of the slit diaphragm. *Journal of the American Society of Nephrology* **10**, 2440–2445.

Van Lieburg, A. and Monnens, L. (2001). Persistent arterial hypotension after bilateral nephrectomy in a 4-month-old infant. *Pediatric Nephrology* **16**, 604–605.

Wickelgren, I. (1999). First components found for key kidney filter. *Science* **286**, 225–226.

Winn, M. P. *et al.* (1999a). Linkage of a gene causing familial focal segmental glomerulosclerosis to chromosome 11 and further evidence of genetic heterogeneity. *Journal of the American Society of Nephrology* **10**, A2241.

Winn, M. P. *et al.* (1999b). Clinical and genetic heterogeneity in familial focal segmental glomerulosclerosis. *Kidney International* **55**, 1241–1246.

16.5 Inherited metabolic diseases of the kidney

16.5.1 Cystinosis

Michael Broyer and Marie-Claire Gubler

Cystinosis is a generalized lysosomal storage disease, autosomal and recessive. The lysosomal cystine accumulation leads to cellular dysfunction of many organs, the most serious being renal involvement. Two phenotypic forms are discerned: the nephropathic form, by far the most common, usually starting in infancy and, more rarely, in adolescence (the juvenile form), and the non-nephropathic or benign form, exceptionally reported in adults. This chapter concerns essentially the nephropathic infantile form.

Historical background

Abderhalden, a chemist from Berlin, reported in 1903 the autopsy of a child who died from inanition at 21 months, whose liver and spleen were loaded with cystine crystals, and who had two sibs who died similarly (Abderhalden 1903); this is supposedly the first reported case of cystinosis. Lignac (1924) reported the autopsy of three cases of children who had severe rickets, renal failure, and dwarfism with cystine deposits in different organs. Between 1931 and 1934, Fanconi (1931) and other paediatricians reported patients with failure to thrive, rickets, glycosuria, proteinuria, and hypophosphataemia, and the term 'Fanconi syndrome' was subsequently coined for alluding to proximal tubular losses. The first detailed study of a large series of patients with Fanconi syndrome and cystine storage was reported by Bickel *et al.* (1952). The next important step was the localization of the cystine storage within cell organelles by Schneider *et al.* (1967), and at the same time the description of a simple cystine assay for the diagnosis. The intralysosomal localization was ascertained by electron microscopy (Patrick and Lake 1968). Subsequently Steinherz *et al.* (1982) showed that the basic defect was the absence of cystine transport out of the lysosome. The last developments concerned the mapping of the gene on chromosome 17 (McDowell *et al.* 1996) and its identification (Town *et al.* 1998). A major step was the report of the *in vitro* and *in vivo* (Thoene *et al.* 1976) effectiveness of cysteamine in decreasing the cystine content of patients' cells, followed 10 years later by the report of the clinical effectiveness of this drug (Gahl *et al.* 1987a).

Epidemiology

Cystinosis is a rare disease. In France, a recent exhaustive study found a mean incidence of 1/167,000 between the years 1975 and 1994 (Cochat *et al.* 1999). This is close to the results of other studies in Europe, 1/179,000 in Germany (Manz and Gretz 1985), for example. In the United States, incidence is estimated around one in 200,000 (Gahl *et al.* 1995). The disease is not restricted to Caucasians and has been reported in Africans (Sochett *et al.* 1984) and Asians (Okami *et al.* 1992).

Clinical presentation of the nephropathic infantile form

First clinical symptoms

Usually, the first 3–6 months of life are symptom-free. The first symptoms mostly develop before the age of 1 year (Broyer *et al.* 1981). They include anorexia, vomiting, polyuria, and constipation, which may be apparently isolated; bouts of fever accompanied by dehydration may also be observed. Failure to thrive becomes obvious with almost constant flattening of the weight curve between 6 and 12 months. If the diagnosis is delayed, severe rickets develops after 10–18 months in spite of regular vitamin D supplementation. Blond hair and a fair complexion with difficulty of tanning after exposure to the sun are often noted in Caucasian cystinotic children. Involvement of the eye is also a primary symptom of cystinosis, starting with photophobia, which usually appears between 2 or 3 years of age associated with cystine crystal deposits. The diagnosis can immediately be suspected if both glucose and proteins are found in the urine but only confirmed by leucocyte cystine assay.

Renal signs and symptoms

When the disease becomes symptomatic, the full expression of Fanconi syndrome is generally present at first examination, but some of the following tubular losses may be absent, including normoglycaemic glycosuria, tubular proteinuria almost constant with massive excretion of β2-microglobulin and lysozyme, hyperphosphaturia with phosphate tubular reabsorption rate below 80 per cent, and hypophosphataemia. Excessive losses of potassium and sodium may lead to hypokalaemia and hyponatraemia. Loss of bicarbonate usually causes severe hyperchloraemic acidosis which may be classified as proximal tubular acidosis with a reabsorption threshold less than 15 mmol/l. The generalized aminoaciduria with urinary loss of α-aminated nitrogen of the order of 10–30 mg/kg/day, is asymptomatic except for the loss of carnitine which may cause carnitine depletion both in plasma and muscle with possible muscle dysfunction (Gahl *et al.* 1988a). Hypercalciuria, often massive, may reach 10 mg/kg body weight (BW) per day. Hypouricaemia, a hallmark of proximal tubulopathy, is typically found due to a defect

2368	 THE PATIENT WITH INHERITED DISEASE

of uric acid reabsorption. Increased organic aciduria with a large excretion of pyroglutamic acid is usual (Rizzo et al. 1999).

A severe concentrating defect develops simultaneously, leading rapidly to a polyuria of 2–5 l/day. Urine of cystinotic patients is characteristically pale and cloudy with a peculiar odour, probably due to aminoaciduria.

The general reabsorptive defect of the proximal tubule may explain severe hydroelectrolyte imbalance, which may be life-threatening. Lithiasis has been reported in rare cases, related to the high urinary excretion of urate, calcium, and organic acids, and nephrocalcinosis may be observed, generally in relation to inadequate supplements of phosphate and/or vitamin D (Theodoropoulos et al. 1995). At this stage, glomerular filtration rate remains normal. The natural history of the disease is marked by a progressive decline of glomerular filtration rate from the age of 4–6 years, eventually progressing to endstage renal failure (ESRF) between 6 and 12 years of age. In a retrospective multicentre European study, Manz and Gretz (1994) examined the progression of renal failure in a group of 205 patients with cystinosis not treated with cysteamine. Mean age at the start of renal replacement therapy was 9.6 years but can occur earlier (Schnaper et al. 1992). Van't Hoff et al. (1995) even reported an 18-month-old infant presenting with chronic renal failure without Fanconi syndrome. Of note, as glomerular filtration rate deteriorates, tubular wasting diminishes. At ESRF, severe renal hypertension may have developed.

When started early, treatment with cysteamine can delay the age of onset of renal failure. Markello et al. (1993) studied change in creatinine clearance in 76 children presenting with cystinosis. In 17 of these subjects, treatment with cysteamine was begun before the age of 2 years, and properly followed for a mean duration of 7.1 years. None of these children developed renal failure and mean creatinine clearance was 57 ± 20 ml/min/1.73 m^2. Treatment was inadequate in 32 other children, either as a result of poor compliance or because therapy was started after the age of 2 years. Twenty-one of these cases went on to develop endstage renal disease (ESRD) and the mean creatinine clearance at last examination was 12.4 ± 7.7 ml/min/1.73 m^2. Finally, of 27 children previously followed-up who had never received the treatment, 16 developed ESRD and the mean creatinine clearance was 8 ± 4.8 ml/min/1.73 m^2 for a mean age of 8.3 ± 1.9 years. The conclusion clearly favoured the early administration of cysteamine in these patients. In another series of 16 patients treated with cysteamine, plasma creatinine was significantly lower at 6 and 8 years compared to a historical group (Van't Hoff and Gretz 1995). The importance of starting cysteamine as soon as possible was also shown by the privileged observation of a cystinotic newborn given cysteamine from day 15 of life who remained almost free of symptoms at the age of 7 years (Da Silva et al. 1985) as well as 10 years later (Gahl et al. 1995). However, other cases treated early developed Fanconi syndrome (Gradus et al. 1986). These different outcomes are possibly related, among other factors, to genetic heterogeneity. Our own experience in children treated with cysteamine would support this hypothesis. Of 20 children over 10 years old followed in our institution in whom cysteamine treatment was instituted before the age of 33 months, five reached ESRF between 11 and 12 years of age and two at the ages of 21 and 23 years. At least two of the youngest were poorly compliant; 13 remained on conservative treatment with mean serum creatinine levels of 128, 207, and 159 µmol/l in the age groups 10–14, 15–20, and 20–23 years, respectively. Treatment with cysteamine is considered to have no effect upon proximal tubule dysfunction. We studied this effect in 17 children in whom treatment had been instituted before the age of 33 months (Broyer et al. 1994). In five of the 17 subjects, glycosuria was no longer seen at the age of 3 years, and in general, remained low. Rates of phosphate reabsorption increased under treatment with cysteamine, rising from a mean value of 39 per cent at 2 years to 70 per cent at around the age of 9–10 years. The treatment, however, had no effect upon tubular proteinuria, or other tubular losses.

Renal pathology

Pathological changes are progressive. They were absent in one 21-week-old cystinotic fetus, even at the ultrastructural level (Gubler et al. 1999). They are usually observed after 1 or 2 years of age, but have been recently described in two 5- and 6-month-old cystinotic patients (Mahoney and Striker 2000). The most striking feature is the marked heterogeneity in the shape and size of proximal tubule sections (Spear 1973). Tubular cells are very irregular, with the presence within the same tubular section of flat and very large cells (Fig. 1). Focal disappearance of the brush border is frequent. Nuclei are also strikingly irregular in number, shape, size, and distribution within cell cytoplasm. Multinucleate giant cell transformation of podocytes is also a distinctive, although inconstant, lesion in cystinosis (Waldherr et al. 1982). Cystine crystals are predominantly interstitial, and are usually absent from tubular cells, except in very young infants (Spear 1973). Between polarizing filters, or by phase contrast microscopy, they appear as refractive rectangular white crystals. By electron microscopy, they are angular, either empty or containing a flocculent material, and usually limited by a single unit membrane (Waldherr et al. 1982). Marked hypertrophy of the juxtaglomerular apparatus is associated

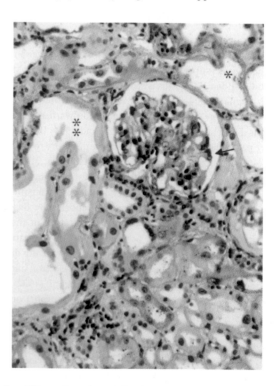

Fig. 1 Renal biopsy. Periodic acid–Schiff stain. There is a marked heterogeneity in the shape and size of proximal tubule sections. The same heterogeneity is seen at the cellular level with diffuse cell atrophy in some sections (*) and irregular alternation of flat and very large cells in others (**). Nuclei are also strikingly irregular in number, size, and distribution within cell cytoplasm. Multinuclear podocytes are focally seen (arrow).

in most patients (Gubler *et al.* 1999). In juvenile-type cystinosis, glomeruli show multinucleate podocytes, whereas tubules have a normal structure (Waldherr *et al.* 1982).

Degenerative changes occur with age. They consist of focal interstitial fibrosis, tubular atrophy, and arteriolar thickening. Glomeruli are long preserved but an increase in mesangial matrix and focal lesions, lined by large and vacuolized podocytes and involving part or all of the tuft, are observed late in the course of the disease (Gubler *et al.* 1999).

Endstage kidneys are strikingly atrophic, weighing no more than 8–10 g each. Except for medullary collecting ducts, tubular structures disappear almost completely, and glomeruli progress to small, sclerotic acellular masses, closely packed together. The arteries have a tortuous course. They are thickened and frequently obstructed by subendothelial fibrosis. Strong renin expression is constant in preglomerular arteries and at the vascular pole of sclerotic glomeruli. In all cases, abundant cystine crystals, located within interstitial foam cells, are concentrated as clusters at the corticomedullary junction, making long linear streaks in the medulla. Thus, atrophy, severe vascular changes, the presence of cystine crystals, and occasional multinucleate podocytes are characteristic of endstage cystinotic kidneys (Gubler *et al.* 1999).

Other tissues and organ involvements

The advent of renal replacement therapy and transplantation has uncovered the continued cystine accumulation in extrarenal organs and has emphasized the multisystemic nature of cystinosis, which may additionally involve the eyes, thyroid, liver, spleen, pancreas, muscle, and central nervous system (CNS) (Broyer *et al.* 1987; Gahl 1987b; Theodoropoulos *et al.* 1993).

Eyes

The corneal localization of cystine crystals can be diagnosed by slit-lamp examination, which is often difficult because of photophobia and the young age of patients. The corneal aspect of cystinosis is considered to be pathognomonic. It can be observed very early in life and is almost constant after 12–16 months. It consists of fine gold-coloured, needle-shaped crystals. The corneal surface (epithelium) is first involved. The peripheral cornea is infiltrated before the centre. The degree of crystal accumulation may be assessed by means of a scoring system and in patients not receiving topical cysteamine this score increases linearly from the age of 16 months to adolescence, reaching a plateau (Gahl *et al.* 2000). Photophobia, watering, and blepharospasm may become disabling; these symptoms are often associated with erosion of corneal epithelium, leading eventually to keratopathy. There are also fundus abnormalities with typical retinopathy characterized by patchy retinal depigmentation and subsequent alteration of the retinogram (Kaiser-Kupfer *et al.* 1986). Sight may be progressively reduced, leading to blindness in a few patients. Glaucoma has also been reported and it was confirmed recently by ultrasound biomicroscopy that cystinotic patients are predisposed to this complication (Mungan *et al.* 2000). Treatment with topical cysteamine is effective in preventing and removing crystals in the cornea (Gahl *et al.* 2000) and early oral cysteamine is also probably effective in preventing the retinopathy.

Endocrine disturbances

Hypothyroidism

Thyroid dysfunction usually appears between 8 and 12 years of age, but it may be earlier or later. It is rarely overt with clinical symptoms but rather discovered by systematic assessment of thyroid function (Lucky *et al.* 1977; Theodoropoulos *et al.* 1993) and it may be partly responsible for the growth impairment. Cysteamine has been reported to delay or prevent thyroid dysfunction (Kimonis *et al.* 1995).

Gonadal function

Abnormalities in the pituitary testicular axis with a low plasma testosterone and high follicle-stimulating hormone (FSH)/luteinizing hormone (LH) level (Chik *et al.* 1993; Tete and Broyer 1999) seem common in male patients with cystinosis. They may preclude full pubertal development being attained. Female patients exhibit pubertal delay but seem to have more normal gonadal functions, and successful pregnancies have been reported (Reiss *et al.* 1988; Andrews *et al.* 1994).

Endocrine pancreas

Postoperative hyperglycaemia and permanent insulin-dependent diabetes have been reported in several series of cystinotic patients after kidney transplantation (Bakchine *et al.* 1984); in patients not treated by cysteamine, 50 per cent had diabetes, according to the World Health Organization (WHO) definition (Robert *et al.* 1999). This diabetes is characterized by a slow progressive loss of insulin and C-peptide production (Filler *et al.* 1998). This risk justifies performing glucose tolerance tests at 5-year intervals. Exocrine pancreas is usually not affected except in one reported case with steatorrhoea (Fivusch *et al.* 1988).

Liver and spleen involvement

Hepatomegaly and splenomegaly occurred in one-third to one-half of the cases after 15 years of age who did not receive cysteamine (Broyer *et al.* 1987). Hepatomegaly is related to enlarged Kupffer's cells that transform into large foam cells containing cystine crystals. This enlargement may be the cause of portal hypertension with gastroesophageal varices bleeding. Splenomegaly is also related to the development of foam cells in the red pulp. Haematological symptoms of hypersplenism may be noted. A recent study showed that cysteamine prevented this type of complication (Gagnadoux *et al.* 1999).

Skin

Aside from the difficulty of tanning in fair complexions, a decrease of sweat production with heat intolerance has been reported (Gahl *et al.* 1984). Premature skin ageing was also observed in transplanted patients (Guillet *et al.* 1998).

Muscle

A distinctive myopathy was reported in some patients with generalized muscle atrophy and weakness mainly of distal muscles with more severe involvement of the interossei muscles and the muscles of thenar eminence (Gahl *et al.* 1988b). Pharyngeal and oral dysfunction, including hypotonia, abnormal gag reflex, and throaty or congested voice seem more common (Sonies *et al.* 1990; Trauner *et al.* 2001). Pulmonary dysfunction recently reported in adult patients is related to respiratory muscle alteration and not to a lung disease (Anikster *et al.* 2001).

Central nervous system

Several kinds of neurological complications have been reported in cystinosis. Convulsions may occur at any age, but it is difficult to evaluate the direct responsibility of cystinosis in this complication. A subtle and specific visuoperceptual defect and lower cognitive performances with sometimes subtle impairment of visual memory and tactile recognition were reported recently (Trauner *et al.* 1988; Nicholas *et al.* 1990; Colah and Trauner 1997). Despite these alterations, intellectual and school performances are usually in the normal range. More severe CNS abnormalities with various defects have also been reported (Broyer *et al.* 1987, 1996; Theodoropoulos *et al.* 1993). The clinical symptoms include hypotonia, cerebellar symptoms, development of bilateral pyramidal signs and walking difficulties, and a progressive intellectual deterioration. In other cases, acute ischaemic episodes may occur with haemiplegia or aphasia. This cystinotic encephalopathy was only observed above 19 years of age, and at present it is difficult to know its actual incidence. The effectiveness of cysteamine treatment for the prevention of CNS involvement is not known either. Cysteamine treatment was associated in some cases with an improvement of neurological symptoms (Broyer *et al.* 1996). Brain imaging in cystinosis may show several types of abnormalities. Brain atrophy, calcifications, and abnormal features of white matter on magnetic resonance imaging (MRI) examination are commonly observed after 15–20 years of age (Broyer *et al.* 1987, 1996; Nichols *et al.* 1990).

Diagnostic tests

Cystinosis must be ascertained by the assay of the cell-free cystine content, usually in leucocytes but also in cultured fibroblasts, conjunctiva, or muscle. In patients with nephropathic cystinosis, its level is about 10– 50 times normal (Schneider *et al.* 1968). This assessment raises a number of problems still needing discussion towards consensus. The blood sample collected on CAD (Citric Acid Dextrose) or heparin has to be transported within 24 h at a temperature of 10–20°C to the specialized laboratory. The first step is the sample preparation and handling of the cells in which cystine will be assayed. Then three methods are available for cystine measurement: cystine binding assay, ion exchange chromatography, and high-performance liquid chromatography (HPLC). The assay using a protein-binding technique on white cells is very sensitive and may be carried out on small blood samples. In cystinosis, the level is usually 2–15 nmol of hemicystine/mg proteins; this level is approximately two times higher and probably more accurately determined on polymorphonuclear than on total leucocytes. This technique enables even heterozygous carriers to be detected (Smolin *et al.* 1987) (0.5–1.4 nmol 1/2 cystine/mg protein). The cystine content of control subjects is usually undetectable or less than 0.4. S-labelled cystine incorporation in cultured amniotic cells or chorionic villi enables a prenatal diagnosis in the first trimester to be made (Patrick *et al.* 1987). The diagnosis may also be made by means of molecular genetics; a simple method was reported for detecting deletion in the locus D17 S829 (Forestier *et al.* 1999) found in 76 per cent of patients of European descent. The use of markers close to this locus when a first child is affected could also allow prenatal diagnosis.

Before the availability of the cystine assay, the diagnosis was made on the discovery of cystine rectangular or hexagonal crystals in a bone marrow aspirate or in a renal biopsy handled with special care because of the solubility of cystine.

Treatment

The therapy of nephropathic cystinosis is both symptomatic and specific.

Symptomatic treatment

The tubular losses due to the Fanconi syndrome have to be corrected:

Water. The water intake must be adjusted to diuresis, short-term weight variation, and if necessary the plasma protein concentration. Fluid requirement increases with external temperature and with fever.

Acid–base equilibrium. Sodium and potassium bicarbonate which have a better gastric tolerance than citrate have to be given in order to obtain a plasma bicarbonate level between 21 and 24 mmol/l. This is sometimes difficult and may need large amounts of buffer, up to 10–15 mmol/kg.

Sodium. Sodium losses sometimes remain uncompensated after achieving acid–base equilibrium. This point is documented by a persistent hyponatraemia with failure to thrive.

Potassium. Hypokalaemia requires potassium supplements in order to maintain serum potassium above 3 mmol/l. Four to 10 mmol/kg are usually necessary to achieve this goal. Prescription of amiloride at a dose of 2–5 mg/day may help in some cases.

Phosphorus. Hypophosphataemia must also be corrected with a supplement of sodium/potassium phosphate at a dose of 0.3–1 g/day. The aim is to obtain a plasma phosphate 1.0–1.2 mmol/l. This supplement is often associated with gastric intolerance.

Vitamin D supplementation. Since tubular 1α hydroxylation is diminished in this disease it is justified to give 1α or 1α25-OHD$_3$ (0.10–0.50 μg/day), especially in cases of symptomatic rickets. These prescriptions must be carefully adjusted by regular follow-up of serum calcium.

Carnitine supplementation. Carnitine supplementation at a dose of 100 mg/kg/day in four divided doses has been proposed in order to correct muscle carnitine depletion (Gahl *et al.* 1988a).

All these supplements have to be given regularly in order to replace the losses which are permanent. A good way to achieve this goal is to prepare in advance all the supplements except vitamin D in a bottle containing the usual amount of water for the day. Losses of water, potassium, and sodium may be drastically reduced by the prescription of indomethacin at a dose of 1.5–3 mg/kg in two separate doses (Haycock *et al.* 1982). When renal degradation progresses and the glomerular filtration rate decreases, the drug must be stopped; at this time tubular losses also decrease and the mineral supplements must be adjusted and progressively tapered off in order to avoid overload, especially with sodium and potassium.

Feeding problems may require tube feeding and in some cases continuous or intermittent total parenteral nutrition (Elenberg *et al.* 1998).

Growth stunting, one of the most striking complications of nephropathic cystinosis, was reported to be improved by administration of recombinant growth hormone at a dose of 1 U/kg/week (Wuhl *et al.* 1998).

Renal replacement therapy

There is no specific requirement for cystinotic children at this stage. Haemodialysis or continuous ambulatory peritoneal dialysis (CAPD)/continuous cyclic peritoneal dialysis (CCPD) are both effective and applied according to the circumstances; at this stage mucosal bleeding was reported mainly on haemodialysis (Broyer *et al.* 1981). As for any child with ESRF, kidney transplantation is considered the best approach. Results of kidney transplantation in the European Dialysis and Transplant Association paediatric registry were better than in any other primary renal disease in children (Broyer 1989). After kidney transplantation there is no recurrence of Fanconi syndrome even if cystine crystals are seen in the graft, where they are carried inside macrophages or leucocytes.

Symptomatic treatment of extrarenal complications

Hypothyroidism has to be compensated by L-thyroxine supplementation, also when asymptomatic. Diabetes mellitus may need a rather low dose insulin substitution. Hypogonadism in male patients may justify testosterone administration. Portal hypertension may lead to ascites and bleeding oesophageal varices, rendering a portal bypass necessary. Hypersplenism with permanent leucopenia and/or thrombopenia may be an indication for splenectomy. Ophthalmological treatment must be routinely considered: photophobia and watering may be improved by local symptomatic therapy but, as already stressed, eye drops containing 0.5 per cent cysteamine were able to prevent or remove corneal deposits already present (Gahl et al. 2000). Corneal graft has been rarely performed, with variable results.

Specific therapy

Only one drug, cysteamine (HS-CH2-NH2), has been shown effective *in vitro* and *in vivo* to suppress lysosomal cystine storage (Thoene et al. 1976). Cysteamine enters the lysosome where it cleaves cystine into two cysteines, and combines with one cysteine to form a disulfide which is able to come out of the lysosome by the lysine port. Nevertheless, the prescription of cysteamine raises some problems since its foul odour and taste make its administration unattractive. Cysteamine was first used as chlorhydrate, then as phosphocysteamine with the same efficacy and a supposedly better odour and taste (Smolin et al. 1988). Cysteamine is now commercially available in North America and Europe as cysteamine bitartrate (Cystagon®). These three forms of cysteamine were shown to have the same pharmacokinetic and tolerance profile (Tenneze et al. 1999). The drug should be started as soon as the diagnosis is confirmed (Markello et al. 1993). The dose is progressively increased from 10 to 50 mg/kg/day and eventually adjusted according to cystine assay. The recommended dose is 1.3 g/1 m^2/day. Cysteamine is rapidly absorbed and its maximum effect in leucocytes occurs after 1–2 h and lasts generally no longer than 6 h. Therefore, it has to be given in four separate doses—one every 6 h—in order to obtain the best prevention of cystine accumulation. Careful monitoring of leucocyte/polymorphonuclear cystine content is essential since the response to cysteamine is variable. The cystine content should be determined 6 h after the last dose. The aim is to keep this content under 2, or better, under 1 nmol of half cystine per milligram of protein. The main adverse effects are gastrointestinal intolerance with an increase in acid output and serum gastrin level (Wenner and Murphy 1997) and unpleasant smelling breath. Gastrointestinal intolerance may be prevented by the prescription of omeprazole and bad breath by different small means. Other early reported adverse effects as hyperthermia, lethargy, and rash (Corden et al. 1981) were in fact related to too high initial dosage of the drug. Another potential adverse effect would be the teratogenicity, as shown in the rat (Beckman et al. 1998). Consequently, awaiting further information, the drug should be stopped in case of pregnancy. The good results obtained on the nephropathy also encourage prescribing cysteamine to patients who are at risk of developing extrarenal complications.

Adolescent/juvenile cystinosis

This corresponds to a very rare milder form of the disease with a later clinical onset and delayed evolution to ESRF (Langman et al. 1985; Hory et al. 1994). It represented 4 per cent of the cases of cystinosis retrieved in France (Cochat et al. 1999). The first symptom appears usually after 6–8 years of age. Proteinuria may be misleading because its severity is sometimes in the nephrotic range and associated with focal and segmental hyalinosis. Fanconi syndrome may be absent (Hory et al. 1994) or moderate. The same is true for extrarenal symptoms. ESRF develops usually around 15 years of age or later in most patients. The cystine content of leucocytes has been found similar to that of infantile cases.

Adult benign cystinosis

Adult or benign cystinosis was first reported by Cogan et al. (1957). This exceptional autosomal-recessive disorder is characterized by the presence of cystine crystals in the eye and the bone marrow. Crystals in the cornea are usually found by chance examination or because of photophobia. The level of cystine in leucocytes is intermediate between that of heterozygotes and homozygotes of nephropathic cystinosis. The affected patients are asymptomatic except for the possible ocular signs.

Molecular genetics

Nephropathic cystinosis is an autosomal-recessive disorder. The primary defect which causes the lysosomal accumulation of cystine in many tissues is related to mutations in the CTNS gene (Town et al. 1998). This novel gene consists of 12 exons and encodes a protein of 367 amino acids named cystinosin which has a structure of integral membrane protein with seven membrane-spanning domains. This molecule addressed to the lysosomal membrane by specific sequences (Cherqui et al. 2001) is a H$^+$ driven lysosomal cystine transporter stimulated by the acidic lysosomal pH (Kalatzis et al. 2001). In the original publication of the gene identification (Town et al. 1998), a 65 kb homozygous deletion encompassing exons 1–10 was found in 23 out of 70 patients and all the other patients were either homozygous for a specific truncating mutation or had a heterozygous compound mutation including the gene deletion. This deletion, either homozygous or heterozygous, was found in 76 per cent of patients of European origin (Forestier et al. 1999), and reported in 56 per cent of the 216 alleles from cystinosis patients surveyed in North America (Anikster et al. 1999). It was also reported in African-Americans (Kleta et al. 2001). It was hypothesized as the result of a non-homologous recombination due to a founder effect that occurred in a white individual in the middle of the first millennium AD in central Europe. To date, more than 55 different mutations affecting the CTNS gene have been identified in cystinosis. Recently, additional mutations were reported in the promoter of this gene (Phomphutkul et al. 2001). Looking for phenotype–genotype correlations, it was shown that the infantile form corresponded usually to the lack of the molecule cystinosin or to a truncating mutation on both alleles or to other mutations in the highly conserved amino acids of the homologous proteins found in the yeast and in *Caenorhabditis elegans*, conversely, late onset cystinosis or atypical forms were reported to correspond to mutations in the non-conserved amino acids in the homologous proteins or to the functionally less active part of the protein on the side of the *N*-terminus intralysosomal part. Adult benign cystinosis was also associated with a recurrent small mutation 928 G-A in exon 12 (Kleta *et al.* 2001) and also with mutation in the promoter gene (Phomphotkul *et al.* 2001). A murine homologous of CTNS was identified and a knock-out model recently studied. Despite cystine accumulation in all organs tested, the phenotype of these animals is quite different from the human cystinosis because they have no renal disease at all but similar ocular changes, a bone defect, and behavioural anomalies. This animal model will prove a unique tool for a better understanding of the renal disease and for testing of emerging therapeutics (Cherqui *et al.*).

Why lysosomal cystine accumulation leads to cellular dysfunction remains largely unknown. It was shown that cystine loading of proximal tubular cells *in vitro* was associated with adenosine triphosphate (ATP) depletion (Foreman *et al.* 1987) and with inhibition of Na$^+$-dependent transporters (Cetinkaya *et al.* 2002), and this could possibly explain the proximal tubular defect and maybe other tissue derangements.

References

Abderhalden, E. (1903). Familiäre cystindiathese. *Hoppe-Seylers Zeitschrift für Physiologische Chemie* **38**, 557–564.

Andrews, P. A., Sachs, S. H., and Vant'Hoff, W. (1994). Successful pregnancy in cystinosis. *Journal of the American Medical Association* **272**, 1327–1328.

Anikster, Y. *et al.* (1999). Identification and detection of the common 65 kb deletion breakpoint in the nephropathic cystinosis gene. *Molecular Genetics and Metabolism* **66**, 111–116.

Anikster, Y. *et al.* (2001). Pulmonary dysfunction in adults with nephropathic cystinosis. *Chest* **119**, 394–401.

Bakchine, H. *et al.* (1984). Diabète induit par les corticoïdes chez 6 enfants après transplantation rénale. *Archives Françaises de Pédiatrie* **41**, 261–264.

Beckman, D. A., Mullin, J. J., and Assadi, F. K. (1988). Developmental toxicity of cysteamine in the rat: effects on embryo-fetal development. *Teratology* **58**, 96–102.

Bickel, H. *et al.* (1952). Cystine storage disease with aminoaciduria and dwarfism (Lignac–Fanconi disease). *Acta Pediatrica* **42**, 171–237.

Broyer, M. (1989). On behalf of the EDTA registry committee. Kidney transplantation in children, data from the EDTA registry. *Transplantation Proceedings* **21**, 1985–1988.

Broyer, M., Guillot, M., Gubler, M. C., and Habib, R. (1981). Infantile cystinosis: a reappraisal of early and late symptoms. *Advances in Nephrology* **10**, 137–166.

Broyer, M., Tete, M. J., and Gubler, M. C. (1987). Late symptoms in infantile cystinosis. *Pediatric Nephrology* **1**, 519–524.

Broyer, M., Tete, M. J., and Jean, G. traitement de la cystinose par la cysteamine. In *Journées Parisiennes de Pédiatrie* Vol. 1, pp. 301–307. Paris: Flammarion Médecine Sciences, 1994.

Broyer, M. *et al.* (1996). Clinical polymorphism of cystinosis encephalopathy. Results of treatment with cysteamine. *Journal of Inherited Metabolic Diseases* **19**, 65–75.

Cetinkaya, I. *et al.* (2002). Inhibition of Na$^+$ dependent transporters in cystine loaded human renal cell: electrophysiological studies on the Fanconi syndrome of cystinosis. *Journal of the American Society of Nephrology* **13**, 2085–2093.

Cherqui, S., Kalatzis, V., Trugnan, G., and Antignac, C. (2001). The targetting of cystinosin to the lysosomal membrane requires a tyrosine based signal and a novel sorting motif. *Journal of Biological Chemistry* **276**, 13314–13321.

Cherqui, S. *et al.* (2002). Intralysosomal cystine accumulation in mice lacking cystinosin the protein defective in cystinosis. *Molecular and Cellular Biology* **22**, 7622–7632.

Chik, C. L., Friedman, A., Merriam, G. R., and Gahl, W. A. (1993). Pituitary-testicular function in nephropathic cystinosis. *Annals of Internal Medicine* **119**, 568–575.

Cochat, P., Cordier, B., Lacote, C., and Saïd, M. H. Cystinosis epidemiology in France. In *Cystinosis* Vol. 1 (ed. M. Broyer), pp. 28–35. Paris: Elsevier, 1999.

Cogan, D. G. *et al.* (1957). Cystinosis in a adult. *Journal of the American Medical Association* **164**, 394.

Colah, S. and Trauner, D. A. (1997). Tactile recognition in infantile nephropathic cystinosis. *Developmental Medicine and Child Neurology* **39**, 409–413.

Corden, B. J., Schulman, J. D., Schneider, J. A., and Thoene, J. G. (1981). Adverse reactions to oral cysteamine use in nephropathic cystinosis. *Developmental Pharmacology and Therapeutics* **3**, 25–30.

Da Silva, V. A. *et al.* (1985). Long term teatment of infantile nephropathic cystinosis with cysteamine. *New England Journal of Medicine* **313**, 1460–1463.

Elenberg, E., Norling, L. L., Kleinman, R. E., and Ingelfinger, J. R. (1998). Feeding problems in cystinosis. *Pediatric Nephrology* **12**, 365–370.

Fanconi, G. (1931). Die nicht diabetischen gkycosurien und hyperglycamien des altern kindes. *Jahresbericht Kinderkeilkunde* **133**, 257.

Filler, G. *et al.* (1998). Slow deteriorating insulin secretion and C-peptide production characterizes diabetes mellitus in infantile cystinosis. *European Journal of Pediatrics* **157**, 738–742.

Fivusch, B., Flick, J., and Gahl, W. A. (1988). Pancreatic exocrine insufficiency in a patient with nephropathic cystinosis. *Journal of Pediatrics* **112**, 49–51.

Foreman, J. W. *et al.* (1987). Effect of cystine dimethyl ester on renal solute handling and isolated renal tubule transport in the rat: a new model of the Fanconi syndrome. *Metabolism* **36**, 1185–1191.

Forestier, L. *et al.* (1999). Molecular characteristics of CTNS deletions in nephropathic cystinosis: development of a PCR-based detection assay. *American Journal of Human Genetics* **65**, 353–359.

Gagnadoux, M. F. *et al.* Hepatosplenic disorders in nephropathic cystinosis. In *Cystinosis* Vol. 1 (ed. M. Broyer), pp. 70–74. Paris: Elsevier, 1999.

Gahl, W. A., Hubbard, V. S., and Orloff, S. (1984). Decreased sweat production in cystinosis. *Journal of Pediatrics* **104**, 904–905.

Gahl, W. A. *et al.* (1987a). Cysteamine therapy for children with nephropathic cystinosis. *New England Journal of Medicine* **316**, 971–977.

Gahl, W. A. *et al.* (1987b). Complications of nephropathic cystinosis after renal failure. *Pediatric Nephrology* **1**, 260–268.

Gahl, W. A. *et al.* (1988a). Oral carnitine therapy in children with cystinosis and renal Fanconi syndrome. *Journal of Clinical Investigation* **81**, 549–560.

Gahl, W. A., Dalakas, M., Charnas, L., and Chen, K. (1988b). Myopathy and cystine storage in muscles in a patient with nephropathic cystinosis. *New England Journal of Medicine* **319**, 1461–1464.

Gahl, W. A., Schneider, J. A., and Aula, P. P. Lysosomal transport disorders: cystinosis and sialic acid storage disorders. In *The Metabolic and Molecular Bases of Inherited Diseases* Vol. III, 7th edn. (ed. C. R. Seriver *et al.*), pp. 3763–3797. New York: McGrawHill, 1995.

Gahl, W. A. *et al.* (2000). Corneal crystals in nephropathic cystinosis: natural history and treatment with cysteamine eyedrops. *Molecular Genetics and Metabolism* **71**, 100–120.

Gradus, D. B. E. *et al.* (1986). Treatment of infantile cystinosis with cysteamine. *New England Journal of Medicine* **314**, 1319–1320.

Gubler, M. C., Lacoste, M., Sich, M., and Broyer, M. The pathology of the kidney in cystinosis. In *Cystinosis* Vol. 1 (ed. M. Broyer), pp. 42–48. Paris: Elsevier, 1999.

Guillet, G. *et al.* (1998). Skin storage of cystine and premature skin ageing in cystinosis. *Lancet* **352**, 1444–1445.

Haycock, G. B., Al-dahhan, J., Mak, R. H. K., and Chantler, C. (1982). Effect of indomethacin on clinical progress and renal function in cystinosis. *Archives of Disease in Childhood* **57**, 934–939.

Hory, B., Billerey, C., Royer, J., and Saint, Hillier, Y. (1994). Glomerular lesions in juvenile cystinosis: report of 2 cases. *Clinical Nephrology* **42**, 327–330.

Kaiser-Kupfer, M. I., Caruso, R. C., Monkler, D. S., and Gahl, W. A. (1986). Long-term ocular manifestations in nephropathic cystinosis. *Archives of Ophthalmology* 104, 706–711.

Kalatzis, V., Cherqui, S., Antignac, C., and Gasnier, B. (2001). Cystinosin, the protein defective in cystinosis is a H^+ driven lysosomal transporter. *EMBO Journal* 20, 5940–5949.

Kimonis, V. E. *et al.* (1995). Effects of early cysteamine therapy on thyroid function and growth in nephropathic cystinosis. *Journal of Clinical Endocrinology and Metabolism* 80, 3257–3261.

Kleta, R. *et al.* (2001). CTNS mutations in African American patients with cystinosis. *Molecular Genetics and Metabolism* 74, 332–337.

Langman, C. B., Moore, E. S., Thoene, J. G., and Schneider, J. A. (1985). Renal failure in a sibship with late onset cystinosis. *Journal of Pediatrics* 107, 755.

Lignac, G. O. E. (1924). Uber Störung des Cystinstoffwe'chsels bei Kindern. *Deutsches Archiv für Klinische Medizin* 125, 139–150.

Lucky, A. W. *et al.* Endocrine studies in cystinosis: compensated primary hypothyroidism. *Journal of Pediatrics* 91, 204–210.

Mahoney, C. P. and Striker, G. E. (2000). Early development of the renal lesions in infantile cystinosis. *Pediatric Nephrology* 15, 50–56.

Manz, F. and Gretz, N. (1985). Cystinosis in the federal republic of Germany: coordination and analysis of the data. *Journal of Inherited Metabolic Disease* 8, 2–4.

Manz, F. and Gretz, N. (1994). Progression of chronic renal failure in a historical group of patients with nephropathic cystinosis. European Collaborative Study on Cystinosis. *Pediatric Nephrology* 8, 466–471.

Markello, T. C., Bernardini, I. M., and Gahl, W. A. (1993). Improved renal function in children with cystinosis treated with cysteamine. *New England Journal of Medicine* 328, 1157–1162.

McDowell, G. *et al.* (1996). Fine mapping of the cystinosis gene using an integrated genetic and physical map of a region within human chromosome band 17p13. *Biochemical and Molecular Medicine* 58, 135–141.

Mungan, N. *et al.* (2000). Ultrasound biomicroscopy of the eye in cystinosis. *Archives of Ophthalmology* 118, 1329–1333.

Nichols, S., Press, G., Schneider, J., and Trauner, D. (1990). Cortical atrophy and cognitive performance in infantile nephropathic cystinosis. *Pediatric Neurology* 6, 379–381.

Okami, T., Nakajima, M., Higashino, H., and Aoki, T. (1992). Ocular manifestations in a case of infantile cystinosis. *Nippon Ganka Gakkai Zasshi* 96, 538–543.

Patrick, A. D. and Lake, B. D. (1968). Cystinosis: electron microscope evidence of lysosomal storage of cystine in lymph node. *Journal of Pathology* 21, 571.

Patrick, A. D. *et al.* (1987). First trimester diagnosis of cystinosis using intact chorionic villi. *Prenatal Diagnosis* 7, 71–74.

Phomphutkul, C. *et al.* (2001). The promoter of a lysosomal membrane transporter gene CTNS binds Sp1, shares sequences with the promoter of an adjacent gene CARKL and causes cystinosis if mutated in a critical region. *American Journal of Human Genetics* 69, 712–721.

Reiss, R. E., Kuwabara, T., Smith, M. L., and Gahl, W. A. (1988). Successful pregnancy despite placental crystals in a woman with nephropathic cystinosis. *New England Journal of Medicine* 319, 223–226.

Rizzo, C. *et al.* (1999). Pyroglutamic aciduria and nephropathic cystinosis. *Journal of Inherited Metabolic Disease* 22, 224–226.

Robert, J. J. *et al.* (1999). Diabetes mellitus in patients with infantile cystinosis after renal transplantation. *Pediatric Nephrology* 13, 524–529.

Schnaper, H. W. *et al.* (1992). Early occurrence of end-stage renal disease in a patient with infantile nephropathic cystinosis. *Journal of Pediatrics* 120, 575–578.

Schneider, J., Bradley, K., and Seegmiler, J. E. (1967). Increased cystine in leukocytes from individuals homozygous and heterozygous for cystinosis. *Science* 157, 1321–1322.

Schneider, J. A., Wong, V., Bradley, K., and Seegmiler, J. E. (1968). Biochemical comparisons of the adult and childhood forms of cystinosis. *New England Journal of Medicine* 279, 1253–1257.

Smolin, L. A., Clark, K. F., and Schneider, J. A. (1987). An improved method for heterozygote detection of cystinosis, using polymorphonuclear leukocyte. *American Journal of Human Genetics* 41, 266–275.

Smolin, L. A. *et al.* (1988). A comparison of the effectiveness of cysteamine and phosphocysteamine in elevating plasma cysteamine concentration and decreasing leukocyte free cystine in nephropathic cystinosis. *Pediatric Research* 23, 616–620.

Sochett, E. *et al.* (1984). Nephropathic cystinosis in black children. Case reports. *South African Medical Journal* 65, 397–398.

Sonies, B. C. *et al.* (1990). Swallowing dysfunction in nephropathic cystinosis. *New England Journal of Medicine* 323, 565–570.

Spear, G. S. (1973). The proximal tubule and the podocyte in cystinosis. *Nephron* 10, 57–60.

Steinherz, R. *et al.* (1982). Cystine accumulation and clearance by normal and cystinotic leukocytes exposed to cystine dimethyl ester. *Proceedings of the National Academy of Science of the United States of America* 79, 4446–4450.

Tenneze, L. *et al.* (1999). A study of the relative bioavailability of cysteamine hydrochloride, cysteamine bitartrate and phosphocysteamine in healthy adult male volunteers. *British Journal of Clinical Pharmacology* 47, 49–52.

Tete, M. J. and Broyer, M. Thyroid and gonads involvement in cystinosis. In *Cystinosis* Vol. 1 (ed. M. Broyer), pp. 63–69. Paris: Elsevier, 1999.

Theodoropoulos, D. S., Krasnewich, D., Kaiser-Kupfer, M. I., and Gahl, W. A. (1993). Classic nephropathic cystinosis as an adult disease. *Journal of the American Medical Association* 270, 2200–2204.

Theodoropoulos, D. S., Shawker, T. H., Heinrichs, C., and Gahl, W. A. (1995). Medullary nephrocalcinosis in nephropathic cystinosis. *Pediatric Nephrology* 9, 412–418.

Thoene, J. G. *et al.* (1976). Cystinosis intracellular cystine depletion by aminothiols *in vitro* and *in vivo*. *Journal of Clinical Investigation* 58, 180–189.

Town, M. *et al.* (1998). A novel gene encoding an integral membrane protein is mutated in nephropathic cystinosis. *Nature Genetics* 18, 319–324.

Trauner, D. *et al.* (1988). Neurologic and cognitive deficits in children with cystinosis. *Journal of Pediatrics* 112, 912–914.

Trauner, D., Fahmy, R. F., and Mishler, D. A. (2001). Oral motor dysfunction and feeding difficulties in nephropathic cystinosis. *Pediatric Neurology* 24, 365–368.

Van't Hoff, W. and Gretz, N. (1995). The treatment of cystinosis with cysteamine and phosphocysteamine in the United Kingdom and Eire. *Pediatric Nephrology* 9, 685–689.

Van't Hoff, W. G., Lederman, S. E., Waldron, M., and Trompeter, R. S. (1995). Early-onset chronic renal failure as a presentation of infantile nephropathic cystinosis. *Pediatric Nephrology* 9, 483–484.

Waldherr, R., Manz, F., and Hagge, H. (1982). The pathology of the kidney in infantile and adolescent cystinosis. *Verhandlungen der Deutschen Gesellschaft fur Pathologie* 66, 297–303.

Wenner, W. J. and Murphy, J. L. (1997). The effects of cysteamine on the upper gastrointestinal tract of children with cystinosis. *Pediatric Nephrology* 11, 600–603.

Wuhl, E. *et al.* (1998). Treatment with recombinant human growth hormone in short children with nephropathic cystinosis: no evidence for increased deterioration rate of renal function. *Pediatric Research* 43, 484–488.

16.5.2 The primary hyperoxalurias

Pierre Cochat and Marie-Odile Rolland

Primary hyperoxaluria (PH) results from endogenous overproduction of oxalic acid, as opposed to secondary hyperoxaluria which is attributable to increased intestinal absorption or excessive intake of oxalate. Such derangement leads to accumulation of oxalate within the body. The main target organ is the kidney since oxalate cannot be metabolized and is excreted in the urine leading to nephrocalcinosis, recurrent urolithiasis, and subsequent renal impairment. Hyperoxaluria—the hallmark of any kind of PH—is associated with increased urinary excretion of either glycolate in PH1 or L-glycerate in PH2.

Oxalate metabolism (Fig. 1)

Oxalate is a poorly soluble end-product of the metabolism of a number of amino acids, particularly glycine, and of other compounds such as sugars and ascorbic acid. The immediate precursors of oxalate are glyoxylate and glycolate. The main site of synthesis of glyoxylate and oxalate is the liver peroxisome, which can also detoxify glyoxylate by reconversion into glycine, catalysed by alanine : glyoxylate aminotransferase (AGT). In the cytosol, glyoxylate can be converted into oxalate by lactic acid dehydrogenase (LDH); it can also be converted into glycolate by glyoxylate reductase (GR), and into glycine by glutamate : glyoxylate aminotransferase. Glycolate can also be formed from hydroxypyruvate, a catabolite of glucose and fructose. Hydroxypyruvate can be converted into L-glycerate by LDH, and into D-glycerate by hydroxypyruvate reductase (HPR), which also has a GR activity.

Primary hyperoxaluria type 1

PH1 (OMIM 259900)—the most common form of PH—is an autosomal recessive disorder caused by the functional defect of the hepatic,

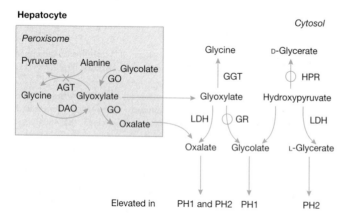

Fig. 1 Major reactions involved in oxalate, glyoxylate, and glycolate metabolism in the human hepatocyte (adapted from Barratt 1999). AGT, alanine: glyoxylate aminotranferase; DAO, D-amino oxidase; GGT, glutamate: glyoxylate aminotransferase; HPR, hydroxypyruvate reductase; LDH, lactate dehydrogenase; ×, metabolic block in PH1; ○, metabolic block in PH2.

peroxisomal, pyridoxal phosphate-dependent enzyme AGT. The disease occurs because AGT activity is undetectable or because AGT is mistargetted to mitochondria, which may explain clinical and enzymatic heterogeneity.

Metabolic derangement (Fig. 1)

PH1 is due to a deficiency of the liver-specific pyridoxal-phosphate-dependent enzyme AGT (EC 2.6.1.44) (Danpure 1986). The resulting decreased transamination of glyoxylate into glycine leads to a subsequent increase in its oxidation to oxalate, a poorly soluble end-product. In patients with a presumptive diagnosis of PH, 10–30 per cent are identified as non-PH1 because AGT activity and immunoreactivity are normal (Danpure 1995; Fargue 2002). Among PH1 patients, 75 per cent have undetectable enzyme activity (*enz*−) and the majority of these also have no immunoreactive protein (cross-reacting material, *crm*−). In the rare *enz*−/*crm*+ patients, a catalytically inactive but immunoreactive AGT is found within the peroxisomes. The remaining PH1 patients have AGT activity in the range of 5–50 per cent of the mean normal activity (*enz*+), and the level of immunoreactive protein parallels the level of enzyme activity (*crm*+) (Danpure 1995). In *enz*+/*crm*+ patients, the disease is caused by a mistargeting of AGT: about 90 per cent of the immunoreactive AGT is localized in the mitochondria instead of in the peroxisomes, where only 10 per cent of the activity is found; almost all patients who are pyridoxine-responsive are in this group (Barratt 1999). Interestingly, human hepatocyte AGT, which is normally exclusively localized within the peroxisomes, is unable to function when diverted to the mitochondria. In addition, patients with a primary peroxisomal disorder—for example, Zellweger syndrome—do not exhibit hyperoxaluria.

A viable mouse model that reproduces derangements associated to human PH1 has been recently developed (Salido *et al.* 2002).

Genetics

PH1 is the most common form of PH (ranging from 1 : 60,000 to 1 : 120,000 live births) (Cochat and Rolland 2000; Leumann and Hoppe 2001). Due to autosomal recessive inheritance, it is much more frequent when parental consanguinity is present, that is, in developing countries (Cochat 1999). Indeed, it is responsible for less than 0.5 per cent of endstage renal failure (ESRF) in children in Europe versus 13 per cent in Tunisia (Cochat and Rolland 2000).

Human liver AGT cDNA and genomic DNA have been cloned and sequenced; the normal AGT gene (*AGXT*) is a single copy gene which maps to chromosome 2q36-q37 (11 exons spanning ~10 kb); the protein contains 392 amino acids and has a molecular mass of 43 kDa (Danpure and Rumsby 1995). Polymorphic variations have been identified; the two best studied polymorphic variants are those encoded by the major *AGXT* allele (80 per cent frequency in the European and North-American populations) and the minor *AGXT* allele, which has a frequency of 20 per cent (Danpure and Rumsby 1995).

Around 40 mutations have been identified so far. Some of them are more frequent and play a role either in enzyme trafficking or in clinical/biochemical phenotype (Danpure and Rumsby 1995; Lumb and Danpure 2000; Nogueira *et al.* 2000; Amoroso 2001; Pirulli *et al.* 2001; Monico *et al.* 2002), for example, Gly82Gln is associated with loss of AGT catalytic activity, Ile244Thr with increased AGT degradation, Gly41Arg with intraperoxisomal AGT aggregation, Gly170Arg with peroxisome-to-mitochondrion mistargetting. Ile244Thr and Gly170Arg mutations are common in European and North-American patients (~40 per cent of mutant alleles) and interact with the Pro11Leu polymorphism. Such a polymorphism has an ~20 per cent allelic frequency and plays an important role in phenotype determination (Lumb and Dampure 2000). The mechanism of action of some mutations has been approached by structural analysis of crystallized variants of AGT (Zhang 2001).

DNA analysis among different ethnic groups has revealed the presence of specific mutations, founder effects and phenotype–genotype correlations among North-African, Japanese, Turkish, and Pakistani populations (Danpure and Rumsby 1995; von Schnackenburg *et al.* 1998; Basmaison *et al.* 2000).

Clinical presentation

PH1 grossly fits five clinical presentations: (a) a rare infantile form with early nephrocalcinosis and kidney failure; (b) a late-onset form with occasional stone passage in late adulthood; (c) the most common form with recurrent urolithiasis and progressive renal failure leading to a diagnosis of PH1 in childhood or adolescence; (d) a rare condition where the diagnosis is given by post-transplantation recurrence; and (e) presymptomatic subjects in whom PH1 is discovered from family history (Cochat and Basmaison 2000).

Renal involvement

PH1 presents with symptoms referable to the urinary tract in more than 90 per cent of the cases: loin pain, haematuria, urinary tract infection, passage of stones, evidence of nephrocalcinosis, uraemia, metabolic acidosis, growth delay, and anaemia. Oxalate exerts a toxic effect on renal epithelial cells and, therefore, leads to direct tubular damage (Scheid *et al.* 1996). However, the most common presentation is stone disease. Calculi—multiple, bilateral, and radio-opaque—are composed of calcium oxalate. Nephrocalcinosis, best demonstrated by ultrasound, is present on plain abdomen X-ray at an advanced stage (Fig. 2). The median age at initial symptoms is 5 years, ranging from birth to the sixth decade; ESRF is reached by the age of 25 years in half of the patients (Cochat and Rolland 2000). The infantile form often presents as a life-threatening condition because of rapid progression to ESRF due to both early oxalate load and immature glomerular filtration rate (GFR): one-half of the patients experience ESRF at the time of diagnosis and 80 per cent develop ESRF by the age of 3 years (Cochat *et al.* 1999).

The association of renal calculi, nephrocalcinosis, and renal impairment strongly suggests PH1.

Extrarenal involvement

When GFR falls to below 30–50 ml/min/1.73 m^2, continued overproduction of oxalate by the liver along with reduced oxalate excretion by the kidneys leads to a critical saturation point for plasma oxalate (Pox > 30–50 µmol/l) so that oxalate deposition occurs in many organs (Morgan *et al.* 1987; Toussaint *et al.* 1993; Monico *et al.* 1999).

Bone is the major compartment of the insoluble oxalate pool and the bone oxalate content is higher (15–910 µmol oxalate/g bony tissue) than among ESRF patients without PH1 (2–9 µmol/g) (Marangella *et al.* 1995b). Calcium oxalate crystals accumulate first in the metaphyseal area and form dense suprametaphyseal bands on X-ray. Later on, oxalate osteopathy leads to pain, erythropoietin-resistant anaemia, and spontaneous fractures (Fig. 3).

Along with the skeleton, systemic involvement includes many organs because of progressive vascular lesions: heart (cardiomyopathy, arrhythmias, heart block), nerves (polyradiculoneuropathy), joints (synovitis, chondrocalcinosis), skin (ulcerating miliary calcium oxalate nodules, livedo reticularis), soft tissues (peripheral gangrene), retina (flecked retinopathy, choroidal neovascularization) (Fig. 4), and other visceral lesions (e.g. intestinal infarction, hypothyroidism) (Cochat and Basmaison 2000).

Systemic involvement—named 'oxalosis'—is responsible for poor quality of life leading to both disability and severe complications. Indeed, PH1 is one of the most life-threatening hereditary renal diseases, mainly in developing countries where the mortality rate may reach 100 per cent in the absence of adequate treatment (Cochat and Rolland 2000).

Diagnosis

Unfortunately, the diagnosis of PH1 is still being often delayed, sometimes for 5–10 years following initial symptoms.

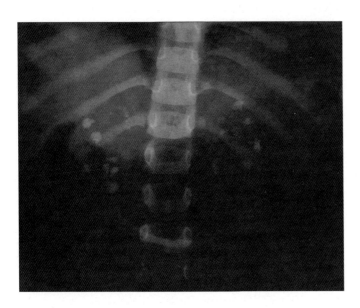

Fig. 2 Plain abdomen X-ray: bilateral nephrocalcinosis in a 5-year-old boy.

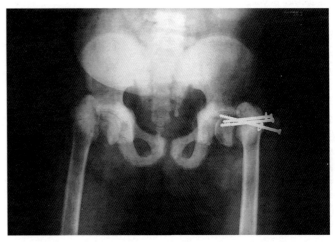

Fig. 3 Plain X-ray: diffuse bone disease and bilateral hip fractures in a 17-year-old boy who underwent two previous renal transplantations in the absence of diagnosis of PH1 in a developing country.

The combination of both clinical and radiological presentation is a strong argument for PH1 in a large number of patients. In addition, family history may provide major additional information.

Physicochemical investigation is of crucial interest in the diagnosis procedure and infrared spectroscopy is helpful for identification and quantitative analysis of stones, showing calcium oxalate monohydrate crystals (type Ic whewellite) (Quy Dao and Dandon 1997). Such crystals can also be identified in urine or tissues (kidney, bone, marrow) by polarized light microscopy or infrared spectroscopy (Figs 5 and 6) (Daudon *et al.* 1998). Fundoscopy may also show flecked retina (Fig. 4).

In patients with normal or significant residual GFR, concomitant hyperoxaluria and hyperglycolaturia are indicative of PH1 (Table 1), but 20–30 per cent of patients do not present with hyperglycoluria (Latta *et al.* 1991). In dialysis patients, the assessment may include plasma oxalate (and/or glycolate): creatinine ratio, and oxalate (and/or glycolate) measurement in dialysate (Gaulier *et al.* 1997).

A definitive diagnosis requires assessment of AGT activity and immunoreactivity in hepatic tissue (from a liver biopsy specimen, minimum of 4 mg). Nevertheless, there is controversial information about the relationship between AGT activity and the severity of the disease (Amoroso *et al.* 2001). However, liver biopsy assessment is mandatory if a liver transplantation is being considered.

In selected populations, a direct molecular diagnosis can be proposed, that is, the search for the Ile244Thr mutation in patients from Maghreb (Basmaison 2000). However, in most Europeans, the search for frequent mutations (e.g. Gly170Arg) cannot currently replace enzymology in the diagnosis of PH1.

Prenatal diagnosis can be performed from DNA obtained from crude chorionic villi (10–12 weeks gestation) or amniocytes (13–17 weeks gestation). It is based on either mutational analysis using PCR amplification or linkage analysis using various intragenic and closely linked extragenic polymorphisms in the *AGXT* gene; in both cases, DNA

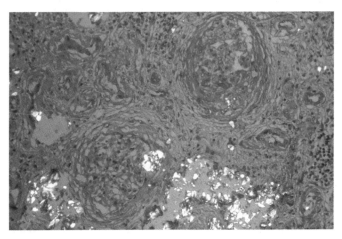

Fig. 6 Renal biopsy in a 30-year-old patient with advanced renal failure (polarized light microscopy): oxalate crystal deposition in tubules, glomeruli and interstitial tissue.

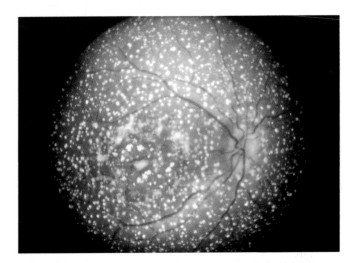

Fig. 4 Fundoscopy in a 13-year-old boy with PH1 showing flecked retina in the absence of visual impairment.

Table 1 Plasma and urine concentrations of oxalate, glycolate, and L-glycerate: normal values (Gaulier 1997; Barratt 1999; Leumann 2001)

Urine		
Oxalate per day		<0.50 mmol/1.73 m^2
Oxalate: creatinine	Age $<$ 1 year	<0.15 mmol/mmol
	1–4 years	<0.13 mmol/mmol
	5–12 years	<0.07 mmol/mmol
	Adult	<0.08 mmol/mmol
Glycolate per day	Child	<0.55 mmol/1.73 m^2
	Adult	<0.26 mmol/1.73 m^2
Glycolate: creatinine	Age $<$ 1 year	<0.07 mmol/mmol
	1–4 years	<0.09 mmol/mmol
	5–12 years	<0.05 mmol/mmol
	Adult	<0.04 mmol/mmol
L-Glycerate: creatinine		<0.03 mmol/mmol
Plasma		
Oxalate	Child	<7.4 μmol/l
	Adult	<5.4 μmol/l
Oxalate: creatinine	Child	<0.19 μmol/μmol
	Adult	<0.06 μmol/μmol

Oxalate (COOH–COOH): 1 mmol = 90 mg.

Glycolate (COOH–CH$_2$OH): 1 mmol = 76 mg.

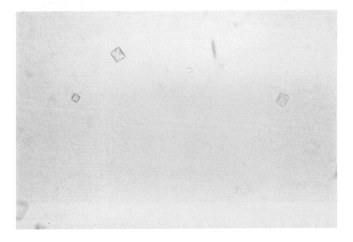

Fig. 5 Urine sediment examination: rhomboaedric calcium oxalate crystals.

from the index case and the parents must be available (Rumsby 1998). Such a procedure allows the identification of normal, affected, and carrier fetuses.

The detection of *AGXT* mutations using simplified reliable technology can be proposed to identify healthy carriers amongst family members, and sometimes for screening of polymorphisms in patients with nephrolithiasis (Pirulli 2001).

Treatment and prognosis

Supportive treatment

Conservative measures should be started as soon as the diagnosis has been made and even suspected. The aims are to decrease oxalate production and to increase the urinary solubility of calcium oxalate. The risk of stone formation is increased when urine oxalate exceeds 0.4–0.6 mmol/l, especially if urine calcium exceeds 4 mmol/l. Therefore, supportive therapy should be adapted to keep concentrations of oxalate and calcium below these limits (Hallson 1988). This should be attempted by giving high fluid intake (>2 l/m^2 per day) and supported by calcium-oxalate crystallization inhibitors. Citrate (potassium or sodium), 100–150 mg/kg per day in 3–4 divided doses (Leumann and Hoppe 2001; Milliner *et al.* 2001), has been shown to be efficient. When it is not available, crystallization inhibition may be obtained by using sodium bicarbonate, magnesium or orthophosphate (Leumann and Hoppe 2001). Diuretics require careful management: frusemide will maintain a high urine output with the risk of an increased calciuria, whereas the diuretic effect of hydrochlorothiazide is less marked but is associated with an appreciable decrease of calcium excretion.

Restriction of dietary oxalate intake (beetroot, strawberries, rhubarb, spinach, coffee, tea, nuts) has limited influence on the disease as oxalate of dietary origin contributes very little to hyperoxaluria in PH (Leumann and Hoppe 2001). Calcium restriction is not recommended, because less calcium would then bind oxalate and form insoluble calcium-oxalate complexes in the gut. Ascorbic acid supplementation is not recommended as it is a precursor of oxalate.

The absence of intestinal oxalate-degrading bacterium *Oxalobacter formigenes* has been found to be associated with hyperoxaluria (Sidhu 1998), so that increased amounts of such a microorganism in the gut by oral route might decrease disposable oxalate.

The main purpose of therapy is to lower both Pox and plasma calcium-oxalate saturation. The effects of conservative measures can be assessed by serial determinations of crystalluria score and calcium oxalate supersaturation software (Jouvet *et al.* 1998; Milliner 2001).

Pyridoxine (cofactor of AGT, see Fig. 1) sensitivity (i.e. >30 per cent reduction of urinary oxalate excretion) is found in 10–40 per cent of patients, so that it must be tested early at a daily dose of 2–5 mg/kg with stepwise increase up to 10–20 mg/kg (Leumann and Hoppe 2001). Response to pyridoxine may delay the progression to ESRF; it can be detected by both oxalate and glycolate measurement and should be tested at any stage of the disease (Danpure and Rumsby 1995; Barratt *et al.* 1999; Milliner *et al.* 2001). However, one should keep in mind that mega-doses of pyridoxine may induce sensory neuropathy. The patients most likely to respond are those with residual AGT activity, but pyridoxine responsiveness is still poorly understood at the molecular level (Marangella 1999).

The treatment of stones should avoid open and percutaneous surgery because further renal lesions will alter GFR. The use of extracorporeal shock wave lithotripsy may be an available option in selected

patients, but the presence of nephrocalcinosis may be responsible for parenchymal damage.

Bilateral nephrectomy is recommended in most patients on renal replacement therapy in order to limit the risk of infection, obstruction and passage of stones.

Renal replacement therapy

Dialysis

Conventional dialysis is unsuitable for patients who have reached ESRF because it cannot clear sufficient amounts of oxalate (Barratt and Danpure 1999). In such patients, Pox ranges between 80–140 μmol/l (normal $<$ 7 μmol/l) (Table 1). Therefore, daily haemodialysis (~8 h per session) using high-flux membranes would be required but such a strategy cannot be routinely used (Yamauchi *et al.* 2001). The challenge is to keep predialysis Pox below 50 μmol/l in order to limit the progression of systemic oxalosis. Conventional long-term haemodialysis is generally contraindicated because it only prolongs a miserable existence: instead of dying quickly from uraemia, patients experience a deterioration in their quality of life and die because of the progression of systemic oxalate deposition. The benefit of (pre-) post-transplantation haemodialysis is still debated and should be limited to patients with either oliguria or severe systemic burden and subsequent long lasting oxalate release from skeleton.

Kidney transplantation

Kidney transplantation allows significant removal of soluble oxalate. However, because the biochemical defect is in the liver, overproduction of oxalate and subsequent deposition in tissues continues unabated. The high rate of urinary oxalate excretion originates from both ongoing oxalate production from the native liver and oxalate deposits in tissues. Due to oxalate accumulation in the graft, isolated kidney transplantation is no longer recommended, because of a 100 per cent recurrence rate leading to poor graft survival (48 per cent at 8 years post-transplantation) and patient quality of life (Cibrik *et al.* 2002). Indeed, renal transplantation does not prevent the progression of skeletal and vascular complications. The chances of a successful transplantation are unrelated to residual AGT activity (Katz *et al.* 1992), but success is improved if the transplantation is performed when there is substantial renal function, that is, a GFR ranging from 20–30 ml/min/1.73 m^2, and in the absence of important extrarenal involvement. In selected patients, good results have been reported after early renal transplantation and vigorous perioperative dialysis (Scheinman 1984; Monico 2001); however, living donors should be avoided because the overall results are poor (Jamieson 1998; Cibrik *et al.* 2002). Isolated kidney transplantation may be regarded as a temporary solution in some countries before managing the patient in a specialized center for further (combined) liver (-kidney) procedure.

Despite previous pyridoxine resistance, it is recommended to retest vitamin B6 following isolated renal transplantation (Monico and Milliner 2001).

Enzyme replacement therapy

Ideally, any kind of transplantation should precede advanced systemic oxalate storage (Cochat and Basmaison 2000; Ellis *et al.* 2001). Further assessment of the oxalate burden needs therefore to be predicted by monitoring sequential GFR, Pox (Table 1), calcium oxalate saturation and systemic involvement (assessment of bone mineral density, bone histology) (Hoppe 1998; Cochat and Rolland 2000; Behnke *et al.* 2001).

Rationale for liver transplantation

Since the liver is the only organ responsible for glyoxylate detoxification by AGT, the excessive production of oxalate will continue as long as the native liver is left in place. Therefore, any form of enzyme replacement will succeed only when the deficient host liver is removed concomitantly (Danpure 1991). Liver transplantation will supply the missing enzyme in the correct organ (liver), cell (hepatocyte), and intracellular compartment (peroxisome) (Danpure 1991; Danpure and Rumsby 1995). The ultimate goal of organ replacement is to change a positive whole-body accretion rate into a negative one by reducing endogenous oxalate synthesis and providing good oxalate clearance via either the native or the transplanted kidney.

Combined liver–kidney transplantation

In Europe, 8–10 combined liver–kidney transplantations per year have been reported in the PH1 Transplant Registry Report; the results are encouraging, as patient survival approximates 80 per cent at 5 years and 65–70 per cent at 10 years (Jamieson 1998). Comparable results have been reported from the United States Renal Data System, with a 76 per cent death-censored graft survival at 8 years post-transplantation (Cibrik 2002). In addition, despite the potential risks for the grafted kidney due to oxalate release from the body stores, kidney survival is about 95 per cent 3 years post-transplantation and the GFR ranges between 40 and 60 ml/min/1.73 m^2 after 5–10 years (Danpure and Rumsby 1991; Jamieson 1998; Ellis *et al.* 2001).

Isolated liver transplantation

Isolated liver transplantation might be the first-choice treatment in selected patients before advanced chronic renal failure has occurred, that is, at a GFR between 60 and 40 ml/min/1.73 m^2 (Cochat 1993). Such a strategy has a strong rationale but raises ethical controversies. Around 20 patients have received an isolated liver transplant without uniformly accepted recommendations, since the course of the disease is unpredictable and a sustained improvement can follow a phase of rapid decrease in GFR (Cochat and Shärer 1993; Ellis *et al.* 2001; Shapiro *et al.* 2001).

Post-transplantation reversal of renal and extrarenal involvement

Deposits of calcium oxalate in tissues can be remobilized according to the accessibility of oxalate burden to the blood stream (Danpure 1991). After combined transplantation, Pox returns to normal before urine oxalate does, and oxaluria can remain elevated as long as several months (Jamieson 1998; Barratt *et al.* 1999; Monico and Milliner 2001). Therefore, there is still a risk of recurrent nephrocalcinosis or renal calculi that might jeopardize graft function. Glycolate, which is soluble and does not accumulate, is excreted in normal amounts immediately after liver transplantation.

Thus, independent of the transplantation strategy, the kidney must be protected against the damage that can be induced by heavy oxalate load suddenly released from tissues. Forced fluid intake (3–5 l/1.73 m^2 per day) supported by diuretics and the use of crystallization inhibitors is the most important strategy. Pox, crystalluria, and calcium oxalate saturation are helpful tools in renal management after combined liver–kidney transplantation (Hoppe *et al.* 1998; Jouvet *et al.* 1998; Gagnadoux *et al.* 2001). The benefit of daily high-efficiency (pre-) post-transplant haemodialysis/filtration is still debated; it will provide a rapid drop in Pox but also an increased risk of urine calcium oxalate supersaturation and therefore should be limited to patients with significant systemic involvement (Hoppe *et al.* 1998; Cochat and Rolland 2000b; Gagnadoux *et al.* 2001).

Combined transplantation should be planned when the GFR ranges between 20 and 40 ml/min/1.73 m^2 because, at this level, oxalate retention increases rapidly (Ellis *et al.* 2001; Shapiro *et al.* 2001). Of course, in patients with ESRF, vigorous haemodialysis should be started and urgent liver–kidney transplantation should be performed. Even at these late stages, damaged organs, such as the skeleton or the heart, do benefit from enzyme replacement (Cochat and Shärer 1993; Gagnadoux *et al.* 2001), which results in an appreciable improvement in quality of life.

Donors for combined liver–kidney transplantation

The type of donor—cadaver or living-related—depends mainly on the physician and the country where the patient is treated (Cochat *et al.* 1999; Nolkemper *et al.* 2000; Nakamura *et al.* 2001). According to the timing of transplantation, a living-related donor may be considered because of the restricted number of potential biorgan cadaveric donors. A living-related donor can be proposed in a pre-emptive procedure using either isolated liver or synchronous liver–kidney transplantation. In patients with ESRD and systemic involvement, a metachronous transplantation procedure might be an option since a first-step liver transplantation will then allow oxalate clearance by vigorous haemodialysis before considering further kidney transplantation from the same (living-related) donor.

Future trends

Although gene therapy has been advocated, many years of research will be required before considering its potential use (Barratt *et al.* 1999).

Different AGT crystal forms have been obtained for some polymorphic variants, and amino acid changes found in these crystals may affect AGT stability (Zhang *et al.* 2001). A better understanding of such changes will allow to design pharmacological agents that will stabilize AGT, thus providing a potential treatment for PH1 without the need for organ transplantation (Danpure, personal communication).

Non-type 1 primary hyperoxaluria

In the presence of overt hyperoxaluria, the pattern of urinary metabolites is indicative but no longer diagnostic of PH. In patients with a clinical picture of PH1, 10–30 per cent have normal AGT activity, that may lead to a diagnosis of PH2 or of another disorder causing hyperoxaluria (Fargue *et al.* 2002). Enzyme activity measurement in a needle liver biopsy can confirm or exclude PH1 and PH2.

Primary hyperoxaluria type 2 (PH2)

PH2 (OMIM 260000) is another rare inherited defect of oxalate metabolism causing raised urine oxalate and L-glycerate.

Metabolic derangement

PH2 is characterized by the absence of an enzyme with GR, HPR, and D-glycerate-dehydrogenase (GD) activities (Fig. 1) (Giafi and Rumsby 1998a; Webster 2000). Analysis of liver and lymphocyte samples from patients with PH2 showed that GR activity was either very low or undetectable while GD activity was reduced in liver but within the normal range in lymphocytes (Giafi and Rumsby 1998b).

Genetics

There is evidence for autosomal recessive transmission and the gene encoding the enzyme glyoxylate-reductase/hydroxypyruvate-reductase (*GRHPR*) has been located on chromosome Iccn (Cramer *et al.* 1999). Several missense, nonsense, and deletion mutations have been identified (Webster 2000).

Clinical presentation

PH2 has been documented in less than 40 patients but there are some unreported cases. Median age at onset of first symptoms is 1–2 years, and the classical presentation is urolithiasis, including haematuria and obstruction. However, stone-forming activity is lower than in PH1; this may be due to greater oxalate excretion and lower concentration of urine citrate and magnesium (Milliner 2001). GFR is usually maintained during childhood and systemic involvement is therefore exceptional (Kemper *et al.* 1997).

Diagnosis

In the presence of hyperoxaluria without hyperglycoluria, a diagnosis of PH2 should be considered, especially when AGT activity is normal. However, hyperoxaluria in PH2 tends to be less pronounced than in PH1 (Milliner *et al.* 2001). The biochemical hallmark is the increased urinary excretion of L-glycerate (Table 1) but the definitive diagnosis requires measurement of GR activity in a liver biopsy (Marangella *et al.* 1995a) as some PH2 patients have normal L-glycericaciduria (Rumsby *et al.* 2001).

Treatment and prognosis

The overall long-term prognosis is better than for PH1. ESRF occurs in 12 per cent of patients, between 23 and 50 years of age. As in PH1, supportive treatment includes high fluid intake, crystallization inhibitors and prevention of complications. Kidney transplantation has been performed in some patients, often leading to recurrence including hyperoxaluria and L-glycerate excretion (Johnson *et al.* 2002). The concept of liver transplantation has therefore been suggested, but more data are needed concerning the tissue distribution of the deficient enzyme and the biochemical impact of hepatic GR/HPR deficiency before such a strategy can be recommended.

Non-type 1 non-type 2 primary hyperoxaluria

There are some isolated reports of PH without AGT or GR/HPR deficiency, and of PH with hyperglycoluria in the absence of AGT deficiency (van Acker *et al.* 1996; Monico and Rumsby 2002). It is therefore likely that there is at least another form of PH yet to be explained; hepatic glycolate-oxidase is a candidate enzyme for a third form of PH.

Conclusion

Patients with either hyperoxaluria or recurrent calcium oxalate urolithiasis should be referred for diagnosis and management to specialist clinical centers with interest and experience in the conditions and access to the appropriate biochemical and molecular biological facilities. Indeed, major advances in biochemistry, enzymology, genetics, and management have been achieved during recent years in PH. Further steps will assess genotype–phenotype relationship and underlying metabolic defects of atypical PH. The ongoing analysis of transplant strategies from multicentre database will improve individual enzyme replacement and subsequent patient survival and quality of life.

References

Amoroso, A. *et al.* (2001). AGXT gene mutations and their influence on clinical heterogeneity of type 1 primary hyperoxaluria. *Journal of the American Society of Nephrology* **12**, 2072–2079.

Barratt, T. M. and Danpure, C. J. Hyperoxaluria. In *Pediatric Nephrology* 4th edn. (ed. T. M. Barratt, E. D. Avner, and W. E. Harmon), pp. 609–619. Baltimore: Williams & Wilkins, 1999.

Basmaison, O., Rolland, M. O., Cochat, P., and Bozon, D. (2000). Identification of 5 novel mutations in the AGXT gene. *Human Mutation* **15**, 577.

Behnke, B., Kemper, M. J., Kruse, H. P., and Muller-Wiefel, D. E. (2001). Bone mineral density in children with primary hyperoxaluria type 1. *Nephrology, Dialysis, Transplantation* **16**, 2236–2239.

Cibrik, D. M., Kaplan, B., Arndorfer, J. A., and Meier-Kriesche, H. U. (2002). Renal allograft survival in patients with oxalosis. *Transplantation* **74**, 707–710.

Cochat, P. and Basmaison, O. (2000). Current approaches to the management of primary hyperoxaluria. *Archives of Diseases in Childhood* **82**, 470–473.

Cochat, P. and Rolland, M. O. Primary hyperoxaluria. In *Inborn Metabolic Diseases and Treatment* 3rd edn. (ed. J. Fernandes, J. M. Saudubray, and G. van den Berghe), pp. 441–446. Heidelberg: Springer Verlag, 2000.

Cochat, P. and Shärer, K. (1993). Should liver transplantation be performed before advanced renal insufficiency in primary hyperoxaluria type 1? *Pediatric Nephrology* **7**, 212–218.

Cochat, P. *et al.* (1999). Primary hyperoxaluria in infants: medical, ethical and economic issues. *Journal of Pediatrics* **135**, 746–750.

Cramer, S. D. *et al.* (1999). The gene encoding hydroxypyruvate reductase (GRHPR) is mutated in patients with primary hyperoxaluria type II. *Human Molecular Genetics* **8**, 2063–2069.

Danpure, C. J. Scientific rationale for hepato-renal transplantation in primary hyperoxaluria type 1. In *Transplantation and Clinical Immunology XXII*. (ed. J. L. Touraine *et al.*), pp. 91–95. Amsterdam: Elsevier, 1991.

Danpure, C. J. and Jennings, P. R. (1986). Peroxisomal alanine : glyoxylate aminotransferase deficiency in primary hyperoxaluria type 1. *FEBS Letters* **201**, 20–24.

Danpure, C. J. and Rumsby, G. Enzymological and molecular genetics of primary hyperoxaluria type 1. Consequences for clinical management. In *Calcium Oxalate in Biological Systems* (ed. S. R. Khan), pp. 189–205. Boca Raton: CRC Press, 1995.

Daudon, M., Estepa, L., Lacour, B., and Jungers, P. (1998). Unusual morphology of calcium oxalate calculi in primary hyperoxaluria. *Journal of Nephrology* **11** (Suppl. 1), 51–55.

Ellis, S. R. *et al.* (2001). Combined liver–kidney transplantation for primary hyperoxaluria in young children. *Nephrology, Dialysis, Transplantation* **16**, 348–354.

Fargue, S., Chevalier-Prost, F., Rolland, M. O., and Cochat, P. (2002). Diagnosis of primary hyperoxaluria type 1: a one-centre experience. *Pediatric Nephrology* **17**, C52.

Gagnadoux, M. F. *et al.* (2001). Long term results of liver–kidney transplantation in children with primary hyperoxaluria. *Pediatric Nephrology* **16**, 946–950.

Gaulier, J. M., Cochat, P., Lardet, G., and Vallon, J. J. (1997). Serum oxalate micro assay using chemiluminescence detection. *Kidney International* **52**, 1700–1703.

Giafi, C. F. and Rumsby, G. (1998a). Kinetic analysis and tissue distribution of human D-glycerate dehydrogenase/glyoxylate reductase and its relevance to the diagnosis of primary hyperoxaluria type 2. *Annals of Clinical Biochemistry* **35**, 104–109.

Giafi, C. F. and Rumsby, G. (1998b). Primary hyperoxaluria type 2: enzymology. *Journal of Nephrology* **11** (Suppl. 1), 29–31.

Hallson, P. C. Oxalate crystalluria. In *Oxalate Metabolism in Relation to Urinary Stone* (ed. G. A. Rose), pp. 131–166. London: Springer Verlag, 1988.

Hoppe, B. *et al.* (1998). Plasma calcium oxalate super saturation in children with primary hyperoxaluria and end-stage renal failure. *Kidney International* **56**, 268–274.

Jamieson, N. V. (1998). The results of combined liver/kidney transplantation for primary hyperoxaluria (PH1) 1984–1997. The European PH1 transplant registry report. European PH1 Transplantation Study Group. *Journal of Nephrology* **11** (Suppl. 1), 36–41.

Johnson, S. A., Rumsby, G., Cregeen, D., and Hulton, S. A. (2002). Primary hyperoxaluria type 2 in children. *Pediatric Nephrology* **17**, 597–601.

Jouvet, P. *et al.* (1998). Crystalluria: a clinically useful investigation in children with primary hyperoxaluria post-transplantation. *Kidney International* **53**, 1412–1416.

Katz, A. *et al.* (1992). Success of kidney transplantation in oxalosis is unrelated to residual hepatic enzyme activity. *Kidney International* **42**, 1408–1411.

Kemper, M. J., Conrad, S., and Müller-Wiefel, D. E. (1997). Primary hyperoxaluria type 2. *European Journal of Pediatrics* **156**, 509–512.

Latta, K. and Brodehl, J. (1991). Primary hyperoxaluria type 1. *European Journal of Pediatrics* **149**, 518–522.

Leumann, E. and Hoppe, B. (2001). The primary hyperoxalurias. *Journal of the American Society of Nephrology* **12**, 1986–1993.

Lumb, M. J. and Danpure, C. J. (2000). Functional synergism between the most common polymorphism in human alanine : glyoxylate aminotransferase and four of the most common disease-causing mutations. *Journal of Biological Chemistry* **275**, 36415–36422.

Marangella, M. (1999). Transplantation strategies in type 1 primary hyperoxaluria: the issue of pyridoxine responsiveness. *Nephrology, Dialysis, Transplantation* **14**, 301–303.

Marangella, M. *et al.* (1995a). Detection of primary hyperoxaluria type 2 (L-glyceric aciduria) in patients with end-stage renal failure. *Nephrology, Dialysis, Transplantation* **10**, 1381–1385.

Marangella, M. *et al.* (1995b). Bony content of oxalate in patients with primary hyperoxaluria or oxalosis-unrelated renal failure. *Kidney International* **48**, 182–187.

Milliner, D. S., Wilson, D. M., and Smith, L. H. (2001). Phenotypic expression of primary hyperoxaluria: comparative features of types I and II. *Kidney International* **59**, 31–36.

Monico, C. G. and Milliner, D. S. (2001). Combined liver–kidney and kidney-alone transplantation in primary hyperoxaluria. *Liver Transplantation* **11**, 954–963.

Monico, C. G. and Rumsby, G. (2002). Molecular genetics of type 1 primary hyperoxaluria. *Sixth European Workshop on Hyperoxaluria*, Hanover.

Monico, C. G., Wilson, D. M., Bergert, J. H., and Milliner, D. S. (1999). Renal oxalate handling and plasma oxalate concentration in patients with chronic renal insufficiency and in patients with primary hyperoxaluria. *Journal of the American Society of Nephrology* **10**, 82A.

Monico, C. G. *et al.* (2002). Potential mechanisms of marked hyperoxaluria not due to primary hyperoxaluria I or II. *Kidney International* **62**, 392–400.

Morgan, S. H., Purkiss, P., Watts, R. W. E., and Mansell, M. A. (1987). Oxalate dynamics in chronic renal failure. Comparison with normal subjects and patients with primary hyperoxaluria. *Nephron* **46**, 253–257.

Nakamura, M. *et al.* (2001). Three cases of sequential liver–kidney transplantation from living related donors. *Nephrology, Dialysis, Transplantation* **16**, 166–168.

Nogueira, P. C. *et al.* (2000). Partial deletion of the AGXT gene (EX1_EX7del): a new genotype in hyperoxaluria type 1. *Human Mutation* **15**, 384–385.

Nolkemper, D. *et al.* (2000). Long-term results of pre-emptive liver transplantation in primary hyperoxaluria type 1. *Pediatric Transplantation* **4**, 177–181.

Pirulli, D. *et al.* (2001). Detection of AGXT gene mutations by denaturing high-performance liquid chromatography for diagnosis of hyperoxaluria type 1. *Clinical Experimental Medicine* **1**, 99–104.

Quy Dao, N. and Daudon, M. *Infrared and Raman Spectra of Calculi*. Paris: Elsevier, 1997.

Rumsby, G. (1998). Experience in prenatal diagnosis of primary hyperoxaluria type 1. *Journal of Nephrology* **11** (Suppl. 1), 13–14.

Rumsby, G., Sharma, A., Cregeen, D. P., and Solomon, L. R. (2001). Primary hyperoxaluria type 2 without L-glyceraciduria: is the disease under-estimated? *Nephrology, Dialysis, Transplantation* **16**, 1697–1699.

Salido, E. *et al.* (1996). Alanine-glyoxylate aminotransferase (*Agxt*) deficient mice: an animal model for the study of primary hyperoxaluria type 1. *Sixth European Workshop on Hyperoxaluria*, Hanover.

Scheid, C. *et al.* (1996). Oxalate toxicity in LLC-PK1 cells: role of free radicals. *Kidney International* **49**, 413–419.

Scheinman, J. I., Najarian, J. S., and Mauer, S. M. (1984). Successful strategies for renal transplantation in primary oxalosis. *Kidney International* **25**, 804–811.

Shapiro, R. *et al.* (2001). Primary hyperoxaluria type 1: improved outcome with timely liver transplantation: a single center report of 36 children. *Transplantation* **72**, 428–432.

Sidhu, H. *et al.* (1998). Absence of *Oxalobacter formigenes* in cystic fibrosis patients: a risk factor for hyperoxaluria. *Lancet* **352**, 1026–1029.

Toussaint, C. *et al.* (1993). Radiological and histological improvement of oxalate osteopathy after combined liver–kidney transplantation in primary hyperoxaluria type 1. *American Journal of Kidney Diseases* **2**, 54–63.

van Acker, K. J. *et al.* (1996). Hyperoxaluria with hyperglycoluria not due to alanine : glyoxylate aminotransferase defect: a novel type of primary hyperoxaluria. *Kidney International* **50**, 1747–1752.

von Schnakenburg, C. *et al.* (1998). Variable presentation of primary hyperoxaluria type 1 in 2 patients homozygous for a novel combined deletion and insertion mutation in exon 8 of the AGXT gene. *Nephron* **78**, 485–488.

Webster, K. E., Ferree, P. M., Holmes, R. P., and Cramer, S. D. (2000). Identification of missense, nonsense, and deletion mutations in the GRHPR gene in patients with primary hyperoxaluria type 2. *Human Genetics* **107**, 176–185.

Yamauchi, T., Quillard, M., Takahashi, S., and Nguyen-Khoa, M. (2001). Oxalate removal by daily dialysis in a patient with primary hyperoxaluria type 1. *Nephrology, Dialysis, Transplantation* **16**, 2407–2411.

Zhang, X., Roe, S. M., Pearl, L. H., and Danpure, C. J. (2001). Crystallization and preliminary crystallographic analysis of human alanine : glyoxylate aminotransferase and its polymorphic variants. *Acta Crystallographica* **57**, 1936–1937.

Foundations dealing with hyperoxaluria

http://www.ohf.org
http://www.airg-france.org

16.5.3 Inherited disorders of purine metabolism and transport

A.M. Marinaki, J. Stewart Cameron, and H. Anne Simmonds

Nephropathy and stones arising from inherited disorders of purine metabolism

A number of inherited genetic metabolic conditions involving defects in the enzymes of purine nucleotide metabolism are known (Fig. 1). Some of these can lead to the overproduction or overexcretion of uric acid and other purine end-products their nephrotoxicity derives from their insolubility and resultant ability of the crystals to initiate stone formation within the urinary tract, or generate inflammation leading to permanent renal damage within renal tissue, sometimes both. These insoluble purines include uric acid, xanthine, and 2,8-dihydroxyadenine (2,8-DHA) in order of decreasing solubility. The two disorders associated with uric acid over-production and excretion, are both X-linked and result from hypoxanthine–guanine phosphoribosyl transferase (HPRT) deficiency or phosphoribosylpyrophosphate synthetase (PRPS) superactivity.

HPRT deficiency and the kidney

HPRT catalyzes the salvage transfer of the phosphoribosyl moiety of PP-ribose-P to hypoxanthine and guanine to form IMP and GMP respectively (Fig. 1). HPRT is a cytoplasmic enzyme with greatest activity in brain and testes (Watts 1985). Its importance in the normal interplay between synthesis and salvage is demonstrated by the gross overproduction of uric acid which results from the inability to recycle either hypoxanthine or guanine in subjects genetically deficient in HPRT, inducing a lack of feedback control of synthesis accompanied by rapid catabolism to uric acid (Wyngaarden and Kelley 1976; Watts 1985; Jinnah and Friedmann 2001).

Genetics and clinical presentation

The gene for HPRT has been cloned and localized to the long arm of the X-chromosome (Xq26–q27.2) (see references in Jinnah et al. 2000; Jinnah and Friedmann 2001). Male hemizygotes carrying the defective gene show a broad spectrum of presentation, these range from the complete enzyme defect the Lesch–Nyhan disease (LND) of severe neurological deficits presenting in infancy to partial defects associated only with uric acid overproduction and its consequences, presenting in adolescence or early adulthood, known as the Kelley–Seegmiller syndrome (KSS) (Wyngaarden and Kelley 1976; Page and Nyhan 1989; Khattak et al. 1998). There is a considerable spectrum of neurological abnormalities of varying degree between these two extremes (Jinnah et al. 2000) related in turn to the different aberrant enzyme proteins, some of which have minor, or only moderately reduced activity with different kinetic properties (Jinnah et al. 2000; Jinnah and Friedmann 2001). These are termed LND variants. A variety of mutations in the gene have been described, the majority being single base substitutions (Jinnah et al. 2000).

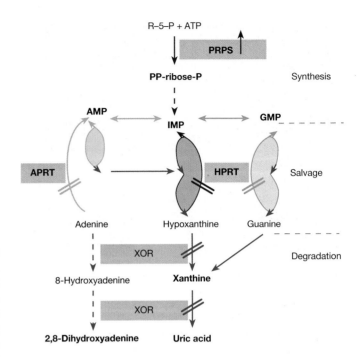

Fig. 1 Purine metabolism in summary; the enzymes HPRT, PRPP synthetase, APRT, and xanthine dehydrogenase (XDH) are indicated, and their inherited absence by double lines. XOR = xanthine oxidoreductase; HPRT = hypoxanthine–guanine phosphoribosyl transferase; APRT = adenine phosphoribosyl transferase; GMP = guanosine monophosphate; IMP = inosine monophosphate; AMP = adenosine monophosphate.

Unfortunately, there is no absolute correlation between the structural changes at the molecular level and the clinical severity of the neurological abnormalities (Jinnah et al. 2000). Although this is an X-linked disorder, LND has been described in females (Ogasawara 1989; Van Bogaert et al. 1992; Aral et al. 1996; de Gregorio et al. 2000), probably arising from an unusually large number of affected versus unaffected cells in the mosaicism which all heterozygotes of sex-linked disorders possess. KSS has also been found in a girl (Sebesta et al. personal communication). Thus, HPRT deficiency should not be ruled out altogether in a female with appropriate symptoms.

All degrees of deficiency may present in the first weeks of life with crystalluria, acute renal failure, and gout sometimes leading to dialysis, transplantation, or death in infancy (Simmonds et al. 1986; Stapleton 1992) (Figs 2 and 3). The severely incapacitating LND is characterized, in addition, by bizarre symptoms which include spasticity with pyramidal tract signs, compulsive self-mutilation, choreoathetosis, and developmental retardation (Watts 1985; McCarthy 1992; Jinnah et al. 2000).

Diagnosis of LND patients is frequently delayed for many years; although self-mutilation is present, such patients have been viewed as having 'cerebral palsy' of unknown cause because plasma urate when measured has been normal, and it is often the renal complications, and sometimes gout secondary to this which have eventually drawn attention to the underlying metabolic defect (McCarthy 1992). The same is true for partial HPRT deficiency (Simmonds et al. 1989; Augoustides-Savvopoulou et al. 2002) (Fig. 4). Although rare, the incidence in the United Kingdom for HPRT deficiency, excluding familial juvenile hyperuricaemic nephropathy (FJHN), is greater than for the other

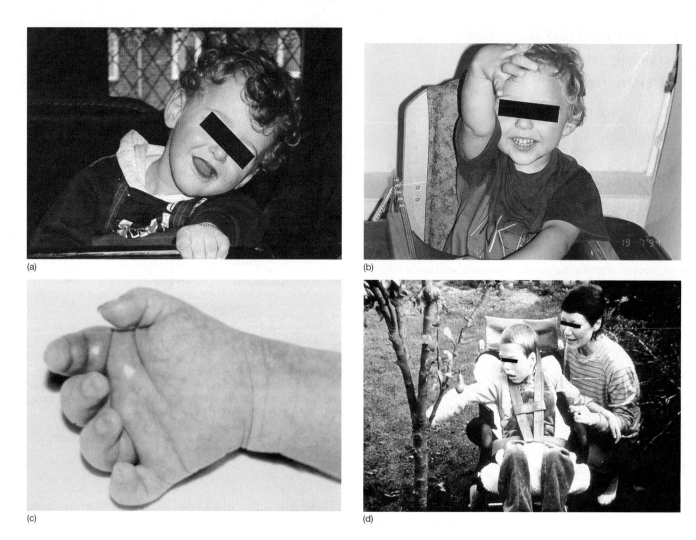

Fig. 2 Patients with the Lesch–Nyhan disease. (a) The boy has had to have all his milk teeth removed to prevent self-mutilation by biting. The dystonic movement is shown by the boy pictured in (b). (c) Acute gout in a 4-week-old baby with the syndrome. (d) The degree of handicap can be severe. Almost all patients with the severe form of the syndrome and major neurological problems die from it in childhood or early adult life.

genetic metabolic purine disorders. Approximately one-third of HPRT deficient patients are new mutations, two-thirds have had severe neurological deficits.

Biochemical diagnosis

Gross overproduction and excretion of uric acid is present in all cases irrespective of the degree of enzyme deficiency, but plasma uric acid may not appear increased until puberty because of the greater renal clearance in children (see Chapter 6.4). Thus, simply measuring plasma uric acid alone could be misleading. In the absence of renal failure, uric acid excretion assessed relative to urinary creatinine is increased two- to fourfold in HPRT-deficient children and adults (Wyngaarden and Kelley 1976) and urinary hypoxanthine excretion is similarly elevated (Simmonds *et al.* 1989; Jinnah and Friedmann 2001).

However, excessive uric acid excretion relative to creatinine may be masked in both children and adults presenting already in acute renal failure (Cameron *et al.* 1984; Simmonds *et al.* 1989). The diagnostic criterion in this situation is the grossly and disproportionately elevated

plasma uric acid (in excess of 1 mmol/l). Renal ultrasound provides the first clue to the correct diagnosis in some neonates by displaying the bright ultrasonogram of crystal nephropathy. Uric acid stones may be the unique manifestation in other cases (see Chapter 6.4).

HPRT deficiency may be confirmed by the low to undetectable concentrations of HPRT in lysed red cells, and is generally associated with an increased adenine phosphoribosyl transferase (APRT) activity (Wyngaarden and Kelley 1976), and since HPRT is undetectable in lysed red cells in the majority of deficient patients, intact cell studies are essential to confirm the phenotype (Page and Nyhan 1989; Jinnah and Friedmann 2001). The fact that up to 30 per cent of cases are new mutations has presented problems for carrier detection, which up till now could not be confirmed with total certainty, either by hair root analysis or biochemical methods (Puig *et al.* 1998). DNA methods for carrier detection are more certain if the mutation is known. Gonosomal mosaicism is possible in non-carrier females with a previous HPRT-deficient child and antenatal testing in subsequent pregnancies should not be precluded. Antenatal diagnosis is possible by direct

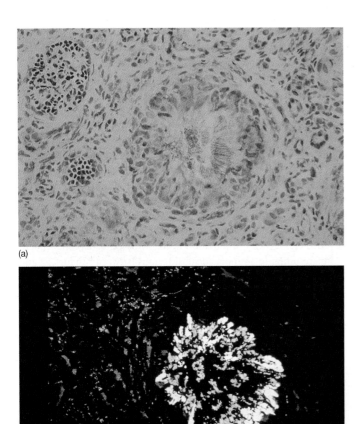

(a)

(b)

Fig. 3 (a) The renal biopsy from the baby illustrated in Fig. 2, showing gross intratubular precipitation of uric acid crystals within the renal tubule which led to acute renal failure. Note that the crystals are surrounded by inflammatory cells. (b) Viewed under polarized light: the uric acid crystals are birefringent.

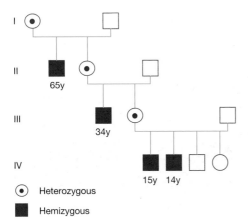

⊙ Heterozygous

■ Hemizygous

Fig. 4 Pedigree of a family with Kelley–Seegmiller syndrome (Augoustides-Savvopoulou et al. 2002), considered to have familial renal disease stretching over two generations until the correct diagnosis followed presentation of two teenage male siblings with urolithiasis.

enzyme assay using chorionic villus sampling in the first trimester, or fetal blood in the second (Page and Nyhan 1989; Simmonds et al. 1991; Jinnah and Friedmann 2001) and by DNA analysis of chorionic villus samples likewise if the mutation is known (Yamada et al. 1996; Torres et al. 2000). Preimplantation diagnosis is now possible (Ray et al. 1999).

Treatment

The elevated uric acid concentrations in either the complete or partial deficiencies may be controlled by a high fluid intake, together with alkali and allopurinol. Allopurinol should be used with care, since urinary oxypurine excretion in all HPRT-deficient patients appears exquisitely sensitive to allopurinol resulting in a rapid increase in concentrations of xanthine, which is extremely insoluble, and unlike that of uric acid which it replaces, the solubility of xanthine is relatively unaltered by alkalinization of the urine. Thus, patients with partial HPRT deficiency and gout may suffer reduction in renal function from xanthine nephropathy when on long-term high-dose allopurinol. The allopurinol metabolite oxipurinol is also relatively insoluble, and both xanthine and oxipurinol calculi have been reported in patients with the LND on long-term allopurinol therapy (Brock et al. 1983; Kenney 1991) (Fig. 5). As in all patients with renal failure or insufficiency, the allopurinol dose must be carefully monitored, and reduced if necessary to no more than 5 mg/kg/24 h in children, or 100 mg/24 h in adults (Simmonds et al. 1989; Simmonds et al. 1991). This is essential to prevent xanthine nephropathy, or, in renal failure the accumulation of oxipurinol—the active drug metabolite—with its attendant risk of bone-marrow depression and other side-effects. Some patients have progressed to ESRD and transplantation, but it should be noted that in such cases azathioprine will be ineffective and mycophenolate mofetil could have catastrophic consequences (Fig. 1). Cyclosporin alone has proved successful.

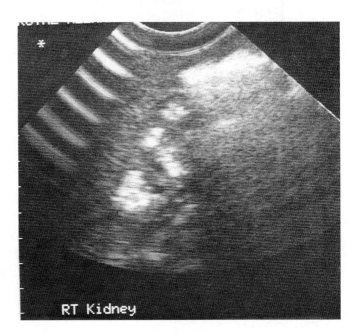

Fig. 5 Ultrasonogram of a patient with long-standing nephrolithiasis from HPRT deficiency. Increased central and medullary echoes are visible from diffuse crystal deposition within the kidney. From Kenney (1991) with permission of the author and publishers.

The long-term prognosis is good in children and adolescents with the partial defect, but patients with LND rarely survive beyond adolescence. Death is usually due to aspiration pneumonia or renal failure (Watts 1985; McCarthy 1992). Sadly, no successful treatment is yet available for the severe neurological complications.

Phosphoribosylpyrophosphate synthetase superactivity

The enzyme PRPS catalyzes the transfer of the pyrophosphate group of ATP to ribose-5-phosphate to form PP-ribose-P (Fig. 1).

Genetics and clinical presentation

As with HPRT deficiency there are two extremes of presentation, the more severe presenting in childhood associated with neurological deficits. Two-thirds of the cases with this rare X-linked disorder have presented only with severe gout or kidney stones in adolescence or early adulthood (Zoref et al. 1975; Becker 2001). Two distinct X-linked loci (PRS1 and PRS2) have been identified for the PRPS genes (Ishizuka et al. 1992; Becker 2001). PRS1 maps to the Xq21-qter

region and PRS2 to the short arm of X (Xp22.3–p22.3). The latter escapes X-chromosome inactivation. A third testis-specific transcript is encoded by another gene on chromosome 7 (Ishizuka et al. 1992). Two PRS associated proteins have been identified in the rat and may play a role in PRS regulation (Kita et al. 1994; Sonada et al. 1997). An association between the kinetic defect and the severity of the phenotypic expression, as in HPRT deficiency, is evident from the finding of patients presenting neonatally or in childhood with severe neurodevelopmental retardation, dysmorphic features, sometimes inherited nerve deafness (Fig. 6), a family history of repeated attacks of bronchopneumonia and death in early infancy, in addition to gross purine overproduction and uric acid crystals in the kidney (Christen et al. 1992; Becker 2001). The diverse phenotypic presentation of defects in PRPS superactivity and altered allosteric regulation is reflected in the genetic heterogeneity of mutation in the PRS1 gene. Six independent points resulting in amino acid substitutions between residues 52 and 192 of the polypeptide have been identified (Becker 2001).

Although this defect is X-linked it should be suspected in any child, female, or young adult of either sex with marked hyperuricaemia and/or hyperuricosuria, but with normal HPRT activity in lysed red

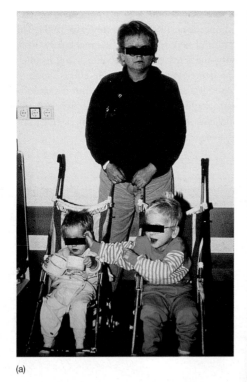

(a)

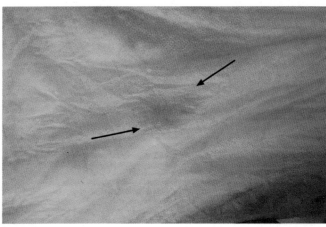

(b)

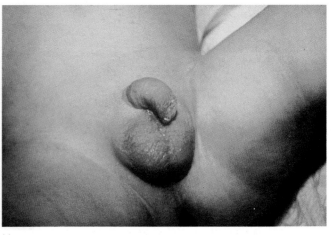

(c)

Fig. 6 (a) Brothers with the juvenile form of PRPS superactivity with their gouty mother. Both have growth, motor, and mental retardation, together with hypotonia. (b) Urate crystals on the nappy (arrow) and (c) the tip of the penis, noticed by the mother. [Patients studied by Christen et al. (1992) with kind permission of Professor F. Hannefeld, University of Göttingen.]

cells (Zoref *et al.* 1975; Becker 2001). Consequently, unlike HPRT deficiency, PRPS overactivity should be considered as a cause of gout in women (Garcia-Pavia *et al.* 2003), particularly in mothers of male children with neurological deficits or urate overproduction. Female carriers may also have sensorineural deafness. As in HPRT deficiency, the first suspicion may derive from the finding of crystals on the diaper or the tip of the penis of a child with the above neurological deficits (Christen *et al.* 1992) (Fig. 6). Recently, PRPS was identified as the underlying cause in a female aged 14 who presented in acute renal failure with a plasma urate greater than 1000 μmol/l (Fairbanks, personal communication). Reported values for PRPS activity have varied widely with the method and cell type used. Patients with the defect have had variant enzymes, insensitive to normal regulation or with catalytic activity two to four times greater than normal (Becker 2001).

Treatment

Prognosis for patients presenting in adolescence is good. Allopurinol, again used with care to avoid xanthine nephropathy, will control plasma uric acid in patients with normal renal function and gout or kidney stones. A high fluid intake and alkalinization of the urine may help and in renal failure the dose must be reduced even further as indicated above. To date, no successful therapy for the associated neurological complications in severe cases has been devised, and death in childhood is frequent.

Adenine phosphoribosyl transferase deficiency and the kidney

Adenine phosphoribosyl transferase is the companion salvage enzyme of HPRT which catalyzes the conversion of adenine to AMP using PP-ribose-P (Fig. 1). Its prime function is the removal of adenine arising as a metabolic waste product from the polyamine pathway. In the congenital absence of APRT, adenine accumulates in quantity and is oxidized by xanthine dehydrogenase (XDH) to 8-hydroxyadenine and then 2,8-DHA (Sahota *et al.* 2001).

Genetics and clinical presentation

Deficiency of APRT is inherited as an autosomal recessive trait (Sahota *et al.* 2001) and the gene is located on chromosome 16 (16q24.3). The chief clinical manifestation is 2,8-DHA urolithiasis and/or nephrotoxicity, both of which relate to the extreme insolubility of 2,8-DHA at any pH, coupled with its high renal clearance: 2,8-DHA is protein bound and is actively secreted by the human kidney. The stones are bluish or putty-coloured and crumbly, rather than yellowish and hard like uric acid (Fig. 7), but often were misidentified as uric acid because of their identical chemical behaviour in giving positive tests in both the colorimetric and murexide reactions.

Two types of defect have been identified, designated type I and type II. Type I subjects are predominantly Caucasian and have no detectable APRT activity in lysed erythrocytes (Sahota *et al.* 2001). Type II defect (erythrocyte lysate APRT activity up to 25 per cent of normal) is found almost exclusively in Japan (Kamatani *et al.* 1992; Deng *et al.* 2001). Differentiation of these two types of defect requires intact cell studies, and correct diagnosis of the type I defect may be masked if a blood transfusion has been essential on admission (Greenwood *et al.* 1982). Molecular analysis has demonstrated that a single mutation involving a substitution of methionine for threonine in position 136, which is part of the putative PP-ribose-P binding site, accounts for approximately 70 per cent of mutant alleles in the Japanese (Kamatani *et al.* 1992).

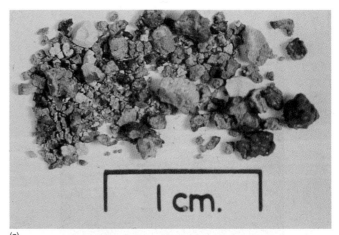
(a)

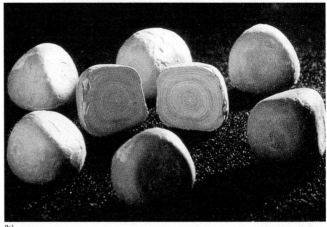
(b)

Fig. 7 The bluish-grey stones of 2,8-dihydroxyadenine (a), compared with the yellowish hard uric acid stones (b). Despite these obvious differences, most chemical tests in clinical use will not distinguish uric acid from 2,8-dihydroxyadenine, although infrared or UV spectroscopy show clearly the difference in the two molecules.

A variety of substitutions, insertions, and deletions have been identified in non-Japanese patients (Chen *et al.* 1991; Menardi *et al.* 1997; Sahota *et al.* 2001).

Clinical symptoms occur only when 2,8-DHA stones or crystals are formed as a consequence of the defect and may vary from benign to life-threatening (Simmonds *et al.* 1976; Greenwood *et al.* 1982; Ceballos-Picot *et al.* 1992; Laxdal 1992; Edvardsson *et al.* 2001; Sahota *et al.* 2001). 2,8-DHA crystalluria is found in all homozygotes, generally without any clinical symptoms (Fig. 8), and is then detected only during family investigations, from the presence of reddish-brown crystals on the diaper, or the characteristic spherical crystals in a urine deposit by light microscopy (Laxdal 1992). At least 15 per cent of cases are asymptomatic. The age of onset of symptoms for both defects has varied from birth to the seventh decade. In those patients with 2,8-DHA urolithiasis, the whole spectrum of symptoms associated with stone formation occur: fever from urinary tract infection, macroscopic haematuria, dysuria, urinary retention, and abdominal colic. Approximately 60 per cent of cases have been male 40 per cent of these being children.

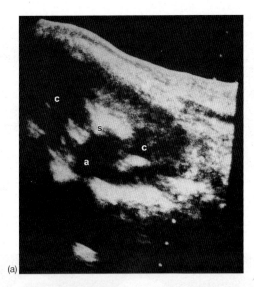

(a)

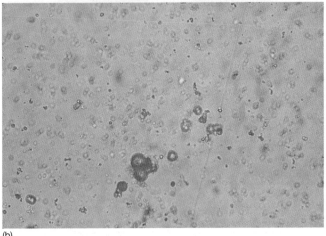

(b)

Fig. 8 (a) Ultrasonogram of 2,8-dihydroxyadenine lithiasis in a girl aged 4.5 years. A large stone(s) is present within the pelvis of the kidney, casting an acoustic shadow (a) and leading to calyceal dilatation (c) [from Greenwood *et al.* (1982) with permission of the authors and publishers]. Patterns of increased echo brightness may be seen also from 2,8-dihydroxyadenine crystal deposition throughout the kidney. (b) Brownish crystals of 2,8-dihydroxyadenine viewed by light microscopy in the urine of a symptomless homozygote for APRT deficiency. These crystals are diagnostic of the condition (Laxdal 1992).

In a number of cases presenting in childhood, acute anuric renal failure first drew attention to the underlying lithiasis (Greenwood *et al.* 1982; Ceballos-Picot *et al.* 1992; Sahota *et al.* 2001). Although this may be reversible, a number of cases have progressed to chronic renal insufficiency requiring maintenance dialysis, and transplantation. In some with a long history of recurrent urolithiasis, the type I defect has been identified only following transplantation (Ceballos-Picot *et al.* 1992) through the finding of microcrystalline deposits at biopsy sometimes with subsequent loss of allograft (Gagné *et al.* 1994; Cassidy *et al.* 2004). The upregulation in expression of adhesion molecules (α-catenin, integrin α3, integrin β6) and platelet-derived growth factor-B in cultured human kidney cells exposed to 2,8-DHA or calcium oxalate monohydrate crystals (Wang *et al.* 2002) may contribute to crystal-induced renal injury by affecting cell–cell or

cell–matrix interactions. The similar histopathology seen in animal models of crystal nephropathy induced by either uric acid, xanthine, or 2,8-DHA may thus represent a general response irrespective of crystal type as suggested by Farebrother *et al.* (1975).

Diet may also play a role in precipitating the clinical symptoms (Greenwood *et al.* 1982). Some foods rich in nucleic acid have a particularly high adenine content. While this is not a problem normally such diets can be potentially lethal to the subjects with this genetic defect because of the consequent overexcretion of 2,8-DHA.

A founder effect is evident from genetic studies in both the Japanese and Icelandic populations which explains the high number of cases recognized (Kamatani *et al.* 1992; Edvardsson *et al.* 2001), but seemingly not in the French (Ceballos-Picot *et al.* 1992). The most likely explanation is that in other countries patients with suspected 'uric acid' lithiasis will be treated effectively with allopurinol—which eliminates the lithogenic 2,8-DHA from the urine—without a correct diagnosis being made. This is regrettable since 2,8-DHA lithiasis is a treatable disorder (see below) and with early recognition and treatment severe renal complications can be avoided and siblings at risk identified.

Diagnosis

Renal ultrasound [Fig. 8(a)] provided the first clue to the underlying crystal nephropathy in one child presenting in coma in acute renal failure (Greenwood *et al.* 1982). In some cases of urolithiasis it has taken more than 50 years before the exact nature of the stone was recognized and appropriate treatment given. Recently, more rapid appropriate diagnosis and better knowledge of the disease has shortened the time from recognition of the urolithiasis to correct diagnosis.

Evaluation of plasma and urine uric acid may assist in distinguishing this type of stone from the two defects above, subjects with complete APRT deficiency generally having normal amounts of uric acid in plasma and urine (Sahota *et al.* 2001). Total urinary purine endproduct (uric acid + precursor oxypurines + adenine derivatives) on a low purine diet has also been normal (0.05–0.1 mmol/kg/24 h), with adenine metabolites constituting approximately 20–30 per cent of this total. Three different adenine metabolites are excreted in the urine: adenine, 8-hydroxyadenine, and 2,8-DHA in the approximate proportion of 1.0 : 0.03 : 1.5. Characteristic crystals of 2,8-DHA in the urine are diagnostic (Laxdal 1992).

Treatment

Treatment with allopurinol is highly effective, immediately and in the long term (Sahota *et al.* 2001), with the same proviso relating to allopurinol dose reduction in renal failure, mentioned in discussion of HPRT deficiency above. Unlike uric acid, alkali will not increase the solubility of 2,8-DHA and evidence from several families suggests its use may be contraindicated (Stone and Simmonds 1991). As mentioned above, if renal failure occurs because of late diagnosis renal transplantation can be successful. The allograft, of course, remains at risk, and recipients will continue to need treatment with allopurinol; therefore, if azathioprine is used as part of the immunosuppressive regime, the dose of both should be reduced (up to 200 mg for allopurinol and 25 per cent of the daily dose for azathioprine).

Hereditary xanthinuria

In hereditary xanthinuria a recessively inherited deficiency of the enzyme XOR results in an inability to degrade hypoxanthine and xanthine to uric acid (Fig. 1) and leads to the accumulation of xanthine and to a lesser extent hypoxanthine in place of uric acid. Xanthine concentrations in plasma and especially in urine are increased. The nephrotoxicity of this purine, like 2,8-DHA, is due to its insolubility at pH 5.0 which, unlike uric acid, can only be doubled, by alkalinizing the urine. Hypoxanthine in contrast is very soluble and poses no problem.

Genetics and clinical presentation

The XOR gene has been cloned and mapped to chromosome 2p22 (Rytkönen *et al.* 1995; Xu *et al.* 1996; Raivio *et al.* 2001) and nonsense, missense, or frame shift mutations found in patients with classical type 1 xanthinuria (Ichida *et al.* 1997; Levartovsky *et al.* 2000; Sakamoto *et al.* 2001). Although in the past the genetic defect was considered rare and supposed generally to affect adults, it is now evident that this is not so. In most homozygotes uric acid is virtually undetectable in plasma and urine on a purine-free diet, and is replaced in the urine by xanthine and, to a lesser extent, hypoxanthine in a ratio of 3–4 : 1. The preferential excretion of xanthine is due to the extensive normal recycling of hypoxanthine by the salvage pathway for which xanthine is not an effective substrate in humans *in vivo*. The potential toxicity of xanthine in xanthinuric subjects relates to its high renal clearance by filtration with little or no tubular reabsorption (Simmonds *et al.* 1986; Raivio *et al.* 2001). In homozygotes with normal renal function, plasma xanthine concentrations range from 10 to 40 μmol/l (normal < 1 μmol/l) resulting in urinary xanthine concentrations of up to 2 mmol/l, generally well in excess of the solubility of xanthine in urine (0.9 mmol/l), even at pH 7.0 (Raivio *et al.* 2001).

Consequently, the potential for precipitation in the kidney or urinary tract is high, particularly in an infant with a history of vomiting, diarrhoea, or recurrent infection, and eventually can lead to tubular blockage and acute renal failure. More than 100 cases have been reported and males predominate over females (Raivio *et al.* 2001). Xanthine stones were first recognized by Marcet at Guy's Hospital London in 1817, whilst xanthinuria—the first inherited purine disorder to be identified—was found in a girl aged 4.5 years by Dent and Philpot (1954), presenting with haematuria and renal stones.

Approximately 40 per cent of the patients with classical xanthinuria have presented with symptoms that could be attributed directly to the defect—irritability, haematuria, urinary tract infection, renal colic, crystalluria, acute renal failure, or urolithiasis. Although the age of onset of nephrotoxicity has varied from childhood to the eighth decade, nearly half of the cases presenting with urolithiasis have been children of 10 years or less (Carpenter *et al.* 1986; Fildes 1989; Bradbury *et al.* 1995; Raivio *et al.* 2001). Symptoms present from birth have included persistent emesis, poor weight gain, and urinary tract infection, whilst irritability, sleeplessness, and gross haematuria have also been noted. Multiple small xanthine stones were removed from the pelvis and ureters of a 9-month-old child presenting with obstructive renal failure and severe dysmorphism (Bradbury *et al.* 1995) (Fig. 9). In some patients the renal damage has led to clubbing of the calyces of the kidney, hydronephrosis, and chronic renal failure. Two children under 6 years have had renal tubular acidosis and hypercalciuria, which was considered secondary to the renal injury in one, but discounted in the other because of similar symptoms in a non-xanthinuric sibling (Fildes 1989). These findings underline the need to add xanthine, as well as 2,8-DHA urolithiasis, to the list of possible causes of persistent urinary tract infection, haematuria, or acute renal failure in children as well as adults.

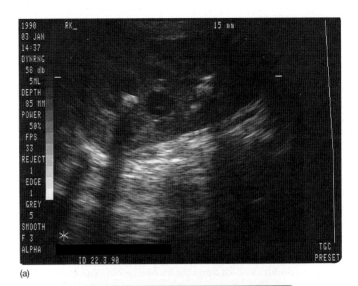

(a)

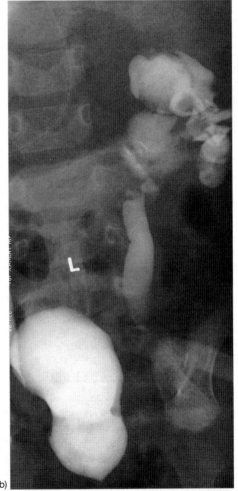

(b)

Fig. 9 (a) Renal ultrasound showing a hydronephrotic right kidney with echo-dense material and acoustic shadowing in a child with xanthinuria. (b) Left radiocontrast nephrotogram from the same patient showing multiple ureteric calculi. (With kind permission of Dr M. Bradbury, Division of Paediatics and Child Health, University of Leeds.)

Diagnosis

Even for this 'classical' xanthinuria, diagnosis is often difficult if stones are not present, especially in infants presenting in acute renal failure. Here again renal ultrasound may first draw attention to the underlying crystal nephropathy (Bradbury *et al.* 1995). The possibility of classical xanthinuria must be considered as the underlying cause of irritability or acute renal failure, especially if there is a history of haematuria, or red-brown deposits on the diaper. A number of patients have been reported in whom renal damage has been severe, leading in some to endstage renal failure, nephrectomy, and even death (Maynard and Benson 1988; Raivio *et al.* 2001). Adults with the more serious renal complications frequently have a history of recurrent urolithiasis dating back to early childhood. Plasma xanthine concentrations up to 243 μmol/l (normal < 1 μmol/l) were found in one such patient in terminal uraemia (Simmonds *et al.* 1984). Xanthine lithiasis, like uric acid lithiasis, is climate dependent, being much more prevalent (associated with more severe renal complications) in countries which fringe the Mediterranean (Salti *et al.* 1992).

Combined xanthine oxidoreductase–aldehyde oxidase deficiency

Xanthinuria, as well as resulting from an isolated deficiency of XOR (type I deficiency), may also arise from, a dual deficiency of XOR and the related enzyme aldehyde oxidase (type II deficiency) (Reiter *et al.* 1990). Aldehyde oxidase, like XOR, is a molybdenum-containing enzyme (Hille and Massey 1985) and a defect in the synthesis of the sulfide ligand of the common molybdenum cofactor, which deletes the activity of XOR and aldehyde oxidase, but leaves the activity of sulfite oxidase intact was proposed in type II subjects (Wahl *et al.* 1982). Indeed, this has been confirmed in recent studies which identified a non-sense mutation in the gene encoding molybdenum cofactor sulfurase, the enzyme catalyzing the sulfuration of the desulfo molybdenum cofactor has been found in a patient with type II xanthinuria (Ichida *et al.* 2001).

This dual deficiency may account for up to 50 per cent of cases with supposed 'classical' xanthinuria (Reiter *et al.* 1990). These subjects are at special risk for drugs that are normally metabolized by aldehyde oxidase, including allopurinol, azathioprine, cyclophosphamide, methotrexate, and quinine (Beedham 1987). Severe haematological toxicity occurred in an undiagnosed type II xanthinuric patient receiving full-dose azathioprine following renal transplantation (Hillebrand and Reiter 1991).

Deficiency of molybdenum-associated cofactor

Patients with a second clinically distinct type of xanthinuria have generally presented in the neonatal period with intractable seizures (Johnson and Duran 2001). These infants have a deficiency of all three enzymes, xanthine oxidoreductase, aldehyde oxidase, and sulfite oxidase, due to the absence of a common molybdenum-containing cofactor (MoCo) essential for all three. As a result, the more severe clinical features of sulfite oxidase deficiency (severe neonatal fitting, microcephaly, and other specific neurological deficits, plus ocular lens dislocation and characteristically high MRI signal on T_2 imaging in the lenticular nuclei) overshadow those of classical xanthinuria (Johnson and Duran 2001).

On the basis of cell culture studies, MoCo deficient patients are divided into complementation groups A or B, reflecting the underlying genetic basis of the disorder (Reiss 2000). The majority of patients fall into Group A and are characterized by a defect in the MOCS1 gene. MOCS1 encodes a bicistronic transcript synthesizing the two enzymes necessary for the first two steps of the MoCo biosynthetic pathway (Reiss *et al.* 1998). Complementation Group B is associated with mutation in MOCS2, a second bicistronic gene, encoding two subunits of molybdopterin synthase (Reiss *et al.* 1999). A defect in the neurotransmitter receptor-clustering protein gephyrin catalyzing the insertion of molybdenum into molybdopterin has recently been reported in a single MoCo deficient patient (Reiss *et al.* 2000). This novel form of MoCo deficiency might respond to molybdate supplementation (Reiss *et al.* 2001).

Hitherto, it was considered that most children with the cofactor disorder will die within the first year of life. However, as with other genetic disorders, those with the most catastrophic mutations are the first to be recognized, and patients presenting later are now being reported (Johnson and Duran 2001). These cases have some uric acid in plasma and urine, together with increased urinary xanthine and hypoxanthine concentrations (Johnson *et al.* 1988; Kavukcu *et al.* 2000; Johnson and Duran 2001) and could have been missed if plasma alone was screened. Infants surviving the neonatal period may develop haematuria due to xanthinuria as the first sign of renal disease and when found with neurological abnormalities and dysmorphology, should alert the clinician to the possibility of MoCo deficiency (Kavukcu *et al.* 2000). Heterogeneity is becoming evident within families, as well as between families, as exemplified by a kindred in which the propositus presented at 12 months with episodes of eye rolling and jerky limb movements. Family screening revealed an otherwise healthy 7-year-old sibling who was attending an eye hospital for dislocated lenses (Hughes *et al.* 1998).

Infants presenting with fits in the neonatal period should always be screened for the cofactor defect. Multiple renal calculi have been observed by ultrasonography.

Treatment

Unfortunately, little can be done for 'classical' xanthinuria types I and II except to limit purine intake and ensure a large output of urine, especially in arid climates. Since the solubility of xanthine is not affected by urinary pH, alkalinization is of no value. There is no treatment for the molybdenum cofactor disorder, but patients respond biochemically to reduction of sulfur in the diet.

Iatrogenic xanthinuria

This problem has been mentioned in Chapter 6.4, but is dealt with here also because the data relate more to xanthine as a toxic purine, although of course this is an acquired state. Xanthinuria and xanthine lithiasis, or crystal-induced acute renal failure, can occur secondary to therapy with allopurinol in situations associated with overproduction of endogenous uric acid, including the tumour lysis syndrome (Ablin *et al.* 1972; Simmonds *et al.* 1986; and see Chapter 6.4).

However, in addition, patients with LND, or partial HPRT deficiency, respond with a particularly rapid rise in xanthine following allopurinol and have presented with xanthine stones, or both acute and chronic xanthine nephropathy (Gomez *et al.* 1978; Brock *et al.* 1983; Simmonds *et al.* 1989). Renal sonography of some LND patients receiving treatment for long periods has shown variable ultrasonographic appearances (Fig. 5) of multiple calculi and increased medullary echogenicity (Kenney 1991). A personal finding of a grossly reduced glomerular filtration rate (GFR) (to 30 per cent) in two brothers with undiagnosed HPRT deficiency treated for 20 years with allopurinol 600 mg per day, in whom uric acid had been virtually replaced by xanthine, underlines the importance of both correct and early diagnosis, and the need to give allopurinol in doses of not more than 300 mg/day; purine metabolites require monitoring in such cases to avoid such unnecessary complications.

Grossly elevated plasma xanthine concentrations (600–700 μmol/l), together with urinary concentrations of nearly 1 mmol/mmol creatinine (normal < 0.01 mmol/mmol creatinine), have also been noted in patients who develop acute renal failure when given allopurinol concomitantly to prevent uric acid nephropathy during aggressive therapy for a variety of malignancies, usually myeloid—the tumour lysis syndrome (Ablin et al. 1972; Simmonds et al. 1986). Treatment should likewise be carefully monitored to ensure a reasonable balance between xanthine and uric acid. The magnitude of the xanthine response in such situations is evident when compared with that of gouty subjects with normal renal function on an equivalent allopurinol dose (300 mg), where the increase in urinary xanthine approximates only 0.1 mmol/mmol creatinine and plasma xanthine concentrations are generally less than 10 μmol/l.

The potential nephrotoxicity of xanthine in humans is supported by experimental studies in pigs fed a purine load in the form of guanine together with allopurinol. This combination precipitated acute renal failure (Farebrother et al. 1975) due to crystalline deposits of xanthine, initially in the distal tubules and collecting ducts, and associated subsequently with extensive tubular epithelial damage and eventual interstitial oedema and inflammation. Studies of the long-term evolution of the renal lesion demonstrated that even such short periods of crystal deposition could cause interstitial scarring as a long-term result leading to severe and permanent renal damage, with no evidence of the crystals that had originally precipitated the lesion.

Deficiency of thiopurine methyl transferase

Although inherited deficiency of this purine enzyme causes no renal consequences as such, it is important in renal transplantation because it is one of the routes by which the active component of azathioprine, 6-mercaptopurine, is metabolized to inactive metabolites. Genetic polymorphism modulates thiopurine methyl transferase (TPMT) enzyme activity and about one in 250–300 individuals will be TPMT deficient homozygotes (Krynetski and Evans 2000; Holme et al. 2002). These individuals are unable to metabolize 6-mercaptopurine normally, with a risk of severe, sometimes fatal, haematological toxicity if treated in usual doses with azathioprine either in transplantation or autoimmune disorders, or with 6-mercaptopurine for haematological malignancies. (Holme et al. 2002). Uraemia induces the enzyme (Weyer et al. 2001).

Disorders of renal urate handling

Hypouricaemia of renal tubular origin

Some children and young adults present either with crystalluria and ureteric colic, or even acute renal failure after exercise, because of genetic alterations in the complex renal tubular handling of urate, which results in a net decrease in urate reabsorption and hypouricaemia (see Chapter 6.4 for details of urate handling in the renal tubule). Excess urinary losses of urate can also occur as one component of a generalized transport abnormality in the proximal tubule (the Fanconi syndrome—see Chapter 5.3), such as that arising from inherited disorders including the Hartnup syndrome, Wilson's disease, cystinosis, galactosaemia, and hereditary fructose intolerance), or as an acquired defect associated

with volume expansion and hyponatraemia in the syndrome of inappropriate secretion of antidiuretic hormone (SIADH) (Sperling 2001) (see Chapter 6.4).

Renal hypouricaemia must, of course, first be distinguished from the hypouricaemia arising from XOR deficiency discussed above, purine nucleoside phosphorylase deficiency, or from ingestion of allopurinol (Stone and Simmonds 1991). Finally, physiological hypouricaemia can occur during pregnancy, mainly in response to volume expansion. Approximately 0.5 per cent of the total population have hypouricaemia from these various causes (Hisatome et al. 1989; Sperling 2001), and the low plasma urate is often detected when multiple plasma analyses are performed.

Isolated hereditary renal hypouricaemia

Clinical manifestations

Hereditary renal hypouricaemia, manifest as hypouricaemia and increased urate clearance (de Vries and Sperling 1979), is due to an isolated defect of tubular handling in subjects with otherwise normal proximal tubular function first described by Praetorius and Kirk (1950), and later by Greene et al. (1972). Most cases arise from mutations in the anion exchanger of the proximal tubule brushborder, URAT-1 (Enomoto et al. 2002). Some patients have no renal symptoms and the condition is an incidental finding, but a number present with acute renal failure or renal colic from crystalluria, haematuria, and/or urinary tract stones of urate or calcium oxalate, presumably the result of the hyperuricosuria (Sperling 2001).

An increasing number of such cases presenting with reversible acute renal failure following exercise have been described since the first report of Erley et al. (1989) (see Ohta 2002 for review of 18 published cases). In the report of Erley et al. (1989) renal biopsy revealed uric acid crystals within the tubules, but this has not been a feature of any subsequent cases. In general, plasma uric acid concentrations have risen to normal during such episodes, and in two cases there was clear hyperuricaemia. In addition, patients presenting with uric acid stones have been reported (Gofrit et al. 1993). A possible role for a deficient antioxidant property of the blood because of the low urate has been postulated. Rhabdomyolysis appears to have played a part in several cases, as judged by increased plasma creatine phosphokinase, but this has been absent in the majority. It is possible that dehydration and lactic acidosis play a part in this association of renal failure on exercise in patients with isolated renal tubular hypouricaemia.

Inheritance

The inheritance in most families is consistent with an autosomal recessive pattern, and in some instances there have been lower plasma urate concentrations in the presumed heterozygotes. In about 30 per cent of the propositi there was associated hypercalciuria, sometimes associated with calcium stones. The majority of patients with isolated renal hypouricaemia and uricosuria have been Israeli non-Ashkenazi Jews or Japanese, which might suggest that, as with APRT deficiency, the genetic defect(s) may be more common in some racial groups. Two cases have been identified in the United Kingdom (unpublished).

Investigations

All other parameters of renal function appear normal and remain so, the only abnormality being an FE_{ur} greater than normal for age and sex. In most patients the FE_{ur} has been between 36 and 85 per cent (Sperling 2001), but in some has actually approached (Matsuda et al. 1982), or exceeded (Akaoka *et al.* 1977) the creatinine clearance (FE$_{ur}$ 88–105 per cent). Studies using pharmacological agents with different postulated modes of action on the complex bidirectional handling of urate in the proximal tubule, such as pyrazinamide, probenecid, and benzbromarone (Shichiri *et al.* 1987; Sperling 2001), have suggested considerable heterogeneity in phenotype despite likely involvement of URAT-1 mutations.

Acquired renal hypouricaemia

This subject is dealt with in Chapter 6.4.

Inherited hyperuricaemia of renal tubular origin

In addition to the genetic purine metabolic defects described above, another genetic defect leading to secondary hyperuricaemia or hyperuricosuria, that can present as acute renal failure in infancy, childhood, or early adult life is glycogen storage disease type I, which results from a deficiency of the enzyme, glucose 6-phosphatase (see Chapter 16.4.2). This disorder must be considered also when there is evidence of overproduction of uric acid in the face of normal purine enzymes. The purine over-production arises from a combination of accelerated ATP breakdown and increased synthesis, the associated lactic acidosis affecting the tubular transport of uric acid (see Chapter 6.4), thereby exaggerating the appearance and severity of hyperuricaemia (Stone and Simmonds 1991).

Familial hyperuricaemia and gout

Hyperuricaemia is also the presenting problem of a genetic disorder which has received little attention until recently, and which affects young males, young females, and even children of either sex. The defect, although first described over 30 years ago (Duncan and Dixon 1960), has been poorly characterized in the past (Calabrese *et al.* 1990; Cameron *et al.* 1993; Bleyer *et al.* 2003). It is now usually termed familial nephropathy with gout or familial juvenile hyperuricaemic nephropathy (FJHN). Onset is commonly in childhood, adolescence, or early adult life, although cases presenting later have been seen, and renal failure is often recognized between 20 and 40 years of age. It has become apparent recently that the considerable variation seen in the FJHN clinical phenotype and similarities in clinical presentation to some families with autosomal dominant medullary cystic kidney disease (ADMCKD) (see Chapter 16.2.2), probably reflects underlying genetic heterogeneity in both disorders.

Nevertheless, the disease, associated sometimes with juvenile onset of gout, and often progressive renal disease is clearly distinguished from the 'primary' gout of the middle-aged male (Berger and Yü 1975) (see Chapter 6.4), and the gouty Polynesian population (Simmonds *et al.* 1994); [Fig. 10(a)] in both of these obesity is an associated characteristic and renal function is usually normal for age.

Genetics and clinical presentation

Autosomal dominant inheritance is suggested by the presentation in consecutive generations, the equal gender ratio and transmission from father to son (Fig. 11). The considerable variation in clinical presentation, even within a family, and overlap between the clinical and pathological definition of FJHN and ADMCKD has complicated the search for the FJHN gene(s) and raised the question of whether FJHN and ADMCKD are the same disease sharing a common genetic cause. This follows identification of a second autosomal dominant medullary

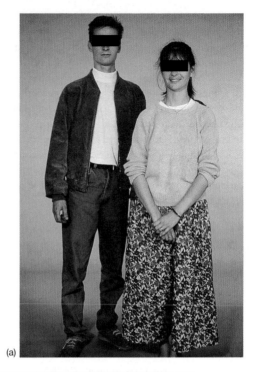

(a)

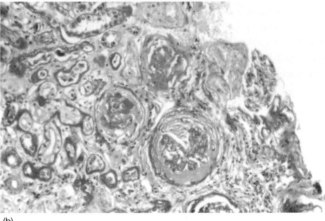

(b)

Fig. 10 (a) A young brother and sister with familial juvenile hyperuricaemic nephropathy, showing the normal slim phenotype in this condition; neither obesity nor dietary indulgence are present and both are normotensive. Their mother and an uncle both had gout and renal failure and she died aged 34 following renal transplantation. (b) Histology of the kidney in familial juvenile hyperuricaemic nephropathy. There is extensive interstitial nephritis and tubular basement membrane thickening, but unlike the Lesch–Nyhan syndrome, there are no visible deposits of urate.

cystic kidney disease locus on chromosome 16p12 designated ADMCKD2 by Scolari *et al.* (1999). The families studied were classified as ADMCKD on the basis of occasional small medullary cysts noted in some, but not all affected patients and typical small kidneys. However, hyperuricaemia and gouty arthritis consistent with a diagnosis of FJHN were also a feature of the clinical presentation. Subsequently, linkage to 16p12 was reported in a large Japanese FJHN family (Kamatani *et al.* 2000) with gouty arthritis, renal failure, and unusually, hypertension (Yakota *et al.* 1991). Linkage to 16p11.2 was shown subsequently in several Czech FJHN

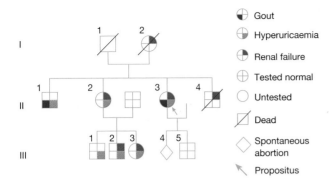

Fig. 11 Family tree of a kindred initially diagnosed as 'familial renal disease' of undescribed type, until the propositus (II$_3$), who had been disproportionately hyperuricaemic for some years, first developed clinical gout at the age of 23 years, followed by her brother (II$_1$), also in his twenties. Of note, two of three apparently healthy children of II$_2$ had diminished renal function (GFR) and hyperuricaemia when they were screened, whilst two subjects in the family have the low FE$_{ur}$ characteristic of familial juvenile hyperuricaemic nephropathy, but normal renal function. These observations strongly suggest that a low FE$_{ur}$ precedes renal dysfunction as well as clinical gout in these subjects and underline the importance of screening healthy members of affected kindreds.

families presenting with hyperuricaemia, decreased FE$_{ur}$, gouty arthritis, and renal insufficiency (Stibůrková et al. 2000, 2003). Studies in a large Belgian family (Dahan et al. 2001) defined the critical region further, and in view of the striking clinical and pathological resemblance between ADMCKD and FJHN, these authors suggested that they might be two closely-related disorders, or even allelic. However in contrast to FJHN many patients with ADMCKD did not show hyperuricaemia, as in the family studied by Hateboer et al. (2001). Examination of candidate genes in the 16p11–12 region led to description by Hart et al. (2002) of mutations in the UMOD gene coding for uromodulin (Tamm-Horsfall protein) in FJHN, a finding confirmed by others in both FJHN (Casari et al. 2003; Turner et al. 2003) and MCKD (Wolf et al. 2003). Twenty five years ago abnormal distribution of uromodulin in interstitial disease had been recorded (Resnick et al. 1978; Zager et al. 1978), and now Dahan et al. (2003) in FJHN and Rampoldi et al. (2003) in MCKD have shown that the mutant forms of uromodulin accumulate within the cells of the thick ascending limb of Henle, accompanied by greatly reduced urinary excretion. However, half to two thirds of the families studied so far do not show UMOD mutations, in addition to the MCKD families of Stavrou et al. (2002) which map to chromosome 1q21. In our own series, only 3 of 13 FJHN families whose UMOD gene exons 4 and 5 have been sequenced showed mutations (Marinaki 2003, unpublished), and one other family had a mutation in the gene for hepatocyte nuclear factor-1β (Bingham et al. 2003). Others have described families not linked to the region of the UMOD gene (Krois et al. 2000; Stibůrková et al. 2000, 2003; Auranen et al. 2001). A further locus at 1q41 has been described in one of our FJHN families, and another from Belgium (Hodaňová et al. 2003 personal communication); thus considerable genetic heterogeneity is present despite the importance of UMOD mutations.

FJHN has been considered rare, based on the reports of isolated kindreds in different countries worldwide. However, more than 50 kindreds have now been studied in the United Kingdom. The condition has often been missed and a diagnosis of 'familial renal disease'

of undetermined type made until an isolated attack of gout, equally rare in renal failure (see Chapter 6.4), appears in one or more family members (Cameron et al. 1991; Moro et al. 1991a). Since gout is an inconsistent feature (Cameron et al. 1993; Puig et al. 1993), the word 'gout' used in earlier descriptions is now usually replaced by 'hyperuricaemia', although gout is clearly an important factor in drawing attention to such kindreds. Importantly, and in contrast to the MCKD diseases, The majority of patients are normotensive, but hypertension may be found and is usually of late onset in those with renal dysfunction (Moro et al. 1991b). When found it must be treated aggressively as untreated hypertension obviously will accelerate the progression of the renal failure.

Diagnosis

There are two biochemical hallmarks for this disease: the first is hyperuricaemia disproportionate to the age, sex, or degree of renal dysfunction; the second is that the degree of renal hypoexcretion of urate is generally extreme with an absence of the usual sex and age differences observed in the normal population; the mean FE$_{ur}$, being only 5.1 per cent—equally low in young men, women, or children (Simmonds et al. 1994; McBride et al. 1995). This value is lower even than the 5.4 per cent found in middle-aged gouty males (see Chapter 6.4) and explains the associated hyperuricaemia and tendency to gout in young females and children in these kindreds (McBride et al. 1997; McBride et al. 1998). This grossly reduced mean FE$_{ur}$ found in affected children is even more striking when compared with the normally high FE$_{ur}$ (range 12–30 per cent) of their healthy counterparts. Another important point is that although this low FE$_{ur}$ increases as renal failure supervenes (see Chapter 6.4) (Bleyer et al. 2003), the increase is much less than in the increment found in the normal population with severe renal disease (see Chapter 6.4). Consequently, in early uraemia the FE$_{ur}$ is normal for a while (Calabrese et al. 1990) and may confuse diagnosis. Obviously, symptomless members of affected families must be screened also, for renal function and urate handling. Ultrasonography of the kidney should be done to detect medullary cysts if present. Hitherto presentation in ADMCKD was considered to be of late onset, but recent publications suggest that they may present at any age (Parvari et al. 2001).

Pathology and pathogenesis

On histology, the kidney usually shows patchy areas of tubular atrophy and fibrosis, with focal interstitial infiltration of lymphocytes and histiocytes and globally sclerosed glomeruli [Fig. 10(b)]. Often associated thickening of the basement membrane in distal tubules and collecting ducts has been observed (Simmonds et al. 1980; Richmond et al. 1981; Puig et al. 1993). These histological features are similar to those reported in families linked to the ADMCKD2 locus (Dahan et al. 2001). However, in a few patients the paucity of features in the biopsy has been remarkable, despite an already significantly reduced renal function. Uric acid crystals have been reported only in three of more than 50 biopsies (Farebrother et al. 1981; Murakami et al. 1990; Reiter et al. 1995), but as discussed in Chapter 6.4, the absence of crystals does not exclude their presence in the past.

The manner in which the renal failure, the low FE$_{ur}$, and hyperuricaemia may relate to one another in FJHN has been the subject of much debate. Urate production is normal as judged by urinary excretion. Lhotta et al. (1998) suggested a gain-of-function mutation of the luminal anion exchanger of the proximal tubule would be consistent with reduced uric acid excretion, dominant inheritance and the observed apoptosis of tubular epithelial cells. However the localization of the URAT-1 gene to chromosome 11 (Enomoto *et al.* 2002) would seem to exclude this possibility. The finding of a reduced FE_{ur} for age and sex preceding a reduction in GFR in otherwise apparently healthy subjects suggests that renal urate hypoexcretion precedes the renal disease (Moro *et al.* 1991a). The beneficial effect of allopurinol (up to 36 years) in 21 kindred members diagnosed and treated sufficiently early that is, before the onset of significant renal disease, provides strong support for this hypothesis (Fairbanks *et al.* 2002). It also suggests that a low FE_{ur} damages the tubules in some way through an increased transtubular flux of urate (Gresser and Zöllner 1991). Alternatively, hyperuricaemia induced in a rat model recently was implicated indirectly in the renal lesion through a crystal-independent mechanism, namely inhibition of nitric oxide synthase (Mazzali *et al.* 2001).

Conversely, it has been suggested that abnormal urate handling may be an early manifestation of an underlying renal disease resulting from abnormal regulation of nephrogenesis, perhaps mediated by a defective G protein-coupled receptor (Dahan *et al.* 2001). A proposal, that the disorder arises from a primary renal vasoconstriction with secondary reduction in FE_{ur} (Puig *et al.* 1998), has a weakness in that measurements of renal vascular resistance (upon which this hypothesis depends) rests on the assumption of normal tubular handling of the *p*-aminohippurate (PAH) used to derive renal plasma flow indirectly. This is an unsafe assumption, when urate and PAH share renal tubular transporters, and renal tubular transport is grossly disturbed.

The genetic heterogeneity described above makes it even more difficult to understand the pathogenesis of the hyperuricaemia. Uromodulin is normally confined to the ascending limb of the loop of Henle, whilst urate exchange is complete in mammals by the end of the proximal tubule. Sodium losses in the ascending limb might lead to hypovolaemia and hence to increased sodium reabsorption (Hart *et al.* 2002; Bleyer *et al.* 2003)(Chapter 6.4), but solute loss is not a feature of FJHN and although hyperuricaemia has been found very rarely in diabetes insipidus and Bartter's syndrome, it is not found in recessive NPH-1 nephronophthisis (Chapter 16.3) in which medullary cysts are associated with profound solute loss. Mutations in other implicated or unknown genes could act through defective trafficking and/or binding of normal uromodulin, but this is unknown at present. Also, the relationship between ADMCKD and FJHN remains obscure: FJHN could be an allelic form of the same disease in which cysts are not visible even on histology, or cysts are missed because of limitations of technology. However there are clinical differences, in particular the greater usual age of onset and the early presence of hypertension in ADMCKD. Further data are needed.

Treatment

The management of FJHN likewise includes areas where there is little disagreement, and others which remain contentious. Aggressive control of blood pressure, where present, is crucial for a successful outcome (Moro *et al.* 1991b). The role of allopurinol in ameliorating the progression of the renal disease has been stressed by some (Richmond *et al.* 1981; Moro *et al.* 1991b; McBride *et al.* 1998), and disputed by others (Yokota *et al.* 1991; Puig *et al.* 1993), However recent studies which confirm the efficacy of allopurinol may explain the above controversy. Efficacy clearly relates to the degree of renal damage at the time of beginning treatment (Fairbanks *et al.* 2002). Importantly, improvement in

GFR has even been noted in the children of the family with the HNF-1β mutation, indicating the importance of allopurinol irrespective of the underlying mutation. If reduced uric acid excretion is due to a gain-of-function mutation of a proximal tubule anion exchanger then treatment with a combination of allopurinol to reduce the renal urate load, and benzbromarone to block the tubular anion exchanger as proposed by Lhotta *et al.* (1998) may be even more beneficial. Indeed, a combination of a uricosuric agent with allopurinol is proving effective in treating hyperuricaemia in FJHN patients in renal failure (Hisatome *et al.* 1996; Lhotta *et al.* 1998; Fairbanks *et al.* 2002). Thus early treatment with allopurinol (possibly with benzbromarone) is essential, irrespective of the underlying genetic defect, but the dose must of course be adjusted for renal function (see Chapter 6.4).

Renal transplantation has been performed in a number of cases. Some 50 per cent have failed. The remainder have retained stable graft function, and free of gout or hyperuricaemia on allopurinol for more than 15 years, as would be expected if this is a disorder of renal urate transport.

References

Ablin, A. *et al.* (1972). Nephropathy, xanthinuria, and orotic aciduria complicating Burkitt's lymphoma treated with chemotherapy and allopurinol. *Metabolism* **21**, 771–775.

Akaoka, I. *et al.* Renal urate secretion in five cases of hypouricemia with an isolated renal defect of urate transport. *Journal of Rheumatology* **4**, 86–94.

Aral, B. *et al.* (1996). Novel nonsense mutation in the hypoxanthine guanine phosphoribosyltransferase gene and nonrandom X-inactivation causing Lesch–Nyhan syndrome in a female patient. *Human Mutation* **7**, 52–58.

Augoustides-Savvopoulou, P. *et al.* (2002). Partial hypoxanthine-guanine phosphoribosyltransferase deficiency as the unsuspected cause of renal disease spanning three generations: a cautionary tale. *Pediatrics* **109**, E17.

Auranen, M. *et al.* (2001). Further evidence for linkage of autosomal-dominant medullary cystic kidney disease on chromosome 1q21. *Kidney International* **60**, 1225–1232.

Becker, M.A. Hyperuricemia and gout. In *The Metabolic and Molecular Basis of Inherited Disease* 8th edn. (ed. C. R. Scriver, A. L. Beaudet, W. S. Sly, and D.Valle), pp. 2513–2535. New York: McGraw Hill, 2001.

Beedham, C. (1987). Molybdenum hydroxylases: biological distribution and substrate-inhibitor specificity. *Progress in Medicinal Chemistry* **24**, 85–127.

Berger, L. and Yü, T.-F. (1975). Renal function in gout. IV. An analysis of 524 gouty subjects including long-term studies. *American Journal of Medicine* **59**, 605–613.

Bleyer, A. J. *et al.* (2003). Clinical characterization of a family with a mutation in the uromodulin (Tamm-Horsfall glycoprotein) gene. *Kidney International* **64**, 36–42.

Bingham, C. *et al.* (2003). Familial juvenile hyperuricemic nephropathy associated with hepatocyte nuclear factor 1β gene. *Kidney International* **63**, 1645–1651.

Bradbury, M. G. *et al.* (1995). Xanthinuria: presentation with acute renal failure in a nine month old girl. *Pediatric Nephrology* **9**, 476–477.

Brock, W. A., Golden, J., and Kaplan, G. W. (1983). Xanthine calculi in the Lesch–Nyhan syndrome. *Journal of Urology* **130**, 157–159.

Calabrese, G. *et al.* (1990). Precocious familial gout with reduced fractional excretion of urate and normal purine enzymes. *Quarterly Journal of Medicine* **75**, 441–450.

Cameron, J. S. *et al.* (1984). Problems of diagnosis in an adolescent with hypoxanthine-guanine phosphoribosyltransferase deficiency. *Advances in Experimental Medicine and Biology* **165A**, 7–13.

Cameron, J. S. Moro, F., and Simmonds, H. A. (1991). What is the pathogenesis of familial juvenile gouty nephropathy? *Advances in Experimental Medicine and Biology* **309A**, 185–191.

Cameron, J. S., Moro, F., and Simmonds, H. A. (1993). Gout, uric acid and purine metabolism in paediatric nephrology. *Pediatric Nephrology* 7, 105–118.

Carpenter, T. O. *et al.* (1986). Hereditary xanthinuria presenting in infancy with nephrolithiasis. *Journal of Pediatrics* 109, 307–309.

Casari, G. and Amoroso, A. (2003). Molecular analysis of uromodulin and SAH genes, positional candidates for autosomal dominant medullary cystic kidney disease linked to 16p12. *Journal of Nephrology* 16, 459.

Cassidy, M. J. D. *et al.* (2004). Diagnosis of adenine phosphoribosyltransferase deficiency as underlying cause of renal failure in a renal transplant recipient. *Nephrology, Dialysis, Transplantation* 19, 736–738.

Ceballos-Picot, I. *et al.* (1992). 2,8-Dihydroxyadenine urolithiasis, an under-diagnosed disease. *Lancet* 339, 1050–1051.

Chen, J. *et al.* (1991). Identification of a single missense mutation in the adenine phosphoribosyltransferase gene from five Icelandic patients and a British patient. *American Journal of Human Genetics* 49, 251–254.

Christen, H.-J. *et al.* (1992). Distinct neurological syndrome in two brothers with hyperuricaemia. *Lancet* 340, 1167–1168.

Christodoulou, K. *et al.* (1998). Chromosome 1 localization of a gene for autosomal dominant medullary cystic kidney disease. *Human Molecular Genetics* 7, 905–911.

Dahan, K. *et al.* (2001). Familial juvenile hyperuricemic nephropathy and autosomal dominant medullary cystic kidney disease type 2: two facets of the same disease? *Journal of the American Society of Nephrology* 12, 2348–2357.

Dahan, K. *et al.* (2003). A cluster of mutations in the UMOD gene causes familial juvenile hyperuricemic nephropathy with abnormal expression of uromodulin. *Journal of the American Society of Nephrology* 14, 2883–2893.

De Gregorio, L. *et al.* (2000). An unexpected affected female patient in a classical Lesch–Nyhan family. *Molecular Genetics and Metabolism* 69, 263–268.

De Vries, A. and Sperling, O. (1979). Inborn hypouricemia due to isolated renal tubular defect. *Biomedicine* 30, 75–80.

Deng, L. *et al.* (2001). 2,8-Dihydroxyadenine urolithiasis in a patient with considerable residual adenine phosphoribosyltransferase activity in cell extracts but with mutations in both copies of APRT. *Molecular Genetics and Metabolism* 72, 260–264.

Dent, C. E. and Philpot, G. R. (1954). Xanthinuria, an inborn error (or deviation) of metabolism. *Lancet* i, 182–185.

Duncan, H. and Dixon, A. St. J. (1960). Gout, familial hyperuricaemia, and renal disease. *Quarterly Journal of Medicine* 29, 127–136.

Edvardsson, V. *et al.* (2001). Clinical features and genotype of adenine phosphoribosyltransferase deficiency in Iceland. *American Journal of Kidney Diseases* 38, 473–480.

Enomoto, A. *et al.* (2002). Molecular identification of a renal urate anion exchanger that regulates blood urate levels. *Nature* 417, 447–452.

Erley, C. M. M. *et al.* (1989). Acute renal failure due to uric acid nephropathy in a patient with renal hypouricaemia. *Klinische Wochenschrift* 67, 308–312.

Farebrother, D. A. *et al.* (1975). Experimental crystal nephropathy (one year study in the pig). *Clinical Nephrology* 4, 243–250.

Farebrother, D. A. *et al.* (1981). Uric acid crystal-induced nephropathy: evidence for a specific renal lesion in a gouty family. *Journal of Pathology* 135, 159–168.

Fairbanks, L. *et al.* (2002). Early treatment with allopurinol in familial juvenile hyperuricaemic nephropathy (FJHN) ameliorates the long-term progression of the disease. *Quarterly Journal of Medicine* 95, 597–607.

Fildes, R. D. (1989). Hereditary xanthinuria with severe urolithiasis occurring in infancy as renal tubular acidosis and hypercalciuria. *Journal of Pediatrics* 115, 277–280.

Gagné, E.-R. *et al.* (1994). Chronic renal failure secondary to 2,8-dihydroxy-adenine deposition: the first report of recurrence in a kidney transplant. *American Journal of Kidney Diseases* 24, 104–107.

Garcia-Pavia, P. *et al.* (2003). Phosphoribosylpyrophosphate synthetase overactivity as a cause of uric acid overproduction in a young woman. *Arthritis & Rheumatism* 48, 2036–2041.

Gofrit, D., Verstandig, A. G., and Pode, D. (1993). Bilateral obstructing ureteral uric acid stone in an infant with hereditary renal hypouricemia. *Journal of Urology* 149, 1506–1507.

Gomez, G. A., Stutzman, L., and Ming Chu, T. (1978). Xanthine nephropathy during chemotherapy in deficiency of hypoxanthine-guanine phosphoribosyltransferase. *Archives of Internal Medicine* 138, 1017–1019.

Greene, M. L. *et al.* (1972). Hypouricemia due to isolated renal tubular defect. Dalmatian dog mutation in man. *American Journal of Medicine* 53, 361–367.

Greenwood, M. C. *et al.* (1982). Renal failure due to 2,8-dihydroxyadenine urolithiasis. *European Journal of Pediatrics* 138, 346–349.

Gresser, U. and Zöllner, N., ed. *Urate Deposition in Man and its Clinical, Consequences.* Berlin: Springer-Verlag, 1991.

Hart, T. C. *et al.* (2002). Mutations of the UMOD gene are responsible for medullary cystic disease 2 and familial juvenile hyperuricaemic nephropathy. *Journal of Medical Genetics* 39, 882–892.

Hateboer, N. *et al.* (2001). Confirmation of a gene locus for medullary cystic kidney disease (MCKD2) on chromosome 16p12. *Kidney International* 60, 1233–1239.

Hille, R. and Massey, V. Molybdenum-containing hydroxylases: xanthine oxidase, aldehyde oxidase, and sulfite oxidase. In *Molybdenum Enzymes* (ed. T. P. Spiro), pp. 443–518. New York: Academic Press, 1985.

Hillebrand, G. and Reiter, S. (1991). Hypourikämie—ein differentialdiagnostisches Probleme. *Internist* 32, 226–229.

Hisanaga, S. *et al.* (1994). Exercise-induced renal failure in a patient with hyperuricosuric hyopuricemia. *Nephron* 66, 475–476.

Hisatome, I. *et al.* (1989). Cause of persistent hypouricemia in outpatients. *Nephron* 51, 13–16.

Hisatome, I. *et al.* (1996). Renal handling of urate in a patient with familial juvenile gouty nephropathy. *Internal Medicine* 35, 564–568.

Holme, S. A. *et al.* (2002). Erythrocyte thiopurine methyltransferase assessment prior to azathioprine use in the UK. *Quarterly Journal of Medicine* 95, 439–449.

Hughes, E. F. *et al.* (1998). Molybdenum cofactor deficiency—phenotypic variability in a family with a late onset variant. *Developmental Medicine and Child Neurology* 40, 57–61.

Ichida, K. *et al.* (1997). Identification of two mutations in human xanthine dehydrogenase gene responsible for classical type I xanthinuria. *Journal of Clinical Investigation* 99, 2391–2397.

Ichida, K. *et al.* (2001). Mutation of human molybdenum cofactor sulfurase gene is responsible for classical xanthinuria type II. *Biochemical and Biophysical Research Communications* 282, 1194–1200.

Ishizuka, T. *et al.* (1992). Promoter regions of the human X-linked housekeeping genes PRPS1 and PRPS2 encoding phosphoribosylpyrophosphate synthetase subunit I and II. *Biochimica Biophysica Acta* 1130, 139–148.

Jinnah, H. A. and Friedmann, T. Lesch–Nyhan disease and its variants. In *The Metabolic and Molecular Basis of Inherited Disease* 8th edn. (ed. C. R. Scriver, A. L. Beaudet, W. S. Sly, and D. Valle), pp. 2537–2570. New York: McGraw Hill, 2001.

Jinnah, H. A. *et al.* (2000). The spectrum of inherited mutations causing HPRT deficiency: 75 new cases and a review of 196 previously reported cases. *Mutation Research* 463, 309–326.

Johnson, J. L. and Duran, M. Molybdenum cofactor deficiency and isolated sulfite oxidase deficiency. In *Metabolic and Molecular Basis of Inherited Disease* 8th edn. (ed. C. R. Scriver, A. L. Beaudet, W. S. Sly, and D. Valle), pp. 3163–3173. New York: McGraw-Hill, 2001.

Johnson, J. L. *et al.* (1988). Molybdenum cofactor deficiency in a patient previously characterised as deficient in sulfite oxidase. *Biochemical Medicine and Metabolic Biology* 40, 86–93.

Kamatani, N. *et al.* (1992). Only three mutations account for almost all defective alleles causing adenine phosphoribosyltransferase deficiency in Japanese patients. *Journal of Clinical Investigation* 90, 130–135.

Kamatani, N. *et al.* (2000). Localization of a gene for familial juvenile hyperuricemic nephropathy causing underexcretion-type gout to 16p12 by genome-wide linkage analysis of a large family. *Arthritis and Rheumatism* **43**, 925–929.

Kavukcu, S. *et al.* (2000). Clinical quiz. Molybdenum cofactor deficiency. *Pediatric Nephrology* **14**, 1145–1147.

Kenney, I. J. (1991). Renal sonography in long standing Lesch–Nyhan syndrome. *Clinical Radiology* **43**, 39–41.

Khattak, F. H., Morris, I. M., and Harris, K. (1998). Kelley–Seegmiller syndrome: a case report and review of the literature. *British Journal of Rheumatology* **37**, 580–581.

Kita, K. *et al.* (1994). A novel 39-kDa phosphoribosylpyrophosphate synthetase-associated protein of rat liver. Cloning, high sequence similarity to the catalytic subunits, and a negative regulatory role. *Journal of Biological Chemistry* **269**, 8334–8340.

Krois, S. *et al.* (2000). Evidence of further genetic heterogeneity in autosomal dominant medullary cystic kidney disease. *Nephrology, Dialysis, Transplantation* **15**, 818.

Krynetski, E. Y. and Evans, W. E. (2000). Genetic polymorphism of thiopurine S-methyltransferase: molecular mechanisms and clinical importance. *Pharmacology* **61**, 136–146.

Laxdal, T. (1992). 2,8-Dihydroxyadenine crystalluria versus urolithiasis. *Lancet* **340**, 184.

Levartovsky, D. *et al.* (2000). XDH gene mutation is the underlying cause of classical xanthinuria: a second report. *Kidney International* **57**, 2215–2120.

Lhotta, K. *et al.* (1998). Apoptosis of tubular epithelial cells in familial juvenile gouty nephropathy. *Nephron* **79**, 340–344.

Matsuda, O. *et al.* (1982). A case of familial renal hypouricaemia associated with increased secretion of para-aminohippurate and idiopathic edema. *Nephron* **30**, 178–186.

Maynard, J. and Benson, P. (1988). Hereditary xanthinuria in 2 Pakistani sisters: asymptomatic in one with beta-thalassemia but causing xanthine stone, obstructive uropathy and hypertension in the other. *Journal of Urology* **139**, 338–339.

Mazzali, M. *et al.* (2001). Elevated uric acid increases blood pressure in the rat by a novel crystal-independent mechanism. *Hypertension* **38**, 1101–1106.

McBride, M. B. *et al.* (1995). Renal urate hypoexcretion in Polynesian women is not as severe as in United Kingdom (UK) women with familial juvenile hyperuricaemic nephropathy. *Advances in Experimental Medicine and Biology* **370**, 35–39.

McBride, M. B., Simmonds, H. A., and Moro, F. (1997). Genetic gout in childhood: familial juvenile hyperuricaemic nephropathy, or 'familial renal disease'? *Journal of Inherited Metabolic Diseases* **20**, 351–353.

McBride, M. B. *et al.* (1998). Efficacy of allopurinol in ameliorating the progression in familial juvenile hyperuricaemic nephropathy (FJHN): a six year update. *Advances in Experimental Medicine and Biology* **431**, 7–11.

McCarthy, G. (1992). Practical aspects of the management of the Lesch–Nyhan syndrome. *British Inherited Metabolic Disease Group Newsletter* **6**, 14–16.

Menardi, C. *et al.* (1997). Human APRT deficiency: indication for multiple origins of the most common Caucasian mutation and detection of a novel type of mutation involving intrastrand-templated repair. *Human Mutation* **10**, 251–255.

Moro, F. *et al.* (1991a). Familial juvenile gouty nephropathy with renal urate hypoexcretion preceding renal disease. *Clinical Nephrology* **35**, 263–269.

Moro, F. *et al.* (1991b). Does allopurinol ameliorate progression in familial juvenile gouty nephropathy (FJGN)? *Advances in Experimental Medicine and Biology* **309A**, 199–202.

Murakami, T. *et al.* (1990). Underexcretory-type hyperuricemia, disproportionate to the reduced glomerular filtration rate, in two boys with mild proteinuria. *Nephron* **56**, 439–442.

Ogasawara, N. *et al.* (1989). Molecular analysis of a female Lesch–Nyhan patient. *Journal of Clinical Investigation* **84**, 1024–1027.

Ohta, T. *et al.* (2002). Exercise-induced acute renal failure with renal hypouricemia: a case report and review of the literature. *Clinical Nephrology* **58**, 313–316.

Page, T. and Nyhan, W. L. (1989). The spectrum of HPRT deficiency: an update. *Advances in Experimental Medicine and Biology* **253A**, 129–133.

Parvari, R. *et al.* (2001). Clinical and genetic characterization of an autosomal dominant nephropathy. *American Journal of Medical Genetics* **99**, 204–209.

Praetorius, E. and Kirk, J. E. (1950). Hypouricemia; with evidence for tubular elimination of uric acid. *Journal of Laboratory and Clinical Medicine* **35**, 865–868.

Puig, J. G. *et al.* (1993). Hereditary nephropathy associated with hyperuricaemia and gout. *Archives of Internal Medicine* **153**, 357–365.

Puig, J. G. *et al.* (1998). Purine metabolism in female heterozygotes for hypoxanthine–guanine phosphoribosyltransferase deficiency. *European Journal of Clinical Investigation* **28**, 950–957.

Raivio, K. O., Saksela, M., and Lapatto, R. Xanthine oxidoreductase—role in human pathophysiology and in hereditary xanthinuria. In *The Metabolic and Molecular Basis of Inherited Disease* 8th edn. (ed. C. R. Scriver, A. L. Beaudet, W. S. Sly, and D. Valle), pp. 2639–2652. New York: McGraw Hill, 2001.

Rampoldi, L. *et al.* (2003). Allelism of MCKD, FJHN and GCKD caused by impairment of uromodulin export dynamics. *Human Medical Genetics* **12**, 3369–3384.

Ray, P. F. *et al.* (1999). Successful preimplantation genetic diagnosis for sex link Lesch–Nyhan syndrome using specific diagnosis. *Prenatal Diagnosis* **19**, 1237–1241.

Reiss, J. *et al.* (1998). Mutations in a polycistronic nuclear gene associated with molybdenum cofactor deficiency. *Nature Genetics* **20**, 51–53.

Reiss, J. *et al.* (1999). Human molybdopterin synthase gene: genomic structure and mutations in molybdenum cofactor deficiency type B. *American Journal of Human Genetics* **64**, 706–711.

Reiss, J. (2000). Genetics of molybdenum cofactor deficiency. *Human Genetics* **106**, 157–163.

Reiss, J. *et al.* (2001). A mutation in the gene for the neurotransmitter receptor-clustering protein gephryn causes a novel form of molybdenum co-factor deficiency. *American Journal of Human Genetics* **68**, 208–213.

Reiter, S. *et al.* (1990). Demonstration of a combined deficiency of xanthine oxidase and aldehyde oxidase in xanthinuric patients not forming oxypurinol. *Clinica Chimica Acta* **187**, 221–234.

Reiter, L., Brown, M.A., and Edmonds, J. (1995). Familial hyperuricemic nephropathy. *American Journal of Kidney Diseases* **25**, 235–241.

Resnick, J. S., Sisson, S., and Vernier, R. L. (1978). Tamm-Horsfall protein: abnormal localization in renal disease. *Laboratory Investigation* **38**, 550–555.

Richmond, J. M. *et al.* (1981). Familial urate nephropathy. *Clinical Nephrology* **16**, 163–168.

Rytkönen, E. M. K. *et al.* (1995). The human gene for xanthine dehydrogenase (XDH) is localized on chromosome band 2p22. *Cytogenetics and Cell Genetics* **68**, 61–63.

Sahota, A. S. *et al.* Adenine phosphoribosyltransferase deficiency and 2,8-dihydroxyadenine lithiasis. In *The Metabolic and Molecular Basis of Inherited Disease* 8th edn. (ed. C. R. Scriver, A. L. Beaudet, W. S. Sly, and D. Valle), pp. 2571–2584. New York: McGraw Hill, 2001.

Sakamoto, N. *et al.* (2001). Identification of a new point mutation in the human xanthine dehydrogenase gene responsible for a case of classical type I xanthinuria. *Human Genetics* **108**, 279–283.

Salti, I. S., Mouradian, M., and Frayha, R. A. (1992). Hereditary xanthinuria. *Arab Journal of Medicine* **1**, 5–12.

Scolari, F. *et al.* (1999). Identification of a new locus for medullary cystic disease, on chromosome 16p12. *American Journal of Human Genetics* **64**, 1655–1660.

Shichiri, M., Iwamoto, H., and Shiigai, T. (1987). Hypouricemia due to increased tubular urate secretion. *Nephron* **45**, 31–34.

Simmonds, H. A., Duley, J. A., and Davies, P. M. (1991). Analysis of purines and pyrimidines in blood, urine and other physiological fluids. In *Techniques in Diagnostic Human Biochemical Genetics. A Laboratory Manual* (ed. F. Hommes), pp. 397–425. New York: Wiley-Liss, 1991.

Simmonds, H. A. *et al.* (1976). The identification of 2,8-dihydroxyadenine, a new component of urinary stones. *Biochemical Journal* **157**, 485–487.

Simmonds, H. A. *et al.* (1980). Renal failure in young subjects with familial gout. *Advances in Experimental Medicine and Biology* **122A**, 15–20.

Simmonds, H. A. *et al.* (1984). Pregnancy in xanthinuria: demonstration of fetal uric acid production? *Journal of Inherited Metabolic Diseases* **7**, 77–79.

Simmonds, H. A. *et al.* (1986). Allopurinol in renal failure and the tumour lysis syndrome. *Clinica Chimica Acta* **160**, 189–195.

Simmonds, H. A. *et al.* (1989). Purine enzyme defects as a cause of acute renal failure in childhood. *Pediatric Nephrology* **3**, 433–437.

Simmonds, H. A. *et al.* (1994). Polynesian women are also at risk for hyperuricaemia and gout because of a defect in renal urate handling. *British Journal of Rheumatology* **33**, 932–937.

Sonoda, T. *et al.* (1997). Cloning and sequencing of rat cDNA for the 41-kDa phosphoribosylpyrophosphate synthetase-associated protein has a high homology to the catalytic subunits and the 39-kDa associated protein. *Biochimica et Biophysica ACTA* **1350**, 6–10.

Sperling, O. (2001). Hereditary renal hypouricaemia. In *The Metabolic and Molecular Basis of Inherited Disease* 8th edn. (ed. R. Scriver, A. L. Beaudet, W. S. Sly, and D. Valle), pp. 5069–5083. New York: McGraw Hill, 2001.

Stapleton, F. B. Uric acid nephropathy. In *Pediatric Nephrology* 2nd edn. (ed. C. M. Edelmann, Jr.), pp. 1647–1659. Boston: Little Brown, 1992.

Stavrou, C. *et al.* (2002). Autosomal-dominant medullary cystic kidney disease type 1: clinical and molecular findings in six large Cypriot families. *Kidney International* **62**, 1385–1394.

Stibůrková, B. *et al.* (2000). Familial juvenile hyperuricemic nephropathy: localization of the gene on chromosome 16p11.2-and evidence for genetic heterogeneity. *American Journal of Human Genetics* **66**, 1989–1994.

Stibůrková, B. *et al.* (2003). Familial juvenile hyperuricaemic nephropathy (FJHN): linkage analysis in 15 families, physical and transcriptional characteristics of the FJHN critical region and analysis of 7 candidate genes. *European Journal of Human Genetics* **11**, 145–154.

Stone, T. W. and Simmonds, H. A. *Purines: Basic and Clinical Aspects*. London: Kluwer, 1991.

Torres, R. J. *et al.* (2000). Molecular basis of hypoxanthine-guanine phosphoribosyltransferase deficiency in thirteen Spanish families. *Human Mutation* **15**, 383.

Turner, J. J. *et al.* (2003). UROMODULIN mutations cause familial juvenile hyperuricemic nephropathy. *Journal of Clinical Endocrinology and Metabolism* **88**, 1398–1401.

Van Bogaert, P. *et al.* (1992) Lesch–Nyhan syndrome in a girl. *Journal of Inherited Metabolic Diseases* **15**, 790–791.

Wahl, R. C. *et al.* (1982). *Drosophila melanogaster* ma-l mutants are defective in the sulfuration of desulfo Mo hydroxylases. *Journal of Biological Chemistry* **257**, 3958–3963.

Wang, L. *et al.* (2002). Induction of α-catenin, integrin α3, integrin β6, and PDGF-B by 2,8-dihydroxyadenine crystals in cultured kidney epithelial cells. *Experimental Nephrology* **10**, 365–373.

Watts, R. W. E. (1985). Defects of tetrahydrobiopterin synthesis and their possible relationship to a disorder of purine metabolism, the Lesch–Nyhan syndrome. *Advances in Enzyme Regulation* **23**, 25–58.

Weyer, N., Koplin, T., Friske, C., and Iven, H. (2001). Human thiopurine-S methyl transferase activity in uremia and after renal transplantation. *European Journal of Clinical Pharmacology* **57**, 129–136.

Wolf, M. T. E. *et al.* (2003). Mutations of the Uromodulin gene in MCKD type 2 patients cluster in exon 4, which encodes three EGF-like domains. *Kidney International* **64**, 1580–1587.

Wyngaarden, J. M. and Kelley, W. N. *Gout and Hyperuricemia*. New York: Grune and Stratton, 1976.

Xu, P., Huecksteadt, T. P., and Hoidal, J. R. (1996). Molecular cloning and characterization of the human xanthine dehydrogenase gene (XDH). *Genomics* **34**, 173–180.

Yakota, N. *et al.* (1991). Autosomal dominantly transmission of gouty arthritis with renal disease in a large Japanese family. *Annals of the Rheumatic Diseases* **50**, 108–111.

Yamada, Y. *et al.* (1996). Molecular analysis of a Japanese family with Lesch–Nyhan syndrome: identification of mutation and prenatal diagnosis. *Clinical Genetics* **50**, 164–167.

Zager, F. A., Cotran, R. S., and Hoyer, J. R. (1978). Pathologic localization of Tamm-Horsfall protein in interstitial deposits in interstitial disease. *Laboratory Investigation* **38**, 52–57.

Zoref, E., de Vries, A., and Sperling, O. (1975). Mutant feedback resistant phosphoribosyl-pyrophosphate synthetase associated with purine overproduction and gout. *Journal of Clinical Investigation* **56**, 1093–1099.

16.6 Renal involvement in tuberous sclerosis and von Hippel–Lindau disease

Hartmut P.H. Neumann, Elizabeth Petri Henske, Othon Iliopoulos, and Sven Glaesker

Involvement of the kidneys is a classical feature of two disorders among those classified as phakomatoses, tuberous sclerosis complex (TSC) and von Hippel–Lindau disease. Both diseases show bilateral renal manifestations and both can be life-threatening due to complications involving the kidneys.

Tuberous sclerosis

Introduction and genetics

TSC is a multiorgan disorder with a prevalence of about 1 : 10,000 (O'Callaghan *et al.* 1998). The signs of TSC can include seizures, mental retardation, and facial angiofibroma. Therefore, in English-speaking countries it was previously called epiloia (epilepsy + anoia). TSC has also been called Bourneville's or Pringle's disease, after the authors of the classical descriptions. TSC has marked clinical variability, and at least 50 per cent of the patients have normal intelligence (Povey *et al.* 1994). Given the awareness of the involvement of many organs (Table 1), the term TSC is now favoured, and the international abbreviation TSC has, therefore, been introduced. TSC is a genetic disorder that has been characterized in detail, by enormous effort made during the past decade. About 30 per cent of patients have relatives affected by TSC, and in these the transmission of the disorder is autosomal dominant. Apparently isolated or sporadic cases are likely to be new mutations. Studies of large families provide evidence of two susceptibility genes for TSC, one named TSC1 on chromosome 9q34 (Fryer *et al.* 1987) and the other named TSC2 on chromosome 16p13 (Kandt *et al.* 1992). The TSC1 gene comprises 20 kb, the transcript 3.4 kb. Twenty-one exons encode a protein of 1164 amino acids named hamartin (van Slegtenhorst *et al.* 1997). The corresponding data for the TSC2 gene are 40 kb, transcript 5.4 kb, 41 exons, and 1784 amino acids forming a protein named tuberin (ETSC 1993).

Multiple lines of evidence indicate that TSC1 and TSC2 are tumour suppressor genes fitting the Knudson 'two hit' model (Knudson 1971). This evidence includes: (a) that germline mutations in TSC1 (van Slegtenhorst *et al.* 1997) and TSC2 (ETSC 1993) are predicted to inactivate protein function and (b) that loss of heterozygosity (LOH) in the TSC1 or TSC2 region occurs in TSC angiomyolipomas, rhabdomyomas, and astrocytomas (Carbonara *et al.* 1994; Green *et al.* 1994a,b; Bjornsson *et al.* 1996; Henske *et al.* 1996). Tuberin and/or hamartin appear to be involved in at least four cellular pathways: (a) vesicular trafficking, (b) cell cycle regulation, (c) steroid hormone function, and (d) cell adhesion via the small GTPase Rho. The *in vivo* significance of these pathways and their contribution to the pathogenesis of lymphangioleiomyomatosis (LAM) are not yet fully understood.

Table 1 Diagnostic criteria for tuberous sclerosis complex (Roach *et al.* 1998)

Primary features
Facial angiofibromas[a]
Multiple ungual fibromas[a]
Cortical tuber (histologically confirmed)
Subependymal nodule or giant-cell astrocytoma (histologically confirmed)
Multiple calcified subependymal nodules protruding into the ventricle (radiographic evidence)
Multiple retinal astrocytomas[a]

Secondary features
Affected first-degree relative
Cardiac rhabdomyoma (histological or radiographic confirmation)
Other retinal hamartoma or achromic patch[a]
Cerebral tubers (radiographic confirmation)
Shagreen patch[a]
Forehead plaque[a]
Pulmonary lymphangiomyomatosis (histological confirmation)
Renal angiomyolipoma (radiographic or histological confirmation)
Renal cysts (histological confirmation)

Tertiary features
Hypomelanotic macules[a]
'Confetti' skin lesions[a]
Renal cysts (radiographic evidence)
Randomly distributed enamel pits in deciduous and/or permanent teeth
Hamartomatous rectal polyps (histological confirmation)
Bone cysts (radiographic evidence)
Pulmonary lymphangiomatosis (radiographic evidence)
Cerebral white matter 'migration tracts' or heterotopias (radiographic evidence)
Gingival fibromas[a]
Hamartoma of other organs (histological confirmation)
Infantile spasms

Definite TSC: Either one primary feature, two secondary features, or one secondary plus two tertiary features
Probable TSC: Either one secondary feature plus one tertiary feature, or three tertiary features
Suspect TSC: Either one secondary feature or two tertiary features

[a] Histological confirmation is not required if the lesion is clinically obvious.

Diagnosis

The diagnosis of TSC is still primarily based on clinical, radiological, and histopathological findings, although genetic testing will likely become more widely used over the next few years. The many findings in TSC, as listed in Table 1, have been ranked according to diagnostic value (Roach *et al.* 1998). Among the lesions that are pathognomonic of TSC are facial angiofibroma, multiple ungual fibromas, and multiple subependymal calcifications revealed by computed tomography (CT) (Fig. 1). Lesions of the kidney (Fig. 2) are only secondary criteria because renal angiomyolipoma and renal cysts occur also as sporadic lesions in individuals not affected by TSC. Currently, the diagnosis of TSC is based on a combination of one to three different lesions, depending on their diagnostic value (Table 1). Molecular genetic analyses require specifically interested laboratories. A first study on more than 200 cases with TSC revealed a sensitivity for finding a mutation of 84 per cent. Of the total mutations, 85 per cent affected the TSC2 gene , whereas 15 per cent the TSC1 gene. Patients with TSC1 are less severely affected regarding occurrence of epileptic seizures, mental retardation, subependymal nodules, cortical tubera, retinal hamartoma, and facial angiofibroma (Dabora *et al.* 2001).

If a diagnosis of TSC is suspected, patients should undergo a detailed standard clinical investigation programme of the brain, eyes, heart, abdomen, and skin (Table 2).

Renal lesions

The principal renal lesions in TSC are angiomyolipomas and cysts (Robbins and Bernstein 1988), which often occur in combination. Renal disease is the most common cause of TSC-related death (Brasier and Henske 1997). Bilateral involvement of the kidneys is typical, but the extent of lesions varies from case to case (Stillwell *et al.* 1987). Angiomyolipomas are present in about 75 per cent of children with TSC by age 10 years (Ewalt *et al.* 1998). Cysts in TSC (Fig. 2) are localized in the renal cortex and show focal concentration (Robbins and Bernstein 1988). Histologically, the cyst epithelium in TSC is often atypical and hyperplastic (Ibrahim *et al.* 1989). Renal angiomyolipomas are hamartomatous lesions consisting of atypical blood vessels, smooth-muscle cells, and fat tissue (Mostofi *et al.* 1981; Fig. 2). Bilateral and multifocal angiomyolipomas are typical of TSC (Neumann *et al.* 1992b). The size varies widely, and growth of lesions is common, with up to 4 cm growth in one year documented. Symptoms include abdominal pain and haematuria. Bilateral angiomyolipoma can cause chronic

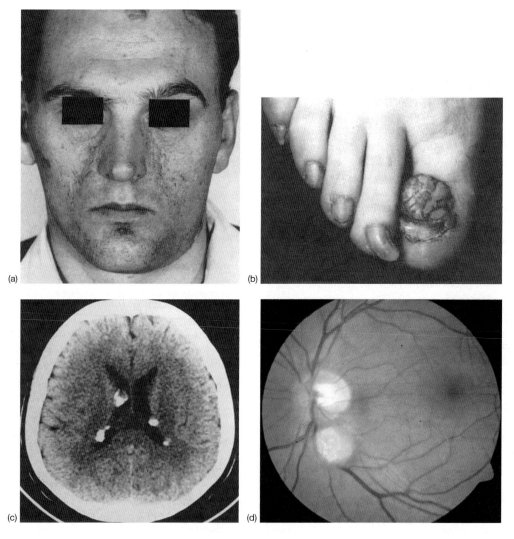

Fig. 1 Extrarenal lesions in tuberous sclerosis complex: (a) facial angiofibroma and forehead plaque, (b) ungual fibroma, (c) subependymal lesions with calcification, and (d) mulberry tumour of the retina.

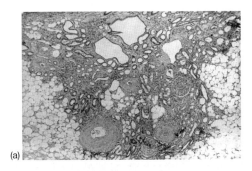
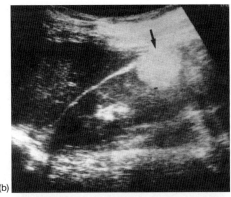
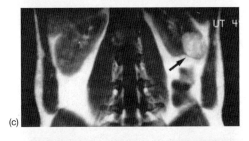
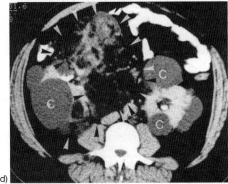

Fig. 2 Renal lesions in tuberous sclerosis complex: (a) histological appearances, (b) ultrasonographic appearances circumscribed, echogenic tumour (angiomyolipoma), (c) MRI circumscribed, predominantly fatty tumour, and (d) CT scan [multiple, bilateral renal cysts (C)] and giant angiomyolipoma; note intravenous contrast-enhanced functioning renal tissue and pelvis.

Table 2 Summary of testing recommendations in tuberous sclerosis complex (Roach *et al.* 1999)

Assessment	Initial testing	Repeat testing
Neuro developmental testing	At diagnosis and at school entry	As indicated
Ophthalmic examination	At diagnosis	As indicated
Electroencephalography	If seizures occur	As indicated for seizure management
Electrocardiography	At diagnosis	As indicated
Echocardiography	If cardiac symptoms occur	If cardiac dysfunction occurs
Renal ultrasonography	At diagnosis	Every 1–3 years
Chest computed tomography	At adulthood (women only)	If pulmonary dysfunction occurs
Cranial computed tomography[a]	At diagnosis	Children/adolescents: every 1–3 years
Cranial magnetic resonance imaging[a]	At diagnosis	Children/adolescents: every 1–3 years

[a] Either cranial computed tomography or magnetic resonance imaging, but usually not both.

unilateral nephrectomy and consecutively progressive deterioration of renal function (Schillinger and Montagnac 1996).

The most life-threatening complication of angiomyolipoma is local bleeding. Haemorrhage usually occurs spontaneously, but can be induced by accident or iatrogenically by diagnostic procedures such as biopsy, and can lead to hypovolaemic shock and even death (Shepherd *et al.* 1991). The radiological appearances of angiomyolipoma are very characteristic (Fig. 2). Echogenicity is a striking finding by ultrasonography. Fat tissue produces typical images on CT, being more easily visualized by CT than by magnetic resonance imaging (MRI). The radiological features are diagnostic for angiomyolipoma (Neumann 1994b); the presence of fat in angiomyolipomas allows differentiation from renal-cell carcinoma. Biopsy is not needed for the diagnosis of angiomyolipomas with typical radiographic features and should be avoided because of the risk of bleeding, which can lead to deterioration of renal function, sometimes necessitating nephrectomy (Neumann 1994b).

There are two major sources of misinterpretation and mismanagement in angiomyolipoma. If angiography is used to 'clarify' the nature of a renal mass, atypical vessels are frequently shown and consequently a malignancy is mistakenly diagnosed. The other pitfall may be small areas of angiomyolipomatous tissue taken as a 'fast cut' during surgery or biopsy, which may be indistinguishable from leiomyosarcoma or liposarcoma because of cellular pleomorphism and giant cells (Mostofi *et al.* 1981). However, sarcoma may occasionally occur in TSC (Fernandez de Sevilla *et al.* 1988). Angiomyolipomatous tissue has also been observed in extrarenal organs such as lymph nodes, but should be interpreted as hamartoma rather than metastases (Bloom *et al.* 1982). Malignant transformation of angiomyolipomas can occur, but is rare. A more common finding is misdiagnosis of atypical epithelioid angiomyolipomas as renal-cell carcinoma, which can be avoided using careful histological and immunophenotypical examination of the tumour. Finally, true metastatic renal-cell carcinoma has, very

renal failure, and some patients require renal replacement therapy (Neumann *et al.* 1995). In such patients, renal transplantation is an established therapy, and worsening of the natural course of TSC due to immunosuppressive drugs has not been observed (Balligand *et al.* 1990). Most patients with TSC and endstage renal failure had previously rarely, been reported in TSC (Ohigashi *et al.* 1991; Washecka and Hanna 1991). The renal-cell carcinomas in TSC are pathologically heterogeneous, including tumours with clear cell, papillary, sarcomatoid, and chromophobe morphology (Bjornsson *et al.* 1996). The clear cell carcinomas in TSC patients lack VHL gene mutations and appear to represent an alternate pathway of renal carcinogenesis.

Optimal management of renal angiomyolipomas has not been established. A number of retrospective studies suggest that the risk of spontaneous bleeding increases as angiomyolipomas increase in size, with 4 cm in diameter often used as an indication of higher risk (De Luca *et al.* 1999). Thorough diagnostic evaluation should be performed to avoid unnecessary resection of benign angiomyolipomas that have either radiographic or histological features of malignancy. Large angiomylipomas have a tendency for spontaneous bleeding which can be effectively treated by embolization in most cases (Mourikis *et al.* 1999). Whenever possible, therapeutic approaches to renal disease in TSC should focus on preserving normal parenchyma.

Extrarenal manifestations

Central nervous system

The clinical signs of involvement of the central nervous system (CNS) in TSC include seizures, autism, and mental retardation. In general, there is a correlation between the extent of cortical lesions and neurological-psychiatric disease. However, patients can lack neurological symptoms despite the presence of typical radiological signs such as subependymal calcifications and cortical tubers. Seizures frequently start within the first months of life with infantile spasms, but other types of epilepsy are also observed (Gomez 1988). Pathologically and radiologically different types of CNS lesions occur. A tuber is a circumscribed deformation of the gyri located especially in the frontal or temporal regions. Subependymal lesions, generally with calcification, are classical signs of TSC (Fig. 1). Giant-cell astrocytomas are mostly found near the foramen of Monro and may cause obstruction of cerebrospinal-fluid pathways leading to hydrocephalus. Heterotopia is a circumscribed neuronal lesion in the white matter (Richardson 1991).

Skin and oral mucosa

Facial angiofibroma (Fig. 1) (frequently called adenoma sebaceum) is found in 70–90 per cent of individuals with TSC (Rogers 1988). Histologically, the symmetrical lesion, mainly of the nose and cheeks, shows fibrosis and ectatic capillaries. Ungual fibroma, also called Koenen tumour, is found in a para- or subungual location, more frequently on toes than fingers (Fig. 2). Hypomelanotic macules occur in all skin areas including hair and eyebrows. The lesions have reduced activity of tyrosinase and decreased melanization, thereby making them easily visible with the Wood's lamp. Shagreen patches are palpable, indurated lesions with an uneven surface, mainly of the lumbosacral region. Forehead, scalp, and facial plaques (Fig. 1) are yellowish-red or brown, elevated lesions. Fibrotic nodules may be seen in the gums.

Eyes

Retinal lesions occur in about 50 per cent of patients with TSC. The classic retinal finding is called a mulberry tumour. It is a prominent, grey or yellowish lesion with characteristic bumps similar to a mulberry (Fig. 1). Another type is flat, semitransparent and white, and is mostly observed in early childhood (Robertson 1988).

Heart

The cardiac manifestation of TSC is rhabdomyoma. The frequently multifocal tumour is usually asymptomatic and regresses over time. Very rarely, it is associated with cardiogenic cerebral embolism, but when symptomatic it is more likely to cause obstruction of cardiac outflow arrhythmia, or valve dysfunction. The lesion may contribute to death of TSC patients in childhood (Shepherd *et al.* 1991).

Pulmonary lymphangioleiomyomatosis

Figure 3 presents a TSC patient who suffered from LAM of the lungs, a condition which can occur sporadically (sporadic LAM) or as a component of TSC. LAM affects almost exclusively young women. Pulmonary parenchymal changes typical of LAM occur in 40 per cent of women

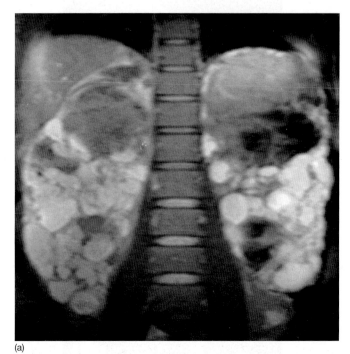

(a)

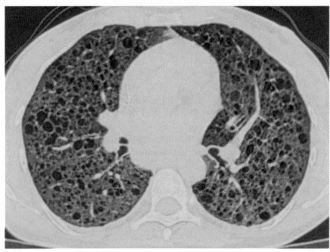

(b)

Fig. 3 A 30-year-old female patient with tuberous sclerosis complex, polycystic kidney disease (a) and pulmonary lymphangioleiomyomatosis (b) (courtesy Professor Müller-Leise, Mönchengladbach).

with TSC (Costello *et al.* 2000). LAM is the third most frequent cause of TSC-related death, after renal disease and brain tumours (Castro *et al.* 1995). While TSC patients have germline mutations in the *TSC1* or *TSC2* genes, sporadic LAM can be caused by somatic *TSC2* gene mutations in the angiomyolipoma and pulmonary LAM cells (Carsillo *et al.* 2000).

The contiguous gene syndrome TSC2–PKD1

Polycystic kidney disease (PKD) accompanied by renal hypertension and chronic renal failure (Mitnick *et al.* 1983) has been described in TSC patients. Such patients have been described genetically with mutations of the *TSC2* gene and the *PKD1* gene, both localized on chromosome 16p13. Clinically they present with progressive renal failure and endstage renal disease in the fourth to sixth decade (Brook Carter *et al.* 1994) (see also Chapter 16.2.2).

Summary

TSC is a multiorgan genetic disorder that has a wide clinical spectrum. At present no curative therapy exists. Nephrologists should be familiar with the radiological findings in order to avoid surgical treatment as far as possible. Local haemorrhage and chronic renal failure are the major renal complications.

von Hippel–Lindau syndrome

Introduction and genetics

Multiple renal cysts, bilateral renal-cell carcinomas, and hypertension due to phaeochromocytoma are some of the principal features of von Hippel–Lindau syndrome, and thus nephrologists may be confronted with this disease.

The diagnosis of von Hippel–Lindau syndrome is currently based on at least two lesions: retinal angiomatosis or haemangioblastoma of the CNS in a particular individual and involvement of one of the frequently affected organs (Figs 4–7) in that patient or a first-degree relative (Neumann 1987). The prevalence of von Hippel–Lindau disease is 1 : 31,000–1 : 53,000 (Neumann 1994a). von Hippel–Lindau syndrome is inherited in an autosomal-dominant fashion. The penetrance is high but not complete by the age of 70. The age at diagnosis of symptomatic patients is mainly the second to fourth decade of life.

The spectrum of renal disease

Renal involvement in von Hippel–Lindau syndrome is characterized by a broad spectrum of manifestations (Figs 4–6). Multiple and bilateral cysts are a frequent finding and are present in about 30 per cent of affected individuals (Neumann 1987). In general, each of the cysts can be identified, and large and small cysts may be present in the same patient; cysts scattered all over the kidneys may rarely mimic the typical images of autosomal-dominant PKD (Chatha *et al.* 2001; Fig. 6). Large single cysts may cause minor abdominal discomfort and occasionally considerable pain. Chronic progressive renal insufficiency are extremely rare in von Hippel–Lindau disease.

The second manifestation of von Hippel–Lindau syndrome in the kidney is renal-cell carcinomas (Figs 4–6). They often present cystic growth patterns (Neumann *et al.* 1998). Symptoms of VHL-associated renal cancer are similar to those of sporadic renal-cell carcinoma but the tumours mostly appear as multilocular and bilateral (Malek *et al.* 1987).

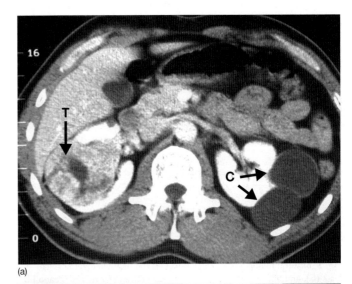

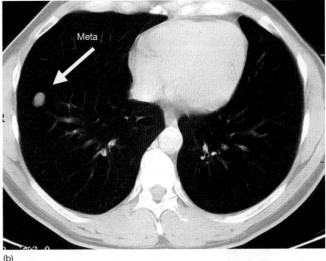

Fig. 4 A 40-year-old patient with von Hippel–Lindau disease: (a) Note a huge tumour (T) of the right kidney and cysts of the left kidney (C) (courtesy Professor Reiser, Munich). (b) Metastasis in the lung of the same patient detected 2 years later.

The clinical course is dominated by metastases in the liver, lungs, and bones and 50 per cent of deaths (Maher *et al.* 1990). Abdominal CT scan, MRI, or ultrasonography may in addition to renal lesions show pancreatic cysts, or rarer pheochromocytomas or pancreatic islet cell tumours.

Patients affected by von Hippel–Lindau syndrome requiring dialysis have a history of renal surgery that finally resulted in bilateral nephrectomy. Renal transplantation has been performed in such patients. Long-term follow-up has shown similar survival and renal functions after 4 years follow-up compared to patients with other underlying diseases (Goldfarb *et al.* 1998).

Nephron sparing surgery is the standard treatment of renal cancer in von Hippel–Lindau disease (Neumann *et al.* 1998). Still under debate is the stage when surgery is indicated. The recommendation of the National Institutes of Health of the United States of America is a size of 3 cm diameter (Walther *et al.* 1999).

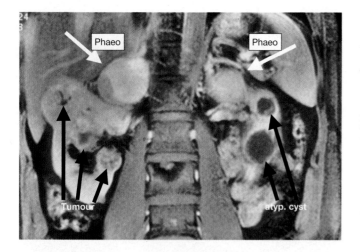

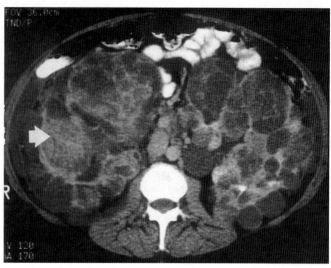

Fig. 5 Bilateral multiple renal carcinoma (T), and multiple atypical renal cysts (C), and bilateral adrenal phaeochromocytomas (arrow and 'Phaeo') in a 36-year-old patient with von Hippel–Lindau disease.

Fig. 6 von Hippel–Lindau disease mimicking PKD. Note abundant renal cysts but also a solid lesion representing a renal tumour. (From Chatha *et al.* 2001.)

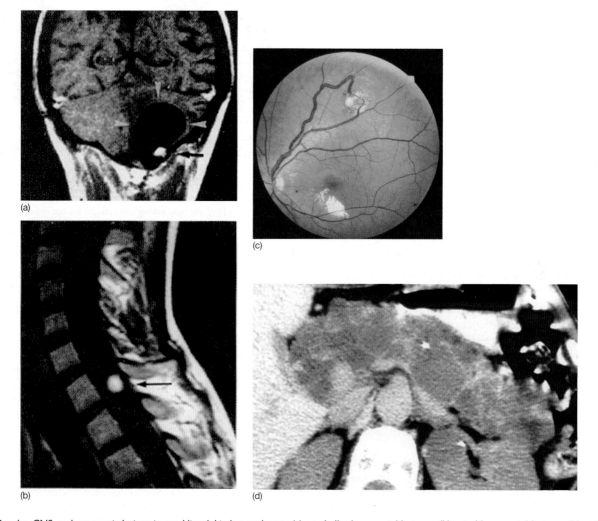

Fig. 7 Occular, CNS, and pancreatic lesions in von Hippel–Lindau syndrome: (a) cerebellar haemangioblastoma, (b) spinal haemangioblastoma, (c) retinal angioma, and (d) multiple pancreatic cysts.

Hypertension due to phaeochromocytoma

Phaeochromocytoma (Fig. 5) is a classical manifestation of the disease and is found in about 15 per cent of affected individuals (Neumann 1987). A peculiar feature of von Hippel–Lindau syndrome is that phaeochromocytoma may be a dominating lesion in some families and absent in others (Neumann and Wiestler 1991). It is of particular interest that about 10 per cent of phaeochromocytomas in the general population are manifestations of the von Hippel–Lindau syndrome (Neumann et al. 2002). These patients frequently present with phaeochromocytoma only but have a positive family history for von Hippel–Lindau disease. von Hippel–Lindau syndrome-associated phaeochromocytomas occur frequently in a multifocal fashion, in both adrenal glands or extra-adrenal paraganglia. The best diagnostic methods were MRI, metaiodobenzylguanidine (MIBG) scintigraphy and 24-h urinary noradrenaline (Neumann et al. 1993). High sensitivity and specificity have also been shown for plasma metanephrine and metanephrine (Eisenhofer et al. 1999). Recently, 18 Fluor DOPA positron emission tomography has been added as a highly sensitive tool for diagnosis of phaechromocytoma (Högerle et al. 2002). Very elegant and now the therapy of choice is laparoscopic adrenal sparing surgery which reveals sufficient adrenal cortex function and a very low relapse rate (Neumann et al. 1999).

Extrarenal and extra-adrenal lesions

An awareness of the complete spectrum of von Hippel–Lindau syndrome-associated lesions is essential for establishing the diagnosis, since patients do not have to have every manifestation in order to be diagnosed with confidence. This knowledge enables the design of screening protocols for patients with renal or adrenal lesions suggestive of the disease, and can influence the choice of treatment for individuals identified as having the syndrome. All parts of the CNS can be affected by haemangioblastomas (Fig. 7a,b); the classical site is the cerebellum, where most of the tumours produce cysts (Lindau tumour) and initiate dysfunction and progressive pressure. Gadolinium-enhanced MRI is the method of choice for detection, and neurological microsurgery has had considerable success. Multifocal haemangioblastomas are very suggestive of von Hippel–Lindau syndrome (Neumann et al. 1992a). Retinal angiomatosis consists of one or more round angiomas with a pair of tortuous feeding vessels (Fig. 7c). The main complication is retinal detachment and impairment of vision, which occurs without any prodromal symptoms. Laser coagulaton is effective, if done before detachment occurs (Schmidt et al. 2000). Pancreatic cysts can also involve the entire organ (Fig. 7d). Epididymal cystadenoma may occur bilaterally and can cause infertility due to obstruction of spermatic ducts. Rare but typical features of von Hippel–Lindau syndrome include also cystadenoma of the braod ligament in females, endolymphatic sac tumour of the inner ear and pancreatic islet cell tumour.

Follow-up

Patients with von Hippel–Lindau syndrome need regular follow-up. As a guideline yearly follow-up investigations are recommended as shown in Table 3.

Genetics

The VHL gene, localized on the short arm of chromosome 3 (3p25–26), was mapped and cloned by positional techniques (Latif et al. 1993). Germline mutations of the VHL gene occur, so far, in

Table 3 Recommended screening programme for von Hippel–Lindau syndrome

Detailed history of the patient and his/her family
Pedigree, operations on brain, spinal cord, eyes, kidneys, adrenal glands, blindness, cancer, early deaths, causes of death[a]
Ophthalmological examination[a]
Blood pressure, catecholamine assay in plasma or 24-h urine[a]
Ultrasonography of the abdomen[a]
MRI scan of the abdomen
MRI of the brain with gadolinium enhancement
Ultrasonography of the testis

[a] Basic programme for children below the age of 10 years.

nearly 100 per cent of the patients presenting with a clinical diagnosis of familial VHL disease (Stolle et al. 1998). Isolated cases can, however, be difficult to diagnose genetically, since they may represent mosaicisms (Sgambati et al. 2000).

Genetic analysis of VHL-associated tumours indicates that VHL is a tumour suppressor gene: in VHL patients, the first allele is inactivated by a germline mutation, followed by deletion of the wild-type allele (LOH in the VHL locus) in all VHL-associated tumours screened so far (Tory et al. 1989; Gnarra et al. 1994). Both VHL alleles are also inactivated in the majority of the sporadic counterparts of VHL-associated tumours.

The gene consists of three exons and codes for at least two isoforms. The largest is a 213 amino acid protein. The second isoform is generated by internal translation of the transcript at methionine 54. Both isoforms are biologically active. The spectrum of germline VHL mutations includes missense and nonsense point mutations, as well as micro-deletions and large deletions. All point mutations occur only downstream of codon 54 and, therefore, inactivate both isoforms. Mutations are distributed over all the exons. They cluster, however, at two 'hotspot areas'; the 3'-end of the first exon and the 5'-end of the third exon. Phenotype–genotype correlations in large families showed a strong correlation of missense mutations with the occurrence of phaeochromocytoma. Families without phaeochromocytoma but with frequent renal involvement are characterized predominantly by large or intragenic deletions, nonsense mutations, splice mutations, and specific missense mutations, different from the ones encountered in phaeochromocytoma-associated disease (Chen et al. 1995). Detection of family-specific germline mutations provides confirmation of the clinical diagnosis as well as the possibility of presymptomatic diagnosis. This facilitates the clinical management of families with the syndrome, since screening and follow-up investigations can be restricted to individuals at risk. A general screening programme for VHL patients is shown in Table 2.

Significant advances were made in our understanding of the crystal structure and function of VHL protein. Resolution of the crystal structure of the protein revealed the presence of two surfaces mediating interactions with other proteins: the alpha and beta domain. The alpha domain brings VHL in stable contact with a multiprotein complex that acts as an E3 ubiquitin ligase. VHL is the receptor of this complex: it employs its beta domain to select the intracellular protein that will be ubiquitinated by the VHL containing complex and targetted for proteasomal destruction. The regulatory subunits of cellular hypoxia-inducible factors (HIFs) are so far regarded as bona fide

Table 4 Differential diagnosis of tuberous sclerosis complex, von Hippel–Lindau disease, and autosomal-dominant polycystic kidney disease

Disease	TSC	VHL	PKD
Renal cysts	Single or multiple	Single or multiple	Polycystic
Renal tumours	Angiomyolipoma	Clear cell cancer	RCC, different types (rare)
Multiple/bilateral tumours	+	+	−
Impaired renal funcion	−	−	+
Pancreatic lesions	−	Multiple cysts, rare: islet cell tumours	Cysts in about 5% of the patients
CNS lesions	Tubera, giant-cell astrocytoma, paraventricular calcifications	Haemangioblastoma (cerebellar, brainstem, spinal)	Cerebral base aneurysm
Hypertension	−	Only if phaeochromocytoma	+

TSC, tuberous sclerosis complex; PKD, polycystic kidney disease; RCC, renal-cell carcinoma.

substrates targetted for destruction by VHL. Inactivation of VHL function leads to constitutive upregulation of HIF and deregulated transcription of HIF inducible genes: these include growth factors (such as transforming growth factor β or TGF β, TGF α, platelet-derived growth factor or PDGF-B) and proangiogenic peptides (such as vascular endothelial growth factor or VEGF). This molecular deregulation may explain the hypervascular nature of VHL-associated tumours. Inactivation of HIF may be a function critical for the ability of VHL to mediate tumour suppression.

Summary

von Hippel–Lindau syndrome should be considered in young patients with multifocal and/or bilateral renal-cell carcinomas and multiple renal cysts. Other patients at risk are those with phaeochromocytoma. Clinical management should be diagnostically intensive, but balanced decisions are needed for therapy and follow-up in asymptomatic patients.

Differential diagnosis of cysts and tumours of the kidneys

In clinical medicine the differential diagnosis of TSC, VHL, and autosomal-dominant PKD seems to be frequently problematic. Table 4 presents an overview with the typical features.

References

Balligand, J.-L. et al. (1990). Outcome of patients with tuberous sclerosis after renal transplantation. *Transplantation* **49**, 515–518.

Bjornsson, J. et al. (1996). 'Tuberous sclerosis-associated renal cell carcinoma. Clinical, pathological, and genetic features'. *American Journal of Pathology* **149**, 1201–1208.

Bloom, D. A. et al. (1982). The signification of lymph nodal involvement in renal angiomyolipoma. *Journal of Urology* **128**, 1292–1295.

Brasier, J. L. and Henske, E. P. (1997). 'Loss of the polycystic kidney disease (PKD1) region of chromosome 16p13 in renal cyst cells supports a loss-of-function model for cyst pathogenesis'. *Journal of Clinical Investigation* **99**, 194–199.

Brook-Carter, P. T. et al. (1994). Deletion of the TSC2 and PKD1 genes associated with severe infantile polycystic kidney disease—a contiguous gene syndrome. *Nature Genetics* **8**, 328–332.

Carbonara, C. et al. (1994). 9q34 Loss of heterozygosity in a tuberous sclerosis astrocytoma suggests a growth suppressor-like activity also for the TSC1 gene. *Human Molecular Genetics* **3**, 1829–1832.

Carsillo, T. et al. (2000). Mutations in the tuberous sclerosis complex gene TSC2 are a cause of sporadic pulmonary lymphangioleiomyomatosis. *Proceedings of the National Academy of Sciences of the United States of America* **97**, 6085–6090.

Castro, M. et al. (1995). Pulmonary tuberous sclerosis. *Chest* **107**, 189–195.

Chatha, R. K. et al. (2001). von Hippel–Lindau disease masquerading as autosomal dominant polycystic kidney disease. *American Journal of Kidney Diseases* **37**, 852–858.

Chen, F. et al. (1995). Germline mutations in the von Hippel–Lindau disease tumour suppressor gene: correlations with phenotype. *Human Mutation* **5**, 66–75.

Costello, L. C. et al. (2000). High frequency of pulmonary lymphangioleiomyomatosis in women with tuberous sclerosis complex. *Mayo Clinic Proceedings* **75**, 591–594.

Dabora, S. L. et al. (2001). Mutational analysis in a cohort of 224 tuberous sclerosis patients indicates increased severity of TSC2, compared with TSC1, disease in multiple organs. *American Journal of Human Genetics* **68**, 64–80.

De Luca, S. et al. (1999). Management of renal angiomyolipoma: a report of 53 cases. *BJU International* **83**, 215–218.

Eisenhofer, G. et al. (1999). Plasma normetanephrine and metanephrine for detecting pheochromocytoma in von Hippel–Lindau disease and multiple endocrine neoplasia type 2. *New England Journal of Medicine* **340**, 1872–1879.

European Chromosome 16 Tuberous Sclerosis Consortium (ETSC) (1993). Identification and characterization of the tuberous sclerosis gene on chromosome 16. *Cell* **75**, 1305–1315.

Ewalt, D. H. et al. (1998). Renal lesion growth in children with tuberous sclerosis complex. *Journal of Urology* **160**, 141–145.

Fernandez de Sevilla, T. et al. (1988). Renal leiomyosarcoma in a patient with tuberous sclerosis. *Urology International* **43**, 62–64.

Fryer, A. E. et al. (1987). Evidence that the gene for tuberous sclerosis is on chromosome 9. *Lancet* **i**, 659–661.

Gnarra, J. R. et al. (1994). Mutations of the VHL tumor suppressor gene in renal carcinoma. *Nature Genetics* **7**, 85–90.

Goldfarb, D. A. et al. (1998). Results of renal transplantation in patients with renal cell carcinoma in von Hippel–Lindau disease. *Transplantation* **64**, 1726–1729.

Gomez, M. R. *Neurologic and Psychiatric Features in Tuberous Sclerosis* 2nd edn. (ed. M. R. Gomez), pp. 21–36. New York, NY: Raven Press, 1988.

Green, A. *et al.* (1994a). The tuberous sclerosis gene on chromosome 9q34 acts as a growth suppressor. *Human Molecular Genetics* **3**, 1833–1834.

Green, A. J. *et al.* (1994b). Loss of heterozygosity on chromosome 16p13.3 in hamartomas from tuberous sclerosis patients. *Nature Genetics* **6**, 193–196.

Henske, E. P. *et al.* (1996). Allelic loss is frequent in tuberous sclerosis kidney lesions but rare in brain lesions. *American Journal of Human Genetics* **59**, 400–406.

Högerle, E. *et al.* (2002). [18]Fluoro-DOPA whole-body positron emission tomography for detection of pheochromocytomas: initial results. *Radiology* **22**, 507–512.

Ibrahim, R. E. *et al.* (1989). Atypical cysts and carcinoma of the kidney in the phacomatoses. *Cancer* **63**, 148–157.

Kandt, R. S. *et al.* (1992). Linkage of an important gene locus for tuberous sclerosis to a chromosome 16 marker for polycystic kidney disease. *Nature Genetics* **2**, 37–41.

Knudson, A. (1971). Mutation and cancer: statistical study of retinoblastoma. *Proceedings of the National Academy of Sciences of the United States of America* **68**, 820–823.

Latif, F. *et al.* (1993). Identification of the von Hippel–Lindau disease tumour suppressor gene. *Science* **260**, 1317–1320.

Maher, E. R. *et al.* (1990). Clinical features and natural history of von Hippel–Lindau disease. *Quarterly Journal of Medicine* **283**, 1151–1163.

Malek, R. S. *et al.* (1987). Renal cell carcinoma in von Hippel–Lindau syndrome. *American Journal of Medicine* **82**, 236–238.

Mitnick, J. S. *et al.* (1983). Cystic renal diseases in tuberous sclerosis. *Radiology* **147**, 85–87.

Mostofi, F. K. *et al. Histological Typing of Kidney Tumours.* Geneva: World Health Organization, 1981.

Mourikis, D. *et al.* (1999). Selective arterial embolization in the management of symptomatic renal angiomyolipomas. *European Journal of Radiology* **32**, 153–159.

Neumann, H. P. H. (1987). Basic criteria for clinical diagnosis and genetic counselling in von Hippel–Lindau syndrome. *Journal of Vascular Diseases* **16**, 220–229.

Neumann, H. P. and Wiestler, O. D. (1991). Clustering of features of von Hippel-Lindau syndrome: evidence for a complex genetic locus. *Lancet* **337**, 1052–1054.

Neumann, H. P. H. (1994a). Pheochromocytoma, multiple endocrine neoplasia type 2, and von Hippel–Lindau disease. *New England Journal of Medicine* **330**, 1091–1092.

Neumann, H. P. H. (1994b). Tuberous sclerosis. *New England Journal of Medicine* **331**, 813.

Neumann, H. P. H. *et al.* (1992a). Central nervous system lesions in von Hippel–Lindau syndrome. *Journal of Neurology, Neurosurgery, and Psychiatry* **55**, 898–901.

Neumann, H. P. H. *et al.* (1992b). Angiomyolipoma of the kidney and tuberous sclerosis. *Journal of the American Society of Nephrology* **3**, 300.

Neumann, H. P. H. *et al.* (1993). Pheochromocytomas, multipe endocrine neoplasia, and von Hippel–Lindau disease. *New England Journal of Medicine* **329**, 1531–1538.

Neumann, H. P. H. *et al.* (1995). Tuberous sclerosis complex with endstage renal failure. *Nephrology, Dialysis, Transplantation* **10**, 343–353.

Neumann, H. P. H. *et al.* (1998). Prevalence, morphology and biology of renal cell carcinoma in von Hippel–Lindau disease compared to sporadic renal cell carcinoma. *Journal of Urology* **160**, 1248–1254.

Neumann, H. P. H. *et al.* (1999). Adrenal-sparing surgery for phaeochromocytoma. *British Journal of Surgery* **86** (1), 94–97.

Neumann, H. P. H. *et al.* (2002). Germline mutations in non-syndromic pheochromocytoma. *New England Journal of Medicine* **346**, 1459–1466.

O'Callaghan, F. J., Shiell, A. W., Osborne, J. P., and Martyn, C. N. (1998). Prevalence of tuberous sclerosis estimated by capture-recapture analysis. *Lancet* **351**, 1490.

Ohigashi, T. *et al.* (1991). Coincidental renal cell carcinoma and renal angiomyolipomas in tuberous sclerosis. *Urology International* **47**, 160–163.

Povey, S. *et al.* (1994). Two loci for tuberous sclerosis one on 9q34 and one on 16p13. *Annals of Human Genetics* **58**, 107–127.

Richardson, E. P. (1991). Pathology of tuberous sclerosis. Neuropathologic aspects. *Annals of the New York Academy of Science* **615**, 128–139.

Roach, E. S. *et al.* (1992). Report of the Diagnostic Criteria Committee of the National Tuberous Sclerosis Association. *Journal of Child Neurology* **7**, 221–224.

Roach, E. S. *et al.* (1998). Tuberous sclerosis complex consensus conference: revised clinical diagnostic criteria. *Journal of Child Neurology* **13**, 624–628.

Roach, E. S. *et al.* (1999). Tuberous Sclerosis Consensus Conference: recommendations for diagnostic evaluation. National Tuberous Sclerosis Association. *Journal of Child Neurology* **14**, 401–407.

Robbins, U. E. and Bernstein, J. Renal involvement in tuberous sclerosis. In *Tuberous Sclerosis* 2nd edn. (ed. M. R. Gomez), pp. 133–146. New York, NY: Raven Press, 1988.

Robertson, D. M. Ophthalmologic findings in tuberous sclerosis. In *Tuberous Sclerosis* 2nd edn. (ed. M. R. Gomez), pp. 89–109. New York, NY: Raven Press, 1988.

Rogers, R. S. Dermatologic manifestations in tuberous sclerosis. In *Tuberous Sclerosis* 2nd edn. (ed. M. R. Gomez), pp. 111–132. New York, NY: Raven Press, 1988.

Schillinger, F. and Montagnac, R. (1996). Chronic renal failure and its treatment in tuberous sclerosis. *Nephrology, Dialysis, Transplantation* **11**, 481–485.

Schmidt, D. *et al.* (2000). Long-term results of laser treatment for retinal angiomatosis in von Hippel–Lindau disease. *European Journal of Medical Research* **5**, 47–58.

Sgambati, M. T. *et al.* (2000). Mosaicism in von Hippel–Lindau disease: lessons from kindreds with germline mutations identified in offsprings with mosaic parents. *American Journal of Human Genetics* **66**, 84–91.

Shepherd, C. W. *et al.* (1991). Causes of death in patients with tuberous sclerosis. *Mayo Clinic Proceedings* **66**, 792–796.

Stillwell, T. S. *et al.* (1987). Renal lesions in tuberous sclerosis. *Journal of Urology* **138**, 477–481.

Stolle, C. *et al.* (1998). Improved detection of germline mutations in von Hippel Lindau disease's tumor suppressor gene. *Human Mutation* **12**, 417–423.

Tory, K. *et al.* (1989). Specific genetic change in tumors associated with von Hippel–Lindau disease. *Journal of the National Cancer Institute* **81**, 1097–1101.

van Slegtenhorst, M. *et al.* (1997). Identification of the tuberous sclerosis gene TSC1 on chromosome 9q34. *Science* **277**, 805–808.

Walther, M. M. *et al.* (1999). Renal cancer in families with hereditary renal cancer: prospective analysis of a tumor size threshold for renal parenchymal sparing surgery. *Journal of Urology* **161**, 1475–1479.

Washecka, R. and Hanna, M. (1991). Malignant renal tumors in tuberous sclerosis. *Urology* **37**, 340–343.

16.7 Some rare syndromes with renal involvement

Jean-Pierre Grünfeld and J. Stewart Cameron

Introduction

There are a large number of rare inherited disorders, in many of which survival is limited and the conditions are rarely, if ever, seen in renal units dealing with adult patients. These conditions are more the subject of specialist paediatric nephrology, and accounts of them have been given by Crawfurd (1988), Gilbert-Barness *et al.* (1989), McKusick (1990), Barness and Opitz (1993), and Clarren (1994). This brief account is confined to inherited disorders which are likely to be encountered, albeit rarely in most cases, in adult clinics and which are not dealt with elsewhere in this book. Rare inherited disorders affecting the glomeruli, including α_1-antitrypsin deficiency, familial dysautonomia, collagen type III nephropathy, and Charcot–Marie–Tooth disease, are dealt with in Chapter 16.4.3.

Alagille syndrome

Alagille syndrome, also called arteriohepatic dysplasia, is an autosomal dominant disorder characterized by abnormal development of liver (paucity of the interlobular bile ducts leading to chronic cholestasis and necessitating liver transplantation in about 20 per cent of the children with the most severe forms), heart (mainly pulmonary artery stenosis or tetralogy of Fallot; major structural congenital heart disease in infancy is associated with increased mortality), skeleton (mainly butterfly vertebrae), eye (mainly posterior embryotoxon), and a peculiar facies. Intracranial bleeding is also a recognized cause of mortality. Vascular abnormalities have been described in various locations, including the central nervous system (CNS) and renal artery. The frequency of Alagille syndrome has been estimated to be approximately 1/70,000 live births. The phenotypic findings are highly variable in severity, from one family to another and within an affected family (Alagille *et al.* 1987; Emerick *et al.* 1999).

Renal abnormalities are found in 40–73 per cent of the patients. Structural anomalies predominate: unilateral renal hypoplasia or agenesis, horseshoe kidney, renal cysts, or urinary tract malformations. The most common functional renal anomaly is renal tubular acidosis (Emerick *et al.* 1999). Glomerular mesangiolipidosis has been described as the consequence of severe chronic cholestasis (Habib *et al.* 1987).

Reversible renal failure may occur in affected infants whereas chronic renal insufficiency progressing to endstage and requiring renal replacement therapy (Shonck *et al.* 1998) may develop in adults. Patients with Alagille syndrome may reach adulthood (Emerick *et al.* 1999), and this disease may occasionally be first diagnosed in adults with mild cholestasis.

Mutations in the JAGGED1 (*Jag1*) gene, located on chromosome 20 p 12, are responsible for Alagille syndrome (Li *et al.* 1997). A high frequency of *de novo* mutations and the possibility of germline mosaicism have been reported (Crosnier *et al.* 1999; Spinner 2001). The gene encodes a ligand for Notch1 receptor, which belongs to the Notch signalling pathway involved in the development of various tissues in *Drosophila, Caenorhabditis elegans*, and vertebrates. *Jag1* is expressed in both ureteric bud derivatives and mesenchyme-derived epithelial structures throughout development of the kidney in human fetus. Variable expressivity of Alagille syndrome is not well explained. Only about 25 per cent of the patients carrying the mutation meet the criteria for 'complete' Alagille syndrome. Patients with partial, mainly cardiac, phenotypes have been described. Patients with prominent renal phenotypes may be found (Spinner *et al.* 1999).

McCright *et al.* (2001) have recently shown that *Notch 2* is involved in kidney, heart, and eye development in mice. In the kidney, *Notch 2* is more specifically required for glomerular morphogenesis and patterning. *Notch 2* and *Jag1* genes are expressed in adjacent cells during glomerular differentiation. The *Jag1* protein is a probable ligand for the *Notch 2* receptor during glomerulogenesis. In addition, mice doubly heterozygous for the *Jag1* null allele and a *Notch 2* hypomorphic allele exhibit developmental abnormalities characteristic of Alagille syndrome. The *Notch 2* gene acts a genetic modifier to interact with a *Jag1* mutation. Thus, similar genetic interactions may occur in Alagille syndrome patients and particular *Notch 2* alleles may influence the severity of Alagille syndrome phenotypes (McCright *et al.* 2002).

Bardet–Biedl syndrome

Renal disease is now recognized as a common feature of this syndrome, which was independently described by Laurence and Moon (1866) and later by Bardet (1920) and Biedl (1922)—hence the unwieldy collection of eponyms. The other common features of the syndrome are polydactyly (Fig. 1a), obesity (Fig. 1b), hypogenitalism in males, mental retardation, spinocerebellar ataxia, nystagmus, and tapetoretinal degeneration (Schachat and Maumenee 1982); skeletal abnormalities, pulmonary stenosis, and deafness are less common. There is some evidence that the Laurence–Moon type, in which neurological features are predominant and polydactyly rare, may be a different, but closely related, syndrome to that described by Bardet and Biedl, since in the latter neurological symptoms and signs such as spastic paraplegia are much rarer and chronic renal failure is relatively common (Greene *et al.* 1989). Another variation is the Alström

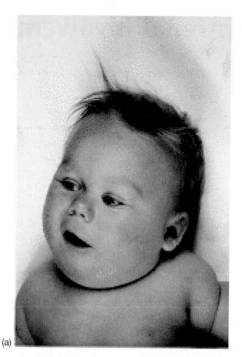

(a)

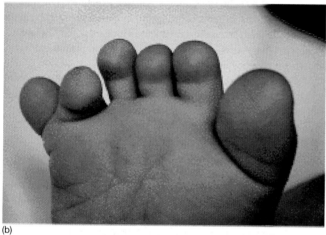

(b)

Fig. 1 The Bardet–Biedl syndrome. (a) Polydactyly and (b) obesity are characteristic features. In some patients, accessory digits may have been removed during childhood, or be only vestigial. Obesity in renal failure in a child or young adult is an important clue to diagnosis. (By courtesy of Professor Sir Cyril Chantler.)

syndrome, in which hypogenitalism is absent but diabetes mellitus and deafness are associated features.

The Bardet–Biedl syndrome (BBS) appears to be genetically heterogenous. BBS is inherited in an autosomal recessive manner. Six BBS loci have been identified: BBS1 on 11q13, BBS2 on 16q21, BBS3 on 3p12, BBS4 on 15q22.2–q23, BBS5 on 2q31, and BBS6 on 20p12, with evidence of at least one more locus. Three BBS genes have been cloned, BBS6, BBS4, and BBS2 (Katsanis *et al.* 2001). Surprisingly, Katsanis *et al.* (2001) have recently demonstrated triallelic inheritance in BBS: among 19 pedigrees with BBS2 mutations, evidence for involvement of another locus occurred in at least nine families. Of the eight outbred pedigrees where BBS6 mutations have been identified, three harboured BBS2 mutations. However, biallelic inheritance (as found

typically in autosomal recessive disorders) may suffice to cause BBS in some families. BBS may not be a single-gene recessive disease but a complex trait requiring three mutant alleles to manifest the phenotype. Triallelic inheritance may represent a transmission model that bridges classical Mendelian disorders with complex traits (Burghes *et al.* 2001).

As with many other recessive disorders, clustering of cases in relatively isolated areas is seen. A high prevalence has been reported in Newfoundland (Parfrey *et al.* 2002) and amongst the Bedouin (Leppert *et al.* 1994). Carriers have been considered to be clinically healthy, but a study of 75 members of one family (Croft and Swift 1990) found a number of clinical and radiological abnormalities in obligate heterozygotes.

Diagnosis is not usually difficult, given the constellation of signs and symptoms, but cases with minor involvement may be missed and accessory digits are often removed. Obesity is a constant feature, and any child with chronic renal disease and obesity should be suspected of having the syndrome (Fralick *et al.* 1990).

Renal disease is particularly common in the Bardet–Biedl variety of the syndrome, to the point where it can be regarded as a cardinal feature affecting 70–95 per cent of patients (Churchill *et al.* 1981; Tieder *et al.* 1982; Harnett *et al.* 1988; Green *et al.* 1989; Parfrey *et al.* 2002). The renal involvement is very variable in nature, but almost all show persistent fetal lobulation, small kidneys with clubbed calyces, and cystic dysplasia. The cysts may communicate with the dilated calyces, causing diagnostic confusion. Thus, an intravenous urogram frequently shows calyceal blunting, calyceal cysts, or diverticula. Prenatal diagnosis has been made by ultrasonography; the kidneys resemble polycystic kidneys (Ritchie *et al.* 1988) and the renal abnormalities are usually present in the neonatal period (Garber and de Bruyn 1991).

Renal histology shows changes of mesangial and interstitial fibrosis, particularly in more advanced cases. Dilated tubules, cysts, and dysplastic features may also be evident. Electron microscopy has shown marked alterations of the glomerular capillary basement membranes with alternate thickening and thinning, and accumulation of fibrillary material in the inner third. These may be the earliest changes since they can be present in kidneys which are otherwise almost normal (Price *et al.* 1981), although this is not the case in all studies (Tieder *et al.* 1982). This finding suggests some similarity with the Alport and nail–patella syndromes (see Chapters 16.4.1 and 16.4.3), and the renal changes are also clearly similar to both nephronophthisis (see Chapter 16.3), which itself may be complicated by tapetoretinal degeneration (Løken–Senior syndrome), and to cystic dysplasia (see Chapter 16.2.1). Thus, the exact nature of the renal lesion in the BBS is as yet unclear.

Clinical signs of both proximal and distal tubular dysfunction are present during childhood, with a reduced concentrating capacity and aminoaciduria (Tieder *et al.* 1982), sometimes leading to polyuria and polydipsia. One case in which cystinuria was present has been described (de Marchi *et al.* 1992) but, presumably, this was coincidental. A full nephrotic syndrome with glomerular changes of focal glomerular sclerosis has also been described (Barakat *et al.* 1990).

Renal failure and hypertension usually supervene during adolescence and early adult life, eventually leading to a need for dialysis (Williams *et al.* 1988; Parfrey *et al.* 2002) or transplantation (Norden *et al.* 1991; Collins *et al.* 1994). Despite the obvious problems faced by such patients and those caring for them, both treatments can be successful. If untreated, renal failure is a common cause of death.

Branchio-oto-renal dysplasia

There are various associations between malformed ears, hearing loss, and renal anomalies (Crawfurd 1988). One of the more common and better delineated of these syndromes is usually called the branchio-oto-renal dysplasia (BOR) syndrome. The gene for this condition has been mapped to chromosome 8q. One family with both the trichor-hinopharyngeal and branchio-oto (BO) syndromes has been reported in which an inherited rearrangement of chromosme 8q involving band 8q13.3 has been documented (Haan *et al.* 1989). Further refined mapping of the gene is consistent with this genetic localization (Kumar *et al.* 1994; Li Ni *et al.* 1994). Subsequently, the gene involved was identified as EYA1 (Abelhak *et al.* 1997). This gene is composed of 17 exons. It is the human homologue of the eya gene, responsible for the 'eyes absent' phenotype in the *Drosophila*. EYA1 mutations have been found in families with BOR or BO syndromes. BOR syndrome has been found to be associated with Duane's syndrome (an ocular motility defect with bilateral retraction of the eyeball and retraction of the palpebra cleft), hydrocephalus and aplasia of the trapezius muscle. This syndrome has been shown previously to be part of the acro-oculorenal syndrome. The genes responsible for BOR syndrome and Duane's syndrome are contiguous (Hardelin *et al.* 1998).

The murine homologue of EYA gene, *Eya1* gene, has been further identified (see review in Hardelin *et al.* 1998). The *Eya1* gene has been inactivated in mice. *Eya1* homozygotes lack ears and kidneys due to defective inductive tissue interactions and apoptotic regression of the organ primordia. *Eya1* homozygosity results in an absence of ureteric bud outgrowth and subsequent failure of metanephric induction. *Gdnf* expression is not detected in the metanephric mesenchyme of homozygous mice. *Eya1* heterozygotes show renal abnormalities and a conductive hearing loss similar to BOR syndrome (Xu *et al.* 1999).

The BOR syndrome is inherited as an autosomal dominant condition; the prevalence about one in 40,000. Patients present with hearing loss; sensorineural, middle-ear, and mixed types have all been described. Branchial fistulas and abnormalities of the pinna (usually described as 'cup-shaped') together with preauricular pits or clefts (Fig. 2) may also be present. Structural renal abnormalities of various types are associated, including renal dysplasia, aplasia, duplication defects, and bladder anomalies (Widdershoven *et al.* 1983). One family with cystic kidneys in the BOR syndrome has been described (Melnick *et al.* 1976). The phenotypic expression varies from family to family, with some having the branchial anomalies and hearing loss without renal dysplasia.

This condition may be more common than is realized. A study of 400 children with hearing problems in Montreal showed 19 with preauricular pits, and four families of nine who consented to further investigation had BOR dysplasia (Fraser *et al.* 1980). The preauricular area should certainly be examined in all patients with renal anomalies or with renal failure of obscure origin and deafness. A number of patients enter end-stage renal disease if the renal anomalies are severe.

Carbohydrate-deficient glycoprotein syndromes

Congenital disorders of glycosylation or carbohydrate-deficient glyco-protein (CDG) syndromes, form a group of autosomal recessive disorders characterized by the abnormal glycosylation of a number of serum glycoproteins (transferrin, haptoglobin, etc.). The most frequent

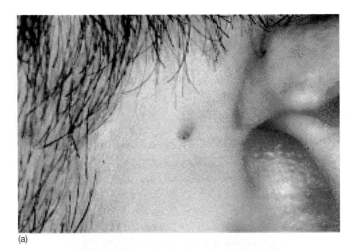
(a)

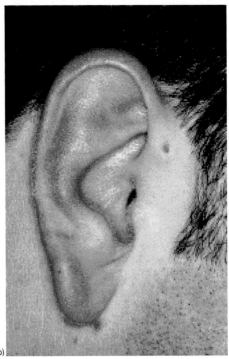
(b)

Fig. 2 Preauricular pits in the branchio-oto-renal syndrome. A variety of pits and clefts can be seen, together with abnormalities of the pinna which may be simplified and cup-shaped.

form is CDGIa which is due to deficient phosphomannose mutase (PMM) activity and mutations of the PMM 2 gene have been identified. Neurological manifestations (psychomotor retardation, cerebellar hypoplasia, strabismus and later neuropathy and retinitis pigmentosa) may be either isolated (this form is generally not fatal) or associated with extraneurological, mostly digestive, manifestations occurring early in life and frequently fatal. The CDGIb form is characterized by phosphomannose isomerase deficiency. It causes enterohepatic disorders with no neurological involvement and this is the only form responding to oral mannose administration. The other CDG types are rare and present as neurological diseases (de Lonlay *et al.* 2001).

Renal involvement found in 20–30 per cent of CDGI patients consists of proximal tubulopathy, hyperechogenicity, and cysts (de Lonlay et al. 2001a). Three cases of a nephrotic syndrome as a part of the CDG syndrome have been described (de Vries et al. 2001). Most cases are diagnosed very early in life, but in the series by de Lonlay et al., the patients ages range from 3.5 months to 19 years.

Cockayne syndrome

Cockayne syndrome is an autosomal recessive disorder characterized by a variety of clinical features of which photosensitivity, precocious senile appearance, poor growth, neurological abnormalities, sensorineural deafness, and pigmentary retinopathy are common (Nance and Berry 1992). The basic lesion appears to be a defect in the repair of DNA after damage, particularly by ultraviolet irradiation (Van Hoffen et al. 1993). Death usually occurs in early life, but some patients survive into adulthood. Renal symptoms consisting of hypertension, mild proteinuria, and declining renal function affect about one in 10 patients. A generalized thickening of the glomerular basement membrane is seen on renal biopsy (Hirooka et al. 1988; Sato et al. 1988).

Cystic fibrosis

Cystic fibrosis is a relatively common recessive inherited condition (one in 19 healthy Caucasian individuals are carriers) arising from mutations in the cystic fibrosis transmembrane conductance regulator gene located at 7q.21.3–22.1 which codes for a cAMP-regulated Cl^- channel in the apical membrane of secretory epithelia (Coutelle et al. 1993). The decrease in volume of secretions is insufficient to explain the very viscid secretions produced from the bronchial glands, and there is also blockage of pancreatic ducts and pancreatic exocrine failure. These viscid bronchial secretions lead to recurrent and persistent pulmonary infections which, until the advent of antibiotics, were usually fatal in childhood. However, an increasing number of patients now survive into their twenties, thirties, and even forties.

In the past, various renal changes were decribed at post mortem (Abramowsky and Swinehart 1982), including amyloidosis and glomerulosclerosis, but more recently it has become evident that proteinuria and glomerulonephritis are rather frequent in these longstanding cases of cystic fibrosis. Whether the glomerulonephritis relates to the underlying disease or to the chronic infections suffered by patients with cystic fibrosis is not clear; the predominant nephritis is IgA nephropathy (Melzi et al. 1991), as in two personal cases, and crescentic nephritis has been seen also. Secondary amyloidosis would be expected and has been recorded (Glenner 1986; McGlennan et al. 1986; Melzi et al. 1991), with a full nephrotic syndrome in some cases (Gaffney et al. 1993) and evolution to renal failure in others (Melzi et al. 1991). In addition, vasculitis has been found in older patients (Finnegan et al. 1989), usually antineutrophil cytoplasmic antibodies (ANCA)-positive and with clinically evident nephritis in three cases. One of Finnegan's patients had Henoch–Schönlein purpura. ANCA have been found in children with cystic fibrosis and infections but without clinical vasculitis (Efthamiou et al. 1991), an interesting observation in view of the controversy as to the pathogenetic significance of these antibodies (see Chapters 4.5.1 and 4.5.3). One-third of patients have hypercalciuria, and microscopic nephrocalcinosis is visible in 90 per cent, including infants (Katz et al. 1988).

Familial hypo/hyperparathyroidism, deafness, and renal disease

Bilous et al. (1992) described a family showing hypoparathyroidism, deafness, and renal disease with an apparently dominant inheritance. The renal component appeared to be dysplasia. This may be a different condition from the family described by Barakat et al. (1977), in which the renal component was a nephrotic syndrome in four siblings; the pattern of inheritance was not clear, but appeared to be recessive.

This syndrome, also called HDR (hypoparathyroidism, sensorineural deafness, and renal anomaly), has been shown to be due to mutations in the GATA3 gene leading to haploinsufficiency. The GATA3 gene (located on the short arm of chromosome 10) belongs to a family of zinc-finger transcription factors that are involved in vertebrate embryonic development. GATA3 is essential in development of parathyroids, auditory system, and kidneys. Of interest, terminal deletions of chromosome 10p result in a Di George-like phenotype that includes hypoparathyroidism, heart defects, immune deficiency, deafness, and renal malformations. Two distinct non-overlapping regions have been identified, the Di George critical region being located more telomeric (Van Esch et al. 2000).

In contrast, Edwards et al. (1989) described a family in which the propositus presented with hypercalcaemia and parathyroid hyperplasia was found. Inheritance was consistent with an autosomal recessive pattern and appeared to be distinct from Alport's syndrome; ocular examination was normal.

Gräsbeck–Imerslund syndrome (proteinuria with vitamin B$_{12}$ malabsorption)

This rare autosomal recessive syndrome (Gräsbeck et al. 1960; Imerslund 1960) presents in infants as a megaloblastic macrocytic anaemia with associated subnephrotic proteinuria, which is usually highly selective (Becker et al. 1977) but has also been reported as nonselective (Rumpelt and Michl 1979), or even of tubular pattern (Geisert et al. 1975). Aminoaciduria may also be present. The syndrome seems to be seen most often in Scandinavia (Nevanlinna 1980), but cases have been reported from Germany (Becker et al. 1977), Israel (Ben Bassat et al. 1969), and elsewhere (Lin et al. 1994) including the United Kingdom (Uttley et al. 1975) and a case from South America (cited by Becker et al. 1977).

Ileal biopsies show a normal morphology and the absorptive defect is confined to vitamin B$_{12}$. Hypertension is absent and the outlook for renal function is benign, but a need for vitamin B$_{12}$ supplementation persists throughout life. Although severe neurological manifestations may be present and respond to parenteral vitamin B$_{12}$ (Salameh et al. 1991), the proteinuria does not change during successful treatment.

The renal histology is variable (Gräsbeck et al. 1960; Becker et al. 1977; Collan et al. 1979; Rumpelt and Michl 1979). Normal glomeruli, mesangial expansion, and 'membranous' nephropathy have been reported on optical microscopy. Podocyte foot process fusion (Becker et al. 1977) and abnormalities of both the capillary basement membrane (Collan et al. 1979) and the podocytes (Rumpelt and Michl 1979) have been described on electron microscopy.

The underlying defect involves cubilin, the intrinsic factor-vitamin B_{12} receptor, located at the apical pole of enterocytes in the terminal ileon. The CUBN gene encoding cubilin is located on the short arm of chromosome 10 and is mutated in patients with Gräsbeck–Imerslund syndrome (Aminoff *et al.* 1999). Cubilin is also coexpressed and colocalized with megalin in the brush border and in the endocytic pathway of renal proximal tubule epithelium, from coated pits to endosomes and lysosomes. During kidney development, both proteins are expressed in S-shaped bodies of the metanephros, and then, cubilin is restricted to proximal tubule (Verroust *et al.* 2000).

Kallmann's syndrome

Kallmann's syndrome is defined by the association of hypogonadotrophic hypogonadism caused by a deficit in gonadotropin-releasing hormone, and anosmia due to atrophy of the olfactory bulbs. Other abnormalities may be found, including neurological symptoms (mirror movements, ocular anomalies, cerebellar syndrome, deafness and pes cavus), high arched palate, labial or palatine cleft, and renal agenesis. The syndrome is genetically heterogeneous. Three modes of transmission have been described: X-linked, autosomal dominant, and autosomal recessive. Mutations in the *KAL-1* gene are responsible for the X-linked form (Hardelin *et al.* 1998). The gene product has been called anosmin-1, a 100-kDa glycoprotein. In this form, unilateral renal agenesis is found in about one third of the patients. Renal agenesis results from defective metanephrogenic blastema induction by the ureteral bud, presumably because of defective branching (Duke *et al.* 1998).

Methylmalonic acidaemia

Methylmalonic acidaemia (MMA) is an autosomal recessive disorder of organic acid metabolism, usually detected during the first year of life. It is due to a defect of methylmalonyl-CoA mutase or of the cofactor, adenosylcobalamin. Defect of the coenzyme may be treated with high pharmacological doses of hydroxycobalamin (vitamin B_{12}) with a consequent reduction in the production of methylmalonate and a less severe clinical course. Infants with B_{12}-unresponsive forms are treated with a low-protein diet, carnitine, and metronidazole.

The revealing symptoms in infancy are hypotomia, vomiting, dehydratation, lethargy, and failure to thrive due to metabolic ketoacidosis and hyperammonaemia. With appropriate treatment an increasing number of children survive and long-term complications may therefore develop. Neurological impairment and mental retardation are found mostly in children with only onset of MMA whereas children with late onset have a normal neurological development. Cardiomyopathy and progressive chronic renal impairment are frequent and serious complications in long-term survivors.

Renal functional impairment is found in 20–60 per cent of B_{12}-resistant adolescents (Baumgarter and Viardot 1995), and also in some B12-sensitive patients (Broyer *et al.* 1974; Baumgarter and Viardot 1995). Renal involvement is related to tubulo-interstitial disease (Broyer *et al.* 1974; Molteni *et al.* 1991). The mechanisms of renal injury are unknown; high urinary concentrations of MMA may exert toxic effects on renal tubular cells. Renal failure further impairs urinary excretion of MMA, aggravating blood retention. Combined liver–kidney transplantation has been successful in a 13.5 year-old boy. Immediately before

surgery, haemodialysis was performed to decrease plasma MMA concentration. Liver transplant provided a new source of methylmalonyl-CoA mutase and corrected MMA (van't Hoff *et al.* 1998). In another 17 year-old female patient, successful kidney transplantation was performed after a 11-month period of haemodialysis. This resulted in normalization in urinary excretion of MMA. The small methylmalonyl-CoA mutase activity present in the transplanted kidney could be sufficient in some cases to ensure normal metabolism of organic acids (Lubrano *et al.* 2001). If need be, restricted protein intake can be associated with kidney transplantation.

Mitochondrial cytopathies with renal involvement*

Until recently, it was believed that these syndromes were rare, confined to childhood, and involved the nervous and muscular systems predominantly. Now it is clear that they may present at any age with manifestations in almost any organ, including the kidney, and often include apparently unrelated manifestations in multiple organs, although a single organ system may be affected for a long period (Johns 1995). It is certain that they are underdiagnosed in many areas of medicine. An area of particular interest in nephrology is tubulointerstitial failure of obscure origin, particularly when followed or accompanied by other apparently bizarre and unrelated manifestations (Szabolcs *et al.* 1994).

Mitochondrial DNA

Human mitochondrial DNA (mtDNA) (Luft 1994; Wallace 1994; Johns 1995) is a closed circular molecule of length 16.5 kb that encodes small (12S) and large (16S) ribosomal RNA (rRNA), 22 transfer RNAs (tRNA), and 13 key subunits of the polypeptide enzymes of the respiratory chain.

The mitochondrial respiratory chain (Fig. 3) is a very complex metabolic pathway comprising about 100 polypeptides. Most of these are encoded by nuclear DNA (nDNA) and only 13 by the mtDNA. mtDNA is transcribed polycystronically and further processed into mature messenger RNAs (mRNAs). At least one of these transcription factors is encoded in nDNA. In addition, nDNA codes for proteins involved in mtDNA replication and repair. Thus, interactions between the nucleus and the mitchondria are expected, and genes encoded within the nucleus and its product may interfere with mtDNA and its gene product. Mutations of nDNA, mtDNA, or both may constitute the genetic basis of mitochondrial diseases.

Mitochondria are the only sources of extranuclear DNA in humans. During egg fertilization, the sperm contributes only its nDNA to the zygote. In contrast, the mother transmits her mtDNA to her offspring and only her daughters can transmit mtDNA to the next generation. Thus, inheritance does not follow conventional Mendelian laws. During cell division, mitochondria are randomly distributed among daughter cells. When an mtDNA mutation arises, it creates an intracellular mixture of normal or wild-type and mutant molecules called heteroplasmy. Subsequently, as the mutant and normal mtDNAs are randomly distributed into daughter cells during mitotic or meiotic replication, a percentage of mutant and normal molecules drifts within the cell towards either pure mutant or pure normal (homoplasmy), whereas others remain heteroplasmic (Rötig *et al.* 1995). The molecular

* In collaboration with Dominique Chauveau.

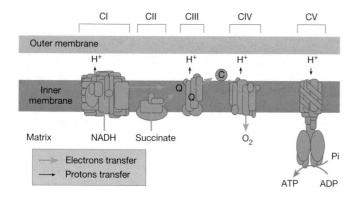

Fig. 3 The respiratory chain. Complexes I–V are coded for partly by mitochondria and partly by nuclear DNA. Complex I (NADH CoQ reductase) oxidizes NADH produced by either the Krebs cycle or fatty acid oxidation. Electrons are transferred to complex IV (cytochrome c oxidase) which oxidizes reduced cytochrome c. Complex V mediates synthesis of ATP. Protons extruded by complexes I, III, and IV accumulate in the intermembrane space and can be used for further ATP synthesis.

mechanisms of clinical heterogeneity in mitochondrial disorders are not elucidated. Heteroplasmy, a threshold effect and accumulation of toxic substrates including lactate beyond respiratory chain defect have all been raised (Leonard and Schapira 2000). The threshold effect refers to the critical number of mutated mtDNA required for the disease to be expressed in different tissues. Since the basic defect is in electron transport in mitochondria the energy supply to cell is insufficient depending on requirement of the tissue on oxidative metabolism.

Mitochondrial cytopathies

Muscles and the CNS are the most commonly affected, and various syndrome complexes have been described (Johns 1995). These include the MERRF syndrome, with myoclonic epilepsy and the histological appearance of 'ragged red fibre' disease in muscles stained with Gomori trichrome, which represent subsarcolemmal collections of abnormal mitochondria. On electron microscopy, the mitochondria appear abnormal, with the appearance of a parking lot seen from the air, with crystalline inclusions. Others have the MELAS syndrome of mitochondrial encephalopathy, lactic acidosis, and stroke-like episodes. Other disorders include the Kearns–Sayre syndrome (external ophthalmoplegia, pigmentary retinopathy, myopathy, and cardiac conduction defects) and Leigh's syndrome (subacute necrotizing encephalomyelopathy). Muscular weakness is particularly prominent after exercise and follows a progressive, sometimes fatal course.

Although mitochondrial cytopathies were first regarded as neuromuscular disorders, a much broader spectrum of clinical features has emerged. Neurosensorial deafness, cardiomyopathy and conduction defects, sideroblastic anaemia or pancytopenia, and diabetes mellitus may be recognized. These different features may occur at different times or synchronously in single patients. Concomitant macular dystrophy may be a clue to the diagnosis (for review of the most common syndromes likely to be encountered, see Luft 1994; Chinnery and Turnbull 1999; Leonard and Schapira 2000).

The renal syndromes of mitochondrial cytopathy are often overlooked (Grünfeld et al. 1996). In childhood with mitochondriopathy, renal involvement may occur at any time, either as a presenting manifestation or late in the course of a multisystemic disorder (Niaudet and Rötig 1997). It encompasses a large spectrum of manifestations. Not surprisingly, in view of the high energy requirement of the renal tubules, proximal tubular dysfunction with de Toni–Debré–Fanconi syndrome is the most frequent presentation and may be recognized neonatally (de Lonlay et al. 2001b). Isolated renal tubular acidosis (Eviatar et al. 1990) and even Bartter-like syndrome (Goto et al. 1990) have been reported. Tubulointerstitial nephritis is also seen (Szabolcs et al. 1994). A variety of mtDNA mutations have been identified in these settings. A minority of children present with heavy-range proteinuria related to focal and segmental glomerulosclerosis and the A3243G point mutation in the leucine^{UUR} tRNA gene (Niaudet and Rötig 1997). Occasionally, myoglobinuria-related acute renal failure is encountered (Hsieh et al. 1996). In adulthood, the A3243G mutation is so far the unique mtDNA mutation responsible for kidney disease. Deafness is almost consistently present at diagnosis of renal involvement, and many patients are misdiagnosed as Alport syndrome. Focal and segmental glomerulosclerosis is the common histological picture (Jansen et al. 1994; Moulonguet-Doleris et al. 2000; Hotta et al. 2001). As for children, renal disease may progress to endstage renal failure, and renal transplantation can be offered. Finally, in two series, as many as 1–6 per cent of Japanese diabetic patients on regular dialysis exhibited the A3243G mutation (Yamagata et al. 2000; Iwasaki et al. 2001).

How to diagnose mitochondrial cytopathies? It should be thought of when facing apparently unrelated organ involvement. Family history is valuable when there is evidence of maternal inheritance. Blood lactate concentration and lactate : pyruvate ratio may be increased at rest or after exercise. Depending on clinical presentation, specific changes on muscle biopsy (red-ragged fibres and succinic dehydrogenase and cytochrome oxydase activities) may be useful. However, biochemical analyses are still the cornerstone to demonstrate involvement of the respiratory chain. Gas chromatography mass spectrometry can demonstrate accumulation of urinary lactate and citric acid cycle intermediates. Study of the respiratory chain complexes in leucocytes or any affected tissue may ultimately be required. Identification of the mtDNA mutation is the next step. However, in the adult patients and some children with suggestive renal presentation, straightforward molecular diagnosis of the A3234G mutation in leucocytes, or in any affected tissue may be offered (Fig. 4).

Finally, as many as 1–2 per cent of patients with isolated diabetes mellitus, mostly non-insulin-dependent, may arise from disease of mtDNA (Ballinger et al. 1992; Froguel and Vionnet 1995). In addition, in a case of early-onset diabetes mellitus, optic atrophy and deafness (Wolfram or DIDMOAD syndrome), a deletion of mtDNA was found (Rötig et al. 1994).

Multicentric osteolysis with nephropathy

Multicentric osteolysis is a group of rare diseases of unknown cause characterized by progressive resorption of bones, primarily in the hands and feet (thus also called acro-osteolysis). The first symptoms usually appear in early childhood and consist of swelling and pain of the wrists, fingers and ankles, simulating arthritic episodes. Subsequently, X-ray films show progressive and symmetric dissolution of bones, starting at the level of carpal bones and metacarpals, then involving foot, elbow, and knee bones. Facial abnormalities (exophtalmos, micrognathia, and triangular shape) are frequently seen.

Typically, nephropathy appears several years after osteolysis has occurred. Proteinuria is the first abnormality, followed by hypertension

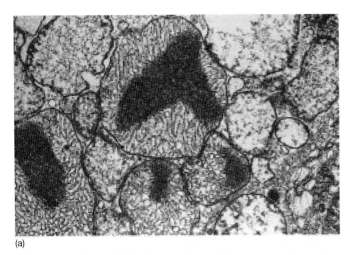

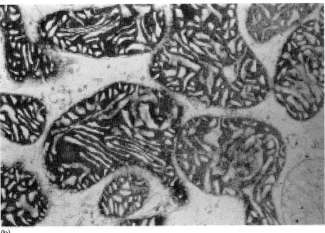

Fig. 4 Abnormal cristas in mitochondria within renal tubular cells in a 7-year-old girl with tubulointerstitial renal disease. Abnormal mitochondria in the tubules on light or electron microscopy may give a clue to the diagnosis of mitochondrial cytopathy in tubulointerstitial disease of apparently obscure origin (magnification 9000×) (reproduced with permission from Szabolcs et al. 1994).

and renal failure (Carnevale *et al.* 1987; Rose *et al.* 1987). Renal biopsy may show focal and segmental glomerulosclerosis. There is no recurrence after kidney transplantation.

The disease is either sporadic, or inherited and genetically heterogeneous (see review in Grünfeld 1998).

The autosomal dominant Hadju–Cheney syndrome encompasses osteolysis of the terminal phalanges, short stature and short neck. Cystic kidney disease is found in about 10 per cent of the cases (Strassburg *et al.* 2001).

Optic nerve disorders and renal disease

Ocular abnormalities have been associated with renal disease in a number of families (Weaver *et al.* 1988; Bron *et al.* 1989). The ocular component has varied from microphthalmos to coloboma, or the optic nerve appearance described as the 'morning glory' optic disc (Torralbo *et al.* 1995) after the flower of that name (*Convolvulus*) (Fig. 5). Renal

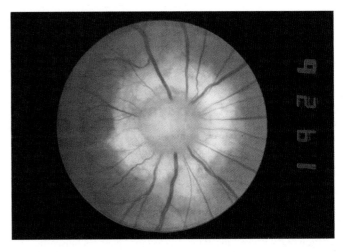

Fig. 5 The 'morning glory' appearance of the optic nerve which may be associated with renal disease, sometimes accompanied by renal failure (by courtesy of Dr David Calver).

failure has ensued in some family members. Interestingly, mutation of the *PAX2* gene has been reported in families (Eccles *et al.* 1999) with optic nerve coloboma, hearing loss, CNS anomalies, renal hypoplasia, vesicoureteral reflux, and progressive renal failure. This gene is normally involved in kidney and eye development (Sanyanusin *et al.* 1995). The renal-coloboma syndrome is an autosomal dominant disorder. PAX2 germline mosaicism has been reported (Amiel *et al.* 2000).

Animal models of renal-coloboma syndrome have been described, including *Krd* and knock-out mice. Heterozygous mice develop various kidney and eye defects. Homozygous knockout mice die at or soon after birth and lack kidneys and ureters (see review in Eccles *et al.* 1999). The major role of *PAX2* in kidney development is discussed in Chapter 17.1.

Mutations of *PAX2* have been looked for in patients with oligomeganephronia, a rare congenital and usually sporadic anomaly. They have been found in only three of nine patients. These three patients had slight abnormalities of the optic disc, in the absence of visual impairment, and therefore belong to the renal-coloboma syndrome (Salomon *et al.* 2001). Eye anomalies are a constant feature of PAX2 mutations but there is a large spectrum of ocular defects ranging from slight optic disc anomalies to microphthalmia (Amiel *et al.* 2000).

Orotic aciduria

This rare condition (Webster *et al.* 1995) arises from defects in one of two multienzymes of pyrimidine synthesis, now usually called multienzyme pyr 5,6 or uridine monophosphate synthase; the two enzymic activities expressed by the single protein are orotidine 5′-monophosphate decarboxylase and orotate phosphoribosyl transferase. Deficiency of either leads to the excretion of large amounts of orotic acid. The condition is inherited as an autosomal recessive pattern, with the gene being located near 3q13.

Clinical manifestations include megaloblastic anaemia, diarrhoea, growth retardation, and cardiac malformations in some patients. The large excretion of very insoluble orotic acid leads to a 'sludge' of crystals within the urinary tract, with colic, haematuria, and obstruction at all levels from the renal pelvis to the urethra, one or more of which have affected about half the reported cases. The urine is clear initially but then throws down a profuse sediment. Treatment with uridine is successful but must be maintained lifelong. A high urine output is also desirable to help solubilize the orotic acid.

Smith–Lemli–Opitz syndrome

Children with this relatively common autosomal recessive syndrome (carrier rate) present with poor growth, microcephaly, various degrees of mental retardation, hypotonia, and incomplete development of the external genitalia in males. Glomerulosclerosis has also been described. The facies is dysmorphic and characteristic (Fig. 6). Other structural anomalies of the gonads, limbs, and digits may be seen in some cases (Pober 1990). It is inherited in an autosomal recessive fashion, but the location of the gene is uncertain. A defect in cholesterol biosynthesis at the 7-dehydrocholesterol to cholest-5-en-3β-ol step has been described (Tint *et al.* 1994), with accumulation of the former and depletion of the latter in plasma and body fluids. How this relates to the clinical manifestations remains obscure, but they could be the result of cholesterol deficiency during fetal development, with lack of 7-dehydrocholesterol for insertion into membranes.

It is interesting that some inhibitors of cholesterol synthesis lead to renal abnormalities in animals (Barbu *et al.* 1988), and about two-thirds of cases show a variety of renal anomalies including dysplasia, hypoplasia, and anomalies of urinary drainage (Cherstvoy *et al.* 1975).

Townes–Brocks syndrome

Townes–Brocks syndrome is an autosomal dominant multiple malformation syndrome characterized by ear anomalies (external auricular

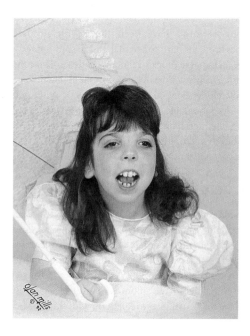

Fig. 6 The Smith–Lemli–Opitz syndrome in a 10-year-old girl. The characteristic facies of upturned nose, micrognathia, and ptosis can be seen. [Case described by Tint *et al.* (1994) with the permission of Dr Ellen Roy Elias, The Floating Hospital for Children, Boston, MA.]

abnormalities, described as 'satyr' on 'lop' ears, and sensorineural hearing loss), limb defects (triphalangeal thumb and polydactyly), anorectal malformations (imperforate anus), and genitourinary anomalies. These include unilateral or bilateral hypoplastic or dysplastic kidneys, renal agenesis, multicystic kidney and various genitourinary tract malformations. Several patients progressed to endstage renal disease. REAR syndrome (renal–ear–anal–radial) has also been a term used to describe this condition (Powell and Michaelis 1999).

Townes–Brocks syndrome is caused by mutations of the zinc finger transcription factor gene *SALL1* (Kohlase *et al.* 1998). The *SALL1* gene is located at 16q12.1. It is a human analogue of spalt (sal) which is a developmental regulation in *Drosophila*. Additional mutations have been subsequently described (Engel *et al.* 2000; Salerno *et al.* 2000). Some phenotypic overlap may exist with the BOR syndrome (Engel *et al.* 2000). It should be stressed, however, that branchial fistulae and cysts are the key diagnostic feature in BOR syndrome whereas they are absent in Townes–Brocks syndrome.

Tubular dysgenesis

Renal tubular dysgenesis is a developmental abnormality of the fetal kidney characterized by the absence of proximal convoluted tubules. It may be observed in the donor in the twin-to-twin transfusion syndrome (Mahieu-Caputo *et al.* 2000) or may be induced by *in utero* inhibition of the renin–angiotensin system by angiotensin-converting enzyme (ACE) inhibitors or AT1 receptor antagonists (Barr and Cohen 1991; Martinovic *et al.* 2001). Renal tubular dysgenesis may also be primary and inherited as an autosomal recessive trait (Allanson *et al.* 1992).

Oligohydramnios is the earliest abnormality, detected at 18–20 weeks of gestation. Fetal kidneys are normal by ultrasonography. Prognosis is very poor. *In utero* fetal death occurs in about 15 per cent of the cases. Most neonates die within hours or days of anuria and respiratory distress. In only two surviving dialysed children, diuresis resumed after a few weeks; residual chronic renal failure persisted. Face deformities of the Potter sequence were found in most cases. Deficient calvarial bone growth leading to wide sutures and large fontanelles have been found in many cases, like in ACE inhibitors-induced disease (Bernstein and Barajas 1994).

Renal pathology is characterized by absence or very reduced number of proximal tubules, presence of primitive tubules, normal differentiation of glomeruli, and diffuse thickening of arteriolar walls. Similar changes are seen in secondary forms of renal tubular dysgenesis, suggesting a congenital or acquired abnormality of the renin–angiotensin system in all these cases.

Velo-cardio-facial (or Shprintzen), Di George, and conotruncal anomaly face syndromes

Interrupted aortic arch, truncus arteriosus, and tetralogy of Fallot with parathyroid and thymic hypoplasia are the classical findings in Di George syndrome (DGS). Velopharyngeal insufficiency and learning disorders with associated conotruncal defects or misalignment ventricular septal defect are seen more commonly in conotruncal anomaly face syndrome and in velo-cardio-facial syndrome (VCFS).

Most affected people have a deletion of chromosome 22q11.2, accounting for the term '22q1.2 deletion syndrome' to describe this entity. The deletion is detected by using commercially available fluorescent *in situ* hybridization (FISH) probes. The deletion can be inherited but more typically occurs as a *de novo* event. It is found in 90 per cent of patients with full DGS phenotype and in 70 per cent of patients with VCFS features. Several genes are located in the deleted region, including the ubiquitin-fusion-degradation-1-like (UFDIL) gene which might be responsible for the DGS phenotype.

Approximately 15 per cent of patients with the DGS/VCFS phenotype have no typical 22q11.2 deletions. They may have atypical deletions, point mutations within the gene, possibly UFDIL, or deletions of 10p. The latter deletions are much less common and lead to the HDR syndrome (see above) with less frequent cardiac defects, more frequent renal anomalies and deafness.

The clinical features encompass cardiovascular defects, immunodeficiency, hypocalcaemic hypoparathyroidism, short stature, hypothyroidism, eye malformations, butterfly vertebrae, palate abnormalities and velopharyngeal incompetence, feeding and speech disorders, and learning disabilities. Structural renal abnormalities have been identified by ultrasound in 37 per cent of deletion-positive patients. Renal insufficiency and renal tubular acidosis have also been reported (see review in Cuneo 2001).

Wiskott–Aldrich syndrome

The principal manifestations of the Wiskott–Aldrich syndrome are immune deficiency and thrombocytopenia, sometimes with purpura, eczema, bloody diarrhoea, and ear infections in boys. Infection and/or bleeding are often fatal in infancy, and survivors may develop leukaemia or lymphoma. In addition, a variety of immune or autoimmune disorders have been described in these patients, including impaired skin graft rejection, but normal T-blast transformation, and raised IgA with low IgM concentrations in serum. The fundamental defect seems to be a disordered expression of a 66-kDa intracellular protein, a small GTPase of the Rho family which interacts with Cdc42, which in turn controls the surface expression of many molecules in immune cells (Featherstone 1996).

Inheritance of this complex syndrome is consistent with an X-linked recessive pattern (Crawfurd 1988, pp. 441–443), and female heterozygotes may show low platelet counts and abnormal platelet function. The gene has been localized to Xp11.22–23 in a region of high gene density (Deray *et al.* 1994).

Renal disease has been described in a number of survivors who may have had an incomplete form of the disease (Spitler *et al.* 1980; De Santo *et al.* 1988–1989). Haematuria casts and proteinuria up to the nephrotic range with concomitant oedema have been noted, but the renal histology has been determined in only a few cases. Gutenberger *et al.* (1970) and Standen *et al.* (1986) described familial thrombocytopenia, increased IgA, and renal disease in several family members. Renal biopsy showed proliferative glomerulonephritis or interstitial nephritis. A patient studied in our unit had a vasculitic picture clinically, which has also been reported in a number of patients without renal involvement. A crescentic glomerulonephritis showing prominent mesangial IgA deposition was present in the renal biopsy, as in the case described by De Santo *et al.* (1988–1989); an evolution into endstage renal failure occurred within 2 years of onset. The patient was later transplanted successfully under minimal immunosuppression (Webb *et al.* 1993).

X-linked granulomatous disease

In two-thirds of patients chronic granulomatous disease is an X-linked condition affecting males in whom the defective gene at Xq 21.1 leads to the absence of a 90-kDa component of cytochrome b. The remaining patients usually have a less severe disease, inherited in an autosomal recessive manner, due to a defect in a cytosolic factor necessary for the respiratory burst. Female heterozygotes carrying the X-linked form of the disease frequently develop systemic lupus erythematosus. The functional defect in both types is defective phagocytosis, associated with impaired chemiluminescence of neutrophils and impaired reduction of the dye nitroblue tetrazolium. Clinical presentation is usually in infancy, with skin sepsis which becomes deeper, resulting in abscess formation, and chronically discharging sinuses from regional lymph nodes.

Alibadi *et al.* (1989) described 50 per cent of the children in their series as having recurrent pyelonephritis associated with retroperitoneal lymphadenitis, granuloma formation, and obstruction. Antibiotics were required to treat the infections, but ureterolysis was necessary in one patient and two had nephrectomies. It is not yet clear whether these findings are typical of other series of this rare inherited disorder, but urinary tract imaging should be performed in any child or young adult presenting with a urinary tract infection. Interstitial cystitis has also been reported (Kontras *et al.* 1971). Sclerosing glomerulonephritis was noted in one family (Dilworth and Mandell 1977).

Zellweger syndrome

Zellweger (cerebro-hepato-renal) syndrome is a childhood autosomal recessive multisystem disorder caused by peroxisomal malfunction. The molecular defects in the diseases of the Zellweger syndrome spectrum are deletions or mutations in *PEX* genes whose gene products, the peroxins (Pex-proteins), are involved in the biogenesis of peroxisomes (Moser 2000).

Infants with Zellweger syndrome are severely hypotonic at birth, have a characteristic face with a tall forehead, hypoplastic supraorbital ridges, and epicanthal folds, and have a combination of neurological, hepatic, renal, cardiac, skeletal, and ocular abnormalities. The renal abnormalities include multiple cortical cysts, proteinuria, and aminoaciduria. The ocular abnormalities include retinal dystrophy and extinguished electroretinograms, lens opacities, and microphtalmos (Garner and Fielder 1990). Death generally occurs within the first year as a result of gross defects of early brain development and major complications.

Heterozygotes have lenticular opacities with curvilinear cortical condensations which may be used for detection of the carrier status. Prenatal diagnosis of Zellweger syndrome can be made.

References

Abelhak, S. *et al.* (1997). A human homologue of the *Drosophila* eyes absent gene underlines branchio-oto-renal (BOR) syndrome and identifies a novel gene family. *Nature Genetics* **15**, 157–164.

Abramovsky, C. R. and Swineheart, G. L. (1982). The nephropathy of cystic fibrosis. *Human Pathology* **13**, 934–939.

Alagille, D., Estrada, A., Hadchouel, M., Gautier, M., Odièvre, M., and Dommergues, J. P. (1987). Syndromic paucity of interlobular bile ducts (Alagille syndrome or arteriohepatic dysplasia): review of 80 cases. *Journal of Pediatrics* **110**, 195–200.

Alibadi, H., Gonzalez, R., and Quie, P. G. (1989). Urinary tract disorders in patients with chronic granulomatous disease. *New England Journal of Medicine* **321**, 706–708.

Allanson, J. E., Hunter, A. G. W., Mettler, G. S., and Jimenez, C. (1992). Renal tubular dysgenesis: a not uncommon autosomal recessive syndrome. A review. *American Journal of Medical Genetics* **43**, 811–814.

Amiel, J. *et al.* (2000). PAX2 mutations in renal-coloboma syndrome: mutational hotspot and germline mosaicism. *European Journal of Genetics* **8**, 820–826.

Aminoff, M. *et al.* (1999). Mutations in CUBN, encoding the intrinsic factor-vitamin B12 receptor, cubilin, cause hereditary megaloblastic anaemia. *Nature Genetics* **21**, 309–313.

Ballinger, S. W. *et al.* (1992). Maternally transmitted diabetes and deafness associated with 10.4 kb mitochondrial DNA deletion. *Nature Genetics* **1**, 11–15.

Barakat, A. Y., Arianas, P., Glick, A. D., and Butler, M. G. (1990). Focal sclerosing glomerulonephritis in a child with Laurence–Moon–Biedl syndrome. *International Journal of Pediatric Urology and Nephrology* **10**, 109–111.

Barakat, A. Y., D'Alabora, J. B., Martin, M. M., and Jose, P. A. (1977). Familial nephrosis, nerve deafness, and hypoparathyroidism. *Journal of Pediatrics* **91**, 61–64.

Barbu, V. *et al.* (1988). Cholesterol prevents the teratogenic effects of AY 9944: importance of timing of cholesterol supplementation to rats. *Journal of Nutrition* **110**, 2310–2312.

Bardet, G. (1920). Sur un syndrome d'obésité infantile avec polydactylie et rétinite pigmentaire (contribution à l'étude des formes cliniques de l'obésité hypophysaire). Thèse, Université de Paris, No. 479.

Barness, E. G. and Opitz, J. M. Renal abnormalities in malformation syndromes. In *Pediatric Kidney Disease* 2nd edn. (ed. C. M. Edelmann, Jr.), pp. 1067–1119. Boston, MA: Little Brown, 1993.

Barr, M. and Cohen, M. M. (1991). ACE inhibitor fetopathy and hypocalvaria. The kidney–skull connection. *Teratology* **44**, 485–495.

Baumgarter, E. R. and Viardot, C. (1995). Long-term follow-up of 77 patients with isolated methylmalonic acidaemia. *Journal of Inherited Metabolism Disease* **18**, 138–142.

Becker, M., Rotthauwe, H. W., Weber, H.-P., and Fischbach, H. (1977). Selective vitamin B12 malabsorption (Imerslund–Gräsbeck syndrome). Studies on gastroenterological and nephrological problems. *European Journal of Pediatrics* **124**, 139–153.

Ben Bassat, J., Feinstein, A., and Ramot, B. (1969). Selective vitamin B12 malabsorption with proteinuria in Israel. *Israel Journal of Medical Sciences* **5**, 62–68.

Bernstein, J. and Barajas, L. (1994). Renal tubular dysgenesis: evidence of abnormality in the renin angiotensin system. *Journal of the American Society of Nephrology* **5**, 224–227.

Biedl, A. (1922). Ein Geschwisterpaar mit adiposo-genitaler Dystrophie. *Deutsche Medizinische Wochenschrift* **48**, 1630.

Bilous, R. W. *et al.* (1992). Brief report: autosomal dominant familial hypoparathyroidism, sensorineural deafness and renal dysplasia. *New England Journal of Medicine* **327**, 1069–1074.

Bron, A. J., Burgess, S. E., Awdry, P. N., Oliver, D., and Arden, G. (1989). Papillo-renal syndrome. An inherited association of optic disc dysplasia and renal disease. Report and review of the literature. *Ophthalmological Paediatrics and Genetics* **10**, 185–198.

Broyer, M., Guesry, P., Burgess, E. A., Charpentier, C, and Lemonnier, A. (1974). Acidémie methyl malonique avec néphropathie hyperuricémique. *Archives Françaises de Pédiatrie* **31**, 543–552.

Burghes, A. H. M., Vaessin, F., and de La Chapelle, A. (2001). The land between Mendelian and multifactorial inheritance. *Science* **293**, 2213–2214.

Carnevale, A., Canun, S., Mendoza, L., and del Castillo, V. (1987). Idiopathic multicentric osteolysis with facial anomalies and nephropathy. *American Journal of Medical Genetics* **26**, 877–886.

Cherstvoy, E. D. *et al.* (1975). The pathological anatomy of the Smith–Lemli–Opitz syndrome. *Clinical Genetics* **7**, 383–387.

Chinnery, P. F. and Turnbull, D. M. (1999). Mitochondrial DNA and disease. *Lancet* **354**, 17–21.

Churchill, D. N., McManamon, P., and Hurley, R. M. (1981). Renal disease—a sixth cardinal feature of the Laurence–Moon–Biedl syndrome. *Clinical Nephrology* **16**, 151–154.

Clarren, S. K. Inherited renal disorders. In *Pediatric Nephrology* 2nd edn. (ed. M. A. Holliday, T. M. Barrett, and E. Avner), pp. 491–514. Boston, MA: Little Brown, 1994.

Collan, Y., Lahdevirta, J., and Jokinen, E. J. (1979). Selective vitamin B12 malabsorption with proteinuria. Renal biopsy study. *Nephron* **23**, 297–303.

Collins, C. M., Mendoza, S. A., Griswold, W. R., Tanney, D., Lieberman, E., and Reznik, V. M. (1994). Pediatric renal transplantation in the Laurence–Moon–Biedl syndrome. *Pediatric Nephrology* **8**, 221–222.

Coutelle, C., Caplen, N., Hart, S., Huxley, C., and Williamson, R. (1993). Gene therapy for cystic fibrosis. *Archives of Disease in Childhood* **68**, 437–443.

Crawfurd, M. D'A. *The Genetics of Renal Tract Disorders*. Oxford University Press, 1988.

Croft, J. B. and Swift, M. (1990). Obesity, hypertension and renal disease in relatives of Bardet–Biedl syndrome. *American Journal of Clinical Genetics* **36**, 37–42.

Crosnier, C. *et al.* (1999). Mutations in JAGGED1 gene are predominantly sporadic in Alagille syndrome. *Gastroenterology* **116**, 1141–1148.

Cuneo, B. F. (2001). 22q11.2 deletion syndrome: DiGeorge, velocardiofacial, and conotruncal anomaly face syndromes. *Current Opinion in Pediatrics* **13**, 465–472.

De Lonlay, P. *et al.* (2001a). A broad spectrum of clinical presentations in congenital disorders of glycosylation I: a series of 26 cases. *Journal of Medical Genetics* **38**, 14–19.

De Lonlay, P. *et al.* (2001b). A mutant mitochondrial respiratory chain assembly protein causes complex III deficiency in patients with tubulopathy, encephalopathy and liver failure. *Nature Genetics* **29**, 57–61.

De Marchi, S., Cecchin, E., and Bartoli, E. (1992). Bardet–Biedl syndrome and cystinuria. *Renal Failure* **14**, 587–590.

Deray, J. M., Ochs, H. D., and Francke, V. (1994). Isolation of a novel gene mutated in Wiskott–Aldrich syndrome. *Cell* **78**, 635–644.

De Santo, N. G. *et al.* (1988–1989). IgA glomerulopathy in Wiskott–Aldrich syndrome. *Child Nephrology and Urology* **9**, 118–120.

De Vries, B. B., van'tHoff, W. G., Surtees, R. A., and Winter, R. M. (2001). Diagnostic dilemmas in four infants with nephrotic syndrome, microcephaly and severe developmental delay. *Clinical Dysmorphological* **10**, 112–121.

Dilworth, J. A. and Mandell, G. L. (1977). Adults with chronic granulomatous disease. *American Journal of Medicine* **63**, 233–243.

Duke, V. *et al.* (1998). Proteinuria, hypertension and chronic renal failure in X-linked Kallmann's syndrome, a defined cause of solitary functioning kidney. *Nephrology, Dialysis, Transplantation* **13**, 1998–2003.

Eccles, M. R. and Schimmenti, L. A. (1999). Renal-coloboma syndrome: a multi-system developmental disorder caused by PAX2 mutations. *Clinical Genetics* **56**, 1–9.

Edwards, B. D., Patton, M. A., Dilly, S. A., and Eastwood, J. B. (1989). A new syndrome of autosomal recessive nephropathy, deafness and hyperparathyroidism. *Journal of Medical Genetics* **26**, 289–293.

Efthamiou, J., Spickett, G., and Lane, D. (1991). Antineutrophil cytoplasmic antibodies, cystic fibrosis and infection. *Lancet* **337**, 1037–1038.

Emerick, K. M., Rand, E. B., Goldmuntz, E., Krantz, I. D., Spinner, N. B., and Piccoli, D. A. (1999). Features of Alagille syndrome in 92 patients: frequency and relation to prognosis. *Hepatology* **29**, 824–829.

Engel, S., Kohlhase, J., and Mc Gaughran, J. (2000). A SALL1 mutation causes a branchio-oto-renal syndrome-like phenotype. *Journal of Medical Genetics* **37**, 460–462.

Eviatar, L. *et al.* (1990). Kears–Sayre syndrome presenting as renal tubular acidosis. *Neurology* **40**, 1761–1763.

Featherstone, C. (1996). How does one gene cause the Wiskott–Aldrich syndrome? *Lancet* **348**, 950.

Finnegan, M. J. *et al.* (1989). Vasculitis complicating cystic fibrosis. *Quarterly Journal of Medicine* **72**, 609–621.

Fralick, R. A., Leichter, H. E., and Sheth, K. J. (1990). Early diagnosis of the Bardet–Biedl syndrome. *Pediatric Nephrology* **4**, 264–265.

Fraser, R. C., Sproule, J. R., and Halal, F. (1980). Frequency of the branchio-oto-renal (BOR) syndrome in children with profound hearing loss. *American Journal of Human Genetics* **7**, 341–349.

Froguel, P. and Vionnet, N. (1995). Genetics of non-insulin dependent diabetes mellitus: from genes to disease. *Advances in Nephrology* **24**, 157–163.

Gaffney, K., Gibbons, D., Keogh, B., and Fitzgerald, M. X. (1993). Amyloidosis complicating cystic fibrosis. *Thorax* **48**, 949–950.

Garber, S. J. and de Bruyn, R. (1991). Laurence–Moon–Bardet–Biedl syndrome: renal ultrasound appearances in the neonate. *British Journal of Radiology* **64**, 631–634.

Garner, A. and Fielder, A. R. Zellweger's syndrome. In *The Eye in Systemic Disease* (ed. D. H. Gold and T. A. Weingeist), pp. 411–413. Philadelphia: J.B. Lippincott, 1990.

Geisert, J., Luckel, J. C., Lutz, D., and Beyer, P. (1975). Les protéinuries de type tubulaire chez l'enfant. *Annales de Pédiatrie* **22**, 297–300.

Gilbert Barness, E. F., Opitz, J. M., and Barness, L. A. Hereditable malformations of the kidney and urinary tract. In *Inheritance of Kidney and Urinary Tract Diseases* (ed. A. Spitzer and E. Avner). Boston, MA: Kluwer, 1989.

Glenner, G. G. (1986). Reactive systemic amyloidosis in cystic fibrosis and other disorders associated with chronic inflammation. *Archives of Pathology and Laboratory Medicine* **110**, 873–874.

Goto, Y., Itami, N., Kajii, N., Tichimaru, H., Endo, M., and Horai, S. (1990). Renal tubular involvement mimicking Bartter syndrome in a patient with Kearns–Sayre syndrome. *Journal of Pediatrics* **116**, 904–910.

Gräsbeck, R., Gordin, R., Kantero, I., and Kühlback, B. (1960). Selective B$_{12}$ malabsorption and proteinuria in young people. *Acta Medica Scandinavica* **167**, 289–296.

Greene, J. S. *et al.* (1989). The cardinal manifestations of Bardet–Biedl syndrome, a form of Laurence–Moon–Biedl syndrome. *New England Journal of Medicine* **321**, 1002–1009.

Grünfeld, J. P. Multicentric osteolysis with nephropathy. In *Inherited Disorders of the Kidney* (ed. S. H. Morgan and J. P. Grünfeld), pp. 349–352. Oxford: Oxford University Press, 1998.

Grünfeld, J. P., Niaudet, P., and Rötig, A. (1996). Renal involvement in mitochondrial cytopathies. *Nephrology, Dialysis, Transplantation* **11**, 760–761.

Gutenberger, J. *et al.* (1970). Familial thrombocytopenia, elevated serum IgA levels and renal disease: report of a kindred. *American Journal of Medicine* **49**, 729–741.

Haan, E. A. *et al.* (1989). Tricho-rhino-phalangeal and branchio-oto syndromes in a family with an inherited rearrangement of chromosome 8a. *American Journal of Medical Genetics* **32**, 490–494.

Habib, R., Dommergues, J. P., Gubler, M. C., Hadchouel, M., Gautier, M., Odièvre, M., and Alagille, D. (1987). Glomerular mesangiolipidosis in Alagille syndrome (arteriohepatic dysplasia). *Pediatric Nephrology* **1**, 455–464.

Hardelin, J. P. *et al.* (1998). Molecular approach to the pathogenesis of renal anomalies in Kallmann's syndrome and in the branchio-oto-renal syndrome. *Advances in Nephrology* **28**, 419–428.

Harnett, J. D. *et al.* (1988). The spectrum of disease in the Laurence–Moon–Biedl syndrome. *New England Journal of Medicine* **319**, 615–618.

Hirooka, M., Hirota, M., and Kamada, M. (1988). Renal lesions on Cockayne syndrome. *Pediatric Nephrology* **2**, 239–243.

Hotta, O., Inoue, C. N., Miyabayashi, S., Furuta, T., Takeuchi, A., and Taguma, Y. (2001). Clinical and pathologic features of focal segmental glomerulosclerosis with mitochondrial tRNALeu (UUR) gene mutation. *Kidney International* **59**, 1236–1243.

Hsieh, F., Gokh, R., and Dworkin, L. (1996). Acute renal failure and the MELAS syndrome, a mitochondrial encephalomyelopathy. *Journal of the American Society of Nephrology* **7**, 647–652.

Imerslund, O. (1960). Idiopathic chronic megaloblastic anaemia in children. *Acta Paediatrica Scandinavica* **49** (Suppl. 119), 1–115.

Iwasaki, N. *et al.* (2001). Prevalence of A-to-G mutation at nucleotide 3243 of the mitochondrial tRNA (Leu(UUR) gene in Japanese patients with diabetes mellitus and end-stage renal disease. *American Journal of Human Genetics* **46**, 330–334.

Jansen, J. J. *et al.* (1997) Mutation in mitochondrial tRNA$^{Leu(UUR)}$ gene associated with progressive kidney disease. *Journal of the American Society of Nephrology* **8**, 1118–1124.

Johns, D. R. (1995). Mitochondrial DNA and disease. *New England Journal of Medicine* **333**, 638–644.

Katsanis, N. *et al.* (2001). Triallelic inheritance in Bardet–Biedl syndrome, a Mendelian recessive disorder. *Science* **293**, 2256–2259.

Katz, S. M., Krueger, L. J., and Falkner, B. (1988). Microscopic nephrocalcinosis in cystic fibrosis. *New England Journal of Medicine* **319**, 263–266.

Kohlhase, J., Wischermann, A., Reichen-Bach, H., Froster, V., and Engel, W. (1998). Mutations in the SALL1 putative transcription factor gene cause Townes–Brocks syndrome. *Nature Genetics* **18**, 81–83.

Kontras, S. B., Bodenbender, J. G., McClare, C. R., and Smoth, J. P. (1971). Interstitial cystitis in chronic granulomatous disease. *Journal of Urology* **105**, 575–578.

Kumar, S. *et al.* (1994). Refining the region of branchio-oto-renal syndrome and defining the flanking markers on chromosome 8q by genetic mapping. *American Journal of Medical Genetics* **55**, 1188–1194.

Laurence, J. Z. and Moon, R. C. (1866). Four cases of retinitis pigmentosa occurring in the same family and accompanied by general imperfection of development. *Ophthalmological Review* **2**, 32–41.

Leonard, J. V. and Schapira, A. H. V. (2000). Mitochondrial respiratory chain disorders I: mitochondrial DNA defects. *Lancet* **355**, 299–304.

Leppert, M. *et al.* (1994). Bardet–Biedl syndrome is linked to DNA markers on chromosome 11q and is genetically heterogenous. *Nature Genetics* **7**, 108–112.

Li, L. *et al.* (1997). Alagille syndrome is caused by mutations in human Jagged1, which encodes a ligand for Notch1. *Nature Genetics* **16**, 243–251.

Li, Ni. *et al.* (1994). Refined localisation of the brachiootorenal syndrome gene by linkage and haplotype analysis. *American Journal of Medical Genetics* **51**, 176–184.

Lin, S. H., Sourial, N. A., Lu, K. C., and Huseh, E. J. (1994). Imerslund–Gräsbeck syndrome in a Chinese family with distinct skin lesions. *Journal of Clinical Pathology* **47**, 956–958.

Lubrano, R. *et al.* (2001). Kidney transplantation in a girl with methylmalonic acidemia and end stage renal failure. *Pediatric Nephrology* **16**, 848–851.

Luft, R. (1994). The development of mitochondrial medicine. *Proceedings of the National Academy of Sciences of the United States of America* **91**, 8731–8738.

Mahieu-Caputo, D. *et al.* (2000). Twin-to-twin transfusion syndrome. Role of the fetal renin–angiotensin system. *American Journal of Pathology* **156**, 629–636.

Martinovic, J. *et al.* (2001). Fetal toxic effects and angiotensin-II-receptor antagonists. Report of three additional cases. *Lancet* **358**, 241–242.

McCright, B., Lozier, J., and Gridley, T. (2002). A mouse model of Alagille syndrome: *Notch 2* as a genetic modifier of *Jag 1* haploinsufficiency. *Development* **129**, 1075–1082.

McCright, B. *et al.* (2001). Defects in development of the kidney, heart and eye vasculature in mice homozygous for a hypomorphic *Notch 2* mutation. *Development* **128**, 491–502.

McGlennan, R. C., Burke, B. A., and Dehner, L. P. (1986). Systemic amyloidosis complicating cystic fibrosis. A retrospective pathologic study. *Archives of Pathology and Laboratory Medicine* **110**, 879–884.

McKusick, V. A. *Mendelian Inheritance in Man. Catalog of Autosomal Dominant, Autosomal Recessive and X-linked Phenotypes.* Philadelphia, PA: Johns Hopkins University Press, 1990.

Melnick, M. *et al.* (1976). Familial branchio-oto-renal dysplasia: a new addition to the branchial arch syndromes. *Clinical Genetics* **9**, 25–34.

Melzi, M. L., Constantini, D., Giani, M., Claris Appiani, A., and Giunta, A. M. (1991). Severe nephropathy in three adolescents with cystic fibrosis. *Archives of Disease in Childhood* **66**, 1444–1447.

Molteni, K. H., Oberley, T. D., Wolff, J. A., and Friedman, A. L. (1991). Progressive renal insufficiency in methylmalonic acidemia. *Pediatric Nephrology* **5**, 323–326.

Moser, H. W. (2000). Molecular genetics of peroxisomal disorders. *Front Biosciences* **5**, D298–D306.

Moulonguet-Doleris, L. *et al.* (2000). Focal segmental glomerulosclerosis associated with mitochondrial cytopathy. *Kidney International* **58**, 1851–1858.

Nance, M. A. and Berry, S. M. (1992). Cockayne syndrome: review of 140 cases. *American Journal of Medical Genetics* **42**, 68–84.

Nevanlinna, H. R. Selective malabsorption of vitamin B$_{12}$. In *Population Structure and Genetic Disorders* (ed. A. W. Eriksson, H. R. Nevanlinna, P. L. Workman, and R. K. Norio), pp. 680–682. London: Academic Press, 1980.

Niaudet, P. and Rötig, A. (1997). The kidney in mitochondrial cytopathies. *Kidney International* **51**, 1000–1007.

Norden, G., Frimans, S., Frisenette-Finch, C., Persson, H., and Karlberg, I. (1991). Renal transplantation in the Bardet–Biedl syndrome, a form of Laurence–Moon–Biedl syndrome. *Nephrology, Dialysis, Transplantation* **6**, 982–983.

Parfrey, P. S., Davidson, W. S., and Green, J. S. (2002). Clinical and genetic epidemiology of inherited renal disease in Newfoundland. *Kidney International* **61**, 1925–1934.

Pober, B. Smith–Lemli–Opitz syndrome. In *Birth Defects Encyclopedia* (ed. M. L. Buyse), pp. 1570–1572. Dover, MA: Blackwell Scientific, 1990.

Powell, C. M. and Michaelis, R. C. Townes–Brocks syndrome. *Journal of Medical Genetics* **36**, 89–93.

Price, D., Gartner, J. G., and Kaplan, B. S. (1981). Ultrastructural changes in the glomerular basement membrane of patients with Laurence–Moon–Biedl–Bardet syndrome. *Clinical Nephrology* **16**, 283–288.

Ritchie, G., Jequier, S., and Lussier-Lazaroff, J. (1988). Prenatal renal ultrasound of Laurence–Moon–Biedl syndrome. *Pediatric Radiology* **19**, 65–66.

Rose, W., Koban, F., Hornak, H., and Bleyl, D. (1987). Traitement d'une insuffisance rénale chronique associée à une acro-ostéolyse héréditaire par hémodialyse itérative. *La Presse Médicale* **16**, 1850–1853.

Rötig, A. *et al.* (1994). Deletion of mitochondrial DNA in a case of early-onset diabetes mellitus, optic atrophy and deafness (Wolfram syndrome, MIM 222300). *Journal of Clinical Investigation* **91**, 1095–1098.

Rötig, A. *et al.* (1995). Renal involvement in the mitochondrial disorders. *Advances in Nephrology* **24**, 367–378.

Rumpelt, H. J. and Michl, W. (1979). Selective vitamin B$_{12}$ malabsorption with proteinuria (Imerslund–Majman–Gräsbeck syndrome): ultrastructural examinations on renal glomeruli. *Clinical Nephrology* **11**, 213–217.

Salameh, M. M., Banda, R. W., and Mohdi, A. A. (1991). Reversal of severe neurological abnormalities after vitamin B$_{12}$ replacement in the Imerslund–Gräsbeck syndrome. *Journal of Neurology* **238**, 349–350.

Salerno, A., Kohlhase, J., and Kaplan, B. S. (2000). Townes–Brocks syndrome and renal dysplasia: a novel mutation in the SALL1 gene. *Pediatric Nephrology* **14**, 25–28.

Salomon, R. *et al.* (2001). PAX2 mutations in oligomeganephronia. *Kidney International* **59**, 457–462.

Sanyanusin, P., Schimmenti, L. A., Ward, T. A., Pierpont, M. E. M., Sullivan, M. J., Dobyns, W. B., and Eccles, M. R. (1995). Mutation of the *PAX2* gene in a family with optic nerve colobomas, renal anomalies and vesicoureteral reflux. *Nature Genetics* **9**, 358–364.

Sato, H., Saito, T., Kurosawa, K., Ootaka, T., Furuyama, T., and Yoshinaga, K. (1988). Renal lesions in Cockayne syndrome. *Clinical Nephrology* **29**, 206–209.

Schachat, A. P. and Maumenee, I. H. (1982). Bardet–Biedl syndrome and related disorders. *Archives of Ophthalmology* **100**, 285–288.

Schonck, M., Hoorntje, S., and Van Hoofff, J. (1998). Renal transplantation in Alagille syndrome. *Nephrology, Dialysis, Transplantation* **13**, 197–199.

Spinner, N. B. (1999). Alagille syndrome and the Notch signaling pathway: new insights into human development. *Gastroenterology* **116**, 1257–1260.

Spinner, N. B. (2001). Jagged1 mutations in Alagille syndrome. *Human Mutation* **17**, 18–33.

Spitler, L. E., Wray, B. B., Mogerman, S., Miller, J. J., O'Reilly, R. J., and Lagios, M. (1980). Nephropathy of the Wiskott–Aldrich syndrome. *Pediatrics* **66**, 391–398.

Standen, G. R., Lillicrap, D. P., Matthews, N., and Bloom, A. L. (1986). Inherited thrombocytopenia, elevated serum IgA and renal disease: identification as a variant of the Wiskott–Aldrich syndrome. *Quarterly Journal of Medicine* **59**, 401–408.

Strassburg, A., Schirg, E., and Ehrich, H. H. H. (2001). A child with polycystic kidney disease: do we have to care about associated malformations? *Nephrology, Dialysis, Transplantation* **16**, 1942–1944.

Szabolcs, M. J. *et al.* (1994). Mitochondrial DNA deletion: a cause of chronic tubulointerstitial nephropathy. *Kidney International* **45**, 1388–1396.

Tieder, M., Levy, M., Gubler, M. C., Gagnadoux, M. F., and Broyer, M. (1982). Renal abnormalities in the Bardet–Biedl syndrome. *International Journal of Pediatric Nephrology* **3**, 199–203.

Tint, G. S. *et al.* (1994). Defective cholesterol biosynthesis associated with the Smith–Lemli–Opitz syndrome. *New England Journal of Medicine* **330**, 107–113.

Torralbo, A., Nebro, S., Remartínez, E., Martínez-Sanz, F., and León, F. (1995). Morning glory optic disc anomaly associated with chronic renal disease. *Nephrology, Dialysis, Transplantation* **10**, 1762–1764.

Uttley, J., MacDonald, M. K., and Uttley, U. (1975). Renal ultrastructure in the Imerslund syndrome. *9th Meeting of the European Society of Paediatric Nephrology*, Cambridge, abstract, p. 58.

Van Esch, H. *et al.* (2000). GATA3 haplo-insufficiency causes human HDR syndrome. *Nature* **406**, 419–422.

Van Hoffen, A., Natarajan, A. T., Mayne, L. V., Van Zeeland, A. A., Mullenders, L. H., and Venema, J. (1993). Deficient repair of the transcribed strand of active genes in Cockayne syndrome. *Nucleic Acids Research* **21**, 5890–5895.

van't Hoff, W. G. *et al.* (1998). Combined liver-kidney tansplantation in methylmalonic acidemia. *Journal of Pediatrics* **132**, 1043–1044.

Verroust, P. J., Kozyraki, R., Hammond, T. G., Moestrup S. K., and Christensen, E. I. (2000). Physiopathologic role of cubilin and megalin. *Advances in Nephrology* **30**, 127–145.

Wallace, D. C. (1994). Mitchondrial DNA sequence variation in human evolution and disease. *Proceedings of the National Academy of Sciences of the United States of America* **91**, 8739–8746.

Weaver, R. G., Cashwell, L. F., Lorentz, W., Whiteman, D., Geisinger, K. R., and Ball, M. (1988). Optic nerve coloboma associated with renal disease. *American Journal of Medical Genetics* **29**, 597–605.

Webb, M. C., Andrews, P. A., Koffman, C. G., and Cameron, J. S. (1993). Renal transplantation in Wiskott–Aldrich syndrome. *Transplantation* **56**, 747–748, 1585.

Webster, D. R., Becroft, D. M. O., and Suttle, D. P. Hereditary orotic aciduria and other disorders of pyrimidine metabolism. In *The Metabolic and Molecular Bases of Inherited Disease* 7th edn. (ed. C. L. Scriver, A. L. Beaudet, W. S. Sly, and D. Valle), pp. 1799–1837. New York: McGraw-Hill, 1995.

Widdershoven, J., Monnens, L., Assmann, K., and Cremers, C. (1983). Renal disorders in the branchio-oto-renal syndrome. *Helvetica Paediatrica Acta* **38**, 654–657.

Williams, B., Jenkins, D., and Walls, J. (1988). Chronic renal failure: an important feature of the Laurence–Moon–Biedl syndrome. *Postgraduate Medical Journal* **64**, 462–464.

Xu, P.-X., Adams, J., Peters, H., Brown, M. C., Heaney, S., and Maas, R. (1999). Eya1-deficient mice lack ears and kidneys and show abnormal apoptosis of organ primordia. *Nature Genetics* **23**, 113–117.

Yamagata, K. *et al.* (2000). Prevalence of japanese dialysis patients with an A-to-G mutation at nucleotide 3243 of the mitochondrial tRNA[Leu(UUR)] gene. *Nephrology, Dialysis, Transplantation* **15**, 385–388.

17

The patient with structural and congenital abnormalities

17.1 The development of the kidney and renal dysplasia

Seppo Vainio

Introduction

The complex structure of the kidney, which is critical for its physiological function, develops during embryogenesis as a result of sequential and reciprocal cell and tissue interactions between epithelial and mesenchymal tissues, namely the epithelial Wolffian duct-derived ureteric bud and the metanephric mesenchyme (Saxén 1987). The mesenchyme develops from the subdomain of the inner tissue layer in the embryo, the mesoderm called the intermediate mesoderm. The kidney is one of the organs in the body that builds its functional unit, the nephron, initially from mesenchymal cells as a result of mesenchymal–epithelial transformation.

The kidney is not only a central organ for excreting most metabolic end-products and controlling the concentrations of the constituents of the body fluids, but due to its mode of development, it is also an excellent model system for investigating many fundamental questions in developmental biology. These include epithelial branching morphogenesis, inductive tissue interactions, differentiation, cell polarization, mesenchymal-to-epithelial transformation, pattern formation, how the segments of the nephron are specified and how nephrons become spatially organized during organogenesis.

The classic work on kidney organogenesis has characterized the cellular fundamentals of kidney development and the gene targeting technique in embryonic stem cells by which the functions of specific genes are inactivated, and work with mice derived from such cells has subsequently begun to reveal the genetic, molecular and cellular mechanisms by which the kidney is assembled. This chapter described the steps involved in kidney morphogenesis and goes on to characterize some of the essential genes that control the early steps.

Assembly of the kidney during development

The adult mammalian kidney, the metanephros, develops mainly from two tissues, the Wolffian duct and the metanephric mesenchyme. Both are derived from the intermediate mesoderm. Prior to the developmental stages in which it gives rise to one of the early tissues of the metanephros, the ureteric bud, the Wolffian duct contributes to the formation of two transient kidney-like organs, called the the pronephros and mesonephros (Fig. 1). The pronephros is apparently non-functional in mammals, but contributes to the development of the second embryonic kidney, the mesonephros. Like the pronephros, the mesonephros is a transient organ and one of its major functions is to provide cells for the developing gonad.

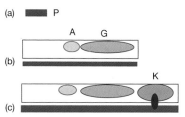

Fig. 1 Organogenesis of the urogenital system. Three kidneys develop during embryogenesis. (a) The pronephros is non-functional and generates the Wolffian duct, which elongates caudally and contributes to the development of the mesonephros. (b) The mesonephros is also a transient organ and plays an important role in generation of the cortical cells of the adrenal gland and the somatic cells of the gonad. (c) Development of the metanephric kidney starts when the ureteric bud forms in the caudal region of the Wolffian duct. Left, anterior; right, posterior; P, pronephros; A, adrenal gland; G, gonad; and K, metanephric kidney.

The initiation of metanephric kidney development is critically dependent on the Wolffian duct once this has extended caudally along the body axis and produced an outgrowth of the ureteric bud (Fig. 1). The ureteric bud is an epithelial tissue that invades the metanephric blastema, around E10.5–11 in the mouse and E35–E37 in humans (Fig. 2). On invading this predetermined mesenchymal tissue, it induces the mesenchymal cells that surround it to condense to form a cap of closely associated cells in the nephrogenic mesenchyme. Even though not yet proven *in vivo*, it is likely that the nephrogenic mesenchmal cells have some stem cells that contribute to the generation of the nephron. The metanephric mesenchyme apparently is capable of producing around 15 epithelial cell types occurring in the kidney.

The stroma is the third tissue type alongside the epithelium and mesenchyme that develops at the periphery of the kidney, and later also in between the ureteric branches. The function of the condensed mesenchymal cells adjacent to the ureteric bud is to induce it to branch, usually forming two new tips, and to begin to form pretubular aggregates at specific spatial positions in the developing kidney which then undergo a mesenchyme-to-epithelial transition to form an epithelial tubule (Fig. 2).

The assembled epithelialized tubule generates the nephron in a number of stages. First it develops into a comma-shaped body, which then becomes an S-shaped body. This in turn will form the glomerulus, proximal tubule, and distal tubule, while the middle part grows into the loop of Henle. The S-shaped body fuses with the ureteric bud, which branches several times during organogenesis (Fig. 3).

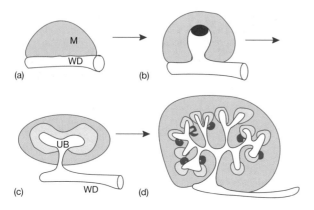

Fig. 2 Early stages of kidney development. (a) Kidney development may be initiated by signals from the nephrogenic mesenchymal cells to induce ureteric bud formation on the Wolffian duct. (b) The ureteric bud invades the metanephric mesenchyme and the tip (in magenta) induces condensation of the kidney mesenchyme. (c) The condensate (blue area) goes on to assemble tubules, whereas the peripheral mesenchyme contributes to the generation of stromal cells. (d) During ureter branching mesenchymal cells are induced in each epithelial tip region (blue areas) in order to initiate epithelial transformation to form nephrons. WD, Wolffian duct; M, metanephric mesenchyme; and UB, ureteric bud.

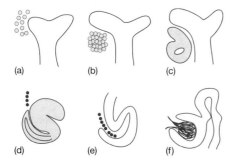

Fig. 3 Steps in nephrogenesis. (a) The condensed mesenchyme (violet area) adjacent to ureteric bud forms a mesenchymal pretubular aggregate, (b) transforms to epithelium and generates the nephron via (c) comma-shaped and (d) S-shaped bodies. The epithelializing body fuses to a branch of the ureteric bud and the endothelial cells migrate in connection with morphogenesis (d) and contribute to glomerulogenesis (e).

Once each ureteric bud has elongated and branched in the course of morphogenesis to generate new epithelial tips, each tip acts as an inductive centre to initiate nephrogenesis. The ureteric bud will generate the duct system that collects the urine into the renal pelvis and urinary bladder, and the process of tubule induction is repeated during its branching to generate approximately the 12,000 nephrons in the mouse kidney and half a million to a million nephrons in its human counterpart. Nephrogenesis is complete by birth in humans, but continues postnatally in the rat and mouse. The endothelial cells, which not only invade the kidney at the initiation of its development but also develop from the kidney mesenchyme, contribute to the formation of the functional nephron (Fig. 3). The early aspects of kidney organogenesis can also be studied *in vitro*, in an organ culture situation (Fig. 4).

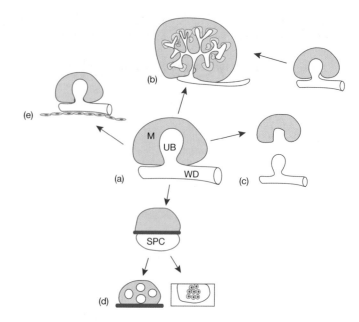

Fig. 4 Organ culture methods for assaying kidney development. Embryonic kidneys can be cultured in several ways *in vitro*. (a) If an E11 mouse organ rudiment consisting of a ureteric bud and mesenchyme is cultured, bud branches and nephrons begin to form within 3–7 days (b). (c) The ureteric bud and kidney mesenchyme can be separated by treating the rudiment enzymatically and cultured together again. Tissues of different genetic backgrounds can also be used. An isolated kidney mesenchyme (c) can be induced with a piece of embryonic dorsal spinal cord (SPC) in a transfilter culture (d). SPC can irreversibly induce a kidney mesenchyme within 24 h, such that the mesenchyme will form tubules in subculture (left). This approach also allows induced mesenchymal cells to be dissociated and reaggregated in a hanging drop assay. Induced mesenchymal cells also form epithelial tubules in such cultures (right). (e) The whole kidney, or the induced mesenchyme, can be placed on a chorioallantois membrane from a developing chick or under the kidney capsule of an adult mouse, whereupon the host will provide the endothelial cells. M, metanephric mesenchyme; UB, ureteric bud; SPC, dorsal part of the spinal cord; and WD, Wolffian duct.

Initiation of kidney development by mesenchymal signals

The results of both classic and more recent studies are consistent with the notion that kidney mesenchyme initiates organogenesis by inducing formation of the ureteric bud (Saxén 1987). However, as it has been seen in some other developing organ systems such as the tooth that the potential to induce morphogenesis resides first in the epithelium, the possibility should also be considered that organogenesis in the kidney may be induced initially by signalling derived from the Wolffian duct prior to outgrowth of the ureteric bud from it. What is known about the genes that determine the metanephric kidney in the first place, and what are the secreted signals that initiate kidney organogenesis?

We have some idea about the sequential interactions that coordinate the formation of the ureteric bud. Some of the genes that are functional during early kidney development are summarized in Table 1. The Wilms' tumour suppressor gene, *Wt1*, encodes a transcription factor that has several isoforms, each of which appears to have a different role in the developing urogenital system that generates the kidney, gonad, and adrenal gland (Schedl and Hastie 2000). *Wt1* was one of the first genes to yield a kidney-related phenotype upon experimental mutation in transgenic mice *in vivo*. The mutant forms of *WT1* can lead to kidney tumours in children and to Wilms' tumour,

Anixidia, genito urinary abnormalities or gonadoblastoma, and mental retardation syndrome, Denys–Drash syndrome, and Frasier syndrome, which involve gonadal and kidney abnormalities, in humans generally (Davies *et al.* 1999; Parker *et al.* 1999).

Wt1 transcripts appear in the condensing metanephric mesenchymal cells. Interestingly, the mesenchyme forms in *Wt1* knock-out mice, but the ureteric bud does not grow out of the Wolffian duct and the metanephric blastema degenerates as a result of apoptosis. As a transcription factor, *Wt1* may contribute to the initiation of kidney development by regulating the expression of secreted factors mediating the mesenchymal signalling required to induce ureter bud formation. Amphiregulin, a member of the epidermal growth factor (egf) family of secreted signals, is one direct target of *Wt1*, but is unlikely to serve as an inductive signal for mesenchyme to epithelium transformation, as blocking of its activity in organ culture with an antibody does not prevent early ureteric bud development, for example (Vainio and Lin 2002). Hence, the precise mechanism by which *Wt1* is involved in the initiation of kidney development remains to be elucidated.

The paired homeobox gene *Pax2* is another gene that has been shown to be critical for kidney morphogenesis, and it is also regulated by *Wt1*. As *Pax2* expression is reduced in the kidney mesenchyme of *Wt1* mutant embryos, these proteins may interact to regulate the initiation of kidney development, although further studies are needed to demonstrate this more directly. Like *Wt1*, there is evidence that *Pax2* may also contribute to the initiation of kidney morphogenesis by controlling the expression of a signalling molecule of the transforming growth factor (tgf)β family, namely glial cell line-derived neurotrophic factor (Gdnf). *Gdnf* expression is lost from kidney mesenchyme in the absence of *Pax2*, which may directly bind to the promoter of *Gdnf*, as it also regulates *Gdnf* transcription *in vitro*, further suggesting a direct interaction between these molecules (Dressler and Woolf 1999; Vainio and Lin 2002). A regulatory element in the *Pax2* gene is sufficient to drive reporter gene expression in the intermediate mesoderm and Wolffian duct derivatives (Fig. 5).

Gene targeting experiments in the mouse have also pointed to a critical role for *Gdnf* in kidney induction. This gene is expressed in the kidney mesenchyme prior to induction of the ureteric bud, and its depletion prevents the bud from forming, indicating that it is an important signal for the induction of ureteric bud outgrowth. Furthermore, as local application of *Gdnf*-releasing beads to the side of the Wolffian duct in organ culture *in vitro* induces supernumerary ureteric buds, *Gdnf* is evidently a significant signal for the induction of

Table 1 Genes that are essential for early kidney development

Gene name	Tissue expressing it[a]	Phenotype
Transcription factors		
Emx2	U, MM	Kidneys, UB, genital tract completely missing
Eya1	MM	Absence of UB growth and failure of MM induction
Foxc1	MM	Two kidneys and double UBs
Foxd1	S	Mutant kidneys are small, few nephrons, fused longitudinally
Pax2	U, MM	Deficient UB outgrowth, MM uninduced
RARα and RARβ2	U, S, MM	Hypoplasia/agenesis
Sall1	MM	Incomplete UB outgrowth, failure
Wt1	MM	MM undergoes irreversible apoptosis tubule formation, apoptosis
Growth factors		
Bmp4	MM	+/− Hypo/dysplastic kidneys, hydroUB, ectopic uterovesical junction, double collecting duct
Bmp7	U, MM	Severe hypoplasia with few nephrons and collecting duct(??)
Fgf7	S	Small kidneys, less UB branches and nephrons
Gdnf	MM	No kidney, as UB bud fails to grow
Wnt4	MM	Failure of kidney tubule formation
Growth factor/receptor		
Gfrα1	U, MM	Kidney agenesis, as with *Ret* and *Gdnf*
Notch2	MM[b]	Glomerular defects
Ret	U	Failure of UB growth
Proteoglycans and their biosynthetic enzymes		
Hs2st	U, MM	Renal agenesis due to lack of U branching and mesenchymal condensation
Glypican3	U, MM	Selective degeneration of medullary collecting duct

[a] Expression at later steps of nephrogenesis not indicated.

[b] In maturing nephron and glomerulae. For original references, see Vainio and Lin 2002.

UB, ureteric bud; MM, metanephric mesenchyme; S, stromal cells.

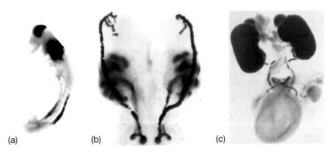

(a)   (b)   (c)

Fig. 5 A promoter for gene expression in the intermediate mesoderm and ureteric bud. A genomic region upstream of the start site of the *Pax2* gene is sufficient to drive reporter (*LacZ*) gene expression in the caudal part of the intermediate mesoderm (a), the Wolffian duct and its derivatives (b), and the ureteric bud and collecting duct (c).

ureteric bud formation and later for the regulation of bud branching. The findings that *Gdnf* is still expressed in *Wt1*-deficient kidneys that lack a ureteric bud and that it does not induce branching in isolated buds suggest that other factors contribute to the regulation of ureteric bud formation alongside *Gdnf* (Sariola 2001; Davies and Fisher 2002).

Apart from *Pax2*, *Gdnf* expression in the kidney mesenchyme may also be regulated by *Eya1*, which is a homologue of the *Drosophila* eyes absent (*Eya*) gene, which encodes yet another transcription factor belonging to the homeobox gene family. A mutation in *Eya* underlies human branchio-oto-renal (BOR) syndrome. As in the case of *Wt1*, *Pax2* and *Gdnf*-mutant embryos, the ureteric bud fails to form in *Eya1* null mouse embryos. The expression of *Gdnf* is also lost in the absence of *Eya1*, but *Pax2* expression persists in the mesenchyme. Hence, *Eya1* may function upstream of *Gdnf* but downstream of *Pax2* in mesenchyme to regulate *Gdnf* expression and the initiation of kidney development (Abdelhak *et al.* 1997; Xu *et al.* 1999).

Recent studies have indicated an essential role for *SallI* in the assembly of the kidney, as *SallI*-deficient embryos exhibit incomplete ureteric bud outgrowth and failure of tubule formation. *SallI* is a mammalian homologue of the Drosophila region-specific homeotic gene *Spalt* (*SalI*) and apparently other genes at the genomic level. Heterozygous *SAL1* mutations in humans lead to Townes–Brocks syndrome, which is an autosomal dominant disease characterized by dysplastic ears, preaxial polydactyly, an imperforate anus and kidney and heart anomalies. Interestingly, even though *SallI* is expressed in the kidney mesenchyme, the mutant mesenchyme can form tubules when induced by spinal cord tissue *in vitro* (see Fig. 4).

Hence, the defect in the knock-out is somehow reflected in the ureteric bud. As *Gdnf*, *Eya1*, and *Wt1* are still expressed in the *SallI* knock-out mesenchyme, *SallI* may be located functionally downstream of these signals, or possibly in a separate pathway (Kohlhase 2000; Nishinakamura *et al.* 2001).

The last of the currently identified genes to be discussed whose function is essential for the induction of kidney development is the transcription factor of the forkhead/winged-helix family *Foxc1*. Like most of the other genes discussed here, *Foxc1* is expressed in the kidney mesenchyme and mutations are associated with Axenfeld–Rieger malformations, involving defects in the eye in humans. *Foxc1* appears to be located at the site where the ureteric bud forms, as double ureteric buds and kidneys can form in *Foxc1*-deficient embryos. *Foxc1* can normally repress *Gdnf* and *Eya1* in the anterior region of the nephric mesenchyme and serve to localize the specific site of ureteric bud formation (Kume *et al.* 2000; Vainio and Lin 2002).

We can conclude that kidney induction involves several different genes, and separate molecular pathways may be involved in the induction process. Some may operate by controlling the expression of *Gdnf*, which is involved in triggering ureteric bud formation. The task is to identify the mediator signals and modes of possible interactions. As many of the essential genes encode likely transcription factors, they may also play a role in determination of the kidney mesenchyme as such. We can also expect to gain further knowledge in the future regarding the mechanisms that position the ureteric bud, this being critical for specifying the site where kidney organogenesis is to be initiated (see also Chapter 16.7).

Formation of the ureteric bud

Formation of the ureteric bud is the first morphological sign of the initiation of kidney development. The process starts with a local thickening of the Wolffian duct at E10.5 in the mouse, after which the ureteric bud invades the adjacent metanephric mesenchyme (Fig. 2). Although information on factors that are involved in ureteric bud growth *in vivo* has accumulated in recent years, we still have a poor understanding of how the elongation and branching steps in the bud are coordinately regulated and what signals synthesized by the bud serve reciprocally to regulate mesenchymal differentiation.

Induction of the ureteric bud

The tyrosine kinase receptor Ret is expressed in the ureteric bud and has been implicated in the control of its proliferation and branching. Several lines of evidence indicate that local mesenchymal expression of Gdnf contributes to ureteric bud induction via this Ret signalling. A coreceptor for c-Ret, Gfra1, has also been identified, which is expressed in the ureteric bud and apparently functions in Gdnf signalling, as its targeted mutation in mice leads to a similar phenotype to that observed in *Ret* and *Gdnf* mutants (Sariola 2001; Davies and Fisher 2002). Ret signalling in renal epithelial cells known as Madine derby canine kidney (MDCK) cells leads to loss of cell adhesion, increased motility and the migration of these cells towards a local source of Gdnf via phosphatidylinositol 3-kinase. This may suggest that the Ret/Gdnf/Gfrα_1 system initiates ureteric budding by promoting its targeting towards the mesenchymal source of Gdnf via a chemoattractive mechanism (Sariola 2001; Vainio and Lin 2002). The details of the signal transduction initiated by the Ret/Gdnf/Gfrα_1 complex remain to be elucidated, however.

Growth and branching of the ureteric bud

Once formed, the Ret/Gdnf/Gfrα_1 system may control ureteric bud growth along with other secreted factors, possibly pleiotophin (HB-GAM) (Sakurai *et al.* 2001) and Bmp4. Pleiotophin is present in the mesenchyme and together with Gndf stimulates the branching of an isolated ureteric bud. Thus, these factors are sufficient for controlling ureteric branching *in vitro*.

Bmp4 is another signal belonging to the tgf superfamily and the bone morphogenetic proteins (Bmp), and it is expressed in the mesenchymal cells that surround the Wolffian duct and ureteric stalk. Hence, it is in the right place to regulate ureteric bud growth.

Bmp4+/− mouse embryos can have a range of developmental abnormalities, some of which affect the kidney, probably being caused by misregulated development of the ureteric bud and being similar to human congenital anomalies of the kidney and urinary tract (CAKUT). In organ culture Bmp4 regulates genes that are expressed by the ureteric bud, and also genes located in the mesenchyme, including *Gndf*, suggesting a more complex mode of function in controlling ureteric bud development (Sariola 2001; Vainio and Lin 2002). Current data point to a role for Bmp4 in kidney development, but the mechanism by which it exercises its effect remains to be demonstrated.

There is evidence for the involvement of other types of molecules as well as secreted signals in the control of ureteric growth and branching, as *in vitro* and *in vivo* data also suggest a role for proteoglycans (PGs). These molecules composed of a core protein and sulfated glycosaminoglycan (GAG) side chains have multiple functions and play a role in growth factor signalling and ECM interactions. Cell surface PGs such as syndecans and glypicans and the enzymes that regulate heparan sulfate (HS) side chain biosynthesis have been implicated in growth factor signalling, for example, that of the fibroblast growth factors (fgfs) and

Wnt/Wg (Wingless) (Selleck 2000; Perrimon and Bernfield 2001). If the GAG chains of PGs are removed or altered *in vitro* by drugs that modify their synthesis, the ureteric bud fails to develop. Interestingly, these modifications can also reverse the action of Bmp4 from inhibition of ureteric bud growth to stimulation of branching, suggesting that PGs play a role in controlling whether the ureteric bud is undergoing growth or generating a branch. The specific effect may be mediated by growth factors that are regulated by the PGs, but their nature currently remains unknown (Vainio and Lin 2002).

The suggestion, even though indirect, of a role for specific PGs in kidney organogenesis came from a mouse mutant heparan sulfate 2-sulfotransferase (*Hs2st*) gene. This encodes an enzyme that catalyzes the 2-0 sulfation of GAGs, which is also essential for interaction of the HS chain with growth factors.

The *Hs2st* gene is first expressed in the ureteric bud, but expression shifts transiently to the mesenchymal cells. Embryos that lack a functional enzyme apparently die perinatally of kidney failure, and analysis has revealed that the initiation of ureteric bud branching and mesenchymal condensation is disturbed. As expected, the expression of genes that mark the epithelial tip of the ureteric bud, such as *Wnt11* (Fig. 6), is lost, and that of *Ret* in the ureteric bud and of *Gdnf* in the mesenchyme is reduced. This can be regarded as suggesting that *Hs2st* may modulate the activity or signals leading to the induction of tubulogenesis in the kidney (Vainio and Lin 2002). Hence, signals that are expressed in either the ureteric bud or the mesenchyme may come to function normally as a result of the activity of PGs modulated by *Hs2st*. Another interpretation would be that *Hs2st* may contribute to kidney development by regulating the interaction of HSPGs with components of the extracellular matrix. Such changes could influence processes such as cell adhesion which are probably required for formation of the condensed kidney mesenchyme.

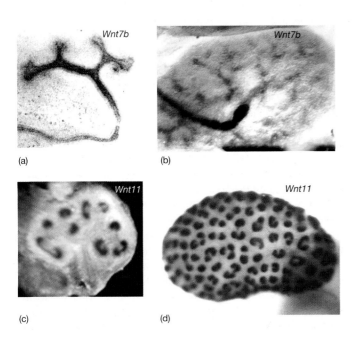

Fig. 6 Expression of *Wnt* genes in the ureteric bud. *Wnt7b* is expressed specifically in the ureteric bud during branching (a) and in the developing collecting duct (b). The *Wnt11* gene is expressed in the epithelial tips of the ureteric bud during branching and is important for kidney development (c, d).

Glypican-3 (*Gpc3*) is a specific PG involved in kidney development that is found in mutant form in humans with Simpson–Golabi–Behmel Syndrome (SGBS) (Grisaru and Rosenblom 2001). Gpc3 is a protein that is not intercalated through the plasma membrane, but is anchored to the membrane by the lipid glycosyl-phosphotidylinositol. *Gpc3* is expressed in the ureteric bud and kidney mesenchyme mainly from E13.5 onwards and appears to have a dual role in the developing kidney. It may control the cellular responses of the collecting duct to growth factors which either stimulate or inhibit its development, as inactivation of its function leads to increased ureteric bud branching in the early stages of kidney development (E12), whereas the distal collecting duct cells proliferate faster than those of the proximal collecting duct at the later stages (E15.5–16.5). Loss of Gpc3 also changes the responses of the kidney to factors such as Bmp2 and 7 that affect ureteric growth and branching in organ culture (Vainio and Lin 2002). Hence, ligands may bind selectively to specific HS sequences and regulate the effect of growth factor signalling in the kidney.

A further interesting feature of Gpc3 is that it is a low affinity receptor for endostatin, a carboxyl-terminal proteolytic cleavage product of the extracellular matrix component type XVIII collagen. Both the collagen and its endostatin fragment are expressed in the ureteric bud, and endostatin applied exogenously under cell culture conditions inhibits the migration response of renal epithelial cells to hepatocyte growth factor and the associated formation of thin processes. Thus, together with its oncogenic receptor c-met, endostatin constitutes another factor that regulates ureteric epithelial branching *in vitro* (Clark and Bertram 1999; Vainio and Lin 2002). The function of endostatin also depends on the presence of Gpc3, and further experiments have suggested a link between these molecules, as blocking of endostatin function with antibodies enhances the outgrowth and branching of isolated ureteric buds *in vitro*, as also seen in Gpc3 knock-out embryos (Vainio and Lin 2002). Hence, endostatin may regulate branching of the ureteric bud via Gpc3 and involve growth factors potentially regulated by Gpc3 that promote branching.

Although the picture of how epithelial growth and branching is regulated is not yet clear, we can list certain critical elements in the process. The Gdnf/Ret signalling system is important for the induction of ureteric budding and its branching, and may be modulated by other factors such as pleiotrophin to contribute to the generation of the specific pattern seen in the ureteric bud tree. Other signals such as fgfs and Wnts may contribute, but this remains to be demonstrated.

Mesenchymal–epithelial transformation and tubulogenesis

One of the aims ever since Grobstein observed that kidney tubule development depends on inductive signals (Saxén 1987) has been to identify the inducers. The traditional view of tubule induction was that mesenchymal cells come into contact with the tips of the ureteric bud and signals expressed by them will induce tubulogenesis. Essential factors for nephrogenesis have now been identified in both the epithelium and the mesenchyme, however, pointing to critical roles for components downstream of that in the ureteric tip.

Inactivation of the function of the *Emx2* gene provided genetic support for the model that maintains that ureteric bud signalling indeed activates kidney tubulogenesis *in vivo*. *Emx2* encodes a homeobox-containing transcription factor which is present first in the ureteric bud, and the bud forms in mutant embryos but organogenesis fails because of a lack of tubules. Although genes such as *Wt1*, *Gdnf*, and *Ret* are expressed in the *Emx2*-deficient mesenchyme, *Wnt4* is not (Miyamoto *et al.* 1997). As will be discussed later, Wnt4 appears to be an important initiating signal for tubulogenesis and lack of its expression is consistent with its critical role in this respect. Thus, *Emx2* may regulate the expression of one or more as yet unidentified ureteric bud-derived inducers in order to trigger tubulogenesis.

Role of Wnt signalling in tubulogenesis

The *Wnt* genes encode a family of secreted signals that are important for key developmental steps during embryogenesis (Huelsken and Birchmeier 2001). Following the discovery in 1994 that *Wnt1* can replace the spinal cord to induce tubules in organ culture assay (Fig. 4), the *Wnts* have been candidates for mediating the induction of tubules in the kidney (Herzlinger *et al.* 1994). However, as *Wnt1* is not normally expressed in the embryonic kidney, its activity must mimic the signalling of some other Wnt that is endogenously expressed in either the kidney mesenchyme or the ureteric bud.

It was also reported in 1994 that *Wnt4* is expressed in differentiating kidney mesenchymal cells, and especially in those cells that will apparently form the nephron (Fig. 7). Indeed, inactivation of its function in mice revealed an essential role in kidney organogenesis. The *Wnt4*-deficient kidney has a clear-cut phenotype, as no tubules are seen, indicating that mesenchymal-to-epithelial transformation has failed (Vainio and Uusitalo 2000). Further experiments also revealed a role for *Wnt4* as an inductive component for tubules, as NIH3T3 mouse cells that expressed *Wnt4* induced tubulogenesis in the kidney mesenchyme *in vitro* (Kispert *et al.* 1998). These cells were also able to reverse the tubulogenesis defect in the *Wnt4*-mutant mesenchyme. Hence, a central role has been detected for *Wnt4*, raising the possibility

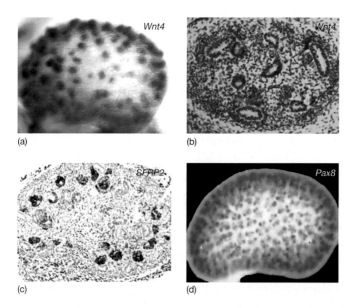

(a)   (b)

(c)   (d)

Fig. 7 Expression of *Wnt4* and some of its target genes during nephrogenesis. (a) and (b) The *Wnt4* gene is expressed in pretubular aggregates whenever these structures generate a nephron. The expression patterns of secreted frizzled-related protein 2 (sFRP2) (c) and the *Pax8* gene (d) correlate with *Wnt4* expression in the developing tubule and may be involved in *Wnt4*-induced tubulogenesis.

that the classic kidney-inducing transfilter assay in which tubulogenesis is induced by coculturing an embryonic kidney with a piece of spinal cord might work because the spinal cord produces a Wnt signal that acts on a downstream tubule-inductive pathway which is normally activated by *Wnt4*. Recently another *Wnt*, *Wnt6*, which has also been shown to be expressed at the tips of the ureteric bud, induced *Wnt4* gene expression and kidney tubules *in vitro*. For these reasons it can be deduced that Wnt6 may function as an epithelial Wnt to trigger tubulogenesis by activating the Wnt4 signal transduction pathway in the mesenchyme (Itäranta *et al.* 2002).

As expected in view of the action of Wnt signalling in the kidney, frizzled receptors for the Wnts are expressed. *Frizzled-4* expression in the chicken correlates with that of *Wnt4* and may function as a receptor for the Wnt4 signal. The expression of secreted frizzled-related protein (sFRP), which can antagonize Wnt signalling by binding the Wnt to activate frizzled receptors, also correlates with *Wnt4* expression in the kidney. Furthermore, *sFRP* expression is also induced in response to Wnt4 signalling and is dependent on its activity. Of the sFRPs, *sFRP1* and *sFRP2* are both expressed in the embryonic kidney, but have different functions, for where sFRP1 may antagonize Wnt signalling, sFRP2 may promote it (Vainio 2003). Hence, the sFRPs may regulate Wnt signalling during kidney development.

Bmp signalling is also involved in tubulogenesis

Apart from the Wnts, evidence is also available to suggest that the Bmps, a subfamily of the *Tgfβ* superfamily of secreted signals, are important developmental regulators of kidney morphogenesis (Hogan 1996). Of the known Bmps, *Bmp7* is the only one that is expressed in the nephrogenic mesenchyme, and embryos that are deficient in this indeed display a phenotype in which the kidney forms normally initially and the ureteric bud branches and comma and S-shaped bodies appear, but nephrogenesis is perturbed from E14.5 onwards (Dudley *et al.* 1995). The expression of genes such as *Pax2*, *Wt1*, and *Wnt4* is reduced in the *Bmp7*-mutant metanephric mesenchyme, and this may be the reason for the increased apoptosis observed in the kidneys of these embryos. The current view is that *Bmp7* functions as a survival factor that prevents apoptosis of the mesenchymal cells and may thus ensure that the kidney mesenchyme does not run out of nephrogenic cells (Reddi 2000). Experimental organ culture results indeed support this idea, as extra *Bmp7* protein prevents metanephric mesenchymal apoptosis. Interestingly, mesenchymal cells are not competent to form tubules even in the presence of extra *Bmp7*, but the growth of stromal cells is induced if Fgf2 is also added to the culture medium (Dudley *et al.* 1999). Based on such findings, it has been proposed that the nephrogenic mesenchyme also secretes signals that promote the proliferation of stromal progenitor cells, which in turn secrete as yet unidentified antidifferentiation and survival signals that control the rate of nephrogenesis.

We can conclude from the analysis of the mouse mutants and other *in vitro* organ culture observations that both epithelial and mesenchymal genes regulate inductive interactions in the kidney (Fig. 8), and that Wnt signalling appears to be critical for tubule induction. We still do not know the nature of the ureteric bud-derived inducer *in vivo*, however, although *in vitro* studies have suggested a role for the leukaemia inhibitory factor (LIF) that is expressed in the ureteric bud as a tubule inducer. In the case of ureter signalling *in vivo*, it may be that one single factor is not sufficient to regulate the diverse functional

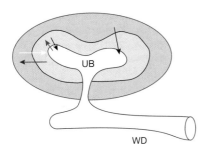

Fig. 8 Inductive interactions in the early embryonic kidney. The tips of the ureteric bud (UB) (blue arrow) secrete signals and initiate the condensation of kidney mesenchymal cells (blue area). The signals involved *in vivo* are not known, but FGFs, TGFα, BMPs, and LIF, which induces kidney tubules *in vitro*, are candidate mediators. Mesenchymal cells, in turn, express signals such as GDNF and pleiotrophin and regulate ureteric bud branching, but initially they control the behaviour of stromal cells at the periphery (magenta arrow). The stromal cells may signal to the tubulogenic cells adjacent to the ureteric bud (white arrow) and to the ureteric bud itself via signals such as retinoic acid (larger black arrow). Most of the signals remain hypothetical at present. *Wnt4* expression in the mesenchyme (blue area) is essential for nephrogenesis, and this signalling induces kidney tubules *in vitro*. WD, Wolffian duct, pink area; stromal zone; and blue area, nephrogenic zone.

tasks of the ureteric bud. The identification of mouse mutants that reveal some essential genes for tubulogenesis, such as *Emx2*, is also expected to help us to find the ureteric bud-derived signals that lead to the induction of nephrogenesis, and in the case of Wnt4 those that regulate tubulogenesis.

The stroma, an important tissue compartment for kidney development

As already noted above, the kidney mesenchyme is likely to generate certain other cell types, such as the stromal cells, which do not participate in the formation of the nephrons or the collecting duct system. Although the manner by which the stromal cells are induced to differentiate in the first place is not known, it is now clear that these cells also perform an important signalling function in kidney organogenesis.

The evidence for the importance of the stroma came from studies of the winged-helix transcription factor *Foxd1* gene (formerly called the *BF2* gene), which proved to be specifically expressed in the stromal cell compartment. Interestingly, inactivation of *Foxd1* function in the mouse generates defects not in the stromal cells but instead in the collecting duct system and the nephrons, which do not express this gene. This finding led to the conclusion that *Foxd1* may regulate kidney development by controlling the expression of a signal emitted by the stromal cells, which then goes on to promote nephrogenesis and ureteric bud branching (Vainio and Lin 2002).

As far as our knowledge of the signals secreted by the stromal cells is concerned, *in vitro* and *in vivo* findings suggest a role for vitamin A, which transduces its signal via the nuclear retinoic acid receptors (Rars). Of the *Rar* genes, *Rarβ2* is expressed only in stromal cells, as also is *Rarα*. Hence, these Rars colocalize only in the stromal cells. That fact that ureteric bud growth is reduced in compound null mouse mutants indicates a role for the vitamin A pathway in the

stroma. Consistent with this reduction, *Ret* expression is lowered in the ureteric bud.

These findings suggest that the stromal cells may secrete a signal such as retinoic acid into the ureteric bud to maintain the expression of *Ret* and in this way contribute to controlling its growth. In support of this, ectopic expression of *Ret* in the ureteric bud in double-mutant embryos rescued kidney development (Batourina *et al.* 2001).

A model can be put forward in which a signalling loop between the stroma, ureteric bud, and kidney mesenchyme may exist to coordinate kidney organogenesis. The possibility remains, however, that stromal signalling may stimulate the activity of the nephrogenic mesenchyme, which then goes on to influence the ureteric bud behaviour via some other reciprocal regulatory signals.

Even though many of the signals that may be expressed by the nephrogenic mesenchyme, stroma, and ureteric bud currently remain hypothetical, there is some evidence to support the notion that Fgf and Wnt signals may be involved. Expression of *Fgf7* has been identified in the stromal cells that surround the ureteric bud and developing collecting duct, and an Fgf7 receptor has been localized in the ureteric bud, suggesting reciprocal signalling. Evidence to suggest a role for Fgf7 came from the analysis of knock-out mice, the kidneys of which have less ureteric branches, smaller collecting ducts and around 30 per cent fewer nephrons. Also, recombinant Fgf7 stimulates the growth of isolated mutant ureteric buds under culture conditions, indicating that Fgf7 indeed functions as a growth factor regulating ureteric bud growth (Vainio and Lin 2002).

Of the Wnts, Wnt2b may similarly play a role in controlling ureteric bud growth, as the gene is present in the perinephric cells upon the initiation of ureteric bud branching. Treatment of isolated ureteric buds with cells expressing *Wnt2b* prior to recombination with freshly separated kidney mesenchyme stimulates the reconstitution of kidney organogenesis in organ culture. These findings suggest that Wnt2b may function as a reciprocal mesenchymal signal regulating early ureteric branching, and knock-out mouse experiments may provide proof of this (Vainio and Lin 2002).

Conclusions and future prospects

The gene targeting approach has been very fruitful in revealing genes that are essential for controlling early kidney development, and it has given us a glimpse of the genetic factors that programme and execute cell and tissue interactions in the course of kidney assembly. Several transcription factors play a role in the initiation of organogenesis, and the question remains as to whether these are involved in specifying the fate of the metanephric blastema by controlling kidney-specific genes. The situation can now be analysed by generating compound mutants, for instance. Methods are now available for rapidly modifying large genomic fragments by homologous recombination to generate mutations in the genome of transgenic mice *in vivo* and to provide further tools for examining kidney development. Hence, we can expect to have access in the near future to more specific ways of studying the functions of other genes specifically during kidney development.

Results obtained with the existing mouse mutants support the hypothesis that kidney development is coordinated by cell signalling between the ureteric bud, nephrogenic mesenchyme, and stroma. The signals secreted by these cell types are largely unknown at present, however, and should be critically addressed, for which purpose cell lines from the kidneys of mouse mutants may prove useful.

As expected, the control of ureteric bud growth and branching involves numerous components, including matrix molecules, growth factors and their receptors, and PGs and their processing enzymes. The details of how molecular interactions between these molecules regulate the pattern of branching and are connected with signalling to the kidney mesenchyme remain to be analysed.

Evidence, nevertheless, exists to suggest a critical role for Wnt signalling in inducing kidney tubules and in the classic model of tubule induction, but we still lack conclusive data on the functional ureteric bud-derived signal/s that control the sequential steps and lead to nephrogenesis *in vivo*. It appears at present that more than one signal is involved, and the current set of mutants that disrupt the initiation of kidney development should allow us to screen these.

References

Abdelhak, S. *et al.* (1997). A human homologue of the Drosophila eyes absent gene underlies branchio-oto-renal (BOR) syndrome and identifies a novel gene family. *Nature Genetics* **15**, 157–614.

Batourina, E. *et al.* (2001). Vitamin A controls epithelial/mesenchymal interactions through Ret expression. *Nature Genetics* **27**, 74–78.

Clark, A. T. and Bertram, J. F. (2000). Molecular regulation of nephron endowment. *American Journal of Physiology* **276**, connection. *Pediatric Nephrology*. **14**, 598–601.

Davies, J. A. and Fisher, C. E. (2002). Genes and proteins in renal development. *Experimental Nephrology* **10**, 102–113.

Davies, R. *et al.* (1999). Multiple roles for the Wilms' tumor suppressor, WT1. *Cancer Research* **59**, 1747–1750.

Dressler, G. R. and Woolf, A. S. (1999). Pax2 in development and renal disease. *International Journal of Developmental Biology* **43**, 463–468.

Dudley, A. T., Godin, R. E., and Robertson, E. J. (1999). Interaction between FGF and BMP signaling pathways regulates development of metanephric mesenchyme. *Genes & Development* **13**, 601–613.

Dudley, A. T., Lyons, K. M., and Robertson, E. J. (1995). A requirement for bone morphogenetic protein-7 during development of the mammalian kidney and eye. *Genes & Development* **9**, 2795–2807.

Grisaru, S. and Rosenblum, N. D. (2001). Glypicans and the biology of renal malformations. *Pediatric Nephrology* **16**, 302–306.

Herzlinger, D. *et al.* (1994). Induction of kidney epithelial morphogenesis by cells expressing Wnt-1. *Developmental Biology* **166**, 815–818.

Hogan, B. L. (1996). Bone morphogenetic proteins in development. *Current Opinion in Genetics and Development* **6**, 432–438.

Huelsken, J. and Birchmeier, W. (2001). New aspects of Wnt signaling pathways in higher vertebrates involved in ureteric bud branching morphogenesis. *Development* **128**, 3283–3293.

Itäranta, P. *et al.* (2002). Wnt-6 is expressed in the ureter bud and induces kidney tubule development *in vitro*. *Genesis* **32**, 259–268.

Kispert, A., Vainio, S., and McMahon, A. P. (1998). Wnt-4 is a mesenchymal signal for epithelial transformation of metanephric mesenchyme in the developing kidney. *Development* **125**, 4225–4234.

Kohlhase, J. (2000). SALL1 mutations in Townes–Brocks syndrome and related disorders. *Human Mutation* **16**, 460–466.

Kume, T., Deng, K., and Hogan, B. L. (2000). Murine forkhead/winged helix genes Foxc1 (Mf1) and Foxc2 (Mfh1) are required for the early organogenesis of the kidney and urinary tract. *Development* **127**, 1387–1395.

Miyamoto, N. *et al.* (1997). Defects of urogenital development in mice lacking Emx2. *Development* **124**, 1653–1664.

Nishinakamura, R. *et al.* (1999). Murine homolog of SALL1 is essential for ureteric bud invasion in organ primordia. *Nature Genetics* **23**, 113–117.

Parker, K. L., Schedl, A., and Schimmer, B. P. (1999). Gene interactions in gonadal development. *Annual Review of Physiology* **61**, 417–433.

Perrimon, N. and Bernfield, M. (2001). Cellular functions of proteoglycans—an overview. *Seminars in Cell Developmental Biology* **12**, 65–67.

Reddi, A. H. (2000). Bone morphogenetic proteins and skeletal development: the kidney-bone connection. *Pediatric Nephrology* **14**, 598–601.

Sakurai, H., Bush, K. T., and Nigam, S. K. (2001). Identification of pleiotrophin as a mesenchymal factor involved in ureteric bud branching morphogenesis. *Development* **128**, 3283–3293.

Sariola, H. (2001). The neurotrophic factors in non-neuronal tissues. *Cellular and Molecular Life Sciences* **58**, 1061–1066.

Saxén, L. *Organogenesis of the Kidney*. Cambridge: Cambridge University Press, 1987.

Schedl, A. and Hastie, N. D. (2000). Cross-talk in kidney development. *Current Opinion in Genetics and Development* **10**, 543–549.

Selleck, S. B. (2000). Proteoglycans and pattern formation: sugar biochemistry meets developmental genetics. *Trends in Genetics* **16**, 206–212.

Vainio, S. (2003). Nephrogenesis regulated by Wnt signalling. *Journal of Nephrology* **16**, 279–285.

Vainio, S. and Lin, Y. (2002). Coordinating early kidney development: lessons from gene targeting. *Nature Reviews Genetics* **7**, 533–543.

Vainio, S. J. and Uusitalo, M. S. (2000). A road to kidney tubules via the Wnt pathway. *Pediatric Nephrology* **15**, 151–156.

Xu, P. X. *et al.* (1999). Eya1-deficient mice lack ears and kidneys and show abnormal apoptosis of organ primordia. *Nature Genetics* **23**, 113–117.

17.2 Vesicoureteric reflux and reflux nephropathy

Kate Verrier Jones

Introduction

Vesicoureteric reflux (VUR) is an abnormality of the junction between the ureter and bladder which is present from birth and associated with an increased risk of urine infections and kidney damage. This type of renal damage was first described as chronic atrophic pyelonephritis, because it was often associated with recurrent or chronic urinary tract infections (UTI) particularly in the preantibiotic era. When a strong association with VUR was demonstrated it became known as reflux nephropathy (RN) or focal renal scarring. More recently, it has become clear that VUR is not always present in children with renal scarring, particularly when scarring is relatively mild (Rushton 1997). Thus it may be more appropriate to describe these focal lesions as chronic pyelonephritis or to use the non-specific descriptive term, focal renal scarring. This chapter is concerned with VUR, its causes and consequences, particularly the associations with UTI and renal damage and the controversies about aetiology, management, and prevention of renal scarring.

Vesicoureteric reflux

Primary VUR is an abnormality of the insertion of the ureter into the bladder that allows retrograde flow of urine from the bladder to the kidney (Hutch 1972). It is present in 1–2 per cent of the population and is almost certainly inherited by an autosomal-dominant mechanism (Report of a meeting of physicians at the Hospital for Sick Children 1996). In children who have been shown to have VUR, the prevalence of VUR demonstrated by radiology decreases with increasing age (Edwards *et al.* 1977; Cardiff–Oxford Bacteriuria Study Group 1979). The importance of VUR is that it is associated with an increased risk of UTI, congenital and acquired renal dysfunction, and other congenital abnormalities including duplex systems, horseshoe kidneys, and ectopic and dysplastic kidneys (Smellie *et al.* 1964; Zerin *et al.* 1993). VUR is not recognized clinically unless imaging investigations are carried out following UTI or antenatally detected renal anomalies, or because of family history of VUR or renal anomalies. The only symptom occasionally attributed to VUR is loin pain, worse with a full bladder or on micturition and relieved when the bladder is empty.

Secondary VUR associated with outflow obstruction or neurogenic bladder is acquired by a different mechanism, primarily related to the increased bladder pressure and subsequent stretching. This is outside the scope of this chapter. Although the aetiology of secondary VUR is different, the consequences are similar with an increased risk of UTI and renal scarring.

Grades of reflux

Reflux has been graded according to the appearance at cystography (International Reflux Study in Children 1985). Grade 1 represents a small degree of VUR into the lower part of an undilated ureter. Grade 2 describes retrograde flow to the renal pelvis in an undilated system and grades 3–5 represent severe VUR into dilated (grade 3) and dilated and tortuous systems (grades 4–5).

Reflux nephropathy

RN is the term used to describe acquired renal scarring in people with VUR (Anonymous 1974) (Fig. 1). Although it is thought that the majority of acquired scars develop following UTIs in early childhood there is increasing evidence that some children with VUR often have congenital dysplastic or hypoplastic kidneys and a few have congenital focal scars without evidence of UTI (Risdon 1993). In these cases there is usually evidence of intrarenal reflux (IRR), although this can be

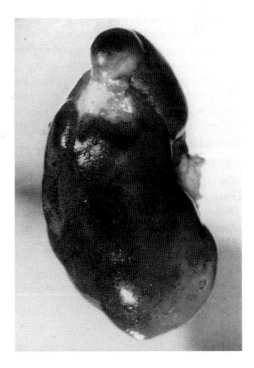

Fig. 1 Kidney removed at postmortem showing a focal scar at the upper pole; reproduced from Clinical Atlas of the Kidney, with permission of Elsevier Science and Professor John Williams.

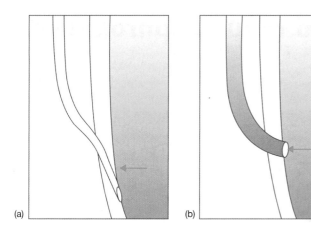

Fig. 2 VUJ: (a) Normal appearance. (b) Showing a refluxing ureter.

missed if appropriate images are not sought (Rolleston *et al.* 1974). RN is associated with reduced renal function, increased proteinuria, complicated pregnancies, hypertension, and chronic renal failure in a few cases (Verrier Jones *et al.* 1989). Understanding the natural history has been made more difficult by the relative insensitivity of ultrasound to the detection of VUR (Mahant *et al.* 2002) or scarring (Smellie and Rigden 1995), the long time lapse between UTI and the development of scars detectable on intravenous urography (IVU) and recent changes in imaging techniques from IVU to ultrasound and ^{99m}Tc dimercaptosuccinic acid (DMSA) scanning.

Anatomy of vesicoureteric junction

The normal anatomy

The normal anatomy of the vesicoureteric junction (VUJ) has been described by Hutch (1972) who gave a detailed account of how the ureter entered the bladder obliquely, with a submucosal and intramural section. Urine does not normally pass in a retrograde direction towards the kidneys because the oblique angle and the submucosal section act as a flap valve. As the bladder expands and the intravesical pressure increases, the submucosal and intramural sections are compressed, closing the valve. The ureteric orifice is usually only seen as a small slit (Fig. 2a).

Anatomy of VUR

In patients with VUR, the ureter enters the bladder at a greater angle, sometimes at 90°. There is only a very short intramural section and little or no submucosal section. In severe cases with high radiological grades the ureter is also dilated and the ureteric orifice is wide open, giving the appearance of a golf-hole orifice. During bladder filling or when exposed to increases in intravesical pressure, the opening widens further allowing large amounts of urine to reflux up towards the kidneys (Fig. 2b). As the child grows the bladder wall becomes thicker and the intramural section lengthens so that VUR tends to become less severe or disappear (Hutch 1961).

Epidemiology

Evidence for the prevalence of these conditions in the community is limited because of the lack of clinical signs or symptoms of VUR or RN. However, much evidence has been gleaned from the routine investigation of children with a history of UTI who are at increased risk of these conditions as well as from children with asymptomatic bacteriuria detected in screening programmes.

Prevalence of VUR in the normal population

The prevalence of VUR has been estimated to be around 1 per cent of the child population (Report of a meeting of physicians at the Hospital for Sick Children 1996). Initially, this was estimated from postmortem studies. Further estimates in recent years were extrapolated from the prevalence in children investigated for VUR because of high risk such as those with a history of UTI, children with a strong family history, and infants studied after antenatal hydronephrosis. In addition, a number of studies have been carried out on healthy children and adults (Table 1).

Postmortem studies

In earlier times the bladder was known to be free of VUR in the majority of cases because water instilled into the bladder at *postmortem* would not usually reflux towards the kidneys when the ureters were cut. The prevalence among people not suffering from UTI or RN was very low.

Imaging studies in normal children

Estimates of the incidence of VUR in healthy individuals has been obtained from studies on healthy volunteers and children earlier in the last century, before the introduction of an ethical approach to investigating healthy individuals including children with unnecessary and invasive tests (Table 1). These studies have been described in detail by Bailey (1979) and Goldraich and Barratt (1987). In addition Booth *et al.* (1975) collected 28 fetal cystograms carried out inadvertently during the course of intrauterine procedures and noted VUR in one fetus in whom VUR was confirmed at 1 year of age. Bailey concluded that VUR was present in between 0.4 and 1.8 per cent of unselected children.

Prevalence of VUR in girls with asymptomatic bacteriuria

Bailey's estimate is compatible with the prevalence of VUR estimated from studies of asymptomatic bacteriuria in girls. Asymptomatic bacteriuria was detected in 1.8 per cent and a third (0.6 per cent of the age-related population) were shown to have VUR (Verrier Jones *et al.* 1986). This is likely to represent an underestimate as asymptomatic bacteriuria is an intermittent condition and will be missed in some girls at a single screening. Girls with VUR and intermittent acute UTIs will not be detected by this type of cross-sectional screening programme. In addition, some girls with VUR do not have either symptomatic or asymptomatic infection at the time of screening. Micturating cystography is thought to have a false-negative rate of up to 15 per cent. Thus, the true prevalence of VUR in schoolgirls could be significantly greater than 0.6 per cent.

Factors causing variation

Age

When serial studies were carried out on children with VUR, VUR was found to improve or disappear with time, although the prevalence among children presenting with first time UTI remains at around

Table 1 Prevalence of VUR in healthy population

Date	Author	Population		Percentage	Comments
1954	Bunge	Children and adults	0/24	0	
1951	Campbell	Children	0/636	0	
1925	Eisendreith et al.	Adults	0/10	0	
		Pregnant women	0/41	0	
1949	Gibson	Children under 12 years	2/43	5	Both children had urological problems
1955	Iannaccone and Panzironi	Infants	1/50	2	VUR not seen on repeat examination
1958	Jones and Headstream	Infants and children	1/100	1	Child had trabeculated bladder
1957	Kjellberg et al.	Infants and children under 13 years	0/101	0	
1965	Litch et al.	Full-term neonates under 2 days old	0/24	0	
1960	Leadbetter et al.	Adult men	0/50	0	
1967	Peters et al.	Preterm neonates under 2.5 kg	0/66	0	
1960	Politano	Children	0/50	0	
1975	Booth et al.	Fetuses	1/28	4	

20–30 per cent. Some of this improvement may be accounted for by the 15 per cent false-negative rate for the detection of VUR on conventional cystography, although some studies have shown a much greater degree of improvement, consistent with maturation of the VUJ with age as described by Hutch (1961).

Gender

Although VUR has been detected more often in girls as a result of investigation following UTIs, there is no evidence that the true prevalence varies between the sexes. The apparent difference is probably related to the mode of presentation to the clinician because the natural history and incidence of UTI is quite different for male and female children. In males UTIs generally occur in the first year of life and VUR, when present, is often more severe than the pattern seen in females. The incidence in girls in the first few months of life is lower than in boys but by 6 months girls experience more UTIs than boys (Lama *et al.* 2000; Nuutinen and Uhari 2001; Cascio *et al.* 2002). In addition, reinfection is much more common in girls than in boys and tends to continue for several years, so that girls come to the attention of general practitioners and paediatricians more often than boys who only occasionally have UTIs or asymptomatic bacteriuria in childhood (Hellström *et al.* 1991).

Race

VUR is said to be uncommon in Black children, but this may be related more to lack of studies than to true ethnic differences.

Prevalence of VUR in high-risk groups

In clinical practice VUR is more common in children with UTIs and infants with antenatal hydronephrosis or a family history of VUR. However, there is no clinical sign that confirms the presence of VUR. In cases where there is a significant risk that VUR is present this can be confirmed by imaging investigations (Kenda *et al.* 1991). Children at risk of VUR are those with UTIs in whom the risk is around one in three (Smellie 1967), those with antenatal hydronephrosis in whom the risk is about one in five (Marra *et al.* 1994), and those with VUR in a first degree relative in whom the risk is around one in two at birth (Aggarwal and Verrier Jones 1989), but falls with age (Kenda and Fettich 1992).

Prevalence of VUR in children with UTIs

The prevalence of VUR in children who have been subjected to imaging investigations following one or more symptomatic UTIs is remarkably consistent at around one in three (Table 2). Similar results were obtained when children were investigated following asymptomatic infection detected in screening programmes. Although the reflux in affected children improves or disappears with time, the prevalence among children investigated following first UTI appears to be independent of age.

Prevalence of VUR in children with antenatal hydronephrosis

In studies carried out because of antenatal hydronephrosis there is a predominance of males because antenatal hydronephrosis is seen more often in boys. VUR is present in around 20 per cent of boys and girls, but there is no evidence for a sex difference for prevalence of VUR within each of the gender groups (Marra *et al.* 1994).

Prevalence of reflux nephropathy (renal scarring)

The true prevalence of renal scarring is unknown but can be estimated from a variety of sources indirectly. It is likely that the prevalence is changing with time since acquired scarring is thought to develop as a result of untreated UTIs in very early childhood. With the advent of

Table 2 Prevalence of VUR in people with UTI

Date	Author	Population	VUR	Percentage	Comments
2002	Cascio et al.	95 infants admitted to hospital with UTI	19/95	33	Patients with antenatal abnormalities excluded
2001	Deshpande and Verrier Jones	Total infants	17/50	34	Audit of an unselected sample. Patients admitted to hospital had significantly more scarring than patients managed at home who were generally less severely unwell
		Inpatients	14/39	36	
		Outpatients	3/11	27	
1996	Dick and Feldman	Systematic review	225/1219	17	Populations studies in unselected children after UTIs. Range of prevalence of VUR 8–40%
1989	Marild et al.	124 Swedish children aged 0.2–6 years with concomitant disease	34/112	30	Children with UTI, with and without concomitant disease diagnosed
		Reflux grade 1–2	26/112	23	
		Reflux grade ≥ 3	8/112	7	
2000	Martinell et al.	111 Swedish girls with acute pyelonephritis followed for 13–38 years	67/106	63	A selected group of high-risk children with recurrent UTI, VUR, or renal scarring
		Women with scarred kidneys	42/52	82	
		Women without scarring	21/55	38	
2000	Verrier Jones et al.	National audit involving 422 children	109/304	36	Unselected sample of children under 2 years admitted to hospital
1973	Savage et al.	Girls aged 5 with asymptomatic bacteriuria	36/104	35	
		VUR grade 1	4/45	9	45 refluxing ureters
		VUR grade 2	32/45	70	
		VUR grade 3	9/45	20	

antibiotics, and, more recently, improvements in the diagnosis of UTI in infants and young children, fewer infants are likely to be left with undiagnosed and untreated UTIs. While it is difficult to prove this there is some indirect evidence from the literature. In particular, it is now rare for a child to be chronically ill due to infected urine.

Imaging in high-risk groups

Estimates of the prevalence of renal scarring can be made from the study of high-risk groups such as those with a history of UTI or asymptomatic bacteriuria. As there is no reliable physical sign and no simple, non-invasive test for renal scarring, estimates are all indirect. A number of classic studies were carried out describing the pathological and radiological appearances of the typical focal pyelonephritic scar (Weiss and Parker 1939) but it is relatively difficult to relate these observations to the population as a whole. In contrast, using studies on girls with asymptomatic bacteriuria, which was detected by screening large populations, it is possible to estimate the minimum prevalence rate in girls from the cases detected (Table 3). Since asymptomatic bacteriuria was present in around 1.8 per cent of the school girl population and a quarter had scarred kidneys, the minimum prevalence in the 1970s was 0.4 per cent. In boys scars tend to be detected earlier, and tend to be less common but more severe in terms of renal function deficit.

Ultrasound of healthy children

In a study of kidney size in children, Verrier Jones et al. (1993) found scars in 4/1000 children giving an estimate of 0.4 per cent. However,

ultrasound is relatively insensitive at detection of small scars and this may be an underestimate. This figure is comparable to that calculated from studies in girls with asymptomatic bacteriuria.

Age and gender

As renal scarring is an acquired and irreversible condition the prevalence within the population as a whole must increase with increasing age. However, because young age at first UTI is an important risk factor for scar formation, individual studies looking at the prevalence of scarring in children of different ages may show the opposite effect. This is because children, usually girls, having their first UTI at 6 years are less likely to have scarring than children who have UTI in the first year of life. Similarly, infant boys have a high risk of UTI in the first few months of life. Many of the boys with severe VUR develop their first UTI at this age and are investigated. First UTIs and recurrent UTIs are relatively uncommon in boys after the first year, and when these occur they are often in boys with normal urinary tracts.

The prevalence of focal scars is lower in boys than in girls reflecting the different clinical presentations. There is a higher risk of scarred kidneys in infant boys who also have a higher incidence of grade V dilating VUR. In girls focal scars predominate and these are thought to be acquired later in some cases (Wennerstrom et al. 2000). This difference is related to the different epidemiology of UTI in the two sexes. Consequently, boys demonstrate a different pattern of scarring with a higher risk of small or globally scarred kidneys (Risdon 1993). In practice, it is not possible to differentiate clinically between kidneys

Table 3 Prevalence of scarring

Date	Author	Population	Scars	Percentage	Comments
1997[a]	Coulthard *et al.*	Children with UTI > 16 years	133/2842	4.7	A population study that includes
		Boys		4.4	inpatients and outpatients
		Girls		4.8	
2001[b]	Deshpande and Verrier Jones	Children having first investigations after one or more UTIs			An unselected group of children referred to as inpatients and outpatients because of UTI
		Total	14/127	11	
		<1 year inpatient	7/42	17	
		<1 year outpatient	0/10	0	
		1–7 years inpatient	6/18	33	
		1–7 years outpatient	1/54	2	
1996[c]	Dick and Feldman	Systematic review of the value of imaging	46/702	6	Variable methods for assessing scars Range 1.6–15%
1989[b]	Marild *et al.*	124 Swedish children aged 0.2–6 years with concomitant disease	10/117	9	
2000[b]	Martinell *et al.*	111 Swedish girls with acute pyelonephritis followed for 13–38 years			
		Initial study mean age 7 years total scars	38/107	36	
		Unilateral scarring	31/107	29	
		Bilateral scarring	7/107	7	
		Final study mean age 22 years total scars	51/107	48	
		Unilateral scarring	37/107	35	
		Bilateral scarring	14/107	13	
2000[a]	Royal College of Paediatrics and Child Health	Children under 2 years with UTI admitted to hospital	34/245	14	
2000[a]	Wennerstrom *et al.*	Children < 15 years following first UTI	74/1221	6	

[a] Intravenous pyelography.

[b] DMSA scans.

[c] UTI, urinary tract infection.

that are small as a result of early childhood UTI and those that are small as a result of congenital dysplasia. This has increased the difficulty of understanding the aetiology of RN.

New scars

New scars have rarely been seen to develop after 4 years of age (Vernon *et al.* 1997) except in children who already have evidence of scarring and VUR. In children with scarred kidneys there is a significant risk of further scarring (Aggarwal *et al.* 1991; Martinell *et al.* 2000). Smellie *et al.* (1985) described 87 children with new scars collected from several centres in the United Kingdom over a wide time period. When new scars occurred they were often associated with severe VUR, recurrent pyelonephritis, and delays in treatment. Wennerstrom *et al.* (2000) showed that girls with acquired renal scarring had significantly more UTIs than those who did not demonstrate progressive scarring. To some extent the lack of evidence of new scars may reflect the fact that new scars can only be seen if repeat imaging studies are carried out. There is no clinical marker for this problem unless complications develop.

National differences

In Sweden sick children are usually assessed at a children's hospital and the diagnosis of UTI in infants has been made promptly for over 50 years. In the United Kingdom the average age of diagnosis of UTI is significantly higher than in Sweden (Jodal and Winberg 1987). The incidence of RN causing chronic renal failure in Swedish children has fallen to almost zero (Helin and Winberg 1980) in contrast to 20–30 per cent in the United Kingdom. Although it is tempting to attribute this to the better management of UTIs in infants and children under 2 years of age (van der Voort *et al.* 1997; Verrier Jones 1999), it is also possible that the difference is related to differences in classification of causes of renal failure.

Radiological diagnosis of VUR and renal scarring

The standard test for the diagnosis and grading of VUR is the micturating cystourethrogram. Other imaging tests have been developed to test for VUR using less invasive methods, either to reduce the radiation dose or to avoid the need for catheterization. Each test has advantages and disadvantages.

Initially IVU was the test for renal scarring and this was used extensively for clinical practice and research until ^{99m}Tc DMSA scans became widely available in the 1980s. Unfortunately, these two tests do not provide identical information and it is difficult to relate experience gathered from IVU to experience with DMSA scans which appear to be more sensitive at scar detection.

Micturating cystourethrogram

This test involves the introduction of a urethral catheter using a sterile technique. Radio-opaque contrast is introduced into the bladder over a few minutes. The method was described in depth by the International Reflux Study Group (International Reflux Study in Children 1985). VUR is recognized when contrast flows up the ureters in a retrograde direction either during the filling phase or during micturition (Fig. 3). It is important to note the appearance of the bladder, since bladder abnormalities, mainly neurogenic bladder, may cause secondary VUR. Similarly, views of the bladder neck and urethra will identify outflow obstruction which is also a cause of secondary VUR. This test has been regarded as the gold standard for the detection of VUR although serial studies have shown a high false-negative rate.

Factors affecting the result

There are a number of factors that can affect the outcome of the cystogram, including the filling rate, the bladder pressure, sedation used, number of cycles performed, extent of screening, and use of general anaesthetic. This is a difficult procedure which should be carried out by a radiologist and nurse experienced in carrying out this test in small children. There are a number of factors that are thought to result in false-negative results (Friedland 1979).

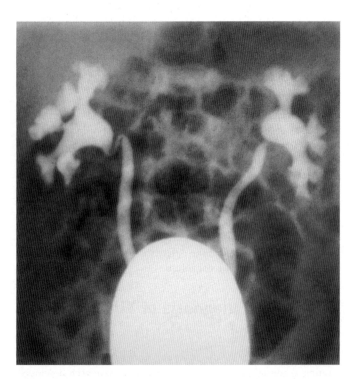

Fig. 3 Micturating cystogram in an infant showing bilateral grade 3 reflux.

In order to standardize the methods used, the International Reflux Study Group published a set of standards to be used by study participants. These standards have been adopted by many specialist children's centres and go some way in reducing the wide variation in practice seen previously. Even using standardized techniques, the estimated false-negative rate is in the region of 15 per cent (International Reflux Study in Children 1985). Contrary to popular belief, there is no evidence that delaying the cystogram for 6 weeks after the presenting UTI is necessary (Craig et al. 1997).

Micturating cystography causes significant distress, particularly after the first 12 months. Repeat investigations are particularly disliked by children and their parents because of physical pain and psychological distress (Phillips et al. 1998).

Risk of UTI following cystography

There is a small but significant risk of introducing UTI at the time of catheterization because it is difficult to ensure sterility around the urethral orifice, particularly in a struggling child. This risk can be reduced, but not completely eliminated, by the use of prophylactic antibiotics around the time of catheterization. In a study in the Northern region in newborn infants, no cases were recorded although no prophylaxis was used, and UTIs in infants may be missed easily or may have been diagnosed and treated but not notified to the study coordinators (Scott et al. 1997). In the Portsmouth area several boys (10 per cent) developed UTIs following cystography (Hallett et al. 1976).

Grades of VUR

Reflux has been graded using a variety of classifications. The system used most often is the International Grading System developed in 1983 by doctors participating in the International Reflux Study. In this classification, VUR was graded using a I–V system (International Reflux Study in Children 1985). Grade I, indicates reflux into the lower part of an undilated ureter; grade II, reflux into an undilated pelvicaliceal collecting system; grade III, reflux into a mildly dilated system; grade IV describes reflux into a dilated and tortuous system; and grade V indicates a very dilated and tortuous system (Fig. 4). Other systems widely used were the Medical Research Council (MRC) grading system (Medical Research Council Bacteriuria Committee 1979).

Intrarenal reflux

This condition, where contrast enters the renal parenchyma by pyelotubular back flow during cystography, is only seen in infants with severe VUR, grade IV or V. It is recognized during conventional cystography only if the upper tract is screened and images taken during active reflux (Fig. 5). It can easily be missed. Areas of renal cortex shown to have pyelotubular back flow have often correlated with areas of focal renal scarring even in the absence of UTI.

Radionucleide studies

Isotope scanning to detect VUR was favoured because of the lower radiation dose involved. However, they do not provide the clear anatomical views obtained from conventional cystography and intravenous pyelography.

Direct nucleide cystography

Direct nucleide cystography can be carried out using a radiolabelled colloid instilled into the bladder following catheterization. The technique is relatively straightforward but VUR cannot be graded by the conventional radiological method although the amount of refluxing isotope can be measured giving a different type of quantification (Conway and Cohn 1994).

Indirect cystography

Indirect cystography can be carried out following the intravenous injection of ^{99m}Tc dimethyl triethyl penta-acetic acid (DTPA) or

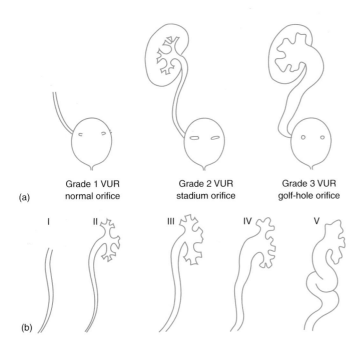

(a) Grade 1 VUR normal orifice Grade 2 VUR stadium orifice Grade 3 VUR golf-hole orifice

(b)

Fig. 4 Diagram of two reflux grading systems: (a) Medical Research Council classification. (b) International grading system.

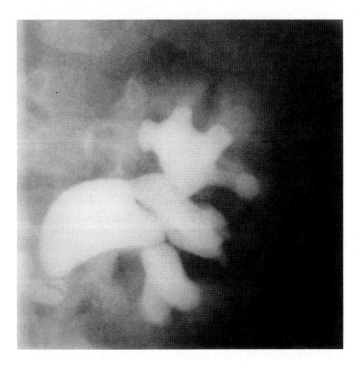

Fig. 5 View of left kidney taken during micturating cystography to show widespread intrarenal reflux.

megalamine (MAG3) (Fig. 6a and b). These isotopes are bound to water soluble substances that are cleared by the kidney and enter the renal pelvis without influence by the tubules. They pass down the urinary tract to the bladder over a period of 2–3 h. Once most of the isotope has been cleared, the child is asked to pass urine while the gamma camera records activity over regions of interest around the kidneys and ureters. If VUR is present, there will be a temporary increase of activity over the kidneys or mid-ureters coincident with the loss of isotope from the bladder. This test avoids the need for catheterization with the associated trauma and infection risk but the success rate depends on the degree of co-operation of the child and other local factors. In some centres it is more sensitive than conventional cystography (Merrick *et al.* 1977).

Ultrasound

Unfortunately, conventional ultrasound is unable to detect VUR (Mahant *et al.* 2002); however, if contrast is used it is possible to

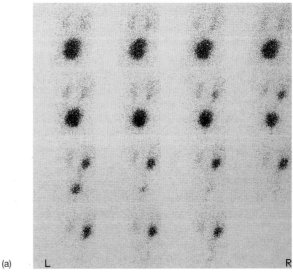

(a) L   R

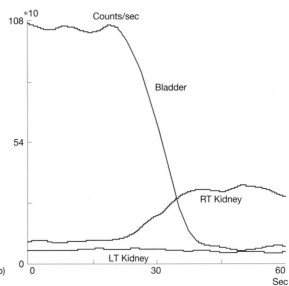

(b)

Fig. 6 Indirect cystogram showing: (a) Sequence of images over 30 min. (b) Counts over the bladder showing an increase in counts over the kidney during bladder emptying.

demonstrate VUR with reasonable accuracy in experienced hands. This has the advantage of avoiding radiation but still requires the use of a catheter. Stable ultrasound contrast media are now available for this technique; however, views of the urethra are not adequate for detailed examination of this area, for example, in the exclusion of ure-thral valves (Darge 2002). Others have had some success with colour Doppler, but this is not widely accepted as a reliable method.

Imaging of reflux nephropathy

Like VUR, RN is a silent condition, only recognized during life if appropriate imaging investigations are carried out. At one time it was considered essential to attempt to identify all scars in children follow-ing the first UTI. However, the disadvantages of overlooking a small scar are relatively small and the cost of ensuring that all scars are detected relatively high in terms of medical resources, stress, and inconvenience to the child and family (Phillips *et al.* 1996; Chambers 1997).

Ultrasound

Although ultrasound is carried out regularly in children following the diagnosis of UTI, it is neither sensitive nor specific for the diagnosis of renal scarring (Stokland *et al.* 1994; Smellie and Rigden 1995). Polar scars, when seen on ultrasound are usually confirmed on other imag-ing tests if they are carried out. It is often difficult to differentiate between a focal scar seen at the mid-pole and an indentation due to a duplex system (Fig. 7). The main disadvantage of ultrasound is that small or developing scars cannot be seen. The report of a normal ultra-sound does not rule out a scar in a young child although this technique is reported to be more reliable for the detection of scars in adults.

Intravenous urography

This was the method used for obtaining views of the renal parenchyma and collecting system for several decades. All the early studies of the aetiology of RN were carried out using this technique. Smellie *et al.* (1964) described classic focal scars, defined as areas of thinned cortex overlying distorted or dilated calices (Fig. 8). Some kidneys showed multiple focal scars, while others, particularly in young boys were smooth and small with relatively preserved calices. The normal renal length using intravenous pyelography and standard views was 3.5–4 vertebral bodies long (Hodson *et al.* 1975). This was a useful way to assess kidney size in growing children.

When bilateral scarring is present, the normal tissue between scarred areas is often hypertrophied, exaggerating the indentations due to focal scarring. Occasionally these hypertrophied areas have been mistaken for tumours. Bilateral scarring is sometimes associated with a significant reduction in renal function. In this situation higher doses of contrast medium are required to demonstrate the renal parenchyma, and tomography may be required to show the kidneys clearly.

The collecting system can be seen within the kidney after a few minutes. The healthy renal calyx should show sharp pointed edges. In the presence of higher grades of VUR the calices lose these sharp points so that they appear to have rounded edges or a blown out or irregular appearance. The ureter is not normally seen to fill through-out its length at pyelography; however, in the presence of VUR of grade 3 or more the diameter of the ureter often exceeds 10 mm and the ureter may be seen as a continuous column. It is not possible to diagnose VUR on pyelography although the features described above may favour the presence of this condition.

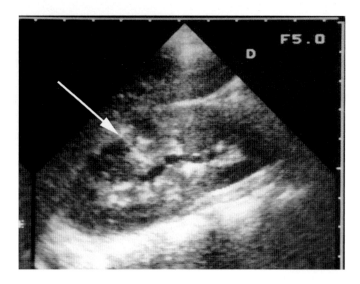

Fig. 7 Ultrasound scan showing a focal scar.

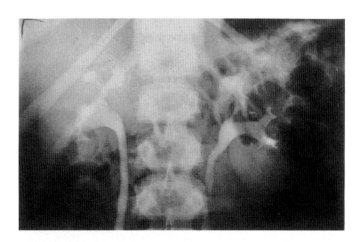

Fig. 8 Intravenous urogram showing significant scarring of the right upper pole. The two upper pole calices are distorted and blunted and the overlying cortex is only 3 mm thick. In contrast, the lower pole shows normal calices with sharp points and the renal cortex is 20 mm thick. The left upper pole is also scarred but the renal cortex is not clearly seen because of overlying bowel gas. Both ureters are unusually full and consistent with VUR.

Dimercaptosuccinic acid scans

Technetium 99m DMSA scans were introduced routinely around 1988. The isotope is normally taken up by the healthy proximal tubules but is not taken up by damaged tubules (Fig. 9). This test has the advant-age over intravenous pyelography as it involves less radiation and is a safer test with less risk of allergic reaction. As the study takes place 2–4 h after the injection it is easier to organize and gain the child's co-operation; however, if the child moves during imaging, the process can be repeated without further injection or radiation. Not only can small focal scars be detected readily as filling defects around the edge of the kidney, but acute focal inflammation due to acute pyelonephritis can also be seen quite clearly.

Unfortunately, it is not possible to differentiate with certainty between acute lesions and permanent scarring so that considerable

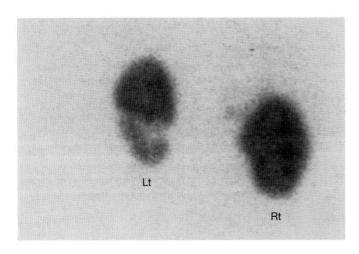

Fig. 9 Technetium 99m DMSA scan showing a small area of loss of cortex at the right upper pole and significant scarring of the left lower pole. Isotope scans are generally counted from the back resulting in a reversal of right and left compared with IVU.

care must be taken to document the date of the most recent infection at the time of the scan. The change from conventional radiography to isotope scanning has complicated the long- and short-term studies on natural history which now appear to produce conflicting results (Smellie and Rigden 1995).

Other imaging techniques

Although renal scarring can be seen on magnetic resonance imaging (MRI) scans or computed tomography, these methods are not used routinely for establishing the diagnosis since the other methods described are more convenient and more readily available. MRI with contrast has been used to demonstrate VUR though this is largely a research tool at present.

Relationship of reflux and reflux nephropathy with UTI

From a clinical point of view VUR is important because it appears to predispose towards the development of both UTI and renal scarring. While VUR is estimated to be present in less than 1 per cent of the population as a whole, the prevalence of VUR in children with a history of UTI is 20–30 per cent and the prevalence of VUR in children with renal scarring is around 40–80 per cent (Tables 1–3). Furthermore, the higher the grade of VUR the greater the risk of scarring.

VUR as a host susceptibility factor for UTI and scarring

VUR may be a predisposing host factor for UTI because bacteria reaching the bladder via the urethra are not eliminated in the usual way during micturition. In the presence of VUR, some infected urine may be pushed up the ureter, only to return to the bladder when it relaxes after completion of micturition, thus providing a sump of residual urine. This increases the opportunity for invading bacteria to become established causing UTI. In addition, infected urine can easily

reach the kidney if VUR is present causing acute pyelonephritis. Finally, the high pressures generated in the bladder are not usually transmitted to the kidneys because the competent VUJ normally prevents transmission of pressure up the ureter. In the presence of VUR, high pressures generated during micturition will be transmitted directly to the kidney which may be damaged by back pressure, particularly if the urine is also infected. In the presence of IRR, infected urine can be introduced into the collecting system and tubules, further increasing the risk of illness and renal damage.

Genetics of VUR

The inherited tendency for VUR has emerged over the last 30 years. The genetic nature of this condition was not immediately obvious because VUR is not recognized clinically and only discovered if a search is undertaken specifically to elicit this condition. The disappearance of VUR with increasing age is another factor that makes genetic studies particularly difficult in this condition. One of the first families to be described is a family from South Wales with five daughters all of whom had UTIs, VUR, and scarring. Three had their ureters reimplanted because of recurrent UTIs and one developed endstage renal failure. Subsequently, several families have been described. Following the identification of an index case the prevalence of VUR in family members falls with age and both sexes are affected equally when investigation is carried out for genetic purposes rather than as part of the investigation of UTI (Kenda and Zupancic 1994). Initially, studies suggested that the inheritance may be multifactorial or dominant with incomplete penetrance. However, when newborn babies are studied in families with an affected first-degree relative, the incidence of affected babies is in the region of 50 per cent with both sexes affected equally, with examples of male and female transmission, consistent with an autosomal-dominant inheritance mechanism (Aggarwal and Verrier Jones 1989).

Reflux nephropathy

Concern about VUR is directly related to the observation that many children with VUR developed significant and progressive renal damage. This damage progressed during childhood and was related to persistence of VUR and intercurrent UTIs. The damage has been regarded as potentially preventable in the majority of cases based on the observation that it is usually detected following UTIs, often in children who also have severe VUR. New scars have sometimes been seen to develop in previously unscarred kidneys when serial imaging studies have been carried out (Table 4).

The term reflux nephropathy was adopted to describe scarred kidneys detected radiologically on investigation for causes of hypertension, renal failure, or following UTI. The term was used because VUR was demonstrated in the majority of cases and was thought to be an important aetiological factor. Previously, this condition was called chronic atrophic pyelonephritis. More recently, the term focal renal scarring has been used as there is some doubt about whether all pyelonephritic scarring is associated with infection and VUR. The aetiology of small smooth scarred kidneys has also been questioned and there is good evidence that dysplastic kidneys are associated with VUR in a large proportion of cases, calling into question the

Table 4 Incidence of new or progressive scars

Date	Author	Population	New scars	Percentage	Comments
1982	Arze et al.	85 adults with chronic pyelonephritis	10/85	11	Four women were said to have had an improvement in appearance of scars
1979	Cardiff–Oxford Bacteriuria Study Group	208 girls with asymptomatic bacteriuria	12/208	5.7	Bacteriuria detected by screening in schools. New and progressive scarring only occurred in girls with scarred kidneys. Follow-up over 4 years
		44 girls with scarred kidneys	12/44	22	
2000	Martinell et al.	111 Swedish girls with acute pyelonephritis followed for 13–38 years			A selected group of patients with recurrent infections, reflux, or scarring followed for a prolonged period
		Progressive scarring	23/107	13.5	
		New scars	13/107	12.1	
		Worsening scars	10/107	9.3	
		Total number of subjects with scars after follow-up	51/107	47.7	
1985	Smellie et al.	74 infants and children who developed new or progressive scars after delays in diagnosis and treatment or prophylaxis	74		A selected group of patients who were found to have new or progressive scarring identified over 20 years
1998	Smellie et al.	226 adults with renal scarring, VUR, and UTI followed for 10–35 years	12/226	5	11 acquired before the introduction of careful medical monitoring
1997	Naseer and Steinhardt	1426 children with acute pyelonephritis	31/1426	2.1	Scars developed in spite of medical care
		Dysfunctional voiding and scars among 31 girls with new scars	24/31	77	Dysfunctional voiding was present in the majority of children with new scars
		Surgery and progressive scarring	17/31	55	Scars developed inspite of ureteric reimplantation in 17/31 children
1997	Vernon et al.	Children with UTI ≥ 3.4 years	5/209	2.4	Age at time of first scan
		Children with UTI > 4 years	0/220	0	Age at time of first scan
2000	Wennerstrom et al.	367/545 children having repeat IVU	40/367	11	All children had recurrent pyelonephritis, VUR, or renal scarring
		Acquired scars in boys	3/84	4	
		Acquired scars in girls	37/283	13	
		Initial VUR grade 0	12/457	2.5	
		Initial VUR grades 1–2	17/176	10	
		Initial VUR grade 3	11/54	20	
1992	Weiss et al.	132 infants and children with VUR and UTI	30/132	26	The US limb of the International Reflux Study
		Medical treatment new or progressive scars	31/65		
		Children having surgical treatment developing new or progressive scars	24/51		
1983	Winter et al.	4000 children with UTIs over 15 years in Canada	37/4000	1	78% of those with new scars had had episodes of prolonged or inadequately treated episodes of acute pyelonephritis
			26/37	32	Children with VUR who developed scars in previously normal kidneys

assumptions about aetiology and the supposition that RN can always be prevented (Risdon 1993). Developmental anomalies associated with VUR may occur in relation to recognized syndromes or as a result of other intrauterine events (Woolf 1997).

Gross anatomy

Pathologists have recognized chronic pyelonephritis for many years and Weiss and Parker (1939) described over a 100 cases. Many of their cases had died young and had evidence of recurrent episodes of acute pyelonephritis, hypertension, anaemia, short stature, rickets, and in women, complicated pregnancies.

Chronic pyelonephritic kidneys are generally smaller and lighter than normal and the outer surface shows one or more contracted fibrotic areas (Fig. 1). The condition may be bilateral. The cut surface of the kidney shows wedge-shaped areas of fibrosis extending from the renal pelvis to the outer surface which is puckered and indented over the scar. The calyx is usually distorted and dilated and the cortical width is reduced. Some kidneys show several scarred areas or are globally reduced in size with universally thin cortex and generalized caliceal dilatation. There may be some abnormal areas showing signs of congenital dysplasia. The collecting system may show evidence of recent infection, although this is less common now that antibiotics are widely available and UTIs are generally treated effectively and promptly. In adults, renal calculi may be present but this is relatively uncommon in children.

Histology

The histological features have been described in detail by Heptinstall (1983). The features represent the permanent renal damage seen as a result of previous acute infection of the renal parenchyma, described as acute pyelonephritis. Focal areas of interstitial fibrosis and tubular atrophy can be seen with a patchy lymphocytic infiltrate. In affected areas glomeruli are sparse and some show signs of ischaemia or sclerosis (Fig. 10). Periglomerular fibrosis is typical of this condition. In some cases, particularly in boys, there may be evidence of renal dysplasia, suggesting that some of the renal abnormalities have been present from before birth. In a few cases there may, in addition, be evidence of active infection seen as bacteria and pus cells in the renal pelvis and tubules or evidence of acute inflammation of the kidney parenchyma with polymorph infiltration. With the widespread availability of antibiotics and careful preparation of patients for surgery,

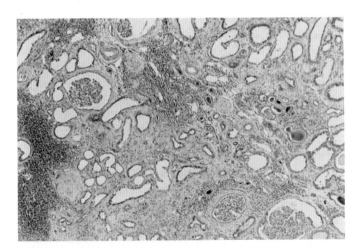

Fig. 10 Area of chronic pyelonephritis from a kidney removed because of reflux, poor function, and recurrent infection. This shows loss of the normal kidney architecture combined with fibrosis and lymphocytic infiltration typical of RN. The normal tubular architecture has almost completely disappeared and has been replaced by abnormal interstitium. Some remaining tubules contain homogenous material giving a thyroid-like appearance. One of the glomeruli is sclerosed, one shows focal sclerosis, and two are relatively preserved but show periglomerular fibrosis (courtesy of Professor G. Williams).

poorly functioning kidneys which are removed because of hypertension or in association with reflux or obstruction rarely show signs of acute infection now.

Pathogenesis of reflux nephropathy

Hypotheses about the causes of RN have been based on observational clinical studies and animal work. Detailed and accurate information in humans has been difficult to obtain because the development of lesions can only be detected during life if sequential and invasive imaging studies are carried out.

Focal lesions visible on ultrasound or pyelography are thought to develop slowly over months or years and the time course for progression to chronic renal failure may continue for several decades. In contrast, the abnormalities seen on DMSA scans can be seen during and immediately after the infective episode. It is likely that the predisposition to this disease starts before birth with the development of VUR in susceptible individuals. Abnormal kidney development is likely to be a factor and dysplastic kidneys are known to be associated with VUR (Woolf 1997).

Evidence from clinical studies

The radiological features of chronic pyelonephritis were described in detail by Hodson and Edwards (1960). They noted, in particular, the characteristic features of the kidneys on IVU and the frequent observation of VUR seen at cystography. The commonest sites for scarring at the upper and lower poles corresponded to the sites for compound papillae that are more likely to allow IRR. This corresponds with observations in animal studies. A number of other studies followed, all of which demonstrated a high incidence of VUR and renal scarring in children with UTIs (Table 1). Although the prevalence of scarring varied between studies, a number of consistent observations were made.

The prevalence of scarring in children with UTIs varied from 4 to 25 per cent, the highest levels being seen in schoolgirls with asymptomatic bacteriuria. In these girls, the prevalence of scarring at initial assessment was similar to the prevalence at final assessment 4–10 years later, suggesting that the vast majority of scars had already developed either as a result of the first diagnosed UTI or before this time, before the initial assessment. This may be because UTIs in early childhood were not detected or treated.

ACE gene polymorphism

Ozen et al. (1999) found that in patients with renal scarring there was an increase in the prevalence of the DD genotype coding for deletion of the ACE gene in Turkish patients. However, Cho and Lee (2002) and Dudley et al. (2002) were unable to confirm this observation in children in Korea or Bristol.

Acute inflammation

The presence of bacteria with certain virulence factors, for example, p fimbria, can trigger an inflammatory response by inducing the influx of polymorphs and the release of inflammatory cytokines. Rolle et al. (2002) recently demonstrated that in children with reflux, nitric oxide may play a significant role in initiating renal damage.

Progression of scarring

It has been postulated that small scars, developing after the first UTI may scar by fibrosis, distorting the collecting duct orifices in the surrounding area, making them more vulnerable to IRR. This could be a mechanism for extension of existing scars.

Screening for asymptomatic bacteriuria

Following the description of chronic pyelonephritis, and its association with VUR and UTI, there was a hypothesis that chronic, unrecognized infection might cause progressive renal damage. Several studies were carried out first in adults and later in children. Large screening programmes were set up in the United Kingdom and the United States and these showed that bacteriuria was common in women but rare in men. Studies in adults showed a relatively low prevalence of RN and little evidence of progressive disease. Subsequently, a second wave of screening programmes was set up aiming to look at the situation in children (Savage et al. 1973). The prevalence of abnormalities is shown in Table 2. Although there was a significant rate of kidney and urinary tract abnormalities with scarring in up to 25 per cent and VUR in over 30 per cent, very few new scars were seen to develop. No child over 4 years with normal kidneys developed scars in spite of exposure, in some cases, to untreated bacteriuria for many years in combination with persistent VUR (Cardiff–Oxford Bacteriuria Study Group 1979). In all these age groups bacteriuria was significantly more common in females than in males, consistent with the observation that focal scarring is seen more often in females.

In a study in infants, asymptomatic infection was found more often in boys. None of the affected infants developed scars although a small number became unwell and were treated for symptomatic infection. The prevalence of abnormalities was relatively low (Wettergren et al. 1990).

Age and renal scarring

Winberg observed the epidemiology of UTIs in childhood in the 1950s. He demonstrated that the commonest age for the first UTI was in the first 2 years of life. He also noted the development of new scars in infants and young children using IVU (Winberg et al. 1975). Subsequently, Berg and Johansson (1983) showed that children who experienced UTIs in infancy were at greater risk of reduced renal function. Vernon et al. (1997) used DMSA scans to show that new scars were unlikely to develop in children over 4 years.

Reflux and renal scarring

The prevalence of VUR in children with scarred kidneys varies from 50 to 80 per cent. Slightly lower rates have been found recently in studies using DMSA scans. Undoubtedly VUR will be overlooked in some children with scars because of the limitations of cystography with a false-negative rate of up to 15 per cent. New evidence suggests that children who develop acute pyelonephritis due to certain p fimbriate organisms develop permanent scars detectable on DMSA scans in the absence of VUR. However, children with these late-onset lesions have not been shown to progress to endstage renal failure.

Diagnosis of UTIs in children under 2 years

In the first 2 years of life, UTI is very common but not easily recognized in the absence of localizing signs in babies in nappies (van der Voort et al. 1997). There is a strong possibility that UTIs in the first years are overlooked and that many infants and toddlers in the United Kingdom with non-specific illnesses managed as viral infections or upper respiratory tract infections have unrecognized UTIs (Jadresic et al. 1993). Similar results were demonstrated by the South Bedfordshire Practitioner's Group (1990) who showed that the recommended steps

were followed in only half of the children demonstrated to have renal scarring. Further evidence for this came from examination of the microbiology database in South Wales. This showed that no samples were collected from infants in primary care over a period of several years and very few were collected from children between 1 and 2 years old.

Additional evidence was obtained by retrospective examination of General Practitioners' (GP) records of children later shown to have UTIs. This showed that children diagnosed with UTIs had previously visited their doctor with non-specific illnesses twice as often as controls (van der Voort et al. 2003). Furthermore, two of the index cases with scars had had laboratory evidence of UTIs filed in the notes but had not been diagnosed according to the medical records or received treatment. Lack of suitable training and facilities in primary care in the United Kingdom for the collection of urine and diagnosis of UTI in infants and toddlers undoubtedly continue to contribute to the development of renal scarring (Verrier Jones 1999). Shaw and Gorelick (1999) also demonstrated the importance of screening for UTI in febrile children in the emergency department.

New scars

Although new scars have been seen to develop relatively infrequently this is hardly surprising since new scars will only be recognized if serial imaging studies are carried out in a susceptible individual (Table 4). Smellie et al. (1985, 1994) studied the circumstances surrounding the development of new scars in two groups of children. She noted that they tended to develop in children with delays in diagnosis and treatment of UTI, children with recurrent UTI, and those with high grades of VUR. She also noted that thorough investigation had not been carried out initially and prophylaxis had not been used at an early stage. A prospective study of this problem would be very difficult to organize for logistic and ethical reasons.

The incidence of new scars appears to fall with increasing age and this led to the assumption that a young or growing kidney was more vulnerable to damage due to UTI than an adult kidney. However, little evidence to support this maturation theory has been produced. This relationship between new scars and young age may reflect the fact that the first opportunities for UTI start soon after birth. Those who are most vulnerable to UTIs and renal damage because of risk factors such as VUR tend to get UTIs earlier than those who are less susceptible who, on average, get their first UTI later. Since VUR seems to be a risk factor for both UTI and scarring and tends to improve or disappear with age, this may be an explanation for the observation that new scars rarely develop in older children.

The tendency for scarring in the early years may be compounded by the difficulty in establishing the diagnosis of UTIs in infants and toddlers (van der Voort et al. 1997; Verrier Jones 1999). This hypothesis has important implications for management since the use of prophylaxis in early childhood to reduce the risk of UTI may simply postpone the time of the first or second UTI and the risk of damage may still be present when prophylaxis is stopped. This has been discussed by Coulthard (2002) following publication of a series of clinical and animal experiments that support his hypothesis. In one study, Howie et al. (2002) demonstrated new scars in adult transplanted kidneys following exposure to UTI and VUR.

Evidence from animal studies

Hodson first demonstrated the characteristic lesions of RN in studies in baby pigs exposed to reflux and infection (Hodson and Kincaid

Smith 1979). Further studies carried out by Ransley and Risdon (1974) using minipigs showed that focal scars could be produced in the presence of reflux and infection and that the size of the scars could be significantly reduced if antibiotic treatment was started soon after the infection became established. They examined the shape of the renal papillae and noted that scars developed in areas of the renal parenchyma overlying compound papillae but not in areas overlying simple convex papillae. They also demonstrated that IRR could be demonstrated in the parts of the cortex draining into compound papillae where scars subsequently developed. They used their observations to postulate that progression of scarring could develop around the edges of the scarred area. As further fibrosis and shrinkage occurred they suggested that the slit like openings of collecting ducts on the convex surfaces might become distorted and allow IRR to occur around the edges of existing scars.

In recent studies using adult minipigs, Coulthard *et al.* (2002) showed that mature kidneys in this model could develop scarring when exposed to VUR and UTI, supporting his hypothesis that the reason new scars are rarely seen in older children is because vulnerable kidneys have usually sustained the first damage at a younger age, when the risk of UTI and VUR is greatest.

Clinical features of reflux nephropathy

There are generally no symptoms directly attributable to the presence of RN which is usually recognized only when imaging tests are carried out because of detection of UTI or a complication such as hypertension, stones, or renal failure. In the United Kingdom RN was one of the commonest causes of chronic renal failure accounting for up to 20 per cent of children and 8 per cent of women. It must be regarded as an important and potentially preventable cause of endstage renal failure. The initial damage appears to be due to UTI and VUR in early childhood, whereas progression to endstage renal failure is due to a separate mechanism involving glomerular hyperfiltration and the development of progressive glomerulosclerosis.

Effect on renal function

As the affected areas of the kidney are non-functional, more detailed assessment generally demonstrates a wide range of abnormalities secondary to glomerular and tubular damage and loss of functioning renal tissue.

Glomerular filtration rate

The serum creatinine and urea are usually within the normal range and the glomerular filtration rate (GFR) may be within normal limits although usually towards the lower end of the range. This is because RN is usually a unilateral condition and the reduced function of the scarred kidney is masked by compensatory hypertrophy of the opposite kidney. When the GFR of each kidney was measured separately using DTPA the function of scarred kidneys was only 31 ml/min/1.73 m^2 compared with 62 ml/min/1.73 m^2 for normal kidneys. The mean GFR for girls with scarring was 99 ml/min/1.73 m^2 compared with 119 ml/min/1.73 m^2 for girls with normal kidneys. Although this represents a loss of functional reserve, this has relatively little effect on everyday adult life, except in pregnancy. However, the effect on health in old age, when GFR tends to decline is yet to be determined (Verrier Jones *et al.* 1982).

Tubular function

During acute infection there is a significant increase in production of markers of inflammation and enzymes which leak out into the urine (Goonasekera *et al.* 1996a). Smolkin *et al.* (2002) demonstrated a significant increase in urine procalcitonin which may prove clinically useful for establishing the diagnosis in infants and children. There is a loss of concentrating capacity due to loss of function of the loop of Henle. In the presence of reduced GFR there is an increased osmotic load in the remaining tubules and therefore the maximum tubular reabsorption of electrolytes and glucose is reduced. Some of the tubular abnormalities seen may represent direct tubular damage in addition.

Some children and young adults appear to have relative salt wasting, and low-normal blood pressure is also seen in some cases, with a tendency to become dehydrated easily when fluids are withheld for surgery or during episodes of gastroenteritis.

Proteinuria

In association with reduction of GFR there is an increase in urinary total protein and microalbumin from an early stage. Yoshiara *et al.* (1993) showed that the glomeruli from kidneys damaged by RN were larger than normal. Similar observations were made by nephrologists in Melbourne who linked this observation to heavy proteinuria, hypertension, and progressive renal failure (El-Khatib *et al.* 1991; Becker and Kincaid-Smith 1993). In advanced cases of RN heavy proteinuria has been observed, occasionally in the nephrotic range. Increasing proteinuria is an indication of deteriorating renal function and heralds the onset of endstage renal failure. These observations fit with the early observations of Weiss and Parker (1939). The use of effective antihypertensive treatment to maintain blood pressure well within the normal range is recommended, preferably with angiotensin-converting enzyme (ACE) inhibitors.

Hypertension

Hypertension has been described in up to a fifth of people with RN. The incidence is relatively low in those with unilateral scarring but occurs in over half of those with bilateral scarring at some stage (Jacobson *et al.* 1989; Martinell *et al.* 1995). It is particularly common in those approaching endstage. Hypertension undoubtedly hastens the deterioration of renal function and adequate treatment is recommended to slow progression. While the hypertension seen in patients with very poor function is generally related to sodium and water overload, in people with unilateral scarring or relatively good renal function hypertension is likely to be due to dysfunction of the renin–angiotensin system (Goonasekera *et al.* 1996b). The juxtaglomerular apparatus adjacent to areas of scarring is at risk of ischaemia and may result in an inappropriate production of renin locally. This can be confirmed by identifying raised levels in the appropriate branch of the renal vein.

Stones

Renal calculi develop in a small but significant proportion of infants with VUR and RN and in a significant number of adults. Some show evidence of idiopathic hypercalciuria in addition to UTI and VUR. Presentation may be varied, passing gravel, severe renal colic, staghorn calculus, persisting or relapsing infection, or obstruction. Stones are often associated with severely damaged kidneys with poor drainage. Surgery or lithotripsy is often required.

Chronic renal failure

RN is an important cause of chronic renal failure and may be the most common preventable cause in children and adults. Precise estimates of the prevalence are difficult because of the problem of establishing the diagnosis accurately once the kidneys have failed. It is likely that changing medical practice has resulted in a reduction in the number of children and young adults reaching endstage due to this condition, but it is likely to account for a significant proportion of cases in the elderly, particularly those born before 1940, when antibiotics became available, or 1960 when knowledge of UTIs in babies started to develop.

Treatment of reflux and prevention of scarring

The management of reflux and prevention of RN has centred around attempts to eliminate VUR and/or to prevent UTIs after the first infection has been diagnosed (Arant 1991). More recently attempts have been made to identify at-risk infants through antenatal screening using ultrasound, followed by imaging soon after birth. In spite of many years of research and large numbers of reported case series, there is little convincing evidence of the value of these strategies. Guidelines for the management of UTI and the prevention of scarring were published in 1991 by the Royal College of Physicians and the traditional view of management is published in a review in the Drugs and Therapeutics Bulletin (Anonymous 1997).

The fashion for surgery to correct VUR started as soon as VUR was identified as an abnormality linked with UTIs and renal scarring. It was hoped that elimination of VUR would result in reduction of UTIs and less risk of renal scarring. In the past decade, the introduction of an endoscopic technique with a submucosal injection (STING) has become popular.

Reimplantation of the ureter

Politano and Leadbetter (1958) described a successful method for surgical reimplantation which eliminated VUR in the majority of cases. Subsequently, Cohen and others described different methods and refinements that reduced the rates of complications and failure to eliminate VUR (Cohen 1975). When carried out by experienced paediatric surgeons, reimplantation is an operation with a high success rate and low complication rate. However, in less experienced hands there is a high risk of complications in the youngest children and those with the highest grades of VUR (O'Donnell 1990). It is now possible to correct VUR using minimally invasive surgery.

Effect on VUR

Surgical correction of VUR is extremely effective at eliminating VUR, particularly using modern techniques. This encouraging outcome must be balanced against the risks of surgery and anaesthesia, the need for serial cystograms immediately before and several months after surgery, and the disappointing results of successful surgery in terms of lack of effect on risk of UTI and failure to prevent renal scarring (Winberg 1994).

Complications

Complications of surgery include obstruction at the lower end of the ureter, urinary leak, acute pyelonephritis in the postoperative period, and other predictable risks of surgery and anaesthesia. These risks are reduced if surgery is carried out by an experienced paediatric urologist with full back up of a paediatric centre with a paediatric anaesthetist and paediatric radiology facilities. Carefully planned pre- and postoperative routines help to minimize these risks.

Infection

It is important to ensure that the urine is sterile at the time of surgery and most surgeons use broad-spectrum intravenous antibiotics to cover the perioperative period. If surgery is carried out on a child with infection of the urinary tract there is a risk of both acute pyelonephritis and septicaemia. A child who is found to have infected urine at the preoperative assessment should be treated for at least 5 days prior to surgery to ensure that the urine is sterile. If the urine infection caused an acute illness, additional time is required for complete resolution of inflammation. However, in children with very frequent infections there is a difficult balance to consider. Acute pyelonephritis following surgery is relatively common if prophylaxis is not used and is associated with the development of new scars (Olbing et al. 1992).

Complications in infants

Surgical and anaesthetic risks are higher in infancy and there is a view that surgery in the first year of life carries a risk of damaging bladder function. Most infants are managed medically until after 12 months.

Effect on scarring

Current theories of the pathogenesis of scarring suggest that very early childhood infections are most likely to cause scarring and the risk of progressive scarring becomes less with time. Very few new scars have been detected with onset after 4 years. This may be because the kidney becomes less vulnerable to permanent damage with increasing age. The diagnosis of UTI in children becomes much easier after 2 years and the prevalence and severity of VUR declines. In children who have already experienced UTIs, the humoral and cellular response to UTI is altered and may be less likely to cause acute inflammation and damage.

In uncontrolled studies of surgical management, patients often do better after surgery than before surgery. This may be because of the relationship with age stated above and the fact that patients may be better managed after the problem has come to medical attention.

Two large controlled studies, The Birmingham Study and the International Study, both failed to demonstrate any significant benefit from surgical and medical management of VUR (Birmingham Reflux Study Group 1987; Smellie et al. 1992) (Fig. 11). However, both these studies have limitations. Patients were recruited in infancy and childhood after one or more presenting UTIs. Thus, in both groups, there were many scars before randomization and surgery. The number of new scars in both groups was much smaller than the number present at the start; neither study included a control limb without treatment, and there were no clear indications about what arrangements were in place to detect and treat acute intercurrent infections. The possibility that renal scarring can be reduced by prophylaxis of infants detected with VUR at birth needs evaluation in a well-designed and adequately powered controlled study.

Effect of surgery on urinary tract infection

Even after successful surgery, the incidence of UTI appears to be unaffected (Jodal et al. 1992). Some children continue to have acute symptomatic UTIs while others are prone to asymptomatic bacteriuria with

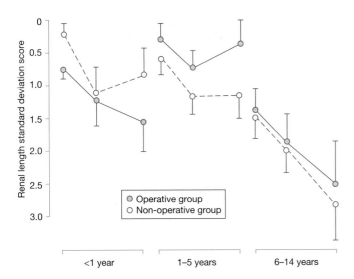

Fig. 11 Change in GFR at 2 and 5 years in operated and non-operated children who participated in the Birmingham Reflux Study. There is no significant difference in renal function between the two groups at any time. *British Medical Journal* (1989) **295**, 237–241. With permission from the BMJ Publishing group and Professor R.H.R. White.

minimal symptoms. However, there is evidence of a reduction in the incidence of acute pyelonephritis after the first 6 months. In the immediate postoperative period, there is a significant risk of acute pyelonephritis which may occur in up to 10 per cent of cases in some series and tends to be associated with a high risk of new scars. This risk declines over the first 6 months after surgery. There is anecdotal experience that children with VUR and recurrent acute pyelonephritis may have a significant improvement in symptoms and well being after successful surgery. The major indication for surgery in children in the United Kingdom is from within this group.

Subureteric injection

The submucosal injection of Teflon has been described by O'Donnell and Puri (1986). This simple procedure required the injection of a small amount of material immediately below the ureteric orifice, to create a small mound. This can change the shape of the ureteric orifice and prevent the reflux of urine. This technique is successful in about 80 per cent of the cases, but the effect may not last in every case. Some patients have the procedure repeated with further benefit.

After the method was first introduced there was concern about the risk of Teflon embolization to remote parts of the body with granuloma formation. Subsequently, collagen was used as an alternative. This material appears to be safer but not so durable and an increasing number have required repeat injections. Complications are relatively infrequent and include infection and obstruction. Some surgeons regard this as the preferred method of managing VUR. Evidence of reduction in risk of UTI or scarring is not available.

Circumcision

There is accumulating evidence of the subprepucial area in male infants as an important source of infecting organisms. In populations with a high rate of circumcision there is a low rate of UTI in male infants with a difference in risk of over 10-fold. Circumcision has been recommended in male infants with abnormal urinary tracts to reduce the risk of UTI although it is not clear how effective this strategy is in preventing UTI or renal scarring in this high-risk group.

Other surgical management

From time to time a nephrectomy may be required, particularly if there are continuing problems with infection or hypertension in a poorly functioning kidney. Stones may be removed surgically or using percutaneous techniques or lithotripsy.

Medical management

Long-term low-dose prophylaxis has been the method of choice for preventing renal scarring in the United Kingdom for children with UTIs and VUR for several decades.

Little attention has focused on the difficulty in diagnosing UTIs in infants in primary care although this may represent an important area where practice could be improved and renal scarring prevented. Even in hospital practice the diagnosis of UTI in infants and toddlers is difficult and time consuming. The use of non-invasive methods of urine collection combined with conventional urine culture has been shown to be slow and inaccurate. In a national audit carried out by the Royal College of Paediatrics and Child Health (2000), the methods used in laboratories across the country were often unsuitable for rapid diagnosis and very insensitive to the problems of urine collection in infancy. A significant number of affected infants and toddlers appeared to have had their diagnosis overlooked when the laboratory test was positive. Other medical methods suggested to reduce the risk of infection, scarring, or pain have been considered but there is little evidence to support their use. Until rapid methods of diagnosis are validated in very young children there will continue to be delays in diagnosis and treatment and any attempt to evaluate prophylaxis or surgery is unlikely to give useful results.

Acute management

Most clinicians favour the use of intravenous antibiotics for the initial management of UTI and the prevention of scarring. However, in a large prospective controlled study there was no evidence of superiority of 10 days of intravenous therapy compared with 3 days of intravenous therapy followed by oral therapy (Benador *et al.* 2001). However, a systematic review of short versus long courses of treatment for lower-tract infections showed that shorter courses were more likely to be followed by persistence of infected urine although the symptoms resolved equally well and the risk of symptomatic recurrence was unaffected (Michael *et al.* 2002).

Prophylaxis

The majority of UTIs reach the urinary tract via the urethra. These infections are generally easy to treat if the child is given an appropriate antibiotic. The theory of prophylaxis is that the normally sterile urinary tract receives a daily flush of broad spectrum antibiotic which eliminates any invading bacteria. Antibiotics are traditionally given in the evening so that they remain in the bladder for as long as possible, overnight. In infants and toddlers who are not toilet trained the need to give the dose in the evening is less clear.

The recommended antibiotics are trimethoprim 1–2 mg/kg or nitrofurantoin 0.5–1 mg/kg. Unfortunately, there is increasing resistance to trimethoprim and breakthrough infection is now common.

Nitrofurantoin is probably superior to trimethoprim because acquired resistance is rare. However, certain bacteria including *proteus* and *pseudomonas* species are generally not sensitive. Nitrofurantoin is bitter tasting and inclined to cause nausea and vomiting in some children.

Although there have been some small studies that suggest that prophylaxis is effective in reducing the risk of reinfection, in a recent systematic review there was insufficient evidence for its effectiveness in children with urinary tract abnormalities and no evidence that it can prevent renal scarring (Williams *et al.* 2001). In addition, there are frequently mild side-effects and complications and occasionally severe complications (Uhari *et al.* 1996). When this is combined with the effect on the environment of widespread, long-term use of antibiotics, it makes the case for well designed studies all the more pressing.

When breakthrough infections occur it is important to look at the sensitivity of the organism since breakthrough with a sensitive organism indicates non-compliance and breakthrough with a resistant organism may indicate that the prophylactic agent is losing effectiveness because the child is colonized with resistant organisms. In children with voiding dysfunction, breakthrough infections are more common (Hellerstein and Nickell 2002). The small but significant risk of complications of medication must be taken into account as well as the long-term risk to the community of widespread use of antimicrobial agents (Williams *et al.* 2001).

Alternative medical measures

Alternative measures have addressed the mechanical and hydrodynamic aspects, bacterial colonization, and the urinary environment with anecdotal success in selected cases.

Bladder emptying

Regular bladder emptying is thought to be important in the prevention of recurrent UTIs in children with VUR. Some children with VUR have dysfunctional bladders and others are inclined to put off trips to the toilet for prolonged periods. Bladder dysfunction is thought to contribute to UTIs, VUR, and renal scarring (Naseer and Steinhardt 1997).

Double micturition

Bladder emptying may be incomplete in children with VUR because urine is forced up the ureters during bladder contraction at the time of micturition only to return to the bladder when bladder emptying is complete. This predisposes to bacterial colonization of the bladder because the normal washing out of invading bacteria is incomplete. Double and treble micturition is the term used when a patient is asked to wait after passing urine and to try to empty the bladder a second or third time to ensure complete bladder emptying.

Constipation

Severe constipation is associated with dilatation of the urinary tract, VUR, incomplete bladder emptying, and recurrent UTIs. A vigorous approach to the treatment of constipation is helpful in some cases. Urinary tract dilatation may resolve after adequate treatment has been maintained for several months (Pery *et al.* 1988; Dohil *et al.* 1994).

Hygiene

Suggestions include wiping the bottom from front to back after defaecation, avoiding bubble bath, avoiding highly scented or irritant soaps and careful washing and drying. Some doctors thought that the agents altering surface tension in bubble bath and shampoo might increase the ability for bacteria to ascend the urinary tract, thus increasing the risk of ascending UTI, although this theory has not been tested.

Cranberry juice

Cranberry juice has been recommended for its ability to prevent UTIs and relieve symptoms. There is preliminary evidence of a substance that interferes with the function of bacterial fimbria. Although a small effect has been demonstrated in some studies, a systematic review failed to find evidence of significant effect. However, it remains a safe and simple remedy available over the counter.

Alteration of urine composition

Advice to drink plenty of water may be based on the fact that a very low urine osmolality is less favourable to bacterial growth. Similarly there have been attempts to prevent infection by altering the urine pH using Mandelamine or *Potassium Citrate Mixture*. Neither of these forms of treatment have been of proven benefit in prevention of infection although potassium citrate solution has a role in reducing symptoms.

Changing bacterial flora

Lactobacilli present in live yoghurt is a normal commensal in the adult female. It has been suggested that live yoghurt will increase the colonization of the genital area by lactobacilli and decrease the prevalence of *Escherichia coli*. Even when applied locally it is difficult to produce a sustained effect.

Avoid unnecessary antibiotics

There is an increased risk of infection after a course of antibiotics given for any reason, which seems to be related to the change in perineal flora that follows treatment. In the Cardiff Bacteriuria Study, girls who had frequent changes of infecting organisms were more likely to develop new scars (Olling *et al.* 1981). It was postulated that a symbiotic relationship develops between the host and the bacteria in the urine after the strain has colonized the urinary tract and the acute inflammation has settled. The persisting bacteria undergo changes in phenotype and are less likely to cause acute symptoms but are better able to survive in the urinary tract.

Pregnancy

Pregnancy is a period of physiological stress when underlying health problems may be exposed. El-Khatib *et al.* (1987) showed that pregnancy in women with reflux and RN was complicated by UTI, hypertension, and proteinuria.

Hypertension

A case–control study showed that women with scars and a past history of asymptomatic bacteriuria were three times more likely to develop hypertension during the latter part of pregnancy than women with a past history of asymptomatic bacteriuria without scars or healthy controls. As a result they were much more likely to undergo induction of labour and forceps delivery or caesarian section (McGladdery *et al.* 1992).

Effect on renal function

Becker *et al.* (1986) found that in women with RN and hypertension their renal function deteriorated significantly during pregnancy.

However, other studies have indicated a more favourable outcome (Martinell *et al.* 1990).

Relationship of pregnancy to urinary tract infection

UTIs are common in women during pregnancy and particularly common in women with a past history of UTIs, VUR, or RN. The persistence of VUR into adult life has also been associated with increased risk of UTIs in some studies. While some UTIs in pregnancy may be asymptomatic or associated with lower tract symptoms, some women have experienced acute pyelonephritis which in turn brings other risks to the pregnancy. Acute pyelonephritis is more common in the latter part of pregnancy. Women with RN are at increased risk of UTI in pregnancy, but women with a history of UTI, without VUR or renal scarring are at similar risk (McGladdery *et al.* 1992).

Anaemia

Women with asymptomatic bacteriuria are at increased risk of anaemia. This may be because of a higher risk of anaemia in the subgroup with scarring, particularly those with reduced renal function.

Effect of reflux and scarring on the infant

Infants born to mothers with VUR and renal scarring are at increased risk of several problems largely related to the health of the mother. Women with hypertension and proteinuria during the second trimester tend to produce low birth weight infants. If severe, hypertension may result in convulsions and intrauterine death. Women with impaired renal function with a GFR below 50 per cent of normal tend to have particularly difficult pregnancies. Hypertension may require medication and beta-blockers have been associated with low birth weight. ACE inhibitors are teratogenic and, therefore, contraindicated in those planning a family.

Severe infection such as acute pyelonephritis may precipitate preterm delivery. Infants of mothers who have had acute pyelonephritis have lower Apgar scores than controls and have an increased risk of Gram-negative infections including septicaemia and UTI in the first few weeks of life.

Screening for VUR

There are a number of situations where it has become the practice to screen for the presence of VUR in apparently healthy children. These situations are discussed below. Whether or not this practice is beneficial to the individual or cost effective has now been questioned. Only systematic reviews and carefully designed studies will answer this question.

Imaging after urinary tract infection

Unlike the situation following bacterial infections of the respiratory tract, it has become usual practice in Western countries to refer children for imaging of the urinary tract following one or more UTIs. The rationale for this practice is that there is a markedly increased incidence of congenital abnormalities and acquired scarring in these children. In a systematic review, Dick and Feldman (1996) were unable to identify any studies that demonstrated that route imaging had an

impact on the development of renal scars or other clinical outcomes in children after their first UTI. Others have questioned this practice from an economic perspective (Stark 1997) and from the child's perspective (Chambers 1997).

The commonest congenital anomaly is VUR which is present in a third of children with UTIs. This figure appears to be relatively unaltered by the severity, presence or absence of symptoms, age, or sex. This is discussed earlier in the section 'Prevalence'.

Other important anomalies are those associated with obstruction, such as urethral valves, pelviureteric junction obstruction, vesicoureteric obstruction, and ureterocoele. The presence of small kidneys or a solitary kidney is worthy of note and indicates the need to assess renal function. Other congenital anomalies are of lesser medical importance, for example, a duplex system is commonly found but, only occasionally, of pathological significance. Other congenital anomalies such as horseshoe kidney or crossed renal ectopia are often associated with VUR, obstruction, or reduced renal function; in the absence of these problems they are of little significance.

There is no evidence that routine imaging of healthy children following the first UTI is beneficial. The incidence of anomalies in children in Cardiff who were investigated in line with published guidelines was only 2 per cent among those who were not ill enough to be admitted to hospital, but 15 per cent of those who were admitted were shown to have renal scars. This suggests that imaging should be focused more closely on those children with severe presenting illness or recurrent infection (Deshpande and Verrier Jones 2001). This could release resources to improve the diagnosis and early treatment of acutely ill infants, thus reducing the development of scarring associated with the first UTI.

Distress caused by investigations

There are several observational studies that have shown that imaging tests cause acute distress and sometimes result in prolonged anxiety. The drawbacks of such tests must be carefully balanced against the chance of revealing a treatable problem (Phillips *et al.* 1996).

Antenatal hydronephrosis

Antenatal ultrasound introduced two decades ago has now become a routine procedure although we do not know to what extent it is valuable or prevents avoidable infection or renal damage. One of the most common observations is hydronephrosis, seen at about 18 weeks gestation and often present again at a second scan in the third trimester. VUR is present in around one in five of these infants when they are investigated soon after birth. However, the extent to which it is important to know the anatomical details is unclear. A hydronephrosis of greater that 30 mm carries a high risk of obstruction and should be thoroughly investigated. High grades of VUR are not always associated with significant dilatation on ultrasound so that some cases can be missed. When a postnatal ultrasound scan is carried out it is usual to wait for several days since the low-urine output in the first day or two means that the collecting system may not be visualized if the scan is done too soon.

Familial VUR

Infants born to parents with VUR or renal scarring carry a one in two risk of having VUR (Scott *et al.* 1997). Since the greatest risk of renal scarring is following UTI in infancy, there is some logic to screening these high-risk infants for the presence of VUR soon after birth. Furthermore, the incidence of VUR is highest at this age and the infant is too young to remember the investigation and any associated discomfort if the test is carried out soon after birth. Affected infants are usually given long-term, low-dose prophylaxis with trimethoprim or nitrofurantoin. As these agents are not licensed for use in the neonate some paediatricians use cephalosporins. Alternatively, infants may be managed without prophylaxis but with care and attention for the development of fever that may be due to UTI. Early treatment of UTIs may be just as valuable as the use of long-term low-dose prophylaxis.

Imaging high-risk infants

At one time it was recommended that infants with risk factors such as low-set ears or single umbilical arteries should undergo imaging tests. This practice is no longer justified in completely healthy babies. If tests are carried out, ultrasound is easier to justify as it is safe and non-invasive. The disadvantage is that it cannot detect VUR or small scars. Infants with congenital anomalies and syndromes are at increased risk of congenital renal anomalies including VUR. In a recent survey of congenital renal anomalies in the Newcastle region, Scott found a high risk of serious renal anomalies among fetuses that died or in pregnancies that were terminated because of antenatal renal anomalies (Scott 2002).

References

Aggarwal, V. K. and Verrier Jones, K. (1989). Vesicoureteric reflux: screening of first degree relatives. *Archives of Disease in Childhood* 64, 1538–1541.

Aggarwal, V. K., Verrier Jones, K., Asscher, A. W., Evans, C., and Williams, L. A. (1991). Covert bacteriuria: long term follow-up. *Archives of Disease in Childhood* 66, 1284–1286.

Anonymous (1974). V.U.R. + I.R.R. = C.P.N.? *Lancet* 2, 1120–1121.

Anonymous (1997). The management of urinary tract infection in children. *Drugs and Therapeutics Bulletin* 35 (9), 65–69.

Arant, B. S., Jr. (1991). Vesicoureteric reflux and renal injury. *American Journal of Kidney Diseases* 17, 491–511.

Arze, R. S., Ramos, J. M., Owen, J. P., Morley, A. R., Elliott, R. W., Wilkinson, R., Ward, M. K., and Kerr, D. N. (1982). The natural history of chronic pyelonephritis in the adult. *Quarterly Journal of Medicine* 51 (204), 396–410.

Bailey, R. R. Vesicoureteric reflux in healthy infants and children. In *Reflux Nephropathy* (ed. J. Hodson and P. Kincaid-Smith), pp. 57–61. New York, NY: Masson, 1979.

Becker, G. J. and Kincaid-Smith, P. (1993). Reflux nephropathy: the glomerular lesion and progression of renal failure. *Pediatric Nephrology* 7, 365–369.

Becker, G. J., Ihle, B. U., Fairley, K. F., Bastos, M., and Kincaid-Smith, P. (1986). Effect of pregnancy on moderate renal failure in reflux nephropathy. *British Medical Journal* 292, 796–798.

Benador, D., Neuhaus, T. J., Papazyan, J.-P., Willi, U. V., Engel-Bicik, I., Nadal, D., Slosman, D., Mermillod, B., and Girardin, E. (2001). Randomised controlled trial of three day versus 10 day intravenous antibiotics in acute pyelonephritis: effect on renal scarring. *Archives of Disease in Childhood* 84, 241–246.

Berg, U. B. and Johansson, S. B. (1983). Age as a main determinant of renal functional damage in urinary tract infection. *Archives of Disease in Childhood* 58, 963–969.

Birmingham Reflux Study Group (1987). Prospective trial of operative versus non-operative treatment of severe vesicoureteric reflux in children: five years' observation. *British Medical Journal* 295, 237–241.

Booth, E. J., Bell, T. E., and McLain, C. (1975). Fetal vesicoureteral reflux. *Journal of Urology* 113, 258.

Bunge, R. G. (1954). Further observations with delayed cystograms. *Journal of Urology* 71, 427–434.

Campbell, M. *Clinical Pediatric Urology*. Philadelphia, PA: Saunders, 1951.

Cardiff–Oxford Bacteriuria Study Group (1979). Long-term effects of bacteriuria on the urinary tract in schoolgirls. *Radiology* 132, 343–350.

Cascio, S., Chertin, B., Yoneda, A., Rolle, U., Kelleher, J., and Puri, P. (2002). Acute renal damage in infants after first urinary tract infection. *Pediatric Nephrology* 17, 503–505.

Chambers, T. (1997). Commentary on article by H Stark. An essay on the consequences of childhood urinary tract infection. *Pediatric Nephrology* 11, 178–179.

Cho, S. J. and Lee, S. J. (2002). ACE gene polymorphism and renal scar in children with acute pyelonephritis. *Pediatric Nephrology* 17, 491–495.

Cohen, S. J. (1975). Ureterozystoneostomie: eine neue antirefluxtechnik. *Aktuelle Urologie* 6, 1.

Conway, J. J. and Cohn, R. A. (1994). Evolving role of nuclear medicine for the diagnosis and management of urinary tract infection. *Journal of Pediatrics* 124, 87–90.

Coulthard, M. (2002). Do kidneys outgrow the risk of reflux nephropathy? *Pediatric Nephrology* 17, 477–480.

Coulthard, M. G., Flecknell, P., Orr, M., Manus, D., and O'Donnell, M. (2002). Renal scarring caused by vesicoureteric reflux and urinary infection: a study in pigs. *Pediatric Nephrology* 17, 481–484.

Coulthard, M. G., Lambert, H. J., and Keir, M. J. (1997). Occurrence of renal scars in children after their first referral for urinary tract infection. *British Medical Journal* 315, 918–919.

Craig, J. C., Knight, J. F., Sureshkumar, P., Lam, A., Onikul, E., and Roy, L. P. (1997). Vesicoureteric reflux and timing of micturating cystourethrography after urinary tract infection. *Archives of Disease in Childhood* 76, 275–277.

Darge, K. (2002). Diagnosis of vesicoureteral reflux with ultrasonography. *Pediatric Nephrology* 17, 52–60.

Deshpande, P. V. and Verrier Jones, K. (2001). An audit of RCP guidelines on DMSA scanning after urinary tract infection. *Archives of Disease in Childhood* 84, 324–327.

Dick, P. D. and Feldman, W. (1996). Routine diagnostic imaging for childhood urinary tract infections: a systematic overview. *Journal of Pediatrics* 128, 15–22.

Dohil, R., Roberts, E., Verrier Jones, K., and Jenkins, H. R. (1994). Constipation and reversible urinary tract abnormalities. *Archives of Disease in Childhood* 70, 56–57.

Dudley, J., Johnston, A., Gardner, A., and McGraw, M. (2002). The deletion polymorphism of the ACE gene is not an independent risk factor for renal scarring in children with vesico-ureteric reflux. *Nephrology, Dialysis, Transplantation* 17, 625–645.

Edwards, D., Normand, I. C. S., Prescod, N., and Smellie, J. (1977). Disappearance of vesicoureteric reflux during long-term prophylaxis of urinary tract infection in children. *British Medical Journal* 2, 285–288.

Eisendreith, D. N., Katz, H., and Glasser, J. M. (1925). Bladder reflux; a clinical and experimental study. *Journal of American Medical Association* 85, 1121–1125.

El-Khatib, M. T., Becker, G. J., and Kincaid-Smith, P. S. Complications associated with pregnancy in patients with reflux nephropathy. In *Abstract Xth International Society of Nephrology*, p. 113. Oxford: Alden Press, 1987.

El-Khatib, M. T., Becker, G. J., and Kincaid-Smith, P. S. (1991). Reflux nephropathy and primary vesicoureteric reflux in adults. *Quarterly Journal of Medicine* 77, 1241–1253.

Friedland, G. W. The voiding cystourethrogram: an unreliable examination. In *Reflux Nephropathy* (ed. J. Hodson and P. Kincaid-Smith), p. 99. New York, NY: Masson Publishing USA Inc., 1979.

Gibson, H. M. (1949). Ureteral reflux in the normal child. *Journal of Urology* 62, 40–43.

Goldraich, N. P. and Barratt, T. M. Vesicoureteric reflux and renal scarring. In *Paediatric Nephrology* 2nd edn. (ed. T. M. Barratt, M. A. Holliday, and R. L. Vernier), pp. 647–666. Baltimore, MD: Williams & Wilkins, 1987.

Goonasekera, C. D. A., Shah, V., and Dillon, M. J. (1996a). Tubular proteinuria in reflux nephropathy: post ureteric re-implantation. *Pediatric Nephrology* **10**, 559–563.

Goonasekera, C. D. A., Shah, V., Wade, A. M., Barratt, T. M., and Dillon, M. J. (1996b). 15-year follow-up of renin and blood pressure in reflux nephropathy. *Lancet* **347**, 640–643.

Hallett, R. J., Paed, L., and Maskell, R. (1976). Urinary infection in boys. A 3 year prospective study. *Lancet* **II**, 1107–1110.

Helin, I. and Winberg, J. (1980). Chronic renal failure in Swedish children. *Acta Paediatrica Scandinavica* **69**, 607–611.

Hellerstein, S. and Nickell, H. (2002). Prophylactic antibiotics in children at risk for urinary tract infection. *Pediatric Nephrology* **17**, 506–510.

Hellström, A., Hanson, E., Hansson, S., Hjälmas, K., and Jodal, U. (1991). Association between urinary symptoms at 7 years old and previous urinary tract infection. *Archives of Disease in Childhood* **66**, 232–234.

Heptinstall, R. H. *Pathology of the Kidney* Vol. III, 3rd edn., pp. 1327–1381. Boston, NY: Little Brown & Co, 1983.

Hodson, C. J. and Edwards, D. (1960). Chronic pyelonephritis and vesicoureteric reflux. *Clinical Radiology* **2**, 219–231.

Hodson, J. and Kincaid Smith, P., ed. *Reflux Nephropathy.* New York, Paris, Barcelona, Milan, Mexico City, Rio de Janeiro: Masson Publishing USA, Inc., 1979.

Hodson, C. J., Davies, Z., and Prescod, A. (1975). Renal parenchymal radiographic measurements in infants and children. *Pediatric Radiology* **3**, 16–19.

Howie, A. J., Buist, L. J., and Coulthard, M. G. (2002). Reflux nephropathy in transplants. *Pediatric Nephrology* **17**, 485–490.

Hutch, J. A. (1961). Theory of maturation of the intravesical ureter. *Journal of Urology* **86**, 534.

Hutch, J. A. *Anatomy and Physiology of the Bladder, Trigone and Urethra.* London: Butterworth, 1972.

Iannaccone, G. and Panzironi, P. E. (1955). Ureteral reflux in normal infants. *Acta Radiological Diagnosis* **44**, 451–456.

International Reflux Study in Children (1985). International system of radiographic grading of vesicoureteric reflux. *Pediatric Radiology* **15**, 105–109.

Jacobson, S. H., Eklöf, O., Eriksson, C. G., Lins, L.-E., Tidgren, B., and Winberg, J. (1989). Development of hypertension and uraemia after pyelonephritis in childhood: 27 year follow up. *British Medical Journal* **299**, 703–706.

Jadresic, L., Cartwright, K., Cowie, N., Witcombe, B., and Stevens, D. (1993). Investigation of urinary tract infection in childhood. *British Medical Journal* **307**, 761–764.

Jodal, U. and Winberg, J. (1987). Management of children with unobstructed urinary tract infection. *Pediatric Nephrology* **1**, 647–656.

Jodal, U. *et al.* (1992). Infection pattern in children with vesicoureteral reflux randomly allocated to operation or long-term antibacterial prophylaxis. *Journal of Urology* **148**, 1650–1652.

Jones, B. W. and Headstream, J. W. (1958). Vesicoureteral reflux in children. *Journal of Urology* **80**, 114.

Kenda, R. B. and Fettich, J. J. (1992). Vesicoureteric reflux and renal scars in asymptomatic siblings of children with reflux. *Archives of Disease in Childhood* **67**, 506–508.

Kenda, R. B. and Zupancic, Z. (1994). Ultrasound screening of older asymptomatic siblings of children with vesicoureteral reflux: is it beneficial? *Pediatric Radiology* **24**, 14–16.

Kenda, R. B., Kenig, T., and Budihna, N. (1991). Detecting vesicoureteral reflux in asymptomatic siblings of children with reflux by direct radionuclide cystography. *European Journal of Pediatrics* **150**, 735–737.

Kjellberg, S. R., Ericsson, N. O., and Rudhe, U. Selected aspects of urinary tract infection. In *The Lower Urinary Tract in Childhood: Some Correlated Clinical and Roentgenologic Observations* p. 182. Stockholm: Almqvist & Wiksell, 1957.

Lama, G., Russo, M., De Rosa, E., Mansi, L., Piscitelli, A., Luongo, I., and Salsano, M. E. (2000). Primary vesicoureteric reflux and renal damage in the first year of life. *Pediatric Nephrology* **15**, 205–210.

Leadbetter, G. W., Duxbury, J. H., and Dreyfuss, J. R. (1960). Absence of vesicoureteral reflux in normal adult males. *Journal of Urology* **84**, 69–70.

Litch, R., Jr., Howerton, L. W., and Davis, L. A., ed. Progress in pyelonephritis, p. 645. Philadelphia, PA: FA Davis, 1965.

Mahant, S., Friedman, J., and MacArthur, C. (2002). Renal ultrasound findings and vesicoureteral reflux in children hospitalised with urinary tract infections. *Archives of Disease in Childhood* **86**, 419–421.

Marild, S., Hellstrom, M., Jodal, U., and Svanborg Eden, C. (1989). Fever, bacteriuria and concomitant disease in children with urinary tract infection. *Paediatric Infectious Disease Journal* **8**, 36–42.

Marra, G., Barbieri, G., Moioli, C., Assael, B. M., Grumieri, G., and Caccamo, M. L. (1994). Mild fetal hydronephrosis indicating vesicoureteric reflux. *Archives of Disease in Childhood* **70**, F147–F150.

Martinell, J., Claesson, I., Lidin-Janson, G., and Jodal, U. (1995). Urinary infection, reflux and renal scarring in females continuously followed for 13–38 years. *Pediatric Nephrology* **9**, 131–136.

Martinell, J., Hansson, S., Claesson, I., Jacobsson, B., Lidin-Janson, G., and Jodal, U. (2000). Detection of urographic scars in girls with pyelonephritis followed for 30 years. *Pediatric Nephrology* **14**, 1006–1010.

Martinell, J., Jodal, U., and Lidin-Janson, G. (1990). Pregnancies in women with and without renal scarring after urinary infections in childhood. *British Medical Journal* **300**, 840–844.

McGladdery, S. L., Aparicio, S., Verrier Jones, K., Roberts, R., and Sacks, S. H. (1992). Outcome of pregnancy in an Oxford–Cardiff cohort of women with previous bacteriuria. *Quarterly Journal of Medicine* **84**, 533–539.

Medical Research Council Bacteriuria Committee (1979). Recommended terminology of urinary tract infection. *British Medical Journal* **2**, 717–719.

Merrick, M. V., Uttley, W. S., and Wild, R. (1977). A comparison of two techniques for detecting vesico-ureteric reflux. *British Journal of Radiology* **50**, 792–795.

Michael, M., Hodson, E. M., Craig, J. C., Martin, S., and Moyer, V. A. (2002). Short compared with standard duration of antibiotic treatment for urinary tract infection: a systematic review of randomised controlled trials. *Archives of Disease in Childhood* **87**, 118–123.

Naseer, S. R. and Steinhardt, G. F. (1997). New renal scars in children with urinary tract infections, vesicoureteral reflux and voiding dysfunction: a prospective evaluation. *Journal of Urology* **158** (2), 566–568.

Nuutinen, M. and Uhari, M. (2001). Recurrence and follow-up after urinary tract infection under the age of 1 year. *Pediatric Nephrology* **16**, 69–72.

O'Donnell, B. (1990). Controversies in therapeutics. Management of urinary tract infection and vesicoureteric reflux in children. The case for surgery. *British Medical Journal* **300**, 1393–1394.

O'Donnell, B. and Puri, P. (1986). Endoscopic correction of primary vesicoureteric reflux: results in 94 ureters. *British Medical Journal* **2**, 1404–1406.

Olbing, H., Claesson, I., Ebel, K. D., and Seppanen, U. (1992). Renal scars and parenchymal thinning in children with vesicoureteric reflux: a 5-year report of the International Reflux Study in Children (European Branch). *Journal of Urology* **148**, 1653–1656.

Olling, S., Verrier Jones, K., Mackenzie, R., Verrier Jones, E. R., Hanson, L. A., and Asscher, A. W. (1981). A four year follow up of schoolgirls with untreated covert bacteriuria: bacteriological aspects. *Clinical Nephrology* **16**, 169–171.

Ozen, S. *et al.* (1999). Implications of certain genetic polymorphisms in scarring in vesicoureteric reflux: importance of ACE polymorphism. *American Journal of Kidney Diseases* **34** (1), 140–145.

Pery, M., Kaftori, J. K., and Alon, U. (1988). False uroradiologic pathology in children with urinary tract infection and faecal impaction. *Child Nephrology and Urology* **9**, 349–352.

Peters, P. C., Johnson, D. E., and Jackson, J. H. (1967). Incidence of vesicouretal reflux in the premature child. *Journal of Urology* **97**, 259–260.

Phillips, D., Watson, A. R., and Collier, J. (1996). Distress and radiological investigations of the urinary tract in children. *European Journal of Pediatrics* **155**, 684–687.

Phillips, D. A., Watson, A. R., and MacKinlay, D. (1998). Distress and the micturating cystourethrogram: does preparation help? *Acta Paediatrica Scandinavica* **87**, 175–179.

Politano, V. A. (1960). Vesicoureteral reflux in children. *Journal of American Medical Association* **172**, 1252–1256.

Politano, V. A. and Leadbetter, W. F. (1958). An operative technique for the correction of V.U.R. *Journal of Urology* **79**, 932.

Ransley, P. G. and Risdon, R. A. (1974). Renal papillae and intrarenal reflux in the pig. *Lancet* **2**, 1114.

Report of a meeting of physicians at the Hospital for Sick Children, Great Ormond Street, London (1996). Vesicoureteric reflux: all in the genes? *Lancet* **348**, 725–728.

Report of a Working Group of the Research Unit, Royal College of Physicians (1991). Guidelines for the management of acute urinary tract infection in childhood. *Journal of the Royal College of Physicians of London* **25** (1), 36–42.

Risdon, R. A. (1993). The small scarred kidney in childhood. *Pediatric Nephrology* **7**, 361–364.

Rolle, U., Shima, H., and Puri, P. (2002). Nitric oxide, enhanced by macrophage stimulating factor, mediates renal damage in reflux nephropathy. *Kidney International* **62**, 507–513.

Rolleston, G. L., Maling, T. M. J., and Hodson, C. J. (1974). Intrarenal reflux and the scarred kidney. *Archives of Disease in Childhood* **49**, 531–539.

Rushton, H. (1997). UTI in children—epidemiology, evaluation and management. *Pediatric Clinics of North America* **44** (5), 1133–1169.

Savage, D. C. L., Wilson, M. I., McHardy, M., Dewar, D. A. E., and Fee, W. M. (1973). Covert bacteriuria of childhood: a clinical and epidemiological study. *Archives of Disease in Childhood* **48**, 8–20.

Scott, J. E. S. (2002). Fetal, perinatal and infant death with congenital renal anomalies. *Archives of Disease in Childhood* **87**, 114–117.

Scott, J. E. S., Swallow, V., Coulthard, M. G., Lambert, H. J., and Lee, R. E. J. (1997). Screening of newborn babies for familial ureteric reflux. *Lancet* **350**, 396–400.

Shaw, K. and Gorelick, M. (1999). Urinary tract infection in the pediatric patient. *Pediatric Clinics of North America* **46**, 1111–1124.

Smellie, J. M. (1967). Medical aspects of urinary infection in children. *Journal of the Royal College of Physicians of London* **1** (2), 189–196.

Smellie, J. M. and Rigden, S. P. A. (1995). Pitfalls in the investigation of children with urinary tract infection. *Archives of Disease in Childhood* **72**, 251–258.

Smellie, J. M., Hodson, C. J., Edwards, D., and Normand, I. C. S. (1964). Clinical and radiological features of urinary infection in childhood. *British Medical Journal* **2**, 1222–1226.

Smellie, J. M., Poulton, A., and Prescod, N. P. (1994). Retrospective study of children with renal scarring associated with reflux and urinary infection. *British Medical Journal* **308**, 1193–1196.

Smellie, J. M., Prescod, N. P., Shaw, P. J., Risdon, R. A., and Bryant, T. N. (1998). Childhood reflux and urinary infections: a follow-up of 10–41 years in 226 adults. *Pediatric Nephrology* **12**, 727–736.

Smellie, J. M., Ransley, P. G., Normand, I. C. S., Prescod, N., and Edwards, D. (1985). Development of new renal scars; a collaborative study. *British Medical Journal* **290**, 1957–1960.

Smellie, J. M., Tamminen-Mobius, T., Olbing, H., Claesson, I., Wikstad, I., Jodal, U., and Seppanen, U. (1992). Five-year study of medical or surgical treatment in children with severe reflux: radiological renal findings. *Pediatric Nephrology* **6**, 223–230.

Smolkin, V., Koren, A., Raz, R., Colonder, R., Sakran, W., and Halevy, R. (2002). Procalcitonin as a marker of acute pyelonephritis in infants and children. *Pediatric Nephrology* **17**, 409–412.

South Bedfordshire Practitioners' Group (1990). Development of renal scars in children: missed opportunities in management. *British Medical Journal* **301**, 1082–1084.

Stark, H. (1997). Urinary tract infections in girls: the cost-effectiveness of currently recommended investigative routines. *Pediatric Nephrology* **11**, 174–177.

Stokland, E., Hellström, M., Hansson, S., Jodal, U., Odén, A., and Jacobsson, B. (1994). Reliability of ultrasonography in identification of reflux nephropathy in children. *British Medical Journal* **309**, 235–239.

Uhari, M., Nuutinen, M., Turtinen, M. D., and Turtinen, J. (1996). Adverse reactions in children during long term antimicrobial therapy. *The Pediatric Infections Disease Journal* **15**, 404–408.

van der Voort, J., Edwards, A., Roberts, R., and Verrier Jones, K. (1997). The struggle to diagnose UTI in children under two in primary care. *Family Practice* **14**, 44–48.

van der Voort, J. H., Edwards, A. G., Roberts, R., Newcombe, R. G., and Verrier Jones, K. (2002). The frequency of visits to the GP before the diagnosis of the first UTI: have UTIs been missed? *Archives of Disease in Childhood* **87**, 530–533.

Vernon, S. J., Coulthard, M. G., Lambert, H. J., Keir, M. J., and Matthews, J. N. S. (1997). New renal scarring in children who at age 3 and 4 years had had normal scans with dimercaptosuccinic acid: follow up study. *British Medical Journal* **315**, 905–908.

Verrier Jones, K. (1999). Under-diagnosis of UTIs in early childhood. *Trends in Urology and Sexual Health* 4 September/October, 13–16.

Verrier Jones, K., Asscher, A. W., Verrier Jones, E. R., Mattholie, K., Leach, K. G., and Thompson, M. (1982). Glomerular filtration rate in schoolgirls with covert bacteriuria. *British Medical Journal* **285**, 1037–1310.

Verrier Jones, K., Asscher, A. W., and Verrier Jones, E. R. Covert infection in childhood. In *Microbial Diseases in Nephrology* (ed. A. W. Asscher and W. Brumfitt), pp. 225–241. New York, NY: Wiley, 1986.

Verrier Jones, K., Hockley, B., Scrivener, R., and Pollock, J. I. Summary of diagnosis and management of urinary tract infections in children under two years: assessment of practice against published guidelines. *Report of the Research Unit of the Royal College of Paediatrics and Child Health*, 2000.

Verrier Jones, K., Sacks, S., Roberts, R., and Asscher, A. W. Covert bacteriuria: long term outcome and effect on subsequent pregnancy. In *Host Parasite Interactions in Urinary Tract Infection* (ed. E. S. Kass and C. Svanborg Eden), pp. 26–33. Chicago, IL: University of Chicago Press, 1989.

Verrier Jones, K., Roberts, E., Mathew, S., and Hayward, C. (1993). Prevalence of urinary tract abnormalities in healthy children. *British Journal of Radiology* **66**, 628–629.

Weiss, S. and Parker, F. (1939). Pyelonephritis: it's relation to vascular lesions and to arterial hypertension. *Medicina Interna* **18**, 221–315.

Weiss, R., Duckett, J., and Spitzer, A. (1992). Results of a randomized clinical trial of medical versus surgical management of infants and children with grades 3 and 4 primary vesicoureteric reflux (United States). The International Reflux Study in Children. *Journal of Urology* **148**, 1667–1673.

Wennerstrom, M., Hansson, S., Jodal, U., and Stokland, E. (2000). Primary and acquired renal scarring in boys and girls with urinary tract infection. *Journal of Pediatrics* **136**, 30–34.

Wettergren, B., Hellstrom, M., Stockland, E., and Jodal, U. (1990). Six year follow up of infants with bacteriuria on screening. *British Medical Journal* **301**, 845–848.

Williams, G., Lee, A., and Craig, J. (2001). Antibiotics for the prevention of urinary tract infection in children: a systematic review of randomised controlled trials. *Journal of Pediatrics* **138**, 868–874.

Winberg, J. (1994). Management of primary vesico-ureteric reflux in children—operation ineffective in preventing progressive renal damage. *Infection* **22**, S4–S7.

Winberg, J., Bergström, T., and Jacobsson, B. (1975). Morbidity, age and sex distribution, recurrences and renal scarring in symptomatic urinary tract infection in childhood. *Kidney International* **8**, S-101–S-106.

Winter, A. L., Hardy, B. E., Alton, D. J., Arbus, G. S., and Churchill, B. M. (1983). Acquired renal scars in children. *Journal of Urology* **129**, 1190–1194.

Woolf, A. S. (1997). Multiple causes of human kidney malformations. *Archives of Disease in Childhood* **77**, 471–477.

Yoshiara, S., White, R. H. R., Raafat, F., Smith, N. C., and Shah, K. J. (1993). Glomerular morphometry in reflux nephropathy: functional and radiological correlations. *Pediatric Nephrology* **7**, 15–22.

Zerin, J. M., Ritchey, M. L., and Chang, A. C. H. (1993). Incidental vesicoureteral reflux in neonates with antenatally detected hydronephrosis and other renal abnormalities. *Radiology* **187**, 157–160.

17.3 The patient with urinary tract obstruction

Muhammad Magdi Yaqoob and Islam Junaid

Introduction

Hydronephrosis, obstructive uropathy, and obstructive nephropathy are terms commonly used to describe obstruction of the urinary tract and its consequences (Campbell 1963). Obstructive nephropathy can be manifested clinically as a sudden or gradual and insidious decrease in renal function. The decrease can be halted and even reversed if the obstruction is relieved. Thus, obstructive uropathy differs from most other diseases affecting the kidney in that it is potentially curable. Obstruction can be due to anatomic or functional abnormalities of the urethra, bladder, ureter, or renal pelvis (Campbell 1963). These abnormalities can be congenital or acquired. Obstructive uropathy also can occur during the course of diseases extrinsic to the urinary tract (Campbell 1963).

Although dilatation of the outflow system proximal to the site of obstruction is a characteristic finding, widening of the ureter and/or pelvicalyceal system does not necessarily indicate the presence of obstruction. Causes of such anatomical abnormality in the absence of obstruction are listed in Table 1.

Obstruction may be partial or complete, unilateral or bilateral. Bilateral obstruction, or obstruction of a single kidney, is a greater threat to the patient than unilateral obstruction. Obstruction associated with infection is a greater threat to kidney function and to life than obstruction in the absence of infection. Since it is common, and often reversible, obstruction of the urinary tract should be considered in every uraemic patient, whether acute or chronic.

Table 1 Causes of non-obstructive collecting system dilatation

Anatomical variants
Large major calyx
Extrarenal pelvis
Distensible system after relief of obstruction
Pregnancy
Megacalyces

Congenital anomalies
Vesicoureteric reflux (due to abnormality of ureteric insertion into bladder)

Acquired anomalies
Reflux after ileal loop diversion, after renal transplantation

Calyceal pathology
Tuberculosis
Calyceal cyst
Papillary necrosis

Incidence

The incidence, prevalence, and cost of obstructive uropathy are difficult to estimate because obstruction can occur in the setting of a wide variety of diseases that may warrant hospitalization or surgical intervention. Obstructive uropathy has a bimodal destruction in humans. Common in childhood, it is due mainly to congenital anomalies of the urinary tact (see Chapter 17.4). Its incidence then declines with age until late adulthood. At the age of 60–65 years, the incidence rises, particularly in men, because of the increased occurrence of prostate disease (Campbell 1963). Urinary tract obstruction was present in 3.8 per cent of a large series of routine autopsies (Bell 1946) and in 25 per cent of autopsies carried out upon uraemic patients (Keuhnelian *et al.* 1964). In 1985, in the United States, 397,100 hospital discharges were coded as obstructive uropathy. Approximately 166 patients per 100,000 population had a presumptive diagnosis of obstructive uropathy on admission to hospitals in the United States (NKUDAB 1990). Among men with renal and urologic disorders, obstructive uropathy ranked fourth at hospital discharge (242 patients/100,000 discharges). In women with renal and urological problems, obstructive uropathy ranked sixth as a diagnosis at hospital discharge (94 patients/100,000 discharges). A survey in Stirling (Scotland) identified the number of men aged 40–79 years with symptomatic benign prostatic hypertrophy (BPH) defined as a prostate size more than 20 g with urinary symptoms (total symptom score $\geq$ 11) and/or a maximum urinary flow rate less than 15 ml/s. It appeared that 25 per cent of men had symptomatic BPH (Garraway *et al.* 1991). Approximately 2.5 million men fall in this category in the United Kingdom currently and the number is expected to grow by almost 50 per cent by 2025. The number of consultations and prescriptions for medical therapy for symptomatic BPH has increased considerably during the 1990s whereas the number of surgical procedures performed on an annual basis has remained stable at around 40,000 cases/year accounting for 70 million Euro/year (McNicholas 1999).

During the 5 years from 1989 to 1993, 4869 patients with the diagnosis of obstructive nephropathy began treatment for endstage renal disease (ESRD) in the United States (USRDS 1996). During this period, obstructive nephropathy accounted for 2 per cent of the patients being treated under the Medicare program for ESRD (USRDS 1996). An additional 35 patients (0.1 per cent) with the diagnosis of 'congenital obstructive uropathy' were treated for ESRD during the same period (USRDS 1996). Among the 4869 patients with obstructive nephropathy being treated for ESRD, approximately 7 per cent were younger than 20 years of age, 36 per cent were between the ages of 20 and 64 years, and 57 per cent were older than 64 years. Males comprised approximately 74 per cent of patients with obstructive nephropathy being treated for ESRD. In terms of racial origin, approximately 81 per cent of the patients were White, 16 per cent African Americans, 2 per cent of Asian descent, and 1 per cent Native Americans (USRDS 1996).

Urinary tract obstruction is a common cause of ESRD in children (Peters 1997). Obstruction of the urinary tract in early gestation can cause renal dysplasia; obstruction occurring in late gestation or after birth can cause irreversible loss of renal function (Peters 1997). New ultrasound techniques developed in the last 15 years have made possible the diagnosis of obstructive uropathy in the fetus. In the adult, the incidence and causes of obstructive uropathy vary with the gender and age of the patient. Calculi and pelviureteric junctional obstruction are common causes of unilateral obstruction, while prostatic enlargement, stone disease, and bladder and pelvic tumours account for about 75 per cent of cases of bilateral obstruction in developed countries. Wide geographic variations occur in the relative incidence of some causes of obstruction, for example, schistosomiasis (see Chapter 7.4).

Causes

Obstruction may be caused by lesions within the lumen or the wall of the urinary tract or by pressure from outside (Table 2).

Upper tract obstruction owing to lesions within the lumen

Calculi are the most common cause of urinary tract obstruction in the young adult male, calcium oxalate stones being most frequently responsible (see Section 8), and the incidence of such obstruction in males is two to three times that in females. Common sites for impaction of stones are in the calyx, at the pelviureteric junction, at the pelvic brim, near the posterior pelvis (especially in females, where pelvic blood vessels and the broad ligament cross the ureter anteriorly), and at the vesicoureteric junction. Stones smaller than 0.5 cm in diameter usually pass spontaneously.

A less common cause of intraluminal upper tract obstruction is papillary necrosis with passage of a sloughed papilla, such as occurs in diabetics, patients with papillary necrosis due to analgesic abuse (see Chapter 6.2), and those with sickle cell disease and trait (see Chapter 6.2). A calcified sloughed papilla in the urinary tract may mimic an opaque calculus, although the characteristic triangular shape of the opacity and the presence of a relevant underlying condition should alert the clinician to the correct diagnosis.

Upper tract obstruction owing to lesions within the wall

Functional obstructions

These result from failure of normal peristalsis through a segment or segments of the urinary tract. Although this may result from a decrease or absence of either circular or longitudinal smooth muscle fibres, in many cases no gross histological abnormalities are present (Whitaker 1975). Typically, obstruction is seen at the pelviureteric junction and this is the most common cause of urinary tract obstruction in childhood. Before the age of 1 year, pelviureteric junction obstruction is usually bilateral; thereafter unilateral obstruction is much more common. The condition may be diagnosed *in utero*, but peak incidence is at age 5, and at least 20 per cent of reported cases occur in adults over the age of 30 years.

A functional defect of the vesicoureteric junction (congenital megaureter) is the second most common cause of intramural obstruction in childhood, but is uncommon in adults. Males are more often affected than females, especially in childhood. Early studies reported a preponderance of circular smooth muscle fibres with a reduction in longitudinal fibres, and the disease was claimed to be analogous to Hirschsprung's disease of the colon. Earlier studies indicated, simply, a reduction in the number of muscle fibres and an increase in collagen fibres, together with preservation of the nerve ganglia (McLaughlin *et al.* 1973), making the analogy with Hirschsprung's disease invalid. However more recent studies have shown segmental upregulation of transforming growth factor-β (TGF-β), in longitudinal muscle layer suggesting segmental developmental delay of the terminal ureter (Jung *et al.* 2000a).

Anatomical obstructions

Intramural anatomical abnormalities are a less common cause of upper urinary tract obstruction. Ureteric strictures following surgery or radiotherapy should be uncommon. They occur in about 1 per cent of patients in the United Kingdom. Strictures have been reported in association with analgesic nephropathy and as a consequence of the

Table 2 Some causes of urinary tract obstruction

Within the lumen	Within the wall	Pressure from outside
Calculus	Pelviureteric neuromuscular dysfunction (congenital, 10% bilateral)	Pelviureteric compression (bands, aberrant vessels)
Blood clot		
Sloughed papilla (diabetes, analgesic abuse, sickle cell disease)	Ureteric stricture (tuberculosis, especially after treatment; calculous)	Tumours, e.g. retroperitoneal growths or glands, carcinoma of colon, diverticulitis, aortic aneurysm
	Ureterovesical stricture (congenital, ureterocele, calculous, schistosomiasis)	
Tumour of renal pelvis or ureter		Retroperitoneal fibrosis
Bladder tumour	Congenital megaureter	Accidental ligation of ureter
	Congenital bladder neck obstruction	Pancreatitis
	Neurogenic bladder	Retrocaval ureter (right-sided obstruction)
	Urethral stricture (calculous, gonococcal, after instrumentation)	Crohn's disease
		Chronic granulomatous disease
	Congenital urethral valve	Prostatic obstruction
	Pinhole meatus	Tumours in pelvis, e.g. carcinoma of cervix
		Phimosis

treatment of diseases directly involving the ureter, such as tuberculosis, where healing by fibrosis occurs.

Upper tract obstruction owing to pressure from outside

Disease of the reproductive system is the most common cause of such obstruction: pelvic malignancies, particularly carcinoma of cervix, are the most common cause in females. Some would argue that the most common cause of 'obstruction' in women is pregnancy: dilatation of the ureter to the level of the pelvic brim is frequently seen in women who have been pregnant (Dure-Smith 1968) and renographic examination carried out just before termination of pregnancy reveals abnormalities on the right side in almost 70 per cent of patients and on the left in 50 per cent. Urographic examination after pregnancy does not show dilatation of renal pelvis or calyces (Fig. 1) and the system is seen to empty on a full-length postmicturition film (Fig. 2), which is evidence against the presence of obstruction, at any rate after delivery. Approximately one-third of women with asymptomatic bacteriuria in pregnancy develop acute pyelonephritis, compared to only 1–2 per cent of non-pregnant females. The relationship, if any, between this fact and the anatomical changes seen in pregnancy is unclear. Presently, sonography, using both B-mode and Colour Doppler, has the potential to demonstrate the physiological compression of the ureters at the pelvic brim. Magnetic resonance urography, with strong T-2 weighted sequences, may also show the site and type of obstruction without contrast agent administration (Grenier et al. 2000).

Diseases of the retroperitoneal space, particularly tumour invasion from cervix, prostate, bladder, colon, ovary, and uterus, commonly cause obstruction. In retroperitoneal fibrosis (see below), it is unclear whether obstruction results from extrinsic compression or failure of peristalsis resulting from encasement of the ureter within a fibrous exoskeleton. That the latter may be the case is suggested by the fact that contrast medium injected into the lower ureter typically passes freely up to the pelvicalyceal system despite the presence of clinical, radiological, and isotopic evidence of functional urinary tract obstruction.

Less common causes include abnormalities of the vascular system and inflammatory bowel disease. The most common vascular cause is abdominal aortic aneurysm, particularly if associated with periaortic fibrosis; aneurysms of external and common iliac arteries rarely cause ureteric compression. The 'retrocaval' ureter, in which the right ureter passes behind the vena cava, resulting in ureteric compression, is another congenital cause of urinary tract obstruction of this type. The condition is more common in men. Examples of inflammatory bowel disease causing obstruction by extrinsic compression include Crohn's disease, diverticulitis, and chronic pancreatitis, especially when pseudocysts develop.

Lower tract obstruction owing to lesions within the lumen

Urethral calculi and blood clots developing after instrumentation or surgery, for example, are causes of lower tract obstruction within the lumen of the outflow tract. Both are very uncommon.

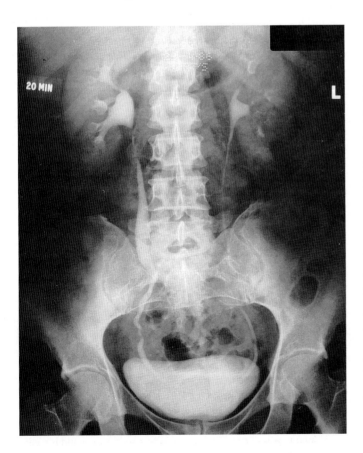

Fig. 1 Right ureter dilated to level of pelvic brim after pregnancy. Note absence of dilatation of renal pelvis and calyces.

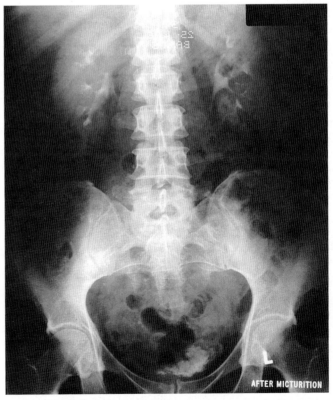

Fig. 2 Same patient as in Fig. 1, after voiding radiograph. Note good emptying of right ureter.

Lower tract obstruction owing to lesions within the wall

Functional

Functional obstruction may occur at the bladder neck and at the level of the distal sphincter owing to a failure of coordination between bladder contraction and sphincter relaxation. Whatever the cause, the bladder reacts to obstruction in one of two ways: either the wall becomes increasingly compliant or the opposite occurs and detrusor hypertrophy results in low compliance. The details of bladder muscle mechanics have been well reviewed (Schäfer 1985). Common causes of functional obstruction to outflow from the bladder (neuropathic or neurogenic bladder) include diabetes mellitus, multiple sclerosis, and spinal cord injuries. The most common cause in childhood is meningomyelocele. In the elderly, cerebrovascular disease and advanced Parkinson's disease and multiple system atrophy are often associated with functional bladder outflow obstruction and in some patients, particularly women, a psychological component appears to exist. Sometimes the cause is obscure. Certain drugs, including those which exhibit antimuscarinic activity, such as tricyclic antidepressants, and calcium-channel-blocking activity, have pharmacological effects on the bladder which provoke urinary retention (Whitfield 1977).

Anatomical

Urethral strictures following repeated instrumentation or surgery or gonococcal infections are common causes of lower tract obstruction resulting from wall lesions, as are urethral tumours and lesions prolapsing from within the bladder, for example, ureterocele. In children, urethral valves may be responsible for such obstruction (see Chapter 17.4).

Causes of lower tract obstruction owing to extrinsic pressure

In men, by far the most common causes are benign prostatic enlargement and prostatic cancer. In women, pelvic malignancy is a common cause; less common causes include uterine fibroids and complete procidentia.

It is important to realize that all causes of lower tract obstruction may also result in upper tract obstruction.

Acute and chronic obstructions

To the clinician, the first and most important question is whether urinary tract obstruction is of recent onset (acute obstruction) or longstanding (chronic obstruction). Since the pathophysiological changes, clinical features, approach to investigation, and management differ in important respects in acute versus chronic obstruction, they will be considered separately.

Acute upper tract obstruction

Normal ureteric peristalsis

Urine flows from kidney to bladder as a result of ureteric and pelvic peristalsis, the effects of gravity, and the pressure of glomerular filtration. Peristalsis is vital for the transport of urine down the ureter, and normally generates high pressures within the lumen, sufficient to propel urine down the ureter without the transmission of the increased pressure to the renal parenchyma. Baseline ureteric pressure is similar to that in the renal pelvis, but during this process increases to values between 10 and 25 mmHg. These pressures are not transmitted to the renal pelvis, where pressure is seldom greater than 4 mmHg.

Effects of acute ureteric obstruction

In the normal dog, pressure within the ureter more than doubles when the ureteric lumen is occluded during peristalsis; similar changes occur in ureteric wall tension. Three minutes after acute ureteric obstruction, baseline and peak pressures and wall tensions are about twice the control values (Rose and Gillenwater 1973). Between 5 and 20 min after induction of obstruction, baseline pressure and wall tensions increase further and approximate to peak values. At 1 h there is a threefold increase in baseline and peak pressures and wall tensions compared with control values; baseline and peak values for pressure and tension do not differ. At this point, occlusion of the ureter does not occur, and pressures generated by ureteric wall tension are transmitted to the renal pelvis and parenchyma. Any further increase in pressure results in dilatation of the ureter.

Renal response to ureteric obstruction

Most of the information about the consequences of urinary tract obstruction on kidney function and structure has been derived from the functional, biochemical, and histological studies in experimental animals. The effect of an increase in pressure within the ureter at the level of the nephron depends upon the degree of obstruction (whether complete or incomplete), whether or not obstruction is unilateral or bilateral, and the duration of obstruction (see review by Klahr 1991).

In the rat (Gillenwater 1986), pressure within the renal tubule shortly after occlusion of the ureter depends upon the state of hydration of the animal. In the hydropenic rat, intratubular pressure does not increase after occlusion of the ureter; if a solute diuresis is induced or if saline is administered intravenously, intratubular pressure increases, eventually approximating to glomerular filtration pressure. Intratubular pressure then declines progressively over the next 24 h. Whether pressures remain elevated thereafter depends upon the volume state of the animal and whether obstruction is bilateral or unilateral.

Unilateral obstruction has a less marked effect upon intratubular pressure than bilateral ureteric obstruction. In the former case, intratubular pressure approximates to normal 24 h after induction of ureteric obstruction. If obstruction is bilateral, intratubular pressures remain high at this time.

Effects of ureteric obstruction upon renal blood flow

Blood flow to the kidney declines after acute ureteric obstruction. Experimental induction of ureteric obstruction in man would be unethical. In clinical practice, the time of onset of obstruction is seldom known with precision. Methods of measurement of renal blood flow such as clearance of *p*-aminohippurate are indirect and depend upon tubular function, which is itself affected by urinary tract obstruction. For these reasons, the effect of ureteric obstruction upon renal blood flow in man is unclear.

The relationship between changes in ureteral pressure and renal blood flow with time is interesting. Three phases are discernible (Fig. 3). Acute ureteral obstruction causes a transient rise in blood flow to the kidney, followed by progressive vasoconstriction. This initial increase in renal blood flow is due to afferent arteriolar vasodilatation and is mediated by intrarenal mechanisms, as indicated by its occurrence in the denervated kidney and in the isolated perfused kidney. The decrease in

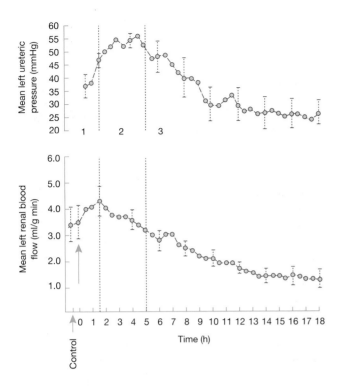

Fig. 3 The relationship between ipsilateral renal blood flow and ureteric pressure during experimental ureteric occlusion in the dog. In phase 1, renal blood flow and ureteric pressure increases. In phase 2, blood flow declines while ureteric pressure continues to increase. In phase 3, both renal blood flow and ureteric pressure decline. Arrow indicates time of ureteric occlusion. Mean ± standard error, $n = 5$ (reprinted with permission from Moody *et al.* 1975).

afferent arteriolar resistance results in an increased glomerular capillary pressure, which partially offsets the decrease in net filtration pressure resulting from the increase in proximal tubular pressure. Thus, in the initial phases of acute obstruction, single nephron glomerular filtration rate (GFR) is maintained at approximately 80 per cent of preobstruction values despite the marked increase in proximal tubular pressure. Most evidence indicates that local production of eicosanoids, mainly prostacyclin and PGE2, may account for the increased renal blood flow observed after the onset of obstruction. This increase in blood flow is eliminated by indomethcin administration (Blackshear *et al.* 1979). Usually after 3–5 h after the obstruction, there is an increase in intrarenal resistance due to vasoconstriction of afferent arterioles. The increase in resistance is mediated by angiotensin II, thromboxane A2, antidiuretic hormone (ADH), and impaired production of nitric oxide (Yarger 1980; Klahr 1991). Thereafter, in phase 3, renal blood flow continues to diminish and ureteric pressure returns towards or to normal. In phase 3, an increase in vascular resistance at the preglomerular level is thought to occur. Elegant micropuncture studies in the rat (Arendshorst *et al.* 1974) support this notion: obstruction of a single nephron for 24 h in an otherwise normal kidney decreases stop-flow pressure, reflecting a reduction in transcapillary pressure due to an increase in preglomerular vascular resistance. At 4 weeks, blood flow is about one-third that of the contralateral unobstructed kidney.

Acute histopathological changes

Acute obstruction results in increased ureteric pressure and decreased renal blood flow, and may be complicated by bacterial infection. The increase in intraluminal pressure and dilatation of the system proximal to the site of obstruction result in compression of the renal substance. The ducts of Bellini are affected first. In the early phase of obstruction, the kidney becomes oedematous and haemorrhagic.

Histologically, tubular dilatation initially affects mainly the collecting duct and distal tubular segments. Bowman's space may be dilated.

Clinical features

Acute upper tract obstruction typically gives rise to pain in the flank, which may radiate to the iliac fossa, inguinal region, testis, or labium. The pain may be dull or sharp, intermittent or persistent, though waxing and waning in intensity. It may be provoked by a high fluid intake, alcohol, or diuretics, measures which increase urinary volume and distend the collecting system: this is particularly noticeable when obstruction occurs at the pelviureteric junction. Loin tenderness may be detected and an enlarged kidney felt. Upper urinary tract infection with malaise, fever, and symptoms and signs of septicaemia may dominate the clinical picture.

Complete anuria is strongly suggestive of complete bilateral obstruction or complete obstruction of a single kidney. The differential diagnosis includes bilateral total renal cortical necrosis, acute anuric glomerulonephritis, and bilateral renal arterial occlusion. Intermittent anuria indicates the presence of intermittent complete obstruction.

Investigation

The investigation of acute obstruction must allow the site and cause to be identified rapidly, accurately, safely, and as economically as possible.

Imaging

Intravenous urography

Emergency intravenous urography (IVU) (see Chapter 1.6.1) is our preferred method of investigating the patient with suspected acute upper tract obstruction (Cattell *et al.* 1989). It will confirm the diagnosis and will usually demonstrate the site, cause, and degree of obstruction, providing invaluable guidance for management. Ultrasonography (Chapter 1.6.1i), although demonstrating dilatation, cannot visualize the ureters adequately (Denton *et al.* 1984; Webb *et al.* 1984).

The initial sequence of intravenous urograms must include full-length and coned renal plain films. The plain film must be examined carefully for opaque calculi along the line of the ureter—calculi overlying bone is easily missed (Figs 4 and 5). Some obstructing calculi are very small and only faintly calcified or non-opaque. Ureteric calculi within the bony pelvis are often impossible to distinguish from calcified phleboliths on the plain film. A large dose of contrast, usually of low osmolality (see Chapter 1.6.1), should be given to compensate for the lack of preparation of the patient.

Since contrast medium enters the pelvicalyceal system and ureter slowly, opacification of the system and ureter may never be seen in severe acute obstruction. In most instances, filling of the pelvicalyceal system and ureter to the level of obstruction can be demonstrated on delayed films (Figs 6 and 7). In acute ureteric obstruction the pelvicalyceal system and ureter may be only slightly dilated. Occasionally, the only abnormality may be a ureter, which remains full throughout its length to the level of the vesicoureteric junction, with this finding persisting on the full-length postmicturition film. Acute obstruction is

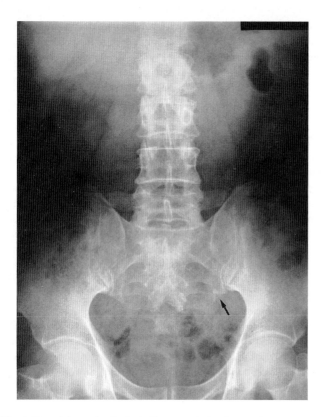

Fig. 4 Plain abdominal radiograph. Opaque calculus (arrowed) medial to left lower sacroiliac joint is easy to overlook.

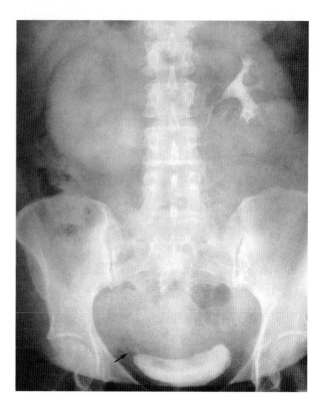

Fig. 6 Obstruction owing to opaque calculus at right vesicoureteric junction (arrowed). A nephrogram but no pyelogram is seen on the right 10 min after contrast injection.

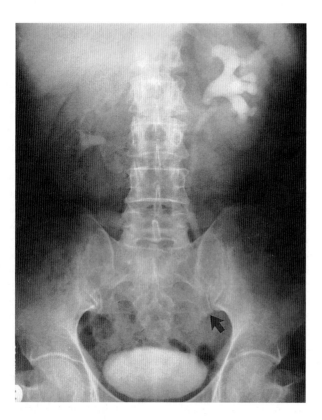

Fig. 5 Same patient as in Fig. 4, after contrast radiograph. Note dilatation of collecting system and ureter to the level of the calculus.

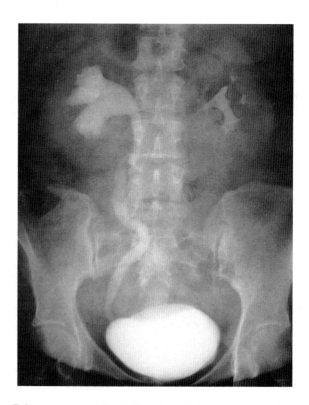

Fig. 7 Same patient as in Fig. 6. Film taken 1 h after contrast injection. Dilatation of pelvicalyceal system and ureter to the level of the obstructing calculus is now seen. Delayed films may need to be taken as much as 24 or even 48 h after contrast anjection to define the situation in some patients.

characterized by increased excretion of contrast medium by the liver, leading to gallbladder opacification on delayed films.

When typical obstructive changes are present, with a ureter dilated down to a calcified opacity, diagnosis is simple. If there is an obstructed nephrogram or dilatation of the pelvicalyceal system and ureter but no radiodense calculus is seen, diagnosis is more difficult. If the history is of recent-onset pain, the likely diagnostic possibilities are: recent passage of an opaque stone, uric acid stone, acute pelviureteric junction obstruction, blood clot, or sloughed papilla.

The presence of a uric acid stone may be suggested by a previous history of such stones, a personal or family history of gout, or clinical circumstances associated with uric acid stone formation, such as cytotoxic drug therapy or chronic small bowel disease. Urography shows uric acid stones as lucent filling defects. Similar filling defects may also occur with transitional cell tumours or blood clots. Since most ureteric stones pass spontaneously, investigation of a possible transitional cell tumour or blood clot should be delayed. If a persistent lucency is present, computed tomography (CT) scanning may be very helpful.

Acute idiopathic pelviureteric junction obstruction should be suspected if there is a large soft tissue density inferomedial to the kidney on the plain film produced by the distended pelvis. This usually fills on delayed films of the urogram with no filling of the ureter.

Clot colic is always associated with macroscopic haematuria. When clot colic is suspected, the urogram should be repeated after 2 weeks, by which time the clot should have lysed and any underlying lucent filling defect can be seen. Such patients require further investigation to define the cause of bleeding.

Sloughed papillae occur in patients with papillary necrosis. Typically, abnormal calyces are seen in both kidneys, but papillary necrosis may occasionally be unilateral, usually as a result of a previous episode of infection associated with unilateral obstruction, especially in diabetics. Occasionally, calcified papillae may mimic stones.

Ultrasonography (see Chapter 1.6.1i)

Ultrasound is less useful than urography in acute obstruction of the upper tract (Denton et al. 1984; Webb et al. 1984). It can define dilatation of the intrarenal collecting system in the upper third of the ureter, but dilatation of the middle and lower thirds of the ureter is not easily detectable ultrasonically and the dilated ureter cannot usually be followed to the level of obstruction. However, colour and pulsed Doppler can sometimes detect the presence or absence of ureteral jets to diagnose ureteric obstruction (Webb 2000).

Ultrasound may be used to investigate patients with acute obstruction if they are pregnant or have a history of contrast allergy. The risk of contrast nephrotoxicity in diabetics with moderate to severe renal impairment and in patients with myelomatosis is currently considered a relative contraindication to IVU: ultrasonography, therefore, has a primary role in the investigation of such patients.

Antegrade and retrograde pyelography and ureterography

If the site of obstruction is not demonstrated by IVU, antegrade or retrograde examination may be helpful. Both techniques can be initiated as a method of diagnosis but then extended to provide a therapeutic role by providing drainage.

CT scanning (see Chapter 1.6.1v)

Unenhanced CT confers major diagnostic benefits, and is a fast, well-tolerated technique. Its accompanying higher effective radiation dose

is recognized (Homer et al. 2001). Unenhanced spiral CT is more effective than IVU in identifying ureteric calculi and is equally effective in detecting urinary obstruction (Wong et al. 2001).

Magnetic resonance urography

The comparatively new development is magnetic resonance (MR) urography using half-Fourier acquisition single-shot turbo spin-echo (HASTE) imaging. It accurately and rapidly shows the level and degree of ureteric obstruction. It can be used to differentiate between acute and chronic obstructions on the basis of its ability to show perirenal fluid (Regan et al. 1996). Although IVU is likely to remain the standard procedure for imaging the upper tract, MR urography enhanced by gadolinium and frusemide may be helpful if there is a dilated system with no excretory function, in pregnant women, in children, and in those with contrast medium allergy (Jung et al. 2000b).

Use of radionuclides (see Chapter 1.6.1vii)

The presence of a calculus does not necessarily mean that the kidney is obstructed, which requires emergency decompression. For renal colic, clinical selection, KUB radiography, and even positive helical CT findings are known to have a low positive predictive value (35, 32 and 56 per cent, respectively) (Sfakianakis et al. 2000). Technetium-mercaptoacetyltriglycine (MAG-3) radioisotope scan can be used to differentiate obstructed from unobstructed kidneys. In one study, 80 patients presenting with acute renal colic and positive helical CT were differentiated into obstructed, 56.5 per cent (32.5 per cent partially obstructed, 24 per cent completely obstructed), and 43.5 per cent without obstruction (21 per cent without any indication of recent obstruction and 22.5 per cent unobstructed but with kidney dysfunction due to spontaneous decompression), using MAG-3 renogram (Sfakianakis et al. 2000).

Management of acute upper tract obstruction

Stones

The majority of patients presenting to an accident and emergency department with renal and ureteric colic will have a stone in the lower third of the ureter, often in that portion of the ureter lying within the bladder wall. Such patients can be managed conservatively, since the stone has already passed through two areas of relative ureteric narrowing; the pelviureteric junction, and the site at which the ureter crosses the bifurcation of the common iliac artery. A conservative policy is likely to prove successful if the stone is 5 mm or less in its maximum diameter. It is unusual for acute episodes of colic to persist for more than 72 h.

Patients with ureteric colic are usually admitted to hospital, although this is unnecessary in many cases since the only medical requirement is the provision of regular analgesia, which can be parental, oral, or rectal.

Although it has long been argued that morphine should be avoided as an analgesic as it may provoke ureteric spasm, there is no evidence that therapeutic doses of morphine have this effect. Pethidine may provoke nausea and vomiting, particularly when administered parentally, but since nausea and vomiting frequently accompany colic, it is difficult to disentangle the effects of such treatment from the effects of colic alone. Very satisfactory pain relief can often be obtained using nonsteroidal anti-inflammatory agents administered orally or per rectum.

With the advent of new, less invasive methods of surgical management of ureteric stones, there is a tendency to intervene earlier. Using ultrasound, stones can be imaged in the intramural ureter by using the full bladder as an acoustic window. Since most stones at that site will pass spontaneously, the extent to which lithotripsy will hasten the process is difficult to establish. Stones in the upper third of the ureter can only be imaged accurately by ultrasound if there is ureteric dilatation above the stone. Using a lithotripter, which incorporates the additional facility of radiological imaging, stones almost anywhere in the ureter can be imaged and treated. Stone-free rates after *in situ* extracorporeal shock-wave lithotripsy (ESWL) have been reported to range from 81 to 96 per cent (Hendrikx *et al.* 1990; Danuser *et al.* 1993). However, it is generally accepted that the success rate of ESWL when treating ureteric calculi is less than when treating renal calculi (Wainstein and Reznick 1994). The reason for this is possibly that disimpaction of the fragmented stone is more difficult within the ureter than in the kidney (Mueller *et al.* 1993). A larger number of shock waves at a higher voltage and an increased number of repeat sessions are required when a stone is within the ureter rather than in the kidney. Some controversy remains whether upper ureteric stones should be manipulated back into the kidney before ESWL. The value of a JJ stent inserted alongside an impacted ureteric stone in both aiding fragmentation and enhancing the passage of stone fragments is now debated.

Endoscopic manoeuvres, which are usually performed under general anaesthesia, are reserved for those patients with persistent colic. These techniques are described more fully in Chapter 8.3.

Drainage of an obstructed system

If there is clinical evidence of infection above an obstruction, drainage must be established as a matter of urgency (Davis 1943). The diagnosis is a clinical one. The patient will be pyrexial and the degree of loin tenderness will be greater than when obstruction is not associated with infection. Examination of bladder urine may be unhelpful, since ureteric obstruction may prevent red and white blood cells and organisms from reaching the lower urinary tract. Leucocytosis may be present but this is not invariably the case, especially in the elderly.

The choice between antegrade and retrograde interventions will depend on the facilities and expertise available. In most specialist centres, there is a clear preference for the insertion of an antegrade needle nephrostomy percutaneously under local anaesthetic. In a dilated high-pressure system, the procedure is usually easy. Such a system may be used to provide drainage for weeks, or even months, if necessary. If excretion of intravenous contrast has outlined renal anatomy, renal puncture may be guided radiographically. In non-opacified systems, the initial puncture may be better directed under ultrasound control using a fine needle. The collecting system is then outlined with contrast and an accurate transparenchymal calyceal puncture can be placed, usually through a lower calyx.

A retrograde ureteric catheter, in contrast, can be relied on to provide drainage at best only for a matter of days. Occasionally, a retrograde catheter cannot be passed beyond the obstruction and the diagnostic role of retrograde ureterography cannot then be extended to a therapeutic one.

Other causes of acute obstruction

The two other most common causes are sloughed papillae and blood clots. The principles of management vary very little from those already outlined for ureteric stones. However, greater attention must be paid in the acute phase to the underlying cause. In the patient with papillary necrosis, infection is a more common accompaniment of obstruction

and surgical intervention, usually with a percutaneous needle nephrostomy, is required more often. When colic results from blood clot, treatment of the underlying cause may be necessary at an early stage. Renal parenchymal tumours and transitional cell tumours of the collecting system may both cause persistent bleeding and colic, and ablative open surgery is usually required. More difficulty is encountered when bleeding occurs from a non-malignant cause. An arteriovenous fistula, whether spontaneous or traumatic, may be embolized with every prospect of success. The most difficult cause of recurrent bleeding to manage is that associated with papillary necrosis in sickle cell trait or disease (see Chapter 4.11). Antifibrinolytic agents may be of value, but administration of such treatment during active bleeding may produce hard rubbery clots, which fill the collecting system and require surgical removal.

Acute obstruction in the lower urinary tract

Pathophysiology (Gillenwater 1978; Klahr 1982)

The mechanical efficiency of smooth muscle fibres is reduced when they become overstretched. As bladder outflow obstruction increases, a point is reached when acute urinary retention will result. Factors which may precipitate acute retention include a sudden diuresis such as that occurs after alcohol ingestion or diuretic therapy for heart failure, urinary tract infection, and drugs which have pharmacological effects upon the bladder, provoking retention, such as those with antimuscarinic and calcium-channel-blocking activity.

Clinical features

Acute urinary retention is often preceded by a history of symptoms of bladder outflow obstruction with hesitancy, diminished forcefulness of the urinary stream, and terminal dribbling. Acute retention is typically associated with severe suprapubic pain, but this may be absent if acute retention is superimposed on chronic retention or if there is an underlying neuropathy.

A potential clinical pitfall is the failure to recognize that patients who have an epidural anaesthetic may develop painless acute retention of urine. Most modalities of bladder sensation are mediated via sacral parasympathetic nerves. The pain from bladder overdistension is sympathetically mediated and will be abolished by a high epidural reaching to D10. Obstetricians need to be particularly alert to this problem.

Pre-existing obstruction may have provoked changes in the bladder such as muscle wall hypertrophy, sacculation, and diverticulum formation: these in turn predispose to persistence of lower urinary tract infection once acquired, and occasionally to bladder stones. Epididymo-orchitis may occur.

Investigation

Most patients presenting with acute urinary retention require no investigation before treatment. Suprapubic pain coexisting with a bladder which is palpably or percussibly distended above the level of the symphysis pubis is sufficient evidence for immediate catheterization.

If doubt about the diagnosis exists, an ultrasound examination will confirm or refute the presence of a distended bladder. Transrectal ultrasound of the prostate can demonstrate both the size of the gland and to some extent the benign or malignant nature of the enlargement. Such an investigation is not indicated in the acute situation but would be of potential benefit after the relief of obstruction.

An ascending urethrogram may be indicated if an attempt at urethral catheterization proves unsuccessful. This is done as an elective procedure after bladder drainage has been secured by suprapubic catheterization.

Management

The bladder may be catheterized *per urethram* or suprapubically. In women, catheterization *per urethram* typically presents no difficulty. A hypospadiac external urethral meatus may be difficult to locate on the anterior vaginal wall.

Urethral catheterization may present more difficulty in men. Too many male urethras are subjected to unnecessary trauma with very significant subsequent morbidity owing both to ignorance of the correct technique of catheterization and of the anatomy. If one attempt to pass a standard 18 French Foley catheter fails, the patient should be catheterized suprapubically. Only an experienced operator should pass a urethral catheter on an introducer. Commercially produced suprapubic catheters are available for insertion under local anaesthetic. Each is accompanied by very adequate instructions for use. If doubt or difficulty exists, the help of a urologist should be sought.

Chronic upper tract obstruction

Chronic ureteric obstruction

Three months after production of experimental obstruction in dogs, baseline ureteric wall tension is increased, and there is no difference between baseline and peak values of wall tension, peak values being measured during ureteric occlusion (Rose and Gillenwater 1973). By contrast, baseline and peak pressures within the ureteric lumen are not significantly different from control values. In chronic obstruction, therefore, normal intraluminal pressures are maintained as a consequence of ureteric dilatation.

These experimental findings suggest that the major component of kidney damage due to obstruction occurs soon after its onset. Certainly, in humans, the greatest measured ureteric pressures have been found during acute obstruction (as high as 50 mmHg during the passage of a stone) and there appears to be an inverse relationship between pressure within the renal pelvis measured in patients with complete obstruction and time. The notion that chronic obstruction with dilatation of the ureter may be relatively benign is supported by the observation that patients with urinary tract obstruction due to congenital anomalies lose renal function only slowly.

Effects of chronic ureteric obstruction upon the kidney

As mentioned above, the ducts of Bellini are first affected by dilatation of the system proximal to the site of obstruction. Subsequently, other papillary structures are affected and ultimately compression of renal cortical tissue occurs with thinning of the renal parenchyma. Enlargement of the kidney occurs in association with dilatation of the renal pelvis. Atrophy of the renal parenchyma with reduction in size of the kidney (obstructive atrophy) is believed to result from the effects of compression of the renal parenchyma and from prolonged renal ischaemia. Slowly progressive partial obstruction tends to result in gross dilatation of the collecting system, dilated calyces, and renal pelvis being surrounded by only a thin rim of renal parenchyma. In acute complete obstruction, dilatation tends to be less marked.

Mechanisms of progression of renal failure in chronic obstruction

The mechanisms underlying the progression of renal disease to ESRD in humans after an initial insult are not well understood. Several studies indicate that tubulointerstitial changes, not glomerular pathology, correlate better with decrements in GFR in a variety of renal disease (Risdon *et al.* 1968; Yaqoob *et al.* 1994). Renal tubular cells produce an array of growth factors, vasoactive peptides, proteases, and cytokines (Eddy 1996; Yaqoob 1997), the action of which might in turn be modulated by the extracellular matrix. The importance of the extracellular matrix acting as an interface between cells and their environment is now widely accepted, as is the role of the matrix in conditioning the events that occur within the cell. Adherence of cells to matrix can induce cells to make cytokines, which, in turn, might induce cells to alter their matrix. Such interactions likely play an important role in inflammation and scarring within the tubulointerstitium. These observations suggest that the tubulointerstitium and derangements of this anatomic compartment contribute importantly to the progression of chronic renal disease.

A number of renal diseases can cause tubulointerstitial pathology. These structural changes of the tubulointerstitial space are often considered secondary to glomerular lesions. However, certain renal diseases, notably obstructive uropathy, are characterized by primary tubulointerstitial pathology and subsequent involvement of glomerular structures.

Obstructive uropathy can cause major changes in the tubulointerstitial compartment of the kidney (Fig. 8). Renal interstitial fibrosis is a common consequence of long-standing obstructive uropathy. Fibrosis likely develops due to an imbalance between extracellular matrix synthesis and deposition and matrix synthesis and deposition and matrix degradation.

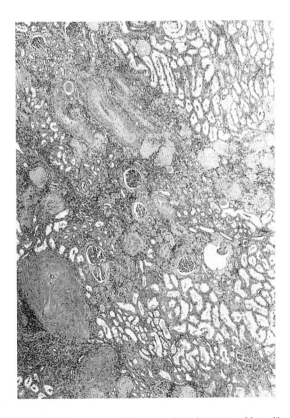

Fig. 8 Histological appearances in long-standing obstruction. Note dilated tubules, interstitial fibrosis, vessel wall thickening, and global sclerosis of some glomeruli.

Angiotensin II plays a pivotal role in the progression of renal disease, including obstructive nephropathy (review by Klahr 2001). Increasing levels of angiotensin II in obstructive nephropathy upregulate the expression of several factors: TGF-β1, tumour necrosis factor-α, platelet-derived growth factor, insulin-like growth factor (IGF-1), osteopontin, vascular cell adhesion molecule-1, monocyte chemoattractant peptide-1, and intercellular adhesion molecule-1, among others. Local production of TGF-β, by intrinsic renal cells or by macrophages invading the kidney, is a key mediator of renal fibrosis. Activation of TGF-β stimulates endothelin production. Endothelin, in turn, is a potent stimulus for fibrogenesis. Oxidative stress, fuelled, in part, by angiotensin II, upregulates the expression of adhesion molecules, chemoattractant compounds, and cytokines. Nuclear factor-κB (NF-κB) is involved in the transcriptional regulation of genes present in several organs, including the kidney. NF-κB is activated in the setting of ureteral obstruction. Administration of angiotensin-converting enzyme (ACE) inhibitors decreased significantly the activation of NF-κB in obstructed kidney (Morrissey and Klahr 1997). Moreover, Schanstra et al. (2002) have shown in elegant experiments that ACE inhibitors attenuate interstitial fibrosis due to increased local bradykinin concentration. Bradykinin receptor B2 knockout mice developed increased interstitial fibrosis following unilateral ureteral obstruction but this fibrosis was reduced in B2 receptor overexpressing transgenic rats. Bradykinin mediates its effect by increasing plasminogen activators and metalloprotease-2.

Sustained obstructive nephropathy leads to distinct patterns of cell proliferation and apoptosis in the tubular, interstitial, and glomerular cells (reviewed by Truong et al. 1998). In many experimental models, tubular cell apoptosis develops quickly after ureteric ligation, peaks between 7 and 24 days postobstruction, and tapers thereafter. Apoptosis initially involved the dilated collecting ducts, but subsequently spreads to other tubules. Tubular cell apoptosis, a probably accounts for renal tissue loss because a direct correlation between its degree and the decline in dry kidney weight is well documented. Pronounced tubular cell proliferation occurs shortly after ureter ligation, peaks at about day 6, and quickly subsides to baseline. Because the peak of tubular cell proliferation immediately precedes the onset of tubular cell apoptosis, a pathologic link may exist between the two processes. Interstitial cell apoptosis occurs with an increasing frequency throughout the course of chronic obstruction. Interstitial cell proliferation appears in a bimodal pattern with the early peak coinciding with that of tubular cell proliferation and consisting mostly of fibroblasts, whereas the later peak consists mostly of inflammatory cells. Glomerular cell and proliferation is not different from control, which explains, in part, the structural integrity of the glomeruli throughout the disease course. Although the general pathways of cell apoptosis and proliferation are well known, the molecular control of these processes in obstructive uropathy is poorly understood. In addition, whether apoptosis or proliferation of tubular and interstitial cells is differentially regulated remains to be studied. However, several molecules known to be overexpressed in kidney with obstructive uropathy may modulate cell apoptosis and proliferation. The relevant functions of these molecules include induction of apoptosis (angiotensin II, reactive oxygen species, caspases), inhibition of the cell cycle (TGF-β, p21) inhibition of apoptosis [epidermal growth factor (EGF), IGF, bcl-2, osteopontin] or promotion of interstitial fibroblast proliferation (platelet-derived growth factor). Studies in neonatal rats indicate that chronic ureteral obstruction decreases the expression of EGF. Replacement of this factor decreased

apoptosis. The administration of IGF-1 also lessened the tubular and interstitial pathologies in the setting of ureteral obstruction. Moreover, urinary tract obstruction in mice induced tubular and interstitial cellular apoptosis in parallel with an increased expression of caspases. Among the evaluated caspases, increased renal caspase 3 activity implied its central role in apoptosis associated with urinary obstruction (Truong et al. 2001).

A number of pharmacological interventions that ameliorate the increased expansion of the interstitial volume, decrease the expression of TGF-β, and downregulate the production of extracellular matrix and the infiltration of the interstitium by macrophages have been described in the experimental settings. Drugs used include ACE inhibitors, administration of arginine (by increasing NO production due to endothelial and neuronal nitric oxide synthase) (Morrissey et al. 1996; Huang et al. 2000), administration of osteogenic protein-1 (by inhibition of apoptosis of tubular cells) (Hruska et al. 2000), and pirfenidone (PFD; Shionogi Research Laboratories, Osaka, Japan and Marnac, Dallas, TX: new compound which prevents or reverses ECM accumulation) (Shimizu et al. 1998). It is likely that in the next decade advances in genetic manipulations and new drug therapies may forestall the development of fibrosis in the setting of urinary tract obstruction (Chevalier 2000; Klahr 2001).

Effects of obstruction on renal function

Glomerular filtration rate before release of obstruction

Little precise information is available about the effects of urinary tract obstruction on the human GFR for some of the reasons given earlier in relation to knowledge about renal blood flow after development of obstruction in humans. However, it is clear from animal models that ureteric obstruction results in a marked reduction in GFR. In both models of complete obstruction (unilateral or bilateral ureteral ligation), the decrease in the whole kidney GFR seen is due to both a decrease in single nephron GFR and in the number of filtering nephrons. The decrease in single nephron GFR is due to decrease in plasma flow rate per nephron, a decrease in net hydrostatic pressure, and a decrease in the filtration coefficient due to decrease in the surface area available for filtration. Three major vasoconstrictors of the renal circulation, angiotensin II, thromboxane A2, and ADH play a role in the decrease of plasma flow rate per nephron as well as decrease in the filtration coefficient by causing mesangial cell contraction (Blackshear 1979; Yarger et al. 1980; Reyes et al. 1991). Administration of inhibitors of these mediators before the onset of obstruction attenuate changes resulting from ureteral obstruction. Moreover, inhibition of the 5-lipoxygenase pathway (generator of leukotrienes) in vivo ameliorates decline in GFR due to ureteral obstruction (Klahr 1991).

Tubular function before release of obstruction

The most common abnormalities in chronic partial ureteric obstruction are disturbances in renal tubular function. As would be expected from the histopathological findings, distal tubular function is more strikingly disturbed than proximal tubular function.

A characteristic feature of patients with chronic partial ureteric obstruction is an impaired ability to concentrate urine. The concentration defect is resistant to administration of ADH and is thus an example of nephrogenic diabetes insipidus. Animal experiments indicate that production of cyclic adenosine monophosphate (cAMP) and translocation of aquaporin II to the apical surface of the collecting tubular cells in response to vasopressin is reduced in chronic partial obstruction, and this may, at least in part, explain the concentration defect (Frokiaer 1996).

Most animal experiments that have examined the effects of ureteric obstruction upon renal tubular function have been performed after acute obstruction has been induced. In dogs, acute unilateral ureteric obstruction produced by elevation of the ureter reduces urine flow and both absolute and fractional sodium and water reabsorption. Similar results have been obtained in the rat following 30 h of acute incomplete obstruction (Abbrecht and Malvin 1960; Suki *et al.* 1966). In this model, micropuncture experiments reveal increased fluid reabsorption in the proximal tubule, perhaps as a result of prolongation of nephron transit time. More chronic ureteric obstruction in the dog reduces the capacity to reabsorb sodium and water (Suki *et al.* 1966).

Since ureteric obstruction affects distal segments of the nephron more than proximal segments, an acidification defect is associated with chronic partial ureteric obstruction in man (Berlyne 1961). In many patients with obstructive nephropathy, urinary pH is inappropriately high for any degree of metabolic acidosis. This distal renal tubular acidosis is present in both unilateral and bilateral ureteric obstruction, and may be associated with hyperkalaemia (Batlle *et al.* 1981).

Glomerular filtration rate and renal blood flow after release of obstruction

In man, the relationship between duration of obstruction and the extent of recovery of renal function after its reversal is unknown, and surprisingly few data have been published. Such studies that do exist (Olbrich *et al.* 1957; Zetterstrom *et al.* 1958; Edvall 1959; Better *et al.* 1973; Gillenwater *et al.* 1975) indicate that renal blood flow increases after relief of obstruction and GFR either remains the same or increases, but no extensive study has been performed in man in which the duration of obstruction has been correlated with the degree of recovery of GFR. There is no reason to doubt that the extent of recovery depends upon whether obstruction is partial or complete, the duration of obstruction, and whether or not obstruction is complicated by bacterial infection.

The relationship between the duration of obstruction and recovery of function has been more clearly defined in experimental animals. Unilateral ureteric ligation was performed in dogs (Kerr 1954). GFR was measured preoperatively and the GFR of each kidney was assumed to be 50 per cent of the overall GFR. When the ligature was removed after 1 week of complete obstruction, the ipsilateral GFR was found to be 25 per cent of the ipsilateral control value and 16 per cent of that of the contralateral kidney measured at the same time. This discrepancy resulted from a compensatory increase in function of the non-obstructed kidney during the week of complete obstruction of its partner. Improvement in GFR of the previously obstructed kidney continued up to, but not beyond, 2 months after release of obstruction, but complete recovery never occurred, the maximum improvement being only to 50 per cent of the GFR of the non-operated kidney. Changes in effective renal plasma flow measured by *p*-aminohippurate clearance paralleled changes in GFR, so the filtration fraction remained unchanged.

Renal blood flow is decreased following relief of bilateral or unilateral ureteric obstruction: whether this results from a redistribution of blood flow within the kidney is uncertain. Most studies in dogs and rats indicate that cortical blood flow is markedly reduced, whereas inner medullary blood flow is normal or increased. It has been postulated that the reduction in cortical flow may, at least in part, result from intrarenal hormonal changes. The fact that production of the vasoconstrictor thromboxane A_2 can more easily be stimulated in the hydronephrotic kidneys of rabbits than in normal rabbit kidneys is consistent with this notion.

Renal tubular function after release of obstruction (postobstructive diuresis)

Renal tubular function after release of obstruction depends, in part, upon whether obstruction was unilateral or bilateral. In man, large diuresis and natriuresis often follow release of complete bilateral obstruction. Factors determining this include the state of hydration prior to release of obstruction—in salt- and water-overloaded patients a more profound diuresis and natriuresis is to be expected; the osmotic diuretic effect of retained, relatively poorly reabsorbable solutes such as urea; accumulation of humoral agents such as atrial natriuretic factor prior to relief of obstruction; and a reduction in tubular reabsorptive capacity for sodium and water resulting from intrinsic tubular damage.

Only this last factor would operate in unilateral obstruction and salt and water diuresis following relief of such obstruction does not present a clinical problem in humans. The relative contribution of the factors listed has not been clearly established in man, but the problem has been studied extensively in experimental animals.

Studies of sodium balance before, during, and after bilateral ureteric obstruction in the rat and in sham-operated controls (McDougal and Wright 1972) show that the increase in sodium and water excretion after relief of obstruction is not simply a consequence of volume expansion. Since it occurs in the face of a marked decline in GFR, it must result, in this model at least, from a reduction in tubular reabsorption of sodium and water. Experimental production of the same degree of uraemia as that produced by bilateral ureteric ligation in the rat followed by its release also induces an increase in sodium and water excretion, but nowhere near the same extent as is seen following relief of obstruction.

Changes in blood atrial natriuretic factor in experimentally induced obstruction have been less studied. Initial observations indicate that atrial natriuretic factor concentrations are markedly increased in acute bilateral obstruction, but the significance of this remains to be elucidated. The problem has, so far, been less studied in humans.

The diuresis that occurs following relief of unilateral obstruction is very much less than that seen after relief of bilateral obstruction. In man, fractional sodium and water excretion after release of unilateral obstruction usually increase, despite the marked decrease in GFR of the obstructed kidney, but are of a much lower order of magnitude than is seen after release of bilateral obstruction. This discrepancy appears, in part, to result from a greater delivery of tubular fluid from cortical nephrons after release of bilateral obstruction. A number of observations support this hypothesis. First, phosphate reabsorption is greater in the postobstructed kidney than in the normal kidney (Better *et al.* 1975). Since phosphate is reabsorbed proximally, this suggests that there may also be an increase in proximal sodium and water reabsorption in this segment in the postobstructive kidney. Second, micropuncture experiments show that sodium and water reabsorption in proximal and distal tubular segments of surface nephrons is greater after release of unilateral ureteric obstruction than after release of bilateral ureteric obstruction. Impaired ability to concentrate the urine is regularly seen after release of urinary tract obstruction. This defect is not responsive to ADH and may result from decreased production of ADH-dependent cAMP production or impaired apical translocation of aquaporin 2 in the postobstructive kidney (Frokiaer 1996). In addition, decreased hypertonicity of the medullary interstitium due to reduced Na^+,K^+-ATPase activity in the outer medulla, increased prostaglandin synthesis, and increased medullary blood flow may also contribute to this defect (Klahr 1997).

Acid excretion is impaired after release of bilateral and unilateral ureteric obstruction in both man and experimental animals: studies of unilateral obstruction provide a more valid indicator of the effect of obstruction upon the kidney since the complicating factors associated with uraemia are absent. After release of unilateral obstruction, urine pH from the postobstructed kidney tends to be greater than 7.0 and the response to an acid load is reduced or absent. Micropuncture experiments reveal no reduction in reabsorption of bicarbonate in proximal or distal segments of surface nephrons and urinary P_{CO_2} remains low after bicarbonate loading. These observations indicate that the acidification defect in the rat results either from impaired secretion of hydrogen ions into distal tubules and collecting ducts of surface nephrons or from reduced bicarbonate reabsorption in juxtamedullary nephrons, or both. A reduction in distal hydrogen ion secretion is likely to be the dominant or main factor as shown by recent observations of reduced H-ATPase pumps in the apical surface of intercalated cells in the obstructed kidney (Sabatini and Kurtzman 1990).

Phosphate handling after release of obstruction

The reabsorption of phosphate by the postobstructed kidney depends on both the duration of the obstruction and whether the obstruction is unilateral or bilateral. In man, there is a dissociation between phosphate and sodium reabsorption following release of unilateral ureteric obstruction, phosphate reabsorption being increased (Better *et al.* 1975) and sodium reabsorption decreased. In rats, release of obstruction after 24 h is followed by a modest increase in phosphate excretion from the control kidney but a much-reduced excretion of phosphate from the postobstructive organ. The increased excretion of phosphate by the control kidney is abolished by prior parathyroidectomy. The likely explanation for reduced phosphate excretion by the postobstructive kidney is a combination of a marked reduction in single nephron GFR and filtered load of phosphate, together with increased proximal reabsorption of salt and water which would greatly decrease delivery of phosphate to the parathormone (PTH)-sensitive sites located more distally in the nephron. In this model, there is a marked increase in fractional excretion of magnesium by the postobstructive kidney, probably due to a decrease in reabsorption of salt and water, as well as magnesium, by the thick ascending limb of the loop of Henle. Human hypomagnesaemia has been reported following relief of bilateral ureteric obstruction (see Chapter 2.5). However, after release of bilateral ureteral obstruction of 24 h duration, phosphate excretion parallels sodium and water excretion (Beck 1979). This increase is not affected by parathyroidectomy and cannot be accounted for by an increase in ECF volume. This increased phosphate excretion can be abolished by dietary restriction of phosphate implying increased filtrate load of phosphate as the main determinant of this defect in bilateral ureteral obstruction.

Hormonal changes induced by obstruction

Erythropoietin

Plasma erythopoietin is low in humans with renal failure due to obstructive uropathy, but neither the degree of anaemia nor the degree of depression of erythropoietin concentrations is known to differ from that occurring in chronic renal failure of similar severity and different aetiology.

Vitamin D metabolism

Anatomical considerations suggest that renal 1-hydroxylase activity might be particularly severely affected in chronic obstruction. However, scant data are available in respect of vitamin D metabolites and vitamin D metabolism in renal failure associated with obstruction compared with renal failure of similar degree but of different aetiologies.

An impression exists that osteomalacia may be more common in patients with renal failure due to obstruction, but the fact that such renal failure is very slowly progressive may account for this (see Chapter 11.3.8).

Hypertension and the renin–angiotensin system

Hypertension is more common in patients with bilateral urinary tract obstruction than in normal individuals matched for age and gender. The prevalence of hypertension resulting from unilateral obstruction is unknown.

An increase in total exchangeable sodium has been demonstrated in chronic bilateral upper tract obstruction and blood pressure frequently returns to normal with correction of obstruction. Patients of this sort appear to have a volume-dependent form of hypertension consequent upon salt and water retention. Concentrations of renin in renal and peripheral veins are normal.

Chronic unilateral urinary tract obstruction, peripheral vein renin concentrations are usually normal or low despite the presence of hypertension, suggesting that chronic unilateral obstruction is not a cause of renin-dependent hypertension.

Atrial natriuretic peptide

Atrial natriuretic peptide release is augmented in patients with bilateral ureteric obstruction and uraemia, probably owing to salt and water overload, and this may contribute to the postobstructive diuresis and natriuresis which occurs after surgical correction of the problem.

Clinical features (Gillenwater 1982)

Patients may present with flank or abdominal pain, renal failure, or both; the symptoms and signs of urinary tract infection and septicaemia may be superimposed. Rarely, presentation is with erythraemia or hypertension and their complications. A proportion of patients are asymptomatic, obstruction being found during investigation of some other condition such as haematuria, urinary infection, or hypertension.

Polyuria often occurs in chronic partial obstruction owing to impairment of renal tubular concentrating capacity. Intermittent anuria and polyuria indicate intermittent complete and partial obstruction.

Investigations

Obstruction must be excluded early in all patients with unexplained renal failure. In patients with known renal disease, rapid deterioration in renal function unexplained by the primary renal problem also demands investigation. Relapsing urinary tract infections should also raise the possibility of an associated obstructing lesion. The diagnosis of partial obstruction should not be discounted simply because urine volume is normal or increased.

The history should include questions relating to analgesic abuse (associated with papillary necrosis, transitional cell tumours, and periureteric fibrosis) and vitamin D consumption (associated with calculus formation). Ingestion of methysergide and other drugs may be associated with retroperitoneal fibrosis. A history or family history of gout, diabetes, or renal stone formation should be obtained.

The choice of imaging depends upon the mode of presentation. IVU is the method of choice in patients with loin pain since it best diagnoses the more common causes—calculous obstruction and idiopathic pelviureteric junction obstruction. Initial investigation of the patient with unexplained impairment of renal function should include ultrasonography, together with plain abdominal radiographs and renal tomography to screen for urinary tract calculi. Tomography may be necessary to detect low-density calculi. Small unobstructed kidneys will be demonstrated in about 50 per cent of patients (Fig. 9) and other means of detecting upper tract dilatation will be unnecessary. Since ultrasound cannot distinguish between an obstructed distended system and a baggy, low-pressure dilated system, an abnormality on ultrasound will prompt further definitive investigation. The cost and limited availability of CT means that it is not the method of choice to detect obstruction; scintigraphy is not recommended as the first investigation in suspected obstruction but is useful in defining whether dilatation shown by other methods is obstructive.

Intravenous urography

A high dose of contrast will need to be administered to patients with renal failure and tomograms and delayed films should be taken as necessary. Films taken immediately after contrast injection will show a dilated pelvicalyceal system as a lucent 'negative pyelogram' surrounded by opacified parenchyma. Later films usually show filling of the dilated pelvicalyceal system and ureter (Fig. 10). Tomography may be necessary to show the faint opacification of dilated calyces. Definition of the dilated ureter may be poor.

In very long-standing obstruction, generalized thinning of the renal parenchyma (obstructive atrophy) is seen. This is typically diffuse and symmetrical and there is associated generalized calyceal dilatation.

CT scanning

On CT, the dilated collecting system appears as a multiloculate fluid collection of water density in the renal sinus. It is possible to distinguish the intrarenal collecting system from the extrarenal portion of the pelvis; this is important since obstruction can only be diagnosed on CT when there is dilatation of the intrarenal collecting system. A prominent extrarenal pelvis may be a normal variant. The whole-dilated

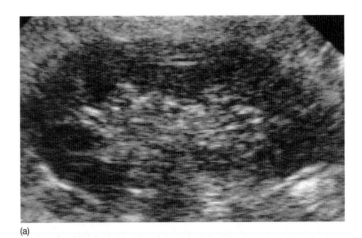
(a)

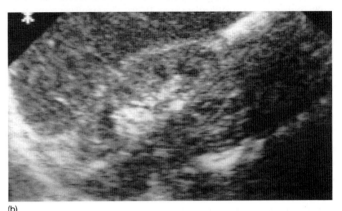
(b)

Fig. 9 (a) Ultrasound scan showing normal right kidney. (b) Ultrasound scans showing, for comparison, small unobstructed right kidney.

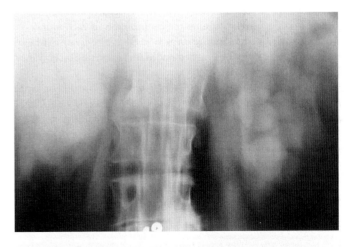

Fig. 10 High-dose intravenous urogram in chronic bilateral obstruction. Note dilated systems seen as lucent negative pyelograms.

ureter is well shown on CT. The main use of CT in the investigation of chronic upper tract obstruction is in defining the cause (Fig. 11).

Scintigraphy

Scintigraphy provides functional evidence of obstruction (Whitfield *et al.* 1981). A radioactive tracer is injected and serial images and computer data record its passage through the kidney. The first passage of the bolus of radioactivity reflects renal perfusion; later images provide information on renal uptake, excretion, and drainage. ^{99}Tc^m-diethylaminetriaminepentaacetic acid (DTPA) and ^{99}Tc^m-methylene diphosphonate are frequently used and are excreted purely by glomerular filtration.

An increase in pressure in the collecting system, sufficient to result in impaired renal function, delays parenchymal clearance of tracer and emptying of the collecting system. On whole-kidney renograms, the time–activity curve fails to decline after the initial intake peak or continues to increase. This does not enable a distinction to be made between obstructive nephropathy, in which parenchymal transit time is prolonged, and retention of tracer within a large, baggy, low-pressure, unobstructed collecting system.

A dynamic renal scintigram performed during diuresis may be of value in this situation (Whitfield *et al.* 1979). The standard procedure is to give frusemide (furosemide) 0.5 mg/kg intravenously immediately after voiding, when a routine scintigram has raised the possibility of obstruction. Time–activity curves obtained over the renal pelvic area immediately after injection of frusemide show no significant change in the renogram. In normal subjects, this is then followed by a rapid reduction in activity, the half-time of this rapid slope being less than 8 min; in the presence of obstruction the half-time exceeds 16 min. It is necessary for the patient to void the bladder before and after the frusemide scintigram to allow measurement of the response to the diuretic. A poor response may result from poor renal function or dehydration rather than from obstruction. In the presence of massive pelvic dilatation, washout may not be observed, and under these circumstances the test is uninterpretable.

Although scintigraphy has been used to screen for obstruction in patients with unexplained impairment of renal function, ultrasonography is preferable in most centres. Radionuclide methods are of particular value in differentiating obstructive nephropathy from the prolongation of transit time associated with a baggy, dilated but unobstructed system and in defining the contribution of each kidney to overall uptake function. A decision as to whether conservative surgery or nephrectomy should be carried out in unilateral obstruction may be much facilitated by the latter examination.

IVU and CT may both provide some limited information on renal function, whereas ultrasound provides none. An immediate nephrogram after intravenous injection of iodine-containing contrast medium, which increases in density with time, is indicative of obstruction of recent onset.

Antegrade and retrograde studies

These are of particular value in defining the site and nature of obstruction following contrast injection and may be a prelude to definitive treatment.

Pressure flow studies

Pressure flow studies were popularized by Whitaker in the late 1960s and early 1970s (Whitaker 1979, 1990; Whitaker and Buxton-Thomas 1984). It is an invasive test with a small risk of provoking infection; second, the technique investigates the collecting system and gives no information on parenchymal function; and third, it is not readily repeatable. With the advent of more sophisticated renography, this test has a limited place in the investigation of obstruction.

Significant incomplete chronic upper urinary tract obstruction

It may be very difficult to tell whether a given degree of partial or intermittent obstruction is impairing or potentially impairing renal function or causing symptoms: symptoms may be present in the absence of deleterious effects upon renal function and the converse may also be true. Different methods of diagnosing obstruction define subtly different pathological features of the condition and a valid correlation between the results of different investigations cannot invariably be made. Incomplete obstruction is clinically important if it causes deterioration in kidney function, which can be halted or corrected by intervention or symptoms, which are improved thereby. In patients with one kidney or those with bilateral partial obstruction, a decline in serial measurements of GFR attributable to obstruction may define the situation. There may be a similar change in uptake of radionuclides in unilateral obstruction. Other proposed methods of detecting significant incomplete obstruction are given in Table 3. Strict validation of these methods would require them to be carried out in patients with supposed obstruction who would then be allocated randomly to intervention or no intervention. Deterioration in function predicted by each of the methods by comparison with matched controls would provide validation. This study is never likely to be done.

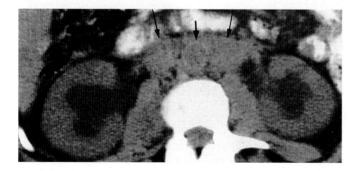

Fig. 11 CT scan in a patient with bilateral urinary tract obstruction due to prostatic cancer. Tumour tissue is clearly delineated on the scan (arrowed).

Table 3 Detection of significant incomplete obstruction

Introduction of a needle into the renal pelvis with direct measurement of the pressure developing after infusion of fluid at a known flow rate (antegrade pressure flow measurement)

Urographic observation of the degree of distension of the renal pelvis induced by intravenous frusemide (frusemide urography)

Observation of the effect of intravenous frusemide upon the isotope renogram (frusemide renography)

Comparison of activity/time curves after injection of ^{99}Tc^m-DTPA in whole kidney versus renal pelvis (retention function analysis)

Measurement of the nephron transit time of a non-reabsorbable tracer (outflow obstruction may increase the transit time)

Differential diagnosis of non-obstructive collecting system dilatation

A number of non-obstructive conditions may cause collecting system dilatation (Table 1). Ultrasound is usually unable to differentiate obstructive from non-obstructive dilatation because of its inability to show calyceal detail, differentiate an intrarenal from an extrarenal pelvis, and demonstrate the ureter. CT is also a poor indicator of whether dilatation is obstructive or non-obstructive, although it can identify cases of dilatation that are due to an extrarenal pelvis. IVU is of value in this connection.

Extrarenal pelvis may mimic pelviureteric junctional obstruction. If frusemide is administered after the 20-min full-length contrast radiograph, contrast medium will have washed out of the affected side on a full-length film 15-min later. In the presence of pelviureteric junctional obstruction the contrast is retained and the pelvicalyceal system increases in size.

Megacalyces are readily identified on urography. The renal cortex is normal and calyceal infundibula, pelvis, and ureter are normal with no evidence of obstruction (Fig. 12).

Vesicoureteric reflux may be associated with dilatation of the ureters; the pelvicalyceal system may also be dilated in severe reflux. The presence of reflux on urography is suggested by the degree of dilatation varying at different times during the examination, by dilatation which is greatest from the vesicoureteric junction upwards, and by a postmicturition film which shows a large bladder residual, representing urine that has refluxed into the ureters during voiding and drained back into the bladder thereafter.

The decision of whether an operation is indicated for idiopathic pelviureteric junctional obstruction may be facilitated by frusemide urography (Fig. 13) or frusemide scintigraphy. In some patients, the urographic findings are unremarkable during asymptomatic periods, while emergency IVU during an episode of pain may define the condition.

Management

The aim of management is to relieve symptoms, improve or conserve renal function, and avoid complications such as septicaemia. Important surgical advances in the past decade include the increasing use of ureteric stents to provide short-term or even long-term relief of obstruction.

Obstruction is the most readily reversible cause of chronic renal failure. Acute obstruction caused by ureteric stones commonly

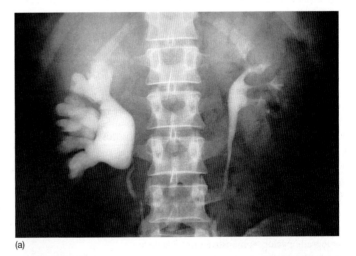

(a)

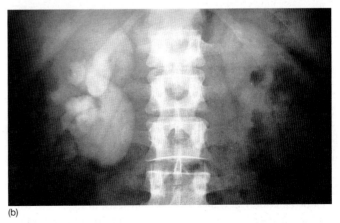

(b)

Fig. 12 Right-sided megacalyces—a normal variant. Note normal renal cortex, calyceal infundibula, pelvis, and ureter with no evidence of obstruction.

Fig. 13 (a) Right-sided pelviureteric obstruction. (b) Same urogram as in (a) 15 min after intravenous injection of frusemide. Note increase in size of pelvicalyceal system, indicating significant pelviureteric junction obstruction.

resolves spontaneously; however, the longer a stone remains in the same position within the ureter the less likely it is that a conservative policy will be successful. The surgical management of ureteric stones is described in Chapter 8.3.

Probably the second most common cause of chronic obstruction in adults is pelviureteric junction obstruction. The Anderson–Hynes pyeloplasty gives very satisfactory results and provides the gold standard against which other open and endoscopic techniques (such as endopyelotomy) must be assessed (Whitfield *et al.* 1983; Wickham and Kellet 1983).

Idiopathic obstruction at the pelviureteric junction may present in childhood. Obstructed megaureter and ureteric obstruction secondary to a ureterocele are also more common in children than in adults. Since all three congenital anomalies cause pelvicalyceal dilatation, it is becoming increasingly common for obstruction to be diagnosed *in utero*. Treatment of the obstruction *in utero* by the insertion of a nephrostomy tube has been reported: it is too early to know whether such early intervention will prove to have long-term benefits (see Chapter 17.4), but at the moment it seems on balance best to wait until immediately after delivery to investigate and relieve the problem (Elder *et al.* 1987).

Ureteric obstruction can occur in a transplanted kidney, most commonly at the site of the ureteroneocystostomy but sometimes more proximally in the ureter. Vesicoureteric stenosis is caused by ischaemia of the ureter, but it is never possible to define whether this ischaemia is associated with rejection or a result of poor vascularization following donor nephrectomy. More proximal ureteric obstruction may be due to mechanical kinking of the ureter, or occasionally to extrinsic compression by a lymphocele. Irrespective of the site and cause of the obstruction, the diagnosis presents special problems. The possibility of obstruction is raised either because of deteriorating renal function or because ultrasound during routine follow-up demonstrates increasing collecting system dilatation. The differential diagnosis includes rejection, cyclosporin nephrotoxicity, and arterial insufficiency. An obstruction may be demonstrated by IVU and/or antegrade pyelography. Retrograde studies are usually difficult and not infrequently impossible, and since, in the case of stenosis at a ureteroneocystostomy, they involve passing a catheter across the segment of ureter under suspicion, the investigation is only indicated if IVU and antegrade pyelography prove unsatisfactory.

Renal survival after reversal of chronic obstruction in humans

Long-term renal outcome following decompression of the chronic obstructive uropathy has rarely been studied. In one study (McClelland 1993), 67 patients referred between 1978 and 1991 with benign obstructive uropathy were analysed for risk factors associated with thezdevelopment of ESRD. During follow-up (median 58 months), 30 patients developed ESRD. Ten presented with advanced renal failure requiring dialysis therapy and 20 patients progressed to ESRD after a mean period of 25 months. In 22 of the remaining 37 patients, progressive renal failure was noted with a median rate of decline in GFR of 3 ml/min/year (range 0.9–9 ml/min/year). In 15 patients with stable renal function, plasma creatinine was lower postdecompression (261 versus 507 μmol/l, $p < 0.01$) compared to the progressive group. Persistent proteinuria greater than 1.0 g/day occurred in 3 out of 15 stable patients compared to 15 out of 22 in the progressive group

($p < 0.01$). Hypertension was equally common in both groups. Despite the patient profile [median age of whole cohort 69 years (range 25–88 years)], actuarial 5 years patient survival was 73 per cent. It was concluded that chronic obstructive uropathy with critical renal insufficiency is an important cause of ESRD especially in patients with proteinuria. While progression was common even after relief of obstruction, patient survival was good, in spite of poor renal outcome. It remains to be seen whether ACE inhibitors, AT1 receptor blockers, and endothelin receptors blockers will improve renal survival in obstructive uropathy.

Pelviureteric junction obstruction

A percutaneous procedure for managing pelviureteric junctional obstruction was first described by Wickham and Kellet (1983). Subsequent experience has confirmed the usefulness of the technique, but there is no consensus on the indications. We advocate that patients with secondary pelviureteric junction stenosis in association with stones, infection, or previous surgery should be offered the operation, whereas those with primary idiopathic obstruction are better treated by an open Anderson–Hynes pyeloplasty.

Malignant obstruction

A wide variety of tumours may cause ureteric obstruction, either by local spread (cervix, prostate, bladder), or secondary to para-aortic nodal enlargement (lymphoma, testicular tumours). The diagnosis rests upon the same investigations as for any other cause of chronic obstruction, but the treatment will vary widely, depending on the cause. An aggressive or radical approach is almost always indicated in a patient who has received no previous treatment for the underlying malignancy. Unilateral or bilateral percutaneous nephrostomies may be necessary to cover the period of time during which chemotherapy or radiotherapy are given with the expectation of controlling the tumour. More difficulty arises when ureteric obstruction is due to recurrent tumour, when the potential benefits of chemotherapy and radiotherapy are significantly less and patients may be facing debilitating treatment for an advancing malignant disease, the prognosis of which is poor. To be confined by nephrostomy drainage for what remains of the patient's life significantly diminishes the quality of life, but may be right in certain circumstances. A percutaneously placed pigtail nephrostomy, which can be inserted under local anaesthetic, has a tendency to fall out or to be pulled out. Open surgery can be avoided by the use of a ring nephrostomy inserted percutaneously under general anaesthesia: this provides secure long-term drainage, for years if necessary.

Obstruction in patients with urinary diversion

There are many reasons for diverting the urine into an isolated loop of ileum or colon. One of the recognized complications is stenosis at the site of anastomosis between the bowel and ureter(s).

The thin muscle wall of the ileum means that it is not possible to fashion an antireflux anastomosis between the bowel and the ureter when diverting the urine into an ileal conduit; a loopogram (a radiograph carried out after injection of contrast into an ideal loop) will normally therefore show bilateral ureteric reflux. The absence of reflux is strong evidence of a stenosis at the ureteroileal junction. An antireflux anastomosis can be achieved when the ureters are placed into either an isolated colonic segment or into the sigmoid colon, as in a ureterosigmoidostomy. In such circumstances the diagnosis of obstruction must be made using techniques applicable to all chronic upper urinary tract obstructions. Although the site of anastomosis can be identified by colonoscopy, obstruction cannot be identified, unless, as may happen, a tumour has developed at the site of anastomosis, when colonoscopy is the method of choice for diagnosis.

Idiopathic retroperitoneal fibrosis (periaortitis)

In this condition, the ureters become embedded in dense fibrous tissue, with resultant unilateral or bilateral obstruction, usually at the junction between the middle and lower thirds of the ureter (Baker *et al.* 1988). The condition is progressive: initially, the fibrous tissue is fairly cellular, later becoming relatively acellular (Mitchinson 1970). The mechanism by which obstruction occurs is unclear, not least because of the frequent observation that contrast medium injected into the lower ureter may pass freely up to the pelvicalyceal system despite the presence of clinical, radiological, and isotopic evidence of functional urinary tract obstruction. The condition was first described in the French literature (Albarran 1905) and the classic description came from Ormond (1948).

Pathogenesis

'Retroperitoneal fibrosis' is an unfortunate term, since there are many causes of fibrosis in the retroperitoneal area and because it is anatomically misleading and says nothing about pathogenesis. Evidence has now accumulated to suggest that the condition is an autoimmune periaortitis. The periaortic nature of the condition has long been known to surgeons and pathologists, and this has been further emphasized by the advent of CT scanning (Fig. 14). In many ways the term 'periaortitis' is, therefore, preferable to retroperitoneal fibrosis.

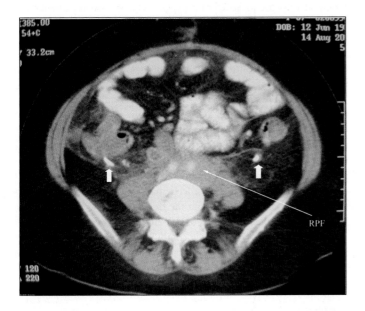

Fig. 14 CT scan in idiopathic retroperitoneal fibrosis (periaortitis) causing urinary tract obstruction. Note aortic calcification and the periaortic nature of the mass.

Histologically, atheroma, medial thinning, splits in the media, and an increase in the adventitia, which contains an inflammatory infiltrate, are seen. These findings are present to some extent in the aortas of some patients with advanced atherosclerosis who have not suffered a clinical illness and who may reasonably be classified as having 'subclinical periaortitis'. The fibrous tissue itself contains macrophages and plasma cells but not polymorphs.

It now seems likely that periaortic fibrosis is an autoimmune response to leakage of material derived from atheromatous plaques in the diseased aorta (Demko *et al.* 1997). The substance ceroid, an insoluble polymer of oxidized lipid and lipoprotein, which may be synthesized artificially by oxidizing low density lipoprotein, may be involved in the reaction: it is found in atheromatous plaques and is identified by staining with oil-red-O (Parums *et al.* 1986). Parums and Mitchinson (1990) detected circulating antibodies to oxidized low density lipoprotein and to ceroid extracted from human atheroma in patients with periaortitis and other disease states. When these results were compared with findings in normal individuals, there was no difference in the antibody titre between patients with ischaemic heart disease and normal controls, but highly significant increases in antibody titre in patients with chronic periaortitis. Stored serum obtained from individuals subsequently shown at autopsy to have had subclinical periaortitis also showed significantly increased antibody titres compared with controls.

It seems reasonable to hypothesize that chronic periaortitis has an autoimmune aetiology in which the allergen is a component of ceroid, probably oxidized low density lipoprotein, produced in human atheroma, and that a specific immune response involves T cells and plasma cells which secrete IgG, macrophages, and eosinophils. These cells release inflammatory mediators, including cytokines, growth factors and profibrogenic substances; thus, resulting in fibroblast proliferation and fibrosis.

Clinical features

The condition is two times as common in men as in women. Patients' ages range from the third to the ninth decade, but peak incidence occurs in the sixth and seventh decades of life: in one series of 60 patients (Baker *et al.* 1988) the mean age of the group was 56 years. The clinical manifestations of this disorder vary with the stage of presentation. Early stage is characterized by pain described as dull, non-colicky, and occurring in a girdle distribution in over 90 per cent of patients (Utz *et al.* 1966). The discomfort is unaffected by posture, level of activity, defecation, or micturition increases with time. Non-steroidal anti-inflammatory drugs, more than narcotics provide symptom relief because of the inflammatory nature of the lesion. Symptoms referable to the urinary tract are usually absent during the early stage. Subsequently, increasing urinary obstruction may result in alteration in urine volume, flank pain, and, with time, the symptoms of uraemia may predominate. Examination is usually unremarkable apart from hypertension, which is found in over 50 per cent of patients (Pryor *et al.* 1983). Oedema, a palpable kidney, and hydrocele are found in less than 10 per cent of patients. Other less common presentations result from fibrotic impingement of the inferior vena cava or the arterial system resulting in lower limb thrombophlebitis, claudication, and intestinal ischaemia (Demko *et al.* 1997). The majority of patients have a normochromic, normocytic anaemia and an increased erythrocyte sedimentation rate (ESR), but a significant minority are normal in one or both of these respects. Proteinuria is present in only a minority of patients and significant bacteriuria is even less common (Baker et al. 1988). The typical patient with this condition is a middle-aged man with flank or abdominal pain, no abnormality or only hypertension on examination, who is uraemic, anaemic, abacteriuric, with negative findings on urinalysis, a raised ESR, and no exotic associated conditions. Erdheim–Chester disease is a rare non-Langerhans cell histiocytosis which is characterized by osteosclerosis, exophthalmos, and diabetes insipidus. Retroperitoneal involvement is found in approximately 20–30 per cent cases. It can mimic retroperitoneal fibrosis but is characterized by xanthogranulomatous infiltration by foamy histiocytes nested in fibrosis (Veyssier-Belot et al. 1996).

Diagnosis

Periaortic fibrosis is clearly more common than hitherto appreciated, if one takes into account subclinical forms of the condition. Even overt idiopathic retroperitoneal fibrosis is, in all probability, much more common than is generally thought. Diagnostic delay is the rule; in one series (Baker et al. 1988), 6–12 months, or even longer, elapsed from the onset of symptoms to diagnosis. Perhaps for this reason bilateral rather than unilateral upper tract obstruction was present in the majority of patients.

When taking the history, enquiry should be made about possible presence of one of the secondary causes of retroperitoneal fibrosis, including malignancy, connective tissue disease, and use of relevant drugs such as methysergide (Graham et al. 1966), β-blockers, methyldopa (Pryor et al. 1983), and bromocriptine, which is another ergot-like drug (Bowler et al. 1986). Koep and Zuidemia (1997) have reviewed retroperitoneal fibrosis associated findings in 491 patients (Table 4). Ultrasonography, isotopic methods, and the IVU will reveal findings typical of urinary tract obstruction, and the latter may show medial deviation of the ureters. This last finding may also be present in normal subjects and is an unreliable guide to diagnosis. CT scanning will show the periaortic mass (Fig. 14). MR imaging in retroperitoneal fibrosis produces findings comparable to those with CT scanning. An advantage of MR imaging is the ability to display the pathological process in multiple planes (transverse, coronal, sagittal).

Table 4 Associated findings in 491 patients with retroperitoneal fibrosis

Findings	% of patients
Idiopathic	67.8
Methysergide exposure	12.4
All malignancies	7.9
Mediastinal fibrosis	3.3
Periaortic inflammation-arteritis	2.4
Mesenteric fibrosis	2.0
Sclerosing cholangitis	1.6
Abdominal aortic aneurysm	1.8
Crohn's disease	1.2
Thrombophlebitis	1.0
Reidel's thyroiditis	0.8
Other	5.3

Data from Keop and Zuidemia (1977).

The differential diagnosis includes lymphoma (in which case splenomegaly and lymphadenopathy may be seen on CT scanning or MR imaging) and various forms of cancer, including that of bladder, bowel, and cervix (Arrive 1989).

A histological diagnosis should be obtained if at all possible, and laparotomy is required in order to obtain a sufficiently large sample to exclude lymphoma and cancer with confidence. Conversely, CT-guided needle biopsy of a mass may be sufficient to diagnose lymphoma or carcinoma with confidence (Whelan et al. 1991).

Management

Management is empirical and controversial since controlled trials of treatment are lacking. Corticosteroid therapy, with or without temporary relief of obstruction by insertion of ureteric stents, ureterolysis alone, and ureterolysis followed by steroid therapy to shrink the periaortic mass and maintain remission have all been used. Corticosteroid therapy alone may correct obstruction (Baker et al. 1988; Higgins et al. 1988), but is by no means invariably effective (Baker et al. 1988). Ureterolysis alone may correct obstruction in the long term but is sometimes associated with recurrence of obstruction or the development of obstruction in a previously unobstructed kidney. Surgical relief of obstruction by ureterolysis followed by long-term corticosteroid therapy (prednisolone 20 mg daily commenced when sutures are removed) has proved a reliable and successful strategy (Baker et al. 1988). When bilateral obstruction is present, bilateral ureterolysis followed by steroid therapy is preferable to unilateral ureterolysis with reliance upon corticosteroid therapy to free the contralateral side, since this is sometimes unsuccessful. Ureterolysis of kidneys shown to be non-functioning on high-dose excretion urography or by appropriate radionuclide techniques is usually unsuccessful in restoring useful renal function (Baker et al. 1988). A reasonable policy for management would seem to be to perform unilateral or bilateral ureterolysis, as appropriate, followed by corticosteroid therapy in patients fit for operation and able to take steroids safely. Surgery alone should be employed in those with a particular contraindication to corticosteroid treatment, such as the presence of a peptic ulcer. Steroid therapy alone (methylprednisolone 500 mg intravenously daily for 3 days, followed by prednisolone 20 mg daily), with or without insertion of ureteric stents, should be reserved for patients unfit for ureterolysis. A dramatic response to steroid treatment sometimes occurs, a marked diuresis being seen within 24 h of commencing treatment.

Since the antioestrogen drug, tamoxifen, may result in the regression of desmoid tumours (which are benign fibrotic tumours), some clinicians have used and reported anecdotally positive responses to this agent among patients with retroperitoneal fibrosis (Bourouma et al. 1997; Ozener et al. 1997). Although differences exist in the pathobiology of retroperitoneal fibrosis and desmoid tumours and the mechanism of action of tamoxifen in this disorder remains unclear, additional controlled evaluation of tamoxifen in the treatment of the former seems warranted given the relative lack of side-effects with this drug therapy.

Another possible approach is combination therapy consisting of steroids and mycophenolate. In a case report, the administration of prednisolone and mycophenolate (2 g/day) resulted in remission in a patient with anuric renal failure (Grotz et al. 1998).

Prognosis

The older and the more uraemic the patient at the time of presentation, the worse is the prognosis. Nevertheless, if treated appropriately, most patients do well (Hem and Mathisen 1984; Alexopoulos et al. 1987; Baker et al. 1988).

Follow-up

In some patients long-term remission is achieved by surgery alone. In those receiving maintenance prednisolone, the drug dose can be reduced progressively and in some patients long-term remission occurs after complete withdrawal of corticosteroid therapy. In one series of 60 patients, 10 relapsed more than 5 years after the time of diagnosis when steroid therapy had been stopped, in that ESR increased to an abnormal level, and obstruction and diminished renal function redeveloped. Five patients relapsed as much as 10 years after the onset of the disease. Lifelong follow-up is therefore mandatory. The best way to monitor such patients is not certain. Clinical assessment, serial measurement of ESR, and assessment of renal function, together with imaging to detect redevelopment of obstruction, seem appropriate. Reduction in the size of the periaortic mass can be detected on serial CT scanning, but residual periaortic tissue is seen frequently, even after steroid therapy, and the usefulness of CT in monitoring disease activity is limited (Brooks et al. 1987; Brooks 1990).

Periaortitis in the absence of ureteric obstruction

The use of CT scanning in the investigation of abdominal pain allows an increasing number of patients with periaortitis to be identified before the onset of urinary tract obstruction. Management is controversial. The development of bilateral ureteric obstruction with severe uraemia within 3 months of diagnosis (at which time renal function was normal and the ureters unobstructed) has occurred in at least one patient (Baker et al. 1992). Until more is known of the natural history of the disease in such patients, it would seem prudent to obtain a histological diagnosis at open operation and to consider corticosteroid therapy to shrink the mass. Whether an attempt to reduce the risk of ureteric obstruction by insertion of stents or displacement of the ureters from the mass at the time of operation should be carried out is unclear.

Chronic inflammatory bowel disease

In addition to problems with urolithiasis discussed in Chapter 8.2, chronic inflammatory bowel disease is associated with chronic and unsuspected urinary tract obstruction in 7–27 per cent of patients (10–15 per cent in most published series; Present et al. 1969; Fleckenstein et al. 1977). The obstruction is nearly always right sided in patients with Crohn's disease, and a valuable clue to its existence is pain radiating down from the right iliac fossa into the right leg. The ureter is usually involved in an inflammatory mass. In contrast, in patients with ulcerative colitis, the disease may occur on either side and nearly always follows colectomy.

An ultrasound examination of the urinary tract to detect obstruction should therefore be a part of the annual review in patients with chronic inflammatory bowel disease.

Chronic granulomatous disease

This is a rather rare inherited condition, usually X-linked, in which bacterial oxidative killing after phagocytosis is defective. There is no respiratory burst and bacteria, particularly *Staphylococcus aureus* and other catalase-positive organisms, can survive intracellularly. Apart from superficial sepsis, which is obvious from birth, deep chronic granulomatous sepsis may occur, with or without external discharging sinuses. A high proportion of survivors have urinary tract obstruction due to granulomas involving the ureters (Allabadi et al. 1990).

Chronic lower urinary tract obstruction (see also Chapter 18.5)

Pathophysiology

In adults, chronic outflow obstruction to the bladder is most commonly due to benign prostatic hypertrophy. Prostatic malignancy and urethral strictures may also be responsible. In children, posterior urethral valves and urethral strictures are most often the cause. Such organic causes are easy to understand, but functional obstruction may occur at the bladder neck and at the level of the distal sphincter owing to a failure of coordination between bladder contraction and sphincter relaxation. The bladder wall may become increasingly compliant or the opposite may occur: this is of significance to the urologist, since patients with poorly compliant bladders fare much better after removal of the obstruction than those with highly compliant bladders. The highly compliant bladder tends not to be associated with upper tract dilatation, whereas the high pressure that exists within a bladder of low compliance may be transmitted to the upper tracts and may be the cause of renal impairment, which on occasion will be severe. The relief of bladder outflow obstruction associated with upper urinary tract dilatation may provoke a postoperative diuresis and subsequent electrolyte imbalance.

Clinical features

There are no pathognomonic clinical features that differentiate high pressure and low pressure chronic retention; the condition is painless in both cases. In each, if the residual urine volume is sufficient the bladder may be palpably distended. The size and consistency of the prostate is variable.

Investigation

In one series of patients presenting with acute retention of urine, approximately half had low-compliance and half had high-compliance bladders. Investigation is aimed at demonstrating associated pathology such as urinary tract infection, upper tract dilatation, stones, and renal impairment, and at defining the severity of bladder outflow obstruction.

A urine culture is also essential. In most centres, ultrasonography of the upper and lower urinary tract, together with a plain abdominal radiograph and a urinary flow rate measurement, have replaced the intravenous urogram. Full urodynamic investigations, with combined videopressure cystourethrography are only necessary in the presence of a neuropathy. Serum biochemistry and routine haematology are also required, but the measurement of acid phosphatase and prostatic-specific antigen levels is indicated only if there is clinical evidence of prostatic malignancy.

Management

The management of chronic bladder outflow obstruction is outside the scope of this chapter and is the remit of the urologist. However, prostatic obstruction represents the most common cause of uraemia in middle-aged and elderly males (Sacks et al. 1989; Feest et al. 1993). This is of great importance, since it is one of the few potentially reversible causes of chronic renal failure in this group. In many patients who present as uraemic emergencies, renal function improves but considerable renal impairment remains (plasma creatinine 300–700 μmol/l, GFR 10–30 ml/min). It is striking that the renal function of such patients may remain unchanged even over many years at this compromised level (Ghose 1990).

Acknowledgements

We acknowledge Dr L. R. I. Baker and Mr W. H. Whitfield for providing the original framework of this chapter.

References

Abbrecht, P. H. and Malvin, R. L. (1960). Flow rate of urine as a determinant of renal countercurrent multiplier systems. *American Journal of Physiology* **199**, 919–922.

Albarran, J. (1905). Retention rénale par peri-urétérite. Libération externe de l'urétère. *Comptes Rendus de l'Association Française d'Urologie* **9**, 511–517.

Alexopoulos, E. et al. (1987). Idiopathic retroperitoneal fibrosis: a long term follow up study. *European Urology* **13**, 313–317.

Allabadi, H., Gonzalez, K., and Quie, P. G. (1990). Urinary tract disorders in chronic granulomatous disease. *New England Journal of Medicine* **321**, 706–708.

Arendshorst, W. J., Finn, W. F., and Gottschalk, C. W. (1974). Nephron stop-flow pressure response to obstruction for 24 h in the rat kidney. *Journal of Clinical Investigation* **53**, 1497–1500.

Arrive, T., Hricak, H., Tavares, N. J., and Miller, T. R. (1989). Malignant versus non-malignant retroperitoneal fibrosis: differentiation with MR imaging. *Radiology* **172**, 139–143.

Baker, L. R. I., Croxson, R., Khader, N., Reznek, R. H., Al Rukhaimi, M., and Wickham, J. E. A. (1992). Rate of development of ureteric obstruction in idiopathic retroperitoneal fibrosis (periaortitis). *British Journal of Urology* **69**, 102–105.

Baker, L. R. I. et al. (1988). Idiopathic retroperitoneal fibrosis. A retrospective analysis of 60 cases. *British Journal of Urology* **60**, 497–503.

Batlle, D. C., Arruda, J. A. L., and Kurtzman, N. A. (1981). Hyperkalaemic distal renal tubular acidosis associated with obstructive uropathy. *New England Journal of Medicine* **304**, 373–380.

Beck, N. (1979). Phosphaturia after release of bilateral ureteral obstruction in rats. *American Journal of Physiology* **237**, F14–F19.

Bell, E. *Renal Diseases*. Philadelphia: Lea and Febiger, 1946.

Berlyne, G. M. (1961). Distal tubular function in chronic hydronephrosis. *Quarterly Journal of Medicine* **30**, 339–355.

Better, O. S., Arieff, A. I., Massry, S. G., Kleeman, C. R., and Maxwell, M. H. (1973). Studies on renal function after relief of complete unilateral ureteral obstruction of three months' duration in man. *American Journal of Medicine* **54**, 234–240.

Better, O. S., Tuma, S., Shimeon, K., and Chaimovitz, C. (1975). Enhanced renal tubular reabsorption of phosphate. *Archives of Internal Medicine* **135**, 245–248.

Blackshear, J. L., Edwards, B. S., and Knox, P. G. (1979). Autoregulation of renal blood flow: effects of indomethacin and ureteral pressure. *Mineral Electrolyte Metabolism* **2**, 130–136.

Bourouma, R., Chevet, D., Michel, F., Cercueil, J. P., Arnould, L., and Rifle, G. (1997). Treatment of idiopathic retroperitoneal fibrosis with tamoxifen. *Nephrology, Dialysis, Transplantation* **12**, 2407–2410.

Bowler, J. V., Ormerod, I. F., and Legg, J. (1986). Retroperitoneal fibrosis and bromocriptine. *Lancet* **2**, 466.

Brooks, A. P. (1990). Computed tomography of idiopathic retroperitoneal fibrosis ('periaortitis'): variants, variations, patterns and pitfalls. *Clinical Radiology* **42**, 75–79.

Brooks, A. P., Reznek, R. H., Webb, J. A. W., and Baker, L. R. I. (1987). Computed tomography in the follow-up of idiopathic retroperitoneal fibrosis. *Clinical Radiology* **38**, 597–601.

Campbell, M. F. Urinary obstruction. In *Textbook of Urology* 2nd edn. (ed. M. F. Campbell), pp. 1916–1938. Philadelphia: W.B. Saunders, 1963.

Cattell, W. R., Webb, J. A. W., and Hilson, A. J. W. Urinary tract obstruction. In *Clinical Renal Imaging*, pp. 90–107. Chichester: John Wiley and Sons, 1989.

Chevalier, R. L. (2000). Obstructive nephropathy: lesson from cystic kidney disease. *Nephron* **84**, 6–12.

Danuser, H., Ackermann, D. K., Marth, D. C., Studer, A. E., and Zingg, E. J. (1993). Extracorporeal shock wave lithotripsy *in situ* or after push-up for upper ureteral calculi: a prospective randomised trial. *Journal of Urology* **150**, 824–826.

Davis, D. M. (1943). Intubated ureterotomy: new operations for ureteral and ureteropelvic stricture. *Surgery, Gynecology, and Obstetrics* **76**, 513–517.

Demko, T. M., Diamond, J. R., and Groff, J. (1997). Obstructive uropathy as a result of retroperitoneal fibrosis: a review of its pathogenesis and associations. *Journal of the American Society of Nephrology* **8**, 684–688.

Denton, T., Cochlin, D. L., and Evans, C. (1984). The value of ultrasound in previously undiagnosed renal failure. *British Journal of Radiology* **57**, 673–675.

Dure-Smith, P. Ureteric dilatation: its anatomic basis, and relation to sex and pregnancy. In *Urinary Tract Infection* (ed. F. O'Grady and W. Brumfitt), pp. 172–175. London: Oxford University Press, 1968.

Eddy, A. A. (1996). Molecular insights into renal interstitial fibrosis. *Journal of the American Society of Nephrology* **7**, 2495–2508.

Edvall, C. A. (1959). Influence of ureteral obstruction (hydronephrosis) on renal function in man. *Journal of Applied Physiology* **14**, 855–858.

Elder, J. S., Duckett, J. W., and Snyder, H. M. (1987). Intervention for fetal obstructive uropathy: has it been effective? *Lancet* **2**, 1007–1010.

Feest, T. G., Round, A., and Hamad, S. (1993). Incidence of severe acute renal failure in adults: results of a community based study. *British Medical Journal* **306**, 481–483.

Fleckenstein, P., Knudsen, L., Pedersen, E. B., Marcussen, J., and Jarnum, S. (1977). Obstructive uropathy in inflammatory bowel disease. *Scandinavian Journal of Gastroenterology* **12**, 519–523.

Frokiaer, J., Marples, D., Knepper, M. A., and Nielsen, S. (1996). Bilateral obstruction downregulates expression of vasopressin-sensitive AQP-2 water channel in rat kidney. *American Journal of Physiology* **270**, F657–F666.

Garraway, W. M., Collins, G. N., and Lee, R. (1991). High prevalance of benign prostatic hypertrophy in the community. *Lancet* **338**, 469–471.

Ghose, R. R. (1990). Prolonged recovery of renal function after prostatectomy for prostatic outflow obstruction. *British Medical Journal* **300**, 1376–1377.

Gillenwater, J. Y. The pathophysiology of urinary obstruction. In *Campbell's Urology* 4th edn. Vol. I (ed. J. H. Harrison, R. F. Gittes, A. D. Perlmutter, T. A. Stamey, and P. C. Walsh), pp. 377–414. Philadelphia: W.B. Saunders, 1978.

Gillenwater, J. Y. (1982). Clinical aspects of urinary tract obstruction. *Seminars in Nephrology* **2**, 46–54.

Gillenwater, J. Y. The pathophysiology of urinary obstruction. In *Campbell's Urology* 5th edn. (ed. P. C. Walsh, R. F. Gittes, A. D. Perlmutter, and T. A. Stamey), p. 554. Philadelphia: W.B. Saunders, 1986.

Gillenwater, J. Y., Westervelt, F. B., Vaughan, E. D., and Howards, S. S. (1975). Renal function after release of chronic unilateral hydronephrosis in man. *Kidney International* **7**, 179–186.

Graham, J. R., Suby, J. I., Le Compte, P. R., and Sandowsky, N. L. (1966). Fibrotic disorders associated with methysergide therapy for headache. *New England Journal of Medicine* **274**, 359–368.

Grenier, N., Pariente, J. L., Trillaud, H., Soussette, C., and Douws, C. (2000). Dilatation of the collecting system during pregnancy: physiologic versus obstructive dilatation. *European Radiology* **10**, 271–279.

Grotz, W., Von Zedwitz, I., Andre, M., and Scollmeyer, P. (1998). Treatment of retroperitoneal fibrosis by mycophenolate mofetil and corticosteroids. *Lancet* **352**, 1195.

Hem, E. and Mathisen, W. (1984). Retroperitoneal fibrosis: a follow-up study. *European Urology* **10**, 43–47.

Hendrikx, A. J. M., Bierkens, A. F., Oosterhof, G. O. N., and Debruyne, F. M. J. (1990). Treatment of proximal and mid-ureteral calculi: a randomised trial of *in situ* and push back extracorporeal lithotripsy. *Journal of Endourology* **4**, 353–361.

Higgins, P. M., Bennett-Jones, D. N., Naish, P. F., and Aber, G. M. (1988). Non-operative management of retroperitoneal fibrosis. *British Journal of Surgery* **75**, 573–577.

Homer, J. A., Davies-Payne, D. L., and Peddinti, B. S. (2001). Randomised prospective comparison of non-contrast enhanced helical computed tomography and intravenous urography in the diagnosis of acute ureteric colic. *Australasian Radiology* **45**, 285–290.

Hruska, K. A., Guo, G., Wozniek, M., Martin, D., Miller, S., Liapis, S., Loveday, K., Klahr, S., Sampath, T. K., and Morrissey, J. J. (2000). Osteogenic protein-1 (OP-1) prevents renal fibrogenesis associated with ureteral obstruction. *American Journal of Physiology* **279**, F130–F143.

Huang, A., Palmer, L. S., Hom, D., Valderrama, E., and Trachtman, H. (2000). The role of nitric oxide in obstructive nephropathy. *Journal of Urology* **163**, 1276–1281.

Jung, P., Brauers, A., Nolte-Ernsting, C. A., Jakse, G., and Gunther, R. W. (2000a). Segmental up-regulation of transforming growth factor-beta in the pathogenesis of primary megaureter. An immunohistochemical study. *British Journal of Urology International* **80**, 946–949.

Jung, P., Brauers, A., Nolte-Ernsting, C. A., Jakse, G., and Gunther, R. W. (2000b). Magnetic resonance urography enhanced by gadolinium and diuretic: a comparison with conventional urography in diagnosing the cause of ureteric obstruction. *British Journal of Urology International* **86**, 960–965.

Kerr, W. S. (1954). Effect of complete ureteral obstruction for one week on kidney function. *Journal of Applied Physiology* **6**, 762–772.

Keuhnelian, J. G., Bartone, F., and Marshall, V. F. (1964). Practical considerations from autopsies in uraemic patients. *Journal of Urology* **91**, 467–473.

Klahr, S. (1982). Obstructive uropathy. *Seminars in Nephrology* **2**, 1–73.

Klahr, S. (1991). New insights into the consequences and mechanisms of renal impairment in obstructive nephropathy. *Seminars in Dialysis* **18**, 689–699.

Klahr, S. Obstructive nephropathy: pathophysiology and management. In *Renal and Electrolyte Disorders* 5th edn. (ed. R. W. Schrier), pp. 544–589. Lippincott-Raven, 1997.

Klahr, S. (2001). Urinary tract obstruction. *Seminars in Nephrology* **21**, 133–145.

Koep, L. and Zuidemia, G. D. (1997). The clinical significance of retroperitoneal fibrosis. *Surgery* **81**, 250–257.

McClelland, P., Yaqoob, M., Williams, P. S., Rustom, R., and Bone, J. M. (1993). Obstructive uropathy and progression of renal failure. *Nephrology, Dialysis, Transplantation* **8**, 952A.

McDougal, W. S. and Wright, F. S. (1972). Defect in proximal and distal sodium transport in post-obstructive diuresis. *Kidney International* **2**, 304–317.

McLaughlin, A. P., Pfister, R. C., Leadbetter, W. F., Salztein, S. L., and Kessler, W. O. (1973). The pathology of primary megaloureter. *Journal of Urology* **109**, 805–811.

McNicholas, T. A. (1999). Management of symptomatic BPH in UK: who is treated and how? *European Urology* **36** (Suppl. 3), 33–39.

Mitchinson, M. J. (1970). The pathology of retroperitoneal fibrosis. *Journal of Clinical Pathology* **23**, 681–689.

Moody, T. E., Vaughn, E. D., and Gillenwater, J. Y. (1975). Relationship between renal blood flow and ureteral pressure during 18 hours of total unilateral occlusion. *Investigative Urology* **13**, 246–251.

Morrissey, J. J. and Klahr, S. (1997). Enalapril decreases NF-κB activation in the kidney with ureteral obstruction. *Kidney International* **52**, 926–933.

Morrissey, J. J., Ishidoya, S., McCracken, R., and Klahr, S. (1996). Nitric oxide ameliorates the tubulointerstitial fibrosis of obstructive nephropathy. *Kidney International* **7**, 2202–2212.

Mueller, S. C., Wilbert, D., Grine, W. B., Jenkins, J. M., and Jordan, W. R. (1993). Low energy lithotripsy with the lithostar: treatment results with 19962 renal and ureteric calculi. *Journal of Urology* **149**, 1419–1424.

National Kidney, Urologic Diseases Advisory Board. The scope and impact of kidney and urologic diseases, in long range plan (Chapter 1). Washington, DC: National Institutes of Health, NIH publication, #90–563, pp. 7–35, 1990.

Olbrich, O., Woodford-Williams, E., Irvine, R. E., and Webster, D. (1957). Renal function in prostatism. *Lancet* **i**, 1322–1324.

Ormond, J. K. (1948). Bilateral ureteral obstruction due to envelopment and compression by an inflammatory process. *Journal of Urology* **59**, 1072–1079.

Ozener, C., Kiris, S., Lawrence, R., Ilker, Y., and Akoglu, E. (1997). Potential beneficial effect of tamoxifen in retroperitoneal fibrosis. *Nephrology, Dialysis, Transplantation* **12**, 2166–2168.

Parums, D. V. and Mitchinson, M. J. (1990). Serum antibodies to oxidised LDL and ceroid in chronic periaortitis. *Archives of Pathology and Laboratory Medicine* **114**, 383–387.

Parums, D. V., Chadwick, D. R., and Mitchinson, M. J. (1986). The localisation of immunoglobulin in chronic periaortitis. *Atherosclerosis* **61**, 117–123.

Peters, C. A. (1997). Obstruction of the fetal urinary tract. *Journal of the American Society of Nephrology* **8**, 653–663.

Present, D. H., Rabinowitz, J. G., Banks, P. A., and Janowitz, H. D. (1969). Obstructive hydronephrosis. A frequent but seldom recognized complication of granulomatous disease of the bowel. *New England Journal of Medicine* **280**, 523–528.

Pryor, J. P., Castle, W. M., Dukes, D. C., Smith, J. C., Watson, M. E., and Williams, J. L. (1983). Do beta adrenoceptor blocking drugs cause retroperitoneal fibrosis? *British Medical Journal* **287**, 639–642.

Regan, F., Bohlman, M. E., Khazan, R., and Schultz-Haakh, H. (1996). MR Urography using HASTE imaging in the assessment of ureteric obstruction. *American Journal of Roentgenology* **167**, 1115–1120.

Reyes, A. A., Robertson, G., and Klahr, S. (1991). Role of vasopressin in rats with bilateral ureteral obstruction. *Proceeding of the Society of Experimental Biology and Medicine* **197**, 49–55.

Risdon, R. A., Sloper, J. C., and de Wardener, H. E. (1968). Relationship between renal function and histological changes found in renal biopsy specimens from patients with persistent glomerulonephritis. *Lancet* **1**, 363–366.

Rose, G. R. and Gillenwater, J. Y. (1973). Pathophysiology of ureteral obstruction. *American Journal of Physiology* **255**, 830–837.

Sabatini, S. and Kurtzman, N. A. (1990). Enzyme activity in obstrutive uropathy: basis for salt wastage and the acidification defect. *Kidney International* **37**, 79–84.

Sacks, S. H., Aparicio, S. A. J. R., Bevan, A., Oliver, D. O., Will, E. J., and Davison, A. M. (1989). Late renal failure due to prostatic outflow obstruction: a preventable disease. *British Medical Journal* **298**, 156–159.

Schäfer, W. (1985). Urethral resistance? Urodynamic concepts of physiological and pathological bladder outlet function during voiding. *Neurourology and Urodynamics* **4**, 161–201.

Schanstra, J. P., Neau, E., Drogoz, P., Gomez, M. A. A., Novoa, J. M. L., Calise, D., Pecher, C., Bader, M., Girolamai, J. P., and Bascands, J. L. (2002). *In vivo* bradykinin B2 receptor activation reduces renal fibrosis. *Journal of Clinical Investigation* **110**, 371–379.

Sfakianakis, G. N., Cohen, D. J., Braunstein, R. H., Leveillee, R. J., Lerner, I., Bird, V. G., Sfakianakis, E., Georgiou, M. F., Block, N. L., and Lynne, C. M. (2000). MAG-3-F0 scintigraphy in decision making for emergency intervention in renal colic after helical CT positive for a urolith. *Journal of Nuclear Medicine* **41**, 1813–1822.

Shimizu, T., Kuroda, T., Hata, S., Fukagawa, M., Margolin, S. B., and Kurokowa, K. (1998). Pirfenidone improves renal function and fibrosis in the post-obstructed kidney. *Kidney International* **54**, 99–109.

Suki, W., Eknoyan, G., Rector, F. C., and Seldin, D. W. (1966). Patterns of nephron perfusion in acute and chronic hydronephrosis. *Journal of Clinical Investigation* **45**, 122–131.

Truong, L. D., Choi, Y. L., Tsao, C. C., Ayala, G., Sheikh-Hamad, D., Nassar, G., and Suki, W. A. (2001). Renal apoptosis in chronic obstructive uropathy: the roles of caspases. *Kidney International* **60**, 924–934.

Truong, L. D., Sheikh-Hamad, D., Chakraborty, S., and Suki, W. A. (1998). Cell apoptosis and proliferation in obstructive uropathy. *Seminars in Nephrology* **6**, 641–651.

United States Renal Data System (1996). Annual data report II. Incidence and prevalence of ESRD. *American Journal of Kidney Diseases* **18** (Suppl. 2), S34–S47.

Utz, D. C. and Henry, J. D. (1966). Retroperitoneal fibrosis. *Medical Clinics North America* **50**, 1091–1099.

Veyssier-Belot, C., Cacoub, P., Caparros-Lefebvre, D., Weehsler, J., Brun, B., Remy, M., Wallaert, B., Petit, H., Grimaldi, A., Weehsler, B., and Godeau, P. (1996). Erdheim–Chester disease. Clinical and radiologic characteristics of 59 cases. *Medicine (Baltimore)* **75**, 157–169.

Wainstein, M. A. and Reznick, M. I. (1994). Technical and experimental innovations in the treatment of urinary calculi. *Current Opinion in Urology* **4**, 217–222.

Weatherall, D., Ledingham, J. G. G., and Warrell, D., ed. *Oxford Textbook of Medicine* 1st edn. Oxford: Oxford University Press, 1987.

Webb, J. A. (2000). Ultrasonography and Doppler studies in the diagnosis of renal obstruction. *British Journal of Urology* **86** (Suppl. 1), 25–32.

Webb, J. A. W., Reznek, R. H., White, F. E., Cattell, W. R., Kelsey Fry, I., and Baker, L. R. I. (1984). Can ultrasound and computed tomography replace high-dose urography in patients with impaired renal function? *Quarterly Journal of Medicine* **211**, 411–425.

Whelan, J. S., Reznek, R. H., Daniell, S. J. N., Norton, A. J., Lister, T. A., and Rohatiner, A. Z. S. (1991). Computed tomography (CT) and ultrasound (US) guided core biopsy in the management of non-Hodgkin's lymphoma. *British Journal of Cancer* **63**, 460–462.

Whitaker, R. H. (1975). Some observations and theories on the wide ureter and hydronephrosis. *British Journal of Urology* **47**, 377–385.

Whitaker, R. H. (1979). The Whitaker test. *Urological Clinics of North America* **6**, 529–539.

Whitaker, R. H. (1990). The diagnosis of upper urinary tract obstruction. *Postgraduate Medical Journal* **66** (Suppl. 1), 25–30.

Whitaker, R. H. and Buxton-Thomas, M. (1984). A comparison of pressure flow studies and renography in equivocal upper urinary tract obstruction. *Journal of Urology* **131**, 446–449.

Whitfield, H. N. (1977). Clinical implications of lower urinary tract pharmacology. *Urological Research* **5**, 51–54.

Whitfield, H. N., Britton, K. E., Hendry, W. F., and Wickham, J. E. A. (1979). Frusemide intravenous urography in the diagnosis of pelvi-ureteric junction obstruction. *British Journal of Urology* **51**, 445–448.

Whitfield, H. N., Britton, K. E., Nimmon, C. C., Hendry, W. F., Wallace, D. M. A., and Wickham, J. E. A. (1981). Renal transit time measurements in the diagnosis of ureteric obstruction. *British Journal of Urology* **53**, 500–503.

Whitfield, H. N., Mills, V., Miller, R. A., and Wickham, J. E. A. (1983). Percutaneous pyelolysis: an alternative to pyeloplasty. *British Journal of Urology* **55**, 93–96.

Wickham, J. E. A. and Kellet, M. J. (1983). Percutaneous pyelolysis. *European Urology* **9**, 122–124.

Wong, S. K., Ng, L. G., Tan, B. S., Cheng, C. W., Chee, C. T., Chan, L. P., and Lo, H. G. (2001). Acute renal colic: value of unenhanced spiral computed tomography compared with intravenous urography. *Annals of the Academy of Medicine, Singapore* **30**, 568–572.

Yaqoob, M., King, A., McClelland, P., McDicken, I., and Bell, G. M. (1994). Relationship between hydrocarbon exposure and nephropathology in primary glomerulonephritis. *Nephrology, Dialysis, Transplantation* **9**, 1575–1579.

Yaqoob, M. M., Alkhunaizi, A. M., Edelstein, C. L., Conger, J. D., and Schrier, R. W. Acute renal failure: pathogenesis, diagnosis and management. In *Renal and Electrolyte Disorders* 5th edn. (ed. R. W. Schrier), pp. 449–506. Lippincott-Raven, 1997.

Yarger, W. E., Schocken, D. D., and Harris, R. J. (1980). Obstructive nephropathy in the rat: possible roles for the renin angiotensin system, prostaglandins, thromboxanes in post-obstructive renal function. *Journal of Clinical Investigation* **65**, 400–412.

Zetterstrom, R., Ericson, N. O., and Winberg, J. (1958). Separate renal function studies in predominantly unilateral hydronephrosis. *Acta Paediatrica Scandinavica* **47**, 540–548.

17.4 Congenital abnormalities of the urinary tract

Wolfgang Rascher and Wolfgang H. Rösch

Introduction

Malformation of the urinary tract is among the most common of all congenital malformations: in one large study of 245,000 necropsies the prevalence of renal anomalies was 1/650 (Ashley and Mostofi 1960), and more than one-third of all malformations diagnosed by prenatal ultrasonography affect the urinary tract (Grisoni *et al.* 1986; Helin and Persson 1986; Grupe 1987). Prior to the common use of prenatal ultrasound these anomalies were undetected until complications in childhood prompted investigation.

The management of congenital anomalies of the urinary tract has changed dramatically. Children with severe uropathies have a much better prognosis when diagnosed antenatally and treated in early infancy rather than later in life, when complications have occurred. This is particularly true when severe infections of the obstructed urinary tract can be prevented. However, the question remains, whether this also applies to mild or moderate uropathies or renal anomalies. Many clinically insignificant abnormalities of the urinary tract are nowadays evident on ultrasonography before delivery and, frequently, no specific treatment is necessary. Incorrect fetal diagnosis, parental anxiety, and unnecessary postnatal diagnostic evaluation and intervention may limit the above-mentioned advantage. Ultrasound screening of the newborn urinary tract has little value in detecting vesicoureteric reflux.

Antenatal and early postnatal diagnosis has changed diagnostic and therapeutic strategies, since the approaches and indications for surgery derived from experience with symptomatic older children are not necessarily applicable to asymptomatic neonates.

Embryology of the fetal urinary system

Development of the urinary system

The urinary system develops from the cloaca and the intermediate mesoderm. Two sets of tubular systems develop into the fetal kidney and subsequently degenerate: the first set, the pronephros, fuses caudally into the pronephric duct which extends into the cloaca. In the fourth embryonic week the pronephros contacts the mesonephric tubules and degenerates, while the ducts become the mesonephric duct. In the human embryo the mesonephric duct also degenerates. A branch of the mesonephric duct near its junction with the cloaca, the ureteric bud, and the metanephros begin to develop into the final renal system within the fifth week postconception (Fig. 1). Nephrons are formed from the interaction of elements of the mesonephros (ureteric bud) and the

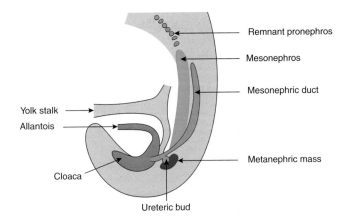

Fig. 1 Development of the fetal urinary system, shown in a 5-week-old fetus. The metanephric mass and the ureteric bud constitute the primordium of metanephros, the final human renal development (modified from Langman 1969).

metanephros: the ureteral bud begins to divide around the sixth week and the third to fifth generation of ureteral bud branches, which appear at about 8 weeks, differentiate into nephrons. This is associated with attachment of a nephron vesicle to the terminal branches of the dividing bud. As the ureteric bud extends, the metanephric mass of mesoderm (metanephric blastema) condenses into the metanephros. The ureteric bud branches successively to form the ureter, pelvis, calyces, and the collecting tubules. The metanephric blastema forms the glomeruli and the upper part of the nephrons. The first nephrons form at about 8 weeks postconception, and branching of the collecting system and nephron formation continues into the fifteenth to twentieth week. The last generation of collecting ducts formed continues to grow centrifugally and to induce nephrons until 32 weeks. The last period of renal development is between 32 and 36 weeks, when ampullae disappear and signal the end of nephron formation. Increases in renal mass that occur during this period (threefold increase in size) result from glomerular, interstitial, and tubular growth, particularly growth of the proximal tubule.

Differentiation of the urinary tract occurs in parallel with the early stages of metanephric development. The mesonephric duct communicates with the allantois and the cloaca at the fifth week of fetal life, when the ureteral bud appears. The urinary system separates from the rectum at about the sixth week, when the urorectal fold forms the septum which divides the urinary system from the primitive gut. The formation of a separate opening of the metanephric duct into the bladder occurs by the seventh week and becomes the vesicoureteral opening. The remainder of the allantois forms the fibrous cord known as the urachus which connects the bladder with the umbilicus. The fetal ureter does not open into the bladder until about the ninth week, which corresponds to the estimated time of onset of fetal renal function.

Separation of the urinary and genital systems

The separation of the urinary tract from the genital system differs in the male and in the female. The Y chromosome, particularly a 35 kb sex-related Y chromosome region (SRY), induces the primordial gonad into the masculine gonad; in the absence of the Y chromosome, the gonad becomes the ovary (Wolf et al. 1992). The gonadal development of the male and the female embryo does not start before the seventh week. In the 6-week-old undifferentiated embryo, two tubular systems exist: first, the mesonephric duct or Wolffian duct, from the mesonephros to the cloaca, and the Müllerian duct, which runs parallel to the mesonephric duct and also joins the cloaca. In the male, regression of the Müllerian duct is induced by Müllerian inhibitory factor, produced by the fetal testis and by the differentiation of the mesonephric duct into the Wolffian ducts. The latter form the convoluted duct of the epididymis and the caudal portion forms the ductus deferens. This process begins during the seventh to eighth weeks.

In the female, the two Müllerian ducts are maintained, and their distal segments join in the midline to form a single cord by the end of the eighth week. The uterovaginal cord opens into the urogenital sinus; that part of the urogenital sinus caudal to the opening to the Müllerian duct forms the vaginal vestibule and contributes to the lower part of the vagina in the female. In the male, this part forms a part of the prostatic membranous urethra. By 12–13 weeks, the median septum of the fused urogenital sinus is resorbed and the uterus, cervix, and part of the vagina evolve. The Wolffian duct regresses nearly completely.

The kidney of the newborn (see also Chapter 1.4)

Development of structure

The kidney of the normal newborn differs both morphologically and histologically from the mature organ. The external surface of the newborn kidney is lobulated, showing the underlying structural organization. With cortical growth, these lobulations are obliterated, so that the surface of the kidney becomes smooth. The last generations of nephrons induced are located in the subcapsular region of the cortex and can serve as an anatomical index of gestational age since nephron induction ceases at about 26 weeks of gestation. The anatomical dimensions of the nephron in the kidney at birth differ from those in adults (Fetterman et al. 1965): the glomerular diameter in the newborn is about one-third of that of an adult, while that of the proximal tubule is only one-tenth of that in adults. The variation in size between the individual nephrons from the same level of the cortex, the so-called nephron heterogeneity, is another characteristic of the newborn kidney. The variation between the length of the shortest and longest proximal tubule in infants is elevenfold and in adults twofold. Variations in glomerular size are less than those of the tubules, and are related to their location in the cortex. The mean intraglomerular

diameter is 1.26 mm in the least mature glomeruli of the outer cortex, 1.73 mm in the middle, and in the inner cortex the mature glomeruli are 2.46 mm in diameter (Fetterman et al. 1965). In the mature kidney, mean glomerular diameter is the same at all levels. The heterogeneity of glomeruli and nephrons at birth is a consequence of the centripetal pattern of nephron formation during fetal life. The most mature units are located within the inner cortex, the least mature nephrons in the outer cortex. The heterogeneity of size, characteristic of the nephrons of the newborn kidney, disappears by the end of the first year of life.

Development of renal function

In adult life blood flow to the kidneys accounts for 20–30 per cent of cardiac output, but during the prenatal period the perfusion is very low: the kidneys of 10–20-week-old human fetuses will receive 3–7 per cent of cardiac output (Rudolph et al. 1971). Although the human embryo produces urine from the twelfth week of gestation, the role of the kidneys in the maintenance of fetal homeostasis is minor compared to that of the placenta.

Immediately after birth, renal blood flow and glomerular filtration rate (GFR) are low and correlate with gestational age; they then increase gradually. GFR doubles within 2 weeks, reaching adult values, corrected for surface area, between 1 and 2 years of age (Aperia et al. 1975). The rate of maturation is similar in term and preterm infants (Fawer et al. 1979).

Development of tubular function

Close cell to cell contact between ureter epithelium and metanephric mesenchyme is required for transformation of mesenchymal cells into epithelial tubules. The molecular events include multiple signals (e.g. wnt-4) to regulate tubulogenesis (Müller and Brändli 1999). The development of sodium chloride reabsorption is an indicator of kidney maturation (Barac-Nieto and Spitzer 1988): premature infants sometimes lose more sodium and chloride than mature infants (Sulyok et al. 1979). In the first week of life, distal fractional sodium reabsorption is only 70 per cent, but improves over the next week, indicating a rapid development of sodium-conserving mechanisms, such as the renin–angiotensin–aldosterone system (Sulyok et al. 1979). The newborn kidney is limited in its ability to excrete an acute sodium load, although there is a normal natriuresis in the first week of life, resulting in a reduction of the extracelluar fluid volume (Rascher and Sulyok 1994). Activation of atrial natriuretic peptide may contribute to sodium homeostasis in the first weeks of life, particularly after sodium loading (Tulassay et al. 1986).

The capacity for potassium excretion, a function of the activity of Na^+,K^+-ATPase, is low at birth and increases in early postnatal life as potassium intake and excretion increase (Schwartz and Evan 1984). The newborn kidney is unable to concentrate urine to the same extent as the mature organ. Since secretion of, and the end-organ responsiveness to, antidiuretic hormone are well developed during early development of the human collecting duct (Abramow and Dratwa 1974), the delay in the ability to concentrate urine maximally is the result of inadequate generation and maintenance of a hypertonic medulla rather than failure of the collecting tubules to permit water reabsorption and subsequent concentration of tubular fluid.

Development of urine production

Fetal urine production starts at about the ninth week of gestation, when the ureter opens into the bladder. Production of adequate quantities of urine and sodium reabsorption start between 12 and 15 weeks of gestation. After the first trimester, fetal urinary output is a major source of amniotic fluid (Lotgering and Wallenburg 1986); consequently, absence or marked depression of urinary output is associated with severe oligohydramnios. The changing biochemical characteristics of the amniotic fluid throughout pregnancy are attributed to fetal maturation: changing urea and creatinine concentrations and the reduction in sodium concentration and osmolality near term may reflect maturation of renal function (Abramovich 1978). Increased concentrations of sodium, chloride, potassium, and high osmolality of fetal urine indicate poor renal tubular function (Crombleholme et al. 1988; Nicolini et al. 1992) and a decline in microprotein concentration in the amniotic fluid during pregnancy appears to correlate with with the maturing resorptive capacity of proximal tubular cells (Freedman et al. 1997). Various fetal urinary parameters have been reported as a marker of fetal renal function, however, sufficient information requires multiple aspirations (Johnson et al. 1995; Müller et al. 1996).

Micturition occurs within 24 h of birth in 92 per cent of newborns, and within 48 h in 99 per cent (Guignard 1987). A healthy infant excretes urine at a rate of 15–30 ml/kg/24 h during the first 2 days of life and between 25 and 120 ml/kg/24 h in the next 4 days.

Causes of urinary tract and kidney malformations

Studies of cell–matrix interactions during renal organogenesis provided convincing evidence that extracellular matrix glycoproteins and their receptors play an important role during kidney development (Müller and Brändli 1999). The molecular basis of congenital urinary and kidney malformations has been extensively studied in genetically engineered null-mutant mice (Woolf 2001). In humans various mutations have been associated with kidney and urinary tract malformations (see syndromes with a renal component—Tables 5–10), but these syndromes are relatively rare and it is a common clinical experience that most cases of kidney and urinary tract malformations are sporadic. However, in some families non-syndromic urinary tract malformations appear to be inherited, suggesting specific mutations have caused the disorder.

Animal experiments suggest that angiotensin is an important factor for urinary tract development, since interruption of the angiotensin II type 1 A and 1 B receptor or of the angiotensinogen gene affects the normal development of the renal medulla and delay glomerular maturation (Tsuchida et al. 1998). Pharmacological inhibition of angiotensin II affects renal function in early postnatal life of rodents (Tufro-McReddie et al. 1995). Null mutations of the angiotensin II type 2 receptor gene located on the X chromosome lead to various urinary tract malformations in male mice (renal dysplasia, hypoplasia, hydronephrosis, and vesicoureteric reflux) (Nishimura et al. 1999). Delayed apoptosis of mesenchymal cells during the developing urinary tract has been suggested as cause for the phenotype, but the final phenotype also depends on modifying genes or non-genetic factors. In patients with multicystic dysplastic kidneys and/or pelviureteral obstruction an association of a polymorphism of intron 1 of the AT2 gene has been described (Ile A-13326 transition) occurring in 19–42 per cent of healthy subjects and in 74–77 per cent of the patients (Nishimura et al. 1999). A similar association with this polymorphism has been reported in patients with obstructive megaureters (Hohenfellner et al. 1999).

Primary vesicoureteric reflux may have a genetic basis with the inheritance in many kindreds appearing to be dominant with variable penetrance and expression (Feather et al. 1996, 2000).

Clinical presentation and diagnosis

Obstetric ultrasound and antenatal diagnosis

Prenatal ultrasonographic screening identifies many fetal abnormalities, including neural tube defects, congenital heart defects, intestinal obstruction, abdominal wall defects, diaphragmatic hernias, abnormalities of the central nervous system, and renal and urinary tract anomalies.

Severe renal diseases often present with reduced amounts of amniotic fluid, since this is derived mainly from fetal urine (Peipert and Donnenfeld 1991). Reduced urine production due to severe obstructive uropathy or renal agenesis is associated with early oligohydramnios and strongly associated with an adverse outcome (Moore et al. 1989), particulary when it occurs during early gestation (Mandell et al. 1992). Fetal compression due to a deficiency of amniotic fluid results in a recognizable constellation of clinical findings, including skeletal abnormalities, characteristic facies, pulmonary hypoplasia, and perinatal death due to respiratory insufficiency (Potter's sequence). When this complication occurs before 28 weeks of gestation it is associated with pulmonary hypoplasia: a deficiency of amniotic fluid prevents normal fetal lung expansion, probably because of external compression (Wigglesworth et al. 1981).

Since fluid-filled masses are easily detected by ultrasound, obstructive uropathy and renal cystic disease are often found fortuitously in the fetus. Anomalies of the kidney and the urinary tract are the most common malformations diagnosed prenatally. An epidemiological study of approximately 12,000 pregnant women in Malmö, Sweden, found an overall prevalence of fetal malformations of 0.5 per cent, about 50 per cent of which were urinary tract anomalies (Helin and Persson 1986). In recently published series the prevalence of urinary tract malformations detected by prenatal ultrasonography ranged between 0.1 and 0.9 per cent (Grisoni et al. 1986; Helin and Persson 1986; Smith et al. 1987; Gunn et al. 1988; Thomas and Gordon 1989; Rosendahl 1990; Scott and Renwick 1993). Approximately one in every 1000 routine examinations will, however, reveal some urinary tract abnormality. Although this is somewhat less than the estimated prevalence of congenital renal or urological abnormalities in the general population (1/650) (Ashley and Mostofi 1960), it includes the most important ones.

Although normal fetal kidneys can sometimes be identified by ultrasound in the sixteenth week of gestation, the adrenals are large and may be a source of misinterpretation. After 32 weeks of gestation, both kidneys can usually be visualized during maternal ultrasonography. The fetal bladder can be seen between 12 and 15 weeks' gestation, when active urine production begins. The cyclical increases in size and emptying can often be seen during an examination. Repeat examinations will demonstrate adequate bladder filling.

Fetal hydronephrosis may be transitory, disappearing postnatally or even later in life with a good and stable renal function (Homsy *et al.* 1990; Johnson *et al.* 1991; Koff 2000). The problem today is not the detection of hydronephrosis, but the early decision on the clinical relevance of the observed pelvic and caliceal dilatation. Classification of severity of pre- and postnatal diagnosed hydronephrosis is given in Table 1.

Potential errors in the prenatal diagnosis

In most, but not all cases, the diagnosis reached by prenatal ultrasonography agrees with that established postnatally. The rate of errors in the prenatal diagnosis of renal and urinary tract anomalies reaches 30 per cent in large series or reviews (Helin and Persson 1986; Grupe 1987; Clarke *et al.* 1989; DeWolf *et al.* 1989). Differentiation between hydronephrosis due to obstruction at the pelviureteric junction and a multicystic–dysplastic kidney may be difficult. Physiological dilatation of the renal pelvis, which may be present in up to 20 per cent of third-trimester fetuses, may also lead to an incorrect diagnosis and possibly to inappropriate therapy (Colodny 1987; Grupe 1987). Hydronephrosis and ureteric dilatation secondary to vesicoureteric reflux have been misinterpreted as obstructive uropathy, while urethral atresia or dilated posterior urethra in the prune-belly syndrome may be mistaken for posterior urethral valves. The renal pyramids are more sonolucent in the fetus than in children and adolescents, and this can be misinterpreted as hydronephrosis or renal cystic disease. Enlargement of the stomach produced by duodenal atresia can be confused with pelviureteric junction obstruction (Sanders and Graham 1982).

Although the anatomical details of urinary tract anomalies can be defined reliably by ultrasonographic examination, only limited information is provided about renal function and urodynamics. Dilatation of the renal pelvis and/or the ureter(s) can be demonstrated accurately, but obstruction can only be deduced from indirect findings, such as reduced renal mass, oligohydramnios, or prolonged absence of urine in the bladder. The degree of dilatation depends on urine flow rate and does not correlate with the severity of the underlying uropathy: minor dilatation of the fetal renal pelvis may progress to severe obstruction requiring postnatal surgical correction, while gross dilatation may resolve completely.

The best indicator of the severity of renal disease appears to be the time at which oligohydramnios develops: before 20 weeks of gestation oligohydramnios due to markedly impaired renal function has a poor prognosis, with death due to pulmonary hypoplasia occurring within hours of birth (Woodard and Parrott 1987; Moore *et al.* 1989; Mandell *et al.* 1992). When oligohydramnios develops after 32 weeks of gestation, pulmonary development is completed and lung function will be normal. Since the majority of fetuses with suspected hydronephrosis proved to be normal, parents should not be unduly alarmed by the physician (Johnson *et al.* 1991; Najmaldin *et al.* 1991; Koff and Campbell 1994).

Clinical presentation in symptomatic children

Few significant urinary tract anomalies are not detected by prenatal ultrasound, and these present mainly as severe urinary tract infections in infants or young children. Newborns and small infants may present with acute renal failure and septicaemia (Gonzalez and Sheldon 1982), with symptoms of poor feeding, failure to thrive, pale colour, and perhaps fever, vomiting, and slow weight gain. A small number of patients, especially the younger ones, are referred in an extremely poor clinical condition, characterized by dehydration with polyuria due to an acute tubular concentration defect as a consequence of severe infection. Severe electrolyte disturbances are often present, combined with renal failure. Hyponatraemia, hyperkalaemia, and prerenal failure are the consequences of salt-losing due to aldosterone resistance resembling an adrenal disorder (Batlle *et al.* 1981; Heijden *et al.* 1985; Melzi *et al.* 1995).

Flank pain is often associated with acute obstruction, and macroscopic haematuria sometimes occurs after mild trauma or when stones have formed within the obstructed kidney. In newborns, obstruction of the pelviureteric junction is usually associated with an abdominal mass, and most commonly presents as urinary tract infection, which is a potentially serious complication.

Micturition disturbances usually point to obstruction of the bladder outlet, such as posterior urethral valves (in boys) and ectopic ureteroceles (dribbling incontinence) in girls. In the sick neonate, and in symptomatic infants and children, ultrasound examination is by far the best initial investigation.

Diagnostic approach

Fetal urinary tract anomalies detected prenatally can be monitored by ultrasound and delivery carried out at a centre where expert neonatal, nephrological, and urological care is available. The first postnatal physical examination is often normal, but may reveal abdominal masses due to hydronephrosis and/or megaureter. Absent abdominal muscle wall (prune-belly) syndrome and enlarged kidneys or bladder may also be diagnosed. A neural tube defect or absent os sacrum may indicate neurogenic bladder disease.

Renal and urinary tract ultrasonography

After the physical examination has been completed ultrasonography should be performed. A prenatal diagnosis of hydronephrosis is often not substantiated shortly after birth: this may be related to the physiological oliguria seen 1 or 2 days after birth. If ultrasound examinations are repeated during normal diuresis, some days after birth, hydronephrosis will reappear if the urinary tract is obstructed (Fig. 2).

A realistic interpretation of an ultrasound examination is important since it provides only anatomical information: dilatation of the urinary tract, for example, is not necessarily induced by obstruction. In addition to dilatation of the renal pelvis and the ureter, bladder filling and bladder wall thickness can be determined by ultrasound. Assessment

Table 1 Classification of severity of prenatal and postnatal diagnosed hydronephrosis (modified according to Grignon *et al.* 1986 and Homsy *et al.* 1990)

	Size of renal pelvis (cm)	Calyceal dilatation	Renal parenchyma
Group I	1	Physiological	Normal
Group II	1–1.5	Normal calyces	Normal
Group III	>1.5	Slight dilatation	Normal
Group IV	>1.5	Moderate dilatation	>0.5 cm
Group V	>1.5	Severe dilatation	<0.5 cm Cortical atrophy

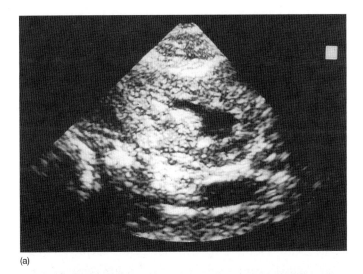

(a)

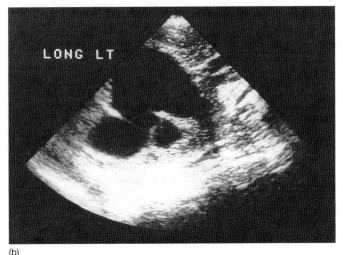

(b)

Fig. 2 Postnatal sonography of the kidney at day 1 (a) and day 7 (b). Note that during physiological oliguria at the first day after birth renal ultrasound is normal, whereas after 7 days during normal diuresis severe hydronephrosis is demonstrable.

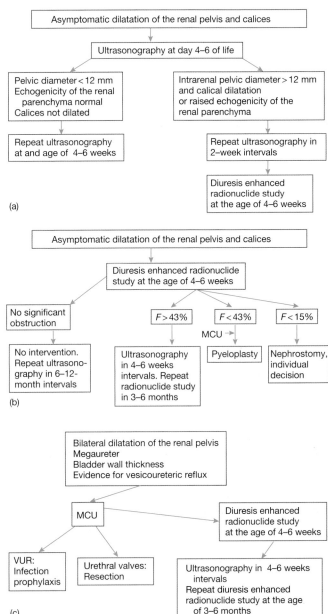

Fig. 3 Postnatal evaluation and suggested treatment of newborns and infants with prenatally detected possible urinary tract obstruction. Adapted from a consensus of German paediatricians, paediatric urologists, paediatric surgeons, paediatric radiologists, including nuclear medicine (Beetz *et al.* 2002). Figure (a) refers to diagnostic approach and (b) of possible treatment decision in upper urinary tract dilatation, whereas (c) presents the approach to lower urinary tract obstruction and pathology. VUR, vesicoureteric reflux; MCU, micturation cystourethrography.

of the function of the renal parenchyma by ultrasound is limited. Ultrasound often suggests the definite diagnosis, and complementary radiological and radionuclide imaging serve only to differentiate between dilatation without significant obstruction and obstruction which has to be corrected. If unilateral hydronephrosis is present, the course should be monitored in weekly or biweekly intervals and after 4–6 weeks radionuclide imaging is indicated (Fig. 3). Diagnostic procedures should also indicate functional renal mass and GFR.

Micturating cystourethrography

Micturating cystourethrography should be performed in patients with bladder wall thickness (urethral valves in boys), unilateral or bilateral dilated ureters, when variable degrees of hydronephrosis are suggestive for vesicoureteric reflux and before corrective surgery (to exclude vesicoureteric reflux). Micturating cystourethrography is independent of the degree of renal function and gives valuable information regarding the lower urinary tract (bladder outflow) and whether vesicoureteric reflux is present. The combination of ultrasound and micturating

cystourethrography allows adequate morphological evaluation in patients with lower urinary tract malformation. It permits appropriate management to be instituted immediately after birth. Routine micturating cystourethrography is not necessary in most cases with unilateral hydronephrosis (Misra *et al.* 1999; Beetz *et al.* 2002).

Further imaging may be planned when the neonate is stable and clinical, laboratory, and radiological findings have been evaluated. This usually provides information about the function of the kidneys and the urodynamics (Reinberg and Gonzalez 1987; Parkhouse and Barratt 1988).

Technetium-99m-dimercaptosuccinic acid scan

The [^{99}Tc^m]dimercaptosuccinic acid (DMSA) scan is an example of a 'static' renal scan and is a useful means of evaluating functional renal parenchyma. The isotope binds to functioning proximal tubular cells. This scan has an important role in identifying small, poorly functioning or non-functioning kidneys (e.g. multicystic–dysplastic kidneys, unilateral renal agenesis) and in obtaining information about individual renal function. It is a useful method for establishing whether a small kidney is worth conserving or whether nephrectomy is appropriate. It also identifies important functional changes due to segmental renal scars in children with vesicoureteric reflux.

In the newborn period, the [^{99}Tc^m]DMSA scan is characterized by a high background activity and relatively low fixation of the isotope in the renal tubules. Since renal function doubles during the first week of age, radionuclide studies should not be performed before the age of 4–6 weeks. As shown in Fig. 4, residual renal function, indicating that a pelviureteric junction obstruction is correctable, can be demonstrated.

Dynamic radionuclide nephrography

Other radioisotopes used to evaluate renal function include [^{99}Tc^m]diethylenetriaminepentaacetic acid (DTPA), for the assessment of glomerular function, and radio-iodine-o-iodohippuric acid ([^{123}I/^{131}I]hippuran) and [^{99}Tc^m]mercaptoacetyltriglycine ([^{99}Tc^m]-MAG3). DTPA is extracted by glomerular filtration only, while the other substances (e.g. [^{123}I]hippuran) is also actively secreted in normal kidneys by proximal tubular secretion (80 per cent). The high extraction rate of more than 80 per cent during each passage through the kidney, compared to 20 per cent for DTPA is of advantage.

Dynamic radionuclide nephrography usually performed with [^{99}Tc^m]MAG3 under basal conditions does not reliably discriminate between obstructive and non-obstructive dilatation, since the radionuclide is retained in the renal pelvis in both conditions. However, when diuresis is enhanced by intravenous fluid load, followed by intravenous frusemide (0.5–1.0 mg/kg) administered 20 min after injection of the radionuclide, important additional urodynamic information can be obtained [diuresis-enhanced radionuclide nephrography (Fig. 5)]. It is important that dynamic radionuclide nephrographies are performed with an empty bladder in order to exclude an obstruction at the ureterovesical junction. In infants this requires the use of an indwelling bladder catheter that is not clamped. Adequate hydration is necessary to yield a reliable examination (Sukhai et al. 1985; Rascher et al. 1992; Steiner et al. 1999) (Table 2).

Intravenous urography

Intravenous urography is only seldom needed and should only be used to answer specific questions. The most common indication is to provide certain anatomical details important for further management. Intravenous urography remains the best investigation if detailed anatomy of the pelvicalyceal system is required. It also provides a good basis for assessing renal size and identifying segmental renal scars and is important in confirming a duplex system or a ureterocele suspected on ultrasonography. In case of significant urinary tract obstruction, early films may show a 'negative' pyelogram. Late films demonstrate retained contrast medium within the renal pelvis and the ureter.

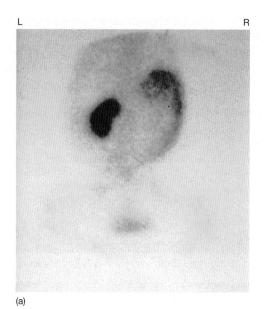

(a)

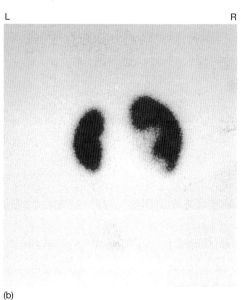

(b)

Fig. 4 [^{99}Tc^m]DMSA uptake scan in a 3-week-old newborn with massive hydronephrosis due to right pelviureteric junction obstruction. The left kidney is normal with increased function (60%, on the left). The right kidney has reduced renal function (40%) with a dilated renal pelvis shown as a negative defect (a). Note the relatively high background activity seen in neonates. [^{99}Tc^m]DMSA uptake scan after corrective surgery appears to be normal (b).

Since the kidney does not concentrate urine adequately immediately after birth, the kidneys may not be clearly visualized within the first few weeks of life, and this investigation should therefore be performed after 4–6 weeks of life. As is the case with dynamic radionuclide nephrography, intravenous urography should be performed with an empty bladder, particularly if obstruction at the ureterovesical junction is suspected.

Magnetic resonance imaging

Magnetic resonance imaging (MRI) has been recently introduced to evaluate morphological and functional information on the kidneys and the urinary tract (Rohrschneider et al. 2000; Rohrschneider and

Stegen 2001). For morphological assessment magnetic resonance urography is based upon *T*2-weighted sequences imaging the fluid-filled spaces of the dilated urinary system. The static fluid produce a high signal not only in the urinary tract, but also other fluid containing structures are imaged. Dynamic MRI allows reliable assessment of individual renal function and urinary excretion. The combination of static and dynamic magnetic resonance urography is used for simultaneous evaluation of morphology and function. Animal studies have shown that respiratory-triggered sequences after gadolinium-DTPA and frusemide application show comparable results as known for diuresis-enhanced radionuclide nephrography (Rohrschneider *et al.* 2000).

Pressure flow studies (Whitaker test)

Antegrade perfusion pressure flow studies (Whitaker 1979) are relatively complex and invasive and no longer used to differentiate between urodynamically minor dilatation and severe obstruction needing correction immediately. It is difficult to standardize the method, particularly in a dilated capacitance systems. Only in selected cases (e.g. enlarged system postoperatively) it can be performed.

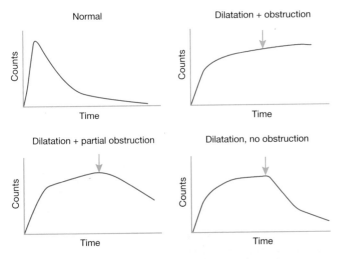

Fig. 5 Possible responses to diuresis-enhanced radionuclide nephrography with [^{99}Tc^m]MAG3 in children with urinary tract dilatation. Arrows indicate frusemide administration (0.5 mg/kg intravenously).

Table 2 Diuresis-enhanced dynamic radionuclide nephrography

Adequate hydration	
In older children	Oral fluid intake of 20 ml/kg 2–3 h prior to radionuclide nephrography
In infants	Intravenous fluid load with half normal saline (0.45% NaCl, 2.5% glucose) solution 4 h prior to radionuclide nephrography in a dose of 20 ml/kg/4 h Normal milk intake should be given (15–25 ml/kg in 4 h) by mouth. If oral fluid intake is stopped (e.g. sedation) add 15–25 ml/kg half-normal saline intravenously
Frusemide injection	
	Twenty minutes following IV injection of the tracer ([^{123}I]hippuran or [^{99}Tc^m]MAG3) add frusemide IV in a dose of 0.5 mg/kg

If vesicoureteric reflux or megaureter is suspected, the study should be done with indwelling open bladder catheter

Maldevelopment

The terminology used for various types of maldevelopment, malformation, and cystic and dysplastic kidneys is confusing. The classification of cystic kidneys according to Potter (1972) was derived from a developmental anatomical and histological approach, and is not related to urodynamic and clinical findings. The definitions developed by Bernstein (1971, 1976) provide the best accepted and most rational basis for the classification of clinicopathological correlations (Zerres *et al.* 1984) (Table 3). Correlations between time of manifestation of the disturbance and the extent of renal development are shown in Table 4.

Table 3 The classification of clinicopathological correlations of maldevelopment

Renal agenesis	Absence of the kidney or an identifiable metanephric structure
Renal hypoplasia	Significantly reduced renal mass without evidence for maldevelopment of the parenchyma
Renal dysplasia	Abnormal differentiation of the renal parenchyma with the development of abnormal structures, including primitive ducts surrounded by collars of connective tissue, metaplastic cartilage, a variety of non-specific malformations such as preglomeruli of the fetal type, and reduced branching of the collecting ducts with cystic dilatations and primitive tubules
Renal aplasia	Severe dysplasia with an extremely small kidney, sometimes identifiable only by histological examination
Renal multicystic dysplasia	Severe cystic dysplasia with extremely enlarged kidney full of cystic structures. It occurs as an isolated non-hereditary renal lesion in response to ureteral atresia (Potter type II) and in response to urethral obstruction (Potter type IV)
Polycystic kidney disease	Diffuse cystic changes in both kidneys without other evidence for parenchymal maldevelopment. It occurs as an autosomal recessive disorder (Potter type I) and as autosomal dominant (Potter type III)

Table 4 Relationship between time of manifestation and the extent of renal maldevelopment (according to Zerres *et al.* 1984)

Time of manifestation of the disturbance	Extent of renal maldevelopment
Prior to union between the metanephric blastema and ureteral bud	Renal agenesis
After union	Hypoplasia/multicystic dysplasia (Potter type II)
In a largely completed stage of renal development	Cystic dysplasia (e.g. with urethral obstruction)
Immediately before or after completion of renal development	Hydronephrosis

Congenital absence of the kidney

Renal agenesis is caused by a failure of the ureteral bud to communicate with the metanephric blastema, and represents a disturbance at a very early stage of development, generally before the fifth week of gestation. Unilateral agenesis is relatively common and is increasingly diagnosed by ultrasound. However, occasionally ultrasonography misses a very small kidney, particularly if it is displaced into the pelvis. Consequently the diagnosis of renal agenesis should be confirmed by a radionuclide scan with [^{99}Tc^m]DMSA, which will show an absence of functional renal tissue. It is also important to exclude any congenital abnormality of the remaining kidney (Atiyeh *et al.* 1992). Serial ultrasonographic examinations will show the development of compensatory hypertrophy in this single kidney. Renal function should also be monitored regularly.

Although renal agenesis and dysplasia have not been considered as hereditary diseases, it is of value examining families with bilateral renal agenesis and/or dysplasia (Roodhooft *et al.* 1984). These authors performed ultrasonographic examination of 71 parents and 40 siblings of 41 index patients with these conditions and found asymptomatic renal malformation in 9 per cent of these subjects at risk. Unilateral renal agenesis was found in 4.5 per cent of family members, compared to a prevalence of only 0.3 per cent in the control population.

Bilateral renal agenesis is very rare and always fatal. The pregnancy is always complicated by oligohydramnios after 16 weeks of gestation, when fetal urine normally begins to make a significant contribution to the volume of amniotic fluid. The severe oligohydramnios leads to the 'Potter sequence' of events, characterized by pulmonary hypoplasia and a characteristic facial appearance (Potter's facies), with flattening of the profile and the nose, low-set ears, underdeveloped chin, and a prominent fold of skin. These are the consequence of compression of the face in the restricted amniotic space lacking an adequate fluid volume. These infants die usually within hours of birth as a result of pulmonary hypoplasia, probably caused by simple compression. Skeletal deformations are caused by intrauterine lack of movement resulting from oligohydramnios (Woodard and Parrott 1987).

The diagnosis of bilateral agenesis can be made by the twentieth week, when ultrasound shows absence of the kidneys. Previously, failure to demonstrate the bladder 1 or 2 h after administration of intravenous frusemide to the mother was considered confirmatory (Wladimiroff 1975). Installation of artificial amniotic fluid may be helpful in pregnancies complicated by oligohydramnios; failure to demonstrate filling of the kidneys and bladder confirms renal agenesis (Gembruch and Hansmann 1988).

Renal hypoplasia

Renal hypoplasia is a rare condition in which the kidney is small, possibly due to inadequate branching of the ureteral bud and a decreased number of nephrons, but histologically normal. The prognosis is good when there is contralateral hypertrophy. Kidneys which are labelled hypoplastic are sometimes histologically dysplastic: follow-up examinations should include measurement of blood pressure and renal function and assessment of renal growth by ultrasonography.

Oligomeganephronic hypoplasia is a congenital non-familial form of bilateral hypoplasia that usually leads to progressive renal failure during childhood. Children present with polyuria and dehydration due to a renal concentration defect, and with failure to thrive and renal insufficiency. The kidneys are small, with a markedly reduced number of nephrons. Each nephron, glomerulus, and tubule is enlarged.

Ectopic kidneys

A simple ectopic kidney is occasionally encountered in childhood, usually as an incidental finding during abdominal sonography, and may be palpable as a mass within the iliac fossa. Although all anomalous kidneys are more prone to disease than normal ones, simple ectopia is seldom responsible for symptoms. The fused pelvic kidney in which the whole mass lies in front of the os sacrum may well give rise to diagnostic problems. The solitary pelvic kidney is often associated with complications such as hydronephrosis due to pelviureteric junction obstruction.

Like other renal abnormalities, horseshoe kidney, in which the lower poles are fixed together, may be found in children with no relevant complaint. It is sometimes associated with other congenital abnormalities (Wilson and Azmy 1986) and is a recognized feature of Turner's syndrome (Lippe *et al.* 1988). Hydronephrosis is the most common complication of a horseshoe kidney and of malrotated kidneys.

If both kidneys lie on the same side of the abdomen, they are almost always fused, with the malpositioned lying below and medial to the normal one; vesicoureteric reflux is the most important pathological feature (Fig. 6).

Renal dysplasia (including multicystic dysplasia)

The term dysplasia is used to describe a specific type of parenchymal maldevelopment. Dysplastic kidneys contain microscopic abnormalities

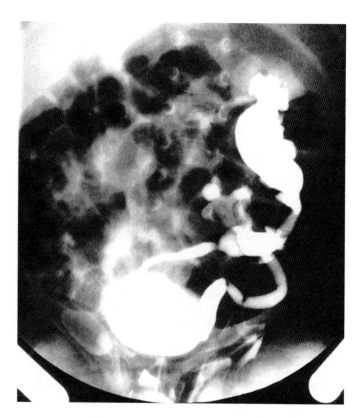

Fig. 6 Vesicoureteric reflux in a 1-month-old boy with crossed ectopia.

that have been attributed to the persistence of mesonephric tissue, developmental arrests, and faulty differentiation leading to persistence of primitive or fetal structures (Bernstein 1971). Potter (1972) separated normal or enlarged kidneys (multicystic–dysplastic kidney disease, type IIa) from small kidneys with reduced size and a few small cysts (type IIb).

The term multicystic kidney disease is generally used to describe dysplastic, usually non-functional kidneys with many large cysts, nearly always associated with ureteral atresia. The presenting sign of multicystic kidney is usually a unilateral mass, resembling severe hydronephrosis. The incidence of multicystic–dysplastic kidneys have been estimated about 1 : 4000 (Shah and Glassberg 2001). Although multicystic kidneys are usually unilateral, bilateral dysplasia may seldom occur, and abnormalities of the contralateral kidney may be present in up to 30 per cent of patients (Atiyeh et al. 1992), making it important to investigate the function and structure of the contralateral kidney. The most useful criteria for ultrasound identification of multicystic kidney are the presence of interfaces between the cysts, non-medial location of the largest cyst, the multiplicity of cysts, the absence of an identifiable renal sinus, and the absence of parenchymal tissue (Stuck et al. 1982) (Fig. 7). The DMSA scan demonstrates non-functioning of the kidney and the method of choice to differentiate multicystic–dysplastic kidney from pelviureteral junction obstruction. Occasionally radionuclide nephrography may fail to diagnose multicystic kidneys (Carey and Howards 1988), and histological examination reveals the exact diagnosis.

The micturating cystourethrogram may show a blind-ending ureter on the side of the multicystic kidney and, occasionally vesicoureteric reflux in the normal contralateral kidney. The outcome in children with unilateral lesions and a normal contralateral kidney is excellent since the contralateral kidney develops compensatory hypertrophy. Surgical removal of the unilateral mass has been advocated for many years, because of an anticipated risk of hypertension and malignancy (Javadpour et al. 1974). If a multicystic kidney is clearly differentiated from a solid and potentially malignant renal mass, conservative management is possible, since most cases regress spontaneously (Shah and Glassberg 2001). However, surgical exploration should be undertaken

in any patient with significant volumes of tissue. If the renal diagnosis of the multicystic kidney disease is clear, conservative management with sequential renal ultrasound examination, observation of arterial blood pressure, and renal function is as good as surgical removal (Gordon et al. 1988; Mentser et al. 1994; Shah and Glassberg 2001).

Disorders of urinary transport

Conditions causing obstruction of the urinary tract are the most important disorders of urinary transport, since they constitute the major avoidable cause of chronic renal failure. Dilatation of the urinary tract is a characteristic consequence of obstructed transport of urine, although it cannot be assumed to be always caused by obstruction: various other factors are associated with dilatation, including high-grade vesicoureteric reflux, maldevelopment, polyuria, and infection. Dilatation of the renal pelvis and ureter alone cannot be accepted as unequivocal evidence of obstruction; this is further substantiated by the fact that the ureteric dilatation may persist even after satisfactory surgical correction of the obstruction. Diagnostic procedures therefore have to differentiate between significant urinary tract obstruction and dilatation without significant obstruction.

Under normal conditions, intrarenal pressure is greatest at the glomerular tuft and gradually diminishes along the nephron. Resting pressures in the renal pelvis are of the order of 4 cm H_2O, increasing to 10 cm H_2O during contractions (O'Reilly 1986). High intrapelvic pressures occur only transiently in sudden acute obstruction and may reach 50–60 cm H_2O: these values will depend not only on the speed of onset and the degree of obstruction, but also on the capacity and compliance of the obstructed segment. Dilatation of a compliant tract will absorb and damp down potential pressure elevation, making resting pressure similar in normal and hydronephrotic obstructed kidneys in the antidiuretic state. However, during high flow rates the pressure in the obstructed kidney may increase dramatically. For filtration across the glomerulus, the pressure gradient between the lumen of the glomerular capillaries and the lumen of the proximal tubules must be maintained: flow is impeded in the ureter or renal pelvis, and the resulting increase in pressure is transferred to the collecting ducts and the tubules with consequent disturbance of nephron function. Early tubular dysfunction causes later abnormalities of glomerular filtration.

Animal models of partial pelviureteric junction obstruction develop progressive hydronephrosis. After some weeks of variable increases in intrapelvic pressure, there is a tendency for pressure to decrease to normal. Since the human renal pelvis accommodates to increasing volume and maintains relatively low intrapelvic pressures (Koff 1985), hydronephrosis is a compensatory mechanism which actually protects obstructed kidneys from further overdistension of the renal pelvis, from pathologically high intrarenal pelvic pressures, and from progressive renal deterioration. This is achieved by acquired changes in compliance, pelvic capacity, and renal function.

The pathophysiological process which leads to renal function impairment in patients with obstructed kidneys is only partially understood (Awazu et al. 1989). Pressure–flow studies suggest an increase in pressure in Bowman's space is generally a transient phenomenon and plays only a minor role in depression of the GFR; this is primarily due to a reduction in plasma flow. As well as early distribution of the blood flow and GFR from the outer to the inner cortex, which occurs in the

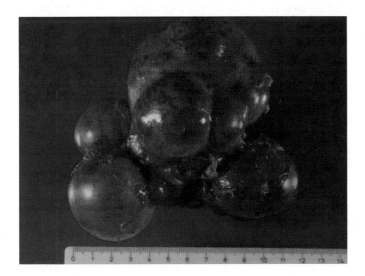

Fig. 7 Anatomical appearance of multicystic dysplasia.

acute phase, the chronic phase is characterized by a loss of function of the deeper nephrons. Hormonal mechanisms have been identified as being responsible for this marked reduction in plasma flow (Klahr *et al.* 1988; Awazu *et al.* 1989). Profound changes in the metabolism of arachidonic acid to vasodilator prostaglandins and vasoconstrictor thromboxanes have been attributed to changes in GFR. Activation of the renin–angiotensin system also contributes to lower GFR and to vasoconstriction in obstructed kidneys. Chronic ureteric obstruction in the fetus may interfere with renal morphogenesis, resulting in irreversible dysplastic changes; when present in early postnatal development it interferes with functional maturation of the kidney and arrest of renal growth (Chevalier *et al.* 1987).

Definition of obstruction

It is difficult to define urinary tract obstruction reliably. It can be defined as the inability of the urinary tract to clear urine from the nephron at an appropriate rate, leading to disturbances in the normal pressure–flow relationship in the urinary tract with the consequence of disturbances of nephron function and renal impairment. The increase in pressure transmits the effects of obstruction back to the kidney, resulting in the renal function impairment, which is part of the fundamental definition of obstruction. The predominant site of injury in obstructive uropathy is the distal nephron. Urinary concentration is impaired early, and sometimes severely, producing polyuria and hyposthenuria (Winberg 1959).

Relief of obstruction and renal function

In contrast to the sparse data on renal blood flow and GFR, ample information is available on tubular abnormalities after relief of obstruction in man. After prolonged obstruction, recovery of GFR in animals is impaired (Kerr 1956). In both humans and animals, release of chronic bilateral obstruction produces a dramatic increase in the absolute amount of urinary sodium and water (Ghazali and Barratt 1974). Although the sudden increase in GFR in combination with impaired tubular reabsorption of sodium and water is likely to be responsible for the observed natriuresis and diuresis, hormonal mechanisms may also contribute. In contrast to the usual antidiuretic response to surgery, infants with obstructive uropathy may suffer clinical deterioration on the first day after relief of obstructive uropathy, which can be prevented by infusion of increasing amounts of sodium and water.

Diagnosis of obstruction

Dilatation does not necessarily imply obstruction. Therefore, clinicians have to demonstrate significant obstruction prior to surgical correction. On dynamic radioisotope nephrography by [$^{99}Tc^m$]MAG3, uptake of the radioisotope by the kidney is decreased and renal transit time prolonged. The most important feature of significant obstruction is retention and delayed removal of activity from the renal pelvis, which cannot be influenced by enhanced diuresis (Fig. 5). If radioisotope nephrography reveals a significant frusemide-induced wash-out of radioisotope, a significant obstruction can be ruled out. Although excretory urography is not the method of choice demonstrating urodynamically significant obstruction, the hallmark of significant urinary tract obstruction is a delayed, increasingly dense, prolonged nephrogram. Early films may show a 'negative' pyelogram; later the

pelvis shows dilated calyces which fill sluggishly with contrast medium. Late films consistently demonstrate retained contrast medium within the renal pelvis and the ureter. Up to now there is no single method that clearly differentiates between obstruction and ectasia (dilatation without obstruction). A continuum occurs between both conditions.

Pelviureteric junction obstruction

Pelviureteric junction obstruction (idiopathic hydronephrosis) is one of the most frequent causes of obstructive uropathy in children. The condition is usually congenital and may have a mechanical basis, due to increasing stenosis or external compression (adhesions, aberrant lower-pole vessels, persisting fetal folds).

With the advent of prenatal ultrasonography, many more cases of hydronephrosis are detected in utero and the diagnosis can be confirmed in asymptomatic neonates (Grignon *et al.* 1986; Homsy *et al.* 1990). Diagnostic procedures have to differentiate between significant obstruction at the pelviureteric junction, which requires surgical correction, and ectasia of the renal pelvis, in which intervention is not indicated. Watchful waiting with repetitive radionuclide studies is the best approach to avoid unnecessary surgery (Aslan *et al.* 1998; Koff 2000; Ulman *et al.* 2000).

In a prospective study of 112 patients (142 kidneys) with congenital hydronephrosis due to ureteropelvic junction obstruction, postnatal management was guided by initial renal function as determined by [$^{99}Tc^m$]DTPA scan (Ransley *et al.* 1990). Independent of the result of the diuretic study, renal function was divided into three groups: renal function greater than 40 per cent was defined as good; renal function of 20–39 per cent, moderate; and less than 20 per cent was defined as poor. In this study 77 per cent of patients with good function had stable or even improved renal function, whereas 23 per cent of patients with initially good function underwent pyeloplasty because of symptoms or decrease in function. No operation was necessary if pelvic diameter was less than 12 mm. When impairment of renal function was used as the criterion to perform surgery, only seven of 104 infants needed operative treatment (Koff and Campbell 1994).

Absolute indications for surgical relief of obstruction include impairment of renal function, pyelonephritis, urolithiasis, and pain. Relative indications for surgical corrections are reduced renal function and a renal pelvic diameter of greater 3 cm and dilated calices (Aslan *et al.* 1998). In newborns and small infants primary correction of the pelviureteric junction by pyeloplasty using the method of Anderson–Hynes is the most frequently chosen procedure. Emergency surgery is not indicated in a neonate with pelviureteric junction obstruction and good renal function: if primary correction is planned within the first months of life, prior percutaneous nephrostomy is not indicated. Preliminary temporary urinary diversion with percutaneous insertion of a nephrostomy catheter is only rarely necessary, for example if there is severe infection of the obstructed kidney.

Older children present with an abdominal mass or with pain in the flank, haematuria secondary to mild trauma, or urinary tract infection. Hypertension is rare, but occurs occasionally, sometimes temporarily after surgical correction.

Ureterovesical junction obstruction

Obstruction at the ureterovesical junction results in ureteric dilatation (megaureter) and hydronephrosis. The obstructive megaureter is associated with a segment of the lower ureter that fails to transport the urine adequately to the bladder. Delayed or reduced recanalization of the ureteral lumen has been suggested as pathogenetic mechanisms (Ruano-Gil *et al.* 1975).

Three other conditions have to be differentiated from an obstructive ureter: the refluxing ureter, the refluxing and obstructive ureter, and the non-refluxing and non-obstructive ureter (primary megaureter) (King 1980). The obstructive megaureter may present in early childhood with acute pyelonephritis and sometimes with haematuria, although it is usually diagnosed prenatally by ultrasonography.

Micturating cystourethrography will exclude vesicoureteric reflux and bladder outflow obstruction: the presence of the former does not exclude obstruction. Dynamic radioisotope is important to demonstrate significant obstruction and renal function impairment. As with pelviureteric junction obstruction, renal damage, pyelonephritis, urolithiasis, and pain are absolute indications for surgical correction.

Obstructive megaureter is treated by excision of the stenotic segment and reimplantation of the ureter with an antireflux technique. Since the results of surgery are not satisfactory in the neonatal period and early infancy, temporary high urinary diversion either by distal loop cutaneoureterostomy, by the Sober procedure, or by pyelocutaneostomy is indicated. If the obstruction is still present in these children after 1 year of age, the ureter should be reimplanted in the bladder and the ureterostomy can be closed. Spontaneous relief of obstruction appears to be possible in primary obstructed megaureter. The non-obstructive, non-refluxing primary megaureter has a tendency to heal. Whereas some authors report a high incidence of corrective surgery (Peters *et al.* 1989; Vereecken and Proesmans 1999), others advocate observational management (Lettgen *et al.* 1993; Liu *et al.* 1994). In a series of 53 newborns with 67 megaureters 23 (34 per cent) resolved spontaneously and 33 (49 per cent) persisted. Surgical correction was done in three ureters because of urinary tract infections and in eight because of deteriorating renal function (Liu *et al.* 1994). Ureteral diameter of less than 6 mm quantified by ultrasonography had a good, and diameters greater than 10 mm had a bad prognosis. Drainage on dynamic renography correlated best with outcome. Thus, the majority of patients with primary megaureter does not require surgical intervention (Liu *et al.* 1994). Antibiotic treatment of urinary tract infections and antibiotic prophylaxis is recommended. Reinfection prophylaxis should be given for at least 6 months.

Posterior urethral valves

Congenital posterior urethral valves are the most common cause of severe subvesical obstruction in the male infant. Valves, which appear as mucosal folds in the posterior urethra below the verumontanum, cause dilatation of the proximal urethra and bladder wall hypertrophy and trabeculation. As a consequence of subvesical obstruction and bladder hypertrophy, bilateral hydronephrosis and megaureters may develop. Early obstruction during renal development may result in severe renal dysplasia (Henneberry and Stephens 1980). According to Potter (1972) cystic dysplasia type IV occurs as a result of urethral occlusion (Table 3).

The principal microscopic abnormality is the presence of subcapsular cysts, the walls of which are usually lined either by cells similar to the epithelial portion of the glomeruli or a structure similar to that of the primitive Bowman's capsule. Varying numbers of normal nephrons are found.

Urinary extravasation may occur in the perinatal period, resulting in perirenal urinoma or urinary ascites (Cass *et al.* 1981; Greenfield *et al.* 1982). Extravasation is usually associated with reasonably good kidney function as the leak protects the kidney from the deleterious effect of back pressure (Fig. 8).

Bilateral hydronephrosis due to posterior urethral valves is frequently detected by routine ultrasonography in pregnancy. After birth, ultrasonography shows massive bladder wall hypertrophy, although the presence of detrusor hypertrophy means that the bladder capacity is often not increased. Micturating cystourethrography is the next diagnostic step: radiographs must be taken in lateral or oblique views in the male. In most patients secondary vesicoureteric reflux is present (Fig. 9).

When there is severe dysplasia and poor renal function, oligohydramnios may develop during pregnancy and pulmonary hypoplasia causes problems immediately after birth. In children with renal failure, polyuria, electrolyte disturbances, and renal acidosis may be the presenting sign. Later in life, acute urinary tract infection and renal failure are the most important presenting signs in children with posterior urethral valves (Gonzalez and Sheldon 1982).

After diagnosis by micturating urethrocystography, electrolyte disturbances, dehydration, acute renal failure, and infection should be treated prior to surgical resection. The bladder should be drained by an indwelling catheter and early endoscopic resection performed as soon as the clinical condition allows. Valves are often difficult to

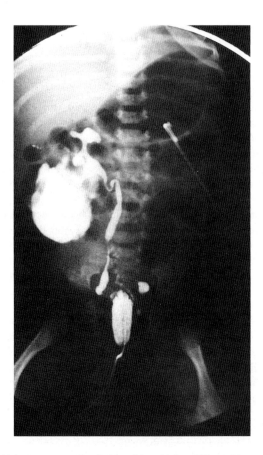

Fig. 8 Urinary extravasation (urinoma) in a **14-day-old boy** with posterior urethral valves. Note that extravasation has prevented dilation of the right renal pelvis and the right ureter. A percutaneous nephrostomy catheter has been placed into the left renal pelvis.

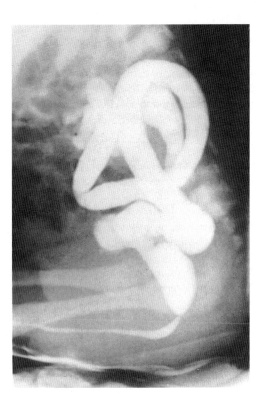

Fig. 9 Bilateral vesicoureteric reflux in a 3-week-old boy with posterior urethral valves. Note the prestenotic enlargement of the posterior urethra.

visualize during cystoscopy since irrigation fluid opens them in a retrograde direction.

In patients with severe hydronephrosis and renal insufficiency, temporary high urinary diversion, such as percutaneous nephrostomy, ureterocutaneostomy by the Sober technique, loop cutaneoureterostomy, or pyelocutaneostomy may be indicated. Renal function and electrolyte homeostasis should be monitored carefully after relief of obstruction; natriuresis and polyuria often develop, and sodium and fluid loss must be replaced.

Despite adequate early treatment, many children develop chronic renal failure due to renal dysplasia (Tejani *et al.* 1986; Parkhouse *et al.* 1988). The prognosis is better in patients with unilateral or no reflux than in those with high-grade bilateral reflux (Johnston 1979). Recently, a better prognosis has been attributed to the combination of posterior urethral valves and large congenital bladder diverticula, and to urinary extravasation with or without urinary ascites (Rittenberg *et al.* 1988). In these cases, the transmission of high pressure to the functioning nephrons is partially prevented (Fig. 8). Renal transplantation is successful in those children with endstage renal disease, although abnormal bladder function may affect graft survival (Reinberg *et al.* 1988). However, a valve bladder *per se* does not affect outcome of renal transplantation (Groenewegen *et al.* 1993; Rajagopalan *et al.* 1994). Bladder dysfunction is an important consequence of posterior urethral valve disease (Peters *et al.* 1990).

Antenatal surgery in fetal obstructive uropathy is still experimental and definite indications for vesicoamniotic shunting have not yet been developed. It may be beneficial in exceptional cases, since complications have been frequent, and the results of neonatal surgical relief are good (Elder *et al.* 1987; Evans *et al.* 1989; Thomas 1990; Quintero *et al.* 1995).

The neurogenic bladder

The most common type of neurogenic bladder in childhood is that associated with meningomyelocele. There is no good correlation between the level of meningomyelocele and the type of neurogenic bladder that develops. In general, the children are born with a normal upper urinary tract. The aim of management is to avoid impairment of renal function due to vesicoureteric reflux, obstruction, increased back pressure, and pyelonephritis. Constant surveillance of kidney function is therefore required. Furthermore, it is important to preserve bladder capacity and to allow bladder growth.

Children with bladder decompensation are at high risk of developing obstructive lesions of the kidney, whether the antagonist activity of the sphincter is markedly increased or the detrusor contractility is reduced. Ultrasonic examination of the kidney and the bladder is very useful in the examination of children with neurogenic bladder. Besides micturating cystourethrography, cystomanometry (urodynamics) is essential in infancy. If vesicoureteric reflux is present, increased intravesical pressure is directly transmitted to the kidneys and, in combination with acute pyelonephritis, may destroy kidney parenchyma. The ultimate therapeutic aim is complete bladder emptying. Ultrasound is helpful in demonstrating a distended bladder and assessing residual volume. Complete bladder emptying with no residual urine can only be guaranteed if normal bladder outflow resistance can be achieved. Pharmacological intervention by α-adrenoceptor blockade with phenoxybenzamine is not sufficient and intermittent catheterization (Joseph *et al.* 1989), often in combination with anticholinergic drugs (oxybutynin 0.4–0.6 mg/kg orally) is the method of choice (Goessl *et al.* 1998; van Gool *et al.* 2001). Oxybutynin is also effective when administered intravesically (Haverkamp *et al.* 2001). In selected cases cutaneous vesicostomy can be performed.

Antireflux surgery is not indicated as long as increased intravesical pressure and outflow obstruction persist, since the thickened bladder wall contributes to a high complication rate, with persistence of reflux or obstruction at the ureterovesical level. Antireflux surgery can be performed in patients with normal bladder wall thickness and intravesical pressure without an increased incidence of complications. In patients without residual urine and with normal intravesical pressure, there is no increased risk for the upper urinary tract and the kidneys: urine incontinence is the major problem in these patients (Borzyskowski and Mundy 1988).

Tethered cord syndrome

Compared to children with meningomyelocele, disturbances of ascension of the spinal cord relative to the vertebral column is seldom the cause of a neurogenic bladder. In these patients, the conus medullaris is deep and fixed in the lumbar channel, sometimes associated with lipomeningocele.

Newborns often present with characteristic skin lesions in the lumbosacral region (dermal sinus, haemangioma, hypertrichosis) (Albright *et al.* 1989). During development these children develop progressive neurological disturbances with bladder dysfunction, scoliosis, and foot deformities.

In the first month of life, the spinal cord can be evaluated sonographically, since ossification of the vertebrae is not complete. However, even at this age and in later life, magnetic resonance tomography is the method of choice (Hall *et al.* 1988). Detachment of the caudal spinal cord from adhesions is the most important aim of surgery, particularly if pain or neurological disturbances exist or progress.

Prune-belly syndrome

Absence of the abdominal musculature, urinary tract dilatation, and bilateral undescended testes is known as prune-belly syndrome (Eagle and Barrett 1950; Greskovich and Nyberg 1988; Rascher *et al.* 2001) (Fig. 10).

There is a broad spectrum of malformations, with severe dilatation of the urinary tract as a consequence of aplasia of the musculature. The pathogenic mechanism is completely different from that of dilatation as consequence of supra- or infravesical obstruction. Some patients with prune-belly syndrome have a real obstruction, such as urethral aplasia with oligohydramnios syndrome. The prognosis of the malformations depends upon the degree of renal dysplasia (Duckett and Snow 1986; Rascher *et al.* 2001).

Treatment of prune-belly syndrome is primarily conservative and surgical management is seldom required. Since massive bladder distension and megaureter often promote urinary tract infection, antibiotic prophylaxis is often logical and highly effective. Conservative management is more efficient than extensive and aggressive surgical approach such as urinary diversion or ureteric remodelling (Duckett and Snow 1986; Burbige *et al.* 1987). Current practice is to correct the cryptorchism surgically.

Duplication of the urinary tract

Embryological aspects

Anomalies of the ureter and its orifice are best explained by disturbances of embryological development. The pathological states of the ureter are best understood as anomalies of origin or division of the

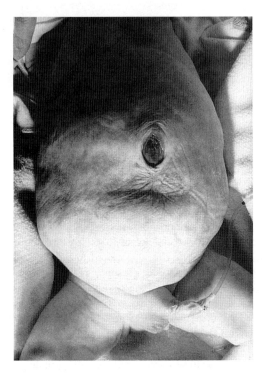

Fig. 10 Clinical appearance of the syndrome of absence of the abdominal musculature, urinary tract dilatation, and bilateral undescended testes (prune-belly syndrome).

ureteric bud. If the ureteric bud bifurcates after its origin, but arises at a normal site, an incomplete ureteral duplication with a Y-ureter will develop. Complete ureteral duplication occurs if there are two ureteric buds, one in the normal location and the other in a low position. The normal bud ends in a normal site on the trigone in the bladder and is normally non-refluxing. The lower bud, representing the ureter of the lower pole of the kidney ends as a lateral orifice and a short submucosal tunnel. The lower-pole ureter is, therefore, often associated with vesicoureteric reflux. If there are two ureteral buds, one with a normal location and one with a high position, the second ureter is incorporated into the developing bladder, ending more distally and medial to the normal one. Thus, this upper-pole ureter ends ectopically.

Ureteroceles, which are cystic dilatations of the terminal segments of the ureter, are caused by maldevelopment of the caudal ureter. Abnormal persistence of a two-cell ureteral membrane, or a delay of the establishment of the lumen of the ureteric bud with that of the mesonephric duct, has also been postulated as a mechanism (Tanagho 1976; Snyder 1987). It has long been recognized that ectopic ureters and those with ureteroceles frequently drain the upper pole and are often associated with dysplastic or non-functional renal tissue: this may be related to an anomalous origin of the ureteric bud from the mesonephric duct (Mackie and Stephens 1975). These authors suggest that the central zone of the metanephric blastema reaching a ureteric bud, arising from a normal location of the mesonephric duct, has a greater potential for normal renal development than a ureteric bud arising above or below this central zone, which is associated with a major risk that dysplasia or hypoplasia will develop.

Ureteral duplication

Duplication of the ureter and the renal pelvis is a common anomaly with an incidence of approximately 0.8 per cent (Snyder 1987); unilateral duplication is six times more frequent than bilateral. If duplication has been detected in a patient, the likelihood of another sibling with duplication rises to one in eight (Atwell *et al.* 1974). However, ureteral duplication is often an incidental finding not associated with a pathological state. Children with ureteral duplication often have vesicoureteric reflux (Privett *et al.* 1976). The spontaneous disappearance of reflux is less common in duplicate ureters than in patients with a single ureter.

Ureterocele

Ureteroceles are often associated with an upper-pole ureter of the kidney with complete ureteral duplication. The ureterocele may vary in size and very large ones may fill nearly the entire bladder (Fig. 11).

When ureteroceles are associated with obstruction, megaureter, and hydronephrosis, mostly of the upper pole, they can be identified prenatally by ultrasonography. Otherwise, the common presentation of a child with a ureterocele is urinary tract infection. Diagnosis of ureteroceles can be made by ultrasonography or by intravenous urography.

Treatment consists of transurethral incision of the ureterocele (Jayanthi and Koff 1999). In case of vesicoureteric reflux reimplantation of the ureter may be indicated. In 80–95 per cent of intravesical ureteroceles only transureteral incision is a sufficient treatment on long-term range, whereas in ectopic ureteroceles 65–100 per cent of the ureters require reconstruction (upper-pole resection with ureterectomy, reimplantation of the ureter, or pelvic floor reconstruction).

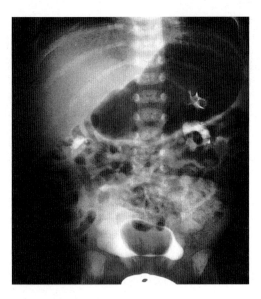

Fig. 11 Huge ureterocele in a 3-week-old boy with bilateral duplication of renal pelvis and ureters. Ultrasonography revealed hydronephrosis of the upper pole and megaureter of the corresponding ureter.

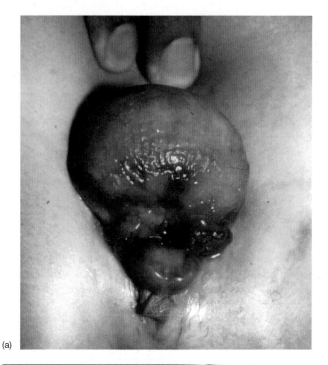

(a)

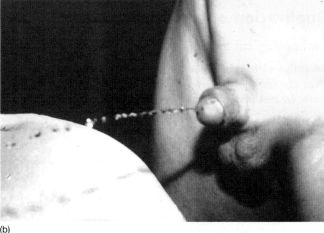

(b)

Fig. 12 Clinical presentation of a newborn boy with bladder exstrophy and epispadias: (a) prior to and (b) after corrective surgery.

Ectopic ureters

An ectopic ureter does not open at the normal site at the corner of the trigone. Ectopic ureters are five times more common in females than in boys. In females, more than 80 per cent of the ectopic ureters belong to the upper pole of a duplex system. In males an ectopic ureter drains a single system more frequently (Cooper and Snyder 2001). Mildly ectopic ureters do not cause any symptoms or problems. Extravesical ectopic ureters, which can cause urinary incontinence in girls, are of clinical importance. If the ectopic ureter drains distally to the sphincter, there is a history of continuous dripping incontinence in combination with an otherwise normal voiding pattern (Malek *et al.* 1972; Gill 1980). Besides intensive examination to demonstrate a duplex system, commonly associated with very poor function of the upper pole, determination of urine osmolality from normally voided urine (high urine osmolality during antidiuresis) and osmolality in the dribbling urine (low osmolality during antidiuresis) is helpful for establishing the diagnosis.

Sometimes the ectopic ureter can be identified retrovesically as a megaureter by ultrasonography. Treatment consists of upper-pole resection, or, if there is salvageable renal parenchyma, implantation of the aberrant ureter into the contralateral ureter or bladder.

In boys, the extravesical ectopic ureter does not open distally to the external sphincter and does not cause dribbling incontinence, but the ectopic ureter may induce epididymitis, when it opens into the seminal vesicle.

The bladder exstrophy–epispadias complex

Exstrophy of the bladder is part of a spectrum of conditions resulting from abnormal development of the cloacal membrane. There are basically three types of syndrome: (a) classical bladder exstrophy, (b) cloacal exstrophy, and (c) penile epispadias.

Because the entire exstrophy group represents a spectrum of anomalies, it is not surprising that transitions between these types have been reported. All of these abnormalities are rare. Bladder exstrophy occurs between one out of 10,000 and one of 30,000 live births, epispadias in one of 1,20,000 births and cloacal exstrophy only in one of 200,000–4,00,000 births. Classical bladder exstrophy is always associated with epispadias (Fig. 12) and severe musculoskeletal defects caused by a widened pubic symphysis. Basically two approaches of management have evolved: (a) cystectomy and permanent urinary diversion, either external, internal, or combined (Stein *et al.* 1999); (b) anatomic reconstruction. This may be by planned single (Schrott 1995, 2001; Grady and Mitchell 1999) or multiple stages (Gearhart 2001) including closure of the bladder, posterior urethra, and abdominal wall with or without pelvic osteotomy, epispadias repair, and bladder neck reconstruction.

Today most centres in the world are emphasizing anatomical reconstruction. At the Department of Urology University of Erlangen-Nuremberg we have successfully used single stage procedure in more than 120 primary cases since 1983. While all of these approaches have merit and supporters, the quality and size of the bladder template, appropriate patient selection, and experience of the surgeon and supporting staff will ultimately determine the outcome in a particular child.

Syndromes with a renal component

Renal abnormalities occur in a large number of malformation syndromes (Gilli *et al.* 1987; Clarren 1994). Although primarily of interest to paediatric nephrologists and geneticists, these syndromes are increasingly a matter of concern for 'adult' nephrologists: improved management in childhood, as in the prune-belly syndrome, prolongs survival into adult life and hence into the care of the adult team; knowledge of the full range of problems of a condition such as Lawrence–Moon–Biedl syndrome has a bearing on the strategy of management of endstage renal failure in such patients; an awareness of the range of malformation syndromes facilitates the diagnosis of the renal disorder in those conditions, such as the branchio-oto-renal syndrome, in which the extrarenal manifestations may be more subtle; and recognition of a syndrome may have implications for genetic counselling.

Congenital renal abnormalities may occur in multisystem disorders such as chromosomal abnormalities, teratogenic embryopathies, and generalized tissue dysplasias. They may be determined by single gene effects, by the consequence of an ill-defined polygenic effect, or not be genetically determined at all.

Renal anomalies may entrain further abnormalities: the Potter sequence in which renal agenesis is associated with oligohydramnios, pulmonary hypoplasia, abnormal facies, crumpled ears, talipes equinovarus, and congenital dislocation of the hips; and the prune-belly syndrome in which a transient urethral obstruction of prostatic hypoplasia causes megacystis–megaureter, renal dysplasia, absent abdominal wall musculature, and cryptorchidism.

The classic reference list for syndromes of congenital disorders is Jones (1988), and for genetically determined disorders in general is the McKusick catalogue (McKusick 1994). Several recent texts are available on the genetics of renal and urinary tract disorders (Barakat *et al.* 1986; Crawford 1988; Spitzer and Avner 1989; Clarren 1994). Gilli lists 282 syndromes with a renal component (Gilli *et al.* 1987), and Tables 5–10 list the most important inheritable multisystem disorders with renal involvement (Gilbert-Barness *et al.* 1989).

Table 5 Autosomal dominant mutations

Condition	Abnormalities of kidney and urinary tract	Associated abnormalities
Bilateral renal agenesis, unilateral renal agenesis, hereditary renal dysplasia	Unilateral agenesis with contralateral hypoplasia, or dysplasia, bilateral renal agenesis	None
Familial hydronephrosis	Unilateral or bilateral hydronephrosis with or without pelviureteric junction obstruction, contralateral renal agenesis	None
Tuberous sclerosis	Polycystic kidney disease, renal angiomyolipomas	Epilepsy, mental retardation, hamartomas, skin lesions, angiofibromas, intraventricular calcifications
von Hippel–Lindau disease	Cystic kidneys, cytoadenomas of epididymis, renal carcinoma, pancreatic cysts	Angiomatous lesions of retina and brain; pancreatic cysts
Peutz–Jegher's syndrome	Polycystic kidney disease	Intestinal polyposis, mucosal pigmentation
Alagille syndrome (arteriohepatic dysplasia)	Marked arterionephrosclerosis with diffuse calcinosis, single kidney, small kidneys, and renal artery	Distinctive phenotype, vertebral anomalies (butterfly vertebrae), peripheral pulmonary stenosis, mental and growth retardation, neonatal cholestasis
Nail-patella (hereditary onychoosteodysplasia) syndrome	Thickening of glomerular basement membranes, mesangial hypercellularity, glomerular sclerosis with tubular atrophy and interstitial fibrosis, segmental sclerosis, cortical atrophy and chronic nephritis, focal deposits of IgM and/or complement. Collagen fibres within basement membrane of glomeruli, collagen fibres in mesangium	Onychodysplasia, fingers and toes, small or absent patellae, iliac spurs, iris heterochromia, malformation of radius
Branchio-oto-renal syndrome	Sharply tapered superior poles and blunting of calyces, hypoplasia	Preauricular pits, branchial fistulas, hearing loss

(Continued)

Table 5 Continued

Condition	Abnormalities of kidney and urinary tract	Associated abnormalities
Opitz–Frias syndrome (G or dysplasia hypospadias syndrome)	Duplication of renal pelvis and ureters, vesicoureteric reflux, hypospadias	Deglutition difficulty, stridorous respiration, weak, hoarse cry, hypertelorism, abnormalities of laryngotracheobronchial tree
Townes–Brocks syndrome (thumb, auricular, anal, and renal anomalies)	Renal hypoplasia, vesicoureteric reflux, and posterior urethral valves	Thumb, auricular, and anal anomalies, congenital heart defects, anomalies in external organs
Myotonic dystrophy and polycystic kidney disease	Polycystic kidney disease	Cleft lip and palate, congenital heart defect, deafness, epilepsy, malformations, limb neurofibromatosis, eye defects
Ectodactyly–ectodermal dysplasia–cleft syndrome	Unilateral renal agenesis	Cleft-like palate, ectodermal dysplasia, deafness, small malformed ears
Ochoa syndrome	Hydronephrosis and hydroureter, intravesical stenosis of ureter, abnormal calibre of the urethra, urethral valves	Peculiar facies and gestures while smiling and crying
Brachmann–de Lange syndrome[a]	Hypoplastic, cystic, and dysplastic kidneys, hypospadias	Shortness of stature, mental retardation, microbrachiocephaly, bushy eyebrows and synophys, hirsutism, phocomelia, cardiac and gastrointestinal defects
Familial amyloid nephropathy (Andrade syndrome with polyneuropathy; Van Allen syndrome with neuropathy and peptic ulcer)	Amyloid nephropathy, vascular renal atrophy due to renal amyloidosis	Neuropathy involving lower limbs, peptic ulcer

[a] Familial occurrence, but autosomal dominant in some cases seems likely. Empiric recurrence risk low.

Reproduced with minor modifications from Gilbert-Barness et al. (1989) with permission from Kluwer Academic Publishers and the authors.

Table 6 Autosomal recessive mutations

Condition	Abnormalities of kidney and urinary tract	Associated abnormalities
Meckel syndrome	Polycystic kidneys with occasional gigantic renal enlargement, vascular anomalies, hydronephrosis, cystic dysplastic kidneys and portal fibrosis, agenesis, atresia of ureters, duplication of ureters, horseshoe kidney	Polydactyly, occipital encephalocele, CNS malformations, ocular anomalies, cleft palate, congenital heart defects, cysts of liver and pancreas
Goldston syndrome (facio-auriculovertebral syndrome)	Cystic dysplasia	Defects of vermis of cerebellum, Dandy–Walker anomaly
Miranda syndrome	Cystic dysplasia with dysplasia of liver	Severe malformations of CNS, intrahepatic fibromuscular proliferation
Smith–Lemli–Opitz syndrome	Cystic dysplasia, malformation of renal artery, unilateral renal hypoplasia, nephrosclerosis, polycystic renal disease, hypospadias, perineal urethral opening, cleft of scrotum, cryptorchidism	Mental retardation, microcephaly, hypotonia, incomplete development of external genitalia, minor anomalies of face, hands, and feet
Lissencephaly type II	Unilateral agenesis, cystic kidneys, micromulticystic kidneys	Obstructive hydrocephalus agyria and CNS abnormalities, Dandy–Walker malformation

(Continued)

Table 6 Continued

Condition	Abnormalities of kidney and urinary tract	Associated abnormalities
Bardet–Biedl syndrome	Tubulointerstitial nephropathy with medullary cystic disease, occasional glomerular sclerosis, occasional cystic disease, dysplasia, caliectasis, renal failure	Tapetoretinal degeneration, obesity, mental retardation, hypogenitalism, polydactyly, syndactyly, anal atresia, anomalies of skull, congenital heart defects, deafness
Cockayne syndrome	Glomerular sclerosis, tubular atrophy, interstitial fibrosis, immune deposits, nephrotic syndrome	Microcephaly, senile-like changes, retinal degeneration, hearing defect, photosensitivity
Drash syndrome	Nephropathy (rapidly progressive glomerulonephritis and malignant nephrosclerosis), diffuse mesangial sclerosis, Wilms' tumour	Ambiguous genitalia, pseudohermaphroditism, streak gonads, gonadoblastoma
Johanson–Blizzard syndrome	Caliectasia, hydronephrosis, and single urogenital orifice	Aplasia nasal alae, hypothyroidism, dwarfism, mental retardation, midline scalp defect, absent permanent teeth
Roberts syndrome	Horseshoe kidney and ureteral and single urogenital orifice	Phocomelia-like limb deficiency, growth retardation, eye anomalies, haemangiomas, hypoplastic nasal cartilages
Winter syndrome (renal, genital, and middle-ear anomalies)	Unilateral agenesis or hypoplasia, bilateral agenesis	Middle-ear anomalies, internal genital malformations
TAR syndrome (radial aplasia-thrombocytopenia)	Unilateral renal agenesis, hypospadias, and transposition of penis and scrotum	Thrombocytopenia, leukaemoid granulocytosis, anaemia, limb defects, congenital heart defects
Hydrocephalus syndrome	Unilateral renal agenesis, hypoplasia of left kidney, cysts	Hydrocephalus, micrognathia, polydactyly, abnormal lobation of lungs, microphthalmia, cleft lip/palate, facial anomalies
Fryns syndrome	Kidney cysts	Facial and CNS anomalies, pulmonary hypoplasia, distal limb anomalies, cleft palate, diaphragmatic hernia
Oro-facial-digital syndrome type I	Polycystic kidneys and liver	Webbing between buccal mucous membrane and alveolar ridge, partial clefts in the mid-upper lip, tongue, and alveolar ridges, dental abnormalities, hypoplasia of alar cartilages, asymmetric shortening of digits with clinodactyly, syndactyly, dry scalp, and variable mental deficiency
Senior–Løken syndrome	Nephronophthisis	Tapetoretinal degeneration
Familial Mediterranean fever	Renal amyloidosis	Recurrent fever
Osteochondrodysplasia		
Asphyxiating thoracic dystrophy	Tubulointerstitial nephropathy with tubular dysfunction and progressive renal insufficiency in children surviving infancy; occasional dysplasia and diffuse cystic disease in newborns; frequent biliary dysgenesis	Contracted thorax, short limbs, biliary dysgenesis, portal fibrosis
Short-rib polydactyly syndrome type I (Saldino–Noonan type)	Cystic dysplasia, hypoplasia of ureters	Dwarfism, thoracic dystrophy, polydactyly, short limbs

(Continued)

Table 6 Continued

Condition	Abnormalities of kidney and urinary tract	Associated abnormalities
Short-rib polydactyly syndrome type II (Majewski type)	Cystic dysplasia	Dwarfism, polydactyly, syndactyly, cleft lip/palate, narrow throax
Elejalde syndrome (acrocephalo-polydactylous dysplasia)	Severe bilateral cystic dysplasia	Gigantism, polydactyly, acrocephaly, excessive connective tissue (subcutaneous and visceral)
Peroxisomal disorders		
Zellweger (cerebro–hepatorenal) syndrome	Focal cortical, glomerular, and tubular cysts, cystic dysplasia, altered metanephric duct remnants, persistent fetal lobulations, horseshoe kidney, urethral duplication	Growth retardation, characteristic facial appearance, hypotonia, congenital heart defects, hepatic siderosis, cirrhosis, and CNS abnormalities
Hyperpipecolic acidaemia	Renal tubular ectasia	Growth retardation, hypotonia, hepatomegaly, cirrhosis with glycogen storage, CNS abnormalities (protein and cerebellar demyelination)
Glutaric acidaemia type II	Bilateral cystic kidneys, cystic dysplasia	'Sweaty feet' odour, CNS abnormalities, retinal bile duct hypoplasia, cholestasis
Neonatally lethal adrenoleucodystrophy	Renal microcysts	CNS and adrenal abnormalities, retinal pigmentary degeneration anomalies
Chondrodysplasia calcificans punctata, rhizomelic type	Micromulticystic kidneys with small glomerular and tubular cysts	Symmetrical shortness of the humeri and femora, punctate epiphyseal calcifications, metaphyseal abnormalities, severe psychomotor retardation, microcephaly, cataracts

Reproduced with minor modifications from Gilbert-Barness *et al.* (1989) with permission from Kluwer Academic Publishers and the authors.

Table 7 X-linked recessive mutations

Condition	Abnormalities of kidney and urinary tract	Associated abnormalities
Oculo-cerebro-renal syndrome (Lowe)	Renal tubular defect mainly of the proximal tubule (Fanconi syndrome)	Metal retardation, glaucoma, cataracts, hypoplastio–dysplastic kidneys
Orofacial digital syndrome	Diffuse cystic disease, sometimes glomerulocystic disease	Webbing between buccal mucosa and alveolar ridge, clefts of lip, teeth anomalies, asymmetric short digits, hypoplasia of alar cartilages
Swyer syndrome (46, XY gonadal dysgenesis)	Glomerulosclerosis with tubular atrophy and interstitial fibrosis	Gonadal dysgenesis, dysgenetic gonads, gonadoblastoma
Daentl syndrome	Duplication of left renal artery, disparity in size of kidneys, persistent fetal lobulations, lipid-laden cells in glomeruli, progressive focal glomerulosclerosis, nephrotic syndrome	Hydrocephalus, thin skin, blue sclerae, growth retardation, abnormal T-lymphocyte function
Goeminne syndrome (congenital muscular torticollis, multiple keloids, cryptorchidism, and renal dysplasia)	Renal dysplasia, chronic pyelonephritis with hypertension	Torticollis, multiple keloids, cryptorchidism, seminiferous tubule failure, multiple cutaneous naevi, varicose veins
Kallmann syndrome (congenital anosmia, hypogonadism, and unilateral renal agenesis)[a]	Unilateral renal agenesis	Congenital anosmia, hypogonadism, cryptorchidism

[a] Some cases may be autosomal dominant with variable expression or autosomal recessive genetic heterogeneity is likely.

Reproduced with minor modifications from Gilbert-Barness *et al.* (1989) with permission from Kluwer Academic Publishers and the authors.

Table 8 Usually sporadic mutations

Condition	Abnormalities of kidney and urinary tract	Associated abnormalities
Goldenhar complex (facio-auriculo-vertebral syndrome)	Pelvic deformity, anomalous renal artery, unilateral cystic dysplasia, duplication	Microtia, preauricular tags, deafness, vertebral anomalies
Klippel–Trenaunay–Weber dysplasia (angio-osteohypertrophy)	Diffuse bilateral nephroblastomatosis	Unilateral limb hypertrophy, cutaneous haemangiomas, varicose veins, osseus and soft tissue hypertrophy, thrombocytopenia, visceral angiomatosis
Wiedemann–Beckwith syndrome[a]	Enlarged kidneys, persistent glomerulogenesis, diffuse bilateral nephroblastomastosis, metanephric hamartomas, hydronephrosis and hydroureters, Wilms' tumour, duplication of collecting system, dysmorphogenetic kidneys, disorganized renal parenchyma with fissures and abnormal lobulations, corticomedullary disarray, sponge kidney	Macrosomia, macroglossia, hypoglycaemia, omphalocele
Williams syndrome	Renal artery stenosis, degenerative renal disease, small penis	Mental retardation, supravalvular aortic stenosis, partial anodontia
Rubinstein–Taybi syndrome	Duplication of kidneys and ureter, absence of kidney, hydronephrosis, abnormality of bladder shape, bladder diverticulum, posterior urethral valves	Mental and motor retardation, broad terminal phalanges of thumbs and great toes, short stature, characteristic facial appearance
Russell–Silver syndrome	Bilateral chronic pyelonephritis, urethral pelvic obstruction with severe reflux	Short stature, hemihypertrophy, elevated urinary gonadotrophins, craniofacial dysostosis
Urinary obstruction sequences[b] (genetics depends on aetiology)	Obstructive lesions	Oligohydramnios, Potter phenotype, pulmonary hypoplasia
Prune-belly sequence[c] and related defects	Developmental dysplasia of smooth muscle of urinary tract, hydroureters and hydronephrosis, urethral or bladder neck obstruction, renal dysplasia, megalourethra, megacystis, megaureters	Dysplasia of the abdominal muscle
Associations		
VATER association and variants	Renal dysplasia or agenesis, persistent urachus, renal ectopia, hypospadias, caudally displaced dysplastic penis, vesicoureteric reflux, pelviureteric junction obstruction, cross-fused ectopia	Vertebral and cardiac anomalies, tracheo-oesophageal fistula, anal stenosis, radial dysplasia
MURCS association	Renal agenesis or ectopy, absence of both kidneys, ureters and renal arteries, renal aplasia	Vertebral defects, absent vagina and uterus
CHARGE association	Duplicated upper pole of one kidney, hydronephrosis, unilateral renal agenesis	Coloboma, choanal atresia, cardiac, genital, and ear defects
Schisis association	Defects of urinary tract, renal agenesis	Neural tube defects, oral clefts, omphalocele, diaphragmatic hernia, cardiac defects, limb deficiencies

[a] Usually sporadic: familial cases, delayed mutation of an unstable premutated autosomal dominant gene.

[b] Familial occurrence of posterior urethral valves has been reported.

[c] Inheritance unknown: unstable autosomal dominant or X-linked premutation.

Reproduced with minor modifications from Gilbert-Barness et al. (1989) with permission from Kluwer Academic Publishers and the authors.

Table 9 Teratogenic abnormalities

Condition	Abnormalities of kidney and urinary tract	Associated abnormalities
Fetal alcohol syndrome	Small rotated kidneys, hydronephrosis. Unilateral renal agenesis	Prenatal and postnatal growth retardation, microcephaly, short palpebral fissures, typical phenotype, limb defects, congenital cardiac defects
Diabetic embryopathy	Renal agenesis and renal dysplasia	Brain, heart, and skeletal anomalies, caudal regression syndrome
Warfarin embryopathy	Unilateral renal agenesis, abnormal urinary tract	Nasal hypoplasia, stippled epiphyses, CNS and eye abnormalities
Thalidomide embryopathy	Renal agenesis, hypoplasia, hydronephrosis, horseshoe kidney, cystic dysplasia, renal ectopia, anomalies of rotation	Limb deficiency—phocomelia, heart, intestinal eye and ear anomalies, genitourinary anomalies

Reproduced with minor modifications from Gilbert-Barness et al. (1989) with permission from Kluwer Academic Publishers and the authors.

Table 10 Chromosomal abnormalities[a]

Condition	Abnormalities of kidney and urinary tract
Autosomal	
Trisomy 21—Down syndrome	Renal dysplasia, nodular renal blastema, persistent fetal lobulation, retardation of maturation of the nephrogenic zone of cortex, haemangiomata, stricture of the pelviureteric junction, hydronephrosis, focal cystic malformation of collecting tubules, immature glomeruli
Trisomy 18 syndrome (Edwards)	Cystic dysplasia, horseshoe kidneys, ureteral duplication, renal duplication, renal agenesis, renal ectopy, renal glomerulosclerosis and cystic tubules, persistent metanephric blastema, micromulticystic kidneys, retention of fetal lobulation, Wilms' tumour
Trisomy 13 syndrome (Patau)	Duplication of kidneys and ureters, unilateral renal agenesis, stenosis of prostatic urethra, excessive renal arteries and veins, excessive fetal lobulations, cystic dysplasia, segmental cystic dysplasia, cystic dilatation of collecting system, hydronephrosis, pelviureteric junction atresia, Wilms' tumour
Trisomy 8 syndrome	Obstructive uropathy with hydronephrosis, posterior urethral valves with hydroureters and hydronephrosis, horseshoe kidney
Trisomy 9 syndrome	Bilateral cystic dysplastic kidneys, atresia of proximal ureters, rudimentary atretic urinary bladder, microcysts of kidneys, double ureters, bladder diverticulum
Triploidy	Micromulticystic kidneys, hypoplasia, hydronephrosis, cryptorchidism, hypospadias, labia majora-like structures
Deletions	
5p [del(5p)] syndrome	Unilateral renal agenesis and other abnormalities
11p [del(11p)] syndrome	Wilms' tumour, sometimes bilateral, disorganization of renal parenchyma, medullary origin of Wilms' tumour, aniridia
Sex chromosome abnormalities	
45,X (Ullrich–Turner) syndrome	Horseshoe kidneys, double or clubbed renal pelvis, hypoplasia, hydronephrosis, bifid ureters, duplication of kidneys and/or ureters, unilateral renal agenesis, malrotation
47,XYY syndrome	Microcysts of kidneys, thin ureters, small bladder, cystic dysplastic kidneys
47,XXY, 48,XXXY, and 49,XXXXY (Kleinfelter syndromes)	Cryptorchidism, small testes, and hypoplastic scrotum in males. No renal parenchymal abnormalities, hydronephrosis, hydroureter, and ureterocele
Chromosome abnormalities in renal-cell carcinoma	Abnormal calyceal collecting system, unilateral aplasia, cystic kidneys, renal dysplasia

[a] Associated malformations in these disorders include multiple congenital anomalies, minor anomalies, mild malformations, and frequently a typical phenotype.

Reproduced with minor modifications from Gilbert-Barness et al. (1989) with permission from Kluwer Academic Publishers and the authors.

References

Abramovich, D. R. The volume of amniotic fluid and its regulating factors. In *Amniotic Fluid: Research and Clinical Application* (ed. D. Fairweather and T. Eshes), pp. 31–49. Amsterdam: Excerpta Medica, 1978.

Abramow, M. and Dratwa, M. (1974). Effect of vasopressin on the isolated human collecting duct. *Nature* **250**, 492–493.

Albright, A. L., Gartner, J. C., and Wiener, E. S. (1989). Lumbar cutaneous hemangiomas as indicators of tethered spinal cords. *Pediatrics* **83**, 977–980.

Aperia, A., Broberger, O., Thodenius, U., and Zetterström, R. (1975). Development of renal control of salt and fluid homeostasis during the first year of life. *Acta Paediatrica Scandinavica* **64**, 393–398.

Ashley, D. J. B. and Mostofi, F. K. (1960). Renal agenesis and dysgenesis. *Journal of Urology* **83**, 211–230.

Aslan, A. R., Kogan, B. A., and Mandell, J. (1998). Neonatal hydronephrosis. *Current Opinion in Urology* **8**, 495–500.

Atiyeh, B., Husmann, D., and Baum, M. (1992). Contralateral renal abnormalities in multicystic–dysplastic kidney disease. *Journal of Pediatrics* **121**, 65–67.

Atwell, J. D., Cook, P. L., Howell, C. J., Hyde, I., and Parker, B. C. (1974). Familial incidence of bifid and double ureters. *Archives of Disease in Childhood* **49**, 390–396.

Awazu, M., Barakat, A. Y., Chevalier, R. L., and Ichikawa, I. (1989). The cause of uremia in obstructed kidneys. *Journal of Pediatrics* **114**, 179–186.

Barac-Nieto, M. and Spitzer, A. (1988). The relationship between renal metabolism and proximal tubule transport during ontogeny. *Pediatric Nephrology* **2**, 356–367.

Barakat, A. Y., Der Kaloustian, V. M., Mufarrij, A. A., and Birbari, A. E. *The Kidney in Genetic Disease.* Edinburgh: Churchill Livingstone, 1986.

Batlle, D. C., Arruda, J. A. L., and Kurtzman, N. A. (1981). Hyperkalemic distal renal tubular acidosis associated with obstructive uropathy. *New England Journal of Medicine* **304**, 373–380.

Beetz, R., Bökenkamp, A., Brandis, M., Hoyer, P., John, U., Kemper, M. J., Kirschstein, M., Kuwertz-Bröcking, E., Misselwitz, J., Müller-Wiefel, D. E., and Rascher, W. (2002). Diagnostik bei konnatalen Dilatationen der Harnwege. *Monatsschrift für Kinderheilkunde* **150**, 76–84.

Bernstein, J. (1971). The morphogenesis of renal parenchymal maldevelopment (renal dysplasia). *Pediatric Clinics of North America* **18**, 395–407.

Bernstein, J. A classification of renal cysts. In *Cystic Disease of the Kidney* (ed. K. D. Gardner), pp. 7–30. New York: Wiley and Sons, 1976.

Borzyskowski, M. and Mundy, A. (1988). The management of the neuropathic bladder in childhood. *Pediatric Nephrology* **2**, 56–66.

Burbige, K. A., Amodio, J., Berdon, W. E., Hensle, T. W., Blanc, W., and Lattimer, J. K. (1987). Prune belly syndrome: 35 years of experience. *Journal of Urology* **137**, 86–90.

Carey, P. O. and Howards, S. J. (1988). Multicystic dysplastic kidneys and diagnostic confusion on renal scan. *Journal of Urology* **139**, 83–84.

Cass, A. S., Khan, A. U., Smith, S., and Godek, C. (1981). Neonatal perirenal urinary extravasation with posterior urethral valves. *Urology* **18**, 258–261.

Chevalier, R. L., Sturgill, B. C., Jones, C. E., and Kaiser, D. L. (1987). Morphologic correlates of renal growth arrest in neonatal partial ureteral obstruction. *Pediatric Research* **21**, 338–346.

Clarke, N. W., Gough, D. C. S., and Cohen, S. J. (1989). Neonatal urological ultrasound: diagnostic inaccuracies and pitfalls. *Archives of Disease in Childhood* **64**, 578–580.

Clarren, S. R. Malformation of the renal system. In *Pediatric Nephrology* 3rd edn. (ed. M. A. Holliday, T. M. Barratt, E. D. Avner, and B. A. Kogon), pp. 491–514. Baltimore: Williams and Wilkins, 1994.

Colodny, A. V. (1987). Antenatal diagnosis and management of urinary abnormalities. *Pediatric Clinics of North America* **34**, 1365–1381.

Cooper, C. S. and Snyder, H. M., III. Ureteral duplication, ectopy and ureteroceles. In *Pediatric Urology* (ed. J. P. Gearhardt, R. C. Rink, and P. D. E. Mouriquand), pp. 430–449. Philadelphia: Saunders Company, 2001.

Crawford, M. D'A. *The Genetics of Renal Tract Disorders.* Oxford: Oxford University Press, 1988.

Crombleholme, T. M., Harrison, M. R., Longaker, M. T., and Langer, J. C. (1988). Prenatal diagnosis and management of bilateral hydronephrosis. *Pediatric Nephrology* **2**, 334–342.

De Wolf, D., Keuppens, F., Temmerman, M., Verboven, M., Deneyer, M., Delree, M., and Sacre-Smits, L. (1989). Antenatal diagnosis of urological disorders by ultrasound: a critical review. *European Journal of Pediatrics* **149**, 62–64.

Duckett, J. W. and Snow, B. W. Prune-belly-syndrome. In *Kinderurologie in Klinik und Praxis* (ed. R. Hohenfellner, J. W. Thüroff, and H. Schulte-Wissermann), pp. 348–365. Stuttgart: Thième, 1986.

Eagle, J. F. and Barrett, G. S. (1950). Congenital deficiency of abdominal musculature with associated genitourinary abnormalities, a syndrome; reports of 9 cases. *Pediatrics* **6**, 721–736.

Elder, J. S., Duckett, J. W., Jr., and Snyder, H. M. (1987). Intervention of fetal obstructive uropathy: has it been effective? *Lancet* **ii**, 1007–1010.

Evans, M. I., Drugan, A., Manning, F. A., and Harrison, M. R. (1989). Fetal surgery in the 1990s. *American Journal of Disease in Childhood* **143**, 1431–1436.

Fawer, C. L., Torrado, A., and Guignard, J. P. (1979). Maturation of renal function in full-term and premature neonates. *Helvetica Paediatrica Acta* **34**, 11–21.

Feather, S., Woolf, A. S., Gordon, I., Risdon, R. A., Vernier-Jones, K., and Aysleen-Green, A. (1996). Vesicoureteric reflux: all in the genes? *Lancet* **348**, 725–728.

Feather, S. A., Malcolm, S., Woolf, A. S., Wright, V., Blaydon, D., Reid, C. J., Flinter, F. A., Proesmans, W., Devriendt, K., Carter, J., Warwicker, P., Goodship, T. H., and Goodship, J. A. (2000). Primary, nonsyndromic vesicoureteric reflux and its nephropathy is genetically heterogeneous, with a locus on chromosome 1. *American Journal of Human Genetics* **66**, 1420–1425.

Fetterman, G. H., Shaploch, N. A., Phillip, N. S., and Gregg, H. S. (1965). Glomerular development in the kidney as an index of maturity. *Pediatrics* **35**, 601–619.

Freedman, A. L., Bukowski, T. P., Smith, C. A., Evans, S. M., Gonzalez, R., and Johnson, M. P. (1997). Use of urinary beta-2-microgloblin to predict severe renal damage in fetal obstructive uropathy. *Fetal Diagnosis and Therapy* **12**, 1–6.

Gearhart, J. P. The bladder exstrophy-epispadias-cloacal exstrophy complex. In *Pediatric Urology* (ed. J. P. Gearhardt, R. C. Rink, and P. D. E. Mouriquand), pp. 511–546. Philadelphia: Saunders Company, 2001.

Gembruch, U. and Hansmann, M. (1988). Artificial instillation of amniotic fluid as a new technique for the diagnostic evaluation of cases of oligohydramnois. *Prenatal Diagnosis* **8**, 33–45.

Ghazali, S. and Barratt, T. M. (1974). Sodium excretion after relief of urinary tract obstruction in children. *British Journal of Urology* **46**, 163–167.

Gilbert-Barness, E. F., Opitz, J. M., and Barness, L. A. Heritable malformations of the kidney and urinary tract. In *Inheritance of Kidney and Urinary Tract Diseases* (ed. A. Spitzer and E. D. Avner). Boston: Kluwer Academic Publishers, 1989.

Gill, B. (1980). Ureteric ectopy in children. *British Journal of Urology* **52**, 257–263.

Gilli, G., Berry, G., and Berry, A. C. Syndromes with a renal component. In *Paediatric Nephrology* 2nd edn. (ed. M. A. Holliday, T. M. Barratt, and R. L. Vernier), pp. 384–404. Baltimore: Williams and Wilkins, 1987.

Goessl, C., Knipsel, H. H., Fiedler, U., Harle, B., Steffen-Wilke, K., and Miller, K. (1998). Urodynamic effects of oral oxybutinin chloride in children with meningomyelocele and detrusor hyperreflexia. *Urology* **51**, 94–98.

Gonzalez, R. and Sheldon, C. A. (1982). Septic obstruction and uremia in the newborn. *Urologic Clinics of North America* **9**, 297–303.

Gordon, A. C., Thomas, D. F. M., Arthur, R. J., and Irving, H. C. (1988). Multicystic dysplastic kidney: is nephrectomy still appropriate? *Journal of Urology* **140**, 1231–1234.

Grady, R. W. and Mitchell, M. E. (1999). Complete primary repair of exstrophy. *Journal of Urology* **162**, 1415–1420.

Greenfield, S. P., Hensle, T. W., Berdon, W. E., and Geringer, A. M. (1982). Urinary extravasation in the newborn male with posterior urethral valves. *Journal of Pediatric Surgery* **17**, 751–756.

Greskovich, F. J. and Nyberg, L. M. (1988). The prune belly syndrome: a review of its etiology, defects, treatment and prognosis. *Journal of Urology* **140**, 707–712.

Grignon, A. *et al.* (1986). Uretero-pelvic junction stenosis: antenatal ultrasonographic diagnosis, postnatal investigation and follow-up. *Radiology* **160**, 649–651.

Grisoni, I. R., Gauderer, M. W. I., Wolfson, R. N., and Izant, R. J. (1986). Antenatal ultrasonography: the experience in a high risk perinatal center. *Journal of Pediatric Surgery* **21**, 358–361.

Groenewegen, A. A., Sukhai, R. N., Nauta, J., Scholtmeyer, R. J., and Nijman R. J. (1993) Results of renal transplantation in boys treated for posterior urethral valves. *Journal of Urology* **149**, 1517–1520.

Grupe, W. E. (1987). The dilemma of intrauterine diagnosis of congenital renal disease. *Pediatric Clinics of North America* **34**, 629–638.

Guignard J. P. Neonatal nephrology. In *Pediatric Nephrology* 2nd edn. (ed. M. A. Holliday, T. M. Barratt, and R. L. Vernier), pp. 921–944. Baltimore: Williams and Wilkins, 1987.

Gunn, T. R., Mora, J. D., and Pease, P. (1988). Outcome after antenatal diagnosis of upper urinary tract dilatation by ultrasonography. *Archives of Disease in Childhood* 63, 1240–1243.

Hall, W. A., Albright, A. L., and Brunberg, I. A. (1988). Diagnosis of tethered cords by magnetic resonance imaging. *Surgical Neurology* 30, 60–64.

Haverkamp, A., Staehler, G., Gerner, H. J., and Dorsam, J. (2001). Dosage escalation of intravesical oxybutinin in the treatment of neurogenic bladder patients. *Spinal Cord* 38, 250–254.

Heijden, A. J. V. D., Versteegh, F. G. A., Wolff, E. D., Sukkai, R. N., and Scholtmeijer, R. J. (1985). Acute tubular dysfunction in infants with obstructive uropathy. *Acta Paediatrica Scandinavica* 74, 589–594.

Helin, I. and Persson, P. (1986). Prenatal diagnosis of urinary tract abnormalities by ultrasound. *Pediatrics* 78, 879–883.

Henneberry, M. D. and Stephens, F. D. (1980). Renal hypoplasia and dysplasia in infants with posterior urethral valves. *Journal of Urology* 123, 912–915.

Hohenfellner, K., Hunley, T. E., Schloemer, C., Brenner, W., Yerkes, E., Zepp, F., Brock, J. W., and Kon, V. (1999). Angiotensin type 2 receptor is important in the normal development of the ureter. *Pediatric Nephrology* 13, 187–191.

Homsy, Y. L., Saad, F., Laberge, I., Williot, P., and Pison, C. (1990). Transitorial hydronephrosis of the newborn and infant. *Journal of Urology* 144, 579–583.

Javadpour, N., Dellon, A. L., and Kumpe, D. A. (1974). Multilocular cystic disease in adults, imitators of renal cell carcinoma. *Urology* 1, 596–599.

Jayanthi, V. R. and Koff, S. A. (1999). Long-term outcome of transurethral puncture of ectopic ureteroceles: initial success and late problems. *Journal of Urology* 162, 1077–1080.

Johnson, C. E., Elder, J. S., Judge, N. E., Adeeb, F. N., Grisoni, E. R., and Fattlar, D. C. (1991). The accuracy of antenatal ultrasonography in identifying renal abnormalities. *American Journal of Diseases in Children* 146, 1181–1184.

Johnson, M. P., Corsi, P., Bradfield, W., Hume, R. F., Smith, C., Flake A. W., Qureshi, F., and Evans, M. I. (1995). Sequential urinalysis improves evaluation of fetal renal function in obstructive uropathy. *American Journal of Obstetrics and Gynecology* 173, 59–65.

Johnston, J. H. (1979). Vesico-ureteric reflux with urethral valves. *British Journal of Urology* 51, 100–104.

Jones, K. L. *Smith's Recognisable Patterns of Human Malformation* 4th edn. Philadelphia: W. B. Saunders, 1988.

Joseph, D. B., Bauer, S. B., Colodny, A. H., Mandell, J., and Retik, A. B. (1989). Clean, intermittent catheterization of infants with neurogenic bladder. *Pediatrics* 84, 78–82.

Kerr, W. S. (1956). Effects of complete ureteral obstruction in dogs on kidney function. *American Journal of Physiology* 184, 521–526.

King, L. R. (1980). Megaloureter: definition, diagnosis and management. *Journal of Urology* 123, 222–223.

Klahr, S., Harris, K., and Purkerson, M. L. (1988). Effects of obstruction on renal functions. *Pediatric Nephrology* 2, 34–42.

Koff, S. A. (1985). Pressure volume relationship in human hydronephrosis. *Urology* 25, 256–258.

Koff, S. A. (2000). Postnatal management of antenatal hydronephrosis using an observational approach. *Urology* 55, 609–611.

Koff, S. A. and Campbell, K. (1994). Nonoperative management of unilateral neonatal hydronephrosis: natural history of poorly functioning kidneys. *Journal of Urology* 152, 593–595.

Langman, J. *Medical Embryology* 2nd edn. Baltimore: Williams and Wilkins, 1969.

Lettgen, B., Kröpfl, D., Bonzel, K. E., Meyer-Schwickerath, M., and Rascher, W. (1993). Primary obstructed megaureter in neonates. Treatment by temporary uretero-cutaneostomy. *British Journal of Urology* 72, 826–829.

Lippe, B., Geffner, M. E., Dietrich, R. B., Boechat, M. I., and Kangarloo, H. (1988). Renal malformations in patients with Turner syndrome: imaging in 141 patients. *Pediatrics* 82, 852–856.

Lotgering, F. and Wallenburg, H. C. S. (1986). Mechanisms of production and clearance of amniotic fluid. *Seminars in Perinatology* 10, 94–102.

Liu, H. Y., Dhillon, H. K., Yeung, C. K., Diamond, D. A., Duffy, P. G., and Ransley, P. G. (1994). Clinical outcome and management of prenatally diagnosed primary megaureters. *Journal of Urology* 152, 614–617.

Mackie, G. G. and Stephens, F. D. (1975). Duplex kidneys: a correlation of renal dyslasia with position of the ureteral orifice. *Journal of Urology* 114, 274–280.

Malek, R. S., Kelalis, P. P., Stickler, G. B., and Burke, E. C. (1972). Observations on ureteral ectopy in children. *Journal of Urology* 107, 308–313.

Mandell, J., Peters, C. A., Estroff, J. A., and Benacerraf, B. R. (1992). Late onset severe oligohydramnios associated with genitourinary abnormalities. *Journal of Urology* 148, 515–518.

McKusick, V. A. *Mendelian Inheritance in Man* 11th edn. Baltimore: Johns Hopkins University Press, 1994.

Melzi, M. *et al.* (1995). Acute pyelonephritis as a cause of hyponatremia/hyperkalemia in young infants with urinary tract malformations. *Pediatric Infectious Diseases Journal* 14, 56–59.

Mentser, M., Mahan, J., and Koff, S. (1994). Multicystic dysplastic kidney. *Pediatric Nephrology* 8, 113–115.

Misra, D., Kempley, S. T., and Hird, M. F. (1999). Are patients with antenatally diagnosed hydronephrosis being over-investigated and overtreated? *European Journal of Pediatric Surgery* 9, 303–306.

Moore, T. R., Longo, J., Leopold, G. R., Casola, G., and Gosink, B. B. (1989). The reliability and predictive value of an amniotic fluid scoring system in severe second-trimester oligohydramnios. *Obstetrics and Gynecology* 73, 739–742.

Müller, U. and Brändli, A. W. (1999). Cell adhesion molecules and extracellular-matrix constituents in kidney development and diesease. *Journal of Cell Science* 112, 3855–3867.

Müller, F., Dommergues, M., Bussières, L., Lortat-Jacob, S., Loirat, C., Oury, J. F., Aigrain, Y., Niaudet, P., Aegerter, P., and Diumez, Y. (1996). Development of human renal function: reference intervals for 10 biochemical markers in fetal urine. *Clinical Chemistry* 42, 1855–1869.

Murnaghan, G. F. (1957). Experimental investigation of the dynamics of the normal and dilated ureter. *British Journal of Urology* 29, 403–409.

Najmaldin, A. S., Burge, D. M., and Atwell, J. D. (1991). Outcome of antenatally diagnosed pelviureteric junction hydronephrosis. *British Journal of Urology* 67, 96–99.

Nicolini, U., Fisk, N. M., Rodeck, C. H., and Beacham, J. (1992). Fetal urine biochemistry: an index of renal maturation and dysfunction. *British Journal of Obstetrics and Gynaecology* 99, 46–50.

Nishimura, H., Yerkes, E., Hohenfellner, K., Miyazaki, Y., Ma, J., Hunley, T. E., Yoshida, H., Ichiki, T., Threadgill, D., Phillips, J. A., III, Hogan, B. M., Fogo, A., Brock, J. W., III, Inagami, T., and Ichikawa, I. (1999). Role of angiotensin type 2 receptor gene in congenital anomalies of the kidney and urinary tract, CAKUT, of mice and man. *Molecular Cell* 3, 1–10.

O'Reilly, P. H. Introduction and general consideration. In *Obstructive Uropathy* (ed. P. H. O'Reilly), pp. 3–12. Berlin: Springer, 1986.

Parkhouse, H. F. and Barratt, T. M. (1988). Investigation of the dilated urinary tract. *Pediatric Nephrology* 2, 43–47.

Parkhouse, H. F., Barratt, T. M., Dillon, M. J., Duffy, P. G., Fay, J., Ransley, P. G., Woodhouse, C. R., and Williams, D. I. (1988). Long-term outcome of boys with posterior urethral valves. *British Journal of Urology* 62, 59–62.

Peipert, J. F. and Donnenfeld, A. E. (1991). Oligohydramnios: a review. *Obstetrical and Gynecological Surgery* 46, 325–339.

Peters, C. A., Bolkier, M., Bauer, S. B., Hendren, W. H., Colodny, A. H., Mandell, J., and Retik, A. B. (1990). The urodynamic consequences of posterior urethral valves. *Journal of Urology* 144, 122–126.

Peters, C. A., Mandell, J., Lebowitz, R. L., Colodny, A. H., Bauer, S. B., Hendren, W. H., and Retik, A. B. (1989). Congenital obstructed megaureters in early infancy: diagnosis and treatment. *Journal of Urology* 142, 641–645.

Potter, E. L. *Normal and Abnormal Development of the Kidney*. Chicago: Year Book, Medical Publishers, 1972.

Privett, J. T. J., Jeans, W. D., and Roylance, J. (1976). The incidence and importance of renal duplication. *Clinical Radiology* **27**, 521–530.

Quintero, R. A., Hume, R., Smith, C., Johnson, M. P., Cotton, D. B., Romero, R., and Evans, M. I. (1995). Percutaneous fetal cystoscopy and endoscopic fulguration of posterior urethral valves. *American Journal of Obstetrics and Gynecology* **172**, 206–209.

Rajagopalan, P. R., Hanevold, C. D., Orak, J. D., Cofer, J. B., Bromberg, J. S., Baliga, P., and Fitts, C. T. (1994). Valve bladder does not affect the outcome of renal transplants in children with renal failure due to posterior urethral valves. *Transplantation Proceedings* **26**, 115–116.

Ransley, P. G., Dhillon, H. K., Gordon, I., Duffy, P. G., Dillon, M. J., and Barratt, T. M. (1990). The postnatal managemant of hydronephrosis diagnosed by prenatal ultrasound. *Journal of Urology* **144**, 584–587.

Rascher, W. and Sulyok, E. Current issues of sodium and fluid homeostasis in the preterm and term newborn. In *Pediatric Nephrology, Pediatric and Adolescent Medicine* Vol. 5 (ed. A. Drukker and A. B. Gruskin), pp. 40–51. Basel: Karger, 1994.

Rascher, W., Bonzel, K. E., Guth-Tougelidis, B., Kröpfl, D., Meyer-Schwickerath, M., and Reiners, C. (1992). Angeborene Fehlbildungen des Harntrakts. Rationelle postpartale Diagnostik. *Monatsschrift für Kinderheilkunde* **140**, 78–83.

Rascher, W., Rupprecht, T., and Rösch, W. Prune belly syndrome. In *Pediatric Uroradiology* (ed. R. Fotter), pp. 177–184. Heidelberg: Springer, 2001.

Reinberg, Y. and Gonzalez, R. (1987). Upper urinary tract obstruction in children: current controversies in diagnosis. *Pediatric Clinics of North America* **34**, 1291–1304.

Reinberg, Y., Gonzales, R., Fryd, D., Maurer, S. M., and Najarian, J. S. (1988). The outcome of renal transplantation in children with posterior urethral valves. *Journal of Urology* **140**, 1491–1493.

Rittenberg, M. H., Hulbert, W. C., Snyder, H. M., and Duckett, J. W. (1988). Protective factors in posterior urethral valves. *Journal of Urology* **140**, 993–996.

Rohrschneider, W. K. and Stegen, P. Magnetic resonance imaging. In *Pediatric Uroradiology* (ed. R. Fotter), pp. 15–26. Heidelberg: Springer, 2001.

Rohrschneider, W. K., Becker, K., Hoffend, J., Clorius, J. H., Darge, K., Kooijman, H., and Tröger, J. (2000). Combined static-dynamic MR-urography for the simultaneous evaluation of morphology and function in urinary tract obstruction. II. Findings in experimentally induced ureteric stenosis. Evaluation of the *Pediatric Radiology* **30**, 523–532.

Roodhooft, A. M., Birnholz, J. C., and Holmes, L. B. (1984). Familial nature of congenital absence and severe dysgenesis of both kidneys. *New England Journal of Medicine* **310**, 1341–1345.

Rosendahl, H. (1990). Ultrasound screening for fetal urinary tract malformations: a prospective study in a general population. *European Journal of Obstetrics and Gynecology* **36**, 27–33.

Ruano-Gil, D., Coca-Payeras, A., and Tejedo-Mateu, A. (1975). Obstruction and normal recanalization of the ureter in the human embryo. Its relation to congenital ureteric obstruction. *European Urology* **1**, 287–293.

Rudolph, A. M., Heymann, M. A., Teramo, W., Barrett, C. T., and Raila, N. C. (1971). Studies on the circulation of the prenatal human fetus. *Pediatric Research* **5**, 452–465.

Sanders, R. and Graham, D. (1982). Twelve cases of hydronephrosis *in utero* diagnosed by ultrasonography. *Journal of Ultrasound Medicine* **1**, 341–348.

Schrott, K. M. (1995). Reconstruction of bladder exstophy in a single-stage. *Pediatrik Cerrahi Dergisi* **9/1**, 253–260.

Schrott, K. M. Blasenekstrophie. In *Kinderurologie* (ed. A. Sigel and R. H. Ringert), pp. 435–260. Heidelberg: Springer, 2001.

Schwartz, G. J. and Evan, A. P. (1984). Development of solute transport in rabbit proximal tubule. III. Na–K-ATPase activity. *American Journal of Physiology* **246**, F845–F852.

Scott, J. E. and Renwick, M. (1993). Urological anomalies in the northern region fetal abnormality survey. *Archives of Disease in Childhood* **68**, 22–26.

Shah, S. I. and Glassberg, K. I. Multicystic dysplastic kidney disease. In *Urology* (ed. J. P. Gearhardt, R. C. Rink, and P. D. E. Mouriquand), pp. 279–287. Philadelphia: Saunders Company, 2001.

Smith, D., Eggington, J. A., and Brookfield, D. S. K. (1987). Detection of abnormality of fetal urinary tract as a predictor of renal tract disease. *British Medical Journal* **294**, 27–28.

Snyder, H. M. C. The duplex system, ectopic ureter, and ureterocele. In *Pediatric Nephrology* 2nd edn. (ed. M. A. Holliday, T. M. Barratt, and R. L. Vernier), pp. 681–690. Baltimore: Williams and Wilkins, 1987.

Spitzer, A. and Avner, E. D. *Inheritance of Kidney and Urinary Tract Diseases*. Boston: Kluwer Academic Publishers, 1989.

Stein, R., Fisch, M., Black, P., and Hohenfellner, R. (1999). Strategies for reconstruction after unsuccessful or unsatisfactory primary treatment of patients with bladder exstrophy or incontinent epispadias. *Journal of Urology* **161**, 1934–1941.

Steiner, D., Steiss, J. O., Klett, R., Miller, J., Bauer, R., Weidner, W., and Rascher, W. (1999). The value of renal scintigraphy during controlled diuresis in children with hydronephrosis. *European Journal of Nuclear Medicine* **26**, 18–21.

Stuck, K. J., Koff, S. A., and Silver, T. M. (1982). Ultrasonic features of multicystic dysplastic kidney: expanded diagnostic criteria. *Radiology* **143**, 217–221.

Sukhai, R. N., Kooy, P. P. M., Wolff, E. D., Scholtmeijer, R. J., and van der Heijden, A. J. (1985). Evaluation of obstructive uropathy in children. ^{99m}Tc-DTPA renography studies under conditions of maximal diuresis. *British Journal of Urology* **57**, 124–129.

Sulyok, E., Varga, F., Gyöy, E., and Csaba, I. F. (1979). Post-natal development of renal sodium handling in premature infants. *Journal of Pediatrics* **95**, 787–792.

Tanagho, E. A. (1976). Embryologic basis for lower ureteral anomalies: a hypothesis. *Urology* **7**, 451–464.

Tejani, A., Butt, K., Glassberg, K., Prince, A., and Gurumurthy, K. (1986). Predictors of eventual end-stage renal disease in children with posterior urethral valves. *Journal of Urology* **136**, 857–860.

Thomas, D. F. M. (1990). Fetal uropathy. *British Journal of Urology* **66**, 225–231.

Thomas, D. F. M. and Gordon, A. C. (1989). Management of prenatally diagnosed uropathies. *Archives of Disease in Childhood* **64**, 58–63.

Tsuchida, S., Matsusaka, T., Chen, X., Okubo, S., Niimura, F., Nishimura, H., Fogo, A., Utsunomiya, H., Inagami, T., and Ichikawa, I. (1998). Murine double nullizygotes of the angiotensin type 1A and 1B receptor genes duplicate severe abnormal phenotypes of angiotensinogen nullizygotes. *Journal of Clinical Investigation* **101**, 755–760.

Tufro-McReddie, A., Romano, L. M., Harris, J. M., Ferder, L., and Gomez, R. A. (1995). Angiotensin II regulates nephrogenesis and renal vascular development. *American Journal of Physiology* **269**, F110–F115.

Tulassay, T., Rascher, W., Seyberth, H. W., Lang, R. E., Toth, M., and Sulyok, E. (1986). Role of atrial natriuretic peptide in sodium homeostasis in premature infants. *Journal of Pediatrics* **109**, 1023–1027.

Ulman, I., Jayanthi, V. R., and Koff, S. A. (2000). The long-term followup of newborns with severe unilateral hydronephrosis initially treated nonoperatively. *Journal of Urology* **164**, 1101–1105.

Van Gool, J. D., Dik, P., and de Jong, T. P. (2001). Bladder-sphincter dysfunction in meningomyelocele. *European Journal of Pediatrics* **160**, 414–420.

Vereecken R. L. and Proesmans, W. (1999) A review of ninety-two obstructive megaureters in children. *European Urology* **36**, 342–347.

Whitaker, R. H. (1979). The Whitaker test. *Urologic Clinics of North America* **6**, 529–539.

Wigglesworth, J. S., Desai, R., and Guerrini, P. (1981). Fetal lung hypoplasia: biochemical and structural variations and their possible significance. *Archives of Disease in Childhood* **56**, 606–615.

Wilson, C. and Azmy, A. F. (1986). Horseshoe kidney in children. *British Journal of Urology* **58**, 361–363.

Winberg, J. (1959). Renal function in water-losing syndrome due to lower urinary tract obstruction before and after treatment. *Acta Paediatrica Scandinavica* **48**, 149–163.

Wladimiroff, J. W. (1975). Effect of furosemide on fetal urine production. *British Journal of Obstetrics and Gynecology* **82**, 221–224.

Wolf, U., Schempp, W., and Scherer, G. (1992). Molecular biology of the human Y-chromosome. *Reviews of Physiology, Biochemistry, and Pharmacology* **121**, 148–213.

Woodard, J. R. and Parrott, T. S. Neonatal urology. In *Pediatric Nephrology* 2nd edn. (ed. M. A. Holliday, T. M. Barratt, and R. L. Vernier), pp. 945–961. Baltimore: Williams and Wilkins, 1987.

Woolf, A. S. Genes, urinary tract development and human disease. In *Pediatric Urology* (ed. J. P. Gearhardt, R. C. Rink, and P. D. E. Mouriquand), pp. 225–236. Philadelphia: Saunders Company, 2001.

Zerres, K., Völpel, M. C., and Weiss, H. (1984). Cystic kidneys. *Human Genetics* **68**, 104–135.

17.5 Medullary sponge kidney

J. Stewart Cameron

Definition, pathology, and epidemiology

Today, medullary 'sponge' kidney (MSK) is principally a diagnosis made or suggested by radiological examination or by ultrasonography, eventhough the earliest descriptions were of pathological specimens. Although often discussed together with cystic diseases of the kidney, this condition is a congenital ectasia of the distal collecting tubules with enlargement of the affected pyramids, either diffusely throughout both kidneys, only in one kidney, or variably in different papillae (Fig. 1). The changes do not resemble those of a sea sponge (Kuiper 1976), nor is the disease truly cystic, but the name 'sponge kidney' is easily remembered and is now accepted in the literature in all languages (e.g. rein en éponge, rene a spugna, etc.). In some European countries it is better known as Cacchi–Ricci disease, after two associates of G Lenarduzzi of Genoa (who first described the radiological appearance

in 1938) who, in turn, defined the disease comprehensively in 1948 (Cacchi and Ricci 1949).

Its pathogenesis is not clear; although MSK appears to be congenital, there is no clear inheritance and it rarely presents in childhood (Patriquin and O'Regan 1985). Today, it is best seen as one manifestation of a complex of congenital growth-related disorders which include some renal tumours and other renal malformations (Fig. 2). MSK must be distinguished carefully from other true medullary cystic diseases, especially medullary cystic kidney disease (MCKD, nephronophthisis, see Chapter 16.3). Abeshouse and Abeshouse (1960) and Ekström *et al.* (1959) described and collected over 150 cases from personal experience and the literature, and Yendt (1990, 1993) reported on 140 personal cases; these series, and those of Kuiper (1976), Harrison and Rose (1979), and Thomas *et al.* (2000), form the main published database. Jungers and Grünfeld (2001) also draw on a personal unpublished series of 179 patients seen from 1973 to 1999 in their comprehensive review.

The prevalence is not exactly known, since the earliest visible radiographic feature, a 'blush' of the papilla, is a subjective observation. In several series of intravenous urographies (IVUs) (Palubinskas 1963; Mayall 1970), about 0.5 per cent have been suggested to have definite MSK, whilst up to a further 1 per cent in Palubinskas' series showed a papillary 'blush'. This only, of course, tells us the prevalence in those submitted to an IVU examination, for whatever reason, and no series of autopsies has been examined from this point of view. From Mayall's study (1970), an estimated prevalence of not less than 1 : 20,000 total

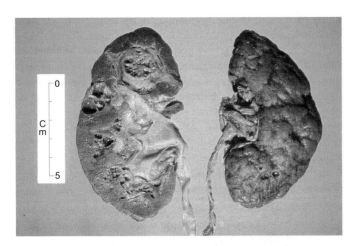

Fig. 1 Postmortem specimen of 'sponge' kidneys, found incidentally in a woman of 64 years. On the left, the cut surface shows marked enlargement and change within all papillae, but variably between papillae, three of four show extensive change and one much less obvious abnormality; this is characteristic of the condition. The 'cyst-like' appearance of the papillae is easily visible, although the 'cysts' are, in fact, ectatic collecting ducts (see text). Over the very dilated ducts of the upper medial calyx, the cortex is thinned and scarred, presumably as a result of repeated infections. The surface of the kidney (right) shows considerable pitting and scarring, especially the depressed scar lying over the upper medial calyx already mentioned; such scarring is unusual, and renal function is usually well preserved. In this patient, the renal scarring may have been related to embolic phenomena complicating rheumatic mitral valve disease.

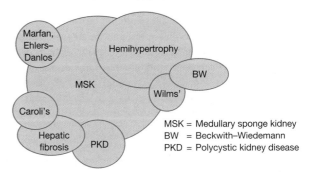

Fig. 2 A Venn diagram to show the relations between the major associations of medullary sponge kidney.

population was suggested. The gender incidence is approximately equal, and there is no obvious racial preponderance. The age at presentation is usually 20–45 years, but a clinical onset in childhood, although unusual, is well recorded (Habib *et al.* 1969; Patriquin and O'Regan 1985; see also Kuiper 1976) (and see Fig. 7). Of patients presenting with nephrolithiasis, about 3–5 per cent will show MSK (O'Neill *et al.* 1981; Wikström *et al.* 1983), although much greater proportions (from 15 to over 20 per cent) have been reported more recently (Yendt 1993; Thomas *et al.* 2000). The proportion depends very much on the intensity of investigation, on the interpretation of the papillary 'blush' (see below), and the nature of the referred population with specialist units and stone clinics in general seeing a higher proportion of repetitive stone formers and unusual cases.

Pathologically, the changes in MSK are confined (as the name suggests) to the medulla (Ekstrom *et al.* 1959; Pyrah 1966). The tubules are dilated with numerous small cysts, which communicate with the collecting tubules or directly with the minor calyces. The cysts are lined with columnar or cuboidal, occasionally by transitional or squamous epithelium. Associated abnormalities of the urinary tract are common (Ekström *et al.* 1959), providing further evidence for the congenital nature of the condition (see below). Seventy per cent of the concretions in the medulla consist of apatite, but the urinary stones are usually calcium oxalate (see below), which makes up the remaining 30 per cent of concretions (Yendt 1993). The reasons for this discrepancy are not clear.

Table 1 Inherited/congenital conditions associated with medullary 'sponge' kidney

Hemihypertrophy
Beckwith–Wiedemann disease
Caroli syndrome
Hepatic fibrosis
Autosomal dominant polycystic kidney disease
Congenital pyloric stenosis
Arterial fibromuscular dysplasia
Marfan syndrome
Ehlers–Danlos syndrome
Osteopenia
Anodontia
Parathyroid adenoma
Joubert syndrome
Horseshoe kidney, and minor urological abnormalities (e.g. renal ectopia, ureteral duplication, malrotation)
Pyeloureteritis cystica
Young's syndrome (immotile cilia)

Conditions associated with medullary 'sponge' kidneys

It is interesting and a little puzzling that none of Abeshouse's large collected series up to 1960 were reported as having any associated abnormality, but an increasing number of clinical associations have been reported since 1965 (Table 1 and Fig. 2), and most recent series report a proportion with one or another of these. These associated conditions are of great interest and practical importance, both because of their implications for screening and management, and because of the light they may throw in the still obscure aetiology of MSK. Some of these are discussed further below in the section on pathogenesis.

The most important of these associated conditions is *hemihypertrophy* (Fig. 3), which is present in as many as one-fourth of cases (Harris *et al.* 1981; Indridason *et al.* 1996; Jungers and Grünfeld 2001; Rommel and Pirson 2001) whilst of those with hemihypertrophy, 5–10 per cent present also with MSK. Hemihypertrophy itself is associated also with Wilms' tumour (Rommel and Pirson 2001), adrenocortical neoplasms, and hepatoblastoma, and the first two have been associated as a triad with MSK. Again, about one in eight of patients with the Beckwith–Wiedemann syndrome had some degree of asymmetric hypertrophy, rising to 40 per cent in those with associated tumours. Chesney *et al.* (1989) have even suggested that MSK and hemihypertrophy represents a *forme fruste* of the Beckwith–Wiedemann syndrome.

The other complex group of conditions associated with MSK includes *hepatic fibrosis* and *autosomal dominant polycystic kidney*. Several patients have been reported in whom clear evidence of MSK was present together with cortical cysts of autosomal adult polycystic kidney disease (ADPKD) (Anderson *et al.* 1990; Jungers and Grünfeld 2001). ADPKD is known to be associated with frequent stone formation,

up to some 20 per cent of cases in some series (see Chapter 16.2.2), and some of these patients will be found to have abnormal medullary pyramids. A number patients have been described also with complicated patterns of renal cyst formation in both cortex and medulla which are difficult to classify (Jungers and Grünfeld 2001). *Hepatic fibrosis* and portal tract dilatation is associated with MSK in about two-thirds of patients (Kerr *et al.* 1962), whilst *Caroli's syndrome* of segmental intrahepatic cystic dilatation of ducts, often associated with congenital hepatic fibrosis, is usually inherited in a recessive fashion and has been reported in several patients with MSK (Mrowka *et al.* 1996; Wiesner *et al.* 1997; Pinto *et al.* 1998). The clinical implication of this is that MSK patients should have echography of their liver.

The other associated conditions listed in Table 1 and shown in Fig. 2 are relatively uncommon, but of note is the fact that some of them form syndromes of local tissue hypertrophy, analogous to that found in the medullary collecting ducts of the kidney.

Clinical features

MSK is symptomless *per se*, but it is complicated by urinary tract infections and renal colic from calculi, which suggest the diagnosis. Renal colic from stones is the most frequent presenting symptom (Ekström *et al.* 1959) and many of the complications of the stones are major features of the disease. Microscopic haematuria is almost always present while gross haematuria is present in 10–20 per cent of patients (Betts and O'Reilly 1992) and may be exacerbated by exercise or infections to macroscopic amounts. Macroscopic haematuria may occur, however, in the absence of either infection or of stones. Minor proteinuria may be present, but amounts greater than a trace should raise suspicion of another diagnosis, for example, renal tuberculosis. Excess white cells, amounting to pyuria, may be present varying according to

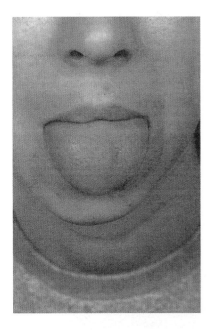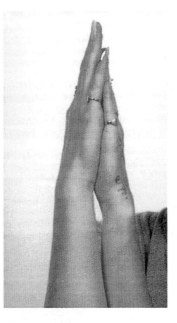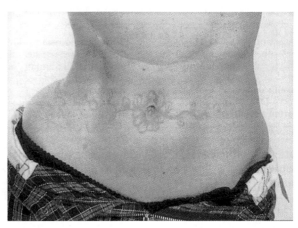

Fig. 3 A patient who had medullary cystic disease, hemihypertrophy, and had been treated in childhood for a Wilms' tumour. Hypertrophy of the right side of the tongue (left), the right hand (middle), and leg (right)—the pelvis is tilted and there is scoliosis because one leg is longer. Note also the scar from a childhood operation for removal of a Wilms' tumour. The kidney on the affected side was larger also [from Rommel and Pirson (2001) with permission].

whether the urine is infected or not. Coincident hypertension is difficult to assess, since some cases are found from radiology performed as part of the investigation of high blood pressure. There is no good evidence that MSK predisposes to hypertension.

Glomerular function is normal unless urinary tract obstruction is present, but this can occur in a number of patients, such as in Granberg's series (1971). This study also revealed a reduced renal extraction of *p*-aminohippurate. Concentrating ability is usually modestly reduced, but one of the most characteristic features of MSK is that urinary acidification is subnormal in the majority of cases, with a consequent acidosis (Granberg *et al.* 1971; Higashihara *et al.* 1984; Osther *et al.* 1988, 1994). This renal tubular acidosis is usually incomplete and sometimes absent. It can, however, be severe enough to retard growth in children (Sluysmans *et al.* 1987) and associated potassium loss has led to intermittent paralysis. The exact relationship between the tubular acidosis and the ectasia is complex and not yet clear, and may not simply represent the result of general damage to distal tubular cells in the ectatic tubules (Jungers and Grünfeld 2001).

Hypercalciuria and hypocitraturia are present in about 30–50 per cent of patients including 26 per cent of women, who otherwise hardly ever suffer idiopathic hypercalciuria (Yendt 1993; Osther *et al.* 1994; Thomas *et al.* 2000). The mechanism of the hypercalciuria is unclear: it seems unlikely that calcium excretion will be increased directly by damage in a lesion predominantly affecting the collecting ducts. Some patients have an absorptive hypercalciuria (O'Neill *et al.* 1981), but most do not (Maschio *et al.* 1982). Although calcium losses might be expected to lead to parathyroid stimulation, the data are inconclusive overall (Maschio *et al.* 1982; Yendt 1993), although a small proportion of patients with associated parathyroid adenomas may be identified (Diouf *et al.* 2000). Urinary cyclic AMP excretion is usually normal. Hyperoxaluria is present also in 64 per cent of cases (Thomas *et al.* 2000) and low urinary magnesium in many (Yagisawa *et al.* 2001). There is also an increased rejection of filtered sodium (Granberg *et al.* 1971).

Table 2 Radiographic features of medullary sponge kidney

Constant features	
Plain film	Normal or enlarged (30%) kidneys
Excretory urography	Changes limited to medullary pyramids
	Ectatic tubules/cysts fill with contrast before calyceal opacification
	Filling of tubules/cysts without compression
	Persistence of medullary contrast even in late films
	Appearance constant in repeated examinations
Variable features	
Plain film	Medullary calcification 40–60%, minute to 5 mm
Excretory urography	Changes unilateral 23%, bilateral 77%
	One pyramid (25%), few (34%), multiple (36%), and all (27%)
	Pattern may vary from 'blush' to rays to cysts
	Free calculi in tract, especially in those with colic
	Enlargement of affected pyramids
	Non-communicating cysts give 'blistered' look to papillary tip
	Urinary tract dilatation and renal scarring
	Cortical cysts
	Deep medullary cavities

Adapted with some modifications and additions from Kuiper (1976).

Radiological features (see Table 2)

The diagnosis of MSK remains essentially a radiographic one. Antegrade visualization of the papilla by contrast media leads in the mildest cases to a blush, in more obvious cases linear radiations, and finally in the florid disease to the outlining of cystic dilatation of the collecting ducts, which of course communicate with the calyces (Figs 4–7), giving the 'bouquet' or 'bunch of grapes' appearance. Gedroyc and Saxton (1988) point out that some patients may have cortical cysts and cavities deep

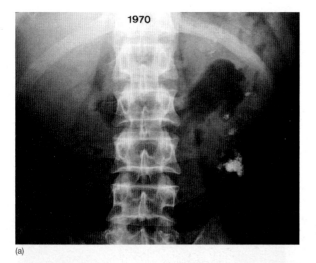

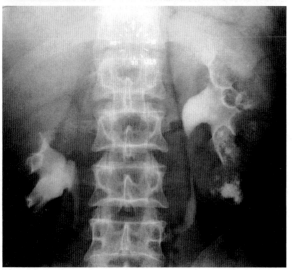

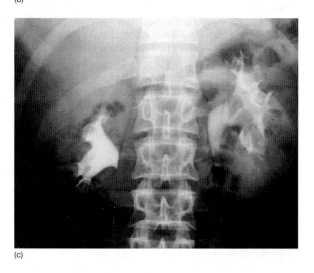

Fig. 4 The plain film (a) and IVU appearances (b) of gross changes of medullary sponge kidney in a patient who presented with renal colic and microscopic haematuria. Six years previously (c) the changes had been much less evident, showing their evolution over a short period. Note that only minor changes are present in the right kidney; such asymmetry is usual in medullary sponge kidney, and may be associated with hemihypertrophy (by courtesy of Dr H.M. Saxton, Department of Radiology, Guy's Hospital, London).

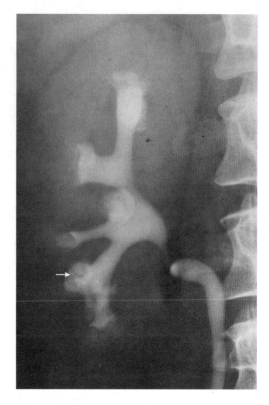

Fig. 5 Less severe forms of the disease, with changes confined to the papillary tip (arrow) (by courtesy of Dr H.M. Saxton, Department of Radiology, Guy's Hospital, London).

in the medulla, thus widening the spectrum of changes. Use of modern low osmolality contrast media does not apparently increase the incidence of medullary cavities detected (Ginalski *et al.* 1992). In more long-standing cases, plain radiography shows multiple small calculi within the substance of the enlarged papillae (Fig. 4).

Other imaging techniques

These have relatively a small place in diagnosis and management of MSK. On *ultrasonography*, the medullary calcification is easily visible; in earlier cases without calcification the papillae may appear 'bright' on ultrasound. In many cases the diagnosis is clear, but in some a difficult differential diagnosis is from renal tuberculosis, distal renal tubular acidosis with nephrocalcinosis, papillary necrosis from sickling, diabetes mellitus or analgesic abuse, calyceal diverticula, and finally from medullary cystic disease (nephronophthisis) with hepatic fibrosis (see Chapter 16.3). One problem is that several of these conditions have been seen to coexist with sponge kidney changes (see Kuiper 1976 for review).

Computed axial tomography was evaluated by Ginalski *et al.* (1991). Although better at picking up small medullary calcifications, it was less satisfactory than intravenous urography for detecting cavities. It may be of particular use also when abscesses or neoplasia complicate the lesion.

Clinical course

The clinical course is generally benign as far as evolution into renal failure is concerned, but occasional patients develop renal failure from

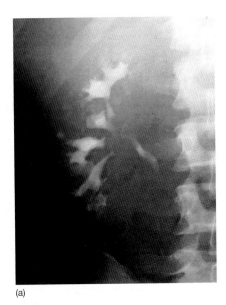
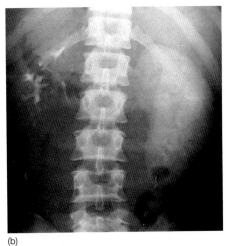

(a)   (b)

Fig. 6 (a) A more irregular pattern with some large medullary cavities. In (b) the left kidney is obstructed by a calculus jammed in the lower ureter and shows a prominent dense persistent nephrogram (by courtesy of Dr H.M. Saxton, Department of Radiology, Guy's Hospital, London).

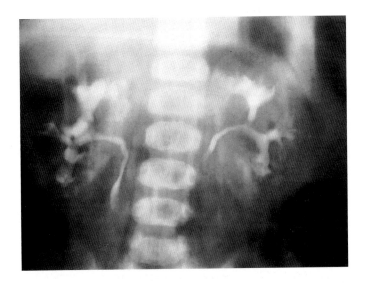

Fig. 7 Medullary sponge kidneys that caused haematuria in a 6-year-old boy (by courtesy of Dr H.M. Saxton, Department of Radiology, Guy's Hospital, London).

pyelonephritis, interstitial nephritis, and calculi (Murisasco *et al.* 1971; Pesce *et al.* 1995). There may be considerable nuisance or even major problems to the patient from recurrent urinary infections and from repeated episodes of calculi, ureteric colic, and episodes of urinary tract obstruction. Infections are commoner in female patients. In some, dozens of small stones may be passed over many years. These days, surgery is rarely required to remove the stones and since the size of the intrapapillary cavities is small, eventually almost all can pass through the urinary tract. Complete obstruction of a kidney is rare and renal failure is also rare but may supervene from obstruction or, occasionally, formation of infected struvite staghorn calculi.

Pathogenesis

The pathogenesis remains unknown. Most authors regard it as a congenital condition, probably present in mild form from birth, even though it rather rarely presents in childhood. In addition, there are a few families in which more than one sibling has been affected (e.g. Murisasco *et al.* 1971); Kuiper (1976) collected 29 patients from such reports, and occasional families with more than one generation affected have been reported (Kuiper 1976) such as the family reported by Jungers and Grünfeld (2001), with seven members affected over three generations, suggesting an autosomal dominant pattern of inheritance. There is growing evidence that MSK represents a disorder of local hypertrophy, located in the collecting ducts as demonstrated by Potter using nephron microdissection, and the several associations with other congenital or hereditary conditions (Fig. 3) provide clues as to possible aetiology. The Beckwith–Wiedemann syndrome, which includes macroglossia and organomegaly, is known to be associated with a locus on chromosome 11p15 and abnormalities of insulin-like growth factor II (IGF II), whilst IGF I has an important role in bone formation. Proesmans *et al.* (2000) suggest that increased IGF II and decrease in IGF I might explain the features of their 12-year-old patient, who had anodontia and osteopenia as well as MSK (Langman 2000), and some other associations in Table 1 also represent conditions with local hypertrophy. Rommel and Pirson (2001) also described a patient with MSK and hemihypertrophy, who had had a Wilms' tumour removed during childhood, a double coincidence noted previously in only two MSK patients. Wilms' tumour (see Chapter 18.2) is associated with alterations in the WT-1 gene at 11p13, and it may occur together with the Beckwith–Wiedemann syndrome (0.2 per cent of cases) and hemihypertrophy (2.5 per cent of cases). Diouf *et al.* (2000) described in contrast an adult patient with hyperparathyroidism and a thyroid nodule as well as MSK, who had a codon 634 mutation in the RET gene on chromosome 10q11.2, which is associated very strongly with multiple endocrine neoplasia type 2A.

The subsequent pathogenesis of the clinical manifestations, once ectasia is present, is easier to understand. Apart from obstruction with stasis and infection, the hypercalciuria, hyperoxaluria, high urinary pH, low urinary magnesium, and hypocitraturia of the syndrome will all favour hydroxyapatite stone formation (see Chapter 8.2), but in only one-fourth of cases are the stones made of this, half being whewellite (calcium oxalate monohydrate), the remainder being almost all wedellite (calcium oxalate dihydrate) (Jungers and Grünfeld 2001). Intrauterine obstruction of tubules by calcium had even been suggested by Deck in 1965 as a possible aetiological mechanism for the condition itself, but there is no evidence to support this concept.

Treatment

No treatment affects the number or presence of the ectatic tubules. A high fluid intake (>2 l/24 h) throughout the day and night both to avoid calculus formation and prevent infections has been recommended by most authors, as well as other measures designed to inhibit the formation of calcium oxalate stones (see Chapter 8.3); a low-animal protein diet should be taken. Thiazides are usually effective in reducing urinary calcium excretion even when hyperabsorption of calcium is present. Potassium citrate may be useful in those with impaired acidification and is preferable to bicarbonate because many patients also have low citrate excretion. Long-term antibiotic treatment may be needed in a few patients with recurrent infections since these can lead on to renal impairment. Obstruction of the urinary tract or major intrarenal sepsis will need treatment on their own merits, should they arise which is rare. Established stones of adequate size usually can be treated by lithotripsy, with or without prior stenting (Chen *et al.* 1993; Nakada *et al.* 1993; Vandeuysen and Baert 1993), but prophylactic attempts to destroy medullary calcifications have not been effective in some hands (Nakada *et al.* 1993; Vandeuysen and Baert 1993) although others recommend this course (Holmes *et al.* 1992). In some patients percutaneous surgery or removal of ureteric stones may be necessary. However, there is a high likelihood of residual stones and further problems compared with stones in the presence of other malformations (Gallucci *et al.* 2001).

References

Abeshouse, B. S. and Abeshouse, G. A. (1960). Sponge kidney: a review of the literature and a report of five cases. *Journal of Urology* **84**, 252–267.

Anderson, J. E. M., Steens, R. D., and Hurst, P. E. (1990). Polycystic disease of the kidney coexisting with medullary sponge kidney. *Australasian Radiology* **34**, 341–343.

Betts, C. D. and O'Reilly, P. H. (1992). Profound haemorrhage causing acute obstruction in medullary sponge kidneys. *British Journal of Urology* **70**, 449–450.

Cacchi, R. and Ricci, V. (1949). Sur une rare maladie kystique multiple des pyramides rénales, le 'rein en éponge'. *Journal d'Urologie* **55**, 497–517.

Chen, W. C., Lee, Y. H., Huang, T. K., Chen, M. T., and Chang, L. S. (1993). Experience using extra corporeal shock-wave lithotripsy to treat calculi in problem kidneys. *Urologia Internationalis* **51**, 32–38.

Chesney, R. W., Kaufman, R., Stapleton, F. B., and Rivas, M. L. (1989). Association of medullary sponge kidney and medullary dysplasia in Beckwith–Wiedemann syndrome. *Journal of Pediatrics* **115**, 761–764.

Diouf, B. *et al.* (2000). Association of medullary sponge kidney disease and multiple endocrine dysplasia type IIA due to RET gene mutation: is there a causal relationship? *Nephrology, Dialysis, Transplantation* **15**, 2062–2066.

Ekström, T., Engfeldt, B., Lagergren, C., and Lindvall, N. *Medullary Sponge Kidney*. Stockholm: Almqvist and Wiksell, 1959.

Gallucci, M. *et al.* (2001). Extracorporeal shock wave lithotripsy in ureteral and kidney malformations. *Urologia Internationalis* **66**, 61–65.

Gedroyc, W. M. and Saxton, H. M. (1988). More medullary sponge kidney variants. *Clinical Radiology* **39**, 423–425.

Ginalski, J. M., Schnyder, P., Portmann, L., and Jaeger, P. (1991). Medullary sponge kidney on axial computed tomography. *European Journal of Radiology* **12**, 104–107.

Ginalski, J. M., Speigel, T., and Jaeger, P. (1992). Use of low osmolality contrast media does not increase prevalence of medullary sponge kidney. *Radiology* **182**, 311–314.

Granberg, P. O., Lagergren, C., and Theve, N. O. (1971). Renal function studies in medullary sponge kidney. *Scandinavian Journal of Urology and Nephrology* **5**, 177–180.

Habib, R., Mouzet Mazza, M. T., Courtecuisse, V., and Royer, P. (1969). L'ectasie tubulaire précalicielle chez l'enfant. *Annales de Pédiatrie* **12**, 288–298.

Harris, R. E., Fuchs, E. F., and Kaempf, M. J. (1981). Medullary sponge kidney and congenital hemihypertrophy: case report and review of the literature. *Journal of Urology* **126**, 676–678.

Harrison, A. R. and Rose, G. A. (1979). Medullary sponge kidney. *Urological Research* **7**, 197–207.

Higashihara, E. *et al.* (1984). Medullary sponge kidney and renal acidification defect. *Kidney International* **25**, 453–459.

Holmes, S. A. *et al.* (1992). The use of extracorporeal shock wave lithotripsy for medullary sponge kidney. *British Journal of Urology* **70**, 352–354.

Indridason, O. S., Thomas, L., and Berkoben, M. (1996). Medullary sponge kidney associated with congenital hemihypertrophy. *Journal of the American Society of Nephrology* **7**, 1123–1130.

Jungers, P. and Grünfeld, J.-P. Medullary sponge kidney. In *Strauss and Welt's Diseases of the Kidney* 7th edn. (ed. R. W. Schrier), pp. 521–546. Boston: Little Brown, 2001.

Kerr, D. N. S., Warrick, C. K., and Hart-Mercer, J. (1962). A lesion resembling medullary sponge kidney in patients with congenital hepatic fibrosis. *Clinical Radiology* **13**, 85–91.

Kuiper, J. J. Medullary sponge kidney. In *Cystic Diseases of the Kidney* (ed. K. D. Gardner), pp. 151–171. New York: John Wiley, 1976.

Langman, C. B. (2000). Commentary on the paper of Proesmans *et al.* *Pediatric Nephrology* **14**, 263–265.

Maschio, G. *et al.* (1982). Medullary sponge kidney and hyperparathyroidism—a puzzling association. *American Journal of Nephrology* **2**, 77–84.

Mayall, G. F. (1970). The incidence of medullary sponge kidney. *Clinical Radiology* **21**, 171–174.

Mrowka, C., Adam, G., Sieberth, H. G., and Matern, S. (1996). Caroli's syndrome asscoiated with medullary sponge kidney and nephrocalcinosis. *Nephrology, Dialysis, Transplantation* **11**, 1142–1145.

Murisasco, A. *et al.* (1971). L'ectasie canaliculaire précalicielle. *Presse Médicale* **79**, 2367–2370.

Nakada, S. Y., Erturk, E., Monaghan, J., and Cockett, A. T. (1993). The role of extracorporeal shock wave lithotripsy in treatment of urolithiasis in patients with medullary sponge kidney. *Urology* **41**, 331–333.

O'Neill, M., Breslau, N. A., and Pak, C. Y. C. (1981). Metabolic evaluation of nephrolithiasis in patients with medullary sponge kidney. *Journal of the American Medical Association* **245**, 1233–1236.

Osther, P. J., Hansen, A. B., and Rohl, H. F. (1988). Renal acidification defects in medullary sponge kidney. *British Journal of Urology* **61**, 322–324.

Osther, P. J., Mathiasen, H., Hansen, A. B., and Nissen, H. M. (1994). Urinary acidification and urinary excretion of calcium and citrate in women with bilateral medullary sponge kidney. *Urologia Internationalis* **52**, 126–130.

Palubinskas, A. J. (1963). Renal pyramidal opacification in excretory urography and its relation to medullary sponge kidney. *Radiology* **81**, 963–970.

Patriquin, H. B. and O'Regan, S. (1985). Medullary sponge kidney in childhood. *American Journal of Roentgenology* **145**, 315–319.

Pesce, C. *et al.* (1995). Rene a spugna midollare con grave compromissione della funzionalità renale. *Pediatria Medica e Chirurgica* **17**, 65–67.

Pinto, R. B. *et al.* (1998). Caroli's disease: report of 10 cases in children and adolescents in Southern Brazil. *Journal of Pediatric Surgery* **33**, 1531–1535.

Proesmans, W., Van Molhem, S., and Latour, L. (2000). A 16-year old boy with medullary sponge kidneys, osteoporosis, and premature loss of teeth. *Pediatric Nephrology* **14**, 259–262.

Pyrah, L. N. (1966). Medullary sponge kidney. *Journal of Urology* **95**, 274–283.

Rommel, D. and Pirson, Y. (2001). Medullary sponge kidney—part of a congenital syndrome. *Nephrology, Dialysis, Transplantation* **16**, 634–636.

Sluysmans, T., Vanoverschelde, J. P., and Malvaux, P. (1987). Growth failure associated with medullary sponge kidney due to incomplete renal tubular acidosis type 1. *European Journal of Paediatrics* **146**, 78–80.

Thomas, E., Witte Y., Thomas, J., and Arvis, G. (2000). Maladie de Cacchi et Ricci: remarques radiologiques, epidémiologiques et biologiques. *Progrès en Urologie* **10**, 29–35.

Vandeuysen, H. and Baert, L. (1993). Prophylactic use of extracorporeal shock wave lithotripsy in management of nephrocalcinosis. *British Journal of Urology* **71**, 392–395.

Wiesner, W., Kohler, A., and Hauser, M. (1997). Cystic enlarged intrahepatic bile ducts, congenital liver fibrosis and sponge kidney: Caroli syndrome. *Schweizerische Rundsch Medizinische Praxis* **86**, 1035–1037.

Wikström, B. *et al.* (1983). Ambulatory diagnostic evaluation of 389 recurrent stone formers. A proposal for clinical classification and investigation. *Klinische Wochenschrift* **61**, 85–90.

Yagisawa, T. *et al.* (2001). Contributory metabolic factors in the development of nephrolithiasis in patients with medullary sponge kidney. *American Journal of Kidney Diseases* **37**, 1140–1143.

Yendt, E. R. Medullary sponge kidney. In *Cystic Renal Diseases* (ed. K. D. Gardner), pp. 379–391. Dordrecht: Kluwer Scientific, 1990.

Yendt, E. R. Medullary sponge kidney. In *Strauss and Welt's Diseases of the Kidney* 5th edn. (ed. R. W. Schrier and C. M. Gottschalk), pp. 573–582. Boston: Little Brown, 1993.

18

The patient with malignancy of the kidney and urinary tract

18.1 Renal carcinoma and other tumours

Manuel Urrutia Avisrror

Introduction

Most kidney malignancies are tumours of epithelial origin whose incidence will show a steady increase, particularly in industrialized countries, owing to a combination of the effects of population ageing and the improvement and increased efficiency of the early detection of malignant diseases.

This chapter is an updated summary of the most important features of the epidemiology, cytogenetics, histological patterns, clinical presentation, and the available therapeutic options for the management of both localized and disseminated disease of renal cell carcinoma (RCC). In a significant number of cases, specialists in both nephrology and oncology contribute to diagnosis and clinical management which explains why it merits inclusion in any textbook dealing with kidney diseases.

Epidemiology and aetiology of kidney cancer

Demographic factors

The approach of considering adenocarcinoma of the kidney separately from tumours of the renal pelvis has provided more information about the influence of age, gender, race, and other environmental and geographical factors on the true prevalence of the disease.

Incidence rates are closely related to ageing, as demonstrated by the steady increase in frequency with each passing decade after the age of 30 (De Reiijke *et al.* 1987), as illustrated in Fig. 1.

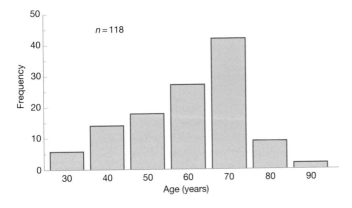

Fig. 1 Age distribution of 118 cases of renal cell carcinoma studied in the Urology Department of the Hospital Clinico Universitario de Salamanca.

Gender is also important, as the reported incidence is 2.5 to 4 times greater in males than in females when the cumulative frequency curves are corrected for gender.

Race does not appear to play a major role, as only small fluctuations have been observed in large epidemiological studies performed in countries whose population contains a variety of ethnic groups, such as the United States.

Heredity is also important as shown by several reports of tumours in consecutive generations of the same family (Brinton 1960). Where specific cytogenetic findings have been described, the greatest effect is in people with blood group A, and in certain inherited conditions including polycystic disease, von Hippel–Lindau disease, and colour blindness (Griffin *et al.* 1967).

Environmental factors are important as shown by comparing the age-adjusted incidence rates. Increased rates are observed in Denmark, Sweden, Norway, New Zealand, and Hawaii (Paganini-Hill *et al.* 1983); countries with intermediate incidence include continental United States and most of Western Europe, and the lowest rates are observed in Japan, China, and India. Comparative analysis reveals that the highest frequencies of malignant tumours of the kidney are found in the industrialized countries and appear to be associated with urbanization, food intake, habits, and exposure to different environmental and industrial carcinogenic agents. Recently, epidemiological studies have found an increased risk of renal cancer associated with female obesity (Mellemgard *et al.* 1994), the use of diuretics (Weinman 1993), and chronic haemodialysis treatment (Ishikawa 1993).

Aetiological factors

The aetiology of renal cancer in humans remains obscure although a large number of hypotheses have been postulated and many possible carcinogenic agents have been proposed. However, most of these theories are based on extrapolations of observations in animal models.

Physical and chemical agents

The only physical agent known to induce renal adenocarcinoma and squamous cell carcinoma of the pelvis is the radioactive compound Thorotrast, a weak α emitter which was used many years ago as a contrast medium for retrograde pyelographic studies.

Since Sempronj and Morelli (1939) induced experimental adenocarcinoma in rats by systemic administration of β-anthraquinoline, several exogenous chemical carcinogens have been linked to renal adenocarcinoma, including aromatic amines and amides, N-nitroso compounds, aliphatic compounds, heavy metals, agents used for chemotherapeutic treatment of malignancies, and natural organic compounds.

Chronic exposure to cadmium, a metal known to be oncogenic and widely employed in the manufacture of various products, such as plastic stabilizers, pigments, and batteries, may be a risk factor (Elinder 1985). A case–control study demonstrated an increase of the relative risk of 2.5 for persons with increased exposure to this metal, possibly related to the inhibition of different zinc-containing enzyme systems with a regulatory action on cell growth.

The carcinogenic effect of lead has been demonstrated by experiment and renal tumours have also been found in wild rats living in suburban areas where the soil has a high lead content. In humans, Paganini-Hill et al. (1980) observed a slight increase in death due to kidney cancer (6/1.6) in a cohort study of newspaper web workers with chronic exposure to the lead pigments contained in coloured ink. Follow-up studies of people exposed to lead vapour inhalation failed to demonstrate a significant increased incidence of malignant renal tumours compared with the general population (see also Chapter 6.5).

Asbestos has a proven carcinogenic effect in man and has also been incriminated as a risk factor in kidney cancer Maclure (1987) .

Among natural organic compounds, aflotoxins B_1 and B_2 produced by *Aspergillus flavus*, a fungus that contaminates a variety of foodstuffs, may cause human renal tumours because they contain lactones which have been shown to induce both renal adenocarcinoma and carcinoma of the renal pelvis in rats. Other natural compounds identified as potent renal carcinogens include cyscain, streptozotocin, daunomycin, and ochratoxin A (see also Chapter 6.8).

Habits

Tobacco smoking is probably the only exposure factor that can be consistently linked to renal cell cancer (Kreiger et al. 1993) and may account for the differences between the incidence rates in males and females. Dimethylnitrosamine and cadmium present in cigarette smoke have been postulated as the aetiological agents on the basis of their known ability to produce experimental kidney tumours in rodents.

Phenacetin-containing analgesics have been reported as significant risk factors for tumours of the renal pelvis, but the possible association with kidney adenocarcinoma has not been convincingly demonstrated. A relative risk of 10 for developing renal cancer has been reported for both short-term and long-term daily users compared with never users (see also Chapter 6.2). Weinman (1993) has reported an increased risk of RCC associated with the chronic use of diuretics.

Hormones

Tumours that are histologically similar to human renal adenocarcinoma are produced by prolonged administration of large doses of oestrogens to male and spayed female hamsters. Tumour induction is inhibited by concurrent administration of testosterone, progesterone, deoxycorticosterone, bromoergocryptin, 20-methyl cholanthrene, and nafoxidine, and the induction period is reduced if the animals undergo unilateral nephrectomy before oestrogen treatment. Human renal adenocarcinoma can be considered as a hormone-related tumour on the basis of its greater frequency of occurrence in males compared to females—a theory supported by the recent finding of hormone receptors in normal kidney tissue and renal tumours. Nevertheless, the relationship with the hormonal environment remains controversial.

Viruses

A viral aetiology for renal adenocarcinoma is postulated on the basis of the identification in human renal tumours of specific antigens for the herpes simplex virus, which have been implicated in the aetiology of a well-differentiated adenocarcinoma in the North American leopard frog (Grannoff 1973).

Genetics of renal cell carcinoma

There has been a significant increase in our understanding of the genetic basis of RCC in recent years. A wide range of chromosomal abnormalities in both hereditary and sporadic RCC tumour cells have been identified.

Genetic and clinical studies of patients with a family history of kidney cancer suggest that there are at least two different types of hereditary RCC.

The first type is characterized by a constitutional translocation of chromosome 3 to chromosome 8, specifically [t(3:8) p(14.24.13)] (Li et al. 1993), although a constitutional translocation of chromosome 3 to chromosome 6 [t(3:6)(p13:q25.1)] and a non-constitutional translocation of chromosome 3 to chromosome 11 have also been reported (Kovacs and Brusa 1989). Recently, Zbar et al. (1994) described a three-generation family affected with multiple papillary RCC; cytogenetic studies demonstrated that the disorder was not linked to polymorphic markers on chromosome 3p or loss of heterozygosity on 3p in the tumour cells, suggesting that a genetic mechanism different from the known hereditary syndromes might be involved.

The second type of familial tumour is linked with von Hippel–Lindau disease, an inherited autosomal dominant multifocal syndrome frequently associated with renal cysts and RCC. Cytogenetic studies in patients with von Hippel–Lindau disease and concomitant renal cell tumours have demonstrated chromosomal deletions in the 3p13–p26 region (Gnarra et al. 1993). It is likely that renal cysts, which are present in about 50 per cent of the patients, are the site of initiation of RCC and that, although von Hippel–Lindau disease maps to the 3p25–p26 region, the onset of kidney cancer associated with this condition is due to a second mutation of the linked sporadic gene that controls manifestations of von Hippel–Lindau disease (see also Chapter 16.6).

The most consistent cytogenetic finding in sporadic renal cell tumours is deletion of the short arm of chromosome 3. This observation provides evidence for the presence of tumour-suppressor genes which have been mapped in the 3p21–p26 and 3p13–p24 regions, whose loss promotes the initiation of tumour growth (Kohno et al. 1993; Presti et al. 1993; Foster et al. 1994). Deletion of chromosome 3p is not correlated with the histological type or stage of the disease, but it is absent in most papillary RCCs and all oncocytic tumours (Presti et al. 1992). Papillary tumours appear to arise through a different genetic mechanism which may involve a gain of chromosomes 7 and 17. Allelic losses on chromosome 17p have been related to tumour grade and tumour progression (Presti et al. 1992; Presti et al. 1993). A number of authors have studied the association of p53 mutations, an antioncogene located on chromosome 17p, and sporadic RCC with inconclusive and discrepant results (Saya et al. 1991; Horesovsky et al. 1993; Uchida et al. 1993). Some findings suggest that abnormalities of p53 may be involved in the progression of RCC and in both carcinogenesis and the progression of transitional cell carcinomas (Reiter et al. 1993; Suzuki and Tamura 1993). Other reported chromosomal anomalies in RCC include trisomies of chromosomes 5, 7, 10, and 18, loss of the Y chromosome, and an extra X chromosome (Casalone et al. 1992; Sugao et al. 1992).

Classification of renal epithelial tumours

In 1997, international consensus was reached on a new histological classification of renal epithelial neoplasms, based on the combination of both microscopic appearance and cytogenetic features. This new classification, commonly referred to as the Heidelberg system, has contributed to clarify some aspects of tumour histogenesis.

Papillary renal cell carcinomas

These account for approximately 5 per cent of all RCCs and the term should be applied only if genetic abnormalities are found, irrespective of the presence of prominent papillae in the histological specimen. Papillary RCC frequently presents as a large well-defined mass surrounded by a thick wall, sometimes cystic-like due to extensive haemorrhagic and necrotic changes in the tumour. The cells are arranged in a complex tubulopapillary pattern intermixed with a stroma showing abundant clusters of macrophage cells. Hypovascularity or avascularity and extensive calcification of the capsule are other unique features (Matsumoto et al. 1992). The most outstanding cytogenetic characteristic is that, unlike most RCCs, chromosome 3p is not deleted. Genotype abnormalities reported so far include trisomies or tetrasomies of chromosome 7, trisomy of chromosomes 16 and 17 (Henn et al. 1993; Hughson et al. 1993), and a translocation breakpoint in chromosome Xp11 (Meloni et al. 1993; Sinke et al. 1993; Suijkerbuijk et al. 1993). A hereditary form of papillary RCC which has not been linked to loss of heterozygosity at locus 3p has been described in a three-generation family, suggesting the presence of a RCC gene not located on 3p that would predispose for the development of renal cell cancers with a distinct histological appearance (Zbar et al. 1994). Retention of chromosome 3 would also explain a more benign biological behaviour.

Chromophobe renal carcinoma

This histological subtype was first described in 1985, and has a reported incidence of 5 per cent of all epithelial renal tumours. Together with papillary carcinoma, it is considered to have a less agressive behaviour than conventional clear cell carcinoma, and some consider it to be the malignant counterpart of renal oncocytoma.

They usually present as large circumscribed masses with a greyishtan cut surface. The tumour cells are predominantly clear, but some eosinophilic cells may also be observed. Structurally, these cells are similar to the intercalated cells of the cortical collecting ducts, and histochemical studies provide strong evidence for derivation from the collecting ducts of the nephron (Gerharz et al. 1993). Genetically, this subtype seems to be correlated with a loss of constitutional heterozygosity at chromosomal regions 3p, 5q, 17p, and 17q, an association not found in other types of RCCs (Kovacs et al. 1992). Other reported cytogenetic anomalies include polysomy of chromosome 7, trisomies of chromosomes 12, 16, 18, 19, structural abnormalities of chromosome11q, and telomeric associations (van den Berg et al. 1993).

Collecting duct carcinoma

This uncommon tumour, first described by Fleming and Lewi (1986), accounts for only 0.4 per cent of all RCCs. Typically, the central part of the kidney appears as a greyish-white infiltrating mass with the bulk of the lesion located in the medulla. Histochemical studies demonstrate that these tumours originate from the collecting tubules as they generally express high-molecular-weight cytokeratines and lectines. Histochemical studies are useful for differentiating collecting duct carcinomas from high-grade transitional tumours of the renal pelvis, with which they are sometimes confused owing to their common embryological origin. Generally, collecting duct carcinomas show a highly aggressive clinical course with early metastasis and death.

Conventional (clear cell) renal carcinoma

This is the most frequent of all renal epithelial neoplasms (70 per cent). It presents with a similar frequency in both kidneys; bilateral tumours are found in 0.5–1.5 per cent of patients, and multicentric tumours in the same kidney have been reported in approximately 4.5 per cent of patients (Table 1).

The gross pathological features observed are related in some way to the morphological and histochemical characteristics of the tumour cells, and the blood supply of the tumour mass. In section, viable tumours have a lobular appearance with a glistening surface whose colour typically ranges from pale yellow to orange if the lipid content in the tumour cells is high or a greyish tone if the lipid content is poor. Large tumours may outgrow their own blood supply, giving rise to necrotic areas with a cystic or gelatinous appearance.

The tumour is often separated from the surrounding parenchyma by a rim of condensed connective tissue that forms a pseudocapsule (Fig. 2). Large and advanced tumours frequently infiltrate the perinephric fat and the collecting system, and they may extend to the lumen of the renal and caval veins and the tumour may reach the level of the right atrium.

When examined with the light microscope (Fig. 3), the bulk of the tumour is composed of fairly uniform cuboidal or columnar cells with small round nuclei, a clear cytoplasm, because of its high content of cholesterol, lipids, and glycogen that are eluted during routine processing, and sparse cytoplasmic organelles. The second most common is the granular cell type (Fig. 4) with a bright eosinophilic and

Table 1 Pathological findings in RCC (n = 118)

	n	**Percentage**
Affected side		
Right	56	47.5
Left	62	52.5
Location		
Upper	32	27.1
Middle	49	41.5
Lower	37	31.4
Cell type		
Clear	102	86.5
Granular	11	9.3
Spindle	5	4.2
Histological type		
Solid	49	41.5
Tubular	34	28.9
Papillary	22	18.6
Mixed	13	11.0
Cell differentiation		
Well differentiated	70	59.3
Poorly differentiated	48	40.7

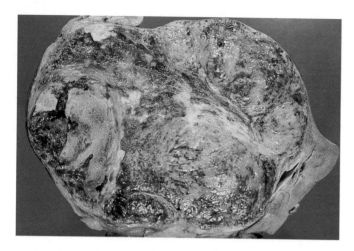

Fig. 2 Cross-section of a typical clear cell carcinoma of the kidney. The tumour has a lobular appearance and is delimited from the surrounding parenchyma by a pseudocapsule composed of a rim of condensed connective tissue.

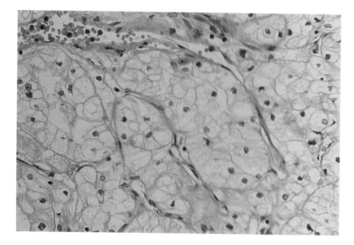

Fig. 3 RCC; clear cell type with clear cytoplasm and small nuclei. (Illustration kindly provided by Michael Dunnill.)

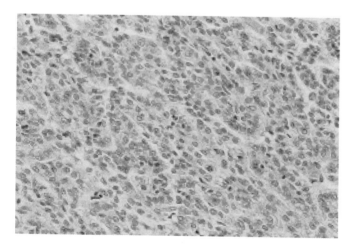

Fig. 4 RCC; granular type showing a typical cell pattern with eosinophilic granular cytoplasm. (Illustration kindly provided by Michael Dunnill.)

granular cytoplasm owing to the large content of organelles, principally mitochondria, and a more developed Golgi apparatus and endoplasmic reticulum.

Unclassified renal carcinoma

This represents less than 2 per cent of all tumours. This category is reserved for those epithelial neoplasms that lack the criteria to be included in the previously described subtypes, such as the sarcomatoid type, where the bulk of the tumour is composed of spindle cells whose epithelial origin can be demonstrated by histochemical studies, where the most consistent finding is a positive reactivity to anticytokeratines AE1/AER; a positive reaction to epithelial membrane antigen, vimentin, and actin is less frequently observed (Bird *et al.* 1991; Auger *et al.* 1993; DeLong *et al.* 1993). Spindle cell carcinomas always have a high grade of malignancy and a poor prognosis. Tetu *et al.* (1987) first reported four cases of a small-cell type of renal carcinoma which presented as large necrotic tumours with highly aggressive behaviour.

Histological grading

The histological grade in most of the malignant tumours has an important impact on long-term survival and many classifications have been developed based upon cell type, differentiation, and pattern arrangement (Thoenes *et al.* 1986). The four-tier grading system proposed by Furhan (1982) is based exlusively on nuclear features and has gained wide acceptance in the United States, but like other systems has limitations and controversies.

A promising approach to an objective grading of tumour cells was the introduction of computer based morphometric analysis of the tumour cells (Pound *et al.* 1993; Unger *et al.* 1993) or by DNA flow cytometry. Using the latter method, Rauschmeier *et al.* (1983) found that grade 1 tumours have a DNA distribution pattern similar to that of normal cells; in grade 2 tumours the DNA distribution is also unimodal but with a significant number of tetraploid cells, whereas grade 3 tumours show a bimodal distribution. In a series of 206 samples of reclassified grade 1 and grade 2 clear cell renal carcinomas, Rainwater *et al.* (1987) reported a 60 per cent normal DNA histogram pattern in grade 1 tumours and a 67 per cent abnormal pattern in grade 2 tumours, which correlated well with subsequent development of distant metastases irrespective of tumour grade and stage. Studies reported in the last 3 years contradict these initial findings and have seriously questioned the value of DNA flow cytometry as a real prognostic factor in the outcome of the disease. Heterogeneity between different samples of a given tumour (Nakano *et al.* 1993), its use as a single predictor (Lanigan *et al.* 1993), and the high cost of the technique are some of the arguments against its routine use in the clinical assessment of RCC.

An alternative to DNA flow cytometry is nuclear morphometry using computer-assisted image anlaysis. We have developed a module for the NIH-Image public domain program that performs fully automated morphometric analysis. This module has been applied in a series of 64 patients with RCCs to assess the predictive value of different morphometric parameters in predicting the probability of survival after nephrectomy (Urrutia *et al.* 2001).[1] The results are presented later in this chapter.

---

[1] A copy of this program (only for MacOS) can be obtained by e-mail request to urrutia@usal.es

Routes of dissemination

Renal cancer spreads via lymphogenous, haematogenous, and lymphohaematogenous routes, and also by direct extension through the renal capsule to adjacent structures. The frequency of both metastatic spread and direct extension correlates with the size of the original tumour. At the time of nephrectomy, up to 40 per cent of the patients may have invasion of the capsule and the perinephric fat, 36 per cent may have renal vein involvement, and approximately 40 per cent may have unsuspected distant metastases.

Lymphatic spread principally involves the hilum and regional lymph nodes followed in descending order by the retroperitoneal, abdominal, mediastinal, supraclavicular, cervical, axillary, and inguinal lymph nodes.

Haematogenous spread is the most prominent route and accounts for the many unusual metastatic sites observed in clinical practice. It is preceded by an extension of the tumour to the renal vein followed by further embolic dissemination to the lungs and axial skeleton. About 55 per cent of metastases appear in the lung, followed in descending order by lymph nodes, liver, bone, adrenal gland, the opposite kidney, and brain. Less common metastatic sites are the spleen, intestinal tract, skin, pancreas, thyroid, corpus cavernosum, bile duct, ovary, parotid, and Bartholin's glands (Leiman et al. 1986). Retrograde venous embolization to pelvic structures via the left spermatic or ovarian vein, which is closely connected to the main renal vein, provides another route for haematogenous spread of the tumour to the genitourinary organs (ureter, bladder, penis, epidydimis, testis, ovary, and vagina).

In lymphohaematogenous spread, the tumour cells bypass the liver and reach the lung via the thoracic duct, the superior vena cava, and the pulmonary circulation.

Staging of renal cancer

There are two main staging systems for renal carcinomas. The first by Robson (1969) gained wide acceptance in Europe and the United States. The features defining the four different stages (Table 2) of this system are based upon pathological findings; therefore, its accuracy is strongly influenced by the extent of the operative procedure.

An alternative classification introduced by the International Union Against Cancer is based on the TNM categories applied to other tumours (Table 3) . As the definition of the categories in the TNM system is based on preoperative information obtained from the different diagnostic methods available to the clinician, initially, this system added little to the reliability of staging renal tumours. The main drawback was the lack of specific tumour markers and the need to use computed tomography (CT) or magnetic resonance imaging (MRI) for an accurate assessment of the size of the tumour, the extent of regional lymph node involvement, and distant metastasis. However, CT and MRI equipment is now available in most hospitals, and this has contributed to the increasing popularity of this system.

Table 2 Staging of renal adenocarcinoma

Stage I (A)	Tumour confined within the kidney capsule
Stage II (B)	Invasion of the perinephric fat, but the tumour is still confined within Gerota's fascia
Stage III (C)	Involvement of regional node and/or renal vein cava
Stage IV (D)	Involvement of adjacent organs and distant metastases

After Robson et al. 1969.

Clinical presentation

Many textbooks and medical publications refer to renal adenocarcinoma as the 'internist tumour' or the 'great imitator in medicine' because it is incorrectly assumed that the early clinical symptoms are non-urological. Nevertheless, a review of the most significant series published reveals that, although the classic urological triad of haematuria, flank pain, and palpable mass is found in only 11–16 per cent of patients, at least one component is reported as an isolated symptom in more than 50 per cent of the cases and two are found in about one-third of all patients (Table 4). Other symptoms, such as asthenia, anaemia, increased erythrocyte sedimentation ratio, or thrombocytosis, cannot be considered as characteristic of RCC because they are also observed in advanced tumours of different origin.

Urological symptoms

Haematuria

Haematuria is by the far the most frequent presenting symptom and was observed in 65 per cent of our patients. The haematuria is

Table 3 TNM staging of RCC

TNM category		Equivalence
T1	<2.5 cm, limited to kidney	Robson I (A)
T2	>2.5 cm, limited to kidney	Robson I (A)
T3a	Perinephric invasion	Robson II (B)
T3b	Major veins invasion	Robson III (C)
T4	Invasion beyond Gerota's fascia	Robson IV (D)
N1	Single, <2 cm	Robson III (C)
N2	Single, 2–5 cm	Robson III (C)
N3	Multiple, <5 cm	Robson III (C)
	Multiple, >5 cm	Robson III (C)
M+	Distant metastases	Robson IV (D)

Table 4 Clinical findings in RCC (n = 118)

Symptom	n	Percentage
Haematuria	76	64.4
Pain	56	47.5
Palpable mass	29	24.6
Fever	16	13.6
Hypertension	15	12.7
Increased erythrocyte sedimentation rate	47	39.8
Anaemia	43	36.4
Erythrocytosis	4	3.4
Thrombocytosis	13	11.0
Hepatic dysfunction	5	4.2
Amyloidosis	1	0.8

characteristically gross, painless, total, and intermittent in nature, although some instances of microhaematuria may be observed. These symptoms are the most important diagnostic signs that can be used to differentiate on a clinical basis from haematuria originating at another site in the lower urinary tract. Another useful sign in patients with gross haematuria is the presence in freshly voided urine of worm-like clots, corresponding to casts of the ureter. In clinical practice, any haematuria with these features should be considered a renal tumour until demonstrated otherwise.

Pain

Pain is usually a late and inconstant symptom, with a reported frequency ranging from 20 to more than 45 per cent of patients. In the majority, the pain is dull and continuous and is due to progressive distension of the fibrous renal capsule. The passage of clots may produce an acute ureteric obstruction which gives rise to symptoms typical of renal colic. The differentiating sign is that haematuria is preceded by pain in acute ureteric obstruction by urinary calculi, whereas with renal tumours pain always follows haematuria.

Palpable mass

A palpable mass is a late symptom and is only observed in advanced tumours. This clinical sign has been reported with a frequency that varies from less than 6 to more than 50 per cent. In our experience, a palpable mass was detected in about 25 per cent of our patients and always corresponded to very large tumours or tumours of the lower pole of the kidney.

Varicocoele of acute onset in an adult patient in the absence of other major symptoms should always draw attention to the possibility of a renal tumour. This symptom is due to the obstruction of the spermatic or caval vein by tumour thrombi.

Less than 5 per cent of patients have presenting symptoms directly related to local or distant metastases, even though metastases are detected in up to 30 per cent of patients at the time of diagnosis. Solitary soft tissue metastases may arise in any organ, but the lung, bone, brain, and liver are the most frequent. Other symptoms related to metastases or local extension of the tumour include hepatomegaly, enlarged left supraclavicular lymph nodes, pathological fractures, haemoptysis, and priapism.

Non-urological symptoms

Non-specific systemic manifestations present a challenge to clinicans and in some instances may delay diagnosis and treatment for a significant period of time or may lead to extensive medical examination before their link with renal cancer is established. They are known to be dependent on humoral or endocrinal activity of the tumour, and some serve as useful clinical markers of tumour activity since they usually disappear if the surgical excision of the tumour is complete but may reappear with the development of metastases or local recurrence.

These paraneoplastic syndromes have been classified into three main groups.

Non-specific syndromes

Metabolic syndromes

Asthenia, anorexia, and weight loss form a clinical triad that is common to all malignant tumours in advanced stages. These symptoms are related to a systemic toxic effect mediated by unknown factors released by the tumour cells. Immunological reaction of the host, severe pain, and a specific malabsorption mechanism have also been implicated in the presentation of these symptoms.

Fever in association with renal cell tumours and in the absence of systemic infection has been reported in about 20 per cent of the cases, and is the first symptom in 3 per cent of patients. Some authors claim that the triad of haematuria, pain, and fever is even more frequent than the classical urological triad described above. The occurrence of fever is related to the liberation of an endogenous pyrogen by the tumour cells or by leucocytes within the tumour, but necrosis, haemorrhage, and local infection of the tumour may also play a role. Fever disappears after nephrectomy, and its persistence or recurrence should always be regarded as indicative of residual tumour or the development of metastases.

Haematological syndromes

Anaemia of normochromic–normocytic type is a common feature, particularly in advanced tumours. Its aetiology remains unclear, but the ferrokinetic patterns found in non-metastatic disease exhibit some features of ineffective erythropoiesis. An extrarenal triad of fever, anaemia, and hyperhaptoglobinaemia has been described in association with renal adenocarcinoma, and these findings seem to discount the possibility of a microangiopathic anaemia as the aetiological factor.

Increased erythrocyte sedimentation ratio is a common non-specific haemotological finding. We have not found any correlation between increased erythrocyte sedimentation ratio and the tumour cell type as reported by others. Other non-specific haematological findings include thrombocytosis, which, unlike other tumours, seems to be unrelated to bone marrow infiltration.

Biochemical syndromes

Reversible hepatic dysfunction has been described in patients with renal adenocarcinoma. This syndrome is characterized by the following clinical and biochemical features: non-tender non-nodular hepatomegaly, increased serum bilirubin, bromsulfthalein retention, increased alkaline phosphatase, increased α_2-globulin, and hypoprothrombinaemia. The histological background is a mild reactive hepatitis characterized by Kupffer cell hyperplasia, with or without fatty changes, and portal triaditis. Its pathogenesis remains uncertain, although an increased lysosomal activity in liver cells has been postulated. This syndrome is not pathognomonic of renal adenocarcinoma and we have observed a similar syndrome in patients with metastatic prostatic cancer. Characteristically, the syndrome reverses after nephrectomy in the absence of metastases.

Amyloidosis is associated with renal carcinoma in 3–5 per cent of all patients and always indicates a poor prognosis. The amyloid deposits generally involve the liver, kidneys, spleen, and adrenal gland, and do not regress after nephrectomy. The aetiology is unknown, but hyperimmunization of the host to his or her own slow-growing tumour has been postulated and seems to be supported by the finding of a marked plasmocytic response in the bone marrow of the affected patients.

Specific syndromes

Hypertension is a prominent symptom and is detected in about 20–40 per cent of all patients. It is probable that in some cases this symptom depends upon the secretion of renin or a renin-like substance by the tumour because there are reports of hypertension with elevated serum renin that are relieved by nephrectomy. In other patients, however, the role played by this substance is controversial since its frequency is about that expected for the age group and is no greater than that in patients with benign lesions or without renal disease. Increased renin unrelated to blood pressure has been reported in about one-third of the patients with high-grade and high-stage tumours, and this feature seems to be associated with a poor prognosis. Other factors which may contribute to hypertension include polycythaemia, arteriovenous shunts, and hypercalcaemia.

Polycythaemia has been reported in renal carcinoma with an incidence ranging from 1.8 to 6 per cent. The term 'erythrocytaemia' seems more appropriate for this condition because a constant feature is the increase of the total red cell mass related to an increased secretion of erythropoietin or an erythropoietin-like substance. The mechanisms postulated to explain the elevated erythropoietin in renal carcinoma include local ischaemia, mechanical stimulation of the juxtaglomerular apparatus by tumour growth, ectopic production of erythropoietin or an erythropoietin-like substance, and substrate activation by a substance produced by the tumour cells. Ischaemia and mechanical stimulation are unlikely to be factors promoting the increased secretion of erythropoietin because elevated concentrations are also observed after nephrectomy in patients who develop local recurrence or metastases. The rather low proportion of patients with erythrocytaemia is noteworthy if we take into account that up to 63 per cent of all patients may have increased erythropoietin.

Hypercalcaemia due to production of a parathyroid-hormone-like substance by the tumour cells and unrelated to osteolytic metastases may also be detected. Clinically, hypercalcaemia may present as an isolated laboratory finding or associated with a severe and rapidly progressive syndrome with symptoms of polyuria, polydipsia, dysphagia, constipation, muscular weakness, mental depression, and hypokalaemic alkalosis. Serum concentrations return to normal after nephrectomy and reappear with the development of local recurrence or metastases.

Various endocrine disorders related to ectopic production of gonadotrophin hormones by the tumour have also been reported in association with renal adenocarcinoma. Male patients with elevated human chorionic gonadotrophin may present with loss of libido, gynaecomastia, or feminization; in women the revealing symptoms are amenorrhoea and hirsutism. Gonadotrophins return to normal after nephrectomy in the absence of metastatic disease.

Miscellaneous syndromes

In addition to the specific and non-specific syndromes discussed above, a broad range of clinical conditions have been associated with renal adenocarcinoma. However, only a few of them, including neuromyopathy, salt-losing nephritis, leukaemoid reaction, and gastrointestinal disorders, have been specifically correlated with tumour development.

Biological markers

Substances other than those associated with specific syndromes may be of use in detecting relapses or monitoring the response to treatment of renal carcinoma. Non-specific biological markers investigated so far include carcinoembryonic antigen, urinary polyamines, prostaglandins, and acute phase reactant proteins.

Increased serum prostaglandin E has also been reported in patients with lung metastases, and it has been proposed as a non-specific marker of pulmonary involvement.

Among acute phase reactants, increased haptoglobin has been reported in 14 of 16 patients with localized tumours and in six patients with distant metastases (Vickers 1974). A further increase after nephrectomy is diagnostic of recurrence.

Increased phosphohexose isomerase and lactate dehydrogenase activity in the plasma, reflecting glycolytic activity within the tumour, may also be observed in advanced tumours and metastatic disease. Elevated serum alkaline phosphatase activity may occur as an isolated abnormality or associated with bone metastases. In our experience, the increased activity of this enzyme in the absence of a concomitant hepatic disease is the best non-specific biological marker for the detection of early bone metastases, and when combined with radionuclide scanning with [99]Tc[m]-diposphonate its diagnostic reliability is increased to almost absolute levels (Urrutia et al. 1977).

Differential diagnosis of kidney adenocarcinoma

A solid mass in the kidney, particularly in older patients, is most likely to be a renal carcinoma. Nevertheless, in clinical practice there are other tumours or tumour-like conditions which may mimic renal adenocarcinoma, and a diagnosis is only possible after surgical removal.

Renal oncocytoma

Renal oncocytomas are essentially benign solid tumours composed entirely of oncocytes (Fig. 5). These cells probably arise from the distal tubules, and are rich in mitochondria but have few other cytoplasmic organelles. The incidence of oncocytoma ranges from 5 to 15 per cent of all solid renal masses; only one instance of bilateral tumours has been reported.

Oncocytomas are usually large tumours with a tan brown colouration and a well-developed capsule; they rarely infiltrate the surrounding renal parenchyma, perinephric fat, or renal vein. Clinically, the presenting symptoms do not differ from those observed in renal cancer, although some authors suggest that the absence of haematuria is a characteristic clinical feature.

The diagnosis may be suspected preoperatively if the following arteriographic signs are present: a 'spokewheel' configuration of the vessels, a homogenous nephrogram phase, and a smooth sharp margin with a central lucent area. In large oncocytomas a low-density area due to central fibrosis may be observed on CT, but this sign is not

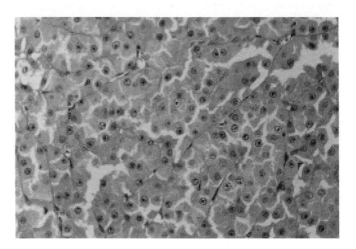

Fig. 5 Renal oncocytoma. (Illustration kindly provided by Michael Dunnill.)

pathognomonic and only an expert pathologist can establish the diagnosis reliably.

Lieber *et al.* (1981) reported that six of 28 oncocytomas categorized as grade 2 developed metastases. More recently, Lewi *et al.* (1986) found an 18 per cent incidence of metastatic disease in a series of 22 patients, with an overall 5 year survival rate of 65 per cent. However, Lieber (1993) was unable to determine whether the few cases reported in the literature were classic renal oncocytomas or high-grade oncocytic or granular cell cancers.

Angiomyolipoma (see also Chapter 16.6)

Angiomyolipomas are tumours composed of heterotopic mesenchymal tissue which were initially described in association with the tuberous sclerosis complex. They represent less than 0.01 per cent of all kidney tumours available for pathological study. Their incidence is 2.6 times greater in females than in males, and the mean age of presentation is 41 years (Farrow *et al.* 1968).

The gross features of large solitary tumours are highly characteristic. They appear as a smooth or irregular protuberant mass with a cut surface ranging from yellow to grey (Fig. 6). Generally, the growth is expansive, but local invasion to the perirenal structures or extracapsular extension may be observed; reports of malignant angiomyolipomas are based more on this invasive behaviour than on distant metastases. The frequency of bilateral or multiple tumours is not well established, but they are more frequent in patients with the tuberous sclerosis complex.

The histological appearance is fairly constant (Fig. 7), consisting of a variable admixture of adult adipose tissue and smooth muscle. The vascular component of the tumour consists of thick-walled tortuous blood vessels that frequently exhibit subintimal fibrosis, hyalinization of media, and lack of normal elastic membranes.

Clinically, angiomyolipoma may present in isolation or in association with the triad of mental retardation, epilepsy, and adenoma sebaceum in patients with the tuberous sclerosis complex. In the majority of the cases, it is asymptomatic and represents an incidental finding in autopsies or routine radiological explorations. Symptoms are related to the size of the tumour and the invasion of adjacent structures. The most frequent is a dull flank pain or diffuse abdominal discomfort;

some patients may have a sudden acute flank pain associated with a palpable abdominal mass and symptoms of acute anaemia. This syndrome, the Wunderlich triad, may be a life-threatening condition and is caused by the spontaneous rupture of large highly vascularized tumours in the retroperitoneal space.

Unlike kidney adenocarcinoma, haematuria is not a common feature in angiomyolipoma because of the expansive rather than infiltrative growth; hence, its frequency is related to the tumour size.

In some patients, systemic hypertension with increased peripheral renin activity may be the initial symptom and hypertension reverses after nephrectomy if a vascular component is involved in its aetiology.

Radiological exploration gives non-specific signs of a mass developed in the kidney that in some instances may show radiolucent areas and calcification. Angiomyolipoma should be suspected if ultrasonography reveals a solid mass with high-density echoes (Fig. 8). CT provides a conclusive diagnosis owing to the low attenuation values

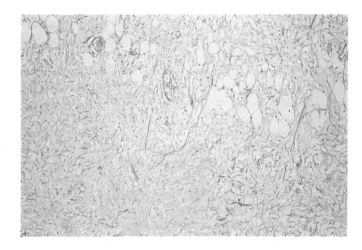

Fig. 7 Typical histological pattern of angiomyolipoma. The tumour is predominantly composed of mature adipose tissue intermixed with solid sheets of smooth muscle.

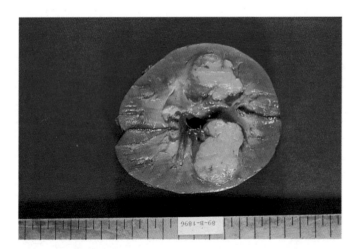

Fig. 6 Solitary angiomyolipoma of the kidney. The tumour appears as a smooth yellowish mass due to the high proportion of fatty tissue.

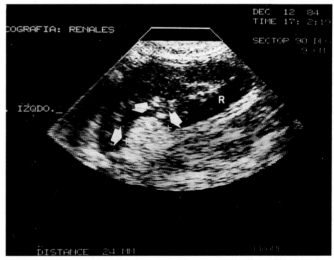

Fig. 8 Ultrasonographic aspect of angiomyolipoma. The typical finding is of a sharply delimited solid mass with high-density echoes, similar to that observed in the renal sinus.

related to the high fat content. Selective angiography may demonstrate signs resembling those observed in malignant epithelial tumours; the presence of tortuous curled vessels together with multisacculated pseudoaneurysms, the absence of arteriovenous shunts, and the presence of circumferential peripheral vessels with a whorled onion-peel appearance are distinct findings that may be suggestive of angiomyolipoma.

The treatment of large symptomatic tumours is partial or total nephrectomy. Conservative surgery is mandatory in patients with solitary kidney or large bilateral tumours, even in the presence of acute haemorrhage. Postoperative radiation and/or chemotherapy are not necessary because of their benign nature.

Malignant mesenchymal tumours

Malignant mesenchymal tumours account for only 2–3 per cent of all renal tumours and are found in no more than 0.1 per cent of autopsies.

Leiomyosarcoma is the most frequent tumour in this group. Its incidence increases with advancing age, more frequently in women than in men. The microscopic features are the same as those of leiomyosarcoma at other sites, showing interlacing fascicles of spindle-shaped cells in well-differentiated tumours; nuclear pleomorphism, cellular atypia, and increased mitotic activity are observed in poorly differentiated tumours. Clinically, patients may present with the typical triad of haematuria, pain, and an abdominal mass in advanced tumours, or any combination of these signs. Radiologically, they are almost indistinguishable from renal carcinoma. Selective arteriography of the kidney may demonstrate either hypervascular or hypovascular patterns with absence of arteriovenous shunts; the latter was observed in the only case of leiomyosarcoma of our series.

The only available treatment is radical nephrectomy, since these tumours are not amenable to radiotherapy or chemotherapy. The prognosis is poor, with a high incidence of short-term local recurrence and distant metastases.

Liposarcoma is the second most frequent of all the malignant renal mesenchymal tumours. They are usually large multilobular tumours arising from the periphery of the cortex or beneath the renal capsule and often extending into the perirenal fat. Metastases are rarely observed and local recurrence is unusual. The histological appearance is similar to that of liposarcomas located elsewhere in the body. Urography shows a radiolucent mass that displaces the kidney, and selective arteriography usually demonstrates an avascular pattern. Surgical excision is best, but no consistent data about long-term survival are available. Postoperative radiotherapy may give some benefits because sarcomas located in soft tissue are very sensitive to this treatment.

Rhabdomyosarcoma of the kidney is a highly malignant tumour of striated muscle whose real incidence is not known. Pure rhabdomyosarcomas are usually reported in adults and rarely in children. Some authors classify these tumours as nephroblastomas with an overgrowth of malignant striated muscle, but most likely they arise from undifferentiated mesenchymal cells with a capacity to differentiate into a variety of malignant mesenchymal tissues. A combination of immunohistochemistry and electron microscopy is needed for a reliable diagnosis of primary rhabdomyosarcoma of the kidney (Grignon *et al.* 1988).

Xanthogranulomatous pyelonephritis (see also Chapter 7.3)

Xanthogranulomatous pyelonephritis is a chronically inflammatory tumour-like condition, often associated with obstruction, calculi, and infection of the upper urinary tract, which may simulate renal adenocarcinoma clinically, morphologically, and radiologically.

The non-specific granulomatous reaction is generally nodular and expansive, and is produced by proliferation of interstitial macrophages with a high cytoplasmic content in neutral lipid and phospholipid. In advanced cases, the tumour may replace the renal parenchyma partially or totally and eventually infiltrate the perinephric fat and retroperitoneum. Less frequently, there may be a diffuse renal involvement.

Grossly, the cut surface is bright yellow to orange because of the large lipid content (Fig. 9). Histologically, the tumour may be confused by the non-expert with the clear cell type of renal carcinoma, but the lesions are characterized by typical multinucleated giant cells and the presence of cholesterol clefts (Fig. 10).

Xanthogranulomatous pyelonephritis lacks specific clinical and radiological features, but its frequent association with calculi, chronic obstruction, and recurrent urinary infection may serve as a useful diagnostic guide. A characteristic finding in the diffuse type is a small renal artery with spreading intrarenal vessels and an irregular spotty nephrogram (Fig. 11).

The treatment is nephrectomy, but this may be rather difficult in some cases because of the perinephric and retroperitoneal involvement.

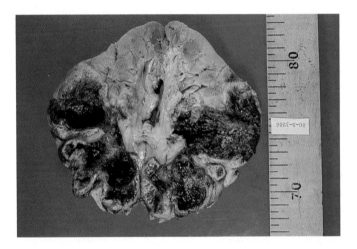

Fig. 9 Macroscopic aspect of a xanthogranulomatous pyelonephritis in a kidney with chronic obstruction.

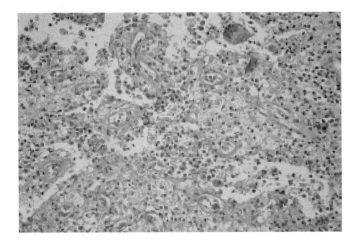

Fig. 10 Histology of Fig. 9. Observe the non-specific granulomatous reaction by macrophages with a high cytoplasmic content in lipids and plasmatic cells.

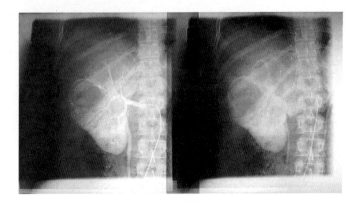

Fig. 11 Arteriography of Fig. 9, which simulated a kidney mass at IVU.

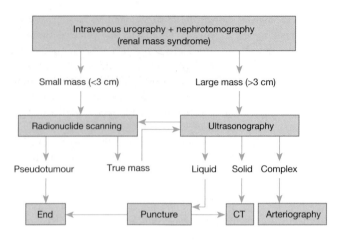

Fig. 12 Stepwise algorithm for the differential diagnosis of renal masses.

Diagnostic procedure

Combination of excretory urography and selective arteriography with the new non-invasive techniques of radionuclide scanning, ultrasonography, CT, and MRI has improved the diagnostic accuracy of renal tumours to almost absolute levels. Figure 12 shows one of the flow diagrams suggested for the diagnosis of suspected renal masses. It is a stepwise algorithm whose purpose is to minimize costs and risks to the patient whilst maximizing the diagnostic reliability (Montero *et al.* 1987).

Excretory urography and nephrotomography

Plain films of the abdomen, which must always be obtained before intravenous pyelograms, may give non-specific signs of mottled calcification or an alteration of the kidney contour in large tumours.

In about 90 per cent of the cases excretory urography shows a space-occupying lesion with distortion of the excretory system. Oblique and standard anteroposterior projections should be routinely obtained to minimize the possibility that a mass in the anterior or posterior surface of the kidney is overlooked.

Nephrotomography is of great help in assessing whether the mass is solid or liquid. Typically, a cystic mass is radiolucent, sharply demarcated from the adjacent parenchyma, and surrounded by a thin wall if it extends beyond the renal cortex. Some authors consider the typical 'beak-like' shape of the parenchyma at the site where the cyst protrudes from the kidney surface to be a pathognomic sign, but it may also be observed in poorly vascularized or slow-growing tumours.

Radionuclide scanning

The next step depends upon both the radiological appearance and the size of the detected mass. Radionuclide scanning with $^{99}Tc^m$-diethylenetriaminepentaacetic acid or $^{99}Tc^m$-glucoheptonate single-photon renal scintigraphy are probably the best methods for the differentiation of small renal masses from congenital or acquired tumour-like conditions, such as fetal lobation, septa of Bertin, and congenital hypertrophy of the upper lip of the renal sinus. The most frequent acquired pseudotumours are nodules of hypertrophied tissue developed in kidneys with chronic pyelonephritis. The conditions are differentiated as follows: there is uptake of radionuclide contrast in normal kidney tissue, whereas true masses lack isotopic activity and appear as a 'cold spot' in the kidney image.

Bone scans with $^{99}Tc^m$-diphosphonate provide a very sensitive method for the early detection of bone metastases, which are usually overlooked in conventional radiological exploration because a bone structural involvement of at least 40–45 per cent is needed for the metastatic lesion to become evident (Urrutia *et al.* 1977).

Ultrasonography

Masses of diameter greater than 3 cm should always undergo a grey-scale ultrasonographic examination. In our experience this method has a diagnostic accuracy of 99.4 per cent for cystic lesions compared with 78.6 per cent with excretory urography alone (Gomez Zancajo 1987).

In the B-mode scan, simple renal cysts are identified by three sonographic features: sonolucency, even at high gain settings, a sharply defined appearance of the far wall, and acoustic enhancement of the back wall, whose intensity is directly related to the cyst diameter. Conversely, solid masses show attenuation of the ultrasonic beam, presence of scattered echoes within the mass, whose number and intensity are closely related to tissue pattern and mass vascularity, and lack of acoustic enhancement of the back wall (Fig. 13). The first and last signs are better demonstrated using the A-mode scan with different gain settings. Pathological conditions that may mimic cystic lesions at ultrasonography include abscesses, cystic tumours, haemorrhagic cysts, and papillary cystoadenocarcinoma.

Cyst puncture with ultrasonographic guidance followed by chemical and/or cytological analysis of the aspirate has a 100 per cent diagnostic accuracy for simple cyst lesions.

Ultrasonography is also a valuable diagnostic tool for detecting caval or cavoatrial invasion by the tumour and eliminates the false-positive results associated with venocavography (Giuliani *et al.* 1987).

Renal angiography

A decade ago selective renal arteriography was the only reliable approach to the diagnosis of renal masses. However, the development of ultrasonography and CT has limited its application to those cases where these methods give equivocal or complex images. Angiography is also indicated when the urologist requests a preoperative assessment of

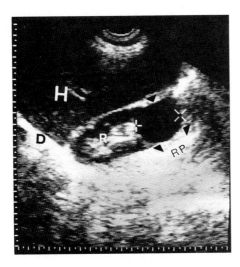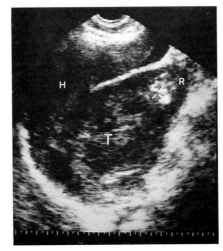

Fig. 13 Sonographic features of a cystic (left) and a solid (right) renal mass.

the vascular pattern in extended and highly vascularized tumours or when transcatheter embolization is planned as part of the therapeutic management. Angiographic findings in hypervascular kidney tumours are increased diameter of the main renal artery, displacement and/or amputation of the intrarenal branches, a neovascular pattern with tortuous vessels, microaneurysms and arteriovenous shunts, giving a typical image of diffuse tumour blush with pooling and puddling of contrast media, and early filling of the renal vein as a result of extensive arteriovenous shunts (Fig. 14). The signs described above may also be present with inflammatory abscesses and chronic haematoma. When the tumour extends beyond the limits of the kidney, a parasitic blood supply arising from the lumbar, phrenic, inferior suprarenal, and gonadal arteries may sometimes be observed. Kidney masses with a hypovascular pattern are a characteristic finding in large tumours outgrowing their blood supply, some mesenchymal tumours, metastatic tumours, lymphoma, spindle cell carcinoma, and infiltrating tumours of the excretory system.

Digital subtraction angiography (DSA) by intra-arterial injection provides information similar to that obtained with conventional arteriography. Intravenous DSA has only of an 80 per cent accuracy for the diagnosis of solid renal masses. The inguinal approach is a less traumatic method than aortography because it allows inferior vena cavography and intravenous aortography with one injection of contrast medium and does not require patient hospitalization.

Computed tomography

CT has a 100 per cent diagnostic accuracy for angiomyolipomas because of their high fat content, which gives low attenuation values (−20 to −80) that are not observed in other kidney tumours. Its diagnostic reliability for cystic and solid masses is the same as that of ultrasonography. Solid masses have attenuation values that are approximately the same as normal parenchyma, and cystic masses show a similar attenuation to water. The attenuation value of solid masses is enhanced after perfusion of contrast medium, but this enhancement is not observed in cystic lesions (Hattery *et al.* 1976).

In addition to its intrinsic diagnostic value, CT is probably one of the most sensitive and least expensive imaging methods for detecting early recurrence after nephrectomy, metastases in the liver, lung, brain,

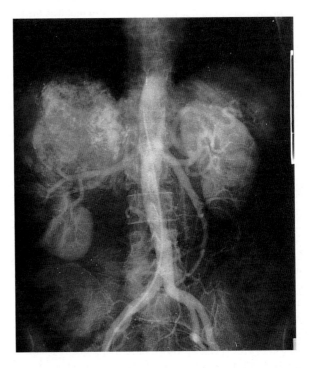

Fig. 14 Arteriography shows a hypervascularized mass in the upper pole of the right kidney. The patient presented with symptoms of fever of unknown origin and hypertension.

or retroperitoneal lymph nodes, and extension of the tumour into the renal or caval vein.

Magnetic resonance imaging

The new technique of magnetic resonance T1 contrast scans is more effective than ultrasonography in the study of renal masses. It provides better differentiation of solid from cystic lesions than CT contrast scans, and also gives good resolution of metastatic lymph nodes and isolated bone metastases. T2 contrast scans provide the best identification of the tumour pseudocapsule, renal vein involvement, and characterization of papillary adenocarcinoma (Karstaedt *et al.* 1986).

Treatment of renal carcinoma

Surgical treatment

Radical nephrectomy

Surgical removal of the tumourous kidney with perinephric fat, regional lymph nodes, and the adrenal gland is considered to be the best available therapeutic option for RCC (Robson *et al.* 1969) although randomized studies have not clearly demonstrated increased survival rates when compared with simple nephrectomy.

In small tumours or tumours located at the lower pole of the kidney, nephrectomy is usually performed by a midline, subcostal, or flank incision. When preoperative assessment demonstrates a large upper-pole tumour or an extension of the tumour into the caval vein, a thoracoabdominal approach (Mortensen 1948), a bilateral subcostal incision, or a midline incision with splitting of the sternum is preferable for better control of the vascular pedicle and the great vessels.

Early identification and control of the vascular pedicle without excessive kidney manipulation has been advocated to prevent the spread of metastases but it is more important to mobilize the kidney in the safest and easiest way (Couillard and deVere White 1993) because early control of the renal vessels does not prevent the formation of tumour emboli.

In large hypervascular tumours, preoperative transcatheter embolization of the kidney with an autologous or inert material (e.g. muscle, gelatin foam, metallic coils, cyanoacrylates, pure ethanol, or sodium tetradecyl sulfate) may prevent excessive bleeding at the time of operation (Alferez and Diaz-Alferez 1980; Konchanin *et al.* 1987). If the purpose of embolization is limited to the control of bleeding, a temporary balloon occlusion of the renal artery, until the pedicle is ligated, is preferred. Side-effects and complications associated with preoperative embolization of the kidney include severe lumbar pain, fever, systemic hypertension, acute renal failure, and ectopic embolization which limit the use of this procedure to the palliative treatment of advanced tumours or to facilitate the removal of large masses.

Caval involvement is detected in about 5–10 per cent of all patients at the time of diagnosis, and in up to 39 per cent tumour thrombi may extend into the right atrium. The best available procedure which reduces the perioperative risk of tumour embolization or uncontrollable haemorrhage is the removal of the kidney and tumour thrombus under extracorporeal circulation (Staehler *et al.* 1994; Kaplan *et al.* 2002).

The role played by regional lymphadenectomy in an attempt to improve the prognosis of the patients with renal carcinoma is controversial and is a matter of debate in urological literature.

Nephron-sparing nephrectomy

Partial nephrectomy or tumour enucleation is becoming increasingly accepted for the surgical treatment of unilateral low-volume primary renal cell tumours in the presence of a normal contralateral kidney. Reported survival rates in large series after long-term follow-up are very similar to those found in radical nephrectomy (Zincke *et al.* 1985; Novick 1987; Campbell *et al.* 1994). The most important argument against this approach, which remains controversial, is the risk of local recurrence (Brkovic *et al.* 1994).

There is a general reluctance to perform bilateral nephrectomy followed by transplantation in patients with bilateral tumours because of the negative effects of immunosuppressive therapy. The best approach is the radical removal of the kidney lodging the larger mass followed by partial nephrectomy or tumorectomy of the remaining kidney.

Wickham (1975) and Novick *et al.* (1977) have reviewed the natural history and therapeutic options for tumours occurring in solitary kidneys. In general terms, the prognosis is poor for patients who have undergone nephrectomy of the contralateral kidney because of a previous renal tumour or those with asynchronous tumours that have recurred within 5 years of the original nephrectomy. The best option in such cases is still *in situ* surgery, except for large middle-pole tumours where bench surgery and autotransplantation are mandatory.

Surgery for metastasis and local recurrence

The use of aggressive surgical treatment for solitary metastases, and selected cases where there are a small number of foci of disease, is generally accepted because it is possible to obtain long-term survival, or even cure, in a proportion of patients (Lieber 1983; Kjaer 1987). Asynchronous metastases which have been removed surgically have a better prognosis than solitary metastases excised at the time of nephrectomy (O'Dea *et al.* 1978). Tumour-reductive surgery is useless in disseminated metastatic spread, but should be considered if the purpose is to improve the patient's quality of life or if there is significant bleeding and arterial embolization is not feasible.

Local recurrence after radical nephrectomy has been detected with increased frequency (up to 37 per cent) owing to routine follow-up CT scans. Neither lymphadenectomy nor adjuvant radiotherapy appear to be useful procedures for preventing local recurrence after surgery for advanced tumours. Surgical excision of isolated local recurrence, whenever feasible, has been advocated as the best available option, but experience is rather limited, with only 11 patients in the largest series (Esrig *et al.* 1992).

Radiotherapy

Radiotherapy as the sole modality has no place in the treatment of renal adenocarcinoma because of low radiosensitivity. A number of randomized clinical trials performed on a significant number of patients (Finney 1973; van der Werf-Messing 1973; Juusela *et al.* 1977) have clearly demonstrated that postoperative radiation therapy as an adjuvant of radical nephrectomy has neither benefit nor bearing on survival or on local recurrence. Despite low radiosensitivity, some believe that radiotherapy should always be used postoperatively to minimize the risk of local recurrences when, at the time of surgery, the tumour extends beyond the kidney or there are firm presumptions of residual tumour after radical nephrectomy. However, it should be noted that, in addition to the null effects, postoperative irradiation is associated with an unacceptable rate of complications (Kjaer *et al.* 1987).

Preoperative radiotherapy may achieve a mass reduction in about 50 per cent of the cases, making feasible the surgical excision of otherwise inoperable tumours.

Radiotherapy may also be beneficial as an adjuvant of surgery in the treatment of selected solitary metastases (Maor *et al.* 1988), and in the control of severe pain and haemorrhage due to tumour growth.

Management of metastatic renal carcinoma

The prognosis for patients with clinically detectable distant metastases (stage IV) at presentation is poor. In this group of patients, which may account for up to 30 per cent of all newly diagnosed tumours (Riches 1964), the outcome is unpredictable and most will die within a few months as a result of disseminated disease. The choice of procedure is a matter of clinical experience.

Surgical approach

Radical nephrectomy in the presence of metastatic disease is a controversial issue, partial or total removal of the primary tumour is probably the best initial treatment. We believe that the increased mortality and morbidity and the extent of local spread, such that the complete excision of the primary tumour and the regional lymph nodes is not feasible, are not valid arguments against using this procedure in view of the benefits that can be obtained in terms of the prolongation of survival or improvement in the quality of life.

The rationale for nephrectomy in metastatic disease is the reduction of tumour burden which, in a few cases, may result in the partial or complete regression of distant metastases and enhance the efficacy of adjuvant immunotherapy or systemic chemotherapy. Nephrectomy is also beneficial when the patient develops severe symptoms attributable to the primary tumour, such as pain which cannot be controlled by opiates, prominent paraneoplastic syndromes, and gross life-threatening haematuria.

Embolization

Angiographic embolization of the renal artery and its branches has been proposed as a suitable alternative to nephrectomy in the management of metastatic disease. The infarction that follows embolization is believed to promote the release of tumour-specific antigens which increase the immune response of the patient.

A more effective approach seems to be the combination of angiographic embolization with nephrectomy, but the results of trials reported to date show that the mean survival times are quite similar to those from series where no treatment was given (Flanigan 1987). The best survival rates with this therapeutic modality appear to be for patients with solitary pulmonary metastases.

Chemotherapy

Renal cancer in the advanced stages is among those urological malignancies where the tumour is refractory to conventional chemotherapy. Experimental laboratory studies suggest that the lack of efficacy of cytotoxic agents is conditioned, in part, by enhanced expression of the multidrug resistance gene *MDR1* with overproduction of the plasma membrane P-glycoprotein 170 by the tumour cells (Fojo *et al.* 1987).

Early clinical trials demonstrated that vinblastine, CCNU, methyl-GAG, adriamycin, and hydroxyurea were the most effective single agents, with objective response rates ranging from 4–28 per cent (Child *et al.* 1983; Garnick 1983). Almost all the available cytotoxic agents have been assessed for advanced RCC, with rather disappointing results. In a recent review of 3502 patients and 72 different chemotherapeutic agents, Yagoda *et al.* (1993) estimated an overall objective response (complete response plus partial response) of only 5.6 per cent, with a 95 per cent confidence interval ranging from 4.8–6.4 per cent. The higher objective response rates are reported for regimens based on floxuridine, 5-fluorouracil, mytomicin C, suramin, vinblastine, and ifosfamide.

Circadian-based infusional chronotherapy with 5-fluour-2-deoxyuridine (floxuridine), the most active single agent, was first reported by Hrushesky *et al.* (1988); the total objective response rate was 37.5 per cent in 24 patients. This modality of chemotherapy allows greater doses of antitumoural drugs with diminished systemic toxicity with respect to continuous infusion or the use of constant rates. Combination of this drug with interferon results in a significant increase in response (Falcone *et al.* 1993).

5-Fluorouracil also shows some activity in RCC which is increased when it is combined with α-interferon (Murphy *et al.* 1992; Sella *et al.* 1992), interleukin-2 (IL-2) plus α-interferon, or IL-2 plus α-interferon plus mytomicin C.

Combination chemotherapy has no distinct advantages over single-agent chemotherapy. The combination of vinblastine and CCNU has increased objective responses rates from 10–19 per cent (Merrin *et al.* 1975; Kuhbock *et al.* 1988), with disease stabilization in up to 62 per cent. They all have been associated with poor or null objective responses. Stebbing *et al.* (2001), has recently reported significant objective partial responses and disease stabilization in a series of 22 patients with advanced tumours treated with a high-dose oral thalidomide regimen, a drug with proven suppressive effects against several cytokines, angiogenic, and growth factors.

A new therapeutic approach based on a combination of cytotoxic agents with drugs such as calcium-channel blockers or clamodulin inhibitors to block or turn off *MDR1* action has given poor preliminary results, but still leaves open the possibility that, in the near future, appropriate pharmacological intervention to reverse multidrug resistance might make renal cell tumours more amenable to chemotherapy. The combination of some chemotherapeutic agents with immunomodulators is another approach that should be studied more extensively since the available data, although limited, suggest a synergistic effect.

Hormone therapy

Experimental and clinical evidence suggests a possible role of steroid hormones in the induction of renal carcinoma. A number of studies have been undertaken to assess the existence of steroid receptors in both normal and tumourous kidney and to determine how this could be used in clinical applications.

Bojar *et al.* (1975) and Concolino *et al.* (1976) first reported the existence of oestrogen and progesterone receptors in normal renal tissue, and soon afterwards they were detected in up to 60 per cent of human renal cell tumours. Androgen receptors have also been detected in normal kidneys and renal cell tumours (Ghanadian *et al.* 1982; Corrales *et al.* 1984).

Preliminary studies (Concolino *et al.* 1978) suggested a greater sensitivity of renal carcinoma to treatment with progestogens in those patients with progesterone receptors in tumour cytosol. Responses obtained in different clinical trials have been generally inconsistent, and some authors have suggested that investigation of the hypothetical hormone dependence of human tumours and the futile attempts to develop hormone therapy have delayed active search for more effective agents.

We studied androgen receptors in 15 patients with renal carcinoma at different clinical stages to determine whether there was any association between the presence of these receptors and the effectiveness of adjuvant medroxyprogesterone therapy (Montero *et al.* 1987). Androgen receptors were detected in 60 per cent of the patients. The clinical outcome of eight patients with receptor levels well above 3 fmol/mg cytosol protein was good to excellent. Of the remaining seven patients, three had low to undetectable receptor levels and followed a downhill course, dying from metastatic disease within a few months. The patient with the highest level of androgen receptors exhibited a spectacular clinical recovery and regression of bone metastases after medroxyprogesterone therapy. This result and the observed trends suggest that medroxyprogesterone may have some value in the adjuvant therapy of renal carcinoma, particularly in those cases where normal to high levels of androgen receptors are detected.

Immunotherapy

The unexpected clinical behaviour of renal cancer strongly suggests that the immune mechanisms of the host participate in the growth of the primary tumour and the development of metastases (Bohm *et al.* 2001). A number of experimental studies of mice with murine renal adenocarcinoma and a strain of transplantable human RCC have demonstrated that the use of cytokines such as α-interferon, γ-interferon, IL-2, and tumour necrosis factor-α, either alone or in combination with radiotherapy, chemotherapy, phytochemicals, or immunostimulators, resulted in a significant inhibition of tumour growth or restitution of tumour-associated immunosuppression (van Dijk *et al.* 1994; Pavone *et al.* 2001). These cytokines have also shown the ability to restore natural killer cell activity and to obtain an adequate lymphokine-activated killer cytotoxicity in humans with advanced RCC (Feruglio *et al.* 1992). In view of these clinical and experimental data, various modalities of both active and adoptive immunotherapy have been tested in metastatic disease, but the results obtained so far are not as promising as expected on the basis of theory. The results obtained using different immunotherapy regimens for the most important series published in the literature are summarized in terms of complete response and partial response in Tables 5 and 6.

Specific immunotherapy

Activation of the host immune response with intradermal BCG injections, tumour cell vaccines, modified autologous tumour extracts, immune RNA, and dendritic cell-based vaccines has been investigated in a number of clinical trials with rather poor and discrepant responses, even for assessment of the same agent (Fowler 1986; Gitlitz *et al.* 2001). Therefore, this modality of immunotherapy should still be considered experimental and not an established procedure in the treatment of RCC.

It has been reported that active immunotherapy with attenuated vaccinia virus AS strain suppresses the growth of renal tumour cells without adverse effects (Arakawa *et al.* 1987). Flavone-8-acetic acid, an immunostimulator drug, has also been proposed as a possible candidate on the basis of its synergic effect with systemic natural killer cells against murine renal cancer (Wiltrout *et al.* 1988; Salup *et al.* 1992). Some authors have reported a significant increase in survival and objective regression of pulmonary metastases with specific immunotherapy using a soluble fraction of autologous tumour injected intradermally with PPD tuberculin or Candida antigen as adjuvant (Tykka *et al.* 1968).

Adoptive immunotherapy

The first attempts at adoptive immunotherapy were made using the technique of serotherapy. However, this was soon changed to the technique of adoptive immunotherapy with transfer factor and immune RNA extracted from lymphoid tissue.

Table 5 Results obtained for interferon-based treatment of advanced RCC

Reference	Regimen	No. of patients	PR	CR	PR + CR (%)
de Kernion *et al.* (1983)	HL-IFN-α	43	1	6	23
Umeda and Nijima (1986)	HLB-IFN-α	73	1	6	14
Umeda and Nijima (1986)	IFN-α 2a	108	2	13	14
Steineck *et al.* (1990)	IFN-α 2a	30	1	1	6
Umeda and Nijima (1986)	IFN-α 2b	45	1	7	18
Creagan *et al.* (1991)	IFN-α 2b	87	1	6	8
Kinney *et al.* (1990)	IFN-β	25	1	4	20
Garnick *et al.* (1988)	IFN-γ	41	1	3	10
Bruntsch *et al.* (1990)	IFN-γ	40	0	1	2
Heider *et al.* (1993)	IFN-γ	25	0	0	0
Hofmockel *et al.* (1993)	IFN-γ	24	1	0	4
Schornagel *et al.* (1989)	IFN-α + VBL	56	0	9	16
Neidhart *et al.* (1991)	IFN-α + VBL	83	3	4	8
Murphy *et al.* (1992)	IFN-α + 5-FU	14	0	0	0
Falcone *et al.* (1993)	IFN-α + FUDR	28	9	1	37

Abbreviations: IFN, interferon; PR, partial response; HL, human leucocyte; VBL, vinblastine; 5-FU, 5-fluorouracil; FUDR, floxuridine.

Another approach is based on the adoptive transfer of lymphokine-activated killer cells combined with recombinant IL-2, which is capable of mediating the regression of cancer in a variety of animal tumour models (Belldegrun *et al.* 1988). After the preliminary report by Rosenberg (1988) of more than 30 per cent of objective remissions in RCC, further clinical trials have found objective response rates ranging from 8 per cent (Mittelman *et al.* 1989) up to 50 per cent (Schoof *et al.* 1993). This combination therapy appears to be more effective in patients with pulmonary metastases, but the possibility of increasing the frequency of brain metastases by damaging the blood–brain barrier should be taken into account (Hayakawa 1992; Fujioka *et al.* 1994). The toxicity associated with lymphokine-activated killer cell therapy is reduced with the simultaneous administration of pentoxifylline and ciprofloxacin (Thompson *et al.* 1993).

Autolymphocyte therapy is a promising new modality of adoptive immunotherapy. The basis of this therapy is the activation of memory T cells in a two-step process. In the first step an autologous cytokine mixture is obtained from peripheral blood mononuclear cells incubated with a monoclonal antibody against the CD3 portion of the T-cell receptor. The second step involves the *ex vivo* activation of memory T cells by incubating peripheral blood mononuclear cells, collected from patients by pheresis, in a medium containing 25 per cent of the cytokine mixture, indomethacin, and cimetidine. These activated T cells are incubated for 5 days, irradiated with 50 rad of

Table 6 Results obtained for IL-2-based treatment of advanced RCC

Reference	Regimen	No. of patients	PR	CR	PR + CR (%)
Atkins et al. (1993)	IL-2 alone	28	3	0	11
Lissoni et al. (1993)	IL-2 alone	30	10	0	33
Lopez et al. (1993)	IL-2 alone	29	3	1	14
Rosenberg et al. (1994)	IL-2 alone	70	20	10	43
Faggiuolo et al. (1992)	IL-2 + IFN-α	23	2	3	22
Atkins et al. (1993)	IL-2 + IFN-α	71	8	4	17
Lipton et al. (1993)	IL-2 + IFN-α	31	7	6	42
Bergmann et al. (1993)	IL-2 + IFN-α	36	7	2	25
Escudier et al. (1993)	IL-2 + IFN-γ	33	7	0	21
Thompson et al. (1992)	IL-2 + LAK cells	42	10	4	33
Weiss et al. (1992)	IL-2 + LAK cells	94	11	5	17
Fujioka et al. (1994)	IL-2 + LAK cells	10	1	1	20
Sosman et al. (1993)	IL-2 + OKT3	29	3	0	10
Pomer et al. (1993)	IL-2 + IFN-α + ATV	40	6	5	28
Belldegrun et al. (1993)	IL-2 + IFN-α + TIL	11	0	3	27
Walther et al. (1993)	IL-2 + cytoreduction	93	11	4	16
Margolin et al. (1994)	IL-4	30	0	0	0

Abbreviations: IFN, interferon; LAK, lymphokine-activated killer; ATV, autologens tumour vaccine; TIL, tumour-infiltrating lymphocyte; IL-4, interleukin 4.

gamma radiation, and reinfused into the patient either alone or with concomitant administration of cimitidine as an immunoadjuvant to further inhibit suppressor T lymphocytes. The reinfusion procedure can be performed in the outpatient clinic. The exact mechanism of action of autolymphocyte therapy is unknown. It has been postulated that different lymphokines secreted by the activated T cells may inhibit tumour growth and that some of these cells may have a direct cytotoxic effect on the tumour cells. Published results regarding the use of autolymphocyte therapy in patients with metastatic RCC appear to demonstrate a twofold increase in survival times with the additional benefits of a satisfactory performance status and minimal toxicity, which in most cases are attributed to the adjuvant therapy with cimetidine (Sawczuk 1993).

Biological response modifiers

Interferons

The introduction of interferons as a variant of non-specific passive immunotherapy for the management of metastatic renal cancer provided some hope in the otherwise uncertain future of this group of patients. Human leucocytic interferon-α and human lymphoblastoid interferon-α have been clinically assessed, and show no significant differences with regard to the rate of objective remissions compared with recombinant interferons (Fujita and Fukushima 1992; Yamada et al. 1993).

An extensive review of the reported data suggests that in renal cell cancer maximal clinical responses (with about 14 per cent of overall objective remissions) are achieved with both lymphoblastoid and recombinant interferon-α preparations and with schedules employing doses between 10×10^6 and 20×10^6 IU/day (Krown 1987). The best response rates (40 per cent) are obtained in patients with lung metastases who are in good general condition. Results in patients with bone, brain, and liver metastases are generally poor.

Side-effects associated with interferon therapy are dose dependent and reversible when administration is discontinued. The most frequent (98 per cent) is an influenza-like syndrome with fever, chills, fatigue, and anorexia.

The results obtained are summarized in Table 5 in terms of percentage of complete and partial responses of the most significant phase I–II clinical trials employing interferon either alone or combined with chemotherapeutic agents.

The results reported by Umeda and Niijima (1986), who used three different interferon preparations administered in different schedules to a total of 226 patients with renal cell cancer, deserve special attention. These authors found that the parameters influencing the response rates included absence of prior chemotherapy or radiotherapy and radical or palliative nephrectomy. They also found that pulmonary metastases are more amenable to interferon therapy than metastases in other organs.

Combinations of interferons with other cytotoxic agents such as 5-fluorouracil, floxuridine, doxorubicin, cyclophosphamide, vinblastine, and cisplatinum have demonstrated synergic or additive effects in both human and animal tumour models (Balkwill 1985).

Interleukin-2

Since 1988, IL-2 has been assessed alone or in combination with α-interferon, lymphokine-activated killer cells, autologous tumour vaccines, tumour-infiltrating lymphocytes, tumour necrosis factor-α, OKT3 and medroxyprogesterone for the treatment of metastatic RCC. (Table 6). The reported results suggest that the best response rates are obtained with regimens that combine IL-2 with α-interferon or with lymphokine-activated killer cells.

Side-effects associated with IL-2 depend upon the dose, the schedule, and the route of administration, being greatest after bolus injection and least severe when it is given subcutaneously (Heinzer et al. 2001; Pavone et al. 2001).

Prognostic factors

In most of the published series, tumour stage is considered to be the most important single independent prognostic factor in determining survival (Dal Bianco et al. 1988; Thrasher and Paulson 1993). In addition to clinical stage, many other factors have been suggested to have a negative influence on survival. These include age, gender, intrinsic morphological features of the original tumour (such as number, location, and size), histological grade, and the type and histological pattern of the individual tumour cells. Some clinical symptoms (weight loss, fever, hepatic dysfunction, erythrocyte sedimentation rate, and hypertension) have also been proposed as features indicating poor prognosis (Sene *et al.* 1992). DNA flow cytometry has limited value as a single prognostic factor owing to tumour heterogeneity (Lanigan *et al.* 1993; Nakano *et al.* 1993). Some morphometric features of the tumour cells have also been found to correlate with survival (Eskelinen *et al.* 1993; Ozer *et al.* 2002).

In this section, we present the results of a preliminary analysis of the influence of both nuclear morphometry parameters and clinical prognostic factors on the probability of survival in a total of 64 patients with renal cell cancer who underwent nephrectomy in our department (Fig. 15). Both, survival and morphometric analysis, were performed using custom programs developed locally (Urrutia 2001; Urrutia *et al.* 2001).[2]

The estimated value for the regression parameters and the results of a global chi-square test for the statistical significance of five different covariates included in a multivariate survival model are summarized in Table 7. These covariates were selected from 10 different size and shape morphometric descriptors and five clinical prognostic factors. Morphometric parameters include the mean and SD of nuclear area, perimeter, minor and major axis, orientation angle, form factor, roundness, ellipticity, compacticity, and nucelar contour index. Clinical prognostic factors include age, gender, histological grade, histological pattern, stage and paraneoplasic syndromes.

We have not found any association of survival with the nuclear area in both univariate and multivariate analysis. This parameter is considered by many authors as the best predictor in terms of recurrence (Pound *et al.* 1993), progression, and survival (Ruiz *et al.* 1995). Delahunt (1994) has also reported the lack of correlation of survival with nuclear area in a series of 178 patients with a follow-up period of 29 years. The observed discrepancies among the studies so far published on nuclear morphometry in renal cell cancer might well be related to a lack of normalization of this method and the known lack of consensus among pathologists regarding the area of the tumour specimen that should be evaluated and submitted to analysis. Collinearity among the different shape parameters, the high intraobserver and interobserver variability when assessing the tumour grade and the lack of experience or knowledge for modelling the risk with complex survival regression models by clinicians would also account for these discrepancies.

Among the clinical and histological parameters evaluted in this study, only the age, clinical stage, and the presence of paraneoplasic syndromes at the time of diagnosis were significantly correlated with survival in a multivariate model. As expected, neither the histological degree nor the histological pattern of the tumour cells seems to have any bearing on survival. Age and gender also do not have a significant influence on prognosis; similar results have been reported by other authors (Flocks and Kadesky 1958; Neves *et al.* 1988).

As can be deduced from Table 7, the biological agressiveness of renal cell tumours seems to depend more on the alterations in the nuclear shape than its size. Another relevant finding of this study is that the morphometric parameters can be used as independent predictors of survival, which is demonstrated by the stability of the

[2] A free copy of both programs can be obtained by e-mail request to urrutia@usal.es

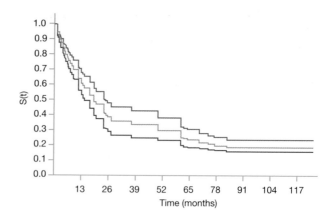

Fig. 15 Cumulative survival function with 95% confidence intervals estimated with a parametric exponential model.

Table 7 Statistical results from a multivariate survival model

Variable	Model 1	Model 2	Model 3
PerimSD	0.960	0.977	1.076
LengthMaxSD	−3.220	−3.274	−0.049
EllipMean	−0.059	−0.060	−0.049
CompMean	106.333	107.095	−87.145
Stage	*	*	−0.286
Paraneoplasic syndrome	*	*	−0.706
Log ML	−96.618	−96.614	−90.363
Prob	0.0001	0.0002	<0.0001
LRT(p)	<0.005	NS	0.001

sign and values of the regression coefficients when the clinical parameters are incorporated in the model.

References

Alferez, C. and Diaz-Alferez, F. Embolizacion en urologia. In *Ponencia al 45 Congreso Nacional de Urologia* (ed. Asociacion Española de Urologia), pp. 154–161. Madrid: ENE Ediciones, 1980.

Arakawa, S., Jr., Hammami, G., Umelu, K., Kamidono, S., Ishigami, J., and Arakawa, S. (1987). Clinical trial of attenuated vaccinia virus AS strain in the treatment of advanced adenocarcinoma. *Journal of Cancer Research and Clinical Oncology* **113**, 95–98.

Atkins, M. B. *et al.* (1993). Randomized phase II trial of high-dose interleukin-2 either alone or in combination with interferon alpha-2b in advanced renal cell carcinoma. *Journal of Clinical Oncology* **11**, 661–670.

Auger, M., Katz, R. L., Sella, A., Ordonez, N. G., Lawrence, D. D., and Ro, J. Y. (1993). Fine-needle aspiration cytology of sarcomatoid renal cell carcinoma: a morphologic and immunocytochemical study of 15 cases. *Diagnostic Cytopathology* **9**, 46–51.

Balkwill, F. R. (1985). Antitumor effects of interferon in animals. *Interferon* **4**, 23–45.

Bell, E. T. *Renal Diseases* 2nd edn. Philadelphia, PA: Lea and Febiger, 1950.

Belldegrun, A., Uppenkamp, I., and Rosenberg, S. A. (1988). Antitumor rectivity of human lymphokine activated killer (LAK) cells against fresh and cultured preparations of renal cell cancer. *Journal of Urology* **139**, 150–155.

Belldegrun, A. *et al.* (1993). Interferon-alpha primed tumor-infiltrating lymphocytes combined with interleukin-2 and interferon-alpha as therapy for metastatic renal cell carcinoma. *Journal of Urology* **150**, 1384–1390.

Bergmann, L. *et al.* (1993). Daily alternating administration of high-dose alpha-2b-interferon and interleukin-2 bolus infusion in metastatic renal cell cancer. A phase II study. *Cancer* **72**, 1733–1742.

Bird, D. J., Semple, J. P., and Seiler, M. W. (1991). Sarcomatoid renal cell carcinoma metastatic to the heart: report of a case. *Ultrastructural Pathology* **15**, 361–366.

Bohm, M., Ittenson, A., Philipp, C., Rohl, F. W., Ansroge, S., and Allhoff, E. P. (2001). Complex perioperative immuno-dysfunction in patients with renal cell carcinoma. *Journal of Urology* **3**, 831–836.

Bojar, H., Balzer, K., Dreyfurst, R., and Staib, W. (1975). Identification and partial characterization of specific estrogen-binding components in human kidney. *Journal of Clinical Chemistry and Clinical Biochemistry* **14**, 515–520.

Brinton, L. F. (1960). Hypernephroma: familial occurrence in one family. *Journal of Internal Medicine* **173**, 888–890.

Brkovic, D., Riedasch, G., Waldherr, R., Rohl, L., and Staehler, G. (1994). Lokale Rezidive nach organerhaltender Nierentumorchirurgie. *Urologe, Ausgabe A* **33**, 104–109.

Bruntsch, U. *et al.* (1990). Phase II study of recombinant human interferon-gamma in metastatic renal cell carcinoma. *Journal of Biologic Response Modifiers* **9**, 335–338.

Campbell, S. C., Novick, A. C., Streem, S. B., Klein, E., and Licht, M. (1994). Complications of nephron sparing surgery for renal tumors. *Journal of Urology* **151**, 1177–1180.

Casalone, R. *et al.* (1992). Significance of the clonal and sporadic chromosome abnormalities in non-neoplastic renal tissue. *Human Genetics* **90**, 71–78.

Child, J. A., Stoter, G., Fossa, S. D., Bono, A. V., de Pauw, M., and the EORTC Urological Group. Chemotherapy of advanced renal cell carcinoma: results of treatment with methyl-glyoxal-bis-guanylhydrazone (methyl-GAG): an EORTC study. In *Cancer of the Prostate and Kidney* (ed. M. Pavone-Macaluso and J. Smith), pp. 693–697. New York. Plenum Press, 1983.

Concolino, G., Marocchi, A., Conti, C., Tenaglia, R., Di Silverio, F., and Conti, C. (1976). Human kidney steroid receptors. *Journal of Steroid Biochemistry* **7**, 831–835.

Concolino, G., Marocchi, A., Conti, C., Tenaglia, R., Di Silverio, F., and Bracci, U. (1978). Human renal carcinoma as a hormone-dependent tumour. *Cancer Research* **38**, 4340–4344.

Corrales, J. K., Pastor, I., Garcia, L. C., Buitrago, J. M., Mercado, F., and Miralles, J. M. (1984). Receptores androgenicos en el riñon humano. Efectos de los niveles circulantes de andro-genos. *Endocrinologia* **71**, 106.

Couillard, D. R. and deVere White, R. W. (1993). Surgery of renal cell carcinoma. *Urologic Clinics of North America* **20**, 263–275.

Creagan, E. T. *et al.* (1991). A randomized prospective assessment of recombinant leukocyte and human interferon with or without aspirin in advanced renal adenocarcinoma. *Journal of Clinical Oncology* **9**, 2104–2109.

Dal Bianco, M., Artibani, W., Bassi, P. F., Pescatori, E., and Pagano, F. (1988). Prognostic factors in renal cell carcinoma. *European Urology* **15**, 73–76.

deKernion, J. B., Srana, J. B., Figlin, R., Lindner, A., and Smith, R. B. (1983). The treatment of renal cell carcinoma with human leukocyte alpha-interferon. *Journal of Urology* **130**, 1063–1066.

Delahunt, B., Becker, R. L., Bethwaite, P. B., and Ribas, J. L. (1994). Computerized nuclear morphometry and survival in renal cell carcinoma: comparison with other prognostic indicators. *Pathology* **26**, 353–358.

DeLong, W., Grignon, D. J., Eberwein, P., Shum, D. T., and Wyatt, J. K. (1993). Sarcomatoid renal cell carcinoma. An immunohistochemical study of 18 cases. *Archives of Pathology and Laboratory Medicine* **117**, 636–640.

De Reijke, T. M., Schlatmann, T. J., and Dabhoiwala, N. F. (1987). Adenocarcinoma of the kidney in childhood. *Urologia Internationalis* **42**, 220–223.

Elinder, C. G. Normal values for cadmium in human tissues, blood and urine in different countries. In *Cadmium and Health: A Toxicological and Epidemiological Appraisal* Vol. 1 (ed. L. Friberg, C. G. Elinder, T. Kjellstrom, and G. F. Nordberg), pp. 81–102. Boca Raton, FL: CRC Press, 1985.

Escudier, B. *et al.* (1993). Combination of interleukin-2 and gamma interferon in metastatic renal cell carcinoma. *European Journal of Cancer* **29**, 724–728.

Eskelinen, M., Lipponen, P., Aitto-Oja, L., Hall, O., and Syrjanen, K. (1993). The value of histoquantitative measurements in prognostic assessment of renal adenocarcinoma. *International Journal of Cancer* **55**, 547–554.

Esrig, D. *et al.* (1992). Experience with fossa recurrence of renal cell carcinoma. *Journal of Urology* **147**, 1491–1494.

Faggiuolo, R. *et al.* (1992). Sc interleukin-2 (rIL2) and alpha interferon (rIFN alpha) in patients with metastatic renal cell cancer (RCC): a phase II study (meeting abstract). *Annals of Oncology* **3**, 140.

Falcone, A. *et al.* (1993). Floxuridine (FUDR) + alpha-2b-interferon (IFN) in metastatic renal carcinoma (MRC): a phase II study (meeting abstract). *Proceedings of the Annual Meeting of the American Society of Clinical Oncology* **12**, A712.

Farrow, G. M., Harrison, E. G., Jr., Utz, D. C., and Jones, D. R. (1968). Renal angiomyolipoma. A clinicopathologic study of 32 cases. *Cancer* **22**, 564–570.

Feruglio, C. *et al.* (1992). Cytotoxic *in vitro* function in patients with metastatic renal cell carcinoma before and after alpha-2b interferon therapy. Effects of activation with recombinant interleukin-2. *Cancer* **69**, 2525–2531.

Finney, R. (1973). An evaluation of postoperative radiotherapy in hypernephroma treatment—a clinical trial. *Cancer* **32**, 1332–1340.

Flanigan, R. C. (1987). The failure of infarction and/or nephrectomy in stage IV renal cancer to influence survival or metastatic regression. *Urologic Clinics of North America* **14**, 757–762.

Fleming, S. and Lewi, H. J. E. (1986). Collecting duct carcinoma of the kidney. *Histopathology* **10**, 1131–1141.

Flocks, R. H. and Kadesky, M. C. (1958). Malignant neoplasms of the kidney, and analysis of 353 patients followed five years or more. *Journal of Urology* **79**, 196–201.

Fojo, A. T., Shen, D. W., Wickley, L. A., Pastan, I., and Gottesman, M. M. (1987). Intrinsic drug resistance in human kidney cancer is associated with expression of a human multidrug-resistance gene. *Journal of Clinical Oncology* **5**, 1922–1927.

Foster, K. *et al.* (1994). Molecular genetic investigation of sporadic renal cell carcinoma: analysis of allele loss on chromosomes 3p, 5q,11p, 17 and 22. *British Journal of Cancer* **69**, 230–240.

Fowler, J. E. (1986). Failure of immunotherapy for metastatic renal cell carcinoma. *Journal of Urology* **135**, 22–25.

Fujioka, T., Nomura, K., Hasegawa, M., Ishikura, K., and Kubo, T. (1994). Combination of lymphokine-activated killer cells and interleukin-2 in treating metastatic renal cell carcinoma. *British Journal of Urology* **73**, 23–31.

Fujita, T. and Fukushima, M. (1992). Interferon therapy for advanced renal cell carcinoma. *Hinyokika Kiyo—Acta Urologica Japonica* **38**, 1293–1298.

Garnick, M. B. Renal cell carcinoma—diagnostic work up and natural history. In *Urologic Cancer* (ed. M. B. Garnick and J. P. Richie), pp. 41–50. New York: Plenum Press, 1983.

Garnick, M. B., Reich, S. D., Maxwell, B., Coval-Goldsmith, S., Richie, J. P., and Rudnick, S. A. (1988). Phase I/II study of recombinant interferon gamma in advanced renal cell carcinoma. *Journal of Urology* **139**, 251–255.

Gerharz, C. D., Moll, R., Storkel, S., Ramp, U., Thoenes, W., and Gabbert, H. E. (1993). Ultrastructural appearance and cytoskeletal architecture of the clear, chromophilic, and chromophobe types of human renal cell carcinoma *in vitro*. *American Journal of Pathology* **142**, 851–859.

Ghanadian, R., Auf, G., Williams, G., and Coleman, P. M. (1982). Steroid receptors in kidney tumours. *Progress in Clinical and Biological Research* **100**, 245–254.

Giuliani, L., Gilberti, C., Martorana, G., Isotta, A., and Neumaier, C. E. (1987). Value of computerized tomography and ultrasonography in the preoperative diagnosis of renal cell carcinoma extending into the inferior vana cava. *European Urology* **13**, 26–30.

Gnarra, J. R. *et al.* (1993). Molecular genetic studies of sporadic and and familial renal cell carcinoma. *Urologic Clinics of North America* **20**, 207–216.

Gomez Zancajo, V. R. (1987). *Valor de la ultrasonografia en el diganostico y seguimiento de las masas renales*. Unpublished D Phil. Thesis, University of Salamanca, Spain.

Grannof, A. (1973). Herpes virus and the Lucke tumour. *Cancer Research* **33**, 1431–1433.

Griffin, J. P., Hughes, G. V., and Peeling, W. B. (1967). A survey of the familial incidence of adenocarcinoma of the kidney. *British Journal of Urology* **39**, 63–66.

Grignon, D. J., McIsaac, G. P., Armstrong, R. F., and Wyatt, J. K. (1988). Primary rhabdomyosarcoma of the kidney. A light microscope, immunohistochemical and electron microscope study. *Cancer* **62**, 2027–2032.

Gtlitz, B. J., Belldegrun, A. S., and Figlin, R. A. (2001). Vaccine and gene therapy of renal cell carcinoma. *Seminars in Urology and Oncology* **2**, 141–147.

Hattery, R. R., Williamson, B., Jr., and Hartman, G. M. (1976). Urinary tract tomography. *Radiological Clinics of North America* **14**, 23–49.

Hayakawa, M. (1992). Lymphokine-activated killer (LAK) therapy for advanced renal cell carcinoma: clinical study on arterial LAK therapy and experimental study on LAK cell activity. *Hinyokika Kiyo—Acta Urologica Japonica* **38**, 1311–1318.

Heider, A., Moritz, T., Elmaagli, A., Kress, M., Seeber, S., and Niederle, N. (1993). Interferon (IFN) gamma in the treatment of metastatic renal cell carcinoma. *Proceedings of the Annual Meeting of the American Society of Clinical Oncology* **12**, A743.

Heinzer, H., Huland, E., and Huland, H. (2001). Systemic chemotherapy and chemoimmunotherapy for metastatic renal cell cancer. *World Journal of Urology* **2**, 111–119.

Henn, W., Zwergel, T., Wullich, B., Thonnes, M., Zang, K. D., and Seitz, G. (1993). Bilateral multicentric papillary renal tumors with heteroclonal origin based on tissue-specific karyotype instability. *Cancer* **72**, 1315–1318.

Hofmockel, G., Wirth, M. P., Heimbach, D., and Frohmuller, H. G. (1993). Results of low dosage cyclic interferon-gamma therapy of metastatic renal cell carcinoma. *Urology* **32**, 290–294.

Horesovsky, G., Recio, L., Everitt, J., Goldsworthy, T., Wolf, D., and Walker, C. (1993). Low frequency of p53 mutations in spontaneous and dimethylnitrosamine-induced renal tumors in Eker rats (meeting abstract). *Proceedings of the Annual Meeting of the American Association for Cancer Research* **34**, A654.

Hrushesky, W. J., von Roemeling, R., Fraley, E. E., and Rabatin, J. T. (1988). Circadian-based infusional chrono-chemotherapy control of progressive metastatic renal cell carcinoma. *Seminars in Surgical Oncology* **4**, 110–115.

Hughson, M. D., Johnson, L. D., Silva, F. G., and Kovacs, G. (1993). Nonpapillary and papillary renal cell carcinoma: a cytogenetic and phenotypic study. *Modern Pathology* **6**, 449–456.

Ishikawa, I. (1993). Renal cell carcinoma in chronic haemodialysis patients—a 1990 questionnaire in Japan. *Kidney International* **41** (Suppl.), 167–169.

Juusela, H., Malmio, K., Alfthan, O., and Oravisto, K. J. (1977). Preoperative irradiation in the treatment of renal adenocarcinoma. *Scandinavian Journal of Urology and Nephrology* **11**, 277–281.

Kaplan, S., Ekici, S., Dogan, R., Demircin, M., Ozen, H., and Pasouglu, I. (2002). Surgical management of renal cell carcinoma with inferior vena cava tumor thrombus. *American Journal of Surgery* **3**, 292–299.

Karstaedt, N., McCullough, D. L., Wolfman, N. T., and Dyer, R. B. (1986). Magnetic resonance imaging of the renal mass. *Journal of Urology* **136**, 566–570.

Kinney, P. *et al.* (1990). Phase II trial of interferon-beta serine in metastatic renal cell carcinoma. *Journal of Clinical Oncology* **8**, 881–885.

Kjaer, M. (1987). The treatment and prognosis of patients with renal adenocarinoma with solitary metastases. 10 year survival results. *International Journal of Radiation, Oncology, Biology, Physics* **13**, 619–621.

Kjaer, M., Frederiksen, P. L., and Engelholm, S. A. (1987). Postoperative radiotherapy in stage II and III renal adenocarcinoma. A randomized trial by the Copenhagen Renal Cancer Study Group. *International Journal of Radiation, Oncology, Biology, Physics* **13**, 665–672.

Kohno, T., Sekine, T., Tobisu, K., Oshimura, M., and Yokota, J. (1993). Chromosome 3p deletion in a renal cell carcinoma cell line established from a patient with von Hippel–Lindau disease. *Japanese Journal of Clinical Oncology* **23**, 226–231.

Konchanin, R. P., Cho, J. K., and Grossman, H. B. (1987). Preoperative devascularization of advanced renal adenocarcinoma using a sclerosing agent. *Journal of Urology* **137**, 199–201.

Kovacs, G. and Brusa, P. (1989). Clonal chromosome aberrations in normal kidney tissue from patients with renal cell carcinoma. *Cancer Genetics and Cytogenetics* **37**, 289–290.

Kovacs, A., Storkel, S., Thoenes, W., and Kovacs, G. (1992). Mitochondrial and chromosomal DNA alterations in human chromphobe renal cell carcinomas. *Journal of Pathology* **167**, 273–277.

Kreiger, N., Marret, L. D., Dodds, L., Hilditch, S., and Darlington, G. A. (1993). Risk factor for renal cell carcinoma: results of a population-based case–control study. *Cancer Causes and Control* **4**, 101–110.

Krown, S. E. (1987). Interferon treatment of renal cell carcinoma: current status and future prospects. *Cancer* **59**, 647–678.

Kuhbock, J. (1988). Survey of chemotherapy of metastatic renal cancer. *Seminars in Surgical Oncology* **4**, 87–90.

Kuhbock, J., Potzi, P., and Madaras, T. (1988). Palliative and adjuvant chemotherapy of metastatic renal cancer. *Seminars in Surgical Oncology* **4**, 116–123.

Lanigan, D., McLean, P. A., Murphy, D. M., Donovan, M. G., Curran, B., and Leader, M. (1993). Ploidy and prognosis in renal carcinoma. *British Journal of Urology* **71**, 21–24.

Leiman, G., Markowitz, S., Veiga-Ferreira, M. M., and Margolius, K. A. (1986). Renal adenocarcinoma presenting with bilateral metastases to Bartholin's glands: primary diagnosis by aspiration cytology. *Diagnostic Cytopathology* **2**, 252–255.

Lewi, H. J. E., Alexander, C. A., and Fleming, S. (1986). Renal oncocytoma. *British Journal of Urology* **58**, 12–15.

Li, F. P., Decker, H. J., Zbar, B., Stanton, V. P., Jr., Kovacs, G., and Seizinger, B. R. (1993). Clinical and genetic studies of renal cell carcinomas in a family with a constitutional chromosome 3; 8 translocation. *Annals of Internal Medicine* **118**, 106–111.

Lieber, M. M. Management of renal cell carcinoma. In *Urological Cancer* (ed. D. G. Skinner), pp. 425–434. New York: Grune and Stratton, 1983.

Lieber, M. M. (1993). Renal oncocytoma. *Urologic Clinics of North America* **20**, 355–359.

Lieber, M. M., Tomera, K. M., and Farrow, G. M. (1981). Renal oncocytoma. *Journal of Urology* **125**, 481–485.

Lipton, A. *et al.* (1993). Interleukin-2 and interferon-alpha-2a outpatient therapy for metastatic renal cell carcinoma. *Journal of Immunotherapy* **13**, 122–129.

Lissoni, P. *et al.* (1993). Immunoterapia con basse dosi di interleuchina-2 per via sottocutanea nel carcinoma renale metastatico. *Archivio Italiano Di Urologia, Andrologia* **65**, 123–128.

Lopez, M. *et al.* (1993). Phase II study of continuous intravenous infusion of recombinant interleukin-2 in patients with advanced renal cell carcinoma. *Annals of Oncology* **4**, 689–691.

Maclure, M. (1987). Asbestos and renal adenocarcinoma: a case–control study. *Environmental Research* **42**, 353–361.

Maor, M. H., Frias, A. E., and Oswald, M. J. (1988). Palliative radiotherapy for brain metastases in renal carcinoma. *Cancer* **62**, 1912–1917.

Margolin, K. *et al.* (1994). Phase II studies of recombinant human interleukin-4 in advanced renal cancer and malignant melanoma. *Journal of Immunotherapy with Emphasis on Tumor Immunology* **15**, 147–153.

Matsumoto, T. *et al.* (1992). Papillary renal cell carcinoma. Report of two cases. *Acta Pathologica Japonica* **42**, 298–303.

Mellemgaard, A., Engholm, G., McLaughlin, J. K., and Olsen, J. H. (1994). Risk factors for renal-cell carcinoma in Denmark III. Role of weight, physical activity, and reproductive factors. *International Journal of Cancer* **56**, 66–71.

Meloni, A. M., Dobbs, R. M., Pontes, J. E., and Sandberg, A. A. (1993). Translocation (X;1) in papillary renal cell carcinoma. A new cytogenetic subtype. *Cancer Genetics and Cytogenetics* **65**, 1–6.

Merrin, C., Mittleman, A., Fanous, A., Wajsman, Z., and Murphy, G. P. (1975). Chemotherapy of advanced renal cell carcinoma with vinblastine and CCNU. *Journal of Urology* **113**, 21–23.

Mittelman, A. *et al.* (1989). Treatment of patients with advanced cancer using multiple long-term cultured lymphokine-activated killer (LAK) cell infusions and recombinant human interleukin-2. *Journal of Biologic Response Modifiers* **8**, 468–478.

Montero, J., Urrutia Avisrror, M., and Corrales, J. Renal malignancies in the elderly. In *Renal Function and Diseases in the Elderly* (ed. J. Macias and S. Cameron), pp. 400–431. London: Butterworth, 1987.

Mortensen, H. (1948). Transthoracic nephrectomy. *Journal of Urology* **113**, 21–23.

Murphy, B. R., Rynard, S. M., Einhorn, L. H., and Loehrer, P. J. (1992). A phase II trial of interferon alpha-2a plus fluorouracil in advanced renal cell carcinoma. A Hoosier Oncology Group study. *Investigational New Drugs* **10**, 225–230.

Nakano, E., Kondoh, M., Okatani, K., Seguchi, T., and Sugao, H. (1993). Flow cytometric analysis of nuclear DNA content of renal cell carcinoma correlated with histologic and clinical features. *Cancer* **72**, 1319–1323.

Neidhart, J. A. *et al.* (1991). Vinblastine fails to improve response of renal cell cancer to interferon alpha n-1: high response rate in patients with pulmonary metastatses. *Journal of Clinical Oncology* **9**, 832–837.

Neves, R. J., Zincke, H., and Taylor, W. F. (1988). Metastatic renal cell cancer and radical nephrectomy, identification of prognostic factors and patient survival. *Journal of Urology* **139**, 1173–1176.

Novick, A. C. (1987). Partial nephrectomy fo renal cell carcinoma. *Urologic Clinics of North America* **14**, 419–433.

Novick, A. C., Steward, B. H., Straffon, R. A., and Banowsky, L. H. (1977). Partial nephrectomy in the treatment of renal adenocarcinoma. *Journal of Urology* **118**, 932–936.

O'Dea, M. J., Zincke, H., Utz, D. C., and Bernatz, P. E. (1978). The treatment of renal cell carcinoma with solitary metastases. *Journal of Urology* **120**, 540–542.

Ozer, E., Yorukoglu, K., Sagol, O., Mungan, U., Demirel, T., Tuzel, E., and Kirkali, Z. (2002). Prognostic significance of nuclear morphometry in renal cell carcinoma. *British Journal of Urology International* **90** (1), 20–25.

Paganini-Hill, A., Glazer, E., Henderson, B. E., and Ross, R. K. (1980). Cause-specific mortality among newspaper web pressman. *Journal of Occupational Medicine* **22**, 542–544.

Paganini-Hill, A., Ross, R. K., and Henderson, B. E. Epidemiology of kidney cancer. In *Urological Cancer* (ed. D. G. Skinner), pp. 383–407. New York: Grune and Stratton, 1983.

Pavone, L., Andrulli, S., Santi, R., Majori, M., and Buzio, C. (2001). Long-term tratment with low doses of interleukin-2 and interpheron-alpha: immunological effects in advanced renal cancer. *Cancer Immunology and Immunotherapy* **2**, 82–86.

Pomer, S., Schuth, R., Schirrmacher, V., and Staehler, G. (1993). Vaccination with modified autologous tumor material and rIL-2/rIFN for treatment of advanced renal cell carcinoma. *Abstracts of 2nd International Congress on Biological Response Modifiers 29–31 January 1993, San Diego, CA*, p. 68.

Pound, C. R., Partin, A. W., Epstein, J. I., Simons, J. W., and Marshall, F. F. (1993). Nuclear morphometry accurately predicts recurrence in clinically localized renal cell carcinoma.*Urology* **42**, 243–248.

Presti, J. C., Cordon-Cardo, C., Jhanwar, S. C., Fair, W. R., and Reuter, V. E. (1992). Clinicopathological correlation of molecular genetic alterations in renal tumors (meeting abstract). *Proceedings of the Annual Meeting of the American Association for Cancer Research* **33**, A2255.

Presti, J. C., Jr., Reuter, V. E., Cordon-Cardo, C., Mazumdar, M., Fair, W. R., and Jhanwar, S. C. (1993). Allelic deletion in renal tumors: histopathological correlations. *Cancer Research* **53**, 5780–5783.

Rainwater, L. M., Hosaka, Y., Farrow, G. M., and Lieberer, M. M. (1987). Well differentiated clear cell renal carcinoma, significance of nuclear deoxyribonucleic acid patterns studied by flow cytometry. *Journal of Urology* **137**, 15–20.

Rauschmeier, H., Hofstadter, F., and Jakse, G. Prognostic relevance of cytologic grading in metastatic renal cell carcinoma. In *Cancer of the Prostate and Kidney* (ed. M. Pavone-Macaluso and J. Smith), pp. 587–593. New York: Plenum Press, 1983.

Reiter, R. E., Anglard, P., Liu, S., Gnarra, J. R., and Linehan, W. M. (1993). Chromosome 17p deletions and p53 mutations in renal cell carcinoma. *Cancer Research* **53**, 3092–3097.

Riches, E. W. Monographs on neoplastic disease. In *Tumours of the Kidney and Ureter* (ed. E. W. Riches), pp. 124–134. Baltimore, MD: Williams and Wilkins, 1964.

Robson, C. J., Churchill, B. M., and Anderson, W. (1969). The results of radical nephrectomy for renal cell carcinoma. *Journal of Urology* **101**, 297–301.

Rosenberg, S. A. (1988). The development of new immunotherapies for the treatment of cancer using interleukin-2. A review. *Annals of Surgery* **208**, 121–135.

Rosenberg, S. A. *et al.* (1994). Treatment of 283 consecutive patients with metastatic melanoma or renal cell cancer using high-dose bolus interleukin-2. *Journal of the American Medical Association* **271**, 907–913.

Ruiz, J. L., Hernandez, M., Martinez, J., Vera, C., and Jimenez, J. F. (1995). Value of morphometry as an independent prognostic factor in renal cell carcinoma. *European Urology* **27**, 54–57.

Salup, R. R., Sicker, D. C., Wolmark, N., Herberman, R. B., and Hakala, T. R. (1992). Chemo-immunotherapy of metastatic murine renal cell carcinoma using flavone acetic acid and interleukin 2. *Journal of Urology* **147**, 1120–1123.

Sawczuk, I. S. (1993). Autolymphocyte therapy in the treatment of metastatic renal cell carcinoma. *Urologic Clinics of North America* **20**, 297–301.

Saya, H. *et al.* (1991). Detection of iatragenic loss of heterozygosity in the p53 gene in human cancers by using PCR-RFLP method (meeting abstract). *Proceedings of the Annual Meeting of the American Association for Cancer Research* **32**, A1783.

Schoof, D. D., Terashima, Y., Batter, S., Douville, L., Richie, J. P., and Eberlein, T. J. (1993). Survival characteristics of metastatic renal cell carcinoma patients treated with lymphokine-activated killer cells plus interleukin-2. *Urology* **41**, 534–539.

Schornagel, J. H. *et al.* (1989). Phase II study of recombinant interferon alpha-2a and vinblastine in advanced renal cell carcinoma. *Journal of Urology* **142**, 253–256.

Sella, A. *et al.* (1992). Phase I study of simultaneously administered recombinant human interleukin-2 (IL-2) with metastatic renal cell cancer (meeting abstract). *Proceedings of the Annual Meeting of the American Association for Cancer Research* **33**, A1597.

Sempronj, A. and Morelli, E. (1939). Carcinoma of the kidney in rats treated with beta-anthraquinoline. *American Journal of Cancer* **35**, 534–537.

Sene, A. P., Hunt, L., McMahon, R. F., and Carroll, R. N. (1992). Renal carcinoma in patients undergoing nephrectomy: analysis of survival and prognostic factors. *British Journal of Urology* **70**, 125–134.

Sinke, R. J. *et al.* (1993). Localization of X chromosome short arm markers relative to synovial sarcoma- and renal adenocarcinoma-associated translocation breakpoints. *Human Genetics* **92**, 305–308.

Sosman, J. A. *et al.* (1993). Phase IB clinical trial of anti-CD3 followed by high-dose bolus interleukin-2 in patients with metastatic melanoma and advanced renal cell carcinoma: clinical and immunologic effects. *Journal of Clinical Oncology* **11**, 1496–1505.

Staehler, G., Drehmer, I., and Pomer, S. (1994). Tumorbefall der Vena cava beim Nierenzellkarzinom. Operationstechnik, Ergebnisse und Prognose. *Urologe, Ausgabe A* **33**, 116–121.

Stebbing, J. et al. (2001). The treatment of advanced renal cell cancer with high-dose oral thalidomide. *British Journal of Cancer* **7**, 953–958.

Steineck, G. et al. (1990). Recombinant leukocyte interferon alpha 2a and Medroxyprogesterone in advanced renal cell carcinoma: a randomized trial. *Acta Oncologica* **29**, 155–162.

Sugao, H. et al. (1992). Cytogenetics of tumor cells from patients witn non-familial renal cell carcinoma. *Urologia Internationalis* **48**, 138–143.

Suijkerbuijk, R. F. et al. (1993). Identification of a yeast artificial chromosome that spans the human papillary renal cell carcinoma-associated t(X;1) breakpoint in Xp11.2. *Cancer Genetics and Cytogenetics* **71**, 164–169.

Suzuki, Y. and Tamura, G. (1993). Mutations of the p53 gene in carcinomas of the urinary system. *Acta Pathologica Japonica* **43**, 745–750.

Tetu, B., Ro, J. Y., Ayala, A. G., Ordoñez, N. G., and Johnson, D. E. (1987). Small cell carcinoma of the kidney. A clinicopathologic, immunohisto-chemical, and ultrastructural study. *Cancer* **60**, 1809–1814.

Thoenes, W., Storkel, S. T., and Rumpelt, H. J. (1986). Histopathology of renal cell tumours (adenomas, oncocytomas and carcinomas). The basic histo-logical and histopathological elements and their use for diagnosis. *Pathological Research and Practice* **181**, 125–143.

Thompson, J. A., Bianco, J., Benyunes, M., Neubauer, M., and Fefer, A. (1993). Pentoxifylline (PTX) and ciprofloxacin (Cipro) reduce the toxicity of high-dose continuous infusion (CIV) IL-2 and LAK cell therapy (meeting abstract). *Proceedings of the Annual Meeting of the American Society of Clinical Oncology* **12**, A946.

Thompson, J. A. et al. (1992). Prolonged continuous IV (CIV) infusion of interleukin-2 and lymphokine-activated killer cell therapy for metastatic renal cell carcinoma (RCC) (meeting abstract). *Proceedings of the Annual Meeting of the American Society of Clinical Oncology* **11**, A824.

Thrasher, J. B. and Paulson, D. F. (1993). Prognostic factors in renal cancer (review). *Urologic Clinics of North America* **20**, 247–262.

Tykka, H., Oravisto, K. J., Lehtonen, T., Sharna, S., and Tallber, T. (1968). Active specific immunotherapy of advanced renal cell carcinoma. *European Urology* **4**, 250–258.

Uchida, T., Wada, C., Shitara, T., Egawa, S., Mashimo, S., and Koshiba, K. (1993). Infrequent involvement of p53 mutations and loss of heterozygos-ity of 17p in the tumorigenesis of renal cell carcinoma. *Journal of Urology* **150**, 1298–1301.

Umeda, T. and Niijma, T. (1986). Phase II study of alpha interferon in renal cell carcinoma. *Cancer* **58**, 1231–1235.

Unger, P. D., Watson, C. W., Liu, Z., and Gil, J. (1993). Morphometric analysis of neoplastic renal aspirates and benign renal tissue. *Analytical and Quantitative Cytology and Histology* **15**, 61–66.

Urrutia, M. (2001). Analysis of survival with parametric and non-parametric models: basics and practical application. *Urologia Integrada y de Investigacion* **4**, 356–382.

Urrutia, M., Montero, J., Grande, J., and Llopis, M. (1977). Fosfatasas y scan oseo en el carcinoma de prostata. *Actas Urologicas Españolas* **4**, 207–212.

Urrutia, M., Tinajas, A., Ludeña, M., Urrutia, M. A., Romani, R., and Lorenzo, M. (2001). Predictive value of the nuclear morphometry in the probability of survival of patients with renal cell carcinoma: preliminary study. *Urologia Integrada y de Investigacion* **4**, 391–407.

van den Berg, E. et al. (1993). Cytogenetic analysis of epithelial renal-cell tumors: relationship with a new histopathological classification. *International Journal of Cancer* **55**, 223–227.

van der Werf-Messing, B. (1973). Carcinoma of the kidney. *Cancer* **32**, 1056–1066.

van Dijk, J. et al. (1994). Therapeutic effects of monoclonal antibody G250, interferons and tumor necrosis factor, in mice with renal-cell carcinoma xenografts. *International Journal of Cancer* **56**, 262–268.

Vickers, M., Jr. (1974). Serum haptoglobins: a preoperative detector of metastatic renal carcinoma. *Journal of Urology* **112**, 310–312.

Walther, M. M. et al. (1993). Cytoreductive surgery prior to interleukin-2-based therapy in patients with metastatic renal cell carcinoma. *Urology* **42**, 250–258.

Weinmann, S. A. (1993). Diuretic use and related risk factors for renal cell cancer. *Disease Abstract International B* **54**, 200.

Weiss, G. R. et al. (1992). A randomized phase II trial of continuous infusion interleukin-2 or bolus injection interleukin-2 plus lymphokine-activated killer cells for advanced renal cell carcinoma. *Journal of Clinical Oncology* **10**, 275–281.

Wickham, J. E. A. (1975). Conservative renal surgery for adenocarcinoma. The place of bench surgery. *British Journal of Urology* **47**, 25–36.

Wiltrout, R. H., Boyd, M. R., Back, T. C., Salup, R. R., Arthur, J. A., and Hornung, R. L. (1988). Flavone-8-acetic acid augments systemic natural killer cell activity and synergizes with IL-2 for treatment of murine renal cancer. *Journal of Immunology* **140**, 3261–3265.

Yagoda, A., Petrylak, D., and Thompson, S. (1993). Cytotoxic chemotherapy for advanced renal cell carcinoma. *Urologic Clinics of North America* **20**, 303–321.

Yamada, Y., Fukatsu, H., Honda, N., Miyagawa, Y., and Segawa, A. (1993). Clinical study of renal cell carcinoma. *Hinyokika Kiyo–Acta Urologica Japonica* **39**, 1197–1203.

Zbar, T. et al. (1994). Hereditary papillary renal cell carcinoma. *Journal of Urology* **151**, 561–566.

Zincke, H., Engen, D. E., and Henning, K. M. (1985). Treatment of renal cell carcinoma by *in situ* partial nephrectomy and extracorporeal operation with autotransplantation. *Mayo Clinic Proceedings* **60**, 651–662.

18.2 Wilms' tumour

Christopher Mitchell

Introduction and definition

Wilms' tumour (WT) (Wilms 1899), the most common genitourinary malignancy of childhood, is a triphasic embryonal neoplasm consisting of varying proportions of blastema, stroma, and epithelium. Although the specific histological appearance was described by Max Wilms in 1899, the eponym is now loosely applied to virtually any malignant tumour arising in the kidney in childhood, some of which are pathologically, clinically, and probably genetically distinct.

Epidemiology

The annual incidence of WT is around eight per million children under the age of 15 years. There are both racial and regional variations in incidence, so that the previously held view that the incidence was constant throughout the world (the 'index' tumour) is not correct (Parkin *et al.* 1988). The risk of developing WT is approximately one in 10,000 live births. The tumour accounts for about 8 per cent of childhood malignancies so, in incidence, ranks fifth among the solid tumours of childhood, after tumours of the central nervous system, lymphoma, neuroblastoma, and soft-tissue sarcoma. The tumour occurs with equal frequency in boys and girls, with a peak incidence in the third year. Although very rare in the neonatal period (Hrabovsky *et al.* 1986), over 75 per cent of children affected are under 4 years of age and at least 90 per cent under 7 years at diagnosis (Breslow and Beckwith 1982; J. Barnes, personal communication; see Fig. 1), with only a very few being diagnosed after the age of 11 years.

Genetics and *WT1* associated nephropathies

WT is essentially a sporadic condition, with only 1–2 per cent of cases being familial. A further 2 per cent of cases occur as part of specific congenital malformation syndromes (see below), which carry a greatly increased risk of WT. Analyses of this latter group of patients resulted in the cloning of the first WT gene *WT1*, together with the realization that WT genetics was considerably more complex than that of retinoblastoma. Currently, there is evidence from a variety of cytogenetic and molecular phenomena for the involvement of at least 10 different genes whose mechanisms of action do not appear always to be those of typical tumour suppressor genes.

Although familial WT is very rare, the existence of such cases has provided indications of location of some of the other genes involved in

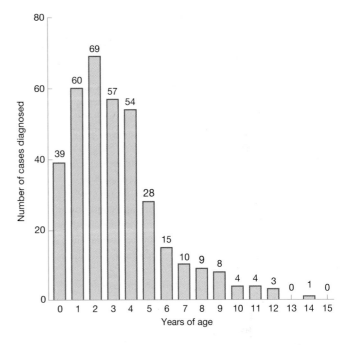

Fig. 1 Proportion of Wilm's tumour cases diagnosed per year of life (United Kingdom Child Cancer study Group data, 361 cases, absolute numbers of cases for each year are given at the top of each bar).

the process of tumourigenesis. So far three loci have been implicated in the development of familial WT, *WT1* at 11p13, *FWT1* on 17q–q21 (Rahman *et al.* 1998), and *FWT2* on 19q13 (McDonald *et al.* 1998), but there is evidence that other loci also exist (Rapley *et al.* 2000).

The *WT1* gene is encoded by 10 exons. The RNA is subject to a complex pattern of alternative splicing (Haber *et al.* 1991) which results in proteins of 45–49 kDa in size. The gene contains functional domains that indicate transcriptional regulatory activity, but the identity of the genes controlled by *WT1* remain unknown. In reconstitution experiments, transient high expression of *WT1* results in the suppression of activity of growth-inducing genes such as early growth response-1 (*EGR1*), insulin-like growth factor-II (*IGF2*), and the A-chain of platelet-derived growth factor (*PDGFA*) (Rauscher 1993). The formation of a *WT1*–p53 complex enhances the transcriptional repression possessed by *WT1* (Mahaswaran *et al.* 1993).

Other tumour-suppressor genes, such as *p53* or *RB1*, are expressed ubiquitously; in contrast, *WT1* has a very restricted pattern of expression. During normal differentiation, *WT1* expression is limited to condensing mesenchyme, renal vesicles, and glomerular epithelium. Expression in podocytes, though, persists into adulthood. Expression of *WT1* within the kidney peaks at about the time of birth and then declines rapidly as the organ achieves its finally differentiated form (Pritchard-Jones *et al.* 1990; Buckler *et al.* 1991). The regions of expression are all thought to be the sites of origin of WT. This differentiation-related expression in the kidney contrasts with the continuous expression seen in mesothelial cells, Sertoli cells of the testes, and granulosa cells of the ovary (Pelletier *et al.* 1991a).

There are three congenital malformation syndromes in which the *WT1* gene exhibits different patterns of mutation. The syndrome of sporadic aniridia, genitourinary anomalies, and mental retardation is known as the AGR triad (Riccardi *et al.* 1978; Francke *et al.* 1979), which is associated with approximately a 50 per cent risk of developing WT (Narahara *et al.* 1984). This contiguous gene syndrome was of great importance in the isolation of the *WT1* gene as virtually all of the AGR patients have a deletion affecting the short arm of chromosome 11, which is visible in cytological preparations. Although the precise extent of each deletion varies, the 11p13 region is always involved. Thus, there is complete loss of one *WT1* allele as part of the deletion. Development of WT usually involves mutation within the remaining *WT1* allele. Patients with the AGR also have a high risk of progression to endstage renal disease (ESRD), compared to patients with isolated WT, a finding which may reflect the effects of the deletion of a single copy of *WT1* on renal development (Breslow *et al.* 2000).

In addition to the AGR triad, the Denys–Drash syndrome (DDS) and Frasier syndrome (FS) are two further rare conditions that often present as severe, early-onset nephrotic syndrome. Both conditions involve intragenic *WT1* mutations and both provide some degree of predisposition to WT. They are described further in the section on *WT1* associated nephropathies.

Not all mutations of *WT1* in WT are homozygous (Little *et al.* 1992). This observation suggests that there may be other genetic loci of importance in Wilms' tumourigenesis, and that, at a genetic level, WT is a heterogeneous disorder, quite unlike retinoblastoma. The existence of genetic loci other than that on chromosome region 11p13 is supported by several other lines of evidence including chromosome studies of tumours, extended observations on loss of heterozygosity (LOH), and studies of genomic imprinting.

The phenomenon of LOH and its occurrence within the chromosome region 11p13 is described in Fig. 2. In some patients the distance over which heterozygosity has been lost is restricted to 11p13, although in others it covers most of the short arm of the chromosome. There is also a group of patients in which the phenomenon is restricted to the 11p15 region (Reeve *et al.* 1989; Wadey *et al.* 1990; Coppes *et al.* 1992a). This locus has now been designated *WT2*. At this point an explanation of genomic imprinting and its relevance to WT is necessary.

During the process that leads to LOH there is, theoretically, an equal chance of the allele of chromosome 11 retained in the tumour being of either maternal or paternal origin. However, it appears that the maternal allele is consistently lost from WTs, with persistence of the paternal allele (Schroeder *et al.* 1987; Williams *et al.* 1989; Pal *et al.* personal communication). By inference, therefore, it is the paternal allele that bears the initiating mutation. These findings suggest the presence of genomic imprinting, an epigenetic phenomenon whereby expression of genes is dependent on their parental origin. It has, for example, been proposed that the maternal genome largely determines

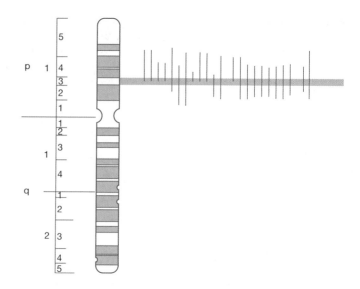

Fig. 2 Extent of chromosome 11 deletions in AGR patients. Chromosome 11 is shown on the left of the figure; deletions are indicated by the vertical bars on the right. The common region of overlap is shown by the solid horizontal line. Many of the deletions end within this region.

embryonic development, whereas the paternal genome largely determines development of the extraembryonic tissues (Hall 1990).

The link between the 11p15 region and WT noted above is further strengthened by its association with the Beckwith–Wiedemann syndrome, which is characterized by visceromegaly, macroglossia, hyperinsulinaemic hypoglycaemia, and a predisposition to a number of different malignancies including WT (Beckwith 1963; Wiedemann 1964). In some patients the overgrowth is asymmetrical, which is recognizable clinically as hemihypertrophy. A few patients with Beckwith–Wiedemann syndrome have been found to have a duplication of part of the short arm of chromosome 11, resulting in triplication of the 11p15 region (Waziri *et al.* 1983; Pueschel and Padre-Mendoza 1984; Turleau *et al.* 1984). The majority of patients have two grossly normal copies of chromosome 11, but both of these copies are paternally derived, a phenomenon termed uniparental isodisomy. In patients with triplication of 11p15 two of the copies are paternal in origin (Grundy *et al.* 1991; Henry *et al.* 1991). These observations suggest that the gene responsible for the Beckwith–Wiedemann syndrome is one that is normally expressed only by the paternal allele. Where both copies of the gene are paternally derived there is double the normal level of expression and the result is the overgrowth that characterizes the syndrome. Thus, the syndrome is an example of a condition caused by inappropriate inheritance of genes that are subject to genomic imprinting. Genetic linkage studies in the rare families with Beckwith–Wiedemann syndrome also indicate that the locus for the condition lies in the chromosome region 11p15 (Koufos *et al.* 1989; Ping *et al.* 1989).

IGF2 is an obvious candidate gene because of its location at chromosome region 11p15, because it is subject to imprinting with expression restricted to the paternal allele, and because it is overexpressed in WT as a consequence of expression from both alleles (Reeve *et al.* 1985; Scott *et al.* 1985; Ogawa *et al.* 1993; Rainier *et al.* 1993).

Perlman syndrome is another, although very rare, condition that constitutes a predisposition to WT. Only 11 children with the condition have been reported in the world literature. A further three cases have been seen at the Hospital for Sick Children in London (Grundy *et al.* personal communication). Superficially, there is a resemblance to the Beckwith–Wiedemann syndrome, but the two conditions are distinct (Grundy *et al.* 1992). Perlman syndrome is characterized by fetal gigantism, a high mortality rate in early life, a distinctive facial appearance, mental retardation, and genitourinary abnormalities including a high risk of developing WT. The syndrome was first recognized as an association between bilateral metanephric hamartomas and nephroblastomatosis in two siblings (Liban and Kozenitsky 1970). Subsequently, similarly affected siblings, one of whom had WT, were reported (Perlman *et al.* 1973, 1974; Neri *et al.* 1984; Greenberg *et al.* 1986; Perlman 1986; Hamel *et al.* 1989). The facial appearance is very characteristic and quite distinct from that seen in Beckwith–Wiedemann syndrome. The features include deep-set eyes, a small, short nose with depressed nasal bridge, an inverted, V-shaped upper lip, and low-set ears. There is macrocephaly, macrosomia, nephromegaly, hepatomegaly, and islet-cell hyperplasia. The neonatal death rate is high (10/14 cases). All four children who survived the neonatal period developed WT, which was bilateral in three of the cases, and a WT was found at autopsy in a fifth patient who died at the age of 4 days. Nephroblastomatosis has been noted in the majority of patients with Perlman syndrome and WT is the only associated malignancy reported so far.

Although Perlman syndrome clearly constitutes a strong predisposition to WT, no cytogenetic or molecular data that indicate the basis of the predisposition have yet been reported.

There are other molecular genetic features discernible in WTs which may be of prognostic significance, but which are described below, in the relevant section.

WT1 associated nephropathies

WT1 plays a major role in renal and genital development as demonstrated by its tissue distribution during development and the absence of kidney and gonads in Wt1 null mice (Kreidberg *et al.* 1993). After birth, *WT1* continues to be expressed in the podocyte and is important in the maintenance of the cell function as indicated by the occurrence of progressive glomerulopathies, with or without WT, in patients presenting specific constitutional mutations of the gene. Moreover, changes in *WT1* expression are observed in patients presenting various types of acquired glomerulopathies characterized by severe podocyte alterations.

No specific glomerular lesions have been described in the contiguous gene syndrome responsible for the AGR triad and the development of WT. However, the risk of progressing to ESRD is higher in AGR patients with the deletion of one copy of *WT1* than in patients with isolated nephroblastoma (Breslow *et al.* 2000). Similarly, increased rate of mortality, due to the progressive development of renal lesions leading to ESRD, has been described in Wt1+/− mice, despite a very slight reduction in the level of *WT1* expression (Guo *et al.* 2002). Regular evaluation of renal function is indicated in AGR patients.

The DDS (Denys *et al.* 1967; Drash *et al.* 1970) consists of male pseudohermaphroditism, a specific form of mesangial sclerosis progressing rapidly to ESRD (Habib *et al.* 1985), and predisposition to WT. The nephropathy, nephrotic syndrome often preceded by isolated proteinuria, is usually discovered before the age of 1 year. It is steroid-resistant, frequently associated with hypertension, and progresses steadily to ESRD, usually before the age of 4 years (Habib *et al.* 1985, 1993). It does not recur after kidney transplantation. Antenatal onset of the disease is rare, but difficult because of a typical manifestations such as oligohydramnios, large hyperechogenic kidneys detected by ultrasonography, and ESRD at birth. All 46, XY patients have either ambiguous genitalia or sex reversal, with dysgenetic tests. Unilateral or bilateral WT may be the first symptom of the disease, or may only be detected after the development of nephrotic syndrome. As a consequence, regular examination of these patients is necessary and prophylactic bilateral nephrectomy should be considered, even in patients without overt tumours, once terminal renal failure is established. Interestingly, an additional feature, diaphragmatic hernia, has been observed in one patient with the complete triad (Devriendt *et al.* 1995), a possible consequence of *WT1* mutation as Wt1 null mice have severe mesothelium anomalies (Kreidberg *et al.* 1993). The syndrome is often incomplete, the constant feature being the glomerular involvement. Patients with a 46,XX karyotype have a normal female phenotype and, recently, it has been shown they may have normal genital development with normal puberty (Jeanpierre *et al.* 1998a). WT does not appear in all patients, probably because of the rapid progression of the nephropathy leading to early death, or because of nephrectomy at the time of ESRD.

The distinctive renal lesion in DDS is diffuse mesangial sclerosis (DMS) (Fig. 3) (Habib *et al.* 1985). In the early stage of the disease, the diagnosis may be difficult: the lesion is characterized by increase in

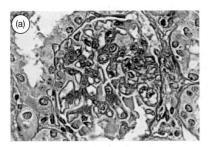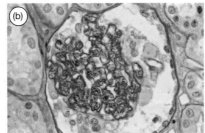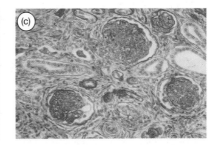

Fig. 3 Diffuse mesangial sclerosis in DDS patients; light microscopy; periodic acid Shiff: (a) ×160: Early glomerular lesion characterized by moderate increase in mesangial matrix and marked podocyte hypertrophy; (b) ×160: fully developed lesion showing accumulation of mesangial material, retraction of the glomerular tuft surrounded by large podocytes; (c) ×80: endstage kidney; all glomeruli are sclerotic and still surrounded by large and vacuolized podocytes; severe tubulointerstitial and arteriolar lesions are associated.

fibrillary mesangial matrix without any mesangial cell proliferation, associated with marked podocyte hypertrophy. The glomerular basement membrane (GBM) looks normal by light microscopy, but segmental thickening and splitting may be seen by electron microscopy. Some mesangial deposits of IgM, C1q, and/or C3 may be present within the mesangial stalks. The fully developed lesion is characterized by a combination of massive enlargement of the mesangial matrix, retraction of the glomerular tuft, and thickening of the capillary walls resulting in reduction in the patency of the capillary lumens. Progression of the disease leads to collapse and complete sclerosis of the glomerular tuft still surrounded by hypertrophied and vacuolated podocytes. At this stage deposits outline the periphery of the tuft. In most patients, the various stages of glomerular lesions coexist in the same specimen. Tubular lesions are constant and characterized by marked proximal tubule dilatation and obstruction by protein casts. They are prominent and diffuse in the antenatal forms of the disease. A peculiar feature, not seen in other glomerulopathies, is the presence of miniature glomeruli in the superficial cortex, a finding consistent with the role of *WT1* in kidney development.

Since the first study of Pelletier *et al.* (1991b), more than 80 germline heterozygous mutations have been reported in patients presenting with complete or incomplete DDS (Baird *et al.* 1992b; Coppes *et al.* 1992b; Jeanpierre *et al.* 1998a,b; Schumacher *et al.* 1998; Koziell *et al.* 1999). As indicated above they are mostly *de novo* missense mutations affecting exon 8 or 9 resulting in changes in the structural organization of zinc finger 2 or 3 and consequently in the DNA binding ability of the *WT1* protein (Little *et al.* 1995). In addition it has been suggested that the mutated protein acts in a dominant negative fashion by dimerization with the wild type protein, an explanation for the severity of DDS compared with the AGR syndrome (Little *et al.* 1993; Reddy *et al.* 1995). In agreement with these *in vitro* findings, absence or reduction of the nuclear expression of WT1 has been observed by immunohistochemistry in podocytes of DDS patients (Yang *et al.* 1999).

In some patients, a glomerulopathy similar to the DDS nephropathy occurs without the other elements of the triad. In some cases, it is an incomplete form of the disease in females without WT, as confirmed by the finding of *WT1* mutation (Jeanpierre *et al.* 1998a). However, isolated DMS could also be the marker of a different entity with autosomal recessive inheritance as suggested by the occurrence in males with normal genitalia, familial incidence and/or parental consanguinity (review in Gubler *et al.* 1999).

FS also results from *WT1* mutation (Barbaux *et al.* 1997) and is characterized by the association of progressive glomerulopathy and male pseudohermaphroditism (Frasier *et al.* 1964; Moorthy *et al.* 1987). At the clinical and morphological levels, however, it is quite distinct from DDS. About 35 cases of the disease have been reported (Kikuchi *et al.* 1997; Klamt *et al.* 1998; Barbosa *et al.* 1999; Demmer *et al.* 1999; Shimoyama *et al.* 2002). Proteinuria is usually the first symptom, detected in childhood or adolescence. It increases progressively with age resulting in nephrotic syndrome resistant to any treatment. ESRD usually occurs between 15 and 35 years of age. Morphological lesions are not specific. Glomeruli may be initially normal, and then focal and segmental glomerular sclerosis/hyalinosis develops, responsible for the progression of the disease. Abnormal genital development characterized by complete male-to-female sex reversal is constant in 46,XY patients. Consequently, it is usually the evaluation of primary amenorrhoea in phenotypic females with nephrotic syndrome that leads to the diagnosis

of FS. Investigation shows infantile internal genitalia and streak gonads, with macroscopic or, more often microscopic gonadoblastoma detected at histological examination of gonads in half of the patients. Tumour recurrence after gonadectomy has not been reported. The risk for developing WT is very low in FS patients, despite their relatively long renal survival. Only one case of nephroblastoma has been reported (Barbosa *et al.* 1999).

In all patients with typical FS, *de novo* point mutations located in the donor splice-site in intron 9 of *WT1* have been identified (Barbaux *et al.* 1997; Kikuchi *et al.* 1997; Klamt *et al.* 1998; Barbosa *et al.* 1999; Demmer *et al.* 1999; Shimoyama *et al.* 2002). They prevent the normal synthesis of *WT1* isoforms containing the short sequence KTS (for lysine, threonine, serine) between zinc fingers 3 and 4, as confirmed by *in vitro* experiments and analysis of tissue from FS patients (Barbaux *et al.* 1997; Kikuchi *et al.* 1997; Klamt *et al.* 1998). The ratio of *WT1* isoforms is normally constant and the +KTS and −KTS isoforms have different regulatory functions. Their imbalance is responsible for podocyte dysfunction and major alteration in male genital development. The requirement of a strict equilibrium between these different isoforms has been further demonstrated in mice expressing only +KTS or only −KTS isoforms (Hammes *et al.* 2001).

Recently, it has been shown that the only clinical expression of the 'Frasier mutation' in 46,XX patients is isolated progressive glomerulopathy with focal and segmental glomerulosclerosis (Klamt *et al.* 1998; Demmer *et al.* 1999; Denamur *et al.* 1999). Patients have a normal female phenotype and normal gonadal functions. One of the XX FS patients achieved normal pregnancy (Denamur *et al.* 1999). Most importantly, her daughter was affected with DDS diagnosed on the finding of early nephrotic syndrome with DMS and of a XY karyotype. This observation underlines the fact that *WT1* germline mutations, even occurring *de novo*, are transmissible. Until recently WT-associated nephropathies were regarded as sporadic diseases. Obviously, XY males with severe genital abnormalities, including dysgenetic testes and streak gonads are sterile. Conversely, most DDS and FS females have normal genital development and now survive because of haemodialysis and renal transplantation. They have a 50 per cent risk of transmitting the mutated gene and the disease to their children. Genetic counselling should be offered to patients with constitutional mutations of *WT1*.

Clinical features

Most children with WT are well and present only because they have an abdominal mass detected by a parent or other person although symptoms such as abdominal pain, haematuria, and fever may sometimes occur. Generally, the contrast with the clinical picture of abdominal neuroblastoma, the major differential diagnosis, is marked. Physical examination should include a search for the stigmata of the various associated conditions, such as hemihypertrophy, Beckwith–Wiedemann syndrome, genital abnormalities, and aniridia. Hypertension, which may arise from excessive renin production, vascular compression by the tumour, or as part of pre-existing renal disease, occurs in a few patients and may be sufficiently severe to require treatment. The blood pressure must, therefore, be measured.

Abdominal examination reveals a smooth, rounded, or lobulated mass arising in the loin; it may be possible to feel the attached normal kidney. The mass is usually ballotable and does not move with respiration, thus allowing distinction from liver or spleen. The previously held view that abdominal examination should not be repeated for fear of tumour rupture or tumour emboli is unfounded. Any metastases present at diagnosis, which are usually pulmonary, will only rarely be detected by clinical examination.

Investigations

The objectives of investigation are to confirm the diagnosis, delineate the extent of the tumour, determine that the contralateral kidney is functional, discover any metastases, and ensure that the child is fit enough to undergo anaesthesia and surgery.

A blood count may detect anaemia resulting from haemorrhage into the tumour; there may also be thrombocytosis in response to haemorrhage. A few patients develop a bleeding diathesis secondary to an acquired form of von Willebrand disease. An incidence of 8 per cent was noted in one study (Coppes et al. 1992b), and so the prothrombin and partial thromboplastin times should be estimated. Further investigations of coagulation may be mandated either by these results or by the clinical state of the patient. Urinalysis, particularly for protein, and measurement of serum electrolytes, urea, and creatinine, should detect any gross abnormalities of renal function. Measurement of urinary catecholamines is essential to exclude neuroblastoma, especially in hypertensive children, if immediate surgery is contemplated. No imaging technique can exclude neuroblastoma with complete accuracy, and some are intrarenal. There are two reasons for taking care to exclude the diagnosis of neuroblastoma: first, immediate surgery may not then be appropriate; and second, catecholamine-secreting tumours pose particular anaesthetic problems, which should be recognized preoperatively. Most centres will now measure catecholamine secretion by a chromatographic method, which renders the previous 'spot' method obsolete, and removes the need for 24 h collections of urine or the use of special diets.

An abdominal ultrasound scan is the imaging investigation of choice for determining the organ of origin, the extent of any spread within the abdomen, the patency of the inferior vena cava, and for detecting any involved lymph nodes. Most centres would also choose to perform a CT or MR scan of the abdomen to further define the anatomy of the tumour. It is important to document normal function of the contralateral kidney before any surgery is contemplated and the excretion of contrast at the end of a CT scan is useful confirmation of function in the contralateral kidney. A dimercaptosuccinic acid (DMSA) scan is an alternative investigation which is particularly valuable in planning surgery for patients with bilateral tumours or those with only a single functioning kidney.

Posteroanterior and lateral chest radiographs are mandatory in the exclusion of pulmonary metastases. The place of CT for the detection of pulmonary metastases in WT remains unclear. A North American study found pulmonary disease by scanning but not by conventional radiography in 11 of 124 children (Willimas et al. 1988), but there was no significant difference in the relapse rate between that small group and the larger number of patients whose lung lesions could be seen on ordinary radiography. The United Kingdom Children's Cancer Study Group reported a number of patients with metastases detected by CT that were not found by conventional radiography (31 out of 142), and found that just over 25 per cent of these patients relapsed (seven out of 31). However, relapses were more common in patients who were otherwise stage I than those who were stages II–V. Overall, four of the

seven patients were salvaged by second-line treatment (including two of three stage I patients) (Owens et al. 1996). These data suggest that the majority of higher-stage patients will have their pulmonary disease adequately treated by their stage-appropriate chemotherapy and need not have their initial treatment intensified. Stage I patients, however, receive so little additional therapy that great care is needed in defining the stage and it is here that CT scanning may be most important.

Postoperatively, other imaging investigations may be indicated by specific histological findings. A ^{99}Tc bone scan is indicated after the diagnosis of the so-called bone-metastasizing renal tumour (also called clear-cell sarcoma; see below). An additional radiological survey of the skeleton is unnecessary. In malignant rhabdoid tumour of the kidney (RTK) a CT scan of the head should be done to exclude the presence of an intracranial second tumour (Bonnin et al. 1984).

Prognostic features

It is important to acknowledge that prognostic factors arise as an artefact of treatment regimens. If treatment was uniformly successful, or a disease uniformly fatal, there would be no prognostic factors. In WT the recognition of prognostic factors has allowed the stratification of treatment, thus enabling the direction of intensive treatment to patients with 'bad risk' disease and the refinement of treatment for patients with 'good risk' disease. The most important prognostic factors in WT are histological appearance and stage (Breslow et al. 1978, 1985, 1986), features first delineated by the series of National WT studies conducted in North America. More recently the possible prognostic significance of a number of molecular genetic factors has been noted; prospective assessment of these factors is now in progress by both the NWTS and SIOP groups.

Pathology

The development of preoperative chemotherapy strategies have led to a reassessment of how the pathological features seen at the time of delayed surgery might have a bearing on prognosis and hence influence subsequent treatment. However, it is easier first to consider the appearances seen in patients having immediate nephrectomy.

Two broad groups of tumours may be recognized by their histological appearances [see Beckwith (1986), for a review]. The majority have classical triphasic tumours, in which epithelial, blastemal, and stromal elements are all present. There is debate about the origin of the stromal elements, which may be a true component of the tumour, but could be a proliferation of normal vascular and connective tissue caused by the proximity of malignant cells. The occasional finding of an undifferentiated sarcomatous stroma weighs against the latter suggestion. The presence of such a stroma is not itself a sign of poor prognosis. Some triphasic tumours may have rhabdomyoblastic differentiation, such that the cells resemble fetal rhabdomyoblasts, often with cross-striations. This appearance is not unfavourable and it must not be confused with the 'malignant RTK', which is a variant with poor prognosis (see below).

The monomorphic epithelial variant, usually found in children less than 1 year of age, is easily recognized as it appears to consist entirely of primitive tubules. This appearance has a very favourable prognosis, as do stage I tumours weighing less than 550 g in patients under 2 years of age (Green *et al.* 1994). Both of these subtypes are effectively treated by nephrectomy only.

The second group of patients are those whose tumours are categorized as one of the unfavourable histologies. Anaplasia is an unfavourable feature occasionally observed in triphasic tumours, where it is characterized by large (greater than four times normal) hyperchromatic nuclei, an increased nuclear : cytoplasmic ratio, and abnormal (e.g. tripolar) mitoses. Anaplasia in WT is often a patchy, focal change, which may escape notice unless a deliberate search is made; including widespread sampling with blocks cut every centimetre across the widest diameter of the tumour. The appearances are often best recognized by scanning the slide at low power.

The other unfavourable histological types are probably distinct tumours, rather than true variants of WT. The bone-metastasizing renal tumour of childhood, or clear-cell sarcoma of the kidney (CCSK) was first reported by Kidd (1970), and it was later separately identified by Marsden and Lawler (1978) from the United Kingdom, and by Beckwith and Palmer (1978) from America: they all describe a distinctive neoplasm with a propensity for skeletal metastasis and aggressive clinical behaviour. The incidence of reported bone metastases was 76 per cent of 38 cases in the British series, and 17 per cent of 75 cases in the American series.

In the third National WT study, the bone-metastasizing tumour comprised nearly 6 per cent of all cases, making it the most frequent form of 'unfavourable' histology. Its age distribution is similar to that of WT. There appears to be a distinct male preponderance for this type both in American and British series, although not as great as originally suggested.

The other unfavourable type is the malignant RTK, recognized by Beckwith and Palmer (1978) in their report from the first National WT study. It is the least common of the unfavourable entities and was found in only 2 per cent of patients entered in the National (American) studies. The age distribution is markedly different to that of WT, with nearly half the patients being diagnosed in the first year of life (see Weeks *et al.* 1989 for review). It is also associated with second primary tumours of various types (usually primitive neuroectodermal tumours) arising in the midline of the posterior intracranial fossa (Bonnin *et al.* 1984). The intracranial tumour may precede or follow the renal tumour. Hypercalcaemia has been reported in a number of cases of malignant rhabdoid tumour (Rousseau-Merck *et al.* 1982; Mitchell *et al.* 1985), but may also occur in congenital mesoblastic nephroma.

Two distinct, low risk entities have been described. The first is congenital mesoblastic nephroma, which is a rare, distinctive tumour of the infantile kidney. It was first recognized as a distinct entity by Bolande *et al.* (1967) [see Bolande (1973), for a review]. There have been reports of local recurrences and metastases but in only one of these was the patient less than 3 months of age. Review of the specimen showed that tumour extended to the margin of resection. There have been other recurrences in patients over 3 months of age; the microscopic appearances were of dense cellularity and numerous mitotic figures. Vascular invasion and tumour rupture have also been associated with an unfavourable outcome. The other low-risk entity is cystic partly differentiated nephroblastoma (CPDN), which is usually seen in children under the age of 2 years. The tumour is composed entirely of cysts and their thin walls, with the septa forming the only 'solid' component of the tumour. The cysts are lined by cuboidal epithelium and the septa contain blastema together with stroma or epithelium. The tumour forms a discrete mass, well demarcated from the non-cystic renal parenchyma. Surgery alone is usually adequate therapy for both of these tumours.

In the SIOP risk assessment system, use is made of the response to chemotherapy, which now consists of four doses of vincristine at weekly intervals and actinomycin D at weeks one and three. Low-risk tumours, as noted above, include mesoblastic nephroma and CPDN. In addition, completely necrotic nephroblastoma is also recognized as a low-risk entity, with 100 per cent survival regardless of stage and hence with no further therapy necessary after resection. The histological criteria for making this diagnosis are the absence of any viable tumour tissue on gross or microscopic examination of multiple blocks, and the presence of regressive or necrotic changes caused by the chemotherapy.

The criteria for histological subtyping of WT established by Beckwith and Palmer state that one component of the tumour must comprise at least 66 per cent of the tumour mass before a subclassification may be assigned. Preoperative chemotherapy may alter the original appearances and often results in the appearance of areas of regression or necrosis. In consequence, the criteria used in subclassification of immediately resected tumours must be adapted to take the chemotherapy induced changes into account. It has been demonstrated that chemotherapy induced changes are prognostically favourable (Zuppan *et al.* 1991; Boccon-Gibod *et al.* 2000). Conversely, the persistence of blastema after chemotherapy indicates chemoresistance and has been shown to be associated with a poor outcome (Weirich *et al.* 2001). Designating intermediate risk tumours involves first assessing the percentage of necrosis or regression that is present. If these changes are present in more than 66 per cent of the tumour, it may then be designated as being of regressive subtype. If the degree of change is less than 66 per cent the tumour may be subtyped according to the predominant histological component, or designated as mixed if there is no predominance. Five entities may be recognized—epithelial, stromal, mixed, regressive, or with focal anaplasia. Each of these entities is of intermediate prognosis.

The high-risk entities include, as noted above, tumours with persistence of blastema, together with diffuse anaplasia, CCSK, and malignant RTK. In order to make a diagnosis of blastemal type nephroblastoma, the viable component must be more than 33 per cent of the tumour mass and at least 66 per cent of the viable areas must be blastema. Other components may also be present in varying amounts. The appearances of diffuse anaplasia, CCSK, and RTK have already been discussed above.

Nephroblastomatosis

Nephroblastomatosis, first described by Hou and Holman (1961), is defined as the persistence of metanephric blastema or its incompletely differentiated derivatives beyond the thirty-sixth week of gestation. It is found commonly in association with WT, with a frequency of 15–30 per cent and also in about 1 per cent of routinely examined perinatal postmortem kidneys in the absence of WT. It is also found in a number of other genetic conditions associated with WT, but in the absence of malignancy [see Beckwith (1986) and Bove and McAdams (1985) for reviews]. These associations have led to the suggestion that nephroblastomatosis is a precursor of WT, a view supported by the finding of a chromosome 11p deletion in nephroblastomatosis tissue from a patient with a normal somatic karyotype (Heidemann *et al.* 1986). Another school of thought is of the opinion that the lesions are a developmental anomaly that may be related to the genesis of WT, but which is neither a precursor of, nor a predisposition to, tumour development.

Beckwith (1986) classifies nephroblastomatosis as intralobar (deep), perilobar (superficial), mixed, and (a rare) panlobar forms. The most common form of nephroblastomatosis is of multiple, small nodules lying superficially in the subcapsular cortex. Occasionally, a continuous subcapsular layer may be formed, which can result in clinically detectable renal enlargement. The lesions of superficial perilobar nephroblastomatosis tend to enlarge with age and to become well differentiated and well defined. Proliferative nodules of monophasic embryonal epithelium may also be seen, with rosetting or a more differentiated tubular or papillary pattern, and prominent mitotic activity. Such lesions can be indistinguishable from WT, hence the name 'Wilms' tumourlets'. The intralobar or deep form of nephroblastomatosis (Machin and McCaughey 1984) is usually a solitary nodule consisting of tubules and blastema. The association with WT is clear, as the lesion is seldom recognized in the absence of a tumour. In these circumstances, the tumours are often multifocal or bilateral, and are usually predominantly stromal or blastemal with minimal epithelial differentiation. The rarest (panlobar) form is bilateral and involves the whole renal parenchyma apart from the medullopelvic area. This variant has not been associated with WT, probably because of limited survival.

Staging systems

Several staging systems have been used for WT, evolving as successive studies have redefined the criteria for each stage. The major contribution to these systems has been from the North American National studies. The current system, in use since the third National study, makes use of the data accumulated in National Wilms' Tumour Study (NWTS 1 and 2) to define five stages, summarized in Table 1. This staging system has been used subsequently in NWTS studies 4 and 5 and also in the United Kingdom Children's Cancer Study Group Wilms' tumour study (UKW) series of studies 1–3.

The use of preoperative chemotherapy has a major impact on the validity of the NWTS staging system. As a consequence, the SIOP group have refined their system, by using a combination of NWTS staging and pathological appearances to account for the implications of early disease response to chemotherapy, to categorize patients into risk groups.

Table 1 National Wilms' Tumour Study III, staging system

Stage	Description
I	Tumour within renal capsule, completely excised
II	Extension outside the renal capsule
III	Extension outside renal capsule, with incomplete surgical excision or loco-regional lymph-node involvement
IV	Metastatic spread to lungs, liver, bones, brain
V	Bilateral tumours

Molecular genetic prognostic factors

Consistent genetic changes have been identified in WTs at chromosome regions 11p13, 11p15, 16q, and 1p. Genes in these regions may be involved in processes such as proliferation, differentiation, or localization, which might affect the behaviour of a tumour. In a study of 232 patients registered in NWTS 3 and 4, Grundy *et al.* (1994) found that LOH of markers on 16q, found in 17.2 per cent of patients with favourable histology or anaplasia, had a significantly lower relapse free and overall survival, even after allowing for stage or histology. LOH for markers at region 1p was found in 11 per cent of the samples, and again was associated with poorer relapse free and overall survival. LOH at 11p or duplication of 1q were not associated with any difference in outcome.

These early results are now being studied in a prospective fashion in the NWTS 5 and SIOP WT 2001 trials; if confirmed these features might be a useful way of further stratifying therapy.

Treatment

Place of treatment

There is overwhelming evidence that WT ought only to be treated in recognized paediatric oncology centres and that there is no place for the casual therapist. Early studies indicated that there was a survival advantage for children treated within a trial or at a specialist centre (Griffel 1977; Lennox *et al.* 1979). Patients not included in a recognized trial, or not treated at a recognized centre, may be overtreated by comparison with current recommendations, being more likely to receive radiotherapy (Pritchard *et al.* 1989). The long-term consequences of radiotherapy, which are outlined below, include the risk of inducing a second malignant neoplasm. Surgeons, radiotherapists, paediatricians, or nephrologists not working in a centre with paediatric oncological expertise who find themselves unexpectedly dealing with a patient with WT should make an urgent referral to an appropriate unit immediately.

Surgery

Timing of surgery

Despite advances in chemotherapy, surgical extirpation is, and almost certainly will remain, the fundamental treatment for WT. Nevertheless, there is now considerable debate about the timing of surgical intervention, the place of percutaneous needle biopsy, and the use of preoperative chemotherapy. North American practice remains steadfastly in favour of immediate surgery followed by adjuvant therapy dictated by the surgical stage. In contrast, the SIOP group in Europe has conducted a series of trials based on the use of preoperative therapy and there is increasing recognition that preoperative treatment may be of benefit in many circumstances. In an attempt to resolve the issues posed by the findings from these two groups, the UKCCSG has conducted a prospective randomized trial comparing immediate surgery with 6 weeks of chemotherapy and delayed surgery (UKW3), the preliminary results of which are included below. Other issues posed by the use of preoperative treatment are considered further in the section on chemotherapy.

There are no generally accepted, absolute contraindications to immediate surgery but there are circumstances in which many surgeons would deem immediate operative intervention less appropriate. The presence of major tumour thrombus in the inferior vena cava will make an operation considerably more risky, and may well necessitate the use of cardiac by-pass if the thrombus is to be removed. It seems illogical to subject a child with disseminated disease to immediate surgery for removal of the primary tumour until control of the metastases has been established. Very large tumours may pose considerable surgical problems, particularly if the tumour is found to be invading other organs such as the liver, spleen, or bowel. It is clear that the vast majority of WTs will respond readily to treatment with vincristine and actinomycin D; in the circumstances outlined above it may well be beneficial to use preoperative chemotherapy to shrink the tumour so as to facilitate the resection.

Accepting that, in some cases, immediate definitive surgery may be inappropriate, the choice facing the clinician will be either to proceed with therapy based solely on the clinicoradiological data, or to subject the patient to a biopsy. Many paediatric oncologists and surgeons feel that a biopsy is unnecessary. However, an analysis of biopsies in UKW3 from 297 patients, thought on clinicoradiological grounds to have WT, confirmed the diagnosis in 266 cases (34). Twenty-two patients (7 per cent) were considered not to have WT by the local pathologist and a further nine cases (making a total of 10 per cent) were found on central review to have either unfavourable histology (4 cases) or other diagnoses (5 cases). Some of these diagnoses were of less common renal tumours such as mesoblastic nephroma or renal cell carcinoma, but others were of non-renal tumours such as neuroblastoma, which may be difficult distinguish to Radiologically. In the SIOP I trial (Lemerle et al. 1976) 21 of 169 randomized patients and in SIOP V (Lemerle et al. 1983) 10 of 164 randomized patients were found to have diagnoses other than WT. Thus, with reliance solely on clinicoradiological features yielding an 8–10 per cent error rate, pretreatment histological confirmation seems essential.

Typically, biopsy in these circumstances will be a closed procedure using a 'Trucut' or similar needle. There are two major concerns about the use of such a procedure:

1. Needle biopsy may not provide a representative sample of the tumour and may fail to reveal unfavourable features such as anaplasia. Preoperative treatment may then mask the unfavourable features in the eventually resected specimen, and result in undertreatment. A review of 266 confirmed WT cases, with no evidence of anaplasia in the biopsy specimen, revealed anaplasia in the nephrectomy specimen in 25 cases. In 10 per cent of the cases confirmed as WT, anaplasia could still be detected in the nephrectomy specimen after the preoperative chemotherapy.

2. Does the process of biopsy in itself render the patients more likely to suffer a subsequent local recurrence? Since a needle biopsy must interrupt the integrity of the renal capsule there is at least a theoretical concern that the procedure might result in local spillage of the tumour along the biopsy track. In the series of patients reported above, no patient suffered such a complication. In the current UKCCSG UKW3 trial only one patient randomized to biopsy had a biopsy track recurrence out of a total of 297 procedures. These data suggest that the risk of recurrence posed to the patient is very minimal.

In the third NWTS 3, 131 children were judged to have primarily unresectable disease. The patients were assigned a pretreatment stage and then treated accordingly. The 4-year survival for this group of patients was only 74 per cent compared to 88 per cent for those patients

having immediate surgery (Ritchey et al. 1994). In the first UKW1, 23 patients (6 per cent of the total number studied) had initially unresectable disease, but instead of being assigned a pretreatment stage were all treated as stage III patients with four-drug chemotherapy and, in those patients with local residual disease after delayed surgery, 30 Gy flank or whole-abdominal irradiation (Pritchard et al. 1995). Unfortunately, the outcome for this small group of patients is not analysed separately from that of the other stage III patients, and so it is impossible to judge the relative merits of these two approaches. The International Society of Paediatric Oncology (SIOP) group has pursued preoperative treatment for many years and has produced persuasive evidence that such a policy improves the stage at the time of surgery. Preliminary data from the UKCCSG UKW3 study supports this view (see below).

Surgical procedure

The three major contraindications to surgery are (a) bilateral disease; (b) a large 'fixed' tumour; and (c) hepatic invasion. In general, 'heroic' surgery is inappropriate, as chemotherapy will shrink tumours very effectively, sparing the child a radical operation with its attendant risks. Particular problems may arise with very large tumours overlying the major blood vessels. Care is needed to avoid the inadvertent ligation of contralateral renal vessels, the superior mesenteric artery, or even the aorta and inferior vena cava. Tumour thrombus in the renal vein or inferior vena cava is usually revealed by preoperative ultrasonography. Occasionally, it is only discovered at operation. In these circumstances the inferior vena cava should be mobilized so that control can be established above and below the thrombus, before removal is attempted.

Chemotherapy

Stratification of therapy, based on the extent of the primary tumour, presence of involved lymph nodes or metastases, and the extent of any tumour spillage at operation, is the key to rational use of chemotherapy. Reduction in therapy for 'good risk' patients and more intensive therapy for 'bad risk' patients results in fewer adverse effects of treatment in the former group, while achieving good survival in the latter.

The first National WT study in North America was the first concerted attempt to analyse postoperative chemotherapy and radiotherapy systematically (D'Angio et al. 1976). That study and its successors (D'Angio et al. 1981, 1989) have been instrumental in devising prognostic stages and in their revision, as has already been noted. Equally important has been the steady progress in delineating optimal treatment within the various disease stages. The major findings in the National series are summarized in Table 2. At the end of the third

Table 2 Major findings in NWTS studies

Stage	RFS	OS	Treatment arm
Stage I	92	97	10 weeks, actinomycin D and Vincristine
Stage II	87	91	15 months, actinomycin D, vincristine, doxorubicin
Stage III	78	86	Actinomycin D, vincristine, doxorubicin, and 10 Gy
Stage IV	72	81	

RFS, relapse-free survival; OS, overall survival.

National study, therapy had been significantly reduced for stage I patients, who appeared to need only 10 weeks of adjuvant chemotherapy and no radiotherapy. In stage II patients, by using a more intensive regimen of vincristine and actinomycin D, neither Adriamycin with its associated cardiotoxicity nor radiotherapy were required. For stage III disease the intensive two-drug regimen was as effective as the three-drug one, and it was possible to reduce radiotherapy from 20 to 10 Gy. The addition of cyclophosphamide to Adriamycin, actinomycin D, and vincristine did not enhance survival of stage IV or 'unfavourable histology' patients. The use of Adriamycin appeared specifically to improve the outlook for patients with bone-metastasizing renal tumour. Strategies for malignant RTK probably ought to be quite different from those used for the other renal tumours of childhood (D'Angio et al. 1989). The outcomes from this trial are summarized in Table 3.

The fourth national study ran from 1986 to 1994; a major objective of this study, apart from the more usual questions of efficacy and toxicity was the cost of treatment. Nine hundred and five children were randomized, either to study the duration of therapy and/or to study single versus divided dose drug administration. Short courses of therapy (6 months) were as effective as long (15 month) ones, and single dose administration of actinomycin D was no more toxic than fractionated dosing, thus confirming the previous finding of a large Brazilian study (de Camargo et al. 1994). Thus, treatment costs can be substantially reduced.

The United Kingdom Children's Cancer Study Group has built its studies in part on the results of these American National studies and also on those of the United Kingdom Medical Research Council trials (Lennox et al. 1979; Morris-Jones et al. 1987). In the UKW1 trial (Pritchard et al. 1995), stage I patients treated with 10 weeks of vincristine at weekly intervals, followed by five three-weekly doses, had a

98 per cent survival at 2 years, suggesting that actinomycin D can be avoided in these patients. In the second Wilms' trial (Mitchell et al. 2000), this treatment was reduced still further to 10 weeks of vincristine at weekly intervals only, without diminution of relapse-free survival. As with the American National studies, the recognition of unfavourable histology and of the adverse impact of lymph-node metastases has led to the use of more aggressive therapy for these patients, with an improvement in their overall survival, so that the current 2 year disease-free survival of patients with unfavourable histology, stages I–III, is around 50 per cent. Results for the second United Kingdom study are given in Table 4 (Mitchell et al. 2000).

Unlike the American or British studies, the cooperative European studies run by SIOP have concentrated on the use of preoperative therapies in an effort to reduce surgical morbidity, particularly tumour rupture. In the first SIOP study, which ran from 1971 to 1974, patients were randomized either to immediate surgery or to preoperative radiotherapy (20 Gy) (Lemerle et al. 1976). The frequency of tumour spillage at operation was significantly reduced by radiotherapy and the stage distribution became skewed towards the more favourable stages. Although there was no difference in the overall survival, recurrence-free survival was better in the rupture-free group. The second SIOP study ran from 1974 to 1976 was non-randomized and observational, to confirm the results of SIOP1. Some patients had immediate surgery at the discretion of the investigator, usually because the tumour was thought to be suitable for primary resection; others received preoperative radiation (20 Gy) and five doses of actinomycin D. Again, a reduced incidence of tumour rupture was found with preoperative treatment.

The fifth SIOP study, which ran from 1977 to 1979, recruited 433 patients (Lemerle et al. 1983) and compared preoperative chemoradiotherapy (20 Gy plus single agent actinomycin D) with preoperative chemotherapy alone, consisting in this instance of two 5 day courses of actinomycin D and four-weekly doses of vincristine. There were no significant differences in freedom from recurrence or overall survival, or in the frequency of tumour spillage, indicating that there was no benefit to adding radiotherapy to the chemotherapy regimen. When the chemotherapy of the fifth SIOP study was compared with the immediate surgery of the first, the skewing of stages towards the more favourable ones was clearly seen. Thus, the proportion of stage I patients increased from 22 to 48 per cent, with a concomitant reduction in the proportion with stage II, node-negative tumours (45–32 per cent) and stage II, node-positive or stage III tumours (33–19 per cent). In the sixth SIOP study (Tournade et al. 1993), all patients received preoperative chemotherapy. Seventeen weeks of therapy in total was as effective as 38 weeks in the treatment of stage I tumours; stage II, node-negative tumours did not benefit from postoperative radiotherapy; and stage node positive and stage III patients benefited from the addition of doxorubicin (Voute et al. 1987). SIOP 9 (Tournade et al. 2001) examined the question of duration of preoperative chemotherapy and showed that 4 weeks was as good as 8 weeks in terms of proportion of stage I patients, intraoperative rupture rate, 2 year EFS, and 5 year OS. The most recent study, SIOP93-01, examined the duration of postoperative chemotherapy in stage I tumours with intermediate risk histology or anaplasia and showed that 4 weeks of postoperative therapy was as good as 18 weeks for stage I patients with intermediate risk histology. There appeared to be no benefit to prolonged postoperative treatment. Reults from SIOP 9 are summarized in Table 5.

Table 3 Outcome for favourable histology, stage I–IV nest arm of NWTS3

Stage	2-year % OS	2-year % EFS	4-year % OS	4-year % EFS
I	98.6	92.3	97.4	91.8
II	97	92.5	94.9	90.1
III	90.9	85.9	90.9	85.9
IV	90.8	80	86.6	77.9

Table 4 UKW2: 2 year and 4 year estimates of survival and event-free survival for 398 FH stratified according to local histology and staging

Stage	Number (%)	2 year % S (95% CI)	2 year % EFS (95% CI)	4 year % S (95% CI)	4 year % EFS (95% CI)
I	136 (34)	96 (91–98)	89 (83–93)	94 (89–97)	87 (80–91)
II	57 (14)	95 (85–98)	82 (72–92)	91 (81–96)	82 (70–90)
III	122 (31)	90 (84–94)	83 (75–88)	84 (77–90)	82 (74–88)
IV	60 (15)	82 (70–89)	72 (59–82)	75 (63–84)	70 (57–80)

Table 5   SIOP 9. 3 Year estimates of survival and event-free survival for 360 trial patients (stages I–III) and 83 stage IV patients

Stage	Number	EFS (%)	OS (%)
I	229	89	95
IIN0	84	74	87
IIN+/III	47	73	91
IV	83	66	77

By extrapolation from these findings it would appear that with the SIOP approach, with a survival rate of 88–92 per cent, only about 20 per cent of patients need radiotherapy; in the third American National study, with similar survival rates, 30 per cent of patients with favourable histology, non-metastatic tumours required radiotherapy (D'Angio 1983).

The third UK Wilms' study examined in a randomized way, the question of whether preoperative chemotherapy improved staging, and thereby led to a reduction in treatment, in effect by early identification of patients with responsive tumours, without any diminution in outcome. Patients deemed at the time of diagnosis to have 'resectable' and localized tumours (i.e. no evidence of metastatic tumours) were randomly assigned either to immediate surgery or to 6 weeks of chemotherapy with vincristine and actinomycin D. In the latter group, surgery was then carried out at about week 6–7 and in both groups the postoperative treatment was based on the NWTS3 stage at the time of surgery. The study proved very difficult to conduct with a very low randomization rate, but over a 10 year period just over 200 patients were randomized. Interim analyses confirmed that histological confirmation of diagnosis was essential, and that there were fewer surgical complications in the preoperatively treated group. It also became clear that vincristine monotherapy was not adequate for stage I patients unless the chest CT was normal at the time of diagnosis. Preliminary analyses of the staging distribution shows that the preoperatively treated group has an excess of stage I and II patients, with a reduction in the proportion of stage III patients, as compared to the immediate surgery group. Overall there is no suggestion of a diminution in outcome. Thus, adoption of this approach will result in an overall reduction in the amount of therapy needed.

Radiotherapy

Paediatric oncological practice is to avoid the use of radiotherapy whenever possible, because of its local deleterious effects on growing tissues. The general trend in WT therapy has been to reduce the dose delivered, as successive trials have indicated that dose reduction does not compromise cure rates and as chemotherapy regimens have been optimized. It should be noted, however, that doxorubicin has generally been used to supplant radiation. There is increasing evidence that this drug, in addition to its short-term effects, may cause a significant long-term incidence of cardiac dysfunction (see below). It may well be that the relative demerits of these two forms of treatment will, in due course, necessitate a reappraisal of their places in the treatment of WT.

At the present time, the generally accepted indication for flank radiation is the presence of a stage III tumour. Data from the third National WT study (D'Angio et al. 1989) suggested that a reduction of

dosage from 20 to 10 Gy did not compromise outcome if three-drug chemotherapy was used. The fourth National study has confirmed that finding.

The need for pulmonary irradiation in patients with lung metastases is a difficult issue and no randomized trial of the need for this form of therapy has ever been carried out. However, comparisons of the results obtained by the various study groups gives some interesting insights.

NWTS 3 employed 12 Gy of whole lung irradiation for stage IV patients, in addition to three- or four-drug chemotherapy. The EFS and OS for these patients were 75 and 82 per cent respectively at 4 years from diagnosis. The contemporary UKW1 recommended radiotherapy only if pulmonary tumours had not resolved after 12 weeks of chemotherapy—thus only 4/40 patients received this therapy. The outcomes of 50 EFS) and 65 per cent (OS) at 6 years are clearly worse. In the subsequent UKW2 pulmonary radiotherapy was recommended for all patients with pulmonary disease at diagnosis; outcomes improved to 70 per cent (EFS) and 75 per cent (OS) at 4 years, figures more in line with the NWTS data. However, of the 59 patients with stage IV disease at diagnosis, only 37 actually received the radiotherapy.

Superficially, therefore, there is a clear case for whole lung radiotherapy in the treatment of lung metastases in WT. The SIOP group, however, have reported survival of over 80 per cent in stage IV patients without systematic use of pulmonary radiotherapy; and 50 per cent of stage IV patients in UKW1 were cured without its use (Pritchard et al. 1995). It is possible that with careful selection of patients and greater use of pulmonary resection, the proportion of patients receiving pulmonary radiotherapy might be reduced without prejudicing their chances of survival, but whether such a development is warranted, given the minimal long-term consequences of 12 Gy of pulmonary radiotherapy, is questionable. A more relevant question might be the identification of patients who could be successfully treated with less doxorubicin, thus obviating the potential long-term side-effects of anthracycline therapy, particularly when given in conjunction with whole lung radiotherapy (Lipshultz et al. 1991; Sorensen et al. 1995). The NWTS concluded that there was a subgroup of stage IV patients who could be successfully treated without doxorubicin. This question may never be adequately resolved. To do so would require not only a randomized trial of the use or not of irradiation, together with standardized chemotherapy, but also very long-term follow-up information on pulmonary and cardiac function, cosmetic defects, and the effects in girls on subseqent breast development and breast feeding.

Special problems

Patients with bilateral tumours or with single kidneys

For these two groups of patients the key is 'conservation of nephrons'. Initial surgery in these circumstances is limited to establishing the histological diagnosis, either by open or closed (trucut) biopsy from both kidneys, because the histology can differ between them. Chemotherapy is then instituted. Once a maximal response has been obtained, the operation is usually bilateral partial nephrectomy. If these procedures will not clear the residual tumour and preserve adequate renal function, then 'bench surgery' has been advocated. Here, the kidney is removed and residual tumour resected; the kidney is then reimplanted. In the presence of extensive nephroblastomatosis, where there could be a subsequent metachronous tumour, it has been suggested that surgery should be conservative (Heidemann et al. 1985). Approaches similar to those outlined for bilateral tumours may be useful in these patients.

Data from SIOP studies (Coppes et al. 1987) show that the highest local stage is important in determining prognosis, and that children with synchronous tumours do better than those with metachronous tumours. In addition, children with metachronous tumours tend to be younger at diagnosis than those with synchronous tumours (13.2 compared to 32.1 months mean age).

Resection of bilateral tumours with preservation of renal function may be impossible in a few children. It may be necessary to remove both kidneys, with renal transplantation after a period of dialysis. This strategy, though, is one of last resort, and should not be contemplated until conventional therapies have clearly failed.

Very occasionally, WT will be found in a patient with a single functioning kidney. Management should follow the guidelines for patients with bilateral tumours, as preservation of normal, functioning renal tissue is critical. Thus, initial chemotherapy with careful monitoring of response and timing of definitive surgery will provide the most favourable result. Immediate nephrectomy followed by dialysis, chemotherapy, and then transplantation would be an option, but one fraught with many additional problems so that it is best avoided if at all possible.

Wilms' tumour in patients with pre-existing renal disease

In these patients, variations in management will be dictated by the type and prognosis of the pre-existing disease. Where there is likely to be inexorable progression to ESRD, there seems little virtue in delaying surgical removal of the tumour and associated kidney. If necessary, dialysis can be instituted to supplement residual renal function. The timing of transplantation is more difficult, but to avoid the complexity of simultaneous cancer chemotherapy and transplantation immunosuppression it seems better to delay transplantation until chemotherapy has been completed and enough time has elapsed for the recurrence of malignancy to be unlikely. In practice, this period would be about 2 years from completion of chemotherapy.

Follow-up and screening investigations

The place of repeated 'screening' investigations in patients with conditions associated with or predisposing to WT has not been established. Often the physicians taking care of such patients are not primarily oncologists, and may not recognize all of the issues involved when making a decision to start screening. Some physicians propose that repeated screening permits earlier detection of clinically occult tumours and leads to an improvement in outcome. Others note that tumours may be clinically detectable only a few weeks after apparently normal (usually ultrasonographic) screening.

There are two separate issues to consider. First, what is the evidence that screening of presymptomatic, predisposed children will lead to earlier detection of tumours? Second, will detection of presymptomatic tumours result in fewer deaths or less treatment-related morbidity (as less therapy would be necessary for lower-stage disease)? Palmer and Evans (1983) reviewed nine patients with WT, known to have aniridia, who had been screened routinely by intravenous urography in an attempt to diagnose their tumours presymptomatically; an unsuspected tumour was detected in only one patient. It was concluded

that urography was inefficient for such screening and suggested that ultrasonography might be better. Green et al. (1993) reviewed data from 3675 patients registered with the National WT study and identified 24 WT patients with aniridia, 19 with Beckwith–Wiedemann syndrome, and 96 with hemihypertrophy. Screening examinations were associated with lower stage at diagnosis in aniridia, but not in the other two conditions. Craft et al. (1995) reviewed 1622 WT patients in the United Kingdom Children's Cancer Registry and found 16 with aniridia, 18 with Beckwith–Wiedemann syndrome, and 18 with hemihypertrophy. There were no significant differences in stage distribution or outcome for any of the three predisposing conditions whether they were not screened, had a tumour detected by screening, or had an interval diagnosis of tumour. At present, therefore, the utility of presymptomatic screening is not proven. Any randomized trial attempting to address this question will require an impracticably long accrual period because of the rarity of the predisposing conditions and the very high cure rates for WT. It seems more sensible to explain to parents that the child has a condition that may predispose to WT, to teach them to examine the child's abdomen, and to encourage them to seek medical advice if they are at all concerned.

During and after treatment, investigation is aimed at detecting early local or distant relapses. Generally, local relapses are less frequent than pulmonary relapse. Typically, chest radiographs should be obtained every 9 weeks during treatment, every 2 months for the first year, and every 3 months for the second year after completion of treatment. Stage IV patients should continue to have chest radiographs at three-monthly intervals for a further year. Screening for local relapse need not be so frequent, and abdominal ultrasonography at completion of treatment and then six-monthly for 2 years is enough. Other sites of relapse are rare, even (despite its name) in bone-metastasizing renal tumour, in which pulmonary metastases are most common. Thus, patients with this tumour need radionucleide bone scans, if at all, only at six-monthly intervals for 2 years.

Patterns and treatment of relapse

With the refinement of initial treatment and the excellent disease free survival, the treatment of relapse has assumed greater importance. In the fifth SIOP study, 54 per cent of all relapses were isolated pulmonary events, the remainder being in other or multiple sites (Lemerle et al. 1983). Sixteen per cent of all relapses involved the abdomen, but only in association with other sites. In the second and third American National WT studies, this site accounted for 58 per cent of all relapses whilst abdominal relapse accounted for a further 29 per cent (Grundy et al. 1989).

Both American and British studies (Grundy et al. 1989; Groote Loonen et al. 1994) have identified factors that indicate an increased likelihood of salvaging relapsed tumours. These factors were tumours with favourable histology that recurred only in the lungs; relapse in the abdomen where radiotherapy had not been included in the primary treatment; relapse that occurred more than 12 months from diagnosis. Each category was associated with a more favourable outcome. Patients with relapsed, 'unfavourable histology' tumours had poor survival regardless of the site or timing of relapse. Nevertheless, the overall survival following relapse was only 24 and 30 per cent in the UK and US series respectively and only 50 and 40 per cent respectively in the 'better' risk patients. Both studies showed that a variety of retrieval strategies were being used, in part dictated by the previous therapy. Subsequently, both groups have introduced standard relapse regimens to provide consistent data on response rates to the agents employed. Apart from the three standard agents—vincristine, actino-mycin D, and doxorubicin—other agents useful in relapse include ifosphamide (52), carboplatin (53), and etoposide (54).

Retrieval therapy is in part dictated by the therapies previously used. Initial surgery may not be necessary for non-irradiated abdominal recurrences of tumours with favourable histology, when radiotherapy and further chemotherapy can be given—an important consideration if the tumour appears not to be resectable. If not previously used, radiotherapy is indicated for multiple pulmonary relapses, and is used in conjunction with salvage chemotherapy. A small number of children with tumours of favourable histology, who developed solitary lung metastases after treatment in NWTS 1, 2, or 3, had a poor outcome with surgery and chemotherapy alone. In the patients who received radiotherapy the addition of surgery did not improve outcome (55), implying that surgery for this group is unnecessary.

The best reported results for relapsed and refractory WT come from the SFOP group. Using a combination of carboplatin and etoposide, response rates of 73 per cent and a survival rate of 33 per cent at 3 years have been obtained (56). All patients with anaplasia responded to this combination. A CCG study suggests that ifosphamide and etoposide may be a more potent combination for the treatment of bone metasta-sizing renal tumours (57).

A total of 51 children with recurrent or chemoresistant Wilms' who have had high-dose chemotherapy with autologous marrow or peripheral blood stem cell reconstitution tumour have been registered with the European Bone Marrow transplant solid tumour registry. Forty-three children underwent the procedure after at least one relapse, or without ever entering a remission. Although a variety of chemotherapy regimens were used, the most common was melphalan, either alone or in combination (with vincristine or BCNU) which was received by 40 patients. Twenty-one patients died after the procedure from progressive disease and three died of respiratory complications. Nineteen patients survive disease-free 2–10 years after the procedure, two are alive with progressive disease, and no follow-up data are available on six (58). The variety of approaches to the treatment of relapsed WT make it impossible to reach firm conclusions about the indications for and best method of administering high dose therapy, but these data suggest that high-dose chemotherapy may offer some chance of cure in patients who are resistant to conventional chemotherapy. Two prospective studies with conditioning regimens containing carboplatin/etoposide/melphalan (59) and thioTEPA/etoposide/cyclophosphamide (60) show encouraging results. Treatment of this type will need to be assessed further and should be undertaken in the future as part of a recognized trial.

Long-term complications of therapy

The majority of short-term toxicity caused by the treatment of WT is predictable according to the various modalities that are used. Thus, neurotoxicity from vincristine, and myelosuppression from doxoru-bicin are both well known and well documented. Seven per cent of patients (27/384) in UKW1 developed clinically significant neuro-toxicity secondary to treatment with vincristine. In eight cases the principal feature was paralytic ileus, and in the other 19 cases peripheral neuropathy varying in severity from mild ptosis to severe foot drop. All patients regained their neurological function. There were 421 episodes of hospitalization necessitated by myelosuppression. In 29 instances the episode was fever in association with neutropenia, and in 13 instances bleeding secondary to thrombocytopenia (Pritchard et al. 1995).

Actinomycin D, which in the past was often given fractionated over a 5 day period, is now more usually given as a single fraction (de Camargo et al. 1993; Green et al. 1995). This change has led to the emergence of an associated hepatopathy characterized by deranged liver function tests and thrombocytopenia. The phenomenon is of variable severity, ranging from a mild elevation in aminotransferase activities and bilirubin, and a mild concurrent fall in platelet count, to a severe disorder with liver failure and disseminated intravascular coagulation which may result in death. It is important to monitor for the occurrence of this condition as it may recur with subsequent courses of actinomycin D. Normally, dose reduction or readopting a fractionated schedule are sufficient to prevent recurrence (Raine et al. 1991; Green et al. 1995).

Concern about the possible long-term cardiotoxicity of anthra-cyclines was heightened by the detection of abnormalities of cardiac function in children who had received only low or moderate doses of anthracyclines (Lipshultz et al. 1991) for the treatment of leukaemia. Although only a minority of patients with WT receives anthracyclines, many will also have received radiation with fields which may encompass part or all of the heart. Twenty-five per cent of 97 patients previously treated for WT, with a mean cumulative anthracycline dose of 303 mg/m^2, had abnormalities of cardiac function compared to a control group with WT who had not received anthracyclines (Sorensen et al. 1995). This incidence of abnormalities is disconcertingly high, but the full relevance of the findings remains unclear, and careful long-term evaluation remains essential. Patients with increased left-ventricular wall stress should probably be advised to avoid extremely strenuous exercise and monitored carefully during pregnancy.

It is often assumed that unilateral nephrectomy has only minimal, if any, long-term morbidity. An evaluation of renal function in a group of long-term WT survivors (more than 13 years off treatment) has shown some evidence of dysfunction of the remaining kidney in 32 per cent. Nineteen percent had chrome EDTA glomerular filtration rates of less than 80 ml/minute/1.73m^2, 11 per cent had hypertension, and 9 per cent had increased urinary albumin excretion. Only 55 per cent of patients had undergone significant compensatory contralateral renal hypertrophy. Children of less than 24 months at the time of diagnosis and those children who had received radiation doses of greater than 1200 cGy to the remaining kidney were most at risk of dysfunction (Levitt et al. 1992). A similar study in adults with solitary kidneys who had undergone partial nephrectomy for a renal malignancy concluded that there was an increased risk of proteinuria, glomerulopathy and progressive renal failure (Novick et al. 1991). Thus, there is a clear case for continuing follow-up with measurements of blood pressure and checks for proteinuria.

The major long-term side-effect of radiotherapy for WT is disturbance of growth. As the radiation field in virtually all children irradiated for this condition is the hemiabdomen, the most obvious disturbance is asymmetrical growth of soft-tissue. As the field includes the full width of the vertebral bodies, there is also a loss in final height. The younger the patient is at the time of irradiation the more severe is the restriction and the more disproportionate they become as adults.

The loss in potential height ranges from 10 cm at the age of 1 year to 7 cm at 5 years.

Prognosis

With the use of modern anaesthetic and surgical techniques and the rational application of combination chemotherapy, the majority of patients with WT will be cured. In part, this is because most patients will present with histologically favourable, low-stage disease, but there have also been genuine advances in chemotherapy, so that the vast majority of WT patients are cured, many with minimal short- or long-term morbidity.

Stage V patients are often treated in a very 'individualized' fashion, and so the available findings are usually those of single centres. Data collected from 22 SIOP centres indicate an overall survival of 64 per cent with a follow-up of 6 years.

Future prospects

The two continuing clinical challenges in WT are to refine therapy in patients with good prognosis, so as to minimize treatment-related morbidity, and to improve therapy for poor-prognosis and relapsing patients, so that their survival improves. Advances in the understanding of the genetic basis of WT may help define more precisely patients with good and poor prognosis than the clinical staging currently in use. Stage I tumours with favourable histology already receive minimal treatment, but the recognition of highly favourable histological or genetic patterns may define a group which needs no adjuvant chemotherapy at all. Preoperative chemotherapy may provide a route to overall reduction of chemotherapy and obviation of radiotherapy. Improvement in the treatment of cases of unfavourable histology awaits the development of novel strategies.

References

Baird, P. N., Santos, A., Groves, N., Jadresic, L., and Cowell, J. K. (1992). Constitutional mutations in the WT1 gene in patients with Denys–Drash syndrome. *Human Molecular Genetics* 1, 301–305.

Barbaux, S., Niaudet, P., Gubler, M. C., Grünfeld, J. P., Jaubert, F., Kuttenn, F., Nihoul-Fékété, C., Souleyreau-Therville, N., Thibaud, E., Fellous, M., and McElreavey, K. (1997). Donor splice site mutations in the WT1 gene are responsible for Frasier syndrome. *Nature Genetics* 17, 467–469.

Barbosa, A. S., Hadjiathanasiou, C. G., Theodoridis, C., Papathanasiou, A., Tar, A., Merksz, M., Gyorvari, B., Sultan, C., Dumas, R., Jaubert, F., Niaudet, P., Moreira-Filho, C. O., Cotinot, C., and Fellous, M. (1999). The same mutation affecting the splicing of WT1 gene is present in Frasier syndrome patients with or without Wilms' tumour. *Human Mutation* 13, 146–153.

Beckwith, J. B. (1963). Extreme cytomegaly of the fetal adrenal cortex, omphalocele, hyperplasia of the kidneys and pancreas, and Leydig cell hyperplasia: another syndrome? Communication to the Western Society for Pediatric Research, November 11.

Beckwith, J. B. Wilms' tumour and other renal tumors of childhood. In *Pathology of Neoplasia in Children and Adolescents* (ed. M. W. B. Finegold), pp. 313–332. Philadelphia: Saunders, 1986.

Beckwith, J. B. and Palmer, N. F. (1978). Histopathology and prognosis of Wilms' tumour: results from the first National Wilms' tumour study. *Cancer* 41, 1937–1948.

Boccon-Gibod, L. *et al.* (2000). Complete necrosis induced by preoperative chemotherapy in Wilms' tumor as an indicator of low risk: report of the International Society of Paediatric Oncology (SIOP) Nephroblastoma Trial and Study 9. *Medical and Pediatric Oncology* 34, 193–200.

Bolande, R. P. (1973). Congenital mesoblastic nephroma of infancy. *Perspectives in Pediatric Pathology* 1, 227–250.

Bolande, R. P., Brough, A. J., and Izant, R. J. (1967). Congenital mesoblastic nephroma of infancy. *Pediatrics* 40, 272–278.

Bonnin, J. M., Rubinstein, L. J., Palmer, N. F., and Beckwith, J. B. (1984). The association of embryonal tumours originating in the kidney and in the brain. A report of seven cases. *Cancer* 54, 2137–2213.

Bove, K. E. and McAdams, A. J. (1985). The nephroblastomatosis complex and its relationship to Wilms' tumour: a clinicopathologic treatise. *Perspectives in Pediatric Pathology* 3, 185–222.

Breslow, N. E. and Beckwith, J. B. (1982). Epidemiological features of Wilms' tumour: results of the National Wilms' Tumour Study. *Journal of the National Cancer Institute* 68, 429–436.

Breslow, N. E. *et al.* (1978). Prognostic factors for patients without metastases at diagnoses. Results of the National Wilms' tumour study. *Cancer* 41, 1577–1589.

Breslow, N. E. *et al.* (1985). Prognostic factors for Wilms' tumour patients with non-metastatic disease at diagnosis. Results of the second National Wilms' tumour study. *Journal of Clinical Oncology* 3, 521–531.

Breslow, N. E. *et al.* (1986). Clinicopathologic features and prognosis for Wilms' tumour patients with metastases at diagnosis. *Cancer* 58, 2501–2511.

Breslow, N. E., Takashima, J. R., Ritchey, M. L., Strong, L. C., and Green, D. M. (2000). Renal failure in the Denys–Drash and Wilms' tumor-aniridia syndromes. *Cancer Research* 60, 430–432.

Buckler, A. J., Pelletier, J., Haber, D. A., Glaser, T., and Housman, D. E. (1991). Isolation, characterization, and expression of the murine Wilms' tumor gene (WT1) during kidney development. *Molecular Cell Biology* 11, 1707–1712.

Coppes, M. J. *et al.* (1987). Prognosis of bilateral Wilms' tumour (BWT) in SIOP 1, 2, and 5. *SIOP Proceedings*, Abstr. 122. SIOP, Jerusalem.

Coppes, M. J. *et al.* (1992a). Loss of heterozygosity mapping in Wilms' tumor indicates the involvement of three distinct regions and a limited role for nondisjunction or mitotic recombination. *Genes Chromosomes and Cancer* 5, 326–334.

Coppes, M. J., Zandvoort, S. W., Sparling, C. R., Poon, A. O., Weitzman, S., and Blanchette, V. S. (1992b). Acquired von Willebrand disease in Wilms' tumour patients. *Journal of Clinical Oncology* 10, 422–427.

Craft, A. W., Parker, L., Stiller, C., and Cole, M. (1995). Screening for Wilms' tumour in patients with aniridia, Beckwith syndrome or hemihypertrophy. *Medical and Pediatric Oncology* 24, 231–234.

D'Angio, G. J. (1983). SIOP and the management of Wilms' tumour. *Journal of Clinical Oncology* 1, 595–596.

D'Angio, G. J. *et al.* (1976). The treatment of Wilms' tumour: results of the first National Wilms' tumour study. *Cancer* 38, 633–646.

D'Angio, G. J. *et al.* (1981). The treatment of Wilms' tumour: results of the second National Wilms' tumour study. *Cancer*, 47, 2302–2311.

D'Angio, G. J. *et al.* (1989). The treatment of Wilms' tumour. Results of the third National Wilms' tumour study. *Cancer* 64, 349–360.

de Camargo, B. and Franco, E. L. (1993). A randomised clinical trial of single-dose versus fractionated-dose dactinomycin in the treatment of Wilms' tumor. *Cancer* 73, 3081–3086.

de Camargo, B. *et al.* (1994). Phase II study of carboplatin as a single drug for relapsed Wilms' tumour: experience of the Brazilian Wilms' Tumour Study Group. *Medical and Pediatric Oncology* 22, 258–260.

Demmer, L., Primack, W., Loik, V., Brown, R., Therville, N., and McElreavey, K. (1999). Frasier syndrome: a cause of focal segmental glomerulosclerosis in a 46, XX female. *Journal of the American Society of Nephrology* 10, 2215–2218.

Denamur, E., Bocquet, N., Mougenot, B., Da Silva, F., Martinat, L., Loirat, C., Elion, J., Bensman, A., and Ronco, P. M. (1999). Mother-to-child transmitted *WT1* splice-site mutation is responsible for distinct glomerular diseases. *Journal of the American Society of Nephrology* **10**, 2219–2223.

Devriendt, K., Deloof, E., Moerman, P., Legius, E., Vanhole, C., de Zegher, F., Proesmans, W., and Devlieger, H. (1995). Diaphragmatic hernia in Denys–Drash syndrome. *American Journal of Medical Genetics* **57**, 97–101.

Denys, P., Malvaux, P., van den Berghe, H., Tanghe, H., and Proestmans, W. (1967). Association d'un syndrome anatomo-pathologique de pseudohermaphroditisme masculin, d'une tumeur de Wilms, d'une nephropathie parenchymateuse et d'un mosaicisme XX/XY. *Archives Francais Pediatrie* **24**, 729–739.

Drash, A., Sherman, F., Hartman, W. H., and Blizzard, R. M. (1970). A syndrome of pseudohermaphroditism, Wilms' tumour, hypertension, and degenerative renal disease. *Journal of Pediatrics* **76**, 585–593.

Francke, U., Holmes, T. B., Atkins, L., and Riccardi, V. M. (1979). Aniridia–Wilms' tumour association; evidence for specific deletion of 11p13. *Cytogenetics and Cell Genetics* **24**, 185–192.

Frasier, S., Bashore, R. A., and Mosier, H. D. (1964). Gonadoblastoma associated with pure gonadal dysgenesis in monozygotic twins. *Journal of Pediatrics* **64**, 740–745.

Green, D. M., Breslow, N. E., Beckwith, J. B., and Norkool, P. (1993). Screening of children with hemihypertrophy, aniridia and Beckwith–Wiedemann syndrome in patients with Wilms' tumor. *Medical and Pediatric Oncology* **21**, 188–192.

Green, D. M., Beckwith, J. B., Weeks, N. M., Moksness, J., Breslow, N. E., and D'Angio, G. J. (1994). The relationship between microstaging variables, age at diagnosis, and tumor weight of children with stage I/favorable histology Wilms' tumor. *Cancer* **74**, 1817–1820.

Green, D. M. *et al.* (1995). Relationship between dose schedule and charges for treatment on national Wilms' tumor study 4. A report from the National Wilms' Tumor Study Group. *Journal of the National Cancer Institute Monographs* **19**, 21–25.

Greenberg, F. *et al.* (1986). The Perlman familial nephroblastomatosis syndrome. *American Journal of Medical Genetics* **24**, 101–110.

Greenberg, F., Copeland, K., and Gresik, M. V. (1988). Expanding the spectrum of the Perlman syndrome. *American Journal of Medical Genetics* **29**, 733–776.

Griffel, M. (1977). Wilms' tumour in New York State: epidemiology and survivorship. *Cancer* **40**, 3140–3145.

Groot-Loonen, J. J., Pinkerton, C. R., Morris-Jones, P. H., and Pritchard, J. (1990). How curable is relapsed Wilms' tumour? *Archives of Disease in Childhood* **65**, 968–970.

Grundy, P., Breslow, N., Green, D. M., Sharples, K., Evans, A. E., and D'Angio, G. J. (1989). Prognostic factors for children with recurrent Wilms' tumour: results from the second and third National Wilms' tumour study. *Journal of Clinical Oncology* **7**, 638–647.

Grundy, P. *et al.* (1991). Chromosome 11 uniparental isodisomy predisposing to embryonal neoplasms. *Lancet* **338**, 1079–1080.

Grundy, P. E. *et al.* (1994). Loss of heterozygosity for chromosomes 16q and 1p in Wilms' tumors predicts an adverse outcome. *Cancer Research* **54**, 2331.

Grundy, R. G., Pritchard, J., Baraitser, M., Risdon, M., and Robards, M. (1992). Perlman and Wiedemann–Beckwith syndromes: two distinct conditions associated with Wilms' tumour. *European Journal of Paediatrics* **151**, 895–898.

Grundy, P. E., Telzerow, P. E., Breslow, N., Moksness, J., Huff, V., and Paterson, M. C. (1994). Loss of heterozygosity for chromosomes 16q and 1p in Wilms' tumors predicts an adverse outcome. *Cancer Research* **54**, 2331–2333.

Gubler, M. C., Yang, Y., Jeanpierre, C., Barbaux, S., and Niaudet, P. (1999). WT1, renal development, and glomerulopathies. *Advances in Nephrology from the Necker Hospital* **29**, 299–315.

Guo, J. K., Menke, A. L., Gubler, M. C., Clarke, A. R., Harrison, D., Hammes, A., Hastie, N. D., and Schedl, A. (2002). WT1 is a key regulator of podocyte function: reduced expression levels cause crescentic glomerulonephritis and mesangial sclerosis. *Human Molecular Genetics* **11**, 651–659.

Haber, D. A., Sohn, R. L., Buckler, A. J., Pelletier, J., Call, K. M., and Housman, D. E. (1991). Alternative splicing and genomic structure of the Wilms' tumor gene *WT1*. *Proceedings of the National Academy of Sciences (USA)* **88**, 9618–9622.

Habib, R., Loirat, C., Gubler, M. C., Niaudet, P., Bensman, A., Levy, M., and Broyer, M. (1985). The nephropathy associated with male pseudohermaphroditism and Wilms' tumor (Drash syndrome): a distinctive glomerular lesion, report of 10 cases. *Clinical Nephrology* **24**, 269–278.

Habib, R., Gubler, M. C., Antignac, C., and Gagnadoux, M. F. (1993). Diffuse mesangial sclerosis: a congenital glomerulopathy with nephrotic syndrome. *Advances in Nephrology* **22**, 43–56.

Hammes, A., Guo, J. K., Lutsch, G., Leheste, J. R., Landrock, D., Ziegler, U., Gubler, M. C., and Schedl, A. (2001). Two splice variants of the Wilms' tumor 1 gene have distinct functions during sex determination and nephron formation. *Cell* **106**, 319–329.

Hall, J. G. (1990). Genomic imprinting: review and relevance to human diseases. *American Journal of Human Genetics* **46**, 857–873.

Hamel, B. C. J., Mannens, M., and Bokkerink, J. P. M. (1989). Perlman syndrome: report of a case and results of molecular studies. *American Journal of Human Genetics* **45**, A48.

Heidemann, R. L., Haase, G. M., Foley, C. L., Wilson, H. L., and Bailey, W. C. (1985). Nephroblastomatosis and Wilms' tumour: clinical experience and management of seven patients. *Cancer* **555**, 1446–1451.

Heidemann, R. L., McGavran, L., and Waldstein, G. (1986). Nephroblastomatosis and deletion of 11p. The potential etiologic relationship to subsequent Wilms' tumour. *American Journal of Pediatric Hematology and Oncology* **8**, 231–234.

Henry, I. *et al.* (1991). Uniparental paternal disomy in a genetic cancer-predisposing syndrome. *Nature* **351**, 665–667.

Hou, L. T. and Holman, R. L. (1961). Bilateral nephroblastomatosis in a premature infant. *Journal of Pathology and Bacteriology* **82**, 249–255.

Hrabovsky, E. E., Othrsen, H. B., deLorimier, A., Kelalis, P., Beckwith, J. B., and Takashima, J. (1986). Wilms' tumour in the neonate: a report from the national Wilms' tumour study. *Journal of Pediatric Surgery* **21**, 385–387.

Jeanpierre, C., Denamur, E., Henry, I., Cabanis, M. O., Luce, S., Cécille, A., Elion, J., Peuchmaur, M., Loirat, C., Niaudet, P., Gubler, M. C., and Junien, C. (1998a). Identification of constitutional *WT1* mutations in patients with isolated diffuse mesangial sclerosis (IDMS) and anlysis of genotype–phenotype correlations using a computerized mutation database. *American Journal of Human Genetics* **62**, 824–833.

Jeanpierre, C., Béroud, C., Niaudet, P., and Junien, C. (1998b). Software and database for the analysis of mutations in the human *WT1* gene. **26**, 273–277.

Kidd, J. M. (1970). Exclusion of certain renal neoplasms from the category of Wilms' tumour. *American Journal of Pathology* **59**, 16a.

Kikuchi, H., Takata, A., Akasaka, Y., Fukuzawa, R., Yoneyama, H., Kurosawa, Y., Honda, M., Kamiyama, Y., and Hata, J. (1998). Do intronic mutations affecting splicing of WT1 exon 9 cause Frasier syndrome? *Journal of Medical Genetics* **35**, 54–48.

Klamt, B., Koziell, A., Poulat, F., Wieacker, P., Scambler, P., Berta, P., and Gessler, M. (1998). Frasier syndrome is caused by defective alternative splicing of WT1 leading to an altered ratio of WT1+/−KTS splice isoforms. *Human Molecular Genetics* **7**, 709–714.

Koufos, A. *et al.* (1989). Familial Wiedemann–Beckwith syndrome and a second Wilms' tumour locus both map to 11p15.5. *American Journal of Human Genetics* **44**, 711–719.

Koziell, A. B., Grundy, R., Barratt, T. M., and Scambler, P. (1999). Evidence for genetic heterogeneity of nephropathic phenotypes associated with Denys–Drash and Frasier syndromes. *American Journal of Human Genetics* **64**, 1778–1781.

Kreidberg, J. A., Sariola, H., Loring, J. M., Maeda, M., Pelletier, J., Housman, D., and Jaenisch, R. (1993). *WT1* is required for early kidney development. *Cell* **74**, 679–691.

Lemerle, J. *et al.* (1976). Preoperative versus post-operative radiotherapy, single versus multiple courses of actinomycin D in the treatment of Wilms' tumours. Preliminary results of a controlled clinical trial conducted by the International Society of Pediatric Oncology (SIOP). *Cancer* **38**, 647–654.

Lemerle, J. *et al.* (1983). Effectiveness of preoperative chemotherapy in Wilms' tumour: results of an International Society of Pediatric Oncology (SIOP) clinical trial. *Journal of Clinical Oncology* **1**, 604–610.

Lennox, E. L., Stiller, C. A., Morris-Jones, P. H., and Kinnier-Wilson, L. M. (1979). Nephroblastoma: treatment during 1970–1973 and the effect on survival of inclusion in the first MRC trial. *British Medical Journal* **2**, 567–569.

Levitt, G. A., Yeomans, E., Dicks-Mireaux, C., Breatnach, F., Kingston, J., and Pritchard, J. (1992). Renal size and function after cure of Wilms' tumour. *British Journal of Cancer* **66**, 877–882.

Liban, E. and Kozenitzky, I. L. (1970). Metanephric hamartomas and nephroblastomatosis in sibs. *Cancer* **25**, 885.

Lipshultz, S. E. *et al.* (1991). Late cardiac effects of doxorubicin therapy for acute lymphoblastic leukaemia in children. *New England Journal of Medicine* **324**, 808–815.

Little, M. H., Prosser, J., Condie, A., Smith, P. J., Van Heyningen, V., and Hastie, N. D. (1992). Zinc finger point mutations within the *WT1* gene in Wilms' tumour patients. *Proceedings of the National Academy of Sciences (USA)* **89**, 4791–4795.

Little, M. H., Williamson, K. A., Mannens, M., Kelsey, A., Gosden, C., Hastie, N. D., and van Heyningen, V. (1993). Evidence that *WT1* mutations in Denys–Drash syndrome patients may act in a dominant-negative fashion. *Human Molecular Genetics* **2** (3), 259–264.

Little, M., Holmes, G., Bickmore, W., Heyningen, V. V., Hastie, N., and Wainwright, B. (1995). DNA binding capacity of the *WT1* protein is abolished by Denys–Drash syndrome *WT1* point mutations. *Human Molecular Genetics* **4** (3), 351–358.

Machin, G. A. and McCaughey, W. T. E. (1984). A new precursor lesion of Wilms' tumour (nephroblastoma): intralobar multifocal nephroblastomatosis. *Histopathology* **8**, 35–53.

McDonald, J. M., Douglass, E. C., Fisher, R., Geiser, C. F., Krill, C. E., Stron, L. C., Virshup, D., and Huff, V. (1998). Linkage of famililail Wilms' tumor predisposition to chromsome 19 and a two-locus model for the etiology of familial tumors. *Cancer Research* **58**, 1387–1390.

Maheswaran, S. *et al.* (1993). Physical and functional interaction between *WT1* and p53 proteins. *Proceedings of the National Academy of Sciences (USA)* **90**, 5100–5104.

Marsden, H. B. and Lawler, W. (1978). Bone-metastasising renal tumour of childhood. *British Journal of Cancer* **38**, 437–441.

Mitchell, C. D., Harvey, W., Gordon, D., Womer, R. B., Dillon, M. J., and Pritchard, J. (1985). Rhabdoid Wilms' tumour and prostaglandin-mediated hypercalcaemia. *European Paediatric Haematology and Oncology* **2**, 153–157.

Mitchell, C. D., Morris-Jones, P., Kelsey, A., Vujanic, G., Marsden, B., Shannon, R., Gornall, P., Owens, C., Taylor, R., Imeson, J., Middleton, H., and Pritchard, J. (2000). The treatment of Wilms' tumour: results of the UKCCSG second Wilms' tumour study. *British Journal of Cancer* **83**, 602–608.

Moorthy, A. V., Chesney, R. W., and Lubinsky, M. (1987). Chronic renal failure and XY gonadal dysgenesis: 'Frasier' syndrome—a commentary on reported cases. *American Journal of Medical Genetics* **3** (Suppl.), 297–302.

Morris-Jones, P., Marsden, H. B., Pearson, D., and Barnes, J. (1987). MRC second nephroblastoma trial, 1974–1978: long-term results. *SIOP Proceedings*, Abstr. 121. SIOP, Jerusalem.

Narahara, K. *et al.* (1984). Regional mapping of catalase and Wilms' tumour–aniridia, genitourinary abnormalities, and mental retardation triad loci to the chromosome segment 11p13.05–p13.06. *Human Genetics* **66**, 181–185.

Neri, G., Martini-Neri, M. E. M., Katz, B. E., and Opitz, J. M. (1984). The Perlman syndrome: familial renal dysplasia with Wilms' tumour, fetal gigantism and multiple congenital anomalies. *American Journal of Medical Genetics* **19**, 195–207.

Novick, C., Gephardt, M. D., Guz, B., Steinmuller, D., and Tubbs, R. R. (1991). Long-term follow-up after partial removal of a solitary kidney. *New England Journal of Medicine* **325**, 1058–1062.

Ogawa, O. *et al.* (1993). Relaxation of insulin-like growth factor II gene imprinting implicated in Wilms' tumour. *Nature* **362**, 749–751.

Owens, C. M., Dicks-Mireaux, C., Burnett, S. J. D., Veys, P. A., and Pritchard, J. (1996). Results of the 2nd Wilms' Tumour Study of the UKCCSG. *American Journal of Radiology* (in press).

Palmer, N. and Evans, A. E. (1983). The association of aniridia and Wilms' tumour: methods of surveillance and diagnosis. *Medical and Pediatric Oncology* **11**, 73–75.

Parkin, D. M., Stiller, C. A., and Draper, G. J. (1988). The international incidence of childhood cancer. *International Journal of Cancer*, **42**, 511–520.

Pelletier, J., Schelling, M., Buckler, A. J., Rogers, A., Haber, D. A., and Housman, D. (1991a). Expression of the Wilms' tumor gene *WT1* in the murine urogenital system. *Genetics and Development* **5**, 1345–1356.

Pelletier, J. *et al.* (1991b). Germline mutations in the Wilms' tumor suppresser gene are associated with abnormal urogenital development in Denys–Drash syndrome. *Cell* **67**, 437–447.

Perlman, M. (1986). Perlman syndrome: familial renal dysplasia with Wilms' tumor, fetal gigantism, and multiple congenital anomalies. *American Journal of Medical Genetics* **25**, 793–795.

Perlman, M., Goldberg, G. M., Bar-Ziv, J., and Danovitch, G. (1973). Renal harmatomas and nephroblastomatosis with fetal gigantism: a familial syndrome. *Journal of Paediatrics* **83**, 414–418.

Perlman, M., Levin, M., and Wittels, B. (1974). Syndrome of fetal gigantism, renal hamartomas, and nephroblastomatosis with Wilms' tumor. *Cancer* **35**, 1212–1217.

Ping, A. J., Reeve, A. E., Law, D. J., Young, M. R., Boehnke, M., and Feinberg, A. P. (1989). Genetic linkage of Beckwith–Wiedemann syndrome to 11p15. *American Journal of Human Genetics* **44**, 720–723.

Pritchard, J., Stiller, C. A., and Lennox, E. L. (1989). Over-treatment of children with Wilms' tumour outside paediatric oncology centres. *British Medical Journal* **299**, 835–836.

Pritchard, J. *et al.* (1995). Results of the United Kingdom Children's Cancer Study Group (UKCCSG) First Wilms' Tumor Study (UKW-1). *Journal of Clinical Oncology* **13**, 124–133.

Pritchard-Jones, K. *et al.* (1990). The candidate Wilms' tumour gene is involved in genitourinary development. *Nature* **346**, 194–197.

Pueschel, S. M. and Padre-Mendoza, T. (1984). Chromosome II and Beckwith–Weidemann syndrome. *Journal of Pediatrics* **104**, 484–485.

Raine, J. *et al.* (1991). Hepatopathy-thrombocytopenia syndrome. A complication of actinomycin-D therapy for Wilms' tumour. *Journal of Clinical Oncology* **9**, 268–273.

Rahman, N. *et al.* (1998). Confirmation of FWT1 as a Wilms' tumour susceptibitlity gene and phenotypic characteristics of Wilms' tumour attributable to FWT1. *Human Genetics* **103**, 547–556.

Rainier, S., Johnson, L. A., Dobry, C. J., Ping, A. J., Grundy, P. E., and Feinberg, A. P. (1993). Relaxation of imprinted genes in human cancer. *Nature* **362**, 747–749.

Rapley, E. A. *et al.* (2000). Evidence for susceptibility genes to familial Wilms' tumour in addition to *WT1*, *FWT1* and *FWT2*. *British Journal of Cancer* **83**, 177–183.

Rauscher, III, F. J. (1993). The *WT1* Wilms' tumor gene product: a developmentally regulated transcription factor in the kidney that functions as a tumor suppressor. *FASEB Journal* **7**, 896–903.

Reddy, J. C., Morris, J. C., Wang, J., English, M. A., Haber, D. A., Shi, Y., and Licht, J. D. (1995). WT1-mediated transcriptional activation is inhibited by dominant negative mutant proteins. *Journal of Biological Chemistry* **270**, 10878–10884.

Reeve, A. E., Eccles, M. R., Wilkins, R. J., Bell, G. I., and Millow, L. J. (1985). Expression of insulin-like growth factor-11 transcripts in Wilms' tumour. *Nature* **317**, 258–260.

Reeve, A. E., Sih, S. A., Raizis, A. M., and Feinberg, A. P. (1989). Loss of alleleic heterozygosity at a second locus on chromosome 11 in sporadic Wilms' tumour cells. *Molecular and Cellular Biology* **9**, 1799–1803.

Riccardi, V. M., Sujansky, E., Smith, A. C., and Francke, U. (1978). Chromosome imbalance in the aniridia–Wilms' tumour association: 11p interstitial deletion. *Pediatrics* **61**, 604–610.

Ritchey, M. L. *et al.* (1994). Management and outcome of inoperable Wilms' tumour—a report of National Wilms' tumour study 3. *Annals of Surgery* **220**, 683–690.

Rousseau-Merck, M. F. *et al.* (1982). An original hypercalcemic infantile renal tumour without bone metastasis: heterotransplantation to nude mice. *Cancer* **50**, 85–93.

Schroeder, W. T. *et al.* (1987). Non-random loss of maternal chromosome 11 alleles in Wilms' tumours. *American Journal of Human Genetics* **40**, 413–420.

Scott, J. *et al.* (1985). Insulin-like growth factor-II gene expression in Wilms' tumour and embryonic tissues. *Nature* **317**, 260–262.

Schumacher, V., Schärer, K., Wühl, E., Altrogge, H., Bonzel, K. E., Guschmann, M., Neuhaus, T. J., Pollastro, R. M., Kuwertz-Broking, E., Bulla, M., Tondera, A. M., Mundel, P., Helmchen, U., Waldherr, R., Weirich, A., and Royer-Pokora, B. (1998). Spectrum of early onset nephrotic syndrome associated with WT1 missense mutations. *Kidney International* **53**, 1594–1600.

Shimoyama, H., Nakajima, M., Naka, H., Park, Y. D., Hori, K., Morikawa, H., and Yoshioka, A. (2002) *European Journal of Pediatrics* **161**, 81–83.

Sorensen, K., Levitt, G., Sebag-Montefiore, D., Bull, C., and Sullivan, I. (1995). Cardiac function in Wilms' tumour survivors (1995). *Journal of Clinical Oncology* **13**, 1546–1556.

Tournade, M. F., Com-Nougue, C., Voute, P. A., Lemerle, J., De Kraker, J., Delemare, J. F. M., Burgers, J. M. V., Habrand, J. L., Moorman, C. G. M., Burger, D., Rey, A., Zucker, J. M., Carli, M., Jereb, B., Bey, P., and Gauthier, B. (1993). Results of the International Society of Paediatric Oncology 6 Wilms' tumor trial and study; a risk adapted therapeutic approach in Wilms' tumor. *Journal of Clinical Oncology* **11**, 1014–1023.

Tournade, M. F., Com-Nougue, C., De Kraker, J., Ludwig, R., Rey, A., Burgers, J. M. V., Sandstedt, B., Godzinski, J., Carli, M., Potter, R., and Zucker, J. M. (2001). Optimal duration of therapy in unilateral and non-metstatic Wilms' tumour in children older than 6 month; Results of the ninth International society of Paediatric Oncology Wilms' tumour trial and study. *Journal of Clinical Oncology*, **19**, 488–500.

Turleau, C., De Grouchy, J., Chavin-Colin, F., Martelli, H., Voyer, M., and Charlas, R. (1984). Trisomy 11p15 and Beckwith–Wiedemann syndrome. A report of two cases. *Human Genetics* **67**, 219–221.

Voute, P. A. *et al.* (1987). Preoperative chemotherapy (CT) as first treatment in children with Wilms' tumour. Results of the SIOP nephroblastoma trials and studies. *SIOP Proceedings*, Abstr. 123. SIOP, Jerusalem.

Wadey, R. B., Pal, N. P., Buckle, B., Yeomans, E., Pritchard, J., and Cowell, J. K. (1990). Loss of heterozygosity in Wilms' tumour involves two distinct regions of chromosome 11. *Oncogene* **5**, 901–907.

Waziri, M., Patil, S. R., Hanson, J. W., and Bartley, J. A. (1983). Abnormality of chromosome 11 in patients with features of Beckwith–Weidemann syndrome. *Journal of Pediatrics* **102**, 873.

Weeks, D. A., Beckwith, J. B., Merau, G. W., and Luckey, D. W. (1989). Rhabdoid tumour of the kidney. A report of 111 cases from the National Wilms' Tumour Study center. *American Journal of Surgical Pathology* **13**, 439–458.

Weirich, A. *et al.* (2001). Clinical impactof histologic subtypes in localised non anaplastic nephroblastoma treated according to trial and study SIOP9/GPOH. **12**, 311–319.

Wiedemann, N. R. (1964). Complexe malformatif familial avec hernie ombilicale et macroglossie: un syndrome nouveau? *Journeau de Genetique Humaine* **13**, 223–232.

Wilimas, J. A., Douglass, E. C., Magill, H. L., Fitch, S., and Hustu, H. O. (1988). Significance of pulmonary computed tomography at diagnosis in Wilms' tumour. *Journal of Clinical Oncology* **6**, 1144–1146.

Williams, J. C., Brown, K. W., Mott, M. G., and Maitland, N. J. (1989). Maternal allele loss in Wilms' tumour. *Lancet* **i**, 283–284.

Wilms, M. *Die Mischgeschwulste der Nieren*, pp. 1–90. Leipzig: Arthur Georgi, 1899.

Yang, Y., Jeanpierre, C., Dressler, G. R., Lacoste, M., Niaudet, P., and Gubler, M. C. (1999). WT1 and PAX-2 podocyte expression in Denys–Drash syndrome and isolated diffuse mesangial sclerosis. *American Journal of Pathology* **54**, 181–192.

Zuppan, C. W., Beckwith, J. B., Weeks, D. A., Luckey, D. W., and Pringle, K. C. (1991). The effects of preoperative chemotherapy on the histologic features of Wilms' tumor. An analysis of cases from the third national Wilms' Tumor Study. *Cancer* **68**, 385–394.

18.3 Tumours of the renal pelvis and ureter

Peter Whelan

Introduction

Tumours of the renal pelvis and ureter are relatively uncommon but both transitional cell carcinoma (TCC) and squamous cell carcinoma may occur and present with haematuria.

Incidence

Transitional cell carcinoma of the renal pelvis comprise between 5 and 7 per cent of all renal malignancies. Because TCC is a multifocal disease, patients presenting initially with bladder TCC have a 2–4 per cent incidence of subsequent upper tract tumours (Lucke and Schumgerger 1957; Nocks *et al.* 1982). The incidence is greater among patients with high recurrence rates, associated carcinoma *in situ*, multiple recurrences, and large volume lesions (Hurle *et al.* 1999), whilst a 20-year longitudinal follow-up of a cohort of 178 patients (Holmang *et al.* 1998) showed only three patients (2 per cent) who developed upper tract lesions over this period.

TCC of the ureter account for 1 per cent of all transitional cell lesions (Bloom 1970).

Patients with involvement of either the renal pelvis alone or the renal pelvis and ureter have a 25–50 per cent chance of subsequently developing a bladder cancer (Murphy *et al.* 1980) and 75 per cent of these lesions appear within the first 3 years. Interestingly, the majority of the bladder lesions develop on the same side as the original tumour whatever treatment has been given.

Patients who undergo radical cystectomy for uncontrolled superficial disease or invasive cancer develop upper urinary tract tumours at an increased rate varying from 2.4 to 8.5 per cent of cases (see Table 1). Factors such as high-grade, high-stage, multifocality, distal ureteric disease, carcinoma *in situ*, and disease in the prostatic urethra are all predisposed to an increased incidence.

Aetiology

Smoking

Studies continue to show a substantial increased risk for the development of upper tract transitional cell tumours in patients who smoke, the risk being considered similar to that for the development of TCC of the bladder. In reported series the proportion of smokers is between 75 and 80 per cent of those with tumours, but it remains difficult to arrive at a relative risk because most newly presenting patients are over 60 and the prevalence for smoking in this age cohort overall is similar to that in the patient group (Booth *et al.* 1980) but whether the dramatic increase in female smoking will mirror in bladder cancer the observed rise in lung cancer remains to be seen.

Table 1 Bladder tumour characteristics of patients with upper urinary tract tumours after cystectomy (from Huguet-Perez *et al.* 2001)

Studies	No. of patients	UUTTS	Superficial	Invasive	High grade	Multi	CIS	Renal	Renal ureter
Balafi *et al.* (1999)	529	16 (3%)	3	13	—	—	10	4	7
Schellhammer and Whitmore (1976)	461	19 (4.1%)	—	—	—	—	—	—	—
Kenworthy *et al.* (1996)	430	11 (2.6%)	6	5	7	4	2	5	6
Zincke *et al.* (1984)	425	14 (3.3%)	9	5	9	11	8	1	4
Markowitz and Skinner (1990)	220	5 (2.4%)	0	5	5	2	2	1	3
Mufti *et al.* (1988)	188	16 (8.5%)	—	—	—	—	—	—	—
Hastie *et al.* (1991)	180	10 (5.5%)	7	3	—	—	4	—	—
Herranz *et al.* (1999)	160	5 (3.1%)	1	4	4	—	0	—	1
Tsuji *et al.* (1996)	61	5 (8.2%)	4	1	4	—	—	—	—
Huguet-Perez *et al.* (2001)	568	26 (4.5%)	11	15	22	22	17	12	15

Inflammation and infection

Chronic inflammation of the renal pelvis has been associated with the development of squamous cell carcinoma of the transitional epithelium. More than half of these patients have an associated calculus, but to put this finding in perspective, less than 1 per cent of all patients with a past history of stones develop tumours in the upper urinary tract and there appears to be no definitive association with the presence of infected stones (i.e. staghorn calculi) and the development of squamous lesions (Clayman et al. 1983). A stone might act as an initiating factor in some patients but there are other mechanisms which are not understood.

Chemical carcinogens

It is generally accepted that certain chemicals, notably B-naphthylamine, are associated with the development of bladder tumours (Case et al. 1959; Hicks 1980). It is probable that an increasing exposure to industrial chemicals, and therefore possible carcinogens, will play an increasing role in raising the incidence of bladder cancer. The relatively low incidence of tumours of the upper urinary tract may be a reflection of the rapid transit of urine through this area, but no studies have been performed to determine whether patients with dilated pelvicalyceal systems or untreated congenital mega ureters, are at greater risk.

Balkan nephropathy

This was first described by Tanchev et al. (1956). It affects the inhabitants of the Danube basin (former Yugoslavia, Romania, and Bulgaria) and has also been reported in Greece. It is associated with the development of tumours of the renal pelvis and ureter (Petkovic et al. 1971) and is a slowly progressive inflammation of the renal interstitium. This process may lead to renal failure. It is of note that bladder involvement is rare and Petkovic et al. (1971) report the ratio between upper tract tumours and bladder tumours as 40 : 1. In view of the aetiology, the patients present special problems with treatment and are referred to later in the discussion of conservative management.

Analgesic nephropathy

Hultergren et al. (1965) reported the development of cancer of the renal pelvis in association with the ingestion of phenacetin containing analgesics. This was subsequently also reported in Australia, but similar associations have not been described from other parts of the world. In the Australian study reported by Mahoney et al. (1977), patients have consumed greater than 5 kg of compound analgesics and there appear to be an association with cigarette smoking as well. In this group, the normal preponderance of males to females was reversed, and between 30 and 50 per cent of the renal pelvic tumours were squamous, although Gittes (1979) reported that these appear to be arising in transitional cell epithelium and may represent squamous metaplasia. The reasons why very few bladder tumours develop as in Balkan nephropathy, remain obscure. The change in use in phenacetin makes it likely that this type of tumour will be seen less and less.

Endstage renal failure

The incidence of TCC is greater in patients with endstage renal disease and is often multifocal (Chew et al. 1995). The underlying aetiology remains obscure but awareness of this possibility and the importance of differentiating it from renal cell carcinoma must always be borne in mind with patients with haematuria.

Staging and grading in pathological assessment

Attempting to stage and grade all urothelial tumours presents similar problems. Four systems originating in America are available for possible use, those described by Broders (1922), Friedman and Ash (1959), Jewitt (1963), and Cummings (1980), whilst the Union International Contre Cancer (UICC; Mostofi et al. 1973) is also a competitor. Gradually, the TNM system has become predominant but this system derives apparently little input from clinical as distinct from pathological data and it is not always as helpful as it might be to clinicians seeking to offer a sensible prognosis.

Histological grading generally meets with agreement but it is open to inter- and even intraobserver error. The long-standing Jewitt (1963) system and the equivalent international consensus conference pathological grades are shown in Fig. 1.

In making a diagnosis, the higher the grade and stage the shorter and worse the prognosis. Unfortunately, when dealing with transitional cell tumours either of the bladder or the upper urinary tract, lesions classified as low grade and low stage, whilst having significantly less chance of killing a patient, nevertheless spread locally and cause distant metastasis that may result in death occasionally (Murphy et al. 1980). At present there is no system of staging and grading sensitive enough to account for these variables, but in general as stated above the higher the grade and stage the worse the prognosis.

Results of any therapy can only be fully evaluated when like is compared to like. As we shall discuss in the section titled 'Treatment', the equivalence or superiority of any new treatment has to have as its base a strict comparative criteria. The near universal acceptance of the UICC stage and grading system, imperfect as it is, has been a major step forward in enabling valid comparisons of therapies to be made.

Symptoms, signs, and screening

Murphy et al. (1980) has shown that for tumours of the renal pelvis, delay between onset of symptoms to presentation for treatment ranged between 1 day and 9 years with a mean in their series of 229 patients of 8.5 months. Gross haematuria was the main common presenting symptom, accounting for 67 per cent of patients and Werth et al. (1981) found similar results; 66 per cent with ureteric neoplasms presented with gross haematuria. Pain was the next most common symptom in the flank or in conjunction with gross haematuria and, therefore, due to clot colic.

Microscopic haematuria led to investigations in 14 per cent of the series of Murphy et al. (1980) and 12 per cent of the series of ureteric tumours (Werth et al. 1981). Other presenting signs and symptoms include pyuria, weight loss, anaemia, unexplained fever, hypertension, renal failure, and calculus disease. Patients with a past history of stone disease usually develop the tumour on the same side as they have had the stone.

In a screening programme for microscopic haematuria involving 3500 men, 21 bladder tumours were found initially (Britton et al. 1990) and subsequent follow-up of these with no visible bladder tumour but positive urine cytology revealed, 6 months after the initial screening, one patient with transitional carcinoma of the renal pelvis (Whelan et al. 1993) (Table 2).

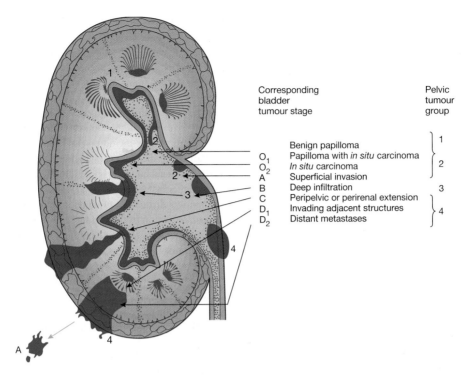

Corresponding bladder tumour stage | Pelvic tumour group

		Pelvic tumour group
	Benign papilloma	1
O_1	Papilloma with *in situ* carcinoma	
O_2	*In situ* carcinoma	2
A^2	Superficial invasion	
B	Deep infiltration	3
C	Peripelvic or perirenal extension	
D_1	Invading adjacent structures	4
D_2	Distant metastases	

Fig. 1 Diagrammatic illustration of the Jewitt (1963) and ICC (TNM) system for classification of tumours of the renal pelvis.

Table 2 Histological grading

Benign	Cells of uniform size, closely resembling normal epithelial cells of the ureter
	No invasion of basement membrane
Malignant	
Grade I	Papillary, well differentiated, few mitoses
Grade II	Less differentiated, irregular cell crowding, atypical nuclei, mitoses
Grade III	More sessile, composed of sheets, cords, and nests of malignant cells
Grade IV	Anaplastic, composed of infiltrating cord cells, exhibiting keratinization and intracellular bridge formation
Stage of invasion	
Stage A	Lesions limited to the mucosa
Stage B	Lesions that invade the muscularis of the ureter
Stage C	Lesions that extend into the periureteral tissues
Stage D	Lesions that exhibit distant metastases

Investigations

Intravenous urography

The majority of cases in TCC of the pelvis or ureter are diagnosed by intravenous urography (IVU); in Zielgelbaum's series (Zielgelbaum *et al.* 1987), all cases were diagnosed by this method, and in most other reported series at least 80 per cent of cases had been diagnosed by this one investigation.

The presence of hydronephrosis with or without hydroureter often defines the bulk of the disease rather than the stage, and in patients who have no obstruction on IVU only 10–15 per cent are subsequently found to have an advanced stage of disease (Bloom 1970), differential diagnosis during this investigation is between blood clot and uric acid stone of sloughed papillae. It is usually the presence of a non-functioning kidney on IVU that leads to further investigations (Babian and Johnson 1980).

Retrograde pyelography

This investigation tends to be used in two circumstances; to confirm the presence of a constant filling defect either in the ureter or renal pelvis, and to investigate patients with a non-functioning kidney. At the time of retrograde studies, selected aspiration for urine cytology has also been incorporated and has helped to confirm the diagnosis especially in high-grade tumours (Grikson and Johansson 1976).

Ultrasonography

This is commonly used as the first investigation of the genitourinary tract especially when impaired renal function is present, and may be helpful in defining non-opaque calculi (i.e. uric acid stones) from other filling defects of the renal pelvis, but it is not specific and cannot differentiate, for example, between slough papillae and transitional cell tumours. Examination of the middle third of the ureter is difficult and the absence of a significant hydroureter, often unhelpful (McCarnon *et al.* 1983).

Computed tomography scanning

Although the early images from computed tomography (CT) scanning were often difficult to interpret and only extensive high-grade and high-stage tumours were definable (Gatewood *et al.* 1982), modern CT scanning can often give excellent views of the renal pelvis and readily differentiate stone from tumour. Spinal CT may also define ureteric lesions; these, however, remain difficult to image completely and whilst this investigation is sometimes helpful it is not definitive.

Magnetic resonance scanning

The efficacy of magnetic resonance (MR) scanning with renal pelvic tumours but again ureteric lesions are often difficult to define and frequently this modality adds little to more simple imaging.

Most upper urinary tract tumours continue to be diagnosed by a combination of intravenous pyelography (IVP) and ascending contrast studies either by means of ascending pyelography or loopography in cases of prior cystectomy. Ureteroscopy is frequently employed but whilst a tissue diagnosis may be obtained and non-opaque calculi differentiated from tumours and *in situ*, because the tumour cannot be adequately staged by this technique, it remains a largely complimentary investigation.

Treatment

Since the report of Kimbal and Ferris (1934), the operation of choice for transitional cell tumours of the upper urinary tract has been total nephroureterectomy with resection of part of the bladder (Figs 2 and 3).

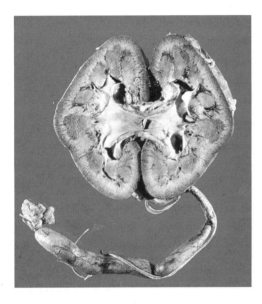

Fig. 2 Nephroureterectomy specimen with resection of part bladder in continuity.

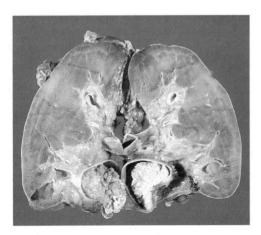

Fig. 3 A bilateral kidney; showing the transitional cell carcinoma in a lower pole calyx.

Most conservative procedures have been for specific reasons and these will be discussed below. Failure to carry out the extensive operation is known to be associated with significant local recurrences. Kaizoe *et al.* (1980) reported an incidence of 64 per cent recurrence at the ureteral stump, following either nephrectomy alone of inadequate nephroureterectomy. An earlier paper by Strong and Pearce (1976), however, found that recurrences of tumour within the bladder was equally frequent whether ureterectomy had been total or not. The majority of reports including the Japanese study (Kaizoe *et al.* 1980) have found an increase in incidence of tumour recurrence in patients who had not adequately excised although in one further large series of 224 patients by Murphy *et al.* (1980), the procedure itself was not an independent favourable prognostic factor. In summary, as in much of surgery, reduction in the incidence of local recurrence is apparent but survival benefit is far more tenuous because of the lack of any prospective trials.

Surgery involves a nephrectomy and ureterectomy with removal of a cuff of bladder incorporating the lower end of the ureter (Fig. 4) and it may be performed via a single incision with the patient in the semi-prone position, or by two incisions one with the patient in a classic kidney posture and the second a lower midline incision with the patient recumbent.

There are no reported differences in outcome following either method, although Skinner (1978) has recommended that lymphadenectomy be incorporated in the nephrectomy. Again, the experiences reported in the literature do not appear to confirm a significant benefit from this additional procedure.

Conservative surgery

Most patients receiving conservative forms of treatment have either a solitary functioning kidney, synchronous bilateral tumours, or renal insufficiency, thereby posing a therapeutic dilemma.

When confronted with patients who have either a previous nephrectomy or have impaired function of the contralateral kidney and in those who have congenital renal agenesis (Vest 1945), efforts should be made to preserve renal function. Most of the reported series date between 1970 and 1984, and this is possible given the average age of the patients (over 60 years) and the greater experience with

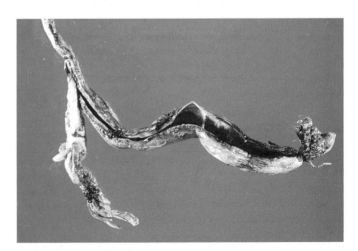

Fig. 4 The lower end of the ureter with a small cuff of bladder, the ureter having been opened longitudinally to reveal a transitional cell tumour of the ureter within.

long-term dialysis support, so that conservative surgery at any price may not now be deemed the best and most satisfactory treatment (Droller 1987).

This concept has been lent weight by more recent series (Hall *et al.* 1998) showing that parenchymal sparing surgery in a further retrospective series of 252 patients showed that tumour stage and type of procedure (complete oblation versus parenchymal sparing) were the only two independent prognostic factors.

In a further subgroup analysis of patients with distal ureteric tumours only, they found that only low-grade, low-stage lesions with a recurrence rate of 13 per cent and no cancer deaths were safe whilst higher stage and grade demonstrated very high recurrence and cancer mortality.

In a thorough review of historical series of open conservative resection and contemporary endoscopic retrograde and percutaneous techniques (Tawfier and Bagley 1997) the ipsilateral recurrence rate for ureteroscopic treatment was 33 per cent in 61 renal tumours and 31 per cent for 144 ureteric tumours in a compilation of reported data with a follow-up ranging from 2 to 132 months. The importance of close follow-up surveillance including interval cystoscopy and ureteroscopy is necessary because of the high number of both ureteric and bladder recurrences.

Although renal preservation with acceptable recurrence and survival rates can be documented after endoscopic procedures for low-grade low-stage tumours, nephroureterectomy still remains the preferred choice and even in patients with compromised renal function especially with high-grade or high-stage disease, serious consideration of total renal ablation needs to be given careful thought and this option should be thoroughly discussed with the patient.

Laparoscopic surgery

With emergence of urological laparoscopic surgery in the last decade, a number of unilateral laparoscopic nephroureterectomies have been performed demonstrating decreased pain and acceleration of patient recuperation (Shalhav *et al.* 1998; McNeil *et al.* 2000).

To perform laparoscopic nephroureterectomy smoothly, the patient must be positioned at 60° oblique to the full lateral flank position for optimum exposure and easier dissection because this enables the surrounding organs to be displaced downwards by gravity. Because the critical and difficult resection of the distal ureter may need open exposure, the use of resection of the transmural distal ureter initially is again being utilized with this procedure. At present, the number of procedures are too few and the follow-up too short to provide any meaningful comparative data. This presents an ideal occasion to compare open operation with laparoscopic operation but non-scientific reasons may yet thwart the truly scientific evaluation of these surgical procedures.

Squamous cell carcinoma

This condition is uncommon and may be associated with chronic infection or the presence of stones (see above). It tends to present in an advanced state and because of this few reports show radical surgery to be effected. The stage can often be better defined using either ultra sonography or CT scanning because the disease is invasive rather than because of any particular properties of the tumour itself. Cytology is rarely of help in the diagnosis because of the concomitant chronic infection, which gives rise to many false-positive results. Prognosis in this condition is gloomy and treatment tends to be aimed at palliation

only. Simple nephrectomy may be helpful as a means to prevent either pain or bleeding. Ureteroscopy and biopsy will enable this condition to be accurately diagnosed and in this manner the patient will be saved from an unnecessary radical procedure.

Summary

TCC of the renal pelvis and ureter is uncommon (a little over 200 cases a year were reported by the BAUS Section of Oncology in the year 2000). It is rare for patients with primary TCC in the bladder to develop upper tract lesions, but conversely it is not uncommon for those presenting with primary upper tract disease, to subsequently develop secondary bladder tumours. The mainstay of investigation remains the IVU, but more accurate visualization, staging, and grading can be obtained using either flexible or ridged nephroureteroscopes taken in conjunction with CT or ultrasounds. In low-grade, low-stage disease there may be a place for local excision either endoscopically or by open operation, but our system of grading and staging does not allow for the biological vagaries of these lesions and the patients put into this category may still die of metastatic disease.

A formal follow-up policy, of those most at risk, that is, high-grade, high-stage tumours with serial CT scanning, has not been evolved and requires at the very least an audit of current practice to see whether within the first 2 years an initial 6 monthly for 12 months and then annually for 1 or 2 years CT scans along with regular check cystoscopies is a useful addition and picks up early recurrent disease.

In the rare cases of patients rendered anephric, they were then supported by dialysis following the operation of nephroureterectomy; there is no information in respect of TCC as to how long a disease-free interval is safe before a transplant is contemplated. In the rare individual cases where this has been confronted, the general guidelines in respect to renal cell carcinoma of a 5-year disease-free interval appears to have been followed, but there is no solid information currently available, on which to base a clinical decision.

A policy of initial radical surgery and careful and conscientious surveillance modified in the light of the initial presenting grade and stage appears to give these patients their best chance of survival.

References

Babian, R. J. and Johnson, D. E. (1980). Primary carcinoma of the ureter. *Journal of Urology* **123**, 357.

Balaji, K. C. *et al.* (1999). Upper tract recurrences following radical cystectomy: an analysis of prognostic factors, recurrence pattern and stage at presentation. *Journal of Urology* **162**, 1603.

Bloom, N. A. (1970). Primary carcinoma of the ureter; a report of 102 cases. *Journal of Urology* **103**, 590.

Booth, C. M., Cameron, U. M., and Pugh, R. C. B. (1980). Urothelial carcinoma of the kidney and ureter. *British Journal of Urology* **52**, 430.

Britton, J. P. *et al.* (1992). A community study of bladder cancer screening by the detection of occult urinary bleeding. *Journal of Urology* **148**, 788–790.

Broders, A. C. (1922). Epithelioma of the genitourinary organs. *American Surgeon* **75**, 574.

Case, R. A. M. *et al.* (1959). Tumour of the urinary bladder as an occupational disease on the rubber industry in England and Wales. *British Journal of Preventative and Social Medicine* **8**, 39.

Chew, K. S. *et al.* (1995). Urological cancers in uremic patients. *American Journal of Kidney Diseases* **25**, 694.

Clayman, R. V., Lange, P. H., and Fralley, E. G. Cancer of the upper urinary tract. In *Principles and Management of Urological Cancer* (ed. N. Javadpoor). Baltimore, MD: Williams & Wilkins, 1983.

Cummings, K. B. (1980). Nephroureterectomy: routine in the management of transitional cell carcinoma of the upper urinary tract. *Urologic Clinics of North America* 7, 569.

Droller, M. J. (1987). Editorial comments. *Journal of Urology* 138, 1148.

Friedman, N. B. and Ash, J. E. Tumours of the urinary bladder. In *Atlas of Tumour Pathology*. Washington, DC: Armed Forces Institute of Pathology, 1959.

Gatewood, J. M. B. *et al.* (1982). Computerised tomography in the diagnosis of transitional cell carcinoma of the kidney. *Journal of Urology* 127, 876.

Gittes, R. F. Tumours of the ureter and renal pelvis. In *Campbell's Urology* 4th edn. (ed. J. H. Harrison, R. F. Gittes, A. Perlmutter, T. A. Stamey, and P. C. Walsh), p. 1010. Philadelphia, PA: Saunders, 1979.

Grikson, O. and Johansson, S. (1976). Urothelial neoplasms of the upper urinary tract. A correlation between cytotoxic and histologic findings in 43 people with urothelial neoplasms of the renal pelvis or ureter. *Acta Cytologica* 20, 20.

Hall, C. M. *et al.* (1998). Prognostic factors, recurrence, and survival of transitional cell carcinoma of the upper urinary tract: a 30-year experiment in 252 patients. *Urology* 52, 594.

Hastie, K. J. *et al.* (1991). Upper tract tumours following cystectomy for bladder cancer. Is routine intervention urography worthwhile? *British Journal of Urology* 67, 29.

Herranz, F. *et al.* (1999). Tumour de urolio superior en pacientes sometidus a cistectomia radial par carcinoma transicional de vejiga. *Atlas Urol. ESP.* 23, 214.

Hicks, R. M. (1980). Multistage carcinogenics I in the urinary bladder. *British Medical Bulletin* 36, 39.

Holmang, S. *et al.* (1998). Long term follow up of a bladder carcinoma cohort. Routine follow up urography is not necessary. *Journal of Urology* 160, 45.

Huguet-Perez, J. *et al.* (2001). Upper tract transitional cell carcinoma following cystectomy for bladder cancer. *European Urology* 40, 318.

Hultergren, N., Largergren, C., and Ljungquist, A. (1965). Carcinoma of the renal pelvis in renal papillary necrosis. *Acta Chirurgica Scandinavica* 130, 314.

Hurle, R. *et al.* (1999). Upper urinary tract tumours developing after treatment of superficial bladder cancer: 7-year follow up of 591 consecutive patents. *Urology* 53, 1144.

Jewitt, H. J. Tumours of the bladder. In *Urology* (ed. M. C. Campbell), p. 1027. Philadelphia, PA: Saunders, 1963.

Kaizoe, T. *et al.* (1980). Transitional cell carcinomas of the bladder in patients with renal pelvic and ureteral cancer. *Journal of Urology* 124, 17.

Kenworthy, P., Tanguay, S., and Diney, C. P. N. (1996). The risk of upper tract recurrence following cystectomy in patients with transitional cell carcinoma involving the distal ureter. *Journal of Urology* 155, 501.

Kimbal, F. N. and Ferris, H. W. (1934). Papillomatous tumour of the renal pelvis associated with similar tumours of the ureter and bladder. Review of the literature and report of two cases. *Journal of Urology* 31, 257.

Lucke, B. and Schumgerger, H. G. Tumours of the kidney, renal pelvis and ureter. In *Atlas of Tumour Pathology* Section 8. Washington, DC: Armed Forces Institute of Pathology, 1957.

Mahoney, J. F. *et al.* (1977). Analgesic abuse, renal parenchymal disease and carcinoma of the kidney and ureter. *Australian and New Zealand Journal of Medicine* 7, 463.

Markowitz, S. B. and Skinner, D. G. (1990). Development of upper tract carcinoma after cystectomy for bladder cancer. *Urology* 36, 20.

McCarnon, J. P., Mullis, C., and Le Vaughan, G. D. (1983). Tumours of the renal pelvis and ureters, comment concepts and management. *Urology* 1, 75.

McNeil, S. A., Chrisuros, M., and Tolley, D. A. (2000). The long-term outcome after laparoscopic nephrectomy. *BJU International* 86, 619.

Mostofi, F. K., Sobin, L. H., and Torloni, H. *Histological Typing of Urinary Bladder Tumours*. Geneva: World Health Organization, 1973.

Mufti, G. R., Grove, T. R., and Riddle, P. R. (1988). Nephroureterectomy after radical cystectomy. *Journal of Urology* 139, 588.

Murphy, D. M., Zincke, H., and Furlow, W. L. (1980). Primary grade 1 transitional cell carcinoma of the renal pelvis and ureter. *Journal of Urology* 123, 629.

Nocks, B. *et al.* (1982). Transitional cell carcinoma of the renal pelvis. *Urology* 12, 479.

Petkovic, S. *et al.* (1971). Tumours of the renal pelvis and ureters. Clinical and aetiologic studies. *J. Urol. Nephrol* 77, 429.

Schellhammer, P. F. and Whitmore, W. F. (1976). Transitional cell carcinoma of the ureter in men having cystectomy for bladder cancer. *Journal of Urology* 115, 56.

Shalhav, A. L. *et al.* (1998). Laparoscopic nephroureterectomy for upper tract transitional cell carcinoma: techniques aspects. *Journal of Endourology* 12, 345.

Skinner, D. G. (1978). Technique of nephroureterectomy with regional lymph node dissection. *Urologic Clinics of North America* 5, 252.

Strong, D. W. and Pearce, H. A. (1976). Recurrent urothelial tumours following surgery for transitional cell carcinoma of the urinary tract. *Cancer* 38, 2173.

Tanchev, I. *et al.* (1956). Prouchavaniia na nefritev v vrachanska okolia. *Savremenaja Medizina* 9, 14.

Tawfier, E. R. and Bagley, D. H. (1997). Upper tract transitional cell carcinoma. *Urology* 50, 321.

Tsuji, Y., Nakamura, H., and Ariyoshi, A. (1996). Upper urinary tract involvement after cystectomy and ileal conduit diversion for primary bladder carcinoma. *European Urology* 29, 216.

Vest, S. A. (1945). Conservative surgery in certain benign tumours of the ureter. *Journal of Urology* 53, 97.

Werth, D. D., Weigel, J. W., and Mebust, W. K. (1981). Primary metastases of the ureter. *Journal of Urology* 125, 628.

Whelan, P. *et al.* (1993). Three year follow-up of bladder tumours found on screening. *British Journal of Urology* 72, 893–896.

Ziegelbaum, M. *et al.* (1987). Conservative surgery for transitional cell carcinoma of the renal pelvis. *Journal of Urology* 138, 1146.

Zincke, H., Garbeff, P. J., and Beahrs, J. R. (1984). Upper urinary tract transitional cell cancer after radical cystectomy for bladder cancer. *Journal of Urology* 31, 50.

18.4 Tumours of the bladder

Robert D. Mills and William H. Turner

Introduction

Over 90 per cent of bladder cancers are urothelial tumours, ranging from well-differentiated papillary lesions not breaching the basement membrane to undifferentiated invasive and potentially metastatic cancers. However, the commonly held view that there are two populations of urothelial bladder tumours, those that behave in a benign way and those that behave like true cancers, is not entirely supported by the facts. Although many invasive cancers present as such, even superficial tumours have a risk, albeit small, of stage and grade progression and hence, ultimately, of death. Furthermore, the disease can affect any part of the urothelium from the renal pelvis to the urethra and recurrence or progression may be remote in time or place from the original tumour. This means that prolonged and careful surveillance of all patients with urothelial tumours is required.

Despite a huge recent increase in the knowledge of the genetic and molecular mechanisms of bladder cancer (O'Brien *et al.* 1995; Knowles 2001; Williams *et al.* 2001), we remain unable to identify with precision those patients with initially superficial disease, who are at risk of subsequent progression.

There is uncertainty about whether surgery or radiotherapy is the most appropriate radical treatment for patients with invasive bladder cancer, although in most countries surgery is used more frequently. This raises the issue of the ideal urinary diversion after radical cystectomy and this is also the subject of debate. The role of chemotherapy as neoadjuvant treatment remains to be clearly defined. International collaborative trials have produced inconclusive results, which are currently being subjected to meta-analysis. Trials of adjuvant chemotherapy are awaited. Potential new prognostic factors are being intensively assessed with a view to targetting chemotherapy at those patients with invasive bladder cancer who are at high risk of relapse. Finally, both the treatment of superficial bladder cancer and the follow-up of all patients with bladder cancer are being reconsidered to try to maximize cost–benefit ratios.

The high incidence of bladder cancer and its unpredictable natural history make it a major challenge for urologists, both in terms of research and clinical practice. In discussing bladder tumours, we outline areas of controversy and will attempt to present opposing views and to indicate our own.

Incidence

In the United States 54,300 new cases and 12,400 deaths from bladder cancer were expected in 2001 (American Cancer Society 2001), and there were 12,080 new cases and 4319 deaths from bladder cancer in England and Wales in 1997 and 1999, respectively (Office for National Statistics 2001). Bladder cancer is up to three times more common in men than in women (Figs 1 and 2) and although bladder tumours are diagnosed most commonly in the 75–79 year age group (Fig. 1), the risk of developing a bladder tumour increases steadily with age (Fig. 2), as does the risk of death from bladder cancer (Fig. 3).

Aetiology and pathogenesis

The causes and development of bladder cancer are complex phenomena, which can only be summarized in this chapter. They have been reviewed at length (Sidransky *et al.* 1992; Aprikian *et al.* 1993; Jones *et al.* 1993; Shirai 1993; Vet *et al.* 1994b; Johansson and Cohen 1997; Williams *et al.* 2001). In general terms, three types of factors can be identified: environmental, genetic, and molecular.

Environmental factors

Environmental substances or conditions implicated as bladder carcinogens are divided into three groups: accepted, suspected, or questionable (Table 1). Most accepted human urothelial carcinogens have been used in industrial settings.

Appreciation of the association between aniline dyes and bladder cancer led to one of the earliest successful interventions by occupational medicine to reduce cancer incidence. 2-Naphthylamine and later, related aromatic amines were shown to be bladder carcinogens (Johansson and Cohen 1997) and industrial exposure was stopped. Industrial carcinogens are still believed to account for about a quarter of bladder cancers.

Cigarette smoke increases the risk of bladder cancer by around threefold (Doll *et al.* 1994) and continued smoking once a diagnosis of bladder cancer is made is associated with a worse disease-associated outcome (Fleshner *et al.* 1999). Urothelial tumours are less strongly associated with cigarette smoking than respiratory tract tumours: nonetheless cigarette smoking may account for up to 60 per cent of all bladder tumours in industrialized and developed countries and is thus the single most important cause of bladder cancer (Brennen *et al.* 2000). How cigarette smoking leads to bladder cancer remains uncertain, but the major classes of potential bladder carcinogens in cigarette smoke are polycyclic aromatic hydrocarbons, aromatic amines, and unsaturated aldehydes (Johansson and Cohen 1997). Aromatic amines, especially 2-naphthylamine, 4-aminobiphenyl, and 4-chloro-*o*-toluidine seem to be associated strongly with cigarette smoking and bladder cancer

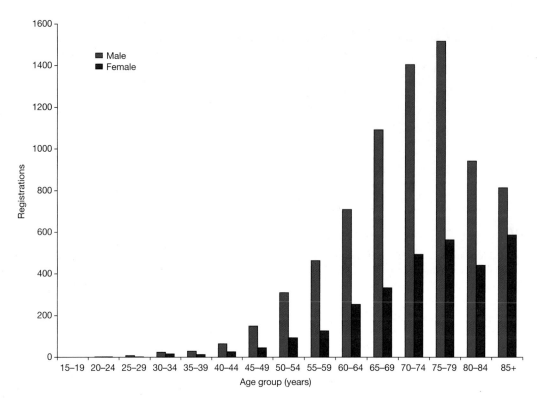

Fig. 1 New cases of malignant bladder tumours in England and Wales in 1998.

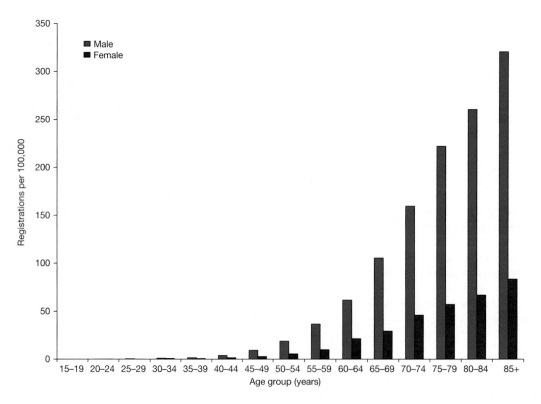

Fig. 2 New cases of malignant bladder tumours per 100,000 population in England and Wales in 1998.

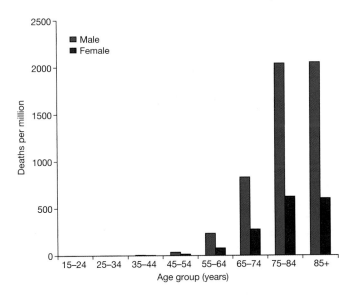

Fig. 3 Deaths from malignant bladder tumours per million population in England and Wales in 1998.

Table 1 Accepted, suspected, and questionable human bladder carcinogens

Accepted
2-Naphthylamine
4-Aminobiphenyl
Benzidine
N,N-bis-(2-chloroethyl)-2-naphthylamine
4-Chloro-o-toluidine
Schistosomia haematobium
Phenacetin
Cyclophosphamide

Suspected
α,β-Unsaturated aldehydes
Nitrosamines
4,4′-Methylene-bis-(2-chloroaniline)
o-Toluidine

Questionable
Caffeine
Saccharine
Cyclamate
Tryptophan

(Shirai 1993). α,β-Unsaturated aldehydes occur throughout the environment and are present in milligram quantities per cigarette. These highly reactive compounds are toxic, mitogenic, and initiate bladder cancer in rats (Johansson and Cohen 1997). Nicotine, its metabolites, or tobacco-specific nitrosamines do not appear to be involved in bladder carcinogenesis.

The next most important condition leading to bladder cancer in global terms is undoubtedly infection with *Schistosomia haematobium* (Johansson and Cohen 1997; Mostafa *et al.* 1999). Carcinogenic nitrosamines are present in the urine of patients with schistosomiasis. However, up to 70 per cent of bladder cancers associated with schistosomiasis are squamous cell carcinomas. This is believed to relate to squamous metaplasia, resulting from a chronic inflammatory response to ova of the schistosome within the bladder wall (Shirai 1993). Indeed

chronic irritation from any source, such as urinary stones or foreign bodies like indwelling catheters, is associated with an increased frequency of urothelial carcinoma: chronic urinary infection is thought to be involved in this process (Shirai 1993; Johansson and Cohen 1997). As with schistosomiasis, the urinary tract neoplasm most often associated with physical irritation from stones or catheters is squamous cell carcinoma, although transitional cell carcinoma is not uncommon.

There is considerable controversy about the urothelial carcinogenicity of caffeine-containing drinks, such as coffee. There is no firm evidence however, that caffeine is mutagenic in humans (Shirai 1993). Cyclophosphamide and phenacetin are the two drugs best known as bladder carcinogens (Shirai 1993). A host of other possible bladder carcinogens has been postulated and investigated (Shirai 1993; Johansson and Cohen 1997), as well as the effect of overall daily fluid intake (Michaud *et al.* 1999; Geoffroy-Perez and Cordier 2001). However, a review of the literature of the carcinogenic effect in humans of agents such as saccharine, tryptophan, and various viruses underlines the inherent problems in current epidemiological methodology, as well as the gaps in our understanding of the nature of human carcinogenesis.

Genetic factors

It is now well established that carcinogenesis in humans is a multistep process (Shirai 1993; Brandau and Bohle 2001), needing at least five steps to lead the disease to metastasis. Each step is represented by a major molecular event, such as a mutation in the cell's genome, deletion of a chromosome, activation of an oncogene, or loss of a suppressor gene's function: a more neoplastic stage is reached with each step. Bladder cancer is a good human model for the study of carcinogenesis, because there are clearly identified chemical carcinogens, associated chromosomal abnormalities and genetic alterations, and the bladder is readily accessible for repeated assessment and tumour sampling (Sidransky *et al.* 1992).

Genetic factors influencing bladder cancer include familial aggregation, genetic polymorphism, the N-acetyltransferase phenotype, activated oncogenes, and chromosomal changes (Shirai 1993). Two patterns of genetic influence are recognized: a very small number of cases of Mendelian autosomal-dominant inheritance and the remaining vast majority of cases, in which there is presumably a multifactorial interaction between environmental and genetic factors. Bladder cancer is associated with HLA polymorphisms and with N-acetyltransferase status. The latter is inherited in an autosomal-recessive manner and probably influences the susceptibility to chemical carcinogens, such as aromatic amines (Vineis *et al.* 2001).

Several chromosomal anomalies have been detected in cytogenetic studies of transitional cell cancer. Numerical aberrations including aneuploidy and chromosome deletions, structural aberrations including isochromosomes, ring chromosomes, and the appearance of abnormal chromosome fragments have been described (Strohmeyer *et al.* 1994). The chromosomes 1–13, 17, and 18 have all been affected (Vet *et al.* 1994b; Simon *et al.* 2000). Restriction fragment length polymorphism analysis has shown loss of heterozygosity at the short arm of chromosome 11 (11p), in the long arm of chromosome 9 (9q), and in 17p, in more than 60 per cent of all bladder cancers (Strohmeyer *et al.* 1994). Although the changes at 9q were stage- and grade-independent, tumour stage and grade correlated with deletion at 17p.

Two kinds of wild-type genes participate in regulation of cell growth and proliferation: proto-oncogenes, which may by activated by point mutation or amplification, and tumour suppressor genes, which may be inactivated by point mutation, rearrangement, or deletion (Sidransky *et al.* 1992). The role, in bladder cancer, of a number of proto-oncogenes and tumour suppressor genes has been studied (Sidransky *et al.* 1992; Steiner *et al.* 1995).

About 10 per cent of bladder cancers have mutations of the proto-oncogene *ras* family, including the *H-ras* and *K-ras* oncogenes (Strohmeyer *et al.* 1994). Whilst it has been suggested that they are not important in the development of the majority of bladder tumours (Sandberg *et al.* 1994), there is contrary evidence that they may indeed represent early steps in the genesis of transitional cell tumours (Burchill *et al.* 1994). Increased expression of the *src* oncogene occurs in low-grade bladder tumours and increased expression of the *c-erb-2* oncogene occurs in tumours of high grade and stage (Sandberg *et al.* 1994). Chromosome 11q carries three oncogenes, which are amplified in up to 20 per cent of bladder cancers, int-2, hst-1, and bcl-1 (Strohmeyer *et al.* 1994). The *c-myc* gene located on 8q encodes a nuclear phosphoprotein that is involved in transcriptional regulation and linked with growth regulation, cell differentiation, and apoptosis. Overexpression of *c-myc* has been detected in up to 50 per cent of both papillary disease and muscle invasive tumours (Schmitz-Drager *et al.* 1997).

The influence of tumour suppressor genes has been studied in transitional cell cancer. The product of the p53 gene, on chromosome 17p, is a nuclear phosphoprotein, which regulates cell growth through induction of cell-cycle arrest, cell differentiation, or apoptosis. The mutant p53 gene protein may allow growth to proceed without restraint, thus increasing the likelihood of tumour formation (Aprikian *et al.* 1993; Keegan *et al.* 1998). Loss of 17p is strongly associated with p53 mutation (Vet *et al.* 1994b) and p53 mutations occur in up to 61 per cent of bladder tumours (Sidransky *et al.* 1992) and p53 nuclear protein accumulation has been shown to correlate with stage and grade (Esrig *et al.* 1993). p53 has been implicated in the genesis of carcinoma *in situ* and early highly malignant lesions, in contrast to those early lesions with loss of chromosome 9, which have been reported to behave in a less malignant way suggesting two separate molecular pathways to bladder cancer (Spruck *et al.* 1994). More recently, however, deletion of chromosomes 9 and 17 has been reported with equal frequency in patients with carcinoma *in situ* and so these changes cannot be regarded as accurate indicators of tumour behaviour (Hartmann *et al.* 2002).

The possible role of p53 as a prognostic factor has been investigated. p53-Positive immunohistochemistry has been reported as an independent prognostic marker for Ta disease (Casetta *et al.* 1997). A correlation was found with outcome in carcinoma *in situ*, and p53 was suggested to be an early event in bladder cancer (Sarkis *et al.* 1994). p53 expression has been shown to be correlated with progression and survival in pT1 tumours (Sarkis *et al.* 1993; Thomas *et al.* 1994; Serth *et al.* 1995; Llopis *et al.* 2000), although, one study suggested that grade was more useful as a prognostic indicator (Thomas *et al.* 1994). However, other studies of patients with pT1 disease managed either endoscopically (Gardiner *et al.* 1994), or by early cystectomy or endoscopically (Shariat *et al.* 2000), showed no correlation with outcome. In invasive tumours, increased p53 expression occurred in one study, but there was no prognostic significance (Vet *et al.* 1994a), whereas in a study of 243 patients after cystectomy for pTa-pT4 disease, p53 expression correlated with an increased risk of recurrence and death (Esrig *et al.* 1994). Studies of p53 status and survival following radiotherapy for muscle invasive disease have also produced contrasting results: Wu *et al.* (1996) found it to be an independent predictor of

survival, whereas Jahnson *et al.* (1995) found no predictive value. A recent review of all published literature on the association of p53 accumulation and prognosis of bladder cancer looked at 3764 patients from 138 studies. No definitive answer was possible from the available data, mainly due to the differing techniques between studies (Schmitz-Drager *et al.* 2000). Prospective studies using standardized techniques are clearly required in order to determine the value of p53 in the clinical management of bladder cancer.

The product of the retinoblastoma (Rb) gene, on 13q, is a nuclear phosphoprotein, which has a central role in cell-cycle regulation through induction of cell-cycle arrest by blocking the E2F family of transcription factors (Keegan *et al.* 1998). Rb gene loss occurs in up to 40 per cent of bladder cancers, particularly high grade and stage tumours (Aprikian *et al.* 1993). Rb mutation and downregulation of Rb protein correlated with decreased 5-year survival in patients with a diverse group of bladder cancers (Cordon-Cardo *et al.* 1992). In a further study of superficial bladder cancer, p53 positivity and Rb negativity alone did not independently predict survival, however, a combination of the two did and was an independent predictor of disease progression (Cordon-Cardo *et al.* 1997). This illustrates the potential value of combining prognostic markers.

Molecular factors

The role in the development of bladder cancer of a number of gene products has been investigated (Vet *et al.* 1994b). Recent evidence suggests that angiogenesis may play an important role in the development of bladder cancer and that different angiogenic pathways characterize superficial and invasive bladder cancers (O'Brien *et al.* 1995; Turner *et al.* 2002). In pT1 tumours, vascular endothelial growth factor expression predicted recurrence at 3 months (O'Brien *et al.* 1995). Angiogenesis was quantitated in muscle invasive disease and correlated with survival, providing as much information as stage (Dickinson *et al.* 1994).

Epidermal growth factor (EGF) is a protein mitogen present in urine. Its receptor (EGFR), the product of the *c-erb* B1 gene (Vet *et al.* 1994b), is a transmembrane protein with tyrosine kinase activity and is involved in cell-growth regulation (Sidransky *et al.* 1992). EGFR is present only in the basal layer of normal urothelium, but throughout the urothelium in transitional cell tumours. Upregulation of EGFR occurs in bladder tumours, particularly those of high stage and grade (Neal *et al.* 1989; Sidransky *et al.* 1992), and correlated with progression and survival in superficial tumours (Lipponen *et al.* 1994) and with progression in a mixed group of tumours (Mellon *et al.* 1995; Ravery *et al.* 1995). EGF levels are consistently low in the urine of patients with bladder tumours of high stage (Kristensen *et al.* 1988), and other possible important ligands, such as transforming growth factor α acting in an autocrine/paracrine mode have been suggested (Mellon *et al.* 1996; Thogersen *et al.* 2001). Overexpression of the oncogene *c-erb* B2, with significant sequence homology to the gene coding for EGFR, correlated with decreased survival in a mixed group of patients with bladder cancer (Sato *et al.* 1992).

E-cadherin is a cell adhesion molecule that acts to maintain epithelial integrity and suppresses invasion in tumour cell lines (Vet *et al.* 1994b). E-cadherin is downregulated in high grade and stage bladder tumours (Bringuier *et al.* 1993) and this correlated with reduced survival time in patients with invasive tumours (Bringuier *et al.* 1993; Byrne *et al.* 2001).

The biology of metastasis is also becoming better understood, with identification of enzymes such as metalloproteinases, which can degrade the extracellular matrix and basement membrane, cytokines, which regulate tumour cell motility, and genes that regulate metastasis (Liu *et al.* 1992; Kanayama 2001).

Pathology

Normal bladder urothelium comprises three to six layers of transitional cells with a tall basal cell layer, intermediate cells, and a surface layer of so-called 'umbrella' cells (Brodsky 1992). The nuclei of the intermediate cells are oval shaped and oriented with the long axis perpendicular to the basement membrane, giving the urothelium its normal appearance and cellular polarity.

Non-malignant urothelial changes

There are a number of urothelial changes which are not frankly malignant, but some of which may be premalignant (Melicow 1974): this is a controversial area, hampered somewhat by inconsistent terminology.

Epithelial hyperplasia is characterized by an increase in the number of cell layers without nuclear or architectural abnormalities. Von Brunn's nests are clusters of benign transitional cells situated in the lamina propria, which probably result from inward bud-like proliferation of the basal cells of the urothelium.

There are a number of urothelial changes which macroscopically (hence cystoscopically) look cystic. Cystitis cystica describes von Brunn's nest that have undergone central liquefaction either by cellular degeneration or active secretion. Cystitis glandularis is similar to cystitis cystica, except that the transitional cell lining of the microcysts has undergone glandular metaplasia. Cystitis glandularis may look papillary at cystoscopy: it is believed to be a precursor of some adenocarcinomas. Cystitis follicularis is a non-neoplastic response to chronic bacterial infection characterized by suburothelial lymphoid follicles. Grossly, cystitis follicularis appears as punctate yellow suburothelial nodules.

Urothelial atypia and dysplasia comprises a spectrum of preneoplastic or premalignant changes that may be responses to inflammation, irritation, or carcinogenic influences. Urothelial dysplasia is characterized morphologically by notched and spherical epithelial cells with enlarged, basally situated nuclei with loss of normal epithelial-cell polarity. Increased numbers of cells or mitoses are not consistent findings. Dysplastic urothelium exhibits morphological changes that are intermediate between normal urothelium and carcinoma *in situ*. In the 1998 World Health Organization/International Society of Urologic Pathology classification of bladder neoplasms, flat intraepithelial lesions of the urinary bladder were categorized as: reactive atypia, atypia of unknown significance, dysplasia, and carcinoma *in situ* (Epstein *et al.* 1998). The first two are not considered to be premalignant, but dysplastic lesions have an increased risk for the development of carcinoma *in situ* and invasive urothelial carcinoma and should, therefore, be followed closely (Cheng *et al.* 2000).

Inverted papillomas are benign proliferative lesions, associated with chronic infection or bladder outlet obstruction. They are frequently localized to the trigone and bladder neck. Trabecular or glandular types of inverted papilloma are described histologically: the glandular type is considered to be preneoplastic. Nephrogenic adenoma is a rare adenomatous-looking tumour which derives its name from its histological similarity to primitive renal collecting tubules. This lesion arises from metaplastic transformation of normal urothelium in response to trauma, infection, or ionizing radiation. The malignant counterpart of nephrogenic adenoma called mesonephric adenocarcinoma has been reported. Mesonephric adenocarcinoma is frequently located in the trigone and bladder neck. Squamous metaplasia is a proliferative lesion in which the normal transitional cell epithelium is replaced by non-keratinizing squamous epithelium. Autopsy studies show that squamous metaplasia occurs in the bladder of nearly 50 per cent of adult women of all ages (usually in the trigone) but in less than 10 per cent of men (Weiner *et al.* 1979). Keratinizing squamous metaplasia, found in 23 per cent of spinal cord injury patients managed with a long-term catheter (Delnay *et al.* 1999), is believed to be premalignant.

Malignant urothelial conditions

Transitional cell carcinoma accounts for up to 95 per cent of bladder carcinomas, squamous carcinoma for less than 3 per cent and adenocarcinoma for less than 2 per cent. In the International Union Against Cancer (UICC) TNM classification (Table 2), three different

Table 2 TNM classification for bladder carcinoma (Sobin and Wittekind 1997)

Primary tumour

Tx	Primary tumour cannot be assessed
T0	No evidence of primary tumour
Ta	Non-invasive papillary carcinoma
Tis	Carcinoma *in situ*: 'flat tumour'
T1	Tumour invades subepithelial connective tissue
T2	Tumour invades into muscle
	T2a tumour invades superficial muscle (inner half)
	T2b tumour invades deep muscle (outer half)
T3	Tumour invades perivesical tissue
	T3a microscopically
	T3b macroscopically
T4	Tumour invades any of the following: prostate, uterus, vagina, pelvic side-wall, abdominal wall
	T4a tumour invades prostate or uterus or vagina
	T4b tumour invades pelvic wall or abdominal wall

Regional lymph nodes

Nx	Regional lymph nodes cannot be assessed
N0	No regional lymph node metastasis
N1	Metastasis in a single lymph node 2 cm or less in greatest dimension
N2	Metastasis in a single lymph node more than 2 cm but not more than 5 cm in greatest dimension, or multiple lymph nodes, none more than 5 cm in greatest dimension
N3	Metastasis in a lymph node > 5 cm in greatest dimension

Metastases

Mx	Distant metastasis cannot be assessed
M0	No distant metastasis
M1	Distant metastasis

Grade

Gx	Grade of differentiation cannot be assessed
G1	Well differentiated
G2	Moderately differentiated
G3–4	Poorly differentiated/undifferentiated

Residual tumour

Rx	Presence of residual tumour cannot be assessed
R0	No residual tumour
R1	Microscopic residual tumour
R2	Macroscopic residual tumour

types of transitional cell carcinoma exist: carcinoma *in situ*, superficial transitional cell carcinoma, and muscle-invasive transitional cell carcinoma.

The histological criteria for making the diagnosis of transitional cell carcinoma include abnormalities in urothelial, cytological, and architectural features. Transitional cell carcinoma differs from normal urothelium by generally having an increased number of epithelial cell layers, papillary folding of the urothelium, abnormalities of nuclear morphology, loss of cellular polarity, abnormalities of the normal cellular maturation from basal to the superficial layers, the presence of giant cells, an increased nuclear to cytoplastic ratio, prominence of nucleoli, and an increased number of mitoses.

Carcinoma *in situ* is characterized by poorly differentiated transitional cell carcinoma confined to the urothelium (Hudson *et al.* 1995). Initially reported in association with invasive bladder cancer, this lesion, which produces histological loss of cellular cohesiveness, widening of intercellular spaces, and nuclear abnormality, has a 40 per cent risk of progression. If it is associated with a papillary tumour, the progression rate is likely to reach 80 per cent. Grossly, carcinoma *in situ* usually appears as an erythematous urothelial lesion. It may, however, be indistinguishable from surrounding unaffected urothelium and thus not apparent at cystoscopy.

Superficial transitional cell carcinoma differs from muscle-invasive carcinoma in that histopathological examination shows no evidence of invasion of the muscle layer (muscularis propria) of the bladder. Based on the UICC TNM classification system (Sobin and Wittekind 1997), bladder tumours are considered to be superficial when they do not invade the lamina propria, stage Ta, or when they show microscopic invasion of the lamina propria, stage T1 (Table 2). Superficial tumours often have a papillary appearance and appear to have a stalk macroscopically; microscopically there is urothelial proliferation and a fibrovascular core (Figs 4–7). About 20 per cent of bladder tumours are muscle-invasive at diagnosis, manifesting diverse patterns of tumour growth, including papillary, nodular, or solid tumours (Figs 8 and 9). Their hallmark is that the muscle layers of the bladder are invaded (T2, at least).

Urothelial tumours are graded cytologically (Carbin *et al.* 1991; Brodsky 1992). Invasive tumours are almost invariably poorly differentiated by any criteria, but the grading of superficial tumours is controversial and can be difficult. It should be remembered that the spectrum of observed cytological changes is continuous, hence the difficulty in trying to allocate an individual tumour to a category of a discontinuous grading system (Oohms *et al.* 1983). A simplified grading system that is less subjective than previous grading has been suggested (Schapers *et al.* 1994). It had prognostic significance, which was useful when stage could not be established accurately.

To decide to what degree a tumour has infiltrated the bladder wall (T stage), the pathologist needs to have muscle included in the specimen and requires a minimum of distortion of the specimen. Biopsies are taken either with cup biopsy forceps, which pinch and tear out a biopsy specimen, or with the electrocautery loop, which cuts away a biopsy. The former technique is less likely to get deep muscle in the biopsy, but will not produce diathermy artefact, whereas the latter can certainly get deep muscle, but may produce diathermy artefact that makes pathological interpretation harder. Indeed, a resection biopsy may sometimes take the full thickness of the bladder wall and the technique requires experience to avoid a perforation, which if in the dome of the bladder, can be a serious complication.

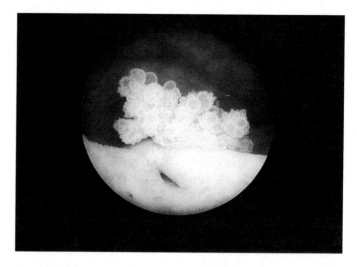

Fig. 4 Papillary appearance of a Ta G1 bladder tumour.

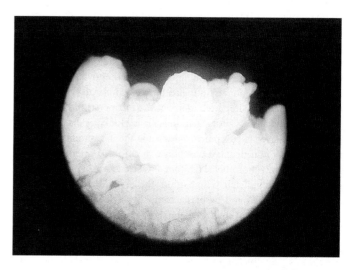

Fig. 5 Papillary appearance of a Ta G1 bladder tumour (close-up).

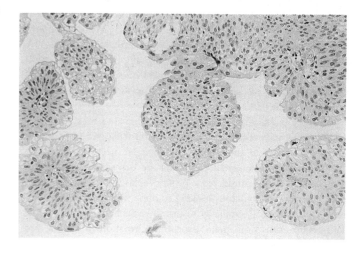

Fig. 6 Microscopic appearance of a Ta G1 bladder tumour.

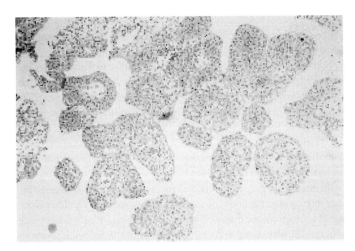

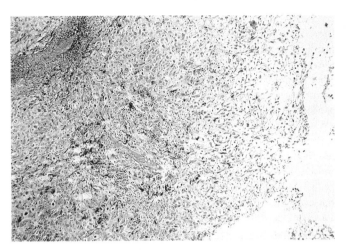

Fig. 9 Microscopic appearance of a invasive poorly differentiated bladder tumour.

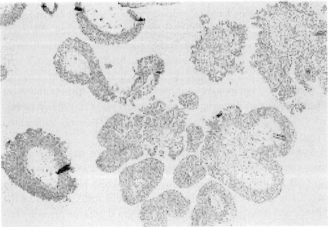

Fig. 7 Microscopic appearance of a Ta G1 bladder tumour.

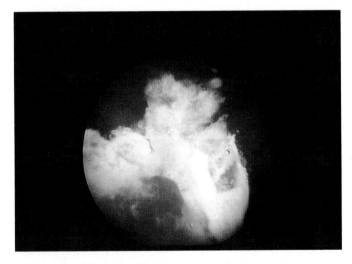

Fig. 8 Solid appearance of an invasive poorly differentiated bladder tumour.

Presentation and diagnosis

Around 80 per cent of patients with bladder tumours present classically with painless macroscopic haematuria, and around 20 per cent present with irritative symptoms with or without haematuria (Wallace *et al.* 1965). The vast majority of patients with macroscopic haematuria present to their family doctor within a week (Wallace *et al.* 1965), and in 10–20 per cent of them, bladder cancer is found (Lynch *et al.* 1994a; Khandra *et al.* 2000). A single episode of macroscopic haematuria requires investigation, even if it resolves: 7 per cent of 112 such patients were found to have bladder cancer (Lynch *et al.* 1994b).

The use of stick testing to detect microscopic haematuria has been studied as a screening tool for bladder cancer and asymptomatic cases are detected in about 5 per cent of a community-based population (Mayfield and Whelan 1998). The incidence increases with age in both sexes and with repeat testing (Tomson and Porter 2002). The yield of investigation of microscopic haematuria depends on the population being studied. Malignancy is more common with increasing age, whereas renal parenchymal disease is more likely in children and young adults (Tomson and Porter 2002). In a population-based study from the Mayo clinic, only 0.5 per cent of subjects with asymptomatic microscopic haematuria had a urological malignancy (Mohr *et al.* 1986). As the specificity is low and the overall costs are high, urine screening is only recommended for those at high risk, such as prior exposure to known bladder carcinogens (Cummings *et al.* 1992). Once asymptomatic microscopic haematuria has been detected, however, a clinical decision has to be made, on discussion with the patient, as to how far investigation should be taken. Many patients may prefer not to be investigated once they understand that the risk of malignancy is small (Del Mar 2000). Irritative symptoms may be prominent in patients with carcinoma *in situ* and this diagnosis should be considered in patients with chronic frequency and dysuria, even without haematuria.

Areas of carcinoma *in situ* or non-papillary invasive tumours may not be apparent macroscopically, therefore, they may not be biopsied and may be missed. Recently, fluorescence cystoscopy using 5-aminolevulinic acid (5-ALA) has been shown to be more sensitive than white light cystoscopy at demonstrating carcinoma *in situ* (Frimberger *et al.* 2000). The technique, however, needs further refinement as there are a number of false-positive lesions. Urinary cytology is of considerable importance in the diagnosis and follow-up of bladder cancer (Ro *et al.* 1992). Urinary cytology is particularly effective at detecting high-grade cellular changes and thus is complementary to cystoscopy, in that it will tend to detect the lesions which may be missed cystoscopically. It also allows cells from throughout the urinary tract to be sampled. Cytology specimens taken at cystoscopy or catheterization may increase the cellular yield, and thus the chance of obtaining malignant cells (Ro *et al.* 1992). The pathologist, however, must know if urine other than voided urine is used, because the increased number of urothelial cells may lead to confusion. For the same reason, details of previous intravesical chemotherapy or radiotherapy should also be given to the pathologist. Other biological markers have been investigated as possible adjuncts in initial diagnosis and surveillance of bladder cancer. These include nuclear matrix protein (NMP22) and bladder tumour antigen (BTA stat and BTA TRAK) assays. Both outperform cytology in the detection of low-grade tumours, however, their specificity is worse. As yet, there is no alternative to cystoscopy for either initial diagnosis or follow-up of bladder cancer (Giannopoulos *et al.* 2000).

All patients with macroscopic haematuria require a cystoscopy and upper urinary tract imaging. The latter may be either an intravenous urography (IVU) or an upper tract ultrasound study. Both IVU and ultrasound have advantages and disadvantages, and neither will detect all upper tract tumours: the yield of tumours will be highest with a combination of ultrasound and IVU and this should, therefore, be regarded as the gold standard (Khandra *et al.* 2000). This is, however, a controversial area. Various options are acceptable provided clinicians appreciate the advantages and disadvantages of the chosen investigations in a particular patient taking into account age and risk factors, such as smoking.

Cystoscopy was traditionally performed under general or regional anaesthesia, although rigid cystoscopy can be done under local anaesthesia. Flexible cystoscopy under local anaesthesia is now standard practice and is better tolerated than rigid cystoscopy: in good hands, both techniques should have similar accuracy. An initial flexible examination spares an anaesthetic to the majority of haematuria patients, who will have no bladder tumour. It also allows patients with a bladder tumour to be directed to a day surgery operating list or an inpatient list, as the size of the tumour dictates or perhaps further staging prior to surgical resection.

Haematuria clinics, a 'one stop' diagnostic service comprising clinical assessment, urine culture and cytology, upper tract imaging, and flexible cystoscopy, have been introduced over recent years. These certainly streamline diagnosis and are popular with patients and urologists (Lynch *et al.* 1994a). Speeding up the process of diagnosis is likely to be important, as there is now evidence that the sooner radical treatment is carried out for muscle-invasive disease the better the outcome (Sanchez-Ortiz *et al.* 2001).

Patients with a suspicious lesion or a cystoscopically obvious bladder tumour require transurethral resection under regional or general anaesthesia: this resection should include bladder muscle to allow the pathologist to assess the T stage of the tumour. Carcinoma *in situ* is suggested by any reddened areas of urothelium and these should be biopsied: urine is also often taken under cystoscopy for cytology and is a sensitive means of detecting carcinoma *in situ* (Hudson *et al.* 1995). Random biopsies of apparently normal urothelium at the time of the initial transurethral resection are probably unnecessary (Kiemeney *et al.* 1994). Before and after resection, a bimanual examination is done to assess whether a mass is present and if so, whether it is mobile or fixed and whether it persists after resection, suggesting deep invasion. Although bimanual examination is subjective, it has been proposed that the presence of a postresection mass has major prognostic significance (Herr 1992a). If the tumour is extensive within the bladder, or

if there is doubt about whether it extends deeply, representative biopsies with muscle are taken and complete resection is not attempted. Subsequent management is dictated by the pathological stage.

The extent of further investigation depends on the pathological stage of the resected tumour. Patients who have superficial lesions that will be managed endoscopically or with intravesical therapy, generally those with Ta lesions, require nothing other than upper tract imaging. Patients with tumours which breach the lamina propria require a second transurethral resection of the site of the original tumour to confirm that no residual tumour exists and that the tumour has not been understaged (Herr 1992b).

Patients who may be candidates for radical treatment require further staging investigation. Local extent can be estimated by either computed tomography or magnetic resonance imaging with the latter being superior (Husband and Reznek 1998), but prior transurethral resection may disrupt tissue planes, making assessment of tumour depth difficult. Reactive pelvic lymphadenopathy may occur after transurethral resection, so any enlarged pelvic lymph nodes (>1 cm) seen with imaging studies may require fine-needle aspiration cytology to exclude metastasis. If this is technically difficult, then a laparoscopic approach may be used. Metastases are sought further by chest radiography. The role of skeletal scintigraphy is controversial: although this is the most sensitive means of detecting bone metastases (See *et al.* 1992), its specificity is low and we reserve bone scanning for patients with raised serum alkaline phosphatase.

Staging is done to establish the indications for treatment and to allow comparison between the results of different series of patients. For both of these reasons it is vital to distinguish between clinically staged and pathologically staged disease (the T stage prefixed by the letters c and p, respectively) because there is a significant error in clinical staging, principally in assessing the depth of local spread and lymph node involvement, and both understaging and overstaging occur (Cummings *et al.* 1992).

Treatment

Superficial tumours

Approximately 80 per cent of bladder cancer patients have superficial tumours at presentation and are generally treated with transurethral resection. Recurrent tumours are treated either by further transurethral resection or by biopsy and cystoscopic fulguration (cystodiathermy). Data on the effects of treatment of superficial tumours by transurethral resection or cystodiathermy or both come from the American National Bladder Cancer Group study (Heney 1992). Recurrence at 12 months in Ta and T1 tumours was around 30 per cent in grade I, 40 per cent in grade II, and 70 per cent in grade III: for Ta tumours together, around 50 per cent recurred at 3 years, compared to 70 per cent of T1 tumours (Heney 1992). Progression rates in Ta and T1 tumours at 3 years were typically 2 per cent for grade I, 10 per cent for grade II, and 45 per cent for grade III: for Ta tumours together 4 per cent progressed, compared to 30 per cent of T1 tumours (Heney 1992). Similar results occurred in the control arm of a European Organisation for Research and Treatment of Cancer (EORTC) study of the treatment of Ta and T1 by intravesical chemotherapy (Oosterlinck *et al.* 1993). Most Ta tumours are grade I, so the risk of progression of Ta tumours overall is very low, but not nil. However, the risk of progression of a T1G3 tumour treated by resection alone is up to 50 per cent (Kaubisch *et al.* 1991).

Intravesical therapy

Adjuvant treatment in the form of intravesical chemotherapy is considered for all new superficial tumours. Patients with superficial tumours who are considered to be at increased risk of tumour recurrence and or progression are considered for either adjuvant intravesical chemotherapy or immunotherapy. This latter group of patients includes those with T1 tumours, G3 tumours, tumours associated with urothelial dysplasia or carcinoma *in situ*, or recurrent Ta G1 or Ta G2 tumours. The principles, techniques, and results of intravesical chemotherapy and immunotherapy have been discussed at length (Richie 1992; Sarosdy 1992; Smith *et al.* 1999; Duque *et al.* 2000).

Intravesical chemotherapy

Several agents have been used for intravesical chemotherapy. Mitomycin C is a high molecular weight antitumour antibiotic that inhibits DNA synthesis and may also lead to DNA cleavage. Doxorubicin (adriamycin) is also a high molecular weight anthracycline antitumour antibiotic that acts by binding to DNA. Epirubicin is a cytotoxic antibiotic structurally related to doxorubicin. Each agent can be used therapeutically, to treat existing tumours particularly if there is extensive superficial tumour that cannot be cleared endoscopically, or prophylactically to reduce the risk of recurrence. Newer intravesical agents such as gemcitibine are continually being evaluated.

Intravesical agents potentially have both local and systemic side-effects: this is apart from the small, but finite risk of repeated urethral catheterization required with some regimes (Thrasher *et al.* 1992). Factors that may influence both local and systemic complications include the concentration of intravesical agent, the exposure time, the pH of the solution, and the integrity of the urothelium. These factors may also affect overall response, for example, epirubicin has optimal activity at pH 8. New drug-delivery techniques such as combinations of chemotherapeutic drugs, sequential chemotherapeutic and immunotherapeutic agents, electromotive drug administration (EMDA), and photosensitizing agents are also being investigated (Witjes *et al.* 2000).

Mitomycin C is minimally absorbed (~1 per cent) by the urothelium, therefore, myelosuppression is rare. The main side-effects are chemical cystitis in up to 30 per cent, leading on occasions (<1 per cent) to a reduced bladder capacity (with its inherent functional consequences) and genital or other skin rashes in about 5 per cent. Doxorubicin is minimally absorbed through the urothelium and myelosuppression is very rare. Local effects are more prominent than with mitomycin C, with chemical cystitis in up to 50 per cent of patients, some of whom develop bladder contracture. Epirubicin has a similar side-effect profile to mitomycin C, producing chemical cystitis in 10–38 per cent and bladder contracture in less than 1 per cent (Ali-el-Dein *et al.* 1997a).

Broadly similar results have been achieved with all the agents used for intravesical chemotherapy, although treatment schedules and side-effects have varied (Lamm 1992; Richie 1992; Duque *et al.* 2000; Nilsson *et al.* 2001). Combined analysis of six EORTC and Medical Research Council (MRC) trials studying the effect of intravesical chemotherapy following TUR found a reduction in short-term (1–3 years) recurrence rate of 20 per cent and an 8 per cent reduction in recurrence rate at 8 years (Pawinski *et al.* 1996). No effect on progression to invasive disease was seen. It is worth pointing out that most of

the controls also received intravesical chemotherapy, albeit delayed. Adjuvant intravesical chemotherapy may be given as a single dose, a single course, or longer-term maintenance therapy. In general, the side-effects of increasing dose outweigh the degree of increased response for newly diagnosed disease. Tolley *et al.* (1996) reported no significant reduction in recurrence rate at 5 years between a single dose (15 per cent) and five doses (23 per cent) of mitomycin C (40 mg). Ali-el-Dein *et al.* (1997b) found no significant difference in recurrence rate at a mean of 32 months using either a single dose of epirubicin (50 mg) or eight doses. Okamura *et al.* (1998) found no significant difference in recurrence rate at 2 years using a 6-week course of epirubicin (40 mg) and maintenance treatment over a year. A criticism of a number of these trials is that they contained a heterogeneous group of patients: those with low risk of recurrence and progression to those with intermediate and high risk. Comparison between trials is also confounded by the use of different doses and schedules. Current standard practice is to give all newly diagnosed patients, with superficial bladder cancer, one dose of an intravesical agent (usually mitomycin C or epirubicin). If histology subsequently suggests high-risk disease, or if the patient develops multiple recurrences, then further intravesical treatment may be considered with a course of intravesical chemotherapy or immunotherapy.

Intravesical bacille Calmette-Guerin therapy

Intravesical BCG (bacille Calmette-Guerin) was introduced by Morales in 1976. Several different strains of BCG have been used, including Pasteur, Tice, Connaught, and Moro: the viability and density of bacilli per milligram of vaccine varies between strains used and between batches of the same strain. The exact mechanism of action of BCG is unknown, however, it is a non-specific immune system stimulant, and it requires an immunocompetent host to be effective. BCG activates macrophages, T-lymphocytes, B-lymphocytes, and natural killer cells: it stimulates lymphokine and interferon production. BCG may be considered as prophylactic therapy for patients who have recurrent Ta G2, Ta G3, or T1 bladder tumours, and who have been rendered tumour-free.

The principal side-effect of intravesical BCG therapy is bladder irritability, which is usually well tolerated by most patients. The most common symptoms are dysuria and urinary frequency, both of which occur in about 90 per cent of patients, haematuria occurs in about 45 per cent, low-grade fever in 24 per cent, malaise in 18 per cent, and nausea in 8 per cent. There is a risk of systemic infection by BCG: this is probably less than 0.5 per cent, but it can be life threatening (Lamm *et al.* 1992). The risk of other systemic complications, such as arthralgia, pneumonia, and rashes, is similar in magnitude to that of systemic sepsis.

A recent review of several prospective randomized clinical trials that have compared the efficacy of intravesical BCG with transurethral resection alone supported the superior efficacy of BCG therapy in reducing recurrence (Shelley 2002). What is not yet clear, however, is the role of intravesical BCG compared to other agents. Several comparisons between chemotherapy and immunotherapy (BCG) have been made in recent years with controversial results. Witjes and colleagues randomized 342 patients to receive BCG or mitomycin C after TUR, and found equal efficacy in reducing recurrence at a median of 7 years, but mitomycin C was more effective in delaying progression in the absence of carcinoma *in situ* (Witjes *et al.* 1998). Malstrom and colleagues found BCG to be superior to mitomycin C for recurrence prophylaxis at a median follow-up of over 5 years, but there was no difference in tumour progression and survival (Malmstrom *et al.* 1999a,b). The American Urological Association Guidelines on early stage bladder cancer (Smith *et al.* 1999), advocate the use of either BCG or mitomycin C, but do not define how to decide on the choice of agents. This is the subject of an ongoing Cochrane review (Shelly *et al.* 2002a,b), but once again, difficulties arise due to heterogeneous patient groups, and different doses and schedules of intravesical agents, as well as strains of BCG.

As with intravesical chemotherapy, the optimum treatment schedule for BCG is unknown. Recent evidence (Lamm *et al.* 2000) has suggested that longer-term maintenance treatment over a 3-year period improves response compared to a standard 6-week course, although, due mainly to side-effects, only 16 per cent of patients were able to complete the maintenance treatment programme.

Carcinoma *in situ*

Review of studies examining the use of intravesical chemotherapy in carcinoma *in situ*, showed that the response is initially around 50 per cent, but that less than 20 per cent of patients remain disease-free at 5 years (Lamm 1992). Patients with carcinoma *in situ*, who are treated with BCG with curative intent, have a response rate of more than 80 per cent (Merz *et al.* 1995). Subsequent positive urine cytology, indicating failure, occurs in about 10–20 per cent of patients, and then invasive disease in the bladder or carcinoma *in situ*, either in the urinary upper tract or in the prostatic urethra has to be suspected (Merz *et al.* 1995). Those who fail early are at high risk of developing invasive disease early.

In general, the treatment of choice of carcinoma *in situ* of the bladder and T1 bladder cancer is intravesical BCG, whereas with recurrent Ta tumours many urologists would use intravesical chemotherapy instead, because of the lower side-effect profile, compared to BCG. It must be stressed that intravesical agents should be regarded as delaying time to recurrence and progression. Whether genuine prevention of progression is possible is still controversial. In one of the longest randomized follow-up studies of TUR alone versus TUR and BCG in high-risk superficial bladder cancer, progression was seen in 53 per cent of both groups at 15 years (Cookson *et al.* 1997). Interpretation was confounded, however, as half of the control group received BCG at a later date. In a separate report from the same institution on patients with exclusively T1G3 disease managed with TUR alone or TUR plus BCG, progression was seen in 65 and 40 per cent ($p = 0.03$), respectively, at a minimum of 15 years follow-up, despite 60 per cent of the control group receiving delayed BCG (Herr *et al.* 1997). This study also shows that in 12 per cent of those with stage progression, this occurred at between 10 and 15 years emphasizing the life-long risk.

Invasive tumours

Unless inappropriate to the patient's general state, invasive tumours are treated radically: this may be either by radical transurethral resection, partial cystectomy, radical cystectomy, or radical radiotherapy (Thrasher *et al.* 1993). Patients who are candidates for radical treatment should have their entire urothelium assessed. Any upper tract urothelial lesion should be managed on its own merits and the distal prostatic urethra is biopsied: invasive cancer or carcinoma *in situ* here is an indication for cystourethrectomy.

If the bladder alone is involved, any of the treatments discussed below may be considered. Whilst radical cystectomy is generally regarded as the gold standard in terms of efficacy, each alternative radical treatment is

bladder preserving and this has steered many clinicians and patients towards these modalities.

Any consideration of the results of treatment of invasive bladder cancer should be made in the light of the general improvement in survival figures from both radiotherapy and from cystectomy over the last three decades. Apart from improvements in techniques of surgery, anaesthesia, and radiotherapy, this is probably also due to more careful preoperative staging, allowing exclusion of patients with metastases and perhaps also due to improved patient and physician awareness of the need to investigate haematuria.

Radical transurethral resection

Radical transurethral resection implies an attempt to clear all tumour from the bladder by endoscopic resection, so that the full thickness of the bladder wall is removed, down to and including some perivesical fat (Herr 1992b). Creating a hole in the bladder by radical transurethral resection is, in skilled hands, less hazardous than might be anticipated, because most of the bladder, except the dome, is extraperitoneal and the bladder heals extremely well with catheter drainage. Radical transurethral resection is probably most appropriate for a patient with a primary, single, small (3 cm or less) T2 tumour, which is at a site where it can be completely resected, such as the base or lateral wall of the bladder. A second resection of the tumour site, quadrantic bladder biopsies, and prostatic urethral biopsies 2–3 weeks after the radical resection are mandatory and must all be negative, otherwise we proceed to cystectomy.

The results of radical transurethral resection of muscle-invasive bladder cancer have been collated by Herr (1992b, 2001): recent data indicate overall 10-year disease specific survival rate of around 75 per cent (Solsona *et al.* 1998; Herr 2001). This is, of course, a highly select group of patients, but compares favourably with cystectomy. The possibility that this can be improved by adjuvant chemoradiotherapy remains to be confirmed, but increases the possibility of bladder-sparing treatment. Overall 5-year survival has been reported as 88 per cent for T2–T3 tumours that were T0 on reresection followed by radiotherapy and cisplatin (Dunst *et al.* 1994).

Partial cystectomy

Partial cystectomy is indicated for solitary tumours situated in the mobile posterior part of the bladder or in the dome and at least 3 cm from the bladder neck, with normal surrounding urothelium allowing resection of a 2–3 cm cuff of bladder (Sweeney *et al.* 1992). The bladder capacity must also be sufficient to avoid producing a small capacity postoperatively. Two particular indications for partial cystectomy are a urachal tumour arising in the dome and a tumour arising in a diverticulum.

The outcome after partial cystectomy has been discussed in detail (Sweeney *et al.* 1992). Recurrence rates were around 60 per cent and overall nearly 10 per cent of patients require conversion to radical cystectomy (Sweeney *et al.* 1992). Five-year survival rates are shown in Table 3 (Novick *et al.* 1976; Brannan *et al.* 1978; Cummings *et al.* 1978; Faysal *et al.* 1979; Merrell *et al.* 1979; Schoborg *et al.* 1979) and are typically 60 per cent for grade 2 disease and 30 per cent for grade 3 disease and 70 per cent for T1 tumours, 55 per cent for T2 tumours, and 20 per cent for T3 tumours.

Although both radical transurethral resection and partial cystectomy are attractive because they preserve the bladder, the restrictive indications are rarely met. The major risk with both modalities alone

Table 3 Five-year survival (%) following partial cystectomy

Author	Grade		
	1	2	3–4
(a) Five-year survival according to grade following partial cystectomy			
Novick et al. (1976)	100	75	40
Brannan et al. (1978)	50	62	55
Cummings et al. (1978)	100	96	32
Schoborg et al. (1979)	75	62	26
Faysal et al. (1979)	100	53	30
Merrell et al. (1979)	78	56	22

Author	pT stage		
	pT1	pT2	pT3
(b) Five-year survival according to stage following partial cystectomy			
Novick et al. (1976)	67	53	20
Brannan et al. (1978)	69	54	33
Cummings et al. (1978)	79	80	6
Schoborg et al. (1979)	69	29	12
Faysal et al. (1979)	58	29	7
Merrell et al. (1979)	100	67	25

Table 4 Five-year survival following radical radiotherapy

Author	T stage	
	≤T2	T3
(a) Local control (%) according to stage following radical radiotherapy		
Cummings (1976)[a]	72	43
Quilty (1986)	—	41
Gospodarowicz (1989)[b]	69	40
Fossa (1993)	—	—
Borgaonkar et al. (2002)	—	—
(b) Five-year survival (%) according to stage following radical radiotherapy		
Cummings (1976)	83	36
Quilty (1986)	—	26
Gospodarowicz (1989)[b]	59	30–52
Fossa (1993)	38[c]	14[d]
Borgaonkar et al. (2002)	48[e]	26

[a] At 21 months.
[b] Cause-specific survival.
[c] T2 and T3a.
[d] T3b.
[e] T2 alone.

is incomplete resection of the primary tumour and failure to identify occult positive lymph node metastases. The former is due mainly to circumferential tumour spread around the bladder wall, which is related to the depth of the tumour. With deep muscle invasion there may be at least 60 per cent circumferential involvement of the bladder microscopically (Baker 1955). Adjuvant treatments may help on both counts, but the absence of prospective randomized studies remains a severe obstacle for urologists to accept such treatments for more than a minority of patients.

Radiotherapy

Radical radiotherapy may not only preserve the bladder, but the function of the preserved bladder may be virtually unaffected by radiotherapy, leaving the patient with no significant postradiotherapy symptoms (Lynch et al. 1992). However, the tumour may not necessarily respond, radiotherapy may indeed disastrously impair bladder function, and a salvage cystectomy for non-responders is a more difficult procedure than a primary cystectomy. It is also likely that the results of lower urinary tract reconstruction after radiotherapy are less good than after primary cystectomy.

Radiotherapy is inappropriate for those with poor pre-existing bladder function, with prior pelvic sepsis or surgery, with inflammatory bowel disease, with bladder diverticula, distended bladders, or upper urinary tract obstruction. Although there have been reports of good results in the treatment of T1G3 disease, this is probably better treated by BCG, and there is no place for radiotherapy in other forms of superficial bladder cancer (Gospodarowicz et al. 1993). A further potential problem is carcinoma *in situ*, which is rarely controlled by radiotherapy and is associated with a high recurrence rate (Gospodarowicz et al. 1993).

There are a number of different radiotherapeutic techniques designed to maximize tumour toxicity and minimize bladder and bowel side-effects: these include accelerated fractionation, hyperfractionation, and

the use of sensitizers or chemotherapy (Wesson 1992). More recently, further refinements in delivery with conformal radiotherapy and intensity-modulated radiotherapy have been developed. The most important prognostic factor, however, is the completeness of trans-urethral resection prior to radiotherapy (Shipley and Rose 1985; Dunst et al. 1994). After radical radiotherapy, meticulous follow-up is required and patients who have failed to respond within 6 months should have a salvage cystectomy. The interpretation of biopsies and cytology may be difficult after radiotherapy, posing further problems in follow-up.

Review of patients following radical radiotherapy shows overall 5-year survival rates of up to 40 per cent and salvage cystectomy rates of around 50 per cent in patients with organ-confined disease (Gospodarowicz et al. 1993). Table 4 shows local control rates and 5-year survival rates according to T stage. No formal comparison of radical radiotherapy against radical cystectomy alone exists. However, comparisons have been made between preoperative radiotherapy and planned cystectomy versus definitive radical radiotherapy and no convincing survival advantage has been shown for either treatment in these studies (Gospodarowicz et al. 1993; Shelley et al. 2001).

Radical cystectomy

Cystectomy is generally indicated for patients with muscle-invasive tumours who are fit for surgery and with no evidence of lymphatic or distant metastases. We judge suitability on biological rather than chronological grounds. All patients for cystectomy, regardless of the planned urinary diversion, are seen by a stoma nurse and wear a stoma bag for 24 h to allow optimal assessment of an ileal conduit site, which is then marked indelibly.

Radical cystectomy involves laparotomy and exclusion of disseminated intra-abdominal disease, pelvic lymphadenectomy, and mobilization and excision of the bladder. In men, the prostate is removed *en bloc*: a potency-preserving technique is often feasible depending on the site of the tumour and probably has no adverse effect on survival (Schlegel *et al.* 1987). Urethrectomy is indicated in patients with either carcinoma or carcinoma *in situ* in distal prostatic urethral biopsies; the overall risk of urethral recurrence if the urethra is preserved is between 4 and 10 per cent.

In women, the uterus, fallopian tubes, and ovaries together with the anterior vaginal wall and the entire urethra are removed *en bloc* unless there is no evidence of tumour at the bladder neck or urethra when reconstruction on to the native urethra may be considered (see below).

Pelvic lymphadenectomy may cure some patients with limited unsuspected pelvic node involvement (Lerner *et al.* 1993), it permits accurate staging and it enables a more anatomical and safer cystectomy. So, despite the lack of randomized controlled data showing a survival advantage, we perform lymphadenectomy, but recognize that it probably only has an impact on survival in those with small volume nodal disease (Mills *et al.* 2001).

The safety of cystectomy has undoubtedly increased over the last 25 years, due particularly to improved perioperative care and aggressive management of complications. Thirty-day mortality should currently be around 2 per cent (Hautmann *et al.* 1993).

Complications with incidences of around 5 per cent include wound infection, pelvic abscess, prolonged ileus, and small bowel obstruction or fistula: pulmonary embolus and myocardial infarction also occur occasionally (Frazier *et al.* 1992). Around 25 per cent of patients have complications (Frazier *et al.* 1992). Morbidity and mortality will probably be higher for departments performing only occasional cystectomies (Birkmeyer *et al.* 2002).

The disadvantages of cystectomy are the perioperative mortality (albeit now low), loss of bladder function, and possibly also continence and potency. In contrast, the cystectomy patient benefits from the greatest likelihood of cure, improved local control, and removal of the possibility of dying with advanced local disease in the bladder, which can be an appalling fate. If the patient has metastases, cystectomy or urinary diversion alone may be considered for symptomatic relief of very troublesome local symptoms, refractory to other measures (Lerner *et al.* 1992).

Current data show overall 5-year survival of around 50 per cent or better following radical cystectomy: Table 5 shows survival in pT stages pT2 and pT3 (Giuliani *et al.* 1985; Malkowicz *et al.* 1990; Pagano *et al.* 1991; Frazier *et al.* 1993; Studer *et al.* 1994; Stein *et al.* 2001; Wijkstrom *et al.* 1998). Survival at 5 years in node-positive patients has been reported to be 20–30 per cent in several series (Roehrborn *et al.* 1991; Lerner *et al.* 1992; Vieweg *et al.* 1999; Mills *et al.* 2001).

Urinary diversion and reconstruction

Following cystectomy, urine can either be diverted into an incontinent stoma (usually an ileal conduit), into a continent urinary reservoir (which is either catheterized regularly by the patient or is controlled by the anal sphincter), or into an orthotopic bladder substitute (a bowel reservoir anastomosed to the urethra, so that the patient voids urethrally). Ileal conduits have been seen as quick and simple procedures, whereas, continent diversions and orthotopic bladder substitutes have been regarded as lengthier and riskier. However, there are clear advantages and disadvantages to all procedures, so careful assessment of each patient is vital to allow an appropriate choice of diversion.

Conduits have been regarded simple and safe in the long-term. The patient need not be motivated and stoma care may be done by a carer. If stoma care fails, the patient simply becomes wet, but the upper

Table 5 Survival (%) according to stage following radical cystectomy

Author	T stage	
	pT2	pT3
Giuliani *et al.* (1985)	56	19
Malkowicz *et al.* (1990)[a]	76	—
Pagano *et al.* (1991)[a]	63	31
Frazier *et al.* (1993)[a]	64	39[b]
Studer *et al.* (1994)	70[c]	40[d]
Wijkstrom *et al.* (1998)	85[e]	50[f]
Stein *et al.* (2001)	89[g]	62[h]

[a] Cause-specific survival.
[b] pT3a, pT3b, and pT4.
[c] pT3a.
[d] pT3b.
[e] Organ confined node-negative disease.
[f] Non-organ confined node-negative disease.
[g] pT2 node-negative disease.
[h] pT3b node-negative disease.

tracts are not at immediate risk: this is a fail-safe method. However, a visible stoma and an external appliance carry psychological morbidity.

Continent diversions and orthotopic bladder substitutes can be made from stomach, ileum, the ileocaecal segment, and either hemicolon (Benson *et al.* 1992; Bachor *et al.* 1993). A continent urinary diversion is an intra-abdominal urinary reservoir. There are a variety of different continence mechanisms for the catheterizable efferent limb. The majority use some form of antireflux mechanism to protect the upper tracts from the combined effects of urinary infection and high reservoir pressure. Orthotopic bladder substitution after radical cystectomy was initially performed in men, however, urethral sparing radical cystectomy in combination with orthotopic bladder substitution is now increasingly performed in selected women (Stenzl *et al.* 2001). Our preference is for a reservoir made from ileum (Studer *et al.* 1995).

Continent diversions and orthotopic bladder substitutes preserve body image better, and orthotopic bladder substitutes allow a more normal voiding habit. Stoma care is not necessary, but patients with a continent urinary reconstruction must be well motivated as their long-term daily input is essential for good functional outcome. Those with continent cutaneous diversion must catheterize their pouch several times each day and bladder substitute patients must understand how to empty their reservoir through pelvic floor relaxation with or without abdominal straining and then do so at regular intervals. The reservoir capacity for continent diversions and orthotopic bladder substitutes should ideally be 500–600 ml and the end-filling pressure should be low, less than 25 cm H_2O (Turner *et al.* 1995). Although continent diversions and orthotopic bladder substitutes that are not emptied may simply leak, they may rupture and are not *invariably* failsafe methods, in contrast to conduits.

The long-term effects of urinary diversions in general include renal impairment due to stone, infection, reflux, or obstruction, gastrointestinal consequences due to bowel resection, metabolic complications due to malabsorption and absorption of urinary solutes through the bowel segment, and tumour formation in the bowel segment. This has been reviewed extensively (Steiner *et al.* 1991; McDougal 1992; Mills and Studer 1999).

Chemotherapy

Chemotherapy has been used to treat two groups of patients with bladder cancer: those with muscle-invasive disease and those with either known spread to pelvic lymph nodes or distant metastases. The use of chemotherapy in bladder cancer, including its use in investigative combinations with other modalities, has been reviewed in detail recently (Sternberg and Calabro 2000; Maluf and Barjorin 2001).

The rationale for treating patients with muscle-invasive disease and no apparent spread at the time of surgery is that most of the subsequent bladder cancer deaths are due to distant metastases presumed to arise from micrometastases present, but undetected at the time of surgery. It has been hypothesized that such micrometastases may theoretically be destroyed by systemic chemotherapy: unfortunately this remains to be demonstrated. In patients with muscle-invasive disease, chemotherapy can be used either before or after surgery, termed neoadjuvant and adjuvant therapy, respectively. The relative merits of neoadjuvant and adjuvant treatments have been discussed at length (Thrasher *et al.* 1993; Natale 2000).

Several chemotherapeutic agents including cisplatin, methotrexate, vinblastine, cyclophosphamide, doxorubicin as well as the newer agents gemcitabine and taxoids have been shown to have significant activity against transitional cell carcinoma when used alone, inducing either a complete or partial response in up to 40 per cent of patients (Scher 1992; Roth *et al.* 1994; Sternberg and Calabro 2000). Unfortunately, most of these responses are only partial and do not last more than 6 months and, therefore, single-agent therapy has been abandoned in favour of combination therapy. Two combinations in particular have been widely used: the three drugs (CMV—cisplatin, methotrexate, and vinblastine) or four drugs (MVAC—methotrexate, vinblastine, doxorubicin, and cisplatin) producing complete responses in up to 30 per cent of cases, although the majority of patients treated, eventually relapse (Sternberg 1993). A great deal of interest is currently focused on combining newer agents with traditional agents or newer agents alone. The combination of gemcitabine and paclitaxel is being compared to MVAC in large randomized trials. Gemcitabine in particular has the advantage of a milder toxicity profile, thus potentially improving quality of life.

The main advantage of neoadjuvant chemotherapy is that theoretically, chemosensitivity may be determined *in vivo* (Scher 1992). The response in the bladder can be assessed by cystoscopy and biopsy and can be used to guide treatment of the primary lesion. Responding patients can be treated to the point of maximal response before definitive local therapy, whereas, patients who fail to respond can be spared the toxicity of further cytotoxic drug administration and referred earlier for definitive local therapy. Disadvantages of this technique, however, are that the response of micrometastases may not in fact parallel that of a responding local tumour, that all patients are exposed to the risks of the initial chemotherapy and definitive local treatment is delayed.

A number of randomized trials of neoadjuvant chemotherapy have been reported, three of which stand out as being of reasonable size: the Nordic I trial, the MRC/EORTC study, and the South Western Oncology Group (SWOG) Intergroup-0080 trial (Malmstrom *et al.* 1996; Anonymous 1999; Natale *et al.* 2001). The combined MRC/ EORTC study is by far the largest with 976 patients. There was no

statistically significant difference in survival between three cycles of neoadjuvant CMV versus no chemotherapy. The study was powered to detect a survival advantage of 10 per cent at 3 years, however, only a 5.5 per cent survival advantage was found ($p = 0.075$) (Anonymous 1999). The Nordic I trial recruited 311 patients and compared two cycles of neoadjuvant doxorubicin and cisplatin and 40 Gy radiotherapy over 5 days followed by cystectomy against radiotherapy or cystectomy alone. There was a 15 per cent improvement in overall survival at 5 years in those with T3a–T4 disease. There was no difference for those with T1 and T2 diseases (Malmstrom *et al.* 1996). This improvement in survival for the T3–T4 subgroup was not confirmed in the Nordic II trial (Malmstrom *et al.* 1999a,b). The SWOG trial included 307 patients randomized to receive three cycles of neoadjuvant MVAC prior to cystectomy versus cystectomy alone. There was a survival benefit of 57 versus 42 per cent at 5 years ($p = 0.04$) in favour of neoadjuvant chemotherapy. At a median follow-up of 7.1 years the median survival was nearly doubled by neoadjuvant MVAC (6.2 versus 3.8 years) (Natale *et al.* 2001). The latter study has been criticized for calculating one-sided p values and failure to use an intention to treat analysis. If a two-sided analysis is performed, the difference in survival no longer remains significant ($p = 0.09$). No trial alone has so far provided sufficient evidence to confirm the benefit of neoadjuvant chemotherapy, however, a meta-analysis by the MRC clinical trials unit using individual patient data from all neoadjuvant chemotherapy trials in bladder cancer is currently being carried out.

Adjuvant chemotherapy is often preferred by urologists, as there is no delay in definitive treatment and further treatment is based on pathological rather than clinical staging. This allows treatment to be tailored to those with the worst prognosis. The main disadvantage with adjuvant chemotherapy is the delay in treatment for occult metastases. It may, in fact, be difficult to administer chemotherapy after cystectomy. The indications for adjuvant chemotherapy have not been standardized: nonetheless, many would offer treatment for nodal or extravesical tumour extension (Scher 1992). Although growth factors, such as granulocyte colony-stimulating factor (GCSF) may reduce the toxicity of regimens currently in use (Sternberg *et al.* 1997), myelosuppression and mucositis remain problems and all regimens are associated with significant morbidity and occasional mortality (Thrasher *et al.* 1993; Anonymous 1999).

Five randomized trials of adjuvant chemotherapy in locally advanced or node-positive bladder cancer exist. Unfortunately interpretation is limited as only small numbers were recruited. Three of these studies suggested that there may be benefit with adjuvant therapy. In one, a prolonged median survival time was recorded for patients receiving cisplatin, doxorubicin, and cyclophosphamide compared to no treatment (Skinner *et al.* 1991). In the second, there was a survival advantage for MVAC or MVEC (epirubicin replacing adriamycin) compared to no treatment (Stöckle *et al.* 1995). In the third study, four cycles of CMV produced a longer relapse-free interval than observation alone (Freiha *et al.* 1996). In the two other studies, Bono and colleagues found no benefit with cisplatin and methotrexate in N0 M0 disease (Bono *et al.* 1989) and Studer and colleagues found no benefit with cisplatin monotherapy following cystectomy for locally advanced, non-metastatic bladder cancer (Studer *et al.* 1994). Single-agent therapy in the latter study would now be regarded as inadequate, although patients were highly selected, resulting in an excellent survival rate for both groups. All studies leave some questions open, and further study in randomized multicentre trials is needed before adjuvant chemotherapy can be considered as standard treatment. The international adjuvant chemotherapy trial coordinated by the EORTC may help to answer whether adjuvant chemotherapy immediately following cystectomy improves survival or not.

We suggest that patients with evidence of metastatic disease at diagnosis should undergo combination chemotherapy, and if there is a complete response of the primary, we offer the patient a salvage cystectomy. This is because both the presence of residual carcinoma in the bladder, despite negative biopsies and cytology, is common and the risk of relapse without cystectomy is high (Scher *et al.* 1988; Splinter *et al.* 1992a,b). Recently 5-year survival as high as 33 per cent has been reported in patients managed by postchemotherapy surgery for suspected or known local residual disease (Dodd *et al.* 1999).

Follow-up

Follow-up is required from the point of view of transitional cell carcinoma, either superficial or invasive, and from the point of view of any form of radical treatment, including the special follow-up which may be needed for urinary diversion after cystectomy.

Urothelial cancer follow-up

Superficial disease

Follow-up of these patients is aimed at detecting recurrences at a resectable stage and trying to detect a recurrence with invasion early to allow more aggressive treatment. Follow-up is tailored to the expected risk of recurrence and progression, with patients being assigned, in general terms, to low- and high-risk groups.

Patients with superficial tumours have traditionally been followed-up by regular cystoscopy under anaesthetic. However, the number of patients with bladder cancer and their frequency of recurrence means that the follow-up of patients with superficial tumours and the treatment of their recurrent superficial lesions has huge cost implications. Changes in healthcare delivery and in the understanding of the behaviour of superficial bladder tumours have led to changes in practice, to try to reduce the need for cystoscopy on an inpatient basis, with attempts to target those patients at high risk of recurrence and progression, so that they receive more intensive follow-up, including adjuvant intravesical therapy, than those at low risk. Flexible cystoscopy enables patients at low risk to be followed-up as outpatients, with admission only required if recurrence is detected.

In general, patients with Ta G1–2 tumours tend to be managed without adjuvant intravesical therapy and with relatively infrequent cystoscopies, whereas those with Ta/1 G2/3 tumours or with carcinoma *in situ* tend to receive adjuvant intravesical therapy and more frequent cystoscopies. It has been suggested that follow-up may be guided by two clinical variables, the number of tumours at presentation and the presence or absence of tumour at cystoscopy 3 months after initial transurethral resection (Parmar *et al.* 1989). These allowed patients to be separated into three groups with low, medium, and high risk of recurrence (Fig. 10), with the advantage that these were objective findings, available to the urologist at the time of cystoscopy. This assessment of the risk of recurrence, combined with the reduction in the rate of recurrence by intravesical chemotherapy, led to further proposed streamlining of superficial bladder cancer follow-up, as shown in Fig. 11 (Hall *et al.* 1994). This is only one possible means of follow-up, and

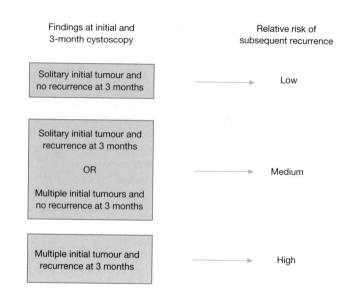

Fig. 10 Assessment of risk of recurrence based on the number of initial tumours and the presence of recurrence at 3 months (Parmar *et al.* 1989).

other protocols could be developed from the same, or similar evidence. Although the evidence on which this proposal was based is clear (Parmar *et al.* 1989), the proposal seems not to have been widely implemented, for reasons that are not clear. Whether it is because setting clinical protocols out on paper makes them look complex to clinicians who actually use similar unwritten protocols routinely, is not known.

Invasive disease

Patients who have had invasive bladder cancer receive more intensive follow-up, because of their high risk of subsequent relapse, although the manner of this depends on which type of radical treatment has been used. It must be stressed that because the impact of treatment on relapse is unproven, early detection does not at present translate into genuinely prolonged survival. Early detection may simply mean that an inevitably fatal relapse is apparent to the patient sooner.

Our follow-up regime for patients after cystectomy aims to detect recurrence in the urethra or upper tracts and distant metastases. Upper tract tumours develop in about 3 per cent of patients after cystectomy, more commonly in those with carcinoma *in situ* of the bladder, involvement of intravesical ureters, or urethral involvement. Careful follow-up of patients with these risk factors is advocated, but the prognosis in patients with upper tract cancer after cystectomy is generally poor. Urethral cytology (Wolinska *et al.* 1977) allows early detection of urethral recurrence and urethrectomy if appropriate. Secondary urethrectomy is indicated in patients who have either overt urethral cancer at the apex of the prostate in their cystoprostatectomy specimen (which should have been diagnosed preoperatively) or those who subsequently develop invasive urethral cancer, particularly when conservative treatment has failed. From the point of view of cancer, our follow-up after cystectomy involves chest radiography and IVU annually for the first 3 years, with subsequent ultrasound assessment of the upper tracts. Urethral lavage is done annually for the first 5 years.

Follow-up after radiotherapy is centred on cystoscopy and examination under anaesthesia to determine whether the primary tumour is eradicated. If this occurs, regular cystoscopic follow-up is combined with chest radiography and IVU to assess the upper tracts. If the

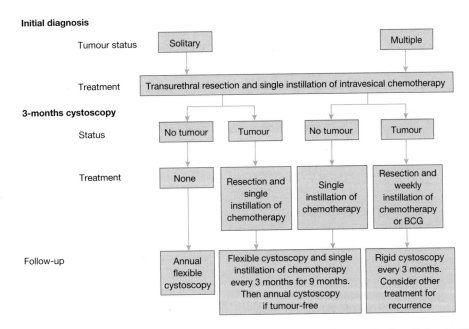

Fig. 11 Proposal for the management of patients with superficial bladder tumours. (Reproduced with permission from Hall *et al.* 1994.)

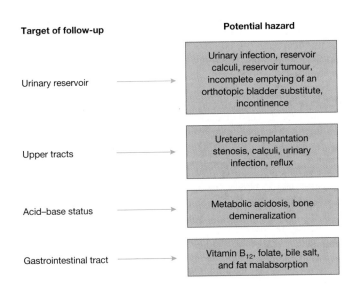

Fig. 12 Follow-up targets for patients with urinary diversion and the possible complications.

primary fails to respond, salvage cystectomy is performed if the patient's general health permits.

Follow-up of urinary diversion

All patients with a urinary diversion require life-long follow-up, because of the potential complications such as ureteric stenosis, renal calculi, urinary infection, electrolyte or acid–base disturbance, fat malabsorption, vitamin B_{12} or folate deficiency, and bone demineralization. The clinically significant risk of some of these complications, in particular bone demineralization, is not yet known, as genuinely long-term follow-up of continent diversion and orthotopic reconstruction is still not available. In addition, follow-up of patients with continent reservoirs or with orthotopic bladder substitutes is necessary to ensure that

continence is satisfactory and that bladder substitute patients have sterile urine, which is voided to completion at regular intervals. The general targets of follow-up after urinary diversion are shown in Fig. 12.

Summary

Bladder tumours are common and represent a considerable urological workload. Only a minority of patients with superficial tumours will suffer progression of disease into the muscle wall of the bladder, but once a tumour has progressed, the patient's prognosis worsens markedly. Considerable attempts are therefore made to try to prevent this, or at least to detect it early, so that radical therapy can be used. For patients with invasive disease, the gold standard of treatment is radical cystectomy, and current methods of lower urinary tract reconstruction permit excellent quality of life after cystectomy. Alternative treatments that preserve the bladder and combinations of these, which may produce equivalent survival to cystectomy, are being investigated. Finally, it seems likely that molecular biological methods will add considerably to our understanding of the biology of the disease and also to our means of managing it.

References

Ali-el-Dein, B. *et al.* (1997a). Intravesical epirubicin versus doxorubicin for superficial bladder tumours (stage pTa and pT1): a randomized prospective study. *Journal of Urology* **158**, 68–73.

Ali-el-Dein, B. *et al.* (1997b). Single dose versus multiple installations of epirubicin as prophylaxis for recurrence after transurethral resection of pTa and pT1 transitional cell bladder tumours: a prospective randomized controlled study. *British Journal of Urology* **79**, 731–735.

American Cancer Society (2001). Cancer facts and figures. www.cancer.org.

Anonymous (1999). Neoadjuvant cisplatin, methotrexate, and vinblastine chemotherapy for muscle-invasive bladder cancer: a randomized controlled trial. *Lancet* **354**, 533–540.

Aprikian, A. G. *et al.* (1993). Biological markers of prognosis in transitional cell carcinoma of the bladder: current concepts. *Seminars in Urology* **11**, 137–144.

Bachor, R. *et al.* (1993). Options in urinary diversion: a review and critical assessment. *Seminars in Urology* **11**, 235–250.

Baker, R. (1955). Correlation of circumferential lymphatic spread of vesical cancer with depth of infiltration: relation to present methods of treatment. *Journal of Urology* **73**, 681–690.

Benson, M. C. *et al.* (1992). Urinary diversion. *Urologic Clinics of North America* **19**, 779–795.

Birkmeyer, J. D. *et al.* (2002). Hospital volume and surgical mortality in the United States. *The New England Journal of Medicine* **346**, 1128–1137.

Bono, A. V. *et al.* (1989). Adjuvant chemotherapy in advanced bladder cancer. Italian Oncologic Group. *Progress in Clinical and Biological Research* **303**, 533–540.

Borgaonkar, S. *et al.* (2002). Radical radiotherapy and salvage cystectomy as the primary management of transitional cell carcinoma of the bladder. Results following the introduction of a CT planning technique. *Clinical Oncology* **14**, 141–147.

Brandau, S. and Bohle, A. (2001). Bladder cancer. I. Molecular and genetic basis of carcinogenesis. *European Urology* **39**, 491–497.

Brannan, W. *et al.* (1978). Partial cystectomy in the treatment of transitional cell carcinoma of the bladder. *Journal of Urology* **119**, 213–215.

Brennen, P. *et al.* (2000). Cigarette smoking and bladder cancer in men: a pooled analysis of 11 case–control studies. *International Journal of Cancer* **86**, 289–294.

Bringuier, P. P. *et al.* (1993). Decreased E-cadherin immunoreactivity correlates with poor survival in patients with bladder tumors. *Cancer Research* **53**, 3241–3245.

Brodsky, G. L. (1992). Pathology of bladder carcinoma. *Hematology/Oncology Clinics of North America* **6**, 59–80.

Burchill, S. A. *et al.* (1994). Frequency of H-ras mutations in human bladder cancer detected by direct sequencing. *British Journal of Urology* **73**, 516–521.

Byrne, R. R. *et al.* (2001). E-cadherin immunostaining of bladder transitional cell carcinoma, carcinoma *in situ* and lymph node metastases with long-term follow-up. *Journal of Urology* **165**, 1473–1479.

Carbin, B. *et al.* (1991). Grading of human urothelial carcinoma based on nuclear atypia and mitotic frequency, II: prognostic importance. *Journal of Urology* **145**, 972–976.

Casetta, G. *et al.* (1997). P53 expression compared with other prognostic factors in OMS grade-1 stage-Ta transitional cell carcinoma of the bladder. *European Urology* **32**, 229–236.

Cheng, L. *et al.* (2000). Flat intraepithelial lesions of the urinary bladder. *Cancer* **88**, 625–631.

Cookson, M. S. *et al.* (1997). The treated natural history of high risk superficial bladder cancer: 15-year outcome. *Journal of Urology* **158**, 62–67.

Cordon-Cardo, C. *et al.* (1992). Altered expression of the retinoblastoma gene product: prognostic indicator in bladder cancer. *Journal of the National Cancer Institute* **84**, 1251–1256.

Cordon-Cardo, C. *et al.* (1997). Cooperative effects of p53 and pRB alterations in primary superficial bladder tumours. *Cancer Research* **57**, 1217–1221.

Cummings, K. B. *et al.* (1976). Observations on definitive cobalt60 radiation for cure in bladder carcinoma: 15-year followup. *Journal of Urology* **115**, 152–154.

Cummings, K. B. *et al.* (1978). Segmental resection in the management of bladder carcinoma. *Journal of Urology* **119**, 56–58.

Cummings K. B. *et al.* (1992). Diagnosis and staging of bladder cancer. *Urologic Clinics of North America* **19**, 455–465.

Del Mar, C. (2000). Evidence based case report. Asymptomatic haematuria . . . in the doctor. *British Medical Journal* **320**, 165–166.

Delnay, K. M. *et al.* (1999). Bladder histological changes associated with chronic indwelling urinary catheter. *Journal of Urology* **161**, 1106–1108.

Dickinson, A. J. *et al.* (1994). Quantification of angiogenesis as an independent predictor of prognosis in invasive bladder carcinomas. *British Journal of Urology* **74**, 762–766.

Dodd, P. M. *et al.* (1999). Outcome of postchemotherapy surgery after treatment with methotrexate, vinblastine, doxorubicin, and cisplatin in patients with unresectable or metastatic transitional cell carcinoma. *Journal of Clinical Oncology* **17**, 2546–2552.

Doll, R. *et al.* (1994). Mortality in relation to smoking: 40 years' observations on male British doctors. *British Medical Journal* **309**, 901–911.

Dunst, J. *et al.* (1994). Organ-sparing treatment of advanced bladder cancer: a 10-year experience. *International Journal of Radiation Oncology, Biology, Physics* **30**, 261–266.

Duque, J. L. F. *et al.* (2000). An overview of the treatment of superficial bladder cancer. *Urologic Clinics of North America* **27**, 125–135.

Epstein, J. I. *et al.* (1998). The World Health Organization/International Society of Urological Pathology consensus classification of urothelial (transitional cell) neoplasms of the urinary bladder. *The American Journal of Surgical Pathology* **22**, 1435–1448.

Esrig, D. *et al.* (1993). p53 nuclear protein accumulation correlates with mutations in the p53 gene, tumor grade, and stage in bladder cancer. *American Journal of Pathology* **143**, 1389–1397.

Esrig, D. *et al.* (1994). Accumulation of nuclear p53 and tumour progression in bladder cancer. *New England Journal of Medicine* **331**, 1259–1264.

Faysal, M. H. *et al.* (1979). Evaluation of partial cystectomy for carcinoma of bladder. *Urology* **14**, 352–356.

Fleshner, N. *et al.* (1999). Influence of smoking status on outcomes in patients with tobacco-associated superficial transitional cell carcinoma (tcc) of the bladder. *Journal of Urology* **161**, 172 (664A).

Fossa, S. D. *et al.* (1993). Bladder cancer definitive radiation therapy of muscle-invasive bladder cancer. A retrospective analysis of 317 patients. *Cancer* **72**, 3036–3043.

Frazier, H. A. *et al.* (1992). Complications of radical cystectomy and urinary diversion: a retrospective review of 675 cases in 2 decades. *Journal of Urology* **148**, 1401–1405.

Frazier, H. A. *et al.* (1993). The value of pathologic factors in predicting cancer-specific survival among patients treated with radical cystectomy for transitional cell carcinoma of the bladder and prostate. *Cancer* **71**, 3993–4001.

Freiha, F. *et al.* (1996). A randomized trial of radical cystectomy versus radical cystectomy plus cisplatin, vinblastine and methotrexate chemotherapy for muscle invasive bladder cancer. *Journal of Urology* **155**, 495–499.

Frimberger, D. *et al.* (2000). Endoscopic fluorescence diagnosis and laser treatment of transitional cell carcinoma of the bladder. *Seminars in Urologic Oncology* **18**, 264–272.

Gardiner, R. A. *et al.* (1994). Immunohistological expression of p53 in primary pT1 transitional cell bladder cancer in relation to tumour progression. *British Journal of Urology* **73**, 526–532.

Geoffrey-Perez, B. and Cordier, S. (2001). Fluid consumption and the risk of bladder cancer: results of multicenter case–control study. *International Journal of Cancer* **93**, 880–887.

Giannopoulos A. *et al.* (2000). Comparative evaluation of the BTAstat test, NMP22, and voided urine cytology in the detection of primary and recurrent bladder tumours. *Urology* **55**, 871–875.

Giuliani, L. *et al.* (1985). Results of radical cystectomy for primary bladder cancer. Retrospective study of more than 200 cases. *Urology* **26**, 243–248.

Gospodarowicz, M. K. *et al.* (1989). Radical radiotherapy for muscle invasive transitional cell carcinoma of the bladder: failure analysis. *Journal of Urology* **142**, 1448–1453.

Gospodarowicz, M. K. *et al.* (1993). A critical review of the role of definitive radiation therapy in bladder cancer. *Seminars in Urology* **11**, 214–226.

Hall, R. R. *et al.* (1994). Proposal for changes in cystoscopic follow up of patients with bladder cancer and adjuvant intravesical chemotherapy. *British Medical Journal* **308**, 257–260.

Hartmann, A. *et al.* (2002). Occurrence of chromosome 9 and p53 alterations in multifocal dysplasia and carcinoma *in situ* of human urinary bladder. *Cancer Research* **62**, 809–818.

Hautmann, R. E. *et al.* (1993). The ileal neobladder: 6 years of experience with more than 200 patients. *Journal of Urology* **150**, 40–45.

Heney, N. M. (1992). Natural history of superficial bladder cancer. Prognostic features and long-term disease course. *Urologic Clinics of North America* **19**, 429–433.

Herr, H. W. (1992a). Staging invasive bladder tumors. *Journal of Surgical Oncology* **51**, 217–220.

Herr, H. W. (1992b). Transurethral resection in regionally advanced bladder cancer. *Urologic Clinics of North America* **19**, 695–700.

Herr, H. W. (2001). Transurethral resection of muscle invasive bladder cancer: 10-year outcome. *Journal of Clinical Oncology* **19**, 89–93.

Herr, H. W. *et al.* (1997). Tumour progression and survival in patients with T1G3 bladder tumours: 15-year outcome. *British Journal of Urology* **80**, 762–765.

Hudson, M. A. *et al.* (1995). Carcinoma *in situ* of the bladder. *Journal of Urology* **153**, 564–572.

Husband, J. E. S and Reznek, R. H., ed. *Imaging in Oncology*. ISIS Medical Media Ltd. Oxford, 1998.

Jahnson, S. *et al.* (1995). p53 and Rb immunostaining in locally advanced bladder cancer: relation to prognostic variables and predictive value for the local response to radical radiotherapy. *European Urology* **28**, 135–142.

Johansson, S. L. and Cohen, S. M. (1997). Epidemiology and etiology of bladder cancer. *Seminars in Surgical Oncology* **13**, 291–298.

Jones, P. A. *et al.* (1993). Pathways of development and progression in bladder cancer: new correlations between clinical observations and molecular mechanisms. *Seminars in Urology* **11**, 177–192.

Kanayama, H. (2001). Matrix metalloproteinases and bladder cancer. *Journal of Medical Investigation* **48**, 31–43.

Kaubisch, S. *et al.* (1991). Stage T1 bladder cancer: grade is the primary determinant for risk of muscle invasion. *Journal of Urology* **146**, 28–31.

Keegan, P. E. *et al.* (1998). p53 and p53-regulated genes in bladder cancer. *British Journal of Urology* **82**, 710–720.

Khandra, M. H. *et al.* (2000). A prospective analysis of 1930 patients with hematuria to evaluate current diagnostic practice. *Journal of Urology* **163**, 524–527.

Kiemeney, L. A. *et al.* (1994). Should random urothelial biopsies be taken from patients with primary superficial bladder cancer? A decision analysis. Members of the Dutch South-East Co-Operative Urological Group. *British Journal of Urology* **73**, 164–171.

Knowles, M. A. (2001). What we could do now: molecular pathology of bladder cancer. *Molecular Pathology* **54**, 215–221.

Kristensen, J. K. *et al.* (1988). Epidermal growth factor in urine from patients with urinary bladder tumours. *European Urology* **14**, 313–314.

Lamm, D. L. (1992). Carcinoma *in situ*. *Urologic Clinics of North America* **19**, 499–508.

Lamm, D. L. *et al.* (1992). Incidence and treatment of complications of bacillus Calmette-Guerin intravesical therapy in superficial bladder cancer. *Journal of Urology* **147**, 596–600.

Lamm, D. L. *et al.* (2000). Maintenance bacillus Calmette-Guerin immunotherapy for recurrent Ta, T1 and carcinoma *in situ* transitional cell carcinoma of the bladder: a randomized southwest oncology group study. *Journal of Urology* **163**, 1124–1129.

Lerner, S. P. *et al.* (1992). Radical cystectomy in regionally advanced bladder cancer. *Urologic Clinics of North America* **19**, 713–723.

Lerner, S. P. *et al.* (1993). The rationale for *en bloc* pelvic lymph node dissection for bladder cancer patients with nodal metastases: long-term results. *Journal of Urology* **149**, 758–764.

Lipponen, P. *et al.* (1994). Expression of epidermal growth factor receptor in bladder cancer as related to established prognostic factors, oncoprotein (c-erbB-2, p53) expression and long-term prognosis. *British Journal of Cancer* **69**, 1120–1125.

Liu, B. C. *et al.* (1992). Biochemistry of bladder cancer invasion and metastasis. Clinical implications. *Urologic Clinics of North America* **19**, 621–627.

Llopis, J. *et al.* (2000). p53 expression predicts progression and poor survival in T1 bladder tumours. *European Urology* **37**, 644–653.

Lynch, T. H. *et al.* (1994a). Rapid diagnostic service for patients with haematuria. *British Journal of Urology* **73**, 147–151.

Lynch, T. H. *et al.* (1994b). Repeat testing for haematuria and underlying urological pathology. *British Journal of Urology* **74**, 730–732.

Lynch, W. J. *et al.* (1992). The quality of life after radical radiotherapy for bladder cancer. *British Journal of Urology* **70**, 519–521.

Malkowicz, S. B. *et al.* (1990). The role of radical cystectomy in the management of high grade superficial bladder cancer (PA, P1, PIS and P2). *Journal of Urology* **144**, 641–645.

Malmstrom, P. U. *et al.* (1996). Five year follow-up of a prospective trial of radical cystectomy and neoadjuvant chemotherapy: Nordic cystectomy trial 1. *Journal of Urology* **155**, 1903–1906.

Malmstrom, P. U. *et al.* (1999a). Neoadjuvant cisplatin-methotrexate chemotherapy of invasive bladder cancer: Nordic trial 2. *European Urology* **35** (Suppl. 2), 60 (238A).

Malmstrom, P. U. *et al.* (1999b). 5-year follow-up of a randomized prospective study comparing mitomycin C and bacillus Calmette-Guerin in patients with superficial bladder carcinoma: Swedish–Norwegian Bladder Cancer Study Group. *Journal of Urology* **161**, 1124–1127.

Maluf, F. C. and Barjorin, D. F. (2001). Chemotherapy in transitional cell carcinoma: the old and the new. *Seminars in Urologic Oncology* **19**, 2–8.

Mayfield, M. P. and Whelan, P. (1998). Bladder tumours detected on screening: results at 7 years. *British Journal of Urology* **82**, 825–828.

McDougal, W. S. (1992). Metabolic complications of urinary intestinal diversion. *Journal of Urology* **147**, 1199–1208.

Melicow, M. M. (1974). Tumors of the bladder: a multifaceted problem. *Journal of Urology* **112**, 467–478.

Mellon, J. *et al.* (1995). Long-term outcome related to epidermal growth factor receptor status in bladder cancer. *Journal of Urology* **153**, 919–925.

Mellon, J. K. *et al.* (1996). Transforming growth factor alpha and epidermal growth factor levels in bladder cancer and their relationship to epidermal growth factor receptors. *British Journal of Cancer* **73**, 654–658.

Merrell, R. W. *et al.* (1979). Bladder carcinoma treated by partial cystectomy: a review of 54 cases. *Journal of Urology* **122**, 471–472.

Merz, V. W. *et al.* (1995). Analysis of early failures after intravesical instillation therapy with bacille Calmette-Guerin for carcinoma *in situ* of the bladder. *British Journal of Urology* **75**, 180–184.

Michaud, D. S. *et al.* (1999). Fluid intake and the risk of bladder cancer in men. *New England Journal of Medicine* **340**, 1390–1397.

Mills, R. D. and Studer, U. E. (1999). Metabolic consequences of continent urinary diversion. *Journal of Urology* **161**, 1057–1066.

Mills, R. D. *et al.* (2001). Pelvic lymph node metastases from bladder cancer: outcome in 83 patients after radical cystectomy and pelvic lymphadenectomy. *Journal of Urology* **166**, 19–23.

Mohr, D. N. *et al.* (1986). Asymptomatic microhaematuria and urologic disease. A population-based study. *Journal of the American Medical Association* **256**, 224–229.

Morales, A. *et al.* (1976). Intracavity Bacillus Calmette-Guerin in the treatment of superficial bladder tumours. *Journal of Urology* **116**, 180–183.

Mostafa, M. H. *et al.* (1999). Relationship between schistosomiasis and bladder cancer. *Clinical Microbiology Reviews* **12**, 97–111.

Natale, R. B. (2000). Adjuvant and neoadjuvant chemotherapy for invasive bladder cancer. *Current Oncology Reports* **2**, 386–393.

Natale, R. B. *et al.* (2001). SWOG 8710 (Int-0800): randomised phase III trial of neoadjuvant MVAC + cystectomy versus cystectomy alone in patients with locally advanced bladder cancer. *Proceedings of the American Society of Clinical Oncology* **20**, 2a (3A).

Neal, D. E. *et al.* (1989). Epidermal growth factor receptor in human bladder cancer: a comparison of immunohistochemistry and ligand binding. *Journal of Urology* **141**, 517–521.

Nilsson, S. *et al.* (2001). A systematic overview of chemotherapy effects in urothelial bladder cancer. *Acta Oncologica* **40**, 371–390.

Novick, A. C. *et al.* (1976). Partial cystectomy in the treatment of primary and secondary carcinoma of the bladder. *Journal of Urology* **116**, 570–574.

O'Brien, T. *et al.* (1995). Different angiogenic pathways characterize superficial and invasive bladder cancer. *Cancer Research* **55**, 510–513.

Office for National Statistics (2001). Cancer trends in England and Wales. www.statistics.gov.uk.

Ooms, E. C. M. *et al.* (1983). Analysis of the performance of pathologists in the gradinf of bladder tumours. *Human Pathology* **14**, 140–143.

Oosterlinck, W. *et al.* (1993). A prospective European Organization for Research and Treatment of Cancer Genitourinary Group randomized trial comparing transurethral resection followed by a single intravesical instillation of epirubicin or water in single stage Ta, T1 papillary carcinoma of the bladder. *Journal of Urology* **149**, 749–752.

Pagano, F. *et al.* (1991). Results of contemporary radical cystectomy for invasive bladder cancer: a clinicopathological study with an emphasis on the inadequacy of the tumor, nodes and metastases classification. *Journal of Urology* **145**, 45–50.

Parmar, M. K. *et al.* (1989). Prognostic factors for recurrence and followup policies in the treatment of superficial bladder cancer: report from the British Medical Research Council Subgroup on Superficial Bladder Cancer (Urological Cancer Working Party). *Journal of Urology* **142**, 284–288.

Pawinski, A. *et al.* (1996). A combined analysis of EORTC and MRC randomized clinical trials for the prophylactic treatment of stage TAT1 bladder cancer. EORTC genitourinary tract cancer cooperative group and the MRC working party on superficial bladder cancer. *Journal of Urology* **156**, 1934–1940.

Quilty, P. M. and Duncan, W. (1986). Primary radical radiotherapy for T3 transitional cell cancer of the bladder: an analysis of survival and control. *International Journal of Radiation Oncology, Biology, Physics* **12**, 853–860.

Ravery, V. *et al.* (1995). Prognostic value of epidermal growth factor-receptor, T138 and T43 expression in bladder cancer. *British Journal of Cancer* **71**, 196–200.

Richie, J. P. (1992). Intravesical chemotherapy. Treatment selection, techniques, and results. *Urologic Clinics of North America* **19**, 521–527.

Ro, J. Y. *et al.* (1992). Cytologic and histologic features of superficial bladder cancer. *Urologic Clinics of North America* **19**, 435–453.

Roehrborn, C. C. *et al.* (1991). Long-term patient survival after cystectomy for regional metastatic transitional cell carcinoma of the bladder. *Journal of Urology* **146**, 36–39.

Roth, B. J. *et al.* (1994). Significant activity of paclitaxel in advanced transitional cell carcinoma of the urothelium: a phase II trial of the Eastern Cooperative Oncology Group. *Journal of Clinical Oncology* **12**, 2264–2270.

Sanchez-Ortiz, R. F. *et al.* (2001). A prolonged interval between the diagnosis of muscle invasion and cystectomy is associated with worse outcome in bladder carcinoma. *Journal of Urology* **165** (Suppl.), 259.

Sandberg, A. A. *et al.* (1994). Review of chromosome studies in urological tumors. II. Cytogenetics and molecular genetics of bladder cancer. *Journal of Urology* **151**, 545–560.

Sarkis, A. S. *et al.* (1993). Nuclear overexpression of p53 protein in transitional cell bladder carcinoma: a marker for disease progression. *Journal of National Cancer Institute* **85**, 53–59.

Sarkis, A. S. *et al.* (1994). Association of P53 nuclear overexpression and tumor progression in carcinoma *in situ* of the bladder. *Journal of Urology* **152**, 388–392.

Sarosdy, M. F. (1992). Principles of intravesical chemotherapy and immunotherapy. *Urologic Clinics of North America* **19**, 509–519.

Sato, K. *et al.* (1992). An immunohistologic evaluation of C-*erb*B-2 gene product in patients with urinary bladder carcinoma. *Cancer* **70**, 2493–2498.

Schapers, R. F. *et al.* (1994). A simplified grading method of transitional cell carcinoma of the urinary bladder: reproducibility, clinical significance and comparison with other prognostic parameters. *British Journal of Urology* **73**, 625–631.

Scher, H. I. (1992). Systemic chemotherapy in regionally advanced bladder cancer. Theoretical considerations and results. *Urologic Clinics of North America* **19**, 747–759.

Scher, H. I. *et al.* (1988). Neoadjuvant M-VAC (methotrexate, vinblastine, doxorubicin and cisplatin) effect on the primary bladder lesion. *Journal of Urology* **139**, 470–474.

Schlegel, P. N. *et al.* (1987). Neuroanatomical approach to radical cystoprostatectomy with preservation of sexual function. *Journal of Urology* **138**, 1402–1406.

Schmitz-Drager, B. J. *et al.* (1997). C-myc in bladder cancer. Clinical findings and analysis of mechanism. *Urological Research* **25** (Suppl. 1), S45–S49.

Schmitz-Drager, B. J. *et al.* (2000). p53 immunohistochemistry as a prognostic marker in bladder cancer. Playground for urology scientists? *European Urology* **38**, 691–699.

Schoborg, T. W. *et al.* (1979). Carcinoma of the bladder treated by segmental resection. *Journal of Urology* **122**, 473–475.

See, W. A. *et al.* (1992). Staging of advanced bladder cancer. Current concepts and pitfalls. *Urologic Clinics of North America* **19**, 663–683.

Serth, J. *et al.* (1995). p53 immunohistochemistry as an independent prognostic factor for superficial transitional cell carcinoma of the bladder. *British Journal of Cancer* **71**, 201–205.

Shariat, S. F. *et al.* (2000). Prognostic value p53 nuclear accumulation and histopathologic features in T1 transitional cell carcinoma of the urinary bladder. *Urology* **56**, 735–740.

Shelley, M. D. (2002). Surgery versus radiotherapy for transitional cell carcinoma. *Cochrane Database of Systematic Reviews* **1**, CD002079, Review.

Shelley, M. D. *et al.* (2002a). Intravesical bacillus Calmette-Guerin versus mitomycin C for Ta and T1 bladder cancer (Protocol for a Cochrane Review). *Cochrane Library* Issue 2.

Shelley, M. D. *et al.* (2002b). Intravesical bacillus Calmette-Guerin in Ta and T1 bladder cancer. *Cochrane Library* Issue 2.

Shipley, W. U. and Rose, M. A. (1985). Bladder cancer: the selection of patients for treatment by full-dose irradiation. *Cancer* **55**, 2278–2284.

Shirai, T. (1993). Etiology of bladder cancer. *Seminars in Urology* **11**, 113–126.

Sidransky, D. *et al.* (1992). Molecular genetics and biochemical mechanisms in bladder cancer. Oncogenes, tumor suppressor genes, and growth factors. *Urologic Clinics of North America* **19**, 629–639.

Simon, R. *et al.* (2000). Patterns of chromosomal imbalances in muscle invasive bladder cancer. *International Journal of Oncology* **17**, 1025–1029.

Skinner, D. G. *et al.* (1984). Contemporary cystectomy with pelvic node dissection compared to preoperative radiation therapy plus cystectomy in management of invasive bladder cancer. *Journal of Urology* **131**, 1069–1072.

Skinner, D. G. *et al.* (1991). The role of adjuvant chemotherapy following cystectomy for invasive bladder cancer: a prospective comparative trial. *Journal of Urology* **145**, 459–464.

Smith, J. A. *et al.* (1999). Bladder cancer clinical guidelines panel summary report on the management of nonmuscle invasive bladder cancer (stages Ta, T1 and Tis). *Journal of Urology* **162**, 1697–1701.

Sobin, L. H. and Wittekind, Ch. *TNM Classification of Malignant Tumours* 5th edn. New York, NY: Wiley-Liss, 1997.

Solsona, E. *et al.* (1998). Feasibility of transurethral resection for muscle infiltrating carcinoma of the bladder: long-term followup of a prospective study. *Journal of Urology* **159**, 95–98.

Splinter, T. A. *et al.* (1992a). A European Organization for Research and Treatment of Cancer—Genitourinary Group phase 2 study of chemotherapy in stage T3-4N0-XM0 transitional cell cancer of the bladder: evaluation of clinical response. *Journal of Urology* **148**, 1793–1796.

Splinter, T. A. *et al.* (1992b). The prognostic value of the pathological response to combination chemotherapy before cystectomy in patients with invasive bladder cancer. European Organization for Research on Treatment of Cancer—Genitourinary Group. *Journal of Urology* **147**, 606–608.

Spruck, C. H., III. *et al.* (1994). Two molecular pathways to transitional cell carcinoma of the bladder. *Cancer Research* **54**, 784–788.

Stein, J. P. *et al.* (2001). Radical cystectomy in the treatment of invasive bladder cancer: long-term results in 1054 patients. *Journal of Clinical Oncology* **19**, 666–675.

Steiner, M. S. *et al.* (1991). Nutritional and gastrointestinal complications of the use of bowel segments in the lower urinary tract. *Urologic Clinics of North America* **18**, 743–754.

Steiner, M. S. *et al.* (1995). Molecular insights into altered cell cycle regulation and genitourinary malignancy. *Urologic Oncology* **1**, 3–17.

Stenzl, A. *et al.* (2001). Urethra-sparing cystectomy and orthotopic urinary diversion in women with malignant pelvic tumors. *Cancer* **92**, 1864–1871.

Sternberg, C. N. (1993). Adjuvant chemotherapy following radical cystectomy. *World Journal of Urology* **11**, 169–174.

Sternberg, C. N. and Calabro, F. (2000). Chemotherapy and management of bladder tumours. *BJU International* **85**, 599–610.

Sternberg, C. N. *et al.* (1997). Interim toxicity analysis of a randomized trial in advanced urothelial tract tumors of high-dose intensity M-VAC chemotherapy (HD-MVAC) and recombinant human granulocyte colony stimulating factor (G-CSF) versus classic M-VAC chemotherapy (EORTC 30924). *Proceedings of the American Society of Clinical Oncology* **16**, 320A.

Stöckle, M. *et al.* (1992). Advanced bladder cancer (stages pT3b, pT4a, pN1 and pN2): improved survival after radical cystectomy and 3 adjuvant cycles of chemotherapy. Results of a controlled prospective study. *Journal of Urology* **148**, 302–306.

Stöckle, M. *et al.* (1995). Adjuvant polychemotherapy of non-organ confined bladder cancer after radical cystectomy revisited: long term results of a controlled prospective study and further clinical experience. *Journal of Urology* **153**, 47–52.

Strohmeyer, T. G. *et al.* (1994). Proto-oncogenes and tumor suppressor genes in human urological malignancies. *Journal of Urology* **151**, 1479–1497.

Studer, U. E. *et al.* (1994). Adjuvant cisplatin chemotherapy following cystectomy for bladder cancer: results of a prospective randomized trial. *Journal of Urology* **152**, 81–84.

Studer, U. E. *et al.* (1995). The ileal orthotopic bladder. *Urology* **45**, 185–189.

Sweeney, P. *et al.* (1992). Partial cystectomy. *Urologic Clinics of North America* **19**, 701–711.

Thogersen, V. B. *et al.* (2001). A subclass of HER1 ligands are prognostic markers for survival in bladder cancer patients. *Cancer Research* **15**, 6227–6233.

Thomas, D. J. *et al.* (1994). P53 expression, ploidy and progression in pT1 transitional cell carcinoma of the bladder. *British Journal of Urology* **73**, 533–537.

Thrasher, J. B. *et al.* (1992). Complications of intravesical chemotherapy. *Urologic Clinics of North America* **19**, 529–539.

Thrasher, J. B. *et al.* (1993). Current management of invasive and metastatic transitional cell carcinoma of the bladder. *Journal of Urology* **149**, 957–972.

Tompson, C. and Porter, T. (2002). Asymptomatic microscopic or dipstick haematuria in adults: which investigation for which patients? A review of the evidence. *BJU International* **90**, 185–198.

Turner, K. J. *et al.* (2002). The hypoxia-inducible genes VEGF and CA9 are differentially regulated in superficial vs invasive bladder cancer. *British Journal of Cancer* **86**, 1276–1282.

Turner, W. H. *et al.* (1995). Continent urinary diversion—reservoir considerations. *Current Opinion in Urology* **5**, 119–122.

Vet, J. A. *et al.* (1994a). p53 mutations have no additional prognostic value over stage in bladder cancer. *British Journal of Cancer* **70**, 496–500.

Vet, J. A. M. *et al.* (1994b). Molecular prognostic factors in bladder cancer. *World Journal of Urology* **12**, 84–88.

Vieweg, J. *et al.* (1999). Pelvic lymph node dissection can be curative in patients with node positive bladder cancer. *Journal of Urology* **161**, 449–454.

Vineis, P. *et al.* (2001). Current smoking, occupation, *N*-acetyltransferase-2 and bladder cancer: a pooled analysis of genotype-based studies. *Cancer Epidemiology, Biomarkers & Prevention* **10**, 1249–1252.

Wallace, D. M. *et al.* (1965). Delay in treating bladder tumours. *Lancet* **ii**, 332–334.

Weiner, D. P. *et al.* (1979). The prevalence and significance of Brunn's nests, cystitis cystica and squamous metaplasia in normal bladders. *Journal of Urology* **122**, 317–321.

Wesson, M. F. (1992). Radiation therapy in regionally advanced bladder cancer. *Urologic Clinics of North America* **19**, 725–734.

Wijkstrom, H. *et al.* (1998). Evaluation of clinical staging before cystectomy in transitional cell carcinoma: a long-term follow-up of 276 consecutive patients. *British Journal of Urology* **81**, 686–691.

Williams, S. G. *et al.* (2001). Molecular markers for the diagnosis, staging and prognosis of bladder cancer. *Oncology* **15**, 1461–1470.

Witjes, J. A. *et al.* (1998). Long-term follow-up of an EORTC randomized prospective trial comparing intravesical bacilli Calmette-Guerin RIVM and mitomycin C in superficial bladder cancer. *Urology* **52**, 403–410.

Witjes, J. A. *et al.* (2000). Management of superficial bladder cancer with intravesical chemotherapy: an update. *Urology* **56**, 19–21.

Wolinska, W. H. *et al.* (1977). Urethral cytology following cystectomy for bladder carcinoma. *American Journal of Surgical Pathology* **1**, 225–234.

Wu, C. S. *et al.* (1996). Prognostic value of p53 in muscle-invasive bladder cancer treatment with preoperative radiotherapy. *Urology* **47**, 305–310.

18.5 Tumours of the prostate

Philip H. Smith

Introduction

Although all urological tumours have their idiosyncrasies and offer a therapeutic challenge, carcinoma of the prostate must be one of the most difficult to understand as increasing knowledge seems to complicate rather than to simplify the central issue of curing the patient. Fifty years ago diagnosis was simple and the newly introduced concept of oestrogen therapy offered hope of success. The recognition that oral oestrogen therapy in large doses was hazardous led to the introduction of many newer treatments. None of these used alone has been shown to be superior but the combination of an antigonadotrophic agent with an antiandrogen may offer a few months increased survival.

In the early 1980s, interest in radical prostatectomy for patients with 'localized' cancer was reawakened by the introduction of the nerve-sparing procedure, which offered the hope of the preservation of sexual potency. This hope led to increasingly early diagnosis and to the development of screening programmes. The 'diagnostic epidemic' of the 1980s with a marked increase in surgical intervention has been followed by a reduction in mortality since the mid-1990s. The significance of this is still under consideration by clinicians and by epidemiologists. At the moment it seems likely that early diagnosis employing serum prostate specific antigen (PSA) estimations with subsequent radical treatment may reduce mortality in patients whose lesions are poorly differentiated, whilst only impairing quality of life for those whose lesions are well or moderately differentiated.

The underlying issue

Although clinical carcinoma of the prostate is largely a condition of elderly people, histological changes consistent with prostatic cancer are found in 30 per cent of those aged 40–50 years (Sakr *et al.* 1993) and in 50 per cent or more of those over 50 years. Fortunately, symptomatic (clinical) cancer of the prostate develops in only a small percentage of the patients with histological changes whilst the competing forces of mortality ensure that only one-fourth to one-third will die of, rather than with, their disease.

Prostate cancer is now the most common and second most fatal cancer in men in the United States and it is likely to become the most common tumour diagnosed in the western world within the next 20 years as the population ages and as reductions in the death rates from other tumours and diseases continue. To the urologist, prostate cancer is a big challenge. To the doctor concerned with public health it is only one of many conditions that threaten quality of life and life itself, since for every man who dies of prostate cancer, three die of accidents, five

Table 1 Leading causes of male deaths in the United States

Coronary artery disease	770,000
Lung cancer	149,000
Strokes	144,000
Accidents	92,000
Diabetes	48,000
Prostate cancer	35,000
Suicide	31,000

After Woolf (1994).

of strokes, and 20 of heart disease (Table 1). It is for the medical profession and for others in society to strike the balance between the urologist's natural concern and the wider perspective of those responsible for public health and for the allocation of medical resources.

Diagnosis

Prostate cancer classically presented with urinary symptoms of obstruction or bladder irritability and a prostate which felt 'craggy' and hard on rectal examination. The diagnosis was not difficult; frequently the patient also had pain from bony metastases.

Now, as a consequence of public education and concern, patients are increasingly 'screened' by the use of the PSA test which results in many tumours being diagnosed at a time when the patient is asymptomatic and the prostate feels benign (Category T1c disease). Such patients have a life expectancy of between 17 and 18 years and represent a much different population from those diagnosed 20 years ago.

Diagnosis is confirmed by transrectal ultrasonography with multiple biopsies, particularly of hypoechoic areas (Fig. 1). Prognostic factors include the tumour grade (Fig. 2), the nodal status, the presence and extent of bony metastases and the effect of therapy upon the level of PSA, especially where this is initially above normal. Examples of needle biopsies are shown in Fig. 3 and of prostatic intraepithelial neoplasia in Fig. 4. Spread of tumour is often by invasion of perineural tissue and/or of blood vessels. Examples of each are seen in Figs 5 and 6. A metastasis to bone marrow is seen in Fig. 7.

The serum PSA gives a good indication of the likelihood of involvement of tissues beyond the prostate. If the PSA is greater than 10 ng/ml local spread is likely and if greater than 20 ng/ml a bone scan may be useful to evaluate the presence and significance of any bony metastases (Fig. 8).

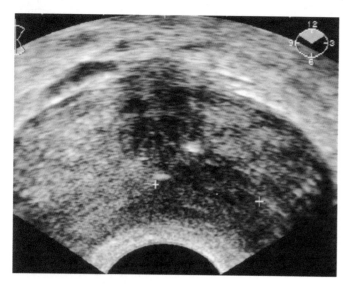

Fig. 1 Transrectal ultrasonogram showing a hypoechoic area consistent with carcinoma of the prostate.

Once the extent of the disease has been determined and categorized, the most appropriate treatment can be considered. Many patients with a PSA of less than 10 ng/ml will opt for radical treatment including radical prostatectomy or radical radiotherapy since lymph node involvement in such patients is rare and bony metastasis most unlikely.

Other patients, particularly those whose PSA is at or within the upper range of normal (4 ng/ml) may opt for deferred treatment with monitoring of the PSA in the first instance. The more advanced and symptomatic patient is likely to opt for hormonal therapy. In such patients the likely outcome can be predicted by repeated PSA tests. If the PSA declines to normal, clinical relapse is unlikely for 2 years (Cooper *et al.* 1990) (Fig. 9). If the PSA remains elevated, if the patient's urinary symptoms or any pain related to metastases do not resolve, or if new lesions occur soon after the start of treatment, progression, and early death are to be expected. During follow-up, bone scans are unlikely to be necessary in the absence of symptoms suggestive of bone involvement.

Screening for prostatic cancer

The introduction of nerve-sparing radical prostatectomy (Walsh and Mostwin 1984) reawakened the interest of the urologist in the concept of curative excision of the primary lesion with retention of sexual function and thus with less impairment of quality of life. Since that time tens of thousands of radical prostatectomies have been undertaken with curative intent.

Within the last decade, PSA testing has become established as the method for earlier diagnosis in patients with symptoms and in those attending for routine health evaluation. Given that diagnosis by PSA testing is followed by a life expectation of 15–20 years before death from prostate cancer can be expected, the wisdom of extending such testing to population screening is open to continuing debate. It is generally accepted that such benefit as will occur is most likely to be seen in men between the ages of 50 and 70 years who, if they are to be screened, must understand that diagnosis followed by radical treatment is likely

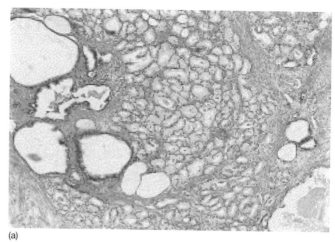

(a)

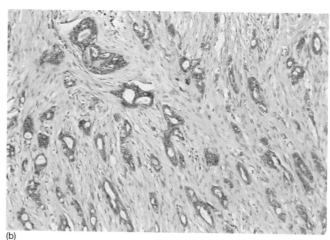

(b)

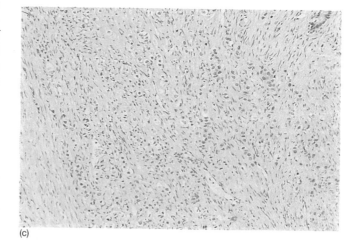

(c)

Fig. 2 (a) Invasive prostatic carcinoma Gleason Grade 1. A circumscribed nodule of rather uniformly-sized neoplastic glands. (b) Invasive prostatic carcinoma Gleason Grade 3. Neoplastic glands showing variation in size and shape and having a markedly infiltrative pattern. (c) Invasive prostatic carcinoma Gleason Grade 5. An undifferentiated sheet of malignant cells with no attempt at glandular formation characterizes this highly aggressive tumour. (Figures 2–7 kindly provided by Dr K. MacLennan, Department of Pathology, St James's University Hospital NHS Trust, Leeds, UK.)

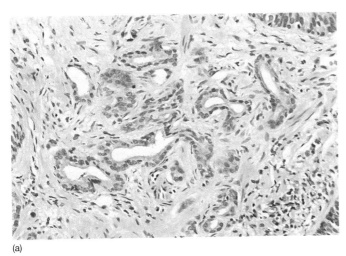

(a)

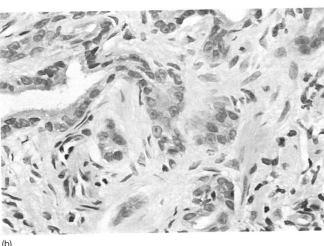

(b)

Fig. 3 (a) Needle biopsy of prostate showing the presence of an invasive carcinoma. The neoplastic glands show marked variation in size and shape and demonstrate an infiltrative pattern within the stroma. (b) At high power prominent nucleoli are seen within the neoplastic glands.

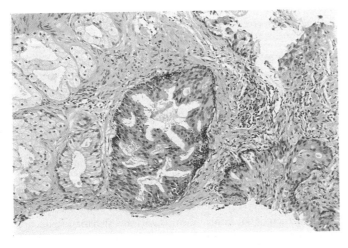

Fig. 4 High-grade prostatic intraepithelial neoplasia. Basophilic gland showing preservation of the normal prostatic architecture, lined by hypercellular micropapillary proliferations.

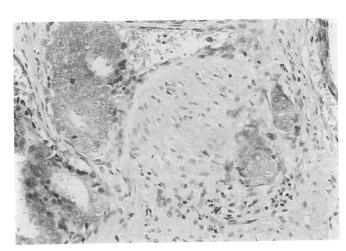

Fig. 5 Perineural spread of prostatic carcinoma. A small nerve trunk shows the presence of neoplastic glands within the perineural space.

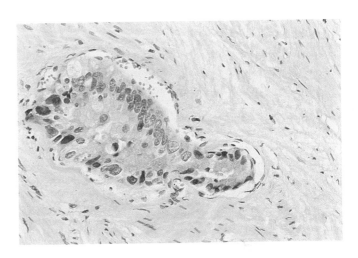

Fig. 6 Intravascular tumour embolus. A dilated vascular channel containing red cells with an embolus of prostatic carcinoma.

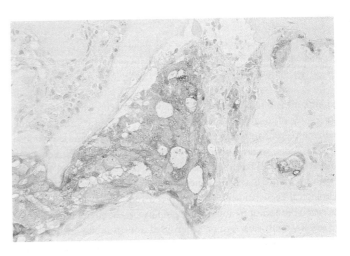

Fig. 7 Bone marrow trephine biopsy containing an area of metastatic prostatic carcinoma here stained for prostate specific antigen using the immunoalkaline phosphatase technique.

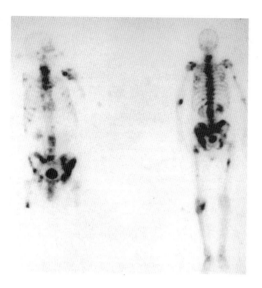

Fig. 8 Bone scan showing extensive 'hot spots' due to bony metastases from carcinoma of the prostate.

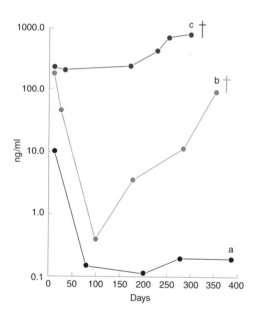

Fig. 9 The relation between PSA and clinical outcome after treatment. (a) A good response with prolonged survival. (b) and (c) If PSA does not fall to normal levels or does not fall at all prolonged survival is unlikely.

to impair their quality of life, at least to some extent, whilst offering no guarantee of long-term cure. With age the forces of competing mortality also come into play and those considering screening should also consider that, whilst 50 per cent of men over the age of 50 years may have histological changes of this condition, only 3 per cent will die of it.

In the United States, the American Cancer Society and the American Urological Association now recommend routine screening for males between the ages of 50 and 70 years. In Europe, the advice is conflicting; in some countries screening is favoured and in others including the United Kingdom it is not currently recommended. The continuing debate has led to the development of the European Randomized Study for Screening of Prostate Cancer (ERSPC) led by Professor Schroder in Rotterdam.

In the ERSPC trial more than 180,000 men aged 55–69 have been randomized since 1994 to screening or control arms in this study which recruits from centres in Belgium, Finland, Italy, The Netherlands, Spain, and Sweden. Men in the control group are offered screening by PSA followed by biopsy if this is abnormal. Treatment of any cancers found is determined by the patient and his or her urologist in consultation. Whilst the majority opt for radical prostatectomy or radical radiotherapy some prefer watchful waiting in the first instance—effectively deferred therapy consequent upon a further rise in the PSA. The first clinical evaluation of this study will take place in 2004. The development and implementation of this study has involved cooperation between urologists, doctors in public health, and epidemiologists and has emphasized to the urologists involved the complexity and expense of any population screening study. The issue is particularly difficult in patients with prostate cancer where it is recognized that the benefit of any form of radical treatment is reflected in improved survival only at more than 10 years after treatment.

Radical treatment of prostatic cancer

Background

It is sensible to consider radical surgical treatment for those lesions believed to be confined within the prostatic capsule. The clinical classification of adenocarcinomas of the prostate is shown in Table 2. Though lymph node involvement and bone metastases can be assessed before surgery, the presence of extracapsular extension or involvement of the seminal vesicles, also factors of adverse prognostic significance, can only be definitively determined by the pathologist. It is therefore not possible to restrict surgical excision only to those patients for whom all the known prognostic factors are favourable. The radiation oncologist must also treat patients whose disease has extended beyond the prostatic capsule. However, unlike the surgeon, the radiation oncologist will never be able to separate patients into those with and those without extracapsular invasion or involvement of the seminal vesicles—a point that should be borne in mind when considering the reported outcomes of surgery and radiotherapy. In addition it should be recognized that the complications of these two forms of treatment are different in that more patients receiving radical prostatectomy are likely to be incontinent or impotent whilst complications relating to bowel function are more frequent in men receiving radiotherapy (Potosky *et al.* 2000).

Radiotherapy

1. *External-beam irradiation* offers the prospect of control of the primary tumour without the risks and side-effects of surgical intervention. The dose that can be administered is limited by the need to avoid damage to the adjacent normal tissue. The experience of Bagshaw *et al.* (1990) and of Hanks (1988) and Perez *et al.* (1988) suggested that useful local control could be obtained. Bagshaw *et al.* (1990) reported upon 1031 patients irradiated before the end of 1988, and noted that the survival for those with incidental (impalpable) carcinoma was identical to that of the age-matched population of Californian men. There was a systematic reduction in survival with increase in stage. For those patients with category T1a–T2a ('coincidentally diagnosed tumour' extending to those with 'tumour apparently confined to one lobe with distortion of the capsule'), survival was approximately 90 per cent at 5 years,

80 per cent at 10 years, and 70 per cent at 15 years. The investigators remark that the survival figures are very similar to those of certain surgical series reported elsewhere.

2. *Brachytherapy* involves the placement of radioactive seeds of palladium-103 or iodine-125 (with a half-life of 17 and 60 days respectively) directly into the prostate using ultrasound guided needles via a preplanned perineal template. The technique has become increasingly popular within the last decade and is recommended with or without external beam boosting for patients with a life expectation of 10 years or more, clinically gland-confined disease, the ability to tolerate spinal or general anaesthesia and a prostate lesser than 40 cm³ in size. Occasionally, neoadjuvant antiandrogen or antigonadotrophin therapy is employed to 'downsize' larger glands prior to implantation. This technique allows the delivery of 115–145 Gy directly to the prostate. Disease free survival rates at 10 years of 60 per cent following brachytherapy alone and 76 per cent following external beam radiotherapy boosting have been reported (Doggett 2000).

3. *Three-dimensional conformal and intensity modulated radiation therapy*. These techniques have been increasingly investigated since 1988. Three-dimensional (3D) conformal radiotherapy, using multileaf collimators to 'conform' the high dose target volume to the shape of the gland is now widely available. Intensity modulated radiotherapy (IMRT) is in its infancy but holds much promise in its ability to irradiate the tumour-bearing tissues to higher dose with increased sparing of the surrounding normal tissues. Advanced imaging allows for tumour and normal organ segmentation and increased dosages can be administered with no increase in toxicity. Zelefsky *et al.* (2001) have recently reported the results on 1100 such patients with clinical stage T1c–T3 prostate cancer treated between October 1988 and December 1998 using this technique. Cohorts of patients were treated with escalating doses of 64.8, 70.2, 75.6, 81, and eventually 86.4 Gy. A 3-month course of neoadjuvant complete androgen deprivation was given to 427 patients with large volume prostates to decrease prostate size prior to therapy. No other therapy was given following radiation. At a median follow-up of 60 months overall (24–142) and a median follow-up of 69 months for those receiving the high dosage (75.6 Gy or more) it has been established that the 5-year actuarial PSA relapse-free survival and the incidence of toxicity were dose related. The 5-year PSA relapse-free survival rates and positive biopsy rates 2.5 years or greater after treatment are shown in Table 3.

Following external beam irradiation the main hazard is to the bowel, the urethra, and the base of the bladder. After a conventional course of radiotherapy the majority of men have a degree of bowel dysfunction and some 10 per cent of patients have troublesome radiation proctitis requiring medical intervention. Telangiectases in the base of the bladder as a result of the radiation give rise to a tendency to haematuria or to such fibrosis in the region of the prostatic urethra that difficulties in micturition arise. In addition, the radiation therapy does not always 'sterilize' the prostate and positive biopsy rates of 68 per cent at two or more years subsequent to treatment have been reported by Freiha (1989), suggesting that total control of the disease has not been achieved. Nonetheless, survival is good despite the fact that radiation therapists are always working at a disadvantage since, unlike surgeons, they can hardly decline to offer their form of therapy and, as Colvert *et al.* (1995) have observed, 'If radiation oncologists had the luxury of excluding poor prognostic factors such as high

Table 2 TMN clinical classification of adenocarcinomas of the prostate (adapted by Sobin and Wittekind 1997)

T—Primary tumour
TX Primary tumour cannot be found
T0 No evidence of primary tumour
T1 Clinically inapparent tumour not palpable or visible by imaging
    T1a Tumour incidental histological finding in 5% or less of tissue esected
    T1b Tumour incidental histological finding in more than 5% of tissue resected
    T1c Tumour identified by needle biopsy (e.g. because of elevated PSA)
T2 Tumour confined within the prostate[a]
    T2a Tumour involves one lobe
    T2b Tumour involves both lobes
T3 Tumour extends through the prostatic capsule[b]
    T3a Extracapsular extension (unilateral or bilateral)
    T3b Tumour invades seminal vesicle(s)
T4 Tumour is fixed or invades adjacent structures other than seminal vesicles: bladder neck, external sphincter, rectum, levator muscles, and/or pelvic wall

N—Regional lymph nodes
NX Regional lymph nodes cannot be assessed
N0 No regional lymph node metastasis
N1 Regional lymph node metastasis

M—Distant metastasis
MX Distant metastasis cannot be assessed
M0 No distant metastasis
M1 Distant metastasis
    M1a Non-regional lymph node(s)
    M1b Bone(s)
    M1c Other site(s)

[a] Tumour found in one or both lobes by needle biopsy, but not palpable or visible by imaging, is classified as T1c.

[b] Invasion into the prostatic apex or into (but not beyond) the prostatic capsule is not classified as T3, but as T2.

Notes:
1. When more than one site of metastasis is present, the most advanced category should be used.
2. T categories—physical examination, imaging, endoscopy, biopsy, and biochemcial tests; N categories—physical examination and imaging; M categories—physical examination, imaging, skeletal studies, and biochemical tests.
3. The regional lymph nodes are the nodes of the true pelvis, which essentially are the pelvic nodes below the bifurcation of the common iliac arteries. Laterality does not affect the N classification.

Table 3 5-year PSA relapse free rates following intensity modulated conformal radiotherapy in 100 patients with T1c–T3 prostate cancer (Zelefsky *et al.* 2001)

Risk group[a]	Overall	Dose (Gy)		Significance
		64.8–70.2	75.6–86.4	
Favourable	85% (±4)	77 (±8)	90 (±7)	$p = 0.05$
Intermediate	58% (±6)	50 (±8)	70 (±6)	$p = 0.001$
Unfavourable	38% (±6)	21 (±8)	47 (±6)	$p = 0.002$

[a] Based on PSA, Gleason score and clinical stage.

Figures in bracket represent the 95% confidence intervals.

grade, advanced stage, and high initial PSA a dramatic improvement in results would be demonstrated'.

Following brachytherapy Han *et al.* (2001) report that approximately one-third of patients develop urinary retention and require catheterization for a short time, whilst 5 per cent develop radiation proctitis.

The use of intensity modulated radiation has been associated with less toxicity than the same dose of 3D conformal radiation therapy. IMRT did not affect the incidence of urinary toxicity.

Radical prostatectomy

Olsson and Goluboff (1994) have shown that in the United States medicare programme alone the number of radical operations increased from 7028 in 1987 to 39,157 in 1992. Over 100,000 such operations are now being done annually in the United States. Though described as a radical operation, it is probably better thought of as a total prostatectomy with nerve-sparing, where practical, since wide excision of the primary is impossible given its position in relation to adjacent organs and the urologist's recognition that capsular penetration is common.

Earlier diagnosis leads to an increasing use of radical surgery (or radical radiotherapy) in patients who will in any case survive 10 years or more. Though radical prostatectomy does decrease the tumour load, is likely to improve the survival of patients with poorly differentiated tumours localized to the prostate and may have some impact on disease specific survival 15 or more years after diagnosis not all patients will be cured. All that can be stated at the moment is that evidence of biochemical recurrence following radical prostatectomy (a rise in PSA to 0.4 ng/ml or above) is seen in 25–30 per cent of patients within 10 years. What will happen to these patients in the next 10 years remains to be seen. All have had a major operation and all have some impairment of their quality of life from the time of the operative procedure, particularly with respect to urinary continence and sexual function. In addition, a small number will develop difficulty with micturition due to stenosis at the anastomosis between the urethra and bladder. On the other hand, if the primary tumour remains *in situ* 5 per cent of patients have trouble from it at some later stage leading to the need for further transurethral resection or to problems from infiltration of the perineum or adjacent organs. Some surgeons have therefore advised total prostatectomy for patients whose tumours are known to have breached the capsule and even for those with limited evidence of node-positive disease. It has been suggested that such patients could subsequently receive hormone therapy to minimize complications and perhaps prolong life. Others have suggested that a preoperative course of hormonal therapy may shrink the prostate to an extent that surgical excision will be both simpler and more effective. The outcome of such therapy remains to be determined.

Outcome of radical treatment

An optimistic finding has been the recent recognition that the mortality rate from carcinoma of the prostate in the United States and in certain European countries has been falling during the last decade (Smart 1997; Boyle *et al.* 2001). A reduction in overall mortality following PSA detection with subsequent radical treatment would not be expected at such an early stage even if the treatment is curative. It remains to be seen whether other factors are contributing to this phenomenon; also whether the reduction will be maintained.

Watchful waiting

Since the majority of prostatic cancers are of no clinical significance it has been suggested that it might be proper to follow-up patients with apparently localized prostatic cancer without therapy in the first instance. This approach is controversial, but in no way impairs the patient's quality of life during the period in which surveillance allows one to judge by repeated digital rectal examination, PSA, and transurethral ultrasonography, whether progression is likely and thus whether the disease is significant. The arguments against such an approach depend upon the success of intervention. Those in favour rely upon the preponderance of latent tumours.

The 'watchful waiting' concept was originally suggested by the Veterans Administration Cooperative Urological Research Group (1967). More recently, interest has centred on the studies of Johansson and Adolfsson (Adolfsson *et al.* 1994; Johansson 1994). In these series of 172 patients (with T1–T3 NXM0 disease) and 223 patients (with T0–T2 NXM0 disease), respectively, there is long-term follow-up. More than half the patients in each group have now died, but the cause-specific death rates were low in that 20 per cent of the patients died of prostate cancer after 10 years in the study of Adolfsson and after 15 years in that of Johansson. In these series, patients were given treatment when progression occurred (as is the case when there is progression despite radiotherapy or total prostatectomy).

These survival figures are not dissimilar to those for radiotherapy or total prostatectomy (Bagshaw *et al.* 1994; Zincke *et al.* 1994) although it must be admitted that most of Johansson's patients had well differentiated disease. Bagshaw *et al.* (1994) quoted the outcome for 377 patients with category T1 or T2a with negative lymph nodes and Zincke *et al.* (1994) the outcomes for patients with category T2c or less, noting that 'clinical stage did not significantly affect survival but tumour grade was associated'. These patients were not diagnosed as a result of PSA screening and it may be that the earlier diagnosis which is now possible will lead to real improvement in overall survival with a reduction in disease-specific mortality.

The concept of watchful waiting has been investigated in two randomized collaborative trials—one in the United Kingdom under the auspices of the Medical Research Council (MRC) (Coordinator Professor Kirk of Glasgow) and another in Europe organized by the urological group of the European Organization for Research on the Treatment of Cancer (EORTC) (Coordinator Professor Studer of Bern). In the MRC study, 938 patients with non-metastatic disease or those with metastases, but without symptoms were randomized to immediate or delayed treatment with orchidectomy or luteinizing hormone-releasing hormone (LHRH) therapy. In the EORTC Study, 1002 patients without metastases who were unsuitable for, or who refused, radical prostatectomy were randomized to immediate or deferred antigonadotrophic therapy (Fig. 10). Both studies are now closed to recruitment, but neither has had its final analysis.

Treatment of disseminated disease

In the hope that the reader is now increasingly uncertain we can turn to the management of the patient whose disease has extended beyond the prostate. Here the current situation is also confusing and the outlook even less satisfactory, since there has been little real progress in 50 years. At that time the recognition that orchidectomy or the use of

MRC trial (coordinator—D. Kirk, Glasgow, UK)

Entry criteria
- Carcinoma of prostate previously untreated
- No metastases or metastases without symptoms

Randomization
- Immediate or deferred orchidectomy or LHRH therapy
  In the deferred case the definition of progression and thus the
  decision to treat is left to the patient and his urologist

Recruitment
- 938 patients

EORTC trial (protocol 30891; coordinator—U. Studer, Bern, Switzerland)

Entry criteria
- Asymptomatic T0–4 M0 prostatic cancer

Randomization
- Immediate or delayed orchidectomy or depot LHRH with 2-week
  cyproterone acetate

Recruitment
- 1002 patients

The aim of these trials is to determine the total period of
symptom-free survival

Fig. 10 Randomized trials of early and deferred therapy for prostatic cancer.

Table 4 Results of some phase III randomized clinical trials in patients with advanced prostatic cancer

Patients	Treatment	Outcome (survival)
Monotherapy		
Protocol 30761	CPA 250 mg daily	NS
T2–4 M0, TX M1	MPA	
	DES 1 mg t.d.s.	
Protocol 30762	EST	NS
T2–4 M0, TX M1	DES 1 mg t.d.s.	
Androgen ablation		
Protocol 30805	Orchidectomy	NS
TX, NX, M1	DES 1 mg daily	
	Orchidectomy +	
	CPA 50 mg t.d.s.	
Protocol 30843	Orchidectomy	NS
TX, NX, M1	Buserelin (+CPA for	
	2 weeks only)	
	Buserelin + CPA 50 mg	
	t.d.s. continuously	
Protocol 30853	Orchidectomy	7-month survival
TX, NX, M1	Zoladex 3.6 mg every	advantage for
	28 days + flutamide	goserelin +
	250 mg t.d.s.	flutamide

t.d.s., three times a day; CPA, cyproterone acetate; DES, stilboestrol; EST, estramustine phosphate; MPA, medroxyprogesterone acetate; NS, no significant difference.

After Smith et al. (1986).

oestrogen could relieve symptoms in patients with advanced disease (Huggins and Hodges 1941) offered great hope and transformed the lives of many. When hormone therapy failed, the dose was increased, and in 1970 Ferguson was recommending stilboestrol, 100 mg daily, for routine management (Ferguson 1970).

In 1967, the Veterans Administration Cooperative Urological Research Group reported upon the cardiovascular side-effects of stilboestrol, 5 mg daily, and from that time there has been an active search for alternative treatments (Veterans Administration Cooperative Urological Research Group 1967). The antiandrogens (both steroidal and non-steroidal) and the LHRH analogues (LHRH agonists) have become available and have been used alone and in combination. In addition, the combination of an oestrogen with a derivative of nitrogen mustard (estramustine) has also been suggested as of value, whilst in the United States other cytotoxic agents were also considered and evaluated by the National Prostatic Cancer Project. The antiandrogens and the LHRH analogues have been tested as monotherapy against the more conventional agents in trials containing several hundred rather than several thousand patients. None has been shown to be superior to stilboestrol (Table 4). Recently, an LHRH *antagonist* has become available. This agent avoids the 'flare' phenomenon of the agonists and deserves further study (Pessis *et al.* 2001).

Labrie *et al.* (1984) reported remarkable results from the combination of an LHRH analogue with an antiandrogen. This form of treatment, now known as total or maximal-androgen blockade has been increasingly regarded as the best, despite the fact that nobody has been able to repeat Labrie's original results. Crawford *et al.* (1989) did demonstrate a 25 per cent increase in survival when the combination therapy was compared with LHRH treatment alone; the benefit was most marked for those with minimal disease (metastases confined to the axial skeleton) and was absent in those with extensive disease and poor performance status. Similar results were found in an EORTC

study (protocol 30853—Coordinator Professor Denis of Antwerp) in which the combined therapy was compared with orchidectomy (Denis *et al.* 1993). However, in this study only 19 per cent of the patients who progressed after orchidectomy were offered an antiandrogen, which even at that time would have been considered as one of the treatments of preference for those in relapse.

The popularity of the combination therapy was in part because the drugs were new, in part to facilitation by the pharmaceutical companies (who have a natural interest in promoting the sales of their newer and expensive compounds), and in part to the feeling that, although the survival advantage was minimal, everything that could be done had been done. This feeling will be of particular importance where medicolegal aspects loom large. From the clinical point of view the advantage is minimal, since it is of the order of a few months; the patient is also exposed to the side-effects of two forms of therapy rather than one. Further, the treatment does not provide a cure. The cost of the modern combined therapy is up to 10 times that of stilboestrol, 1 mg daily (Table 5), and the community must decide whether it is best served by such additional expenditure.

The argument is always that oestrogens have such cardiovascular toxicity that it is no longer ethical to use them. In fact, this toxicity is variable, ranging from 2.7 to 16 per cent in simultaneous studies (Pavone *et al.* 1986; Smith *et al.* 1986). Although Robinson (1993) observed more cardiovascular deaths after stilboestrol when compared with orchidectomy or total androgen blockade, the overall survival of the patients was no worse—they merely died of cardiovascular problems rather than from prostate cancer.

Not everyone feels strongly opposed to oestrogen therapy and the Swedish Prostatic Cancer Cooperative Group recently reported a study

Table 5 Cost of 28 days' hormonal treatment for patients with prostate cancer

	Price (£. p)
Stilboestrol 1 mg daily + aspirin 75 mg	24.00
Cyproterone acetate 100 mg t.d.s.	96.70
Cyproterone acetate 50 mg t.d.s.	48.30
Flutamide 250 mg t.d.s.	77.07
Goserelin injection 3.6 mg	122.27
Goserelin injection 10.8 mg[a]	366.81
Goserelin + cyproterone 50 mg t.d.s.	170.57
Goserelin + flutamide 250 mg t.d.s.	199.34
Biclutamide 150 mg	240.00

[a] This injection lasts 3 months.

of 197 patients with high grade and high stage prostate cancer randomized to estramustine phosphate or diethyl stilboestrol (Hedlund *et al.* 1996). They found that stilboestrol 'had relatively good effect in this very aggressive form of prostate cancer'.

The continuing confusion led to a meta-analysis of relevant studies of monotherapy versus total androgen blockade (Prostate Cancer Triallists Collaborative Group 2000). This demonstrated that combination therapy whether including or excluding cyproterone acetate was likely to lead to a benefit of only 2–3 months in terms of survival from combined therapy. Knowing that the case against oestrogen is flimsy, that the advantage of total androgen blockade is limited and that there is as yet no information on whether monotherapy followed by the addition of the other component of androgen blockade on progression (sequential therapy) is worse than the use of combination therapy at the outset, one may also wonder whether intermittent treatment may also be practical in the patient who shows an initial response to treatment.

Intermittent therapy

There are now at least three separate trials of intermittent therapy in which treatment is stopped in patients who respond clinically and by PSA reduction to initial therapy to be restarted following a significant subsequent rise in PSA. Of these one is in the United States (ECOG), one in the EORTC, and one in Southern Europe. The South European study (Fig. 11) has randomized 626 patients to continuous or intermittent therapy and is now closed to recruitment.

This concept is of considerable clinical, scientific, and economic importance and results are awaited with interest.

Relapse after hormonal therapy

After initially successful treatment, relapse is almost inevitable if the patient lives long enough. Evidence of progression reflected in an increase in serum PSA will be apparent at least 6–9 months before the patient develops changes on a bone scan or symptoms from bony metastases or other problems. Change of treatment may involve the

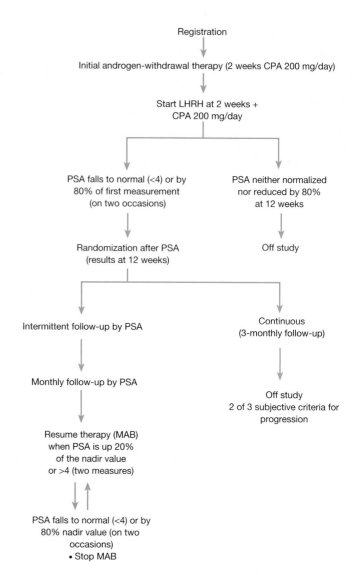

Fig. 11 Randomized trial of intermittent versus continuous total androgen blockade (coordinator Professor Calais da Silva, Portugal). CPA, cyproterone acetate; LHRH, luteinizing-hormone releasing hormone; MAB, nitrogen mustard, adriamycin, bleomycin; PSA, prostate-specific antigen.

addition of an antiandrogen or antigonadotrophic agent if monotherapy has been given, or consideration of the use of steroids, suramin, or cytotoxic agents if total androgen blockade has been employed.

The situation has been made more complex following the recognition of the flutamide withdrawal syndrome (Dupont *et al.* 1993; Kelly and Scher 1993; Sartor *et al.* 1994) and by the suggestion from the UK Medicines Control Agency that cyproterone acetate should be restricted to short courses to cover testosterone flare associated with LHRH agonists, for the treatment of hot flushes after orchidectomy or LHRH agonists, or for patients who have not responded to, or who are intolerant of, other treatments.

Some clinicians prefer to change treatment at the first (biochemical) sign of relapse; others do so only when the patient develops symptoms. Whatever the approach adopted, it is rare for a patient to live for more than a year once symptomatic progression has been seen, since all secondary forms of therapy are also palliative.

Secondary hormonal treatment

In managing the individual patient in whom there are signs of progression the first step is to assy the plasma testosterone as a measure of compliance, since not all patients take their tablets regularly and not every patient responds in the same way to a given form of treatment.

Where there is progression despite the fact that the plasma testosterone is in the castrate range, the alternative forms of treatment include castration or LHRH analogue therapy for the patient who has been managed initially with an antiandrogen, the addition of an antiandrogen in those treated in the first instance with an antigonadotrophic agent, and cessation of flutamide therapy in those treated by total androgen blockade including this agent. Treatment with prednisone may also offer palliation.

Cytotoxic chemotherapy

Though cytotoxic chemotherapy is effective in many tumours are is little evidence of its activity in patients with prostatic cancer. The National Prostatic Cancer Project published results of trials of hormone and chemotherapy, but as the figures included stable disease the claims were over-optimistic. Low-dose adriamycin (10 mg/m^2 weekly), epirubicin and mitomycin C (15 mg/m^2 6-weekly) have brought symptomatic relief with some objective response and minimal toxicity (Jones *et al.* 1986; Delaere *et al.* 1992). More recently a combination of mitoxantrone and prednisone has been shown to be more effective in reducing symptoms and improving quality of life than prednisone alone (Tannock *et al.* 1996; Osoba *et al.* 1999; Dowling *et al.* 2000). This combination has now been approved by the Food and Drug Administration for palliation of advanced prostate cancer.

Prevention

Any condition that is common is better prevented than cured. This is especially the case when treatment is expensive and the outcome is uncertain—as it is in patients with prostate cancer.

Some of the factors known to be associated with the development of prostate cancer include ageing, race, a family history—and the production of androgens. The first three factors are out of the individual's control and few men would be willing to accept a significant reduction of their androgen production in the hope of preventing prostate cancer perhaps 10–20 years in the future.

However, other factors of importance may include the level of 5-alpha reductase activity, a diet high in animal fats, sexual behaviour, and environmental factors. Inhibition of 5-alpha reductase reduces the amount of free testosterone available to the prostate cells. Finasteride inhibits 5-alpha reductase and a randomized trial in the United States is currently comparing the effect of prophylactic finasteride or placebo in 18,000 middle-aged males.

The importance of dietary factors can be seen from the lower incidence of prostate cancer in China, Japan, and the Mediterranean countries where the intake of cereals, fresh fruit, and raw vegetables is higher than in Northern Europe or the United States where the preference, at least in the past, has been for red meat and animal fat. It has yet to be determined whether sexual activity or sexual infection are key factors in the development of prostate cancer. However, given that it is known that prostate cancer does not occur in eunuchs and has a lower incidence in those who are celibate, it may be that the condom will come to be seen as protecting not only against infection, but also against prostate cancer. Environmental factors may include exposure to cadmium, employment in the nuclear power industry and farming.

Clearly much work still needs to be done. In the meantime a diet low in red meat and animal fats, high in cereals, fresh fruit, and vegetables may be of great benefit to the younger man, especially if combined with a cautious approach to sexual relationships (Denis 1996; Kirkby *et al.* 1996; Boyle 1997; Matlaga *et al.* 2001; Tymchuk *et al.* 2001).

Treatment of specific problems

No single agent has yet become established as 'best treatment' for the management of the patient in relapse and emphasis tends to be placed upon the problems that the patient has, including obstructive symptoms, bone pain, anaemia, and uraemia.

Obstruction

It is always possible to carry out a further transurethral resection because of regrowth of the primary tumour, but it is less easy to guarantee that the patient will not become incontinent since the tumour commonly extends to involve the external sphincter. In these circumstances, relief of obstruction also damages the sphincter and impairs continence.

Bone pain

The management of bone pain is complex. Areas that are localized can be dealt with by single-fraction irradiation (using 8 Gy) or by hemibody irradiation (Zelefsky *et al.* 1989). More recently it has been suggested that strontium-89 may be more effective (Porter *et al.* 1993) and clinical trials are now also being undertaken of the possible value of sodium clodronate in reducing the morbidity from skeletal complications and in controlling pain from bony metastases in a study coordinated by the MRC in London.

Where bony metastases are likely to lead to pathological fractures orthopaedic intervention is desirable and in those vertebral lesions giving rise to spinal cord compression, dexamethasone is indicated immediately with early surgical decompression (or palliative radiotherapy in those unfit for surgery). In a patient in whom such a problem is not associated with extensive metastases elsewhere, survival may be prolonged.

Anaemia

A patient developing anaemia usually has extensive bone marrow infiltration but can be maintained for several months by repeated transfusions.

Uraemia

In the patient developing fatigue and lassitude because of an increase in creatinine associated with ureteric obstruction, treatment may be helpful at the time of first diagnosis but is rarely of benefit if the patient has already been treated effectively with hormones. It is sometimes possible to stent such ureters and always possible to undertake a percutaneous nephrostomy. The improvement is usually transient as the disease progresses. Most urologists do not recommend intervention in the patient who has relapsed. In this group of patients the prime consideration is the relief of symptoms, since life cannot be prolonged for more than a few months. It is the quality of this period of survival that is of prime importance.

Analgesics

Once the patient is needing analgesics more or less continuously, it is important that he be seen by a physician with a particular interest in the management of patients with terminal cancer in order that the best techniques for pain control can be offered. In the United Kingdom, patients are usually referred to a hospice at this stage as here they can find the expertise they need.

Despite all the modern advances, many patients with prostatic cancer do progress and all urologists, in conjunction with their colleagues in radiation oncology and in palliative care, have experience of managing the difficult problems that arise.

Conclusion

This chapter has been written in a way that attempts to draw the attention of the reader to the limitations facing the surgeon and physician in helping patients to come to terms with their disease process, which it seems cannot yet be cured. The changes in clinical approach have so far brought minor rather than major benefit to the individual patient over the last 25 years. The central issue concerns radical prostatectomy and whether it is capable of curing those with localized disease. If it can do so, and if the patient with latent cancer can be separated from those whose cancer will progress, great strides will be made. For the patient with more advanced disease, it is clear that one form of hormonal therapy is not dramatically superior to another, that all hormonal treatment alone or in combination is palliative and that intermittent therapy may be appropriate. Cytotoxic chemotherapy has not yet found an established place in this condition.

When clinical symptoms develop, the illness is often prolonged and very distressing to patient, family, and those who provide medical and nursing help. Perhaps the main advances have been made by the radiation oncologist and the physician interested in palliative care, both of whom can now provide much more effective care for patients whose disease is progressing despite all treatment. New forms of therapy are urgently required.

References

Adolfsson, J. *et al.* (1994). Deferred treatment of clinically localised low grade prostate cancer: the experience from a prospective series at the Karolinska Hospital. *Journal of Urology* 152, 1757–1760.

Bagshaw, M. A. *et al.* (1990). Radiation therapy for localised prostate cancer. Justification by long term follow up. *Urologic Clinics of North America* 17, 787–802.

Bagshaw, M. A., Cox, R. S., and Hancock, S. C. (1994). Control of prostate cancer with radiotherapy: long term results. *Journal of Urology* 152, 1781–1785.

Boyle, P. Epidemiology and natural history of prostate cancer. In *Proceedings of the First International Consultation on Prostate Cancer* (ed. G. Murphy, L. Denis, K. Griffith, S. Khoury, C. Chatelain, and A. T. Cockett), pp. 1–29. Paris: SCI, 1997.

Boyle, P. *et al.* (2001). Trends in prostate cancer mortality worldwide: results of a systematic analysis. *Journal of Urology* 165 (5), 61.

Colvert, K. T. *et al.* Radiation therapy for patients with T1 and T2a(b1) prostate cancer: selection yields high success rates maintained more than 10 years after treatment. In *Proceedings of 4th International Symposium on Recent Advances of Urological Cancer Diagnosis and Treatment* (ed. G. Murphy, S. Khoury, C. Chatelain, and L. Denis), pp. 214–220. Paris: SCI, 1995.

Cooper, E. H. *et al.* (1990). Prostate specific antigen and the prediction of prognosis in metastatic prostatic cancer. *Cancer* 66 (Suppl.), 1025–1028.

Crawford, E. D. *et al.* (1989). A controlled trial of leuprolide with and without flutamide in prostatic carcinoma. *New England Journal of Medicine* 321, 429–434.

Delaere, K. P. J. *et al.* (1992). Phase II study of epirubicin in advanced hormone resistant prostatic cancer. *British Journal of Urology* 70, 641–642.

Denis, L. J. (1996). Health care resources should be targeted to chemoprevention in prostate cancer: the argument for. *European Urology* 29 (Suppl. 2), 13–16.

Denis, L. J. *et al.* (1993). Goserelin acetate and flutamide versus bilateral orchidectomy: a phase III EORTC trial (30853). *Urology* 42, 119–129.

Doggett, S. W. What is the role of interstitial brachytherapy? In *Prostate Cancer* (ed. W. Bowsher), pp. 178–191, 2000.

Dowling, *et al.* (2000). Prostate specific antigen response to mitoxantrone and prednisone in patients with refractory prostate cancer: prognostic factors and generalisability of a multi-center trial. The clinical practice. *Journal of Urology* 163, 1481–1485.

Dupont, A. *et al.* (1993). Response to flutamide withdrawal in advanced cancer in progression under combination therapy. *Journal of Urology* 150, 908–913.

Ferguson, J. D. (1970). Cancer of the prostate II. *British Medical Journal* 4, 539–540.

Freiha, F. A. Carcinoma of the prostate—non-metastatic disease. In *Combination Therapy in Urological Malignancy* (ed. P. H. Smith), pp. 119–141. London: Springer-Verlag, 1989.

Han, B. H. *et al.* (2001). Patient reported complications after prostate brachytherapy. *Journal of Urology* 166, 953–957.

Handley, M. R. and Stuart, M. E. (1994). The use of prostate specific antigen for prostate cancer screening: a managed care perspective. *Journal of Urology* 152, 1689–1692.

Hanks, G. E. (1988). External beam radiotherapy for clinically localised prostate cancer: patterns of care studies in the United States. *Monographs of the National Cancer Institute* 7, 75–84.

Hedlund, P. O. *et al.* (1996). Treatment of high grade, high stage prostate cancer with estramustine phosphate or diethylstilboestrol. *Scandinavian Journal of Urology and Nephrology* 31, 168–172.

Huggins, C. and Hodges, C. V. (1941). Studies on prostate cancer. 1. The effect of castration, of estrogens and of androgen injection on serum phosphatase in metastatic carcinoma of the prostate. *Cancer Research* 1, 293–297.

Johansson, J. E. (1994). Expectant management of early stage prostatic cancer: Swedish experience. *Journal of Urology* 152, 1753–1756.

Jones, W. G. *et al.* (1986). Mitomycin C in the treatment of metastatic prostate cancer: report on an EORTC phase II study. *World Journal of Urology* 4, 182–185.

Kelly, W. K. and Scher, H. I. (1993). Prostatic specific antigen decline after antiandrogen withdrawal: the flutamide withdrawal syndrome. *Journal of Urology* 149, 607–609.

Kirby, R. S., Brawer, M. K., and Denis, L. J. *Prostate Cancer* pp. 7–12. Oxford: Health Press Ltd., 1996.

Labrie, F. *et al.* (1984). Combined treatment with LHRH agonist and pure antiandrogen in advanced carcinoma of the prostate. *Lancet* ii, 1090.

Matlaga, B., Hall, M. C., Stindt, D., and Torti, F. M. (2001). Response of hormone refractory prostate cancer to lycopene. *Journal of Urology* 166, 613.

Medical Research Council Prostate Cancer Working Party Investigators Group (1997). Immediate versus deferred treatment for advanced prostatic cancer: initial results of the Medical Research trial. *British Journal of Urology* 79, 235–246.

Olsson, C. A. and Goluboff, E. T. (1994). Detection and treatment of prostate cancer: perspective of the urologist. *Journal of Urology* **152**, 1695–1699.

Osoba, D. *et al.* (1999). Health-related quality of life in men with metastatic prostate cancer treated with prednisone alone or mitoxantrone and prednisone. *Journal of Clinical Oncology* **17**, 1651–1653.

Pavone, M. *et al.* (1986). Comparison of diethylstilboestrol, cyproterone acetate and medroxyprogesterone acetate in the treatment of advanced prostate cancer: final analysis of phase III trial of the EORTC GU group. *Journal of Urology* **136**, 624–631.

Perez, C. A. *et al.* (1988). Definitive radiation therapy in carcinoma of the prostate localised to the pelvis: experience at the Mallinkrodt Institute of Radiology. *Monographs of the National Cancer Institute* **7**, 85–94.

Pessis, *et al.* (2001). Monotherapy with a new GNRH antagonist, Abarelix Depot (A–D), results in more rapid testosterone (T) suppression without an initial surge compared with leuoprolide acetate (L) plus Bicalutamide (B): results of a multicenter phase III study. *Journal of Urology* **165** (5), 685A, 166.

Porter, A. T. *et al.* (1993). Results of a randomised phase III trial to evaluate the efficacy of strontium-89 adjuvant to local field external beam irradiation in the management of endocrine resistant metastatic prostate cancer. *International Journal of Radiation Oncology, Biology, Physics* **25**, 805–813.

Potosky, A. L. *et al.* (2000). Health outcomes after prostatectomy or radiotherapy for prostate cancer: results from the cancer prostate outcomes study. *Journal of the National Cancer Institute* **92**, 1582–1592.

Prostate Cancer Triallists Collaborative Group (2000). Maximum androgen blockade in advanced prostate cancer: an overview of the randomised trials. *Lancet* **355**, 1491–1498.

Robinson, M. R. G. (1993). A further analysis of European Organisation for Research on Treatment of Cancer protocol 30805, orchidectomy versus orchidectomy plus cyproterone acetate versus low dose diethylstilboestrol. *Cancer* **72** (Suppl.), 3858–3862.

Sakr, W. A. *et al.* (1993). The frequency of carcinoma and intraepithelial neoplasia of the prostate in young male patients. *Journal of Urology* **150**, 379–385.

Sartor, O. *et al.* (1994). Surprising activity of flutamide withdrawal, when combined with aminoglutethimide, in treatment of 'hormone refractory' prostate cancer. *Journal of the National Cancer Institute* **86**, 222–227.

Smart, C. R. (1997). The results of prostate carcinoma screening in the US as reflected in the surveillance, epidemiology and end results program. *Cancer* **80**, 1835–1844.

Smith, P. H. *et al.* (1986). A comparison of the effect of diethylstilboestrol with low dose estramustine phosphate in treatment of advanced prostate cancer: final analysis of a phase III trial of the European Organisation for Research on the Treatment of Cancer. *Journal of Urology* **136**, 619–623.

Tannock, I. F. *et al.* (1996). Chemotherapy with mitoxantrone plus prednisone or prednisone alone for symptomatic hormone-resistant prostate cancer: a Canadian randomized trial with palliative end points. *Journal of Clinical Oncology* **14**, 1756–1764.

Tymchuk, C. N., Barnard, R. J., Heber, D., and Aronson, W. J. (2001). Evidence of an inhibitory effect of diet and exercise on prostate cancer cell growth. *Journal of Urology* **166**, 1185–1189.

Veterans Administration Cooperative Urological Research Group (1967). Treatment and survival of patients with cancer of the prostate. *Surgery, Gynecology and Obstetrics* **24**, 1011–1017.

Walsh, P. C. and Mostwin, J. L. (1984). Radical prostatectomy and cystoprostatectomy with preservation of potency: results using a new nerve sparing technique. *British Journal of Urology* **56**, 694–697.

Wolf, S. H. (1994). Public health perspective: the health policy implications of screening for prostatic cancer. *Journal of Urology* **152**, 1685–1688.

Zelefsky, M. J. *et al.* (1989). Palliative hemiskeletal irradiation for widespread metastatic prostate cancer. *International Journal of Radiation Oncology, Biology, Physics* **17**, 1281–1285.

Zelefsky, M. J. *et al.* (2001). High dose radiation delivered by intensity modulated conformal radiotherapy improves the outcome of localised prostate cancer. *Journal of Urology* **166**, 876–881.

Zincke, H. *et al.* (1994). Long term (15 years) results after radical prostatectomy for clinically localised (stage 2C or lower) prostate cancer. *Journal of Urology* **152**, 1850–1857.

19

Pharmacology and drug use in kidney patients

19

Pharmacology and drug
use in kidney patients

19.1 Drug-induced nephropathies

Marc E. De Broe

Introduction

Drugs are an infrequent cause of community-acquired acute renal failure (ARF). However, drugs share the spotlight with renal hypoxia as the leading aetiologic factor for hospital-acquired ARF (Nolan and Anderson 1998; Vijayan and Miller 1998). With the increasing capacity of the medical establishment to treat the most serious life-threatening conditions, the in-hospital exposure to nephrotoxic drugs will increase as will the risk of drug-induced ARF.

The incidence of in-hospital ARF, attributed to drug nephrotoxicity, is estimated at between 18 and 33 per cent of cases (Rasmussen and Ibels 1982; Hou *et al.* 1983; Kleinknecht *et al.* 1986; Kaufman *et al.* 1991; Bennett and Porter 1993; Baraldi *et al.* 1998).

In a 1-year survey of 2175 cases of ARF, 398 (18.3 per cent) were considered to be drug-induced (Kleinknecht *et al.* 1986). Antibiotics were the most frequently cited drugs, followed by analgesics, nonsteroidal anti-inflammatory drugs (NSAIDs), and contrast media. More than half of the patients had non-oliguric ARF. The mortality rate was 12.6 per cent, which is much lower than in patients who develop ARF in the setting of surgery and trauma. At 6-month follow-up post-ARF, 47.7 per cent were fully recovered, 15.3 per cent had regained previous renal function, and 23.1 per cent had some degree of residual renal impairment. Chronic haemodialysis was required in only 2 patients (0.5 per cent). Residual renal impairment was more frequent in older and oliguric patients, in those with previous chronic renal insufficiency, those who received antibiotics, and those whose ARF period was prolonged. The percentage of residual renal impairment is higher than that reported in the series of Davidman *et al.* (1991) or Pru *et al.* (1982), but is in accordance with that found 5 years later in the same country

(Fleury *et al.* 1990) and is supported by an earlier report from the European Dialysis and Transplant Association (Wing *et al.* 1983). When Schwarz *et al.* (2000) analysed the outcome of drug-induced acute interstitial nephritis, 60 per cent of NSAID induced acute interstitial nephritis representing the majority of the cases were left with some degree of chronic renal insufficiency.

Table 1 summarizes the incidence of drug-induced ARF reported for the last two decades. As can be seen, the incidence of ARF due to contrast media and antibiotics has declined while, two new categories of offending agents have appeared, for example, NSAIDs and angiotensin- converting enzyme (ACE) inhibitors. The susceptibility of the kidney to nephrotoxic injury has several reasons (Fig. 1). Renal blood flow (25 per cent of the resting cardiac output) exceeds 1000 ml/min = 3.5 ml/g of renal tissue/min. Compared to the majority of other tissues, except the brain, this results in a 50 times higher rate of drug delivery. In addition, the important oxygen supply required to support active ion and solute transport result in the fact that any change in blood flow and/or oxygen deprivation may have dramatic effects. In particular, acute tubular necrosis involving thick ascending limb of Henle is a prominent manifestation of a sudden reduction in renal blood flow with accompanying hypoxia. This anatomic site is especially vulnerable to oxygen deprivation due to the marginal oxygen balance that results from a high oxygen consumption related to the acive NaCl reabsortion and the limited blood supply due to the anatomic structure of the vasa recti (Heyman *et al.* 1991).

The kidney has the greatest endothelial surface per gram of tissue and possesses the highest capillary hydrostatic pressure favouring trapping of circulating antigen and *in situ* immune complex formation. Tubular transport and other renal metabolic processes utilize

Table 1 Incidence of acute renal failure due to drugs and contrast media

Authors	Year	N	% acute renal failure due to					
			Antibiotics	**Contrast agents**	**Analgesics**	**NSAIDs**	**ACE inhibitors**	**Total**
Rasmussen and Ibels (1982)	1982	143	11	11	—	—	—	22
Hou *et al.* (1983)	1983	129	7	12	—	—	—	20
Frankel *et al.* (1983)	1984	64	8	5	—	—	—	19
Kleinknecht *et al.* (1986)	1986	2175	6	2	4	3	0.5	18
Fleury *et al.* (1990)	1990	700	5	2	3	3	3	21
Kaufman *et al.* (1991)	1991	100	3	—	—	1	6	19
Baraldi *et al.* (1998)	1998	109	5	2	—	22	7	36

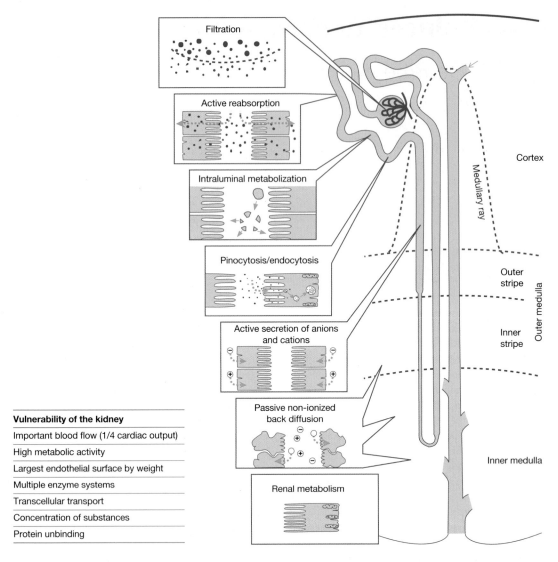

Fig. 1 Schematic representation and main localization along the nephron of the various patterns of drugs and xenobiotic handling by the kidney (De Broe and Roch-Ramel 1998).

considerable oxygen and are susceptible to the action of metabolic inhibitors. The kidney is the only place where highly protein-bound drugs are unbound, traverse the tubular cells and either accumulate within the proximal tubular epithelium and/or reach the tubular lumen. An abundance of tubular epithelial enzymes involved in the tubular transport systems can be blocked, particularly in view of the highly concentrated solutes in the tubular fluid that may reach urinary/plasma concentration ratios exceeding 1000 in some cases.

In the distal part of the nephron, urine is concentrated and the likelihood of crystalline precipitation increases substantially, particularly if urinary pH favours decreased solubility. As the urinary concentrating process also involves the counter-current mechanism, solute concentrations in the medullary interstitium reach values several times higher than tissues elsewhere in the body. Finally, during the process of renal excretion, a particular drug may undergo bioactivation towards reactive metabolites (Rush *et al.* 1984).

The kidney possesses several mechanisms for the renal handling excretion of drugs and xenobiotics; all of them may contribute to a certain extent to drug nephrotoxicity (Fig. 1). Numerous, if not the

majority of, drugs and xenobiotics are handled/eliminated, at least partly, by the kidney. For their handling/elimination by the kidney, they use one or, in most cases, two, or even more mechanisms. In addition, many other polar metabolites are formed by metabolism or conjugates by the liver, which are then excreted by the kidney.

The organic ion-transport system is instrumental in the intracellular accumulation of nephrotoxic cephalosporins due to the lower transport capacity of the lumenal membrane when compared to the basolateral membrane (Tune 1993). Another way in which proximal tubular transport is implicated in nephrotoxicity involves glutathione S-conjugates of xenobiotics. Once transported into the cell, these xenobiotic conjugates undergo biotransformation to electrophils, which then bind to macro-ophilic sites of intracellular macromolecules such as DNA. A third way in which a particular type of renal handling plays a central role in the nephrotoxic effect of a particular class of drugs aminoglycosides is the megalin mediated binding-endocytosis and lysosomal trapping of aminoglycosides (Sandoval *et al.* 2000). The mechanisms by which drugs and chemicals may damage the kidney are listed in Table 2.

Table 2 Mechanisms of renal toxicity of drugs (Nolan and Anderson 1998; Schwarz et al. 2000)

Reduction in renal perfusion through alteration of intrarenal haemodynamics
NSAID, ACE inhibitors, cyclosporine, contrast media, norepinephrine, angiotensin receptor blockers, diuretics, interleukins, cocaine, mitomycin C, tacrolimus, oestrogen, quinine

Acute tubular necrosis
Antibiotics: aminoglycosides, cephaloridine, cephalothin, amphotericin B, rifampicin, vancomycin, foscarnet, pentamidine
NSAIDs, glafenin, contrast media, acetaminophen, cyclosporine, cisplatin, IV immune globulin, dextran, maltose, sucrose, mannitol, heavy metals

Acute interstitial nephritis with or without glomerulopathy
Antibiotics: ciprofloxacin, methicillin, penicillin G, ampicillin, cephalothin, oxacillin, rifampicin
NSAIDs, glafenin, ASA, fenoprofen, naproxen, phenylbutazone, piroxicam, tolemetin, zomepirac, contrast media, sulfonamides, thiazides, phenytoin, furosemide, allopurinol, cimetidine, omeprazole, phenindione

Tubular obstruction
Sulfonamides, methotrexate, methoxyflurane, glafenin, triamterene, ticrynafen, acyclovir, ethylene glycol, protease inhibitors

Haeme pigment-induced toxicity (rhabdomyolysis)
Cocaine, ethanol, lovastatin

Hypersensitivity angiitis
Penicillin G, ampicillin, sulfonamides

Thrombotic microangiopathy/haemolytic–uraemic syndrome
Cyclosporine, oral contraceptives, mitomycin C, cocaine, quinine

Non-steroidal anti-inflammatory drugs

Individuals who have normal renal function and are properly hydrated, are not at risk for developing adverse renal effects of NSAIDs. NSAID-induced deterioration of renal function depends on the specific drug, the dose and duration of pharmacological effect, and particularly, the state of health of the recipient. Patients who have prostaglandin-dependent states associated with comorbid diseases, such as high-renin states or chronic renal failure, are especially susceptible to NSAID-induced renal toxicities. Renal prostaglandins, by initiating by counter-regulatory vasodilatation, are crucial in maintaining the perfusion in individuals with parenchymal renal disease and renal impairment, and when circulating volume is decreased, such as dehydrated patients, patients with severe heart disease (congestive heart failure), severe liver disease (cirrhosis), nephrotic syndrome (low-oncotic pressure) and in the elderly population (>80), and in individuals with parenchymal renal disease and renal impairment.

The renal syndromes associated with NSAIDs are the consequence of inhibition of cyclo-oxygenase (COX), which modifies the compensatory actions of prostaglandins (Fig. 2, Table 3). This modifies the compensatory actions of prostaglandins and consequently leads to a fall in both renal blood flow and glomerular filtration rate with concomitant abnormal water and salt retention. In addition, nephrotic syndrome and tubular interstitial disease can complicate NSAID use in exceptional cases.

Water retention, secondary to NSAIDs, is manifest as hyponatriaemia and occurs when the basal prostaglandin antagonism of

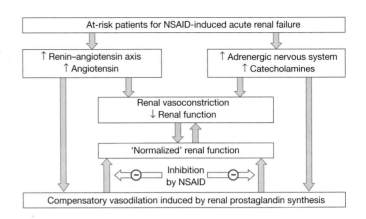

Fig. 2 Disruption of compensatory vasodilation response (Whelton and Watson 1998).

antidiuretic hormone is removed allowing a modified water reabsorption in the collecting duct of the kidney. When this action is coupled with NSAID induced enhanced sodium chloride reabsorption in the thick ascending limb of Henle, free-water clearance is virtually eliminated causing profound hyponatriaemia. The decrease in the response to loop diuretics is mediated both by removing the inhibition of sodium chloride reabsorption and the increase in medullary blood flow causing a reduction in the renal concentration capacity. The net result is that the concurrent use of NSAIDs may blunt the diuresis induced by loop diuretics.

Oedema due to NSAID-induced sodium retention usually occurs in susceptible individuals within the first week of therapy. Furthermore, these effects are reversible when the drug is discontinued. Clinically evident peripheral oedema occurs in up to 5 per cent of the patients.

Hyperkalaemia is an unusual complication of NSAID ingestion, presumably because of the multiple factors that are capable of maintaining potassium homeostasis even in the absence of prostaglandins. However, NSAID-induced hyperkalaemia may occur in up to 46 per cent of high-risk individuals, but is reversible upon discontinuation of therapy. Patients at risk to develop hyperkalaemia include those with pre-existing renal impairment, cardiac failure, diabetes, multiple myeloma, concomitant potassium supplementation, potassium sparing diuretic therapy, or taking an ACE inhibitor.

NSAID-induced ARF deterioration occurs in the setting of severe vasoconstrictive renal ischaemia and can be attributed to interruption of the delicate balance. Between are hormonally mediated pressor mechanisms and prostaglandin-associated vasodilatory effects. During NSAID inhibition of renal prostaglandin synthesis, unopposed vasoconstriction occurs because regulatory vasodilation has been eliminated. Risk factors for these rather frequent complications of the use of NSAID are listed in Table 4.

The rare complication of nephrotic syndrome—acute interstitial nephritis of NSAID use—may develop at any time during treatment, but typically occurs months or even years after the therapy has been initiated and generally resolves upon discontinuation of therapy.

In spite of the nephrotic range proteinuria, the most impressive histopathological finding in NSAID-induced nephrotic syndrome involves the interstitium and tubules. A focal infiltrate can be found around the proximal distal tubules. While this infiltrate consists primarily of cytotoxic T-lymphocytes, it also contains other T-cells, some

Table 3 Effects of NSAIDs on the kidney (adapted from Whelton 2000)

Syndrome	Mechanisms	Risk factors
Sodium retention and oedema	$\downarrow$ PG, $\downarrow$ RBF, $\downarrow$ GFR, $\uparrow$ Chloride absorption $\uparrow$ Antidiuretic hormone $\downarrow$ Natriuretic effect of loop diuretics	NSAID use, hepatic disease, renal disease, HTN, DM, diuretic use, circulatory compromise, dehydration, advanced age
Hyperkalaemia	$\downarrow$ PG, $\downarrow$ RAA axis activity, $\downarrow$ K$^+$ delivery to renal tubule $\downarrow$ Cellular uptake of K$^+$	Renal disease, CHF, type 2 DM, multiple myeloma, use of K$^+$ supplements, K$^+$ sparing diuretics, ACE inhibitors
Acute renal failure	$\downarrow$ PG, $\downarrow$ RBF, $\downarrow$ GFR haemodynamic disruption	CHF, renal disease, hepatic disease, diuretic use, advanced age, dehydration, SLE, shock, sepsis, hyper-reninaemia, hyperaldosteronaemia
Nephrotic syndrome/ proteinuria/ interstitial nephritis[a]	$\uparrow$ Recruitment and activation of lymphocytes, likely through leukotriene formation, affecting glomerular and peritubular permeability	Fenoprofen use, possibly female gender, advanced age
Renal papillary necrosis[a]/ chronic interstitial nephritis	Direct toxicity $\downarrow$ PG	Massive NSAID ingestion Dehydration

NSAID, nonsteroidal anti-inflammatory drugs; PG, prostaglandin; RBF, renal blood flow; GFR, glomerular filtration rate; HTN, hypertension: DM, diabetes mellitus; K$^+$, potassium; RAA, renin–angiotensin–aldosterone; CHF, congestive heart failure; ACE, angiotensin-converting enzyme; SLE, systemic lupus erythematosis.

[a] Distinctly unusual.

Table 4 *At risk* patients for NSAID-induced acute renal failure

Severe heart disease (congestive heart failure)

Severe liver disease (cirrhosis)

Nephrotic syndrome (low oncotic pressure)

Chronic renal disease

Elderly population (age 80 or $>$)

Dehydration (protracted—several days)

B-cells and plasma cells. Changes in the glomerulus in these patients were minimal and resembled those of classical minimal change glomerulonephritis with marked epithelial foot process fusion.

NSAID-induced acute interstitial nephritis is a recognized cause of ARF, the frequency of which seems to be increasing. In a recent report by Schwarz *et al.* (2000), of 64 biopsy proven cases of acute interstitial nephritis, 85 per cent were drug-induced. The responsible drugs included antibiotics, analgesics, NSAIDs, and diuretics. Permanent renal insufficiency (moderate to severe), was observed in 26 per cent of these cases, 65 per cent of them after NSAID-intake. Risk factors for the development of persistent renal failure after acute renal failure due to NSAIDs are pre-existing renal damage, long intake of causative drugs, slow oligosymptomatic disease development (less oliguria) and histological signs of tubular atrophy, interstitial granuloma, and pronounced interstitial infiltration. The better the drug in question is

tolerated without acute symptoms, the longer the intake before diagnosis, and the worse the prognosis of renal insufficiency. This could mean that asymptomatic chronic drug intake with persistent subacute interstitial nephritis results in chronic interstitial nephritis.

Renal papillary necrosis is an extremely unusual and not very well proven clinical event during intake of massive amounts of NSAIDS.

Is the prolonged use of NSAID-associated with renal papillary necrosis or chronic renal failure?

In contrast to the rather well characterized acute effects of NSAIDs on the kidney, the chronic effects are less well documented. Although renal papillary necrosis and chronic renal failure can occur after prolonged use of NSAIDs, the actual risk of these serious complications is not known. The epidemiologic data are controversial. In the case–control study by Perneger *et al.* (1994), the risk of endstage renal disease was 8.8 in subjects who had taken 5000 or more doses of NSAIDs in their lifetime, as compared with those who had taken fewer than 1000 pills. These data, however, are based on a flawed study design in which case patients or proxies were not consistent; odds ratio was 0.6 for subjects with a cumulative dose of 1000–4999 pills, and the limited number of exposed control individuals. Sandler *et al.* (1991) reported that the odds ratio for chronic renal disease was 2.1 (95% confidence interval, 1.1–4.1) in daily users of NSAIDs, but surprisingly, this risk was limited to men older than 65 years. After adjustment for the use of other analgesics, the odds ratio for this group was 10.0 (95% confidence interval, 1.2–82.7). The high proportion of proxy interviews primarily with spouses might have biased the results especially in younger adults and woman. In contrast, Nuyts *et al.* (1995) in a Belgian case–control study investigating occupational risk factors for chronic renal failure in 272 patients with chronic renal failure of all types and matched controls found that regular use of NSAIDs was not associated with an increased risk (odds ratio, 0.94; 95% confidence interval, 0.60–1.48). Renal papillary necrosis has been induced experimentally by NSAIDs in animals, although the severity of the effects varies from one product to another and is increased by caffeine (Zambraski 1995). In a prospective, uncontrolled comparison of intravenous urography, sonography, and computed tomography (CT) in 259 patients who had taken 1000–26,000 doses of NSAIDs as the sole or predominant analgesic in their lifetime, papillary necrosis was found in 38 patients. Only 65 per cent of these patients had renal functional impairment (Segasothy et al. 1996). These interesting observations, however, need further investigation. The frequency of renal papillary necrosis as a primary or contributing cause of endstage renal disease in the context of chronic NSAID use remains unknown, and the medical imaging techniques best suited for the diagnosis of this disease are not in wide use (Elseviers et al. 1995).

The most recent advance in NSAID pharmacology are agents that specifically block the COX-2 isoform while sparing the effect of COX-1 related activities (Fig. 3). These drugs have been designated by the WHO as a new pharmacological category of NSAIDs, namely the 'coxibs' (Lipsky et al. 1998). By blocking COX-2, the intent is to spare toxicity in organs such as the gut and kidney, thereby increase their utility, especially in elderly patients (Fig. 2). Both the currently available COX-2 specific inhibitors, that is, celecoxib and rofecoxib, have established their safety advantage with respect to clinically important reductions in gastrointestinal toxicity and platelet-sparing characteristics (Lipsky et al. 1998; Cryer et al. 1999; Langman et al. 1999; Bombardier et al. 2000; Goldstein et al. 2000; Leese et al. 2000; Silverstein et al. 2000; Verburg et al. 2001). Bleeding complications are seen with aspirin and traditional NSAIDs have essentially been eliminated. However, the clinical impact of coxibs upon renal and cardiovascular function is an area of evolving information, especially now that it is known that the COX-2 isoenzyme is expressed within the human kidney. Case reports have now clearly established that COX-2 inhibitors may cause decrease in glomerular filtration rate, increase in sodium retention, peripheral oedema, increase in systolic blood pressure and increase in serum potassium concentration. The same caution should be exercised with use of COX-2 inhibitors in patients who are at risk of adverse effects with NSAIDs.

Inhibitors of the renin–angiotensin system

Soon after the release of this useful class of antihypertensive drugs, the syndrome of functional acute renal insufficiency was described as a class effect. This phenomenon was first observed in patients with renal artery stenosis, particularly when the entire renal mass was affected, as in bilateral renal artery stenosis or in renal transplants with stenosis to a solitary kidney (Hricik et al. 1983). Acute renal dysfunction appears to be related to loss of postglomerular efferent arteriolar vascular tone and, in general, is reversible after withdrawing the ACE inhibitor (Textor 1990).

In addition, ACE inhibition treatment has been associated exceptionally with membranous glomerulopathy and an acute interstitial nephritis with eosinophilia (Smith et al. 1989; Opie 1992). The former renal side-effect of these drugs seems to be restricted to patients with pre-existing renal disease who use high doses of the drug.

Inhibition of the ACE kinase II results in at least two important effects (Fig. 4): depletion of angiotensin II and accumulation of bradykinin (de Jong and Woods 1998). The role of the latter effect on renal perfusion pressure is not clear.

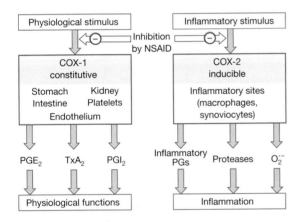

Fig. 3 Cyclo-oxygenase and prostaglandin synthesis (Mitchell et al. 1994).

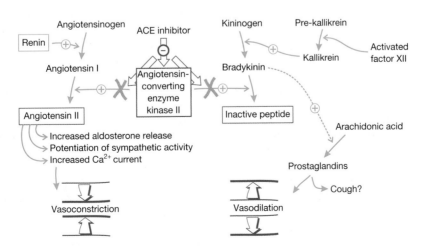

Fig. 4 Renin, converting enzyme, and vascular tone (adapted from Opie 1992).

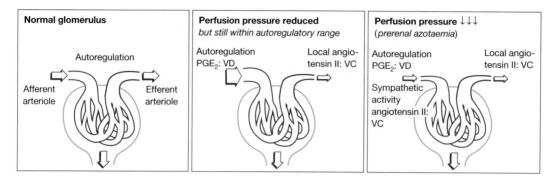

Fig. 5 Renal haemodynamics in normal and hypoperfusion conditions (VD, vasodilation; VC, vasoconstriction).

To understand the angiotensin I-converting enzyme inhibitor-induced drop in glomerular filtration rate, it is important to understand the physiological role of the renin–angiotensin system in the regulation of renal haemodynamics (Fig. 5). When renal perfusion drops, renin is released into the plasma and lymph by the juxtaglomerular cells of the kidneys. Renin cleaves angiotensinogen to form angiotensin I, which is cleaved further by converting enzyme to form angiotensin II, the principal effector molecule in this system. Angiotensin II participates in glomerular filtration rate regulation in at least two ways. First, angiotensin II increases arterial pressure—directly and acutely by causing vasoconstriction and more 'chronically' by increasing body fluid volumes through stimulation of renal sodium retention; directly through an effect on the tubules, as well as by stimulating thirst and indirectly via aldosterone. Second, angiotensin II preferentially constricts the efferent arteriole, thus helping to preserve glomerular capillary hydrostatic pressure and, consequently, glomerular filtration rate.

When arterial pressure or body fluid volumes are sensed as subnormal, the renin–angiotensin system is activated and plasma renin activity and angiotensin II levels increase. This may occur in the context of clinical settings such as renal artery stenosis, dietary sodium restriction or sodium depletion as during diuretic therapy, congestive heart failure, cirrhosis, and nephrotic syndrome. When activated, this renin–angiotensin system plays an important role in the maintenance of glomerular pressure and filtration through preferential angiotensin II-mediated constriction of the efferent arteriole. Thus, under such conditions the kidney becomes sensitive to the effects of blockade of the renin–angiotensin system by angiotensin I-converting enzyme inhibitor or angiotensin II receptor antagonist.

The highest incidence of renal failure in patients treated with ACE inhibitors was associated with bilateral renovascular disease (Textor 1990). In patients with already compromised renal function and congestive heart failure, the incidence of serious changes in serum creatinine during ACE inhibition depends on the severity of the pretreatment heart failure and renal failure.

Volume management, dose reduction, use of relative short-acting ACE inhibitors, diuretic holiday for some days before initiating treatment, and avoidance of concurrent use of NSAIDs (hyperkalaemia) are among the appropriate measures for patients at risk.

Since most ACE inhibitors are eliminated via renal excretion, it should be emphasized that the dose of the drug has to be adjusted for renal function. In patients with renal failure, the ACE inhibitor should be started at very low doses and should be titrated only gradually. The acute and sometimes severe fall in glomerular filtration rate during ACE inhibitor treatment in patients with renal disease, a caricatural

functional response of angiotensin II dependent kidney, should be considered separately from the expected beneficial effects of ACE inhibition or angiotensin II receptor blockade to prevent the progress of renal function decline as documented by several clinical studies (Bjorck *et al.* 1990; Lewis *et al.* 1993; Maschio *et al.* 1996; Brenner *et al.* 2001; Lewis *et al.* 2001; Parving *et al.* 2001).

The most commonly reported fetal side-effect of ACE inhibition is second to third trimester onset of oligohydramnios and growth retardation, followed by delivery of an infant whose neonatal course is complicated by prolonged and often profound hypotension and anuria (Rosa *et al.* 1989). Hence, ACE inhibitors should not be used during pregnancy. Once the possible physiological mechanisms of these side effects had been elucidated, it became increasingly clear that these effects could also be used to extend the diagnostic and therapeutical armamentarium of today's medicine.

In contrast to the more acute and severe fall in glomerular filtration rate as discussed earlier, the fall in filtration in patients with renal parenchymal disease and impaired renal function, generally is rather small, and mostly not diagnosed as such if less sensitive methods such as changes in serum creatinine are used.

ACE inhibition indeed have been found to lower urinary protein excretion in patients with renal disease of various origins. Both in patients with asymptomatic proteinuria and in patients with frank nephrotic syndrome, a fall in proteinuria with a rise in serum albumin has been described (Taguma *et al.* 1985; Reams and Bauer 1986; Heeg *et al.* 1987, 1989; Bjorck *et al.* 1990). It has been argued that this improvement in the urinary protein leakage is the consequence of the renal haemodynamic effect of the ACE inhibitor, since blood pressure lowering with other antihypertensive does not result in a fall in proteinuria (Heeg *et al.* 1987, 1989). In addition, the effects of ACE inhibition or angiotensin II receptor antagonism to block the growth-promoting capacity of angiotensin II adds to the beneficial effects of renin–angiotensin blockade. In the last few years, the beneficial effects of both ACE inhibition and angiotensin II receptor antagonists to prevent the progressive renal function decline in both type I (Lewis *et al.* 1993) and type II (Brenner *et al.* 2001; Lewis *et al.* 2001; Parving *et al.* 2001) diabetic nephropathy as well as in non-diabetic nephropathies (Maschio *et al.* 1996; The GISEN Group 1997; Ruggenenti *et al.* 1999; Jafar *et al.* 2001) has been well documented.

Radiocontrast agents

The use of iodinated contrast media continues to be a common cause of hospital-acquired ARF and its development increases the in-hospital mortality significantly (Porter 1994a; Levy *et al.* 1996). Contrast media-induced nephropathy is defined as an otherwise unexplained acute deterioration of renal function after intravascular administration of contrast media.

Next to changes in glomerular filtration rate or serum creatinine levels, an increase in urinary enzyme excretion seems also to be a sensitive marker of tubular alteration after contrast media exposure (Bettmann 1991; Hunter and Kind 1992). However, no conclusive relationship has been demonstrated between the detection of enzymes in urine and the fall in glomerular filtration rate (Donadio *et al.* 1988; Hunter and Kind 1992; Porter 1994b; Erley *et al.* 1999).

All currently used water-soluble contrast media are based on the tri-iodinated benzene ring. The first high osmolar contrast media (1500 mOsm/kg) contained an ionizing carboxyl group with a cation, usually sodium. In the 1970s, a new generation of ratio 3 monomeric non-ionic, low osmolar contrast media was introduced (iohexol, iopromide 700 mOsm/kg). These low osmolar contrast media cause less injection-associated pain and lower acute toxicity in animals. In the 1980s and 1990s, the ratio 6 dimeric contrast media were developed, based on two tri-iodinated benzene rings, with the absence of a carboxyl group and with a high number of hydroxyl groups (iodixanol, iotralan). Non-ionic dimeric contrast media are hypo-osmolar and are presented as iso-osmolar solution, containing electrolytes (Ca^{2+} and Na^+ ions). Low osmolar contrast media are now first choice, at least in at-risk patients. Worldwide, low osmolar contrast media are used in 75 per cent of the patients. The use of iso-osmolar contrast media, which theoretically should be even less toxic than low osmolar contrast media, is increasing. However, in spite of improvements in the chemical structure of contrast media, they remain the third leading cause of hospital-aquired ARF in the 1990s (Krämer *et al.* 1999).

Mostly, the increase in serum creatinine starts 24–48 h after contrast media exposure, peaks after 3–5 days, and returns to baseline 7–10 days after. Except for patients with a higher degree of renal function impairment, contrast media-induced nephropathy presents as a non-oliguric form of acute renal failure.

Morphological changes were observed mainly as vacuolar changes in the proximal convoluted tubular cells (Moreau *et al.* 1975; Dobrota *et al.* 1995; Tervahartiala *et al.* 1997). These morphological changes parallel the increases in urinary enzyme excretion (Moreau *et al.* 1975; Battenfeld *et al.* 1991), but a strong relationship to renal function impairment after contrast media has not been demonstrated (Heyman *et al.* 1988).

In patients without any risk factor, the incidence is less than 1 per cent despite the use of up to 800 ml of contrast media (Rosovsky *et al.* 1996). In patients at high risk, the frequency of contrast media-induced nephropathy has been reported to increase in the last few years, which seems to be related to the wider use of diagnostic and therapeutic interventions in elderly and critically ill patients (Rudnicki *et al.* 1996).

Pathogenesis

Contrast media attenuates both renal haemodynamics and renal tubular function (Heyman *et al.* 1994). After injection of contrast media there is a transient increase, followed by a more prolonged decrease in renal blood flow (Caldicott *et al.* 1970; Katzberg *et al.* 1977; Bakris and Burnett 1985). To date, only endothelin and adenosine have been shown to play a role as important vasoactive substances mediating in chronic media induced nephropathy.

Experimental studies in a variety of animal models of ARF reveal a consistent nephroprotective effect of adenosine antagonism (Osswald *et al.* 1979; Bidani and Churchill 1983; Lin *et al.* 1986, 1988; Bidani *et al.* 1987; Gouyon and Guignard 1988; Deray *et al.* 1990; Rossi *et al.* 1990).

Prevention—risk factors

The major risk factors for contrast media induced nephropathy are summarized in Table 5.

Experimental radiocontrast-induced renal failure requires various preceding stresses, including subtotal nephrectomy, dehydration, congestive heart failure, inhibition of nitric oxide, or prostaglandin synthesis. The major risk factors for radiocontrast nephropathy in humans are: high doses of contrast media, pre-existing renal failure especially in diabetes mellitus patients, dehydration or decreased effective arterial volume (congestive heart failure, cirrhosis, and nephrotic syndrome), as well as other factors favouring prerenal failure including ACE inhibitors and NSAIDs (Murphy *et al.* 2000); multiple myeloma may not be an independent risk factor (McCarthy and Becker 1992). Non-ionic, low-osmolality media should be considered at least in patients with a serum creatinine greater than 1.6 mg/dl (Rudnick *et al.* 1995).

A very recent study demonstrated that spiral computed tomographic angiography performed for the detection of renal artery stenosis is not associated with an increased risk for contrast media nephropathy compared with intra-arterial digital substraction angiography despite a greater dose of intravenous administered contrast media in computed tomographic angiography (Lufft *et al.* 2002).

The rationale for a better prevention of radiocontrast nephropathy is built on pathogenesis.

The first strategy to offset the increase of renal vascular resistance was the use of dopamine. A few studies reported a beneficial effect (Hans *et al.* 1990; Kapoor *et al.* 1996), especially in patients with the highest serum creatinine levels (Hans *et al.* 1998). However, most studies were inconclusive (Weisberg *et al.* 1993; Abizaid *et al.* 1999), or even reported a negative effect in patients with peripheral vascular disease (Gare *et al.* 1999). Adrenergic blockade was also ineffective in an experimental model (Duarte *et al.* 1998).

Table 5 Risk factors for contrast media-induced nephropathy

Confirmed	Suspected	Disproved
Decrease in effective arterial volume		
Concurrent use of nephrotoxic drugs		
Chronic renal failure	Hypertension	Myeloma
Diabetic nephropathy	Generalized atherosclerosis	Diabetes without nephropathy
Severe congestive heart failure	Abnormal liver function tests	
Amount and frequency of contrast media	Hyperuricaemia	
Volume depletion/ hypotension	Proteinuria	
High osmolar contrast media		

More specific vasodilator treatments have been tested. Increased endothelin levels were confirmed in humans injected with radiocontrast media, with a compensatory increase in ANP levels (Clarck *et al.* 1997). However, endothelin receptor antagonism with an ET_A/ET_B blocker exacerbated radiocontrast nephropathy (Wang *et al.* 2000) and ANP administration had no effect (Kurnik *et al.* 1998).

Adenosine A1 receptor antagonists exhibited some beneficial effects in experimental radiocontrast nephropathies (Erley *et al.* 1997; Pollock *et al.* 1997; Yao *et al.* 2001). An early clinical study claimed that theophylline, a non-specific adenosine receptor antagonist, prevented the small fall in glomerular filtration rate and effective renal plasma flow seen in the placebo-treated group (Erley *et al.* 1994). However, two recent large trials using theophylline were negative (Abizaid *et al.* 1999; Erley *et al.* 1999).

Prostaglandin E1 was used in a randomized study and had a marginally beneficial effect (Koch *et al.* 2000), with only borderline significance after statistical adjustment (Sketch *et al.* 2001).

Decreased nitric oxide formation has been confirmed in humans injected with radiocontrast media (Dzgoeva *et al.* 1999). L-Arginine administration aiming at increasing nitric oxide levels was effective in an experimental model (Andrade *et al.* 1998); however, intra-arterial delivery before and after the procedure may be difficult in clinical practice.

Dialysis has no proven benefit in regard to a prevention of contrast media-induced nephropathy in azotaemic patients. Due to their vasodilating effect and in the hope of preventing calcium overload in the tubular cells (Bakris and Burnett 1985), calcium channel blockers have been used in both experimental (Deray *et al.* 1990), and clinical studies (Osswald *et al.* 1975; Russo *et al.* 1990; Neumayer *et al.* 1993). Despite early promising results, large prospective trials failed to observe a beneficial effect regarding the decline in glomerular filtration rate after contrast media exposure (Khoury *et al.* 1995; Carraro *et al.* 1996; Spangberg Viklund *et al.* 1996). Taken together a prophylactic value of calcium channel blockers (either short or long acting) has not been proven.

Tepel *et al.* (2000) recently published the first clinical trial using acetylcysteine (1200 mg of acetylcysteine per day, given orally in divided doses on the day before and on the day of the administration of the radiocontrast agent) in order to prevent the decline in renal function in patients with moderate renal insufficiency, who were undergoing CT. A close look at the data does not show unequivocal benefit of acetylcysteine in this setting as the placebo group did not show a significant decline in renal function after contrast media exposure, and the significant difference between both groups resulted from an unexplained decline in creatinine levels in the acetylcysteine group compared to stable creatinine levels in the placebo group. Therefore, these data should be confirmed in a larger number of patients and in patients with a more seriously compromised renal function before acetylcysteine can be considered a potentially useful drug for prevention of chronic media induced nephropathy.

Cisplatin

The clinical use of cisplatin, an important and widely used anticancer drug, is often complicated by nephrotoxicity and ototoxicity, gastrointestinal disturbances, and immunosuppression. Early clinical trials with cisplatin in cancer patients found a striking number of cases of persistent azotaemia and acute renal failure. Incidence of the renal side-effects has been largely reduced in recent years because of preventive measures.

The vulnerability of the kidney during cisplatin treatment is almost certainly linked to its primary role in the excretion of the drug.

Pathogenesis

Cisplatin goes along with reduction of renal plasma flow, occurring before any change in glomerular filtration rate suggesting and increased renal vascular resistance. In addition, tubular dysfunctions is evidenced by several brush border enzymes appearing in the urine of patients after cisplatin administration. Electrolyte disturbances, such as hypomagnesaemia, hypocalcaemia, and hypokalaemia are frequently observed in cisplatin treated patients. Polyuria that often accompanies administration and occurs in two distant phases, urinary osmolality initially falls over the first 24 and 48 hours. This early polyuria usually ameliorates spontaneously. The second phase of increased urinary volume occurs between 72 and 96 h after cisplatin administration. Cisplatin may also induce an incomplete distal tubule acidosis by altering the cellular respiration leading to changes in tubular handling of hydrogen, magnesium, potassium, and calcium balance. Acute tubular necrosis and acute interstitial nephritis has been described with cisplatin treatment. After prolonged administration, chronic renal failure may appear without any particular characteristics. The relationship between cisplatin DNA binding to renal cytotoxicity is not clear. Nevertheless, studies in cells whose repair processes are deficient show that cisplatin is especially toxic in them (Fraval *et al.* 1978), making such a possibility likely. From a theoretical point of view, it is conceivable that since nephrotoxic acute renal failure requires replacement to damaged tubular cells with new ones, the recovery phase of an acute tubular nephrotoxicity due to cisplatin might be influenced by this cisplatin DNA binding. The kidney is the principal excretory organ of cisplatin.

In addition to glomerular filtration of the unbound part of cisplatin, there is an particular S3-segment cisplatin accumulation which may involve, although it is still not clear, transport or binding to components of the organic based transport system. Cisplatin is excreted, largely unchanged, in the kidney. On the other hand, once in the renal cell, cisplatin undergoes biotransformation. In addition to binding cell macromolecules, a large portion (30–50 per cent) of total cell platinum is in a form whose molecular weight is below 500 Da and whose chromatographic behaviour is different from cisplatin. The cisplatin DNA adducts cause errors during DNA replication, which lead to mutation, especially G $\rightarrow$ T transversions. Such mutations may be responsible for second malignancies that arise after cisplatin therapy. A very recent paper provides evidence that tumour necrosis factor-α (TNF-α) is a critical factor in chemokine and cytokine expression and renal injury in a murine model of cisplatin nephrotoxicity (Ramesh and Reeves 2002).

Prevention—risk factors

Several attempts have been made to reduce nephrotoxicity by either coadministration of 'renoprotective' compounds, alternative methods of administration, or by developing analogues with an improved therapeutic index. There seems to be no reason to advocate for the use of diuretics in prevention of cisplatin-induced nephrotoxicity based on several clinical investigations. Prior hydration with hypertonic salt seems to reduce cisplatin-induced ARF. The increase in chloride concentration in the urine that occurs after hypertonic salt infusion may reduce the conversion of cisplatin to toxic aquated metabolites, a process known to be sensitive to chloride ion concentration. The use hypertonic saline was introduced several years ago in the clinic and resulted in a clear decrease in incidence of nephrotoxicity after cisplatin. Furthermore, compared to bolus dose, fractionation or continuous infusion of the total dose of cisplatin over 3–5 days is equally effective from the therapeutic standpoint but spares renal function (Salem *et al.* 1984).

The administration of nephrotoxic drugs such as aminoglycosides, NSAIDs, or iodinated contrast media simultaneously with cisplatin should be avoided, since cumulative toxicity has been demonstrated (Gonzalez-Vitale *et al.* 1978). An impressive list of compounds has been used to decrease cisplatin toxicity (antinatriuretic factor, glycine, diethyldithiocarbamate, calcium channel blockers, cimetidine, sodium thiosulfate, glutathione, and other sulfidryl compounds). Among them, only sodium thiosulfate has received a significant clinical application and has been reported to reduce the renal toxicity of cisplatin administered. However, controversies still exists as to the effect of sodium thiosulfate on cisplatin antitumour activity.

The high incidence of nephrotoxicity of the currently used inorganic platinum compounds stresses the importance of undertaking research to identify platinum complexes that would have less nephrotoxicity as comparable antitumour properties.

Carboplatin was developed to avoid the nephrotoxicity of cisplatin and was initially considered as less nephrotoxic. However, several studies have shown comparable nephrotoxicity of carboplatin and cisplatin.

Interleukin-2

Renal toxicity, the main limiting adverse effect of interleukin-2 administration, often prompts physicians to discontinue or reduce the dose, especially in the aged and subjects with reduced renal function. Clinical studies have characterized a reversible syndrome associated with interleukin-2 administration that consists of hypotension, oliguria, fluid retention, azotaemia, and a very low urinary excretion of sodium (Webb *et al.* 1988; Philip *et al.* 1989). It has been ascribed to the so-called 'vascular leak syndrome'. Based on experimental studies, this syndrome is thought to occur due to a primary increase in the vascular permeability with consequent shifting of proteinaceous intravascular fluid into the interstitium of multiple organs, along with hypoalbuminaemia and reduction of the intravascular volume (Rosenstein *et al.* 1986). Because of this, the ARF after interleukin-2 administration was initially considered to be secondary to the 'vascular leak syndrome'. However, subsequent studies in cancer patients with interleukin-2 continuous infusion have reported renal failure occurring in patients with stable haemodynamics (Ponce *et al.* 1993).

Acute interstitial nephritis characterized by parenchymal infiltration with T-lymphocytes has also been reported (Feinfeld *et al.* 1991) in a few patients. It has been suggested that acute tubular nephritis could be the result of a cytotoxic lymphocyte-mediated reaction induced by the interleukin-2 treatment (Valsveld *et al.* 1993).

5-Aminosalicylic acid

Definition—epidemiology

Over the past few years, an association between the use of 5-aminosalicylic acid (5-ASA) in patients with chronic inflammatory bowel disease (IBD) and the development of a particular type of chronic tubulointerstitial nephritis has been suggested.

For many years, sulfasalazine, an azo compound derived from sulfapyridine and 5-ASA, the latter being the pharmacologically active moiety, was the only valuable non-corticosteroid drug in the treatment of IBD. Since the therapeutically inactive sulfapyridine moiety was largely responsible for the mainly haematological side-effects of sulfasalazine, this stimulated the development of new 5-ASA formulations (mesalazine, olsalazine, balsalazine) for topical and oral use. In the last decade, these new 5-ASA products replaced sulfasalazine as the first-line therapy for mildly to moderately active IBD. However, a literature search revealed 17 published cases of renal impairment associated with 5-ASA therapy in patients with IBD, and in several it was shown that this did not recover completely upon stopping the drug, even after a follow-up period of several years. In a retrospective study, nephrologists reported 40 patients with IBD showing renal impairment, including 15 cases with interstitial nephritis and previous use of 5-ASA. Stimulated by these findings, we started a European prospective registration study aiming to register all patients with IBD and renal impairment and to control for a possible association with 5-ASA therapy. A cohort of 1449 IBD patients seen during one year in the outpatient clinic of 28 European departments of gastroenterology was investigated. A possible association of the observed renal impairment with 5-ASA therapy can only be suspected in two to five patients with an undetermined renal diagnosis resulting in a frequency ranging from 1.3 to 3.3 per 1000 patients. Results of this study are comparable with the frequency for chronic renal lesions of less than 2 per 1000 patients estimated by World *et al.* (1996) based on published results of clinical trials ($n = 449$ patients).

However, determining the cause of renal disease in those with IBD is not straightforward. The most frequent renal complications are oxalate stones and their consequences, such as pyelonephritis, hydronephrosis, and (in the long-term) amyloidosis. Chronic IBD is also associated with glomerulonephritis: minimal-change glomerulonephritis, membranous, membranoproliferative, focal glomerulosclerosis, and proliferative crescentic glomerulonephritis have all been reported. As for many drugs, reversible, acute interstitial nephritis has been exceptionally seen with the use of 5-ASA compounds. In view of this complexity, the association of 5-ASA and chronic interstitial nephritis in patients with IBD can be difficult to interpret, since renal involvement may be an extraintestinal manifestation of the underlying disease. However, the particular form of chronic tubulointerstitial nephritis in patients with IBD treated with 5-ASA is characterized by an important cellular infiltration of the interstitium with macrophages, T cells, and also B cells.

Pathogenesis and pathology

That 5-ASA causes renal disease is supported by the number of case reports appearing in the recent literature of patients with IBD using 5-ASA as their only medication, the improvement (at least partially) of impaired renal function upon stopping the drug, and a worsening after resuming 5-ASA use. Furthermore, the molecular structure of 5-ASA is very close to that of salicylic acid, phenacetin, and aminophenol, drugs with well-documented nephrotoxic potential. Calder *et al.* (1972) found that necrosis of the proximal convoluted tubules and papillary necrosis developed in rats after a single intravenous injection of 5-ASA at doses of 1.4, 2.8, and 5.7 mmol/kg body weight (high pharmacological doses). The mechanism of renal damage, possibly caused by 5-ASA itself, may be analogous to that of salicylates by inducing hypoxia of renal tissues, either by uncoupling oxidative phosphorylation in renal mitochondria, by inhibiting the synthesis of renal prostaglandins, or by rendering the kidney susceptible to oxidative damage by reducing renal glutathione concentration by inhibition of the pentose phosphate shunt.

In contrast to the classical 'analgesic nephropathy', papillary necrosis is not observed with 5-ASA. The presence of an extensive T- and B-cell infiltration (even granulomas) surrounding atrophic tubules suggest cell mediated immune response such as T-cell response against an autoantigen modified by the drug.

Clinical expression

An intriguing aspect of this type of toxic nephropathy is the documented persistence of the inflammation of the renal interstitium even several months/years after onset of the drug intake. The disease is more prevalent in men, with a male : female ratio of 15 : 2. The age of reported cases ranged from 14 to 45 years. By contrast with analgesic nephropathy, where renal lesions are only observed after several years of analgesic abuse, interstitial nephritis associated to 5-ASA was already observed during the first year of treatment in seven of 17 reported cases, most of whom had started 5-ASA therapy with documented normal renal function. In several cases, particularly in those in which there is a delayed diagnosis of renal damage, recovery of renal function does not occur, and some needed renal replacement therapy.

Diagnosis—treatment

Since this type of chronic tubulointerstitial nephritis produces few, if any, symptoms, and if diagnosed at later stage progresses to irreversible chronic endstage renal disease, serum creatinine should be measured in any patient with inflammatory bowel disease treated with 5-ASA at the start of the treatment, every 3 months for the remainder of the first year, and annually thereafter. The use of concurrent immunosuppressive therapy, as is the case in severe forms of chronic IBD, may necessitate extension to the period of intensive renal function monitoring. If serum creatinine increases, a renal biopsy is the only way to demonstrate the type of renal disease involved.

Chinese herbs

In 1992, physicians in Belgium noted an increasing number of women presenting with renal failure, often near endstage, following their exposure to a slimming regimen containing Chinese herbs. An initial survey of seven nephrology centres in Brussels identified 14 women under the age of 50 who had presented with advanced renal failure due to biopsy-proven, chronic tubulointerstitial nephritis over a 3-year period; nine of whom had been exposed to the same slimming regimen. As of early 2000, a total of more than 120 cases had been identified. The epidemiology is unknown, as is the risk for the development of severe renal damage, but the recent publication of case reports from several countries in Europe and Asia would seem to indicate that the incidence of herbal medicine nephrotoxicity is more common than previously thought.

Pathogenesis

The pathogenesis of Chinese herbal nephropathy is incompletely understood. A plant nephrotoxin, aristolochic acid (AA), has been proposed as a possible aetiologic agent. Support for this hypothesis is provided by findings in animal models of disease (Cosyns et al. 2001; Debelle et al. 2002). In a first study, rabbits were given intraperitoneal injections of AA (0.1 mg AA/kg 5 days a week for 17–21 months) (Cosyns et al. 2001). Histological examination of the kidneys and genitourinary tract revealed renal hypocellular interstitial fibrosis, and atypical and malignant uroepithelial cells.

In a more recent study (Debelle et al. 2002), the daily subcutaneous administration of 10 mg/kg of AA to salt depleted rats induce after 35 days renal failure associated with tubular atrophy and interstitial fibrosis. In some of the rats, a papillary urothelial carcinoma of the pelvis was found.

AA (0.15 mg/tablet) has been used as an immunomodulatory drug for 20 years in Germany by thousands of patients, sometimes in doses comparable to that found in Chinese herb slimming regimens; despite this exposure, during that period there is no report relating chronic tubulointerstitial nephritis to the use of AA in this clinical setting.

In addition to AA, patients with Chinese herb nephropathy also received the appetite suppressants, fenfluramine and diethylpropion; agents with vasoconstrictive properties and diuretics at low dose (De Broe 1999a).

Together, these observations suggest that the relatively fast-developing chronic tubulointerstitial renal disease may have been caused by combined exposure to a potent nephrotoxic substance, that is, AA, and to renal vasoconstrictors, fenfluramine/diethylpropion, associated with clinical risk factors such as volume depletion. The type of renal insult observed with this major potential nephrotoxic substance expressing this renal effect in association with a number of risk factors is also observed with several other drugs such as ACE inhibitors, NSAIDs, radiographic contrast media, lithium, etc. The findings of Debelle and his colleagues (Debelle et al. 2002) of the necessity to induce a stimulated intrarenal renin–angiotensin system in order to obtain fibrointerstitial lesions are in line with the combined exposure concept observed with several potential nephrotoxins.

Another uncertain factor is why only some patients exposed to the same herbal preparations develop renal disease. Women appear to be at greater risk than men. Other possibly important factors include toxin dose, batch-to-batch variability in toxin content, individual differences in toxin metabolism, and a genetically determined predisposition toward nephrotoxicity and/or carcinogenesis (Diamond and Pallone 1994).

In one of the two studies showing a link between Chinese herbal nephropathy and carcinogenesis, an increased dose of AA was associated with an enhanced risk of carcinoma (Nortier et al. 2000). Tissue samples revealed AA related DNA adducts, indicating a possible mechanism underlying the development of malignancy. The presence of these adducts was noted by Lord et al. (2001) reporting two patients with urolithelial malignancy and Chinese herbal nephropathy.

Another possible factor is the abnormal function of p53, a known tumour suppressor gene. In the second study showing a link between the nephropathy and carcinogenesis, all atypical cells were found to overexpress this protein, thereby suggesting the presence of a mutation in the gene (Cosyns et al. 1999).

In view of the important role of AA in the pathogenesis of this tubulointerstitial disease 'Aristolochia nephropathy' should thus preferably replace the previously used term of 'Chinese herb nephropathy'.

Presentation and prognosis

Affected patients typically present with renal insufficiency with other findings associated with primary tubulointerstitial disease. The blood pressure is either normal or only mildly elevated, protein excretion is only moderately increased (<1.5 g/day), and the urine sediment reveals only a few red and white cells. The elevation in protein excretion consists of both albumin and low molecular weight proteins that are filtered and then reabsorbed by the intact proximal tubule (Kabanda *et al.* 1995). Thus, tubular dysfunction contributes to the proteinuria.

The plasma creatinine concentration at presentation ranged from 1.4 to 12.7 mg/dl (123–1122 μmol/l) (Depierreux *et al.* 1994). Follow-up studies have revealed relatively stable renal function in most patients with an initial plasma creatinine concentration below 2 mg/dl (176 μmol/l) (Reginster *et al.* 1997). However, progressive renal failure resulting in eventual dialysis or transplantation may ensue in patients with more severe disease even if further exposure to Chinese herbs is prevented.

The risk for progressive disease increases with the duration of exposure.

An extremely similar clinical and pathologic process has been reported in a group of patients from Taiwan who had ingested a selection of uncontrolled traditional Chinese herbs that differed from those of the slimming regimen (Yang *et al.* 2000). Despite discontinuation of these remedies, progressive renal failure was common. Although the exact relation between this disorder and traditional Chinese herbal nephropathy associated with the slimming regimen is unclear, toxins common to different herbal remedies may cause interstitial renal fibrosis (Vanherweghem 2000).

Treatment

There is no proven effective therapy for this disorder which typically presents with marked interstitial fibrosis but not prominent inflammation. An uncontrolled study suggested that corticosteroids may slow the rate of loss of renal function (Vanherweghem *et al.* 1996).

The high incidence of cellular atypia of the genitourinary tract suggests that, at a minimum, these patients should undergo regular surveillance for abnormal urinary cytologies. Whether more aggressive management strategies, such as bilateral native nephroureterectomies (particularly in those undergoing renal transplantation), are required is unclear. Findings from a recent report support the more aggressive option (Cosyns *et al.* 1999).

Renal transplantation is an effective modality for those who progress to end-stage renal disease. One report noted no recurrence in five such patients (Reginster *et al.* 1997).

Lithium

Lithium is used extensively in the treatment of manic-depressive psychosis. Different forms of renal effects/injury have been described: most frequently nephrogenic diabetes insipidus, but also acute renal failure, renal tubular acidosis, chronic interstitial nephritis, nephrotic syndrome,

and focal–segmental glomerular sclerosis/global glomerular sclerosis. Hyperparathyroidism is rarely observed in lithium-treated patients.

Pathogenesis and pathology

Lithium is eliminated from the body almost entirely by the kidney, being filtered at the glomerulus and reabsorbed in the proximal tubule, resulting in a clearance of one-third of the normal creatinine clearance. It moves in and out of cells only slowly and accumulates in the kidney, particularly in the collecting tubule, entering these cells through sodium channels in the lumenal membrane. Its principal toxicity relates to distal tubular function, where inhibition of adenylate cyclase and generation of cyclic AMP results in downregulation of aquaporin-2, the collecting tubule water channel, and a decrease in antidiuretic hormone receptor density, leading to resistance to antidiuretic hormone. Hence, a defective concentrating capacity ensues. Further effects compound this. A low intracellular level of cyclic AMP leads to increased cellular levels of glycogen observed in kidney biopsy specimens from patients taking lithium, as does the fact that lithium also directly inhibits enzymes involved in glycogen breakdown. The ensuing glycogen storage may interfere with distal tubular function and be responsible for the observation that polyuria and polydipsia in lithium-treated patients is due to nephrogenic diabetes insipidus.

The tubular defect in the distal nephron can also impair the ability to maximally acidify the urine. A lithium-induced decrease in the activity of the H^+-ATPase pump in the collecting tubule may be responsible for this defect.

Lithium treatment has been aetiologically related to parathyroid hypertrophy and hyperfunction, the latter seeming to be due to an upward resetting of the level at which the plasma calcium concentration depresses parathyroid hormone (PTH) release. Persistent hypercalcaemia (in 5–10 per cent of the patients) may exacerbate both the concentrating defect and the interstitial nephritis seen in lithium-treated patients.

Renal biopsies from patients taking lithium show a specific histological lesion in the distal tubule and collecting duct. On light microscopy, there is swelling and vacuolization in cells associated with a considerable accumulation of periodic acid-Schiff (PAS)-positive glycogen. This is present in all renal biopsies from patients taking lithium, it appears within days after the administration of lithium and disappears when lithium ingestion is ceased.

Hestbech *et al.* (1977) were the first to suggest that progressive chronic interstitial lesions occurred in the kidneys of patients receiving lithium. However, a controlled study showed no difference between biopsies from patients taking lithium and those from a group of patients who had affective disorders but were not doing so. Specifically, there was no difference in the incidence of glomerular sclerosis, interstitial fibrosis, tubular atrophy, cast formation, or interstitial volume, but there was a significant increase in the number of microcysts in the lithium-treated patients. One reason why it has been difficult to answer the nature of lithium-induced chronic renal damage has been the lack, until recently, of an animal model in which lesions similar to those noted in human biopsies could be demonstrated. However, a recent study on lithium nephrotoxicity carried out in the rabbit showed clear-cut evidence of progressive histological and functional impairment, with the development of significant interstitial fibrosis, tubular atrophy, glomerular sclerosis, and cystic tubular lesions. A recent publication by Markowitz *et al.* (2000) revealed a chronic tubulointerstitial nephropathy in

100 per cent of 24 patients having received lithium for several years, associated with cortical and medullary tubular cysts or dilatation. There was also a surprisingly high prevalence of focal segmental glomerulosclerosis and global glomerulosclerosis, sometimes of equivalent severity to the chronic tubulointerstitial disease. Despite discontinuing lithium treatment, seven of nine patients with initial serum creatinine values above 2.5 mg/dl progressed to endstage renal disease. Nevertheless, an answer to the question as to whether or not chronic lithium therapy causes chronic interstitial nephritis still needs more hard data.

Clinical features

Chronic poisoning can occur in patients whose lithium dosage has been increased or in those with a decreased effective circulating volume, decreased sodium intake, diabetes mellitus, gastroenteritis, and renal failure, resulting in increased lithium reabsorption, hence increase in serum lithium levels (Table 6). Symptoms associated are related to plasma levels of lithium (Table 7).

Table 6 Drug interactions with lithium

Salt depletion strongly impairs renal elimination of lithium	
Salt loading increases absolute and fractional lithium clearance	
Diuretics	
Acetazolamide	Increased lithium clearance
Thiazides	Increased plasma lithium level due to decreased lithium clearance
Amiloride	Usually no change in plasma lithium level; may be used to treat lithium-induced polyuria
Non-steroidal anti-inflammatory drugs	Increased plasma lithium level due to decreased renal lithium clearance (exceptions are aspirin and sulindac)
Bronchodilators (aminophylline, theophylline)	Decreased plasma lithium level due to increased renal lithium clearance
Angiotensin-converting enzyme inhibitors	May increase plasma lithium level
Cyclosporin	Decreased lithium clearance

Table 7 Signs and symptoms of toxic effects of lithium

Toxic effect	Plasma lithium level	Signs and symptoms
Mild	1–1.5 mmol/l	Impaired concentration, lethargy, irritability, muscle weakness, tremor, slurred speech, nausea
Moderate	1.6–2.5 mmol/l	Diorientation, confusion, drowsiness, restlessness, unsteady gait, coarse tremor, dysarthria, muscle fasciculation, vomiting
Severe	>2.5 mmol/l	Impaired consciousness (with progression to coma), delirium, ataxia, generalized fasciculations, extrapyramidal symptoms, convulsions, impaired renal function

Chronic lithium poisoning is frequently associated with electrocardiogram changes including ST-segment depression and inverted T-waves in the lateral precordial leads. Lithium is concentrated within the thyroid and inhibits thyroid synthesis and release causing hypothyroidism and hypothermia. It may also cause thyrotoxicosis and hyperthermia. Symptoms of hypercalcaemia may also be present, such as exacerbating the concentrative defect already present in these patients. The classical symptoms observed in the context of glomerular lesions such as minimal change or focal glomerulus sclerosis can be seen. Proteinuria generally begins within 1.5 and 10 months after the onset of therapy and completely or partially resolves in most patients, 1, 2, or 4 weeks after lithium is discontinued. In several patients, reinstitution of lithium leads to recurrent nephrosis.

Diagnosis—treatment

Polyuria and polydispsia due to nephrogenic diabetes insipidus and other acute manifestations of the effect of lithium on the kidney usually disappear rapidly if lithium is withdrawn. The decision about management, however, usually revolves around relative benefit of the lithium in controlling and preventing the manifestation of manic-depressive psychosis and disadvantage to the patient of the major side-effect of lithium, namely, polyuria. In most cases, lithium is so clearly beneficial that the polyuria is accepted as a side-effect and lithium is continued. It is likely that the serum concentration of lithium is important, and that the renal damage is more likely to occur if the serum concentration is consistently high or if repeated lithium toxicity occurs. The serum lithium concentration should thus be monitored carefully (at least every 3 months) and maintained at the lowest level that will provide adequate control of the manic depressive psychosis.

Much more difficult to handle is the situation where a patient on long-term lithium therapy is found to have impaired renal function for which there is no obvious alternative cause. As stated above, renal failure may progress even if lithium therapy is withdrawn, and in some patients the discontinuation of lithium can lead to a devastating deterioration in their psychiatric condition. The decision as to whether or not to discontinue lithium should therefore be made after frank and open discussion, admitting all uncertainties, with the patient, psychiatric colleagues, and (if appropriate) relatives/carers.

ARF, with or without oliguria, can be associated with lithium treatment. In this case, ARF can be considered a prerenal type; consequently, it resolves rapidly with appropriate fluid therapy. Indeed, the histological appearance in such cases is remarkable for its lack of significant abnormalities. For conditions that stimulate sodium retention and, consequently, lithium reabsorption, such as low salt intake and loss of body fluid by way of vomiting, diarrhoea, or diuretics, decreasing lithium clearance should be avoided (Table 1). With any acute illness, particularly one associated with gastrointestinal symptoms such as diarrhoea, lithium blood levels should be closely monitored and the dose adjusted when necessary. Indeed, most episodes of acute lithium intoxication are largely predictable, and thus avoidable, provided that precautions are taken (Table 7).

Removing lithium from the body as soon as possible is the mainstay of treating lithium intoxication. With preserved renal function, excretion can be increased by use of frusemide, up to 40 mg/h, obviously under close monitoring for excessive losses of sodium and water induced by this loop diuretic. When renal function is impaired in association with severe toxicity, extracorporeal extraction is the most efficient way to decrease serum lithium levels. One should, however, remember that lithium leaves the cells slowly and that plasma levels rebound after haemodialysis is stopped, so that longer dialysis treatment at more frequent intervals is required.

Aminoglycosides

Nephrotoxicity and otovestibular toxicity remain frequent side-effects that seriously limit the use of aminoglycosides, a still important class of antibiotics. Aminoglycosides are highly charged, polycationic, hydrophilic drugs that cross biological membranes to a little extent, if at all (Kaloyanides and Pastoriza-Munoz 1980; Lietman 1985). They are not metabolized but are eliminated, unchanged, almost entirely by the kidneys. Aminoglycosides are filtered by the glomerulus at a rate almost equal to that of water. After entering the lumenal fluid of proximal renal tubule, a small but toxicologically important portion of the filtered drug is reabsorbed and stored in the proximal tubule cells. The major transport of aminoglycosides into proximal tubule cells involves interaction with acidic, negatively charged phospholipid-binding sites at the level of the brush border membrane. After charge-mediated

binding, the drug is taken up into the cell in small invaginations of the cell membrane, a process in which megalin plays a role (Molitoris 1997; Schmitz *et al.* 2001). Within 1 h of injection, the drug is located at the apical cytoplasmic vacuoles, called endocytotic vesicles. These vesicles fuse with lysosomes, sequestering the unchanged aminoglycosides inside those organelles. A small part (20 per cent) of the internalized aminoglycosides is shuttled to the Golgi complex (Sandoval *et al.* 2000). Once trapped in the lysosomes of proximal tubule cells, aminoglycosides electrostatically attached to anionic membrane phospholipids interfere with the normal action of some enzymes (i.e. phospholipases and sphingomyelinase). In parallel with enzyme inhibition, undigested phospholipids originating from the turnover of cell membranes accumulate in lysosomes, where they are normally digested. The overal result is lysosomal phospholipidosis due to non-specific accumulation of polar phospholipids as 'myeloid bodies', so called for their typical electron microscopic appearance (De Broe 1985) (Fig. 6).

Figure 6 shows the ultrastructural appearance of proximal tubule cells in aminoglycoside-treated patients (4 days of therapeutic doses). Lysosomes (large arrow) contain dense lamellar and concentric structures. Brush border, mitochondria (small arrows) and peroxisomes are

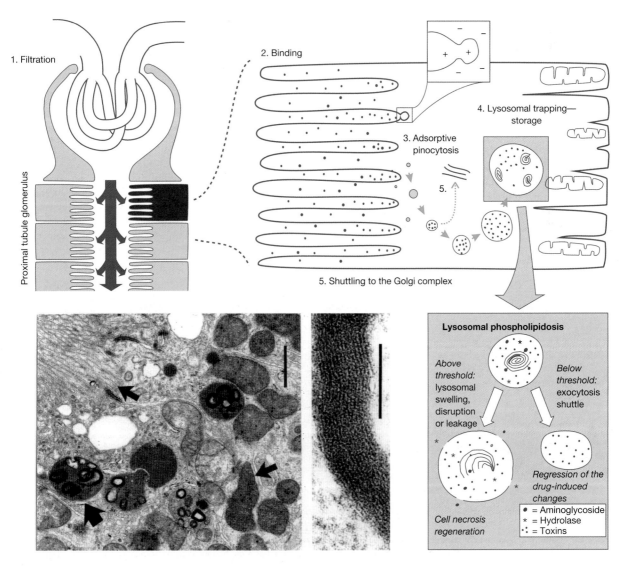

Fig. 6 Renal handling of aminoglycosides, resulting in lysosomal phospholipidosis and cell death (De Broe 1999b).

unaltered. At higher mangification, the structures in lysosomes show a periodic pattern. The bar in A represents 1 μm, in part B, 0.1 μm (De Broe *et al.* 1984).

Figure 6 shows the relationship between constant serum levels and concomitant renal cortical accumulation of gentamicin after a 6 h intravenous infusion in rats. The rate of accumulation is expressed in micrograms of aminoglycoside per gram of wet kidney cortex per hour, due to the linear accumulation in function of time. Each point represents one rat whose aminoglycosides were measured in both kidneys at the end of the infusion and the serum levels assayed twice during the infusion (Giuliano *et al.* 1986).

In rats, nephrotoxicity of gentamicin is more pronounced when the total daily dose is administered by continuous infusion rather than as a single injection. Thus, a given daily dose of drug does not produce the same degree of toxicity when it is given by different routes. Indeed, renal cortical uptake is 'less efficient' at high serum concentration than at low ones. A single injection results in high peak serum levels that overcome the saturation limits of the renal uptake mechanism. The high plasma concentrations are followed by fast elimination and, finally, absence of drug for a while. This contrasts with continuous low serum levels obtained with more frequent dosing when the uptake at the level of the renal cortex is not only more efficient but remains available throughout the treatment period (V_{max}—maximum velocity) (Fig. 7).

Two trials in humans found that the dosage schedule had a critical effect on renal uptake of gentamicin, netilmicin (Verpooten *et al.* 1989), amikacin, and tobramycin (De Broe *et al.* 1991). Subjects were patients with normal renal function (serum creatinine concentration between 0.9 and 1.2 mg/dl, proteinuria lower than 300 mg/24 h) who had renal cancer and submitted to nephrectomy. Before surgery, patients received gentamicin (4.5 mg/kg/day), netilmicin (5 mg/kg/day), amikacin (15 mg/kg/day), or tobramycin (4.5 mg/kg/day) as a single injection or as a continuous intravenous infusion over 24 h. The single-injection schedule resulted in 30–50 per cent lower cortical drug concentrations of netilmicin, gentamicin, and amikacin as compared with continuous infusion. For tobramycin, no difference in renal accumulation could be found, indicating the linear cortical uptake of this particular aminoglycoside

(Giuliano *et al.* 1986). These data, which supported decreased nephrotoxic potential of single-dose regimens, coincided with new insights in the antibacterial action of aminoglycosides (concentration-dependent killing of Gram-negative bacteria and prolonged postantibiotic effect) (Bennett *et al.* 1979). In a recent overview including all available information, Barclay *et al.* (1999) came to the conclusion that, to date, no controlled trials have compared methods of dose-individualization. In addition to a slight overall improvement in efficacy, once-daily administration has resulted in a small reduction in nephrotoxicity. In the studies using more sensitive measures of toxicity, the differences in toxicity were greater, strenghtening the case for once-daily administration. Therapeutic drug monitoring is probably required with once-daily administration.

In Table 8, risk factors for aminoglycoside nephrotoxicity are summarized. Several risk factors have been identified and classified as

Table 8 Risk factors for aminoglycoside nephrotoxicity

Patient-related factors	Aminoglycoside-related factors	Other drugs
Older age[a]	Recent aminoglycoside therapy	Amphotericin B
Pre-existing renal disease		Cephalosporins
Female gender	Larger doses[a]	Cisplatin
Magnesium, potassium, or calcium deficiency[a]	Treatment for 3 days or more[a]	Clindamycin
Intravascular volume depletion[a]		Cyclosporin
Hypotension[a]	Dose regimen[a]	Foscarnet
Hepatorenal syndrome		Frusemide
Sepsis syndrome		Piperacillin
		Radiocontrast agents
		Thyroid hormone

[a] Similar to experimental data.

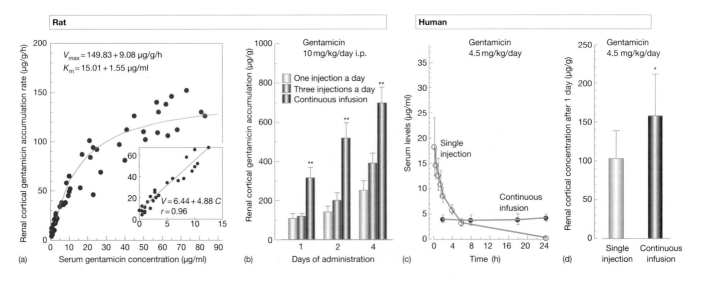

Fig. 7 Non-linear relationship between constant serum levels and concomitant renal cortical accumulation of an aminoglycoside (a). This renal handling pattern results in a higher cortical concentration when the aminoglycoside is administered as a continuous infusion compared to a single injection (b). The same characteristics are observed in humans (c, d). * = $p < 0.05$; ** = $p < 0.01$.

Table 9 Prevention of aminoglycoside nephrotoxicity

Identify risk factor
Patient related
Drug related
Other drugs
Give single daily dose of gentamicin, netilmicin, or amikacin
Reduce the treatment course as much as possible
Avoid giving nephrotoxic drugs concurrently
Make interval between aminoglycoside courses as long as possible
Calculate glomerular filtration rate out of serum creatinine concentration

patient related, aminoglycoside related, or related to concurrent administration of certain drugs.

The usual recommended aminoglycoside dose may be excessive for older patients because of decreased renal function and decreased regenerative capacity of a damaged kidney. Pre-existing renal disease clearly can expose patients to inadvertent overdosing if careful dose adjustment is not performed. Hypomagnesaemia, hypokalaemia, and calcium deficiency may be predisposing risk factors for consequences of aminoglycoside-induced damage (Moore *et al.* 1984). Liver disease is an important clinical risk factor for aminoglycoside nephrotoxicity, particularly in patients with cholestasis (Moore *et al.* 1984). Acute or chronic endotoxaemia amplifies the nephrotoxic potential of the aminoglycosides (Zager 1988).

Prevention (Table 9)

Coadministration of other potentially nephrotoxic drugs enhances or accelerates the nephrotoxicity of aminoglycosides. Comprehension of the pharmacokinetics and renal cell biological effects of aminoglycosides, allows identification of aminoglycoside-related nephrotoxicity risk factors and makes possible secondary prevention of this important clinical nephrotoxicity.

References

Abizaid, A. S. *et al.* (1999). Effects of dopamine and aminophylline on contrast-induced acute renal failure after coronary angioplasty in patients with preexisting renal insufficiency. *American Journal of Cardiology* **83** (2), 260–263, A5.

Andrade, L., Campos, S. B., and Seguro, A. C. (1998). Hypercholesterolemia aggravates radiocontrast nephrotoxicity: protective role of arginine. *Kidney International* **53**, 1736–1742.

Bakris, G. L. and Burnett, J. C. J. (1985). A role for calcium in radiocontrast-induced reductions in renal hemodynamics. *Kidney International* **27**, 465–468.

Baraldi, A. *et al.* (1998). Acute renal failure of medical type in an elderly population. *Nephrology, Dialysis, Transplantation* **13** (Suppl. 7), 25–29.

Barclay, M. L., Kirkpatrick, C. M., and Begg, E. J. (1999). Once daily aminoglycoside therapy. Is it less toxic than multiple daily doses and how should it be monitored? *Clinical Pharmacokinetics* **36** (2), 89–98.

Battenfeld, R. *et al.* (1991). Ioxaglate-induced light and electron microscopic alterations in the renal proximal tubular epithelium of rats. *Investigative Radiology* **26**, 35–39.

Bennett, W. M. and Porter, G. A. Overview of clinical nephrotoxicity. In *Toxicology of the Kidney* (ed. I. B. Hook and R. S. Goldstein), pp. 61–97. New York: Raven Press, 1993.

Bennett, W. M. *et al.* (1979). The influence of dosage regimen on experimental gentamicin nephrotoxicity: dissociation of peak serum levels from renal failure. *Journal of Infectious Diseases* **140** (4), 576–580.

Bettmann, M. A. (1991). The evaluation of contrast-related renal failure. *American Journal of Roentgenology* **157**, 66–68.

Bidani, A. K. and Churchill, P. C. (1983). Aminophylline ameliorates glycerol-induced acute renal failure in rats. *Canadian Journal of Physiology and Pharmacology* **61**, 567–571.

Bidani, A. K., Churchill, P. C., and Packer, W. (1987). Theophylline-induced protection in myoglobinuric acute renal failure: further characterization. *Canadian Journal of Physiology and Pharmacology* **65**, 42–45.

Bjorck, S. *et al.* (1990). Contrasting effects of enalapril and metoprolol on proteinuria in diabetic nephropathy. *British Medical Journal* **300**, 904–907.

Bombardier, C. *et al.* (2000). Comparison of upper gastrointestinal toxicity of rofecoxib and naproxen in patients with rheumatoid arthritis. *New England Journal of Medicine* **343**, 1520–1528.

Brenner, B. M. *et al.* (2001). Effects of losartan on renal and cardiovascular outcomes in patients with type 2 diabetes and nephropathy. *New England Journal of Medicine* **345**, 861–869.

Calder, I. C. *et al.* (1972). Nephrotoxic lesions from 5-aminosalicylic acid. *British Medical Journal* **1**, 152–154.

Caldicott, W. J., Hollenberg, N. K., and Abrams, H. L. (1970). Characteristics of response of renal vascular bed to contrast media. Evidence for vasoconstriction induced by renin-angiotensin system. *Investigative Radiology* **5**, 539–547.

Carraro, M. *et al.* (1996). Dose effect of nitrendipine on urinary enzymes and microproteins following non-ionic radiocontrast administration. *Nephrology, Dialysis, Transplantation* **11**, 444–448.

Clarck, B. A., Kim, D., and Epstein, F. H. (1997). Endothelin and atrial natriuretic peptide levels following radiocontrast exposure in humans. *American Journal of Kidney Diseases* **30**, 82–86.

Cosyns, J. P. *et al.* (1999). Urothelial lesions in Chinese-herb nephropathy. *American Journal of Kidney Diseases* **33** (6), 1011–1017.

Cosyns, J. P. *et al.* (2001). Chronic aristolochic acid toxicity in rabbits: a model of Chinese herbs nephropathy? *Kidney International* **59** (6), 2164–2173.

Cryer, B. *et al.* (1999). *In vivo* effects of rofecoxib, a new cyclooxygenase (COX)-inhibitor, on gastric mucosal prostaglandin (PG) and serum thromboxane (TXB2) synthesis in healthy humans. *Gastroenterology* **116**, G0611.

Davidman, M. *et al.* (1991). Iatrogenic renal disease. *Archives of Internal Medicine* **151**, 1809–1812.

Debelle, F. D. *et al.* (2002). Aristolochic acids induce chronic renal failure with interstitial fibrosis in salt-depleted rats. *Journal of the American Society of Nephrology* **13**, 431–436.

De Broe, M. E. Prevention of aminoglycoside nephrotoxicity. In *Proceedings EDTA–ERA* (ed. A. M. Davison and P. J. Guillou), pp. 959–973. London: Baillière Tindal, 1985.

De Broe, M. E. (1999a). On a nephrotoxic and carcinogenic slimming regiment. *American Journal of Kidney Diseases* **33**, 1171–1173.

De Broe, M. E. Renal injury due to environmental toxins, drugs, and contrast agents. In *Atlas of Diseases of the Kidney* (series ed. R. W. Schrier; ed. T. Berl and J. B. Bonventre), pp. 11.1–11.16. Philadelphia: Current Medicine, 1999b (http://www.kidneyatlas.org/book1/adk1_11.pdf).

De Broe, M. E. and Roch-Ramel, F. Renal handling of drugs and xenobiotics. In *Clinical Nephrotoxins—Renal Injury from Drugs and Chemicals* (ed. M. E. De Broe, G. A. Porter, W. M. Bennett, and G. A. Verpooten), pp. 13–30. Dordrecht: Kluwer Academic Publishers, 1998.

De Broe, M. E., Verbist, L., and Verpooten, G. A. (1991). Influence of dosage schedule on renal cortical accumulation of amikacin and tobramycin in man. *Journal of Antimicrobial Chemotherapy* **27** (Suppl. C), 41–47.

De Broe, M. E. *et al.* (1984). Early effects of gentamicin, tobramycin and amikacin on the human kidney. A prospective, comparative study. *Kidney International* **25**, 643–652.

de Jong, P. E. and Woods, L. L. Renal injury from angiotensin I converting enzyme inhibitors. In *Clinical Nephrotoxins—Renal Injury from Drugs and Chemicals* (ed. M. E. De Broe, G. A. Porter, W. M. Bennett, and G. A. Verpooten), pp. 239–250. Dordrecht: Kluwer Academic Publishers, 1998.

Depierreux, M., Van Damme, B., Vanden Houte, K., and Vanherweghem, J. L. (1994). Pathologic aspects of a newly described nephropathy related to the prolonged use of Chinese herbs. *American Journal of Kidney Diseases* 24, 172–180.

Deray, G. *et al.* (1990). A role for adenosine calcium and ischemia in radio-contrast-induced intrarenal vasoconstriction. *American Journal of Nephrology* 10, 316–322.

Diamond, J. R. and Pallone, T. L. (1994). Acute interstitial nephritis following use of Tung Shueh pills. *American Journal of Kidney Diseases* 24, 219–221.

Dobrota, M. *et al.* (1995). Biochemical and morphological effects of contrast media on the kidney. *Acta Radiology* (Suppl.) 399, 196–203.

Donadio, C. *et al.* (1988). Glomerular and tubular effects of ionic and nonionic contrast media (diatrizoate and iopamidol). *Contributions to Nephrology* 68, 212–219.

Duarte, C. G., Zhang, J., and Ellis, S. (1998). Effects of radiocontrast and endothelin administration on systolic blood pressure and renal damage in male spontaneously hypertensive and Wistar Kyoto rats with phentolamine-induced adrenergic blockade. *Investigative Radiology* 33, 104–112.

Dzgoeva, F. U. *et al.* (1999). Decrease in kidney nitric oxide formation detected by electron paramagnetic resonance in acute renal failure due to contrast media. *Nephron* 81, 441.

Elseviers, M. M. *et al.* (1995). High diagnostic performance of CT scan for analgesic nephropathy in patients with incipient to severe renal failure. *Kidney International* 48, 1316–1323.

Erley, C. M. *et al.* (1994). Adenosine antagonist theophylline prevents the reduction of glomerular filtration rate after contrast media application. *Kidney International* 45, 1425–1431.

Erley, C. M. *et al.* (1997). Prevention of radiocontrast-induced nephropathy by adenosine antagonists in rats with chronic nitric oxide deficiency. *Journal of the American Society of Nephrology* 8, 1125–1132.

Erley, C. M. *et al.* (1999). Prevention of radiocontrast-media-induced nephropathy in patients with preexisting renal insufficiency by hydration in combination with the adenosine antagonist theophylline. *Nephrology, Dialysis, Transplantation* 14, 1146–1149.

Feinfeld, D. A. *et al.* (1991). Interstitial nephritis in a patient receiving adoptive immunotherapy with recombinant interleukin-2 and lymphokine-activated killer cells. *American Journal of Nephrology* 11 (6), 489–492.

Fleury, D., Vanhille, P., Pallot, I. L., and Kleinknecht, D. (1990). Drug induced acute renal failure: a preventable disease linked to drug misuse. *Kidney International* 3, 1238.

Frankel, M. C., Weinstein, A. M., and Stenzel, K. H. (1983). Prognostic patterns in acute renal failure: the New York Hospital, 1981–1982. *Clinical Experimental Dialysis Apheresis* 7, 1457.

Fraval, H. N. A., Rawlings, C. J., and Roberts, J. J. (1978). Increased sensitivity of UV repair deficient human cells to DNA bound platinum products which unlike thymine dimers are not recognized by an endonuclease extracted from *Micrococcus leuteus. Mutation Research* 51, 121–132.

Gare, M. *et al.* (1999). The renal effect of low-dose dopamine in high-risk patients undergoing coronary angiography. *Journal of the American College of Cardiology* 34, 1682–1688.

Giuliano, R. A. *et al.* (1986). *In vivo* uptake kinetics of aminoglycosides in the kidney cortex of rats. *Journal of Pharmacology and Experimental Therapeutics* 236, 470–475.

Goldstein, J. L. *et al.* (2000). Reduced risk of upper gastrointestinal ulcer complications with celecoxib, a novel COX-2 inhibitor. *American Journal of Gastroenterology* 95, 1681–1690.

Gonzalez-Vitale, J. C., Hayes, D. M., Cvitkovic, E., and Sternberg, S. S. (1978). Acute renal failure after cis-dichlorodiammineplatinum(II) and gentamicin-cephalothin therapies. *Cancer Treatment Reports* 62 (5), 693–698.

Gouyon, J. B. and Guignard, J. P. (1988). Theophylline prevents the hypoxemia-induced renal hemodynamic changes in rabbits. *Kidney International* 33, 1078–1083.

Hans, B. *et al.* (1990). Renal functional response to dopamine during and after arteriography in patients with chronic renal insufficiency. *Radiology* 176, 651–654.

Hans, S. S. *et al.* (1998). Effect of dopamine on renal function after arteriography in patients with pre-existing renal insufficiency. *American Surgeon* 64, 432–436.

Heeg, J. E., de Jong, P. E., van der Hem, G. K., and de Zeeuw, D. (1987). Reduction of proteinuria by angiotensin converting enzyme inhibition. *Kidney International* 32, 78–83.

Heeg, J. E., de Jong, P. E., van der Hem, G. K., and de Zeeuw, D. (1989). Efficacy and variability of the antiproteinuric effect of ACE inhibition by lisinopril. *Kidney International* 36, 272–279.

Hestbech, J., Hansen, H. E., Amdisen, A., and Olsen, S. (1977). Chronic renal lesions following long-term treatment with lithium. *Kidney International* 12, 205–213.

Heyman, S. N., Rosen, S., and Brezis, M. (1994). Radiocontrast nephropathy: a paradigm for the synergism between toxic and hypoxic insults in the kidney. *Experimental Nephrology* 2, 153–157.

Heyman, S. N. *et al.* (1988). Acute renal failure with selective medullary injury in the rat. *Journal of Clinical Investigation* 82, 401–412.

Heyman, S. N. *et al.* (1991). Early renal medullary hypoxic injury from radiocontrast and indomethacin. *Kidney International* 40, 632–642.

Hou, S. H. *et al.* (1983). Hospital-acquired renal insufficiency: a prospective study. *American Journal of Medicine* 74, 243–248.

Hricik, D. E. *et al.* (1983). Captopril-induced functional renal insufficiency in patients with bilateral renal artery stenosis or renal artery stenosis in a solitary kidney. *New England Journal of Medicine* 308, 373–376.

Hunter, J. V. and Kind, P. R. N. (1992). Nonionic iodinated contrast media: potential renal damage assessed with enzymuria. *Radiology* 183, 101–104.

Jafar, T. *et al.* (2001). Angiotensin-converting enzyme inhibitors and progression of nondiabetic renal disease: a meta-analysis of patient-level data. *Annals of Internal Medicine* 135, 73–77.

Kabanda, A. *et al.* (1995). Low molecular weight proteinuria in Chinese herbs nephropathy. *Kidney International* 48, 1571–1576.

Kaloyanides, G. J. and Pastoriza-Munoz, E. (1980). Aminoglycoside nephrotoxicity. *Kidney International* 18, 571–582.

Kapoor, A. *et al.* (1996). Use of dopamine in prevention of contrast induced acute renal failure. A randomised study. *International Journal of Cardiology* 53, 233–236.

Katzberg, R. W. *et al.* (1977). Renal renin and hemodynamic responses to selective renal artery catheterization and angiography. *Investigative Radiology* 12, 381–388.

Kaufman, J., Dhakal, M., Patel, B., and Hamburger, R. (1991). Community-acquired acute renal failure. *American Journal of Kidney Diseases* 17, 191–198.

Khoury, Z. *et al.* (1995). The effect of prophylactic nifedipine on renal function in patients administered contrast media. *Pharmacotherapy* 15, 59–65.

Kleinknecht, D., Landais, P., and Goldfarb, B. (1986). Les insuffisances renales aigues associees 11 des medicaments OU 11 des produits de contraste iodes. Resultats d'une enquete cooperative multicentrique de la société de Néphrologie. *Néphrologie* 7, 41–46.

Koch, J. A., Plum, J., Graensee, B., and Modder, U. (2000). Prostaglandin E1: a new agent for the prevention of renal dysfunction in high risk patients caused by radiocontrast media? PEG1 Study Group. *Nephrology, Dialysis, Transplantation* 15, 43–49.

Krämer, B. K., Kammerl, M., Schweda, F., and Schreiber, M. (1999). A primer in radiocontrast-induced nephropathy. *Nephrology, Dialysis, Transplantation* 14, 2830–2834.

Kurnik, B. R. *et al.* (1998). Prospective study of atrial natriuretic peptide for the prevention of radiocontrast induced nephropathy. *American Journal of Kidney Diseases* 31, 674–680.

Langman, M. J. *et al.* (1999). Adverse upper gastrointestinal effects of rofecoxib compared with NSAIDs. *Journal of the American Medical Association* 282, 1929–1933.

Leese, P. T. *et al.* (2000). Effects of celecoxib, a new cyclooxygenase-2 inhibitor, on platelet function in healthy adults: a randomized controlled trial. *Journal of Clinical Pharmacology* **40**, 124–132.

Levy, E. M., Viscoli, C. M., and Horwitz, R. I. (1996). The effect of acute renal failure on mortality: a cohort analysis. *Journal of the American Medical Association* **275**, 1489–1494.

Lewis, E. J., Hunsicker, L. G., Bain, R. P., and Rohde, R. D. (1993). The effect of angiotensin-converting-enzyme inhibition on diabetic nephropathy. *New England Journal of Medicine* **329**, 1456–1462.

Lewis, E. J. *et al.* (2001). Renoprotective effect of the angiotensin-receptor antagonist irbesartan in patients with nephropathy due to type 2 diabetes. *New England Journal of Medicine* **345**, 851–859.

Lietman, S. Aminoglycosides and spectinoycin: aminocylitols. In *Principles and Practice of Infectious Diseases* 2nd edn., Part I (ed. G. L. Mandel, R. G. Doublas Jr., and J. E. Bennett), pp. 192–206. New York: John Wiley & Sons, 1985.

Lin, J. J., Churchill, P. C., and Bidani, A. K. (1986). Effect of theophylline on the initiation phase of postischemic acute renal failure in rats. *Journal of Laboratory and Clinical Medicine* **108**, 150–154.

Lin, J. J., Churchill, P. C., and Bidani, A. K. (1988). Theophylline in rats during maintenance phase of post-ischemic acute renal failure. *Kidney International* **33**, 24–28.

Lipsky, P. E. *et al.* (1998). The classification of cyclooxygenase inhibitors. *Journal of Rheumatology* **25**, 2298–2303.

Lord, G. M. *et al.* (2001). Urothelial malignant disease and Chinese herbal nephropathy. *Lancet* **358**, 1515–1516.

Lufft, V. *et al.* (2002). Contrast media nephropathy: intravenous CT angiography versus intraarterial digital substraction angiography in renal artery stenosis: a prospective randomized trial. *American Journal of Kidney Diseases* **40**, 236–242.

Markowitz, G. S. *et al.* (2000). Lithium nephrotoxicity: a progressive combined glomerular and tubulointerstitial nephropathy. *Journal of the American Society of Nephrology* **11**, 1439–1448.

Maschio, G. *et al.* (1996). Effect of the angiotensin-converting-enzyme inhibitor benazepril on the progression of chronic renal insufficiency. *New England Journal of Medicine* **334**, 939–945.

McCarthy, C. S. and Becker, J. A. (1992). Multiple myeloma and contrast media. *Radiology* **183**, 519–521.

Mitchell, J. A. *et al.* (1994). Selectivity of nonsteroidal antiinflammatory drugs as inhibitors of constitutive and inducible cyclooxygenase. *Proceedings of the National Academy of Sciences USA* **90**, 11693–11697.

Molitoris, B. A. (1997). Cell biology of aminoglycoside nephrotoxicity: newer aspects. *Current Opinion in Nephrology and Hypertension* **6**, 384–388.

Moore, R. D., Smith, C. R., Lipsky, J. J., Mellits, E. D., and Lietman, P. S. (1984). Risk factors for nephrotoxicity in patients treated with aminoglycosides. *Annals of Internal Medicine* **100** (3), 352–357.

Moreau, J. F. *et al.* (1975). Osmotic nephrosis induced by water soluble triiodinated contrast media in man. *Radiology* **115**, 329–336.

Murphy, S. W., Barrett, B. J., and Parfrey, P. S. (2000). Contrast nephropathy. *Journal of the American Society of Nephrology* **11**, 177–182.

Neumayer, H. H., Gellert, J., and Luft, F. C. (1993). Calcium antagonists and renal protection. *Renal Failure* **15**, 353–358.

Nolan, C. R. and Anderson, R. J. (1998). Hospital—acquired acute renal failure. *Journal of the American Society of Nephrology* **9**, 710–718.

Nortier, J. L. *et al.* (2000). Urothelial carcinoma associated with the use of a Chinese herb (Aristolochia fangchi). *New England Journal of Medicine* **342**, 1686–1692.

Nuyts, G. D. *et al.* (1995). New occupational risk factors for chronic renal failure. *Lancet* **346**, 7–11.

Opie, L. H. The renin–angiotensin–aldosterone system and otehr proposed sites of action of angiotensin-converting enzyme inhibitors. In *Angiotensin Converting Enzyme Inhibitors—Scientific Basis for Clinical Use* 2nd ed. (ed. L. Hopie), pp. 1–22. New York: Wiley-Liss, 1992.

Osswald, H., Helminger, I., Jendralski, A., and Abrar, B. (1979). Improvement of renal function by theophylline in the acute renal failure of the rat. *Naunyn-Schmiedeberg's Archives of Pharmacology* **307**, R47 (abstract).

Osswald, H., Schmitz, H. J., and Heidenreich, O. (1975). Adenosine response of the rat kidney after saline loading, sodium restriction and hemorrhagia. *Pflugers Archives* **357**, 323–333.

Parving, H. H. *et al.* (2001). The effect of irbesartan on the development of diabetic nephropathy in patients with type 2 diabetes. *New England Journal of Medicine* **345**, 870–878.

Perneger, T. V., Whelton, P. K., and Klag, M. J. (1994). Risk of kidney failure associated with the used of acetaminophen, aspirin, and nonsteroidal anti-inflammatory drugs. *New England Journal of Medicine* **331**, 1675–1679.

Philip, T. *et al.* (1989). Interleukine-2 with and without LAK cells in renal cell carcinoma: the Lyon first-year experience with 20 patients. *Cancer Treatment Reviews* **13** (Suppl. A), 91–104.

Pollock, D. M., Polakowsky, J. S., Wegner, C. D., and Opgenorth, T. H. (1997). Beneficial effect of ETA receptor blockade in a rat model of radiocontrast-induced nephropathy. *Renal Failure* **19**, 753–761.

Ponce, P. *et al.* (1993). Renal toxicity mediated by continuous infusion of recombinant interleukin-2. *Nephron* **64** (1), 114–118.

Porter, G. A. (1994a). Contrast-associated nephropathy: presentation, pathophysiology and management. *Mineral and Electrolyte Metabolism* **20**, 232–243.

Porter, G. A. (1994b). Urinary biomarkers and nephrotoxicity. *Mineral and Electrolyte Metabolism* **20**, 181–186.

Pru, C., Ebben, J., and Kjellstrand, C. (1982). Chronic renal failure after acute tubular necrosis. *Kidney International* **21**, 176.

Ramesh, G. and Reeves, W. B. (2002). TNF-α mediates chemokine and cytokine expression and renal injury in cisplatin nephrotoxicity. *Journal of Clinical Investigation* **110**, 835–842.

Rasmussen, H. H. and Ibels, L. S. (1982). Acute renal failure: multi variant analysis of causes and risk factors. *American Journal of Medicine* **73**, 211–218.

Reams, G. P. and Bauer, J. H. (1986). Effect of enalapril in subjects with hypertension associated with moderate to severe renal dysfunction. *Archives of Internal Medicine* **146**, 2145–2148.

Reginster, F., Jadoul, M., and van Ypersele de Strihou, C. (1997). Chinese herbs nephropathy presentation, natural history and fate after transplantation. *Nephrology, Dialysis, Transplantation* **12**, 81–86.

Rosa, F. W. *et al.* (1989). Neonatal anuria with maternal angiotensin-converting enzyme inhibition. *Obstetrics and Gynecology* **74**, 371–374.

Rosenstein, M., Ettinghausen, S. E., and Rosenberg, S. A. (1986). Extravasation of intravascular fluid wediated by the systemic administration of recombinant interleukin-2. *Journal of Immunology* **137**, 1735–1742.

Rosovsky, M. A. *et al.* (1996). High-dose administration of nonionic contrast media: a retrospective review. *Radiology* **200**, 119–122.

Rossi, N. *et al.* (1990). The role of adenosine in HgCl$_2$-induced acute renal failure in rats. *American Journal of Physiology* **258**, F1554–1560.

Rudnick, M. R. *et al.* (1995). Nephrotoxicity of ionic and nonionic contrast media in 1196 patients: a randomized trial. The Iohexol Cooperative Study. *Kidney International* **47**, 254–261.

Rudnicki, M., Berns, J. S., Cohen, R. M., and Goldfarb, S. (1996). Contrast media-associated nephrotoxicity. *Current Opinions in Nephrology and Hypertension* **5**, 127–133.

Ruggenenti, P. *et al.* (1999). Renoprotective properties of ACE-inhibition in non-diabetic nephropathies with non-nephrotic proteinuria. *Lancet* **354**, 359–364.

Rush, G. F., Smith, J. H., Newton, J. F., and Hook, J. B. (1984). Chemically induced nephrotoxicity: role of metabolic activation. *Critical Reviews in Toxicology* **13**, 99–160.

Russo, D., Testa, A., Volpe, L. D., and Sansone, G. (1990). Randomised prospective study on renal effects of two different contrast media in humans: protective role of a calcium channel blocker. *Nephron* **55**, 254–257.

Salem, P., Khalyl, M., Jabboury, K., and Hashimi, L. (1984). Cisdiaminedichloroplatinium [II] by a 5-day continuous infusion. *Cancer* **53**, 837–840.

Sandler, D. P., Burr, F. R., and Weinberg, C. R. (1991). Nonsteroidal anti-inflammatory drugs and the risk of chronic renal disease. *Annals of Internal Medicine* **115**, 165–172.

Sandoval, R. M., Dunn, K. W., and Molitoris, B. A. (2000). Gentamicin traffics rapidly and directly to the Golgi complex in LLC-PK(1) cells. *American Journal of Physiology, Renal Physiology* **279** (5), F884–F890.

Schmitz, C., Hilpert, J., Jacobsen, C., Boensch, C., Christensen, E. I., Luft, F. C., and Willnow, T. E. (2001). Megalin deficiency offers protection from renal aminoglycoside accumulation. *Journal of Biological Chemistry* **277**, 618–622.

Schwarz, A. *et al.* (2000). The outcome of acute interstitial nephritis: risk factors for the transition from acute to chronic interstitial nephritis. *Clinical Nephrology* **54**, 179–190.

Segasothy, M., Samad, S. A., Zulfigar, A., and Bennett, W. M. (1996). Chronic renal disease and papillary necrosis associated with long-term use of nonsteroidal anti-inflammatory drugs as the sole or predominate analgesic. *American Journal of Kidney Diseases* **24**, 17–24.

Silverstein, F. E. *et al.* (2000). Gastrointestinal toxicity with celecoxib versus nonsteroidal anti-inflammatory drugs for osteoarthritis and rheumatoid arthritis. The CLASS study: a randomized controlled trial. *Journal of the American Medical Association* **284**, 1247–1255.

Sketch, M. H. J. *et al.* (2001). Prevention of contrast media-induced renal dysfunction with prostaglandin E1: a randomized, double-blind, placebo-controlled study. *American Journal of Therapeutics* **8**, 155–162.

Smith, W. R., Neil, J., Cusham, W. C., and Butkus, D. E. (1989). Captopril associated acute interstitial nephritis. *American Journal of Nephrology* **9**, 230–235.

Spangberg Viklund, B. *et al.* (1996). Does prophylactic treatment with felodipine, a calcium antagonist, prevent low-osmolar contrast-induced renal dysfunction in hydrated diabetic and nondiabetic patients with normal or moderately reduced renal function? *Scandinavian Journal of Urology and Nephrology* **30**, 63–68.

Taguma, Y. *et al.* (1985). Effect of captopril on heavy proteinuria in azotemic diabetes. *New England Journal of Medicine* **313**, 1617–1620.

Tepel, M. *et al.* (2000). Prevention of radiographic-contrast-agent-induced reductions in renal function by acetylcysteine. *New England Journal of Medicine* **343**, 180–184.

Tervahartiala, P. *et al.* (1997). Structural changes in the renal proximal tubular cells induced by iodinated contrast media. *Nephron* **76**, 96–102.

Textor, S. C. (1990). ACE inhibitors in renovascular hypertension. *Cardiovascular Drugs and Therapy* **4**, 229–235.

The GISEN Group (Gruppo Italiano di Studi Epidemiologici in Nefrologia) (1997). Randomised placebo-controlled trial of effect of ramipril on decline in glomerular filtration rate and risk of terminal renal failure in proteinuric, non-diabetic nephropathy. *Lancet* **349**, 1857–1863.

Tune, B. The nephrotoxicity of cephalosporin antibiotics (1993). Structure-activity relationship. *Community Toxicology* **1**, 145–157.

Valsveld, L. T. *et al.* (1993). Possible role for cytotoxic lymphocytes in the pathogenesis of acute interstitial nephritis after recombinant interleukin-2

treatment for renal cell cancer. *Cancer Immunology, Immunotherapy* **36** (3), 210–213.

Vanherweghem, J. L. (2000). Nephropathy and herbal medicine. *American Journal of Kidney Diseases* **35**, 330–332.

Vanherweghem, J. L., Abramowicz, D., Tielemans, C., and Depierreux, M. (1996). Effects of steroids on the progression of renal failure in chronic interstitial renal fibrosis: a pilot study in Chinese herbs nephropathy. *American Journal of Kidney Diseases* **27**, 209–215.

Verburg, K. M. *et al.* (2001). COX-2–specific inhibitors: definition of a new therapeutic concept. *American Journal of Therapeutics* **8**, 49–64.

Verpooten, G. A. *et al.* (1989). Once-daily dosing decreases renal accumulation of gentamicin and netilmicin. *Clinical Pharmacology and Therapeutics* **45**, 22–27.

Vijayan, A. and Miller, S. B. (1998). Acute renal failure: prevention and non-dialytic therapy. *Seminars in Nephrology* **18**, 523–532.

Wang, A. *et al.* (2000). Exacerbation of radiocontrast nephrotoxicity by endothelin receptor antagonism. *Kidney International* **57**, 1675–1680.

Webb, D. E. *et al.* (1988). Metabolic and renal effects of interleukin-2 immunotherapy for metastatic cancer. *Clinical Nephrology* **30** (3), 141–145.

Weisberg, L. S., Kurnik, P. B., and Kurnik, B. R. (1993). Dopamine and renal blood flow in radiocontrast-induced nephropathy in humans. *Renal Failure* **15**, 61–68.

Whelton, A. (2000). Renal and related cardiovascular effects of conventional and COX-2 specific NSAIDs and non-NSAID analgesics. *American Journal of Therapeutics* **7**, 63–74.

Whelton, A. and Watson, A. J. Nonsteroidal anti-inflammatory drugs: effectson kidney function. In *Clinical Nephrotoxins—Renal Injury from Drugs and Chemicals* (ed. M. E. De Broe, G. A. Porter, W. M. Bennett, and G. A. Verpooten), pp. 203–216. Dordrecht: Kluwer Academic Publishers, 1998.

Wing, A. J. *et al.* (1983). Combined report on regular dialysis and transplantation in Europe XIII acute (reversible) renal failure. *Proceedings of the European Dialysis and Transplantation Association* **20**, 64–71.

World, M. J., Stevens, P. E., Ashton, M. A., and Rainford, D. J. (1996). Mesalazine-associated interstitial nephritis. *Nephrology, Dialysis, Transplantation* **11**, 614–621.

Yang, C.-S., Lin, C.-H., Chang, S.-H., and Hsu, H.-C. (2000). Rapidly progressive fibrosing interstitial nephritis associated with Chinese herbal drugs. *American Journal of Kidney Diseases* **35**, 313–318.

Yao, K., Heyne, N., Erley, C. M., Risler, T., and Osswald, H. (2001). The selective adenosine A1 receptor antagonist KW-3902 prevents radiocontrast media-induced nephropathy in rats with chronic nitric oxide deficiency. *European Journal of Pharmacology* **414**, 99–104.

Zager, R. A. (1988). A focus of tissue necrosis increases renal susceptibility to gentamicin administration. *Kidney International* **33**, 84–90.

Zambraski, E. J. (1995). The effects of nonsteroidal anti-inflammatory drugs on renal function: experimental studies in animals. *Seminars in Nephrology* **15**, 205–213.

19.2 Handling of drugs in kidney disease

D.J.S. Carmichael

Introduction

Many drugs and their metabolites are excreted by the kidney by glomerular filtration, tubular secretion, or in some cases both. Renal impairment has a significant effect on clearance of these drugs, with important clinical consequences. These are most obvious in patients with overt renal failure; more subtle forms of renal dysfunction may also be important and are extremely common, most notably as a result of ageing (see Chapter 1.5). Patients on renal replacement therapy are often taking a large number of drugs of increasing complexity and possible interaction. There is also an increased use of antihypertensive agents, lipid lowering drugs, and drugs such as bisphosphonates and antimicrobials to counteract or prevent adverse effects of corticosteroids and immunosuppressive agents, in routine nephrological practice. Although in theory changes in dosage and dose interval of all drugs, which are affected by renal impairment, should be considered, in practice dose adjustment is necessary for relatively few drugs, the most important of which are those with a narrow therapeutic index or adverse effects related to drug or metabolite accumulation. The corollary is that drugs are often prescribed in greater doses than are necessary to achieve therapeutic plasma concentrations. This is less likely to occur when the drug is started at a low dose and titrated against a therapeutic effect (antihypertensives).

Although renal impairment has its most important effect upon excretion, other aspects of pharmacokinetics (absorption, distribution including protein binding, metabolism, and renal haemodynamics) and pharmacodynamics may be altered.

The major determinant of alteration in dosage of a drug is the change in clearance, which can be estimated by measuring the glomerular filtration rate (GFR) (Dettli 1983). However, tubular secretion of drugs (Reidenberg 1985) does not always change in parallel with GFR. There may also be independent alterations in pharmacokinetics due to extrarenal factors (Gibaldi 1977; Hinderling 2001). There are many handbooks (some in electronic form), which provide guidelines for the adjustment of dosage in renal impairment. Many of these data are derived from measurement or estimation of changes in clearance, half-life ($t_{1/2}$) and volume of distribution (V_d). However, the determination of these pharmacokinetic variables is very model-dependent and their application has limitations. Many assumptions are made in calculating half-lives; particularly that a drug follows first order kinetics. It has even been suggested that calculated half-lives are often wrong (Wright and Boddy 2001), but may still be a useful guide to prescribing. Despite these reservations it is valid to know how a particular drug is handled in the presence of renal impairment. This information should be used in conjunction with drug history and pharmacodynamic endpoints. Consequently, the guidelines should only be regarded as useful approximations. They cannot be expected to overcome the major errors made when prescribing in renal disease, namely

(1) ignorance of renal impairment before a drug is prescribed;

(2) ignorance of how a drug is cleared from the body;

(3) failure to monitor therapeutic and adverse effects.

This chapter considers the basic pharmacokinetic changes that occur in the presence of impaired renal function and how they affect drug usage. The effects of haemodialysis, haemofiltration, haemodiafiltration, and peritoneal dialysis (PD) are considered. Common therapeutic problems, with an emphasis on newer drugs, in patients with impaired renal function are illustrated.

Pharmacokinetics

Absorption

Gastrointestinal

Ammonia production occurs in the stomach in chronic renal failure, concomitant with urea accumulation and hydrolysis. Ammonia buffers hydrochloric acid, causing an increase in gastric pH. Consequently, there may be reduced absorption of drugs such as ferrous sulfate, folic acid, pindolol, and cloxacillin whose absorption is greater at acid pH. Aluminium hydroxide, which is used as a phosphate binding agent may also bind several drugs including ciprofloxacin, aspirin, and iron, and therefore should not be administered simultaneously with these agents. Ascorbic acid given with ferrous sulfate may aid the absorption although oral iron is prescribed less frequently with the widespread use of intravenous iron preparations in patients on erythropoietin. Most drugs are absorbed in the proximal small intestines, D-xylose absorption is reduced by renal failure (Craig *et al.* 1983), but malabsorption of drugs does not appear to be a major problem in uraemia. Diuretic resistance is reported to occur in the nephrotic syndrome and with congestive cardiac failure as a consequence of poor intestinal absorption (Huang *et al.* 1980; Odlind and Beerman 1980), although more probable explanations such as binding to tubular protein or reduction in renal blood flow seem more likely (Wilcox 2002).

Peritoneal

The peritoneum is used as an absorptive surface during PD in patients with peritonitis. The transfer of some antibiotics is bidirectional although it is primarily from the peritoneum to the circulation;

absorption of gentamicin is unidirectional from peritoneum to plasma (Somani *et al.* 1982). The investigation of drug clearance in PD is discussed separately below. Although the peritoneum can be used for the administration of insulin, this practice is now less common. There are several confounding factors. Balducci (1982) observed that insulin was better absorbed from an empty peritoneum, concluding that the presence of dialysate reduced absorption by lowering the insulin concentration in the PD fluid. PD such as continuous cycling dialysis (Diaz-Buxo 2000), and use of different dialysate solutions are also important (Williams *et al.* 2000). Apart from the inconvenience of administration in these circumstances, such use of intraperitoneal insulin becomes uneconomical (Quellhorst 2002). Insulin absorption may vary from patient to patient (38 per cent range 17–66 per cent) with the variation not accounted for by changes in membrane transport characteristics (Fine *et al.* 2000). During peritonitis insulin requirements may decline as absorption increases with mesothelial damage.

Distribution

Protein binding is affected by renal impairment, which is accompanied by increased concentrations in plasma of a number of acidic compounds that compete for binding sites on albumin and other plasma proteins (Reidenberg 1983; Tillement *et al.* 1983). Some of these have been identified: indoxyl sulfate and 2-hydroxyhippuric acid (Bowmer and Lindup 1982), 3-carboxy-4-methyl-5propyl-2-furanpropanoic acid which inhibits phenytoin binding (Mahuchi and Nakahashi 1988), 2-hydroxybenzoylglycine (Lichtenwalner and Suh 1983), and free fatty acids (Bowmer and Lindup 1982). Serum albumin concentration is low in patients with the nephrotic syndrome and may also decline in cachectic patients and in elderly people, reducing the number of drug-binding sites. As a consequence, the proportion of free to bound drug is increased, and there is greater fluctuations in the free drug concentration following the administration of each dose. This could be responsible for an increased susceptibility to adverse drug reactions (Lewis *et al.* 1971; Gugler and Azarnoff 1983). The binding of a variety of drugs has been evaluated in renal impairment *in vivo* and *in vitro* (Table 1) (Biaski 1980; Gulyassy and Depner 1983; Reidenberg 1983; Tillement *et al.* 1983; Webb *et al.* 1986; Kapstein *et al.* 1987; Vanholder *et al.* 1988) but few appear to be of clinical significance.

Routine measurement of the plasma drug concentration includes both bound and unbound (free) drug. Binding of phenytoin to plasma protein is reduced in direct proportion to the reduction in GFR (Brater 1994). The proportion of free (active) drug increases for a fixed total plasma concentration. Furthermore, this free fraction can be removed by dialysis (Dasgupta and Abu-Alfa 1992). These factors should be noted when prescribing phenytoin; any adjustments should be small (50 mg at a time) to avoid adverse effects. Tissue binding of digoxin (and consequently its volume of distribution) declines in renal failure and a smaller loading dose is needed. The effect of reduced digoxin clearance as GFR diminishes is even more important, and a lower maintenance dose is required than in patients with normal renal function. Monitoring the plasma concentration is often of use especially if digoxin is being used for its inotropic action (which is relatively difficult to gauge clinically), in contrast to its effect on ventricular response in patients with atrial fibrillation. In the anephric patient, the elimination of digoxin by non-renal mechanisms usually permits a dose of approximately 0.125 mg on alternate days (Kuop *et al.* 1975). Volume of distribution may alter in renal failure because of fluid retention and expansion of the circulating blood volume, alteration in protein and tissue binding, and alterations in the proportion of fat and muscle in the body. In the elderly, fat increases as a proportion of total body weight by approximately 25 per cent in men and 40 per cent in women, and this leads to an increase in volume of distribution for lipid-soluble drugs (Herman *et al.* 1985; Hammerstein *et al.* 1998; Joest *et al.* 1999).

Metabolism

The majority of drugs are excreted by the kidney either as the original compound or after metabolism in the liver to more polar (water-soluble) substances. Uraemia may affect drug metabolism (Gibson 1986) and reduces the non-renal clearance of drugs such as acyclovir, aztreonam, moxolactam, cefotaxime, captopril, cimetidine, and metoclopramide. This alteration in clearance is minor in comparison to the retention in renal impairment of metabolites that have therapeutic or adverse effects (Table 2) (Palmer and Lasseter 1975; Verbreeck *et al.* 1981; Drayer 1983). Measurements of plasma drug concentrations for therapeutic monitoring

Table 1 Alteration in drug binding in renal impairment

Reduced	Unaltered	Increased
Theophylline	Indomethacin	Imipramine
Phenytoin	Metoclopramide	
Methotrexate	Trimethoprim	
Diazepam	D-Tubocurarine	
Frusemide	Quinidine	
Dicloxacillin	Dapsone	
Warfarin		
Barbiturates		
Clofibrate		
Salicylates		
Morphine		

Table 2 Parent drugs, metabolites, and possible adverse effects

Drug	Metabolite	Effect of metabolite
Allopurinol	Oxypurinol	Causes rashes
Clofibrate	Chloro phenoxy-isobutyric acid	Muscle damage, neuropathy
Nitroprusside	Thiocyanate	Toxic symptoms
Primodone	Phenobarbitone	Active drug
Procainamide	N-acetyl procainamide	Antiarrhythmic
Sulfonamides	Acetylsulfonamides	Rashes
Pethidine	Norpethidine	Causes seizures
Morphine	Morphine-6-glucuronide	Prolongs analgesia
Codeine	Morphine	Prolongs analgesia and respiratory depression
Propoxyphene	Norpropoxyphene	Cardiotoxic
Acebutalol	N-acetyl analogue	Confers selectivity
Nitrofurantoin	Nitrofuratoin metabolite	Peripheral neuropathy

must be interpreted cautiously. Not only is there the possibility of the free fraction of the drug being altered (as discussed above in the case of phenytoin), but assays of imperfect specificity may also detect accumulating metabolites (active or inactive) confounding interpretation. It is of significance when metabolites of drugs are retained in the plasma in the presence of renal impairment. The retention of these metabolites appears to reduce the proportion of active drug available; for example, the area under the curve for celecoxib specific cyclo-oxygenase 2 inhibitor (COX-2 inhibitor) is reduced in renal impairment (Davies *et al.* 2000). The situation may be more complex. Mycophenotic and mycophenolic acid (MPA), the active form of mycophenolate mofetil (MMF) is avidly protein bound and only the free portion is active. This binding may be reduced in uraemia and in addition MPA may also be displaced by its metabolite MPA-glucuronide (MPAG), which is renally excreted and therefore retained in the presence of renal impairment (Meier-Kriesche *et al.* 2000). Metabolites may not only cause adverse effects but also indirectly affect drug concentrations.

Renal failure may reduce drug metabolism, for instance, the conversion of sulindac to its sulfide metabolite is reduced in uraemia (Gibson *et al.* 1987), which has been invoked as a partial explanation for the lower incidence of adverse effects as compared to indomethacin (Berg and Talseth 1985).

The kidney synthesizes $1,25(OH)_2$ vitamin D_3 from its precursor $25(OH)D_3$. In chronic renal impairment this metabolism is reduced. Metabolism of $24,25-(OH)_2D_3$ is also affected. The synthetic analogue $1-\alpha(OH)D_3$ is converted to $1,25(OH)D_3$, *in vivo* and is used therapeutically.

Presystemic ('first pass') metabolism by the liver of some drugs such as propranolol and cimetidine may be reduced in renal impairment causing increases in plasma concentrations.

Renal excretion

Renal excretion of drugs depends upon

(1) filtration;

(2) active tubular secretion and reabsorption;

(3) passive diffusion.

Renal clearance of drugs can be expressed as function of GFR, the fraction of the drug that is unbound or free in plasma, secretion, and reabsorption (Gibaldi 1984). Compounds with a molecular weight below 60,000 Da are filtered to a variable extent (depending on molecular size) through the glomerulus unless they are protein bound, in which case only the unbound portion is filtered.

$$Cl_R = f_u \times GFR + secretion - reabsorption$$

where, Cl_R is the renal clearance and f_u the fraction of unbound drug (available for filtration). Therefore, if Cl_R is lower than $GFR \times f_u$, then reabsorption (usually passive) must be taking place, and if Cl_R is greater than $GFR \times f_u$ then secretion must be taking place.

Compounds with a molecular mass of less than 60,000 Da are filtered through the glomerulus to a variable extent, depending on molecular size, unless they are protein bound when only the unbound portion is altered. Non-polar (lipid soluble) drugs diffuse readily across tubular cells, whereas polar (water soluble) compounds do not. Since less than 1 per cent of the volume filtered is usually excreted as urine, drugs in tubular fluid become concentrated relative to plasma

as water is reabsorbed. Polar drugs generally remain in the tubular fluid and are excreted in the urine, while non-polar drugs are reabsorbed by passive diffusion down their concentration gradient into plasma. Some polar drugs are eliminated in the urine as a result of active or facilitated transport mechanisms that transport organic acids or bases.

Many drugs are metabolized, primarily in the liver, to produce more polar compounds, which cannot be passively reabsorbed and so are eliminated in the urine. However, there may be reduced clearance of these metabolites, which could have therapeutic or adverse effects (see Table 2).

Organic acids (e.g. penicillins, cephalosporins, salicylates, frusemide, and thiazides) and organic bases (e.g. amiloride, procainamide, and quinidine) have active tubular secretion. In addition, some drugs interact to inhibit tubular secretion of others (e.g. probenecid with penicillins, with cephalosporins, and with frusemide). Elimination of organic acids (AH) or bases (B) is affected by the H^+ ion concentration of the tubular fluid with any change of urinary pH that favours ionization leading to more drug excretion:

$$pK_B$$
$$H^+ + B \rightleftarrows BH^+$$
$$AH \rightleftarrows H^+ + A^-$$
$$pK_A$$

The amount of ionized drug at any particular pH is determined by its pK. The pK is the pH at which 50 per cent of the drug is ionized. If an organic acid has a pK_A less than 7.5, making the urine alkaline (i.e. increasing its pH) increases the amount of ionized drug (A^-) and therefore its excretion. The converse is true for organic bases with a pK_B greater than 7.5, which are eliminated as the charged (BH^+) form favoured by acid pH. The excretions of salicylates (weak acids) and amphetamines (weak bases) exemplify these principles and underlie the rationale for alkaline diuresis in the treatment of salicylate poisoning. Drugs present in tubular fluid may affect the excretion of other compounds: for example, aspirin and paracetamol reduce the excretion of methotrexate (Reidenberg 1985). A low protein diet reduces the acidity of the urine and may thereby lead to increased reabsorption of oxypurinol, a metabolite of allopurinol that is thought to be responsible for some of the adverse side effects of allopurinol (Berlinger *et al.* 1985; Kitt *et al.* 1989).

Although it is a simplification to disregard the tubular handling of drugs in renal impairment, both filtration and secretion of drugs appear to fall in parallel and in proportion to GFR. The most important aspect of prescribing in renal disease is awareness of the existence of renal impairment and of changes in renal function.

Measurement of glomerular filtration

Some measure of GFR is needed. In practice, the measurement of endogenous creatinine clearance or the estimation of creatinine clearance from a single plasma or serum measurement, with adjustment for body weight, age, and gender, is usually sufficient, provided their limitations are noted. Timed urine collections are not always accurate even in hospital and very often patients have already been started on drug therapy before the result is known. The main limitation of plasma creatinine as an estimate of GFR is the presence of changing renal function (e.g. acute renal failure) since there is a considerable lag between change in GFR and the consequent increase in plasma creatinine concentration. In elderly individuals in particular, some measurement or estimate of GFR is important, as creatinine production is reduced and, therefore, the serum creatinine may seriously underestimate the degree of renal impairment. Both GFR and effective renal plasma flow decline with age.

In pharmacokinetic handbooks the degree of renal impairment will often be defined as mild (GFR > 50 ml/min), moderate (GFR > 20 to <50 ml/min), or severe (GFR < 20 ml/min). This can act as a guide when estimating dose reduction or changes.

Drug kinetics

Most drugs that are eliminated by the kidney display first-order kinetics (Dettli 1983). This means that the rate of removal is proportional to the concentration of the drug. The elimination rate constant k_e is the proportion of the total amount of drug removed per unit time.

This can be expressed by the equation:

$$\frac{dC}{dt} = -k_e c.$$

Integrating from $t = 0$ to $t = t$ yields

$$C_1 = C_0 \, e^{-k_e t}$$

where k_e is the elimination constant, C_0 is the drug concentration at t_0, and C_1 is the drug concentration at t_1. Since, this is a simple exponential decline it gives rise to a straight line when the concentration is plotted on a semilogarithmic plot against time (Fig. 1). The half-life ($t_{1/2}$) of a drug is the time for its plasma concentration to fall by half after absorption and distribution are complete. It is useful in determining dosage interval, drug accumulation (both extent of accumulation and time taken to reach steady state), and persistence of drug after dosing is stopped. It is inversely related to k_e:

$$t_{\frac{1}{2}} = \frac{0.693}{k_e} \quad (0.693 = \ln 2).$$

The clearance of a drug depends upon $t_{1/2}$ (k_e) and the volume of distribution (V_d). V_d does not usually correspond to a real volume, although for a drug confined exclusively to the plasma, it would approximate the plasma volume. In practice, drugs are distributed through a larger space than this and V_d is a constant with units of

volume that relate the amount of drug in the body (units of mass) to the measured plasma concentration (units mass/volume):

$$V_d = \frac{m}{C_p}$$

where m is the mass of the drug in the body and C_p is the plasma concentration. V_d thus represents an apparent volume, which the drug would have distributed in to produce the measured plasma concentration. The volume of distribution itself may be affected by protein and tissue binding of drugs, changes in intravascular and extravascular fluid volumes and lean body mass. The clearance of a drug is related to k_e and V_d.

$$Clearance = k_e \times V_d = \frac{0.693 V_d}{t_{\frac{1}{2}}}.$$

Clearance (Cl) can be used to calculate the steady-state concentration of a drug (C_{ss}) that can be anticipated in response to any particular dosage regimen. At steady state the rate at which a drug enters the plasma is equal to the rate at which it leaves:

$$Rate \; in = \frac{F \times dose}{dose \; interval}$$

where F is the fraction reaching the circulation (assumed to be 1.0–100 per cent, for intravenous administration) and

$$Rate \; out = C_{ss} \times Cl,$$

where C_{ss} is the plasma concentration at steady state. By substituting the above equation we obtain

$$C_{ss} = \frac{F \times dose \times t_{\frac{1}{2}}}{dose \; interval \times 0.693 \times V_d}.$$

From these relations it can be seen that C_{ss} will increase with a longer $t_{1/2}$ and a smaller volume of distribution. C_{ss} can be reduced either by lowering the dose or by increasing the dose interval. The relationship between the elimination of a drug in the presence of renal impairment and normal renal function can be estimated. This estimate which has been calculated for a number of drugs can be used to gauge the appropriate reduction in dose or increase in dose interval compared to a standard regimen,

$$Q_r = \frac{k_e}{k_n}$$

where Q_r is the elimination rate fraction, k_e is the actual elimination rate constant, and k_n is the elimination rate constant if the GFR was 100 ml/min.

The difference between k_e and k_n is only clinically important in renal impairment when non-renal elimination accounts for less than 50 per cent of the total elimination, provided that the non-renal elimination is not reduced markedly by other means.

The expected reduction in dose of a drug necessitated by renal impairment can be calculated in terms of Q_r

$$D_t = D_n \times Q_r$$

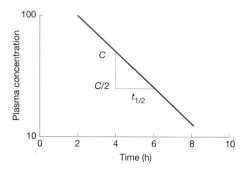

Fig. 1 Plot of log concentration of a drug against time to demonstrate the half-life of a drug.

where D_t is the dose in renal failure and D_n is the dose assuming normal renal function. Alternatively, the dosage interval can be prolonged by the same proportion:

$$I_r = \frac{I_p}{Q_r}$$

where I_r is the dose interval in renal failure and I_n is the dose assuming normal renal function. Either way, the dose/unit time is the same and is less than that in patients with normal renal function. In practice, the decision whether to reduce the dose or prolong the dose interval is not always equivalent. An example is the use of aminoglycoside antibiotics, which must achieve a threshold peak concentration in order to kill bacteria effectively. In consequence, small but frequent doses may fail to achieve efficacy, whereas the same total dose delivered less frequently may achieve the desired therapeutic effect without leading to accumulation and toxicity. Continuous infusion of gentamicin provided the same plateau concentration as a bolus dose, but produced more cortical binding in nephrectomy specimens and by inference more tubular toxicity (Verpooten *et al.* 1989). The Q_r value has been estimated for many drugs and nomograms have been constructed as guides to correct dosages. These assume that other factors such as non-renal elimination and volume of distribution remain constant in the presence of reduced or changing renal function, limiting their precision. However, they can be extremely useful at the start of therapy, which can be modified subsequently on the basis of actual, that is individual, plasma concentrations.

Pharmacodynamics

Pharmacodynamics is defined as the biochemical and physiological effects of drugs and the mechanisms of action. It is unclear how this process is affected and to what extent by renal impairment. The basic principles of pharmacodynamics are illustrated as follows:

$$\text{Drug [D]} + \text{Receptor [R]} = \underset{k_2}{\overset{k_1}{\rightleftarrows}} \text{DR} \rightarrow \text{Effect}$$

$$\text{Effect} = \frac{\text{Maximal effect [D]}}{K_D + [D]}$$

where [D] is the concentration of free drug and $K_D = k_2/k_1$ the dissociation constant.

$$\text{Fraction of receptors occupied} = \frac{[D]}{(K_D + [D])}$$

The effect is absent when [D] = 0, half maximal when [D] = K_D, and maximal as [D] > K_D.

There are different shapes of potency curves concave both upwards and downwards; linear and sigmoid. However, any concentration effect may be distorted if the action of a drug is multifactorial as will be the case with antihypertensives when it is likely that more than a single receptor is involved. The steepness of a curve will affect not only the efficacy but also the adverse effects of the drug. Drug interactions occurring at a receptor level will also have a pharmacodynamic basis.

Renal haemodynamics

Renal blood flow will only exert an independent effect on the excretion of drugs once the GFR has declined. A rapid reduction in drug clearance may result from acute renal failure associated with hypovolaemia. Non-steroidal anti-inflammatory agents may also alter GFR by inhibiting prostaglandin synthesis (Schrier and Conger 1986). This is more likely to occur in the presence of infection, particularly pyelonephritis, or dehydration, or saline depletion. Antibiotic treatment in these circumstances, often before renal function has been assessed, may produce additional difficulties. Angiotensin-converting enzyme (ACE) inhibitors and angiotensin receptor antagonists (blockers) may diminish GFR by lowering glomerular efferent arteriolar tone under certain circumstances such as dehydration or renovascular disease. Amphotericin renal toxicity may be related to vasoconstriction (Sawaya *et al.* 1991).

Dialysis and haemofiltration

The clearance of drugs by haemodialysis and haemofiltration follows first-order kinetics (Bohler *et al.* 1999). The rate of removal can be calculated from the law of conservation of matter using the equation:

$$\text{Cl}_d = \frac{Q \times (A - V)}{V}$$

where Cl_d is the dialysis or haemofilter clearance, Q the blood flow, A the blood concentration entering the dialysers, and V the blood concentration leaving the dialyser. A modification of this equation is necessary for drug concentrations measured in plasma as the blood flow here represents the whole blood. It should also be noted that blood pump flow rates may overestimate actual blood flow through dialysis needles or dialysis catheters. Since it is not always possible to obtain measurements of drug plasma concentrations in individual cases, an estimate of drug clearance can be obtained by use of the sieving coefficient(s) (Bickley 1988).

This coefficient is the proportion of the drug (or solute) that will cross the membrane and should be constant for a particular drug and membrane.

The expression for the sieving coefficient has been simplified:

$$S = \frac{C_{uf}}{C_{arterial}}$$

where C_{uf} is the concentration in filtrate and $C_{arterial}$ is the concentration in blood entering the filter. This value can be used to calculate the clearance and is more applicable to haemofiltration, as ultrafiltrate volumes are known:

$$\text{Cl} = S \times \text{UFR}_{avg}$$

where UFR_{avg} is the average ultrafiltration rate per unit time. This value can be substituted into the formula for calculating drug dosages in renal impairment discussed above, including, where necessary, non-renal elimination.

The factors given in Table 3 should be considered. The clearance of a drug depends on its molecular weight (and size) and protein binding (Gibson and Nelson 1983). Haemofilters have a pore size of 0.01 µm and artificial kidneys for haemodialysis 0.001 µm. In haemofiltration, drugs with a molecular weight less than that of inulin (5200 Da) will pass through, in haemodialysis most drugs with a molecular weight of less than 500 Da (which includes most antibiotics) will be cleared, but drugs such as vancomycin (1800 Da), amphotericin (960 Da), and erythromycin (734 Da) behave differently with respect to haemofiltration/haemodialysis. Joos *et al.* (1996), Golper and Marx (1998), Keller *et al.* (1999), and Pea and Furlanut (2001) have reviewed the clearance of

Table 3 Factors influencing clearance of drugs

Properties of the drug
Molecular weight
Protein binding
Volume of distribution

Delivery of drug to the filter
Blood flow to the filter
Blood flow within the filter

Properties of the filter
Volume of distribution
Pore size
Surface area

drugs and particularly antibiotics to ensure therapeutic but non-toxic levels. Heavily protein bound drugs, even with a lower molecular weight (propranolol 259 Da) will not be filtered, but drugs which are displaced from binding sites in the presence of renal impairment will become available for filtration. Water soluble drugs pass through filters more readily than those which are fat soluble. The other differences between the different techniques of haemodialysis, haemodiafiltration, and intermittent and continuous haemofiltration are dealt with in other texts. Digoxin and antidepressants are examples of drugs with a large volume of distribution, which will have low plasma concentrations and, therefore, little of the drug is available for filtration. There are differences, other than pore size, between haemodialysis and haemofiltration. In haemodialysis, clearance is by diffusion with a concentration between the dialysate and plasma. Therefore, drugs of a low molecular mass will be cleared more than in haemofiltration where there is no concentration gradient and clearance is by convection. Drug clearance will be optimal (whichever system is used) the greater the blood flow to the artificial filter, provided the filter does not become clotted or the membrane pores obstructed by protein, which may occur in prolonged continuous haemofiltration. Haemodialysis is performed for short periods and it is usually sufficient to administer drugs, which are cleared by dialysis at the end of treatment, in a dose adjusted to take into consideration absent or diminished renal function. These principles apply, if automated, high blood flow (300–400 ml/min), large filtrate-volume (up to 80 ml/min), and short duration haemofiltration (with more efficient clearance of drugs with higher molecular mass than by haemodialysis) are employed. In the more usual form of haemofiltration (either arteriovenous or venous to venous) blood flow rates and, therefore, filtration rates are much lower, and drug clearance is very slow. However, because it is continuous and may be used for several days, net clearance may be high and supplemental doses may be needed.

Peritoneal dialysis

PD clears drugs very much less efficiently than haemodialysis/filtration. This may allow maintenance of therapeutic levels with less frequent dosing (e.g. vancomycin). Clearance studies as well as indicating whether the study is performed in conventional continuous ambulatory peritoneal dialysis (CAPD) or automatic PD (APD) should account for any residual renal function (Taylor *et al.* 1996; Brophy and Mueller 1997; Elwell *et al.* 2000). The excellent study on intravenous tobramycin and cefazolin (Manley *et al.* 2000) illustrates the principles.

A combination of APD (three dwell periods over 8 h) followed by two periods of CAPD exchange (8 h each) were employed over a 24 h period following intravenous administration of the drugs with measurement of dialysate and serum concentration. These values were applied to a monoexponential model to provide a combination of measured and derived clearance estimations. The serum elimination constant k_e for the automated dwells was calculated from measurements at the start and end of dwell periods and derived for the conventional PD periods. This not only allowed confirmation that single intravenous dosing provided sufficient intraperitoneal concentration, but it was also possible to predict the peritoneal concentrations that would have followed had the drug had been given intraperitoneally. Guidelines for the administration of intraperitoneal antibiotics are available (Keane *et al.* 1996) and suggest that for most intraperitoneal antibiotics a dwell period of at least 4 h is needed, therefore, requiring an additional antibiotic exchange. The same guidelines recommend an increment of 25 per cent for those with residual function.

Poisoning

Haemodialysis, PD, haemofiltration, and haemoperfusion have all been used to eliminate poisons and drugs in overdose from the body (Toxbase 2002). Similar principles apply to those for the handling of drugs in therapeutic dialysis and filtration. A substance which has a low V_d, low protein binding and is unipolar will be cleared more efficiently.

PD is very slow but can be used to clear alcohols, salicylate, and lithium if haemodialysis or filtration is unavailable.

Haemodialysis

All toxins of 100–2000 Da can be removed using conventional filters and preferably bicarbonate buffering as many toxins will cause acidosis. However, there may be rebound of plasma levels of a substance after a period of treatment and continuous haemofiltration following haemodialysis may be needed. Thallium poisoning may need prolonged treatment over several days.

High flux membranes used in continuous haemo- and haemodiafiltration will remove larger sized molecules (10,000 Da). Clearance of any substance may be overestimated if it is only removed from plasma—measurements are usually of plasma concentration—rather than if it is removed from red blood cells also.

Haemoperfusion

This technique relies on the affinity of the adsorbent for a toxin. Activated charcoal or polystyrene exchange resins are used in a column arranged like an artificial kidney. It is possible to combine haemoperfusion preceding filtration or dialysis in series. This is particularly useful for toxins with a low V_d. Heparin may be adsorbed onto the perfusion column and up to 2000 units per hour may be needed.

Drugs

Drug prescribing

When a drug with clinically important renal excretion is prescribed in the presence of renal impairment, the dose can be adjusted in two main ways. Either the size of each dose or the frequency of administration can be reduced. Plasma drug concentrations can be used to confirm that the initial adjustment of dosage is correct in that particular individual. Steady-state concentrations of anticonvulsants, digoxin, and theophylline can be measured after the equivalent of five half-lives of the drug. For antibiotics such as gentamicin, the peak and trough concentrations taken after the first day's administration is essential and continued monitoring is required if renal function is impaired or changing.

Significant reduction in dosage is more likely to lead to subtherapeutic plasma concentrations. A combination of modest reduction in dosage with less frequent administration is suitable for most drugs. Dose adjustments must be kept simple and clear since unfamiliar dosages and the administration of drugs at odd times may result in error.

Antimicrobials

Many antimicrobial agents are excreted by the kidney. With the exception of aminoglycosides and vancomycin, most have a wide therapeutic index and little or no dose adjustment is usually made until the GFR is less than 20 ml/min. Although larger doses than strictly necessary are frequently used, this is not unreasonable in seriously ill patients in whom the priority must be to provide adequate plasma concentrations. Special consideration should be given to patients with acute changes in renal function, as adverse effects may occur before it is realized that renal function is impaired. Antimicrobials that are removed by dialysis should be administered after dialysis, or a supplemental dose given at that time.

Penicillins

Adjustments of dose for the commonly used penicillins are given in Table 4. Fractions of usual doses are shown rather than the absolute dose. Piperacillin is cited as an example of broad-spectrum injectable penicillin with antipseudomonas activity; azlocillin (Aletta *et al.* 1980) and ticarcillin (Parry and Neu 1979) require similar dose adjustment. Piperacillin has been combined with tazobactam and ticarcillin with clavulanic acid to confer penicillinase resistance. Tazobactam metabolites accumulate in renal impairment and dose reduction is required; the metabolite is partially cleared by haemodialysis and PD (Halstenson *et al.* 1994).

Cephalosporins

Although there are few absolute indications for this multifarious class of drugs, they are particularly useful as broad-spectrum antibiotics in patients with impaired or changing renal function as less toxic alternatives to aminoglycosides. Cephalexin and cephradine, which are active when given by mouth, can be used in normal dose until the GFR is less than 10 ml/min, at which the daily dose is halved. The combination of loop diuretic and cefuroxime requires caution. In this situation, ceftazidime appears to be a safer alternative (Walstad *et al.* 1988). Cefuroxime is often prescribed in excessive doses (Walstad *et al.* 1983). Cefotaxime, ceftazidime, and the newer cefoxitin can also be adjusted by increasing the dose interval to once a day if GFR is less than 10 ml/min. Ceftriaxone and cetizosime should be treated like cefuroxime by dose reduction. Dose adjustments are shown in Table 5.

Aminoglycosides

Even in mild renal failure an adjustment of dose is needed for the aminoglycosides. Furthermore, they are inherently nephrotoxic, and their use may worsen renal impairment and cause ototoxicity. Several factors make nephrotoxicity more likely: previous or prolonged treatment, hypovolaemia, dehydration, concomitant administration of diuretics, hypokalaemia, and hypomagnesaemia (Humes 1988) and there may be particular problems in the elderly (Raveh *et al.* 2002). Obstructive jaundice also increases the risk (Desai and Tsang 1988). The simplest way to prevent aminoglycoside toxicity is to avoid their use altogether in patients with any suspicion of renal impairment. Of the available aminoglycosides, tobramycin is marginally less nephrotoxic than gentamicin (Smith *et al.* 1980) and netilmicin appears to be less ototoxic than tobramycin (Lerner *et al.* 1983).

There are many nomograms and other guidelines for dose adjustment of aminoglycosides for patients with renal impairment (Bennett 1990), but each method has drawbacks. Dose adjustment may take two forms. Reduction of the dose (given at the usual interval) may lead to an increased likelihood of subtherapeutic peak plasma concentrations. If only the dose interval is increased, then subtherapeutic plasma concentrations are more likely to occur over longer periods. Whichever method is used, an adequate loading dose (1–1.5 mg/kg for gentamicin) is required. A combination of both methods with frequent peak measurements (taken 1 h after intravenous dosing) and trough measurements (immediately before the next dose) is optimal. Such measurements should be made daily when alterations in renal function are anticipated and two to three times a week under other circumstances. The dose regimen is adjusted to produce peak plasma concentrations of gentamicin between 6 and 10 mg/l and trough concentrations not exceeding 2 mg/l, doses and therapeutic concentrations are shown in Table 6.

An alternative and now favoured method is to give a single daily dose starting with 5 mg/kg (Hustinx and Hoepelman 1993; Barclay *et al.* 1999) with daily measurement, when renal function is changing,

Table 4 Penicillin dose adjustment

Drug	Dose reduction	Comments
Flucloxacillin	Nil	Dose seldom adjusted
Ampicillin		Dose seldom adjusted
Amoxycillin + clavulinic acid	GFR < 20 ml/min	Half normal dose posthaemodialysis
Benzylpenicillin	GFR < 20 ml/min	Daily dose should not exceed 20 mU
Piperacillin	GFR 20–50 ml/min Half normal dose GFR < 20 ml/min One-third to one-half the normal dose	Half normal dose posthaemodialysis

Table 5 Cephalosporin dose adjustment

Drug	GFR (ml/min)	Dose reduction
Cefotaxime	20–50	One-fifth to one-half the normal dose
Ceftazidime	20–50	One-fifth to one-half the normal dose
Cefuroxime	20–50	One-fifth to one-half the normal dose
Cefotaxime	<20	One-tenth to one-fifth the normal dose
Ceftazidime	<20	One-tenth to one-fifth the normal dose
Cefuroxime	<20	One-tenth to one-fifth the normal dose

Table 6 Doses and therapeutic plasma concentrations of aminoglycosides

Drug	Usual daily dose	Therapeutic concentration	
		Peak (mg/l)	Trough (mg/l)
Gentamycin	2–5 mg/kg	5–10	<2.5
Tobramycin	2–5 mg/kg	5–10	<2.5
Netilmycin	2–5 mg/kg	5–10	<2.5
Amikacin	10–30 μg/kg	20–30	<10
Kanamycin	10–30 μg/kg	20–30	<10

Peak concentration measured 1 h post injection.

Trough concentration immediately before next dose.

Usual daily dose is administered eight hourly.

Netilmycin dose can be increased to 7.5 mg/kg/day in severe infections but with careful therapeutic monitoring.

of trough drug concentration. The rationale behind this concept is that peak values need to be high to achieve bactericidal activity, particularly in the presence of neutropenia. The nephrotoxic effects will be less because trough concentrations are low (see above; Verpooten *et al.* 1989).

Vancomycin

Vancomycin is used extensively in patients with staphylococcal infections. It is indicated in the treatment of epidemic methicillin-resistant strains and is used in the treatment of peritonitis in CAPD, which is often caused by *Staphylococcus epidermidis*. It is used for intravenous-line sepsis, particularly in patients in the intensive care unit. The target steady-state plasma concentration is approximately 15 mg/l (Brown and Mauro 1988). Vancomycin is excreted by the kidney and the dose interval should be increased in renal impairment. In endstage renal failure a loading dose of 1.5 mg/kg may maintain therapeutic levels for some days. Measurement of plasma drug concentration can be used to determine the timing of subsequent doses. The drug is not cleared by dialysis except with high-flux, and to a lesser extent cupraphane, dialysers (Bohler *et al.* 1992). There is insignificant clearance in haemofiltration or haemodiafiltration unless high blood flow is used (Davies *et al.* 1992). Vancomycin can still be given in the last hour of dialysis (Edell *et al.* 1988) or during haemofiltration with the above considerations.

In the treatment of peritonitis in CAPD a single dose of 500 mg intravenously can be given every fifth day to produce satisfactory therapeutic levels (Whitby *et al.* 1987). Alternatively, the drug can be administered intraperitoneally (Beaman *et al.* 1989) to produce adequate therapeutic concentrations and satisfactory treatment of peritonitis.

Teicoplanin

This antibiotic is a glycopeptide related to vancomycin. It is used intravenously but can also be given intraperitoneally and reportedly enters the bloodstream but does not cross back into the peritoneal cavity. In renal failure the half-life is approximately three times that in normal individuals (Bonati *et al.* 1987). After a loading dose of 400 mg the maintenance dose of 200 mg/day should be reduced after 3 days, even in mild renal impairment. There is virtually no clearance by PD or haemodialysis (Hoffer *et al.* 1991; Wilson 2000). Following a loading dose of 800 mg a haemodialysis patient can be given 400 mg on days 8 and 15 to complete a course of treatment.

Linezolid is an oxazolidinone and is also active against MRSA. It should be treated as a monoamine oxidase inhibitor with respect to potential interactions. The dose requires reduction if the GFR falls below 30 ml/min and the drug is cleared by haemodialysis.

Aztreonam

Aztreonam is a monocyclic β-lactam. It has a wide spectrum of activity against Gram-negative organisms. It is usually given in a dose of 1 g eight-hourly. However, the dose should be reduced in renal impairment (Gerig *et al.* 1984; Fillastre *et al.* 1985). If the GFR is less than 10 ml/min a loading dose of 1 g is given, followed by a maintenance dose of 250 mg eight-hourly. Aztreonam is haemodialysed and half the usual dose is given as a supplement after dialysis. It can be used in peritonitis in CAPD (Gerig *et al.* 1984) (1 g intravenously followed by 500 mg intraperitoneally six-hourly).

Carbapenems

Imipenem and meropenem are examples of these newer broad-spectrum antibiotics. Imipenem is combined with cilastin to prevent inactivation in the kidney and is more likely to induce seizures (Mouton *et al.* 2000). Dosage adjustment is required with renal impairment, with particular accumulation with cilastin, and both are cleared by haemodialysis or filtration (Fillastre and Singlas 1991; Thalhammer and Horl 2000).

Macrolides

Erythromycin, clarithromycin, and azithromycin are often used in upper respiratory-tract infections (including mycoplasma, psittacosis, and legionnaire's disease) and soft tissue infections. They are particularly useful in patients who are allergic to penicillin. They are handled differently in the presence of renal impairment. Erythromycin and azithromycin need no dose adjustment but clarithromycin needs dose reduction if the GFR falls below 30 ml/min. They are not haemodialysed to any significant extent (Periti *et al.* 1989). They will all interfere with cyclosporin by inhibiting its metabolism and may, therefore, cause cyclosporin toxicity in transplant recipients.

Tetracyclines

All the tetracyclines, with the exception of minocycline and doxycycline, are excreted renally. Plasma half-lives are markedly prolonged (up to 100 h) in renal impairment and as they are antianabolic there is a concentration-related increase in blood urea, which itself may cause an osmotic diuresis. This emphasizes the importance of a measure of GFR independent of blood urea (e.g. plasma creatinine) in patients with potential renal impairment before prescribing these drugs. Doxycycline or minocycline can be used cautiously in patients with renal impairment, but the other tetracyclines are contraindicated. Doxycycline does have some renal clearance but hepatic clearance increases with renal impairment, partly because there is a reduction in binding to plasma proteins and red blood cells (Houin *et al.* 1983). It is not dialysed and no dose adjustments are needed in patients on dialysis. Demeclocycline is a non-physiological vasopressin antagonist and is used in the treatment of the syndrome of inappropriate ADH secretion.

Metronidazole

Metronidazole is used against anaerobic bacteria and against protozoa including *Trichomonas* spp. and *Entamoeba histolytica*. It is given in usual doses to patients with renal impairment. It is dialysed (Somogyi *et al.* 1983) and a supplemental dose (half the usual dose) is required after dialysis.

Sulfonamides, trimethoprim, and cotrimoxazole

The use of sulfonamides as single agents has largely been superseded. They are eliminated by acetylation followed by renal excretion, and acetylated metabolites (which have no antibacterial activity) cause crystalluria and tubular damage. Most sulfonamide usage is currently accounted for by cotrimoxazole (sulfamethoxozole 400 mg and trimethoprim 80 mg). However, it is now appreciated that trimethoprim as a single agent alone is effective for most urinary infections that were previously treated with cotrimoxazole, thus avoiding the toxicity of the sulfonamide. Sulfamethoxazole and trimethoprim display similar renal excretion, except at extremes of urinary pH. Alkaline urine promotes sulfamethoxazole excretion, acid urine trimethoprim (Craig and Kunin 1973). It is doubtful if this is clinically important. In the presence of renal impairment (GFR < 20 ml/min) one-half the usual dose may be used. A supplement of one-half the normal dose is given after dialysis.

Much greater doses of cotrimoxazole are needed in the treatment of *Pneumocystis carinii* infection, the risk of adverse effects being balanced against the seriousness of the condition in patients who often have impaired renal function. The dose is trimethoprim 20 mg/sulfamethoxazole 100 mg/kg body weight per day divided into two or more doses. The plasma concentration should be maintained at approximately 5–8 μg/l measured after five doses and can by achieved by lower maintenance doses.

Fluoroquinolones

Ciprofloracin is the first and most widely used of this group of drugs and although related to nalidixic acid, differs from it in that it can be prescribed for urinary infections in patients with renal impairment. It is particularly useful in the treatment of antibiotic-resistant Gram-negative organisms, including *Pseudomonas aeruginosa*. Unlike other antibiotics effective against *Pseudomonas*, it is available as both oral and intravenous preparations. It can also be used in the treatment of peritonitis in CAPD (Fleming *et al.* 1987) for which it can be given orally (500 mg six-hourly or 750 mg 12-hourly). Renal excretion exceeds the GFR, and in patients with normal renal function approximately 60 per cent is cleared by the kidneys (Roberts and Williams 1989). It is recommended that the dose should be reduced (except as above) in renal impairment (500–750 mg/day maximum); however, the proportion that is eliminated by the kidney is reduced in renal failure (Singlas *et al.* 1987) as a result of an increase in hepatic clearance and of secretion through the bowel wall (Roberts and Williams 1989). Ciprofloxacin is not significantly removed by haemodialysis but is removed by haemofiltration (Davies *et al.* 1992). Ofloxacin and levofloxacin appear to behave differently when the GFR falls below 35 ml/min they are not removed by dialysis (Fillastre 1990; Bellman *et al.* 2002).

Antimicrobials in urinary tract infections

It is essential that agents reach therapeutic concentrations in the urine or renal parenchyma. Nitrofurantoin and nalidixic acid are used in the treatment of cystitis, but are of limited use in pyelonephritis. If there is renal impairment, nalidixic acid will not reach sufficient urinary concentrations. In addition, nitrofurantoin causes peripheral neuropathy in patients with impaired renal function. There is little value in the use of urinary antiseptics such as hexamine.

Tuberculosis

Tuberculosis can be a difficult therapeutic problem in patients with renal failure. Rifampicin (Fabre *et al.* 1983) and isoniazid (Gold *et al.* 1976) can be given in the usual dosage. Neither is cleared significantly by dialysis. Pyridoxine should be given with isoniazid to prevent peripheral neuropathy (Cuss *et al.* 1986). The plasma half-life of ethambutol is, however, prolonged in renal impairment (Andrew 1980; Lee *et al.* 1980). If the GFR is less than 30 ml/min, the dose should be 10–15 mg/kg per day with a further reduction to 4 mg/kg daily if the GFR is less than 10 ml/min. Although 10 mg/kg daily has been used at these levels of GFR, cases of optic atrophy have been reported (Andrew 1980). Ethambutol is not dialysed to any significant extent. Pyrazinamide should be given at reduced dose (10–15 mg/kg) (Cuss *et al.* 1986). Capreomycin (Lehmann *et al.* 1988), a second-line drug, can be used in isoniazid or streptomycin resistance but is itself nephrotoxic and ototoxic but can be given in a single dose of 500 mg. With repeated transplant patients on cyclosporin, rifampicin cannot be used as it reduces the concentration of cyclosporin very substantially as a result of hepatic enzyme induction (Allen *et al.* 1985).

The necessity to use more than three agents will be dictated by the nature and severity of the infection. Treatment may need to be prolonged to between 9 and 12 months in uraemic or immunosuppressed patients, in contrast to the shorter courses that are preferred in patients with normal renal function.

Antiviral agents

Acyclovir, valacyclovir, and ganciclovir are all eliminated by the kidney and adjustments are needed in patients with renal impairment. Valacyclovir is better absorbed after oral administration. In herpes zoster infections and herpes simplex encephalitis, acyclovir is required in huge doses, which may themselves cause renal impairment particularly if the patient is dehydrated. Adverse effects including cerebral irritation, ataxia, and myoclonus which can be avoided with dose reduction (Fletcher *et al.* 1988; Lake *et al.* 1988). The intravenous dose should be reduced stepwise from 800 mg daily at a GFR of less than 10 ml/min. In patients on haemodialysis a loading dose of 400 mg followed by 200 mg 12-hourly and a supplemental dose of 400 mg postdialysis achieves therapeutic concentrations (Almond *et al.* 1995); a single daily dose of 800 mg is sufficient in patients on CAPD (Stathoulopoulou *et al.* 1995).

Ganciclovir is active against cytomegalovirus. The dose should be reduced from 5 mg/kg 12-hourly to 2.5 mg/kg 24-hourly, if the GFR is less than 25 ml/min. A single dose of 1.25 mg/kg can be given after dialysis (Faulds and Heel 1990).

Foscarnet is used to treat cytomegalovirus retinitis in patients with acquired immune deficiency. It cannot be used if the serum creatinine exceeds 250 μmol/l. Adequate hydration and adjustment from 200 mg/kg per day in patients with normal renal function to 20 mg/kg per day at a creatinine of 250 μmol/l are required.

Antiviral use in HIV patients is complex particularly in the context of renal impairment (Jayasekara *et al.* 1999; Izzedine *et al.* 2001). Both reviews discuss a number of drugs including lamivudine, zidovudine (nucleoside reverse transcriptase inhibitors), and abacavir (a protease inhibitor).

Lamivudine is 70 per cent excreted, unchanged in the urine and dose adjustment is required. Trimethoprim, which may be required simultaneously decreases clearance, but without a reciprocal effect (Johnson *et al.* 1999).

Zanamivir in indicated to treat influenza in at-risk patients, which would probably include those on immunosuppression. Although the drug is renally excreted, it is safe to use at the usual doses, 20 mg/day by inhalation (Cass *et al.* 1999).

Zidovudine

Zidovudine is used in patients with the human immunodeficiency virus. It is a basic substance and undergoes glucuronidation and is eliminated by the kidney by tubular secretion. The dose should be reduced in patients with renal impairment. Probenecid will block the glucuronidation of the drug and will partially block the tubular excretion of this metabolite (Kornhauser *et al.* 1989) but will not block the tubular excretion of zidovudine itself. The drug is cleared by haemodialysis (Deray *et al.* 1988).

Interferons

This class of agents has antiviral activity, but may also be used in patients with malignancy or autoimmune diseases, often in circumstances where there may be renal impairment. Interferon-α is metabolized in the kidney (to a greater extent than interferon-β or γ), but has negligible renal excretion (Wills 1990). The dose does not require adjustment but there are reports of adverse effects including development of the nephrotic syndrome.

Antifungal agents

Crystalline amphotericin is nephrotoxic and should be used with great caution in patients with existing renal impairment (Bates 2001). Its toxicity may be caused in part by vasoconstriction (Sawaya *et al.* 1991) and its adverse effects may be amelioriated by sodium supplementation. Amphotericin encapsulated in liposomes (liposomal amphotericin) is thought to be less toxic (Boswell 1998), although that view has been questioned (Graybill 1996).

Both forms will cause hypokalaemia and hypomagnesaemia. The protein binding of ampholericin is reduced in renal impairment and low plasma concentrations need interpretation accordingly. The protein binding remains sufficient to prevent significant removal by dialysis (Block and Bennett 1974).

Flucytosine

Flucytosine clearance follows the GFR (Daneshmend and Warnock 1983) and the dose should be reduced progressively from roughly one-half the usual dose with a GFR of 50 ml/min to one-fourth with a GFR below 20 ml/min with monitoring of the individual plasma concentrations. It is cleared by haemodialysis and half the dose should be given postdialysis. As it is excreted by the kidney it is useful in fungal pyelonephritis and urinary infections. It should be used in conjunction with another antifungal agent to avoid development of resistance.

Imidazoles

Ketoconazole, miconazole The oral absorption of ketoconazole is reduced in patients with renal impairment (Daneshmend and Warnock 1983). Both miconazole and ketoconazole are extensively metabolized and can be used in the usual dosage despite renal impairment (Lewi *et al.* 1976). Ketoconazole, given by mouth, achieves therapeutic concentrations in the peritonitis of CAPD (Johnson *et al.* 1985). Neither ketoconazole nor miconazole should be used with cyclosporin as they induce metabolizing enzymes causing plasma concentrations of cyclosporin to decline substantially.

Fluconazole Fluconazole is used in candida and cryptococcal infections. It is also used prophylactically in immunocompromised patients.

Unlike the other imidazoles, its elimination is dependent upon GFR; thus, it should be reduced to one-half the usual dose—400 mg on the first day followed by 100 mg once daily after the first day of therapy in patients with a GFR of less than 50 ml/min; with normal renal function it achieves a high urine concentration. It is removed by dialysis and is given as a single dose after each treatment (Oono *et al.* 1992). Information of its effects on cyclosporin, causing an increased plasma concentration, is conflicting and may be dose-dependent; cyclosporin concentration requires careful monitoring (Stockley 1994). It should be assumed that hetoconazole will interfere with both cyclosporin and tacrolimus drug concentrations.

Griseofulvin

Griseofulvin can be given in usual dosage to patients with renal impairment. It does not interfere with cyclosporin.

Antiprotozoal agents

Malaria

Up-to-date information as to the likely pattern of resistance in different parts of the world may be sought from local reference laboratories.

Severe and complicated malaria Quinine may be given by slow intravenous infusion to patients severely ill with *Plasmodium falciparum* infection. It should be given in usual dosage (White 1985) to patients with chronic renal impairment. If acute renal failure develops as a complication of the disease, then the dose may need to be reduced after 2–3 days. It is not removed by haemodialysis or PD and can be given every 24 h. If the patient is on haemofiltration, which does partially clear the drug it should be given every 8–12 h. Quinidine is also active and available in parenteral form. It is given as an alternative to quinine in similar doses by slow intravenous infusion with monitoring of the electrocardiogram and blood pressure.

Uncomplicated malaria *P. falciparum* infection is treated with quinine in usual dosage (White 1985). Tetracycline is often given to patients with normal renal function to enhance the curative effect of quinine, but only doxycycline is appropriate in this regard in patients with renal impairment. Fansider (pyrimethamine with sulfadoxine) is given following quinine, but caution should be exercised, as for any sulfa-containing drug, in renal impairment.

Infection with *P. vivax*, *P. ovale*, and *P. malariae* can be treated with chloroquine. The dose is reduced by one-half if the GFR is less than 50 ml/min and to one-fourth if the GFR is less than 10 ml/min. Primaquine can be given in the usual doses to achieve a radical cure with elimination of hepatic forms.

Prophylaxis Chloroquine (usual dose 300 mg/week) can be given to patients with renal impairment. Proguanil (usual dose 200 mg daily) should be given at one-half the usual dose if the GFR is below 10 ml/min.

Patients with multisystem failure

Many of the most complex prescribing problems arise in patients with acute renal failure particularly if this occurs as part of multisystem failure perhaps in a patient requiring artificial ventilation and some form of renal replacement therapy.

Neuromuscular blocking agents

Succinylcholine is rapidly hydrolyzed by plasma cholinesterase. No dose adjustment is needed. For more prolonged paralysis use atracurium, which is degraded by non-enzymatic Hofmann elimination independent of renal or hepatic function. It is removed by dialysis and haemofiltration and the dose titrated to produce a therapeutic effect (Ward *et al.* 1987). Avoid tubocurarine, gallamine, alcuronium, pancuronium, and vecuronium (Caldwell *et al.* 1988; Lynam *et al.* 1988). Aminoglycosides, which accumulate in renal impairment without monitoring and appropriate dose adjustment (see above), are themselves weak, non-polarizing, neuromuscular blocking agents (particularly if there is hypokalaemia) and may interact to produce prolonged paralysis.

Anaesthetic and sedating agents

Inhalation anaesthetics and injectable anaesthetics such as propofol are used in the usual dosage in patients with renal impairment. Fentanyl and alfentanyl require no dose adjustment (Chauvin *et al.* 1987a; Meuldermans *et al.* 1988), but may have prolonged effects if there is concomitant hepatic dysfunction. The potency of thiopentone (Dundee and Richards 1954), which is cleared by non-renal means, and other barbiturates is increased in uraemia by a direct effect of uraemia upon the central nervous system (Danhof *et al.* 1984; Dingemanse 1988; Lynam *et al.* 1988). The pharmacokinetic effect does not warrant precise dose adjustment. Diazepam has metabolites which accumulate and midazolam is preferable with dosage reduction if the GFR falls below 10 ml/min. Phenothiazines, butyrophenones, and heminevrin are given in usual doses. Despite the minor changes in patients with renal impairment, it is well recognized that patients may have prolonged periods of sedation and confusion following mechanical ventilation.

Narcotic analgesics

Opiates are affected by renal failure and retention of metabolites can produce adverse effects (Davies *et al.* 1996). Reduced intermittent doses, epidural administration, or low dose continuous infusions reduce the incidence of adverse effects. Diamorphine is metabolized into morphine and then to morphine-3-glucuronide and morphine-6-glucuronide (Guay *et al.* 1988), both of which accumulate to prolong both analgesia and respiratory depression (Chauvin *et al.* 1987b; Sawe *et al.* 1987; Sear 1988; Wolff *et al.* 1988). Morphine and its metabolites are removed somewhat more by haemofiltration than by dialysis. Pethidine (meperidine) is converted to norpethidine (normeperidine), which accumulates and can cause seizures (Szeto *et al.* 1977). Papaveretum is a mixture of alkaloids of opium including morphine, codeine, noscapine, and papaverene; its use is not recommended.

Treatment of shock

Cardiac inotropes are used in normal dosage, although renal vasoconstriction may be deleterious so the minimum effective dose of adrenaline, noradrenaline, dobutamine, or dopamine should be used. They are not affected by haemodialysis or filtration. Dopamine in low doses (2.5–5 μg/kg per min) is a renal vasodilator. Intravenous nitrates are given in normal dosage. Sodium nitroprusside may be used in the management of hypertension or left ventricular failure. It is metabolized to sodium thiocyanate (Palmer and Lasseter 1975), which is eliminated by the kidney, and so may accumulate in renal failure, causing toxicity. It is removed by haemodialysis or PD. In liver failure the detoxification of cyanide to thiocyanate may be impaired so the use of sodium nitroprusside should be avoided in this circumstance. Plasma concentrations greater than 10 mg/dl produce nausea, anorexia, and fatigue; levels greater than 20 mg/dl may be fatal.

Activated protein C, drotrecogin α (activated), has shown promising results in the treatment of severe sepsis (Ely *et al.* 2002). Experience in severe renal impairment is limited, but there appear to be no dosage adjustments required as the drug is rapidly deactivated in the plasma (Macias *et al.* 2002).

Antiarrhythmics

In patients with abnormal renal function it is advisable to keep treatment simple. Most antiarrhythmic drugs are used without dose modification: for example, lignocaine and verapamil. Digoxin is a notable exception with a lower loading and maintenance dose than usual. Flecainide and disopyramide require dosage reduction. Amiodarone requires a lower maintenance dose (100 mg daily) when the GFR falls below 20 ml/min (Latini *et al.* 1984).

Drugs acting on the central nervous system

Drugs acting on the central nervous system may have a prolonged effect not only because of changes in pharmacokinetics but also because of increased sensitivity as a consequence of uraemia.

Antidepressants

The data on antidepressant drugs is conflicting. All drugs should be used with caution. Tricyclics are given in usual dosage. Fluoxetine, paroxetine, and other SSRIs have been used widely in patients on dialysis although dosage reductions are advised. It is best to avoid citalopram and venlafaxine.

Lithium

Lithium is used primarily in affective disorders. It is filtered and then reabsorbed, mainly in the proximal tubule. The dose should be reduced in renal impairment with careful monitoring of plasma concentration. In sodium depletion (e.g. with chronic thiazide diuretic use) tubular reabsorption of lithium is increased, leading to higher plasma concentrations and toxicity. The effect of non-steroidal anti-inflammatory drugs (NSAIDs) on renal haemodynamics may also be important. Lithium itself is a cause of chronic tubulointerstitial damage.

Major tranquillizers

No dose change is required when phenothiazines or butyrophenones are used in patients with renal impairment. Newer drugs such as clozapine, rispiridone, and sulpiride should be used with caution.

Minor tranquillizers

Benzodiazepines can be prescribed in usual dosage. Diazepam and chlordiazepoxide have active metabolites which may accumulate. Short acting drugs, such as nitrazepam and temazepam may avoid hangover the morning after use as night sedation.

Anticonvulsants

Phenytoin and valproic acid are both highly protein-bound. The protein binding of phenytoin declines in proportion to the GFR (Mahuchi and Nakahashi 1988; Brater 1994). The unbound (free or active components) will be proportionately greater for a given plasma concentration as the GFR declines and this will have the effect of lowering the therapeutic range (see above). Changes in the protein binding of valproic acid are not clinically important (Vanholder et al. 1988). Both drugs are prescribed in usual dosage with renal impairment and neither is dialysed (Adler et al. 1975). Carbamazepine is prescribed in the usual doses (Gulyassy and Depner 1983). Newer anticonvulsants include lamotrigine, which needs no dose adjustment, but both vigabatrin (reduced from the usual 2–3 g/day when the GFR is < 60 ml/min) and gabapentin (1200 mg/day reduced to 300 mg on alternate days) need dose reduction. Adverse effects are more common with vigabratin in patients with renal impairment, even with appropriate dose adjustment.

Weaker analgesics

Codeine and dihydrocodeine, although weaker analgesics, still have the potential to cause severe respiratory depression in some patients, likewise dextropropoxyphene (combined with paracetamol as coproxamol). Its metabolite norproxyphene, which accumulates in renal failure, sometimes causes cardiac toxicity.

Buprenorphine is metabolized in the liver and does not appear to have any important toxic metabolites.

Non-narcotic analgesics

Paracetamol (which in overdosage is an important cause of acute renal failure) is excreted in small amounts by glomerular filtration with some passive tubular reabsorption (Prescott et al. 1989). The majority of the drug is metabolized and the glucuronide and sulfide metabolites, which are subject to active tubular secretion, accumulate in renal impairment. There is some regeneration of the parent compound. Despite this, paracetamol is used in usual doses. Aspirin has the disadvantage of causing gastric damage and increasing the bleeding diathesis of patients with renal failure. Renal elimination of its metabolite salicylate is enhanced in alkaline urine (see above).

Antihistamines

Terfenadine should be avoided because of prolongation of the QT-interval perhaps made more likely in renal impairment. Prochlorperazine and chlorpheniramine are used in usual dosage but may cause drowsiness.

Cardiac failure and oedema

Diuretics

Spironolactone, triamterene, and amiloride, all potassium sparing diuretics, should be avoided or used with extreme caution in renal impairment because of the danger of hyperkalaemia. The same applies for combination diuretics such as 'Moduretic' (amiloride and hydrochlorothiazide) or 'Dyazide' (triamterene and hydrochlorothiazide). Thiazides apart from metolazone (a quinolone) become less effective if the GFR is below 25 ml/min. 'Diuretic resistance' is reported in chronic renal impairment, congestive cardiac failure, and nephritic syndrome. Wilcox (2002) in his review notes that reduction in renal blood flow, which may be relevant, will result in less delivery of diuretic to the site of action. Increasing the dose of loop diuretics may improve this, but will not overcome the increased distal reabsorption of sodium, which may occur in oedematous staes. It is for this reason that thiazides, including metolazone, by acting downstream to the loop diuretics will exert an additive or synergistic effect. In the nephrotic syndrome the V_d

of loop diuretics as the serum albumin, to which they are highly bound, concentration falls. The drug diffuses into the extracellular space and is unavailable for glomerular filtration thereby preventing it reaching its intratubular site of action. However, the drug will remain bound to filtered, tubular, protein which may limit its bioavailability. Different strategies to overcome this problem include reported success of administration of the loop diuretic with albumin (Inone et al. 1987; Na et al. 2001); or attempts to displace furosemide from its binding site with sulfioxazole which was unsuccessful (Agarwal et al. 2000). Severe sodium and water depletion can occur in diuretic therapy and volume depletion itself may affect renal haemodynamics with secondary effects upon renal function and concomitant drug therapy.

Angiotensin-converting enzyme inhibitors

Whether ACE inhibitors are being used to treat cardiac failure or hypertension the same precautions apply. Starting doses should be low and increased slowly with careful monitoring of serum creatinine and potassium. Particular caution is necessary if these drugs are used in combination with diuretics or in other high renin states (e.g. volume depletion), when marked hypotension ('first dose effect') may be anticipated. Caution is also necessary when there is (or may be) a possibility of renal artery stenosis, both because of the risk of hypotension and also because of reduced GFR in the affected kidney(s). They should generally not be used with potassium sparing diuretics because of the added risk of hyperkalaemia. All are eliminated by the kidney which accounts for the reduced dose usually required in the elderly (Drummer et al. 1987; Duchin et al. 1987; Kelly et al. 1988; Thomson et al. 1989). Exactly the same advice pertains to angiotensin II receptor antagonists with candersartan (Gleiter and Monke 2002) and losartan (Sica et al. 2000) as examples.

Hypertension

Problems should be avoidable by titration of a low starting dose of any drug to produce the required therapeutic effect. Thiazides are less effective as the GFR falls and a loop diuretic is often given in combination with other agents.

β-Blockers

Atenolol, bisoprolol, pindolol, nadolol, and sotalol are all excreted by the kidney and reduced doses may be needed. The metabolites of acebutolol may accumulate. Other β-blockers are prescribed unchanged.

Vasodilators, calcium channel blockers, and α-blockers

No dose adjustment is needed for any of these drugs. Minoxidil therapy often requires concomitant use of a loop diuretic.

Centrally acting agents

α-Methyl dopa, clonidine are given in usual doses and titrated for their effect, but moxonidine may require dose reduction.

Lipid lowering agents

Hyperlipidaemia is found in patients with the nephrotic syndrome, in most patients with chronic renal failure, and in many patients with functioning renal transplants. Diet should be used to control these abnormalities but drug treatment may be needed. The anion-exchange resins (e.g. colestipol) and 3-hydroxy-3-methylglutaryl coenzyme A-reductase (HMG-CoA reductase) inhibitors (e.g. simvastatin, atorvostatin, and pravastatin) can be given in usual doses, with the exception of fluvastatin, for which the dose is reduced in both renal impairment and the nephrotic syndrome (Appel-Dingemanse 2002). Cerivastatin has been withdrawn because of an increased incidence of myopathy and myositis, which remains an important adverse effect of other statins particularly if given in the presence of renal impairment or with cyclosporin or gemfibrizol. The fibrates (gemfibrizol, bezafibrate) can be used with dose reduction at GFR less than 20 ml/min. There is no role for the use of clofibrate because of its potential to cause peripheral neuropathy.

Thrombolytics, anticoagulants, and haemostatics

Streptokinase, anistreplase, and alteplase can all be used in patients with renal impairment with acute myocardial infarction but the potential risks of haemorrhage have to be weighed against the advantages. They can be given to transplant patients. Urokinase and alteplase can be used in usual dosages to declot dialysis catheters.

Anticoagulants and antiplatelet agents

Warfarin is used in normal dosage (Van Peer et al. 1978) and its effect monitored by measuring prothrombin time in the usual way. It is highly protein bound and, therefore, not dialysed. It may be subject to displacement from protein binding sites with consequent reduction in volume of distribution. In nephrotic patients, hypoalbuminaemia leads to increased sensitivity to warfarin. Unfractionated (standard) heparin is administered intravenously by infusion in usual dosage. There is now widespread use of low molecular weight heparins (e.g. enoxaparin, tinzaparin) both as prophylaxis and in treatment of thromboembolic disease. The dose is administered subcutaneously and usually prescribed without monitoring of its effect. Sanderlink (2002) demonstrated in a study of subjects with normal renal function and varying degrees of renal impairment that absorption (measured by anti-Xa activity) was unchanged but that the elimination half-life was prolonged significantly in those with a GFR less than 30 ml/min, and that this was more evident with repeated dosing. The anti-Xa exposure was significantly increased. It is, therefore, recommended that the dose should be reduced by half in severe renal impairment. Prophylactic aspirin is given in the usual low dose (75–150 mg daily), but clodiprogel dosage should be reduced.

Prostacyclin is used to prevent platelet aggregation in artificial kidneys and haemofilters. It is also used as a vasodilator with particular effects upon the pulmonary circulation. It is rapidly hydrolyzed and, therefore, not affected by renal impairment.

Tranexamic acid completely inhibits the activation of plasminogen to plasmin, but the dose should be reduced and the dose interval prolonged in renal failure (Foster et al. 1990). Ureteric obstruction by blood clot has been reported in patients with massive haemorrhage from the upper renal tract.

Diabetes mellitus

Insulin

Insulin requirements fall with declining renal function, probably as a consequence of reduced metabolism of insulin by the kidney in both acute and chronic renal failure. The glucose concentration of dialysate in haemodialysis will determine whether insulin adjustments are needed; in critical care when patients may be fed enterally or parenterally or haemofiltration insulin may be required as a continuous infusion.

The absorption of insulin in PD has been discussed previously and may be very variable.

Oral hypoglycaemic agents

Gliclazide, gliquidone, and glipizide are the safest drugs to use although dose reduction may be needed if GFR is below 10 ml/min. Other sulfonylureas, particularly chloropramide with its long half-life, should be avoided. Metformin, a biguanide, should not be used if the GFR falls below 20 ml/min, as there is a high risk of lactic acidosis. Metformin induced lactic acidosis may require haemofiltration with bicarbonate as the buffer; haemodialysis may increase metformin clearance in these circumstances (Lalau et al. 1989). The thiazolidinediones, rosiglitazone, and pioglitazone require no dose adjustment. Acarbose should be avoided in renal impairment.

Insulin requirements fall with declining renal function, probably as a consequence of reduced metabolism of insulin by the kidney in both acute and chronic renal failure. In patients on haemodialysis it is often necessary to give supplemental insulin during treatment. The same situation applies in patients on haemofiltration in acute renal failure, particularly if they are being fed parenterally, and in continuous arteriovenous haemodialysis (CAVHD) when the dialysate is a glucose based solution. Non-diabetic patients may require insulin temporarily under these circumstances. Patients on CAPD may need a change in insulin preparation and adjustment in the frequency and route of administration. The intraperitoneal requirement is approximately 50 per cent of intravenous requirements.

Asthma

β-Agonists administered by inhalation, oral, or parenteral routes need no adjustment in patients with renal impairment. Although tobuterol is an exception. Aminophylline and theophylline can be given in usual doses, but metabolites may accumulate (Kraan et al. 1988) and theophylline levels may be falsely raised (Nanji et al. 1988). The leukotrione antagonist montelukast can be used without dosage reduction, although it is recommended that the dose is reduced in moderate to severe renal impairment (BNF 2002). Dekhuijzen and Koopmans (2002) advise that this is not necessary.

Gastrointestinal drugs

H₂-antagonists and antiulcer drugs

There is an increased risk of confusional states with cimetidine in patients with impaired renal function. Cimetidine is cleared by the liver, but metabolites accumulate if the GFR is less than 20 ml/min (Bjaeldager et al. 1980). Ranitidine is preferable in this situation, but it should be noted that it interferes with creatinine secretion and increases plasma creatinine. It is partly cleared by the kidneys (Roberts 1984) and the dose should be halved when the GFR is less than 10 ml/min. It is dialysed (Gladziwa et al. 1988), and a supplemental dose is needed after dialysis. Approximately one-third of a 50 mg dose is cleared by a single exchange in CAPD (Sica *et al.* 1987) and a 150 mg twice daily dose can be used safely. It is commonly given to patients requiring artificial ventilation to reduce the risk of stress ulceration. In these circumstances, 25 mg twice or thrice daily intravenously is sufficient. No supplemental dose is needed during haemofiltration even though 20 per cent may be removed during 20 l of exchange. Omeprazole and misoprostol are given in usual doses. Misoprostol may cause reductions in GFR through haemodynamic changes in the kidney.

Hyperuricaemia

Allopurinol

Allopurinol is metabolized to oxypurinol, which is retained in renal impairment and may be responsible for some of the adverse effects including rashes, bone marrow depression, and gastrointestinal upset. The dose should be reduced to 100 mg/day when the GFR is less than 20 ml/min, and in haemodialysis patients the dose is given after treatment. Allopurinol interferes with the metabolism of 6-mercaptopurine (an active metabolite of azathioprine) causing accumulation and toxicity (e.g. leucopenia). Treatment of gout in transplant patients is difficult (Braun 2000; Fam 2001). Reduction in the dose of azathioprine is one step but occasionally the drug has to be stopped altogether. Unfortunately, cyclosporin increases serum uric acid concentrations and probenecid may have to be used. Benzbromazone (another uricosuric) has been used in mild and moderate renal impairment, but is only available on a named patient basis in the United Kingdom although it is available in Europe, South Africa, and Japan.

Uricosuric agents

Uric acid is excreted most efficiently in alkaline urine. This may be achieved with potassium citrate, with care to avoid hyperkalaemia, but in advanced renal failure the urine is relentlessly acidic in pH.

Probenecid

Probenecid inhibits secretion of acids in the proximal tubule and prevents reabsorption of urate from the tubular lumen. It prolongs the effect of penicillins, cephalosporins, naproxen, indomethacin, methotrexate, and sulfonylureas (all of which are weak acids), causing accumulation and the potential for toxicity. It also inhibits tubular secretion (and hence activity) of frusemide and bumetanide. It also inhibits liver uptake and, hence, glucuronidation of several drugs including zidovudine (see under antivirals).

Colchicine

Colchicine has been partly replaced by NSAIDs for the treatment of acute gout. However, it remains valuable in patients in whom NSAID are undesirable (e.g. peptic ulcer disease, cardiac failure, renal impairment) with no dose adjustments.

Losartan has been found to act so as to lower serum uric acid concentrations in renal transplant patients (Yamamoto 2000; Kamper 2001). It acts by increasing urinary excretion of uric acid and xanthine as well as oxypurinol. This may be useful as an adjunct to its other indications.

Anti-inflammatory agents

NSAIDs including aspirin inhibit prostaglandin synthesis by inhibition of cyclo-oxygenase. The principal renal prostaglandins in man are PGE_2 and PGI_2 each of which is vasodilator and natriuretic (Dunn 1983). In addition to effects on renal blood flow prostaglandins also influence tubular ion transport directly. In healthy individuals inhibition of cyclo-oxygenase has no detectable effect on renal function, but in patients with cardiac failure, nephrotic syndrome, liver disease, glomerulonephritis, and other renal disease cyclo-oxygenase inhibitors predictably cause a reversible fall in GFR which can be severe. They also cause fluid retention. They may also cause hyperkalaemia. There is evidence that sulindac causes less inhibition of renal cyclo-oxygenase than a dose of ibuprofen that is equi-effective on extrarenal tissues; sulindac may cause less renal impairment than other NSAIDs. Aspirin may also spare cyclo-oxygenase in the kidney to some extent. The clinical relevance of these observations remains uncertain and caution is needed in severe renal impairment for all of this group of drugs. The newer inhibitors of COX-2 are thought to have less gastrointestinal side-effects than other NSAIDs, but will have the same effects upon renal function (Swan *et al.* 2000). Celecoxib is also heavily protein bound. It is eliminated after metabolism to carboxylic acid and glucuronide metabolites and excreted in the faeces and urine. There are no adjustments required in renal impairment (Davies *et al.* 2000).

Indomethacin, azapropazone, and diflunisal have important renal excretion, whereas most other NSAIDs are eliminated by metabolism. Diflunisal is less protein bound in the presence of renal impairment, although the clinical importance of this is slight (Verbreeck and De Schepper 1980; Eriksonn *et al.* 1989). Sulindac has an active sulfide metabolite (Gibson *et al.* 1987), but in renal impairment this metabolism is reduced (Diskin *et al.* 1988; Nesher *et al.* 1988). It has been reported to have fewer side-effects than indomethacin (Berg and Talseth 1985; Nesher *et al.* 1988). The NSAIDs are highly protein bound and are not removed by dialysis.

Corticosteroids and immunosuppressive agents

Prednisone and prednisolone are not eliminated by the kidney. However, in theory, the dose should be reduced when patients have advanced uraemia (Bergrem 1983) as hepatic clearance is reduced (Bianchetti *et al.* 1976). Bergrem confirms that usual doses of prednisolone can be used in patients with the nephritic syndrome. Hypoalbuminaemia reduces the number of binding sites on plasma protein, but the increase in steroid side-effects reported by Lewis *et al.* (1971) failed to account for other factors such as underlying disease and renal dysfunction. Methylprednisolone is cleared by haemodialysis, and should be given after dialysis (Sherlock and Letteri 1977).

Azathioprine accumulates in renal impairment and the dose should be reduced from a maximum of 3 to 1 mg/kg/day if the GFR falls below 10 ml/min (Schusziara *et al.* 1986). Allopurinol prevents the metabolism of 6-mercaptopurine; the active metabolite of azathioprine, and the combination should be avoided. The metabolism of azathioprine has a genetic variability. Hypoxanthine guanine phosphoro101 transferase (HPRT) oxidation by xanthine oxidase shows little variability, but inactivation via methylation by thiopurine methyl transferase (TPMT) is variable. Estimates show that 11 per cent of the population has low TPMT activity with one in 300 with a very low level. This appears to have aroused less interest in renal physicians than in other specialities (Holme *et al.* 2002). Monitoring of white blood count concentration may not always predict toxicity.

Cyclophosphamide is used in a variety of vasculitic conditions often intravenously. The dosing schedules vary, but up to 1 g every 2 weeks may be given as induction therapy. The dose should be reduced stepwise according to estimations of the GFR with half the usual dose administered in severe renal failure. As it is removed by haemodialysis it should be administered postdialysis (Haubitz *et al.* 2002).

Methotrexate is used frequently in rheumatological disorders (rheumatoid arthritis, psoriatic arthropathy, systemic lupus erythematosus), usually as a small weekly dose. It should be noted that the drug is a weak acid and eliminated by proximal tubular secretion, which can be blocked by salicylates or NSAID. There are also reports of interaction, causing increased serum levels, when higher doses are used in conjunction with amoxycillin (Ronchera *et al.* 1993), and vancomycin although the mechanism was less clear (Blum *et al.* 2002).

Cyclosporin is a highly lipid soluble drug, which is exclusively bound to plasma proteins and has a large volume of distribution. It is metabolized by the liver via the cytochrome P-450 system by mono- and di-hydroxylation as well as *N*-demethylation. Only minor amounts are excreted in the urine as parent drug or metabolites. Renal impairment does not affect the metabolism. However, since many other drugs may be prescribed to patients taking cyclosporin therapy several important interactions may occur. These will both increase plasma concentration and, therefore, increase the risk of nephrotoxicity or reduce plasma concentrations and increase the risk of transplant organ rejection. Aminoglycosides may have an additive effect upon the nephrotoxicity itself. Drugs affecting the cytochrome P-450 system are listed in Table 7.

Tacrolimus (Wallemacq and Vereeck 2001) and sirolimus (MacDonald *et al.* 2000) can be regarded as behaving in a similar fashion to cyclosporin.

MMF converted to its active metabolite MPA has been discussed in the section on pharmacokinetics. Careful monitoring of plasma concentrations and therapeutic effects are needed particularly in renal impairment (MacPhee *et al.* 2000).

Miscellaneous drugs

Acetazolamide

Acetazolamide may produce electrolyte disturbance particularly in renal impairment and in the elderly (Chapron *et al.* 1989). Its use should be avoided or carefully monitored.

Table 7 Drugs affecting cytochrome P-450 system

Inhibitors	Inducers
Ketaconazole	Rifampicin
Erythromycin	Phenytoin
Oral contraceptives	Phenobarbitone
Methylprednisolone	Carbamazepine
Diltiazem	Sodium valproate
Nicardipine	
Verapamil	
Cimetidine	

Biphosphonates

It is appropriate to use intravenous disodium pamidronate or etidronate in hypercalcaemia associated with malignancy even with renal failure. The likely outcome is an improvement in renal function particularly if other measures such as sodium and water depletion are addressed. Biphosphonates (with the exception of alendronic acid) can be used to treat postmenopausal or corticosteroid induced osteoporosis and Paget's disease. Pamidronate has been used effectively and safely after renal transplantation (Fan *et al.* 2000). Doses should be reduced in moderate renal impairment Mitchell *et al.* 2000). Etidronate if combined with calcium supplementation may cause hypercalcaemia.

Sildenafil

Sildenafil is used for erectile dysfunction, and can be used with dose reduction to 25 mg (half the usual dose) if the GFR falls below 30 ml/min (Miurhead *et al.* 2002).

Amfebutamone

Amfebutamone (bupropion), used as an aid to smoking cessation, is recommended in a daily dose of 140 mg, but there is no information on its use in patients on dialysis.

Summary

1. Always check the method of elimination of any drug before prescribing in the presence of known or suspected renal impairment.

2. Monitor any changes in renal function.

3. Look out for any adverse or side-effects.

References

Adler, D. S., Martin, E., Gambertoglio, J. G., Tozer, T. N., and Spire, J.-P. (1975). Haemodialysis of phenytoin in a uraemic patient. *Clinical Pharmacology and Therapeutics* **18**, 65–69.

Agarwal, R., Gorski, J. C., Sundblad, K., and Brater, D. C. (2000). Urinary protein binding does not affect response to furosemide in patients with nephrotic syndrome. *Journal of the American Society of Nephrology* **11**, 1100–1105.

Aletta, J. M., Francke, E. F., and Neu, H. C. (1980). Intravenous azlocillin kinetics in patients on long-term haemodialysis. *Clinical Pharmacology and Therapeutics* **27**, 563–566.

Allen, R. D. M., Hunnisett, A. G., and Morris, P. J. (1985). Cyclosporin and rifampicin in renal transplantation. *Lancet* I, 980.

Almond, M. K., Fan, S., Dhillon, S., Pollock, A. M., and Raftery, M. J. (1995). Avoiding acyclovir neurotoxicity in patients with chronic renal failure undergoing haemodialysis. *Nephron* **69**, 428–432.

Andrew, O. T. (1980). Tuberculosis in patients with end-stage renal failure. *American Journal of Medicine* **68**, 59–65.

Appel-Dingemanse, S., Smith, T., and Merz, M. (2002). Pharmacokinetics of fluvastatin in subjects with renal impairment and nephrotic syndrome. *Journal of Clinical Pharmacology* **42**, 312–318.

Balducci, M., Slama, D. G., Rottembourg, J., Baumelou, A., and Delage, A. (1981). Intraperitoneal insulin in uraemic diabetics undergoing continuous ambulatory peritoneal dialysis. *British Medical Journal* **283**, 1021–1023.

Barclay, M. L., Kirkpatrick, C. M. J., and Begg, E. J. (1999). Once daily aminoglycoside therapy. *Clinical Pharmacokinetics* **36**, 89–98.

Bates, D. W. *et al.* (2001). Correlates of acute renal failure in patients receiving parenteral amphotericin B. *Kidney International* **60**, 1452–1459.

Beaman, M., Soalro, L., McGonigle, R. J. S., Michael, A., and Adu, D. (1989). Vancomycin and ceftazidime in the treatment of CAPD peritonitis. *Nephron* **51**, 51–55.

Bellman, R. *et al.* (2002). Elimination of levofloxacin in critically ill patients with renal failure: influence of continuous veno-venous hemofiltration. *International Journal of Clinical Pharmacology and Therapeutics* **40**, 142–149.

Bennett, W. H. Guide to drug dosage in renal failure. In *Clinical Pharmacokinetics. Drug Data Handbook* (ed. G. J. Mammen), pp. 31–84. Hong Kong: ADIS, 1990.

Berg, J. K. and Talseth, T. (1985). Acute renal effects of sulindac and indomethacin in chronic renal failure. *Clinical Pharmacology and Therapeutics* **37**, 325–329.

Berlinger, W. G., Park, G. D., and Spector, R. (1985). The effect of dietary protein and the clearance of allopurinol and oxypurinol. *New England Journal of Medicine* **313**, 771–776.

Bergrem, H. (1983). Pharmacokinetics and protein binding of prednisolone in patients with nephritic syndrome and patients undergoing haemodialysis. *Kidney International* **23**, 876–881.

Bianchetti, G. *et al.* (1976). Pharmacokinetics and effects of propranololin terminal uraemic patients and in patients undergoing regular dialysis treatment. *Clinical Pharmacokinetics* **1**, 373–384.

Biaski, S. K. (1980). Disease induced changes in plasma binding of basic drug. *Clinical Pharmacokinetics* **5**, 246–262.

Bickley, S. K. (1988). Drug dosing during continuous arteriovenous haemofiltration. *Clinical Pharmacy* **7**, 198–206.

Bjaeldager, P. A. L., Jensen, J. B., and Larsen, N.-E. (1980). Elimination of oral cimetidine in chronic renal failure and during haemodialysis. *British Journal of Clinical Pharmacology* **9**, 585–592.

Block, E. R. and Bennett, J. E. (1974). Flucytosine and Amphotericin B: haemodialysis effects on plasma concentration and clearance. *Annals of Internal Medicine* **80**, 613–617.

Blum, R., Seymour, J. F., and Toner, G. (2002). Significant impairment of high-dose methotrexate clearance following vancomycin administration in the absence of overt renal impairment. *Annals of Oncology* **13**, 327–330.

Bohler, J. *et al.* (1987). Rebound of plasma vancomycin levels after haemodialysis with highly permeable membranes. *European Journal of Clinical Pharmacology* **42**, 635–639.

Bohler, J., Donauer, J., and Keller, F. (1999). Pharmacokinetic principles during continuous renal replacement therapy: drugs and dosage. *Kidney International* **72**, S24–S28.

Bonati, M. *et al.* (1987). Teicoplanin pharmacokinetics in patients with chronic renal failure. *Clinical Pharmacokinetics* **12**, 292–301.

Bowmer, C. J. and Lindup, W. E. (1982). Decreased drug binding in uraemia: effect of indoxyl sulphate and other endogenous substances on the binding of drugs and dyes in human albumin. *Biochemical Pharmacology* **31**, 319–323.

Brater, D. C. *Handbook of Drug Use in Patients with Renal Disease* 6th edn. *Improved Therapeutics*, Indianapolis, USA, 1994.

Braun, W. E. (2000). Modification of the treatment of gout in renal transplant recipients. *Transplant Proceedings* **32**, 199.

Brophy, D. F. and Mueller, B. A. (1997). Automated peritoneal dialysis: new implications for pharmacists. *Annals of Pharmacotherapeutics* **31**, 756–764.

Brown, D. L. and Mauro, L. S. (1988). Vancomycin dosing chart for use in patients with renal impairment. *American Journal of Kidney Diseases* **11**, 15–19.

Caldwell, J. E. *et al.* (1988). Pipercuronium and pancuronium: comparison of pharmacokinetics and duration of action. *British Journal of Anaesthesia* **61**, 693–697.

Cass, L. M., Efthymiopoulos, C., Marsh, J., and Bye, A. (1999). Effect of renal impairment on the pharmocokinetics of intravenous zanamivir. *Clinical Pharmacokinetics* **36**, 513–519.

Chapron, D. J., Gomolin, I. H., and Sweeney, K. R. (1989). Acetazolamide blood concentrations are excessive in the elderly: propensity for acidosis and relationship to renal function. *Journal of Clinical Pharmacology* **29**, 348–353.

Chauvin, M., Lebrault, C., Levron, J. C., and Duvaldestin, P. (1987a). Pharmacokinetics of alfentanil in chronic renal failure. *Anaesthetics and Analgesia* **66**, 53–56.

Chauvin, M., Sandouk, P., Scherrmann, J. M., Farinotti, R., Strumza, P., and Duvaldestin, P. (1987b). Morphine pharmacokinetics in renal failure. *Anaesthiology* **66**, 327–331.

Craig, R., Murphy, T., and Gibson, T. P. (1983). Kinetic analysis of D-xylose absorption in normal subjects and in patients with chronic renal insufficiency. *Journal of Laboratory and Clinical Medicine* **101**, 496–506.

Craig, W. A. and Kunin, C. M. (1973). Trimethoprim-sulfamethoxazole: pharmacodynamic effects of urinary pH and impaired renal function. *Annals of Internal Medicine* **78**, 491–497.

Cuss, F. M. C., Carmichael, D. J. S., Allington, A., and Hulme, B. (1986). Tuberculosis in renal failure: a high incidence in patients born in the third world. *Clinical Nephrology* **25**, 129–133.

Daneshmend, T. K. and Warnock, D. W. (1983). Clinical pharmacokinetics of antifungal drugs. *Clinical Pharmacokinetics* **8**, 17–42.

Danhof, M., Hisaoka, M., and Levy, G. (1984). Kinetics of drug action in disease states II. Effect of experimental renal dysfunction on phenobarbital concentration in rats at onset of loss of righting reflex. *Journal of Pharmacology and Experimental Therapeutics* **230**, 627–631.

Dasgupta, A. and Abu-Alfa, A. (1992). Increased free phenytoin concentrations in predialysis serum compared to post dialysis serum inpatients with uraemia treated with haemodialysis; role of uraemic compounds. *American Journal of Clinical Pathology* **98**, 19–25.

Davies, G., Kingswood, C., and Street, M. (1996). Pharmacokinetics of opioids in renal dysfunction. *Clinical Pharmacokinetics* **31**, 410–422.

Davies, N. M., McLachlan, A. J., Day, R. O., and Williams, K. M. (2000). Clinical pharmacokinetics and pharmacodynamics of celecoxib: a selective cyclo-oxygenase-2 inhibitor. *Clinical Pharmacokinetics* **38**, 225–242.

Davies, S. P., Azadian, B. S., Kox, W. J., and Brown, E. A. (1992). Pharmacokinetics of ciprofloxacin and vancomycin in patients with acute renal failure treated by continuous haemodialysis. *Nephrology, Dialysis, Transplantation* **7**, 848–854.

Dekluijzen, P. W. and Koopmans, P. P. (2002). Pharmacokinetic profile of zafirlukast. *Clinical Pharmacokinetics* **41**, 105–114.

Deray, G. *et al.* (1988). Pharmacokinetics of zidovudine in a patient on maintenance haemodialysis. *New England Journal of Medicine* **319**, 1606–1607.

Desai, T. K. and Tsang, T.-K. (1988). Aminoglycoside nephrotoxicity in obstructive jaundice. *American Journal of Medicine* **85**, 47–50.

Dettli, L. Drug dosage in renal disease. In *Handbook of Clinical Pharmacokinetics* Section III (ed. M. Gibaldi and L. Prescott), pp. 261–276. Balgowlah, Australia: ADIS Health Science Press, 1983.

Diaz-Buxo, J. A. (2000). Use of intraperitoneal insulin with CCPD. *Seminars in Dialysis* **13**, 207.

Dingemanse, J., Polhuijs, M., and Danhof, M. (1988). Altered pharmacokinetic–pharmacodynamic relationship of heptabarbital in experimental renal failure in rats. *Journal of Pharmacology and Experimental Therapeutics* **246**, 371.

Diskin, C. J., Ravis, W., Campagna, K. D., and Clark, C. R. (1988). Pharmacokinetics of sulindac in ESRD. *Nephron* **50**, 397.

Drayer, D. E. Pharmacologically active drug metabolites: therapeutic and toxic activities, plasma and urine data in man, accumulation in renal failure. In *Handbook of Clinical Pharmacokinetics* (ed. M. Gibaldi and L. Prescott), pp. 114–132. Balgowlah, Australia: ADIS Health Science Press, 1983.

Drummer, O. H., Workman, B. S., Miach, P. J., Jarrett, B., and Lovis, W. J. (1987). The pharmacokinetics of captopril and captopril disulfide conjugates in uraemic patients on maintenance dialysis: comparison with patients with normal renal function. *European Journal of Clinical Pharmacology* **3**, 267–271.

Duchin, K. L., Pierides, A. M., Heald, A., Singhvi, S. M., and Rommel, A. J. (1984). Elimination kinetics of captopril in patients with renal failure. *Kidney International* **25**, 942–948.

Dundee, J. W. and Richards, R. K. (1954). Effect of azotemia upon the action of intravenous barbiturate anesthesia. *Anesthesiology* **15**, 333–346.

Dunn, M. J. Renal prostaglandins. In *Renal Endocrinology* (ed. M. J. Dunn), pp. 1–74. Baltimore: Williams and Wilkins, 1983.

Edell, L. S., Westby, G. R., and Gould, S. R. (1988). An improved method of vancomycin administration to dialysis patients. *Clinical Nephrology* **29**, 86–87.

Elwell, R. J., Bailie, G. R., and Manley, H. J. (2000). Correlation of intraperitoneal antibiotic pharmacokinetics and peritoneal membrane transport characteristics. *Peritoneal Dialysis International* **20**, 694–698.

Ely, E. W., Bernard, G. R., and Lensing, A. W. (2002). Activated protein C for severe sepsis. *New England Journal of Medicine* **347**, 1036–1037.

Eriksson, R. K., Wahlin-Boll, E., Odar-Cederlof, I., Lindholm, L., and Melander, A. (1989). Influence of renal failure, rheumatoid arthritis and old age on the pharmacokinetics of diflunisal. *European Journal of Clinical Pharmacology* **36**, 165–174.

Fabre, J., Fox, H. M., Dayer, P., and Balant, L. Differences in kinetic properties of drugs: implications as to the selection of a particular drug for use in patients with renal failure, with special emphasis on antibiotics and beta adrenoceptor blocking agents. In *Handbook of Clinical Pharmacokinetics* Section III (ed. M. Gibaldi and L. Prescott), pp. 233–260. Balgowlah, Australia: ADIS Health Science Press, 1988.

Fam, A. G. (2001). Difficult gout and new approaches for control of hyperuricaemia in the allopurinol-allergic patient. *Current Rheumatology Reports* **3**, 29–35.

Fan, S. L.-S., Almond, M. K., Ball, E., Evans, K., and Cunningham, J. (2000). Pamidronate therapy as prevention of bone loss following renal transplantation. *Kidney International* **57**, 684–690.

Faulds, D. and Heal, R. C. (1990). Ganciclovir; a review of antiviral activity, pharmacokinetic properties and therapeutic efficacy in cytomegalovirus infections. *Drugs* **39**, 597–638.

Fillastre, J. P. *et al.* (1990). Pharmacokinetics of quinolones in renal insufficiency. *Journal of Antimicrobial Chemotherapy* **26**, 551.

Fillastre, J. P. *et al.* (1985). Pharmacokinetics of aztreonam in patients with chronic renal failure. *Clinical Pharmacokinetics* **10**, S91–S100.

Fillastre, J.-P. and Singlas, E. (1991). Pharmacokinetics of newer drugs with renal impairment (Part I). *Clinical Pharmacokinetics* **20**, 293–310.

Fine, A., Parry, D., Ariano, R., and Dent, W. (2000). Marked variation in peritoneal insulin absorption in peritoneal dialysis. *Peritoneal Dialysis International* **20**, 652–655.

Fleming, L. W., Morland, T. A., Scott, A. C., Stewart, W. K., and White, L. O. (1987). Ciprofloxacin in plasma and peritoneal dialysate after oral therapy in patients on continuous ambulatory peritoneal dialysis. *Journal of Antimicrobial Chemotherapy* **19**, 493–503.

Fletcher, C. V., Chinnock, B. J., Chace, B., and Balfour, H. H. (1988). Pharmacokinetics and safety of high-dose oral acyclovir for suppression of cytomegalovirus disease after renal transplantation. *Clinical Pharmacology and Therapeutics* **44**, 158–163.

Foster, G. R. *et al.* (1990). Extensive crescent formation with antifibrinolytic therapy in a case of diffuse endocapillary glomerulonephritis. *Nephrology, Dialysis, Transplantation* **5**, 512–514.

Gerig, J. S., Bolton, N. D., Swabb, E. A., Scheld, M., and Bolton, W. K. (1984). Effect of haemodialysis and peritoneal dialysis on aztreonam pharmacokinetics. *Kidney International* **26**, 308–318.

Gibaldi, M. *Biopharmaceutics and Clinical Pharmacokinetics*. Philadelphia: Lea and Febiger, 1984.

Gibson, T. P. (1986). Renal disease and drug metabolism: an overview. *American Journal of Kidney Diseases* **8**, 7–17.

Gibson, T. P. and Nelson, H. A. Drug kinetics and artificial kidneys. In *Handbook of Clinical Pharmacokinetics* (ed. M. Gibaldi and L. Prescott), pp. 301–324. Balgowlah, Australia: ADIS Health Science Press, 1983.

Gladziwa, U. (1988). Pharmacokinetics of ranitidine in patients undergoing haemofiltration. *European Journal of Clinical Pharmacology* **35**, 427–430.

Gleiter, C. H. and Monke, K. E. (2002). Clinical pharmacokinetics of candesartan. *Clinical Pharmacokinetics* **41**, 7–17.

Gold, C. H., Buchanan, N., Tringham, V., Viljoen, M., Strickwold, B., and Moodley, G. P. (1976). Isoniazid pharmacokinetics in patients in chronic renal failure. *Clinical Nephrology* **6**, 365–369.

Golper, T. A. and Marx, M. A. (1998). Drug dosing adjustments during continuous renal replacement therapies. *Kidney International* **66**, S165–S168.

Graybill, J. R. (1996). Lipid formulations for amphotericin B. Does the emperor need new clothes? *Annals of Internal Medicine* **124**, 921–923.

Guay, D. R. *et al.* (1988). Pharmacokinetics and pharmacodynamics of codeine in end-stage renal disease. *Clinical Pharmacology and Therapeutics* **43**, 63–71.

Gugler, R. and Azarnoff, D. L. Drug protein binding and the nephritic syndrome. In *Handbook of Clinical Pharmacokinetics* (ed. M. Gibaldi and L. Prescott), pp. 96–108. Balgowlah, Australia: ADIS Health Science Press, 1983.

Gulyassy, P. F. and Depner, T. A. (1983). Impaired binding of drugs and ligands in renal diseases. *American Journal of Kidney Diseases* **2**, 578–601.

Halstenson, C. E. *et al.* (1994). Pharmacokinetics of tazobactam MI metabolite after administration of piperacillin/tazobactam in subjects with renal impairment. *Journal of Clinical Pharmacology* **34**, 1208–1217.

Hammertstein, A., Derendorf, H., and Lowenthal, D. T. (1998). Pharmacokinetic and pharmacodynamic changes in the elderly. *Clinical Pharmacokinetics* **35**, 49–64.

Haubitz, M. *et al.* (2002). Cyclophosphamide pharmacokinetics in patients with renal insufficiency. *Kidney International* **61**, 1495–1501.

Herman, R. J., McAllister, C. B., Branch, R. A., and Wilkinson, G. R. (1985). Effects of age on meperidine disposition. *Clinical Pharmacology and Therapeutics* **37**, 19–24.

Hinderling, P. H. (2001). Biased estimates of nonrenal clearance. *Journal of Pharmacology Science* **90**, 960–966.

Hoffer, D., Koeppe, P., and Naumann, E. (1991). Pharmacokinetics of teicoplanin in haemodialysis patients. *Infection* **19**, 324–327.

Holme, S. A., Duley, J. A., Sanderson, J., Routledge, P. A., and Anstey, A. V. (2002). Erythrocyte thiopurine methyl transferase assessment prior to azathroprine use in the UK. *Quarterly Journal of Medicine* **95**, 439–444.

Houin, G., Brunner, F., Nebout, T., Cherfasni, M., Lagrue, G., and Tillement, J. P. (1983). The effects of chronic renal insufficiency on the pharmacokinetics of doxycycline in man. *British Journal of Clinical Pharmacology* **16**, 245–252.

Huang, C. M., Atkinson, A. J., Levin, M., Levin, N. W., and Quintanilla, A. (1974). Pharmacokinetics of furosemide in advanced renal failure. *Clinical Pharmacology and Therapeutics* **16**, 659–666.

Humes, H. D. (1988). Aminoglycoside nephrotoxicity. *Kidney International* **33**, 900–911.

Hustinx, W. M. N. and Hoepelman, I. M. (1993). Aminoglycoside dosage regimens: is once a day enough? *Clinical Pharmacokinetics* **25**, 427–432.

Inone, D. *et al.* (1987). Coadministration of albumin and furosemide in patients with the nephrotic syndrome. *Kidney International* **32**, 198–203.

Izzedine, H., Lannay-Vacher, V., Baumelon, A., and Deray, G. (2001). An appraisal of antiretroviral drugs in haemodialysis. *Kidney International* **60**, 821–830.

Jayasekara, D. *et al.* (1999). Antiviral therapy for HIV patients with renal insufficiency. *Journal of Acquired Immune Deficiency Syndrome* **21**, 384–392.

Joest, M., Ritz, E., and Mutschler, E. (1999). Renal handling of drugs in the healthy elderly. *European Journal of Clinical Pharmacology* **55**, 205–211.

Johnson, R. J., Blair, A. D., and Ahmed, S. (1985). Ketoconazole kinetics in chronic peritoneal dialysis. *Clinical Pharmacology and Therapeutics* **37**, 325–329.

Johnson, M. A., Moore, K. H., Yuen, G. J., Bye, A., and Pakes, G. (1999). Clinical pharmocokinetics of lamivudine. *Clinical Pharmacokinetics* **36**, 41–66.

Joos, B., Schmidli, M., and Keusch, G. (1996). Pharmacokinetics of antimicrobial agents in anuric patients during continous venovenous haemofiltration. *Nephrology, Dialysis, Transplantation* **11**, 1582–1585.

Kamper, A. L. and Nielsen, A. H. (2001). Uricosuric effect of losartan in patients with renal transplants. *Transplantation* **27**, 671–674.

Kapstein, E. M., Chang, E. I., Egodage, P. M., Nicoloff, J. T., and Massry, S. G. (1987). Thyroxine transfer and distribution in critical nonthyroidal illnesses, chronic renal failure and chronic ethanol abuse. *Journal of Clinical Endocrinology and Metabolism* **65**, 606–616.

Keane, W. F. *et al.* (1996). Peritoneal dialysis-related peritonitis treatment recommendations: 1996 update. *Peritoneal Dialysis International* **16**, 557–573.

Keller, E., Hoppe-Seyler, G., and Schollmeyer, P. (1982). Disposition and diuretic effect of furosemide in the nephrotic syndrome. *Clinical Pharmacology and Therapeutics* **32**, 442–449.

Keller, F., Bohler, J., Czock, D., Zellner, D., and Mertz, A. K. (1999). Individualized drug dosage in patients treated with continuous hemofiltration. *Kidney International* **72**, S29–S31.

Kelly, J. G., Doyle, G. D., Carmody, M., Glover, D. R., and Cooper, W. D. (1988). Pharmacokinetics of lisinopril, enalapril and enalaprilat in renal failure: effects of haemodialysis. *British Journal of Clinical Pharmacology* **26**, 781–786.

Kitt, T. M., Park, G. D., Spector, R., and Tsalikian, E. (1989). Reduced renal clearance of oxypurinol during a 400 calorie protein-free diet. *Journal of Clinical Pharmacology* **29**, 65–71.

Kornhauser, D. M. *et al.* (1989). Probenecid and zidovudine metabolism. *Lancet* **2**, 473–475.

Kraan, J. *et al.* (1988). The pharmacokinetics of theophylline and enprofylline in patients with liver cirrhosis and in patients with chronic renal disease. *European Journal of Clinical Pharmacology* **35**, 357–362.

Kuop, J. R., Jusko, W. J., Elwood, C. M., and Kohli, R. K. (1975). Digoxin pharmacokinetics: role of renal failure in dosage regimen design. *Clinical Pharmacology and Therapeutics* **18**, 9–21.

Lake, K. D., Fletcher, C. V., Love, K. R., Brown, D. C., Joyce, L. D., and Pritzker, M. R. (1988). Ganciclovir pharmacokinetics during renal impairment. *Antimicrobial Agents and Chemotherapy* **32**, 1899–1900.

Lalau, J. D. *et al.* (1989). Hemodialysis in the treatment of lactic acidosis in diabetics treated by metformin: a study of metformin elimination. *Clinical Pharmacology, Therapy and Toxicology* **27**, 285–288.

Latini, R., Tognoni, G., and Kates, R. E. (1984). Clinical pharmacokinetics of amiodarone. *Clinical Pharmacokinetics* **9**, 136–156.

Lee, C. S., Marbury, T. C., and Benet, L. Z. (1980). Clearance calculations in haemodialysis: application to blood, plasma and dialysate measurements for ethambutol. *Journal of Pharmacokinetics and Biopharmaceuticals* **8**, 69–81.

Lehmann, C. R. *et al.* (1988). Capreomycin kinetics in renal impairment and clearance by hemodialysis. *American Review of Respiratory Disease* **138**, 1312–1313.

Lerner, A. M. *et al.* (1983). Randomized, controlled trial of the comparative efficacy, auditory toxicity and nephrotoxicity of tobramycin and netilmycin. *Lancet* **2**, 1123–1126.

Lewi, P. J. *et al.* (1976). Pharmacokinetic profile of intravenous miconazole in man. Comparison of normal subjects and patients with renal insufficiency. *European Journal of Clinical Pharmacology* **10**, 49–54.

Lewis, G. P., Jusko, W. J., and Burke, C. W. (1971). Prednisolone side-effects and serum protein levels. *Lancet* **2**, 778–780.

Lichtenwalmer, D. M. and Suh, B. (1983). Isolation and chemical characterization of 2-hydroxybenzoylglycine as a drug binding inhibitor in uraemia. *Journal of Chemical Investigation* **71**, 1289–1296.

Lynam, D. P. *et al.* (1988). The pharmacokinetics of vecuronium in patients anesthetized with isoflurane with normal renal function or with renal failure. *Anesthesiology* **69**, 227–231.

MacDonald, A., Scarola, J., Burke, J. T., and Zimmerman, J. J. (2000). Clinical pharmacokinetics and therapeutic monitoring of sirolimus. *Clinical Therapeutics* **22**, B101–B121.

MacPhee, I. A. *et al.* (2000). Pharmacokinetics of mycophenolate mofetil in patients with end-stage renal failure. *Kidney International* **57**, 1164–1168.

Macias, W. L., Dhainhault, J. F., and Yan, S. C. (2002). Pharmacokinetic–pharmacodynamic analysis of drotrecogin alfa (activated) in patients with severe sepsis. *Clinical Pharmacology and Therapeutics* **72**, 391–402.

Mahuchi, H. and Nakahashi, H. (1988). A major inhibitor of phenytoin binding to serum protein in uraemia. *Nephron* **48**, 310–314.

Manley, H. J., Bailie, G. R., Frye, R., Hess, L. D., and McGoldrick, M. D. (2000). Pharmacokinetics of intermittent intravenous cefazolin and tobramycin in patients with automated peritoneal dialysis. *Journal of the American Society of Nephrology* **11**, 1310–1316.

Meier-Kriesche, H. U., Shaw, L. M., Korecka, M., and Kaplan, B. (2000). Pharmacokinetics of mycophenolic acid in renal insufficiency. *Therapeutic Drug Monitoring* **22**, 27–30.

Meuldermans, W. *et al.* (1988). Alfentanil pharmacokinetics and metabolism in humans. *Anesthesiology* **69**, 527–534.

Mitchell, D. Y. *et al.* (2000). Effect of renal function on risedronate pharmacokinetics after a single oral dose. *British Journal of Clinical Pharmacology* **49**, 215–222.

Mouton, J. W., Touzw, D. J., Horrevortz, A. M., and Vinks, A. A. (2000). Comparative pharmacokinetics of the carbapenems: clinical implications. *Clinical Pharmacokinetics* **39**, 185–201.

Muirhead, G. J., Wilner, K., Colburn, W., Haug-Pihale, G., and Rouviex, B. (2002). The effects of age and renal and hepatic impairment on the pharmacokinetics of sildenafil. *British Journal of Clinical Pharmacology* **53**, 21S–30S.

Na, K. Y. *et al.* (2001). Does albumin preinfusion potentiate diuretic action of furosemide in patients with nephrotic syndrome? *Journal of the Korean Medical Scociety* **16**, 448–454.

Nanji, A. A. and Greenway, D. C. (1988). Falsely raised plasma theophylline concentrations in renal failure. *European Journal of Clinical Pharmacology* **34**, 309–310.

Nesher, G., Zimran, A., and Hershko, C. (1988). Reduced incidence of hyperkalaemia and azotaemia in patients receiving sulindac compared with indomethacin. *Nephron* **48**, 291–295.

Nilsen, O. G., Aasarod, K., Wideroe, T. E., and Guentert, T. W. (2001). Single- and multiple-dose pharmacokinetics, kidney tolerability and plasma protein binding of tenoxicam in renally impaired patients and healthy volunteers. *Pharmacology Toxicology* **89**, 265–272.

Odlind, B. G. and Beerman, B. (1980). Diuretic resistance reduced bioavailability and effect of oral frusemide. *British Medical Journal* **280**, 1577.

Oono, S., Tabec, K., Tetsuka, T., and Asano, Y. (1992). The pharmacokinetics of fluconazole during haemodialysis in uraemic patients. *European Journal of Clinical Pharmacology* **42**, 667–669.

Palmer, R. F. and Lasseter, K. C. (1975). Sodium nitroprusside. *New England Journal of Medicine* **292**, 294–297.

Parry, M. F. and Neu, H. C. (1976). Pharmacokinetics of ticarcillin in patients with abnormal renal function. *Journal of Infectious Diseases* **133**, 46–49.

Pea, F. and Furlanut, M. (2001). Pharmacokinetic aspects of treating infections in the intensive care unit. *Clinical Pharmacokinetics* **40**, 833–868.

Periti, P., Mazzei, T., Mini, E., and Norelli, A. (1989). Clinical pharmacokinetic properties of the macrolide antibiotics. Effects of age and various pathophysiological states. Part 1. *Clinical Pharmacokinetics* **16**, 193–214.

Prescott, L. F., Speirs, G. C., Critchley, J. A. J. H., Temple, R. M., and Winney, R. J. (1989). Paracetamol disposition and metabolite kinetics in patients with chronic renal failure. *European Journal of Clinical Pharmacology* **36**, 291–297.

Quelhorst, E. (2002). Insulin therapy during peritoneal dialysis: pros and cons of various forms of administration. *Journal of the American Society of Nephrology* **13**, S92–S96.

Raveh, D. *et al.* (2002). Risk factors for nephrotoxicity in elderly patients receiving once-daily aminoglycosides. *Quarterly Journal of Medicine* **95** (5), 291–297.

Reidenberg, M. M. The binding of drugs to plasma proteins from patients with poor renal function. In *Handbook of Clinical Pharmacokinetics* (ed. M. Gibaldi and L. Prescott), pp. 89–95. Balgowlah, Australia: ADIS Health Science Press, 1983.

Reidenberg, M. M. (1985). Kidney function and drug action. *New England Journal of Medicine* 313, 816–818.

Roberts, C. J. C. (1984). Clinical pharmacokinetics of ranitidine. *Clinical Pharmacokinetics* 9, 211–221.

Roberts, D. E. and Williams, J. D. (1989). Ciprofloxacin in renal failure. *Antimicrobial Agents and Chemotherapy* 23, 820–823.

Ronchera, C. L. *et al.* (1993). Pharmacokinetic interaction between high dose methotrexate and amoxycillin. *Therapeutic Drug Monitoring* 15, 375–379.

Sanderink, G. J. *et al.* (2002). Pharmacokinetics and pharmacodynamics of prophylactic dose of enoxaparin once daily over 4 days in patients with renal impairment. *Thrombosis Research* 105, 225–231.

Sawaya, B. P. *et al.* (1991). Direct vasoconstriction as a possible cause for amphotericin B induced nephrotoxicity in rats. *Journal of Clinical Investigation* 87, 2097–2107.

Sawe, J. *et al.* (1987). Kinetics of morphine in patients in renal failure. *European Journal of Pharmacology* 32, 377–382.

Schrier, R. W. and Conger, J. D. Acute renal failure: pathogenesis, diagnosis and management. In *Renal and Electrolyte Disorders* 3rd edn. (ed. R. W. Schrier), pp. 423–460. New York: Little Brown and Company, 1986.

Schusziarra, V. *et al.* (1986). Pharmacokinetics of azathioprine under haemodialysis. *International Journal of Clinical Pharmacology and Therapeutics* 14, 298–302.

Sear, J. W. (1988). Drug metabolites in anaesthetic practice—are they important. *British Journal of Anaesthesia* 61, 525–526.

Sherlock, J. E. and Letteri, J. M. (1977). Effect of haemodialysis on methylprednisolone plasma levels. *Nephron* 18, 208–211.

Sica, D. A., Conistock, T., Harford, A., and Eshelman, F. (1987). Ranitidine pharmacokinetics in continuous ambulatory peritoneal dialysis. *European Journal of Clinical Pharmacology* 32, 587–591.

Sica, D. A., Halstenon, C. E., Gehr, T. W., and Keane, W. F. (2000). Pharmacokinetics and blood pressure response of losartan in end-stage renal failure. *Clinical Pharmacokinetics* 38, 519–526.

Singlas, E., Taburet, A. M., Landru, I., Albin, H., and Ryckelinck, J. P. (1987). Pharmacokinetics of ciprofloxacin tablets in renal failure: influence of haemodialysis. *European Journal of Clinical Pharmacology* 31, 589–593.

Smith, C. R. *et al.* (1980). Comparison of the nephrotoxicity and auditory toxicity of gentamicin and tobramycin. *New England Journal of Medicine* 302, 1106–1109.

Somani, P., Shapiro, R. S., Stockard, H., and Higgins, J. T. (1982). Unidirectional absorption of gentamycin from the peritoneum during continuous ambulatory peritoneal dialysis. *Clinical Pharmacology and Therapeutics* 32, 113–121.

Somogyi, A., Kong, C., Sabto, J., Gurr, F. W., Spicer, W. J., and McLean, A. J. (1983). Disposition and removal of metronidazole in patients undergoing haemodialysis. *European Journal of Clinical Pharmacology* 25, 683–687.

Stathoulopoulou, F., Almond, M. K., Dhillon, S., and Raftery, M. J. (1995). Clinical pharmacokinetics of oral acyclovir in patients on continuous ambulatory peritoneal dialysis. *Nephron* 69, 428–432.

Stockley, L. H. (1994). *Drug Interactions* pp. 589–614. Oxford: Blackwell Scientific Publications, 1994.

Swan, S. K. *et al.* (2000). Effect of cyclooxygenase-2 inhibition on renal function in elderly persons receiving a low-salt diet. A randomized controlled trial. *Annals of Internal Medicine* 133, 1–15.

Szeto, H. H., Inturissi, C. E., Honde, R., Saal, S., Cheigh, J., and Reidenberg, M. M. (1977). Accumulation of normeperidine, an active metabolite of meperidine in patients with renal failure. *Annals of Internal Medicine* 86, 738–741.

Taylor, C. A., Abdel-Rahman, E., Zimmermann, S. W., and Johnson, C. A. (1996). Clinical pharmacokinetics during continuous ambulatory peritoneal dialysis. *Clinical Pharmacokinetics* 31, 293–308.

Toxbase (2000). http://www.spib.axl.co.uk/toxbaseindex.htm.

Thalhammer, F. and Horl, W. H. (2000). Pharmacokinetics of meropenem in patients with renal failure and patients receiving renal replacement therapy. *Clinical Pharmacokinetics* 39, 271–279.

Tillement, J. P., Lhoste, F., and Guidicelli, J. F. Diseases and drug protein binding. In *Handbook of Clinical Pharmacokinetics* (ed. M. Gibaldi and L. Prescott), pp. 57–69. Balgowlah, Australia: ADIS Health Science Press, 1983.

Vanholder, R., Van Landschoot, N., De Swet, R., Schoots, A., and Ringoir, S. (1988). Drug protein binding in chronic renal failure: evaluation of nine drugs. *Kidney International* 33, 996–1004.

Van Peer, A., Belpaire, F., and Bogaert, M. (1978). Warfarin elimination and responsiveness in patients with renal dysfunction. *Journal of Clinical Pharmacology* 18, 84–88.

Verbeeck, R. K. and De Scheffer, P. J. (1980). Influence of chronic renal failure and hemodialysis on diflunisal plasma protein binding. *Clinical Pharmacology and Therapeutics* 27, 628–635.

Verbeeck, R. K., Branch, R. A., and Wilkinson, G. R. (1981). Drug metabolites in renal failure: pharmacokinetic and clinical implications. *Clinical Pharmacokinetics* 6, 329–345.

Verpooten, G. A., Giuliano, R. A., Verbist, L., Eestermans, G., and De Broe, M. E. (1989). Once-daily dosing decreases renal accumulation of gentamicin and netilmicin. *Clinical Pharmacology and Therapeutics* 45, 22–27.

Vinik, H. R., Reves, J. G., Greenblatt, D. J., Abernethy, D. R., and Smith, L. R. (1983). The pharmacokinetics of midazolam in chronic renal failure patients. *Anesthesiology* 59, 390–394.

Wallemacq, P. E. and Vereeck, R. K. (2001). Comparative clinical pharmacokinetics of tacrolimus in paediatric and adult patients. *Clinical Pharmacokinetics* 40, 283–295.

Walstad, R. A., Nilson, O. G., and Berg, K. J. (1983). Pharmacokinetics and clinical effects of cefuroxime in patients with severe renal insufficiency. *European Journal of Clinical Pharmacology* 24, 391–398.

Walstad, R. A., Dahl, K., Hellum, K. B., and Thurmann-Nielsen, E. (1988). The pharmacokinetics of ceftazidime in patients with impaired renal function and concurrent frusemide therapy. *European Journal of Clinical Pharmacology* 35, 273–279.

Ward, S., Boheimer, N., Weatherley, B. C., Simmonds, R. J., and Dopson, T. A. (1987). Pharmacokinetics of atracurium and its metabolites in patients with normal renal function, and patients in renal failure. *British Journal of Anaesthesia* 59, 697–706.

Webb, D., Buss, D. C., Fifield, R., Bateman, N., and Routledge, P. A. (1986). The plasma protein binding of metoclopramide in health and renal disease. *British Journal of Clinical Pharmacology* 21, 334–336.

Whitby, M., Edwards, R., Aston, E., and Finch, R. G. (1987). Pharmacokinetics of single dose of intravenous vancomycin in CAPD peritonitis. *Journal of Antimicrobial Chemotherapy* 19, 351–357.

White, N. J. (1985). Clinical pharmacokinetics of antimalarial drugs. *Clinical Pharmacokinetics* 10, 187–215.

Wilcox, C. S. (2002). New insights into diuretic use in patients with chronic renal disease. *Journal of the American Society of Nephrology* 13, 798–805.

Williams, P. *et al.* (2000). Insulin efficacy with a new bicarbonate/lactate peritoneal dialysis solution. *Peritoneal Dialysis International* 20, 467–469.

Wills, R. J. (1990). Clinical pharmacokinetics of interferons. *Clinical Pharmacokinetics* 19, 390–399.

Wilson, A. P. (2000). Clinical pharmacokinetics of teicoplanin. *Clinical Pharmacokinetics* 39, 167–183.

Wolff, J., Bigler, D., Christensen, C. B., Rasmussen, S. N., Andersen, H. B., and Tonnesen, K. H. (1988). Influence of renal function on the elimination of morphine and morphine glucuronides. *European Journal of Clinical Pharmacology* 34, 353–357.

Wright, J. G. and Boddy, A. V. (2001). All half-lives are wrong, but some half-lives are useful. *Clinical Pharmacokinetics* 40, 237–244.

Wright, M. R. *et al.* (1988). Effect of haemodialysis on metoclopramide kinetics in patients with severe renal failure. *British Journal of Clinical Pharmacology* 26, 474–477.

Yamamoto, T., Moriwaki, Y., Takahashi, S., Tsutsumi, Z., and Hada, T. (2000). Effect of losartan potassium, an angiotensin II receptor antagonist, on renal excretion of oxypurinol and purine bases. *Journal of Rheumatology* **27**, 2232–2236.

Additional reading

Bellisant, E., Sebilla, V., and Vaintand, G. (1998). Methodological issues in pharmacokinetic-pharmacodynamic modeling. *Clinical Pharmacokinetics* **35**, 151–166.

Benet, L. Z., Kroetz, D. L., and Sheiner, L. B. Pharmacokinetics: the dynamics of drug, absorption, distribution, and elimination. In *Goodman and Gilman's The Pharmacological Basis of Therapeutics* Section I (ed. J. G. Hardman and L. E. Limberd), pp. 3–28. New York: McGraw-Hill, 1996.

Ibrahim, S. *et al.* (2000). Clinical pharmacology studies in patients with renal impairment: past experience and regulatory perspectives. *Journal of Clinical Pharmacology* **40**, 31–38.

Keller, F., Giehl, M., Frankewitsch, T., and Zellner, D. (1995). Pharmacokinetics and drug dosage adjustment in renal impairment. *Nephrology, Dialysis, Transplantation* **10**, 1516–1521.

19.3 Action and clinical use of diuretics

Rainer Greger, Florian Lang, Katarina Sebekova, and August Heidland

Cellular mechanisms of action of diuretics

Diuretics are pharmacological tools to reduce the extracellular fluid volume (ECV) by increasing urinary solute and water excretion (Seldin and Giebisch 1997). To this end diuretics inhibit renal tubular reabsorption of NaCl and water. A variety of diuretics are in use targetting different cellular transport mechanisms and thus leading to distinct effects on urinary electrolyte and water excretion. All diuretics enhance urinary Na^+ and water excretion but they differ in efficacy and their effect on the urinary excretion of other electrolytes. Optimal clinical use of diuretics requires that these differences are understood and that the cellular mechanisms involved are known. With the exception of osmotic diuresis, all diuretic drugs now in use exert their effect by targetting primarily a single molecule. Thus, the primary effect of the diuretic is well defined. However, the altered delivery of fluid and electrolytes to nephron segments distal from the primary site of action may alter transport properties in those segments, thus significantly modifying the diuretic action. In addition and probably more important, the contraction of ECV induced by the diuretic triggers regulatory mechanisms aiming at the enhancement of renal tubular Na^+ and electrolyte reabsorption. Thus, the clinical effect of diuretics differs significantly from what were expected in view of the primary mechanism. In this section, the tubular transport mechanisms accounting for the primary and secondary cellular mechanisms of action shall be described. Figure 1 provides an overview of the major renal tubular transport mechanisms participating in diuretic action.

Carbonic anhydrase inhibitors—proximal diuretics

The proximal nephron usually reclaims some 60–70 per cent of filtered water, Na^+, K^+, and Cl^-, more than 90 per cent of filtered HCO_3^-, and almost 100 per cent of organic solutes such as glucose and amino acids (Burckhardt and Greger 1992).

The driving force for Na^+ transport across the apical cell membrane is created by the Na^+,K^+-ATPase at the basolateral cell membrane, which expels three Na^+ ions from the cell towards the blood side in exchange for the cellular uptake of two K^+ ions, the process being fuelled by the hydrolysis of adenosine triphosphate (ATP). Na^+ uptake across the lumenal membrane is mainly due to $Na^+–H^+$ exchange, mediated by the NHE3 isoform (Biemesderfer et al. 1993). The rate of exchange is regulated by a pH sensing site which increases the turnover rate whenever the cytosolic pH becomes acidic (Kinsella and Aronson 1980).

A smaller proportion of Na^+ uptake occurs through cotransport with solutes such as D-glucose, amino acids, or phosphate. A small amount of Na^+ is reabsorbed via selective ion channels (Gögelein and Greger 1986).

The secretion of H^+ via NHE3 titrates filtered HCO_3^- leading to the formation of carbonic acid (H_2CO_3). H_2CO_3 is then dehydrated by carbonic anhydrase at the lumenal cell membrane (Lang et al. 1978). The CO_2 thus produced enters the cell across the lumenal cell membrane and within the cell is rehydrated to carbonic acid which dissociates to produce H^+ and HCO_3^- ions. The H^+ are utilized for H^+ secretion by the NHE3, the HCO_3^- leaves the cell across the basolateral cell membrane mainly via Na^+, $(HCO_3^-)_3$ cotransport (Romero 2001). The Na^+ taken up in exchange for H^+ is further pumped out by the Na^+,K^+-ATPase. The net effect is the reabsorption of Na^+ and HCO_3^-.

A very important feature of the proximal nephron is further extremely high permeability of its paracellular shunt pathway. The tight junctions and lateral spaces are highly permeable to water and small ions. Thus, the epithelium cannot sustain any substantial ionic or osmotic gradient. Similarly, the transepithelial electrical potential is only approximately 1 mV (Frömter and Gessner 1974). These properties mean that very small osmotic gradients across the epithelium will lead to substantial fluxes of water. As Fig. 1(a) shows, the combination of large transcellular reabsorptive fluxes and a high paracellular permeability is specifically suited to 'bulk' transport, but it will not enable the epithelium to generate large ionic gradients.

The reabsorption of HCO_3^- and Na^+ leads to a small osmotic gradient driving water reabsorption (Schafer et al. 1974). The water reabsorption leads to increase of the Cl^- concentration in the tubule fluid. Driven by the (small) chemical gradient, Cl^- diffuses out of the lumen and thus creates a small lumen-positive potential difference across the epithelium. This lumen-positive potential drives Na^+ from lumen to blood. Moreover, Na^+ and Cl^- reabsorption are favoured by water flux (solvent drag). The large fraction of passive Na^+ and Cl^- absorption is energetically advantageous, since ATP is only consumed during transcellular transport. In a very simplified analysis (Greger 1987) one can deduce that given a Na^+,K^+-ATPase stoichiometry of three Na^+/ATP, up to 9 mol of Na^+ can be reabsorbed with the breakdown of only 1 mol of ATP.

The continued secretion of H^+ and reabsorption of HCO_3^- requires rapid dehydration of lumenal carbonic acid and rapid formation of carbonic acid in the cell. Both depend on the respective activities of carbonic anhydrase. Carbonic anhydrase inhibitors (Fig. 2a), such as acetazolamide, inhibit the cytosolic as well as the membrane-bound enzyme and thus reduce the reabsorption of HCO_3^-. In the proximal

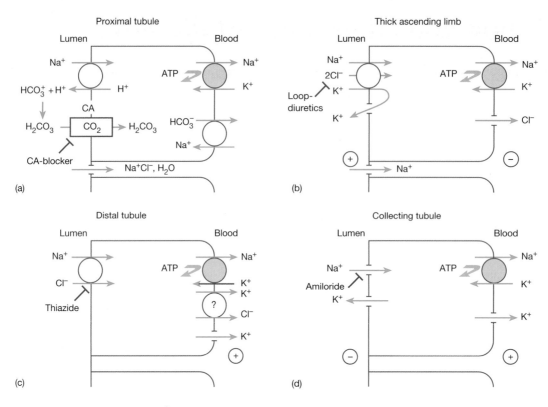

Fig. 1 Simplified schemes for the mechanisms of Na^+, Cl^-, and H_2O transport in the nephron segments. $\bigcirc$ = carrier, $\bullet$ = primary active pump, $+$ = ion channel. (a) Proximal tubule. Note that transcellular transport involves mostly Na^+ and HCO_3^-. Much Na^+, and most of the Cl^- and H_2O is reabsorbed via the paracellular shunt pathway. CA-blocker = blocker of the carbonic anhydrase. (b) Thick ascending limb of the loop of Henle. The entire Cl^- flux is across the cell. Half of the Na^+ is transported across the cell, the other half is reabsorbed across the paracellular shunt pathway. The driving force for this latter component comes from the lumen-positive transepithelial voltage. Loop diuretics such as frusemide bind to one of the Cl^--binding sites of the $Na^+,2Cl^-,K^+$-cotransporter. (c) Distal tubule. The entire NaCl reabsorption occurs across the cell. Thiazides block the Na^+Cl^--cotransporter. (d) Principal cell of the collecting tubule. The entire Na^+ reabsorption occurs across the cell. The extent of K^+ secretion depends on the Na^+ reabsorption in as much as Na^+ depolarizes the lumenal cell membrane and increases the driving force for K^+ exit into the lumen. Amiloride blocks the lumenal Na^+ channel. The reabsorption of Na^+ exceeds the secretion of K^+. Electroneutrality is maintained by Cl^- reabsorption involving Cl^- channels (not shown).

nephron they inhibit the generation of CO_2 at the lumenal membrane, the production of carbonic acid in the cell, and the carrier-mediated exit of HCO_3^- across the basolateral membrane, reducing HCO_3^- and Na^+ reabsorption. Despite impaired H^+ secretion carbonic anhydrase inhibitors lead to an acidic lumenal fluid due to accumulation of carbonic acid (Lang et al. 1978). In later tubule segments the lumenal pH is turned alkaline due to delayed formation of CO_2 and consumption of H^+. The increase in tubule fluid pH in later tubule segments may reduce the reabsorption of weak organic acids, and thus increase their renal elimination.

Carbonic anhydrase is not limited to the proximal tubule but is expressed as well in loop of Henle, distal tubule, and collecting duct. The contribution of these nephron segments to the diuresis following carbonic anhydrase inhibition is, however, small.

Following administration of carbonic anhydrase inhibitors the inhibition of proximal tubular HCO_3^- reabsorption is incomplete, other Na^+ coupled transport processes are still operative, and the proximal natriuretic and diuretic response is blunted by augmented reabsorption in the more distal nephron segments. The enhanced delivery of NaCl to the macula densa decreases the glomerular filtration rate (GFR) via glomerulotubular feedback (Osswald and Vallon 1998). Hence, the diuretic and natriuretic effect of carbonic anhydrase

inhibitors is modest. The increased urinary loss of HCO_3^- produces a metabolic acidosis which further blunts the diuretic activity of carbonic anhydrase inhibitors.

More recently, a specific inhibitor of NHE3 has been developed (Hropot et al. 2001). Its effect should be similar to that of carbonic anhydrase inhibitors. Unlike carbonic anhydrase inhibitors, however, NHE3 inhibitors are expected to alkalinize proximal tubular fluid and to interfere with NHE3 functions other than H^+ secretion, such as protein reabsorption (Gekle et al. 1999).

Inhibitors of the $Na^+,2Cl^-,K^+$-cotransporter—loop diuretics

The thick ascending limb of the loop of Henle reabsorbs up to 30 per cent of the filtered load of Na^+ and Cl^-. Some K^+ is also reabsorbed at this site, along with substantial amounts of Ca^{2+} and Mg^{2+}. Due to the absence of water channels in the lumenal membrane, water permeability of this nephron segment is low and very little water is reabsorbed (Greger 1985a). This means that the tubule fluid at the end of the thick ascending limb is hypotonic, while the reabsorbed fluid is hypertonic. This hypertonic reabsorptive process feeds the countercurrent system, which enables the kidney to excrete concentrated urine. During

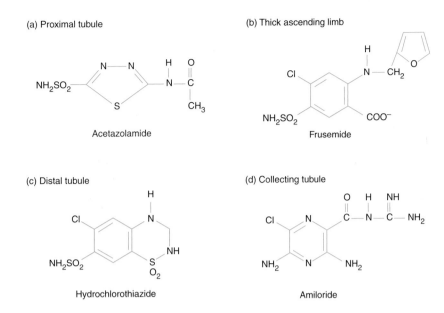

Fig. 2 Structural formula of several diuretics. The carbonic anhydrase inhibitor, acetazolamide, acts mainly in the proximal tubule. Its target is the carbonic anhydrase in the lumenal membrane and in the cell, as well as the HCO_3^- exit system across the basolateral membrane (cf. Fig. 1). Frusemide is one example of an inhibitor of the $Na^+,2Cl^-,K^+$-cotransporter in the thick ascending limb of the loop of Henle. It binds to one of the Cl^--binding sites of this carrier. Hydrochlorothiazide acts by binding to the NaCl carrier in the lumenal membrane of the distal tubule. Amiloride blocks the Na^+ channels in the principal cell of the collecting duct.

water diuresis, this same mechanism generates a tubular fluid with low Na^+ and Cl^- concentrations, allowing the excretion of a dilute urine.

The basic mechanism responsible for Na^+ and Cl^- reabsorption in the thick ascending limb of the loop of Henle (Greger 1985a) is depicted in Fig. 1(b). The reabsorptive process is fuelled by the Na^+,K^+-ATPase localized in the basolateral membrane. The uptake of Na^+ across the lumenal membrane occurs via a cotransport system which couples the uptake of Na^+ to that of Cl^- and K^+. Hence, after determination of its stoichiometry, this cotransporter was labelled the $Na^+,2Cl^-,K^+$-carrier (Greger and Schlatter 1981; Geck and Heinz 1986). The cloned molecule has been labelled BSC1 or NKCC2 (Gamba et al. 1994; Payne and Forbush 1994). The K^+ taken up across the lumenal membrane almost completely recycles across the same membrane through renal outer medullary K^+ channels (ROMK) (Bleich et al. 1990; Hebert 1998). Cl^- leaves the cell through the basolateral Cl^- channels ClCKb (Kieferle et al. 1994) and presumably via a KCl-cotransport system (Greger et al. 1990). To become functional, the Cl-channels (ClCKb) need the subunit barttin (Estevez et al. 2001; Waldegger et al. 2002). The recycling of K^+ to the lumen and the basolateral exit of Cl^- to the blood side creates a lumen-positive transepithelial potential difference of some 6–15 mV. The paracellular shunt pathway in this nephron segment is far less permeable than that of the proximal nephron. The tight junctions are more complex, with more strands, are only permeable to small ions, and are also cation-selective (Greger 1985a). Nevertheless the lumen-positive potential leads to a substantial reabsorptive flux of Na^+ via the paracellular route. In total, six Cl^- ions are moved across the cell, while three Na^+ ions are extruded by the Na^+,K^+-ATPase and another three Na^+ ions are reabsorbed through the paracellular pathway. Given the poor water permeability of this nephron segment, little water will follow the reabsorptive flux of NaCl, thus generating a dilute lumenal fluid.

By binding at (one) Cl^- binding site of the $Na^+,2Cl^-,K^+$-carrier, frusemide-type loop diuretics (Fig. 2b) inhibit the lumenal uptake of these ions, and, therefore, the reabsorption of NaCl (Greger and Schlatter 1983; Greger 1985b; Lohrmann et al. 1992). The structure–activity relationship of many of these compounds has been explored and, as a result, the minimum requirements of a molecule which will bind to and inhibit the $Na^+,2Cl^-,K^+$-carrier have been defined (Schlatter et al. 1983; Wittner et al. 1987; Lohrmann et al. 1994). All diuretics belonging to this group (e.g. frusemide, bumetanide, piretanide, torasemide, azosemide) are effective from the lumenal side of the membrane and have the same mechanism of action. Inspection of Fig. 1(b) indicates that the thick ascending limb cells have a grossly reduced Na^+,K^+-ATPase activity, and thus reduced ATP consumption, in the presence of loop diuretics. This effect can be used in vitro to preserve this tissue and it may be useful clinically in the prophylaxis of acute renal failure (Brezis et al. 1984a,b; Greger 1985a, 1987; Greger and Wangemann 1987; Lohrmann et al. 1994) (see Chapter 8.4).

The diuresis and natriuresis produced by loop diuretics may reach as much as 20–30 per cent of the filtered load. If the K^+ recycling in the thick ascending limb is incomplete in the normal state, loop diuretics will increase the load of lumenal K^+ delivered to the distal tubule. In addition to this effect the increased distal load of NaCl will lead to an increased secretion of K^+ and protons in the distal nephron (see below): hypokalaemia is, therefore, a predictable effect of all loop diuretics. Since at least part of the Ca^{2+} and Mg^{2+} reabsorption in the thick ascending limb of the loop of Henle is paracellular and voltage driven (Greger 1985a; Wittner et al. 1993), loop diuretics will, by abolishing the transepithelial potential difference, reduce the reabsorption of these divalent cations and enhance their excretion.

The onset of the natriuretic and diuretic effect of these drugs is very rapid and the loss of salt and water may be substantial. If the volume loss is not matched by adequate repletion, hyper-reninaemia and a reduction in GFR are predictable consequences. When volume contraction is induced by loop diuretics, urate reabsorption is increased in the loop of Henle (Lang *et al.* 1977), thus leading to hyperuricaemia.

A feedback response normally reduces single nephron filtration rate in response to increased NaCl delivery to the macula densa by the tubular fluid: this is paralysed by loop diuretics which block the $Na^+,2Cl^-,K^+$-carrier in the apical membrane of the macula densa cells (Schlatter *et al.* 1989; Schlatter 1993). Loop diuretics have little effect in nephron segments other than the thick ascending limb of the loop of Henle, although some proximal effect has been reported, probably due to the weak inhibition of carbonic anhydrase by this class of substances.

Inhibitors of early distal NaCl reabsorption—thiazide diuretics

The early distal tubule, that is the nephron segment which follows the thick ascending limb, reabsorbs some 10 per cent of the filtered load of the NaCl by mechanisms which are depicted in Fig. 1(c) (Greger 1988). The reabsorption is fuelled by the basolateral Na^+,K^+-ATPase, and the uptake of Na^+ proceeds by the NaCl cotransport system NCC (Gamba *et al.* 1993). The transepithelial electrical potential difference at this nephron site is slightly lumen-negative.

Thiazide diuretics (Fig. 2c) apparently interact with the NaCl cotransporter. This cotransporter shows some similarity with the $Na^+,2Cl^-,K^+$-cotransporter with respect to their postulated tertiary structures (Gamba *et al.* 1993, 1994; Payne and Forbush 1994), but they are clearly distinct on the basis of their primary structures and also with respect to their functional properties. Thiazide diuretics inhibit lumenal uptake of Na^+ and Cl^- in the distal tubule and have no effect in the thick ascending limb of the loop of Henle (Schlatter *et al.* 1983; Velázquez and Wright 1986; Fanestil *et al.* 1990). Conversely, loop diuretics do not inhibit the NaCl cotransporter present in the distal tubule (Schlatter *et al.* 1983). Thiazides are less potent than loop diuretics, but more potent than the other diuretics. As they produce a substantial increase in distal tubule NaCl load they cause kaliuresis. In addition to their effect in the early distal tubule these substances all have some inhibitory effect in the proximal nephron, probably due to the inhibition of carbonic anhydrase. It should be kept in mind that this class of substances was originally discovered in the search for more potent carbonic anhydrase inhibitors. Thiazides reduce the GFR even in the presence of adequate hydration, although the mechanism of this is not known.

Thiazide diuretics, unlike loop diuretics, reduce the excretion of Ca^{2+} (Costanzo and Windhager 1978). Ca^{2+} reabsorption in distal tubule cells is accomplished by entry via the lumenal Ca^{2+} channels ECaC (Hoenderop *et al.* 2002) and exit at least in part via basolateral $Na^+–Ca^{2+}$ exchange and Ca^{2+}-ATPase (Friedman and Gesek 1993; Hoenderop *et al.* 2002). It is speculated that inhibition of NaCl cotransport lowers cytosolic Na^+ concentration thus enhancing the driving force for basolateral $Na^+–Ca^{2+}$ exchange. The subsequent decrease of cytosolic Ca^{2+} then disinhibits the Ca^{2+} channel in the lumenal membrane.

Sodium channel blockers in the collecting duct—K^+-sparing diuretics

Only a very small percentage of filtered Na^+ is reclaimed in the collecting duct system, and the cellular mechanism of this process is

shown in Fig. 1(d). The active extrusion of Na^+ again occurs via the Na^+,K^+-ATPase, while the uptake of Na^+ across the lumenal membrane proceeds via the Na^+ selective channel ENaC (Lingueglia *et al.* 1993; Canessa *et al.* 1994). Na^+ entry through the Na^+ channels is paralleled by K^+ exit through K^+ channels (Hunter *et al.* 1986; Frindt and Palmer 1987; Schlatter *et al.* 1989) such as ROMK (Moral *et al.* 2001). The extent to which Na^+ is reabsorbed will determine the K^+ secretory flux, simply because the uptake of Na^+ depolarizes the lumenal membrane, and depolarization increases the driving force for K^+ secretion (Schafer *et al.* 1990). Hence, K^+ loss will be augmented whenever the distal delivery of NaCl is increased. The paracellular pathway in this nephron segment is rather tight, and allows the establishment of large ionic and electrical gradients. Unlike the transport mechanisms in the proximal nephron or the thick ascending limb of the loop of Henle, one molecule of ATP is consumed for the reabsorption of only three Na^+ ions, making this transport mechanism energetically more costly as compared to that in the other nephron segments (Burckhardt and Greger 1992). The mechanism of Cl^- reabsorption in this nephron segment is still a matter of debate (Schlatter and Schafer 1988). The regulation of Na^+ reabsorption in the principal cell is under the control of mineralocorticoids and, at least in some species, also under the more acute control of arginine vasopressin (AVP). Both hormones increase the reabsorption of Na^+ (Schlatter 1989).

The Na^+ reabsorption in the collecting duct can be blocked by amiloride (Li and Lindemann 1983; Palmer and Frindt 1987) and triamterene (Busch *et al.* 1996). By blocking the Na^+ channel, these substances indirectly reduce K^+ secretion through the lumenal K^+ channels; they are, therefore, natriuretic and antikaliuretic. The natriuresis is only moderate, and the specific importance of these substances is their antikaliuretic effect. In hyperaldosteronism, a comparable effect can also be achieved with aldosterone antagonists such as spironolactone (Shakelton *et al.* 1986; Fanestil 1988). Clinical doses of amiloride or triamterene act specifically on the collecting duct. Very high concentrations are required to inhibit other transporters such as the $Na^+–H^+$ exchanger.

Stimulation of water excretion—osmotic diuresis

To enhance water excretion, all diuretics have to interfere with renal tubular water reabsorption. Renal tubular water reabsorption depends in large part on movement of water through water channels (Preston and Agre 1991; Agre *et al.* 1993). The driving force is an osmotic gradient, built up by solute transport across the tubular epithelia. At least in theory, water excretion could be pharmacologically enhanced by interference with the function of the water channels or by dissipation of the osmotic gradient.

Insertion of water channels into the apical cell membrane of connecting tubule, cortical and medullary collecting duct is under control of ADH through V_2 receptors (Gonzalez *et al.* 1997). Inhibitors of the V_2 receptors have been shown to induce the expected water diuresis (Yamamura *et al.* 1992; Ohnishi *et al.* 1993).

All diuretics now in use enhance renal water excretion by decreasing the osmotic gradient. The diuretics discussed above do so by primarily inhibiting tubular transport. Osmotic diuretics primarily affect the osmotic gradient. Substances used for this purpose, such as mannitol, are freely filtered at the glomerulus and are not reabsorbed by the tubule; hence their tubular concentration increases as water is reabsorbed. The increased lumenal concentration of poorly absorbable mannitol decreases the osmotic gradient created by solute reabsorption. With this in mind, the mannitol should be most effective in the terminal nephron segments where the mannitol concentration is highest. However, mannitol mainly impedes reabsorption in proximal tubule and thin descending limb of Henle's loop (Okusa and Ellison 2000). The particular efficacy in these nephron segments is due to their leakiness preventing the builtup of larger osmotic gradients. At increasing lumenal mannitol concentrations, the lumenal NaCl concentration must be lowered to maintain an osmotic gradient driving water from lumen to blood. As discussed above, the tight junctions of proximal tubules are highly permeable to Na^+. Any decrease of the lumenal Na^+ concentration creates a chemical gradient driving Na^+ from blood to lumen and thus impedes Na^+ reabsorption. The decrease of Na^+ reabsorption adds to lumenal osmolarity and contributes to the osmotic diuresis. The impairment of net Na^+ reabsorption leads to natriuresis on top of diuresis.

The diuresis following mannitol infusion is compounded by renal vasodilation leading to washout of the renal medullary hypertonicity and thus breakdown of the osmotic gradient driving water reabsorption in collecting duct (Nashat et al. 1969; Lang 1987). The vasodilation is at least partially due to prostacyclin (Johnston et al. 1981) and atrial natriuretic peptide (ANP) (Yamasaki et al. 1988). Mannitol may increase the GFR (Better et al. 1997), an effect again mediated in part by ANP.

Organ specificity and drug interactions of diuretics

The above section has dealt with the cellular mechanisms of Na^+ and water reabsorption and the mechanisms by which the different groups of diuretics interfere with this reabsorption. In the following discussion we shall briefly address the questions of (a) why diuretics are kidney-specific, (b) how other drugs may modify the diuretic action, and (c) how the different groups of diuretics may be combined.

Why are diuretics organ specific? The organ specificity of diuretics is surprising, since they act on transport proteins, many of which are present in organs other than the kidney. For example, the $Na^+, 2Cl^-, K^+$-cotransporter has been found in intestine, excretory glands, inner ear epithelium, red blood cells, neuronal cells, and smooth muscle cells. Na^+ channels occur in the intestine, respiratory epithelium, and glandular ducts, and carbonic anhydrase is present in many polar and apolar cells. Why should inhibitors of these transport proteins have effects on the kidney but little if any systemic action? One reason for organ specific action is that the functionally similar transport systems present in the kidney and in other organs are not identical at the molecular level and may thus bear different drug sensitivity (Gamba et al. 1994; Payne and Forbush 1994). More importantly, however, organ specificity is the result of drug accumulation in the lumenal fluid due to water reabsorption and due to drug secretion by the proximal nephron. The basolateral cell pole of the proximal tubule possesses transporters which take up organic anions such as p-aminohippurate and drugs such as diuretics, causing them to accumulate within the tubule cell (Ullrich et al. 1989). Other transporters then transfer the drugs into the lumenal fluid. The combination of water reabsorption and drug secretion leads to a drug concentration in the tubule fluid which may be more than 10 times larger than that of the plasma.

Clinically used doses, will, therefore, affect the transporters in the lumenal membrane of the tubule before those of any other organ. In some disease states, where secretion in the proximal tubule may be defective, much greater doses of, for example, a loop diuretic are required to achieve a diuretic response, and serious side-effects such as ototoxicity may occur, since endolymph secretion in the inner ear is inhibited (Marcus et al. 1987).

Drugs interfering with the secretion of diuretics

Many drugs can interfere with the secretion of diuretics. Amongst these, probenecid has been studied in some detail. Probenecid markedly reduces the diuretic response to a previously effective dose of a loop diuretic. All loop diuretics are affected (Braitsch et al. 1990) and the secretion of these different diuretics in the proximal tubule is equally inhibited by a given dose of probenecid. One would predict that all drugs which are weak organic acids would potentially reduce the effectiveness of loop diuretics and produce a reduced renal excretion rate. On the other hand, loop diuretics might reduce the renal clearance of these weak organic acids. Unfortunately, very few experimental data are available regarding this issue.

Combination of diuretics

Since different diuretics act at different nephron sites, one might predict that the effects of combinations of two diuretics from different groups would be additive. The response is usually more than additive; a fraction of the diuretic response exerted at the level of the loop of Henle will be blunted by increased reabsorption in more distal tubule segments. If the loop diuretic is now combined with a thiazide, this compensatory reabsorption is eliminated by the diuretic response to the second drug. The same phenomenon can be looked at from a different perspective: if a small load is delivered to a certain tubule segment, the diuretic response in this segment can only be minimal. If, for example, the flow rate at the end of the proximal tubule is reduced by volume contraction, the effect of a loop diuretic will be much less than it is in volume expansion, when the end-proximal flow rate is increased.

Choice and combination of diuretics will be discussed more explicitly in the subsequent sections; it is sufficient to state here that the adverse effects of threatening hypokalaemia, which may be caused by loop diuretics and thiazides, can be compensated for by concomitant use of potassium-sparing diuretics such as amiloride or triamterene.

Clinical use of diuretics

Arterial hypertension

Thiazide diuretics have long been considered to be the 'cornerstone' in the antihypertensive therapy and are still recommended as initial treatment by 'The Seventh Report of the National Committee on Detection, Evaluation and Treatment of High Blood Pressure' (The JNC VII Report 2003) for most patients with uncomplicated hypertension—either alone or in combination with one of the other classes (ACE inhibitors, angiotensin II receptor blockers, β-blockers, calcium channel blockers). Their blood-pressure-lowering effect is particularly pronounced in the elderly (Amery et al. 1985), in Afro-Americans (Veterans Administrative Cooperative Study Group on Antihypertensive Agents 1982a), in systolic hypertension (SHEP Cooperative Research Group

1991), in low renin states (Bühler *et al.* 1985), and in volume-dependent hypertension (renal parenchymal and steroid-induced hypertension). In general, thiazides are more effective antihypertensives than loop diuretics (Araoye *et al.* 1978) except in renal insufficiency (creatinine > 25 mg/l or >220 μmol/l). If not chosen as the first drug (for instance in type I diabetes or high-renin hypertension), diuretics are useful second-step drugs to be added to other regimens when these are insufficient.

Mechanisms of antihypertensive action

Diuretics initially lower the arterial blood pressure by reducing plasma volume and cardiac output, although total peripheral vascular resistance is enhanced. With continued diuretic treatment, plasma volume and cardiac output tend to return towards pretreatment values, while total peripheral vascular resistance decreases (Tarazi *et al.* 1970). The mechanism of this 'reversed autoregulatory response', which requires a sustained mild decrease of extra- and intravascular fluid volume (Tobian 1974; Shah *et al.* 1978), is still incompletely understood. The following potential mechanisms are discussed:

(1) normalization of enhanced intracellular Na^+ and Ca^{2+} concentrations (Erne *et al.* 1984);

(2) decreased vascular responsiveness to vasoconstrictors such as angiotensin II and noradrenaline (Weidmann *et al.* 1983a);

(3) increased formation of vasodilating prostaglandins (Scherer and Weber 1979; Webster and Dollery 1980);

(4) decrease of the endogenous digitalis-like natriuretic hormone (Na^+,K^+-ATPase inhibitor) with its vasoconstrictor properties (Hamlyn *et al.* 1991); and

(5) K^+ channel opening effects in resistance arteries (Calder *et al.* 1994).

Counteracting mechanisms

The diuretic-induced salt and water loss activates several neurohormonal systems, such as the sympathetic adrenergic nervous system, the renin–angiotensin–aldosterone system (RAAS), and vasopressin (Heidland and Hennemann 1969; Luke *et al.* 1979; Weidmann *et al.* 1983a; Burnier and Brunner 1992; Petersen and Di Bona *et al.* 1993). These counter-regulatory mechanisms enhance total peripheral vascular resistance and stimulate tubular Na^+ reabsorption. In particular, activation of the RAAS limits the blood-pressure-lowering effect. Thus, hypertensive patients who fail to respond to diuretics have a greater increase of renin or angiotensin II than those who do respond (Leonetti *et al.* 1978; Vaughan *et al.* 1978; Gavras *et al.* 1981). In line with this observation is the enhanced blood-pressure-lowering effect of the additional application of angiotensin-converting enzyme (ACE) inhibitors (Brunner *et al.* 1980).

The antihypertensive action of diuretics is also limited by K^+ depletion (Krishna *et al.* 1989), via not clearly understood mechanisms such as constriction of resistance vessels (Haddy 1975), Na^+ retention (Welt *et al.* 1960), and/or elevation of plasma renin (Tannen 1983). Correction of diuretic-induced hypokalaemia may reduce the blood pressure (Kaplan *et al.* 1985).

Therapeutic approach of diuretic therapy in hypertension: dosage considerations and combined therapy

In the past, the high dose of diuretics contributed to various metabolic side-effects. In fact, the dose–response curve of the antihypertensive action of thiazides is flatter than that for their diuretic effects, probably due to activation of counter-regulatory mechanisms. Thus, the maximum antihypertensive effect of bendrofluazide was achieved from 1.25 mg daily, while the administration of 2.5, 5, and 10 mg, respectively, exerted a dose-related reduction in plasma K^+ concentrations without a relevant additional antihypertensive action (Carlsen *et al.* 1990). The least blood-pressure-lowering daily doses of other diuretics are: for indapamide (1.5 mg), chlorthalidone and hydrochlorothiazide (12.5 mg), spironolactone (75 mg) (Campbell *et al.* 1985; McVeigh *et al.* 1988; Knauf and Mutschler 1993b; Weidmann 2001), and the loop diuretic torasemide (2.5 and 5 mg, respectively) (Baumgart *et al.* 1990). Combined administration of K^+-losing and K^+-sparing diuretics can produce additive effects (Myers 1987). The blood-pressure-lowering action of diuretics is potentiated by modulating the compensatory increase of angiotensin II and—in part—aldosterone by coadministration of an ACE inhibitor (Brunner *et al.* 1990). This combination also allows a better tolerance, due to dose reduction and fewer adverse effects, resulting also in a better compliance. Recently, first data were published about the add-on therapy with eplerenone, a selective aldosterone antagonist in hypertensive patients, inadequately controlled on ACE inhibitor or angiotensin receptor blocker alone (Krum *et al.* 2002).

Effects of diuretics on morbidity and mortality in hypertension

The benefits of diuretics on deaths from stroke, renal failure, coronary heart disease, or congestive heart failure (CHF) were clearly demonstrated for malignant hypertension (Harrington *et al.* 1959; Sokolow and Perloff 1960) as well as in severe hypertension (diastolic blood pressure 115–129 mmHg), in controlled studies (Veterans Administration Cooperative Study Group on Antihypertensive Agents 1972). Concerning mild to moderate hypertension (diastolic blood pressure 90–114 mmHg), a meta-analysis of 14 unconfounded randomized trials of antihypertensive drugs (chiefly diuretics and β-blockers) demonstrated that a decreased diastolic blood pressure of 5–6 mmHg within a treatment period of 5 years, reduces total cardiovascular mortality by 21 per cent, the incidence of stroke by 42 per cent, and the fatal and non-fatal coronary events by 14 per cent (Collins *et al.* 1990). Thus the benefits relating to coronary heart disease were less than expected, since epidemiological evidence suggests that long-term diastolic blood pressure reduction of 5–6 mmHg decreases events resulting from coronary heart disease by approximately 20–25 per cent (MacMahon *et al.* 1990). The discrepancy may be due to the short duration of individual trials. Moreover, some cardiotoxicity of diuretics has been discussed. In a meta-analysis from 14 large-scale studies this assumption was supported (Hoes *et al.* 1994). They showed that non-K^+-sparing diuretics seem to increase the risk of arrhythmias and sudden cardiac death, at least in a subgroup of hypertensive patients with clinical evidence of heart disease—probably due to a diuretic-induced K^+- and Mg^{2+}-depletion.

On the other hand, in three trials in elderly patients with hypertension, in which the diuretic-induced electrolyte disturbances were minimized by coadministration of the K^+-sparing diuretic amiloride or by K^+ supplementation, the data was more positive. The incidence of fatal coronary heart disease was reduced in the Systolic Hypertension in the Elderly Program (SHEP Cooperative Research Group 1991) (including 4736 patients) by 27 per cent, in the Swedish Trial in Old Patients (STOP, Dahlöf *et al.* 1991) (including 1627 patients) by 50 per cent, and in the Medical Research Council (MRC) trial in older adults (MRC Working Party 1992) (including 4396 patients) by 44 per cent. Thus, an impressive reduction in the incidence of coronary events or sudden death was achieved in the elderly by minimizing the diuretic-induced hypokalaemia.

In the Antihypertensive and Lipid-Lowering Treatment to Prevent Heart Attack Trial (ALLHAT 2002), a randomized double-blind study with a total of 33,357 participants, it was shown that thiazide diuretics are superior in preventing one or more major forms of cardiovascular disease events than ACE inhibitors, β-blockers, and calcium channel blockers. However, this study was criticized for its heterogenous population, whereby a high number of African-Americans were included. This subgroup is known to respond to antihypertensive therapy with diuretics and ACE inhibitors differently than Caucasians. Similar data to the ALLHAT study were obtained in a network meta-analysis from 42 clinical trials that included 192,478 patients, randomized to seven major treatment strategies including placebo, diuretics, β-blockers, ACE inhibitors, calcium channel blockers, α-blockers, and angiotensin II receptor blockers. Low-dose diuretics were the most effective first-line treatment for preventing the occurrence of cardiovascular disease morbidity and mortality (Psaty et al. 2003). Contrary to these data, in an Australian prospective, randomized trial with 6083 elderly subjects with hypertension (age 65– 84 years), ACE inhibitors were shown to lead to better outcomes than treatment with diuretic agents, despite similar reductions of blood pressure (Lindon et al. 2003). Finally, in an evaluation of seven sets of prospectively designed overviews with data from 29 randomized trials ($n = 162,341$), treatment with any commonly used antihypertensive regimen reduced the risk of total major cardiovascular events. Larger reductions in blood pressure produced larger reductions in risk (Blood Pressure Lowering Treatment Trialists' Collaboration 2003). With regard to these last mentioned data, the European Society of Hypertension as well as the German League Against High Blood Pressure still do not view diuretics as the first-line of antihypertensive therapy, in comparison to the newer drugs. However, they recommend an early combination of diuretics with ACE inhibitors, angiotensin II receptor blockers or calcium channel blockers and β-blockers.

Congestive heart failure

Reduction of effective arterial blood volume (EABV) due to a low cardiac output or a relative vasodilation in high output cardiac insufficiency are key factors leading to salt and water retention in CHF (Schrier 1988). To restore the disturbed volume homeostasis, the activated baroreceptors trigger at least four efferent pathways of volume regulation: the catecholamine cascade, the RAAS, the non-osmotic release of AVP and endothelin. All these substances enhance Na^+ and fluid retention indirectly through renal haemodynamic as well as directly by tubule effects (Martin and Schrier 1997). On the contrary, various vasodilators and natriuretic compounds, such as atriopeptins (ANP; and brain natriuretic peptide, BNP) and endothelial factors (nitric oxide and prostaglandins) are activated to overcome these effects (Martin and Schrier 1997).

Pharmacokinetics and pharmacodynamics in congestive heart failure

In patients with CHF and preserved renal function, the delivery of loop diuretics to the urine is not disturbed. However, their pharmacodynamics may be markedly impaired. Thus, the relationship between fractional excretion of Na^+ (FE_{Na}) and urinary excretion of the diuretic is shifted downwards and to the right (Brater et al. 1984; Brater 1994). This impaired response is caused by hyperreabsorption in the proximal tubule with decreased delivery of Na^+ to the loop of Henle as well as an increased Na^+ reabsorption in the distal tubule and collecting duct, in part due to hyperaldosteronism. After long-term administration

of loop diuretics, the increased delivery of Na^+ to the distal tubule serves as a stimulus for cell hypertrophy with consequent Na^+ hyperreabsorption (Kaissling and Stanton 1987).

Acute effects of diuretics

In patients with acute myocardial infarction (with or without left ventricular failure) or with chronic heart failure the immediate haemodynamic action of loop diuretics is characterized by reduced pulmonary wedge pressure, a reduction in cardiac index and a sharp increase in systemic vascular resistance (Nelson et al. 1983; Fiehring and Achhammer 1990). Left ventricular end-diastolic pressure is reduced due to a lowered preload, in particular in patients, who are on the steep portion of the Frank–Starling curve (Parmley 1985). In severe left ventricular failure and acute pulmonary congestion due to myocardial infarction intravenous administration of loop diuretics improved left ventricular filling pressure (Dikshit et al. 1973) due to an increased venous capacitance, possibly partly mediated by prostaglandins, released by the kidney (Bourland et al. 1977). This 'internal phlebotomy' is further augmented by the ensuing diuresis. An opposite effect may occur in patients with severe CHF (NYHA III–IV), in whom intravenous administration of frusemide promoted a reversible vasoconstriction and transient myocardial dysfunction, probably due to a decreased EABV with subsequent activation of the 'neurohormonal axis' (Francis et al. 1985).

Chronic effects of diuretics

In long-term diuretic treatment of CHF, cardiac output is either decreased, unaltered, or even slightly enhanced, due to afterload reduction by diminished total peripheral vascular resistance (Nishijma et al. 1984; Podszus and Piesche 1990). Echocardiographically there may be an improvement in fractional shortening with a reduction in cardiac volume (Haerer et al. 1990). Pulmonary wedge pressure was shown to be markedly decreased (Silke 1993). Exercise tolerance tests demonstrate either reduction in cardiac work or increased tolerance (Fiehring and Achhammer 1990; Haerer et al. 1990). Clinical improvement of patients with CHF (frequently by about one NYHA class) is mostly caused by a reduction in respiratory work due to decreased pulmonary fluid content and improved compliance (Biddle and Yu 1979; Düsing and Piesche 1990). Successful treatment of CHF by diuretics is associated with a progressive decline of elevated plasma concentrations of ANP (Anderson et al. 1988) while RAAS may be further activated (Ikram et al. 1980).

Recommendations for clinical use

In CHF, ACE inhibitors are the recommended first-line therapy. In mild CHF the majority of patients with overhydration and pulmonary congestion can be managed by dietary Na^+ restriction and coadministration of thiazide diuretics. If the diuretic response is suboptimal, loop diuretics become necessary. In severe heart failure, increasing doses of loop diuretics, in potential combination with thiazide diuretics, are required (Channer et al. 1994). Also coadministration of K^+-sparing diuretics (triamterene, amiloride, and spironolactone) may prove useful, since these agents inhibit Na^+ reabsorption and secretion of potassium and hydrogen ions in the late distal tubule and collecting duct. In patients who are resistant to thiazide therapy, combined treatment with repeated ceiling doses of loop diuretics or continuous infusion of frusemide has been successful (van Meyel et al. 1993).

Recently, aldosterone antagonism is recommended in patients with advanced heart failure (NYHA III–IV), in addition to ACE inhibitors and diuretics (Task Force Report 2001). The rationale for this therapy is the ability of aldosterone to induce potassium and magnesium depletion, sympathetic activation, and progressive cardiac fibrosis, independently of blood pressure. ACE inhibitors and angiotensin II type I receptor antagonists as a rule do not lead to suppression of elevated aldosterone levels sufficiently. In the Randomized Aldactone Evaluation Study (RALES) the effects of the mineralocorticoid receptor antagonist spironolactone (25–50 mg/day) were investigated. After mean follow-up of 24 months, a 30 per cent reduction of deaths from all causes and 25 per cent lower hospitalizations, compared to placebo, was achieved. Prerequisite for this combined therapy is serum potassium less than 5.0 mmol/l and creatinine less than 250 μmol/l, with regular check-ups (at first after 1 week) (Pitt *et al.* 1999).

The adverse effects of spironolactone (painful gynaecomastia, impotence, and menstrual disturbances) are probably prevented by the newly developed, more selective aldosterone antagonist eplerenone, which has much less affinity to other steroid receptors (progesterone, androgens) than spironolactone and exerts cardiovascular protective actions (Deylan *et al.* 2000; Brown 2003).

Potential coadministration of thiamine

Long-term diuretic therapy may induce a subclinical thiamine deficiency due to increased urinary loss of this vitamin. In some patients with moderate to severe CHF, thiamine repletion was shown to improve left ventricular function and biochemical evidence of thiamine deficiency (Shimon *et al.* 1995).

Haemofiltration and haemodialysis in endstage chronic heart failure with therapy refractory oedema

In patients with complete refractoriness to combined diuretic therapy and ACE inhibitors, fluid removal by repeated haemofiltration, regular haemodialysis treatment, or continuous ambulatory peritoneal dialysis may prolong survival for several months or even years (Dormans *et al.* 1996; Iorio *et al.* 1997).

Liver cirrhosis and ascites

In liver cirrhosis, blood pressure and peripheral vascular resistance are lowered, while cardiac output is enhanced. There is a relative underfilling of the arterial circulation, due to the effects of an excessive production of nitric oxide, with activation of the baroreceptors and subsequent neurohormonal stimulation (RAAS, sympathetic nervous system, vasopressin) (Schrier *et al.* 1988). The concept of 'underfilling' is supported by the demonstration of a markedly reduced (−25 per cent) central blood volume (Henriksen *et al.* 1989), as well as the diuretic effect of central volume expansion due to head-out water immersion (Epstein 1978), implantation of a peritoneal–venous shunt (Epstein 1982), and albumin infusion. Furthermore, activation of the 'neurohormonal axis' with elevated plasma concentrations of noradrenaline, angiotensin II, and vasopressin (in advanced stages) (Epstein *et al.* 1977; Bichet *et al.* 1982), in the presence of a normal plasma concentration of ANP (Gerbes *et al.* 1985), underlines the role of hypovolaemia. Hyperaldosteronism is often, albeit not always, found in cirrhosis: besides elevated levels, normal and even reduced concentrations have been reported (Epstein *et al.* 1977; Wernze *et al.* 1978). In the pathogenesis of cirrhotic ascites, several local and systemic factors are involved, such as portal hypertension (due to intrahepatic sinusoidal obstruction), renal Na^+ and water retention, enhanced lymph production in the liver and intestinal tract (Witte *et al.* 1980).

As a consequence of the decreased EABV, neurohormonal activation, renal vasoconstriction, and tubular hyperreabsorption of Na^+ result. Of particular importance is the impaired capacity to excrete solute-free water, which favours the development of a dilutional hyponatraemia.

Using the Li^+ clearance method, proximal Na^+ reabsorption may increase from 60 per cent up to 85 per cent of the filtered load (Gatta *et al.* 1991). The avid Na^+ reabsorption may lower FE_{Na} to less than 0.2 per cent, which indicates a diuretic-resistant state (Knauf *et al.* 1990; Knauf and Mutschler 1997).

Therapeutic approach

Treatment is indicated in patients suffering from ascites-induced symptoms such as tense ascites, dyspnoea, anorexia, gastro-oesophageal reflux, abdominal hernias, and risk of spontaneous bacterial peritonitis (Maharaj 1988). The following sequential treatment is recommended: bed rest and reduced Na^+ intake, aldosterone antagonists, thiazides, loop diuretics, and plasma expanders with large volume parasynthesis.

Before diuretic therapy is introduced, a rigid reduction of dietary salt intake (~3 g NaCl/day) with fluid restriction in hyponatraemia (1–1.5 l/day) combined with bed rest for at least 4 days is recommended. Recumbency enhances Na^+ and fluid excretion by increasing central blood volume and alleviates the activated RAAS and sympathetic nervous system. About 10 per cent of patients may benefit from this regimen. However, if an adequate response (reduction in body weight by 400 g/day for 4 days) (Gerbes 1993) is not achieved, administration of diuretics will be required.

Aldosterone antagonists (spironolactone or potassium canrenoate) should be prescribed with regard to the increased plasma aldosterone concentrations and/or the enhanced sensitivity of the renal tubule to aldosterone (Suki *et al.* 1985). Spironolactone is absorbed from the intestinal tract (about 70 per cent), and subsequently metabolized in the liver, followed by enterohepatic circulation (Sungaila *et al.* 1992). Three to four days are needed to achieve a steady state. Spironolactone binds to aldosterone receptors mainly located in the cytoplasm of collecting duct cells and antagonizes the hormonal action in a competitive manner. The effective dose depends on the degree of hyperaldosteronism (Bernardi *et al.* 1985) and varies between 50 and 400 mg/day. In a multicentre trial spironolactone was effective in about 70 per cent of the patients (Bernardi *et al.* 1993). As an alternative to spironolactone, amiloride (15–30 mg daily) has been suggested (Yamada and Reynolds 1970); however, there are no controlled studies as yet. Administration of triamterene is complicated by its impaired hepatic metabolism in liver cirrhosis (Knauf and Mutschler 1997).

In releasing hepatic ascites, thiazide and loop diuretics are less effective than aldosterone antagonists (50–70 per cent), due to both altered pharmacokinetics and pharmacodynamics (Perez-Ayuso *et al.* 1983). A decreased delivery of frusemide to the urine may be caused not only by a decline of GFR but also by an impaired secretion of the diuretic in the proximal tubule (Pinzani *et al.* 1987). Furthermore, enhanced Na^+ reabsorption in the proximal and distal tubule contributes to diuretic resistance. While the effectiveness of other loop diuretics such as piretanide and bumetanide is comparable to that of frusemide, torasemide may induce a greater diuretic effect due to its impaired hepatic metabolism, with elevated blood concentrations (Brunner *et al.* 1988; Gentilini *et al.* 1994). Also the postulated antialdosterone properties of torasemide may contribute to its greater natriuretic potency (Uchida *et al.* 1991). The diuretic response of loop and thiazide diuretics is improved by the coadministration of spironolactone. Generally, the natriuretic effects of diuretics are greater in recumbency than in the upright position, which should be taken into account, particularly in diuretic resistance.

Recently, the administration of a non-peptide V2 receptor peptide antagonist has been shown to restore the impaired water excretion in cirrhotic rats (Tsuboi et al. 1994). In addition, this compound suppressed the increased expression of the water channel Aquaporin (AQP2) in cirrhotic rats (Fujita et al. 1995).

Plasma expanders

Diuretic resistance finally results from a progressive decrease of EABV, with a consequent impairment of renal perfusion and enhanced tubular Na^+ reabsorption. Furthermore, activation of the RAAS and sympathetic nervous system may play a contributory role. In these patients intravenous administration of salt-poor albumin (20–25 g) may improve the diuretic response. This procedure is of particular importance when large-volume paracentesis is performed as an effective alternative therapy (Quintero et al. 1985). A peritoneovenous shunt has been proposed for patients resistant to diuretics, which improves systemic and renal haemodynamics (Stasssen and McCullough 1985), but unfortunately is associated with a high rate of severe complications.

Specific complications of diuretic therapy and guidelines for optimal therapy

Administration of diuretics (in particular loop diuretics) may result in a multitude of electrolyte disturbances such as hyponatraemia, hypokalaemia, and hypochloraemic alkalosis (Sherlock et al. 1966). Aldosterone antagonists may induce hyperkalaemia and metabolic acidosis due to interference with hydrogen ions and K^+ secretion in the collecting duct. Furthermore, hypotension, prerenal azotaemia (pseudohepatorenal syndrome), and encephalopathy are frequently precipitated by diuretic therapy (Naranjo et al. 1979). Great care should be taken in the monitoring of plasma K^+ concentration, since diuretics may induce profound hypokalaemia (Epstein 1984), which stimulates ammonia production (Gabazda and Hall 1966) and thereby contributes to hepatic encephalopathy. With regard to these facts, Sherlock (1981) stated pithily that 'the patient is better wet and wise than dry and demented'.

Many complications result from the limited capacity of fluid reabsorption from the peritoneal cavity into the general circulation. Therefore, the daily weight loss should not exceed 300–500 g (Shear et al. 1970). Patients with additional peripheral oedema, in whom a weight loss of up to 1 kg/day may be acceptable, are an exception (Pockros and Reynolds 1986).

Nephrotic oedema

In the past, the key role of reduced EABV (underfilling) in the genesis of fluid and Na^+ retention in nephrotic oedema has been overestimated. Thus, in line with nephrotic animals (Kaysen et al. 1985), in the majority of nephrotic patients a normal (or even increased) plasma volume (Dorhout Mees et al. 1979; Geers et al. 1984) has been measured which fits to a normal (or suppressed) activity of the RAAS (Brown et al. 1982). The risk of excessive capillary fluid filtration in hypoalbuminaemic states seems to be counterbalanced by the lowered tissue oncotic pressure (Koomans et al. 1986; Manning 1987). The reduced EABV seems to be limited to a minority of patients with severe hypoalbuminaemia associated with a capillary leakage, such as minimal change glomerulopathy (Lagrue et al. 1975; Meltzer et al. 1979; Koomans et al. 1986). In the latter group, in addition to stimulation of the RAAS and adrenergic nervous system, an enhanced non-osmotic release of AVP has been demonstrated (Usberti et al. 1984; Rascher et al. 1986; Tulassay et al. 1987). However, overactivity of the renal nerve in nephrotic rats (DiBona et al. 1988) may also occur in the absence of volume contraction as a consequence of the renal disease.

The most important factor for the development of nephrotic oedema seems to be a primary defect of renal Na^+ excretion, leading to expansion of plasma volume and a subsequent 'overflow' in the peripheral capillaries. The experimental proof of this concept is demonstrated in the unilateral nephrosis model of rats, where Na^+ retention is confined to the diseased kidney (Ichikawa et al. 1983). The mechanisms involved in renal Na^+ retention concern, besides a potentially reduced GFR, an enhanced Na^+ reabsorption in the distal nephron (Ichikawa et al. 1983). On the other hand, in the proximal tubule, Na^+ reabsorption is unchanged or decreased, due to reduced protein concentration in the peritubular capillaries. The RAAS does not play a key role in Na^+ retention, in contrast to the effects of an activated adrenergic system (reviewed by Palmer and Alpern 1997). In addition, resistance to the action of ANP has been found (Humphreys 1994) due to an accelerated breakdown of the normally produced cyclic guanosine monophosphate (cGMP) (Morgan et al. 1989).

Management of nephrotic oedema

Dietary Na^+ intake should be restricted to about 50 mmol/day, corresponding to a diet with no added salt. Effects of head-out water immersion are only moderate, due to the normal or an enhanced central blood volume. If diuretics are indicated, patients with preserved GFR will respond to thiazides. Spironolactone was shown to exert at least a short-term effect (Shapiro et al. 1990). Response to loop diuretics is frequently decreased due to altered pharmacokinetics. In hypoalbuminaemia the renal clearance of active frusemide is diminished, while its metabolism in the proximal tubule to the inactive glucunoride is enhanced (Pichette et al. 1996). Moreover, the volume distribution of loop diuretics is augmented with a decreased delivery of the diuretic to the kidney. In addition, bio-availability of the free diuretic in tubular fluid at its site of action may be reduced, due to binding with filtered albumin (Green and Mirkin 1980). In perfusion studies, addition of albumin to tubular fluid blunts the response to frusemide, while agents that interfere with the albumin binding restore the diuretic effect (Kirchner et al. 1991).

In addition, pharmacodynamic resistance may be induced by enhanced distal tubular and occasionally proximal Na^+ reabsorption (Kirchner et al. 1992). As a consequence, most patients with drug resistance need greater doses of loop diuretics. If their response is insufficient, a combination with a distal (thiazide) or, exceptionally, a proximal (acetazolamide) acting diuretic should be attempted. In truly resistant cases, continuous infusion of loop diuretics and/or intravenous administration of salt-poor hyperoncotic albumin can be employed (Davison et al. 1974). However, infused albumin is rapidly excreted into the urine due to an increase in the glomerular barrier size selectivity in glomerular disease (Shemesh et al. 1986). Furthermore, in a retrospective analysis in patients with minimal change glomerulopathy, albumin infusions appeared to prolong the nephrotic stage as well as to increase the risk of its relapse (Yoshimura et al. 1992a,b). These data are in line with the administration of albumin to rats with puromycin nephrotic syndrome, which induced glomerular epithelial injury with detachment of the foot processes and a decreased recovery of the anionic charge (Yoshimura et al. 1992a,b).

Finally, haemofiltration has been employed successfully as an alternative approach in diuretic-resistant patients with nephrotic oedema (Fauchald et al. 1985).

Chronic renal failure

In chronic renal failure, as an adaptive mechanism for the decrease of GFR and Na^+ filtered load, the FE_{Na} increases progressively (magnification phenomenon, Bricker et al. 1978). Nevertheless, the maximal capacity for Na^+ excretion is impaired, favouring an expansion of ECV (Beretta-Piccoli et al. 1976), followed by vascular congestion, peripheral and pulmonary oedema, and even CHF. Positive Na^+ balance results at least in part from a relative or absolute activation of the adrenergic system and RAAS, while enhanced plasma ANP and ouabain-like activity (Hamlyn et al. 1991) favour Na^+ excretion.

Dietary salt and fluid restriction, together with diuretics, are used chiefly for treatment of oedema, salt-dependent hypertension, metabolic acidosis, and hyperkalaemia. Correction of Na^+ balance also seems to be of importance, since Na^+ is a trophic factor for the kidney (Dworkin et al. 1990) and left ventricle (Schmieder et al. 1988), independently of systemic blood pressure. Loop diuretics are the drugs of choice, since they maintain their efficacy in advanced renal failure. They enhance fluid and Na^+ delivery to the distal nephron, resulting in an enhanced excretion of potassium and hydrogen ions, in particular in the presence of secondary hyperaldosteronism. Unlike thiazides (Knauf et al. 1994), they do not suppress GFR, probably by abolishing the tubular–glomerular feedback (TGF) response (Schnermann and Briggs 1985) by inhibition of the Na^+,$2Cl^-$,K^+-cotransporter in the macula densa cells (Schlatter et al. 1989). In patients with advanced chronic renal failure (GFR about 5 ml/min) high doses of frusemide still exert a diuretic effect associated with a transient rise of inulin and p-aminohippuric acid clearance (Heidland et al. 1972; Scherzer et al. 1987).

Altered determinants of diuretic response in chronic renal failure

Pharmacokinetic factors

Oral bio-availability of loop diuretics (approximately 50 per cent for frusemide and 80 per cent for bumetanide and torasemide) is unchanged in chronic renal failure. However, their renal clearance is markedly diminished in proportion to the decreased GFR. In contrast to their renal clearance, the non-renal elimination of bumetanide and torasemide, undergoing hepatic metabolism by the cytochrome P-450 system, is unchanged. The plasma clearance of frusemide, however, is prolonged (Völker et al. 1987; Knauf and Mutschler 1991), probably due to an impaired glucuronidation, which takes place in the kidney rather than in the liver (Hammarlund-Udenaes and Benet 1989). Normally, half of the intravenously administered dose of frusemide is eliminated by glucuronidation, while the other half is secreted into the tubular lumen.

Delivery of loop diuretics from the blood to the organic anion secretory pathway in the proximal tubule is reduced as consequence of decreased renal perfusion and a wider ECV distribution in hypoalbuminaemia (due to reduced protein binding). Furthermore, in renal failure their secretion by the organic anion transport system is inhibited (Rose et al. 1976) by accumulated organic anions (Spustova et al. 1988),

including urates and effects of metabolic acidosis. Finally, access of secreted loop diuretics to their site of action in the thick ascending limb of the loop of Henle may be impaired by intraluminal binding to filtered albumin (Kirchner et al. 1990) (Table 1).

Pharmacodynamic factors

As GFR decreases the absolute Na^+ excretion (UV_{Na}) following loop diuretics is progressively diminished. Nevertheless, the FE_{Na} is not impaired and may even exceed the normal response (Heidland et al. 1969a,b; Brater et al. 1986). Similarly, when relating the fractional clearance of loop diuretics with their diuretic effect (FE_{Na}), an upward shift of the plateau to the left is obtained, indicating an increased intrinsic response of the remaining nephrons. This exaggerated action in chronic renal failure may be explained by an enhanced Na^+ delivery and reabsorption in the loop segment, due to glomerular hyperfiltration and decreased proximal tubule reabsorption following hypervolaemia (Fig. 3).

Adaptive mechanisms (braking phenomenon)

Postdiuretic fluid and Na^+ retention limit their response and can compensate for the entire Na^+ loss (Wilcox et al. 1983). It may be caused by Na^+-retaining hormones as well as an upregulation of the ion transporter along the thick ascending limb. To overcome the effects of the rebound action, loop diuretics have to be administered repeatedly in most instances. Furthermore, after prolonged therapy, relative resistance to loop diuretics develops as consequence of structural and functional changes in distal nephron segments. Due to the chronically increased Na^+ delivery—in the presence of elevated plasma aldosterone levels—cell hypertrophy of the distal and convoluted tubule and collecting duct occurs (Kaissling et al. 1985; Ellison et al. 1989), associated with an increased number of thiazide-sensitive NaCl cotransporters at the apical membrane (Chen and Vaughn 1990) and of Na^+,K^+-ATPase pumps at the basolateral membrane (Le Hir et al. 1982). Consequently, the hypertrophic cells reabsorb more Na^+ than normal cells (Kaissling and Stanton 1987). Such an intranephronal compensation may also occur in humans, since coadministration of thiazide diuretics increases the efficacy of loop diuretics in a supra-additive fashion (Loon et al. 1989; Fliser et al. 1994; Knauf and Mutschler 1997).

Recently, a novel adenosine type I receptor (AI) antagonist has been developed which inhibits Na^+ reabsorption in the proximal tubule

Table 1 Partial resistance to loop diuretics in chronic renal failure (modified according to Ritz et al. 1994a; Wilcox 2002)

Pharmacokinetic causes (diminished delivery of the active drug to the loop of Henle)

Decreased delivery due to reduced renal blood flow and enlarged volume of distribution (decreased drug binding in hypoalbuminaemia)

Impaired diuretic secretion in the proximal tubule due to metabolic acidosis and competition of the organic anion transport system (OAT-1) by accumulated organic anions including urate

Intratubular binding of the secreted diuretic to filtered albumin

Pharmacodynamic causes

Reduced number of functioning nephrons and decreased Na^+ filtered load

'Braking' phenomenon due to a rebound effect and/or intraperitoneal compensation

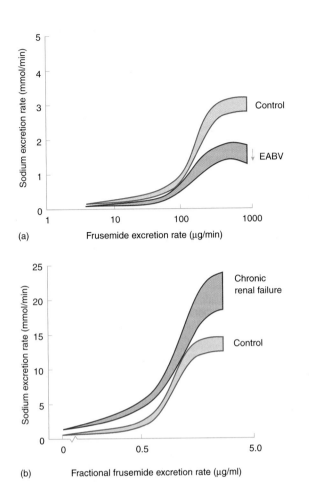

Fig. 3 (a) Relationship between urinary delivery of an intravenous loop diuretic and the natriuretic response in normal controls, in patients with chronic renal failure, and in renal failure patients with reduced effective arterial blood volume (EABV). (b) Relationship between the fractional delivery of a loop diuretic into the urine [urinary excretion rate (µg/ml)] divided by the creatinine clearance (ml/min), and the fractional excretion of sodium (modified after Brater *et al.* 1984, 1986; Knauf and Mutschler 1997, with permission).

with a concomitant rise of GFR, while TGF is blocked (Wilcox *et al.* 1999). Furthermore, intravenous administration of a low dose ANP in chronic renal failure patients was shown to increase sodium excretion, associated with a marked rise of urinary cGMP, while aldosterone levels were suppressed (Conte *et al.* 1997). The exaggerated tubular response to ANP was explained with a lower renal catabolism of the infused hormone.

Consequences for patient management

The maximal effective dose of frusemide is 160–200 mg IV (Brater *et al.* 1986). In view of the potential ototoxicity, higher doses of frusemide should be avoided (Heidland and Wigand 1970). Promising alternatives to frusemide in chronic renal failure are torasemide and bumetanide (Kampf and Baethke 1980; Marone *et al.* 1984; Andreucci *et al.* 1990). Unfortunately, long-term therapy with high doses of muzolimine in chronic renal failure was complicated by severe neurological disturbances and encephalomyelopathy (Daul *et al.* 1987).

Following repeated administration of ceiling doses of diuretics, the maximal effective urinary concentration may not always be optimal due to an initial overshoot and subsequent undershoot. With continuous intravenous administration, however, the urine concentration of the diuretic can be kept at the plateau of its dose–response curve, resulting in greater efficacy (Rudy *et al.* 1991).

In moderate renal insufficiency, combinations of low doses of loop and thiazide diuretics are more effective than high-dose monotherapy (Wollam *et al.* 1982; Knauf and Mutschler 1993b; Ritz *et al.* 1994). Thiazides not only obliterate the resistance and rebound antinatriuresis and resistance to prolonged loop diuretic administration, but also attenuate the enhanced Ca^{2+} excretion, induced by loop diuretics. However, thiazides given alone or in combination reduce the GFR due to blockade of TGF, in particular in the presence of volume depletion (Wollam *et al.* 1982).

To overcome the partial resistance to loop diuretics in chronic renal failure three approaches are recommended:

(1) intermittent use of higher doses of loop diuretics (5–10 times the therapeutic dosage in normal subjects);

(2) combination of loop and thiazide diuretics with sequential blockade of the nephron; and

(3) continuous administration of the diuretic by intravenous perfusion.

Diuretic therapy in maintenance dialysis patients with residual renal function

Loop diuretics do not slow the loss of renal function in chronic renal insufficiency, as demonstrated in a controlled clinical trial in patients treated on continuous peritoneal dialysis (Medcalf *et al.* 2001). High doses of loop diuretics may have some role in the control of fluid balance in selected patients on haemodialysis with residual renal function (Verenstraeten *et al.* 1975; Weisschedel *et al.* 1983). They may permit greater amounts of beverages, minimize dangerous weight gain in the interdialytic interval, and thereby reduce the hypotensive responses due to dialytic fluid removal. In short-term studies (3 months) a doubling of the residual urine production was shown in patients with a mean residual creatinine clearance of 1.9 ml/min (van Olden *et al.* 1993).

Diuretics in acute renal failure

Mannitol

Experimental studies and mechanisms of action

Prophylactic, and in some studies therapeutic, administration of mannitol ameliorated acute renal failure after aortic clamping, renal artery obstruction, noradrenaline, glycerol, methaemoglobin, myoglobin, cisplatin, and amphotericin B (reviewed by Levinsky and Bernhard 1988; Shilliday and Allison 1994). One or more of the following mechanisms may be involved:

(1) prevention and relief of tubule obstruction due to debris and protein precipitates following an increased intratubule flow rate (Burke *et al.* 1980);

(2) lessening of endothelial and epithelial cell swelling (Flores *et al.* 1972);

(3) protection of mitochondrial function (Schrier *et al.* 1984);

(4) scavenging of free oxygen radicals (Freeman and Crapo 1982); and

(5) renal vasodilation due to the combined effects of increased prostaglandin formation (Johnston *et al.* 1981), inhibition of renin release (Vander and Miller 1964), and enhanced secretion of ANP (Gianello *et al.* 1989).

Clinical studies (see also Section 10)

Prophylactic administration of hypertonic mannitol in adult patients undergoing cardiopulmonary surgery exerted no benefits (Yeboah *et al.* 1972). In contrast, postoperatively in children, a faster decline of elevated creatinine was reported in a prospective trial (Rigden *et al.* 1984). In vascular (aortic) surgery, benefits over adequate hydration were only reported in an uncontrolled (Powers *et al.* 1964), but not in a controlled trial (Beall *et al.* 1963). Some benefits of mannitol were observed in uncontrolled studies in the prevention of toxic nephropathies due to cisplatin, amphotericin B, and radiocontrast media (reviewed by Lieberthal and Levinsky 1991), as well as in crush-induced rhabdomyolysis, in comorbidity with alkalization (Eneas *et al.* 1979; Ron *et al.* 1984; Better and Stein 1990). In recipients of cadaveric kidney transplants, the incidence of acute renal failure was either reduced (Weimar *et al.* 1983) or not influenced (Lachance and Barry 1985).

When summarizing the anecdotal observations and the multitude of uncontrolled and controlled studies, the benefits of hypertonic mannitol therapy in prevention and treatment of incipient clinical acute renal failure are still 'not proven' (Shilliday and Allison 1994).

Performance of mannitol therapy

When treating oliguric patients, the initial dose of hypertonic mannitol should not exceed 12–25 g. If renal function does not respond, therapy should be stopped to prevent the risk of hypervolaemia and acute left ventricular failure.

Loop diuretics in acute renal failure

In ischaemic or toxic acute renal failure damage of the thick ascending limb is an early event and probably induced by an insufficient oxygen supply (Heyman *et al.* 1988), since the substrate supply and the transport processes of this nephron segment are closely linked (Wittner *et al.* 1984). In incipient acute renal failure, loop diuretics may preserve energy expenditure and oxygen consumption by suppressing the chloride reabsorptive work (Brezis *et al.* 1984a,b, 1985; Greger and Wangemann 1987). Benefits of loop diuretics may be achieved by the following mechanisms:

(1) reduction of transport activity of the thick ascending limb of the loop of Henle (production of a 'resting state');

(2) prevention or removal of obstructing casts by an enhanced intratubule flow rate;

(3) renal vasodilatation due to increased prostaglandins (Mackay *et al.* 1984);

(4) inhibition of TGF (Wright and Schnermann 1974), which may be activated in acute renal failure due to enhanced Na^+ delivery to the macula densa following reduced Na^+ reabsorption in the proximal tubule.

Animal experiments

Effects of loop diuretics in experimental acute renal failure are less consistent than those of mannitol. In noradrenaline-induced acute renal failure in dogs frusemide improved renal function (Patak *et al.* 1979). However, the data in rat models of ischaemic acute renal failure are controversial (Kramer *et al.* 1980b). In toxic acute renal failure in rats, improved renal function was observed in the following models: mercuric chloride (Thiel *et al.* 1976), cisplatin (Pera *et al.* 1979), and radiocontrast media combined with indomethacin (Heyman *et al.* 1989). A detrimental effect was observed in glycerol (Greven and Klein 1976), cephaloridine, and aminoglycosides-induced renal failure (Hewitt 1977).

Loop diuretics in clinical acute renal failure

Prophylactic treatment of high-risk patients after open heart or vascular surgery was either ineffective (Abel *et al.* 1976) or beneficial (Nuutinen *et al.* 1978). Radiocontrast media-induced acute renal failure was lessened in an uncontrolled study (Oguagha *et al.* 1981). According to Lieberthal and Levinsky (1991), prophylactic administration of loop diuretics, although not proven, may be performed in high-risk settings (cardiovascular surgery, rapid intravascular haemolysis, rhabdomyolysis, radiocontrast media administration, acute hyperuricaemia, and cisplatin therapy), if conventional volume therapy does not result in an increased urine output (>2–3 l/day).

Loop diuretics also may reverse oliguria in incipient acute renal failure, and thereby facilitate the management of fluid balance disorders. Whether the prognosis of developing acute renal failure can be improved is unknown.

In established acute renal failure, administration of large doses of frusemide in controlled and uncontrolled studies showed no improved mortality (Cantarovich *et al.* 1973; Kleinknecht *et al.* 1976; Brown *et al.* 1986), even after infusion into the renal artery (Epstein *et al.* 1975). A beneficial action was only demonstrated in one study in patients with less severe acute renal failure (Anderson *et al.* 1977).

Combination of dopamine and loop diuretics

Dopamine in low doses (1–5 μg/kg body weight/min) increases renal blood flow, GFR, and Na^+ excretion (McDonald *et al.* 1964); and is assumed to reduce the incidence of postoperative acute renal failure (Polsen *et al.* 1987; Schwarz *et al.* 1988). In incipient acute renal failure, resistance to high doses of loop diuretics or hypertonic mannitol, addition of dopamine was reported to increase urine flow and possibly GFR (Lindner 1983; Graziani *et al.* 1984; Hörl *et al.* 1989). However, low doses of dopamine may cause adverse cardiac effects and has been disappointing in enhancing the response to frusemide in patients with heart failure (Vargo *et al.* 1996; Powers *et al.* 1999).

Atrial natriuretic peptide

ANP increases GFR, due to preglomerular vasodilation, and enhances Na^+ excretion, probably by closing lumenal Na^+ channels in the collecting duct. In the rat, intrarenal arterial or intravenous infusion of ANP (or the residue peptide atriopeptin) can reverse ischaemic and toxic acute renal failure (Heidbreder *et al.* 1986, 1988; Shaw *et al.* 1987; Schafferhans *et al.* 1988); in particular combined treatment with dopamine (which prevents an ANP-induced hypotension) appeared promising (Conger *et al.* 1989).

Meanwhile preliminary reports of the use of ANP in the prevention and treatment of clinical acute renal failure have appeared. In a controlled study in patients with established intrinsic acute renal failure,

ANP enhanced GFR and reduced the need of haemodialysis treatment (Rahman *et al.* 1994). In contrast, Götz *et al.* (1989) could not find any benefit in 13 patients with dopamine- and frusemide-resistant acute renal failure. Also, two studies of cadaveric kidney transplantation failed to show any consistant benefit from ANP on the incidence of acute renal failure (Smits *et al.* 1989; Sands *et al.* 1991). However, urodilatin, the kidney-borne analogue of circulating ANP, was reported to reduce the incidence of acute renal failure after heart (Hummel *et al.* 1993) and liver transplantation (Cedidi *et al.* 1994). However, there is a need for large, controlled studies.

Idiopathic oedema

Idiopathic oedema is characterized by recurring attacks of generalized oedema in women of childbearing age. In its pathogenesis, an abnormal homeostatic response to upright posture (a weight gain of about 1 kg/day) is implicated, due to an activation of the RAAS and/or the sympathetic nervous system (Greenberg and Puschett 1991).

In many patients the syndrome is aggravated by diuretics. If this treatment is stopped, there is a protracted rebound retention of Na^+ and water, reinforcing again the patient's perception of an apparent 'need' for diuretics (MacGregor *et al.* 1979). Basics of therapy are low Na^+ diet and, if unavoidable, spironolactone or low-dose thiazide diuretics on an alternate day basis (Greenberg and Puschett 1991). When diuretics are stopped, rebound Na^+ retention can be avoided with consequent restriction of salt intake (Missouris *et al.* 1992).

Brain oedema

Hypertonic mannitol has been used to reduce cerebral swelling, since it increases serum osmolality and does not cross the normal blood brain barrier. Its intravenous infusion results in expansion of plasma volume, reduction of blood viscosity, reactive constriction of pial arteries, and an augmented cerebral blood flow, which may improve the metabolism of the brain, with a concomitant efflux of water to the interstitial space. Mannitol has to be applied in a bolus-like fashion, since its continuous infusion may result in the penetration of the damaged tissue with adverse effects (Cruz *et al.* 2001). Benefits of mannitol were recently shown in a randomized, controlled clinical study in acute traumatic brain injury (Schrot and Muizelaar 2002).

Other indications of diuretic therapy

Use of carbonic anhydrase inhibitors

Glaucoma is the most common indication for the use of carbonic anhydrase inhibitors. Reduction of intraocular pressure is achieved by inhibition of fluid secretion in the anterior chamber (Wistrand 1984). Its local application may reduce its systemic side-effects. Acetazolamide-induced urinary alkalinization via bicarbonaturia may ameliorate acute urate and pigment nephropathy and enhance the clearance of weak organic acids (such as barbiturates) due to reduced non-ionic back diffusion (Conger 1977). However, acetazolamide is obsolete in salicylate toxicity, since the complicating metabolic acidosis favours an accumulation of the protonated and lipophilic form of salicylic acid in the central nervous system (Gabow *et al.* 1978). Acetazolamide has also been suggested for cancer patients receiving high doses of methotrexate, in order to improve its poor solubility in acidic urine (Shamash *et al.* 1991).

Treatment of metabolic alkalosis

Acetazolamide improves metabolic alkalosis caused by thiazide or loop diuretics and glucocorticoids (Miller and Berns 1977) (see Chapter 2.6), as well as hypercapnia in patients with left ventricular dysfunction or cor pulmonale, in whom saline administration is contraindicated (Berger and Warnock 1986). Furthermore, K^+-sparing drugs are beneficial in the treatment of metabolic alkalosis.

Acute mountain sickness

Untrained lowlanders when climbing to altitudes of more than 3000 m may develop posthypercapnic alkalosis with marked fluid retention and pulmonary and cerebral oedema. Acetazolamide was reported to improve these symptoms (Greene *et al.* 1981; Larson *et al.* 1982).

Therapeutic use of thiazides

Calcium nephrolithiasis (see also Chapter 8.2): thiazide diuretics decrease Ca^{2+} excretion by about 20–50 per cent. The effect is enhanced by low and abolished by high Na^+ intake (Yendt and Cohanim 1978). Ca^{2+} retention is induced both by volume contraction (with consequent increased Ca^{2+} reabsorption along the proximal and distal tubulus) and by an intrinsic action on distal tubule cells (with activation of the basolateral Na^+–Ca^{2+} exchange). In addition, thiazides may reduce oxalate excretion (Ahlstrand *et al.* 1984), probably due to a decreased oxalate absorption in the distal colon (Hatch and Vaziri 1994). Owing to these actions, thiazides reduce stone formation in idiopathic hypercalciuria (Coe 1981; Lemieux 1986; Mortensen *et al.* 1986; Coe *et al.* 1988), in normocalciuric individuals (Yendt and Cohanim 1978; Baggio *et al.* 1986), and in absorptive hyperoxaluria (Yendt and Cohanim 1986).

Thiazides and bone mineralization

Long-term thiazide treatment has been associated with enhanced bone mineralization in elderly hypertensives (Wasnich *et al.* 1983) and a lower incidence of femoral neck fractures (Hale *et al.* 1984; Rashiq and Logan 1986; LaCroix *et al.* 1990). A small number of observations suggests a preventive effect in steroid-induced osteoporosis (Condon *et al.* 1978).

Diuretic therapy of diabetes insipidus

In patients with diabetes insipidus (pituitary and renal type) polyuria and polydipsia can be improved by thiazides and salt restriction (Crawford *et al.* 1960; Lant and Wilson 1971). This is achieved by the combined effects of reduced GFR, enhanced proximal Na^+ reabsorption, and inhibition of the renal diluting mechanism. In Li^+-induced diabetes insipidus, amiloride has been advocated because it ameliorates the resistance to ADH by inhibiting the entry of Li^+ into the principal cells of the distal nephron (Batlle *et al.* 1982). Combination of thiazides and amiloride may be more antidiuretic than thiazides alone in patients with diabetes insipidus.

Treatment of hypercalcaemia

Loop diuretics inhibit NaCl as well as Ca^{2+} and Mg^{2+} reabsorption in the thick ascending limb of the loop of Henle and may lower plasma Ca^{2+} in hypercalcaemia (Suki *et al.* 1970). However, in emergency hypercalcaemia, the first step of treatment is repletion of body Na^+ and ECV by infusion of several litres of saline. Persistent volume contraction will otherwise reduce the calciuric effect of loop diuretics. Currently, administration of biphosphonates is the therapy of choice in hypercalcaemia.

Diuretics in renal tubular acidosis

In distal renal tubule acidosis (type I) no pH gradient can be generated in the distal nephron (see Chapter 5.3). Loop diuretics have been used successfully to increase proton secretion. Prolonged treatment results in normalization of metabolic acidosis, regression of osteomalacia, and a potential retardation of the progressive course of nephrocalcinosis (Györy and Edwards 1971; Heidbreder et al. 1982). The beneficial effect is explained by an increased Na^+ delivery to the distal nephron, leading to enhanced Na^+ reabsorption and consequent generation of a negative voltage in the lumen (Hropot et al. 1985).

In proximal renal tubule acidosis (type II) thiazide diuretics prevent HCO_3^- wasting due to reduced GFR and increased proximal tubule Na^+ and HCO_3^- reabsorption. Even in patients with the full expression of type II renal tubular acidosis, bicarbonaturia, metabolic acidosis, hypophosphataemia, and rickets can be corrected (Rampini et al. 1968; Santos-Atherton and Frank 1986).

Hyperkalaemic renal tubular acidosis (type IV) is caused either by aldosterone deficiency [due to ACE-inhibitor therapy, hyporeninism, or diabetes mellitus (De Fronzo 1980)], resistance to the action of aldosterone (pseudohypoaldosteronism type I and II, Schambelan et al. 1981) or a H^+ secretion defect. Loop diuretics are beneficial due to an enhanced distal Na^+ delivery and stimulated aldosterone secretion following volume contraction (Rastogi et al. 1985). In a subgroup of patients with type IV tubular acidosis, hydrogen ion secretion may not respond due to an 'irreversible voltage-dependent defect' (Batlle et al. 1981). Effectiveness of loop diuretics can be assessed easily by monitoring the urine pH after drug administration (Tarka et al. 1983).

Diuretics and the syndrome of inappropriate antidiuretic hormone secretion

Basic treatment of the syndrome of inappropriate antidiuretic hormone (SIADH) secretion is fluid restriction. In some cases ADH antagonists such as demeclocycline, Li^+, or the non-peptide AVP antagonist OPC-31260 (Fujisawa et al. 1993) may be effective. In its long-term management, loop diuretics and generous dietary Na^+ intake have been recommended (Decaux et al. 1981). Loop diuretics prevent the ADH-induced concentration of the urine by blocking NaCl reabsorption in the thick ascending limb. In acute hyponatraemic states the combination of frusemide and hypertonic saline has been used (Hantman et al. 1973).

Diuretics in intoxications

Forced diuresis with administration of large volumes of electrolyte solution and loop diuretics increases the renal excretion of many drugs and poisons, such as salicylates, long-acting barbiturates, ethylene glycol, and thallium (Lameijer and van Zwieten 1978). Since bromide and iodide may be reabsorbed to some extent by the thick ascending limb (Walser and Rahill 1966), halide intoxications can also be treated by loop diuretics in a specific fashion.

Loop diuretics in asthma

Inhaled frusemide has been reported to protect asthmatic subjects against a wide range of bronchoconstrictor challenges, including exercise, nebulized distilled water, and adenosine 5′-monophosphate, but not by directly acting agonists such as histamine and methacholine (Bianco et al. 1988, 1989; Robuschi et al. 1988; Pavord et al. 1992). The effect seems to be mediated by inhibition of fluid and salt secretion in airway epithelia (Widdicombe et al. 1983) and the concomitant production of inhibitory prostanoids (enhanced synthesis of prostaglandin E_2). However, this therapeutic approach has found only limited acceptance and is not clinically used at present.

Adverse haemodynamic and metabolic reactions to diuretics

Volume depletion

Mild volume depletion during diuretic therapy is normally well tolerated. However, in patients with impaired cardiac reflexes (such as occur in diabetics and in the elderly), as well as in those with reduced EABV (CHF and liver cirrhosis), clinical signs of hypovolaemia such as orthostatic hypotension may occur.

Adverse biochemical correlates are (a) metabolic alkalosis, (b) metabolic acidosis, (c) hyponatraemia, (d) hypokalaemia, (e) hypomagnesaemia, (f) hyperkalaemia, (g) disturbed calcium homeostasis, (h) hyperuricaemia, (i) enhanced serum creatinine and urea/creatinine ratio, (j) hyperglycaemia, and (k) hyperlipidaemia.

Metabolic alkalosis

Diuretic-induced contraction of ECV causes an increased bicarbonate reabsorption in the proximal and distal tubule probably via stimulation of the Na^+/H^+ antiporter activity by a direct effect of the diuretic (Capasso et al. 1997) as well as indirectly by angiotensin II. Moreover, diuretics can enhance urinary proton excretion directly, as in the case of loop diuretics, and indirectly due to secondary hyperaldosteronism. Another mediator of metabolic alkalosis may be a diuretic-induced hypokalaemia, with a shift of H^+ from ECV to the intracellular compartment, in exchange for K^+.

Metabolic acidosis

Carbonic anhydrase inhibitors cause a moderate metabolic acidosis by impairing HCO_3^- reabsorption in the proximal tubule. In the elderly, severe metabolic acidosis may develop in proportion to the blood concentrations of acetazolamide. Interestingly, the diuretic may induce metabolic acidosis even in patients without functioning kidneys, probably by an impairment of parathormone-mediated bone buffering of acids (De Marchi and Cecchin 1990). Metabolic acidosis, induced by K^+-sparing diuretics (amiloride, triamterene, spironolactone, and eplerenone), is caused by a reduced H^+ secretion in the connecting duct. In addition, K^+ retention and hyperkalaemia may contribute to metabolic acidosis by diminishing ammonia production and net acid excretion.

Hyponatraemia

Hyponatraemia is common after administration of diuretics, but rarely of clinical significance. However, occasionally a life-threatening extreme hyponatraemia (about 100 mmol/l) may occur (Ashraf et al. 1981). Hyponatraemia is a typical complication in older people, particularly elderly women (Friedman et al. 1989; Sonnenblick et al. 1993), as well as in patients with decreased EABV (CHF and hepatic cirrhosis) (Schrier and Berl 1980).

Most commonly hyponatraemia is induced by thiazides or thiazide-like diuretics alone or in combination with K^+-sparing diuretics, while loop diuretics represent a rare cause (Sonnenblick et al. 1993). In most patients hyponatraemia occurs within the first 2 weeks or even within 24 h of diuretic administration (Friedman *et al.* 1989; Baglin *et al.* 1995).

Mechanism of hyponatraemia

Hyponatraemia only develops when the tonicity of urine exceeds that of the fluid intake. Correspondingly, in most cases urine is inappropriately concentrated. The following factors may be involved:

1. Impaired free water excretion: thiazides reduce renal diluting ability by both decreased distal fluid delivery (due to reduced GFR and enhanced proximal fluid reabsorption) and inhibition of Na^+ reabsorption in the cortical diluting segment.

2. Inappropriate (enhanced) secretion of ADH (Horowitz *et al.* 1972) due to diuretic-induced hypovolaemia (non-osmotic release). An exaggerated response will occur in patients with pre-existing contraction of EABV.

3. Unrestricted fluid intake (Schrier and Berl 1980; Gross *et al.* 1988). Thiazides may even exert a dipsogenic effect in some elderly subjects (Kone *et al.* 1986) or psychotic patients (Emsley and Gledhill 1984). The risk for hyponatraemia can be identified by using a single challenge dose of a thiazide diuretic. In predisposed subjects, a decreased plasma Na^+ combined with weight gain has been observed within 6 h (Friedman *et al.* 1989).

4. Concomitant drug therapy: water intake may be increased by drugs which either stimulate thirst (tricyclic antidepressants) or have ADH-like effects [chlorpropamide, non-steroidal anti-inflammatory agents (NSAIDs)].

Management of diuretic-induced hyponatraemia involves withdrawal of the drug (and prevention of its later resumption), restriction of fluid intake (<1 l/day) and, if necessary, Na^+ and K^+ repletion (Ayus 1986). If Na^+ depletion is severe and symptomatic, slow infusion of isotonic saline may be useful to enhance plasma Na^+ by about 1 mmol/l/h in the first hours, but not more than 25 mmol/l within the first 2 days. The target of treatment is a plasma Na^+ of 130 mmol/l (Arieff 1993).

Hypokalaemia

All diuretics acting proximal to the cortical collecting duct induce kaliuresis and may reduce plasma K^+. Approximately 50 per cent of patients treated with conventional doses of thiazides have a K^+ concentration less than 3.5 mmol/l, and 7 per cent less than 3.0 mmol/l (Morgan and Davidson 1980). Total body K^+ varies considerably: a decline (5–10 per cent), no change, or an initial decline followed by a return to normal have been reported (Tannen 1985). A recent meta-analysis of 23 studies clearly verifies that total body K^+ decreases (Singh *et al.* 1992). The following factors may be involved:

(1) Enhanced K^+ secretion due to an increased lumenal flow rate and Na^+ delivery to the K^+ secretory sites in the colleting duct.

(2) Hypovolaemia-mediated stimulation of aldosterone and glucocorticoid secretion.

(3) Metabolic alkalosis due to both enhanced bicarbonate reabsorption following volume contraction and urinary losses of protons, which aggravate and maintain hypokalaemia (in part by a shift of K^+ into cells).

(4) Dietary Na^+ intake: both high and low Na^+ intake stimulate urinary K^+ excretion, while moderate Na^+ restriction (60–90 mmol/day) minimizes K^+ loss (Tannen 1985).

(5) Type, dose, and half-life of the diuretic: thiazides are more kaliuretic than loop diuretics, both at the peak diuresis (higher K^+/Na^+ ratio) and in the postdiuretic period (Knauf and Mutschler 1993a). Furthermore, urinary K^+ loss is directly proportional to dose (Venkata *et al.* 1981; Carlsen *et al.* 1990) and half-life of the diuretic (Tweeddale *et al.* 1977).

(6) Diuretic-induced hypomagnesaemia may result in K^+ wasting by yet unidentified mechanisms.

Clinical consequences of diuretic-induced hypokalaemia

Arrhythmias, sudden death, and stroke In short-term studies using the Holter monitor, both an association and no relationship have been reported. However, several long-term intervention trials suggest that diuretic therapy does increase the number and complexity of ventricular premature beats (MRC trial, Framingham study, Levy *et al.* 1987)—in particular in patients with pre-existing coronary heart disease (Caralis *et al.* 1984) or acute myocardial infarction (Solomon 1984). It is important to know that plasma catecholamines, by enhancing cellular uptake of K^+, can aggravate hypokalaemia (Struthers *et al.* 1983). Furthermore, hypokalaemia-induced arrhythmias are more likely in patients treated with cardiac glycosides, in particular with concomitant Mg^{2+} depletion.

The use of high doses of thiazide diuretics has been incriminated as a cause of an enhanced incidence of sudden death in three intervention trials (Oslo-study, Holme *et al.* 1984; MRFIT 1985; MRC Working Party on Mild Hypertension 1988), but this remains controversial and unproven. Enhanced mortality (3.8-fold) after thiazide therapy has been reported in one retrospective analysis in hypertensive diabetics (Warram *et al.* 1991). However, there are doubts about the validity of the dates. K^+ depletion has been linked to hypertension and stroke (Kaplan *et al.* 1985).

Management of hypokalaemia

The first step is its prevention by use of low doses of diuretics. Urinary K^+ losses can further be reduced by:

(1) moderate Na^+ restriction (to about 60–90 mmol/day);

(2) K^+ (and Mg^{2+})-sparing diuretics (Dykner and Wester 1984); and

(3) administration of ACE inhibitors (Griffing *et al.* 1983), on angiotensin II type 1 receptor antagonists.

Potassium chloride supplements (approximately 40 mmol/day) carry the risk of mucosal ulceration if their passage through the intestine is slow. Achievement of a positive K^+ balance seems to be of particular interest with regard to recent provocative data suggesting a 'vasculoprotective' effect of K^+ in rats (Tobian 1988) and man (Khaw and Barrett-Connor 1987).

In four intervention trials, in which thiazide-induced hypokalaemia was avoided either by K^+-sparing drugs or K^+ supplementation, a clear reduction of sudden death from coronary heart disease was shown (EWPHE trial, Amery *et al.* 1985; STOP-trial, Dahlöf *et al.* 1991; SHEP Cooperative Research Group 1991; MRC Working Party 1992). A similar decline was recently demonstrated in a population-based case–control study in hypertensive patients, receiving low doses of thiazides in combination with K^+-sparing drugs (Siscovik *et al.* 1994).

Hypomagnesaemia

Single doses of loop diuretics cause an acute, short-lived increase in Mg^{2+} excretion, followed by a compensatory retention, whereas thiazides have a slower but prolonged action (Knauf and Mutschler 1993a). The effects of long-term diuretic therapy on plasma and tissue Mg^{2+} concentration are controversial. In a meta-analysis of 15 studies with an 'adequate' control group lasting longer than 6 weeks, reductions (-10 per cent) and increases ($+6$ per cent) of plasma Mg^{2+} were reported (Davies and Fraser 1993). However, in the elderly and in CHF, reduced plasma and tissue Mg^{2+} concentrations, partly paralleled by a concomitant K^+ loss, have been observed in some (but not all) studies (Lim and Jacob 1972; Dykner and Wester 1979). Mg^{2+} depletion may be an independent stimulus to cardiac arrhythmias, and may cause an enhanced renal K^+ loss. Interestingly K^+ deficiency may fail to respond to K^+ supplementation if Mg^{2+} depletion is not corrected (Dykner and Wester 1979).

Hyperkalaemia

K^+-sparing diuretics (spironolactone, eplerenone, amiloride, or triamterene) occasionally may induce severe and possibly lethal hyperkalaemia (Mor et al. 1983; Akbarpour et al. 1985). Risk factors are:

(1) impaired renal function (GFR < 50 ml/min);

(2) diabetes mellitus (in particular with type IV renal tubular acidosis); and

(3) drug therapy that predisposes to hyperkalaemia, (potassium chloride, ACE inhibitors, angiotensin II type 1 receptor antagonists, β-blockers, NSAIDs, and heparin).

Diuretics and calcium homeostasis

Chronic administration of thiazides enhance Ca^{2+} absorption along the proximal and distal tubule, due to a mild volume depletion as well as by an activation of basolateral $Na^+–Ca^{2+}$ exchange in the distal nephron. Decreased urinary Ca^{2+} excretion is accompanied by a slightly reduced intestinal Ca^{2+} absorption (Bushinsky et al. 1984). The net effect is a positive Ca^{2+} balance. Some data indicate that thiazides potentiate the renal effects of parathormone by enhancing the formation of lumenal cell membrane Ca^{2+} channels, which are important for distal tubule Ca^{2+} absorption (Shimizu et al. 1991). In addition, thiazides may have effects on bone because they can increase serum Ca^{2+} levels in patients on maintenance haemodialysis (Kopple et al. 1970). The incidence of hypercalcaemia in subjects taking higher doses of thiazides has been estimated to be about 12 per cent (Mallette 1992). Besides generation of a de novo hypercalcaemia, thiazides may worsen or make overt the hypercalcaemia from primary hyperparathyroidism, vitamin D treatment, and malignancy (Malette 1992). Thus serum Ca^{2+} concentration should be confirmed as normal before starting thiazide therapy and should be monitored repeatedly in the following months.

Loop diuretics on the other hand reduce Ca^{2+} reabsorption in the thick ascending limb and hence increase urinary Ca^{2+} excretion. Chronic therapy can lead to calcium stones and—depending on the dosage—also to medullary nephrocalcinosis regardless of age, although the risk is higher in preterm infants (Hufnagle et al. 1982; Kim et al. 2002). Due to their calciuric effects, loop diuretics seem to be an important determinant of plasma intact parathormone level (Reichel et al. 1992). There are also reports of increased immunoreactive parathormone in frusemide-treated patients with CHF, and kidney transplants (Elmgreen et al. 1980; Petit et al. 1988; Bittar et al. 1989). Even short-term administration of loop diuretics in healthy subjects increased plasma parathormone transiently, although plasma ionized Ca^{2+} was unchanged (Reichel et al. 1992).

Glucose intolerance

Diuretics impair glucose tolerance dose-dependently. In the MRC trial on mild hypertension (MRC 1981) high doses of bendrofluazide (10 mg daily) over 3 years induced a four times greater incidence of glucose intolerance than in the placebo group. A lesser frequency (increase by a factor of 2–3) was achieved when lower doses of diuretics were used (EWPHE trial, Amery et al. 1985; MRC Working Party 1992). In a 10-week placebo-controlled parallel group study of bendrofluazide (1.25–10 mg daily) blood glucose increased by 7 per cent after 10 mg, while 1.25 mg exerted no adverse effect (Carlsen et al. 1990). In a 14-year follow-up study of diuretic treatment in hypertensives, only 1 per cent developed clinical diabetes (Murphy et al. 1982). Worsening of glucose tolerance seems to be more pronounced after administration of the long-acting diuretic, chlorthalidone (Tweeddale et al. 1977), while the effects of loop diuretics seem to be less marked (Feely and O'Byrne 1990).

Occasionally thiazides and loop diuretics can induce a severe hyperosmolar non-ketotic syndrome (Curtis et al. 1972; Khaleeli and Wyman 1978). Indapamide (1.5 mg/day) and K^+-sparing drugs seem to be neutral on glucose tolerance. Fortunately, the diabetogenic effects may be reversible when diuretics are discontinued (MRC 1981; Murphy et al. 1982), although not immediately (Pollare et al. 1989). Combinations with β-blockers may exaggerate the glucose intolerance induced by thiazides (Dornhorst et al. 1985).

Pathogenesis

Glucose intolerance is related to diuretic-induced hypokalaemia (Sundberg et al. 1982). Its central role is also emphasized by its amelioration after K^+ supplementation (Sundberg et al. 1982; Helderman et al. 1983). Even small reductions of plasma K^+ concentration (-0.28 mmol/l) within the normal range may be associated with decreased insulin sensitivity (Pollare et al. 1989). K^+ depletion may also inhibit pancreatic insulin secretion (Grünfeld and Chappell 1983), but the frequent occurrence of hyperinsulinaemia underlines the importance of insulin resistance. This may also be induced by activation of the sympathetic adrenergic system by diuretics (Heidland and Hennemann 1969; Luke et al. 1979).

In vitro diuretics may directly interfere with glucose utilization in rat diaphragms (Dzurik et al. 1993) and isolated rat adipocytes (Jacobs et al. 1984) and may also interfere with pancreatic insulin secretion (in vitro and in vivo) (Frumann 1981), possibly by inhibition of chloride channels (Sandström and Sehlin 1988) or by activation of ATP-sensitive K^+ channels. In rats thiazides increase hepatic glucose production by enhancing glycogenolysis (Senft et al. 1966) due to inhibition of hepatic phosphodiesterase and increased cyclic adenosine monophosphate (cAMP) formation (Hoskins and Jackson 1978).

Implications for therapy

Despite their potential adverse effects on insulin resistance, diuretics have been successfully used in patients with type 1 and type 2 diabetes to enhance the antihypertensive abilities of ACE inhibitors and angiotensin receptor blockers. In particular, with regard to expansion of the ECV in diabetics, diuretics act in a complementary way and contributed to a decline of proteinuria and the retardation of the progressive renal disease. The clear dose dependency of glucose intolerance underlines the need for treatment with the lowest effective doses (Carlsen et al. 1990; Harper et al. 1994), especially in combination with ACE inhibitors. In the JNC VII Report (2003), low-dose diuretics in combination with ACE inhibitors are still recommended in patients with diabetes mellitus.

Hyperlipidaemia

Incidence of hyperlipidaemia during diuretic therapy

Short-term administration of thiazide and loop diuretics dose-dependently increases the concentration of total triglycerides, the major apoproteins (A_1 and A_2), total cholesterol, and low-density lipoprotein-cholesterol (LDL-C) as well as very low-density lipoprotein-cholesterol (VLDL-C), whereas the concentration of high-density lipoprotein-cholesterol (HDL-C) is not altered or is slightly reduced (Greenberg et al. 1984; Pollare et al. 1989). Table 2 summarizes data obtained by Ames (1986).

Whether these effects disappear with chronic use of diuretics is controversial. After long-term therapy cholesterol concentrations have been reported to be close to baseline values (Helgeland et al. 1978; Hypertension Detection and Follow-Up Program Cooperative Group 1979; Amery et al. 1982; Veterans Administration Cooperative Study Group on Antihypertensive Agents 1982b; Greenberg et al. 1984) or slightly elevated even after 9 years of diuretic treatment (Weinberger 1985; Middecke et al. 1987; Skarfors et al. 1989). Cessation of thiazide therapy in a long-term study (5–6 years) decreased total cholesterol (−7 per cent) and LDL-C (−12 per cent) (Holzgreve 1992).

Changes in lipid metabolism caused by various diuretics are not uniform. Indapamide (2.5 mg/day) had no effect on triglycerides or LDL-C (Weidmann et al. 1981), but increased HDL-C (Meyer-Sabellek et al. 1985). Also, K^+-sparing diuretics, as well as their combination with (low doses of) thiazides, are largely neutral with regard to plasma lipids (Amery et al. 1982; Weidmann et al. 1992).

Possible mechanisms

The mechanisms of diuretic-induced dyslipidaemia are still unclear. A causal role of hypokalaemia seems likely, at least by inducing insulin resistance and hyperinsulinaemia, which promotes hypertriglyceridaemia and slightly lowers HDL-C (Ferrari and Weidmann 1990). In addition, volume depletion as well as diuretic-induced stimulation of the sympathic–adrenergic system (Heidland and Hennemann 1969; Weidmann et al. 1983b) may promote lipolysis (Keller et al. 1989), enhance hepatic synthesis of cholesterol, and impair lipoprotein lipase activity as well as the LDL-receptor-mediated catabolism. Also, sex hormones seem to be of importance. Thus postmenopausal but not premenopausal women show lipid changes during diuretic therapy (Boehringer et al. 1982).

Diuretic effects on renal function

Hyperuricaemia

A dose-dependent increase in uricaemia (about 70 μmol/l) has been reported in 50–75 per cent of diuretic-treated hypertensives (Shutske and Allen 1984). However, the prevalence of clinical gouty arthritis is

no more than 2 per cent (Beevers et al. 1971). Nevertheless gout should be a relative contraindication. Diuretic-induced hyperuricaemia occurs through increased urate reabsorption in the proximal tubule, caused by volume contraction and activation of the RAAS. Administration of an ACE inhibitor or the angiotensin II receptor I antagonist losartan prevents or reverses hyperuricaemia (Weinberger 1989; Nakashima et al. 1992).

Renal haemodynamics

Short-term administration of thiazides and carbonic anhydrase inhibitors decreases GFR (Crosley et al. 1960; Heidland et al. 1964), due to ECV depletion and an activation of the TGF system (Tucker et al. 1978). When diuretic-induced volume depletion is severe, a marked decline of renal function can result in a reversible acute renal failure, in particular after coadministration of ACE inhibitors (Hogg and Hillis 1986).

In rats diuretic-induced volume depletion causes a marked azotaemia, due to both reduced GFR and enhanced urea nitrogen production following increased proteolysis (Kamm et al. 1987).

After prolonged antihypertensive therapy with thiazides in essential hypertension, impaired renal function occasionally may return to pretreatment values (van Brummelen 1979; Loon et al. 1989). In patients with severe hypertension, long-term administration of thiazides slowed the decline in GFR (Veterans Administration Cooperative Study Group on Antihypertensive Agents 1972). In diabetic nephropathy either a retarded (Parving et al. 1985) or an accelerated decline of GFR (Walker et al. 1987) has been reported. In the EWPHE trial occasional renal impairment occurred (two cases per 1000 treatment years) in patients receiving the combination of hydrochlorothiazide and triamterene (Amery et al. 1985). In a long-term study (2 years) in hypertensive patients with impaired renal function, administration of hydrochlorothiazide was associated with a decrease in creatinine clearance (−17 per cent), while indapamide therapy was associated with an increase (+28.5 per cent, Madkour et al. 1995). During chronic loop diuretic therapy in patients with renal insufficiency, an increase in blood urea nitrogen has been observed (Dal Canton et al. 1985), probably due to a hypovolaemia-mediated enhanced back diffusion of urea. In idiopathic oedema, long-term frusemide treatment was associated with a dose-dependent decline in GFR and tubule interstitial changes (Shichiri et al. 1984).

Following mannitol treatment of traumatic brain oedema, several cases of acute renal failure were reported and explained by a mannitol intoxication with ECV expansion, cellular desiccation, hyponatraemia, and high osmolar gap (Dorman et al. 1990).

Acute interstitial nephritis associated with diuretic therapy

Thiazides, frusemide, and chlorthalidone can produce an acute interstitial nephritis (Lyons et al. 1973; Fuller et al. 1976), occasionally with granulomas (Ten et al. 1988). In particular, combination with triamterene has been more commonly implicated (Enriquez et al. 1995).

Table 2 Changes in blood lipids after short-term hydrochlorothiazide therapy

	Total triglycerides	Total cholesterol	VLDL-cholesterol	LDL-cholesterol	HDL-cholesterol
Range of increase (%)	4–37	4–30	7–65	7–29	
Mean increase (%)	23	6.5	28	15	0

Data of Ames (1986).

Diuretic-induced acute interstitial nephritis usually resolves after stopping the drug. However, occasionally renal impairment persists (Enriquez *et al.* 1995). The finding of granulomas in drug-induced acute interstitial nephritis may be an indication for treatment with steroids.

Diuretic-induced ototoxicity

Clinical observations

Transient as well as permanent hearing losses and deafness have been described in patients with uraemia after ethacrynic acid therapy (Pillay *et al.* 1969). Also, intravenous administration of high doses of frusemide (0.6–1.0 g/40 min) induced acute hearing losses (up to 30 dB and more), which were reversible within some hours (Heidland and Wigand 1970). In the past, cases of permanent deafness, even after a low oral daily dose of frusemide (200 mg or less) have been reported (Quick and Hoppe 1975; Gallagher and Jones 1979). Loop diuretics are particularly harmful if given together with aminoglycosides.

Pathogenesis of diuretic-induced ototoxicity

Loop diuretics inhibit the $Na^+,2Cl^-,K^+$-cotransporter in the stria vascularis, reduce K^+ secretion into the endolymph (Marcus *et al.* 1987), and cause (similar to aminoglycosides) a depletion of glutathione (Hoffmann *et al.* 1988). The ototoxic potential of equipotent doses of bumetanide and piretanide seems to be less than that of frusemide and ethacrynic acids in dogs, guinea-pigs, cats (Jung and Schön 1979; Brown 1981), and in clinical studies (Tazel 1981).

Diuretic-induced pancreatitis

There are several case reports that frusemide may induce an acute pancreatitis (Buchanan and Cane 1977; Stenvinkel and Alvestrand 1988).

Urinary voiding

In elderly patients with a reduced urinary bladder capacity brisk diuresis can result in an acute urinary retention or urinary incontinence.

Diuretic-induced skin reactions

Cases of chronic photosensitivity as well as skin eruptions resembling subacute lupus erythematosus, attributed to hydrochlorothiazide therapy (Reed *et al.* 1985; Robinson *et al.* 1985), have been reported.

Sexual function

A high incidence of male impotence (23 per cent) was reported in the MRC trial (MRC 1981) after intense doses of bendrofluazide (10 mg/day). In the MRFIT study (Grimm *et al.* 1985), sexual activity was also decreased (25 per cent). However, in the control group the incidence of sexual dysfunction (16 per cent) was rather high. In the multicentre randomized controlled trial (TAIM study, Wassertheil-Smoller *et al.* 1991), chlorthalidone (25 mg/day) adversely affected sexual function in approximately 25 per cent of patients. Interestingly, this problem was prevented in chlorthalidone recipients who followed a weight reduction diet. Disturbances of sexual function are observed not only after thiazides but also after spironolactone administration (Overdiek and Merkus 1986). During indapamide administration, sexual function was reported to remain unchanged.

Diuretics and the risk of renal cell carcinoma

In a careful analysis (of nine case–control studies in 4985 patients) and three cohort investigations (in 805 cases from renal cell carcinoma), from a follow-up (of a total of 1,226,229 patients), an association

between diuretic therapy and renal cell carcinoma has been found. Especially affected were women after a long-term diuretic therapy (at least 15 years) with a high dose of thiazides (50–100 mg) (Grossmann *et al.* 1999). To date it is unknown whether low-dose diuretic therapy, in particular in combination with ACE inhibitors, is associated with a comparable cancer risk. In at least one case–control study with ACE inhibitors, cancer risk was less than in the general population during long-term therapy (Collins *et al.* 1990).

Specific toxicity

Acetazolamide

In elderly patients acetazolamide (250–1000 mg/day) may induce moderate acidaemia (pH 7.21–7.29) in about 35 per cent of the patients and occasionally with a severe form (pH 7.15, Heller *et al.* 1985). In patients with liver cirrhosis, carbonic anhydrase inhibitors may cause hepatic encephalopathy due to increased formation of ammonia. After prolonged use of acetazolamide nephrocalcinosis and apatite stones may develop due to the combined effects of phosphaturia, hypercalciuria (caused by systemic acidosis) and an alkaline urine pH (in which calcium phosphate salts are poorly soluble).

Spironolactone

Long-term therapy with the aldosterone antagonist spironolactone may be complicated by painful gynaecomastia (Overdiek and Merkus 1986), menstrual disturbances (Hutchinson 1985), and male impotence (due to decreased biosynthesis of testosterone, Overdiek and Merkus 1986), following its concomitant binding to androgen and progesterone receptors. In the rat, chronic administration of the aldosterone antagonist canrenoate (but not spironolactone) caused a dose-related increase in myelocytic leukaemia and breast cancer, as well as testicular and thyroid adenomas (Lumb *et al.* 1978). These complications are probably due to one or more metabolites of canrenoate, which are not formed from spironolactone (Oppermann *et al.* 1988). Analysis using specific high-performance liquid chromatography has shown that canrenone accounts for 20–25 per cent of the fluorimetric metabolites of spironolactone in man (Abshagen *et al.* 1990).

The recently developed eplerenone is the first available selective aldosterone blocker without binding affinity to androgen and progesterone receptors.

Triamterene

Triamterene is poorly water-soluble and can precipitate in the urine, resulting in red-brown deposits, red-brown crystals, and casts. Occasionally, triamterene-induced nephrolithiasis has been reported (Ettinger and Weil 1979). In many cases, however, triamterene and its metabolites seem to be simply incorporated into stones as innocent bystanders (Anonymous 1985). A controlled study failed to show an increased incidence of renal calculi in association with triamterene therapy (Jick *et al.* 1982).

Interactions with other drugs

Non-steroidal anti-inflammatory drugs and diuretics: interactions and adverse reactions

NSAIDs interfere with both the pharmacokinetics and pharmacodynamics of loop diuretics. As organic anions, they compete for proximal tubule secretion and shift their dose–response curve to the right (Chennavasin *et al.* 1980, also cf. above). With exception of the selective extrarenal cyclo-oxygenase inhibitor, sulindac, NSAIDs impair the natriuresis induced by loop diuretics (Patak *et al.* 1975) due to both haemodynamic and tubule (at the cells of the thick ascending limb) effects. Prostaglandins reduce Na^+ reabsorption in the thick ascending limb (Higashihara *et al.* 1979) and are also involved in the renal hyper-circulation caused by loop diuretics (Mackay *et al.* 1984). Concerning thiazide diuresis, either no effect (Favre *et al.* 1983) or a reduced response (Kramer *et al.* 1980a) has been reported.

Simultaneous use of NSAIDs and K^+-sparing diuretics may cause acute renal failure in healthy subjects (Anonymous 1986) and in particular in the elderly (Favre *et al.* 1983). In addition, they enhance the risk of hyperkalaemia when GFR is reduced. Control of hypertension by diuretics is impaired by NSAIDs. Indomethacin attenuates the blood-pressure-lowering action of thiazides (Watkins *et al.* 1980), while coadministration of naproxen or piroxicam may even increase the blood pressure (Wong *et al.* 1986).

Angiotensin-converting enzyme inhibition and diuretics

Acute renal failure is not an unusual complication of ACE-inhibitor therapy. The main precipitating factor is Na^+ depletion due to diuretics or dietary Na^+ restriction, whether or not a stenosis of large renal vessels is present (Hricik 1985; Packer *et al.* 1987). In many (but not all) cases, renal function improves after stopping the diuretics and correction of the Na^+ deficit, even if the ACE inhibitor is continued (Bridoux *et al.* 1992). Acute deterioration of renal function may be explained by both a reduced tone of glomerular efferent arterioles (Blythe 1983) and a potentially decreased production of glomerular prostaglandins in the presence of Na^+ depletion (Podjarny *et al.* 1988). Simultaneous administration of ACE inhibitors and K^+-sparing diuretics can cause abrupt and severe hyperkalaemia, occasionally leading to complete heart block (Lakhani 1986).

Allopurinol and diuretics

Adverse reactions to allopurinol (toxic epidermal necrolysis and hypersensitivity syndrome) seem to occur more often in patients taking thiazides (Anonymous 1985; Aubock and Fritsch 1985). Net excretion of the active metabolite oxipurinol (although not of the parent allopurinol) is very sensitive to volume contraction.

Lithium and diuretics

Loop and K^+-sparing diuretics enhance the renal clearance of Li^+ by reducing its tubule reabsorption. On the other hand, they lower its renal clearance due to volume contraction (Petersen *et al.* 1974; Singer 1981; Greger 1990). The net effect may cause Li^+ toxicity; serum Li^+ concentration should be closely monitored when diuretic therapy is commenced.

Cardiac glycosides and diuretics

K^+-losing diuretics enhance the risk of cardiac arrhythmias in patients on glycoside therapy. The most probable explanation is their competition with glycosides for the same binding site on Na^+,K^+-ATPase. Hence, hypokalaemia shifts the dose response to glycosides to the left (Norgaard *et al.* 1981).

Antibiotics and diuretics

The ototoxic effect of aminoglycosides (gentamicin, kanamycin) and the nephrotoxic potential of the first- and second-generation cephalosporins may be enhanced by loop diuretics (Brummett *et al.* 1981).

References

Abel, R. M. *et al.* (1976). Acute postoperative renal failure in cardiac surgical patients. *Journal of Surgical Research* **20**, 341–348.

Abshagen, U., Besenfelder, E., Endele, R., Koch, K., and Neubert, B. (1990). Kinetics of canrenone after single and multiple doses of spironolactone. *European Journal of Clinical Pharmacology* **16**, 255–262.

Agre, P. *et al.* (1993). Aquaporin CHIP: the archetypal molecular water channel. *American Journal of Physiology* **265**, F463–F476.

Ahlstrand, C., Tiselius, H. G., Larsson, L., and Hellgren, E. (1984). Clinical experience with long-term bendroflumethiazide treatment in calcium oxalate stone formers. *British Journal of Urology* **56**, 255–262.

Akbarpour, F., Afrasiabi, A., and Vaziri, N. D. (1985). Severe hyperkalemia caused by indomethacin and potassium supplementation. *Southern Medical Journal* **78**, 756–757.

Amery, A. *et al.* (1982). Influence of antihypertensive therapy on serum cholesterol in elderly hypertensive patients. *Acta Cardiologica* **37**, 235–244.

Amery, A. *et al.* (1985). Mortality and morbidity results from the European Working Party on High Blood Pressure in the Elderly Trial. *Lancet* i, 1349–1354.

Ames, R. P. (1986). The effect of antihypertensive drugs on serum lipids and lipoproteins. I. Diuretics. *Drugs* **32**, 260–278.

Anderson, J. V., Woodruff, P. W., and Bloom, S. R. (1988). The effect of treatment of congestive heart failure on plasma atrial natriuretic peptide concentration: a longitudinal study. *British Heart Journal* **59**, 207–211.

Anderson, R. J., Linas, S. L., Burns, S., Henrichs, L., Miller, T. R., Gabow, P. A., and Schrier, R. W. (1977). Nonoliguric acute renal failure. *New England Journal of Medicine* **296**, 1134–1138.

Andreucci, V. E. *et al.* (1990). Efficacy of IV torasemide in the treatment of acute and chronic high grade renal failure. *Progress in Pharmacology and Clinical Pharmacology* **8** (1), 229–238.

Anonymous (1985). Treatment of gout. *Drug and Therapeutics Bulletin* **23**, 47–48.

Anonymous (1986). Triamterene and the kidney. *Lancet* **1**, 424.

Araoye, M. A. *et al.* (1978). Furosemide compared with hydrochlorothiazide. Long-term treatment of hypertension. *Journal of the American Medical Association* **240**, 1863–1866.

Arieff, A. I. (1993). Management of hyponatremia. *British Medical Journal* **307**, 305–306.

Ashraf, N., Locksley, R., and Arieff, A. I. (1981). Thiazide-induced hyponatremia associated with death or neurologic damage in outpatients. *American Journal of Medicine* **70**, 1163–1168.

Aubock, J. and Fritsch, P. (1985). Asymptomatic hyperuricaemia and allopurinol induced toxic epidermal necrolysis. *British Medical Journal* **290**, 1969.

Ayus, J. C. (1986). Diuretic-induced hyponatremia. *Archives of Internal Medicine* **146**, 1295–1296.

Baggio, B., Gambaro, G., Marcini, F., Cicerello, E., Tenconi, R., Clementi, M., and Borsatti, A. (1986). An inheritable anomaly of red-cell oxalate transport in 'primary' calcium nephrolithiasis correctable with diuretics. *New England Journal of Medicine* **314**, 599–604.

Baglin, A., Boulard, J. C., Hanslik, T., and Prinseau, J. (1995). Metabolic adverse reactions to diuretics. Clinical relevance to elderly patients. *Drug Safety* **12** (3), 161–167.

Batlle, C., Arruda, J. A. L., and Kurtzman, N. A. (1981). Hyperkalemic distal renal tubular acidosis associated with obstructive uropathy. *New England Journal of Medicine* **304**, 373–380.

Batlle, D., Gavira, M., Grupp, M., Arradu, J. A. L., Wynn, J., and Kurtzman, N. A. (1982). Distal nephron function in patients receiving chronic lithium therapy. *Kidney International* **21**, 477–485.

Baumgart, P., Walger, P., van Eiff, M., and Achhammer, I. (1990). Long-term efficacy and tolerance of torasemide in hypertension. *Progress in Pharmacology and Clinical Pharmacology* **8**, 169–181.

Beall, A. C., Holman, M. R., Morris, G. C., and De Bakey, M. (1963). Mannitol induced osmotic diuresis during vascular surgery. Renal haemodynamic effects. *Archives of Surgery* **86**, 34–42.

Beevers, D. G., Hamilton, M., and Harpur, J. E. (1971). The long-term, treatment of hypertension with thiazide diuretics. *Postgraduate Medical Journal* **47**, 639–643.

Beretta-Piccoli, C., Weidmann, P., De Chatel, R., and Reubi, F. (1976). Hypertension associated with early stage kidney disease: complementary roles of circulating renin, the body sodium, volume state and duration of hypertension. *American Journal of Medicine* **61**, 739–747.

Berger, B. E. and Warnock, D. G. Mechanism of action and clinical use of diuretics. In *The Kidney* 3rd edn. (ed. B. M. Brenner and F. C. Rector), pp. 433–455. Philadelphia: Saunders, 1986.

Bernardi, M., Laffi, G., Salvagnini, M., Azzena, G., Bonato, S., Marra, F., Trevisani, F., Gasbarrini, G., Naccarato, R., and Gentilini, P. (1993). Efficacy and safety of the stepped care medical treatment of ascites in liver cirrhosis: a randomized controlled clinical trial comparing two diets with different sodium content. *Liver* **13** (3), 156–162.

Bernardi, M., Servadei, D., Trevisani, F., Rusticali, A. G., and Gasbarrini, G. (1985). Importance of plasma aldosterone concentration on the natriuretic effect of spironolactone in patients with liver cirrhosis and ascites. *Digestion* **31**, 189–193.

Better, O. S. and Stein, J. H. (1990). Early management of shock and prophylaxis of acute renal failure in traumatic rhabdomyolysis. *New England Journal of Medicine* **322**, 825–828.

Better, O. S., Rubinstein, I., Winaver, J. M., and Knochel, J. P. (1997). Mannitol therapy revisited (1940–1997). *Kidney International* **52**, 886–894.

Bianco, S., Pieroni, M. G., Refini, R. M., Rottoli, L., and Sostini, P. (1989). Protective effect of inhaled furosemide on allergen-induced early and late asthmatic reactions. *New England Journal of Medicine* **321**, 1069–1073.

Bianco, S., Vaghi, A., Robuschi, M., and Pasargiklian, M. (1988). Prevention of exercise-induced bronchoconstriction by inhaled furosemide. *Lancet* **ii**, 252–255.

Bichet, D. G., Van Putten, V. J., and Schrier, R. W. (1982). Potential role of increased sympathetic activity in impaired sodium and water excretion in cirrhotic patients. *New England Journal of Medicine* **307**, 1552–1557.

Biddle, T. L. and Yu, P. N. (1979). Effect of furosemide on hemodynamics and lung water in acute pulmonary edema secondary to myocardial infarction. *American Journal of Cardiology* **43**, 86–90.

Biemesderfer, D. *et al.* (1993). NHE3: a Na^+/H^+ exchanger isoform of renal brush border. *American Journal of Physiology* **265**, F736–F742.

Bittar, A. E. *et al.* (1989). Hyperparathyroidism, hypertension and loop diuretic medication in renal transplant patients. *Nephrology, Dialysis, Transplantation* **4**, 740–744.

Bleich, M., Schlatter, E., and Greger, R. (1990). The luminal K channel of the thick ascending limb of Henle's loop. *Pflügers Archiv* **415**, 449–460.

Blood Pressure Lowering Treatment Trialists' Collaboration (2003). Effects of different blood-pressure-lowering regimens on major cardiovascular events: results of prospectively-designed overviews of randomised trials. *Lancet* **362**, 1527–1534.

Blythe, W. B. (1983). Captopril and renal autoregulations. *New England Journal of Medicine* **308**, 390–391.

Boehringer, K., Weidmann, P., Mordasini, R., Schiffl, H., Bachmann, C., and Risen, U. (1982). Menopause-dependant plasma lipoprotein alterations in diuretic-treated women. *Annals of Internal Medicine* **97**, 206–209.

Bourland, W. A., Day, D. K., and Williamson, H. E. (1977). The role of the kidney in the early nondiuretic action of furosemide to reduce elevated left atrial pressure in the hypervolemic dog. *Journal of Pharmacology and Experimental Therapeutics* **201**, 221–229.

Braitsch, R., Lohrmann, E., and Greger, R. Effect of probenecid on loop diuretic induced saluresis and diuresis. In *Diuretics III, Chemistry,*

Pharmacology, and Clinical Applications (ed. J. Puschett), pp. 137–139. New York: Elsevier, 1990.

Brater, D. C. (1994). Pharmacokinetics of loop diuretics in congestive heart failure. *British Heart Journal* **72** (Suppl.), 40–43.

Brater, D. C., Anderson, S. A., and Brown-Cartwright, D. (1986). Response to furosemide in chronic renal insufficiency. Rationale for limited doses. *Clinical Pharmacology and Therapeutics* **40**, 134–139.

Brater, D. C., Day, B., Burdette, A., and Anderson, S. (1984). Bumetanide and furosemide in heart failure. *Kidney International* **26**, 183–189.

Brezis, M., Rosen, S., Silva, P., and Epstein, F. H. (1984a). Selective vulnerability of the thick ascending limb to anoxia in the isolated perfused kidney. *Journal of Clinical Investigation* **73**, 182–189.

Brezis, M., Rosen, S., Silva, P., and Epstein, F. H. (1984b). Renal ischaemia: a new perspective. *Kidney International* **26**, 375–383.

Brezis, M. *et al.* (1985). Disparate mechanisms for hypoxic cell injury in different nephron segments. Studies in the isolated perfused rat kidney. *Journal of Clinical Investigation* **76**, 1796–1806.

Bricker, N. S. *et al.* (1978). 'Magnification phenomenon' in chronic renal disease. *New England Journal of Medicine* **299**, 1287–1293.

Bridoux, F. *et al.* (1992). Acute renal failure after the use of angiotensin-converting enzyme inhibitors in patients without renal artery stenosis. *Nephrology, Dialysis, Transplantation* **7**, 100–104.

Brown, C. B., Ogg, C. S., and Cameron, J. S. (1986). High dose furosemide in acute renal failure: a controlled trial. *Clinical Nephrology* **15**, 90–96.

Brown, E. A. *et al.* (1982). Evidence that some mechanism other than the renin system causes sodium retention in nephrotic syndrome. *Lancet* **2**, 1237–1240.

Brown, R. D. (1981). Comparisons of the acute effects of i.v. furosemide and bumetanide on the cochlear action potential (N1) and on the AC cochlear poten 6 kHz in cats, dogs and the guinea pig. *Scandinavian Audiology* **14** (Suppl.), 71–84.

Brown, N. J. (2003). Eplerenone cardiovascular protection. *Circulation* **107**, 2512–2518.

Brummett, R. E., Bendrick, T., and Himes, D. (1981). Comparative ototoxicity of bumetanide and furosemide when used in combination with kanamycin. *Journal of Clinical Pharmacology* **21**, 628–636.

Brunner, G. *et al.* (1988). Comparison of diuretic effects and pharmacokinetics of torasemide and furosemide after a single dose in patients with hydropically decompensated cirrhosis of the liver. *Drug Research* **38**, 176–179.

Brunner, H. R., Gavras, H., and Waeber, B. (1980). Enhancement by diuretics of the antihypertensive action of long-term angiotensin converting enzyme blockade. *Clinical and Experimental Hypertension* **2**, 639–657.

Brunner, H. R. *et al.* (1990). Treating in individual hypertensive patients: considerations on dose, sequential monotherapy and drug combination. *Journal of Hypertension* **8**, 3–11.

Buchanan, N. and Cane, R. D. (1977). Frusemide-induced pancreatitis. *British Medical Journal* **2**, 1417.

Bühler, F. R., Bolli, P., Kiowski, W., and Müller, F. B. (1985). Relevance of the renin–angiotensin–aldosterone system for effectiveness and adversity of antihypertensive treatment. *Progress in Pharmacology* **6**, 33–44.

Burckhardt, G. and Greger, R. Principles of electrolyte transport across plasma membranes of renal tubular cells. In *Handbook of Physiology Section on Renal Physiology* (ed. E. E. Windhager), pp. 639–657. Rockville: American Physiological Society, 1992.

Burke, T. J., Cronin, R. E., Duchin, K. L., Peterson, R. L., and Schrier, R. W. (1980). Ischaemia and tubule obstruction during acute renal failure in dogs—mannitol protection. *American Journal of Physiology* **238**, F305–F314.

Burnier, M. and Brunner, H. R. (1992). Neurohormonal consequences of diuretics in different cardiovascular syndromes. *European Heart Journal* **13** (Suppl. G), 28–33.

Busch, A. E. *et al.* (1996). Blockade of epithelial Na^+ channels by triamterenes—underlying mechanisms and molecular basis. *Pflügers Archiv* **432**, 760–766.

Bushinsky, D. A., Favus, M. J., and Coe, F. L. (1984). Mechanism of chronic hypocalciuria with chlorthalidone: reduced calcium absorption. *American Journal of Physiology* **247**, F746–F752.

Calder, J. A., Schachter, M., and Sever, P. S. (1994). Potassium channel opening properties of thiazide diuretics in isolated guinea pig resistance arteries. *Journal of Cardiovascular Pharmacology* **24**, 158–164.

Campbell, D. B., Lowe, S., Taylor, D., Turner, P., and Walsh, N. (1985). A fresh approach to the evaluation of antihypertensive agents. *Hypertension* **7** (Suppl. II), 143–151.

Canessa, C. M., Schild, L., Buell, G., Thoreus, B., Gautschi, I., Nonsberger, J. D., and Rossier, B. C. (1994). Amiloride-sensitive epithelial Na^+ channel is made of three homologous subunits. *Nature* **367**, 463–467.

Cantarovich, F., Galli, C., and Benedetti, L. (1973). High dose furosemide in established acute renal failure. *British Medical Journal* **4**, 449–450.

Capasso, G., Pica, A., Saviano, C., Rizzo, M., Mascolo, N., and DeSanto, N. (1997). Clinical complications of diuretic therapy. *Kidney International* **51** (Suppl. 59), S16–S20.

Caralis, P. C., Materson, B. J., and Perez-Stable, E. (1984). Potassium and diuretic-induced ventricular arrhythmias in ambulatory hypertensive patients. *Mineral Electrolyte Metabolism* **10**, 148–154.

Carlsen, J. E., Kober, L., Torp-Pedersen, C., and Johannsen, P. (1990). Relation between dose of bendrofluazide, antihypertensive effect, and adverse biochemical effects. *British Medical Journal* **300**, 975–978.

Cedidi, C., Meyer, M., and Kuse, E. R. (1994). Urodilatin: a new approach for the treatment of therapy-resistant acute renal failure after liver transplantation. *European Journal of Clinical Investigation* **24** (9), 632–639.

Channer, K. S., McLean, K. A., Lawson-Matthew, P., and Richardson, M. (1994). Combination diuretic treatment in severe heart failure: a randomised controlled trial. *British Heart Journal* **71**, 146–150.

Chen, Z. F. and Vaughn, D. J. (1990). Effects of diuretic treatment and of dietary sodium on renal binding of 3H-metolazone. *Journal of the American Society of Nephrology* **1**, 91–98.

Chennavasin, P., Seiwell, R., and Brater, D. C. (1980). Pharmacokinetic-dynamic analysis of the indomethacin–furosemide interaction in man. *Journal of Pharmacology and Experimental Therapeutics* **215**, 77–81.

Coe, F. L. (1981). Prevention of kidney stones. *American Journal of Medicine* **71**, 514–516.

Coe, F. L., Parks, J. H., Bushinsk, D. A., Langman, C. B., and Favus, M. J. (1988). Chlorthalidone promotes mineral retention in patients with idiopathic hypercalciuria. *Kidney International* **33**, 1140–1146.

Collins, R. et al. (1990). Blood pressure, stroke, and coronary heart disease. Part 2, short-term reductions in blood pressure: overview of randomized drug trials in their epidemiology context. *Lancet* **335**, 827–838.

Condon, J. P., Nassim, J. R., Dent, C. F., Hilb, A., and Stainthorpe, E. M. (1978). Possible prevention of treatment of steroid-induced osteoporosis. *Postgraduate Medical Journal* **54**, 249–252.

Conger, J. D. (1977). Intrarenal dynamics in the pathogenesis and prevention of acute urate nephropathy. *Journal of Clinical Investigation* **59**, 786.

Conger, J. D., Falk, S. A., Yuan, B. H., and Schrier, R. W. (1989). Atrial natriuretic peptide and dopamine in a rat model of ischemic acute renal failure. *Kidney International* **35**, 1126–1132.

Conte, G., Bellizzi, V., Cianciaruso, B., Minutolo, R., Fuiano, G., and De Nicola, L. (1997). Physiologic role and diuretic efficacy of atrial natriuretic peptide in health and chronic renal disease. *Kidney International* **51** (Suppl. 59), S28–S32.

Costanzo, L. S. and Windhager, E. E. (1978). Calcium and sodium transport by the distal convoluted tubule of the rat. *American Journal of Physiology* **235**, F492–F506.

Crawford, J. D., Kennedy, G. C., and Hill, L. E. (1960). Clinical results of treatment of diabetes insipidus with drugs of the chlorothiazide series. *New England Journal of Medicine* **262**, 737–743.

Crosley, A. P., Jr., Cullen, R. C., White, D., Fresman, J. F., Castillo, C. A., and Rowe, G. G. (1960). Studies on the mechanism of action of chlorothiazide in cardiac and renal diseases. I. Acute effects on renal and systemic hemodynamics and metabolism. *Journal of Laboratory and Clinical Medicine* **55**, 182–190.

Cruz, J., Minoja, G., and Okuchis, K. (2001). The novel clinical benefits of emergency megadose mannitol for rapidly deteriorating patients with bilaterally unreactive pupils: a randomised trial. *Neurosurgery* **49**, 864–871.

Curtis, J. et al. (1972). Chlorothalidone induced hyperosmolar hyperglycemic, nonketotic coma. *Journal of the American Medical Association* **220**, 1592–1593.

Dahlöf, N. et al. (1991). Morbidity and mortality in the Swedish Trial in Old Patients with Hypertension (STOP-Hypertension). *Lancet* **338**, 1281–1285.

Dal Canton, A., Fuiaho, G., Conte, G., Terribile, M., Sabbatini, M., Cianciaruso, B., and Andreucci, V. E. (1985). Mechanism of increased plasma urea after diuretic therapy in uremic patients. *Clinical Science* **68**, 255–261.

Daul, A., Graben, N., and Bock, K. D. (1987). Neuromyeloenzephalopathie nach hochdosierter Muzolimintherapie bei Dialysepatienten. *Münchener Medizinische Wochenschrift* **129**, 542–543.

Davies, D. L. and Fraser, R. (1993). Do diuretics cause magnesium deficiency? *British Journal of Clinical Pharmacology* **36**, 1–10.

Davison, A. M., Lambie, A. T., Verth, A. H., and Cash, J. D. (1974). Salt-poor human albumin in management of nephrotic syndrome. *British Medical Journal* **1**, 481–484.

Decaux, G., Waterlot, Y., Genette, F., and Mockel, J. (1981). Treatment of the syndrome of inappropriate secretion of antidiuretic hormone with furosemide. *New England Journal of Medicine* **304**, 329–330.

De Fronzo, R. A. (1980). Hyperkalemia and hyporeninemic hypoaldosteronism. *Kidney International* **17**, 118–134.

Delyan, J. A., Rocha, R., Cook, C. S., Tobert, D. S., Levin, S., Roniker, R., Workman, D. L., Sing, Y. I., and Whelihan, B. (2000). Eplerenone, a selective aldosterone receptor antagonist (SARA). *Cardiovascular Drug Review* **19**, 185–200.

De Marchi, S. and Cecchin, E. (1990). Severe metabolic acidosis and disturbances of calcium metabolism induced by acetazolamide in patients on haemodialysis. *Clinical Science* **78**, 295–302.

DiBona, G. F., Herman, P. J., and Sawin, L. L. (1988). Neural control of renal function in edema forming states. *American Journal of Physiology* **254**, R1017–R1024.

Dikshit, K., Vyden, J. K., Forrester, J. S., Chatterjee, K., Prakash, R., and Swan, H. J. C. (1973). Renal and extra-renal hemodynamic effects of furosemide in congestive heart failure after myocardial infarction. *New England Journal of Medicine* **288**, 1087–1090.

Dorhout Mees, E. J. et al. (1979). Observations on edema formation in the nephrotic syndrome in adults with minimal lesions. *American Journal of Medicine* **67**, 378–384.

Dorman, H. R., Sondheimer, J. H., and Cadnapaphornchai, P. (1990). Mannitol-induced acute renal failure. *Medicine* **69** (3), 153–159.

Dormans, T. P. L., Huige, R. M. C., and Gerlag, P. G. G. (1996). Chronic intermittent haemofiltration and haemodialysis in end stage chronic heart failure with oedema refractory to high dose frusemide. *Heart* **75**, 349–351.

Dornhorst, A., Powell, S. H., and Pensky, J. (1985). Aggravation by propranolol of hyperglycemic effect of hydrochlorothiazide in type II diabetics without alteration of insulin secretion. *Lancet* **i**, 687–690.

Düsing, R. and Piesche, L. (1990). Second-line therapy of congestive heart failure with torasemide. *Progress in Pharmacology and Clinical Pharmacology* **8**, 105–120.

Dworkin, L. D. et al. (1990). Effects of nifedipine and enalapril on glomerular injury in rats with deoxycorticosterone-salt hypertension. *American Journal of Physiology* **259**, F598–F604.

Dykner, T. and Wester, P. O. (1979). Ventricular extrasystoles and intracellular electrolytes before and after potassium and magnesium infusion in hypokalemic patients on diuretic treatment. *American Heart Journal* **97**, 12–18.

Dykner, T. and Wester, P. O. (1984). Intracellular magnesium loss after diuretic administration. *Drugs* 28 (Suppl. 1), 161–166.

Dzurik, R., Fedellsova, V., Dzurikova, V., and Spustova, V. (1993). Diuretics in the treatment of hypertension. *Vnitrni Lekarstvi* 39, 909–915.

Ellison, D. H., Velázquez, H., and Wright, F. S. (1989). Adaptation of the distal convoluted tubule of the rat: structural and functional effects of dietary salt intake and chronic diuretic infusion. *Journal of Clinical Investigation* 83, 113–126.

Elmgreen, J. *et al.* (1980). Elevated parathyroid hormone concentration during treatment with high ceiling diuretics. *European Journal of Clinical Pharmacology* 18, 363–364.

Emsley, R. A. and Gledhill, R. F. (1984). Thiazides, compulsive water drinking and hyponatraemic encephalopathy. *Journal of Neurology, Neurosurgery and Psychiatry* 47, 886–887.

Eneas, J. F., Schoenfeld, P. Y., and Humphreys, M. H. (1979). The effect of infusion of mannitol-sodium bicarbonate on the clinical course of myoglobinuria. *Archives of Internal Medicine* 139, 801–805.

Enriquez, R. *et al.* (1995). Granulomatous interstitial nephritis associated with hydrochlorothiazide/amiloride. *American Journal of Nephrology* 15, 270–273.

Epstein, F. H. (1982). Underfilling versus overflow in hepatic ascites. *New England Journal of Medicine* 307, 1577–1579.

Epstein, M. (1978). Renal effects of head-out water immersion in man: implications for an understanding of volume homeostasis. *Physiological Review* 58, 529–581.

Epstein, M. Therapy in renal disorders in liver disease. In *Therapy of Renal Diseases and Related Disorders* (ed. W. N. Suki and S. G. Massry), pp. 335–346. Boston: Martinus Nijhoff Publishers, 1984.

Epstein, M., Levinson, R., Sancho, J., Haber, E., and Re, R. (1977). Characterization of the renin–aldosterone system in decompensated cirrhosis. *Circulation Research* 41, 818–829.

Epstein, M., Schneider, N. S., and Befeler, B. (1975). Effect of intrarenal furosemide on renal function and intrarenal hemodynamics in acute renal failure. *American Journal of Medicine* 58, 510–516.

Erne, P., Bolli, P., Bürgisser, E., and Bühler, F. R. (1984). Correlation of platelet calcium with blood pressure. Effect of antihypertensive therapy. *New England Journal of Medicine* 310, 1084–1088.

Estevez, R., Boettger, T., Stein, V., Birkenhager, R., Otto, E., Hildebrandt, F., and Jentsch, T. J. (2001). Barttin is a Cl$^-$ channel beta-subunit crucial for renal Cl$^-$ reabsorption and inner ear K$^+$ secretion. *Nature* 414, 558–561.

Ettinger, B. and Weil, E. (1979). Triamterene-induced nephrolithiasis. *Annals of Internal Medicine* 91, 745–746.

Fanestil, D. D. (1988). Mechanism of action of aldosterone blockers. *Seminars in Nephrology* 8, 249–263.

Fanestil, D. D., Tran, J. M., Vaughn, D. A., Maciejewski, A. R., and Beaumont, K. Investigations of the metazolone receptor. In *Diuretics III, Chemistry, Pharmacology, and Clinical Applications* (ed. J. Puschett), pp. 195–204. New York: Elsevier, 1990.

Fauchald, P., Noddeland, H., and Norseth, J. (1985). An evaluation of ultrafiltration as treatment of diuretic-resistant oedema in nephrotic syndrome. *Acta Medica Scandinavica* 17, 127–131.

Favre, L., Glasson, P. H., Riondel, A., and Vallotton, M. B. (1983). Interaction of diuretics and non-steroidal anti-inflammatory drugs in man. *Clinical Science* 64, 407–415.

Feely, J. and O'Byrne, S. (1990). Effects of drugs on glucose tolerance in non-insulin-dependent diabetics (part I). *Drugs* 40, 6–18.

Ferrari, P. and Weidmann, P. (1990). Insulin sensitivity in humans: alterations during drug administration and in essential hypertension. *Mineral Electrolyte Metabolism* 16, 16–24.

Fiehring, H. and Achhammer, I. (1990). Influence of 10 mg torasemide IV and 20 mg furosemide i.v. on the intracardiac pressures in patients with heart failure at rest and during exercise. *Progress in Pharmacology and Clinical Pharmacology* 8 (1), 97–104.

Fliser, D., Schröter, M., Neubeck, M., and Ritz, E. (1994). Coadministration of thiazides increases the efficacy of loop diuretics even in patients with advanced renal failure. *Kidney International* 46, 482–488.

Flores, J., DiBona, D. R., Beck, C. H., and Leaf, A. (1972). The role of cell swelling in ischemic renal damage and the protective effect of hypertonic solute. *Journal of Clinical Investigation* 51, 118–126.

Francis, G. S., Siegel, R. M., Goldsmith, S. R., Olivari, M. T., Levine, B., and Cohn, J. N. (1985). Acute vasoconstrictor response to intravenous furosemide in patients with chronic congestive heart failure. *Annals of Internal Medicine* 103, 1–6.

Freeman, B. A. and Crapo, J. D. (1982). Free radicals and tissue injury. *Laboratory Investigation* 47, 412–426.

Friedman, E., Shadel, M., Halkin, H., and Farfel, Z. (1989). Thiazide-induced hyponatraemia. Reproducibility by single dose rechallenge and an analysis of pathogenesis. *Internal Medicine* 110, 24–30.

Friedman, P. A. and Gesek, F. A. (1993). Calcium transport in renal epithelial cells. *American Journal of Physiology* 264, F181–F198.

Frindt, G. and Palmer, L. G. (1987). Ca-activated K channels in apical membrane of mammalian CCT, and their role in K secretion. *American Journal of Physiology* 252, F458–F467.

Frömter, E. and Gessner, K. (1974). Free-flow potential profile along the rat kidney proximal tubule. *Pflügers Archiv* 351, 69–83.

Frumann, B. L. (1981). Impairment of glucose tolerance produced by diuretics and other drugs. *Pharmacology and Therapeutics* 12, 613–649.

Fujisawa, G., Ishikawa, S., Tsuboi, Y., Okada, K., and Saito, T. (1993). Therapeutic efficacy of non-peptide ADH antagonist OPC-31260 in SIADH rats. *Kidney International* 44, 19–23.

Fujita, N., Ishikawa, S. E., Sasaki, S., Fujisawa, G., Fushimi, K., Marumo, F., and Saito, T. (1995). Role of water channel AQP-CD in water retention in SIADH and cirrhotic rats. *American Journal of Physiology* 269, F926–F931.

Fuller, T. J., Barcenas, C. G., and White, M. G. (1976). Diuretic-induced interstitial nephritis. Occurrence in a patient with membranous glomerulonephritis. *Journal of the American Medical Association* 235, 1998–1999.

Gabazda, G. J. and Hall, P. W. (1966). Relation of potassium depletion to renal ammonium metabolism and hepatic coma. *Medicine* 45, 481–490.

Gabow, P. A., Anderson, R. J., Potts, D. E., and Schrier, R. W. (1978). Acid–base disturbances in the salicylate-intoxicated adult. *Archives of Internal Medicine* 138, 1481–1493.

Gallagher, K. L. and Jones, J. K. (1979). Furosemide induced ototoxicity. *Annals of Internal Medicine* 91, 744–745.

Gamba, G. *et al.* (1993). Primary structure and functional expression of a cDNA encoding the thiazide-sensitive, electroneutral sodium–chloride cotransporter. *Proceedings of the National Academy of Sciences USA* 90, 2749–2753.

Gamba, G. *et al.* (1994). Molecular cloning, primary structure, and characterization of two members of the mammalian electroneutral sodium–(potassium)–chloride cotransporter family expressed in kidney. *Journal of Biological Chemistry* 269, 17713–17722.

Gatta, A. *et al.* (1991). A pathophysiological interpretation of unresponsiveness to spironolactone in a stepped-care approach to the diuretic treatment of ascites in nonazotemic cirrhotic patients. *Hepatology* 14, 231–236.

Gavras, H. *et al.* (1981). Role of reactive hyperreninemia in blood pressure changes induced by sodium depletion in patients with refractory hypertension. *Hypertension* 3, 441–447.

Geck, P. and Heinz, E. (1986). The Na–K–2Cl cotransport system. *Journal of Membrane Biology* 91, 97–105.

Geers, A. B. *et al.* (1984). Plasma and blood volumes in patients with the nephrotic syndrome. *Nephron* 38, 170–173.

Gekle, M., Drumm, K., Mildenberger, S., Freudinger, R., Gassner, B., and Silbernagl, S. (1999). Inhibition of Na$^+$–H$^+$ exchange impairs receptor-mediated albumin endocytosis in renal proximal tubule-derived epithelial cells from opossum. *Journal of Physiology* 520, 709–721.

Gentilini, P. *et al.* (1994). Pathogenesis and treatment of ascites in hepatic cirrhosis. *Cardiology* 84 (Suppl. 2), 68–79.

Gerbes, A. L. (1993). Medical treatment of ascites in cirrhosis. *Journal of Hepatology* **17** (Suppl. 2), S4–S9.

Gerbes, A. L., Arendt, R. M., Ritter, D., Jungst, D., Zahringer, J., and Paumgartner, G. (1985). Plasma atrial natriuretic factor in patients with cirrhosis. *New England Journal of Medicine* **313**, 1609–1610.

Gianello, P. *et al.* (1989). Evidence that atrial natriuretic factor is the humoral factor by which volume loading or mannitol infusion produces an improved renal function after acute ischemia. *Transplantation* **48**, 9–14.

Gögelein, H. and Greger, R. (1986). Na selective channels in the apical membrane of rabbit late proximal tubules (pars recta). *Pflügers Archiv* **406**, 198–203.

Gonzalez, C. B., Figueroa, C. D., Reyes, C. E., Caorsi, C. E., Troncoso, S., and Menzel, D. (1997). Immunolocalization of V1 vasopressin receptors in the rat kidney using anti-receptor antibodies. *Kidney International* **52**, 1206–1215.

Götz, R. *et al.* (1989). Acute renal failure in the intensive care unit: are there benefits of atrial natriuretic factor in dopamine/furosemide resistant acute renal failure? *Kidney International* **35**, 282 (abstract).

Graziani, G. *et al.* (1984). Dopamine and furosemide in oliguric acute renal failure. *Nephron* **37**, 39–42.

Green, T. P. and Mirkin, B. L. (1980). Resistance of proteinuric rats to furosemide: urinary drug protein binding as a determinant of drug effect. *Life Science* **26**, 623–630.

Greenberg, A. and Puschett, B. Idiopathic edema. In *Therapy of Renal Diseases and Related Disorders* 2nd edn. (ed. W. N. Suki and S. G. Massry), pp. 27–44. Boston: Kluwer Academic Publishers, 1991.

Greenberg, G., Brennan, P. J., and Miall, W. E. (1984). Effects of diuretic and beta-blocker therapy in the Medical Research Council Trial (MRC). *American Journal of Medicine* **76**, 45–51.

Greene, M. K., Kerr, A. M., McIntosh, I. B., and Prescott, R. J. (1981). Acetazolamide in prevention of acute mountain sickness: a double-blind controlled cross-over study. *British Medical Journal* **283**, 811–818.

Greger, R. (1985a). Ion transport mechanisms in thick ascending limb of Henle's loop of mammalian nephron. *Physiological Reviews* **65**, 760–797.

Greger, R. (1985b). Wirkung von Schleifendiuretika auf zellulärer Ebene. *Nieren- und Hochdruckkrankheiten* **14**, 217–220.

Greger, R. (1987). Pathophysiologie der renalen Ischämie. *Zeitschrift für Kardiologie* **76**, 81–86.

Greger, R. (1988). Chloride transport in thick ascending limb, distal convolution, and collecting duct. *Annual Review of Physiology* **50**, 111–122.

Greger, R. (1990). Possible sites of lithium transport in the nephron. *Kidney International* **37**, S26–S30.

Greger, R. and Schlatter, E. (1981). Presence of luminal K, a prerequisite for active NaCl transport in the thick ascending limb of Henle's loop of rabbit kidney. *Pflügers Archiv* **392**, 92–94.

Greger, R. and Schlatter, E. (1983). Cellular mechanism of the action of loop diuretics on the thick ascending limb of Henle's loop. *Klinische Wochenschrift* **61**, 1019–1027.

Greger, R. and Wangemann, Ph. (1987). Loop diuretics. *Renal Physiology* **10**, 174–183.

Greger, R., Bleich, M., and Schlatter, E. (1990). Ion channels in the thick ascending limb of Henle's loop. *Renal Physiology and Biochemistry* **13**, 37–50.

Greven, J. and Klein, H. (1976). Renal effects of furosemide in glycerol-induced acute renal failure of the rat. *Pflügers Archiv* **365**, 81–87.

Griffing, G. T., Sindler, B. H., Areccgia, S. A., and Melby, J. C. (1983). Reversal of diuretic-induced secondary hyperaldosteronism and hypokalaemia by Enalapril (MK421): a new angiotensin converting enzyme inhibitor. *Metabolism: Clinical and Experimental* **32**, 711–716.

Grimm, R. H., Cohen, J. D., McFate Smith, W., Falvo-Gerard, L., and Neaton, J. D. (1985). Hypertension management in the multiple risk factor intervention trial (MRFIT) (1985). *Archives of Internal Medicine* **145**, 1191.

Gross, P. *et al.* (1988). Role of diuretics, hormonal derangements, and clinical setting of hyponatremia in medical patients. *Klinische Wochenschrift* **66**, 662–669.

Grossmann, E., Messerli, F. H., and Goldbourt, U. (1999). Does diuretic therapy increase the risk of renal cell carcinoma in women? *American Journal of Cardiology* **83**, 1090–1093.

Grünfeld, C. and Chappell, D. A. (1983). Hypokalemia and diabetes mellitus. *American Journal of Medicine* **75**, 553–554.

Györy, A. Z. and Edwards, K. D. C. (1971). Effect of mersalyl, ethacrynic acid and sodium sulfate infusion on urinary acidification in hereditary renal tubular acidosis. *Medical Journal of Australia* **2**, 940–945.

Haddy, F. J. (1975). Potassium and blood vessels. *Life Sciences* **16**, 1489–1498.

Haerer, W. *et al.* (1990). Acute and chronic effects of a diuretic monotherapy with piretanide in congestive heart failure—a placebo-controlled trial. *Cardiovascular Drugs Therapy* **4**, 515–522.

Hale, W. E., Stewart, R. B., and Marks, R. G. (1984). Thiazide and fractures of bone. *New England Journal of Medicine* **310**, 926–927.

Hamlyn, J. M. *et al.* (1991). Identification and characterization of a ouabain-like compound from human plasma. *Proceedings of the National Academy of Sciences USA* **88**, 6259–6263.

Hammarlund-Udenaes, M. and Benet, L. Z. (1989). Furosemide pharmacokinetics and pharmacodynamics in health and disease—an update. *Journal of Pharmacokinetics and Biopharmaceutics* **17**, 1–46.

Hantman, D., Rossier, B., Zohlman, R., and Schrier, R. (1973). Rapid correction of hyponatremia in the syndrome of inappropriate secretion of antidiuretic hormone. *Annals of Internal Medicine* **78**, 870–875.

Harper, R. *et al.* (1994). Effects of low dose versus conventional dose thiazide diuretic on insulin action in essential hypertension. *British Medical Journal* **309**, 226–230.

Harrington, M., Kincaid-Smith, P., and McMichael, J. (1959). Results of treatment of malignant hypertension. *British Medical Journal* **ii**, 969–989.

Hatch, M. and Vaziri, N. D. (1994). Do thiazides reduce intestinal oxalate absorption? A study *in vitro* using rabbit colon. *Clinical Science* **86**, 353–357.

Hebert, S. C. (1998). Roles of Na–K–2Cl and Na–Cl cotransporters and ROMK potassium channels in urinary concentrating mechanism. *American Journal of Physiology* **275**, F325–F327.

Heidbreder, E., Hennemann, H., Krempien, B., and Heidland A. (1982). Salidiuretische Behandlung der renal-tubulären Acidose und ihrer Komplikationen. *Deutsche Medizinische Wochenschrift* **97**, 1504–1507.

Heidbreder, E. *et al.* (1986). Toxic renal failure in the rat: beneficial effect of atrial natriuretic factor. *Klinische Wochenschrift* **64** (Suppl. IV), 78–82.

Heidbreder, E. *et al.* (1988). Uranyl nitrate-induced acute renal failure in rats: effect of atrial natriuretic peptide on renal function. *Kidney International* **34** (Suppl. 25), S79–S82.

Heidland, A. and Hennemann, H. M. (1969). Aktivierung des sympathicoadrenalen Systems nach Diuretika. Beziehungen zum salidiuretischem Effekt und Glomerulumfiltrat. *Klinische Wochenschrift* **47**, 518–524.

Heidland, A. and Wigand, M. E. (1970). Einfluß hoher Furosemiddosen auf die Gehörfunktion bei Urämie. *Klinische Wochenschrift* **48**, 1052–1056.

Heidland, A., Hennemann, H., and Wigand, M. E. Dosiswirkung und optimale Infusionsgeschwindigkeit hoher Furosemidgaben bei terminaler Niereninsuffizienz. In *Medikamentöse Therapie bei Nierenerkrankungen* (ed. R. Kluthe), pp. 221–228. Stuttgart: Georg Thieme Verlag, 1972.

Heidland, A., Klütsch, K., Schneider, K. W., and Suzuki, F. (1964). Thiaziddiuretika und Nierenfunktion bei Hypertonie und kardialer Dekompensation. *Klinische Wochenschrift* **42**, 831–833.

Heidland, A. *et al.* The influence of diuretics on the fractional fluid and electrolyte excretion in renal insufficiency. In *Renal Transport and Diuretics* (ed. K. Thurau and H. Jahrmärker), pp. 395–403. Berlin: Springer Verlag, 1969a.

Heidland, A., Klütsch, K., Moormann, A., and Hennemann, H. (1969b). Möglichkeiten und Grenzen hochdosierter Diuretikatherapie bei hydropischer Niereninsuffizienz. *Deutsche Medizinische Wochenschrift* **94**, 1568–1574.

Helgeland, A., Hjermann, I., Leren, P., Enger, S., and Holms, I. (1978). High density lipoprotein cholesterol and antihypertensive drugs: the Oslo Study. *British Medical Journal* **2**, 403–408.

Heller, I., Halvey, J., Cohen, S., and Theodor, E. (1985). Significant metabolic acidosis induced by acetazolamide. *Archives of Internal Medicine* **145**, 1815–1817.

Henriksen, J. H., Bendtsen, F., Sorasen, T. A., Stadenger, C., and Rhing-Labon, H. (1989). Reduced central blood volume in cirrhosis. *Gastroenterology* **97**, 1506–1513.

Hewitt, W. L. (1977). Reflections on the clinical pharmacology of gentamicin. *Acta Pathologica Microbiologica Scandinavica* **214** (Suppl. B81), 151–153.

Heyman, S. N., Brezis, M., and Reubinoff, C. A. (1988). Acute kidney failure with selective renal medullary injury. *Journal of Clinical Investigation* **82**, 401–412.

Heyman, S. N., Brezis, M., Greenfeld, Z., and Rosen, S. (1989). Protective role of furosemide and saline in radiocontrast-induced acute renal failure in the rat. *American Journal of Kidney Diseases* **4–5**, 377–385.

Higashihara, E., Stokes, J. B., Kokko, J. P., Campbell, W. B., and Dubose, T. D. (1979). Cortical and papillary micropuncture examination of chloride transport in segments of the rat kidney during inhibition of prostaglandin production—possible role of prostaglandins in the chloruresis of acute volume expansion. *Journal of Clinical Investigation* **64**, 1277–1287.

Hoenderop, J. G., Nilius, B., and Bindels, R. J. (2002). Molecular mechanism of active Ca^{2+} reabsorption in the distal nephron. *Annual Review of Physiology* **64**, 529–549.

Hoes, A. W., Grobbee, D. E., Peet, T. M., and Lubsen, J. (1994). Do non-potassium sparing diuretics increase the risk of sudden cardiac death in hypertensive patients? Recent evidence. *Drugs* **47** (5), 711–733.

Hoffman, D. W., Jones-King, K. L., Whitworth, C. A., and Rybak, L. P. (1988). Potentiation of ototoxicity by glutathione depletion. *Annals of Otology, Rhinology, and Laryngology* **57**, 36–41.

Hogg, K. J. and Hillis, W. S. (1986). Captopril/metolazone induced renal failure. *Lancet* **i**, 501–502.

Holme, I. *et al.* (1984). Treatment of mild hypertension with diuretics: the importance of ECG abnormalities in the Oslo Study and in MRFIT. *Journal of the American Medical Association* **251**, 1298–1299.

Holzgreve, H. (1992). Where now the diuretics in antihypertensive treatment? *European Heart Journal* **13** (Suppl. G), 104–108.

Hörl, W. H., Müller, V., and Heidbreder, E. (1989). Verlauf und Prognose bei postoperativem und posttraumatischem akuten Nierenversagen. *Medizinische Welt* **40**, 616–619.

Horowitz, J., Keynan, A., and Ben-Ishay, D. (1972). A syndrome of inappropriate ADH secretion induced by cyclothiazide. *Journal of Clinical Pharmacology and New Drugs* **12**, 337–341.

Hoskins, B. and Jackson, C. M. (1978). The mechanism of chlorothiazide-induced carbohydrate intolerance. *Journal of Pharmacology and Experimental Therapeutics* **206**, 423–430.

Hricik, D. E. (1985). Captopril-induced renal insufficiency and the role of sodium balance. *Annals of Internal Medicine* **103**, 222–223.

Hropot, M., Fowler, N., Karlmark, B., and Giebisch, G. (1985). Tubular action of diuretics: distal effects on electrolyte transport and acidification. *Kidney International* **28**, 477–489.

Hropot, M., Juretschke, H. P., Langer, K. H., and Schwark, J. R. (2001). S3226, a novel NHE3 inhibitor, attenuates ischemia-induced acute renal failure in rats. *Kidney International* **60**, 2283–2289.

Hufnagle, K. G. *et al.* (1982). Renal calcification: a complication of long-term frusemide therapy. *Pediatrics* **70**, 360–363.

Hummel, M. *et al.* (1993). Urodilatin, a new therapy to prevent kidney failure after heart transplantation. *Journal of Heart Lung Transplant* **12** (2), 209–217.

Humphreys, H. (1994). Mechanisms and management of nephrotic edema. *Kidney International* **45**, 266–281.

Hunter, M., Lopes, A. G., Boulpaep, E., and Giebisch, G. H. (1986). Regulation of single potassium ion channels from apical membrane of rabbit collecting tubule. *American Journal of Physiology* **251**, F725–F733.

Hutchinson, W. D. (1985). Amenorrhoea after treatment with spironolactone and hydroflumethiazide. *British Medical Journal* **291**, 1094.

Hypertension Detection and Follow-up Program Cooperative Group (1979). Five year findings of the Hypertension Detection and Follow-up Program: II. Mortality by race, sex and age. *Journal of the American Medical Association* **42**, 2572–2577.

Ichikawa, I. *et al.* (1983). Role for intrarenal mechanism in the impaired salt excretion of experimental nephrotic syndrome. *Journal of Clinical Investigation* **71**, 91–103.

Ikram, H., Chan, W., Espiner, E. A., and Nicholls, M. E. (1980). Haemodynamic and humoral responses in acute and chronic frusemide therapy in congestive heart failure. *Clinical Science* **59**, 443–449.

Iorio, L., Simonelli, R., Nacca, R. G., and DeSanto, L. S. (1997). Daily hemofiltration in severe heart failure. *Kidney International* **51** (Suppl. 59), S62–S65.

Jacobs, D. B., Mookerja, B. K., and Jang, C. Y. (1984). Furosemide inhibits glucose transport in isolated rat adipocytes via direct inactivation of carrier proteins. *Journal of Clinical Investigation* **74**, 1679–1685.

Jick, H., Dinan, B. J., and Hunter, J. R. (1982). Triamterene and renal stones. *Journal of Urology* **27**, 224–225.

Johnston, P. A., Bernard, D. B., Perrin, N. S., and Levinsky, N. G. (1981). Prostaglandins mediate the vasodilatory effect of mannitol in the hypo-perfused rat kidney. *Journal of Clinical Investigation* **68**, 127–133.

Jung, W. and Schön, F. (1979). Effects of modern loop diuretics on the inner ear. A quantitative evaluation using computer techniques. *Archives of Otorhinolaryngology* **224**, 143–147.

Kaissling, B. and Stanton, B. A. (1987). Adaptation of distal tubuli and collecting duct to increased sodium delivery. I. Ultrastructure. *American Journal of Physiology* **225**, F910–F915.

Kaissling, B., Bachmann, S., and Kriz, W. (1985). Structural adaptation of the distal convoluted tubule to prolonged frusemide treatment. *American Journal of Physiology* **248**, F374–F381.

Kamm, D. E., Wu, L., and Kuchmy, B. L. (1987). Contribution of the urea appearance rate to diuretic-induced azotemia in the rat. *Kidney International* **32**, 47–56.

Kampf, V. D. and Baethke, R. (1980). The diuretic acitivity of bumetanide in a controlled comparison with furosemide in patients with various degrees of impaired renal function. *Arzneimittelforschung* **30**, 1015–1018.

Kaplan, N. M., Carnegie, A., Raskin, P., Heller, J. A., and Simmons, M. (1985). Potassium supplementation in hypertensive patients with diuretic-induced hypokalemia. *New England Journal of Medicine* **312**, 746–749.

Kaysen, G. A. *et al.* (1985). Plasma volume expansion is necessary for edema formation in the rat with Heymann nephritis. *American Journal of Physiology* **248**, F247–F253.

Keller, U., Weiss, M., and Stauffacher, W. (1989). Contribution of α- and β-receptors to ketogenic and lipolytic effects of norepinephrine in humans. *Diabetes* **38**, 454–459.

Khaleeli, A. A. and Wyman, A. L. (1978). Hyperosmolar non-ketotic diabetic coma induced by furosemide in modest dosage. *Postgraduate Medical Journal* **54**, 43–44.

Khaw, K. T. and Barrett-Connor, E. (1987). Dietary potassium and stroke-associated mortality: a 12 year prospective population study. *New England Journal of Medicine* **316**, 235–240.

Kieferle, S., Fong, P., Bens, M., Vandewalle, A., and Jentsch, T. J. (1994). Two highly homologous members of the ClC chloride channel family in both rat and human kidney. *Proceedings of the National Academy of Sciences USA* **91**, 6943–6947.

Kim, G., Kim, B., Kim, M., Chung, S., Han, H., Ryu, J., Lee, Y., Lee, K., Lee, J., Huh, W., and Oh, H. (2002). Medullary nephrocalcinosis associated with long-term furosemide abuse in adults. *Nephrology, Dialysis, Transplantation* **16**, 2303–2309.

Kinsella, J. L. and Aronson, P. S. (1980). Properties of the Na–H exchanger in renal microvillus membrane vesicles. *American Journal of Physiology* **238**, F461–F469.

Kirchner, K. A., Voelker, J. R., and Brater, D. C. (1990). Intratubular albumin blunts the response to furosemide—a mechanism for diuretic resistance in the nephrotic syndrome. *Journal of Pharmacology and Experimental Therapeutics* **252**, 1097–1101.

Kirchner, K. A., Voelker, J. R., and Brater, D. C. (1991). Binding inhibitors restore furosemide potency in tubule fluid containing albumin. *Kidney International* **40**, 418–424.

Kirchner, K. A., Voelker, J. R., and Brater, D. C. (1992). Tubular resistance to furosemide contributes to the attenuated diuretic response in nephrotic rats. *Journal of the American Society of Nephrology* **2**, 1201–1207.

Kleinknecht, D., Ganeval, D., Gonzalez-Duque, L. A., and Fermanian, J. (1976). Furosemide in acute oliguric renal failure: a controlled trial. *Nephron* **17**, 51–58.

Knauf, H. and Mutschler, E. (1991). Pharmacodynamic and kinetic considerations on diuretics as a basis of differential therapy. *Klinische Wochenschrift* **69**, 239–250.

Knauf, H. and Mutschler, E. K$^+$ loss induced by diuretics. In *Diuretics IV* (ed. J. B. Puschett), pp. 253–256. Amsterdam: Elsevier, 1993a.

Knauf, H. and Mutschler, E. (1993b). Low-dose segmental blockade of the nephron rather than high-dose diuretic monotherapy. *European Journal of Clinical Pharmacology* **44** (Suppl. 1), S63–S68.

Knauf, H. and Mutschler, E. (1997). Sequential nephron blockade breaks resistance to diuretics in edematous states. *Journal of Cardiovascular Pharmacology* **29** (3), 367–372.

Knauf, H., Cawello Schmidt, G., and Mutschler, E. (1994). The saluretic effect of the thiazide diuretic bumetizide in relation to the glomerular filtration rate. *European Journal of Clinical Pharmacology* **46**, 9–13.

Knauf, H. *et al.* (1990). Prediction of diuretic mobilization of cirrhotic ascites by pretreatment fractional sodium excretion. *Klinische Wochenschrift* **68**, 545–551.

Kone, B., Gimenez, L., and Watson, A. J. (1986). Thiazide-induced hyponatriemia. *Southern Medical Journal* **79**, 1456–1457.

Koomans, H. A. *et al.* (1986). Lowered tissue-fluid oncotic pressure protects the blood volume in the nephrotic syndrome. *Nephron* **42**, 317–322.

Kopple, J. D. *et al.* (1970). Thiazide-induced rise in serum calcium and magnesium in patients on maintenance haemodialysis. *Annals of Internal Medicine* **72**, 895–901.

Kramer, H. J., Schumann, J., Wasserman, C., and Dusing, R. (1980b). Protaglandin-independent protection by furosemide from oliguric ischemic renal failure in conscious rats. *Kidney International* **17**, 455–464.

Kramer, H. J. *et al.* (1980a). Interactions of conventional and antikaliuretic diuretics with the renal prostaglandin system. *Clinical Science* **59**, 67–70.

Krishna, G. G., Müller, E., and Kapoor, S. (1989). Increased blood pressure during potassium depletion in normotensive men. *New England Journal of Medicine* **320**, 1177–1182.

Krum, H., Nolly, H., Workman D., He, W., Roniker, B., Krause, S., and Fakouhi, K. (2002). Efficacy of eplerenone added to renin–angiotensin blockade in hypertensive patients. *Hypertension* **40**, 117–123.

Lachance, S. L. and Barry, J. M. (1985). Effect of furosemide on dialysis requirement following cadaveric kidney transplantation. *Journal of Urology* **133**, 950–953.

LaCroix, A. Z. *et al.* (1990). Thiazide diuretic agents and the incidence of hip fracture. *New England Journal of Medicine* **322**, 286–290.

Lagrue, G. *et al.* (1975). A vascular permeability factor elaborated from lymphocytes. I. Demonstration in patients with nephrotic syndrome. *Biomedicine* **23**, 37–40.

Lakhani, M. (1986). Complete heart block induced by hyperkalaemia associated with treatment with a combination of captopril and spironolactone. *British Medical Journal* **293**, 271.

Lameijer, W. and van Zwieten, P. A. (1978). Accelerated elimination of thallium in rat due to subchronic treatment with furosemide. *Archives of Toxicology* **40**, 7–16.

Lang, F. (1987). Osmotic diuresis. *Renal Physiology* **10**, 160–173.

Lang, F., Greger, R., and Deetjen, P. Effect of diuretics on uric acid metabolism and excretion. In *Diuretics in Research and Clinics* (ed. W. Siegenthaler, R. Beckerhoff, and W. Vetter), pp. 213–224. Stuttgart: Thieme, 1977.

Lang, F., Quehenberger, P., Greger, R., and Oberleithner, H. (1978). Effect of benzolamide on luminal pH in proximal convoluted tubules of the rat kidney. *Pflügers Archiv* **375**, 39–43.

Lant, A. F. and Wilson, G. M. (1971). Long-term therapy of diabetes insipidus with oral benzothiadiazine and phthalmidine diuretics. *Clinical Science* **40**, 497–511.

Larson, E. B., Roach, R. C., Schoene, R. B., and Hornbein, T. F. (1982). Acute mountain sickness and acetazolamide: clincial efficacy and effect on ventilation. *Journal of the American Medical Association* **248**, 328–332.

Le Hir, M., Kaissling, B., and Dubach, U. C. (1982). Distal tubular segments in the rabbit kidney after adaptation to altered Na- and K-intake. Changes in Na$^+$–K$^+$-ATPase activity. *Cell and Tissue Research* **224**, 493–504.

Lemieux, G. (1986). Treatment of idiopathic hypercalciuria with indapamide. *Canadian Medical Association Journal* **135**, 119–121.

Leonetti, G. *et al.* (1978). Relationship between the hypotensive and renin-stimulating actions of diuretic therapy in hypertensive patients. *Clinical Science and Molecular Medicine* **55**, 307s–309s.

Levinsky, N. G. and Bernard, D. B. Mannitol and loop diuretics in acute renal failure. In *Acute Renal Failure* (ed. B. Brenner and J. M. Lazarus), pp. 841–856. Edinburgh: Churchill Livingstone, 1988.

Levy, D. *et al.* (1987). Risk of ventricular arrhythmias in left ventricular hypertrophy: the Framingham Heart Study. *American Journal of Cardiology* **60**, 560–565.

Li, H.-Y. and Lindemann, B. (1983). Competitive blocking of epithelial sodium channels by organic cations: the relationship between macroscopic and microscopic inhibition constants. *Journal of Membrane Biology* **76**, 235–251.

Lieberthal, W. and Levinsky, N. G. (1991). Treatment of acute tubular necrosis. *Seminars in Nephrology* **10**, 571–583.

Lim, P. and Jacob, E. (1972). Magnesium deficiency in patients on long-term diuretic therapy for heart failure. *British Medical Journal* **3**, 620–622.

Lindner, A. (1983). Synergism of dopamine and furosemide in diuretic resistant oliguric acute renal failure. *Nephron* **33**, 121–126.

Lindon, M. H. *et al.* (2003). Comparison of outcomes with angiotensin-converting-enzyme inhibitors and diuretics for hypertension in the elderly. *New England Journal of Medicine* **348** (7), 583–592.

Linguegglia, E., Voilley, N., Waldmann, R., Lazdunski, M., and Barbry, P. (1993). Expression cloning of an epithelial amiloride-sensitive Na$^+$ channel. *FEBS Letters* **318**, 95–99.

Lohrmann, E., Burhoff, I., and Greger, R. (1994). Tubular effects of the loop diuretic torasemide. *Cardiology* **84** (Suppl.), 135–142.

Lohrmann, E., Masereel, B., Nitschke, R., Pirotte, B., Delarge, J., and Greger, R. (1992). Action of diuretics at the cellular level. *Progress in Pharmacology and Clinical Pharmacology* **9**, 24–32.

Loon, N. R., Wilcox, C. S., and Unwin, R. J. (1989). Mechanism of impaired natriuretic response to furosemide during prolonged therapy. *Kidney International* **36**, 682–689.

Luke, C. R., Ziegler, M. G., Coleman, M. D., and Kopin, I. J. (1979). Hydrochlorothiazide induced sympathetic hyperactivity in hypertensive patients. *Clinical Pharmacology and Therapeutics* **26**, 428–432.

Lumb, G., Newborne, P., Rust, J. H., and Wagner, B. (1978). Effects in animals of chronic administration of spironolactone—a review. *Journal of Environmental Pathology and Toxicology* **1**, 641–660.

Lyons, H. *et al.* (1973). Allergic interstitial nephritis causing reversible renal failure in four patients with idiopathic nephrotic syndrome. *New England Journal of Medicine* **288**, 124–128.

MacGregor, G. A. *et al.* (1979). Is 'idiopathic' oedema idiopathic? *Lancet* **i**, 397–400.

Mackay, G., Miur, A. L., and Watson, M. L. (1984). Contribution of prostaglandins to the systemic and renal vascular responses to furosemide in normal man. *British Journal Clinical Pharmacology* **17**, 513–519.

MacMahon, S. *et al.* (1990). Blood pressure, stroke, and coronary heart disease: part I. Prolonged differences in blood pressure: prospective observational studies corrected for the regression dilution bias. *Lancet* **335**, 765–774.

Madkour, H. *et al.* (1995). Comparison between the effects of indapamide and hydrochlorothiazide on creatinine clearance in patients with impaired renal function and hypertension. *American Journal of Nephrology* **15**, 251–255.

Maharaj, B. (1988). Diuretics in cirrhotic ascites. *Progress in Pharmacology* **63**, 245–266.

Mallette, L. E. (1992). The hypercalcemias. *Seminars in Nephrology* **12**, 159–190.

Manning, R. D. (1987). Effects of hypoproteinemia on renal hemodynamics, arterial pressure and fluid volume. *American Journal of Physiology* **252**, F91–F98.

Marcus, D. C., Marcus, N. Y., and Greger, R. (1987). Sidedness of action of loop diuretics and ouabain on nonsensory cells of utricle: a micro-Ussing chamber for inner ear tissues. *Hearing Research* **30**, 55–64.

Marone, C., Reubi, F. C., and Lahn, W. (1984). Comparison of the short-term effects of loop diuretics piretanide and furosemide in patients with renal insufficiency. *European Journal of Clinical Pharmacology* **26**, 413–418.

Martin, P.-Y. and Schrier, R. W. (1997). Sodium and water retention in heart failure: pathogenesis and treatment. *Kidney International* **51** (Suppl. 59), S57–S61.

McDonald, R. H., Goldberg, L. I., McNay, J., and Tuttle, E. P. (1964). Effects of dopamine in man: augmentation of sodium excretion, glomerular filtration rate and renal plasma flow. *Journal of Clinical Investigation* **43**, 1116–1124.

McVeigh, G., Galloway, D., and Johnston, D. (1988). The case for low dose diuretics in hypertension: comparison of low and conventional doses of cyclopenthiazide. *British Medical Journal* **297**, 95–98.

Medcalf, J. F., Harris, K. P., and Walls, J. (2001). Role of diuretics in the preservation of residual renal function in patients on continuous ambulatory peritoneal dialysis. *Kidney International* **59**, 1128–1133.

Meltzer, J. I. *et al.* (1979). Nephrotic syndrome: vasoconstriction and hypervolemic types indicated by renin-sodium profiling. *Annals of Internal Medicine* **91**, 688–696.

Meyer-Sabellek, W., Gotzen, R., Heitz, J., Arntz, H. R., and Schulte, K. L. (1985). Serum lipoprotein levels during long-term treatment of hypertension with indapamide. *Hypertension* **7**, 170–174.

Middecke, M., Weisweiler, P., Schwandt, P., and Holzgreve, H. (1987). Serum lipoproteins during antihypertensive therapy with beta-blockers and diuretics: a controlled long-term comparative trial. *Clinical Cardiology* **10**, 94–98.

Miller, P. D. and Berns, A. S. (1977). Acute metabolic alkalosis perpetuating hypercarbia: a role for acetazolamide in chronic obstructive pulmonary disease. *Journal of the American Medical Association* **238**, 2400–2401.

Missouris, C. G., Cappuccio, F. P., Markandu, N. D., and MacGregor, G. A. (1992). Diuretics and oedema: how to avoid rebound sodium retention. *Lancet* **339**, 1546.

Mor, R., Pitlik, S., and Rosenfeld, J. B. (1983). Indomethacin- and moduretic-induced hyperkalemia. *Israeli Journal of Medical Sciences* **19**, 535–537.

Moral, Z. *et al.* (2001). Regulation of ROMK1 channels by protein-tyrosine kinase and -tyrosine phosphatase. *Journal of Biological Chemistry* **276**, 7156–7163.

Morgan, D. A. *et al.* (1989). Renal sympathetic nerves attenuate the natriuretic effect of atrial peptide. *Journal of Laboratory and Clinical Medicine* **114**, 538–544.

Morgan, D. B. and Davidson, C. (1980). Hypokalemia and diuretics: an analysis of publications. *British Medical Journal* **280**, 905–908.

Mortensen, J. T., Schultz, A., and Ostergaard, A. H. (1986). Thiazides in the prophylactic treatment of recurrent idiopathic kidney stones. *International Urology and Nephrology* **18**, 265–269.

MRC (1981). Medical Research Council Working Party on Mild to Moderate Hypertension 1981. Adverse reactions to bendrofluazide and propranolol for the treatment of mild hypertension. *Lancet* **ii**, 539–543.

MRC Working Party (1992). Medical Research Council trial of treatment of hypertension in older adults: principal results. *British Medical Journal* **304**, 505–512.

MRC Working Party on Mild Hypertension (1988). Coronary heart disease in the Medical Research Council trial of treatment of mild hypertension. *British Heart Journal* **59**, 364–368.

MRFIT (1985). Multiple Risk Factor Intervention Trial Research Group. Baseline rest electrocardiographic abnormalities, antihypertensive treatment, and mortality in the Multiple Risk Factor Intervention trial. *American Journal of Cardiology* **55**, 1–15.

Murphy, M. B., Lewis, P. J., Kohner, E., Schumer, B., and Dollery, C. T. (1982). Glucose intolerance in hypertensive patients treated with diuretics; a fourteen-year-follow up. *Lancet* **ii**, 1293–1295.

Myers, M. G. (1987). Hydrochlorothiazide with or without amiloride for hypertension in the elderly. A dose titration study. *Archives of Internal Medicine* **147**, 1026–1030.

Nakashima, M., Uematsu, T., Kosuge, K., and Kanamaru, M. (1992). Pilot study of the uricosuric effect of DuP-753, an new angiotensin II receptor antagonist, in healthy subjects. *European Journal of Clinical Pharmacology* **42**, 333–335.

Naranjo, C. A., Pontigo, E., Valdenegro, C., Gonzalez, G., Ruiz, I., and Busto, U. (1979). Furosemide-induced adverse reactions in cirrhosis of the liver. *Clinical Pharmacology and Therapeutics* **25**, 154–160.

Nashat, F. S., Scholefield, F. R., Tappin, J. W., and Wilcox, C. S. (1969). The effects of changes in haematocrit on the intrarenal distribution of blood flow in the dog's kidney. *Journal of Physiology* **201**, 639–655.

Nelson, G. I. C. *et al.* (1983). Haemodynamic effects of frusemide and its influence on repetitive rapid volume loading in acute myocardial infarction. *European Heart Journal* **4**, 706–711.

Nishijma, H. *et al.* (1984). Acute and chronic hemodynamic effects of the basic therapeutic regimen for congestive heart failure. Diuretics, low salt diet and bed rest. *Japanese Heart Journal* **25**, 571–585.

Norgaard, A., Kjeldsen, K., and Clausen, T. (1981). Potassium depletion decreases the number of ^{3}H-ouabain binding sites and the active Na–K transport in skeletal muscle. *Nature* **293**, 739–741.

Nuutinen, L. S., Kairaluoma, M., Tuononen, S., and Larmi, T. K. I. (1978). The effect of furosemide on renal function in open heart surgery. *Journal of Cardiovascular Surgery* **19**, 471–479.

Oguagha, C., Porush, J. G., and Chou, S. Y. Prevention of acute renal failure following infusion intravenous pyelography in patients with chronic renal failure by furosemide. In *Proceedings of the 8th International Congress on Nephrology* p. 293 (abstract). Athens: Karger, 1981.

Ohnishi, A. *et al.* (1993). Potent aquaretic agent. A novel nonpeptide selective vasopressin 2 antagonist (OPC-31260) in men. *Journal of Clinical Investigation* **92**, 2653–2659.

Okusa, M. D. and Ellison, D. H. Physiology and pathophysiology of diuretic action. In *The Kidney: Physiology and Pathophysiology* (ed. D. W. Seldin and G. Giebisch), pp. 2877–2922. New York: Raven Press, 2000.

Oppermann, J. A., Piper, Ch., and Gardiner, P. Spironolactone and potassium canrenoate despite chemical similarities, differing metabolism accounts for different toxicological findings in animals. In *Therapie mit Aldosteronantagonisten* (ed. E. Mutschler), pp. 3–9. München: Urban und Schwarzenberg, 1988.

Osswald, H. and Vallon, V. Tubuloglomerular feedback and its role in acute renal failure. In *Critical Care Nephrology* (ed. C. Ronco and R. Belomo), pp. 613–622. Boston: Kluwer Academic Publishers, 1998.

Overdiek, J. W. P. M. and Merkus, F. W. H. M. (1986). Spironolactone metabolism and gynaecomastia. *Lancet* **i**, 1103.

Packer, M. *et al.* (1987). Functional renal insufficiency during long-term therapy with captopril and enalapril in severe chronic heart failure. *Annals of Internal Medicine* **106**, 346–354.

Palmer, B. F. and Alpern, R. J. (1997). Pathogenesis of edema formation in the nephrotic syndrome. *Kidney International* **51** (Suppl. 59), S21–S27.

Palmer, L. G. and Frindt, G. (1987). Effects of cell Ca and pH on Na channels from rat cortical collecting tubule. *American Journal of Physiology* **253**, F333–F339.

Parmley, W. W. (1985). Pathophysiology of congestive heart failure. *American Journal of Cardiology* 56, 7A–11A.

Parving, H.-H., Andersson, A. R., Hommel, E., and Smidt, U. (1985). Effects of long-term antihypertensive treatment on kidney function in diabetic nephropathy. *Hypertension* 7 (Suppl. 2), 114–117.

Patak, R. V., Fadem, S. Z., Lifschitz, M. D., and Stein, J. H. (1979). Study of factors which modify the development of norepinephrine-induced acute renal failure in the dog. *Kidney International* 15, 227–237.

Patak, R. V., Mookerjee, B. K., Bentzel, C. J., Hysert, P. E., Babej, M., and Lee, J. B. (1975). Antagonism of the effects of furosemide by indomethacin in normal and hypertensive man. *Prostaglandins* 10, 649–658.

Pavord, I. D., Wisniewski, A., and Tattersfield, A. E. (1992). Inhaled frusemide and exercise induced asthma: evidence of a role for inhibitory prostanoids. *Thorax* 47, 797–800.

Payne, J. A. and Forbush, B. (1994). Alternatively spliced isoforms of the putative renal Na–K–Cl cotransporter are differentially distributed within the rabbit kidney. *Proceedings of the National Academy of Sciences, USA* 91, 4544–4548.

Pera, M. F., Zook, B. G., and Harder, H. C. (1979). Effects of mannitol or furosemide diuresis on the nephrotoxicity and physiological disposition of cis-dichlorodiammineplatinum-(II) in rats. *Cancer Research* 39, 1269–1278.

Perez-Ayuso, R. M. *et al.* (1983). Randomized comparative study of efficacy of furosemide versus spironolactone in nonazotemic cirrhosis with ascites. *Gastroenterology* 84, 961–968.

Petersen, J. S. and Di Bona, G. F. Interactions between diuretics and the renal sympathetic nerves. In *Diuretics IV: Chemistry, Pharmacology and Clinical Applications* (ed. J. B. Puschett and A. Greenberg), pp. 161–176. Amsterdam: Elsevier Science Publishers, 1993.

Petersen, V., Hvidt, S., Thompson, K., and Schou, M. (1974). Effect of prolonged thiazide treatment on renal lithium clearance. *British Medical Journal* 3, 143–145.

Petit, W. A. *et al.* (1988). Influence of frusemide on parathyroid hormone levels in hyperparathyroidism. *New England Journal of Medicine* 318, 644–645.

Pichette, V., Geadah, D., and du Souich, P. (1996). The influence of moderate hypoalbuminaemia on the renal metabolism and dynamics of furosemide in the rabbit. *British Journal of Pharmacology* 119, 885–890.

Pillay, V. K. G., Schwartz, F. D., Aimi, K., and Kark, R. M. (1969). Transient and permanent deafness following treatment with ethacrynic acid in renal failure. *Lancet* i, 77–79.

Pinzani, M., Daskalopoulos, G., Laffi, G., Gentilini, P., and Zipser, R. D. (1987). Altered furosemide pharmacokinetics in chronic alcoholic liver disease. *Gastroenterology* 92, 294–298.

Pitt, B., Zannad, F., Remme, W. J., Cody, R., Castaigne, A., Perez, A., Palensky, J., and Wittes, J. (1999). The effect of spironolactone on morbidity and mortality in patients with severe heart failure. *New England Journal of Medicine* 341, 709–717.

Pockros, P. J. and Reynolds, T. B. (1986). Rapid diuresis in patients with ascites from chronic liver disease: the importance of peripheral edema. *Gastroenterology* 90, 1827–1833.

Podjarny, E. *et al.* (1988). Prostanoids in renal failure induced by converting enzyme inhibition in sodium-depleted rats. *American Journal of Physiology* 254, F358–F363.

Podszus, T. and Piesche, L. (1990). Effect of torasemide on pulmonary and cardiac haemodynamics after oral treatment of chronic heart failure. *Progress in Pharmacology and Clinical Pharmacology* 8 (1), 157–166.

Pollare, T., Lithell, M., and Berne, C. (1989). A comparison of the effects of hydrochlorothiazide and captopril on glucose and lipid metabolism in patients with hypertension. *New England Journal of Medicine* 321, 868–873.

Polsen, R. J. *et al.* (1987). The prevention of renal impairment in patients undergoing orthotopic liver grafting by infusion of low dose dopamine. *Anaesthesia* 42, 15–19.

Powers, D. A., Duggan, J., and Brady, H. R. (1999). Renal-dose (low-dose) dopamine for the treatment of sepsis-related and other forms of acute renal failure: ineffective and probably dangerous. *Clinical Experimental Pharmacological Physiology* 26, 523–528.

Powers, S. R., Boba, A., Hostnik, W., and Stein, A. (1964). Prevention of postoperative acute renal failure with mannitol in 100 cases. *Surgery* 35, 15–23.

Preston, G. M. and Agre, P. (1991). Isolation of the cDNA for erythrocyte integral membrane protein of 28 kilodaltons: member of an ancient channel family. *Proceedings of the National Academy of Sciences USA* 88, 11110–11114.

Psaty, B. M. *et al.* (2003). Health outcomes associated with various antihypertensive therapies use as first-line agents: a network meta-analysis. *Journal of the American Medical Association* 289 (19), 2534–2544.

Quick, C. A. and Hoppe, W. (1975). Permanent deafness associated with furosemide administration. *Annals of Otology Rhinology and Laryngology* 84, 94–101.

Quintero, E. *et al.* (1985). Paracentesis versus diuretics in the treatment of cirrhotics with tense ascites. *Lancet* i, 611–612.

Rahman, S. N. *et al.* (1994). Effects of atrial natriuretic peptide in clinical acute renal failure. *Kidney International* 45 (6), 1731–1738.

Rampini, S., Fanconi, A., Illig, R., and Prader, A. (1968). Effect of hydrochlorothiazide on proximal renal tubular acidosis in a patient with idiopathic 'de Toni–Debre–Fanconi syndrome'. *Helvetica Paediatrica Acta* 23, 13–15.

Rascher, W. *et al.* (1986). Diuretic and hormonal responses to head-out water immersion in nephrotic syndrome. *Journal of Pediatrics* 109, 609–614.

Rashiq, S. and Logan, R. F. A. (1986). Role of drugs in fractures of the femoral neck. *British Medical Journal* 292, 861–863.

Rastogi, S., Bayliss, J. M., Nascimento, L., and Arruda, J. A. L. (1985). Hyperkalemic renal tubular acidosis: effect of furosemide in humans and in rats. *Kidney International* 28, 801–807.

Reed, B. R., Huff, J. C., and Jones, S. K. (1985). Subacute cutaneous lupus erythematosus associated with hydrochlorothiazide therapy. *Annals of Internal Medicine* 103, 49.

Reichel, H., Deibert, B., Geberth, S., Schmidt-Gayk, H., and Ritz, E. (1992). Frusemide therapy and intact parathyroid hormone plasma concentrations in chronic renal insufficiency. *Nephrology, Dialysis, Transplantation* 7, 8–15.

Rigden, S. P. *et al.* (1984). The beneficial effect of mannitol on postoperative renal function in children undergoing cardiopulmonary bypass surgery. *Clinical Nephrology* 21, 148–151.

Ritz, E., Fliser, D., Nowicki, M., and Stein, G. (1994). Treatment with high doses of loop diuretics in chronic renal failure. *Nephrology, Dialysis, Transplantation* 9 (Suppl. 3), 40–43.

Robinson, H. N., Morison, W. L., and Hood, A. F. (1985). Thiazide diuretic therapy and chronic photosensitivity. *Archives of Dermatology* 121, 522–523.

Robuschi, M., Vaghi, A., Gambaro, G., Spagnotto, S., and Bianco, S. (1988). Inhaled furosemide (F) is highly effective in preventing ultrasonically nebulized water (UNH:20) bronchoconstriction. *American Review of Respiratory Diseases* 137, 412 (abstract).

Romero, M. F. (2001). The electrogenic Na^+/HCO_3^- cotransporter, NBC. *Journal of the Pancreas* 2, 182–191.

Ron, D., Taitelman, U., Michaelson, M., Sar-Joseph, G., Bursztein, S., and Better, O. S. (1984). Prevention of acute renal failure in traumatic rhabdomyolysis. *Archives of Internal Medicine* 144, 277–280.

Rose, H. J., O'Malley, K., and Pruitt, A. W. (1976). Depression of renal clearance of furosemide in man by azotemia. *Clinical Pharmacology and Therapeutics* 21, 141–146.

Rudy, D. W. *et al.* (1991). Loop diuretics for chronic renal insufficiency: a continuous infusion is more potent than bolus therapy. *Annals of Internal Medicine* 115, 360–366.

Sands, J. M., Neylan, J. F., and Mitch, W. E. (1991). Atrial natriuretic factor does not improve the outcome of cadaveric renal transplantation. *Journal of the American Society of Nephrology* 1, 1082–1086.

Sandström, P. E. and Sehlin, J. (1988). Furosemide reduces insulin release by inhibition of Cl and Ca^{2+} fluxes in beta cells. *American Journal of Physiology* **255**, E591–E596.

Santos-Atherton, D. and Frank, S. (1986). The functional response to furosemide in a case of de Toni–Debre–Fanconi disease. *Acta Endocrinologica Supplementum (Copenhagen)* **279**, 452–457.

Schafer, J. A., Troutman, S. L., and Schlatter, E. (1990). Vasopressin and mineralocorticoid increase apical membrane driving force for K secretion in rat CCD. *American Journal of Physiology* **258**, F199–F210.

Schafferhans, K. *et al.* (1988). Atrial natriuretic peptide in gentamicin-induced acute renal failure. *Kidney International* **34** (Suppl. 25), S101–S103.

Schambelan, M., Sebastian, A., and Rector, F. C., Jr. (1981). Mineralocorticoid-resistant renal hyperkalemia without salt wasting (type II pseudohypoaldosteronism): role of increased chloride reabsorption. *Kidney International* **19**, 716–727.

Scherer, B. and Weber, P. C. (1979). Time dependent changes in prostaglandin excretion in response to furosemide in man. *Clinical Science* **56**, 77–81.

Scherzer, P., Wald, H., and Popovtzer, M. (1987). Enhanced glomerular filtration and Na$^+$–K$^+$-ATPase with furosemide administration. *American Journal of Physiology* **252**, F910–F915.

Schlatter, E. (1989). Antidiuretic hormone regulation of electrolyte transport in the distal nephron. *Renal Physiology and Biochemistry* **12**, 65–84.

Schlatter, E. (1993). Effects of various diuretics on membrane voltage of macula densa cells. Whole-cell patch-clamp experiments. *Pflügers Archiv* **423**, 74–77.

Schlatter, E. and Schafer, J. A. (1988). Intracellular chloride activity in principal cells of rat collecting ducts (CCT). *Pflügers Archiv* **410**, R86 (abstract).

Schlatter, E., Bleich, M., Hirsch, J., and Greger, R. (1993). pH-sensitive K$^+$ channels in the distal nephron. *Nephrology, Dialysis, Transplantation* **8**, 488–490.

Schlatter, E., Greger, R., and Weidtke, C. (1983). Effect of 'high ceiling' diuretics on active salt transport in the cortical thick ascending limb of Henle's loop of rabbit kidney. Correlation of chemical structure and inhibitory potency. *Pflügers Archiv* **396**, 210–217.

Schlatter, E., Salomonsson, M., Persson, A. E. G., and Greger, R. (1989). Macula densa cells sense luminal NaCl concentration via the furosemide sensitive Na–2Cl–K cotransporter. *Pflügers Archiv* **414**, 286–290.

Schmieder, R. E., Messerli, F. H., Garavaglia, G. E., and Nunez, B. D. (1988). Dietary salt intake: a determinant of cardiac involvement in essential hypertension. *Circulation* **78**, 951–965.

Schnermann, J. and Briggs, P. Function of the juxtaglomerular apparatus: Local control of glomerular hemodynamics. In *The Kidney: Physiology and Pathophysiology* (ed. D. Seldin and G. Giebisch), pp. 669–697. New York: Raven, 1985.

Schrier, R. W. (1988). Pathogenesis of sodium and water retention in high-output and low-output cardiac failure, nephrotic syndrome, cirrhosis, and pregnancy (first of two parts). *New England Journal of Medicine* **319**, 1065–1072.

Schrier, R. W. and Berl, T. Disorders of water metabolism. In *Renal and Electrolyte Disorders* (ed. R. W. Schrier), pp. 1–64. Boston: Little Brown, 1980.

Schrier, R. W., Arnold, P. E., Gordon, J. A., and Burke, T. J. (1984). Protection of mitochondrial function by mannitol in ischemic acute renal failure. *American Journal of Physiology* **247**, F365.

Schrier, R. W. *et al.* (1988). Peripheral arterial vasodilatation hypothesis: a proposal for the initiation of renal sodium and water retention in cirrhosis. *Hepatology* **8** (5), 1151–1157.

Schrot, R. J. and Muizelaar, J. P. (2002). Mannitol in acute traumatic brain injury. *The Lancet* **359**, 1633–1634.

Schwartz, L. B., Bissell, M. G., Murphy, M., and Gewertz, B. L. (1988). Renal effects of dopamine in vascular surgical patients. *Journal of Vascular Surgery* **8**, 367–374.

Seldin, D. W. and Giebisch, G. Preface. In *Diuretic Agents: Clinical Physiology and Pharmacology* (ed. D. W. Seldin and G. Giebisch), pp. 1–672. San Diego: Academic Press, 1997.

Senft, G., Losert, W., and Schultz, G. (1966). Ursachen der Störungen des intramuskulären Kohlenhydratstoffwechsels unter dem Einfluß sulfonamidierter Diuretika. *Naunyn-Schmiedebergs Archiv für Pharmakologie und Experimentelle Pathologie* **255**, 369–382.

Shah, S., Khatri, J., and Freis, E. D. (1978). Mechanism of antihypertensive effect of thiazide diuretics. *American Heart Journal* **95**, 611–618.

Shakelton, C. R., Wong, N. L. M., and Sutton, R. A. Distal (potassium-sparing) diuretics. In *Diuretics: Physiology, Pharmacology and Clinical Use* (ed. J. H. Dirks and R. A. L. Sutton), pp. 117–134. Philadelphia: W.B. Saunders, 1986.

Shamash, J., Earl, H., and Souhami, R. (1991). Acetazolamide for alkalinisation of urine in patients receiving high dose methotrexate. *Cancer Chemotherapy and Pharmacology* **28**, 150–151.

Shapiro, M. D. *et al.* (1990). Role of aldosterone in the sodium retention of patients with nephrotic syndrome. *American Journal of Nephrology* **10**, 44–48.

Shaw, S. G. *et al.* (1987). Atrial natriuretic peptide protects against acute ischemic renal failure in the rat. *Journal of Clinical Investigation* **80**, 1232–1237.

Shear, L., Ching, S., and Gabuzda, G. J. (1970). Compartmentalization of ascites and edema in patients with hepatic cirrhosis. *New England Journal of Medicine* **282**, 1391–1396.

Shemesh, O. *et al.* (1986). Effect of colloid volume expansion on glomerular barrier size-selectivity in humans. *Kidney International* **29**, 916–923.

SHEP Cooperative Research Group (1991). Prevention of stroke by antihypertensive drug treatment in older persons with isolated systolic hypertension. Final results of the Systolic Hypertension in the Elderly Program (SHEP). *Journal of the American Medical Association* **265**, 3255–3264.

Sherlock, S. Ascites. In *Diseases of the Liver and Biliary System* 6th edn. (ed. S. Sherlock), pp. 116–133. Oxford: Blackwell Scientific Publications, 1981.

Sherlock, S., Senewiratne, B., Scott, T. A., and Walker, J. G. (1966). Complications of diuretic therapy in hepatic cirrhosis. *Lancet* i, 1049–1053.

Shichiri, M., Shiigai, T., and Takeuchi, J. (1984). Long-term furosemide treatment in idiopathic edema. *Archives of Internal Medicine* **144**, 2161–2164.

Shilliday, I. and Allison, M. E. (1994). Diuretics in acute renal failure. *Renal Failure* **16** (1), 3–17.

Shimizu, T. *et al.* (1991). Interaction of trichlormethiazide or amiloride with PTH in stimulating calcium absorption in the rabbit connecting tubule. *American Journal of Physiology* **261**, F36–F43.

Shimon, I., Almog, S., Vered, Z., Seligmann, H., Shefi, M., Peleg, E., Rosenthal, T., Motro, M., Halkin, H., and Ezra, D. (1995). Improved left ventricular function after thiamine supplementation in patients with congestive heart failure receiving long-term furosemide therapy. *The American Journal of Medicine* **98**, 485–490.

Shutske, G. M. and Allen, R. C. Diuretics in hypertension: whence and whither. In *Hypertension: Physiological Basis and Treatment* (ed. H. Ong and J. Lewis), pp. 123–192. New York: Academic Press, 1984.

Silke, B. (1993). Central hemodynamic effects of diuretic therapy in chronic heart failure. *Cardiovascular Drugs and Therapy* **7**, 45–53.

Singer, I. (1981). Lithium and the kidney. *Kidney International* **19**, 374–387.

Singh, B. N. *et al.* (1992). Diuretic-induced potassium and magnesium deficiency: relation to drug-induced QT prolongation, cardiac arrhythmias and sudden death. *Journal of Hypertension* **10**, 301–316.

Siscovick, D. S. *et al.* (1994). Diuretic therapy for hypertension and the risk of primary cardiac arrest. *New England Journal of Medicine* **330**, 1852–1857.

Skarfors, E. T., Lithell, H. O., Selinus, I., and Aberg, H. (1989). Do antihypertensive drugs precipitate diabetes in predisposed men? *British Medical Journal* **298**, 1147–1152.

Smits, P. *et al.* (1989). The effect of human atrial natriuretic peptide on the incidence of acute renal failure in cadaveric kidney transplantation. *Transplantation International* **2**, 73–77.

Sokolow, M. and Perloff, D. (1960). Five-year survival of consecutive patients with malignant hypertension treated with antihypertensive agents. *American Journal of Cardiology* **6**, 858–863.

Solomon, R. J. (1984). Ventricular arrhythmias in patients with myocardial infarction and ischemia. Relationships to serum potassium and magnesium. *Drugs* **28** (Suppl. 1), 66–76.

Sonnenblick, M., Friedlander, Y., and Rosin, A. J. (1993). Diuretic-induced severe hyponatremia. Review and analysis of 129 reported patients. *Chest* **103**, 601–606.

Spustova, V., Gerykova, M., and Dzurik, R. (1988). Serum hippurate accumulation and urinary excretion in renal insufficiency. *Biochemia Clinica Bohemoslovaka* **17**, 205–212.

Stassen, W. N. and McCullough, A. J. (1985). Management of ascites. *Seminars in Liver Disease* **5**, 291–307.

Stenvinkel, P. and Alvestrand, A. (1988). Loop-diuretic-induced pancreatitis with rechallenge in a patient with malignant hypertension and renal insufficiency. *Acta Medica Scandinavica* **224**, 89–91.

Struthers, A. D., Whitesmith, R., and Reid, J. L. (1983). Prior thiazide diuretic treatment increases adrenaline-induced hypokalemia. *Lancet* **i**, 1358–1360.

Suki, W. N., Stinebaugh, B. J., Frommer, J. P., and Eknoyan, G. Physiology of diuretic action. In *The Kidney: Physiology and Pathophysiology* (ed. D. W. Seldin and G. Giebisch), pp. 2127–2162. New York: Raven Press, 1985.

Suki, W. N., Yuin, J. J., and VonMinden, M. (1970). Acute treatment of hypercalcemia with furosemide. *New England Journal of Medicine* **283**, 836–840.

Sundberg, S., Salo, H., and Gordin, A. (1982). Effect of low dose diuretics on plasma and blood cell electrolytes, plasma uric acid and blood glucose. *Acta Medica Scandinavica* **668**, 95–101.

Sungaila, I. *et al.* (1992). Spironolactone, pharmacokinetics and pharmacodynamics in patients with cirrhotic ascites. *Gastroenterology* **102**, 1680–1685.

Tannen, R. (1985). Diuretic-induced hypokalemia. *Kidney International* **28**, 988–1000.

Tannen, R. L. (1983). Effects of potassium on blood pressure control. *Annals of Internal Medicine* **98**, 773–780.

Tarazi, R. C., Dustan, H. P., and Fröhlich, E. D. (1970). Long-term thiazide therapy in essential hypertension. *Circulation* **41**, 709–717.

Tarka, J., Kurtzman, N. A., and Batlle, D. C. (1983). Clinical assessment of urinary acidification using a short test with oral furosemide. *Kidney International* **23**, 737 (abstract).

Task Force Report (2001). Guidelines for the diagnosis and treatment of chronic heart failure. *European Heart Journal* **22**, 1527–1560.

Tazel, J. H. (1981). Comparison of adverse reactions to bumetanide and furosemide. *Journal of Clinical Pharmacology* **21**, 615–619.

Ten, R. M. *et al.* (1988). Acute interstitial nephritis: immunologic and clinical aspects. *Mayo Clinic Proceedings* **63**, 921–930.

The Antihypertensive and Lipid-Lowering Treatment to Prevent Heart Attack Trial (ALLHAT) (2002). Major outcomes in high-risk hypertensive patients randomized to angiotensin-converting enzyme inhibitor or calcium channel blocker versus diuretic. *Journal of the American Medical Association* **288** (23), 2981–2997.

The JNC 7 Report (2003). The Seventh Report of the Joint National Committee on Prevention, Detection, Evaluation, and Treatment of High Blood Pressure. *Journal of the American Medical Association* **283** (19), 2560–2572.

Thiel, G. *et al.* (1976). Protection of rat kidney against $HgCl_2$-induced acute renal failure by induction of high urine flow without renin suppression. *Kidney International* **10**, S191–S200.

Tobian, L. (1974). Hypertension and the kidney. *Archives of Internal Medicine* **133**, 959–967.

Tobian, L. (1988). The Volhard lecture: potassium and sodium in hypertension. *Journal of Hypertension* **6** (Suppl. 4), 12–24.

Tsuboi, Y., Ishikawa, S. E., Fujisawa, G., Okada, K., and Saito, T. (1994). Therapeutic efficacy of the non-peptide AVP antagonist OPC-31260 in cirrhotic rats. *Kidney International* **46**, 237–244.

Tucker, B. J., Steiner, R. W., Gushwa, L. C., and Blantz, R. C. (1978). Studies on the tubuloglomerular feedback system in the rat. The mechanism of reduction in filtration rate with benzolamide. *Journal of Clinical Investigation* **62**, 993–1004.

Tulassay, T. *et al.* (1987). Atrial natriuretic peptide and other vasoactive hormones in nephrotic syndrome. *Kidney International* **31**, 1391–1395.

Tweeddale, M. G., Ogilvie, R. I., and Ruedy, J. (1977). Antihypertensive and biochemical effects of chlorthalidone. *Clinical Pharmacology and Therapeutics* **22**, 519–527.

Uchida, T. M. *et al.* (1991). Anti-aldosteronergic effect of torasemide. *European Journal of Pharmacology* **205**, 145–150.

Ullrich, K. J., Rumrich, G., and Klöss, S. (1989). Contraluminal organic anion and cation transport in the proximal renal tubule: V. Interaction with sulfamoyl- and phenoxy diuretics, and with β-lactam antibiotics. *Kidney International* **36**, 78–88.

Usberti, M. *et al.* (1984). Role of plasma vasopressin in the impairment of water excretion in nephrotic syndrome. *Kidney International* **25**, 422–429.

van Brummelen, P., Woerlee, M., and Schalekamp, M. A. D. H. (1979). Long-term versus short-term effects of hydrochlorothiazide on renal haemodynamics in essential hypertension. *Clinical Science* **56**, 463–469.

Vander, A. J. and Miller, R. (1964). Control of renin secretion in the anesthetized dog. *American Journal of Physiology* **207**, 537–546.

van Meyel, J. J. M., Smits, P., Gerlag, P. G. G., Russel, F. G. M., and Gribnau, F. W. J. Continuous infusion of furosemide in the treatment of severe congestive heart failure and diuretic resistance. In *Diuretics IV: Chemistry, Pharmacology and Clinical Applications* (ed. J. B. Puschett and A. Greenberg), pp. 445–448. Amsterdam: Elsevier Science Publishers, 1993.

van Olden, R. W., van Meyel, J. J. M., and Gerlag, P. G. G. Acute and long-term efficiency of high-dose furosemide in haemodialysis patients with residual renal function. In *Diuretics IV* (ed. J. B. Puschett and A. Greenberg), pp. 117–119. Amsterdam: Elsevier Science Publishers, 1993.

Vargo, D. L., Brater, D. C., Rudy, D. W., and Swan, S. K. (1996). Dopamine does not enhance furosemide-induced natriuresis in patients with congestive heart failure. *Journal of the American Society of Nephrology* **7**, 1032–1037.

Vaughan, E. D., Jr. *et al.* (1978). The renin response to diuretic therapy: a limitation of antihypertensive potential. *Circulation Research* **421**, 376–381.

Velázquez, H. and Wright, F. S. (1986). Effects of diuretic drugs on Na, Cl and K transport by rat renal distal tubule. *American Journal of Physiology* **250**, F1013–F1023.

Venkata, C., Ram, S., Garrett, N., and Kaplan, N. M. (1981). Moderate sodium restriction and various diuretics in the treatment of hypertension: Effects of potassium wastage and blood pressure control. *Archives of Internal Medicine* **141**, 1015–1019.

Verenstraeten, P. J. C., Dupis, F., and Toussaint, C. (1975). Effects of large doses of furosemide in endstage chronic renal failure. *Nephron* **14**, 333–338.

Veterans Administration Cooperative Study Group on Antihypertensive Agents (1972). Effects of treatment on morbidity in hypertension: III. Influence of age, diastolic pressure and prior cardiovascular disease: further analysis of side effects. *Circulation* **45**, 991–1004.

Veterans Administration Cooperative Study Group on Antihypertensive Agents (1982a). Comparison of propranolol and hydrochlorothiazide for the initial treatment of hypertension. I. Results of short-term titration with emphasis on racial differences in response. *Journal of the American Medical Association* **248**, 1996–2003.

Veterans Administration Cooperative Study Group on Antihypertensive Agents (1982b). Comparison of propranolol and hydrochlorothiazide for the initial treatment of hypertension II. Results of long-term therapy. *Journal of the American Medical Association* **248**, 2004–2011.

Völker, J. R. *et al.* (1987). Comparison of loop diuretics in patients with chronic renal insufficiency. *Kidney International* **32**, 572–578.

Waldegger, S. *et al.* (2002). Barttin increases surface expression and changes current properties of ClC–K channels. *Pflügers Archiv* **444**, 411–418.

Walker, W. G., Hermann, J., Yin, D. P., Murphy, R. P., and Patz, A. (1987). Diuretics accelerate diabetic nephropathy in hypertensive insulin-dependent and non-insulin-dependent subjects. *Clinical Research* **35**, 663A.

Walser, M. and Rahill, W. J. (1966). Renal tubular reabsorption of bromides compared with chlorides. *Clinical Science* **30**, 191–208.

Warram, J. H. *et al.* (1991). Excess mortality associated with diuretics in diabetes mellitus. *Archives of Internal Medicine* **151**, 1350–1356.

Wasnich, R. D., Benfante, R. J., Yanok, K., Heilburn, L., and Vogel, J. M. (1983). Thiazide effect on the mineral content of bone. *New England Journal of Medicine* **309**, 344–347.

Wassertheil-Smoller, S., Blaufox, M. D., and Oberman, A. (1991). Effect of antihypertensives on sexual function and quality of life: The TAIM Study. *Archives of Internal Medicine* **114**, 613–620.

Watkins, J., Carl-Abbot, E., Hensby, C. N., Webster, J., and Dollery, C. T. (1980). Attenuation of hypotensive effect of propranolol and thiazide diuretics by indomethacin. *British Medical Journal* **281**, 702–705.

Webster, J. A. and Dollery, C. T. (1980). Antihypertensive action of bendroflumethiazide: increased prostacyclin production. *Clinical Pharmacology and Therapeutics* **28**, 751–758.

Weidmann, P. (2001). Metabolic profile of indapamide sustained-release in patients with hypertension: data from three randomised double-blind studies. *Drug Safety* **24** (15), 1155–1165.

Weidmann, P., Beretta, C., Link, L., Blanchet, M. G., and Boehring, K. (1983a). Cardiovascular counterregulation during sympathetic inhibition in normal subjects and patients with mild hypertension. *Hypertension* **5**, 873–880.

Weidmann, P. *et al.* (1983b). Antihypertensive mechanism of diuretic treatment with chlorthalidone. Complementary roles of sympathetic axis and sodium. *Kidney International* **23**, 320–325.

Weidmann, P., De Courten, M., and Ferrari, P. (1992). Effect of diuretics on the plasma lipid profile. *European Heart Journal* **13** (Suppl. G), 61–67.

Weidmann, P., Meier, A., Mordasani, R., Riesen, W., Bachmann, C., and Peheim, E. (1981). Diuretic treatment and serum lipoproteins: effect of tienilic acid and indapamide. *Klinische Wochenschrift* **59**, 343–346.

Weimar, W. *et al.* (1983). A controlled study on the effect of mannitol on immediate renal function after cadaver donor kidney transplantation. *Transplantation* **35**, 99–101.

Weinberger, M. H. (1985). Antihypertensive therapy and lipids: evidence, mechanisms, and implications. *Archives of Internal Medicine* **145**, 1102–1105.

Weinberger, M. H. (1989). Angiotensin converting enzyme inhibitors enhance the antihypertensive efficacy of diuretics and blunt or prevent adverse metabolic effects. *Journal of Cardiovascular Pharmacology* **13** (Suppl. 3), S1–S4.

Weisschedel, E., Grussendorf, M., and Ritz, E. (1983). Diuretic effect of muzolimine in advanced renal failure. *Clinical Nephrology* **19**, 51–53.

Welt, L. G., Hollander, W., Jr., and Blythe, W. B. (1960). The consequences of potassium depletion. *Journal of Chronic Diseases* **11**, 213–254.

Wernze, H., Spech, H. I., and Müller, G. (1978). Studies on the activity of the renin–angiotensin–aldosterone system (RAAS) in patients with cirrhosis of the liver. *Klinische Wochenschrift* **56**, 389–397.

Widdicombe, J. H., Nathanson, I. T., and Higland, E. (1983). Effects of 'loop' diuretics on ion transport by dog tracheal epithelium. *American Journal of Physiology* **245**, C388–C396.

Wilcox, C. S. (2002). New insights into diuretic use in patients with chronic renal disease. *Journal of the American Society of Nephrology* **13**, 798–805.

Wilcox, C. S., Welch, W. J., Schreiner, G. F., and Belardinelli, L. (1999). Natriuretic and diuretic actions of a highly selective adenosine A_1 receptor antagonist. *Journal of the American Society of Nephrology* **10**, 714–720.

Wilcox, C. S. *et al.* (1983). Response of the kidney to furosemide I: effects of salt intake and renal compensation. *Journal of Laboratory and Clinical Medicine* **102**, 450–458.

Wistrand, P. J. (1984). The use of carbonic anhydrase inhibitors in ophthalmology and clinical medicine. *Proceedings of the New York Academy of Science* **429**, 609–619.

Witte, C. L., Witte, M. H., and Dumont, A. E. (1980). Lymph imbalance in the genesis and perpetuation of the ascites syndrome in hepatic cirrhosis. *Gastroenterology* **78**, 1059–1068.

Wittner, M., Di Stefano, A., Wangemann, P., Delarge, J., Liegeois, J. F., and Greger, R. (1987). Analogues of torasemide—structure function relationships. Experiments in the thick ascending limb of the loop of Henle of rabbit nephron. *Pflügers Archiv* **408**, 54–62.

Wittner, M., Mandon, B., Roinel, N., De Rouffignac, C., and Di Stefano, A. (1993). Hormonal stimulation of Ca^{2+} and Mg^{2+} transport in the cortical thick ascending limb of Henle's loop of the mouse: evidence for a change in the paracellular pathway permeability. *Pflügers Archiv* **423**, 387–396.

Wittner, M., Weidtke, C., Schlatter, E., DiStefano, A., and Greger, R. (1984). Substrate utilization in the isolated perfused cortical thick ascending limb of rabbit nephron. *Pflügers Archiv* **402**, 52–62.

Wollam, G. L., Tarazi, R. C., Bravo, E. L., and Dustan, H. P. (1982). Diuretic potency of combined hydrochlorothiazide and furosemide therapy in azotemia. *American Journal of Medicine* **72**, 929–938.

Wong, D. G., Spence, J. D., Lamki, L., Freemen, D., and McDonald, J. W. (1986). Effect of non-steroidal anti-inflammatory drugs on control of hypertension by beta-blockers and diuretics. *Lancet* **i**, 997–1001.

Wright, F. S. and Schnermann, J. (1974). Interference with the feedback control of glomerular filtration rate by furosemide, triflocin and cyanide. *Journal of Clinical Investigation* **53**, 1695–1708.

Yamada, S. and Reynolds, T. B. (1970). Amiloride (MK–870), a new antikaliuretic diuretic. *Gastroenterology* **59**, 833–841.

Yamamura, Y. *et al.* (1992). Characterization of a novel aquaretic agent, OPC-31260, as an orally effective, nonpeptide vasopressin V2 receptor antagonist. *British Journal of Pharmacology* **105**, 787–791.

Yamasaki, Y., Nishiuchi, T., Kojima, A., Saito, H., and Saito, S. (1988). Effects of an oral water load and intravenous administration of isotonic glucose, hypertonic saline, mannitol and furosemide on the release of atrial natriuretic peptide in men. *Acta Endocrinology (Copenhagen)* **119**, 269–276.

Yeboah, E. D., Petrie, A., and Pead, J. L. (1972). Acute renal failure and open heart surgery. *British Medical Journal* **1**, 415–418.

Yendt, E. R. and Cohanim, M. (1978). Prevention of calcium stones with thiazides. *Kidney International* **13**, 397–409.

Yendt, E. R. and Cohanim, M. (1986). Absorptive hyperoxaluria: a new clinical entity-successful treatment with hydrochlorothiazide. *Clinical and Investigative Medicine* **9**, 44–50.

Yoshimura, A. *et al.* (1992a). Aggravation of minimal change nephrotic syndrome by administration of human albumin. *Clinical Nephrology* **37** (3), 109–114.

Yoshimura, A. *et al.* (1992b). Studies in the mechanism by which albumin infusion exacerbates nephrotic syndrome. *Journal of the American Society of Nephrology* **4** (3), 644 (abstract).

Index

Page numbers in **bold** refer to major sections of the text.
Page numbers in *italics* refer to pages on which tables may be found.

antidiuretic hormone (ADH) (continued)
  in new born 66
  release, complete suppression 223
  secretion 215
    in humans 215
    inhibitory effect 215
    non-osmotic hypersecretion 1565
  urinary clearances 418
anti-DNA antibodies 811
  influence of sequence and structure, on the
    binding of 811
  pathogenicity of 811
anti-dsDNA antibody 191
antiendothelial cell antibodies (AECA) 745
antifibrillarin 847
antifungal therapy 646, 1187, 1192
  with DEC 646
  pre-emptive 1192
    in renal failure 1187
      dose modification of 1187
antifungal agents and strategies 1192
anti-GBM antibodies see antiglomerular basement
    membrane antibodies
anti-GBM disease see antiglomerular basement
    membrane disease
antigen 174, 476–7, 531
  amyloid 174
  captured 184
  capture ELISA 183
  fibrin-related 476
  intrinsic glomerular 189
  presentation of 588, 1176
    helper T cells 589
  putative 531
  specificity 477
  streptococcal 189
  surface 349
  viral amyloid 174
antigenaemia 531, 2098, 2157
  chronic 531
antigen–antibody immune complexes,
    localization 601
antigenic signal 2051, 2052, 2057
antigen-presenting cells (APCs) 490,
    1176, 2049
antigen-specific lymphocytes 490
antiglobulin, mixed cryoglobulinaemia 797
antiglomerular basement membrane (anti-GBM)
    antibodies 188, 190, 201, 416, 584, 586, 595,
    748, 2124
  de novo anti-GBM nephritis 2124
  disease see antiglomerular basement
    membrane disease
  in patients with RPGN 190
  regular assessment 190
  renal biopsies 560
antiglomerular basement membrane (anti-GBM)
    disease 188, 202, 549, 565–6, 570–1, 579–81,
    587, 595
  acute interstitial infiltrate in severe crescentic
    nephritis 565
  aetiology 586–7
    environmental triggers 586–7
    inherited susceptibility 586
  with autoimmune diseases 581
  characteristic 566
  clinical features 581–4
    diagnosis of pulmonary haemorrhage 582
    general manifestations 581–2
    other manifestation 584
    pulmonary manifestations 582
    radiological changes 582–3
    renal manifestations 583–4
  definition 579
  diagnosis 584–6
    immunological features 584–5
    pulmonary features 585–6
    renal features 585

antiglomerular basement membrane (anti-GBM)
    disease (continued)
  epidemiology 579–81
    disease associations 580–1
    incidence 579–80
  glomerulonephritis 188, 595
    epitope 189
    in patients with Alport's disease 189
    after transplantation 595
  highly cellular circumferential crescent 571
  pathogenesis 587–9
    epitope of antibodies 588
    glomerular basement membrane 587–8
    Goodpasture antigen 587–8
    Goodpasture antigen derived peptides 588–9
    helper T-cells 589
    pathogenecity 588
    T cell responses to the Goodpasture
      antigen 588
  in renal allograft 560
  after renal transplantation 595
  response 580
  risk 587
  associated with small vessel vasculitis 580
antihistamines 743, 1946, 2610
anti-HLA antibodies 2053
antihypertensive (AH) therapy 849, 1377, 1383, 1405,
    1409, 1704, 1763, 2009, 2062, 2275, 2277
  adverse effects of 1704
  agents (drugs) 173, 1377, 1383, 1410, 1425–6, 1425,
    1761, 2275, 2280
    in childhood 1425
  counteracting mechanisms 2624
  effects of 1405
  emergencies 1411–12
    acute aortic dissection 1411
    acute stroke 1411
    pre-eclampsia 1411
  first-line 2275
  mechanism of action 2624
  neutral renomedullary lipid 1365
  in renal artery stenosis 1383
  selection of 1761
  side-effects of 1763
anti-ICAM-1 antibodies 1458–9
anti-idiotypic regulatory mechanism 2057
anti-IL-2R mAbs 2065–6
  with a CNI, MMF, and steroids 2066
  with CsA and steroids 2065
  with CsA, AZA, and steroids 2065–6
anti inflammatory cytokines 1660, 1666
anti-inflammatory drugs 440, 454, 484, 969,
    2171, 2612
  effects 429
  non-steroidal see non-steroidal
    anti-inflammatory drugs
anti-Jo-1 877
antileprosy drugs 648
antilymphocyte agents 2069
antilymphocyte antibody therapy 2094
antilymphocyte globulin 570
antilymphocyte preparations 2065–6
antimicrobials 2605
  responses 189–90
    antibodies against streptococcal antigens 189
  therapy 1489
antimineralocorticoid effect 2221
anti-MPO reactivity 852
  associated with glomerulonephritis 852
  with renal vasculitis 852
antimuscarinics 2452
antimyeloperoxidase ANCA 563
antinatriuretic hormones 2223–4
antineutrophil antiplasmic antibody (ANCA)/
    antineutrophil cytoplasmic antibody 170, 364, 471,
    559, 616, 745, 775, 852, 1522, 2044, 2124, 2410
  with shunt nephritis 616
  associated vasculitis 2124

antinuclear antibodies (ANA) 186, 192, 706,
    810, 872
  ANA test 191
  autoantibody 846
  titres 192
antinuclear cytoplasmic antibodies (ANCA) 188
antinuclear staining 187
antineutrophil cytoplasmic antibodies 188
antioxidant 429
  acetylcysteine 1699
  capacity, associated with pre-eclampsia 2274
  drug 108
  α-lipoic acid 2197
  strategies 848
  therapy 1460
antiphospholipid antibodies (APLA) 189, 1176, 2250
  anticardiolipin (aCL)
    associated with the antiphospholipid
      syndrome (APS) 189
  idiotypic 1176
  lupus anticoagulant-(LAC) 189
antiphospholipid syndrome (APS) 189, 1558
antiplatelet drugs 531, 1383, 1674, 2014, 2044
  treatment for CKD 1674
antiproliferative activity 2054
antiproteinuric effects 894
antipyrine, aminopyrine 1033
antirejection therapy 2094
antiretroviral therapy 608, 905
  efficacy 608
antirheumatic drugs 861
antirifampicin antibodies, circulating 649
anti-RNAP antibodies 847
anti-RNA polymerase (anti-RNAP) 844
anti-RNAP or -III 844
anti-Ro (SS-A) 872
antisalivary gland antibodies 873
anti-salmonella therapy 645
antischistosomal therapy 645
  chemotherapy 1182–3
  prophylactic 1183
anti-Sm antibody 191
antistaphylococcal agent 1489
antistreptococcal antibodies 189
antistreptolysin O (ASO) 472, 534, 548
antithrombin 2270
  antithrombin III 423, 426, 442
antithrombotic activity 741
anti-thy-1 glomerulonephritis 1648
antithymocyte globulins 2066, 2255
anti-TNF therapy
  with blocking antibodies (infliximab) 570
  soluble receptors (eternacept) 570
    maintenance therapy 570
antitopoisomerase antibodies 847
antitopoisomerase I 187, 844
antitoxin 2238
antitrypanosoma antibodies 650
α1-antitrypsin 423, 472, 528, 563, 747, 751–2, 770,
    790, 793, 1211, 1220, 1346, 1355, 2357–8
  deficiency 2357, 2407
antituberculosis agents 1165
  adverse effects of 1165
antitubular basement membrane disease 1539–40
antitumour necrosis factor therapy, for Wegener's
    granulomatosis 779
antiulcer drugs 2611–12
antiviral therapy 1536, 2040, 2108, 2113
antrafenin, acute interstitial nephritis due to 1534
anuria 4, 69, 1186, 1467, 1469, 2453
  complete obstruction 2453
  in infants 69
anxiety 20
aorta, coarctation 1372
aortic aneurysm 1484
  repair 1390
aortic calcification 2008
aortic clamping time 1637

glomerulus (continued)
  endocapillary proliferation 476, 545
  extracapillary proliferation 1521
  extracellulary matrix synthesis/breakdown 1665
  filtration barrier see glomerular capillaries,
    endothelium; glomerular filtration
  function, impairment leading to cell
    death 381
  haemodynamics in pregnancy in animals
    2215–16
  high proportion of 479
    clinical **479**
    histological prognostic markers 479
  hydrostatic pressure 2215
  injury see glomerular injury
  ischaemia 1533
  juxtamedullary 444
    loss in elderly 74
  leakage of proteins 389–91
    selectivity 389
  leucocyte infiltration *177*, 179
  leucocyte recruitment 373–4, *373*
  lithium effect, histology 1085–6
  mitogen sources
    platelets 531
  molecules summoning leucocytes
    chemokines *374*
    complement 372–3
    lipid chemotactic factors 380
    proinflammatory cytokines 382
  monocyte infiltration 1660
  necrotizing or proliferative disorders 144
  number 175
  obsolescence 180, 1405
    effects of antihypertensive treatment 1405
  oncotic pressure 2215–16
  parietal epithelium **357**
  pathology in 631
  permeability for macromolecules 354–5
  in primary IgA nephropathy 475
  progressive loss of structure 478
  proliferation 377
    increase inhibition 380
    mesangial cells 377
    stimuli *382*
  proteinuria 392–3
  in radiation nephritis 1093
  renal biopsy changes 176–7, *177*
    cellular components 176
    deposits 176–8
  resident cells
    clearance by apoptosis 382
  sieving profile 391
  size in neonates 2472
  stained with haematoxylin 524
  stained with silver methenamine 524
  streptococcal histones 550
    superantigens **550**
  ultrastructure 347–58
  visceral epithelium 350–3
    class II antigen expression 1657
    role in glomerulosclerosis
      development 1657
  wall water permeability 2215
glomerulus blood flow (GBF) 1296, 1301
  autoregulation of 1301
glucagon 242
  in chronic renal failure 1709
  glomerular hyperfiltration in diabetes 670
  increased
    in diabetic ketoacidosis 330–1
    in hyperkalaemia 253–4
  phosphate excretion increase 295
  plasma potassium 242
  role in glucose intolerance 1709
glucocorticoid 245, 295, 439, 451, 516, 734–6, 928,
  934, 1240
  cyclophosphamide 2250

glucocorticoid (continued)
  deficiency 221, 989–90
    isolated 221
  excess 252
  glucocorticoid-mediated 252
  receptor 252, 2053
  remediable hyperaldosteronism 252, 339
glucocorticosteroids **2053**
glucoglycinuria **947**, 952
gluconate 2007
gluconeogenesis
  cAMP action on phosphate transport 294
  in uraemia 1721
glucose 2219–20
  administration, in hyperkalaemia *258*
  alcoholic ketoacidosis treatment 331
  blood, in diabetic ketoacidosis 330–1
  control 2201
  excretion 53, 2225
    changes in **2225**
  homeostasis 967, 1709
    in chronic renal failure 1709
  intestinal transporter (SGLTI) 946, 1480
  intolerance 1965
  metabolism
    glycosuria, osmotic diuresis 232
    Na$^+$–glucose transporter 925, 946
  polymers 1963–4
  reabsorption 53–4
    carriers of 53
    defect in Fanconi's syndrome 967
    entry step 943
    maximal 962
    threshold 54
  reabsorption curve 945
    for normal subjects 945
    patients with types A and B renal
      glycosuria 945
  renal handling of **2219–20**
  in the elderly 81
  threshold 946
  tolerance 242, 948
  tolerance impairment
    growth hormone 1732
    insulin secretion 1709
    uraemic syndrome 1720
  tolerance test 946, 948
  transporters (GLUT) 1453
  urine detection 25
glucose degradation products (GDPs) 1719,
  1957, 2204
glucose–galactose malabsorption 54, 947
glucose–galactose transporter 947
glucose monocarboxylic acid 130
glucose oxidase 25
glucose 6-phosphatase 134, **2351**
  deficiency of 2351
glucose–6–phosphate dehydrogenase, acute renal failure
  due to 1616
glucose tolerance test 242, 948
glucosuria 25, 54
glucotoxicity 1964
glucuronide 419
glue sniffing 905
GLUT1 54
glutamic acid, excretion disorder 952-3
glutamine, metabolism 937, 1776
γ-glutamyl cycle 965–6
γ-glutamyl transferase 1834
γ-glutamyl transpeptidase 2299
glutaraldehyde, recommendations 1931
glutaric acidaemia 2488
glutathione peroxidase (GSH-Px) 1454
  activity 969
glutathione-S-transferase (GST) 1175, 2090
o-glycan side chains, underglycosylation 492
glycaemia **672**, 2203
  control 672

glycation
  advanced end products 1718
  end-products, haemodialysis 1719
  non-enzymatic of proteins, in peritoneal
    dialysis 1957
glycerol 1454
glycine
  protective effect on ischaemic cells 1452
  transport disorder 952
o-glycoforms 489
o-glycosylation 489
glycogenolysis, accelerated 430
glycogen storage disease 2351
glycolate 1208
glycolysis 1451
β2-glycoprotein 189, 1558
glycoproteins
  gp330 (Heymann's antigen) 370
  inhibition of crystallization in urine 1203
glycosaminoglycans 681, 848
  amyloid deposits 681
  inhibition of crystallization in urine 1211
  solubility product (SP) 1199
glycosphingolipid deposition 2346
  hypertrophic obstructive cardiomyopathy 2346
  of transplanted cadaveric kidneys 2349
glycosuria 302, 431, 719, 736, **945–8**, 962, 2220
  causes of **945–6**
  in Fanconi syndrome 719
  finding of 947
    genetics **947**
  with hyperphosphaturia 947
  incidence of 947
  normal glucose reabsorption **945**
  orthoglycaemic 719, 736
  of pregnancy 947–8, 2220
    renal handling of other sugars **2220**
  primary (isolated) renal 946–7
    clinical features **946–7**
    definition **946**
    diagnosis 946–7
    genetics **947**
    incidence 946–7
    pathophysiology **946**
  secondary renal 947–8
    glucoglycinuria 947
    glucose-galactose malabsorption 947
    glycosuria of pregnancy 947–8
    glycosuria with glycinuria 947
    glycosuria with hyperphosphaturia 947
glycosylated haemoglobin, blood pressure control 2250
glycosylation 489, 710, 725
  abnormal **725**
  light-chain 725
glycosyltransferases 489
glycyrrhetinic acid 340
  in carbenoxolone 340
  in chewing tobacco 340
  in licorice 340
glyoxylate aminotransferase (AGT) 2374
glyoxylate reductase (GR) 1208, 2374
glypican-3 (Gpc3) 2425
Goeminne syndrome 2488
gold and D-pencillamine-associated nephropathy 861
Goldblatt hypertension 1333
Goldblatt models 1329
Goldenhar complex (facio-auriculo-vertebral
  syndrome) 2489
gold nephropathy 861
  clinical features 861
  management 861–2
  outcome 862
  prediction 862
gold standards, for diagnosing renovascular
  disease 1695
Goldston syndrome *2316*, *2486*
gonadal development 2472
gonadal hormone, disturbances in 2146

magnetic resonance angiography (MRA) (continued)
  in living donor transplant 161–2
  management 107, 147, 161–2, 2106
magnetic resonance cholangiopancreatography 1575
magnetic resonance imaging (MRI) scans 48, 94, 121–8,
    148, 225, 270, 773, 865, 889, 1188, 1407, 1610,
    2016, 2083, 2111, 2269, 2437, 2476–7, 2509,
    2515–16, 2544
  and renovascular disease 148
  angiography see magnetic resonance
      angiography (MRA)
  breath hold acquisition techniques 121
  contraindications to 121
  conventional angiography 125
  endorectal-coil MR imaging 127
  FOVs (26–30 cm), MRA 125
  gadolinium-based contrast media 124
  indications of 126–8
  iron oxide contrast media 124
  lanthanides and 124
  liver imaging 124
  manganese contrast media 124
  phase-contrast (PC) imaging, velocity encoding value
      (VENC) 124
  prognosis assessment 426
  treatment 2083
    pathophysiology 1610
    unrelated to pregnancy 1610
  urography 125–6
magnetic resonance renography 125
magnetic resonance urography 125–6, 139, 1468, 2455
  static fluid technique 126
maintenance therapy 570, 2157, 2277
  intravascular volume maintenance 1472
  long-term 570
  with steroids 2157
Majewski type syndrome 2488
major basic protein (MBP) 1532
major histocompatibility complex (MHC) 569, 1025,
    1540, 2052
  antigen 2056–7
    dendritic cells 2052
    endothelial cells 2045
    immunogenicity 2065
    murine H2 2065
    restricted T cells 2057
  class I antigens 2052
    presentation and processing 588–9
  class II antigens 2055
    glomerular visceral epithelial cells 1656–7
  Heymann's nephritis 373
  MHC–peptide engagements 2049
  treatment 569
    general considerations 569
malabsorption
  glucose–galactose 946
  intestinal 952
  methionine 949, 952
  phosphate 953
malabsorption syndromes 871
malaise 2279
malakoplakia 142
malaria 2608
  associated glomerulonephritis 642
    molecular mechanisms 642
    management 642
malarial acute renal failure 1617
maleic acid 296
  Fanconi syndrome induction 978
malformations 2473
  causes of 2473
malignancy 222, 509, 629, 1177–9, 1557, 2175–7, 2184
  development of 1179
  frequency 629
  HUS in 1557
  and nephropathy 625, 627
    histological appearance 627
  in patients with nephrotic syndrome, incidence 630

malignant disease 394
  glomerular disease association see under glomerular
      disease
  hypouricaemia 1063
  uric acid clearance 1063, 1097
malignant hypertenion 1403–5
  abysmal prognosis of 1400
  clinical presentation 1406–7
    blood pressure 1406
    heart 1407
    neurological symptoms 1406
    optic funds 1406–7
  conditions predisposing to 1402
  definition of 1399
  development of renal impairment 1401
  family history of 1400
  hypertensive encephalopathy 1407
  in IgA glomerulonephritis 1402
  incidence of 1399–400
  interlobular artery in 1404
  laboratory investigations 1407–8
    haematology 1408
    renin–aldosterone system 1407–8
    urine 1408
  management 1409–12
    antihypertensive emergencies 1411–12
    general principles 1409–11
    prevention 1409
  outcome 1399
    in relation to aetiology 1401
  pathogenesis, roles of 1408–9
    blood pressure 1408
    the endothelium 1408
    genetic factors 1409
    other vasoactive systems 1409
    renin–angiotensin system 1408–9
    vasopressin 1409
  prognosis 1399–400
  proliferative endarteritis 1403
    effects of antihypertensive treatment 1405
    pathology in the organs 1405
  renal function and survival 1400–2
  renal pathology in 1403–5
    afferent arteries 1403–4
    glomeruli 1404
    interlobular arteries 1403
    pathological changes and renal dysfunction 1404–5
    renal pathology and secondary malignant
        hypertension 851, 1399–412, 1754
    tubules and interstitium 1404
  role of genetic factors 1409
  role of other vasoactive systems 1409
  role of vasopressin 1409
  signs and symptoms 1406
malignant hyperthermia 255
malignant melanoma 627, 631, 2108
  treated with Cryptosporidium parvum 627
malignant mesenchymal tumours 2513
malignant nephrosclerosis 1331, 1337, 1404
malignant obstruction 2464
malignant ventricular arrhythmias 323
malingering 404
malnutrition 1795, 1905, 1993–5, 2019, 2201–2
  and inflammation 1965
  assessment/investigation 1965
  dialysis patients 2019
  effect of dialysis 1905
  on haemodialysis 2203
  prevention 2019–20
  see also nutrition
malnutrition and inflammation
  'cytokine driven' 1965
malondialdehyde (MDA) 1454, 1871
malperforant 2197
maltese crosses 31, 33, 2346
maltodextrin 2143
mammalian target of rapamycin (mTOR) 2064
mammary tumours, virus-induced 628

β2M amyloidosis 1861–2, 1865
  β2m modification, β2m production 1865
mandelamine 2444
manic depressive psychosis 2592
mannitol 214, 1459–60, 1476, 1483, 1637, 2087,
    2629–30
  clinical studies 2630
  experimental studies and mechanisms of action 2629
  performance of 2630
  prophylactic 1459
  in the ECF 214
mannose binding lectin (MBL) 185
mannose-binding protein (MBP) 819
maple syrup urine disease 24
marathon runners 221
'march' haemoglobinuria 398
Marfan syndrome 2496
'marginal' donor 2185
marginal kidneys 2185
marking-nut poisoning 1625
Massachussetts Male Aging Study 1741
massive hydration, with isotonic saline 1457
Masson–Goldner stain 1840
Masson trichrome stain 174
mass transfer area coefficient (MTAC) 1959, 1990,
    1997–8
  peritoneal 1997–8
mast cells 478, 1661
  diagnosis 478
  differential diagnosis 478
maternal dehydration, effects on fetus 65
maternal follow-up 2256
  after pregnancy 2256
maternal hypertension 2267
maternal ketoacidosis 65
maternal morbidity 2277
maternal outcome 2265–6
matrix-assisted laser desorption spectroscopy 488
matrix metalloproteinases (MMP) 1027
matrix substance 1205
maturity-onset diabetes of the young (MODY) 966
  genetic/metabolic causes 966
maximal intensity projections (MIPs) 148
  reconstructions 151
maximal reabsorptive capacity (Tm$_G$) 962
maximum reabsorption rate of phosphate 54
m. bulbus spongiosus 1737
MDRD (American Modification of Diet in Renal
    Disease) 1308, 1671
mean arterial blood pressure (MAP) 1321, 1755
  MAP kinases, cascades 1456
mean parenchymal transit time (MPTT) 136, 2462
measles 442, 545, 604
measured urine volume 217
measurement of serum 218
  by flame photometry 218
  by ion-specific electrode 218
mebendazole 10
mechanical injury of glomerulus 375
mechlorethamine 452, 457
Meckel syndrome 2486
meclofenamate 454
median nerve 1888
mediastinal fibrosis 2466
Medical Research Council (MCR) 2624, 2633
Mediterranean FeVer (MEFV) gene 690
medroxyprogesterone 1747, 2517
medulla, renal 1298
medullary carcinoma of the thyroid 273
medullary collecting tubule (MCT) 73
medullary cystic kidney disease (MCKD) 2318,
    2325, 2331
medullary function in infants 66
medullary ischaemia 1448
medullary nephrocalcinosis 144, 955, 1262–3, 1269,
    1272–3
  causes of 1269
    total parenteral nutrition 1269

urolithiasis 54, 111, 118, 302, 1207, 1536, **2249**, 2374
  CT scanning 111
  helical CT for 111
  in hypophosphataemia 54
  recurrent 2374
  techniques 111
    multislice helical CT **111**
    reconstruction techniques **111–12**
urological complications **166, 2083–6**
  in transplant recipients 166
  ureteric obstruction 2084–6
    causes **2084**
    investigaion 2085
    treatment **2085–6**
  urinary leaks 2083–4
    investigation 2083–4
    management **2084**
urological evaluation 2156
uromodulin 2391–2
uropathy 626, 632
  obstructive 626, 632
    indirect effects 626
uropontin, for stone formation 1211
uroradiology *see* imaging
urothelial atypia 2551
urothelial cancer **2549–61**
  clinical prevention 2553–4
  follow-up 2560
  pathology 2551–2
  treatment 2554–60
  urothelial cells 31
urothelial conditions 2551
  malignant 119, 1097, **2551–2**
  non-malignant **2551**
urothelial dysplasia 2551
urothelial malignancies 119, 1097, 2551–2
US renal transplantation experience 853
uterine artery, waveform analysis 2274
uterine cervix 1181
uterine haemorrhage 1608, 1611, 2238

vaccination 603
  in idiopathic nephrotic syndrome 450
vaccines 422–3
  pneumococcal 422
  varicella 423
vaccinia virus, immunotherapy, in renal cell carcinoma 2518
vacuolization, isometric 178
vacuum device **1745**
  to treat erectile impotence 1745
vagina
  examination 11
  female sexual disorders 1747
  menstrual abnormalities 1747
  palpation 18
vaginal delivery 2255
vaginal discharge, in children 18
vaginitis 1117, 1119
  colonization 1119
  treatment 1119
valacyclovir 2607
valganciclovir 2098
valley fever 1191
valproic acid *see* sodium valproate
Valsalva manoeuvre 15
valsalva ratio 1742
valvular heart disease **1782**
  mitral annular calcification
    dialysis 1782
    predisposing factors in dialysis patients 1912
vanadium 1075
Van Allen syndrome 2486
vancomycin 67, 1126, 1536, 1783, 2115, 2156, 2603, **2605–6**
  acute interstitial nephritis 1536

vancomycin *(continued)*
  acute renal failure due to
    elderly 1637
  handling/dosages in renal disease 2606
  renal carbuncle 1126
vardenafil 1744
varicella zoster virus 423, 2113, 2158
  infection in renal transplant recipients 2113
  varicella/chicken pox 423
varicocoele 2510
varicose dilatation, of the vein 1921
vascular access 1712, **1909–23, 2202**
  angiography **1917**
  arteriovenous fistula 1911
  blood flow of 1919
  care of 1915
    needles for puncture, usage, and **1915**
    usage **1915**
  classification of 1909
  comparison of patency rates for various types **1918**
  complications of 1918–21
    aneurysmal/varicose dilatation 1921–2
    infection **1919–20**
    local **1919–21**
    steal syndrome **1920**
    stenosis/occlusion 1919
    systemic **1918**
    venous hypertension 1921
  constructing an external shunt, insertion of cannula 1910
  in diabetic nephropathy 2043
  dialysis 1916–17
  evaluation and examination of **1917**
  factors influencing long-term patency **1918**
  haemodialysis 1910, 1915, 1920
    Cimini-Brescia fistula 1939, 1948, 2171
    results/outcome 1918
    thrombosis complications 1918
  local complications 1919
    infection 1919
    stenosis and occlusion 1919
  long-term results and factors influencing outcome 1918
  selection of type **1910**
  strategies for long-term maintenance **1923**
  suitability for **1712**
  systemic complications **1918**
  timing of formation **1909**
  types **1909–10**
    using a vascular graft 1912
    vascular grafts 1912–14
  see also arteriovenous fistula
vascular access device 1911
  installation of **1911**
vascular anastomosis 2078–9
  alternative techniques of urinary reconstruction 2080
  drainage and closure of the wound 2080
  multiple vessels 2079
  ureteric stents 2080
  urinary drainage 2079–80
vascular atherosclerotic disease 2040
vascular calcifications 2103–4, 2151
  non-myocardial 2151
vascular cell adhesion molecule (VCAMs) 743, 815, 1024, 1533
  VCAM1 477, 1409, 2272
  see also adhesion molecules
vascular complications
  renal transplantation 2089, 2092
vascular congestion, in the corpora cavernosa 884
vascular disease
  in chronic renal failure 399, 423, 426, 1883, 2168
  congestion 884
  damage, principal mechanism 428
  involving the kidney 179
  microangiopathy 1883

vascular disease *(continued)*
  renal allograft recipients 2105
    schematic representation 179
      of the lumen 180
    of the main renal arteries 2168
vascular endothelial growth factor (VEGF)
  in diabetic retinopathy 349, 380, 1656, 1955
vascular endothelium, glycosphingolipid deposits 428, 2347
vascular events, hyperuricaemia association 1068
vascular grafts 1912, 1923
  aneurysm of the **1923**
vascular hyalinosis 1333
vascular hypertrophy, induced by angiotensin II 1323
vascular injury 852, 1075
  eicosanoids suggesting 1075
vascular insufficiency 851
vascular leak syndrome 2589
vascular lesions **179**, 482, 2267, 2272
  of pre-eclampsia 2272
vascular malformation syndromes 1422
  renovascular hypertension 1421
vascular narrowing 850
vascular nephrosclerosis 2168
vascular pedicle injuries 1366
vascular permeability factor (VPF) 449
vascular probe, complications 20
vascular resistance 2216
vascular sclerosis 173, **1659**
  kidney scarring 1659
  progressive 173
vascular sensitivity 2217
vascular sludging 884
  in adult 884
  the corpora cavernosa 884
vascular smooth muscle 215
  proliferative effects 215
vascular stability 846
vascular stenoses 112
  helical CT application 112
  renal vascular stenoses 112
vascular thrombosis 2092, 2156
vascular tissue 741, 1847
vascular volume 1000
vasculitic glomerulonephritis 859
vasculitic inflammation 741–9
  immunopathological aspects of **741**
vasculitis 12, 19, 202, 560, 569, 585, 741, 747–8, **768–74**, 780, 784–5, 859–60, **1053**, 1374
  ACR 1990 criteria, for the classification of 7688
  acute renal failure due to *1465*
  ANCA and classification of **769**
  ANCA-associated 560, 569
  and microscopic polyangiitis 770–85
    clinical and pathological features **770**
    diagnosis **775–7**
    treatment and outcome 777–85
  antineutrophil cytoplasmic antibodies 745, 747–8
    Wegener's granulomatosis 766
    animal models of 747–8
  Chapel Hill consensus criteria for the nomenclature of 768
  in children 774
  clinical presentation 772–4
    alveolar haemorrhage **774**
    cardiac involvement **774**
    cutaneous involvement 773
    eye involvement 773
    gastrointestinal tract **774**
    muscle and joint symptoms 773
    nervous system involvement 773
    non-specific features 772
    renal disease 772
  cryoglobulinaemic 744 *see also* cryoglobulinaemia
  environmental factors **770**
  epidemiology of 769
    aetiological factors 769
    incidence and demography 769

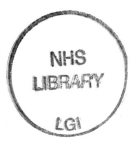